Oxford Textbook of
Palliative Nursing

Oxford Textbook of
Palliative
Nursing

4TH EDITION

Edited by

Betty R. Ferrell, RN, PhD, MA, FAAN, FPCN, CHPN
Professor and Director
Department of Nursing Research and Education
City of Hope Comprehensive Cancer Center
Duarte, California

Nessa Coyle, ACHPN, PhD, FAAN
Consultant
Palliative Care and Clinical Ethics in Oncology
New York, New York

Judith A. Paice, PhD, RN, FAAN
Director of Cancer Pain Program
Division of Hematology-Oncology
Feinberg School of Medicine
Northwestern University
Chicago, Illinois

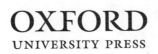

OXFORD
UNIVERSITY PRESS

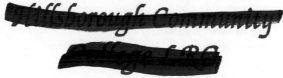

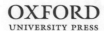

OXFORD
UNIVERSITY PRESS

Oxford University Press is a department of the University of Oxford.
It furthers the University's objective of excellence in research,
scholarship, and education by publishing worldwide.

Oxford   New York
Auckland   Cape Town   Dar es Salaam   Hong Kong   Karachi
Kuala Lumpur   Madrid   Melbourne   Mexico City   Nairobi
New Delhi   Shanghai   Taipei   Toronto

With offices in
Argentina   Austria   Brazil   Chile   Czech Republic   France   Greece
Guatemala   Hungary   Italy   Japan   Poland   Portugal   Singapore
South Korea   Switzerland   Thailand   Turkey   Ukraine   Vietnam

Oxford is a registered trademark of Oxford University Press
in the UK and certain other countries.

Published in the United States of America by
Oxford University Press
198 Madison Avenue, New York, NY 10016

© Oxford University Press 2015

Library of Congress Cataloging-in-Publication Data
Oxford textbook of palliative nursing / edited by Betty R. Ferrell, Nessa Coyle, Judith A. Paice. —
4th edition.
p. ; cm.
Textbook of palliative nursing
Includes bibliographical references and index.
ISBN 978-0-19-933234-2 (alk. paper)
I. Ferrell, Betty, editor.   II. Coyle, Nessa, editor.   III. Paice, Judith A., editor.
IV. Title: Textbook of palliative nursing.
[DNLM: 1. Hospice and Palliative Care Nursing.   2. Terminal Care.   WY 152.3]
RT87.T45
616'.029—dc23
2014012519

9 8 7 6 5 4 3 2

Printed in the United States of America
on acid-free paper

Contents

Preface

Our Heritage, Our Future

The first edition of this Textbook was published in 2001. This was only fourteen years ago, yet it seems like a very long time given the remarkable progress in our field. The previous editions of the book included forewords by those whom we think of as the "godmothers" of palliative care and true pioneers: Cicely Saunders, Florence Wald, and Jeanne Quint Benoliel. The forewords are worth reading in the previous edition if you have not seen them, as their words are a reminder of decades not so long ago when death was not discussed, hospice didn't exist or was a very new idea, and the term "palliative care" was not in our vocabulary. These leaders advocated for excellent palliative care before there were any guidelines, certification, organizations, or educational programs devoted to care of the seriously ill or dying.

This fourth edition of the *Oxford Textbook of Palliative Nursing* represents what we know now to be true. Palliative care is an essential element of our healthcare system and is becoming increasingly significant amidst an aging society and organizations struggling to provide both compassionate and cost-effective care. We also know, as did the pioneers of our field, that nurses are at the center of this care across settings and populations.

This fourth edition of the Textbook is not only longer than the first, it is "deeper" in thought, born of the rich clinical experiences of the authors and the ever-growing evidence base of palliative care. Our predecessors stood on their passion and advocacy, and we are fortunate to now stand on a wealth of knowledge and clinical experience. Our hope with each edition of the Textbook is to capture the science but also the art of caring for seriously ill and dying patients and their families.

We are ever grateful to those who came before to guide the way, those who live this in their daily work and to the future leaders who will continue to build the system that will care for each of us.

Betty R. Ferrell
Nessa Coyle
Judith A. Paice

Acknowledgments

We are deeply indebted to Andrea Hayward, our assistant who coordinated each step of the process of this edition. We also thank the many authors around the world who contributed to this edition. This book is a testament to the universality of nursing care and how knowledgeable, passionate nurses are ever-present in this most sacred time of life.

Contributors

Paula R. Anderson, RN, MN, OCN
Oncology Research Initiatives
University of Texas Southwestern Medical Center
Moncrief Cancer Center
Fort Worth, Texas

Romina Arceo, ANP-C
Nurse Practitioner of Pain and Palliative Care
Department of Pain Medicine and Palliative Care
Mount Sinai Beth Israel
New York, New York

Rev. Pamela Baird, AS
End-of-Life Practitioner
Seasons of Life
Arcadia, California

Marie A. Bakitas, DNSc, APRN, NP-C, AOCN, ACHPN, FAAN
Marie L. O'Koren Endowed Chair and Professor of Nursing
UAB School of Nursing
The University of Alabama at Birmingham
Birmingham, Alabama

Barbara M. Bates-Jensen, PhD, RN, FAAN
Associate Professor of Nursing
School of Nursing and David Geffen School of Medicine
University of California
Los Angeles, California

Vanessa Battista, MS, CPNP, CCRC
Pediatric Nurse Practitioner
The Children's Hospital of Philadelphia
Philadelphia, Pennsylvania

Stacey Berg, MD
Professor of Pediatrics
Baylor College of Medicine
Texas Children's Cancer Center
Houston, Texas

Patricia Berry, PhD, RN, ACHPN, FPCN, FAAN
Professor of Nursing
Director, Hartford Center of Gerontological Nursing Excellence
School of Nursing
Oregon Health and Science University
Portland, Oregon

Barton T. Bobb, MSN, FNP-BC, ACHPN
Palliative Care and Pain Consult Team
VCU Medical Center
Richmond, Virginia

Marilyn Bookbinder, RN, PhD, FPCN
Department of Pain Medicine and Palliative Care
Mount Sinai Beth Israel
New York, New York

Tami Borneman, RN, MSN, CNS, FPCN
Senior Research Specialist
Nursing Research and Education
City of Hope National Medical Center
Duarte, California

Laura Bourdeanu, PhD
Assistant Professor of Nursing
The Sage Colleges
Troy, New York

Mary Bowman, ACNP-BC
Virginia Commonwealth University Health Systems
Richmond, Virginia

Frank Brennan, MD
Palliative Care Physician
Calvary Hospital
Sydney, Australia

Katherine Brown-Saltzman, RN, MA
Clinical Specialist in Palliative Care
UCLA Medical Center
Los Angeles, California

Margaret L. Campbell, PhD, RN, FPCN
Professor of Research
College of Nursing
Wayne State University
Detroit, Michigan

Denice Caraccia Economou, RN, MN, CHPN
Senior Research Specialist
City of Hope National Medical Center
Duarte, California

Joan G. Carpenter, MN, CRNP, NP-C, GNP-BC, ACHPN
Doctor of Philosophy Candidate and Predoctoral Research
  Scholar
College of Nursing
University of Utah
Salt Lake City, Utah
Nurse Practitioner
Coastal Hospice and Palliative Care
Salisbury, Maryland

Brigit Carter, PhD, RN, CCRN
Assistant Professor of Nursing
Duke University Medical Center
Durham, North Carolina

Nathan I. Cherny, MBBS, FRACP, FRCP
Norman Levan Chair of Humanistic Medicine
Associate Professor of Medicine
Department of Medical Oncology
Shaare Zedek Medical Center
Jerusalem, Israel

**John D. Chovan, PhD, DNP, RN, CNP, CNS,
  PMHNP-BC, PMHCNS-BC, ACHPN, AHN-BC**
Department of Nursing
Otterbein University
Mount Carmel Hospice and Palliative Services
Westerville, Ohio

Kimberly Chow, ANP-BC, ACHPN
Palliative Medicine Service
Memorial Sloan-Kettering Cancer Center
New York, New York

Kathleen N. Clifford, MSN, FNP-BC, AOCNP, ACHPN
St. Luke's Mountain States Tumor Institute
Boise, Idaho

Douglas Cluxton, MA, LPC
Bereavement Services
OhioHealth Hospice
Columbus, Ohio

Daniel Cogan, GNP-BC, ACHPN
Director of Palliative Care
Nassau University Medical Center
East Meadow, New York

Audrey Kurash Cohen, MS, CCC-SLP
Clinical Specialist, Speech Language Pathologist
Department of Speech, Language and Swallowing Disorders
Massachusetts General Hospital
Boston, Massachusetts

Peggy Compton, RN, PhD, FAAN
Associate Professor of Nursing
University of California
Los Angeles, California

Stephen R. Connor, PhD
International Palliative Care Consultant
Worldwide Palliative Care Alliance
London, England
Open Society Foundations
New York, New York
Capital Caring
Falls Church, Virginia

Stacie Corcoran, RN, MS
Nurse Leader
Memorial Sloan Kettering Cancer Center
New York, New York

Inge B. Corless, RN, PhD, FAAN
Professor of Nursing
MGH Institute of Health Professions
Boston, Massachusetts

Valerie T. Cotter, DrNP, AGPCNP-BC, FAANP
Advanced Senior Lecturer
Director of Adult-Gerontology Primary Care Nurse
  Practitioner Program
University of Pennsylvania School of Nursing
Philadelphia, Pennsylvania

Patrick J. Coyne, ACHPN, ACNS-BC, FAAN, FPCN
Clinical Director of the Thomas Palliative Care Unit
Virginia Commonwealth University
Massey Cancer Center
Richmond, Virginia

Constance M. Dahlin, ANP-BC, ACHPN, FPCN, FAAN
Director of Professional Practice
Hospice and Palliative Nurses Association
Pittsburgh, Pennsylvania
Palliative Care Specialist and Nurse Practitioner
Beverly, Massachusetts

Barbara J. Daly, PhD, RN, FAAN
The Gertrude Perkins Oliva Professor
  of Oncology Nursing
Frances Payne Bolton School of Nursing
Case Western Reserve University
University Hospitals of Cleveland
Cleveland, Ohio

Betty Davies, RN, CT, PhD, FAAN
Adjunct Professor and Senior Scholar
School of Nursing
University of Victoria
Victoria, Canada

Pamela Stitzlein Davies, MS, ARNP, ACHPN
Nurse Practitioner
Palliative and Supportive Care Service
Seattle Cancer Care Alliance
University of Washington
Seattle, Washington

Henry Ddungu, MD
Medical Consultant
Uganda Cancer Institute/Hutchinson
    Center Cancer Alliance
Kampala, Uganda

Grace E. Dean, PhD, RN
Associate Professor
School of Nursing
Center for Sleep and Respiratory Neurobiology
University of Pennsylvania
Philadelphia, Pennsylvania

Susan Derby, RN, MA, GNP-BC
Memorial Sloan-Kettering Cancer Center
Pain and Palliative Care Service
New York, New York

J. Nicholas Dionne-Odom, MA, MSN, RN
UAB School of Nursing
University of Alabama at Birmingham
Birmingham, Alabama

Julia Downing, PhD, MMed Sci, BN, RGN
Honorary Professor
Makerere University
Kampala, Uganda
Director of Education and Research
International Children's Palliative Care Network
London, United Kingdom

Deborah Dudgeon, MD, FRCPC
W. Ford Connell Professor of Palliative Care Medicine
Departments of Medicine
Oncology and Family Medicine
Queen's University
Kingston, Ontario, Canada

Kathy Egan-City, MA, BSN, RN
President and Executive Director
Millennium Research Institute
San Diego, California

Nancy K. English, PhD, APRN, CS, CHPN
Adjunct Assistant Professor of Nursing
University of Colorado Health Sciences
Aurora, Colorado

Elizabeth Ercolano, RN, MSN, DNSc, AOCNS
Associate Research Scientist
School of Nursing
Yale University
New Haven, Connecticut

Mary Ersek, PhD, RN, FPCN, FAAN
Director, National PROMISE Center
Philadelphia Veterans Affairs Medical Center
Professor of Nursing
University of Pennsylvania
Philadelphia, Pennsylvania

Laura A. Espinosa, RN, MS, PhD
Instructor
The Methodist Hospital Research Institute
Director of Nursing
Methodist West Houston Hospital
Houston, Texas

Tamar Ezer, JD
Deputy director of the Law and Health Initiative
Public Health Program
Open Society Foundations
New York, New York

Iris Cohen Fineberg, PhD, MSW
Associate Professor
Stony Brook School of Social Work
Stony Brook University
Stony Brook, New York

Regina M. Fink, RN, PhD, AOCN, FAAN
Research Nurse Scientist
University of Colorado Hospital
Cordillera, Colorado

Anessa M. Foxwell, MSN, CRNP
Palliative Care Service
Hospital of the University of Pennsylvania
Philadelphia, Pennsylvania

Bonnie Freeman, RN, MSN, ANP-BC, CHPN
Supportive Care Medicine
Pain and Palliative Care Medicine
City of Hope National Medical Center
Duarte, California

Katherine Froggatt, PhD, BSc(Hons)
Professor of Ageing and Palliative Care
International Observatory on End of Life Care
Lancaster University
Lancaster, United Kingdom

Mei R. Fu, PhD, RN, ACNS-BC, FAAN
College of Nursing
New York University
New York, New York

Wayne L. Furman, MD
Department of Oncology
St. Jude Children's Research Hospital
Memphis, Tennessee

Michelle S. Gabriel, RN, MS, ACHPN
Palliative Care Clinical Nurse Specialist
VA Palo Alto Health Care System
Palo Alto, California

Licet Garcia, BA
Clinical Trials Unit Business Manager
Department of Medicine/CARE Center
University of California
Los Angeles, California

Rose A. Gates, RN, PhD, AOCN, NP
Adult Nurse Practitioner
Oncology Rocky Mountain Cancer Center
Colorado Springs, Colorado

Denisse Ruth Parra Giordano, MSN
Assistant Professor of Nursing
Department of Medicine
University of Chile
Ñuñoa, Santiago, Chile

Linda M. Gorman, RN, MN, PMHCNS-BC, CHPN, OCN
Palliative Care Clinical
    Nurse Specialist and Consultant
Los Angeles, California

Marcia Grant, RN, DNSc, FAAN
Professor
Division of Nursing Research and Education
City of Hope National Medical Center
Duarte, California

Deborah Grassman, ARNP
Bay Pines VA Medical Center
St. Petersburg, Florida

Mikel Gray, PhD
Professor of Nursing
Department of Acute and Specialty Care
University of Virginia
Charlottesville, Virginia

Julie Griffie, RN, MSN, ACNS-BC, AOCN
Manager
Nursing Practice
Clinical Cancer Center
Medical College of Wisconsin
Froedtert Hospital
Milwaukee, Wisconsin

Liz Gwyther, MD, MBChB, FCFP, MSc
Senior Lecturer in Palliative Medicine
School of Public Health and Family Medicine
University of Cape Town
Cape Town, South Africa, Africa

Debra E. Heidrich, MSN, RN, ACHPN, AOCN
Palliative Care Clinical Nurse Specialist
Bethesda North Hospital, TriHealth, Inc.
Cincinnati, Ohio

Marjorie J. Hein, MSN
Nurse Practitioner
Nursing Support, Medical Oncology
City of Hope National Medical Center
Duarte, California

Melody Brown Hellsten, DNP, RN, PPCNP-BC, CHPPN
Pediatric Nurse Practitioner
Texas Children's Cancer Center - PACT
Houston, Texas

Pamela S. Hinds, PhD, RN, FAAN
Professor of Pediatrics
The George Washington University
Director of Nursing Research and Quality Outcomes
Associate Director of The Center for Translational Science
Children's National Medical Center
Washington, DC

Marianne Jensen Hjermstad, PhD, MPH, RN
Professor of Palliative Medicine
European Palliative Care Research Centre
Department of Medicine
Norwegian University of Science and Technology
Trondheim University Hospital
Trondheim, Norway

Chi Dang Hornik, PharmD, BCPS
Clinical Specialist in Neonatal Intensive Care
Department of Pharmacy
Duke University Medical Center
Durham, North Carolina

Doris Howell, RN, PhD
RBC Chair
Oncology Nursing Research & Senior Scientist
Ontario Cancer Institute
University Health Network
Lawrence Bloomberg Faculty of Nursing
Toronto, Ontario, Canada

Jayne Huggard, MHSc (Hons), NZRN, Dip Couns., Dip ATE, Cert Grief Couns., CertSupervision, MNZAC
Mercy Hospice
Auckland, New Zealand

Peter K. Huggard, EdD, MPD (Hons), MEd (Couns) (Hons)
Senior Lecturer
Division of Social and Community Health
Faculty of Medical and Health Sciences
University of Auckland
Auckland, New Zealand
Affiliate Research Professor
Idaho State University
Pocatello, Idaho

Anne Hughes, RN, ACHPN, PhD, FAAN
Advanced Practice Nurse
Palliative Care Service
Laguna Honda Hospital and Rehabilitation Center
San Francisco, California

Elizabeth Johnston Taylor, PhD, RN
Associate Professor, School of Nursing
Loma Linda University
Loma Linda, California

Barbara Jones, PhD, MSW
Associate Professor of Social Work
Co-Director of The Institute for Grief, Loss, and Family Survival
The University of Texas at Austin
Austin, Texas

Gloria Juarez, PhD, RN
Assistant Professor of Nursing Research and Education
City of Hope National Medical Center
Duarte, California

Stein Kaasa, PhD, MD
Department of Oncology
St. Olav's Hospital
Trondheim University Hospital
Trondheim, Norway

Boon Han Kim, PhD, RN
Dean and Professor of Information in Clinical Nursing
College of Nursing
Hanyang University
Seongdong-gu, Seoul, South Korea

Hyun Sook Kim, PhD, RN, MSN, MSW
Professor of Social Welfare
Korea National University of Transportation
Jeungpyeong-gun, Chungbuk, South Korea

Kenneth L. Kirsh, PhD
Principal Investigator
Millennium Research Institute
VP of Clinical Research and Advocacy
Millennium Laboratories
San Diego, California

Carl A. Kirton, DNP, RN, ANP-BC, MBA
Chief Nursing Officer
Department of Nursing and Patient Care Services
Lincoln Hospital and Mental Health Center
Bronx, New York

Fatia Kiyange, MSc
Program Director
African Palliative Care Association
Kampala, Uganda

Patti Knight, RN, MSN, CS, CHPN
Palliative Care Unit Patient Manager
Department of Palliative Care and Rehabilitation Medicine
University of Texas MD Anderson Cancer Center
Houston, Texas

Dana Kramer, RN, MS, FNP-BC
Palliative Medicine NP Fellow
Memorial Sloan-Kettering Cancer Center
New York, New York

Kate Kravits, RN, MA
Senior Research Specialist
Division of Nursing Research and Education
City of Hope National Medical Center
Duarte, California

Elizabeth Kvale, MD
Associate Professor
Center for Palliative and Supportive Care
University of Alabama at Birmingham
Birmingham, Alabama

Gwenn LaRagione, RN, BSN, CCM, CHPPN
Nurse Coordinator
The Children's Hospital of Philadelphia
Philadelphia, Pennsylvania

Philip J. Larkin, BSc, MSc, PhD
Professor of Clinical Nursing
School of Nursing, Midwifery and
    Health Systems
University College Dublin
Belfield, Ireland

Bonnie B. Lasinski, MA, PT, CI, CLT-LANA
Clinical Director
Lymphedema Therapy
Woodbury, New York

Mary Layman-Goldstein, RN, MS, ANP-BC, ACHPN
Nurse Practitioner
Memorial Sloan-Kettering Cancer Center
New York, New York

Marcia Levetown, MD, FAAPHM
Principal
HealthCare Communication Associates
Houston, Texas

Rana Limbo, PhD, RN, PMHCNS-BC, CPLC, FAAN
Associate Director of Resolve Through Sharing
Bereavement and Advance Care Planning
    Services
Gundersen Health System
La Crosse, Wisconsin

Ellen A. Liu, MSN
Nurse Practitioner
City of Hope National Medical Center
Duarte, California

Diederik Lohman
Senior Researcher of Health and Human Rights
Human Rights Watch
New York, New York

Henry U. Lu, MD, DABPN
Director of Pain Clinic and Supportive Services
Co-Director of the Center for Palliative Care Education
    and Research
Makati Medical Center
Makati City, Philippines

Laurel J. Lyckholm, MD
Department of Hematology/Oncology
Virginia Commonwealth University
Massey Cancer Center
Richmond, Virginia

Patricia Maani-Fogelman, DNP
Department of Palliative Medicine
Geisinger Medical Center
Danville, Pennsylvania

Pamela Malloy, RN, MN, FPCN
ELNEC Project Director
American Association of Colleges of Nursing (AACN)
Washington, DC

Marianne Matzo, PhD, APRN-CNP, FPCN, FAAN
Professor and Frances E. and A. Earl Ziegler Chair in Palliative
  Care Nursing
Director of Sooner Palliative Care Institute
University of Oklahoma College of Nursing
Director of Survivorship and Supportive Care Center
Adjunct Professor of Geriatric Medicine
Peggy and Charles Stephenson Cancer Center
Oklahoma City, Oklahoma

Terri L. Maxwell, PhD, APRN
Vice President of Clinical Initiatives
Hospice Pharmacia, A Division of excelleRx, Inc.
Philadelphia, Pennsylvania

Polly Mazanec, PhD, ACNP-BC, AOCN, FPCN
Assistant Professor
FPB School of Nursing
Case Western Reserve University
Cleveland, Ohio

Jennifer McAdam, RN, PhD
Associate Professor in Nursing
Samuel Merritt University
Oakland, California

Mary S. McCabe, RN, MA
Director of Cancer Survivorship Program
Memorial Sloan-Kettering Cancer Center
New York, New York

Ruth McCorkle, PhD, RN, FAAN
Florence S. Wald Professor of Nursing and Professor
  of Epidemiology
School of Nursing and School of Public Health
Yale University
Director of Psychosocial Research
Yale Comprehensive Cancer Center
New Haven, Connecticut

Kathleen Michael, PhD, RN, CRRN
Assistant Professor of Nursing
Department of Organizational Systems and Adult Health
University of Maryland
Baltimore, Maryland

Paula Milone-Nuzzo, PhD, RN, FHHC, FAAN
Professor of Nursing
Pennsylvania State University
University Park, Pennsylvania

Pamela A. Minarik, PhD, RN, CNS, FAAN
Professor and Learning Center Faculty Development
Samuel Merritt University School of Nursing
San Francisco Peninsula Learning Center
San Mateo, California

Nicoleta Mitrea, APRN, PhD
Director of Nursing
National Coordinator of Palliative Nursing Education
Hospice Casa Sperantei
Basov, Romania

Beatriz Montes de Oca
Founder and Director
Hospice Cristina A.C.
Guadalajara, Mexico

Robert K. Montgomery, RN, ND
Coordinator of Pain Service
University of Colorado Hospital
Cordillera, Colorado

Xiomara Carmona Montoya, RN
Department of Palliative Care
Pablo Tobón Uribe Hospital
Medellin, Colombia

Betty D. Morgan, PhD, PMHCNS, BC
Associate Professor Emeritus
School of Nursing, College of Health Sciences
University of Massachusetts
Lowell, Massachusetts

Daniela Mosoiu, MD, PhD
Director of Education
Strategy and National Development
Hospice Casa Sperantei
Basov, Romania

Sonni Mun, MD
Adjunct Assistant Professor of Geriatrics and Palliative Medicine
Mount Sinai Hospital
New York, New York

Faith N. Mwangi-Powell, PhD
Chief of Party- USAID-ASSIST Project
University Research Co., LLC
Nairobi, Kenya

Ayda G. Nambayan, RN, DSN
Consultant for Advanced Training and Education
Co-Director of the Center for Palliative Care Education
  and Research
Makati Medical Center
Makati City, Philippines

Leslie Nield-Anderson, ARNP, PhD
Geropsychiatric Consultant
Sunhill Medical Center
Sun City Center, Florida

Linda L. Oakes, MSN, RN
Pain Clinical Nurse Specialist
St. Jude Children's Research Hospital
Memphis, Tennessee

Margaret O'Connor, AM
Emeritus Professor of Nursing
Palliative Care Research Team
School of Nursing and Midwifery
Monash University
Melbourne, Victoria

Edith O'Neil-Page, RN, MSN AOCNS
Palliative Care Clinical Nurse Specialist
UCLA Ronald Reagan Medical Center
Los Angeles, California

Shirley Otis-Green, MSW, LCSW, ACSW, OSW-C
Senior Research Specialist
Department of Population Sciences
Division of Nursing Research and Education
City of Hope National Medical Center
Duarte, California

Joan T. Panke, MA, NP
Palliative Care NP
MedStar Washington Hospital Center
Washington, DC

Jeannie V. Pasacreta, PhD, APRN
CEO
Integrated Mental Health Services, LLC.
Newtown, Connecticut

Steven D. Passik, PhD
Principal Investigator
Millennium Research Institute
VP of Clinical Research and Advocacy
Millennium Laboratories
San Diego, California

Tania Pastrana, MD
Research Scientist
Department of Palliative Medicine
University Hospital Aachen
Aachen, Germany

Sirin Petch, RN
Clinical Nurse
University of California
Los Angeles, California

Richard A. Powell, MA, MSc
Deputy Director Research
HealthCare Chaplaincy
New York, New York

Nancy Preston, PhD, RGN
Senior Lecturer in Palliative Care
International Observatory on End of Life Care
Lancaster University
Lancaster, United Kingdom

Maryjo Prince-Paul, PhD, APRN, ACHPN, FPCN
Assistant Professor of Nursing
Frances Payne Bolton School of Nursing
Case Western Reserve University
Cleveland, Ohio

Kathleen Puntillo, RN, PhD, FAAN, FCCM
Professor Emeritus and Research Scientist
Department of Physiological Nursing
University of California
San Francisco, California

Patrice Rancour, MS, RN, CNS, PMHCNS-BC
Center for Integrative Medicine
The Ohio State University
OSU Center for Integrative Medicine
Columbus, Ohio

Reggie Saldivar, MD
Memorial Sloan-Kettering Cancer Center
Pain and Palliative Care Service
New York, New York

Miguel Antonio Sánchez Cárdenas, PhD, MHSA, RN
National University of Colombia
Bogotá, Colombia

Margaret A. Schwartz, MSN, CNRN, APN
Department of Neurology
Northwestern University
Chicago, Illinois

Susie Seaman, NP, MSN, CWOCN
Sharp Rees-Stealy Wound Clinic
San Diego, California

Terran Sims, RN, MSN, ACNP
Nurse Practitioner
Department of Urology
University of Virginia
Charlottesville, Virginia

Thomas J. Smith, MD, FACP, FASCO
Professor of Palliative Medicine and Oncology
Johns Hopkins Medicine
Baltimore, Maryland

Rose Steele, RN, PhD
Professor of Nursing
York University
Toronto, Ontario, Canada

Virginia Sun, RN, PhD
Assistant Professor of Nursing Research
  and Education
City of Hope National Medical Center
Duarte, California

Ann Syme, RN, PhD
Director of the Research Institute Palliative End of
  Life Care
Covenant Health
Edmonton, Alberta, Canada

Sayaka Takenouchi, RN, PhD, MPH
Assistant Professor of Nursing Science
Kyoto University
Kizugawa City, Kyoto, Japan

Keiko Tamura, RN, PhD, OCNS
Yodogawa Christian Hospital
Higashi Yodogawa-ku, Osaka, Japan

Cheryl Thaxton, RN, MN, CPNP, FNP-BC, CHPPN
Nurse Practitioner-Supportive and Palliative Care Team
Baylor Regional Medical Center at Grapevine
Grapevine, Texas

Roma Tickoo, MD, MPH
Assistant Attending Physician
Pain and Palliative Care Service
Department of Medicine
Memorial Sloan-Kettering Cancer Center
New York, New York

Jennifer A. Tschanz, RN, MSN, FNP, AOCNP
Nurse Practitioner
Department of Hematology Oncology
Naval Medical Center San Diego
San Diego, California

Mary L.S. Vachon, PhD, RN
Psychotherapist in Private Practice
Professor of Psychiatry
University of Toronto
Toronto, Ontario, Canada

Rose Virani, RNC, MHA, OCN, FPCN
Senior Research Specialist/ELNEC Project Director
Division of Nursing Research and Education
City of Hope
Duarte, California

Deborah L. Volker, PhD, RN, AOCN, FAAN
Associate Professor of Nursing
School of Nursing
The University of Texas at Austin
Austin, Texas

Gay Walker, RN, CHPN
Program Development
Community Liaison
Providence TrinityKids Care
Torrance, California

Dorothy Wholihan, DNP, ANP-BC, GNP-BC, ACHPN
Clinical Assistant Professor of Nursing
Coordinator of Palliative Care
New York University
New York, New York

Clareen Wiencek, RN, PhD, CNP, ACHPN
Nurse Manager
Thomas Palliative Care Unit
Massey Cancer Center
Virginia Commonwealth University Health System
Richmond, Virginia

Anne Wilkinson, PhD, MS
Professor and Chair of Palliative and Supportive Care
Western Australia Centre for Cancer and Palliative Care
    Research
School of Nursing and Midwifery
Edith Cowan University
Joondalup, Western Australia

Anna Cathy Williams, RN, BS, PHN
Senior Research Specialist
City of Hope National Medical Center
Duarte, California

Donna J. Wilson, RN, MSN, RRT
Clinical Nurse Specialist/Personal Trainer
Fitness Coordinator
Integrative Medicine Center
Memorial Sloan-Kettering Cancer Center
New York, New York

Deborah Witt Sherman, PhD, APRN, BC, ACHPN, FAAN
Professor of Nursing
College of Nursing and Health Sciences
Florida International University
Miami, Florida

Elaine Wittenberg, PhD
Associate Professor of Nursing Research and Education
City of Hope National Medical Center
Duarte, California

SECTION I

General principles

CHAPTER 1

Introduction to palliative nursing care

Nessa Coyle

> I don't have hope for living. I have hope for dying peacefully and having peace for my family. ... My goal now is to die with dignity and to make it as easy as could be for my family and to have a really spiritual death. ... I gave it a lot of thought. ... I knew I was going to get to that point. ... I really wanted to die right ... to have everybody comfortable and accepting it and know it was time ... the grief would be there but they knew they did everything. ... How you live is important but how you die is important.
>
> A palliative care patient

Key points

- Palliative nursing reflects whole-person care and is integral to all nursing care.

- Providing palliative care depends on the nurse having strong interpersonal skills and clinical knowledge and is informed by respect for the person and the ethical principles of autonomy, beneficence, nonmaleficence, and justice.

- The genuine, warm, and compassionate relationship of a nurse with his or her patient is frequently a healing relationship even in the face of death. It is a combination of state-of-the art clinical competence with fidelity to the patient, the ability to listen and remain present in the face of much suffering and distress, and effective communication.

- It is the nurse who provides much of the care and support to patients and families throughout a disease trajectory and who is more likely to be present at the time of death than any other health professional.

Although nurses have long led the way in caring for those with life-limiting illness and of the dying through their presence, skill, and fidelity,[1] this specialized care has frequently been separated from mainstream healthcare. Now, based on the changing needs of society and the prevalence of chronic and prolonged debilitating illness, there is a growing recognition of the need to integrate palliative care into mainstream healthcare for those with serious or life-threatening illness. This recognition is demonstrated through the continued growth of palliative care teams throughout the United States,[2–5] the recognition of palliative medicine and nursing as areas of subspecialty,[6,7] and the opportunity of hospitals to obtain Advanced Certification in Palliative Care through the Joint Commission of Accreditation of Healthcare Organizations (JCAHO).[8]

This chapter will guide the reader through the major shifts in patterns of disease and treatment that have impacted the delivery of nursing care in the 21st century and the way we die. Various definitions of palliative care will be reviewed and the importance of language in describing palliative care emphasized. The relationship of palliative care to hospice care will be outlined. Finally, the distinctive features of palliative care nursing will be discussed and two case studies will be used to illustrate key aspects of palliative care nursing. We have come a long way in the field of palliative nursing and end-of-life care but still have a long way to go. Examples of nursing leadership in this integral field of nursing are demonstrated throughout the textbook.

Advances in healthcare and the changes in the trajectory of dying in the 21st century

Advances in healthcare in economically developed countries have changed the trajectory of dying. Improved nutrition and sanitation, preventive medicine, widespread vaccination use, the development of broad-spectrum antibiotics, and an emphasis on early detection and treatment of disease have resulted in fewer deaths in infancy and childhood, and fewer deaths from acute illness.[9,10] The combination of a healthier population in many developed countries and effective treatments for disease has resulted in the ability to prolong life. This has led to both benefits and challenges for society.[11] For example, in the United States, more than 70% of those who die each year are 65 years of age or older. The majority of these deaths, however, occur after a long, progressively debilitating chronic illness, such as cancer, cardiac disease, renal disease, or lung disease.[12]

With this changing paradigm of chronic illness, people are living longer with progressive disease and debilitation. Quality of life (QOL) is impacted by a high prevalence of poorly controlled symptoms, psychological and social distress, caregiver burden, and financial stress.[13–16] Sadly, both the burden of illness and access to palliative care are negatively impacted by socioeconomic status and demography. Poverty and minority status are associated with worse access and poorer outcomes.[17–22] In addition, the palliative care needs and end-of-life needs of children have only recently been recognized.[23,24] The field of palliative care nursing has expanded in response to these challenges.[25–28] It has built on the long tradition of hospice care and the models of excellent nursing care within hospice.[1,29,30]

Definitions of palliative care

World Health Organization definition

In recognition of the changing trajectory of dying and the implications for palliative care, the World Health Organization (WHO) modified its 1982 definition of palliative care to the following: "Palliative care is an *approach* to care which improves quality of life of patients and their families facing life-threatening illness, through the prevention, assessment and treatment of pain and other physical, psychological and spiritual problems."[31] This definition emphasizes QOL, not quantity, and affirms that dying is a normal part of the cycle of life.

The new WHO definition broadens the scope of palliative care beyond end-of-life care and suggests that such an approach can be integrated with life-prolonging therapy and should be enhanced as death draws near. In a similar vein, the National Comprehensive Cancer Network (NCCN) developed guidelines to facilitate the "appropriate integration of palliative care into anticancer therapy."[32] The focus of all these efforts is to change the standard practice of palliative care (identified as "too little, too late")—in which there is a distinct separation between diagnosis, treatment, and end-of-life care—to a vision of the future in which there is "front-loading" of palliative care. This means, for example, that at the time of the cancer diagnosis and initiation of treatment, the patient would also have access to psychological counseling, nutrition services, pain management, fatigue management, and cancer rehabilitation.[31] Such a model is appropriate for other chronic diseases as well. MediCaring, a national demonstration project spearheaded by the Center to Improve Care of the Dying, is an example of an attempt to integrate palliative care into medical and disease management for seriously ill patients with cardiac and pulmonary disease who have a life expectancy of between 2 and 3 years. The intent was to make this program a Medicare benefit, as is the case with hospice care.[33,34] Unfortunately, as with many demonstration projects, this remained a concept only and went no further.

Palliative care can also be described as an interdisciplinary or transdisciplinary[35] therapeutic model appropriate for all populations with serious life-threatening illness. A team approach acknowledges the multidimensional concerns of patients and families, which are within the purview of multiple professional disciplines. Symptoms are not only physical but also associated with suffering; life is no longer as it was, and the fragility of life is clear. Suffering may be experienced on a physical, psychological, social, emotional, and spiritual level. The words of a palliative care patient give voice to the interconnection of these domains—the connection between the physical and the spiritual: "I'm terrified of choking to death. I have to talk about it. I have such a fear of dying. I am afraid God is punishing me. I feel without hope."

Palliative care is a simultaneous care model, the palliative care team working alongside the patient's primary physician and other members of the healthcare team. Palliative care is relevant throughout the course of the disease. It provides a continuum of care with end-of-life care and hospice care as a "slice" of palliative care.[36] Palliative care can be provided at a *generalist* level of care—a best practice during the routine care of all patients with serious or life-threatening illness—and at a *specialist* level of care, an interdisciplinary service for patients or families who require a team of professionals with special competencies obtained through education, training, and certification.[7,36,37] All of these definitions of palliative care emphasize the importance of family support. Refer to chapter 66 for information about education and training opportunities for nurses whose goal is to specialize in palliative care.

The relationship of hospice care to palliative care in the United States

The hospice model of care was developed to address the specific needs of the dying and of their families, so long neglected by the medical system of care. The modern hospice movement started in England in 1967 through the work of Dame Cicely Saunders (who was trained as a nurse, a social worker, and a physician) and colleagues at St. Christopher Hospice in London. The hospice movement came to the United States in the mid-1970s, when Dr. Florence Wald, a nursing pioneer, led an interdisciplinary team to create the first American hospice.[1,38]

Hospice care became a Medicare benefit in the 1980s. Patients traditionally followed in hospice programs could no longer receive life-prolonging therapy, and it was required that they be certified by a physician as having a life expectancy of six months or less. This presented a problem for patients living with a chronic debilitating disease, whose life expectancy was unclear or was greater than six months, or who, for a variety of reasons, did not want to be "identified" as a hospice patient. The patient and family-centered care provided through hospice programs was needed, but the rationing of hospice programs (based on prognosis and closeness to death) and the requirement of denying life-prolonging therapies were barriers that deprived many individuals of the benefit of such care.

The palliative care model evolved in the United States from the traditional hospice perspective to address QOL concerns for those patients living for prolonged periods with a progressive, debilitating disease. It recognized the change in the trajectory of dying, in many industrial countries, from that of a relatively short illness leading to death to one involving a progressive and prolonged debilitating illness, frequently associated with multiple factors affecting QOL. It recognized that such factors required skilled and compassionate palliative care interventions, regardless of prognosis, life-prolonging therapy, or closeness to death.[39–41] The impact of incorporating palliative care into the patients' overall medical care is demonstrated by a randomized controlled trial of 151 patients newly diagnosed with metastatic lung cancer who received either usual care plus a palliative care referral or usual care alone. After 12 weeks those with early palliative care had a better QOL, fewer depressive symptoms, less aggressive treatment at end-of-life, and longer survival by three months.[42] The impact of an advanced practice nurse on these patients was also demonstrated.

In looking at the relationship between hospice and palliative care, perhaps hospice can best be described as a program through which palliative care is intensified as an individual moves closer to death. Ideally, patients living with a chronic, debilitating, and progressive disease and their families receive palliative care

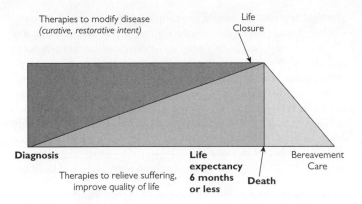

Therapies to modify disease
(curative, restorative intent)

Life Closure

Diagnosis

Therapies to relieve suffering, improve quality of life

Life expectancy 6 months or less

Death

Bereavement Care

Figure 1.1 The continuum of palliative care.

throughout the course of the patients' disease and its treatment. As they come closer to death, they are able to transition seamlessly and without added distress into a hospice program of care (Figure 1.1). Hospice care is provided mainly in the home with short periods of hospitalization for difficult-to-control symptoms or family respite.[43]

The "open access" hospice approach—a blended model between curative and palliative care—endeavored to mainstream hospice care into the current system of palliative care. The goal of open access was to deliver hospice care concurrently with the patient's other treatments, allowing state-of-the-art end-of-life care for a much longer period. The hope was that patients would access hospice earlier and would have the space and support to come to terms with their ambivalence about dying. Eligibility for hospice services would be determined solely by the regulatory requirements.[44] However, open access programs remain the exception because of cost.

In 2011 the Joint Commission of Hospital Accreditation launched an advanced certification for hospital-based palliative care programs that "demonstrate exceptional patient and family-centered care in order to optimize quality of life for patients with serious illness."[8] This was an important acknowledgment of the need for hospitals to provide palliative care for patients with serious illness as part of comprehensive care. By 2012 there were over 1,500 hospital-based palliative care programs in the United States. Hospitals with 300 beds or more were more likely to have such programs (75% of such hospitals) than those with a fewer number of beds (50% of such hospitals).[3] Although the comprehensiveness of the programs varies, a palliative care nurse always plays a central role. The number of hospice programs has also increased. There are over 5,300 such programs in the United States; however less than 50% of patients throughout the United States receive end-of-life care with hospice support.[4] This occurs despite evidence that hospice care is associated with the highest level of family satisfaction among last places of care[45,46] In addition hospice care has been demonstrated to provide quality care at the same time as reducing cost of care.[46,47]

Describing palliative care to patients and families—language matters

The Center to Advance Palliative Care (CAPC) reported data from a public opinion survey on palliative care conducted in 2011.[48] Language was found to influence the acceptability of palliative care to the general public, and, in that vein, palliative care needed to be differentiated from hospice or end-of-life care. The term "serious illness" rather than "advanced disease" made that distinction. Based on their findings, CAPC suggested the following language to describe palliative care:

> Palliative care is specialized medical care for people with serious illness. This type of care is focused on providing patients with relief from symptoms, pain, and stress of serious illness—whatever the diagnosis. The goal is to improve quality of life for both the patient and the family. Palliative care is provided by a team of doctors, nurses and other specialists who work with the patient's other doctors to provide an extra level of support. Palliative care is appropriate at any age and at any stage of a serious illness and can be provided together with curative treatment.[48]

The distinctive features of palliative care nursing

With this as a background, it is important to define the field of palliative care nursing and to recognize how it differs in essence from other areas of nursing care. In this way, nurses can be educated and trained appropriately, and the special nature of such education and training can be recognized. Palliative care nursing reflects a "whole-person" philosophy of care implemented across the life span and across diverse healthcare settings. The patient and family are the unit of care. The goal of palliative nursing is to promote QOL along the illness trajectory through the relief of suffering, and this includes care of the dying and bereavement follow-up for the family and significant others in the patient's life. Relieving suffering and enhancing QOL includes the following: providing effective pain and symptom management; addressing psychosocial and spiritual needs of the patient and family; incorporating cultural values and attitudes into the plan of care; supporting those who are experiencing loss, grief, and bereavement; promoting ethical and legal decision-making; advocating for personal wishes and preferences; using therapeutic communication skills; and facilitating collaborative practice.[49–52]

In addition, in palliative nursing, the "individual" is recognized as a very important part of the healing relationship. The nurse's individual relationship with the patient and family is seen as crucial. This relationship, together with knowledge and skills, is the essence of palliative care nursing and sets it apart from other areas of nursing practice. It is a specialty. However, generalist level palliative care as a therapeutic approach is appropriate for all nurses to practice. It is an integral part of many nurses' daily practice, as is clearly demonstrated in work with the elderly, the neurologically impaired, and infants in the neonatal intensive care unit. Such comprehensive care is practiced every day throughout the world by skilled and compassionate palliative care nurses both individually and as part of a team approach. Specialized education and training, as well as mentoring by seasoned palliative care nurses, is recognized as a needed foundation for specialized palliative care and hospice nursing. Without such training, nurses will inevitably find themselves in situations where they are unable to provide the necessary symptom control and amelioration of suffering for those living with advanced progressive disease and those near death. "I failed to care for him properly because I was ignorant"—these are haunting thoughts, sometimes expressed in words, other times borne silently, by the nurse. Moral distress is the result.

Moral distress occurs when the nurse is aware of a moral problem, acknowledges a moral responsibility, makes a moral judgment about the correct action to take, yet as a result of real or perceived constraints, is unable to take that action.[53–56] Commonly cited sources of moral distress for nurses are continued life supports that are not perceived to be in the best interests of the patient; inadequate communication about end-of-life care between providers, patients, and families; inadequate staffing or staff who are not adequately trained to provide required care; inadequate pain relief for patients; and false hope given to patients and families. Although some moral distress is probably inevitable when working in palliative care and end-of-life care, if not attended to it can result in the individual becoming morally numbed to ethically challenging situations, resulting in demoralization, negativity, and burnout. However, moral distress if recognized can become an instigator of insight, change, and learning rather than a detrimental force.[56]

When under the care of a skilled palliative care nurse, patients and their families struggling to live in the face of progressive, symptomatic, and debilitating disease can be well cared for and supported throughout this process—and find meaning and peace even in the face of death. This is the essence of skilled palliative nursing care—to facilitate the "caring" process through a combination of science, presence, openness, compassion, mindful attention to detail, and teamwork. It remains true, however, that although we have both the knowledge and the art to control the majority of symptoms that occur during the last months, weeks, and days of life, we still have much to learn about how to alleviate the psychological and spiritual distress that comes with life-threatening illness. Listening to the experts—our patients and their families—will help us obtain this necessary knowledge.[14]

Many patients recognize themselves as dying and struggle with this role. To be dying and to care for someone who is dying are two sides of a complex social phenomenon. There are roles and obligations for each person.[10] To be labeled as "dying" affects how others behave toward an individual and how the individual behaves toward self and others.[10] The person is dying, is "becoming dead" (personal communication, Eric Cassell, January 1, 2000), with all that implies at both an individual and a social level. A feeling of failure and futility may pervade the relationship between the patient and a nurse or physician not educated or trained in hospice or palliative care. They may become disengaged, and the potential for growth on the part of both patient and clinician may be lost—"I failed to care for him properly because I was ignorant … the memory haunts me."

The palliative care nurse and the interdisciplinary or transdisciplinary palliative care team: collaborative practice

The composition of teams providing palliative care varies tremendously, depending on the needs of the patients and the resources available.[57,58] The one common denominator is the presence of a nurse and a physician on the team. Regardless of the specific type of palliative care team, it is the nurse who serves as a primary liaison between the team, patient, and family, and who brings the team plan to the bedside, whether that is in the home, the clinic, or the inpatient setting. Because of the close proximity of the nurse to the patient and family through day-to-day observation and care, there is often a shift in the balance of shared decision-making with the patient or surrogate at the end of life from physician to nurse.[59,60] However, continued involvement of the physician in palliative care should still be fostered and encouraged; it is a myth that the physician need be less involved as the goal of care shifts from cure to comfort. Not uncommonly, a physician oriented toward life-prolonging therapies, who has provided care for a given patient over a number of years, may feel lost, helpless, overwhelmed, and uncertain of his or her role in the care of the dying. Yet, the patient and family may feel very close to that physician and have a great need for him or her at this time. Fear of abandonment by the patient, and the physician's desire to "do everything" rather than abandon the patient, may result in inappropriate and harmful treatments being offered and accepted. A nurse who is educated and trained in palliative care and end-of-life care can do much to guide and support the physician during this transition and to redirect or reframe the interventions from "doing everything" toward "doing everything to provide comfort and healing."

Advanced practice palliative care and hospice nurses

Advanced practice palliative care and hospice nurses have pioneered models of palliative nursing care in many different settings in the United States and elsewhere around the world.[61–70] For example, a former critical care nurse may now provide palliative care at an urban/trauma emergency center. Her focus is on patients who are not expected to survive their hospital stay, many of whom are respirator dependent. She may not work as part of a standing palliative care team but has access to the multiple disciplines within the institution, whom she can call on as needed. Another nurse practices at an urban acute care teaching hospital as part of a palliative care team. The patients he works with may not be actively dying, but are in need of symptom management, psychosocial support, grief and bereavement counseling, discharge planning, and/or long-term care planning. Continuity of care is emphasized, as well as education of nursing and medical staff. A third nurse practices at a large inner-city hospital serving a disadvantaged urban population. She heads the interdisciplinary End-of-Life Consultation Service and sees patients and their families concerning pain, grief, and ethical questions.

In contrast, a nurse with expertise in both geriatrics and palliative care works at a university-affiliated geriatric practice. Generally, the patients she serves have advanced chronic illness such as end-stage heart and lung disease, dementia, or cancer. Many of these patients are at risk for "falling through the cracks," as their prognosis and trajectory of dying may be uncertain and they do not fit into established categories for provision of home care. A fifth example is a nurse practitioner who works in a rural primary care practice with an emphasis on palliative care. He focuses on integrating palliative care into traditional health services for an underserved, sparsely populated rural community. As in the case of many senior palliative care nurses, this nurse practitioner mentors graduate and undergraduate students. A last example of this diversity in practice settings is a clinical specialist who practices at a long-term care facility—a setting where palliative-care needs of patients have only recently begun to receive due attention. This nurse's focus is to integrate palliative care into the normal flow of clinical care at the nursing home.

The role of the advanced-practice palliative care nurse is addressed in detail in chapter 62. Other examples of advanced-practice palliative care nursing are illustrated throughout the text, including chapter 70—International Palliative Care Initiatives, reflecting various stages of development.

Palliative care can be seen as a preventive model—preventing unnecessary suffering. By matching care plans to patient goals, palliative care and hospice care provide patients with the care they want and the freedom to avoid unwanted medical interventions. This is illustrated through the following case study.

Case study
Mrs. Gorky, a patient with endometrial cancer

Mrs. Gorky was a 64-year-old woman with advanced endometrial cancer. Her husband had died 10 years earlier of lung cancer. They had no children. She lived alone but had numerous friends, entertained frequently, and had an active social and intellectual life. Mrs. Gorky was initially treated with surgery and chemotherapy, but when her disease advanced on second-line chemotherapy she decided to forgo further disease-focused treatment and concentrate on QOL for whatever time she had left. With some reluctance from the primary service providers, who felt she was "giving up too soon," she was referred to the palliative care service to provide management of pain and other symptoms as well as psychological and social support during the rest of her illness trajectory. This approach to her care gave what she described as a sense of "safety" so that she could continue to live life to the fullest. She completed advance directives and appointed a healthcare agent who knew and respected her goals and values. Mrs. Gorky had a good year with minimal symptoms, when she developed increasing shortness of breath. She was found to have a large tumor compressing her trachea. She chose conservative treatment with steroids, opioids, and low-dose lorazepam. Her symptoms stabilized, and she was able to resume her normal activities. However, it was recognized and accepted by the patient that she was entering the final phase of her life and that a referral to home hospice would provide the necessary support at home. Her wish was to die at home and not be readmitted to the hospital. Mrs. Gorky did ask that she continue to be followed by the palliative care physician and advance practice nurse, with whom she had formed strong relationships, alongside the hospice team. This was arranged, and good communication was established between the palliative care advance practice nurse and hospice team. Mrs. Gorky was followed in the hospice program for 9 months. This required two recertifications of her appropriateness for this level of care. She expressed tremendous gratitude and appreciation for the work of the hospice team, their availability when questions arose, delivery of medications to the house, and the home visits they made. Although she described herself as "nonreligious—an atheist," she spoke of the pleasure she felt in visits from the Buddhist hospice chaplain. Although initially well controlled, her shortness of breath gradually got worse. She became increasingly housebound in the last month of life and accepted increased levels of sedation to control the dyspnea. Hospice provided 24-hour "crisis" care for the last 2 days of her life, and she was able to die peacefully at home. This patient was clear about what she wanted, was articulate and able to make her wishes known, and had the ability to withstand medical pressure to continue in active disease-focused therapy when this was not consistent with her goals and values. Mrs. Gorky benefited from the full spectrum of palliative care including end-of-life care with hospice support. Her goal was achieved through a peaceful death at home. The palliative care nurse played a central role for the patient ensuring continuity of care and communication between the two teams providing her care.

The second case presents a more complicated picture with medical and ethical dilemmas at the heart of the patient and families care. The transition from life-prolonging invasive interventions to QOL as the main focus of care was a difficult process and journey for the family. The advance practice palliative care nurse was instrumental in advocating for the patient and family and clarifying goals of care, which in turn, directed his actual care.

Case study
Robert Day, a patient with a recurrent brain tumor

Robert was a 33-year-old man with a recurrent brain tumor originally diagnosed in 2010.

He was treated with multimodal therapy including surgery, radiation therapy, and both conventional and experimental chemotherapy. Although clinically free of disease, he had progressive and accumulative disease and treatment-related sequela. These included cerebellar ataxia and marked wasting of his legs, chronic headache, intermittent respiratory failure, and impaired swallowing with multiple episodes of aspiration pneumonia.

Other issues included periods of life-threatening sepsis, and severe back pain associated with steroid-induced osteoporosis and collapsed thoracic vertebrae. He had a central line in place for periodic antibiotics, a tracheostomy, and a feeding tube (PEG). Although alert and oriented, Robert was cognitively impaired in memory and concentration. He was assessed as functioning at the level of a 10-year-old. In a 1-year period Robert had six admissions to the cancer center, four of which involved admission to the ICU and ventilator support. In a 1-year period he had spent only 2 months at home, yet that is where he wanted to be. His care at home was mainly provided by his parents—with some home nursing support. His father had recently retired from work to help care for him. This family lived in a one-bedroom apartment—the living room had been converted into a bedroom for Robert. The family's goal of care was that all measures be taken to keep Robert alive including cardiopulmonary resuscitation and that his QOL when home was good. They shared that he had been at death's door several times but had pulled through. When it was time for Robert to leave the hospital yet one more time—the inpatient staff expressed concern that his parents were unrealistic and were not able to take care of him adequately at home. They felt that he belonged in a long-term facility and that home care was an "unsafe" discharge. The palliative care team who had been working with this family for many months, although understanding the concerns of the inpatient staff, supported the patient and family's right to take him home. Prior to discharge home several family meetings were held where goals of care were readdressed. The focus of care changed from prolonging life at any cost to QOL for whatever time Robert had left. The palliative care physician became the physician of record for this young man, who was referred to home hospice with ongoing support from the palliative care advance practice nurse for continuity of care. The inpatient staff expressed agreement with this plan. In the following year Robert had only one 5-day admission to evaluate an acute hearing loss. His gradual deterioration continued, and he died at home under the care of his parents with hospice support. Discussion with the inpatient hospital staff prior to Robert's discharge gave them the opportunity to express the moral distress they experienced in this and similar situations when asked to perform interventions that they felt were not in the best interest of the patient. The palliative care nurse was a guiding voice for the staff, the patient, and the family.

End-of-life care in the United States today: improving but still a long way to go

The inadequacy of care for the dying, who are among the most voiceless and vulnerable in our society, came into national focus during the debates over the past three decades surrounding patient autonomy, the right to die, physician-assisted suicide, and euthanasia. The national dialogue was fueled by the actions of Dr. Jack Kevorkian and his "suicide machine"; the rulings of two US appeals courts on the right to die[71,72]; findings from the Study to Understand Prognoses and Preferences for Outcomes and Risks of Treatments (SUPPORT)[16]; interviews with family caretakers; a review of end-of-life content in nursing and medical texts[73,74]—which reflected minimal to no such content—and the Institute of Medicine's reports on end-of-life care, with its series of recommendations to address deficiencies in care of the chronically ill and dying, both children and adults.[24,75]

Means to a Better End, a report card generated by Last Acts (a Robert Wood Johnson–funded coalition created with almost 1,000 national partner organizations dedicated to end-of-life reform), was the first attempt at a comprehensive report on the state of end-of-life care in the United States.[76] Between August 30 and September 1, 2002, slightly more than 1,000 Americans were surveyed by telephone and asked their opinions regarding the quality of healthcare at the end of life. Three-quarters of those surveyed had suffered the loss of a family member or close friend in the last 5 years. Each of the 50 states and the District of Columbia were represented in the survey and were rated on eight criteria: state advance directive policies, location of death, hospice use, hospital end-of-life care services, care in intensive care units at the end of life, pain among nursing home residents, state pain policies, and the presence of palliative-care-certified nurses and doctors. The findings suggested that, "despite many recent improvements in end-of-life care and greater public awareness about it, Americans had no better than a fair chance of finding good care for their loved ones or for themselves when facing a life-threatening illness." A more recent state-by-state report card suggests although there has been improvement we still have a long way to go.[5]

Activities at the federal, state, and community levels continue to work toward improving access to skilled palliative care and end-of-life care. In addition, philanthropically supported programs to improve care of the dying have been developed at a community level to meet the needs of specific populations or underserved communities. The End-of-Life Nursing Education Consortium (ELNEC) is one such example that has had an ongoing national and international impact on nursing education in palliative care and end-of-life care (www.aacn.nche.edu/elnec).

Another example of a successful philanthropic funding was the Project on Death in America (PDIA), an initiative funded by the Open Society Institute, which was created in 1994 to help transform the experience of dying in the United States. Over the course of nine years, PDIA created funding initiatives in professional and public education, the arts and humanities, research, clinical care, and public policy. In addition a Faculty Scholars Program was initiated and ran from 1995 to 2007. A total of 87 interdisciplinary faculty scholars were selected including advanced practice nurses, educators, and researchers. Over thirty million dollars were invested in supporting their research, education, and program development in hospice and palliative care. The majority of these clinicians, educators, and researchers have gone on to be leaders in the field.[11] Unfortunately, many philanthropically supported programs are unable to self-sustain once the financial support comes to an end.

There are a growing number of palliative care programs being developed within institutions and long-term care facilities[3,29] as well as end-of-life pathways and critical care pathways for the dying.[77,78] These pathways have met with varying levels of acceptance at a clinical level. Home hospice programs that offer palliative care consultation services to the broader patient population are a recent innovation that may improve access to palliative care in nonhospice patients. Board certification in palliative nursing and palliative medicine are also important milestones in recognizing the specific body of knowledge and expertise necessary to practice with competence in this specialty.[7,6]

The Institute of Medicine report on improving care at the end of life[75] suggested that people should be able to achieve a "decent" or "good" death—"one that is free from avoidable distress and suffering for patients, families, and caregivers; in general accord with patients' and families' wishes; and reasonably consistent with clinical, cultural and ethical standards" (p. 24). The report and recommendations focused on the interdisciplinary nature of palliative care. This is an accepted principle in palliative care with a growing literature to support the benefit of an interdisciplinary or transdisciplinary team approach,[57,58] of which nursing is a core discipline. Traditionally, nursing has been at the forefront in the care of patients with chronic and advanced disease, and recent advances in symptom management, combined with the growing awareness of palliative care as a public health issue, have provided the impetus for bringing together this compendium of nursing knowledge.[79,80]

In summary

Progress is being made in the care of the seriously ill and dying, and palliative care nurses have been involved each step of the way. Board certifications in palliative nursing at both the generalist and advanced practice levels have been important milestones, giving recognition to the specific body of knowledge and expertise necessary to practice with competence in this area. However, palliative nursing is a combination of knowledge, skills, and compassion that involves valuing all the characteristics and past experience of a human being. It is an *approach* to care that focuses on the person as well as the disease. It is a way of thinking and an attitude of mind. There is a level of personal human contact with the seriously ill and dying person that goes beyond the tasks and procedures that can so often dominate everyday work. The patient and nurse embark on a journey together shaped by a search for meaning, personal dignity, and control over their lives. It is the nurse who provides much of the burden of care and support throughout a patient's and family's disease trajectory and the one who is more likely to be present at time of death than any other healthcare professional.

> Those who have the strength and the love to sit with a dying patient in the silence that goes beyond words will know that the moment is neither frightening nor painful, but a peaceful cessation of the functioning of the body. ... Watching a peaceful death of a human being reminds us of a falling star; one of a million lights in a vast sky that flares up for a brief moment only to disappear into the endless night forever ... it makes us aware of our finiteness, our limited lifespan.[81]

References

1. Dahlin C, Mazenec P. Building from our past: celebrating 25 years of clinical practice in hospice and palliative nursing. J Hosp Palliat Nurs. 2012;13(65):520–528.
2. National Hospice and Pallative Care Organization. 2010. NHPCO Facts and Figures: Hospice Care in America. Retrieved from http://

www.nhpco.org/files/public.Statistic_Research/hospice_Facts_Figures. Accessed July 23, 2013.

3. Center to Advance Palliative Care (CAPC). 2012. Growth of Palliative Care in U.S. Hospitals: 2012 Snapshot. http://reportcard.capc.org/pdf/capc-growth-analysis-snapshot-2011.pdf. Accessed June 5, 2013.

4. National Hospice and Palliative Care Organization. 2012. NHPCO Facts and Figures: Hospice Care in America. http://www.org/sites/default/public/Statistics_Research/2012_Facts_Figures. Accessed July 24, 2013.

5. Morrison RS, et al. America's care of serious illness: a state-by-state report card on access to palliative care in our nation's hospitals. J Palliat Med. 2011;14(10):1094–1096.

6. Quest TE, Marco CA, Derse AR. Hospice and palliative medicine: new subspecialty, new opportunities. Ann Emerg Med. 2009;54(1):94–102.

7. Martinez JM. Hospice and palliative nursing certification: the journey to defining a new nursing specialty. J Hosp Palliat Nurs. 2011;13(6):S29–S34.

8. The Joint Commission (TJC). Eligibility for Advanced Certification for Palliative Care. http://www.jointcommission.org/certification/eligiblity_palliative_care.aspx. Accessed June 5, 2013.

9. Corr C. Death in modern society. In: Doyle D, Hanks WC, MacDonald N (eds.), Oxford Textbook of Palliative Medicine. 2nd ed. Oxford: Oxford University Press; 1998:31–40.

10. Aries P. Western Attitudes Towards Death: From the Middle Ages to the Present. Baltimore, MD: Johns Hopkins University Press; 1974.

11. Clarke D. Transforming the Culture of Dying: The Work of the Project on Death in America. 2013. New York, NY: Oxford University Press.

12. NCHS Data Brief. Available at: www.cdc.gov/nchs/data/databriefs/db115.htm/ Accessed July 25, 2013.

13. Steinhauser KE, Christakis NA, Clipp EC, McNeilly M, McIntyre L, Tulsky JA. Factors considered inportant at the end of life by patients, family, physicians, and other care providers. JAMA. 2000;284:2476–2482.

14. Coyle N. Suffering in the first person. In: Ferrell BF (ed.), Suffering. Boston: Jones and Bartlett; 1996:29–64.

15. Ferrell BF, Coyle N. The Nature of Suffering and the Goals of Nursing. Oxford: Oxford University Press; 2008.

16. SUPPORT Principal Investigators. A controlled trial to improve care for seriously ill hospitalized patients: the study to understand prognoses and preferences for outcomes and risks of treatment (SUPPORT). JAMA. 1995;274(20):1591–1598.

17. Galea S, et al. Estimated deaths attributable to social factors in the United States. Am J Public Health. 2011;101(8):1456–1465.

18. Hughes A, Davies B, Gudmundsdottir M. "Can you give me respect?" Experiences of the urban poor on a dedicated AIDS nursing home unit. J Assoc Nurses AIDS Care. 2008;19:342–356.

19. Lewis JM, et al. Dying in the margins: understanding palliative care and socioeconomic deprivation in the developed world. J Pain Symptom Manage. 2011;42(1):105–118.

20. Lyckholm LJ, et al. Barriers to effective palliative care for low-income patients in late stages of cancer: report of a study and strategies for defining and conquering the barriers. Nurs Clin North Am. 2010;45(3):399–409.

21. Barnato AE, et al. Racial and ethnic differences in preferences for cnd-of life treatment. J Gen Intern Med. 2009;24(6):695–701.

22. Goldsmith B, Dietrich J, Du Q, Morrison S. Variability in access to hospital palliative care in the United States. J Palliat Med. 2008;11(8):1094–1102.

23. Institute of Medicine. When Children Die: Improving Palliative and End-of-Life Care for Children and Their Families. Washington, DC: National Academy Press; 2003.

24. Berlinger N, Jennings B, Wolf SM. The Hastings Center Guidelines for Decisions on Life-Sustaining Treatment and Care Near the End of Life. Revised and expanded 2nd ed. The Hastings Center. Oxford: Oxford University Press; 2013.

25. The Alliance for Palliative Nursing. The Future of Palliative Care Nursing: The Alliance White Paper. www.the alliancefor excellence. org/DisplayPage.aspx?Title=About%20Us. Assessed July 26, 2013.

26. Institute of Medicine (IOM). The Future of Nursing Leadership: Leading Change, Advancing Health Care. Transformational Models of Nursing Across Different Care Settings. Washington, DC: National Academies Press. http://www.nap.edu/catalog/12956.html

27. Clinical Practice Guidelines for Quality Palliative Care. 3rd ed. Pittsburgh, PA: National Consensus Project for Quality Palliative Care, 2013. Available at: http://www.nationalconsensusproject.org. Accessed June 14, 2013.

28. Hughes, A. Meeting the palliative care needs of the underserved. In Dahlin CM, Lynch MT (eds.), Core Curriculum for the Advanced Practice Hospice and Palliative Care Registered Nurse. 2nd ed. Pittsburgh, PA: Hospice and Palliative Nurses Association; 2013:529–544.

29. Lynch T, Connor S, Clark D. Mapping levels of palliative care development: a global update. J Pain Symptom Manage. 2013;45(6):1094–1106.

30. Institute of Medicine (IOM). 2010. The Future of Nursing: Leading Change, Advancing Health. http://www.iom.edu/Reports/2010/The-Future-of-Nursing-Leading-Change-Advancing-Health.aspx. Accessed June 17, 2013.

31. World Health Organization. 2010. WHO Definition of Palliative Care. http://www.who.int/cancer/palliative/definition/en/. Accessed July 26, 2013.

32. National Comprehensive Cancer Network. 2011. Clinical Practice Guidelines in Oncology: Palliative Care. Retrieved from http://oral-cancerfoundation.org/treatment/pdf/palliative.pdf. Accessed April 28, 2014.

33. Joanne Lynn's Testimony Before the Commission on Long-Term Care, July 17, 2013. Retrieved from http://medicaring.org. Accessed July 24, 2013.

34. MediCaring.org. Website. http://medicaring.org. Accessed July 24, 2013.

35. Grey M, Connolly C. "Coming together, keeping together, working together": interdisciplinary to transdisciplinary research and nursing. Nurs Outlook. 2008;56:102–107.

36. Mazanec OP, Daly BJ, Pitora EF, Kane D, Wile S, Wolen J. A new model of palliative care for oncology patients with advanced disease. J Hosp Palliat Nurs. 2009;11(6):324–331.

37. Lynch MT, Dahlin CM, Hultman T, Coakley E. Palliative care nursing: defining the discipline? J Hosp Palliat Nurs. 2011;13(2):106–111.

38. Wald FS. Hospice care in the United States: a conversation with Florence S. Wald. JAMA. 1999;281:1683–1685.

39. White paper on standards and norms for hospice and palliative care in Europe: part 1. European J of Palliative Care. 2009;16(6):278–289.

40. White paper on standards and norms for hospice and palliative care in Europe: part 2. 2012. European J Palliative Care. 2010;17(1):22–32.

41. Core competencies in palliative care: an EAPC white paper on palliative care education: part 1. European J of Palliative Care. 2013;20(2):86–91.

42. Temel JS, Greer JA, Muzikansky A, et al. Early palliative care for patients with metastatic non-small cell lung cancer. N Engl J Med. 2010;363:733–742.

43. Connor SR. Hospice and Palliative Care: The Essential Guide. 2nd ed. New York, NY: Routledge; 2009.

44. Wright AA, Katz IT. Letting go of the rope: aggressive treatment, hospice care, and open access. N Engl J Med. 2007;357:324–327.

45. Wright AA, Keating NL, Balboni TA, Matulonis UA, Block SD, Prigerson HG. Place of death: correlations with quality of life of patients with cancer and predictors of bereaved caregivers mental health. J Clin Oncol. 2010;28(29):4457–4464.

46. Morrison RS, Penrod JD, Cassel B, Caust-Ellenbogen M, Litke A, Spragens J, Meier DE. Cost savings associated with US hospital palliative care consultation programs. Arch Intern Med. 2008;118(16):1783–1790.

47. Kelley AS, Deb P, Du Q, Carlson MD, Morrison RS. Hospice enrollment saves money for Medicare and improves care quality across a number of different lengths-of-stay. Health Affairs. 2013;32(3): 552–561.

48. 2011 Public Opinion Research on Palliative Care. Retrieved at http://www.capc.org/tools-for-palliative-care-programs/marketing/public-opinion-research/2011.

49. Becker R. Palliative care 1: principles of palliative care nursing and end-of-life care. Nursing Times. 2009;105(13):14–16.

50. Becker R. Palliative care 2: exploring the skills that nurses need to deliver high quality palliative care. Nursing Times. 2009;105(14),18–20.

51. Becker R. Palliative care 3: using palliative nursing skills in clinical practice. Nursing Times. 2009;105:(15),18–21.

52. Dahlin CM. Communication in palliative care: an essential competency for nurses. In: Coyle N, Ferrell BR (eds.), Oxford Textbook of Palliative Nursing. 3rd ed. Oxford: Oxford University Press; 2010:107.

53. Epstein EG, Delgado S. Understanding and addressing moral distress. OJIN: The Online Journal of Issues in Nursing. 2010;15(3): Manuscript 1.

54. Epstein EG, Hemric AB. Moral distress, moral residue and the crescendo effect. J Clin Ethics. 2009;20:330–342.

55. Robinson R. Registered nurses and moral distress. Dimens Crit Care Nurs. 2010;29(5):197–202.

56. Browning AM. CNE article: moral distress and psychological empowerment in critical care nurses caring for adults at end of life. Am J Crit Care. 2013;22(2):143–151.

57. Loscalzo MJ, Von Gunten C. Interdisciplinary team work in palliative care: compassionate expertise for complex illness. In: Chochinov H, Breitbart W (eds.), Handbook of Psychiatry in Palliative Medicine. 2nd ed. New York, NY: Oxford University Press, 2009:172–185.

58. Stark D. Teamwork in palliative care: an integrated approach. In: Altilio T, Otis-Green S (eds.), Oxford Textbook of Palliative Social Work. New York, NY: Oxford University Press; 2011:415–424.

59. Peereboom K, Coyle N. Facilitating goals of care discussions for patients with life-limiting disease: communication strategies for nurses. J Hosp Palliat Nurs. 2012;14:251–258.

60. Lawrence JF. The advance directive prevalence in long-term care: a comparison of relationships between a nurse practitioner healthcare model and a traditional healthcare model. J Amer Acad Nurse Practit. 2009;21:179–185.

61. Lewis R, Neal RD, Williams NH, et al. Nurse-led vs. conventional physician-led follow-up for patients with cancer: systematic review. J Adv Nursing. 2009;65(4):706–723.

62. McCabe MS, Jacobs LA. Clinical update: survivorship care—models and programs. Semin Oncol Nurs. 2012;28(3):e1–e8.

63. Costa L, Poe SS. Nurse-led interdisciplinary teams: challenges and rewards. J Nurs Care Qual. 2008;23:292–295.

64. Bakitas M, Bishop MF, Caron P, Stephens L. Developing successful models of cancer palliative care services. Semin Oncol Nurs. 2010;26:266–284.

65. Deitrick LM, Rockwell EH, Gratz N, et al. Delivering specialized palliative care in the community: a new role for nurse practitioners. ANS Adv Nurs Sci. 2011;34:E23–E36.

66. Bookbinder M, Glajchen M, McHugh M, et al. Nurse practitioner-based models of specialist palliative care at home: sustainability and evaluation of feasibility. J Pain Symptom Manage. 2010 Sep 18. Epub ahead of print.

67. Griffith J, Lyman JA, Blackhall LJ. Providing palliative care in the ambulatory care setting. Clin J Oncol Nurs. 2010;14:171–175.

68. Newhouse RP, Stanik-Hutt J, White KM, et al. Advanced practice nurse outcomes 1990–2008: a systematic review. Nurs Econ. 2011;29:230–250.

69. Prince-Paul M, Burant C, Saltzman JN et al. The effects of integrating an advanced practice palliative care nurse in a community oncology center: a pilot study. J Support Oncol. 2010;8(1):21–27.

70. Nelson JE, Cortez TB, Curtis JR, et al. Integrating palliative care in the ICU: the nurse in a leading role. J Hosp Palliat Nurs. 2011;13(2):89–94.

71. In re Quinlan, 755 A2A 647 (NJ), cert denied, 429 70 NJ 10, 355 A2d 647 (1976).

72. Cruzan v Director, Missouri Department of Health, 497 US 261, 110 S Ct 2841 (1990).

73. Ferrell BR, Virani R, Grant M, Juarez G. Analysis of palliative care content in nursing textbooks. J Palliat Care. 2000;16:39–47.

74. Rabow MW, Hardie GE, Fair JM, McPhee SJ. End-of-life care content in 50 textbooks from multiple specialties. JAMA. 2000; 283:771–778.

75. Field MJ, Cassel CK, eds. Approaching Death: Improving Care at the End of Life. Report of the Institute of Medicine Task Force on End of Life Care. Washington, DC: National Academy of Sciences, 1997.

76. Last Acts. Means to a Better End: A Report Card on Dying in America Today. November 2002. Available at: http://www.rwjf.org/files/publications/other/meansbetterend.pdf. Accessed November 16, 2009.

77. van der Heide A, Veerbeek L, Swart S, van der Mass PJ, van Zuylen L. End of life decision making for cancer patients in different clinical settings and the impact of LCP. J Pain Symptom Manage. 2009;39(1):33–43.

78. Smith D. Development of end of life care pathways for patients with heart failure in a community setting. Int J Palliat Nurs. 2012;18(6): 295–300.

79. Dahlin CR, Lynch MT, eds. Core Curriculum for the Advanced Practice Hospice and Palliative Nurse. 2nd ed. Pittsburgh, PA: HPNA, 2013.

80. National Consensus Project. Clinical Practice Guidelines for Quality Palliative Care. 3rd ed. Pittsburgh, PA: National Consensus Project for Quality Palliative Care; 2013. www.nationalconsensusproject.org. Accessed July 5, 2013.

81. Kubler-Ross, E. On Death and Dying. New York, NY: Touchstone Press; 1969:296.

CHAPTER 2

National consensus project for quality palliative care
Promoting excellence in palliative nursing

Constance M. Dahlin

We need to be keeping more data, recording our expertise and speaking up for ourselves so when people say quality of care, they will also say, quality of nursing.

Susan B. Hassmiller, PhD, RN, FAAN, February 20, 2013

History of the National Consensus Project

National discussion on end-of-life care, death and dying in America, and the poor status of such care in the United States was the backdrop for the National Consensus Project (NCP). In 2001 national leaders in hospice and palliative care convened in New York City to discuss the need for guidelines and standards in palliative care to guide the growth and expansion of palliative care in the United States. Palliative nurses had a prominent presence at the meeting. This laid the foundation for the creation of the National Consensus Project for Quality Palliative Care. It initially consisted of the five foremost national palliative care organizations in the United States at that time: the American Academy of Hospice and Palliative Medicine (AAHPM), the Center to Advance Palliative Care (CAPC), the Hospice and Palliative Nurses Association (HPNA), the National Hospice and Palliative Care Organization (NHPCO), and the Last Acts Partnership for Caring. Each organization had four representatives from their administrative leadership and designated members to participate in the process.[1]

At the outset, the mission of the NCP was to create clinical practice guidelines to improve and ensure the quality of palliative care in the United States. There was a three-pronged goal for the *Clinical Practice Guidelines for Quality Palliative Care*: (1) to promote quality and reduce variation in new and existing programs, (2) develop and encourage continuity of care across settings, and (3) facilitate collaborative partnerships among palliative care programs, community hospices, and a wide range of other healthcare delivery settings.[1]

In developing the palliative care clinical practice guidelines, consensus among project members was essential. The document was created through a multifaceted approach inclusive of scientific evidence, clinical experience, and lastly, expert opinion. First, there was a review of all the international standards and guidelines, most notably from Canada, Australia, Scotland, and Great Britain.[1] Second, there was a review of the specific literature in hospice and palliative care.[1] Finally, there was an inclusive writing process underscoring the importance and potential impact of the project.[1] The NCP members reviewed the document line by line, each line necessitating at least 80% agreement of task force members for inclusion. Upon its completion, over 100 leaders in healthcare reviewed and offered revisions on the document. Finally, 50 liaison organizations agreed to help promote the document.

In 2004, through this consensus process, the first edition of the *Clinical Practice Guidelines for Palliative Care* was published. An executive summary was printed in the *Journal of Palliative Medicine*.[2] The document reviewed the current status of palliative care, delineated eight domains of care (see Box 2.1) and encapsulated the palliative-care-related research organized by domains.[1]

The *Clinical Practice Guidelines* offered a framework for the future of palliative care. Their purpose was to serve as a manual or blueprint to create new programs, guide developing programs, and set high expectations for excellence for existing programs (see Box 2.2 for the history of the development of the *Clinical Practice Guidelines*). Rather than set minimally acceptable practices, the guidelines set ideal practices and goals that palliative care services

---

Box 2.1 Eight domains of care developed by the National Consensus Project

Domain 1: Structure and processes of care
Domain 2: Physical aspects of care
Domain 3: Psychological and psychiatric aspects of care
Domain 4: Social aspects of care
Domain 5: Spiritual, religious, and existential aspects of care
Domain 6: Cultural aspects of care
Domain 7: Care of imminently dying patient
      (*changed in 2013 to care of the patient at the end of life)
Domain 8: Ethical and legal aspects of care

Box 2.2 History of the Clinical Practice Guidelines development

National Consensus Project for Quality Palliative Care

2001 Meeting in New York City of national palliative care leaders.

2002 Clinical guidelines development.

2003 Initial Review by advisory committee.

2003 Release of the first edition of the *Clinical Practice Guidelines for Quality Palliative Care* in March at the Annual Assembly received endorsement by 40 organizations and associations.

2005 Disseminated to 90 organizations and associations.

2006 Served as the basis of NQF's document *A National Framework and Preferred Practices for Palliative and Hospice Care Quality: A Consensus Report.*

2009 Release of second edition of the *Clinical Practice Guidelines for Quality Palliative Care* at the Annual Assembly of the American Academy of Hospice and Palliative Medicine and the Hospice and Palliative Nurses Association. Aspects of Palliative Care featured in review of health care reform under the Obama Administration.

2011 The *Clinical Practice Guidelines for Quality Palliative Care* used as underlying principles for The Joint Commission *Advanced Palliative Care Certification.*

2013 Release of third edition at the Annual Assembly of the American Academy of Hospice and Palliative Medicine and the Hospice and Palliative Nurses Association endorsed by 54 organizations and associations.

---

should strive to attain. Since the guidelines were not associated with any regulatory body or reimbursement process, they were voluntary.[3] There was confidence that the *Clinical Practice Guidelines* would:

♦ Facilitate the development and continuing improvement of clinical palliative care programs providing care to patients and families with life-threatening or debilitating illness.

♦ Establish uniformly accepted definitions of the essential elements in palliative care that promote quality, consistency, and reliability of these services.

♦ Establish national goals for access to quality palliative care.

♦ Foster performance measurement and quality improvement initiatives in palliative care services.

♦ Foster continuity of palliative care across settings (i.e., home, residential care, rehabilitation, hospital, and hospice).[1]

Basic assumptions about palliative care were constructed. First, palliative care services would adhere to established standards and requirements for healthcare quality such as safety, effective leadership, medical record keeping, and error reduction. Second, palliative care programs would observe established professional and organizational codes of ethics. Third, the guidelines would continue to evolve and be revised to integrate changes in professional practice, the evidence base, and healthcare reform. Fourth, the consensus process would continue ensuring representation of a broad range of professionals and disciplines. This process would guarantee that the guidelines would continue to promote

the highest quality of clinical palliative care services across the healthcare continuum. Fifth, there was recognition of specialty palliative care versus primary palliative care. Primary palliative care could be incorporated in any discipline and included basic pain and symptom management and communication skill. Specific palliative care qualifications would continue to be delineated by specialty organizations granting professional credentials and programmatic accreditation. Sixth, there was a core assumption that ongoing professional palliative care education would occur and include the knowledge, attitudes, and skills required to deliver quality palliative care across the domains established in the document.[1]

The response to the document was very positive. The *Clinical Practice Guidelines* were subsequently endorsed by many organizations and broadly disseminated. In fact, the Annual Assembly of the Hospice and Palliative Nurses Association and the American Academy of Hospice and Palliative Medicine in Phoenix, Arizona, was attended by Florence Wald. At the unveiling presentation, Dr. Wald, a pioneer in hospice care in America, stated how proud she was that palliative care had come so far and that she had hoped she would someday be able to see such guidelines. To further awareness of the *Clinical Practice Guidelines*, articles specific to each domain were published in a variety of journals. This included physical aspects of care,[4] psychological aspects of care,[5] social aspects of care,[6] spiritual aspects of care,[7] cultural aspects of care,[8] care of the imminently dying,[9] and ethical and legal aspects of care.[10]

In 2005, the structure of the NCP moved to a collaborative governance structure under the Coalition of Hospice and Palliative Care. In 2006, the National Quality Forum (NQF) used the *Clinical Practice Guidelines* as a basis of their document *A National Framework for Palliative and Hospice Care Quality Measurement and Reporting.*[11] The mission of the NQF is to "improve American healthcare through the endorsement of the consensus-based national standards for measurement and public reporting of healthcare performance data. The goal is to maintain meaningful information about the care delivery such as safety, benefit, patient centeredness, equality, and efficiency of healthcare." The NQF adoption of the guidelines was significant because the goal of their document was to formulate palliative care standards and preferred practices with implications for reimbursement, internal and external quality measurement, regulation, and accreditation.[11] See Appendix 2.1 for a listing of the NCP *Clincial Practice Guidelines* and the corresponding NQF Preferred Practices.

In 2009, five years after the initial release of the *Clinical Practice Guidelines*, the landscape of palliative care had changed. The number of palliative care and hospice programs had substantially grown. Palliative care was being discussed in healthcare reform. It was necessary that the guidelines be updated and kept in concordance with the NQF preferred practices. Moreover, many stakeholders inquired how the conceptual ideas of the *Clinical Practice Guidelines* could be implemented into practice. As part of the commitment to have the guidelines reflect changes in palliative care, healthcare policy, and healthcare research, the guidelines were updated by the four organizational members of the Hospice and Palliative Care Coalition under which the NCP was structured. Coalition organizations included the AAHPM, CAPC, HPNA, and NHPCO.

Within the review process, it was necessary to be certain that all 38 of the NQF preferred practices were reflected within the domains. To broaden the scope of the document, there was appraisal and discussion within special interest focus groups related to palliative care (i.e., pediatrics, social work, oncology, geriatrics).[12] In addition, an updated literature search was performed. To ensure the inclusivity and expansiveness of the guidelines to all settings where palliative care is provided, clarifications were made and sections were further developed.[12] The guidelines were again released at the Annual Assembly of the American Academy of Hospice and Palliative Medicine and the Hospice and Palliative Nurses Association.

From 2009 to 2013, significant maturation within the field of palliative care occurred. Palliative medicine was recognized by the American Board of Medical Specialties, thereby acknowledging palliative medicine as a distinct and well-defined field of medical practice. The numbers of hospice and palliative care programs across the nation with increased representation across healthcare systems and settings grew extensively. Other major developments occurred in the healthcare panorama as well. Healthcare reform within the Patient Protection and Affordable Care Act of 2010 included critical elements of palliative care.[13] A palliative care quality measurement strategy was created within the NQF whereby new quality measures were endorsed and measurement development was enhanced.[14–17] The Joint Commission initiated Advanced Palliative Care Certification in 2011.[18] Finally, published research revealed that early intervention palliative care had demonstrated improved quality of life, decreased psychological symptoms, and perhaps increased survival.[19,20] The NCP guidelines again were updated to reflect the field by a consortium of six key national palliative care organizations: American Academy of Hospice and Palliative Medicine, Center to Advance Palliative Care, Hospice and Palliative Nurses Association, National Association of Social Workers, National Hospice and Palliative Care Organization, and the National Palliative Care Research Center.

National Consensus Project definition of palliative care

In the original edition, the NCP created a definition of palliative care. However, in subsequent editions, in order to promote consistency, the NCP used the palliative care definition used by both the Center for Medicare and Medicaid Services (CMS) and Federal Register, which states:

> Palliative care means patient and family-centered care that optimizes quality of life by anticipating, preventing, and treating suffering. Palliative care throughout the continuum of illness involves addressing physical, intellectual, emotional, social, and spiritual needs and to facilitate patient autonomy, access to information, and choice.[21]

In addition, there are several underlying palliative care tenets delineated by the NCP:[21]

1. Palliative care is patient- and family-centered care.

2. There is comprehensive palliative care with continuity across health settings.

3. Early introduction of palliative care concepts should begin at diagnosis of a serious or life-threatening illness by the primary team. Specialist consultation may be offered as well.

4. Palliative care may be offered concurrently with or independent of curative or life-prolonging care. Patient and family hopes for peace and dignity are supported throughout the course of illness, during the dying process, and after death.

5. Palliative care is interdisciplinary and collaborative. Patients, families, palliative care specialists, and other healthcare providers collaborate and communicate about care needs.

6. Palliative care team members have clinical and communication expertise.

7. The goal of palliative care is the relief of physical, psychological, emotional, and spiritual suffering of patients and families.

8. Palliative care should focus on quality care.

9. There should be equitable access to palliative care services.[21]

The eight domains of the Clinical Practice Guidelines

Structure and Process of Care

This domain addresses the organization of specialty palliative care teams and the necessary processes and procedures for quality care delivery. The criteria emphasize coordinated assessment and continuity of care across healthcare settings. In particular, there is a description of the interdisciplinary team composition, team member qualifications, and necessary education, training, and support. There is attention and emphasis on interdisciplinary team engagement and collaboration with patients and families. Finally, the domain incorporates the new mandates for quality under the Patient Protection and Affordable Care Act.[21]

Physical Aspects of Care

This domain recognizes the multidimensional management of symptoms with pharmacological, interventional, behavioral, and complementary interventions. There is emphasis on the assessment and treatment of physical symptoms using appropriate, validated tools. Finally, there are recommendations for the use of explicit policies for the treatment of pain and symptom management, as well as safe prescribing of controlled medications.[21]

Psychological and Psychiatric Aspects of Care

This domain acknowledges the psychological and psychiatric dimensions of palliative care. It reviews the collaborative assessment process of these diagnoses, similar to the multidimensional approach for physical aspects. It defines essential elements including patient-family communication on assessment, diagnosis, and treatment options in the context of patient and family goals of care. Most significant, this domain now includes required criteria for a bereavement program.[21]

Social Aspects of Care

This domain emphasizes interdisciplinary engagement and collaboration with patients and families to identify, support, and capitalize on patient and family strengths. It defines essential elements of a palliative care social assessment. Notably, it includes the description of the role of the bachelor's- or master's-prepared social work professional.[21]

Spiritual, Religious, and Existential Aspects of Care

This domain has evolved to include a spirituality definition. While simultaneously stressing interdisciplinary responsibility and collaboration in assessment and management of spiritual issues and concerns, there is the emphasis of the use of an appropriately trained chaplain. Requirements for staff training and education in spiritual care are described. Finally, the domain promotes spiritual and religious rituals and practices for comfort and relief.[21]

Cultural Aspects of Care

The development of this domain now includes a definition of required interdisciplinary team culture and cultural competence, highlighting culture as a source of resilience and strength for the patient and family. Cultural and linguistic competence with respect to language, literacy, and linguistically appropriate service delivery is stressed.[21]

Care of the Patient at the End of Life

The title of this domain has changed from Care of the Imminently Dying to Care of the Patient at the End of Life to broaden care to advanced stages of illness through death. In particular, it emphasizes the social, spiritual, and cultural aspects of care, as well as guidance to family, throughout the dying trajectory. It underscores the importance of meticulous assessment and management of pain and other symptoms. Communication, information, and documentation of the signs and symptoms of the dying process, inclusive of the patient, the family, and all other involved health providers is underscored.[21]

Ethical and Legal Aspects of Care

This domain is separated into three sections: advance care planning, ethics, and the legal aspects of care. The responsibility of the palliative care team to promote ongoing goals of care discussions accompanied by completion and documentation of advance care planning is emphasized. Significant is the affirmation and acknowledgment of the frequency and complexity of palliative care ethical and legal issues. Consultation from ethics committees and legal counsel are stressed, as are team competencies in ethical principles and education regarding particular legal aspects of care. There is also emphasis on the understanding of the respective scope of practice issues between team members.[21]

National Consensus Project *Clinical Practice Guidelines*: implications for nursing

Nursing and palliative care are intertwined. Recognition of specialty palliative nursing expertise and assuring the quality of palliative nursing practice are essential to quality palliative care. In the 2011 Institute of Medicine (IOM) report *The Future of Nursing: Leading Change, Advancing Health* acknowledged the essential contributions of nursing at the bedside and in healthcare redesign in its four messages.[22]

1. Nurses should practice to the full extent of their education and training.

2. Nurses should achieve higher levels of education and training through an improved education system that promotes seamless academic progression.

3. Nurses should be full partners, with physicians and other healthcare professionals, in redesigning healthcare in the United States.

4. Effective workforce planning and policymaking require better data collection and information restructure.[22]

The NCP promotes these messages and delineates quality in three areas particularly appropriate for nursing and consistent with the IOM report: professional development, education, and certification. Nurses at all levels can promote consistent roles, job descriptions, and education. The guidelines provide nationally recognized definitions of hospice and palliative care, acknowledging the role of nursing in the interdisciplinary team, and care coordination, thereby promoting practice to the full extent of a nurse's education and training. Since participating NCP members include representation from nursing, hospice, research, palliative care, and social work, they were meant to be inclusive across all settings. The NCP guidelines establish essential elements of specialist palliative care that promote quality, consistency, and reliability of services. This helps define primary palliative nursing versus specialty palliative nursing. Perhaps this will also promote nurses' achievement of higher education and training in academic programs with palliative care.

Moreover, since the NCP guidelines are meant to guide program development and benchmarking, they can assist palliative nurse leaders or coordinators in program development. The NCP guidelines may promote more effective data collection and information gathering by nurses. As nationally recognized guidelines, they can be easily incorporated into a program. Finally, they allow the palliative care nurse to measure his or her program in terms of quality and breadth. Box 2.3 offers an overview of how the guidelines can be implemented for nurses.

The importance of nurse adoption of the *Clinical Practice Guidelines*

There are many important reasons for nurses to adopt the *Clinical Practice Guidelines*. They offer a framework to care, educational areas, and criteria for benchmarking. Nurses practice in a variety of settings that may have palliative care programs. This includes acute care programs, ambulatory care programs, rehabilitation facility programs, community programs, home care programs, hospice programs, long-term care facilities, accountable care organizations, and patient medical homes. As a framework to care, the *Clinical Practice Guidelines* assist nurses in creating quality palliative services or developing quality programs in all of these settings. In particular, the structure for bereavement can promote essential program components in the various domains (e.g., quality improvement processes, bereavement programs, spiritual care, and cultural care). The emphasis on consistency is important, particularly in orientation, job descriptions, and peer review. By assisting programs in developing critical organizational structures and processes, there may be improved staff retention and morale.

As an education tool, the guidelines offer the content for programs and can promote more effective educational programs. The scope of potential topics includes: the focus of orientation, communication, pain and symptom assessment, social/cultural assessment, and spiritual assessment. These areas are important

Box 2.3 Nurse applications of the *Clinical Practice Guidelines*

Domain 1: Structure and Processes of Care

1. All nurses should receive education in primary palliative care in undergraduate, graduate programs, and doctoral programs.

2. All nurses should pursue continuing education in primary palliative care.

3. All nurses should receive an orientation in primary palliative care that includes attitudes, knowledge, and skills in the domains of palliative care. This includes basic pain and symptom assessment and management, basic communication skills around advanced illness, ethical principles, grief and bereavement, family and community resources, and hospice care (both philosophy and eligibility).

4. All nurses, especially specialty hospice and palliative nurses, should work within an interdisciplinary team, which may include a variety of disciplines.

5. Specialty hospice and palliative nurses should have regularly scheduled and organized support for their palliative care work and designated meetings to discuss the work.

6. Specialty hospice and palliative nurses should be certified in hospice and palliative care. Certification is available for the Nursing Assistant, the Licensed Practical/Vocational Nurse, the Registered Nurse, and the Advanced Practice Registered Nurse.

7. All nurses should participate in quality initiatives to improve palliative care.

8. Specialty hospice and palliative nurses should promote continuity in palliative care across health settings and promote hospice as an option.

Domain 2: Physical Aspects of Care

1. All nurses should assess pain, dyspnea, and function using appropriate and consistent tools in patients with serious, life-threatening illness.

2. All nurses should document findings in their care plan.

3. All nurses should follow evidence-based treatment pathways to manage pain and symptoms and reassess as appropriate.

Domain 3: Psychological and Psychiatric Aspects of Care

1. All nurses should assess depression, anxiety, and delirium using appropriate and consistent tools in patients with serious, life-threatening illness.

2. All nurses should document findings in their care plan.

3. All nurses should follow evidence-based treatment pathways to manage psychological symptoms to reassess as appropriate.

4. Specialty hospice and palliative nurses should assess patient and family coping and assist in developing a bereavement plan.

5. Specialty hospice and palliative nurses should participate in the development of structured bereavement programs for palliative care services.

Domain 4: Social Aspects of Care

1. All nurses should review social supports and concerns of patients and family with advanced, serious, or life-threatening illness.

2. Specialty hospice and palliative nurses should assist in development of a comprehensive social care plan that addresses the social, practical, and legal needs of the patients and caregivers, including but not limited to relationships, communication, existing social and cultural networks, decision-making, work and school settings, finances, sexuality/intimacy, caregiver availability/stress, and access to medicines and equipment.

Domain 5: Spiritual, Religious, and Existential Aspects of Care

1. Specialty hospice and palliative nurses should perform a spiritual assessment that includes religious, spiritual, and existential concerns using a structured instrument, and integrate the information obtained from the assessment into the palliative care plan.

2. All nurses should refer patients and families with serious and life-threatening illness to spiritual counselors, chaplains, social community leaders, and religious leaders, as appropriate.

Domain 6: Cultural Aspects of Care

1. All nurses should assist in a cultural assessment as a component of comprehensive palliative and hospice care assessment, including but not limited to locus of decision-making, preferences regarding disclosure of information, truth-telling and

(continued)

Box 2.3 Continued

decision-making, dietary preferences, language, family communication, desire for support measures such as palliative therapies and complementary and alternative medicine, perspectives on death, suffering and grieving, and funeral/burial rituals.

Domain 7: Care of the Patient at the End of Life

1. Specialty hospice and palliative nurses should recognize and review signs and symptoms of dying with the patient, family, and staff. These discussions should be documented.

2. All nurses should assure comfort by treating symptoms of patients at the end of life (e.g., pain, dyspnea, mouth care, skin).

3. All nurses should review any cultural, religious, or pertinent rituals regarding death and after-death care with the patient and family.

4. All nurses should provide post-death support to the family.

5. All nurses should treat the body after death with respect, in accordance with the cultural and religious practices of the family and in accordance with local law.

Domain 8: Ethical and Legal Aspects of Care

1. All nurses should promote and review advance care planning and appropriate documents.

2. All nurses should provide ethical care and work with an ethics committee to develop guidelines to resolve ethical dilemmas.

3. Specialty hospice and palliative nurses should understand the legal aspects of palliative care and seek out legal counsel as necessary.

---

to nurses in all settings. Moreover, the guidelines support the use of research and evidence-based practice. Just as important, the essential aspects of ethical foundations and legal regulations assist the nurse in scope of practice issues and mitigate moral distress by having more clearly delineated processes for conflict resolution.

As benchmarks, the *Clinical Practice Guidelines* assist the nurse and his or her palliative care program in achieving the highest possible quality of care in all health settings by ensuring adherence to the highest standards of care. Their use may result in improved patient outcomes and better compliance with state and federal regulations. Because appropriate resource utilization is a common concern, the emphasis on community assessment and communication across settings and specialties may provide a nursing benchmark. Moreover, the strict description of pain and symptom assessment, management, the use of assessment tools, and evidenced-based practice is significant. These criteria may help with improved patient and family satisfaction in pain and symptom control. Domain 2, Physical Aspects of Care, and Domain 3, Psychological and Psychiatric Aspects of Care, may help organizations meet evidence requirements for the American Nurses Credentialling Center Magnet Status Recognition in the following areas: Structural Empowerment, concerning nursing image and professional development; Exemplary Professional Practice, concerning consultation and resources, autonomy, and interdisciplinary relationships; New Knowledge, Innovation, and Improvements, concerning quality improvement; and Empirical Quality Results, concerning quality of care.[23] They can also facilitate Joint Commission accreditation in the areas of pain management, culturally competent care, and end-of-life care.

Conclusion

The National Consensus Project for Quality Palliative Care's *Clinical Practice Guidelines for Quality Care* is a significant resource. It offers the nurse a framework for quality care in all settings. The *Clinical Practice Guidelines* are appropriate to a range of populations from

neonates to children to adults and older adults; a range of chronic progressive and serious life-threatening illnesses, injuries, and trauma; and a range of vulnerable and underresourced populations (homeless individuals, immigrants, individuals with low income, oppressed racial and ethnic groups, veterans, prisoners, older adults, and individuals with mental illness).[21] Finally, the *Clinical Practice Guidelines* are appropriate for any setting because they facilitate partnerships for caring for patients with debilitating and life-limiting illnesses, and offer support for the nurse in delivering the care, particularly for long-term patients.

References

1. National Consensus Project for Quality Palliative Care. Clinical Practice Guidelines for Quality Palliative Care. Pittsburgh, PA: National Consensus Project for Quality Palliative Care, 2004.

2. American Academy of Hospice and Palliative Medicine, Center to Advance Palliative Care, Hospice and Palliative Nurses Association, Last Acts Partnership, National Hospice and Palliative Care Organization. National Consensus Project for Quality Palliative Care: Clinical Practice Guidelines for Quality Palliative Care, executive summary. J Palliat Med. 2004;7(5):611–627.

3. Ferrell B, Connor S, Cordes A, et al. The national agenda for quality palliative care: The National Consensus Project and the National Quality Forum. J Pain Symptom Manage. 2007;33(6):737–744.

4. Blouin G, Fowler B, C D. The national agenda for quality palliative care: promoting the National Consensus Project's domain of physical symptoms and the National Quality Forum's preferred practices for physical aspects of care. J Pain Palliat Care Pharmacother. 2008;23(3):1–7.

5. Hultman T, Reder ER, Dahlin C. Improving psychological and psychiatric aspects of palliative care: the National Consensus Project and the National Quality Forum preferred practices for palliative and hospice care. Omega. 2008;57(4):323–339.

6. Altilio T, Otis-Green S, Dahlin C. Applying the National Quality Forum preferred practices for palliative and hospice care: a social work perspective. J Soc Work End Life Palliat Care. 2008;4(1):3–16.

7. Scott K, Thiel MM DC. The national agenda for quality palliative care: the essential elements of spirituality in end of life care. Chaplaincy Today. 2008;24(2):15–21.

8. Dahlin C. Promoting culture within pain and palliative care: National Consensus Project guidelines and National Quality Forum preferred practices. The Pain Practitioner. 2007;17(2):7–9.

9. Lynch M, Dahlin C. The National Consensus Project and National Quality Forum preferred practices in care of the imminently dying: implications for nursing. J Hosp Palliat Nurs. 2007; 9(6):316–322.

10. Colby WH, Dahlin C, Lantos J, Carney J, Christopher M. The National Consensus Project for Quality Palliative Care Clinical Practice Guidelines domain 8: ethical and legal aspects of care. HEC Forum. 2010; 22(2):117–131.

11. National Quality Forum. A National Framework and Preferred Practices for Palliative and Hospice Care Quality: A Consensus Report. Washington, DC: National Quality Forum, 2006.

12. National Consensus Project for Quality Palliative Care. Clinical Practice Guidelines for Quality Palliative Care. 2nd ed. Pittsburgh, PA: National Consensus Project for Quality Care, 2009.

13. Patient Protection and Affordable Care Act (PPACA), Public Law 111-148, §2702, Title III (B)(III) Section 3140,124, Stat. 119, 318-319, Consolidating amendments made by Title X of the Act and the Health Care and Education Reconciliation Act of 2010. http://www.gpo.gov/fdsys/pkg/PLAW-111publ148/html/PLAW-111publ148.htm Last updated March 10, 2010. Accessed October 7, 2013.

14. National Quality Forum. 2011. National Quality Forum National Priorities Partnership. http://www.qualityforum.org/Setting_Priorities/NPP/Input_into_the_National_Quality_Strategy.aspx Last updated September 2011. Accessed October 7, 2013.

15. National Quality Forum. 2010. National Quality Forum Endorsed Standards. http://nationalqualityforum.org/Measures_List.aspx. Last updated June 2012. Accessed October 7, 2013.

16. National Quality Forum. Palliative Care and End-of-Life Care: A Consensus Report. Washington, DC: National Quality Forum, 2012. http://www.qualityforum.org/Publications/2012/04/Palliative_Care_and_End-of-Life_Care%E2%80%94A_Consensus_Report.aspx Last updated August 29, 2012. Accessed October 7, 2013.

17. National Quality Forum. Measure Applications Partnership: Performance Measurement Coordination Strategies for Hospice and Palliative Care Final Report. Washington, DC: National Quality Forum, 2012. http://www.qualityforum.org/Publications/2012/06/Performance_Measurement_Coordination_Strategy_for_Hospice_and_Palliative_Care.aspx. Last updated February 8, 2013. Accessed October 7, 2013

18. The Joint Commission. 2011. Advanced Certification in Palliative Care. http://www.jointcommission.org/certification/palliative_care.aspx. Accessed August 31, 2013.

19. Bakitas M, Lyons KD, Hegel MT, et al. Effects of a palliative care intervention on clinical outcomes in patients with advanced cancer: the Project ENABLE II randomized controlled trial. JAMA. 2009;302(7):741–749.

20. Temel J, Greer J, Muzikansky A, et al. Early palliative care for patients with metastatic non-small cell lung cancer. N Engl J Med. 2010;363:733–742.

21. National Consensus Project for Quality Palliative Care. Clinical Practice Guidelines for Quality Palliative Care. 3rd ed. Pittsburgh, PA: National Consensus Project for Quality Palliative Care, 2013.

22. Institute of Medicine. The Future of Nursing: Leading Change, Advancing Health. Washington, DC: National Academies Press, 2011.

23. American Nurses Credentialing Center. Announcing a New Model for ANCC's. Recognition Program©. 2008 Magnet News. http://www.nursecredentialing.org/MagnetModel.aspx#Empirical. Accessed October 7, 2013.

Appendix 2.1

The 2013 National Consensus Project Domains and the corresponding 2006 National Quality Forum Preferred Practices

NCP domains	NQF preferred practices
DOMAIN 1. STRUCTURE AND PROCESSES OF CARE GUIDELINE 1—GENERAL STRUCTURE OF CARE	PREFERRED PRACTICE 1 ♦ Provide palliative and hospice care by an *interdisciplinary team* of skilled palliative care professionals, including, for example, physicians, nurses, social workers, pharmacists, spiritual care counselors, and others who collaborate with primary healthcare professional(s). PREFERRED PRACTICE 2 ♦ Provide access to palliative and hospice care that is responsive to the patient and family *24 hours a day, 7 days a week.*
DOMAIN 1. STRUCTURE AND PROCESSES OF CARE GUIDELINE 1—GENERAL STRUCTURE OF CARE	PREFERRED PRACTICE 3 ♦ Provide *continuing education* to all healthcare professionals on the domains of palliative care and hospice care. PREFERRED PRACTICE 4 ♦ Provide *adequate training and clinical support* to assure that professional staff are confident in their ability to provide palliative care for patients.
DOMAIN 1. STRUCTURE AND PROCESSES OF CARE GUIDELINE 1—GENERAL STRUCTURE OF CARE	PREFERRED PRACTICE 5 ♦ Hospice care and specialized palliative care professionals should be *appropriately trained, credentialed, and/or certified* in their area of expertise.
DOMAIN 1. STRUCTURE AND PROCESSES OF CARE GUIDELINE 2—GENERAL PROCESSES OF CARE	PREFERRED PRACTICE 6 ♦ Formulate, utilize, and regularly review a *timely care plan* based on a *comprehensive interdisciplinary assessment of the values, preferences, goals, and needs of the patient and family* and, to the extent that existing privacy laws permit, ensure that the plan is broadly disseminated, both internally and externally, to all professionals involved in the patient's care. PREFERRED PRACTICE 7 ♦ Ensure that on *transfer between healthcare settings, there is timely and thorough communication* of the patient's goals, preferences, values, and clinical information so that continuity of care and seamless follow-up are assured.

(continued)

NCP domains	NQF preferred practices
DOMAIN 1. STRUCTURE AND PROCESSES OF CARE GUIDELINE 2—GENERAL PROCESSES OF CARE	**PREFERRED PRACTICE 8** ◆ Healthcare professionals should *present hospice as an option to all patients* and families when death within a year would not be surprising, and reintroduce the hospice option as the patient declines. **PREFERRED PRACTICE 9** ◆ Patients and caregivers should be asked by palliative and hospice care programs to *assess physicians'/ healthcare professionals' ability* to discuss hospice as an option.
DOMAIN 1. STRUCTURE AND PROCESSES OF CARE GUIDELINE 2—GENERAL PROCESSES OF CARE	**PREFERRED PRACTICE 10** ◆ Enable patients to make *informed decisions* about their care by educating them on the process of their disease, prognosis, and the benefits and burdens of potential interventions. **PREFERRED PRACTICE 11** ◆ Provide *education and support to families* and unlicensed caregivers based on the patient's individualized care plan to assure safe and appropriate care for the patient.
DOMAIN 2. PHYSICAL ASPECTS OF CARE GUIDELINE 1—ASSESSMENT AND MANAGEMENT OF PAIN AND SYMPTOMS	**PREFERRED PRACTICE 12** ◆ *Measure and document* pain, dyspnea, constipation, and other symptoms using available standardized scales. **PREFERRED PRACTICE 13** ◆ *Assess and manage symptoms* and side effects in a timely, safe, and effective manner to a level acceptable to the patient and family.
DOMAIN 3. PSYCHOLOGICAL AND PSYCHIATRIC ASPECTS OF CARE GUIDELINE 1—ASSESSMENT AND MANAGEMENT OF PSYCHOLOGICAL AND PSYCHIATRIC SYMPTOMS	**PREFERRED PRACTICE 14** ◆ *Measure and document* anxiety, depression, delirium, behavioral disturbances, and other common psychological symptoms using available standardized scales. **PREFERRED PRACTICE 15** ◆ *Manage* anxiety, depression, delirium, behavioral disturbances, and other common psychological symptoms in a *timely, safe, and effective* manner to a level acceptable to the patient and family. **PREFERRED PRACTICE 16** ◆ *Assess and manage psychological reactions* of patients and families to address emotional and functional impairment and loss (including stress, anticipatory grief, and coping) in a regular ongoing fashion.
DOMAIN 3. PSYCHOLOGICAL AND PSYCHIATRIC ASPECTS OF CARE GUIDELINE 2—BEREAVEMENT PROGRAMS	**PREFERRED PRACTICE 17** ◆ *Develop and offer a grief and bereavement care plan* to provide services to patients and families prior to and for at least 13 months after the death of the patient.
DOMAIN 4. SOCIAL ASPECTS OF CARE	**PREFERRED PRACTICE 18** ◆ Conduct *regular patient and family care conferences* with physicians and other appropriate members of the interdisciplinary team to provide information, discuss goals of care, disease prognosis, and advanced care planning, and offer support. **PREFERRED PRACTICE 19** ◆ *Develop and implement a comprehensive social care plan* which addresses the social, practical, and legal needs of the patient and caregivers, including but not limited to: relationships, communication, existing social and cultural networks, decision-making, work and school settings, finances, sexuality/ intimacy, caregiver availability/stress, and access to medicines and equipment.
DOMAIN 5. SPIRITUAL, RELIGIOUS, AND EXISTENTIAL ASPECTS OF CARE GUIDELINE 1—ASSESSMENT	**PREFERRED PRACTICE 20** ◆ Develop and document a plan based on *assessment of religious, spiritual, and existential concerns* using a structured instrument and integrate the information obtained from the assessment into the palliative care plan. **PREFERRED PRACTICE 21** ◆ Provide information about the availability of spiritual care services and make *spiritual care available* either through organizational spiritual counseling or through the patient's own clergy relationships.
DOMAIN 5. SPIRITUAL, RELIGIOUS, AND EXISTENTIAL ASPECTS OF CARE GUIDELINE 2—ELEMENTS OF ASSESSMENT	**PREFERRED PRACTICE 22** ◆ Specialized palliative and hospice care teams should include *spiritual care professionals appropriately trained and certified* in palliative care.
DOMAIN 5. SPIRITUAL, RELIGIOUS, AND EXISTENTIAL ASPECTS OF CARE GUIDELINE 3—FACILITATION OF RITUALS AND PRACTICES	**PREFERRED PRACTICE 23** ◆ Specialized palliative and hospice spiritual care professionals should build *partnerships with community clergy, and provide education and counseling related to end-of-life care.*

(continued)

NCP domains	NQF preferred practices
DOMAIN 6. CULTURAL ASPECTS OF CARE	**PREFERRED PRACTICE 24** ◆ Incorporate *cultural assessment* as a component of comprehensive palliative and hospice care assessment, including, but not limited to: locus of decision-making, preferences regarding disclosure of information, truth telling and decision-making, dietary preferences, language, family communication, desire for support measures such as palliative therapies and complementary and alternative medicine, perspectives on death, suffering and grieving, and funeral/burial rituals. **PREFERRED PRACTICE 25** ◆ Provide professional interpreter services and culturally sensitive materials in the *patient's and family's preferred language*.
DOMAIN 7. CARE OF THE PATIENT AT THE END OF LIFE GUIDELINE 1—IDENTIFICATION, COMMUNICATION, AND MANAGEMENT	**PREFERRED PRACTICE 26** ◆ *Recognize and document the transition to the active dying phase* and *communicate* to the patient, family, and staff the expectation of imminent death. **PREFERRED PRACTICE 27** ◆ The *family is educated* on a timely basis regarding signs and symptoms of *imminent death* in a developmentally, age-, and culturally appropriate manner. **PREFERRED PRACTICE 28** ◆ As part of the ongoing care planning process, routinely ascertain and *document patient and family wishes* about the care setting for *site of death*, and fulfill patient and family preferences when possible. **PREFERRED PRACTICE 29** ◆ Provide *adequate dosage of analgesics* and sedatives as appropriate to achieve patient comfort during the active dying phase and address concerns and fears about using narcotics and of analgesics hastening death.
DOMAIN 7. CARE OF THE PATIENT AT THE END OF LIFE GUIDELINE 3—POSTDEATH CARE	**PREFERRED PRACTICE 30** ◆ *Treat the body post death with respect* according to the cultural and religious practices of the family and in accordance with local law.
DOMAIN 7. CARE OF THE PATIENT AT THE END OF LIFE GUIDELINE 4—BEREAVEMENT PLANNNING	**PREFERRED PRACTICE 31** ◆ *Facilitate effective grieving* by implementing in a timely manner a bereavement care plan after the patient's death, when the family remains the focus of care.
DOMAIN 8. ETHICAL AND LEGAL ASPECTS OF CARE GUIDELINE 1—ADVANCED CARE PLANNING	**PREFERRED PRACTICE 32** ◆ *Document the designated/surrogate decisionmaker* in accordance with state law for every patient in primary, acute, and long-term care and in palliative and hospice care. **PREFERRED PRACTICE 33** ◆ *Document the patient/surrogate preferences* for goals of care, treatment options, and setting of care at first assessment and at frequent intervals as conditions change. **PREFERRED PRACTICE 34** ◆ *Convert the patient treatment goals into medical orders* and ensure that the *information is transferable* and applicable across care settings, including long-term care, emergency medical services, and hospitals, such as the Physician Orders for Life-Sustaining Treatments (*POLST*) Program. **PREFERRED PRACTICE 35** ◆ Make *advance directives and surrogacy designations available* across care settings, while protecting patient privacy and adherence to Health Insurance Portability and Accountability Act (HIPAA) regulations, e.g., by Internet-based registries or electronic personal health records. **PREFERRED PRACTICE 36** ◆ Develop healthcare and *community collaborations to promote advance care planning* and completion of advance directives for all individuals, e.g., Respecting Choices, Community Conversations on Compassionate Care.
DOMAIN 8. ETHICAL AND LEGAL ASPECTS OF CARE GUIDELINE 2—ETHICS IN ADVANCED ILLNESS	**PREFERRED PRACTICE 37** ◆ *Establish or have access to ethics committees* or ethics consultation across care settings to address ethical conflicts at the end of life. **PREFERRED PRACTICE 38** ◆ For minors with decision-making capacity, *document the child's views and preferences for medical care*, including assent for treatment, and give appropriate weight in decision-making. Make appropriate professional staff members available to both the child and the adult decisionmaker for consultation and intervention when the child's wishes differ from those of the adult decisionmaker.

Adapted from The National Consensus Project for Palliative Care 2013 *Clinical Practice Guidelines for Palliative Care* and the National Quality Forum 2006 *A National Framework and Preferred Practices for Palliative and Hospice Care Quality: A Consensus Report.*

CHAPTER 3

Hospital-based palliative care

Patricia Maani-Fogelman and Marie A. Bakitas

I had the pleasure of meeting with you in my mother's room a few weeks ago and wanted to let you know that although it was a very difficult time for me, your patience, listening and compassion really helped put me at ease and your wisdom helped guide me into making some responsible decisions. I really believe that with your help I was able to stand up for what my mother wanted and I did the right thing even though it was the hardest to do. Thank you for all you did for me and for all of the others you assist.

A patient's daughter's note to a palliative medicine nurse practitioner after a consult for her mother

An invasion of armies can be resisted, but not an idea whose time has come.

Victor Hugo

Key points

- The structure, clinical processes, and measurement of outcomes of specialized palliative and hospice services, organized as hospital-based palliative care (HBPC) programs, have grown in sophistication in response to documented, poor end-of-life (EOL) care, growth of the elderly and advanced chronic illness populations, and documented successes of pilot and maturing clinical palliative care programs.

- Standards, guidelines, and other resources are now available to assist health systems to develop, sustain, or expand palliative care services for persons of all ages and stages of illness, along the entire care continuum. All hospitals and healthcare systems should develop palliative care services that are consistent with these standards and the mission, size, and scope of the health system.

- Processes of "best-practice" palliative care should address the right person at the right time and to the appropriate degree. Fundamental processes of HBPC include introduction of palliative care services to patients and their families at the time of diagnosis with life-limiting illness; triggers for palliative care referral; standardized assessment; proactive advance care planning; treatment decision-making; crisis prevention; expert symptom management; attention to psychosocial, spiritual, and physical needs; family care; and bereavement.

- Processes and infrastructures of care should exist "upstream" from palliative care services so that advance care plans documenting patients' values and preferences for care (including proxy decision maker, site of care, symptom management, artificial nutrition and hydration, and resuscitation) can be honored.

- Establishing standardized assessment, measurement, and reporting of patient, family, and institutional outcomes is an essential component of every HBPC program both for program evaluation and research.

- Institutional resources, both internal (e.g., quality improvement and ethics committees) and external (e.g., The Joint Commission [TJC], Center to Advance Palliative Care [CAPC]), can assist with the development or improvement of a high quality, cost-effective HBPC program.

Hospital-based palliative care (HBPC) is a continually evolving moral imperative: the number of Americans living with chronic illness exceeds 90 million, and seven of every 10 Americans die from complications of a chronic illness.[1,2] This burden is significantly higher in the Medicare population where the majority of deaths are attributable to nine diagnoses: congestive heart failure, chronic lung disease, cancer, coronary artery disease, renal failure, peripheral vascular disease, diabetes, chronic liver disease, and dementia.[3] As the 2012 Dartmouth Atlas of Healthcare notes, "Patients with chronic illness in their last two years of life account for about 32% of total Medicare spending, much of it going toward physician and hospital fees associated with repeated hospitalizations."[3] Moving forward with better integration of palliative care in the end-of-life care of inpatients, one must consider the following: What do our patients desire at the end of their lives? Where do they want to spend the time they have left—closer to home, in the hospital, or at home? When medical interventions are deemed medically inappropriate or unlikely to yield a meaningful benefit, do patients want to pursue treatment or cease and desist with transition to a different plan of care?

Comparisons of location of death for Medicare beneficiaries during the period 2005–2009 versus 2000 reveal fewer numbers died in hospital yet use of intensive care unit services and healthcare transitions increased most in the last few weeks of life.[1,3,4] Although research confirms that patients with advanced illness report a preference to die at home, the majority are still dying in the hospital. Care was rarely aligned with reported preferences: among the patients who indicated that they preferred to die at home, the majority (55%) died in the hospital. The evidence demonstrates the vital importance of high-quality delivery of palliative care services within the context of inpatient care, especially when the admission is likely to become the patient's terminal admission. This understandably highlights the importance of pioneering methodologies to end-of-life care to facilitate engagement of patients and their families in early discussions of preferences for end-of-life care in advanced medical illness before catastrophe strikes and aggressive interventions are initiated at end of life.[3–5] Chronic illness and longer life were the legacy of the 20th century. However, the healthcare system did not keep pace with medical advances. The hospital became a common location for a good portion of EOL care despite Americans' stated preference for death at home.[4,5] An analysis of the experience of dying among chronically ill Medicare recipients revealed more hospice care in 2007 than in 2003. Although a percentage of seriously ill patients experienced their final admission in a critical care unit, by and large hospital deaths occurred in non-critical-care units and could have been anticipated for hours or days before death actually occurred. Despite this opportunity to provide comfort measures during the dying process, patients dying in the acute care hospital experienced pain, dyspnea, anxiety, and other distressing symptoms.[6–8] Hospitals were designed primarily to provide acute, episodic care to persons with acute illness rather than comfort and continuity to persons who were not expected to survive a particular disease or episode of illness. Therefore, fundamental system reform and redesign was needed to improve (and possibly prevent) hospital care of persons with life-limiting illness. As Berwick[9] wrote, "Academic medicine has a major opportunity to support the redesign of healthcare systems; it ought to bear part of the burden for accelerating the pace, confidence, and pervasiveness of that change.... 'Where is the randomized trial?' is, for many purposes, the right question, but for many others it is the wrong question, a myopic one. A better one is broader: 'What is everyone learning?'" Asking the question that way will help clinicians and researchers see further in navigating toward improvement. This is a call to action, particularly for nurses, since nursing care is the primary service provided during hospital admission and much of the care and the system that patients experience could be influenced by nurses at all organizational levels. The way nurses learn and share their knowledge will further direct the process of patient care. Most other types of care, such as physician consultation, diagnostic tests, and pharmaceutical treatments, do not generally require inpatient admission.

Hospital-based palliative care programs have begun to change the quality and quantity of hospitalized deaths.[10–11] Nurses have served as leaders and active team members to define, direct, and lead multidisciplinary and interdisciplinary teams and modify efforts at multiple levels of the hospital care system to improve the complex care process for persons with life-limiting illness.[12] Improved palliative care structure, standards for care processes, and measurement of outcomes have begun to come about as a result of the development of HBPC programs. The new millennium marked the "end of the beginning" of the discipline of palliative care.

This chapter provides nursing leaders and others with historical and foundational information on HBPC for the purpose of improving access to high-quality palliative and hospice services for the right person, at the right time, and in the right amount. The chapter begins with two cases. The first case illustrates how

many patients experience life-limiting illness in many of our current health systems. The second case illustrates how serious illness can be experienced differently in a health system with a comprehensive HBPC program. The cases are followed by discussion of a variety of HBPC structures or models, palliative care delivery processes, quality improvement (QI) and outcomes measurement, and future directions in the evolution of HBPC programs. The information contained in this chapter is important for all nurses who care for persons with life-limiting illness, including senior nursing leaders, clinical nurse specialists, nurse practitioners, nurse managers, educators, quality improvement nurses, nurse researchers, and especially nurses on the front lines at the bedsides of patients with serious illness.

Case study

Mrs. O, an 80-year-old female with altered mental status, urosepsis, and respiratory failure

Mrs. O, an 80-year-old female, was admitted to the medical/surgical unit with altered mental status, dehydration, and urinary tract infection. After initial labs and urine cultures were sent, she was started on broad-spectrum antibiotics and intravenous fluids for gentle rehydration. Her past medical history was significant for emphysema, hypertension, and breast cancer in remission since age 50.

Mrs. O developed further confusion, hypotension, agitation, cough, and dyspnea. A chest radiograph reveal bilateral infiltrates, and the medical team ordered supportive oxygen therapy, nebulizer treatments, and transfer to a special care unit for close observation. Labs later confirmed sepsis.

Her respiratory status continued to decline, with increasing oxygen demand, and a face mask was added. As Mrs. O was declining, the resident asked her, "Do you want us to do everything for you, to save your life?" She continuously nodded her head "Yes" to the question. Shortly after this "discussion," Mrs. O suffered a respiratory arrest, received cardiopulmonary resuscitation (CPR) including intubation and mechanical ventilation, and was transferred to the intensive care unit (ICU) in critical condition. No family members were identified to assist the medical team with decision-making.

While she was in the ICU, a Swan-Ganz catheter and central line were inserted, multiple daily blood draws were taken, and Mrs. O remained heavily sedated to prevent dislodging her tubes. Her medical condition progressively deteriorated, and the medical and nursing staff became increasingly frustrated, feeling helpless and not knowing Mrs. O's goals of care. Her primary care physician had not held prior discussions with her and did not have any record of advance directives. After multiple attempts, a cousin from out of state was located who advised the medical team that he did not really have a relationship with the patient and could not make any decisions for her. Over the second week of her ICU stay she arrested again, requiring compressions and defibrillation. She progressed to overwhelming septic shock with multiorgan failure that did not respond to aggressive interventions such as dialysis. On hospital day #20, Mrs. O died in the ICU.

Quality-of-care issues identified in this case

- Discussion of advance directives should take place with patients when they have capacity and are not in crisis.

- Early introduction of palliative care specialists may help to clarify and document patients' goals of care and pain/symptom management preferences.

- Lack of advance planning can result in healthcare provider frustration, fatigue, and moral distress.

- Medical and nursing staff education about advance directives, palliative care, and EOL issues can establish baseline competence levels.

- Unnecessary patient and staff suffering can be minimized if palliative care education, protocols, and policies are in place to support patient identification of goals of care.

Case study

Mr. X, a 47-year-old male Status post (s/p) motor vehicle accident

Mr. X is a 47-year-old male who was driving home from work when he swerved and lost control of his vehicle, which then went down over an embankment, and was entrapped. He was found unconscious by an oncoming driver, who called 911. His Glasgow Coma Score was 6T, and active medical problems upon admission to the Intensive Care/Trauma Unit included subarachnoid hemorrhage, subdural hemorrhage, multiple intraparenchymal hemorrhages, left parieto-occipital scalp laceration, and right upper lung collapse. Electroencephalogram revealed diffuse slowing consistent with encephalopathy without evidence of epileptiform activity. Magnetic resonance imaging (MRI) showed diffuse widespread axonal injury to the brain with large areas of contusion and hemorrhagic transformation.

The palliative care team (PCT) was consulted on admission and was present for initial and all subsequent meetings with the patient's wife and extended family. There was noted conflict between family members with regard to the plan of care and perceptions about Mr. X's preferences. Despite aggressive interventions, Mr. X did not demonstrate any neurological improvement and continued to decline with loss of reflexive maneuvers and ventilator-dependent respiratory failure. The medical teams were in agreement that his prognosis was extremely poor, and he would not recover to a meaningful level of function. Multiple family meetings were held, and his wife shared that her husband would not desire artificial means of support in the event he was not going to make a full and meaningful recovery to independent function (prior-to-admission baseline). His parents and siblings felt everything should be continued and escalated and that life in a nursing home was still better than death. His adult children were conflicted, feeling caught in the struggle between angry grandparents and their mother.

During a family meeting on hospital day #5, the patient's father and brother asked when he would recover to return home. The PCT reviewed with the family that due to the devastating extent of the injuries, he would require continuous custodial care in a skilled facility and he would not regain any independent function. His siblings then replied that would not be an acceptable life for the patient, who was an outdoor enthusiast and enjoyed a very active lifestyle. His parents also agreed with this assessment. His wife and children were in agreement as well. The PCT reviewed the options for Mr. X's plan of care with his spouse and extended family. The family decided to elected terminal extubation and transition to comfort measures and inquired as to how his comfort would be assured, that is, what parameters would be assessed for comfort and how they would be assessed.

Following the meeting, the family asked for immediate extubation with transition to comfort care. The PCT assisted with terminal extubation orders, and the comfort measures order set was started. The patient was medicated prior to extubation and placed on an opioid infusion to assure he remained free of respiratory distress and pain. After extubation, the critical care nurses assisted with personal care and removed all nonessential medical equipment (i.e., ventilator, infusion devices, code cart) from patient's room to allow more room for family to remain with patient. The family returned to the room and remained with the patient until his death.

Quality-of-care issues identified in this case

- The patient was identified early in the traumatic illness.

- Patient and family's values and preferences for care were identified early and integrated into the plan of care.

- A team approach allowed for various members to assist with the patient's diverse needs across the entire episode of illness.

- Palliative care involvement occurred in the hospital setting. Continuity occurred across all settings.

- The patient's preference for location of death was met.

Brief history and definitions of hospital-based palliative care

In 1974, the Royal Victoria Hospital in Montreal, Canada, developed one of the first initiatives in North America to improve HBPC. They developed a palliative care service to meet the needs of hospitalized patients who were terminally ill within the general hospital setting.[13] An integral part of the Royal Victoria Hospital, a 1000-bed teaching hospital affiliated with McGill University, the palliative care service consisted of five complementary clinical components: (1) the Palliative Care Unit, (2) the home care service, (3) the consultation team, (4) the palliative care clinic, and (5) the bereavement follow-up program. Members of an interdisciplinary team were involved with the care of these patients, and the focus was on holistic care with pain control and symptom management.

Three decades later, these basic palliative care concepts were becoming more prevalent in many US hospitals. In the United States, a number of milestones over the past four decades have shaped the evolution of care of the seriously ill (see Box 3.1). In the 1970s, the concept of home-based hospice programs (often volunteer only) migrated to the United States from Europe and Canada. Since that time, a number of professional, medical, societal, and academic endeavors have coalesced in the form of HBPC programs, which adapt and "upstream" many principles of hospice care into mainstream medicine. Although there is no requirement for all healthcare systems to have such a program, palliative care is gradually being recognized as a "standard of care." For organizations that still need convincing, Meier[14-16] the case for implementation of and early involvement of hospital based palliative care: (1) to improve clinical quality of care for seriously ill patients; (2) to increase patient and family satisfaction with care; (3) to meet the demand of a growing, chronically ill, elderly demographic; (4) to serve as "classrooms" for the next

Box 3.1 Milestones in the evolution from home hospice to hospital-based palliative care

1970s: Awareness of hospice philosophy transfers from Great Britain to the United States

- 1976 Karen Ann Quinlan case

1980s: Recognition of aging population, chronic disease demographics, growth of National Institute on Aging and the American Association of Retired Persons

- Passage of Medicare Hospice Benefit
- Recognition of AIDS

1990s: National recognition in the United States of the problem of EOL care

- 1990 Nancy Cruzan case
- 1990–1997 Kevorkian-assisted deaths
- 1991 Patient Self-Determination Act
- 1995—SUPPORT study findings of poor EOL care
- 1997 Legalization of assisted suicide in Oregon
- 1997 Institute of Medicine (IOM) Report: "Approaching Death: Improving Care at the End of Life"
- 1997 Institute for Health Care Improvement (IHI) EOL Breakthrough Collaborative
- 1998 First palliative care APN programs (Ursuline College, New York University)
- 1999 Kevorkian convicted of first-degree murder and imprisoned

2000s: Baby boomers with aging parents achieve positions of leadership and authority (Project on Death in America [pdia] scholars/leaders) entering and legitimizing palliative medicine as a specialty field

- 2001 Institute of Medicine Report "Improving Palliative Care for Cancer"
- Public Broadcasting System (PBS) Bill Moyers Special, "On Our Own Terms"
- 1995–2003 Robert Wood Johnson Foundation funds EOL activities
- Last Acts
- Promoting Excellence in EOL Care
- Partnership for Caring
- Educating Physicians in End-of-Life Care (EPEC)
- End-of-Life Nursing Education Consortium (ELNEC)
- Open Society/Project on Death in America (PDIA)
- Faculty Scholars Program
- 2001 Disseminating End-of-Life Education to Cancer Centers (DELEtCC)
- 2002 Department of Veterans Affairs initiates multiple palliative/EOL programs
- Mayday, Kornfeld sponsor mini-fellowships (Northwestern, Memorial Sloan Kettering, etc.)
- Growth and development of specialty education and organizations
- Shift of professional membership organizations from being homes of the isolated to active change agents in policy, education, and clinical change: HPNA, AAHPM
- Center to Advance Palliative Care & Palliative Care Leadership Centers
- NHPCO, AAHPM, HPNA—membership organizations
- Palliative Medicine achieves ABMS specialty status
- Advanced and NA specialty nursing certification
- Expansion of Harvard course, EPEC, ELNEC, JPM
- Development of (MD) fellowship programs
- 2004 National Consensus Project + 2008 NQF-Quality Guidelines
- 2005 Terry Schiavo case
- Research evidence to support palliative care emerging and developing new funding sources
- NPCRC/ACS Junior Faculty & Pilot Project Awards
- 2008 The Joint Commission considers Palliative Care Certification process
- 2008–2014 California launches 5-year initiative "Spreading Palliative Care in Public Hospitals" to develop HBPC programs
- 2010 *New England Journal of Medicine* landmark study: "Early Palliative Care for Patients with Metastatic Non–Small-Cell Lung Cancer"
- 2011 The Joint Commission launches Palliative Care Certification

generation of clinicians who need to provide better care to the seriously ill; and (5) to provide value-added, cost-effective care in the face of a national healthcare and economic crisis.[17] A recent review of palliative care studies presents a compelling argument that, based on the amount of available evidence, HBPC is state-of-the-art care.

Although much of the data to support the evolution of HBPC have come from care deficits identified in hospitalized patients at the very end of life[1-4]; the goal of HBPC is to improve the quality of life of persons with life-limiting illness much earlier in the course of illness across all settings of healthcare.[10,13,15,16]

A number of definitions of HBPC exist and contain similar elements. In 1990, the World Health Organization defined "palliative care" as care that "seeks to address not only physical pain, but also emotional, social, and spiritual pain to achieve the best possible quality of life for patients and their families. Palliative care extends the principles of hospice care to a broader population that could benefit from receiving this type of care earlier in their illness or disease process."[18] An HBPC program has been defined by the American Hospital Association (AHA) as "an organized program providing specialized medical care, drugs, or therapies for the management of acute or chronic pain and/or the control

of symptoms administered by specially trained physicians and other clinicians; and supportive care services, such as counseling on advance directives, spiritual care, and social services, to patients with advanced disease and their families."[15,16] The Center to Advance Palliative Care (CAPC) defines HBPC as "an interdisciplinary medical team focused on symptom management, intensive patient–physician–family communication, clarifying goals of treatment and coordination of care across health care settings."[14] In Temel's et al. (2010)[19] landmark study, "Early Palliative Care for Patients with Metastatic Non–Small-Cell Lung Cancer," lung cancer patients who received palliative care along with conventional treatment survived 2.7 months longer than patients who received only standard oncological care. Published by the *New England Journal of Medicine*, this study clearly demonstrated the value, need, and importance of palliative medicine interventions for patients with advanced, life-limiting illness.[18]

The good news is that since the AHA survey began to measure the availability of HBPC programs in 2000, there has been a steady growth (see Figure 3.1).[15] This positive movement is tempered by two issues. First, there is wide variability in patients' access to palliative care programs across the United States (see Figure 3.2). In particular, the southern region of the United States, at 41%, has the lowest availability of programs.[20] Second, despite definitions of HBPC, mandatory standards of care do not yet exist; therefore, programs vary in their quality, components, and emphasis on the missions of service, research, and education.

Primary, secondary, and tertiary models of hospital-based palliative care

Promoting HBPC requires a myriad of resources. Depending on the model of palliative care being introduced, the required resources can vary greatly. For example, some changes may require financial support via construction or addition of staff, whereas other changes are less resource intensive. Regardless of the healthcare system and the availability of resources, all healthcare practitioners have the ability to introduce palliative care concepts and use already established resources to develop

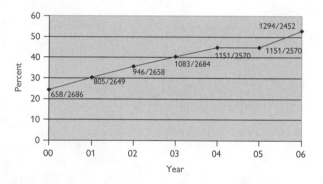

Figure 3.1 Percent of hospitals reporting an HBPC program. Source: Data from Goldsmith, Dietrich, et al. (2008), reference 20.

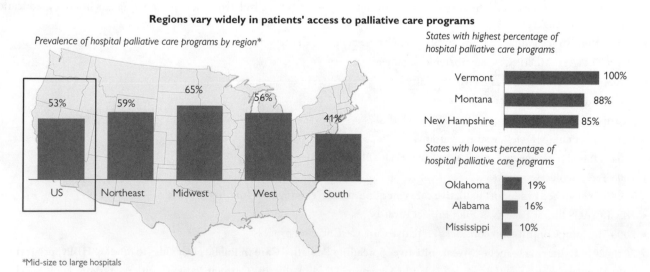

Figure 3.2 Variability in access to palliative care. Source: Nurse Executive Watch, 2008. Reprinted with permission.

or improve their palliative care services. According to von Gunten,[21] "One way that patients and their families will get better care is to ensure that clinical services focusing on the relief of suffering are available in every hospital." [(p. 876)] He suggests that hospitals (and healthcare systems) consider their mission and level of palliative care delivery (e.g., primary, secondary, tertiary), as they do other medical specialties, and incorporate a model of palliative care resources in accordance with that level. Institutions with limited resources may choose a primary model that focuses on enhancing existing services and clinician education, while secondary and tertiary palliative care programs may provide multiple services, including inpatient and/or outpatient consult teams, an inpatient palliative care/hospice unit, and a home care program, all under the jurisdiction of a single hospital system. A full-service approach can ease transitions among different levels of care and has the potential to provide the optimum in seamless palliative care. The CAPC also offers various consensus guidelines for operational and inpatient unit metrics that hospitals can use to measure programs for quality, sustainability, and growth.[20] Table 3.1 lists a variety of different models that have been described by the CAPC. In addition to an extensive manual on developing a program,[21] the CAPC offers a variety of other resources including individual consultation to developing programs via on-site visits and follow up consultations (see "Center to Advance Palliative Care Leadership Centers," below).

Table 3.1 Program model options

Characteristics	Solo practitioner model	Full team model	Geographic model
The following chart is designed to help the planning team assess various options and their potential to provide this care in a manner that best meets hospital and patient needs.			
Philosophy/approach	◆ Consultative service	◆ Consultative service with full team of doctor, ANP or nurse, and social worker assesses and follows patients referred by attending physician	◆ Inpatient program with all patients on designated unit
	◆ Doctor (MD) or advanced nurse practitioner (ANP) provides initial assessment and communication with attending physician, nursing, and social work staff		
			◆ Inpatient staff team (doctor, ANP, social worker, chaplain, therapists specially trained to provide palliative care) manages patients
		◆ Provides advice to primary physician, or may assume all or part of care of patient and/or write patient orders	
	◆ May or may not write patient orders		◆ Staff is trained in palliative care and focuses on creating an inpatient environment supportive of patients and families
	◆ MD or ANP refers patients to needed services (such as social work), discusses needs in conference, and communicates with clinicians		
		◆ Doctor bills fee-for-service as a consultant physician	
			◆ Approach is milieu intensive as well as individual patient focused
		◆ Team refers patient to needed services and discharges to appropriate setting(s), discusses needs in conference, and communicates with all team members	
	◆ Assists patient and family with advance directives and plans for future		◆ Care reimbursed under licensure and guidelines (e.g., acute care)

Table 3.1 (Continued)

Characteristics	Solo practitioner model	Full team model	Geographic model
Service model	◆ MD or ANP receives referrals from attending physician, hospital staff, patient, or family	◆ Team works in unison to coordinate care plan and provide services	◆ Patients referred to palliative care program are screened by team for appropriateness
		◆ Social worker on team may assume role of case manager	◆ Appropriate patients are transferred to service when they meet admission criteria
	◆ All units in hospital deliver palliative care as part of their mission		
		◆ Team develops and uses standing orders to manage patient	◆ Palliative care team assumes responsibility for patient management and discharge planning
	◆ MD or ANP develops protocols for patient care in conjunction with treatment team, educates staff about palliative care and protocols		
		◆ All hospital units deliver palliative care as part of their mission	◆ Patient may be followed on an outpatient basis after discharge
Staffing and budget implications	◆ One FTE MD or ANP	◆ 0.5 to one FTE medical director	◆ 0.5 to one FTE medical director
	◆ 0.2 FTE clerical support	◆ One FTE ANP	◆ One FTE ANP
	◆ Access to and time allotted for social worker, nursing, physical and occupational therapists (PT and OT), and pharmacy to respond to referrals (should be monitored for time requirements)	◆ 0.5 medical social worker	◆ 0.5–1.0 FTE medical social worker
		◆ One FTE clerical support	◆ 0.5–1.0 FTE chaplain
		◆ Access to and time allotted for social work, nursing, PT, OT, and pharmacy to respond to referrals (should be monitored for time requirements)	◆ 0.2 FTE finance person
			◆ Nurse manager
			◆ Inpatient unit staffing
	◆ 0.2 FTE finance person		◆ Preferably, unit is situated where staff are likely to have training in fundamentals of palliative care
	◆ 0.2 FTE medical director (if ANP-led)	◆ 0.2 FTE finance person	
			◆ An allocation of DRG revenues may be required when a patient transfers from another unit to palliative care.
Patient volume thresholds	◆ Patient coordination is intensive, and ANP spends time with patient providing psychosocial support as well as symptom management and family teaching. Staff teaching as well	◆ Number varies, depending on whether patient is transferred to the team for all management	◆ Geographic unit approach allows the institution to designate beds, yet allows the number of beds to flex with patient volume
		◆ Can reach the largest number of patients and does not restrict the number of beds occupied by patients requiring palliative care services	◆ Most efficient staffing with 12 or more beds, preferably in rooms with space for family members to stay and room for staff and family members to meet
	◆ Literature does not define volume but anecdotal reports suggest maximum comfortable caseload of 4 new cases per day and average census of 10 patients/week		

Table 3.1 (Continued)

Characteristics	Solo practitioner model	Full team model	Geographic model
			◆ Because reimbursement is still acute-care oriented, the unit can flex to a capacity deemed appropriate to staffing levels and clinical expertise
Benefits/advantages	◆ Lower start-up costs and financial risk	◆ More medical expertise available	◆ The program has a clinical milieu and staff to support it
	◆ Opportunity to develop a program based on existing patient population	◆ Provides alternative to medical staff who struggle with implementing new skills and knowledge	◆ Greater control over patient care
	◆ Less threatening to medical staff		◆ Higher visibility and influence within the hospital
	◆ Builds on existing programs and services and uses them whenever possible	◆ Consultative service reaches largest number of nurses and physicians through bedside and nursing station teaching and role modeling	
			◆ Inpatient unit can be made patient- and family-friendly
			◆ May be easier to manage overuse of resources, length of stay
		◆ Builds on existing programs and services and uses them whenever possible	◆ Opportunity for philanthropic support more easily developed
			◆ Can convert all or part of an existing unit to minimize additional staffing
Disadvantages/threats	◆ Program rests on one individual's shoulders	◆ Added costs for team with limited, or no, additional revenue	◆ Geographic patient concentration deprives staff in other parts of the hospital from exposure to the service and learning opportunities
	◆ Patient volume quickly limited by workload	◆ Physician must establish rapport with many medical staff members; consultant serves as an advisor to the primary physician, and recommendations may or may not be followed	
			◆ May be viewed as the "death ward," making physicians reluctant to refer patients
	◆ Service effectiveness is dependent on staff knowledge and cooperation		
			◆ Unless beds can be shared efficiently with an adjacent unit, underuse of continuous nursing coverage beds due to low referral volume will translate into losses for the unit
	◆ All units referring patients need to be educated		
		◆ Service effectiveness is dependent on staff knowledge and cooperation	
		◆ All units referring patients need to be educated	

Primary palliative care

Primary palliative care should be available at all hospitals. This level of care requires, at a minimum, clinician education in the basics of pain and symptom management. Primary palliative care refers to a level of care whereby basic skills and competencies are required of all physicians, nurses, and other healthcare practitioners who come in contact with persons with life-limiting illness. The National Consensus Project (NCP), the National Quality Forum (NQF), and the Joint Commission (TJC) have each identified standards that should be addressed in all hospitals and other settings (see later discussion). All practitioners should be competent at this level.

Clinicians can gain the knowledge, attitudes, and skills needed to provide palliative care to their patients through basic palliative care training and clinical practice. There is a growing availability of continuing education, including established formal programs for all disciplines to improve their knowledge of basic palliative care principles. The End-of-Life Nursing Education Consortium (ELNEC) and Education for Physicians on End-of-Life Care (EPEC) are two comprehensive educational programs that can provide such information. Both educational programs are further described later in this chapter and in chapter 66.

Secondary palliative care

Secondary palliative care refers to a model in which all providers have a minimum level of competence and specialists provide palliative care through an interdisciplinary team (IDT), specialized unit, or both. The development and success of these specialized services come about as a result of strong leadership, marketing, and accessibility.[16,19,21] It is not necessary for an IDT or unit to evaluate every patient with palliative care needs who is admitted to the hospital, but these specially trained clinicians are available as a resource and guide for their colleagues.

Tertiary palliative care

Teaching hospitals and academic centers with teams of experts in palliative care are classified as tertiary organizations. A tertiary-level program may serve as a consultant to primary- and secondary-level practices in difficult clinical situations or as model programs to assist developing centers. These centers also serve as training programs for incoming palliative medicine providers, with fellowship programs ranging from 1 to 2 years for both physicians and nurses. Practitioners and institutions involved at the tertiary level of palliative care are also involved in educational and research activities.[21-25] Multidisciplinary training programs for nurses and physicians are an important function of a tertiary center (see below). Tertiary centers also have an obligation to perform research to enhance the evidence base for palliative care.

It is the responsibility of all hospitals and healthcare organizations to be competent, at a minimum, at the primary level of palliative care. Organizations at different levels may choose among different components of care to incorporate into their model. Some components are less resource intense (e.g., staff education, care pathways), while others may require additional allocations of budget and personnel. The latter resources include IDTs, specialized PCUs, outpatient/ambulatory palliative care clinics, and structured outreach or strong relationships with skilled nursing facilities (SNF) and home-based hospice programs.

The inpatient interdisciplinary consult team

A growing literature summarizes the development of palliative care consultation teams within hospitals to offer specialized consultation and expertise to patients, families, and other healthcare providers.[24-27] Dunlop and Hockley published a manual in 1990 and a second edition in 1998 describing the experience in England. They described the movement as one that tries to take the hospice philosophy of care and bring it into the hospital using a consultancy team. A number of US and European hospital-based teams have described their experiences.[28,29] Among the components of successful teams are an interdisciplinary approach, physician and nonphysician referral, rapid response to requested consultations, around-the-clock availability, and ability to follow patients through all care settings.

Interdisciplinary consultation teams can be effective in modeling behaviors that are supportive of appropriate HBPC but they should also recommend infrastructure and organizational changes as part of their approach to consultation. Gathering data about demographic statistics about the location and nature of regular consultations may help to identify the need for particular institutional policies and procedures. For example, if a particular unit or care provider has difficulty managing patients with dyspnea on a regular basis, targeted educational approaches and treatment algorithms or standardized orders may help achieve consistent and long-lasting change. Theoretically, an IDT could "put itself out of business" with such an approach. Conversely, teams may become "stretched too thin" in their attempts to meet the needs of their organization, however, the news remains positive: teams to date have not reported the need to dissolve as an outcome of implementing system changes.

Studies have begun to examine the impact of IDTs on the overall care of hospitalized, seriously ill patients.[30,31] However, this is challenging research and, as in any multicomponent intervention, it is difficult to identify exactly which components or processes of the team are responsible for the outcomes. Valid, reliable measures and multimethod research are likely to be needed to capture this information.[38] Maintaining an IDT can be costly; therefore, it is imperative to continue to evaluate programs and strengthen the evidence base to provide economic justification for many hospitals. A consensus panel has recommended minimum data that should be collected by all consultation services[31] (see "Measurement," later in this chapter).

Inpatient hospice and palliative care units

Some hospitals, faced with the problem of providing high-quality palliative care, have found the development of a specialized unit to be the solution. In the United Kingdom, these units have been developed from preexisting oncology units, as part of another unit, or sometimes in a separate building that is distinct but near the hospital it serves.[30] Hospitals in the United States have varying amounts of experience with opening specialized units for the care of patients with hospice, or palliative care needs.[32-34] An inpatient unit has some advantages and disadvantages. Advantages include the following:

♦ Patients requiring palliative care have a familiar place to go during the exacerbations and remissions that come with progressive disease.[35-39]

◆ Unit staff and policies are under the control and financing of experts trained as a team who are skillful at difficult care and communications.[36-37]

◆ Patients may get palliative care earlier if other care teams see the advantages of this approach and trust that patients will receive good care.[40-43]

Providers who monitor their patients on these units (if allowed) can learn valuable lessons about palliative care that can be carried forward to future patients.[44-48] These future patients may not require admission to the PCU for some types of care. Some disadvantages of creating a PCU include the following:

◆ It can prevent others from learning valuable palliative care techniques if the PCU staff are seen as "specialized" and are secluded in one area.[47-48]

◆ Care providers may come to rely on this expertise instead of learning palliative care techniques themselves.

◆ If PCU transfer includes a transfer of doctors to a palliative care specialist, patients and families may feel abandoned by their primary team in the final hours.

◆ Hospice providers fear loss of the hospice philosophy when a PCU exists in the context of the general hospital.

Outpatient/ambulatory palliative care clinics

In an ideal world, patients with life-limiting illness spend the majority of their time outside of the hospital with only occasional need for attention by a palliative care specialist. Transitions of care are a common area of difficulty for patients with palliative care needs. An outpatient service can serve as an initial point of referral for patients early in their disease process[33] or it may allow a discharged patient to continue to have specialized management of their symptoms and other needs. A number of models of delivering outpatient care exist,[33-36] from a consultative model in which palliative care clinicians participate in other disease-focused outpatient visits (e.g., in clinics serving patients with advanced lung disease, congestive heart failure, cancer, amyotrophic lateral sclerosis [ALS], etc.) to a model in which geographic space is dedicated to palliative care clinicians and patients. Outpatient services are still considered a novel, less frequent service component of HBPC in most organizations, however this has become a recognized service delivery need that is fast growing in demand and popularity across national health systems today.[44-49]

Liaisons with skilled nursing facilities and home hospice

Perhaps one of the most important ways to improve HBPC is to develop strong relationships with other healthcare agencies outside of the hospital, so that alternatives to inpatient admission for palliative care exist. Alternatives such as home hospice care or skilled hospice care within assisted-living centers, free-standing hospices, or specially designated areas in nursing homes or rehabilitation facilities can provide expert palliative and hospice care. However, some areas of the United States lack these options. For example, in some rural areas, healthcare services such as visiting nurses agencies, home care, hospice, and SNFs are sparse, or staff may feel unprepared to care for people who require intensive palliative care. Some visiting nurse and home care agencies may

see so few symptomatic, seriously ill patients that it is difficult for staff to maintain adequate palliative care and hospice expertise in these agencies. There continues to be a need to develop models and strengthen relationships between HBPC programs and community agencies that will provide palliative care services prior to or following hospital palliative care services.[50-59] An area for further growth and exploration is the branching out of palliative care delivery to satellite locations with advanced illness patients such as end-stage renal disease, Class III-IV heart failure patients, and nursing home residents with multiple advanced and complex comorbid medical conditions.

Bereavement services

Improving HBPC does not end with the development of mechanisms to ensure peaceful, pain-free patient death. Although accomplishing this goal is surely a comfort to family and friends, bereavement care for survivors is an important final step in the process of HBPC. Which families are most in need of specific services? Identifying families at the greatest risk has been the topic of palliative care research, particularly in evaluating the quality of palliative care services.[60-66]

Bereavement services for survivors are an important part of the total care plan after the patient's death (see chapters 29 and 60). The NQF preferred practices standard for bereavement care indicates organizations should "Facilitate effective grieving by implementing in a timely manner a bereavement care plan after the patient's death, when the family remains the focus of care."[63] Adverse physical and psychological outcomes of unsupported grief are known to occur during the bereavement period.[67] Because of this, bereavement services are a typical component of the services offered to families when patients die as part of a hospice program. Because not all deaths in the United States have hospice involvement, a large portion of families must rely on bereavement follow-up offered by other care providers. Although historically few hospitals routinely offered bereavement services to families after patients died in the hospital,[61] a growing interest in implementing such programs has come about as a result of implementing HBPC programs.

Bereavement services can address currently unmet needs of survivors, who can benefit from resources that offer information and support in coping with the loss.[63,65-68] Having follow-up contact with decedents' family members can also provide HBPC programs with information about the effectiveness of EOL care. Families' perspectives should be sought about what went well and what could be improved. For example, results of a focus group of bereaved family members indicated that, although the family was quite satisfied with pain management, breathing changes and dyspnea were not anticipated and were very distressing.[69] Hence, this became a target for improving EOL care in one hospital.

Use of family proxy perspectives is an emerging area of research and quality improvement.[70-75] (Measurement issues are described later in this chapter.) Press-Ganey, a healthcare measurement and improvement company that is well known for collecting patient satisfaction data after hospital discharge, now also has a survey to collect family perspectives on the EOL experience in the hospital.[76] This survey asks about topics such as care at the time of death; care provided by nurses, physicians, chaplains, social workers, and others; environment; family care; symptoms; and overall satisfaction with care.

Standardized bereavement care can take many forms and can result in improved family satisfaction with care.[65] These actions might include sending a note of sympathy or establishing some other contact from a staff member, mailing a list of local bereavement resources or a pamphlet, and delaying the time before a hospital bill is mailed out to prevent its coinciding with funeral or memorial services. A variety of bereavement services have been developed for parents that specifically address their needs after the death of an infant or child.[68,77]

Interdisciplinary education: a key component of palliative care

It is imperative that staff that care for patients with life-limiting illness have sufficient and appropriate palliative care knowledge and skills. Organizations with or without HBPC programs should encourage staff members to participate in conferences on EOL and palliative care and also should support them through the continuing education process (e.g., becoming certified in a specialty). The value of improved education is not only in direct patient care, but in the role modeling that takes place. The majority of students in medical, nursing, and other healthcare disciplines receive clinical training for practice in hospitals. However, few hospitals provided role models for teaching palliative care practices. The following is one of several comments made by family members about the insensitive way the act of "pronouncing" the death of their loved one was handled by an inexperienced new medical intern.[56,57,59]

> I was holding his hand when he stopped breathing. I called the nurse, who called the doctor. He went over and looked at him lying in the bed, listened for a heartbeat with his stethoscope and said, "He's dead," and walked out of the room. That's it—not "I'm sorry." No, "Is there anything we can do?" Just, "He's dead." It was painful, and made us think that the staff didn't care.

A study by Ferris and colleagues[58] documented that medical schools devote little time to care of dying patients. A survey of medical interns revealed significant concern and fear about providing these services with no or little supervision. The traditional "See one, do one, teach one" supervisory principle of medical education was ineffective. One resident explained that the pronouncing experience was not one that was perceived as causing harm when performed by the inexperienced. Another stated, "I felt really inadequate, I had absolutely no idea what to do when the nurse called me to pronounce this patient whom I had never met—my first night on call. I was never taught the steps—how long should I listen to the chest to be sure there was no heartbeat; what, if anything else, I should do; what should I say to the family. Thankfully, the death coordinator was there to help me fill out the paperwork." Conversely, in states where nurses are allowed to pronounce deaths, some course work exists to teach a process that gives attention to the family. For resident education, there is a comprehensive, multimedia program called "The Art of Compassionate Death Notification."[59] The program includes a facilitator's guide, manuals for learners, a pocket card of the process, and videos demonstrating communication skills. At our medical center, the residency program conducts real-world patient scenarios where residents are given random patient case scenarios (actors play the role of patients/family) and carry out their evaluation of the case. These scenarios are observed by senior physician reviewers, who then provide feedback to the resident regarding communication technique, body language, and so forth. The focus of such teaching formats is to provide trainees with honest feedback on their ability to navigate real-life scenarios and bring attention to both the areas in which they excel and those in which they need assistance or improvement, such as communication/choice of words, body language, and self-awareness.

The lack of role models for students in the clinical setting is further compounded by the lack of palliative care content in student curricula[81] and major textbooks.[60-62] When major medical and nursing texts were analyzed, they were found to be sorely lacking in the content that would inform students about the basics of palliative symptom management, decision-making, and critical communication skills.[77-80] On a positive note, however, there is evidence that this situation is changing: the growing awareness of and need for palliative care has triggered more incorporation of palliative care-focused content in medical and nursing school curricula and textbooks. Teaching formats have also become more innovative: Ellison and Radecke (2005) conducted an "Issues at the End of Life" course as a joint effort between the office of a university chaplain and a palliative medicine program for college students. This course earned multiple teaching awards for originality, creativity, and collaboration. "Issues at the End of Life" divided the class into sessions focused on religious, spiritual, and theological issues and included guest presenters from Geisinger Medical Center in Danville, Pennsylvania, including physicians, nurses, bioethicists, hospice and social workers, and counselors. The objectives were to demystify aging, illness, and death while enhancing empathy and compassion to promote improved communication skills that could be used across various difficult situations. The most unique element of this course was its service-learning project for the creation of a personal legacy: Each student worked with a designated community member facing EOL issues (due to advanced age, terminal illness, or both) to create a lasting, meaningful record of the person's life. Projects included audio- and video recorded life histories, memory books, and even a quilt made from scraps of symbolic garments such as wedding attire, outfits from special occasions, baby blankets, and baptismal gowns. The course was a brilliant recognition of the common human experience of life and death—highlighting the need for better awareness, recognition, and interventions that offer as much attention at the end of life as one receives throughout life.[63]

Listed here are other creative ways to actively engage learners in palliative care education:

- Arrange for clinician role models to provide lectures to students and faculty.

- Assist with curriculum review of current EOL care training.

- Change elective coursework and clinical work in hospice and palliative care to required status, and include these subjects in other mandatory clinical assignments.

- Use texts that contain clinically relevant palliative care content.

- Include content on ambulatory-based symptom management and decision-making that defines patient preferences for care.

- Encourage students to describe evidence-based approaches to palliative care and to challenge their mentors about approaches and interventions that increase the burden of care without clear patient benefit.

◆ Encourage students to learn from staff role models appropriate ways of communicating bad news and of presenting options that respect patient preferences and values.

◆ Identify opportunities for undergraduate or graduate fellowships in palliative care.

◆ Encourage quality improvement teams to offer students opportunities to participate and to collect data from patients, charts, and staff.

Experienced healthcare providers also have needs for specialty palliative care educational experiences. (See chapter 66 for a detailed discussion on the topic.) Both the nursing and medical professions have embraced the concept of palliative care continuing education, advanced academic training, and certification.

In the area of continuing education, the ELNEC and EPEC are exemplary programs. The ELNEC program is a collaboration of the City of Hope Medical Center and the American Association of Colleges of Nursing, and the program has a variety of curricula for different audiences (undergraduate and graduate nursing faculty, nurses working in critical care, pediatrics, or geriatric settings, etc.). The American Medical Association (AMA) and EPEC programs address similar issues for physicians. Both curricula are widely available as a means to educate practicing nursing and medical staff.

The Harvard Medical School program in palliative care education and practice

Another example of palliative care continuing education is sponsored by the Harvard Medical School Center for Palliative Care. In response to the need for leaders in palliative care education in nursing and medicine, the Harvard program offers intensive learning experiences for physician and nurse educators who wish to become expert in the clinical practice and teaching of comprehensive, interdisciplinary palliative care, as well as to gain expertise in leading and managing improvements in palliative care education and practice at their own institutions. The program includes a special pediatric track. The course is delivered in two sections: Part 1 consists of 7 days of intensive learning, followed by a 6-month interim when participants work on an individual project and contribute to weekly e-mail discussions of problematic clinical, educational, and program development cases presented by other participants through e-mail exchanges. Part 2 is a second 7-day block that includes continued experiential learning and training focused on communication, teaching methods, teamwork, and leadership.

The curriculum features content on how to (1) teach the fundamentals of palliative care (assessment of physical causes of distress, psychosocial and spiritual assessment, ethical and cultural issues, palliative care in geriatric and pediatric populations, depression, and bereavement); (2) communicate at the end of life (understanding the experience of life-threatening illness, delivering bad news, communicating across cultural barriers, family meetings, providing feedback to learners); (3) manage challenges in palliative care education (principles of adult learning, understanding, learning styles, new teaching methodologies); and (4) develop and promote clinical and educational programs in palliative care (assessing institutional structure and culture, evaluating readiness to change, dealing with resistance, developing and financing palliative care programs, and fund-raising strategies).

The course faculty includes physicians, nurses, social workers, and educators from within the Harvard teaching hospitals as well as outside experts. Complete information can be accessed at http://www.hms.harvard.edu/cdi/pallcare/pcep.htm.

Advanced education and certification in palliative care

As standards of care are increasingly applied to HBPC programs, advanced specialty training in palliative care will likely become a requirement. Academic opportunities for education and preparation as an advanced palliative care practitioner currently exist in a number of programs (see chapter 66 for additional details).

Following these programs and other specialized training, nurses may take advanced certification in palliative care through the National Board for Certification of Hospice and Palliative Nurses (NBCHPN). Eligible nurse practitioners and clinical nurse specialists can acquire the credential of ACHPN (Advanced Certified Hospice and Palliative Nurse). Certification exams are also available for registered nurses, licensed vocational nurses, nursing assistants, and nurse administrators. Nationally, hundreds have become board certified as palliative care specialists since the examinations' inception.

A major advance in the field came about in 2007 when the American Board of Medical Specialties (ABMS) voted to approve hospice and palliative medicine as a recognized medical subspecialty. The application to recognize the subspecialty had broad support and was cosponsored by 10 medical specialty boards. As a result, physicians in a number of specialties—including internal medicine, family medicine, pediatrics, psychiatry, neurology, surgery, emergency medicine, and obstetrics and gynecology—are able to seek this certification. Prior to that time, this certification exam was offered by the American Board of Hospice and Palliative Medicine (ABHPM). In the first decade of certification, over 2100 physicians obtained certification from ABHPM. The ABHPM was not recognized by the ABMS, but worked successfully over the course of the decade to persuade the ABMS to recognize hospice and palliative medicine as a medical subspecialty. Although voluntary, this recognition is used by the government, healthcare systems, and insurers as evidence of high standards. There are currently 24 member boards of the ABMS (see www.abms.org). These 24 member boards constitute the officially recognized allopathic specialties of medicine in the United States.

Developing standards for hospital-based palliative care

A number of organizations have worked together to develop standardized palliative care practices.

National Consensus Project

In April 2004, the NCP for Palliative Care released its *Clinical Practice Guidelines for Quality Palliative Care*. An updated second edition of the guidelines was published in 2013. The guidelines, which can be downloaded free of charge (http://www.nationalconsensusproject.org), represent a consensus of four major US palliative care organizations: the American Academy of Hospice and Palliative Medicine, the CAPC, the Hospice and Palliative Nurses Association (HPNA), and the National Hospice and Palliative Care Organization (NHPCO). The guidelines identify core precepts and structures of clinical palliative care programs. Domains of palliative care from the guidelines are listed in Table 3.2. The domains were intended as a framework for HBPC

Table 3.2 National Quality Forum preferred practices organized by National Consensus Project domains of quality palliative care

NCP domains of quality palliative care	NQF preferred practices
1. Structure and processes of care	1. Provide palliative and hospice care by an interdisciplinary team of skilled palliative care professionals, including, for example, physicians, nurses, social workers, pharmacists, spiritual care counselors, and others who collaborate with primary healthcare professional(s). **[4. STAFFING]**
	2. Provide access to palliative and hospice care that is responsive to the patient and family 24 hours a day, 7 days a week. **[3. AVAILABILITY]**
	3. Provide continuing education to all healthcare professionals on the domains of palliative care and hospice care. **[8. EDUCATION]**
	4. Provide adequate training and clinical support to assure that professional staff are confident in their ability to provide palliative care for patients. **[12. STAFF WELLNESS]**
	5. Hospice care and specialized palliative care professionals should be appropriately trained, credentialed, and/or certified in their area of expertise. **[4. STAFFING]**
	6. Formulate, utilize, and regularly review a timely care plan based on a comprehensive interdisciplinary assessment of the values, preferences, goals, and needs of the patient and family and, to the extent that existing privacy laws permit, ensure that the plan is broadly disseminated, both internally and externally, to all professionals involved in the patient's care.
	7. Ensure that upon transfer between healthcare settings, there is timely and thorough communication of the patient's goals, preferences, values, and clinical information so that continuity of care and seamless follow-up are assured. **[11. CONTINUITY OF CARE]**
	8. Healthcare professionals should present hospice as an option to all patients and families when death within a year would not be surprising and should reintroduce the hospice option as the patient declines. **[11. CONTINUITY OF CARE]**
	9. Patients and caregivers should be asked by palliative and hospice care programs to assess physicians'/healthcare professionals' ability to discuss hospice as an option.
	10. Enable patients to make informed decisions about their care by educating them on the process of their disease, prognosis, and the benefits and burdens of potential interventions.
	11. Provide education and support to families and unlicensed caregivers based on the patient's individualized care plan to assure safe and appropriate care for the patient.
2. Physical aspects of care	12. Measure and document pain, dyspnea, constipation, and other symptoms using available standardized scales. **[5. MEASUREMENT & 6. QI]**
	13. Assess and manage symptoms and side effects in a timely, safe, and effective manner to a level that is acceptable to the patient and family. **[5. MEASUREMENT & 6. QI]**
3. Psychological and psychiatric aspects of care	14. Measure and document anxiety, depression, delirium, behavioral disturbances, and other common psychological symptoms using available standardized scales. **[5. MEASUREMENT & 6. QI]**
	15. Manage anxiety, depression, delirium, behavioral disturbances, and other common psychological symptoms in a timely, safe, and effective manner to a level that is acceptable to the patient and family. **[5. MEASUREMENT & 6. QI]**
	16. Assess and manage the psychological reactions of patients and families (including stress, anticipatory grief, and coping) in a regular, ongoing fashion in order to address emotional and functional impairment and loss. **[5. MEASUREMENT & 6. QI]**
	17. Develop and offer a grief and bereavement care plan to provide services to patients and families prior to and for at least 13 months after the death of the patient. **[9. BEREAVEMENT]**
4. Social aspects of care	18. Conduct regular patient and family care conferences with physicians and other appropriate members of the interdisciplinary team to provide information, to discuss goals of care, disease prognosis, and advance care planning and to offer support.
	19. Develop and implement a comprehensive social care plan that addresses the social, practical, and legal needs of the patient and caregivers, including but not limited to relationships, communication, existing social and cultural networks, decision-making, work and school settings, finances, sexuality/intimacy, caregiver availability/stress, and access to medicines and equipment. **[4. STAFFING]**
5. Spiritual, religious, and existential aspects of care	20. Develop and document a plan based on an assessment of religious, spiritual, and existential concerns using a structured instrument, and integrate the information obtained from the assessment into the palliative care plan. **[4. STAFFING]**

(Continued)

Table 3.2 (Continued)

NCP domains of quality palliative care	NQF preferred practices
	21. Provide information about the availability of spiritual care services, and make spiritual care available either through organizational spiritual care counseling or through the patient's own clergy relationships. **[4. STAFFING]**
	22. Specialized palliative and hospice care teams should include spiritual care professionals appropriately trained and certified in palliative care. **[4. STAFFING]**
	23. Specialized palliative and hospice spiritual care professionals should build partnerships with community clergy and provide education and counseling related to EOL care. **[4. STAFFING]**
6. Cultural aspects of care	24. Incorporate cultural assessment as a component of comprehensive palliative and hospice care assessment, including but not limited to locus of decision-making, preferences regarding disclosure of information, truth-telling and decision-making, dietary preferences, language, family communication, desire for support measures such as palliative therapies and complementary and alternative medicine, perspectives on death, suffering, and grieving, and funeral/burial rituals.
	25. Provide professional interpreter services and culturally sensitive materials in the patient's and family's preferred language.
7. Care of the imminently dying patient	26. Recognize and document the transition to the active dying phase, and communicate to the patient, family, and staff the expectation of imminent death.
	27. Educate the family on a timely basis regarding the signs and symptoms of imminent death in an age-appropriate, developmentally appropriate, and culturally appropriate manner.
	28. As part of the ongoing care planning process, routinely ascertain and document patient and family wishes about the care setting for the site of death, and fulfill patient and family preferences when possible. **[11. CONTINUITY OF CARE]**
	29. Provide adequate dosage of analgesics and sedatives as appropriate to achieve patient comfort during the active dying phase, and address concerns and fears about using narcotics and of analgesics hastening death.
	30. Treat the body after death with respect according to the cultural and religious practices of the family and in accordance with local law. **[9. BEREAVEMENT]**
	31. Facilitate effective grieving by implementing in a timely manner a bereavement care plan after the patient's death, when the family remains the focus of care. **[9. BEREAVEMENT]**
8. Ethical and legal aspects of care	32. Document the designated surrogate/decision maker in accordance with state law for every patient in primary, acute, and long-term care and in palliative and hospice care.
	33. Document the patient/surrogate preferences for goals of care, treatment options, and setting of care at first assessment and at frequent intervals as conditions change.
	34. Convert the patient treatment goals into medical orders, and ensure that the information is transferable and applicable across care settings, including long-term care, emergency medical services, and hospital care, through a program such as the Physician Orders for Life-Sustaining Treatment (POLST) program.
	35. Make advance directives and surrogacy designations available across care settings, while protecting patient privacy and adherence to HIPAA regulations, for example, by using Internet-based registries or electronic personal health records.
	36. Develop healthcare and community collaborations to promote advance care planning and the completion of advance directives for all individuals, for example, the Respecting Choices and Community Conversations on Compassionate Care programs.
	37. Establish or have access to ethics committees or ethics consultation across care settings to address ethical conflicts at the end of life.
	38. For minors with decision-making capacity, document the child's views and preferences for medical care, including assent for treatment, and give them appropriate weight in decision-making. Make appropriate professional staff members available to both the child and the adult decision-maker for consultation and intervention when the child's wishes differ from those of the adult decision maker.

*Boldface entries refer to corresponding domain from "Operational Features for Hospital Palliative Care Programs: Consensus Recommendations," Weissman and Meier (2008), reference 65.
Source: http://www.nationalconsensusproject.org/guidelines.pdf and www.qualityforum.org.

programs to develop and evaluate their approaches to delivering comprehensive palliative care services. Although voluntary, one potential outcome for these guidelines is to provide a framework for certification or mandatory accreditation.[66]

National Quality Forum

In 2007, in response to a need for national quality standards, the NQF released a document listing "preferred practices."[63] The NQF collaborated with the NCP in developing these 38 "best practices" or performance measures, which are organized under the NCP eight domains of care (Table 3.2). The practices are evidence-based or endorsed by expert consensus and apply to hospice and palliative care services across all care settings.

The NQF is a nonprofit, public-private partnership organization whose mission is to develop ways to improve the quality of US healthcare. The NQF has representation from national, state, regional, and local organizations representing consumers, public and private insurers, employers, professionals, health plans, accrediting bodies, labor unions, and other organizations representing healthcare research and quality improvement. They rely on or use consensus-building processes to develop national standards for measurement and public reporting of healthcare performance that is safe, timely, beneficial, patient-centered, equitable, and efficient. These standards have served in other areas of care as a method to link performance with reimbursement.

The NQF used the following definition of palliative care to develop the practices: "Palliative care is both a philosophy of care and an organized, highly structured system for delivering care. The goal of palliative care is to prevent and relieve suffering and to support the best possible quality of life for patients and their families, regardless of the stage of the disease or the need for other therapies. Palliative care expands traditional disease-model medical treatments to include the goals of enhancing quality of life for patients and family, optimizing function, helping with decision making, and providing opportunities for personal growth."[66]

Center to Advance Palliative Care

One of the major efforts to improve HBPC programs in the United States is led by the CAPC. Originally formed and funded by a 4-year grant from the Robert Wood Johnson Foundation in 2000, the national center was established at Mount Sinai School of Medicine in New York City. The Aetna Foundation, the Brookdale Foundation, the JEHT Foundation, and the John A. Hartford Foundation also provide support. The Center has a mission to make available to hospitals and health systems nationwide information on how to establish high-quality palliative care services.

The CAPC assists hospitals with the planning, development, and implementation of HBPC programs. In addition to assisting hospitals and other health systems in program development, CAPC facilitates collaboration among hospitals, hospices, and nursing homes; promotes educational initiatives in palliative care; and encourages growth and development of new and innovative mechanisms for financing palliative care programs.[82-84] More recently, they have collaborated on the development of a strong evidence base and palliative care research with the National Palliative Care Research Center (NPCRC, described later in this chapter).

The CAPC has developed six palliative care leadership centers (PCLCs) to assist organizations that wish to learn the practical aspects of developing a palliative care program. The six organizations are Fairview Health Services, Minneapolis, Minnesota; Massey Cancer Center of Virginia Commonwealth University Medical Center, Richmond; Medical College of Wisconsin, Milwaukee; Mount Carmel Health System, Columbus, Ohio; Palliative Care Center of the Bluegrass, Lexington, Kentucky; and University of California, San Francisco. Each represents a different type of healthcare system and palliative care delivery model. They serve as exemplary organizations offering site visits, hands-on training, and technical assistance to support development of palliative care programs nationwide. Further information regarding the PCLCs can be found on the CAPC website (http://www.capc.org).

Building on the work of the NCP and NQF, in 2008 a consensus panel of CAPC staff, consultants, and PCLC faculty convened to determine which operational details were essential for program sustainability and growth for HBPC. They identified "must have" and "should have" elements that are arranged under 12 domains.[67] Each of these activities is described further in Figure 3.3.

The National Palliative Care Research Center

The mission of the NPCRC is to improve care for patients with serious illness and address the needs of their families by promoting palliative care research. In partnership with the CAPC, the NPCRC aims to rapidly translate these findings into clinical practice. The NPCRC uses three mechanisms to accomplish its aims:

- Establish priorities for palliative care research;
- Develop a new generation of researchers in palliative care;
- Coordinate and support studies focused on improving care for patients and families living with serious illness.

The NPCRC, located in New York City, receives direction and technical assistance from the Mount Sinai School of Medicine. Prior to the establishment of the NPCRC, there was no organizing force promoting and facilitating the conduct of palliative care research. Because departments or divisions of palliative medicine do not yet exist in most medical schools, palliative care research is conducted by a small number of highly successful investigators working in isolation at a limited number of universities and clinical settings in the United States.

The NPCRC provides an administrative home to promote intellectual exchange, sharing of resources (e.g., biostatisticians), and access to data from ongoing studies to plan and support new research. Furthermore, the Center takes a collaborative approach to establishing its funding priorities. As such, it is a key force in the development of an evidence base from which standards of HBPC can be developed and measured. (For more information about its activities, see http://www.npcrc.org.)

The Joint Commission

The Joint Commission is one of the paramount accreditation organizations for hospitals and other healthcare organizations. Its purpose is to continuously improve the safety and quality of care provided to the public. The Joint Commission is an independent, not-for-profit organization, and perhaps its most important benefit is that TJC-accredited organizations make a commitment to continuous improvement in patient care. During an accreditation survey, TJC evaluates a group's performance by using a set of standards that cross eight functional areas: (1) rights, responsibilities, and ethics; (2) continuum of care; (3) education and communication; (4) health promotion and disease prevention; (5) leadership; (6) management of human resources; (7) management of information; and (8) improving network performance.[68,69]

In 2004, a specific palliative care focus was introduced within two standards: (1) rights, responsibilities, and ethics and (2) the provision of care, treatment, and services. The goal of the ethics, rights, and responsibilities standard is to improve outcomes by recognizing and respecting the rights of each patient and working in an ethical manner. Care, treatment, and services are to be provided in ways that respect the person and foster dignity. The performance standard states that a patient's family should be involved in the care, treatment, and services if the patient desires. Care, treatment, and services are provided through ongoing assessments of care; meeting the patient's needs; and either successfully discharging the patient or providing referral or transfer of the patient for continuing care.[68] More detailed information is available by contacting TJC or visiting their website at http://www.jcrinc.com.

SYSTEM ASSESSMENT TOOL

Source: Modified from Supportive Care for the Dying:
A Coalition for Compassionate Care

Website: www.careofdying.org

The following is a chart to identify your system's strengths for a hospital-based palliative care program. The characteristics listed are designed to focus on palliative care for patients facing serious illness and their families. These characteristics may be in place in your institution but they may not specifically address palliative care. This tool is to be used during the system assessment as you communicate with direct caregivers, quality and risk management staff, and patients and their families. It is designed to be helpful as you focus on your infrastructure to improve palliative care. Although your institution may not offer all of the characteristics listed, this tool can be used to assess partnerships and other health care resources within your system that make these characteristics available to your staff and people you serve.

SYSTEM CHARACTERISTICS	P = PRESENT NP = NOT PRESENT	RATE ITS EFFECTIVE IMPLEMENTATION 0 = NOT AT ALL 10 = FULLY IMPLEMENTED AND EFFECTIVE	RATE PRIORITY FOR ACTION PLAN 0 = NOT AT ALL 10 = UNDERTAKE WITHIN YEAR
Vision and Management Standards			
Organization's strategic plan and annual objectives include focus on excellence in palliative care			
Performance improvement plans include focus on improvement of all aspects of palliative care for those with serious illnesses			
Educational resources are designated to support development of competencies and practices in palliative care *(See Appendix B, Description of Core Competencies in Palliative Care)*			
Practice Standards (Procedures, Policies, Care Protocol)			
Holistic comfort care or palliative care standard(s) are implemented. Standards specify population to be served			
Interdisciplinary palliative care consult services are available			
Advance care planning supports are available			
Cultural/religious guidelines are integrated			
Organ/tissue donation guidelines are implemented			
Complementary or integrative therapies are supported			

Figure 3.3a Continued

SYSTEM CHARACTERISTICS	P = PRESENT NP = NOT PRESENT	RATE ITS EFFECTIVE IMPLEMENTATION 0 = NOT AT ALL 10 = FULLY IMPLEMENTED AND EFFECTIVE	RATE PRIORITY FOR ACTION PLAN 0 = NOT AT ALL 10 = UNDERTAKE WITHIN YEAR
Spiritual, Religious, and Cultural Standards			
Support is available 24 hours a day for patient, family, and professional caregivers			
Links/communication are established with spiritual care providers			
Bereavement Support Standards			
Active follow-up available for 100% of bereaved families whose loved ones have died within your facility or practice environment 2-4 weeks following death			
Bereavement support groups and 1:1 support available and offered for families and professionals			
Psychosocial and Emotional Standards			
Referral and individual support is available 24 hours for patients/families and professional caregivers			
Support groups for patient/families are available regardless of diagnosis(es)			
Waiting time to join a support group is less than 2 weeks			
Patients/families are given information about support groups			
Communication Standards			
Patient care preferences; values; spiritual, emotional, and relationship needs; and treatment decisions are consistently and accurately communicated across care settings and professional providers			
Patient care preferences are honored across care settings and professional providers			
Frequent physician communication occurs throughout the course of the serious illness			
Communication with community spiritual care providers is routine			
Professional Experiential Education during Orientation and as Continuing Education *Education on palliative care provided for all leadership teams, employed staff and physicians in the following areas:*			
Organization values and strategic objectives			
Ethics			
Palliative care practice standards			
Palliative care quality standards			
Communication			
Grief and bereavement			

Figure 3.3a Continued

SYSTEM CHARACTERISTICS	P = PRESENT NP = NOT PRESENT	RATE ITS EFFECTIVE IMPLEMENTATION 0 = NOT AT ALL 10 = FULLY IMPLEMENTED AND EFFECTIVE	RATE PRIORITY FOR ACTION PLAN 0 = NOT AT ALL 10 = UNDERTAKE WITHIN YEAR
Patient/family supports			
Professional caregiver/staff support			
Spiritual/religious/cultural standards			
Individual performance expectations			
Individual Performance/Competency Standards Established and Monitored at Least Annually (See Appendix B, Description of Core Competencies in Palliative Care)			
Volunteer Program Standards (If Applicable)			
Training program for volunteers required			
Volunteers available to visit seriously ill patients and/or maintain vigil with dying person if appropriate			
Quality Improvement Standards			
Routine feedback from patients, family caregivers, bereaved family members, and community partners is obtained			
Annual objectives and priorities include focus on palliative care and respond to feedback from above			
Employee Support Standards			
Human Resources policies for employees support bereavement leave for those the person defined as close or family and is at least 7 days			
Human resources policies allow others to "give" vacation time or time off to support other employees			
Acuity and patient assignments provide time to "be with" the patient and family throughout the course of the serious or life-threatening illness			
Professional caregiver is supported to attend memorial/funeral service of patients			
Community Network and Partnerships			
Care offered by faith-based ministries (including parish nursing) is coordinated with patient needs			
Hospital partners with formal and informal community organizations to meet support needs for patient and family caregivers			
Hospice/home care services are available and linked to other hospital palliative care services			
Education about accessing palliative care is integrated within schools, workplaces, faith-based organizations, and other community formal and informal gatherings			

Figure 3.3a System assessment tool. Source: modified from "Supportive Care of the Dying: A Coalition for Compassionate Care." http://www.supportivecarecoalition.org/.

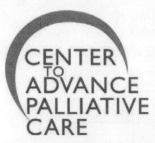

CAPC Development Tool: Palliative Care Decision Checklist

About this Tool

Now that the planning team has collected data, it is time to determine what that data means and whether it makes an effective case for a palliative care program. The following questions are meant to help the planning team in interpreting the data in order to answer these questions.

Palliative Care Decision Checklist

✓ Evidence of Demand for Services
- ❑ Is there an adequate volume of patients with serious and life-threatening illness to support a palliative care program?
- ❑ Would this approach address unmet patient and family needs? (For example, have satisfaction or other surveys showed a need for pain control, better patient-physician communication, improved care planning, or support for bereavement?)

✓ Stakeholder Interest and Support
- ❑ Have key stakeholders voiced an interest in the program/services?
- ❑ Have opponents' viewpoints been weighed and considered?
- ❑ Is there a clear medical staff champion?
- ❑ Is there a clear administrative champion?
- ❑ Do key stakeholders support the proposed program?
- ❑ Are there potential philanthropic supporters of a program?

✓ Potential Impact
- ❑ Does this initiative represent a net gain for the hospital in terms of cost (i.e., management of outlier cases), quality (i.e., better pain and symptom management and fulfillment of JCAHO standards), or market share?
- ❑ Are these net gains valued by the hospital? (For example, is quality a chief concern of management? Is cost avoidance a concept well understood by management?)
- ❑ Will a palliative care program result in measurable improvements in community health status and/or patient quality of life? (For example, would improved continuity of care prompt more referrals from community physicians? Would a program increase use of any of a hospital's affiliated

Figure 3.3b Continued

services, such as hospice or home care? Would this use of affiliated services lower readmissions of patients with low reimbursement DRGs?)

❑ Is the potential impact of the program measured using a method acceptable to the hospital? (For example, if cost avoidance is not well understood by administrators, how can its impact be conveyed – will hiring a certain number of palliative care staff reduce ICU stays by 30%?)

❑ Has available reimbursement been examined for proposed services?

❑ What is the best investment timing -- Is this a good time to propose a) investment or b) cost savings endeavors?

❑ Is there a likely charitable donor or foundation who would finance part of start-up and/or operations?

✓ Other Important Factors

❑ When is the hospital's next JCAHO review?

❑ What is the hospital's budget cycle?

❑ Can the program achieve early and visible "wins" (e.g., patient/physician satisfaction, physician referrals, staff perceiving improved coordination of services)?

❑ Is there a collaborative working relationship between target disease-specific program staffs (e.g., oncology, critical care, cardiology) and palliative care leaders?

❑ Would this program represent a significant point of marketplace differentiation for the hospital?

❑ Is the difference between palliative care and related services such as hospice or geriatrics clear?

The following checklist is partly adapted from the Palliative Care Toolbox developed by Hospital Corporation of America Cancer Care and Oncology Associates Inc.

Figure 3.3b CAPC development tool: palliative care decision checklist.

These standards incorporated a stronger emphasis on palliative care practices within organizations. Hence, organizations are being held accountable for the manner in which they provide appropriate palliative care. It is in the public's best interest that TJC requires organizations to adhere to these provisions for a successful accreditation. In 2008, a process to develop specific "Certification for Palliative Care Programs" was begun, and in 2011 TJC's Advanced Certification Program for Palliative Care was launched: The standards for palliative care certification are built on the NCP's *Clinical Practice Guidelines for Quality Palliative Care* and the NQF's *National Framework and Preferred Practices for Palliative and Hospice Care Quality*. Standards and expectations were developed using experts in palliative care and key stakeholder organizations. The standards are published in the *Palliative Care Certification Manual*.

Chapters address the following issues:

◆ Program management

◆ Provision of care, treatment, and services

◆ Information management

◆ Performance improvement

To be eligible for Advanced Certification for Palliative Care, a palliative care program must:

◆ Be provided within a TJC-accredited hospital. All types of hospitals are eligible, including children's hospitals and long-term acute care hospitals. A dedicated unit or dedicated beds are not required.

◆ Provide the full range of palliative care services to hospitalized patients 24 hours per day, 7 days per week.

• Programs must have team members available to answer phone calls nights/weekend and the ability to come to the hospital to see patients 24/7 when necessary to meet patient/family needs.

• Programs must be able to provide the same level of palliative care services during nights/weekends as during normal weekday hours.

• Programs are not required to have palliative care team members physically present in the hospital 24/7.

◆ Have served a minimum of 10 patients and have at least one active patient at the time of the initial TJC on-site review. Hospice patients are eligible for inclusion in the minimum patient count only if they were receiving inpatient palliative

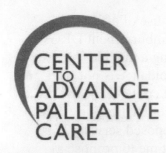

CAPC Development Tool: Needs Assessment Checklist

About this Tool

Determining the needs of your institution is an essential step in securing support for a palliative care program. It ensures that the program will be based upon, and well integrated with, the goals and services of the institution. The questions provided in this palliative care needs assessment checklist are designed to help you design your program effectively when the time comes.

Needs Assessment Checklist

✓ Who does the institution now serve?
Describe the target patient population. Learning about hospital patients and volume will help in estimating patient need, potential case volume, and key specialists vital to gaining support and referrals. This data is usually available from the hospital IT department, billing, and medical records. Identify a colleague in IT who can work with the planning team to obtain this information.

- ❑ Total number of beds in the institution
- ❑ Total number of acute care beds and staffed acute inpatient beds
- ❑ Total number of admissions and Medicare admissions
- ❑ Overall occupancy rate and ICU occupancy rate
- ❑ Average length of stay, Medicare average length of stay, and ICU length of stay
- ❑ Number of patients with a length of stay of more than five days, 10 days, and 20 days. In which diagnostic groupings?
- ❑ Who are the organization's predominant populations and "diagnostic groups" (e.g., how many admissions per year are there for cancer, heart disease, dementia, and other complex, chronic illnesses)?
- ❑ What are the typical/expected admitting problems of seriously ill patients? (Infection, nutritional problems, fractures?)
- ❑ What were the number, diagnoses (Diagnostic Related Group, or "DRGs"), location, and median and mean lengths of stay of adult deaths in the hospital in the last 12-month period for which data were available?
- ❑ How does the information for deceased patients in the hospital compare to patients discharged alive in the same DRG groupings?
- ❑ What is the payer mix for patients who die in the hospital?

Figure 3.3c Continued

✓ <u>What services</u> does the institution currently provide?
Taking inventory of the services the hospital provides will help to identify areas of need. Surveying front-line doctors, nurses, and social workers can provide insight into what services may be missing or fragmented at the patient services level.

- ❑ What services related to palliative care are presently available, such as a pain service or case management program?
- ❑ Is there a hospital survey evaluating patient pain and symptoms? (JCAHO requires regular assessment of symptom distress in hospitalized patients. These data, available from quality or compliance staff, can provide information about care and quality needs critical to successful accreditation. Pain and symptom assessment tools are included in Appendix X.)
- ❑ Is there a hospital satisfaction survey evaluating patient and family satisfaction? (JCAHO mandates hospitals conduct post-discharge consumer satisfaction surveys, which may reveal concerns about "impersonal" experience, untreated pain, delays in treatment, poor communication, poor continuity of care, or other priorities for improvement.)
- ❑ What formal or informal resources address the needs of family caregivers?
- ❑ How are services integrated or coordinated between departments?
- ❑ How does the volume/workload for services coordination (e.g., case management) compare with the volume/workload for direct patient care and medical services?
- ❑ Is there employee frustration with patient care services, nursing recruitment or retention issues? (Employee surveys, particularly of nursing staff, may reveal concerns about quality, frustration with providers, and stress due to time pressures and a complex and vulnerable patient base. Hospital leaders are especially concerned about nurse satisfaction and retention.)
- ❑ What needed services are missing or unavailable for the target patient population when they are inpatients? Identify service gaps.

✓ <u>What does it cost</u> the organization to provide these services?
Hospitals review new clinical program based on potential for revenue generation. Palliative care programs affect the bottom line through some revenue generation but mainly through cost avoidance. They improve management of complex cases, thus achieving more appropriate resource use, earlier patient discharge to more appropriate community settings, and resulting, improved capacity for new admissions and revenues. In addition, because palliative care programs increase patient, family or referring physician loyalty, they increase market share and referrals, and therefore boost revenues. They also lead to substantial philanthropic gifts. Ask the hospital finance department for assistance in collecting the data listed below. Worksheets for analyzing costs and revenues associated with patients that would be served by a palliative care program are included in this section.

- ❑ What does a one-year retrospective analysis of key patient groups show? (Analyze individuals who died as hospital inpatients and inpatients admitted with target chronic illnesses, such as cardiac and renal failure, COPD, and cancer. Identify the most prevalent 10 to 12 diagnostic categories, ICU utilization by diagnosis group, and the most prevalent cancer diagnoses among admissions. Analyses should include each patient's primary diagnosis, age, payer, and length of stay, so as to quantify patient volumes and case mix to help make the case.
- ❑ Are there patients receiving services that cannot be billed because they are indigent? What are the costs associated with these cases?

Figure 3.3c Continued

✓ How much integration with community organizations exists?

Most palliative care programs collaborate with professionals from existing services, both within the hospital and from the wider community. Their missions frequently intersect as they deliver pain management, hospice, rehabilitation medicine, nursing home care, and home health services to their patients. An inventory of available services is important to overall planning. In addition, clinicians affiliated with those programs may be available to assist in developing the palliative care program.

❑ How often do social workers or case managers refer patients to community agencies such as home health agencies or hospices for services?

❑ For which specific services?

❑ What coordination agreements exist (formal and informal)? Does the hospital have an affiliate certified home healthy agency, hospice, or hospice contract? Is there one primary hospice relationship, or many? Are hospital-community agency coordination processes standardized across the institution or are they random?

❑ Do one or more of these agencies have an interest in supporting the need for and development of a palliative care program in the acute care setting?

The above checklist is partly adapted from the Palliative Care Toolbox developed by Hospital Corporation of America Cancer Care and Oncology Associates Inc.

Figure 3.3c CAPC development tool: needs assessment checklist.

care from the program prior to transitioning to hospice care. These patients may be selected for tracer activity during the on-site review with the reviewer focusing on the episode of inpatient palliative care closest to the hospice transition.

◆ Use a standardized method of delivering clinical care based on clinical practice guidelines and/or evidence-based practice.

◆ Direct and coordinate the provision of palliative care, treatment, and services for the program patients (that is, write orders, direct or coordinate activities of the patient care team, and influence composition of the patient care team).

◆ Follow an organized approach supported by an interdisciplinary team of health professionals.

◆ Use performance measurement to improve its performance over time. Four months of performance measure data must be available at the time of the initial on-site certification review. At least two of the four measures must be clinical measures related to or identified in practice guidelines for the program. Measures selected by the program or service should be evidence-based, relevant, valid, and reliable. At this time, TJC is not defining the specific measures that are implemented; the emphasis is on the use of performance measures for improving palliative care services.

◆ Updates on TJC progress on standard development can be obtained from TJC website under "certification programs"[67]: http://www.jointcommission.org/certification/palliative_care.aspx.

Veterans Health Administration initiatives

The US Department of Veterans Affairs (VA) healthcare system has shown leadership in improving palliative and EOL care in their hospitals through multiple initiatives that have been designed or implemented since the early 1990s. In 1992, Secretary Jesse Brown mandated that VA medical centers (VAMCs) establish hospice

consultation teams to respond to the complex palliative care needs of patients with advanced disease. The VA provided training for team members during 1992 and 1993. One team reported success in pain and cost reduction while also undertaking significant institution-wide improvements through education of nurses and house staff and making pain management resources available.[70]

In 1997, the VA began an intensive, system-wide, continuous quality improvement (CQI) initiative to improve pain management. This endeavor resulted from a 1997 survey that found both acute and chronic pain management services to be inconsistent, inaccessible, and nonuniform throughout the system. Two major thrusts formed the basis of the initiative: issuing a system-wide mandate and forming a permanent National Pain Advisory Committee to provide direction and encouragement to the development of the program. Thus, this initiative incorporated two essential elements found in all successful system-wide improvement strategies: an influential champion at the highest level of the organization and a mandate for organizational commitment to this activity. The charge document offered a variety of suggestions for system improvement: making pain more visible by enhancing current measurement and reporting methods (using the "Fifth Vital Sign" approach in all patient contacts in the system); increasing access to pain therapy and increasing professional education about pain; adopting the Agency for Health Care Policy and Research and American Pain Society guidelines for pain management; pursuing research on pain therapies for veterans; distributing and sharing pain management protocols via a central clearinghouse; and exploring methods to maintain cost-effective pain therapy.

Also in 1997, the VA incorporated a palliative care measure in the performance criteria of its regional directors. In this program, performance of the directors is evaluated based on the number of charts that contain information about veterans' preferences regarding various palliative care indicators.[70,72]

In 1998, the Robert Wood Johnson Foundation Last Acts program created a Clinical Palliative Care Faculty leadership program and awarded a 2-year grant to promote development of 30 faculty fellows from VA-affiliated internal medicine training programs. Their goal was to develop curricula to train residents in the care of dying patients, to integrate relevant content into the curricula of residency training programs, and to add internal medicine faculty leaders and innovators to the field of palliative medicine.

In 2001, the VA Hospice and Palliative Care initiative began. This was a two-phase initiative to improve EOL care for veterans. Phase 1 of the project was funded in part by the NHPCO and the Center for Advanced Illness Coordinated Care. This phase of the initiative was designed to accelerate access to hospice and palliative care for veterans. A major product of the program was the Hospice-Veteran Partnership Toolkit. It also created 2.5 full-time equivalent employee positions in geriatrics and extended care to be used for hospice and palliative care presence in the VA system.

In 2004, phase 2 of the project was launched. It was funded in part by Rallying Points and the NHPCO. It built on the success of phase 1 and developed a Hospice-VA Partnership in every state to build an enduring infrastructure for the Accelerated Administrative and Clinical Training Program. In a statement made in 2002 regarding the VA national initiatives, the VA made a clear commitment to improving hospice and palliative care for their patients. The Geriatrics and Long Term Care strategic plan states,[70] "All VAMCs will be required to have designated inpatient beds for hospice and palliative care, or access to these services in the community, and an active hospice and palliative care team for consult, care and placement." Funding continues to be designated to build palliative care consult teams at every facility, to fund new PCUs, and to enhance existing PCUs. For example, in 2009, the New England Network of VAs received awards for three new PCUs and enhancement funding for two existing units. Additional national efforts include partnerships with CAPC, HPNA, NHPCO, and EPEC and ELNEC to provide veteran-specific palliative and EOL education.

As the services have grown, the VA has also taken a leadership role in evaluating these services through the use of the Family Assessment of Treatment at End-of-life (FATE) tool.[72,73] This 32-item tool assesses family members' impressions of care received by the deceased veteran in the last month of life. It includes topics such as well-being and dignity, information and communication, respect for treatment preferences, emotional and spiritual support, management of symptoms, care around the time of death, access to outpatient services, and access to benefits and services after the patient's death.[73] To date this tool has demonstrated improved outcomes at the end of life (as judged by the family member) in those veterans who received specialized palliative care consultations.[71] As a result of these initiatives, nearly 50% of veterans dying in VA facilities received the services of a palliative care team.[74] Together, these initiatives address the need for improvement on multiple fronts and create a momentum in the VA system that can set an example for other large hospital-based systems of care. Also please see chapter 43 on veterans.

Professional societies contribute to palliative care development

Multiple professional societies have made contributions to the development of HBPC generalized or specialty population-specific palliative care standards, guidelines, or consensus statements by raising professional and public awareness of the unique issues of palliative care. A few selected organizations and their initiatives are described in this section.

National Hospice and Palliative Care Organization

The NHPCO was founded in 1978 as the National Hospice Organization. The organization changed its name in February 2000 to include palliative care. Many hospice care programs added palliative care to their names to reflect the range of care and services they provide, as hospice care and palliative care share the same core values and philosophies.

According to its website, the NHPCO is the largest nonprofit membership organization representing hospice and palliative care programs and professionals in the United States. The NHPCO is committed to improving EOL care and expanding access to hospice care with the goal of profoundly enhancing quality of life for people dying in America and their loved ones. The NHPCO advocates for the terminally ill and their families. It also develops public and professional educational programs and materials to enhance understanding and availability of hospice and palliative care; convenes frequent meetings and symposia on emerging issues; provides technical informational resources to its membership; conducts research; monitors congressional and regulatory activities; and works closely with other organizations that share an interest in EOL care.

Hospice and Palliative Nurses Association

The Hospice Nurses Association was incorporated in 1987 to establish a network and support for nurses in this specialty. In 1998, the organization formally added palliative care to its mission to recognize the needs of nurses working in palliative care settings separate from hospice. The HPNA has become the nationally recognized organization providing resources and support for advanced practice nurses, registered nurses, licensed practical nurses, and nursing assistants who care for people with life-limiting and terminal illness. As such, to guide best practices they have developed a number of position statements and standards that are available to members and nonmembers on a variety of topics.

Processes for providing HBPC

While HBPC programs are increasing in number, many organizations are still at the stage of contemplating enhancing palliative resources or developing a program. Such an endeavor requires careful planning, as these programs are not "one size fits all." Patience, persistence, and consensus building are key to successful program development.[20-28] As described earlier, the CAPC has taken a leadership role in assisting organizations of all types to build a successful program that is suited to their unique patient population, resources, and organizational culture.

Particular to integrating palliative care principles into cancer centers through a multiyear grant, the City of Hope developed the Disseminating End of Life Education to Cancer Centers (DELEtCC).[75] In this multiyear project, 2-person teams attended a 3-day workshop conducted by nationally recognized expert faculty to focus on best practices in palliative oncology care. The teams received additional follow-up support and assistance to help ensure successful program implementation. In all, 400 participants from 199 different cancer programs/institutions from 42 states attended one of the four programs.

A complete primer on developing a HBPC program is beyond the scope of this chapter; however, some of the most important care processes are described in this section. Those wishing more complete information are referred to the excellent resources mentioned earlier in the chapter.

Process of program development

Regardless of organizational type, the first step in developing a HBPC program is to perform a system assessment or "organizational scan" to identify existing organizational strengths, resources, potential partnerships, and collaborators.[19] A task force or team of interested clinicians, administrators, and possibly consumers might be a good start. Examples of possible existing resources include clinicians from all disciplines with interest and training in palliative care, existing relationships with hospice, case management, discharge planners, and hospital chaplaincy programs. The needs assessment should determine the hospital focus on length of stay, ventilator days and pharmacy/ancillary costs per day, palliative care leadership based on personal experience or professional interest, pre-existing pain programs, and trustee/philanthropic interest in, and support for, palliative care.

After the system assessment is performed, the second step is to identify areas of need within the organization to highlight where palliative care programs can make the greatest contribution. Many institutions have easy access to data that can help to "build the case" for palliative care. Selling the idea of palliative care to an institution or gaining institutional support is easier when benefits (such as cost savings, efficiency, and improved clinical care) can be shown. Common areas of need that have shown improvement as a result of HBPC programs include pain and symptom management, patient and family satisfaction, nurse retention and satisfaction, bed and ICU capacity, and length of stay. Other outcomes may include pharmacy costs, establishment and strengthening of hospice partnerships, and improving fragmented subspecialty care.

To assist organizations with the complexities of the planning process, the CAPC provides a systems assessment tool and a needs assessment checklist, which can be found at http://www.capc.org/building-a-hospital-based-palliative-care-program/designing/system-assessment.

The process of providing palliative care: developing an interdisciplinary team

The holistic process of providing palliative care to patients and their families is rarely accomplished by one individual or discipline. The IDT is the foundation of the HBPC service and in many ways is unique in contrast to how medical care is traditionally provided. The core IDT typically consists of specially trained palliative care professionals, including physicians, nurses at all levels of training (registered nurses, nursing assistants, and advanced practice nurses [APNs]), social workers, pharmacists, spiritual care counselors, healing arts/complementary practitioners, hospice representatives, and volunteers.[85-90]

Identifying which team member(s) can best serve a patient's needs is a key part of the initial assessment.[91-95] One clinician may be designated to receive initial consults and organize distribution of work for the day. A team may decide that all new consults are seen first by a medical provider: either the physician or the APN. The physician also serves as the medical resource person for other team members and supervises physician learners. Advanced practice nurses may work independently or collaboratively with the attending physician to conduct initial consultations. If resources allow, this may be done together; however, workload and resources may dictate that new consults are divided among the medical providers.

In organizations that support learners, after a period of supervision and observation, it may be that the learner (e.g., fellow, resident, medical or nursing student) conducts an initial chart review and patient and/or family interview and then presents the patient to the physician or APN, after which the pair will revisit the patient. At all times the team should be aware of the patient's energy level and the learner's level of expertise in deciding whether this format is appropriate. During the initial consult psycho/social/spiritual needs are identified and other team members are integrated into the plan of care.[78]

A palliative-care-certified physician and/or APN may be responsible for the initial assessment and day-to-day medical care of most patients. However, depending on the patient's needs, another member of the team might take the lead in care. For example, if the patient's primary concern is physical, then a medical provider may direct the plan of care. If the patient's primary concern is existential in nature, the spiritual care provider may take the lead. Alternatively, if the patient's primary need is for family support, the social worker may be the most active care provider. Healing arts and complementary medicine practitioners and volunteers are also integral members of the IDT.

Healing arts/complementary medicine practitioners are providers from a variety of backgrounds who can provide massage, energy work, or instruction in guided imagery or meditation. Palliative care volunteers are specifically trained to see palliative care patients and are overseen by a volunteer coordinator. They provide presence, active listening, and company for patients and families. Although some tasks are seemingly small, such as reading, playing cards, or running small errands, these are often essential aspects of care from the patient/family perspective.

Pharmacists, healing arts/complementary therapy clinicians, hospice liaisons, and volunteers may or may not be part of the core team in some organizations. For example, even though medication needs may be complex, few teams have a dedicated pharmacist who could round daily with the team. Hence, it may be more realistic to have a pharmacist present during regularly scheduled IDT meetings. Similarly, local hospice liaisons, healing arts/complementary therapy practitioners, and others may only be available to meet with a team weekly.

Nonclinical members of the team including administrative, financial, or practice managers and secretarial support are responsible for holding the IDT together by providing the supportive infrastructure within which the team can operate. These key team members may serve as representatives or liaisons on important institutional committees. Another important function of program administrators is the collection of data for clinical and fiscal evaluation for quality improvement, program justification to the institution, or research. The receptionist/secretarial support may be the first contact for patients and referring clinicians and can become the "face or voice of the program." Individuals selected for these positions should be skilled, patient, and caring to enable them to deal with the stress of people in crisis and urgency of consultations.

After an initial consultation, depending on the patients' needs, they may continue to be seen in follow-up throughout their hospitalization. Some patients may have acute needs (such as uncontrolled pain) that may require them to be seen more than once daily. Other patients may be seen several times a week or weekly or until the goal of the initial consultation is achieved. Some patients may be visited by the medical provider, the spiritual care provider, the healing arts provider, and a volunteer—all on the same day. In the earlier case of Mr. X, visits from the palliative medicine provider and the spiritual care provider, among others, were frequent and provided the family with constant contact and opportunities to discuss concerns and feelings or the simple comfort of another human presence.

Processes to support interdisciplinary team communication

Communication may be the most challenging and crucial aspect of providing palliative care.[78–81] Intrateam communications that are regular and efficient will allow for seamless care to be delivered. Teams will likely explore a variety of mechanisms to achieve optimal communication about not only issues of patient care but also team function. The purpose of regular patient-care-related team meetings is to allow all disciplines to contribute to the development and implementation of comprehensive care plans that reflect the values, preferences, goals, and needs of each individual patient.

Practicing as a true IDT requires significant and ongoing intention and effort. Traditionally the medical model has driven healthcare delivery and, to a large extent, still does. However, in a holistic care model of palliative care, the psycho/social/spiritual care providers should have equal authority and input; for many clinicians, this represents a change in practice. Teams should be mindful of tendencies to become "efficient" that can sometimes lead to a focus only on the medical or physical aspects of care.

Minimally, a weekly face-to-face meeting, in which all IDT members gather, is considered an essential element of team function in order to provide high-quality, coordinated care. During the IDT meeting, active patients are presented and all team members have an opportunity to contribute their expertise in the development of the plan of care. In some cases, weekly meetings may not be enough and a team may choose to meet more frequently. These meetings are also a place to role model for the learners healthy and respectful team interactions that recognize the value and expertise of each team member.

Performing the palliative care consult

A palliative care consult can be initiated in a variety of different ways. Some services (or reimbursement mechanisms) require that a physician initiate the consult, rather than a nurse or other care provider. If someone other than the attending physician requests a consult on a hospitalized patient, it would still be important to include the attending (or primary care) physician in the consult. Ideally a provider-to-provider conversation prior to consultation would review and identify the priority issues. Most services do this before seeing the patient.

When is a consult made?

Consultations should be initiated any time a person with life-limiting illness has physical, psychological, social, or spiritual needs.[81] Palliative care programs began for many reasons, but one of them was to meet the EOL care planning and symptomatic needs of patients who are not yet hospice eligible, either because of life expectancy (greater than 6 months) or because they are receiving active disease-modifying treatment. Palliative care referrals do not hinge on the "less than 6 months" life expectancy as is often the case for hospice referrals. Referring patients with life-limiting illness early is one of the benefits of having a palliative care service.

Some organizations have built-in consult triggers, protocols, or algorithms for specific life-limiting illnesses in which consults are recommended at diagnosis.[82–84] "Automatic referrals" would be generated for all patients who are newly diagnosed with certain types of life-limiting cancers (e.g., pancreatic, brain, stage IIIB and greater lung, liver, etc.).[30–32] Figure 3.4 provides an example of a "trigger tool" used by one of the authors in her practice; this tool was piloted in various settings across the medical center including the adult ICU, inpatient oncology, and general medical surgical floors. Noncancer patient populations that maybe considered for automatic referrals are those with ALS, heart failure, dialysis-dependent renal failure, and those who, regardless of diagnosis, experience frequent hospitalizations. These patient populations are typically highly in need of palliative care services. Careful planning and close collaboration with colleagues is necessary to establish a process for automatic referrals that ensures that the patients that are most in need of palliative care services have them "early and often." Some automatically scheduled palliative care consultations may occur in the outpatient setting or clinic, while some organizations have hospital "triggers" that may alert that primary team that a patient may benefit from these specialized services. Over time, in HBPC programs with high community visibility and/or marketing efforts, it may be common to have patients or family members self-refer.

What is included in the initial palliative care consultation?

The initial consult will lay the foundation for all further interactions with the patient and family. In addition to specialty expertise, the palliative care team may offer the unique resources of presence and time. Much has been written about the importance of setting during the initial consult.[6,92] Making sure there is adequate time to see the patient and family is crucial. If time restrictions are unavoidable, state these constraints at the outset of the consultation. Sitting down during the consultation and making sure everyone who is participating in the consult has a seat is important (see chapter 5 on communication).[79] Depending on the resources available and the composition of the team, an initial consult can occur almost anywhere. For inpatient consults, it is often in the patient's room; for outpatient consults, it may be in the clinic exam room. If resources permit, consults can also be done at patient's homes or in local care facilities. The main concern is an environment that allows for privacy and quiet—often difficult to find in most acute care hospitals.

Patients are generally unfamiliar with the term "palliative care" and/or associate it with hospice care or death. Patients who are early in their disease process may wonder why a consult to this service has been initiated. Establishing the patients' level of understanding and explaining the role and focus of the palliative care team is an important starting point to the consultation. Often patients and families may need reassurance that they are not being "abandoned" by their primary team. Explaining that the palliative care team consults and provides expert guidance to the primary team but does not replace them is important. Providing a clear

PALLIATIVE AND SUPPORTIVE MEDICINE CONSULT (PSMC) TOOL
(Worksheet only. Not part of permanent medical record.)

Medical Record Number: _____ Age: _____ Reason for Admission: _____

To evaluate appropriateness of a PSMC, consider the following criteria:

	SCORING
1) **Would you be surprised if this patient were alive in one year?**	
Yes – Score 3 points	
No – Score 0	
TOTAL SECTION 1 (0 OR 3)	

2) **Basic Disease Process**	Score 2 points each
a. Cancer (metastatic/recurrent)	
b. Advanced COPD (requires home oxygen)	
c. Neurological disease (difficulty swallowing or incontinent)	
d. End-stage renal disease (considering stopping dialysis)	
e. Advanced congestive heart failure (one-block DOE)	
f. >3 hospitalizations or ED visits for incurable disease in past year	
g. Other terminal or incurable disease causing significant symptoms	
TOTAL SECTION 2	

3) **Uncontrollable Symptoms or Clinical Conditions**

Score 2 points each	Score 1 point each	Score 1 point each
a. Pain	e. Anxiety	i. Prolonged vent support
b. Dyspnea	f. Depression	j. Other _____
c. Naesua	g. Weight loss	
d. Bowel obstruction	h. Constipation	
		TOTAL SECTION 3

4) **Anticipated Functional Status of Patient at Time of Discharge** — Score as specified
Using ECOG Performance Status (Eastern Cooperative Oncology Group)

Grade	Scale	Score
0–1	Fully active, able to carry on all pre-disease activities without restriction or restricted in physically strenuous activity but ambulatory and able to carry out work of a light or sedentary nature.	0
2	Ambulatory and capable of most self-care but unable to carry out any work activities. Up and about more than 50% of waking hours.	1
3–4	Capable of only limited self care; confined to bed or chair more than 50% of waking hours or worse.	3
	TOTAL SECTION 4 (0, 1, OR 3)	

5) **Psychosocial issues (patient or family)**	Score 2 points each
a. Need to discuss end of life issues	
b. Need for evaluation for possible hospice referral	
c. Artificial hydration or nutrition requested or considered	
d. Unrealistic goals o rexpectations	
TOTAL SECTION 5	
TOTAL SCORE SECTIONS 1–5	

SCORING GUIDELINES:

TOTAL SCORE ≤ 8	Problem-directed consult, if desired
TOTAL SCORE = 9–11	Consider PSMC
TOTAL SCORE ≥ 12	Strongly consider PSMC

Form completed by _____ Date: _____

Figure 3.4 (Continued)

and confident explanation of services will help everyone know what to expect. Providing a brochure or some written information about what palliative care is and who the team members are can be helpful. Assessing the patient/family knowledge and understanding their current situation is the next step. Healthcare providers often believe that they have done a complete and thorough job in explanations; however, patients are under stress and may need multiple explanations in very simple language before they fully understand their situation.

Next, a complete and thorough assessment is begun. This should include a review of symptoms and physical complaints, as well as an assessment of psychological, emotional, social, and spiritual concerns. Eliciting a clear picture of the patient's social support structure and family relationships is essential, as the contextual issues will often affect, if not drive, decision-making. Exploring what gives meaning to patients' lives and who they are as individuals will help direct care. Do not hesitate to humanize the medical encounter by taking the time to get to know the patient as a whole person—their

PALLIATIVE AND SUPPORTIVE RAPID RESPONSE CONSULT (PMRRC)

(Worksheet only. Not part of permanent medical record.)

Medical Record Number: _____ **Age:** _____ **Reason for Admission:** _____

To evaluate appropriateness of a PMRRC consider the following criteria:

1. Palliative Medicine consult tool score>9 (see page 1)
2. Patient referred from SNF for PEG tube placement with underlying significant dementia or progressive metastatic cancer.
3. Patient older than 75 years old with significant medical problems and: 1. No advanced directive and no surrogate decision maker   2. Advanced directive that lists both do and do not selections   3. Progressive single or multi-system disease with anticipated survival of one year or less and limited therapies available for the underlying disease   4. Family or home caregivers with disparate goals for the patient   5. Patient is full code and has multi-system organ failure, metastatic cancer, or a progressive terminal disease despite treatment or no treatment is planned for the underlying disease
4. Any sub-optimally controlled acute post trauma or post operative pain problem
5. Any patient with cancer and pain
6. Patients or families that are requesting medical treatments for life prolongation or CPR that the primary service believes would be of little or no benefit to the patient.
7. Assistance with medication logistics and discussion of possible hospice referral or comfort care plans for SNF

Figure 3.4 GMC palliative and supportive medicine consult tool and palliative and supportive rapid response consult tool. Developed by Neil Ellison, MD, and Patricia Maani-Fogelman, DNP, Geisinger health system.

hobbies, passions in life, the meaning they attribute to work, and family are all important aspects of learning about a new individual. Assessing and attending to cultural preferences will enhance communication and increase the effectiveness of interventions.

Other areas that are important to assess are goals of care, advance care planning wishes, and treatment decision-making style. Due to time constraints and sometimes lack of skill, these complex issues are often overlooked or only superficially explored by the primary team. Yet they are some of the most important pieces of the puzzle when constructing a plan of care. It is important to find out what the patient/family is hoping for from treatment interventions. This is where the role of nursing advocacy comes in: As the individuals spending the greatest amount of time at the bedside, nurses can often identify the patient/family personal preferences and goals, ascertaining the answers to questions such as "What does getting better mean to you?" Often this issue is ignored when in fact it needs more time and consideration. To the medical team, "getting better" may mean the patient is able to leave the hospital; to the patient it may mean a full recovery or expectation of return to a high level of functionality. The clinical implications of a new disease or advanced illness are not always clear to the patient or family, requiring further review and discussion. Exploring, on the first visit, whether the patient and family have ever considered and/or completed advance directives may elucidate this. Completing advance directives is a structured way of looking at goals of care and what is meaningful when making treatment decisions. Some programs have developed standardized templates that remind the team (and the referring provider) of the important and comprehensive domains of care and intervention that are included in the consultation.

Who should be present at an initial consultation?

While there are times that it is appropriate to conduct a consult without the patient present (e.g., the patient is in coma)—in most cases every effort is made to include the patient. The patient should decide which support members and/or family they want to include. There may be one or more members of the palliative care team present. A member from the referring team may want to attend—but this is less common on initial consult. If a focused family meeting is arranged it is imperative that the referring team be present so all decision makers are in the room together. Family meetings are a large part of palliative care interventions. During the initial consult it may be clear that a family meeting is needed to proceed with discussion about care planning, and on occasion such a meeting may be simultaneously organized as a part of the initial consult. Direct inquiry with the patient will also identify key family/support members desired for any discussions, and efforts should be undertaken to include those identified whenever possible. Conducting a family meeting takes skill and planning—in today's hectic world it is often difficult to coordinate multiple schedules or for family members to reach the hospital due to distance and other concerns. In these instances the use of teleconferencing has become especially helpful. Resources are available to assist inexperienced team members with the important process of organizing and conducting a family meeting.[85]

Continuing the care: day-to-day operations

Patients with serious illness may follow many different paths. Table 3.3 illustrates paths that may be typical in the current "care as usual" for a seriously ill patient, compared with an "ideal" or expected pathway in a healthcare system with an HBPC program. Numerous institutions have studied their processes of care and have created clinical pathways that can help standardize procedures and reduce the variation of care experienced by terminally ill or symptomatic palliative care patients as they traverse the complex healthcare system.[86] Usual components include attention to patient symptoms, as well as family needs at system entry and throughout the course of stay until discharge. Assigning time frames to address needs helps in monitoring progress and tracking outcomes that have been met as well as those that continue to need attention.

Although published guidelines and standards may offer similar suggestions, the road map format of clinical pathways identifies practical and accountable mechanisms to keep patient care moving in the direction of specific identified outcomes. Some pathway forms allow for documentation of variation from the designated path. Analysis of several instances of variation might alert a care team about a potential system "defect" in need of improvement.

Many institutions have implemented standard orders or evidence-based algorithms to guide various aspects of care pertinent to EOL situations. Some of these include limitations of certain types of therapies such as CPR and blood pressure medications.

In addition, preprinted order sheets that outline management of symptoms and side effects such as nausea, constipation, and pain are making it easier for physicians and trainees to reproduce comprehensive plans that do not vary because of individual opinion. These order forms can be valuable teaching tools in a setting of regularly changing care providers. Figure 3.5 shows a sample order sheet and the companion guidelines printed on the reverse for patients who are hospitalized and have a palliative focus of care. Certainly, important considerations in the development of such "recipes" for care include having broad, multidisciplinary, evidence-based input. The process of producing such documents is also potentially a care consensus and learning environment for many teams.

Care pathways and orders also demonstrate what care is provided when a patient is no longer receiving curative care. In cases where curative care ceases, clinicians and patients may believe "there is nothing more to do." Order sheets, algorithms, and care pathways are common in complex acute care situations. Using these same tools, palliative care can demonstrate the complex, aggressive care that can be directed at comfort. The patient and family can have confidence that everything will be done to provide pain management and relief of suffering. Nurses in particular can advocate through development of hospital policy, education, and individual practice for aggressive comfort care. The healthcare team must ensure that a positive approach—focusing on what can be done for patients with life-limiting illness and their families—is implemented. Pathways may go a long way toward reducing variation in care so that delays or unpredictable outcomes are avoided.[103,105,112] At a macro level of cancer care, the National Comprehensive Cancer Network[92] has published a care algorithm

Table 3.3 How hbpc programs might influence "care as usual" for persons with life-limiting illness

Current process of care	Care process with an integrated HBPC
Patient with known life-limiting, chronic illness arrives in emergency department for relief of uncontrolled disease-related symptoms.	Patient with known life-limiting, chronic illness meets criteria and is referred for initial outpatient Palliative Care Team (PCT) Consultation and standardized holistic assessment
	◆ PCT documents and communicates consultation to patient/family & referring team
	◆ Advance directives documents completed including patient's preference for resuscitation status
	◆ Prospective symptom management plan identified
	◆ Community-based resources in place
	◆ Regular PCT follow-up planned in conjunction with other medical appointments when possible (including MSW, chaplain, healing arts providers as appropriate).
ED workup and hospital admission to medical unit.	Patient develops disease-related symptoms, which are managed by PCT staff by phone.
Inpatient/hospitalist medical team continues diagnostic workup.	Patient requires brief, planned hospital admit for symptom relief procedure; continuity of care ensured by preplanned inpatient PCT follow-up over hospitalization.
Patient undergoes tests and procedures. Symptom management per medical team.	Symptoms are assessed using standardized tool & documented. Evidence-based symptom treatment is implemented and symptoms rapidly managed with standardized symptom assessment/management algorithm or pathway. (If patient is approaching EOL and cannot or does not wish to die outside of hospital then Comfort Measures standardized orders are implemented).
Patient's disease process is not able to be reversed. Patient develops acute deterioration and is transferred to the intensive care unit on ventilator.	Discharge plan coordinated by inpatient PCT for patient to have home care (or hospice care) as needed.
After prolonged stay, patient dies in hospital.	Patient dies in preferred site of death. Bereavement care offered to family after the death.

DARTMOUTH-HITCHCOCK MEDICAL CENTER

One Medical Center Drive
Lebanon, New Hampshire 03756

Physician/ARNP Order Sheet
Comfort Measures
Any order preceded by a check box must have the box checked to enable the order. All other orders will be automatically implemented

☐ **DISCONTINUE ALL PREVIOUS ORDERS**

Activity: ☐ OOB as tolerated   ☐ OOB with assistance ☐ Bedrest
Hunger: ☐ Diet as tolerated   ☐ NPO ☐ Other_____
Thirst: ☐ PO Fluids as tol. **IV Fluids:** ☐ No IVF   ☐ Yes_____
Dyspnea: ☐ O$_2$ prn for patient comfort ☐ No Oxygen   ☐ Fan at bedside
Elimination: ☐ Insert Foley Catheter prn
Oral Care: ☐ **per guideline (see reverse)** ☐ **Other**_____
Skin Care: ☐ **per guideline (see reverse)** ☐ **Other**_____

Monitoring:

Vital Signs: ☐ No   ☐ Yes - specify_____

Weight: ☐ No weights   ☐ Yes - specify _____

Labs: ☐ No lab draws   ☐ Yes labs - specify _____

Consider Other Consults (if not already involved): ☐ Palliative Care ☐ Pastoral Care

Medication for Symptom Management
Pain – Scheduled (If PCA use special sheet) :
Pain - Breakthrough:
Dyspnea:
Anxiety/Agitation:
Myoclonus:
Depression:
Sleep Disturbance:
Pruritus:
Fever:
Nausea/Vomiting:
Constipation:
Diarrhea:
Other Orders:

A generic equivalent may be administered when a drug has been prescribed by brand name unless the order states to the contrary.

_____   _____
Physician/ARNP Signature   Date/Time

_____   _____
Print Physician/ARNP Name   Pager or Phone

Secretary Transcribing

Original to the medical record   Yellow copy to Pharmacy   See Other Side
P&T Committee: 7/15/2004 (P-225)   Medical Records: 08/03/2004 Form #1826

Figure 3.5 (Continued)

and extensively detailed "care standards" in its *Palliative Care Clinical Guideline*. This booklet is produced as a professional and patient guide and is available from http://nccn.org.

Documenting palliative care consultations

As in all aspects of healthcare delivery, documentation is the foundation for communicating with other providers, particularly across care settings. As a consultative service, including the primary care providers in the plan of care promotes collegiality and helps assure follow-through. Recommendations for symptom management, identification of goals of care, advance planning and resuscitation wishes, or emotional counseling and support are at the heart of the palliative care assessment and interventions.

An electronic medical record (EMR) may provide an immediate way to share information with all members of the care team.

Guidelines for Comfort Measures Orders

D/C ALL PREVIOUS ORDERS – Assess & reorder existing orders effective for comfort.

Activity: Goal is patient comfort. Activity level and hygiene routine should be based on patient's preference.

Hunger: Goal is to respond to patient's hunger, not to maintain a "normal nutritional intake."

Thirst: Goal is to respond to patient's thirst, which is best accomplished by oral fluids, sips, ice chips, and mouthcare per patient desires, not IV hydration.

IV Fluids Goal is to avoid over-hydration which can lead to discomfort from edema, pulmonary and gastric secretions, and urinary incontinence. A small volume of IV fluid may assist with medication metabolism and delirium.

Dyspnea: Respond to the patient's perception of breathlessness rather than "numerical abnormalities"; i.e. oxygen saturation via pulse oximetry. Interventions include medications (e.g. opioids, antianxiety agents, steroids), scopolamine patch and minimizing IV fluids to decrease secretions; oxygen therapy per nasal cannula prn for patient comfort—avoid face mask.
Fans at Bedside – Fans are available for patient comfort and are often more effective for perception of breathlessness than other interventions.

Elimination: Focus on managing distress from bowel or bladder incontinence. Insert Foley Catheter prn – per patient comfort and desire.

Oral Care: Studies show dry mouth is the most common & distressing symptom in conscious patients at end of life.
Ice chips and sips of fluid prn; humidify oxygen to minimize oral/nasal drying.
Mouth care q 2 hours and prn – sponge oral mucosa and apply lubricant to lips and oral mucosa.

Skin Care: Air mattress, Pressure Sore Prevention Measures per DHMC skin care guidelines.
Incontinent care every 2 hours and prn.

Monitoring: Focus monitoring on the patient's symptoms (e.g. pain) & responses to comfort measures.

Psychosocial Consults: Goal is to provide resources and support through the dying process.

Medication for Symptom Management (Scheduled & PRN):
Pain Management, scheduled and breakthrough: consider PCA/IV/SQ/rectal analgesics.
Dyspnea Management: consider opioids, scopolamine patch, atropine for secretions.
Anxiety/Agitation Management: consider combination of lorazepam (Ativan) & haloperidol (Haldol).
Myoclonus: consider benzodiazepines &/or opioid rotation for myoclonus.
Depression Management: evaluate for antidepressants or methylphenidate.
Sleep Disturbance Management: consider diphenhydramine (Benadryl).
Pruritus Management: consider diphenhydramine (Benadryl) PO/IV.
Fever Management: consider acetaminophen (Tylenol) PO/rectal
Nausea/Vomiting Management: consider prochlorperazine (Compazine), metoclopramide; 5-HT3 antagonist PO/IV.
Constipation Management: consider Narcotic Bowel Orders.
Diarrhea Management: consider diphenoxylate/atropine (Lomotil) or loperamide (Imodium).

Figure 3.5 Comfort measures order sheet. Includes guidelines for care and references for staff education on the back. Source: Dartmouth-Hitchcock Medical Center, June 2004. Used with permission.

Pertinent members with whom the consult should be shared include the primary referral service (if the patient is inpatient), the primary care provider, and other specialties consulting on the patient. Providing a copy of the consultation note, electronically in real time, can assist with the timely communication and implementation of recommendations.

Documentation can also be a vehicle for education that should not be overlooked. Including specifics in the plan of care can help other providers learn aspects of palliative care. For example, breakthrough dosing for pain medications is often underdosed by the primary team. When addressing pain management in the palliative plan of care, noting the total daily opioid use and writing the details of the calculation (10%–20% of total daily need) in print can teach other providers how to prescribe adequate breakthrough medication in the future.

Finally, documenting goals of care, resuscitation wishes and advance care planning in a way that is visible to everyone is a challenge. Patients often complain that they have provided documents or information, such as an advance directive, but at the point of care the information is not easily located. As a quality improvement initiative, our institution created a visible tab embedded in the EMR for advance directives. In this system, important documents (advance directives and Do Not Resuscitate orders) are scanned into the record and are readily available. For patients who have verbally stated wishes but have not completed the official document, a clinician can complete a templated advance care planning note that carries the same force as an official form. This can be completed by any team member and can indicate the durable power of attorney as well as care wishes (e.g., resuscitation wishes, medically administered nutrition/hydration wishes, etc.). The templated notes and actual documents are all located in the same section of the EMR and are accessible to all providers (including in the Emergency Department and physician offices that are part of the medical center system).

Completing the process: transitions of care and continuity

The palliative care team must remember that they are the consultants and ultimately most patients will remain under the guidance of the primary provider. While some referring providers welcome aggressive assistance in care, others may prefer to accept or decline palliative care team recommendations. Talking a case over with the primary team is always preferable to leaving a note in the record.

Continuity is improved dramatically when there is an outpatient as well as an inpatient component of an HBPC. Our outpatient service is managed by a team of APNs and physician providers. All inpatients can be followed in the outpatient setting (when indicated). This provides an opportunity to reinforce or adjust recommendations made while the patient was hospitalized. It also provides an opportunity to explore complex emotional topics or decision-making.

For patients who do not return to the center, providing continuity is difficult. Sending the initial palliative care consult and pertinent notes to the receiving team (including the patient's primary care provider or skilled nursing facility if applicable) is useful. Being open to phone calls or proactively placing a personal call to the receiving provider will help to build bridges to the community and encourage community providers to see the palliative care team as a resource.

Extending the reach of hospital-based palliative care: advance care planning

The Patient Self-Determination Act (PSDA) of 1991 required that hospitals and other organizations receiving Medicare or Medicaid funding provide written information to patients about their rights to make decisions to accept or refuse medical care.[85-86] Further, it stipulated that advance directives, including living wills and appointment of a healthcare proxy, may be used to provide substituted judgment in the event of patients' inability to speak for themselves regarding healthcare decisions. Although this legislation was designed to allow patients to have a durable mechanism to outline their preferences for certain types of treatments, for many years it had little impact on yielding improvements in EOL care.[86] There are several reasons for this. First, not all patients actually choose to complete advance directives. Often, inexperienced personnel distribute the information without providing appropriate explanation of the documents, leading to lack of completion by patients. Even for patients who complete them, the forms may not be specific enough to address the situation in which patients later find themselves. Second, even when a patient has taken the time to thoughtfully complete a document, the healthcare provider may not be aware of it[85-86] or the healthcare proxy may not interpret it as the patient intended.[105]

Staff of HBPC programs can play an important role in patient decision-making with each individual patient and within the larger healthcare system. At an individual patient level, consensus guidelines recommend that patients/families' preferences for surrogate decision makers and treatment goals be documented at the initial assessment and whenever there is a change in the patients' situation.[86] However this task is not complete until the information is both documented in the medical record and shared with the primary team. In addition to documenting the presence of advance directives, for hospitalized patients these wishes must be translated into medical orders (e.g., completion of Do Not Resuscitate forms if the patient prefers not to have this life-sustaining treatment applied). Furthermore, documentation

of these preferences should accompany patients when transitioning to other healthcare settings. Different states have laws about how these orders are documented and transferred among settings. Many states' laws have provisions for patients at home who are dying and do not want to be resuscitated to use home labeling systems such as a "DNR bracelet," sticker, or forms. Some states may have Physician Orders for Life-Sustaining Treatment (POLST) programs to identify ambulatory/outpatient wishes outside of the hospital. (More information on individual state efforts regarding POLST-type programs is available at http://www.ohsu.edu/ethics/polst/about/index.htm.)

Healthcare providers who are not focused on palliative care needs may not gather information about advance directives and patient treatment preferences as an automatic component of their health history (such as identifying and documenting allergies and medications). Therefore, it is not uncommon for providers to be unaware of the presence of the patient's advance directive until the patient is in crisis. Such late awareness can result in patient's making choices under duress that they might not otherwise have made. For example, if the patient experiencing respiratory distress is asked if he "would like everything done" to help him to breathe better—the answer is understandably "yes." If the topic had been discussed earlier in his admission, he would have been provided with comprehensive information regarding his prognosis and probable course of illness, and multiple options for treating dyspnea at EOL (e.g., opioid and oxygen rather than intubation and ventilation). Meeting the patient and family's preferences for EOL care requires advance care planning that occurs early in the course of illness, or preferably in the primary healthcare setting while people are well and healthy. Intensive healthcare provider education on communicating with patients about advance care planning, before a health crisis occurs, is an area where a HBPC program can have influence beyond the bedside of the individual patient.

The case study of Mr. X demonstrates the importance of early palliative care intervention so that advance directives and patient- and family-centered care can be delivered. The introduction of palliative care at the time of diagnosis allowed for appropriate and effective utilization of the palliative care services. When the patient is identified early in the course of illness, the palliative care team can act as a resource for advance care planning, goals of care discussions, bereavement support, pain and symptom management, and psychosocial issues. As the patient nears death, and the goal of care becomes focused more on comfort, the palliative care team will be a familiar member of the care team during a potentially stressful time.

Outcomes and their measurement: the role of quality improvement and research in hospital-based palliative care

Measurement of outcomes is vital to demonstrate quality and to maintain viability and growth of HBPC programs. Although the field is still developing, tools are beginning to emerge to measure care, assist with developing standards of care, and most importantly, bring individual and organizational transparency and accountability to the care that is being delivered. Documentation of less than excellent outcomes may result in the organizational tension needed for change to occur. Such motivation can stimulate improvement and motivation for both administrators and clinicians.

As described earlier in this chapter, a number of organizations such as the CAPC, NQF, and NCP have urged all programs to collect standardized measures across settings. In particular, the CAPC has taken the lead in providing technical assistance in this regard. Resources for business, clinical, quality management, and strategic and financial planning are available on the CAPC website, with link to the actual tools and instruments for measurement and planning of clinical care.

A number of efforts have been initiated to advance the measurement of palliative care outcomes. The Institute of Medicine issued a report in 2007, "Cancer Care for the Whole Patient: Meeting Psychosocial Health Needs."[88] This report requested development of mechanisms to measure quality of care by organizations that are involved in developing and measuring standards of quality. In response, the American Society of Clinical Oncologists (ASCO), recognizing that oncologists had few reliable resources to assess and measure the quality of supportive care delivered in their practices, launched a health plan program developed by its Quality Oncology Practice Initiative (QOPI).[49] Data are collected on a quarterly basis and, if desired, reported by ASCO to insurers. Measurement of data in this fashion not only impacts on the quality of care delivered within an individual program but also promotes evidence-based practices and standardization across settings.

Another national effort, led by the University HealthSystem Consortium (UHC), recommended collection of data for the purpose of academic benchmarking nationally.[89,90] The UHC, comprising over 100 academic medical centers and nearly 200 of their affiliates, is an alliance of US Academic Medical Centers (AMCs), whose goal is to provide resources to support transformational change leading to clinical and operational excellence. Through the consensus of an expert panel and based on other published guidelines, the consortium developed 11 key performance measures and collected data from the 35 centers that agreed to participate—some had palliative care consultation services, others did not. The 11 measures included pain assessment, use of a pain rating scale, pain reduction, bowel regimen, dyspnea assessment and relief, comprehensive assessment, psychosocial assessment, patient/family meeting, documentation of discharge plan and arrangement for discharge services. They found significant variability across these centers, but identified five organizations that were found to be "better performers" overall. However, no organization reached the predetermined 90% benchmark on all parameters, while some hospitals achieved low or 0% achievement of some.[89,90] Despite its limitations, this project demonstrated the importance of measurement of palliative care indicators.

As previously described, the NCP 8 domains and NQF 38 preferred practices are key resources for the development of measures to determine HBPC quality. Although voluntary, the preferred practices were intended to provide a standard of care for which measures could be developed for quality assessment. Other NQF guidelines have become the foundation for accreditation and reimbursement. It is the hope that this same outcome will occur in the palliative care preferred practices.

The CAPC website and a printed technical manual[19] contain tools for measuring HBPC outcomes. When assisting an organization to establish a program, CAPC encourages the incorporation of clinical, financial, operational, and customer metrics.[33]

Table 3.4 Metric categories

Metric domain	Examples
Operational	Patient demographics (diagnosis, age, gender, ethnicity) referring clinician, disposition, hospital length of stay
Clinical	Symptom scores, psychosocial symptom assessment
Customer (patient, family, referring clinicians)	Patient, family, referring clinician satisfaction surveys
Financial	Costs (pre- and post-HBPC consultation), inpatient palliative unit, net loss/gain for inpatient deaths

Source: Data from Weissman, Meier, and Spragens (2008), reference 33.

In 2008, the CAPC convened a consensus panel to discuss which operational metrics should be measured as programs "strive for quality, sustainability and growth" and which metrics can be used to "compare service utilization across settings." The twelve domains of operational data that were agreed on may be used to compare service characteristics and impact within a program or between programs. The four categories of measurement to assure effectiveness and efficiency recommended by CAPC are (1) clinical (pain and symptom control) metrics, (2) program operational measures, (3) customer metrics (satisfaction surveys of patients, families and providers), and (4) financial metrics. Table 3.4 lists some examples of these measurement variables. Examples of actual tools to measure these characteristics are available on the CAPC website mentioned earlier.

Every program should have a plan to measure and monitor its effect on the quality of patient care, ideally from program inception. Some measures will be useful for internal planning for staffing, need for program growth, and productivity goals. These same measures could then be compared to other programs as external benchmarks, especially for newer programs under development. Ultimately, the data collected can be used to assure that high quality palliative care is provided across organizations.[33,65,90]

Economic issues

Despite higher spending per individual on healthcare than any other country, over 50% of caregivers of Americans hospitalized with a life-threatening illness surveyed report suboptimal care.[74] Over 1.5 million Americans die of chronic illness each year, and more than 70% of these are admitted to a hospital during the last 6 months of life.[90,91,93] The number of people over age 85 will double to 10 million by the year 2030. Currently, 23% of Medicare patients with more than four chronic conditions account for 68% of all Medicare spending.[3,93] As the population ages and technology advances, the potential for prolonged care with minimal improvement in quality of life and associated human suffering looms large. The cost to an overburdened healthcare system could be disastrous over the long term. Just because the technology exists does not mean it should be used for everyone. The *Dartmouth Atlas of Health Care* reported that 98% of Medicare decedents spent at least some time in a hospital in the year before death. And of this group, 15%–55% had at least one stay in a critical care unit in the 6 months before death.[112]

Palliative care has been demonstrated to lower costs for both hospitals and payers by reducing hospital lengths of stay as well as pharmacy and procedural costs. Morrison et al. conducted a retrospective study reviewing hospital costs for eight hospitals with established palliative care programs over a 2-year period. Considerable cost savings (cost avoidance) were demonstrated when matching patients who had palliative care team involvement were compared with those patients who did not.

Although it is not the goal of palliative care to reduce costs, several studies have demonstrated this to be the case.[89–94] Reduction in costs by palliative care intervention may occur in multiple ways. Patients and their families are often stressed and burdened by a serious illness. Many times they are not clear about what to expect and may be experiencing the fragmentation of multiple specialty providers giving seemingly conflicting messages. Compounding this is the erroneous societal expectation that medicine is able to fix nearly any health challenge. It is no wonder that patients and families sometimes have unreasonable expectations and are unable to discern the larger picture when functional status is declining and treatment options offer fewer benefits to quality or quantity of life.

In HBPC clinicians may be able to provide the family with "the big picture" of the illness situation. As an "objective" coordinator, the palliative care provider is particularly skilled at summarizing all relevant information and assisting the patient to match treatments with their own personal values and preferences. In so doing, patients and families are better able to apply their personal wishes and goals to the care that is being offered. They may elect to decline certain diagnostics or invasive treatments in favor of those that will provide comfort. Some may choose to not escalate care or perhaps discontinue treatments that were previously initiated. In the setting of a prolonged critical care stay where treatments are no longer resulting in positive progress, a palliative care consult may result in deescalation of disease-modifying care in favor of increasing "low-tech" comfort care. Such changes in treatment can result in reducing suffering of the patient and family and, at times, can also result in significant cost avoidance. Consistent with criteria from the CAPC report card, the palliative care consult may "reduce unwanted, unnecessary and painful interventions."[23]

In the less costly hospital care that occurs in the critical care unit, the palliative care team can assist patients and families to select medical treatments and care that are consistent with their values and preferences. When patients and families have a clear understanding of their prognosis, and realistic information about proposed procedures or treatments, they may wish to decline further hospital care and return home. In some situations when symptom relief procedures or family respite is indicated, palliative care involvement can facilitate timely occurrence of the needed procedures so that time in the hospital is minimized. Not only does this potentially reduce costs, but quality of care is also enhanced.[89–93]

In settings of seemingly futile care or conflict among healthcare providers, patients, and families or among healthcare providers, involvement of palliative care in conjunction with an ethics committee consultation may help achieve more rapid conflict resolution.[48] Cost savings can be accomplished in indirect ways as well. When the palliative care team is involved, they can spend the time at the bedside necessary to manage pain and other symptoms. This is invaluable to an already overburdened primary treating team, who may be working with other patients who also have intensive care needs. Thus, quality of life and satisfaction for the patient and family as well as professional colleagues is enhanced. The palliative care team may also be invaluable in assisting with complex plans for discharge, coordinating care across settings, and enhancing communication between the treating team and the patient and their family.

Influencing institutional, state, and national policy

It is not enough to provide excellent, comprehensive care to just the patients that are referred for consultation. The truly effective HBPC program must seek out ways to influence care for all patients with life-limiting illness by developing an awareness and ability to influence healthcare policy within their institutions, and at a state or national level. The influence should begin within the larger organization in two main ways: (1) by developing policies, procedures, and practices that will guide care of all persons with life-limiting illness within the agency and any affiliates; and (2) by integrating palliative care education and competency standards into basic orientation and continuing (preferably mandatory) staff education. Examples of the former include development of consultation triggers, policies for advance care planning, limitations of life-sustaining treatments, "comfort measures," withdrawal of mechanical ventilation, and standardized pain and symptom assessment and management. This type of influence will likely necessitate regular or ad hoc participation or leadership on institutional practice or ethics committees. Staff orientation has grown in sophistication such that "simulated" patients and learning labs are becoming standard mechanisms for learning basic care skills. Practicing skills of communicating bad news, holding family meetings, and discussing advance care planning are some possible activities that lend themselves to such environments. Similarly, most organizations hold staff accountable for mandatory CPR certification. It would seem reasonable to require mandatory "do not resuscitate" classes in which staff learns effective care to provide when patients are near death but will not be resuscitated. Other educational endeavors include annual presentations at other departments or affiliated agencies' grand rounds on palliative care topics. Also holding annual regional palliative care conferences for professionals or the general public can bring attention to the program.

Acting locally at the state level in legislative or health policy forums can make a big difference in care of patients. Examples of vital work performed at the state level include crafting of advance directive documents and laws, expanding hospice coverage to Medicaid, opioid prescribing laws, and other practice issues. The NQF preferred practices include a recommendation to "develop health care and community collaborations to promote advance care planning and completion of advance directives for all individuals—for example, the Respecting Choices and Community Conversations on Compassionate Care programs."[20] Some states have palliative care or EOL task forces that make policy and legislative recommendations that will enhance care of the seriously ill. For example, in New Hampshire, legislation created an EOL task force in which palliative care clinicians helped revise advance care planning legislation (see http://www.healthynh.com/fhc/ initiatives/performance/eol/endoflifecare.php). Expert input helped improve advance directives forms and incorporate APNs as providers who could write DNR orders among other improvements. Palliative care and survivorship were added as major initiatives to the State Cancer Plan, which mandates some palliative practices for organizations to strive for as well as potential designate grant funds for palliative care focused projects (see http://www.nhcancerplan.org).

In addition to supporting legislative initiatives to improve care, it is just as vital to monitor policy that could have a harmful effect on patient care. For example, overly restrictive prescribing policies can make it difficult for patients in pain to obtain sufficient opioids. Activism around restrictive policies may have direct impact on patients' outcomes. Legislators respect the input of healthcare professionals who are able to provide expert input and "real-life" patient examples to assist in crafting legislation. Meier and Beresford offer a practical summary and multiple examples of ways in which palliative care professionals can contribute to state and national legislation and policy.[96]

Collaborating with local organizations also lends power to individual efforts. For example, the NHPCO, the American Cancer Society, nursing and medical associations, and professional organizations at local, state, or national levels often have lobbyists and resources to assist with legislative efforts. Chapter 66 contains a broader discussion on the nursing role in policy development. However, it is important for HBPC program staff and leaders to keep these initiatives in mind as they develop within a healthcare setting.

Future directions

Despite a strong foothold within mainstream medicine, there is a need for much growth, improvement, and education to sustain and expand palliative care. Calvin Coolidge is quoted as saying, "We cannot do everything at once, but we can do something at once." Box 3.2 lists some future professional and societal issues that need attention. Great strides have been made in providing a solid infrastructure for growth in the form of increasing research evidence, consensus guidelines for practice, reliable and valid outcome measures, and specialty educational/certification standards. These standards need to be widely disseminated and adopted. As more HBPC programs develop, there is likely to be a shortage of specialty-trained personnel and the faculty to educate them. Additional sources of funding and support are needed to continue the current momentum of change.

However, palliative care programs must not remain insular. Good work and rigorous studies need to be disseminated outside of the specialty via "mainstream" healthcare journals and conferences. Continuous outreach education to increase awareness among patients, communities, and all healthcare providers (nursing, physicians, physical therapists, nursing aides, etc.) remains a cornerstone of improving the delivery of palliative medicine. Hospital with PCTs should promote and support their programs and staff in these endeavors and allow the time and space needed to expand palliative care services throughout their communities. External agencies (e.g., TJC) must require mandatory adherence to standards, and those agencies that meet established standards should be properly reimbursed for their performance. Funding for palliative care research, adequate reimbursement, and support for faculty development must become national priorities. Perhaps consumer demand for patient- and family-centered care will be the "tipping point"

Box 3.2 Future growth of hospital-based palliative care
Within specialty
♦ Full/mandatory implementation of NCP + NQF guidelines
♦ Evaluate/expand requirement of palliative care programs to have specialty-certified clinicians
♦ Increase educational funding/support for palliative care specialty education
♦ Increase number of specialty-trained faculty and students
♦ Increase availability of technical support for new programs
External/societal/policy
♦ Publish palliative care studies in top-tier journals
♦ Increase NIH funding for palliative care research
♦ Accreditation requirements for HBPC
♦ Improve fiscal policy for reimbursement for hospice and palliative care services
♦ Develop medical and nursing school departments of palliative care
♦ Faculty career development support
♦ Legislative initiatives that support/promote palliative care and patient-/family-centered care

---

that will make palliative care services an integral part of every organization that touches the lives of persons with life-limiting illness and their families.

As awareness for palliative medicine interventions for the advanced illness patient evolves, it is our moral imperative that provides the clearest rationale: "Be kind whenever possible. It is always possible" (Dalai Lama). In every action taken, let us endeavor to always practice with kindness, and let kindness be the driving force for changing the face of healthcare delivery.

Acknowledgments

The authors acknowledge the following colleagues, who provided important information for the development of this chapter: Neil Ellison, MD (Director, Palliative Medicine Program, Geisinger Health System); Jenna M. Carmichael, PharmD (Geisinger Health System, Clinical Oncology); Jay Horton, ARNP; Sean Morrison, MD; Lisa Morgan (Center for the Advancement of Palliative Care); Lisa Stephens, ARNP (Dartmouth-Hitchcock Palliative Care Team); and Melissa Thompson, RN, CHPN (VAMC: VISN 1 Palliative Care Coordinator).

Patricia Maani-Fogelman especially acknowledges the following individuals for their constant love, encouragement, and faith: Timothy G. Fogelman; Heather D. Tirino; Christopher V. Maani, MD; and Ruby Weller, CRNP.

References

1. Teno JM, Gozalo PL, Bynum JW, et al. Change in end-of-life care for Medicare beneficiaries: site of death, place of care, and health care transitions in 2000, 2005, and 2009. JAMA. 2013;309(5):470–477.

2. Morden NE, Chang C-H, Jacobson JO, Berke EM, Bynum JPW, Murray KM, et al. End-of-life care for Medicare beneficiaries with cancer is highly intensive overall and varies widely. Health Aff. 2012;31(4):786–796.

3. Goodman DC, Esty AR, Fisher ES, Chang C-H. 2011, April 12. Trends and Variation in End-of-Life Care for Medicare Beneficiaries with Severe Chronic Illness: A Report of the Dartmouth Atlas Project. Robert Wood Johnson Foundation. Retrieved from http://www.rwjf.org/en/research-publications/find-rwjf-research/2011/04/trends-and-variation-in-end-of-life-care-for-medicare-beneficiar.html.

4. Smith AK, McCarthy E, Weber E, et al. Half of older Americans seen in emergency department in last month of life: most admitted to hospital, and many die there. Health Aff. 2012;31:1277–1285.

5. Bercovitz A, Decker FH, Jones A, Remsburg RE. End-of-life care in nursing homes: 2004 National Nursing Home Survey. Natl Health Stat Report. 2008;9:1–24.

6. SUPPORT Principal Investigators. A controlled trial to improve care for seriously ill hospitalized patients. JAMA. 1995;274:1591–1598.

7. Bailey FA, Williams BR, Goode PS, Woodby LL, Redden DT, Johnson TM 2nd, et al. Opioid pain medication orders and administration in the last days of life. J Pain Symptom Manage. 2012;44(5):681–691.

8. Lindqvist O, Lundquist G, Dickman A, Bükki J, Lunder U, Hagelin CL, et al. Four essential drugs needed for quality care of the dying: a Delphi-study based international expert consensus opinion. J Palliat Med. 2013;16(1):38–43.

9. Berwick, DM. The science of improvement. JAMA. 2008;299(10):1182–1184.

10. Berlinger N, Jennings B, Wold SM. Guidelines for Decisions on Life-Sustaining Treatment and Care Near the End of Life. New York: Oxford University Press; 2013.

11. Gade G, Venohr I, Conner D, et al. Impact of an inpatient palliative care team: a randomized controlled trial. J Palliat Med. 2008;11:180–190.

12. Smith AK, Thai JN, Bakitas MA, Meier DE, Spragens LH, Temel JS, et al. The diverse landscape of palliative care clinics. J Palliat Med. 2013;16(6):661–668. doi: 10.1089/jpm.2012.0469. Epub 2013 May 10.

13. Ajemian I, Mount B. The Royal Victoria Hospital Manual on Palliative/Hospice Care: A Resource Book. Montreal: Palliative Care Service: Royal Victoria Hospital; 1980.

14. Center to Advance Palliative Care. 2011. 2011 Public Opinion Research on Palliative Care: A Report Based on Research by Public Opinion Strategies. www.capc.org/tools-for-palliativecare-programs/marketing/public-opinion-research/2011-public-opinion-research-on-palliative-care.pdf. Accessed September 25, 2011.

15. Weissman DE, Meier DE. Center to Advance Palliative Care inpatient unit operational metrics: consensus recommendations. J Palliat Med. 2009;12(1):21–25. doi:10.1089/jpm.2008.0210.

16. American Hospital Association. Hospital Statistics. Chicago: Health Forum; 2012, 2013.

17. The National Consensus Project for Quality Palliative Care. 2013. Clinical Practice Guidelines for Quality Palliative Care, Third Edition. http://www.nationalconsensusproject.org.

18. World Health Organization. Cancer Pain Relief and Palliative Care. Geneva: World Health Organization; 1990.

19. Temel JS, Greer JA, Muzikansky A, et al. Early palliative care for patients with metastatic non–small-cell lung cancer. N Engl J Med. 2010;363(8):733–742.

20. Center to Advance Palliative Care, National Palliative Care Research Center. America's Care of Serious Illness: A State-by-State Report Card on Access to Palliative Care in Our Nation's Hospitals. New York: Center to Advance Palliative Care; 2008:34.

21. von Gunten C. Secondary and tertiary palliative care in US hospitals. JAMA. 2002;287:875–881.

22. O'Mahoney S, Blank AE, Zallman L, Selwyn P. The benefits of a hospital-based inpatient palliative care consultation service: preliminary outcome data. J Palliat Med. 2008;8:1033–1039.

23. Center to Advance Palliative Care, National Palliative Care Research Center. Building a Hospital Based Palliative Care Program. Retrieved from www.capc.org/building-a-hospital-based-palliative-care-program. Accessed July 21, 2013.

24. Lorenz KA, Lynn J, Dy SM, et al. Evidence for improving palliative care at the end of life: a systematic review. Ann Intern Med. 2008;148:147–159.

25. Teno JM. Palliative care teams: self-reflection—past, present, and future. J Pain Symptom Manage. 2002;23:94–95.

26. Hanks GW, Robbins M, Sharp D, et al. The imPaCT study: a randomised controlled trial to evaluate a hospital palliative care team. Br J Cancer. 2002;87:733–739.

27. Higginson I, Finlay I, Goodwin D, et al. Do hospital-based palliative teams improve care for patients or families at the end of life? J Pain Symptom Manage. 2001;23:96–106.

28. Dunlop RJ, Hockley JM. Terminal Care Support Teams. New York: Oxford University Press; 1990.

29. Dunlop RJ, Hockley JM. Hospital-Based Palliative Care Teams: The Hospital–Hospice Interface. Vol. 2. 2nd ed. New York: Oxford University Press; 1998.

30. Woitha K, Van Beek K, Ahmed N, Jaspers B, Mollard JM, Ahmedzai SH, et al. Validation of quality indicators for the organization of palliative care: a modified RAND Delphi study in seven European countries (the Europall project). Palliat Med. Epub 2013 July 16.

31. Claessen SJ, Francke AL, Belarbi HE, Pasman HR, van der Putten MJ, Deliens L. A new set of quality indicators for palliative care: process and results of the development trajectory. J Pain Symptom Manage. 2011;42(2):169–182.

32. Zimmermann C, Riechelmann R, Krzyzanowska M, Rodin GC, Tannock I. Effectiveness of specialized palliative care: a systematic review. JAMA. 2008;299:1698–1709.

33. Weissman DE, Meier DE, Spragens LH. Center to Advance Palliative Care palliative care consultation service metrics: consensus recommendations. J Palliat Med. 2008;11:1294–1298.

34. Smith TJ, Coyne P, Cassel B, Penberthy L, Hopson A, Hager MA. A high-volume specialist palliative care unit and team may reduce in-hospital end-of-life care costs. J Palliat Med. 203;6:699–705.

35. Bakitas M, Stevens M, Ahles T, et al. Project ENABLE: a palliative care demonstration project for advanced cancer patients in three settings. J Palliat Med. 2004;7:363–372.

36. Rabow M, Dibble S, Pantilat S, McPhee S. The comprehensive care team: a controlled trial of outpatient palliative medicine consultation. Arch Intern Med. 2004;164:83–91.

37. Byock I, Twohig JS, Merriman M, Collins K. Promoting excellence in end-of-life care: a report on innovative models of palliative care. J Palliat Med. 2006;9:137–151.

38. Follwell M, Burman D, Le LW, et al. Phase II Study of an outpatient palliative care intervention in patients with metastatic cancer. J Clin Oncol. 2009;27:206–213.

39. Rabow MW, Dibble SL, Pantilat SZ, McPhee SJ. The comprehensive care team: a controlled trial of outpatient palliative medicine consultation. Arch Intern Med. 2004;164:83–91.

40. Bakitas M, Lyons K, Hegel M, et al. The project ENABLE II randomized controlled trial to improve palliative care for rural patients with advanced cancer: baseline findings, methodological challenges, and solutions. Palliat Support Care 2009;7:75–86.

41. Wetle T, Shield R, Teno J, Miller SC, Welch L. Family perspectives on end-of-life care experiences in nursing homes. Gerontologist. 2005;45:642–650.

42. Shield RR, Wetle T, Teno J, Miller SC, Welch L. Physicians "missing in action": family perspectives on physician and staffing problems in end-of-life care in the nursing home. J Am Geriatr Soc. 2005;53:1651–1657.

43. Casarett D, Karlawish J, Morales K, Crowley R, Mirsch T, Asch DA. Improving the use of hospice services in nursing homes: a randomized controlled trial. JAMA. 2005;294(2):211–217.

44. Wetle T, Teno J, Shield R, Welch L, Miller SC. End of Life in Nursing Homes: Experiences and Policy Recommendations. Washington, DC: AARP Public Policy Institute; 2004.

45. Zerzan J, Stearns S, Hanson L. Access to palliative care and hospice care in nursing homes. JAMA. 2000;284:2489–2494.

46. Wright AA, Keating NL, Balboni TA, et al. Place of death: correlations with quality of life of patients with cancer and predictors of bereaved caregivers' mental health. J Clin Oncol. 2010;28:4457–4464.

47. Wright A, Zhang B, Ray A, et al. Associations between end-of-life discussions, patient mental health, medical care near death, and caregiver bereavement adjustment. JAMA. 2008;300:1665–1673.

48. National Quality Forum. A National Framework and Preferred Practices for Palliative and Hospice Care Quality: A Consensus Report. Washington, DC: National Quality Forum; 2006.

49. Elwert F, Christakis NA. The effect of widowhood on mortality by the causes of death of both spouses. Am J Public Health. 2008;98:2092–2099.

50. Eggly S, Meert KL, Berger J, Zimmerman J, Anand KJ, Newth CJ, et al. Physicians' conceptualization of "closure" as a benefit of physician-parent follow-up meetings after a child's death in the pediatric intensive care unit. Eunice Kennedy Shriver National Institute of Child Health and Human Development Collaborative; Pediatric Critical Care Research Network. J Palliat Care. 2013;29(2):69–75.

51. Ducharme F, Kergoat MJ, Antoine P, Pasquier F, Coulombe R. The unique experience of spouses in early-onset dementia. Am J Alzheimers Dis Other Demen. Epub 2013 July 2.

52. Eastman P, Le B, Pharaoh A. The establishment and initial outcomes of a palliative care bereavement service. Palliat Med. 2012;26(7):961–962.

53. Finlay E, Shreve S, Cassarett D. Nationwide veterans affairs quality measure for cancer: the family assessment of treatment at end of life. Am J Clin Oncol. 2008;26:3838–3844.

54. Teno J, Clarridge BR, Casey VA, et al. Family perspectives on end-of-life care at the last place of care. JAMA. 2004;291:88–93.

55. Tang ST, McCorkle R. Use of family proxies in quality of life research for cancer patients at the end of life: a literature review. Cancer Invest. 2002;20:1086–1104.

56. Press Ganey Associates. Patient/Family Satisfaction with End-of-Life Care Survey. Available at: http://www.pressganey.com. Accessed January 1, 2009.

57. Macdonald M, Liben S, Carnevale F, et al. Parental perspectives on hospital staff-members' acts of kindness and commemoration after a child's death. Pediatrics. 2005;116:884–890.

58. Ferris TGG, Hallward JA, Ronan L, Billings JA. When the patient dies: a survey of medical housestaff about care after death. J Palliat Med. 1998;1:231–239.

59. Shively P, Midland D, eds. The Art of Compassionate Death Notification. La Crosse, WI: Gundersen Lutheran Medical Foundation; 1999.

60. Ferrell BR, Grant M, Virani R. Strengthening nursing education to improve end-of-life care. Nurs Outlook. 1999;47:252–256.

61. Carron AT, Lynn J, Keaney P. End-of-life care in medical textbooks. Ann Intern Med. 1999;130:82–86.

62. Ferrell BR, Virani R, Grant M. Analysis of end-of-life content in nursing textbooks. Oncol Nurs Forum. 1999;26:869–876.

63. Ellison, NM, Radecke MW. An undergraduate course on palliative medicine and end-of-life issues. J Palliat Med. 2005;8(2):354–361.

64. Center to Advance Palliative Care. Palliative Care Leadership Centers. Available at www.capc.org. Accessed August 21, 2013.

65. Weissman DE, Meier DE. Operational features for hospital palliative care programs: consensus recommendations. J Palliat Med. 2008;11:1189–1194.

66. The Joint Commission. 2008. Comprehensive Accreditation Manual for Hospitals: The Official Handbook (CAMH). Available at http://www.jointcommission.org. Accessed March 17, 2008.

67. The Joint Commission. 2013. Certification for Palliative Care Programs. Available at www.jointcommission.org/CertificationPrograms/Pallative_Care. Accessed June 22, 2013.

68. Hume M. Improving care at the end-of-life. Qual Lett Healthc Lead. 1998;10(10):2–10.

69. Abrahm JL, Callahan J, Rossetti K, Pierre L. The impact of a hospice consultation team on the care of veterans with advanced cancer. J Pain Symptom Manage. 1996;12:23–31.

70. Creating and expanding hospice and palliative care programs in VA, 2002. Available at http://www.va.gov/geriatrics/guide/longtermcare/Hospice_and_Palliative_Care.asp. Accessed August 21, 2013.

71. Casarett D, Pickard A, Bailey FA, et al. Do palliative consultations improve patient outcomes? J Am Geriatr Soc. 2008;56:593–599.

72. Edes T, Shreve S, Cassarett D. Increasing access and quality in Department of Veterans Affairs Care at the end of life: a lesson in change. J Am Geriatr Soc. 2007;55:1645–1649.

73. Grant M, Hanson J, Mullan P, Spolum M, Ferrell B. Disseminating end-of-life education to cancer centers: overview of program and of evaluation. J Cancer Educ. 2007;22:140–148.

74. Epstein R, Street R Jr. Patient-Centered Communication in Cancer Care: Promoting Healing and Reducing Suffering. Bethesda, MD: National Cancer Institute; 2007. NIH Publication No. 07-6225.

75. World Health Organization. 2003. Palliative Care: What Is It? Available at www.who.org. Accessed November 24, 2009.

76. Byock I. Completing the continuum of cancer care: integrating life-prolongation and palliation. CA Cancer J Clin. 2000;50:123–132.

77. Schwartz CE, Wheeler HB, Hammes B, et al. Early intervention in planning end-of-life care with ambulatory geriatric patients: results of a pilot trial. Arch Intern Med. 2002;162:1611–1618.

78. Von Gunten C, Ferris F, Emanuel L. Ensuring competency in end-of-life care: communication and relational skills. JAMA. 2000;284:3051–3057.

79. End of Life/Palliative Education Resource Center. 2008. Fast Fact and Concept #016: Conducting a Family Conference 2nd Edition. Available at http://www.eperc.mcw.edu/fastFact/ff_016.htm. Accessed December 1, 2008.

80. Du Pen S, Du Pen AR, Polissar N, et al. Implementing guidelines for cancer pain management: results of a randomized controlled clinical trial. Am J Clin Oncol. 1999;17:361–370.

81. Stair J. Oncology critical pathways: palliative care: a model example from the Moses Cone Health system. Oncology. 1998;14(2):26–30.

82. Berwick DM. Controlling variation in health care: a consultation from Walter Shewhart. Med Care. 1991;29:1212–1225.

83. Meisel A. The Right to Die. New York: Wiley; 1995, 1998.

84. Teno J, Lynn J, Wenger N, et al. Advance directives for seriously ill hospitalized patients: effectiveness with the patient self-determination act and the SUPPORT intervention. J Am Geriatr Soc. 1997;45:500–507.

85. Sulmasy DP, Terry PB, Weisman CS, et al. The accuracy of substituted judgments in patients with terminal diagnosis. Ann Intern Med. 1998;128:621–629.

86. Institute of Medicine. Cancer Care for the Whole Patient: Meeting Psychosocial Health Needs. Washington, DC: National Academies Press; 2007.

87. Twaddle M, Maxwell T, Cassel J, et al. Palliative care benchmarks from academic medical centers. J Palliat Med. 2007;10:86–98.

88. Dartmouth Institute for Health Policy and Clinical Practice. Tracking Improvement in the Care of Chronically Ill Patients: The Dartmouth Atlas Brief on Medicare Beneficiaries Near the End of Life. Lebanon, NH: Dartmouth Institute for Health Policy and Clinical Practice; 2013.

89. Morrison RS, Penrod JD, Cassel JB, et al. Cost savings associated with US hospital palliative care consultation programs. Arch Intern Med. 2008;168:1783–1790.

90. The Robert Wood Johnson Foundation. 2004. Accounting for the Costs of Caring Through the End of Life: Cost Accounting Peer Workgroup Recommendations to the Field.

91. Solomon M, Romer A, Sellers D. Meeting the Challenge: Improving End-of-Life Care in Managed Care: Access, Accountability, and Cost. Newton, MA: Robert Wood Johnson; 1999.

92. Engelhardt J, McClive-Reed K, Toseland R, Smith TL, Larson DG, Tobin D. Effects of a program for coordinated care of advanced illness on patients, surrogates, and healthcare costs: a randomized trial. Am J Manag Care. 2006;12:93–100.

93. Zhang B, Wright AA, Huskamp HA, et al. Health care costs in the last week of life: associations with end-of-life conversations. Arch Intern Med. 2009;169:480–488.

94. Sweeney L, Halpert A, Waranoff J. Patient-centered management of complex patients can reduce costs without shortening life. Am J Manag Care. 2007;13:84–92.

95. Hughes SL, Cummings J, Weaver F, Manheim L, Braun B, Conrad K. A randomized trial of the cost effectiveness of VA hospital-based home care for the terminally ill. Health Serv Res. 1992;26:801–817.

96. Meier DE, Beresford L. Palliative care professionals contribute to state legislative and policy initiatives. J Palliat Med. 2008;11:1070–1073.

CHAPTER 4

Principles of patient and family assessment

John D. Chovan, Douglas Cluxton, and
Patrice Rancour

> To get to my body, my doctor has to get to my character. He has to go through my soul …
> I'd like my doctor to scan me, to grope for my spirit as well as my prostate. Without such
> recognition, I am nothing but my illness.
>
> Anatole Broyard[1(pp. 40,45)]

Key points

- Comprehensive assessment of the patient and family is essential to planning and implementing palliative nursing care.

- Assessment involves input from the patient, family, and all members of the transdisciplinary team with information shared verbally as well as in the patient's electronic health record.

- Ongoing, detailed, and comprehensive assessment is needed to identify the complex and changing needs and goals of patients facing chronic or life-threatening illness and of their families.

An effective assessment is crucial to establishing an appropriate nursing care plan for the patient and family. The palliative care nursing assessment may vary little from a standard nursing assessment.[2,3] To assess effectively, nurses working at the generalist level and at the advanced level of practice and other members of the transdisciplinary healthcare team must maximize their listening skills and minimize quick judgments. Clinicians must actively explore both their initial hunches and alternative hypotheses to minimize premature closure.[4] Nurses use the therapeutic use of self to engage patients and families during the assessment, including the tools of active listening and the appropriate use of silence.

The goals of the palliative care plan that evolve from the initial and ongoing nursing assessments focus on maximizing quality of life. Ferrell's quality-of-life framework[5] is used to organize the assessment. The four quality-of-life domains in this framework are physical, psychological, social, and spiritual well-being. For the purpose of this chapter, the psychological and social domains are combined into one: the psychosocial domain.

Because the needs of patients and families may change throughout the course of a chronic or life-threatening illness, these quality-of-life assessments are examined here at four critical stages along the illness trajectory: (1) at the time of diagnosis; (2) during treatment, that is, initial treatments and subsequent planned or unplanned treatments; (3) after treatment, that is, when the planned course of treatment is completed or when the patient's goals shift away from treatment; and (4) during active dying.

Effective palliative care assessments are predicated on nurses understanding their thoughts, values, emotions, convictions, and experience with respect to issues commonly arising in palliative nursing care. Eckroth-Bucher reported that "creating an interpersonal environment that heals is possible only if the nurse uses self-awareness skills as a guide in the communication process."[6(p. 308)] Self-awareness has been demonstrated not only to improve quality of care, but also to decrease stress on the part of nurses' patients and patients' families.[7] Box 4.1 comprises some of the issues that palliative care nurses might explore about themselves to enable their effective assessments.

Chronic and life-threatening illnesses

The experiences of seriously ill patients are dynamic in terms of the continuous or episodic declines they face throughout the illness trajectory. These experiences are associated with the trajectory that is characteristic for the particular illness. For example, persons living with dementia experience a slow, gradual decline, frequently at home or in a memory unit of a long-term care facility. Persons living with chronic obstructive pulmonary disease (COPD), on the other hand, experience a gradual decline punctuated by exacerbations requiring hospitalization and treatment, oscillating between a quasi-steady-state of relatively stable symptoms and acute episodes of severe symptomatology. Also, persons with a cancer diagnosis may experience a cure and then be cancer-free for the rest of their lives, or they may experience a recurrence of their disease. Every illness has its distinctive trajectory, but every person's journey along that trajectory is unique.

The focus of care for palliative care patients is an ever-shifting balance between cure and palliation. At diagnosis, the focus is likely to

Box 4.1 Questions for self-awareness prior to palliative nursing assessments

What do I believe about ...?

◆ quality of life

◆ suffering

◆ patient autonomy

◆ pain and treating pain

◆ death and dying

◆ advance directives

◆ code status

◆ organ donation

◆ funerals / burial / cremation

◆ cultures other than my own

◆ the use of:

  ✓ CPR

  ✓ life support / ventilators / tracheostomies

  ✓ artificial nutrition at end of life / feeding tubes (NG, OG, PEG)

  ✓ artificial hydration at end of life

  ✓ drugs that could hasten death

Could I authentically discuss ...?

◆ quality of life

◆ suffering

◆ patient autonomy

◆ pain and treating pain

◆ death and dying

◆ advance directives

◆ code status

◆ organ donation

◆ funerals / burial / cremation

◆ cultures other than my own

◆ the use of:

  ✓ CPR

  ✓ life support / ventilators / tracheostomies

  ✓ artificial nutrition at end of life / feeding tubes (NG, OG, PEG)

  ✓ artificial hydration at end of life

  ✓ drugs that could hasten death

Would I feel comfortable ...?

◆ including my last name when introducing myself to patients and families

◆ asking family members to leave the room if necessary

◆ asking others in the room to let the patient answer my questions without their help

◆ asking questions that are controversial

◆ asking questions that are personal

◆ talking with families of dying or dead patients

◆ touching patients who are dying or dead

be more curative, focusing on minimizing the impact of the disease process on the person, while managing symptoms and optimizing quality of life are secondary foci. But over time, as the illness progresses and the patient declines, the focus shifts and becomes increasingly more palliative, that is, reduction of symptoms and maximizing quality of life become the primary foci, while attempts to impact on the disease process are purely for the sake of comfort. Examples of these kinds of illnesses today include HIV/AIDS; cardiovascular, respiratory, gastrointestinal, hepatic, and renal diseases; diabetes; neurological disorders such as multiple sclerosis, cerebral palsy, amyotrophic lateral sclerosis, Parkinson's disease, and dementia; multiple types of cancer; and sickle cell disease. For some of these illnesses, the focus of medical care may include attempting to extend life through research with the hope of finding a cure.

Noncancer illness accounted for nearly two-thirds (62.3%) of the admissions to hospice in 2011 as reported by the National Hospice and Palliative Care Organization,[8] the distribution of which is listed here:

Persons diagnosed with a chronic or life-threatening illness may repeatedly alter their expectations about the future. Words describing the status of the disease during a cancer illness, for example, include "no evidence of disease," "remission," "partial remission," "stable disease," "recurrence," "relapse," and "metastasis." Noncancer illnesses such as heart failure (HF) and COPD are described by words such as "exacerbation" and "recovery." Patients

Debility unspecified	13.9%
Dementia	12.5%
Heart disease	11.4%
Lung disease	8.5%
Other*	15.9%

*Other included stroke, coma, kidney disease, liver disease, ALS and non-ALS motor neuron disease, and HIV/AIDS.

report experiencing a "roller-coaster ride" in which the hopeful points in better health are often followed by crises with relapse or disease progression. Patients may be told, more than once, that they are likely to die within a short period of time, only to recover and do well for a period of time. As a result, the finality of death may be more difficult when it does occur because up to this point in the patient's trajectory, the disease has always responded to treatment.

Case study

Tarana: background information

Tarana, is a 76-year-old widowed, female patient of Asian Indian descent. She was raised Muslim, but is not completely adherent to her faith. She has been living with heart failure for the last 10 years, which is likely related to her diagnosis at age 40 years of HIV/AIDS and to her therapy with antiretrovirals. Her husband infected her and then took his own life 5 years after diagnosis, leaving Tarana alone with no income and with wavering faith. After being widowed, she raised her twin sons, who are now 40 years old, while living with the family of her less-than-religious younger sister, Krupa, including Krupa's now-32-year-old daughter, Marala.

Patient and family assessment

Introduction to physical assessment

Nurses understand that quality of life is based in part on the severity and impact of physical symptoms. Physical assessment not only provides a baseline of symptoms at one point in time, but also monitors their changes, the emergence of new symptoms, the effectiveness of their treatments, and changes in how they impact on the patient's quality of life. Physical assessment can uncover symptomatology in the psychosocial and spiritual domains as nurses use the therapeutic use of self when assessing and caring for patients and their families.

Physical assessment focuses primarily on organ systems and symptoms related to their functioning. Historical information can come from the electronic health record (EHR) to understand documented details from previous assessments done by others on the transdisciplinary care team, including diagnostic lab results and imaging. Subjective information is collected by talking to the patient and developing a picture of how they view their health and health status. During the interview, the nurse reviews each organ system with the patient to collect data on symptoms. The nurse develops objective information by doing a physical examination. Observing a patient's facial expressions, the nurse may notice nonverbal signs of pain. Auscultating heart sounds can shape an understanding of circulation changes and, thus, ischemic pain. The abdomen can deliver information about bloating and constipation through auscultation and palpation. Percussing the lungs can provide data about respiratory status and, thus, dyspnea.

Physical assessment also includes a determination of functional status. Various scales have been shown to be predictive of survival in specific classes of palliative patients based on an assessment of their functional status. For example, the Palliative Performance Scale (PPS) allows the nurse to assign a number on a 10-point scale (0%–100% in increments of 10%) of functional status based on five observed parameters: ambulation, activity and evidence of disease, self-care, intake, and level of consciousness.[9]

Introduction to psychosocial assessment

Persons diagnosed with a chronic or life-threatening illness experience many losses. Responses to illness, however, vary tremendously among individual patients and family members. In addition, the same person may respond differently at various times during an illness. How a particular patient copes depends on the severity of the illness, the patient's history of coping with stressful life events, and available supports. Some individuals develop coping styles that are more helpful than others when facing a life-threatening illness.

Box 4.1 and Tables 4.1 and 4.2 provide a framework for three key elements of psychosocial assessment: (1) conducting the psychosocial assessment, (2) distinguishing nonpathological grief from depression, and (3) doing a general mental status assessment. Throughout the illness trajectory, nurses use these tools to monitor patient response to illness and treatment.

Nurses assess two very important parameters to assist patients and families to cope in the most functional way possible. These

Table 4.1 Framework for Psychosocial Assessment

Determining the types of losses:

Physical losses	Psychosocial losses	Spiritual losses
Energy	Autonomy	Illusion of predictability/ certainty
Mobility	Sense of mastery	
Body parts	Body image alterations	Illusion of immortality
Body function	Sexuality	Illusion of control
Pain	Relationship changes	Hope for the future
Sexuality	Lifestyle	Time
	Work changes	
	Role function	
	Money	
	Time	

Determining the types of responses to loss:

Observing emotional responses	Identifying coping styles
Anxiety	*Functional:*
Anger	Normal grief work
Denial	Problem-solving
Withdrawal	Humor
Shock	Practicing spiritual rituals
Sadness	*Dysfunctional:*
Bargaining	Aggression
Depression	Fantasy
Acceptance	Minimization
	Addictive behaviors
	Guilt
	Psychosis

Determining personal needs:

Assessing the need for information	Assessing the need for control
Wants to know details	Very high
Wants the overall picture	High
	Moderate/average
Wants minimal information	Low
Wants no information, but wants the family to know	Absent, wants others to decide

Table 4.2 Differentiating normal grief from depression

Parameter	Normal grief	Depression
Course	Self-limiting but recurrent with each additional loss	Frequently not self-limited
Preoccupation	Preoccupied with loss	Self-preoccupied, rumination
Emotions	Emotional states variable	Consistent dysphoria or anhedonia (absence of pleasure)
Sleep	Episodic difficulties sleeping	Insomnia or hypersomnia
Energy	Lack of energy, slight weight loss	Extreme lethargy, weight loss
Losses	Identifies loss	May not identify loss or may deny it
Crying	Crying is evident and provides some relief	Crying absent or persists uncontrollably
Social interaction	Socially responsive to others	Socially unresponsive, isolated
Dreams	Dreams may be vivid	No memory of dreaming
Anger	Open expression of anger	No expression of anger
Intervention	Adaptation does not require professional intervention	Adaptation requires professional treatment

parameters are (1) the need for information and (2) the need for control in making decisions. Observers of exceptional patients—persons who have thrived in spite of their prognosis—have noted that patients who are proactive and assertive information seekers often appear to experience better outcomes than patients who are passive in making decisions.[10] Indicators of a person's need for control may include:

♦ An expressed need for information.

♦ Comfort in asking questions.

♦ A willingness to assert their own needs and wishes relative to the plan of care.

♦ Initiative taken to research print and Internet resources on the illness and treatment.

Table 4.1 provides details for doing a psychosocial assessment. More detailed information on the psychosocial aspects of cancer patients can be found in Holland's *Psycho-Oncology*.[11]

Some patients with advanced disease have been able to integrate their losses in a meaningful way, managing to reconcile and transcend them. An example of such a person is Randy Pausch, a late computer science professor at MIT who reported in his *Last Lecture*[12] on making meaning of living with a terminal diagnosis of cancer. And, of course, while all this is going on with the patient, family members are also going through a myriad of their own responses, which often are at different rates and intensities within the same family unit. Randy Pausch's wife Jai Pausch recounts her journey in *Dream New Dreams*.[13] Refer to chapter 30 of this text, "Supporting Families in Palliative Care."

Grief is a normal reaction to loss, especially a major loss such as one's health. Nurses understand that although persons may be experiencing normal grief, ineffective adaptations or coping can indeed lead to depression.[14] Criteria for depression the *Diagnostic and Statistical Manual of Mental Disorders*, fifth edition (DSM-5),[15] include grieving the loss of a loved one, but only if other criteria for depression are met. In chronic illness, grief is also likely to be recurrent as losses accumulate. This does not make it pathological, but it does form the basis of the roller-coaster phenomenon that many patients describe, which can lead to a more pathological depression.[16,17] Table 4.2 compares normal grief with depression.

In some cases, patients may appear to be having difficulties in coping but the nurse cannot easily identify the specific problem. The nurse may need to make a more thorough mental health screening assessment to determine the most appropriate referral.[18] Key elements in such an assessment are found in Table 4.3. In such instances, a referral to a behavioral health professional may also be warranted. Additional information and tools used to assess for

Table 4.3 General mental health assessment

Appearance	Psychomotor behavior
Hygiene	Gait
Grooming, makeup	Observable symptoms (tics, tremors, perseveration, pilling)
Manner of dress (appropriate, inappropriate)	Movement (akathisias, dyskinesias)
Posture	Coordination
Body language	Compulsions
Mood and affect (congruence)	Energy
Interview behavior	
Specific feelings expressed	**Speech**
Facial expressions	Pressured, slow, rapid
	Goal-oriented, rambling, incoherent, fragmented, coherent
Intellectual ability	Relevant, irrelevant
Attention (distractibility)	Poverty of speech
Concentration	Presence of latencies (delayed ability to respond when conversing)
Concrete/abstract thinking	
Comprehension	
Insight into situation, illness	**Thought patterns**
Judgment	Loose, perseverating
Educational level	Logical, illogical, confused
	Oriented, disoriented
	Poorly organized, well organized
Sensorium/level of consciousness	Tangential, circumstantial
Alert	Preoccupied, obsessed
Drowsy	Paranoid ideas of reference
Somnolent	Delusions
Obtunded	Hallucinations
Stuporous	Blocking, flight of ideas
Unresponsive	Neologisms (made-up words)
	Word salad (meaningless word order)
	Presence of suicidal or homicidal ideation, plan, access to means

emotional distress can be found in chapter 48, "Palliative Care Nursing in the Outpatient Setting."

Introduction to Spiritual Assessment

Although chapter 32, "Spiritual Assessment," provides additional information on collecting information on the spiritual domain, the following discussion illustrates the importance of including the spiritual domain as a component of a comprehensive nursing assessment.

Attempts to define spirituality can often result in feelings of dismay and inadequacy. It is like trying to capture the wind or grasp water. Assessing and addressing the spiritual needs of patients, therefore, can be a formidable challenge. Spirituality may include one's religious identity, beliefs, and practices, but it involves much more. The person without an identified religious affiliation is no less spiritual. Indeed, the desire to speak one's truth, to explore the meaning of one's life and illness, and to maintain hope are all fundamental human quests that reflect the depth of the spirit. Various definitions of spirituality have appeared in the literature over several years. But spirituality is defined by consensus in the palliative care community as "the aspect of humanity that refers to the way individuals seek and express meaning and purpose and the way they experience their connectedness to the moment, to self, to others, to nature, and to the significant or sacred."[19(p. 887)]

The spiritual issues that arise at the time of diagnosis of a serious or life-threatening illness are abundant and varied. As a person progresses through the phases of an illness, he or she is confronted with mortality, limitations, and loss. This frequently leads to questions such as "What is my life's purpose?", "What does all this mean?", "What is the point of my suffering?", "Why me?", and "Is there life after death?" Indeed, Viktor Frankl, in his classic work *Man's Search for Meaning*,[20] affirmed that the quest to find meaning is one of the most characteristically human endeavors. To find meaning in suffering enhances the human spirit and fosters survival.

According to Abraham Maslow's theory,[21] human needs can be placed on a hierarchy that prioritizes them from the most basic physical and survival needs to the more transcendent needs. Thus, a patient's ability and willingness to engage in dialogue about issues of meaning, to discuss successes and regrets, and to express his or her core values may occur only after more fundamental needs are addressed. This reality in no way diminishes the spiritual compared with the physical; rather, it supports the need for a transdisciplinary approach that provides holistic care of the entire person. For example, if a nurse practitioner relieves a young woman's cancer pain and a social worker secures transportation for her to treatments, the patient and her family may be more able to address the vital concerns of her soul. Religious or spiritual advisor consultation may be indicated.

Responding to the spiritual needs of patients and families is not solely the domain of the chaplain, clergy, or other officially designated professionals. All members of the healthcare team share the responsibility of identifying and being sensitive to spiritual concerns. The sensitivity of the nurse to a patient's spiritual concerns improves the quality of palliative care throughout the illness trajectory. When members of the transdisciplinary healthcare team serve as companions to a patient and family during their journey with an illness, they offer vital and life-affirming care.

A patient must not be viewed in isolation, but rather in the context of those who are affected by the illness. The focus of spiritual assessment, therefore, includes not only the patient, but members of the patient's family—however the patient defines his or her family—including people not related to the patient by blood, marriage, or adoption, such as friends, neighbors, their faith community, and unmarried partners. This perspective affirms the power of a systems view, the view that places the patient at the center of care while still being integral to the interdependent and connected family. Spiritual support to family members not only assists them directly but also may contribute to patient comfort secondarily: Comfort may increase as the patient sees his or her loved ones being cared for as well.

The purpose of a spiritual assessment is to increase the healthcare team's knowledge of the patient's and family's sources of strength and areas of concern to prepare for planning quality care that maximizes patient and family quality of life. The methods of assessment include direct questioning, acquiring inferred information, and observing. As with the physical and psychosocial domains, this is most effectively accomplished when a basis of trust has been established. The transdisciplinary team best serves patients' and families' needs when they determine whether the patient is experiencing spiritual distress and desires specialized spiritual care. Patients tend to fall into one of three groups: (1) those who may be experiencing spiritual struggle but are unlikely to request a chaplain's visit; (2) those who would like a visit from a chaplain but may or may not request one and would be dissatisfied if they did not receive one; and (3) those for whom religion and spirituality is not important and who would not want a visit from a chaplain.[22]

The nurse's role historically includes being able to support the patient's spiritual life and concerns. A body of knowledge and cultural practices prescribe and confer the specific role—such as minister, priest, rabbi, or other religious figure—with certain privileges to function as a companion to those patients who are addressing religious and spiritual concerns. Linking the patient with these professionals based on a sensitive screening of needs will enhance the patient's healing and integrative process. The *Religious Struggle Screening Protocol*[22] is a tool to discern among these groups of patients and to respond more effectively to their needs and preferences. It begins with the simple question, "Is religion or spirituality important to you?" There follows an algorithm based on patient responses that leads to specific action steps. Box 4.2 is a summary of the kinds of questions useful for the nurse to ask as part of a spiritual screening.

One of the fundamental principles underlying spiritual assessment (and spiritual care) is the commitment to the value of telling one's story.[23] Alcoholics' Anonymous,[24] a very successful program with spiritual tenets, acknowledges the power of story. This might be paraphrased as follows: in the hearing is the learning, but in the telling is the healing. Park[25] presents the concept of a person's global meaning, their internal mechanism of making sense of the world.

Box 4.2   Spiritual screening questions

- Is religion or spirituality important to you?
- If so, does your religion or spirituality give you comfort?
- If not, has there ever been a time when spirituality or religion was important to you?
- Would you like a visit from a chaplain?

Simple, open-ended questions such as "How is this illness affecting you?" and "How is the illness affecting the way you relate to the world?" provide the opportunity for validation of the patient's global meaning and placing her or his response to the illness within it.

Cultural competence

The Joint Commission (TJC) defines cultural competence as "the ability of health care providers and health care organizations to understand and respond effectively to the cultural and language needs brought by the patient to the health care encounter."[26(p. 1)] Expecting that healthcare professionals will know all of the customs, beliefs, and practices of patients from every culture is unrealistic, of course. All providers, however, should strive for some degree of cultural competence. Reference sources are useful to nurses and other members of the transdisciplinary team in gaining cultural competence.[27]

Nurses and other members of the transdisciplinary healthcare team assess in culturally competent ways when they:

◆ Are aware of one's own ethnicity, biases, and ethnocentrism, the unconscious tendency to assume that one's own worldview is everyone's worldview or is somehow superior.

◆ Convey respect.

◆ Solicit the patient and family as teachers and guides regarding cultural practices.

◆ Ask about the patient's personal preferences, such as food, spiritual beliefs, family relationships, music, communication preferences, and interpersonal customs.

◆ Avoid expectations for any individual to represent his or her whole culture.

◆ Assess the patient's and family's beliefs about illness and treatments.

◆ Respect cultural differences regarding personal space and touch: "Whom do I ask for permission to examine you?" and "May I touch you here?"

◆ Determine needs and desires regarding health-related information: "When I have information to tell you, how much detail do you want to know and to whom do I give it?"

◆ Note and affirm the use of complementary and integrative healthcare practices: "Do you ever consult a healer or a person who provides medicines to persons in your community?"

◆ Are sensitive to the need for interpreter services[28] (Box 4.3) and engage professional interpreters, not relying on family members to interpret.[29]

Box 4.3 Meeting the need for interpreter services

Overview

◆ Medical interpretation can occur with an onsite face-to-face translator, a telephone-based interpreter, or a video-based interpreter over the Internet.

◆ Skills of a medical interpreter are not just the ability to interpret quickly and exactly between two languages, but also the ability to provide a cultural interpretation and context.

◆ A child or family member should not be used as an interpreter for major explanations or decision-making about healthcare. Even adult children may feel uncomfortable speaking with their parents or grandparents about intimate topics. Furthermore, many lay people do not know or understand medical terms in their own language. Informed consent requires that the patient receive accurate information that he or she can understand, before making a healthcare decision.

◆ Use the services of a certified medical interpreter, if possible. See the websites for the International Medical Interpreters Association (http://www.imiaweb.org/) and the National Board of Certification for Medical Interpreters (http://www.certifiedmedicalinterpreters.org/) for more information.

When working with an interpreter in healthcare

◆ Speak directly to the patient, not the interpreter.

◆ Use simple language and ask open-ended questions. Be patient for the answers.

◆ Observe nonverbal communication and inquire of the patient what these might mean.

◆ Ask that any educational information be repeated back to you from the patient.

Services

◆ Several telephone-based interpretation services are available. AT&T and Language Line provides translation services by subscription or on a pay-as-you-go basis (http://www.languageline.com). The partnership is also making interpretation services more accessible via smartphones and has a new video-based interpreting service for ASL, Spanish, Cantonese, Mandarin, and Vietnamese.

◆ RTT Mobile and Sprint have partnered to provide a device for use by emergency responders and hospitals to communicate with persons with limited English proficiency. Called ELSA, the device immediately connects the service provider with an interpreter in the requested language over the Sprint network, enabling instant communication (http://www.rttmobile.com/PR/pr_sprint.html).

◆ Many online, video-based interpretation services are available. Language Access Network (http://www.lan.com) provides a service called MARTI (My Accessible Real-Time Trusted Interpreter). It is HIPPA compliant and available 24/7, 365 days a year by subscription.

Review of the Electronic Health Record

Before meeting a patient or family member, the nurse prepares for the face-to-face encounter. This is done by reviewing the patient's EHR and developing an understanding of the nature of the patient's journey thus far: the initial nursing database. With the advent of the EHR and its emergence in hospitals, clinics, and primary care offices, access to up-to-the-minute patient data supports thorough preparation prior to making face-to-face contact with patients and their families. Also, palliative care patients are often very ill and do not have the energy or patience for, or interest in, answering myriad questions—especially if the questions do not relate to their immediate needs. The nurse conducts individualized assessments based on prioritized symptoms for each patient, therefore, based on the initial review of the EHR.

Beginning the database prior to the initial face-to-face encounter will assist the nurse to focus assessments and increase the effectiveness of the time spent with patients and their families. Frequently, for patients in hospitals and other facilities, the nurse will print portions of the EHR, particularly the face sheet and the most recent history and physical examination, and write on them while building the nursing database from the EHR and also during the face-to-face assessment interview. Electronic tools are under development to minimize reliance on paper, but are not widely available.

Although the three domains are discussed separately in this chapter, the nurse understands that holistic, transdisciplinary care of patients and their families often leads to interweaving of the domains during not only the review of the EHR but also face-to-face assessment encounters.

The nursing review of the EHR should reflect an understanding of the following:

- *Demographic Information*: Note the patient's name and identification number, age, date of birth, gender, ethnicity, primary language, and occupation. The patient's address and phone number may become important for discharge planning and if advance directives (see below) must be completed. Among the demographic information to collect are the names and contact information of any other service providers who have participated in the patient's journey, such as healthcare professionals, home health agencies, and clergy. If in an in-patient context, also note the room number and bed number of the patient.

- *Referral Information*: Note whether the patient was referred for palliative services from another healthcare provider and, if so, the date of the referral and the reason given by the referrer for the consult.

- *Next of Kin and Contact Information*: Note any familial relationships, such as spouse, partner, significant other, children (adults and minors), parents, and anyone else documented in the record. The nurse may want to document these relationships in a genogram (see Figure 4.1) to facilitate sharing of sometimes complex family structures. Some of this information may be documented in the EHR by other contributors of the transdisciplinary team, such as Social Work, Case Management, and Pastoral Care. Although the Health Insurance Portability and Accountability Act of 1996 (HIPAA) requires protection of personal health information, some patients' identities and whereabouts are subject to an extra level of security, such as prisoners, abused persons, and VIPs. This is noted in the nurse's database.

Finally, if two patients on the census have similar names, such as Lucy Walls and Lucia Wells, the nurse notes it.

- *Primary Point of Contact*: Identifying one point of contact for the patient and the associated phone number will facilitate communication between the palliative care team and the family. This person—frequently a spouse, parent, nearest living relative, or eldest child—will often be the designated person for making the healthcare decisions that they know the patient would have made for him or herself. This surrogate decision-maker will often be documented in the EHR as the "Healthcare Power of Attorney," "HCPOA," or "POA" (or sometimes "DPOA" for durable power of attorney). Should a person become unable to speak for themselves without having a designated surrogate to speak for them, most state laws designate a hierarchy of persons who are called on to speak for the patient, such as a court appointed guardian, then a legal spouse, followed by adult children (sometimes as a group), siblings, other family members, and then other interested nonrelated parties. Distinguishing between the person who holds legal authority (power of attorney) for fiscal decision-making and the person who holds legal authority (power of attorney) for healthcare decision-making is important. If it is the same person or if the distinction is not obvious, the nurse clarifies during the interview.

- *Religious Affiliation*: Note the patient's stated religious affiliation and clergy, if indicated. Refer to the spiritual assessment information in this chapter for detailed information.

- *Advance Directives and Code Status*: The Patient Self-Determination Act of 1990 requires all inpatient facilities to ask patients on admission if they have advance directives and, if so, to request a copy of them. Laws regarding advance directives and orders for code status are specific to each state, so the nurse must be familiar with the local laws for advance directives and orders for code status. A national movement to provide a way for the wishes of a patient to be explicitly stated in a single order from a healthcare provider, the POLST (Physician Orders for Life-Sustaining Treatment) Paradigm,[30] is being implemented in various states and municipalities across the country. The presence or absence of advance directives and orders for life-sustaining treatment must be noted. The nurse reviews the documents and notes the patient's wishes as stated in them. If the documents are missing or incomplete, note that the missing data may be acquired during the assessment interview or referred to the resource persons (social worker or chaplain, for example) so designated at the nurse's institution. Also, note if the EHR indicates whether the patient is a registered organ donor.

- *Insurance Coverage*: Patient care within the context of the US healthcare system is often delimited by the patient's resources. For example, Medicaid may have a restricted medication formulary. If the patient does not have adequate insurance coverage, consider a Social Work consult to help the patient access the necessary resources to obtain financial assistance.

- *Recent Health Trajectory*: Nurses may tap several sources of information in the EHR to develop an understanding of the patient's recent health trajectory and current health status. The most recent history and physical examination document (H&P) will describe the patient's diagnosis, history of the present illness, past medical and surgical history, and family and social history, all of which are pertinent to the provision of quality palliative care. It will also serve as a subjective and objective

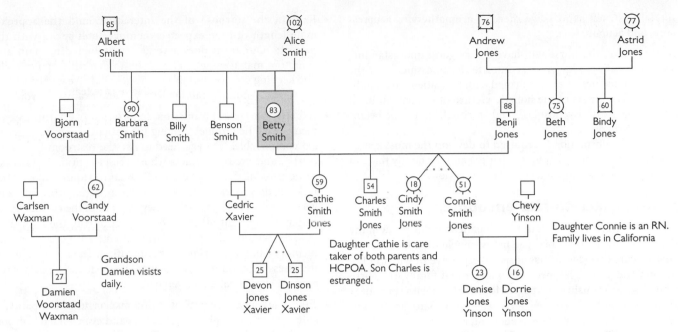

Figure 4.1 An example genogram. Most assessment genograms will be handwritten. Source: Illustration courtesy of John D. Chovan.

snapshot of the physiological state of the patient by organ system at the time the H&P was created as well as a summative impression of the health status of the patient at that time: the subjective review of systems, the functional assessment, and the objective physical examination. The functional assessment is particularly good at helping people not familiar with healthcare jargon to understand the changes in the patient across the illness trajectory, and is typically reflected in the PPS score. The initial findings and plan of medical care are also included. The nurse continues to develop the picture of the patient's current state by reviewing the consultation notes by the other involved services and the recent progress notes, including other medical services and ancillary services, such as case management, dietary, respiratory therapy, physical and occupational therapy, and speech therapy. Note also the use and whereabouts of hearing aids, eyeglasses, and dentures, and the placement of ports, central lines, pacemakers, defibrillators, and implants.

- *Medications*: Review the patient's drug allergies and medications as listed in the EHR (home use and inpatient use), including over-the-counter and herbal preparations. Note if any newly ordered medications relate to the patient's comfort. Make note of medications that are or are not present for key symptoms including pain, dyspnea, anxiety, appetite, nausea, bowel function, and sleep, and for any symptoms mentioned in the H&P or indicated by the results of the diagnostic tests, such as lab results and reports from radiology and pathology. For example, patients with liver or kidney failure may have pruritus; and patients with a newly diagnosed chronic illness may have a depressed mood. Also note if any home medications can induce tolerance. Stopping these medications abruptly could cause the patient to experience discontinuation or withdrawal symptoms.

- *Diagnostic Test Results*: The results of diagnostic tests are important not only to understand the patient's current state but also to understand trends that inform the trajectory of the patient's illness and current symptoms. Trends in vital signs

can indicate improvement or declining status related to infections, oxygenation, and hemodynamic stability. Organ perfusion can be evaluated in part by indicators such as mental status changes, renal function tests, and liver function tests. In turn, functionality of these organs can affect the patient's plan of care. For example, the metabolites of morphine, a commonly used opioid analgesic, are excreted by the kidneys. When renal function is compromised (serum creatinine greater than 2.0 mg/dL, or greater than 1.5 mg/dL in older adults), the metabolites rapidly accumulate. Because they are neurotoxic, they can cause confusion. Drugs that are metabolized by the liver will lose their efficacy with compromised liver function, and the production of albumin—essential for functions such as drug transportation, wound healing, hemostasis, immune function, water and electrolyte balance, and muscle mass—and prealbumin (or transthyretin) can decline or cease. Levels of albumin (20-day half-life) are used to evaluate long-term nutritional status because they are thought to reflect the patient's nutritional status for the past few months. Prealbumin (2-day half-life) levels are thought to reflect nutritional status over the past few days, and because absolute value of prealbumin may be influenced by other factors, trends in the prealbumin level are used to evaluate improvement during a clinical stay rather than specific values. Radiology and pathology reports may provide further information about symptoms and the severity and trajectory of the patient's illness, such as biopsy results, mass effects, and location of spinal compression fractures.

- *Complementary Therapies*: Note the presence or absence of any complementary therapies the patient has used or those symptoms that may be amenable to available complementary therapies: creative/reactive modalities such as music therapy and art therapy; body energy work such as Reiki, Therapeutic Touch, and Healing Touch; introspective modalities such as guided imagery, meditation, and hypnotherapy; and interventional modalities such as massage therapy, aromatherapy, acupressure, and acupuncture.

At this point, the nurse will have a very good understanding of the data that are required to complete the assessment and the information that must be reconfirmed with the patient and family. The initial hypothesis of the holistic picture of the patient in all domains, physical, psychosocial, and spiritual, should be beginning to take shape.

Additional information is required to develop the most appropriate palliative plan of care for the patient and the family that can only be collected through a face-to-face interview.

The initial face-to-face encounter

The nurse is prepared to encounter the patient at any point in the trajectory of their illness because many people do not encounter palliative care services at diagnosis. Irrespective of when in the trajectory the nurse first meets the patient and family, the nurse establishes a relationship and begins to build trust with the patient and family—and other caregivers—as appropriate, at the first meeting and at every subsequent encounter.

Nurses and other members of the transdisciplinary healthcare team establish rapport and build trust when they:

- Find the nurse on the unit who is caring for the patient and ask about any issues the nurse might have become aware of during his or her care for the patient thus far. Note these issues in the database and add them to the list of items for further probing during the patient and family interview.

- Use hand sanitizer or wash their hands within view of the patient and family to demonstrate professionalism and concern for safety.

- Verify that this is the correct patient: Check the armband, if applicable. If the patient is alert, begin the interview, "Good morning. What is your name?" If the patient is not alert, attempt to arouse the patient if possible. If the patient is not responsive, the EHR and/or the family may be the best source of information.

- Introduce themselves to the patient and others in the room with first and last name, role, and how the patient may address her or him: "My name is Jane Doe. I am a nurse practitioner on the palliative care team. Your attending physician Dr. Jones asked our service to see you and I talked with your RN Josh this morning. You may call me Jane."

- Determine how the patient would like to be addressed: first name, last name, title, and/or nickname: "What may I call you?" Do not be surprised if a patient asks to be called something more formal than expected, such as "You may call me Mrs. Jackson," or by an unfamiliar name. Do not hesitate to ask how a name is spelled if in doubt.

- Identify the other persons in the room and their relationship with the patient: "Whom do we have in the room with us, Mrs. Jackson?" Sometimes the patient will introduce the individuals if they can, or the individuals in the room will introduce themselves. The nurse requests elaboration of the relationship between the patient and others in the room as appropriate. Modify the genogram as appropriate.

- Explain the purpose of the interaction and the approximate length of time expected the nurse will spend with the patient: "Our team does several things including pain and symptom management, helping you to determine your goals, and keeping you comfortable in the hospital. We will be spending about 20 minutes talking with you and examining you."

- Ask the patient's permission to proceed with the assessment: "May I continue?", giving the patient an opportunity to get comfortable: "Do you need to use the restroom before we start?", and excusing others whom the patient does not wish to be present during the interview and examination: "Mrs. Jackson, do you want your visitors to stay here during our conversation or would you rather they step out of the room?" Some patients may want others to be present during the interview, to assist with recall—particularly patients with compromised memory—but not during the examination. The nurse modifies the assessment routine to accommodate the focused goals of the assessment and patient preferences.

- Take a seat near the patient, being respectful of the patient's cultural norms for physical closeness and eye contact, "Do you mind if I sit down next to you? So we can talk more comfortably?" Some patient rooms are very small, so the nurse is cognizant of his or her presence in the room and the most appropriate place to be seated to interact with the patient and family.

Completing the nursing database

Now that the nurse has begun to establish rapport and trust with the patient and the patient's family in the room, the nurse completes the nursing database using interview, observation, and assessment techniques drawn from all three domains. Nurses complete the nursing database when they:

- Invite the patient to describe how he or she learned of the illness: "So tell me, Mrs. Jackson, how you learned about your illness."

- Take care not to interrupt the patient too often; use communication techniques such as probing, reflecting, clarifying, responding empathetically, and asking open-ended questions to encourage greater detail if the patient's account is brief or sketchy.

- Proceed through the physical assessment, the psychosocial assessment, and the spiritual assessment (see below).

- Prepare to end the interview when appropriate, thus supporting patient-centered care: ask the patient and the family if they have any unanswered questions for which the nurse might assist with finding the answers, and give them the opportunity to ask about something that is unclear or that they had not had the chance to ask earlier.

- Ask the patient and family if they can think of anything else that the nurse might do for them that would contribute to their comfort, and close the initial interview by summarizing any action items.

- Bid everyone a professional goodbye as appropriate.

An emerging issue that relates to family members' health is genetic testing for familial diseases. The nurse asks patients with diseases that could have a genetic origin whether they would be

---

Box 4.4 Genetic counseling information

National Society of Genetic Counselors (610-872-7608; http://www.nsgc.org) has an extensive listing of genetic counselors in the United States and around the world through the *Find a Genetic Counselor* tool (http://www.nsgc.org/LinkClick. aspx?link=64&tabid=143).

---

interested in receiving more information. Patients or family members who desire more facts will benefit from written materials and referral to an experienced genetic counselor. Box 4.4 provides resource information on genetic counseling. For more information, refer to the American College of Preventive Medicine's *Genetic Testing Clinical Reference for Clinicians*.[31]

Assessment at diagnosis

The palliative care nursing assessment goals at the time of diagnosis are to:

- Determine the baseline health of the patient and family.
- Identify problems for which interventions can be planned with the patient and family that maximize their quality of life.
- Uncover learning needs to guide teaching that promotes optimal self-care.
- Ascertain patient and family strengths to reinforce healthy habits and behaviors for maximizing well-being.
- Discern when the expertise of other healthcare professionals is needed, such as a social worker, registered dietitian, chaplain, or therapist.

Physical assessment at diagnosis

Nurses complete the physical assessment at diagnosis when they:

- Move through the review of systems to verify and to update information in the nursing database.
- Avoid nursing jargon—terminology unfamiliar to the average person—such as the use of abbreviations, acronyms, and short-cut phrases, for example, Q 4 HRS, PO, HS; UTI, CHF, and PEG; and tele, tachy, brady down, and Q-sign.
- Request permission to touch the patient: "Mrs. Jackson, now I would like to examine you. Is that OK?"
- Obtain data by inspection, auscultation, palpation, and percussion; observe and interview the patient as necessary during the examination; and explain each action in advance: "I'm going to listen to your lungs and heart, then your belly." The format, policies, procedures, and expectations of the healthcare agency in which the assessment occurs guide the specific details that are collected and documented. Box 4.5 shows cues to guide the review of systems, Box 4.6 shows cues to guide the functional assessment and PPS score, and Box 4.7 shows cues to guide the head-to-toe physical assessment.
- Assist with the discussion and decision-making about code status using language that does not confuse the patient and family. Such a discussion must be undertaken based on the goals established by the patient in conversation with the members of

---

Box 4.5 Review of systems

General

"In general, how have you been feeling?"
Weight changes
Changes in energy level
Changes in sleeping pattern
Fevers, chills, sweats
Pain: acute, chronic

P—Precipitates/Palliates: What happened when first noticed? What brings it on? What makes it better?

Q—Quality: Aching, burning, cramping, deep, stabbing, throbbing

R—Region/Radiation: Where is the locus of the pain? To where does the pain radiate?

S—Severity: Pain scale, 0 = no pain, 10 = worst ever

  ◆ Acceptable level

  ◆ Getting better, worse, or staying the same

T—Timing: onset, constant or episodic, frequency, duration

U—Understanding: What do you think it means?

Head, eyes, ears, nose, throat (HEENT)

Head, neck

- Head or neck pain—PQRSTU
- Headache—PQRSTU

Eyes

How is your vision?

Changes, pain, discharge

Blurriness

Double vision

Photophobia

Redness

Tiredness

Ears

How is your hearing?

Changes, pain, discharge

Tinnitus

Vertigo

Nose, sinuses

How's your sense of smell?

Changes, pain, discharge

Post nasal drip

Congestion

Obstruction

Throat, mouth

Pain: mouth, tongue, teeth, throat, swallowing— PQRSTU

(continued)

Box 4.5 Continued

- Changes: voice, swallowing, gums
- Sores
- Bleeding

Respiratory

How is your breathing?

Changes

Pain when breathing—PQRSTU

Dyspnea: at rest, on exertion, how far can you walk; tripoding

Cough: productive, quantity, color

Wheezing: on inspiration, on expiration

Cyanosis: lips, fingernails, toenails

Orthopnea: sleep with pillows, how many

Sleep apnea, snoring

Paroxysmal nocturnal dyspnea

Cardiovascular

- Chest pain (CP)—PQRSTU or pressure
- Syncope: how often, for how long
- Palpitations: sense of rapid or irregular heartbeat, how often, for how long
- Lower extremity edema
- Leg pain with or without ambulation—PQRSTU
- Wounds or ulcers in feet, slow healing

Gastrointestinal

- Appetite
- Difficulty swallowing
- Heartburn—PQRSTU
- Food intolerances
- Nausea: how often, for how long, precipitates, palliates
- Vomiting: amount, color, how often, for how long, precipitates, palliates
- Pain: abdominal—PQRSTU
- Abdominal swelling or distention
- Flatulence
- Bowel movements: last BM, normal frequency (daily, Q2D, Q3D); incontinence
- Stool changes: form, frank blood, black & tarry
- Constipation: how often, for how long, precipitates, palliates
- Diarrhea: how often, for how long, precipitates, palliates
- Hemorrhoids

Genitourinary

- Pain—PQRSTU: flank, suprapubic, dysuria
- Frequency
- Urgency
- Hesitancy
- Strength of stream
- Nocturia
- Hematuria
- Urinary incontinence
- Incomplete emptying, still need to urinate when done
- Hair changes: pubic, axillary, other
- Libido: decrease, increase
- Orgasm: changes, anorgasmia
- Fertility problems
- Date of last breast self-exam
- Breast, changes, pain—PQRSTU, discharge

For men:

- Date of last genital self-exam
- Penis: changes, pain—PQRSTU, discharge
- Scrotum: changes, pain—PQRSTU
- Arousal: changes, ED, priapism, pain—PQRSTU
- Intercourse: changes, pain—PQRSTU, inability to complete to satisfaction
- Ejaculation: changes, delay, premature, pain—PQRSTU
- Semen: changes, amount, color, consistency

For women:

- External: changes, pain—PQRSTU, discharge
- Menses: changes, pain—PQRSTU
- Intercourse: changes, pain—PQRSTU, dryness, inability to complete to satisfaction

Musculoskeletal

- Muscle ache—PQRSTU
- Low back pain—PQRSTU
- Pain, swelling, cracking, popping of joints
  - ✓ Upper extremities: shoulders, elbow, wrists fingers
  - ✓ Lower extremities: Hips, knees, ankles, toes
- Bone pain—PQRSTU

Endocrine

- Heat or cold intolerance
- Polyuria, polydipsia, polyphagia
- Changes in distribution of facial hair, body hair

(continued)

Box 4.5 Continued

Immune

- Allergies: respiratory, topical, food
- Any unexplained inflammation
  - ✓ Rubor—erythema
  - ✓ Tumor—swelling
  - ✓ Calor—warmth
  - ✓ Dolor—pain—PQRSTU
  - ✓ Functio laesa—loss of normal function

Hematology/oncology

- Abnormal bleeding or bruising
- New or growing lumps or bumps
- Hypercoagulability

Skin and hair

- Hair: changes (color, texture), loss
- Skin
  - ✓ Lesions: changed size, shape, color
  - ✓ Eruptions, growths
  - ✓ Itching, pain—PQRSTU

Neurological

- Tremors
- Numbness
- Weakness
- Dizziness
- Balance or coordination problems
- Sudden loss of neurological function
- Abrupt loss or change in level of consciousness
- Witnessed seizure activity

Psychiatric

- Mental status changes
- Mood changes
- New worry or anxiety
- Changes in thought patterns
- Memory changes

Box 4.6 Functional assessment

Compare to before the illness, last month, 6 months ago, 1 year ago.

Activities of daily living

- Bathing
- Dressing
- Personal grooming
- Eating
- Transfers
- Toileting
- Continence
- Ambulation

Instrumental activities of daily living

- Shopping
- Meal preparation
- Taking medications
- Housekeeping
- Laundry
- Transportation
- Telephone use/communication
- Managing personal finances

Environment

- Do you live alone?
- Do you feel safe in your neighborhood?
- Can you pay your bills for heat, water, and electric?
- Do you drive or take the bus? Or something else?
- Are you involved in any community activities?

Nutrition, diet

- Appetite
- Foods: favorites, dislikes
- 24-hour food diary recall
- Who buys and prepares your meals?
- Can you afford to purchase food?
- Nutritional balance

Coping

- What kinds of stressors do you face every day?
- Any significant stressors in the past year?
- How do you try to relieve stress?
- Is that helpful?

Exercise

- Type
- Amount

the healthcare team. The discussion should be in the context of the person's health status and an understanding of likely outcomes of an attempt to resuscitate. Possible negative outcomes of an attempt to resuscitate include pain and injuries, such as rib fractures, clavicular fractures, and tracheal bleeding from the trauma of chest compressions. If a patient's health is particularly compromised, include in the discussion the low likelihood that the patient would return to her or his current level of functioning should the resuscitation efforts be successful.[32] If consistent with the patient's goals of care, one way to

Box 4.6 Continued

♦ Warm-up

♦ Monitoring response to exercise

Occupational health

♦ What job do you do now? Or did you do before you retired?

♦ Are any of your health problems related to exposure to something at work?

Abuse—How are things at home?

♦ Domestic violence

♦ Child abuse

♦ Elderly abuse

Perception of health

♦ How do you define health?

♦ How do you view your situation now?

♦ What are your concerns?

introduce the topic to the patient and/or family is, "We hope for the best, but try to prepare for the worst. I would like to ask you a few questions about your thoughts about care at the end of life. Have you thought about this? What would be important for you at the end of your life?" Depending on the patient's or family member's responses, further conversation may be required regarding details, such as the desire for resuscitative efforts (including chest compressions, defibrillation, and intubation)

Box 4.7 Physical examination

General: Observe for patient disposition, acute distress, arousability; manner of dress, posture, body language, diaphoresis.

  Vital Signs: temperature, heart rate, respiratory rate, SpO_2, O_2 rate, O_2 delivery device, vent parameters, SBP/DBP.

  HEENT:

Head	Observe for shape and evidence of trauma.
Eyes	Observe pupils bilat for shape and reaction to light and accommodation, retinal fundi, sclera, icterus, discharge, glasses.
Ear	Observe external ear, ear canal, tympanic membranes bilat, cerumen, discharge, hearing aids.
Nose	Observe for inflammation, obstruction, discharge
Neck	Palpate cervical lymph nodes for stiffness.
Throat	Observe for jugular vein distention (JVD), thyroid location; palpate sublingual lymph nodes, thyroid; observe oropharynx, dentition, dental hygiene, dry or cracked lips. Auscultate carotid pulses bilat.

Respiratory: Observe chest excursion, use of accessory muscles, effort; palpate for tenderness; auscultate breath sounds all lobes anterior/posterior, appreciate adventitious sounds, rales, rhonchi, wheezing; palpate fremitus, crepitus; percuss for dullness.

Cardiovascular: Observe posture, edema, cyanosis, cardiac assist devices; auscultate heart sounds; palpate peripheral pulses (radial, pedal) bilat

Gastrointestinal: Observe for distention, abdominal ascites, ostomy, rectal tube, stool, last BM; auscultate bowel sounds in all four quadrants; palpate superficially and deep; observe for rebound tenderness; percuss for margins of abdominal organs.

Genitourinary: Observe for presence of urine, volume, color.

Musculoskeletal: Observe for spontaneous movements of extremities, muscle strength, spinal flexibility, temperature, deformities; L/R comparisons.

Neurological: Observe for level of consciousness, orientation, grossly intact cranial nerves II–XII, sensation in all extremities, full range of motion (ROM) in extremities, cerebellar reflexes, tremors, Romberg, gait.

Psychiatric: Observe for mood, affect, anxiety, disordered speech, language, delirium, hallucinations, capacity for decision-making, memory, attention span, need for mini mental state exam (MMSE).

Integumentary: Observe for rashes, bruising, wounds, discoloration, mottling, lesions, nevi (ABCD), venous access ports, complexion, makeup.

and for artificial life support (including mechanical ventilation, artificial hydration, and artificial nutrition).

♦ Determine the patient's current PPS score based on observations and collected data about the patient's ambulation, activity and evidence of disease, self-care, intake, and level of consciousness.

♦ Assess and document the overall health of family members. Identification of the major health problems, physical limitations, and physical strengths of family members serves as a basis for care planning. The physical capabilities and constraints of the caregivers available to assist and support the patient may affect the plan of care, especially in relation to the most appropriate setting for care. This information also provides direction for the types of referrals that may be needed to provide care.

Psychosocial assessment at diagnosis

The primary psychosocial feature of a new diagnosis is anticipatory grief. Patient responses and those of their family members to receiving bad news range from shock, disbelief, and denial to anger and fatalism. Statements such as, "I can't believe this is happening to me" or "Why is this happening to us?" are signals to the nurse that the patient and family are grappling heavily with this threat to life as they know it to be. There is already a sense that life will be forever changed. A longing emerges to return to the way things were.

In response to these emotional states, nurses and other members of the transdisciplinary team are most helpful when they:

♦ Normalize the patient's and family's experiences: "Many people share similar reactions to this kind of news."

♦ Use active listening skills to facilitate grief work: "Of all that is happening to you right now, what is the hardest part to deal with?"

♦ Create a safe space for self-disclosure, and build a trust relationship: "No matter what lies ahead, you will not face it alone."

- Develop a collaborative partnership to establish a mutual plan of care: "What would help you the most right now?"

- Respect the patient's or family's use of denial in the service of coping with harsh realities: "It must be hard to believe this is happening."

- Assess the patient's and family's coping styles: "When you have experienced difficult times in the past, how did you get through them?"

- Reinforce strengths. "It sounds like this has helped you before."

- Maximize a sense of control, autonomy, and choice. "It seems you really have a handle on this."

- Assess the patient's need for information: "What do you know about your illness?", "Are you the kind of person who likes to know as much as possible, or do you function on a need-to-know basis only?", "What would you like to know about your illness now?"

- Check the need for clarification: "What did you hear?" or "Summarize in your own words how you understand your situation now."

- Mentor patients and families who have had little experience with the healthcare system, and coach them on having effective conversations with other members of the healthcare team. Suggest that they write down questions and the answers they receive, and teach them ways to navigate the complexities of the healthcare system.

Nurses must always remember that although the patient is feeling strong emotions when they first learn of the diagnosis, the family is also experiencing intense feelings. Similar assessments of family members will help to mobilize resources at critical times. Family members experience their grief reactions at their individual rates throughout the course of the patient's illness. Each family member has his or her own particular coping style and need for information. See chapter 30, "Supporting Families in Palliative Care," for additional information.

Nurses and other members of the transdisciplinary healthcare team assess the psychosocial domain at diagnosis when they:

- Assist in the process of making initial treatment decisions, which can be an opportunity to begin a relationship that will continue to grow. Members of the healthcare team may ask questions such as, "What is most important to you in life?" and "Is quality of life or quantity of life most meaningful?" Assisting the patient and family in identifying and expressing their values will guide them in subsequent decision-making.

- Observe changes in family members' roles and responsibilities. For example, one member of the household may decide to stay at home to care for the loved one and no longer work outside the home, thus eliminating one source of family income, or the adult child may become the caregiver when the parent can no longer take care of herself or himself.

- Identify external community support systems such as a faith community, volunteer organizations, and transportation services.

- Assist the patient and family to identify coping strategies to use while awaiting answers from results of diagnostic tests and procedures. Waiting for results is not only one of the most

---

Box 4.8 Common responses of children to serious illness in the family

- Magical thinking that results in feelings of guilt, for example, "I once told Mommy I wished she were dead."

- Fears of abandonment, especially in younger children

- Fears of contracting the disease

- Anger, withdrawal, being uncooperative, especially in adolescents

- Acting-out behavior with lack of usual attention

- Frustrations with an altered lifestyle because of decreased financial resources, less family fun activities because of the ill person's inability to participate, interruptions in schedule

- Inability to concentrate and focus, especially regarding schoolwork

---

stressful times but also a stressful time that recurs throughout the illness.

- Identify family communication ground rules to seek to improve communication among family members: "Is it OK if we discuss this subject with you and your family?"

- Help the patient and family explore the benefits and burdens of various treatment options when making decisions about the plan of care.

- Assess parental readiness to assist children with their adaptation needs: "How do you plan to tell your children?"

- Assess the coping of children within the family by being aware of their fears and concerns. Box 4.8 describes some common responses of children to having an adult loved one who is ill.

Spiritual assessment at diagnosis

The diagnosis of a serious illness generally brings with it a sense of shock to the patient and family. It may threaten many of their assumptions about life, disrupt their sense of control, and cause them to ask "Why?" At diagnosis, an important nursing assessment is to learn any spiritual practices that might have an impact on the patient and family's healthcare decisions, such as avoiding particular foods, not receiving blood products, and not being touched by a person of the opposite gender. Spiritual goals at this phase are to normalize initial concerns, to provide information that fosters positive coping, to inform the healthcare team of any special spiritual needs, and to encourage the patient and family to seek supportive spiritual resources.

Nurses and the other members of the transdisciplinary healthcare team assess the spiritual domain at diagnosis when they:

- Determine the patient's and family's level of hopefulness or optimism about the future: "What are you hoping for?" or "How do you see the future at this time?"

- Inquire about how the patient and family have dealt with past crises of faith, meaning, or loss: "What helped you get through that?"

- Determine the patient's and family's comfort level in talking about the spiritual life: "Some people need or want to talk about these things; others don't. How is it for you?"

- Inquire about spiritual support persons available to the patient and family, such as a priest, pastor, rabbi, counselor, or spiritual advisor: "Is there a spiritual support person available to you? Does he or she know you are here?"

- Determine the patient's or family's need or desire to speak with a spiritual support person: "Would you like me to contact that spiritual support person for you?"

- Ask about spiritual practices that inform the healthcare team about caring for the patient and family: "Are there any spiritual practices that we should be aware of to help us take better care of you?"

- Ask about spiritual self-care practices to promote healthy coping: "How are you taking care of yourself at this time?"

- Listen for comments from the patient and family regarding the importance of their religious traditions and practices: "Well, she reads the Bible every day, but don't ask her about the last time she went to church."

Case study

Tarana at diagnosis: heart failure

Tarana's heart failure journey began for her when she noticed that her lower legs, ankles, and feet were swelling, causing her to lie down to put her feet up. Krupa commented then that Tarana was walking less spryly when they would go shopping, stopping a bit more frequently than in the past to rest. Tarana was referred to a cardiologist who diagnosed heart failure: ACC/AHA Stage C[33] (NYHA Class II[34]) heart failure, with a left ventricular ejection fraction (LVEF) of 35%. The cardiologist started Tarana on furosemide, carvediol, and lisinopril, and recommended mild exercise, a salt-restricted diet, and a referral to a palliative care advanced practice nurse.

The palliative care assessment goals for Tarana and her family at the time of diagnosis are to:

- Assess Tarana for knowledge about her plan of care and readiness to adhere to the medical plan of care, as well as any roadblocks to doing so.

- Assess Tarana and her family for their need for resources so they can learn about how to live and cope effectively with this lifelong, incurable illness.

- Determine Tarana's and her family's need for supportive encouragement and to screen for depression and challenging behaviors, as well as the need for therapy and antidepressants.

- Assess for available spiritual supports and the need for a chaplaincy referral.

- Assess for readiness to discuss advance directives and the need for appropriate forms.

Assessment during treatment

Reassessments during treatment determine the changes that have occurred since the initial assessment. They occur regularly during scheduled interactions with patients and families, as well as during any emergent crisis.

The palliative care nursing assessment goals during treatment are to:

- Assess the patient's systems in all domains that have a history of, or are at risk for problems, considering both changes from the patient's baseline problems and any side effects of the treatments.

- Identify the current and potential problems to plan early interventions with the patient and family, particularly as they approach decision points regarding treatment.

- Ascertain the need for teaching to prevent, minimize, and manage problems with the goal of maximizing quality of life.

- Identify patient and family strengths, healthy habits, and behaviors to reinforce for maximizing well-being.

- Determine the need for other healthcare professionals' expertise to make appropriate referrals, for example a referral to a physical therapist or a pharmacist.

Physical assessment during treatment

Knowledge of the usual disease process and of the side effects of treatment assists the nurse in focusing reassessments on those body systems most likely to be affected. The nurse begins to build a strategy during the assessment of possible nursing interventions and therapies that might be used to address disease progression and symptoms before they occur or worsen.

In addition to the patient's physical assessment, the nurse makes periodic observations and inquiries about the health of other family members. Documenting any changes in their health problems or physical limitations and physical strengths that might have an impact on the patient's care and the family's overall quality of life is important. The nurse determines the PPS score and also documents changes in PPS score from the last documented assessment. Changes in PPS score have been shown to be better predictors of mortality than simply PPS alone.[33]

Psychosocial assessment during treatment

Once a treatment plan has been initiated, patients often express relief that "something is finally being done." Taking action frequently reduces anxiety. The most important psychosocial intervention at this stage is the amelioration of as many treatment side effects as possible. After basic needs for physical well-being are assessed and symptoms are controlled, the patient is able to explore and meet higher needs, including the needs for belonging, self-esteem, and self-actualization.[21] Patients who are preoccupied with pain and nausea or vomiting have no energy or ability to explore the significance of their illness or their feelings about it. Effective management of physical symptoms is mandatory before the patient can begin to work on integrating the illness experience into the tapestry of his or her life.

After several months or years of treatment, the effects of having a chronic illness may exhaust even the hardiest person. Patients may begin to weigh the benefits versus the burdens of continuing aggressive therapies. Initially, patients will endure almost anything if they believe a cure is possible. As time unfolds, their attitudes may change as they watch their quality of life erode with

Table 4.4 Assessing for anxiety and depression

Signs and symptoms of anxiety	Signs and symptoms of depression
Excessive worry	Sad mood (refer as needed)
Trouble falling or staying asleep	Insomnia and hypersomnia
Irritability, muscle tension	Anhedonia (absence of pleasure)
Restlessness, agitation	Feelings of worthlessness or inappropriate guilt
Unrealistic fears (phobias)	
Obsessions (persistent painful ideas)	Fatigue, decreased energy
Compulsions (repetitive ritualistic acts)	Diminished ability to concentrate, make decisions, or remember
Self-medication	Marked weight loss or weight gain
Anorexia or overeating	Psychomotor retardation
Frequent crying spells, headaches, gastrointestinal upsets, palpitations, shortness of breath	Recurrent thoughts of death, suicidal ideation (lethality assessed by expressed intent, presence of a plan and the means to carry it out, previous attempts, and provision for rescue)
Thoughts interfere with normal activities of daily living	

little prospect of a more curative outcome. Patients may also reprioritize what is most important to them. For example, the Type A personality may find less satisfaction at the office, or the stay-at-home parent may experience a lower level of fulfillment from daily routines around the house. Change, transition, and existential questioning characterize this phase, particularly while preparing to transition to the next phase.[35]

Nurses and other members of the transdisciplinary healthcare team assess the psychosocial domain during treatment when they:

◆ Inquire about the patient's newly emerging identity as a result of the illness: "What activities and which relationships bring you the most joy and meaning?" or "Have you been able to define a new purpose for yourself?"

◆ Assess for signs of anxiety and depression, which remain the two most common psychosocial problems associated with severe illness (Table 4.4); for more information contrasting anxiety and depression, consult Holland's *Psycho-Oncology*.[36–38]

◆ Screen for suicidal ideation in cases of depression: "Have you been feeling so bad that you've been thinking of a way to hurt yourself?", "Do you have a plan for how to do it?", and "Do you have access to what you would use to carry out your plan?"

◆ Determine the need for counseling and possible psychotropic medication to enhance positive coping and comfort.

Spiritual assessment during treatment

With the treatment of a serious illness comes the introduction of an additional stressor to the patient and family. It is important to assess how they incorporate the demands of treatment into their daily routine and how these changes have affected the meaning of their lives. The spiritual goals during treatment are to reinforce positive coping, mobilize existing spiritual resources, invite the patient and family to develop new skills for self-care, update documentation of patient wishes as they evolve, and continue disclosures in an atmosphere of trust.

Nurses and other members of the transdisciplinary healthcare team assess the spiritual domain during treatment when they:

◆ Assess how hope is shifting: "What are your hopes for the future?

◆ Assess the level and quality of support they are receiving, for instance, from other family members, faith community, and neighbors: "What kinds of support do you need?" and "Who is helping you out?"

◆ Explore expressions of anxiety and fear: "What is concerning you the most at this time?"

◆ Assess how the patient and family are coping with the rigors of treatment: "What is the most challenging part of this for you?" and "What is helping you day by day?"

◆ Determine the need for referrals to a chaplain or faith community as needed.

◆ Inquire about the patient and family's definitions of quality of life and the impact of treatment on these aspects of their lives: "What is most important to you in life now?"

◆ Determine their use of spiritual practices such as meditation, relaxation, prayer, or burning incense, for example, and offer assistance in developing them: "What are you doing to take care of your spirit?"

◆ Ask how the patient or family members feel about their current practices: "Are these helpful or not?"

◆ Assess the need for changes in the patient's advance directives and in code status: "Have you thought any more about who you would want to make your healthcare decisions for you if you were not able to make them yourself?", "Have you talked with your family about whether or not you want to be put on a breathing machine if you cannot breathe on your own?", "Do you still want a feeding tube if you need one?", "If you require dialysis to stay alive, do you want it?"

Case study

Tarana during treatment

Tarana often feels very fatigued, short of breath, and not able to do as much as she would like to do, causing her to be hospitalized. Most often she is hospitalized to be treated with IV antibiotics for pneumonia or to have her medications adjusted. Tarana hopes that each hospitalization will provide a final cure. As the years progress, her functional status continues to decline, and she develops atrial fibrillation and other arrhythmias. Her cardiologist adds digoxin to her therapeutic regimen. While in the hospital, her attending physician refers her to the inpatient palliative care team to assist with symptom management. Over time, she begins to question her treatment goals and her faith.

At this most recent hospitalization, Tarana's LVEF is 25% and her arrhythmias are more lethal—episodes of ventricular tachycardia. After a family meeting, she reluctantly agrees to receive an automatic implantable cardioverter-defibrillator (AICD). Before her surgery, the nurse talks with her about "expecting the best but preparing for the worst," yet she "does not want to talk about anything bad happening."

The goals of the palliative care nursing assessment during Tarana's latest hospitalization for treatment are to:

- Assess information needs for treatment decision-making.

- Assess the impact of her current symptoms on her quality of life as well as Tarana's thoughts about what would make her most comfortable.

- Determine Tarana's adherence to her medical plan of care identify roadblocks and possible remediation for those roadblocks.

- Identify Tarana's need for education about her AICD and how it works.

- Address why she does not want to talk about her advance directives.

- Determine the need for a mental health consult for depression and anxiety.

- Assess the need for a chaplain referral to assist with emerging existential issues and threatened faith.

Assessment after treatment

After treatment, the patient embarks on a journey leading to long-term survival, chronic illness, recurrence or exacerbations, or the terminal phases of the illness. The course of treatment for cancer patients is frequently chemotherapy and/or radiation. Once treatment is completed, the patient enters either remission, long-term survival, or a terminal trajectory. Patients with terminal cancer diagnoses and patients with terminal noncancer diagnoses, of course, may at any time decide to stop all attempts to cure the illness and to initiate a completely palliative plan of care, maximizing comfort and quality of life. Sometimes, treatment of an illness during an exacerbation simply does not work. At this point, after treatment is over or the patient stops treatments, the nursing assessment continues to focus on quality of life including patient and family coping.

Because more than 55% of all deaths in America during 2012 occurred without hospice care,[8] patients in this part of their disease trajectory should be assessed frequently to determine if they would be appropriate for hospice, that is, do they meet criteria based on their illness.

The goals of the palliative care nursing assessment after treatment are to:

- Assess the benefits and burdens of all interventions to manage the symptoms remaining from the treatments and/or the disease process.

- Determine the current physical problems that are most distressing to the patient and family to prepare for possible palliative interventions.

- Assess functional status and disease process to determine when a hospice referral is appropriate.

- Assess learning needs about managing problems with the goal of maximizing quality of life.

- Assess patient and family strengths, healthy habits, and behaviors to enhance well-being and to prevent problems.

Survivors are defined as those patients whose diseases are cured, who go into long remissions, who become chronically ill, or who recover from an exacerbation of a chronic illness. These individuals may require some degree of palliative care for the rest of their lives. Examples of survivors likely to require ongoing palliative care include: (1) cancer survivors with graft-versus-host disease (GVHD), irreversible peripheral neuropathies, or structural alterations of the integumentary, gastrointestinal, and genitourinary systems, such as mastectomies, amputations, colostomies, ileostomies, and laryngectomies, and (2) persons with other chronic illnesses who have survived an acute episode and have returned to a chronic phase of their disease process.

Psychosocial issues for survivors include fear of recurrence or exacerbation as well as practical considerations such as insurance and job discrimination. Many patients make major life changes regarding work and relationships as a result of their illness experiences. These patients live with the ramifications of the disease and its treatment for the rest of their lives, even cancer patients who have met criteria for being cured.

Some patients begin to explore in new ways the spiritual foundations and assumptions of their lives. Often, patients relate that in spite of the crisis of an illness and its treatment, the experience resulted in a deepened sense of meaning and gratitude for life. Examples of such growth experiences as a result of surviving cancer can be found in *Cancer as a Turning Point*.[39]

Physical assessment after treatment

The patient is reassessed after treatment to determine the changes that have occurred since previous assessments. Although the focus is on the systems that have been affected and altered by the disease and treatments, assessing the patient from a holistic perspective is even more crucial. Thorough assessment of the residual problems and changes in the patient's body are critical to successful symptom management. Effective management of symptoms with palliative interventions achieves the goal of maximizing the patient's and family's quality of life, whether in long-term survival or during the terminal phase. The PPS is a general scale that is widely applied to patients with life-threatening illnesses. Nurses also use functional assessment tools that are developed for patients living with specific chronic or life-threatening illnesses.

In addition to the patient's physical assessment, nurses continue to make periodic observations and inquiries about the health of other family members. Noting changes in family members' health, physical limitations, and physical strengths is important to ascertain any impact on the patient's care and the family's lifestyle.

Psychosocial assessment after treatment ceases

For those patients who are free of disease, palliative care focuses on post-treatment-related symptoms and fears of recurrence. For others, disease progression or recurrence is most often signaled by the appearance of advancing physical symptoms. When this happens, the patient's worst nightmare has been realized. A recurrence or exacerbation is experienced differently than an initial diagnosis, because the patient is now a veteran of the patient role and may understand all too well what the recurrence or exacerbation means.

Research suggests that a strong correlation exists between caregiver stress and morbidity.[40] This is especially true of caregiver stress that affects blood pressure and mental health stress responses such as chronic depression. For additional information, refer to chapter 30, "Supporting Families in Palliative Care."

Nurses and other members of the transdisciplinary healthcare team assess the psychosocial domain after treatment when they:

- Revisit the quality versus quantity of life preferences as the patient and family weigh the benefits and burdens of further treatment. Beginning these conversations earlier rather than later in the illness helps to make them less threatening and creates an ongoing dialogue that will help the patient, family, and healthcare providers alike when further treatment becomes futile.

- Evaluate the patient's readiness to discuss a transition in emphasis from curative to comfort care only. The patient often signals his or her readiness by statements such as, "I'm getting tired of spending so much time at the hospital" or "I've had it with all of this." Ask: "What has your physician told you that you can expect now?" or "How do you see your future?"

- Explore readiness to set new goals of treatment: "I know you understand that your illness has not responded to the treatments as we had hoped. I'd like to reexamine your healthcare goals with you."

- Assess for family adaptation to stress and coping.

- Revisit the need for advance directives and changes in code status.

- Reevaluate the need for a discussion about hospice if the patient begins to question the efficacy of treatments and present hospice as the gold standard for end-of-life care. A hospice referral should never be made as a gesture indicating that "There is nothing more that we can do for you." The benefits of increased availability of services, such as symptom management, respite opportunities, and bereavement care for the family, should be emphasized.

- Determine the patient's and family's need and interest for education about death and dying.

- Discern the risk factors for complicated bereavement in family members, as described in Box 4.9.

Spiritual assessment after treatment

The main spiritual goal of this phase of illness is to provide the patient and family a "place to stand" to review the past and look toward the future. This encourages grieving past losses, creating a sense of meaning, and consolidating strengths for the days ahead.

Nurses and other members of the transdisciplinary healthcare team assess the spiritual domain after treatment when they:

- Determine the quality and focus of the patient's and family's hopes for the future. Listen for a transition from hoping for a cure to another kind of hope, such as hope for a remission, hope to live until a special family event occurs, and hope for continuing care for their family when the patient cannot care for them. Observe for any barriers to hope or evidence of hopelessness.[41]

- Listen for comments that suggest a crisis of belief and meaning. For example, at recurrence, a patient may feel abandoned or experience an assault on his or her faith. Questions such as "Why?" and "Where is God?" and "Why are my prayers not being answered?" are very common. Nurses respond to these questions by normalizing them and emphasizing that to question God or one's faith can indicate a vitality of faith, not its absence.

- Assess the patient's and family's use of spiritual practices: "What are you doing to feel calmer and more peaceful?" Determine the need for a chaplain referral if the patient or family are interested and open to such an intervention.

- Inquire about the desire for meaningful rituals, such as communion, special prayers, or anointing. Evaluate the need for consulting with the patient's or family's clergy or a chaplain on the healthcare team.

- Assess the level and quality of community supports: "Who is involved in supporting you and your family at this time?" and "Do you think you need any additional help?"

- Listen for indicators of spiritual suffering such as language about unfinished business, regrets, diminished faith, and fears of abandonment, or evidence of relationship discord: "What do you find yourself thinking about at this time?" and "What are your chief concerns or worries?"

- Assess the need and desire of the patient and family to talk about the meaning of the illness, the patient's declining physical condition, and possible death: "Is there something you would like to talk with me about that you are not asking right now?" and "Would you rather talk somewhere away from your loved ones?"

- Assess the patient's and family's need to review critical life incidents, to allow grieving, and to explore beliefs regarding the afterlife: "What do you believe happens to a person at the time of death?"

Box 4.9 Risk factors for complicated bereavement in family members

- Concurrent life crises
- History of other recent or difficult past losses
- Unresolved grief from prior losses
- History of mental illness or substance abuse
- Extreme anger or anxiety
- Marked dependence on the patient
- Age of the patient and the surviving loved ones, developmental phases of the patient and family members
- Limited support within the family's circle or community
- Anticipated situational stressors, such as loss of income, financial strain, lack of confidence in assuming some of the patient's usual responsibilities
- Illnesses among other family members
- Special bereavement needs of children in the family
- The patient's dying process is difficult, as can be indicated by poorly controlled symptoms of pain, shortness of breath, agitation, delirium, or anxiety
- Absence of helpful cultural and/or religious beliefs

> **Box 4.10** Assessing for funeral plans and preferences
>
> * Has the patient and/or family selected a funeral home or a funeral and memorial society?
>
> * Has the patient and/or family decided about the disposition of the body? For example: organ, eye, and/or tissue donation; autopsy; in-earth burial (above ground or below ground); cremation; and/or total body donation to a medical school.
>
> * Has the decision been made regarding a burial or disposition of the ashes? For example: the cemetery, the plot for burial or inurnment, the mausoleum crypt, the columbarium niche, or the location for scattering ashes.
>
> * Does the patient want to make his or her wishes known regarding the type of service, or will the family decide these details? For example: clothes to be buried in, favorite songs to be sung or played, poems to be read, casket or urn selection, open or closed casket.
>
> * A consumer-oriented guide to funeral planning is http://www.funeral-help.com that includes funeral planning software for purchase.

* Determine the need and desire for reconciliation: "Are there people with whom you want or need to speak about anything?" and "Do you find yourself having any regrets?"

* Determine the patient's and family's readiness to talk about the most meaningful, celebratory occurrences in life to foster integrity, life review, and a sense of meaning: For example, "How did you meet your spouse?", "Were your children all born here?", and "Where did you and your other half like to vacation?"

* Assess the patient's and the family's readiness to discuss funeral preferences and plans and desired disposition of the body, as noted in Box 4.10.

* Assess for a referral to hospice for end-of-life care if the death of the patient might be anticipated within the year. Ask other members of the transdisciplinary healthcare team: "Would it surprise you if this person would die within the year?"

Case study

Tarana after treatment

Tarana's hospitalizations for her heart failure occurred about once every three to six months. At this, her most recent hospitalization, she was admitted due to a myocardial infarction. Her LVEF is at about 20%. She is extremely fatigued and tired of all of these hospitalizations, but she wants to make sure to be at her son's upcoming wedding. After talking with her family, she decides that this would be her last hospital admission and that she wants to pursue hospice care at home. She does not change her code status because she wants to have every chance of being at that wedding "even if it means bringing me back from the dead."

The goals of the palliative care nursing assessment after Tarana's treatment are to:

* Reevaluate adherence to activities that could maximize her quality of life.

* Evaluate appropriateness of interventions that could prevent further crises arising from her heart failure.

* Determine the need for relationship building within the family system to reduce everyone's stress levels.

* Establish Tarana's wishes with respect to her advance directives and complete the forms.

* Assess for a referral to hospice.

Assessment during active dying

The goal of hospice is to support the terminally ill patient and family wherever they choose to be. Hospice teams provide palliative care in patients' homes, acute care settings, nursing homes, and specially designed inpatient hospice facilities. Unfortunately, many patients die without the support of hospice services.

The goals of a palliative care nursing assessment when the patient is actively dying are to:

* Observe for signs and symptoms of impending death that could be managed aggressively to promote comfort (Table 4.5).

* Determine the primary source of the patient's and family's suffering to plan interventions to provide relief.

* Identify the primary sources of strength for the patient and family members so that they can be used to provide support.

* Ascertain the patient's and family's need and readiness for teaching about the dying process.

Table 4.5 Common physical symptoms experienced by people who are actively dying

Pain	PQRSTU (see Box 4.4)
Agitation	Nonpurposeful movements associated with increased anxiety
Anorexia	No interest in eating or drinking
Confusion	Disorientation and lack of orderly thought
Delirium	An acute change in consciousness, cognition, and perceptual disturbances that can fluctuate throughout the day
Dyspnea	Shortness of breath
Fatigue	Overwhelming tiredness
Incontinence	Bladder, bowel
Insomnia	Difficulty sleeping
Mottling	Changes in skin color and temperature due to decreasing circulation that progresses from distal to proximal during the last 2–3 hours of life
Restlessness	Uncontrollable increase in motor activity
Skin breakdown	Due to local ischemia secondary to immobility
Terminal secretions	Collection of saliva in the back of the throat that gurgles with each breath

◆ Look for ways to support the patient and family to enhance meaning during this intense experience.

◆ Determine whether the family members and friends who are important to the patient have had the opportunity to visit in person or on the telephone, as desired by the patient and family.

◆ Assess the family to anticipate family members' reactions to the patient's death.

◆ If not in hospice, assess for appropriateness for referral.

Physical assessment during active dying

Physical assessment during the active dying process is highly focused and is limited to determining the cause of any suffering and identifying sources of comfort. Table 4.6 shows common areas to assess in the last few days of a person's life.

In addition to the patient's physical assessment, nurses monitor the health of other family members to prevent and minimize problems that could compromise their health during this very stressful time. Frequently, assessing the family's need to participate in making the patient comfortable can lead to interventions enabling them to do something to help the patient.

Psychosocial assessment during active dying

Many people believe that the transition from life to death is as sacred as the transition experienced at birth. Keeping this in mind, nurses can help to create a safe environment in which patients and families are supported in their relationships and the creation of meaningful moments together. The patient may also still be reviewing his or her life. Common psychosocial characteristics of the person who is actively dying include social withdrawal, decreased attention span, and decreasing ability to concentrate, all culminating in a gradual loss of consciousness. Spiritual experiences such as visions and visitations from deceased relatives or spiritual/religious figures are often viewed as normal and transcendent at this stage of life in those with strong spiritual beliefs. Nurses avoid the tendency to medicalize transcendent experiences and view them as nonaberrant, positive, and an opportunity for making meaning.

During active dying, nurses and other members of the transdisciplinary healthcare team assess the psychosocial domain when they:

◆ Assess the patient's reports of seeing deceased loved ones or visions as normal and not as evidence of confusion or other mental health problems; determine the need for a behavioral health consult to distinguish such experiences from delirium.

◆ Evaluate for the need to support communication among the patient, family members, and close friends, and the need for reminiscing, story-telling, and other familiar ways of relating to each other—for example, through humor and singing.[42,43]

◆ Assess the patient's and family's need and readiness for continued education about death and dying.

◆ Evaluate for the need and readiness of family members to learn that continued touching and talking to the patient is appropriate, even if the patient is unconscious.

◆ Assess for need and readiness of the family members to learn to give permission to the patient to let go and to provide reassurance that the family will remain intact and will learn to deal effectively with the patient's absence.

◆ Observe family members for evidence of poor coping and for the need to make referrals for additional support.

◆ Assess the family members for the need and readiness to learn about organizing visitation shifts that rotate in the face of lengthy and exhausting vigils at the bedside.

◆ Revisit any complementary and alternative therapies that the family might find effective.[44]

Spiritual assessment during active dying

When the patient enters the phase of active dying, spiritual realities often increase in significance. Persons with life-threatening illnesses who participate in spiritual rituals experience feelings of higher existential well-being and less subsequent spiritual strain.[45] The goals of spiritual care during active dying are to:

◆ Facilitate any unfinished business among the patient and significant others, such as discussions with others to express love, regret, forgiveness, and gratitude.

◆ Promote the integrity of the dying person by honoring his or her life. One way to do this is by encouraging reminiscence at the bedside of the patient, recalling the "gifts" the patient bestowed on the family—that is, his or her legacy of values and qualities passed on to survivors.

◆ Assist the patient and family in extracting meaning from the dying experience.

◆ Provide sensitive comfort by being present and listening, or determine the patient's and family's need for privacy.

◆ Provide information regarding hospice, bereavement support groups, or counseling if indicated.

During active dying, nurses and other members of the transdisciplinary healthcare team assess the spiritual domain when they:

◆ Determine the need for different or more frequent visits by the patient's or family's spiritual support person: "Is there anyone I can call to be with you at this time?" and "Are there any meaningful activities or rituals you want to do?"

◆ Inquire about dreams, visions, or unusual experiences such as seeing angels or persons who have died, reports of needing to go home, or awaiting the arrival of a bus or a train, to normalize these if they are disclosed. Ask if these experiences are sources of comfort or fear and encourage further discussion, if appropriate.

◆ Assess for ability to maintain hope by asking, "What are you hoping for at this time?" reassuring the patient and family that they can be hopeful and still acknowledge that death is imminent and that moving toward a transcendent hope is vital. Evaluate for the need to reinforce that although the focus of hope may have been on cure, remission, or an extension of time earlier in the disease trajectory, now hope may be focused on an afterlife, the relief of suffering, or the idea of living on in loved ones' memories.

Table 4.6 Assessment during active dying

General	Symptoms	Are pain and other symptoms well controlled? Would massage, body energy work, or other complementary therapies add to patient's comfort?
	Family	Is everyone present who is supposed to be there? Are family members capable & comfortable with continuing to provide physical care for the patient? Are family members getting enough sleep and rest to maintain their own health? Are additional resources needed to support the family? Would the patient want the family pet in the room or on the bed?
	Location	Is the home the best place for the patient to die? Has the family thought about their comfort in living in the house after their loved one dies there? Is the room too hot or too cold for the patient and for the family in the room?
	Spirit	Does the patient want a particular member of the clergy present? Are they available to be here for the patient and the family? Are there any spiritual or cultural rituals to be done before or immediately after death?
	Help	Does the family know whom to call on a 24-hour basis for advice and support? Does the family know not to call for emergency medical services when the patient dies?
Head & neck	Mind	How important is level of alertness versus control of pain and anxiety which may cause sedation?
	Vision	What objects and people at the bedside provide comfort when seen by the patient? Family photos? Children's drawings? Special objects? Pets? Loved ones sitting nearby? What degree of lighting does the patient prefer? Does darkness increase anxiety? Would scented candles provide solace?
	Hearing	What sounds most comfort the patient? Music? Family chatting nearby? The TV or radio on in the background? Would music thanatology be of comfort? Someone reading to him or her? Silence?
	Smell	What scents does the patient enjoy? Would aromatic lotions be soothing? Are there clothes of a particular person whose scent would be of comfort? Does the patient have favorite colognes or perfumes? If on oxygen, would humidification be of comfort?
	Taste	What are the patient's favorite flavors? Would mouth care to relieve dryness be more acceptable with fruit punch, apple juice, beer, or coffee?
	Mouth	Does the family/caregiver understand how to provide good, frequent mouth and lip care, particularly if the patient is a mouth-breather?
	Face	Does the patient receive comfort from face & head massage or a facial with aromatic salves?
Shoulders & arms	Mechanics	Do the caregivers understand good body alignment and several ways to position the patient comfortably? Are they following good body mechanics when repositioning the patient?
	Soothing	Would applying aromatic lotion to hands and arms comfort the patient and give family members something meaningful to do?
Chest, back, & spine	Lungs	Is the patient at high risk for death rales? Is there a scopolamine patch or other meds in the home for immediate use if noisy respirations begin? Would oxygen help the patient breathe easier?
	Heart	If patient is at home, is the family prepared for the moment of death? For example, do they know NOT to call 911? Do they have a neighbor close by to come and be with them until a healthcare provider arrives?
	Back & spine	Are pain patches in place or do they need to be changed? Does the family know how to boost the patient back up in bed when they slide down?
Legs & feet	Circulation	Are family members interested/concerned with learning the assessment technique of feeling the feet and limbs for coolness and examining for mottling as they progress slowly from the periphery to the center of the body during the last few hours of life?
	Soothing	Would applying aromatic lotion to feet & legs comfort the patient and give family members something meaningful to do?
Abdomen	Bowels	If the patient is incontinent of stool, do family members are comfortable and know how to provide personal hygiene? Do family members know how to use protective pads, adult diapers, pull sheets to keep the patient clean? If stools are frequent, can anti-diarrheals be given?
	Bed	Does the family know how to make an occupied bed, using good body mechanics?
	Skin	Are protective ointments needed to decrease skin breakdown if the incontinence is frequent? Are pressure points up off of the bed?
Pelvis	Urine	If incontinence is present, would inserting a Foley catheter prevent skin irritation & conserve the patient's & family's energies? Is the family comfortable doing this? Are others available to insert the catheter?

◆ Listen for and solicit comments regarding the efficacy of spiritual practices. For instance, if the patient is a person who prays, ask, "Are your prayers bringing you comfort and peace?"

◆ Assess for expressions of fear, panic attacks, or an increase in physical symptoms such as restlessness, agitation, pain, or shortness of breath that may indicate intense spiritual distress. Evaluate for the need for a chaplain's intervention to provide spiritual comfort and to assist the patient in reaching peace, possibly reducing the need for medications.

◆ Determine the need and desire of the patient and family to engage in forgiveness, to express feelings to one another, and to say their good-byes. Assess the need to facilitate phone conversations if the family member or friend cannot be present physically and to educate the family to hold the phone up to the dying patient's ear to hear the voice at the other end, even if the patient cannot move or is comatose.

◆ Assess for a prolonged dying process that may indicate the patient is having difficulty letting go, perhaps due to some unfinished business, an unsaid good-bye, or fears related to dying. Explore with the patient and family what these issues might be and assess for the need for a chaplain referral.

◆ Assess for readiness of the family to celebrate the life of the loved one by acknowledging his or her contributions to family members, close friends, and the community.

◆ Explore the need and desire for additional comfort measures in the environment, such as soothing music, devotional readings, gazing out a window at nature, or increased quiet.

◆ Ask the family about their anticipated needs and preferences at the time of death: "Is there anyone you will want us to call for you?" "What can the healthcare team do to be most supportive?" "Are there specific practices regarding the care of the body that you want the team to carry out?"

Case study

Tarana's death

The morning after the wedding, Marala found Tarana in bed, unresponsive with labored breathing. Her left arm was contracted and the left side of her face was drooping severely. In spite of Tarana's enrollment in hospice, Marala called 911. The EMTs intubated Tarana and brought her to the hospital where she was put on a ventilator. Imaging showed that she had experienced a massive CVA with intracranial bleeding and a significant midline shift. Her prognosis for recovery was poor.

Her family arrived at the hospital. After much family discussion and interaction with the palliative care team, the healthcare power of attorney proceeded to agree to a change in code status as well as to approve a palliative ventilator withdrawal.

Krupa asked to have Tarana's feet pointed toward Mecca and family members took turns reading from the Qu'ran. After receiving the orders from the intensivist nurse practitioner, the nurse deactivated the AICD, premedicated Tarana, and then withdrew the ventilator. After a few hours, Tarana began making rattling noises and began agonal breathing. Krupa expressed that the sounds were very bothersome to her and asked that her sister be placed on oxygen. The nurse requested an order for glycopyrrolate for terminal secretions and initiated humidified oxygen via nasal cannula at a flow rate of 2 liters/minute.

Tarana was moved to a bed on the Acute Palliative Care Unit. The room lights were dimmed and her favorite CD was played quietly in the room. As she declined, the nurse noticed discolorations in her upper and lower extremities, which were partially obscured by her dark skin tone, and taught the family about mottling and about the progressive cold temperature of Tarana's legs. Later than night, Tarana stopped breathing and her heart stopped beating. Tarana died surrounded by her loved ones. The healthcare team who had come to know Tarana and her family over the course of her illness joined the family as they all wept. Tarana's body was prepared for a Muslim burial.

The goals of the palliative care nursing assessment during Tarana's active dying phase are to:

◆ Evaluate Tarana and her family frequently for comfort including the need for extra chairs, the desire for coffee, and reminders to take breaks from time to time.

◆ Assess the environment for factors that are calm and soothing.

◆ Be vigilant for adherence to the patient's religious and cultural preferences in spite of the absence of written advance directives.

◆ Determine the need to resolve conflict about end-of-life care preferences and measures that could be implemented to improve patient and family outcomes.

◆ Discover the need to educate the family on the appropriate response to changes in a dying loved one's status.

◆ Inquire about the family's readiness to learn about the hospice's community grief program.

◆ Determine one's own needs and the staff need for support after caring for a patient for a long time that has now died.

Conclusion: Principles of patient and family assessment

A comprehensive palliative care nursing assessment of the patient and family occurs throughout the trajectory of the illness and is a holistic view that includes the physical, psychosocial, and spiritual domains. Patient and family assessment provides the foundation for mutual goal setting, devising a plan of care, implementing interventions, and evaluating the effectiveness of care. Reassessments are done throughout the patient's illness, looking for changes from previous assessments to ensure that quality of life is maximized in all domains (Box 4.11).

Maximizing quality of life for patients and families is a process. It is a journey that the nurse and all members of the transdisciplinary healthcare team travel alongside of the patient and family. The palliative care nurse understands above all, that irrespective of the phase or focus of the assessment, two of the most important assessment questions that the nurse can ask the patient and family are "What is your greatest concern?" and "How can I be of help?"

Box 4.11 Best practice tip

Clinicians who are in ambulatory settings may find the use of an abbreviated symptom assessment form helpful to track the efficacy of palliative care interventions. Whereas pain is usually plotted along the familiar 0–10 scale, other symptoms such as nausea, vomiting, diarrhea, constipation, fatigue, anxiety, and depression can be quickly evaluated on a flow sheet as, mild, moderate, or severe. Also, the PPS can provide a numerical evaluation of functionality that is quick to record and compare. These kinds of tools assist in transdisciplinary evaluation of symptoms and patient status without requiring paging through lengthy progress notes. In this way, treatment can be highly individualized and more evidence-based.

References

1. Broyard A. Intoxicated by My Illness. New York, NY: Balantine Books; 1992.
2. Potter P, Perry A. Fundamentals of Nursing. 7th ed. St. Louis, MO: Elsevier Mosby; 2013.
3. Jarvis C. Physical Examination and Health Assessment. 6th ed. St. Louis, MO: Saunders; 2011.
4. Norman GR, Eva KW. Diagnostic error and clinical reasoning. Med Educ. 2010;44:94–100.
5. Ferrell B, Koczywas M, Grannis F, Harrington A. Palliative care in lung cancer. Surg Clin North Am. 2011;91(2):403–417. http://dx.doi.org/10.1016/j.suc.2010.12.003.
6. Eckroth-Bucher M. Self-awareness: a review and analysis of a basic nursing concept. Adv Nurs Sci. 2010;33(3):297–309.
7. Gunasekara I, Pentland T, Rodgers T, Patterson S. What makes an excellent mental health nurse? A pragmatic inquiry initiated and conducted by people with lived experience of service use. Int J Ment Health Nurs. 2014;23(2):101–109
8. Facts and Figures: Hospice Care in America. Washington, DC: National Hospice and Palliative Care Organization; 2012. http://www.nhpco.org/sites/default/files/public/Statistics_Research/2012_Facts_Figures.pdf. Accessed June 3, 2013.
9. Maltoni M, Scarpi E, Pittureri C, Martini F, Montanari L, Amaducci E, et al. Prospective comparison of prognostic scores in palliative care cancer populations. Oncologist. 2012;17(3):446–454.
10. Frenkel M, Ari SL, Engebretson J, Peterson N, Maimon Y, Cohen L, et al. Activism among exceptional patients with cancer. Support Care Cancer. 2011;19(8):1125–1132.
11. Holland JC, Breitbart WS, Jacobsen PB, Lederberg MS, Loscalzo MJ, McCorkle R. Psycho-Oncology. 2nd ed. New York, NY: Oxford University Press; 2010.
12. Pausch R. The Last Lecture. New York, NY: Hyperion; 2008.
13. Pausch, J. Dream New Dreams: Reimagining My Life After Loss. New York, NY: Harmony; 2012.
14. Flaskerud J. Grief and depression: are they different? Issues Ment Health Nurs. 2011;32;338–340.
15. American Psychiatric Association. Diagnostic and Statistical Manual of Mental Disorders. 5th ed. Arlington, VA: American Psychiatric Publishing; 2013.
16. Wakefield JC, First MB. Validity of the bereavement exclusion to major depression: does the empirical evidence support the proposal to eliminate the exclusion in DSM-5? World Psychiatry. 2012;11(1):3–10.
17. Wakefield JC. DSM-5 grief scorecard: assessment and outcomes of proposals to pathologize grief. World Psychiatry. 2013;12(2):171–173.
18. Vodermaier A, Linden W, Siu C. Screening for emotional distress in cancer patients: a systematic review of assessment instruments. J Natl Cancer Inst. 2009;101(21):1464–1488.
19. Puchalski C, Ferrell B, Virani R, Otis-Green S, Baird P, Bull J, et al. Improving the quality of spiritual care as a dimension of palliative care: the report of the Consensus Conference. J Palliat Med. 2009;12(10):885–905.
20. Frankl V. Man's Search for Meaning. Boston, MA: Beacon Press; 1959.
21. Maslow AH. Motivation and Personality. 3rd ed. Hummelstown, PA: Scott Foresman-Addison Wesley; 1987.
22. Fitchett, G, Risk, J. Screening for spiritual struggle. J Pastoral Care Counsel. 2009;63(4):1–12.
23. Pethel L, Engel JD. The Palliative Care and Hospice Caregiver's Workbook: Sharing the Journey with the Dying. Oxon, UK: Radcliff; 2010.
24. Lembke A, Humphreys K. What self-help organizations tell us about the syndrome model of addiction. In: Shaffer H, et al. (eds.), APA Addiction Syndrome Handbook, Vol. 2: Recovery, Prevention, and Other Issues. APA handbooks in psychology. Washington, DC: American Psychological Association; 2012:157–168.
25. Park CL. Trauma and meaning making: converging conceptualizations and emerging evidence. In: Hicks JA, Rutledge C. (eds.), The Experience of Meaning in Life: Classical Perspectives, Emerging Themes, and Controversies. New York, NY: Springer; 2013:61–76.
26. The Joint Commission. Advancing Effective Communication, Cultural Competence, and Patient- and Family-Centered Care: A Roadmap for Hospitals. Oakbrook Terrace, IL: The Joint Commission; 2010.
27. Purnell L. Transcultural Healthcare: A Culturally Competent Approach. 4th ed. Philadelphia, PA: FA Davis; 2012.
28. Hadziabdic E, Hjelm K. Working with interpreters: practical advice for use of an interpreter in healthcare. Int J Evid Based Healthc. 2013;11(1):69–76.
29. Hadziabdic E, Albin B, Heikkila K, Hjelm K. Family members' experiences of the use of interpreters in healthcare. Prim Health Care Res Dev. 2013;12:1–14.
30. POLST: Physician Orders for Life Sustaining Treatment Paradigm. Portland, OR: National POLST Paradigm Task Force; 2012. http://www.polst.org. Accessed July 16, 2013.
31. Genetic Testing Clinical Reference for Clinicians. Washington, DC: American College of Preventive Medicine; 2009. http://www.acpm.org/?GeneticTestgClinRef. Accessed June 18, 2013.
32. Yancy CW, Jessup M, Bozkurt B, Masoudi FA, Butler J, McBride PE, et al. ACCF/AHA guideline for the management of heart failure: a report of the American College of Cardiology Foundation/American Heart Association Task Force on Practice Guidelines. J Am Coll Cardiol. 2013;62(16):e147–e239.
33. NYHA Classification—The Stages of Heart Failure. Chevy Chase, MD: Heart Failure Society of America; 2011. http://www.abouthf.org/questions_stages.htm. Accessed June 22, 2013.
34. Chan E, Wu H, Chan Y. Revisiting the Palliative Performance Scale: change in scores during disease trajectory predicts survival. Palliat Med. 2013;27(4):367–374.
35. Rancour P. Using archetypes and transitions theory to assist patients to move from active treatment to survivorship. Clin J Oncol Nurs. 2008;12(6):935–940. doi:10.1188/08.CJON. 935-40.
36. Levin TT, Alici T. Anxiety disorders, In: Holland J, et al. (eds.), Psycho-Oncology. 2nd ed. New York, NY: Oxford University Press; 2010:324–331.
37. Massie MJ. Depressive disorders. In: Holland J et al. (eds.), Psycho-Oncology. 2nd ed. New York, NY: Oxford University Press; 2010:311–318.
38. Pessin H, Amakawa L, Breitbart WS. Suicide. In: Holland J, et al. (eds.), Psycho-Oncology. 2nd ed. New York, NY: Oxford University Press; 2010:319–323.
39. LeShan LL, Achterberg J, Muller W, McElroy SC, Rossman ML. Cancer as a Turning Point, Volume II: From Surviving to Thriving. Louisville, CO: Sounds True; 2008.
40. Li R, Cooper C, Bradley J, Shulman A, Livingston G. Coping strategies and psychological morbidity in family carers of people with dementia: a systematic review and meta-analysis. J Affect Disord. 2012;139(1):1–11. doi:10.1016/j.jad.2011.05.055
41. Knabe HE. The meaning of hope for patients coping with a terminal illness: a review of literature. J Palliative Care Med. 2013;S2:004. doi:10.4172/2165-7386.S2-004
42. Threshold Choir. Santa Rosa, CA: Threshold Choir; 2012. http://thresholdchoir.org. Accessed June 18, 2013.
43. Chalice of Repose Project: The Voice of Music-Thanatology. Mt. Angel, OR: The Chalice of Repose Project; 2013. http://chaliceofrepose.org/. Accessed June 18, 2013.
44. Rancour P. Integrating complementary and alternative therapies into end-of-life care. InTouch: A Hospice and Palliative Care Resource of the Ohio Hospice and Palliative Care Organization. 2008;12:8–10.
45. Park CL, Lim H, Newlon M, Suresh DP, Bliss DE. Dimensions of religiousness and spirituality as predictors of well-being in advanced chronic heart failure patients. J Relig Health. 2014;53(2):579–590.

CHAPTER 5

Communication in palliative care

An essential competency for nurses

Constance M. Dahlin and
Elaine Wittenberg

Communication sets the stage for the therapeutic relationship, providing
the nurse with a context of the patient and the family's individual, unique,
response to illness.[1]

Key points

- Effective communication, the foundation to quality palliative
  care, assures an individualized, respectful approach to care,
  from diagnosis to death, with regard to values, preferences, and
  beliefs.

- The art of nursing communication includes listening, silence,
  presence, and therapeutic use of self to facilitate a patient- and
  family-centered process.

- Communication, a learned skill that establishes the
  nurse-patient relationship, is composed of 20% verbal and 80%
  nonverbal characteristics.

- Nursing communication includes gathering and imparting
  information, providing support, and reassurance, as dictated
  by the individual needs of patients and families.

- Nurses have a direct role in difficult conversations such as
  advance care planning (ACP), delivery of bad news, poor prognosis, or transition to hospice and palliative care.

- Communication is essential in team collaboration and conflict
  management.

Introduction

Communication is the cornerstone of palliative care; it is the
essence of the art and science of palliative nursing.[2] Essential
aspects of nursing communication include caring, collaboration,
continuous presence, fostering of hope, patient advocacy, and support.[2] The National Consensus Project for Quality Palliative Care
Clinical Guidelines for Quality Palliative Care 3rd Edition emphasizes communication as the basis of care in this statement: "The
care plan is based on the identified and expressed preferences,
values, goals, and needs of the patient and family and is developed
with professional guidance and support for patient-family decision
making."[3] To achieve quality care, the process of care-planning
must be accompanied by relief of pain and other distressing symptoms, preparation for death, and the opportunity for life closure.
Thus, effective communication promotes assessment of the physical, psychological, social, and spiritual domains.

Palliative nursing crosses all specialty areas of nursing practice.
Within all populations of patients—pediatrics to geriatrics, medicine to surgery and critical care, myriad diseases and conditions—
there are seriously ill patients who would benefit from palliative
care. Communication is essential to the delivery of quality palliative care. These patients will face difficult physical and psychological symptoms, resulting in poor quality of life and ultimately
death. In some instances, it is not a matter of *if* patients will die;
it is a matter of how and when. A good death is measured by the
degree to which the plan reflects the individuality and the values,
preferences, and beliefs of the patient and their family unit.

Nurses have an important role in the team process and are
essential in promoting optimal communication among the team,
patient, and family. Although some nurses view their role as indirect and limited, the vital role of nurses in palliative care communication is well established.[4] Nurses at all levels of practice
assist patients to define their goals and wishes as well as express
their cultural and religious practices and preferences. Nurses
then play a critical role in advocating for and implementing the
patient's wishes and preferences and communicating these to
family members and other healthcare providers. This role was
initially delineated in 1998 within the American Association of
Colleges of Nursing's document *A Peaceful Death: Recommended
Competencies and Curricular Guidelines for End-of-Life*. One
core competency for end-of-life nursing care is communication.

Nurses should "communicate effectively and compassionately with the patient, family, and health care team members about end-of-life issues."[5]

Since that time, a more active nursing role in communication has evolved, and many nurse organizations endorse full participation of nursing in palliative communication.[4,6] The American Nurses Association (ANA) *Nursing: Scope and Standards of Practice* includes a communication standard stating the nurse's responsibility to assess communication format preferences of patients, families, and colleagues; assess his or her own communication skills; convey information to patients, families, and the interdisciplinary team; maintain communication to promote safe and effective transfers of care; and provide professional perspective in healthcare discussions.[7] Specific to palliative care, ANA delineates the role of the nurse in the position statement *Registered Nurses' Roles and Responsibilities in Providing Expert Care and Counseling at the End of Life.* This statement says, "The counseling a nurse provides regarding end-of-life choices and preferences for individuals facing life-limiting illness, as well as throughout the patient's life span, honors patient autonomy, and helps to prepare individuals and families for difficult decisions that may lie ahead."[8] In addition, "Nurses must advocate for and play an active role in initiating discussions about DNR with patients, families, and members of the health care team" as described in the position statement *Nursing Care and Do Not Resuscitate (DNR) and Allow Natural Death (AND) Decisions.*[9]

The Hospice and Palliative Nursing Association reinforces the integral aspect of communication throughout palliative nursing. In *Palliative Nursing: Scope and Standards of Practice*, the expectation of competency in communication is described in the following:[10]

- The hospice and palliative registered nurse communicates effectively in a variety of formats in all areas of practice.

- The nurse uses effective verbal, nonverbal, and written communication with patients and families, interdisciplinary team members, and the community.

- The hospice and palliative registered nurse communicates with the patient, family, the interdisciplinary team, and healthcare providers regarding patient care and the provision of that care. The nurse facilitates an interdisciplinary process.

A specific registered nurse competency states that the nurse "demonstrates the use of effective verbal, non-verbal, and written communication with patients, families, members of the healthcare team and community in order to therapeutically address and accurately convey the palliative needs of patients and families."[11] Finally, the *HPNA Position Statement: The Nurse's Role in Advanced Care Planning* explains the critical role of the hospice and palliative nurse to advocate, educate, and support a patient's right to self-determination, autonomy, and dignity. Recognizing the diversity in personal, religious, and cultural value systems, the hospice and palliative nurse develops respectful relationships with patients, families, and colleagues.[12] This rapport affords hospice and palliative nurses the unique role of facilitating care throughout the illness trajectory, including providing information about treatment options and facilitating documentation that captures the patients' values, preferences, and beliefs.

Overview

Within their undergraduate education, few nurses receive formal education specific to communication, let alone in palliative care. Yet, nurses rank communication as the most important competency.[13] Over 20 years ago, Degner and Gow described protecting student nurses from death education until they graduated.[14] Although nurses are now exposed to care along the disease trajectory, this phenomenon continues today as nurses still feel unprepared in communication skills.[15,16] This may be more pronounced in an age when there is greater ease and comfort in social media than in face-to-face encounters. In one author's experience (CMD), when young nurses are asked about their communication fears, the themes are consistent with the literature. They include fear about saying the wrong thing, causing emotional distress or sadness that they feel unequipped to manage, showing emotion with patients and families, or not having permission by the clinical team to discuss serious matters.[4,6,16]

Nurses avoid palliative communication experiences, rationalizing that they won't be responsible for the care of seriously ill or dying patients within their chosen patient population. However, this is no longer valid reasoning. The National Consensus Project *Clinical Practice Guidelines* describes patients suitable for palliative care as those with "a broad range of diagnostic categories, living with a persistent or recurring medical condition that adversely affects their daily functioning or will predictably reduce life expectancy."[3] Specifically, these patients include individuals with chronic and life-threatening injuries from accidents or other forms of trauma or stroke; those with congenital injuries, developmental and intellectual conditions leading to dependence on life-sustaining treatments and/or long-term care, supported by others to perform their activities of daily living; those with progressive chronic conditions (e.g., peripheral vascular disease, malignancies, renal or liver failure, stroke with significant functional impairment, advanced heart or lung disease, frailty, various forms of dementia, and neurodegenerative disorders); and vulnerable, underserved, and underresourced populations who develop serious or life-threatening illness (e.g., homeless individuals, immigrants, individuals with low income, oppressed racial and ethnic groups, veterans, prisoners, older adults, and individuals with mental illness).[3] The shift of palliative care from the last few months of life to coping with the actual diagnosis of a serious, life-threatening illness allows more patients to access and benefit from such care. The result is more palliative patients across the health spectrum necessitating greater nursing involvement. Moreover, the diversity of populations and the range of life-limiting illnesses require an array of communication strategies and interventions.

Nursing opportunities for communication arise during patient care including task-related care, personal care, illness education, bad news delivery, assessment of spiritual and religious concerns, in response to physical and psychological distress, and within interdisciplinary collaboration.[17] There are myriad settings beyond the home or the hospital including where care occurs: rehabilitation facilities; ambulatory or outpatient clinics; long-term care facilities; Veterans facilities; correctional facilities; homeless shelters; and mental health settings. Often it is the nurse who is the consistent health provider. It is essential that nurses understand the potential for communication interactions, as well as the challenges. Without effective communication, the patient's experience of suffering is unknown, and effective symptom control is impossible.[18,19]

Historical perspective of communication at the end of life

Communication for seriously ill and dying patients has changed dramatically over the last 150 years. Up until the 19th century, the lack of effective medical therapies for many infections, illnesses, and diseases resulted in deaths at younger ages. Death was a visible phenomenon and part of everyday life. Deaths commonly occurred at home and surrounded by family. Nurses were commonly exposed to disease and death as they often provided private duty care to these patients.

Death and dying then became more invisible as patients moved into hospitals to die. Until the 1960s, the process of death and dying itself went unacknowledged. The patient lay in a hospital bed, clearly failing but with little prospect to voice concerns or feelings about the process. Any discussion about the dying person occurred among healthcare providers and sometimes included a short discussion with family.[20] Thus, people died in isolation, with the possibility of anxiety, fear, and abandonment. Moreover, the indirect communication and lack of truth-telling caused nurses to engage in inauthentic interactions, resulting in moral distress.[20]

From the 1960s to the 1980s, the principles of informed consent and autonomy became valued aspects of healthcare. This meant patients were told the facts about their care whether they wanted this information or not. In the 1990s, the pendulum swung the other way; truth-telling became a central focus of terminal care.[21] Instead of withholding information about a terminal illness, death and dying became an open topic of discussion for patients. However, such conversations were held irrespective of the patient's and family's culture, values, preferences, or beliefs. Active patient participation in healthcare became the underlying value with a hope for greater sense of control and diminished anxiety.

Just as social norms regarding serious illness and death and dying discussions changed, there were changes in theories about communication skills. For a long time, communication skills were considered to be intuitive or inherited traits. Practitioners either had empathetic and effective communication skills or not.[21] Later, it was evident that communication skills, like other healthcare competencies, could be acquired by healthcare providers.[21]

Since 2000, there has been a focus on teaching palliative-care specific communication skills. These skills center on topics such as advance care planning, goals of care, breaking bad news, and family meetings.[18] As the health professional with the most access to patients, nurses are essential in these conversations. They have a realistic perspective of the patient and the family in all domains of care. However, nurses are often left out of difficult conversations, resulting in inconsistency and discontinuity of care. Nurses need to both participate in such conversations and lead them.

Effective communication

Communication is described as a conditional process that supports the patient's individual coping style.[22] It is a central aspect of patient- and family-centered care, whereby the needs of the patient and family dictate care. Communication promotes many critical aspects of care: information sharing; active listening; identification of values, goals, and healthcare preferences; decision-making; offers support and facilitates collaboration.[2,23] Effective communication, as viewed by seriously ill patients and their families, primarily consists of providing accurate information in a sensitive, simple, and straightforward manner, using plain language.

Good communication allows for optimal palliative care, as it is the basis of the relationship.[1,24] Communication grounds a strong nurse-patient relationship that provides a therapeutic basis for the care.[2] Specific nursing behaviors focus on the promotion of information sharing, disclosure, reassurance, presence, facilitation, and dignity.[25,26] Indeed, emotional intelligence may promote more effective communication. Specific abilities include (1) the correct identification of emotions in oneself and others; (2) the use of emotions to facilitate reasoning, understanding emotions; and (3) managing emotions.[27]

Nurse interactions have been described within the following categories: supporting, caring, collaborating, reassuring, fostering hope, and advocating for the patient.[14,26] Research speaks to the various aspects of communication: active listening, presence, eliciting preferences, and facilitating communication choices.[28] There seems to be agreement that the establishment of trust, continuity, and understanding fosters good relationships.[24] Moreover, it is also important that the nurse have a healthy coping style and understanding of timing in communication. Box 5.1 reviews valued communication behaviors.

Creating a patient-centered approach facilitates more effective communication.[22] Research has revealed that patients desire honesty and hope in their healthcare providers. Focusing on quality of life offers hope and meaning to the patient, leaving open the possibility of "miracles," while simultaneously assisting the patient to prepare for losses.[4] Honesty can be achieved through open dialogue and determining patient readiness to discuss serious illness, death, and/or dying.[29] Additionally, discussing outcomes other than cure, such as improved functional status or independence in care needs, focuses care on the current situation.

Box 5.1 Communication behaviors valued by patients and families

Being present and being silent

Being in the moment

Knowing and being comfortable with oneself

Knowing the other person

Connecting

Affirming and valuing

Acknowledging vulnerability

Utilizing intuition

Empathizing and willing to be vulnerable

Providing serenity and silence

Sources: Boreale and Richardson (2011), reference 52; Wittenberg-Lyles et al. (2012), reference 42.

The role of the nurse in palliative care

Within the spectrum of healthcare, nurses are one of the most trusted members of the healthcare team across the spectrum, from diagnosis during treatment and in the final stages of life. Since relief of suffering is the basis of nursing, all nurses practice some aspects of palliative care. Nurses relieve suffering through various communication modalities: availability, presence, empathy, respect, listening and talking, eye contact, smile, warm voice tone, words of comfort, caring, encouragement and even humor, as well as the use of touch.[30] Essentially, this is achieved through therapeutic presence: attending to suffering, affirming the patient's self-worth and dignity, decreasing isolation, facilitating identification and clarification of treatment goals, promoting ACP and enhancing holistic care.[31]

The nurse has a pivotal role in accompanying the patient through this journey and can create a healing environment within a poignant situation. Nurses are often first to identify issues for patients with life-threatening illness. Through direct patient care and constant presence at the bedside, the nurse may have the best opportunity to learn the patient's hopes, fears, dreams, and regrets. He or she has the opportunity to facilitate a process that allows the patients to state their care wishes and the family's ability to hear those wishes. These may be related to advanced care planning, goals of care, conflict between patient and family wishes, and use of life-sustaining measures for patients with life-threatening illnesses.

There are clear elements of communication that patients and families desire that have been demonstrated through research. One study described satisfactory patient communication as compassionate, responsive, and dedicated; while unsatisfactory patient communication was sparse, conflicted, contradictory, and increasing only when things were close to the end.[32] Overall, it appears patients and families wanted consistent and routine communication with a compassionate presence.[33] Required communication skills broadly include effective listening, appropriate nonverbal communication, counseling skills, empathy, and supportiveness.[5] Research revealed that the most beneficial behaviors for families are (1) keeping family informed, (2) providing assurance, (3) being a compassionate presence, (4) facilitating final acts, and (5) honoring dignity.[26] These behaviors reflect both verbal and nonverbal skills. Another study categorized nurses' communication as the following: skills that explore patient concerns, provision of support, enhancing disclosure, educational preparation, and referral, as necessary, for further counseling.[25] Essentially, facilitative styles that reflect the therapeutic use of self and patient-centered care are more beneficial.[22]

There are several levels of communication for the nurse to address. One is day-to-day interactions surrounding the tasks involved in caring for the patient. On a simple level, this may involve small talk, or discussion of basic treatment issues, such as pain medication schedules, activities of daily living, or personal care. Another level is assessment of treatments. The nurse approaches the patient in an open manner to allow the patient to honestly evaluate the response of treatments, hoping to gain more specific information concerning treatment effectiveness, distress, or pain. The third and most complex level of communication is the existential level. This occurs at the level of the patient's deepest sense of self. Communication at this level is sensitive and often nuanced because the existential aspects of end-of-life include disclosure, searching for meaning, and suffering.[19] Exploration at this level can help a patient to live with a life-threatening illness, achieving both quality of life and psychological healing.[34]

Across the palliative care spectrum, communication occurs at critical junctures. Depending on the diagnosis or condition of the patient, such communication may occur over a long or a short period of time. Since 80%–90% of patients who die have a chronic illness, there are usually many opportunities for communication to occur.[3] Within the nurse-patient relationship, Perrin speaks about three stages: introductory, middle, and termination.[35] The introductory phase is where the nurse and the patient learn about each other's styles. The middle phase involves establishing a working relationship in which the work is done, such as pain and symptom management, discussions about the meaning of life, along with legacy work and family work. The final and third phase is termination, in which the nurse and the patient say goodbye to each other either because the patient or nurse is leaving the system or the patient is dying.

The initial communication or introductory phase starts at diagnosis with the introduction of the nurse as a member of the care team. During this period, the nurse assesses the patient's learning styles and information needs, and the patient determines the style of the nurse.[35] The tasks of the nurse include exploring the patient's understanding of his or her illness, eliciting personality and coping styles, and identifying existing documents related to the delegation of surrogate decisionmakers, advance directives, or out of hospital medical orders for life-sustaining treatments. Assessing learning style includes discerning the patient's ability to learn and to understand the seriousness of the illness. These abilities vary according to the age and cognitive development of the patient, as well as literacy, numeracy (capacity for numerical thought and expression), and native language. For children and some older adults, the family or support unit is primarily involved in the information process. The introductory phase leads into the next phase.

The working phase often extends over a long period of time. Supportive care focuses on lifestyle changes from a serious, life-threatening illness, including information on the condition, treatment, and management (pharmacological, nonpharmacological, and interventional).[36] The patient and family establish trust with the nurse, who provides presence, emotional support, and reassurance.[35,36] The nurse has insight into patient and family coping and articulates their concerns or perceptions of care. At this time, according to Pierce, the nurse fulfills three critical communication tasks in end-of-life care: (1) creates an environment conducive to communication, (2) eases interaction between physician and patient, and (3) facilitates interaction between family and patient.[37] Therefore, difficult discussions of bad news require nursing presence at critical conversations. This allows the nurse to offer his or her perspectives of care and facilitates follow-up using similar language and shared information.

As the patient enters the dying process, the termination phase commences. It should be noted that termination may also occur if the patient changes practice settings or the nurse transitions to another position. Nevertheless, the nurse offers continued presence and reassurance in monitoring comfort and providing intensive caring to both the patient and family.[32] Communication between the nurse and the patient and family focuses on support of decision-making, assurance of comfort, relief from pain and symptoms, information about the dying process, and solace in anticipatory grieving. The nurse and the patient are able to come to some closure as the patient dies. Immediately following the death, the nurse has a critical role in providing family support to promote a healthy grief and bereavement process as much as possible.

Nursing presence at any discussions—particularly when important information is conveyed—cannot be overemphasized. The team may need education regarding nursing's pivotal role in patient advocacy, particularly in supporting the patient after difficult conversations. If a primary nurse is not able to participate in important discussions, a nursing colleague may participate to offer a nursing perspective. If this is not possible, it is essential that the team review the specifics about the conversation with the nurse—in particular the news delivered, the phrasing used, and the patient's response. This allows the nurse to provide collaborative follow-up support. Sometimes the nurse may be reticent and wait to be invited, rather than being proactive to participate or facilitate such discussions. This can result in the nurse feeling uninformed, undervalued, ultimately leading to ineffective care.

Although communication seems fairly straightforward, it is actually a complex, continual transactional process that occurs between persons by which information, feelings, and meaning are conveyed through verbal and nonverbal messages.[38] As viewed by multiple goals theory, communication interaction is seen as the exchange of ideas around a task as well as the exchange of ideas around a relationship. In essence, multiple goals theory describes every message as possessing two levels of meaning: the content level and the relationship level.[39,40]

In professional contexts, these can be referred to as the *task* and *relationship* levels. Message content generally concerns the *tasks* of communication—for example, instructing, diagnosing, managing, directing, encouraging, supporting, and so forth. *Relationship* refers both to how people interpret the content of messages and how they understand their shared connection. For example, if a nurse asks a patient, "What is your pain level today?" the content is obviously an inquiry designed to obtain information about the patient's pain. Still, the relationship level of meaning is determined by how these words are spoken. If the nurse is glancing at paperwork or working with medical equipment while she asks this question, and no eye contact is made, or if she is standing in the hallway rather than at the bedside, the patient will likely interpret as a matter of routine communication rather than a genuine inquiry. As a result, no relational components are developed within the exchange.

While the content level of a message is conveyed by the words themselves, the relational level generally is manifested by nonverbal communication. Nonverbal communication includes physical appearance, the nurse's body type and clothing, both of which influence perception. Artifacts, the presence of physical objects and the environmental setting, can be barriers to developing relationships with patients and families. These objects include bedrails, bedside tables, and other medical equipment, which can reduce the emotional connection during conversation. A nurse sitting for a short time at the bedside versus standing at a distance and separated by bedrails can greatly impact communication. Vocalics, the variety of ways that words are spoken including volume, pitch, accent, rate of speech, use of pauses, and tone, also are part of nonverbal communication. The way the voice is used communicates loudly on a relational level. For example, speaking loudly to an elderly patient who has good hearing can be condescending and distance the nurse from the patient. Proxemics, the way space and distance is used during communication, and whether or not it is respected and acknowledged during nursing work can impact relational communication. Finally, haptics, or the use of touch, can be task-related but can also convey relational messages of warmth and caring.

Communication barriers

Communication barriers exist for the patient, the family, and the nurse. For the patient, there are many psychological barriers such as anger, fear, sadness, and helplessness that prevent communication.[23] Patients feel any discussion will cause too much distress for themselves and/or their families. For some patients, communication is not an area of comfort or value, so they may have little interest in processing feelings or information. Cultural factors that affect communication such as language and literacy may exist for the patient. Educational level and health literacy prevents comprehensive communication, particularly when medical language and jargon are used. Depending on socioeconomic status, patients may be overwhelmed with insurance issues, appointments, tests, procedures, and treatments and their cost implications. Patients may engage in a bit of "magical thinking"—that is the fear that talking about something may make it happen. The healthcare environment is often a barrier; the fast-paced, noisy, and unfamiliar atmosphere results in overstimulation limiting communication. Finally, physical limitations such as cognitive, vision, hearing, and speech impairments as well as pain or exhaustion may limit communication.[41]

Families share many of these same barriers. However, there are additional considerations. Families may not understand the full extent of illness and may not know what to discuss. Moreover, families may find it too painful to talk about the advanced state of their loved one's illness as such discussion triggers anticipatory grief and loss. In order to maintain hope, families tend to overestimate the possibility of cure. They also fear future regrets if they do not pursue or demand further curative treatment. Lastly, it is not uncommon that family members have little knowledge of the patient's preferences for types of care. Therefore, their ability to fully participate in decision-making in the context of the patient's preferences is limited.

Circumstantial barriers exist as well.[42] These barriers include time for the nurse to attend to the patient or fully discuss issues. Time is always an issue. The scheduling of patients with layered appointments and tests may allow for little reflective time or time for meaningful discussion. Changes in the patient's condition may prevent full discussion of details, considerations, or future treatment. Families may be uninformed and receiving mixed messages. Situations where information exchange must occur by telephone prevent the nurse from "reading" the family's nonverbal communication.

Communication barriers for nurses include personal, professional, and legal concerns. Nurses may have difficulty or discomfort with communication due to personality, cultural norms, struggles of unresolved grief, fear of their own mortality, or fear of being emotional in front of a patient.[43,44] Lack of education or training, or lack of personal and professional experience with death and dying means they have little exposure to end-of-life communication.[13,45]

Young nurses worry that bringing up issues related to death and dying will cause too much emotional distress to the patient and family.[43,44] Or they may worry they will get in trouble with their colleagues. Other nurses are concerned that talking about palliative issues will result in patient and family conflict.[46] Finally, even though communication is part of the scope of practice and advocacy and information sharing is part of their role, many nurses misperceive palliative care communication as out of their purview.

Consequently, nurses may employ avoidance behaviors surrounding communication. A nurse may focus more on the biomedical aspects, particularly using technical medical jargon, thereby avoiding any elicitation of or response to a patient's thoughts and feelings.[23] The nurse may focus only on the present time, thereby preventing the patient from expressing concerns about a previous time. For example, rather than listening to the patient share concerns from an earlier time, the nurse may stop the conversation by saying, "But how are you now?" Another way of avoiding discussion is to change the focus or the subject. For example, if the patient says, "I am worried about my family," the nurse may divert the conversation by saying, "So, how is your nausea?" Sometimes the nurse may interrupt the conversation by offering advice: "Of course, you will get over this in time. It won't last for too long." Another avoidance technique is responding to a patient's expressed difficulties by stating, "Clearly you need to talk to the social worker about your issues."[47] Or, "this is not my role to discuss this." Finally, nurses and physicians may collude with patients in avoiding any discussions of death and dying, preventing any information-sharing with the patient.[48,49]

The COMFORT model: a model for effective communication

A novel communication training curriculum named COMFORT, an acronym that identifies the basic principles of nurse communication, is offered as a communication framework.[42] Built from evidence-based research in hospice and palliative care settings, the COMFORT curriculum teaches nurses to focus concomitantly on task and relational communication as a way of improving communication and resolving communication challenges. These seven principles include narrative clinical practice (**C-Communicate**), health/cultural literacy (**O-Orientation and Opportunity**), presence in practice (**M-Mindful presence**), the role of family caregivers (**F-Family**), transitions in care (**O-Openings**), patient/family needs (**R-Relating**), and teamwork (**T-Team**). COMFORT is designed to assist nurses with the practice of biopsychosocial and patient-centered communication. The framework is not a linear guide, an algorithm, a protocol, or a rubric for sequential implementation by nurses but rather a set of holistic principles that can be used concurrently and reflectively in the care of patients/families with life-limiting illness.

The COMFORT curriculum is grounded in a narrative approach to communication and champions relationships among nurse, patient, family, and team members to create a collaborative environment for integrated care, from diagnosis to death. In narrative clinical practice, communication is aimed at fostering dialogue as compared with simple information exchange.[50] Nurses are encouraged to communicate in a way that honors the lived experiences of both patient and family and takes into consideration the emergent properties of the patient's life and the conditions in which the information is presented.[50] The goal of COMFORT is to help nurses to initiate conversations about quality of life and end-of-life concerns before death nears. This assures that palliative care is implemented during a patient's treatment process and core concepts of palliative care are integrated into treatment. Each of the seven modules is designed to highlight communication theory and skill development, as detailed below.

C-communicate

Witnessing, a concept within narrative clinical practice, encourages the nurse to be present to and for the patient's story rather than focused on a list of tasks to complete.[51] Narratives are relational events shared and coconstructed by nurse, patient, and family.[51] A narrative approach extends biological care to include the psychosocial concerns and losses of a patient/family. Nurses are taught to elicit the patient/family's story, use person-centered messages that acknowledge emotion, and recognize the communication expectations of patients and families.

O-orientation and opportunity

The COMFORT framework is based on a transactional model of communication, advocating that nurses should adjust their communication style to meet the needs of patients and families. This communication should focus on orienting the patient to life-limiting illness and options for care in an understandable way and articulating what opportunities for treatment and care exist for a patient/family. Accommodating patients and families is a conscious choice. An idea called *convergence* is emphasized. Convergence describes communication that aligns with differences or seeks to understand tensions while not alienating a patient or family by stereotyping, or assuming cultural knowledge or competency. Recognizing opportunities to help orient patients and families to diagnosis and prognosis includes communication skills that gauge health literacy levels, acknowledge vulnerability, and practice cultural humility.

M-mindful presence

Mindfulness and presence are two nonverbal behaviors that clinicians can bring to patients/families when verbal behavior is necessarily limited (maybe due to illness or cultural differences), but that also can be practiced in any patient/family interaction. This involves active listening skills and the ability to witness. Listening is as important as talking.[52] While hearing is purely physiological and doesn't require any effort, listening requires effort and skill to attend, receive, perceive, organize and interpret, and respond to messages.[51] In hospice and palliative care, mindfulness includes relaxing to the immediacy of what is happening, appreciating opposing tensions, perception shifting, seeing what needs to be done, and practicing abiding in the midst of emotions.[53] Mindful presence positions nurses as purposefully attentive to the moment, actively engaged in the here and now, sensitive to context, nonjudgmental, and empathic. This can be accomplished by communicating empathy, engaging in active listening, acknowledging cultural diversity, and employing supportive nonverbal communication.

F-family

Understanding a family climate will aid the nurse in determining the burden and targeting appropriate interventions for the family caregiver(s). The COMFORT framework considers the communication patterns of patient and family, comprising family conversation and family conformity. Family conversation patterns involve the rules that govern appropriate topics for family conversation, determining whether or not family members talk openly about death, dying, illness and how often they speak with each other. Family conformity patterns are directed by an established hierarchy within the family structure and are often defined by a patriarch or matriarch. Hierarchical roles within the family are often emphasized over conversation and disclosure. Noting the role of conversation and conformity can enable teams to best care for families traversing the roughest part of the road in illness. Viewing the family as a system aids in recognition of predictable family communication patterns and allows the nurse to respond and adjust communication to the varying needs of family caregivers.

O-openings

The most difficult moments in practice can sometimes provide a reason to not engage patients and families about transitions in care, changes in place of care, or even talk about the most sensitive subjects like dying, sexuality, and spirituality. It might seem there is a better time, or surely some resolution that will be found on its own. When tension and anxiety is at its peak for patients and families, an opportunity presents itself to connect rather than avoid. COMFORT offers clinical communication tools enabling nurses to engage patients and families at moments of observable tension in the course of care, facilitate self-disclosure, build trust, and better navigate pivotal points of transition across the illness trajectory. By identifying pivotal points of communication in patient/family care, nurses can communicate through tension and facilitate conversations about difficult topics.

R-relating

When responding to patient and family needs, nurses may recognize that statements have multiple meanings and goals. Practicing clinical communication includes an awareness of these multiple goals to better support patient care. The nurse can move beyond what is said to interpret multiple meanings between patients and families, often dependent on relational history, and explore and address more truthful and complex statements. The COMFORT framework encourages nurses to practice complementary disclosure, understand the multiple goals of a patient/family, and work through conflicting goals to help reach understanding about plans of care.

T-team communication

The COMFORT framework explicates the model for interdisciplinary collaboration and highlights the nurse's need to use interpersonal relationship skills to help team members establish mutual respect and trust in order to facilitate collaboration about psychosocial issues. Recognizing how clinical roles contribute to collaboration, distinguishing successful collaboration from group cohesion, and using communication strategies to foster collaboration are emphasized.

Within the framework, Modules C (narrative clinical communication) and F (family) provide beginner level education. Modules O/O (orientation/opportunity), M (mindful presence), and T (team) provide intermediate level communication skills instruction, while O (openings) and R (relating) provide advanced communication skills and are intended for nurses with clinical observation experience. Box 5.2 reviews the COMFORT Model.

Information needs of patients and families

To best provide supportive care to patients and families, it is necessary to understand their information and communication needs. Patients require information around treatment options,

---

Box 5.2 Overview of COMFORT model within family caregivers' communication

1-Seek to understand the role of the primary caregiver
Elicit descriptions and sharing from the caregiver(s) in order to understand the family and experience of care.

OBSERVATIONS TO NOTE:

◆ Who is representing the family?
◆ What is family/family's appearance? Affect?

QUESTIONS TO ASK:

◆ What has been happening with (patient name)?
◆ Will you describe your role as caregiver to (patient name)?

STATEMENTS TO MAKE:

◆ We are glad to have this opportunity to help your family or patient name.
◆ We want to support your family.

2-Learn about the family system
Elicit descriptions and sharing about the family system in order to understand the family and experience of care.

OBSERVATIONS TO NOTE:

◆ What family is present? Is participating?
◆ How is the patient represented by family?

QUESTIONS TO ASK:

◆ How has this illness been difficult for the family?
◆ What would be helpful to your family?

(continued)

Box 5.2 Continued

STATEMENTS TO MAKE:

- Tell me about your family.
- Describe your family members to me.

3-Identify communication deficits between family members

Explore communication deficits by eliciting descriptions and stories about family (e.g., examining strained relationships, handling crisis, and stressful events to reveal points of tension for potential conflict).

OBSERVATIONS TO NOTE:

- Are there any family members that you haven't met?
- Are there patterns of silence among family members?

QUESTIONS TO ASK:

- Has your family experienced another family illness before? Family death? Tragic death?
- Are there family members who don't get along?

STATEMENTS TO MAKE:

- Let me/us know what your family needs.
- Every family is unique with their own story.

4-Listen to patient and family needs

Explore patient/family cultural concerns using talk, silence, and nonverbal immediacy.

OBSERVATIONS TO NOTE:

- Are there specific cultural identities that you can observe?
- What is the family treatment of health professionals? The system?

QUESTIONS TO ASK:

- What things would make (patient) more comfortable? Food? Space?
- How can we make your family more comfortable while you are in the hospital with (patient)?

STATEMENTS TO MAKE:

- We want to be sensitive to every family's cultural values, so we need help in knowing what you need.
- Everyone's background and life experience are so important for us to understand.

5-Share family caregiver typing with team members

Explore family caregiver interventions with team as a result of team exploration and conversation.

OBSERVATIONS TO NOTE:

- Are family members describing the patient's case in a way that is consonant with your understanding?
- What are their family dynamics? Open and direct? Or closed and indirect? A combination?

QUESTIONS TO ASK:

- How are the primary care providers holding up in this family?
- What are your sources of support?

STATEMENTS TO MAKE:

- I would like the opportunity to talk with _____ alone for just a few minutes.
- This is a very difficult situation; you are carrying an immense burden. I look forward to helping you find ways to share that burden.

6-Make plans for family meeting

Elicit team contributions and narratives in order to collaborate about ways in which to prioritize communication and support needs for the family and patient.

OBSERVATIONS TO NOTE:

- What competing issues or health situations are there for this family?
- Is the patient (or their wishes) well represented in current care plans?

QUESTIONS TO ASK:

- What are other team observations about the family's understanding?
- How can we communicate more effectively with this family?

Box 5.2 Continued

STATEMENTS TO MAKE:

- Inform team members: "Previously, this family has experienced xxxxx"
- Inform team members: "Resources for this caregiver are/include xxxxx"

7-Host a family meeting

Host a family meeting early in patient care to share information in a comfortable environment to encourage family members to share thoughts, needs, and feelings.

OBSERVATIONS TO NOTE:

- Where are people sitting? What does their nonverbal communication tell you?
- Are family members taking phone calls during the family meeting? Who is absent?

QUESTIONS TO ASK:

- What are some of the best outcomes you can imagine?
- (family member name), what is most concerning to you?

STATEMENTS TO MAKE:

- Please feel free to interrupt me if you don't understand what I am saying or you need something explained in detail.
- This is a difficult time, and we want to understand your concerns.

8-Offer extended care

Provide, with the team, ongoing evaluation and planning for quality of life dimensions in family care.

OBSERVATIONS TO NOTE:

- What resources does this family have/use?
- Does this family seem fatigued?

QUESTIONS TO ASK:

- Where are you staying? Have you eaten today?
- How are things getting done at home? Do you have someone to help you?

STATEMENTS TO MAKE:

- Ask other team members: "Has anyone considered the caregiver's spiritual needs?"
- To caregiver: I'd like for you to start thinking about what you need and how we could help you.

---

management of symptoms, support from family and friends, fulfillment of family or cultural expectations, attaining meaning, and maintaining dignity and control. Correspondingly, the communication needs for the patient include disease specifics, rationale for care, being listened to, and the opportunity to participate in important discussions.[54] The role of the nurse is to assess the patient's knowledge and concerns in these areas, offer reinforcement of information, and to facilitate information exchange with the rest of the care team. The nurse also guides the patient in understanding the care plan, clarifies team responsibility for specific aspects of care and provides support in the process.

The communication needs of the family and other carers depend on their role in the family system, age, decision-making ability, and other rules within and specific to the family. Often, families need to process information about the illness and understand why the patient became ill.[55] Families also need to understand how the interdisciplinary team works, including the individual team members involved in care, their role in the plan of care, what influences the plan of care, and the site of care.[52] In order for full participation in the patient's care, family communication is essential. Specific themes include reassurance of

the patient's comfort; support in coping with the patient's condition; understanding the evolving care plan; and delineating the current aspect of clinical care. Moreover, families may be very involved in care but have multiple home and work obligations. Therefore, it may be a challenge for family members to participate directly in meetings at the bedside, which may necessitate frequent nursing updates about care. Finally, families may experience a high level of stress from their need for constant updates of information.[54] The nurse has a major role in acknowledging and validating the family's stress and emotions. The willingness to engage in support diminishes feelings of mistrust and promotes team validation.[55]

Situational communication issues arise in palliative care. A common circumstance is when either the family member or the patient requests that the other party not be informed about the extent of seriousness of the situation. If the family is protecting the patient, the nurse should explore the family's reason for withholding information. Such requests may include cultural issues, fear of death, fear that the patient will lose hope and give up, or discomfort with any such discussions. Each concern requires a different approach. If there is a cultural issue, the nurse must explore the cultural mores. If the family states they are fearful, the nurse can explain that most patients want to know their diagnosis so that they can participate in life closure activities and want to determine how to spend their final days. Most importantly, the nurse must assess the patient and determine whether he or she wants to know health information and how much health information he or she wants to know. Finally in this situation, the nurse must honor his or her own integrity. The response to the family who request topics be avoided should include that the nurse won't bring up such topics but if the patient brings up any difficult topics, the nurse will be honest in attending to the conversation.

When the patient is trying to protect the family, the principles of autonomy and confidentiality are paramount. In this situation, the nurse should explore the reasons why the patient is withholding information from the family. Often there may be a past personal history or event rooted in shame, guilt, or lack of acceptance of a lifestyle. The nurse can first provide therapeutic presence in allowing the patient to process this. Additional social work and/or spiritual care support may be necessary. If appropriate, the nurse should explain that if family is to be involved in caregiving, it is helpful to have a full understanding of the patient's illness and comorbid conditions. The patient ultimately has the right to limit information, and the nurse must honor this.

Another challenge is family dynamics. Serious illness results in either effective coping, where the family comes together, or ineffective coping, where the family falls apart. Assessment of both the patient and family reveals consistency in perspectives of family coping. Patient support may be suboptimal if there is inconsistent structure to support the ill person or if family members are overburdened by care. Often, there are conflicted relationships due to abuse, neglect, substance abuse, and past violence. Or relationships may be strained by divorce or separation. These situations are fraught with drama and take the focus away from the patient. The nurse must understand he or she cannot fix these problems. Moreover, these situations necessitate collaboration, Assistance from social work, mental health specialists, and/or addictions personnel is critical. Moreover, the nurse and the team must focus on the tangible health issues at hand.

The role of anxiety in communication

An important phenomenon affecting nurse-patient-family communication is anxiety. Anxiety occurs in both the patient and the nurse, affecting how communication is delivered by the nurse and how it is received by the patient. Pasacreta and colleagues[56] well describe the role of anxiety in receiving communication. Anxiety is a necessary element in everyday life. Indeed, mild anxiety helps most people do their work by being alert to issues, identifying problems, and facilitating creative solutions. Therefore, a mildly anxious person may be able to process information and, in fact, be quite creative. However, a simple preventive health encounter may induce mild anxiety in some patients, allowing them to only process simple basic health information. It is important for the nurse to assess the patient's anxiety and his or her ability to process each interaction.

As health issues become more serious, in particular regarding disease progression, anxiety increases toward a moderate level. A patient's ability to process information becomes selective. At that point, the patient has a heightened awareness and may be thinking of possible bad outcomes including worsening disease. In this case, the nurse supports the patient by allowing him or her to voice fears and concerns and by reiterating information that the team has provided. However, it may only be in small amounts of information.

The highest level is severe anxiety and panic, resulting in total impairment of a patient's ability to process information.[56] This often occurs in the patient when it is communicated that there are no further curative treatment options, a short prognosis, or a terminal diagnosis. In this situation, once the clinician gives the difficult news, the patient may go into shock or panic about the news. He or she is unable to process any further information. Understanding the patient's anxiety level at this point is critical. At this point, the nurse offers acknowledgment of the difficult news the patient has heard, validating reactions and discussing emotions. Nonverbal communication includes therapeutic presence. At this point, the team should refrain from any further information sharing until the patient has time to process the bad news.

Anxiety in the nurse has different ramifications. A nurse may have anxiety in caring for a dying patient. This may be the result of inexperience with death and dying, lack of experience during the actual dying process, or inability to accept the dying process. In some cases, the nurse's anxiety may not interfere with understanding and responding to patient and family cues. In other cases, the nurse may be so focused on tasks they are unable to attend or be present with the patient and family and miss cues. Other factors may effect communication such as the nurse's age proximity to the patient, a patient and family's physical resemblance to the nurse's family or friends, or a similar diagnosis to a loved one in the nurse's family. As the patient's needs escalate or family dynamics escalate, the nurse's anxiety may significantly increase, resulting in communication failures. This may depend on the experience and expertise of the nurse in life-threatening illness. Lastly, a sudden emergency or precipitous decline may cause understandably severe anxiety and emotional distress. Thus, communication skills may become compromised just when they are needed most. Therefore, it is important for the nurse to monitor his or her own anxiety in patient care. More importantly, nurses need to work collaboratively to support each other in these situations. This includes taking breaks, changing assignments, and debriefing difficult cases in real time and afterward as well. Additionally, with collaboration from the interdisciplinary team, the nurse can discern the issues and benefit from sharing the burdens of care.

Core elements of nurse communication

Imparting information

A primary role of the nurse is to impart information, including illness education, medications, or treatment information. By the nature of their scope of practice, advanced practice registered nurses (APRNs) may also offer diagnosis, prognosis, and treatment options. The task of imparting information is complex, because information alone is not enough. Rather, information must be provided within the context of educational level, literacy level, numeracy level, primary language, developmental level, psychological state, and time constraints of a healthcare setting. The patient's educational level and understanding of medical language affects his or her information processing. If a patient hasn't completed high school, he may not understand complex words. If English is a second language, attention must be paid to medical terminology. Developmentally appropriate language refers to the age of the patient and his or her ability to reason. Younger children do not have complex reasoning abilities, whereas adolescents do. Information for pediatric patients and families must meet their particular needs, with modifications to make the language simpler and more concrete. The same is true for those patients with developmental delays or cognitive deficits. The stress of being in a healthcare setting impairs a person's ability to process information. Therefore, imparting information usually means providing information incrementally, at a fifth or sixth grade education level to allow patients and families to best hear and process what is being said.

Case study—imparting information

Joan meets for the first time with Mrs. Rodriguez, the patient, and her partner, George:

JOAN: Hi, I'm the nurse manager on the hospice and palliative care unit. Would you tell me why you would like to see me?

MRS. R: Well, I have been diagnosed as having Alzheimer's. I just have a lot of questions and I need them answered. I just can't believe I've got this disease.

JOAN: OK, would you mind having a seat here? George, please have a seat as well.

MRS. R: I, I just, somehow I just feel like all the tests that they took were, um, not about me, that they were about somebody else. I came back to just find out what I'm supposed to do.

JOAN: OK, let me ask you Mrs. Rodriguez, have you spoken with your doctor?

MRS. R: Well, yeah, she's the one that gave me this diagnosis.

JOAN: OK, and did she give you any information about the progression of the disease?

MRS. R: She just gave me the diagnosis, and she didn't tell me what the progression would be. I don't know anything about it, except that I know that people who have Alzheimer's end up in a wheelchair and in a nursing home slobbering all over themselves.

GEORGE: She doesn't want that.

JOAN: Of course, nobody wants that. Unfortunately, Alzheimer's is a disease that does not have a cure. It progresses slowly. Did your doctor explain that part to you?

MRS. R: She did. But I am healthy. George and I go to the senior center three times a week, we dance. We play bingo. I had a little accident and bumped my head and the tests show that I have Alzheimer's. I just can't believe this.

JOAN: It sounds like this all came on very quickly. Have you had any problems with forgetfulness?

MRS. R: A little. Like misplacing my car keys.

JOAN: It sounds like you may be at the beginning of the disease. Right now, dancing is easy, but it may come to a time when you may have trouble dancing. Did your doctor give you any medication?

MRS. R: Not yet.

JOAN: As the disease progresses, you will likely need medication and you may need someone to help you. Mrs. Rodriguez, with whom do you live?

MRS. R: I live alone.

GEORGE: For now. We planned to move in together in the fall.

JOAN: Moving in together is a big step! How wonderful! George, in what ways do you see yourself helping Mrs. Rodriguez?

The principles of verbal and nonverbal communication are considered essential components of narrative practice. These principles place the person and relationship as central in the interaction. By employing narrative approaches, more emphasis on the role of

Box 5.3 Useful open-ended questions to initiate discussions
How are things going for you?
How are you coping with your illness?
What concerns you about your illness?
What concerns do you have about your illness?
How is treatment going for you?
What concerns you about your treatment?
What worries do you have about your illness or treatment?
What are your hopes in terms of your illness and treatment?
Who are the important people to you?
What relationships are the most important to you?
Who are the people who provide you support?
What gives you meaning in your life?
What gives you joy in your life?
What provides you with the strength to live or cope with each day?
Is there any important or unfinished business you need to attend to?

Sources: Adapted from Dahlin (2010), reference 2; and Buckman (2010), reference 18.

patient and family in the process of communicating can become a reality. Patient-centeredness describes shared opportunities for communicating among all involved parties. Here, Joan gives them opportunity for task and relationship communication: she responds to Mrs. Rodriguez by providing candid information on Alzheimer's disease and discusses George's role (task). Through nonverbal and verbal communication, such as asking the patient and family member to sit down, she can support and comfort both of them as well as reduce their uncertainty (relationship). In facilitating their expression of emotion, Joan is bearing witness to Mrs. Rodriguez's and George's suffering; she is honoring their voices through active listening and messages that recognize and legitimize feelings. Box 5.3 summarizes the nurse's communication role when imparting information to patients and families.

Information gathering

The next role of the nurse is to gather information. The most effective tool in gathering information from patients and families is the use of open-ended questions. Open-ended questions promote both the opportunity and richness to listen to the patient's narrative and observe nonverbal communication. The nurse benefits from the expression of values, priorities of care, coping, life priorities, and spiritual concerns. Closed-ended questions include "yes-or-no" questions or limited response questions and leading questions. The use of closed-ended questions, which usually focus on physical symptoms or history questions, limits the patient's response, thereby inhibiting elaboration, explanations, and clarifications of various topics. Within the time constraints of clinical care, a nurse may not have enough time for a long conversation. However, a few key questions set a tone of a caring relationship. Box 5.3 offers a list of potential questions.

Often important questions are asked but, as the patient starts to answer, the nurse moves the conversation on. When the nurse asks an open-ended question, it is essential to listen to the answer. Otherwise, distraction, unresponsiveness, or lack of acknowledgment is invalidating to the patient and/or family. Resentment may also result if the patient has shared something intimate without receiving acknowledgment of its significance. The next case scenario offers how to gather information.

Case study: gathering information

A palliative care team meets to discuss a patient's plan of care. Previously, a family meeting was held and it was decided that the patient's feeding tube would be removed and he would be sent to another facility closer to his family.

DR. GEORGE: Upon moving him to the facility, we will need to contact Dr. Smith because the patient might begin to actively die.

NURSE SARAH: Do you think he can get better?

DR. GEORGE: No. He has so many comorbidities that his quality of life will be very, very poor.

NURSE SARAH: Well, he said "Amen" when I prayed with him yesterday. I think there's more cognitive activity than we think. I don't see why his daughter is being allowed to make decisions, especially to remove the feeding tube. I believe that he has the ability to make his own decisions and has the right to decide if he wants to die.

DR. GEORGE: Well, there are many things to consider about removing the feeding tube. I know you are not happy with this decision. We will ask him today during rounds.

NURSE SARAH: There are other questions you can ask to determine delirium, and you can ask other questions to see if he is able to make that decision.

DR. GEORGE: Well, yes, we can assess decision-making capacity. That's fine. We can do that. The family may have had that conversation.

NURSE SARAH: I have talked to the family about what happens before and after withdrawal of the feeding tube.

DR. GEORGE: The family doesn't want to see the patient go through that. He cannot feed by himself biologically.

NURSE SARAH: There is still a 10% chance he can go back to gardening, something he enjoyed.

DR. GEORGE: There is no 10% chance he'll go back to that quality of life which he valued the most.

NURSE SARAH: In that case, if it was up me, then let me go. I just wanted to make sure. I will talk to his daughter more and reassure her that the decision is in his best interest.

Interdisciplinary collaboration is the backbone of palliative nursing, as holistic care plans can only emerge from working with other team members. Collaboration consists of interdependence and flexibility wherein team members must work together to accomplish goals. In this case, the nurse and physician team members must agree about the family's decision to withdraw the feeding tube. It will be important that family members receive the same message from both team members. Newly created activities emerge from the collaborative process, as the physician announces that they will assess patient cognition together during rounds after the meeting. This was not previously identified as a task for the team until it emerged from the review of the patient's case. After further discussion, the team members agreed that the goal would be to assist the family with their decision and facilitate the transition in patient placement as best as possible. A final element of interdisciplinary collaboration

is reflection on the team's process and decision-making; although not seen in this case example, it is important for teams to reflect on patient care in lieu of the patient's preferences for care. Quality improvement can emerge from the reflective team process.

Listening

Listening is an active process that requires concentrated presence and attention. This allows better understanding of the patient's journey within the disease trajectory and of how the patient is processing information. During this process, the nurse listens to the patient's story without interrupting: noting his or her specific word choices, and concerns. One helpful technique is to ask an open-ended question, such as "What brought you to the hospital?" or "Tell me about what has been going on?" Specifically, the nurse observes both the spoken verbal content in the patient's responses, focusing on both what is said and what is left unsaid. In addition, the nurse notes speech patterns, tone, rapidity, and coherency. Concurrently, the nurse observes the nonverbal expressions including emotion and accompanying physical movement. All of this will determine distress in the physical, psychological, spiritual and emotional dimensions of care as well as which areas are a priority to address.

The nurse's use of silence is paramount. This allows the nurse to be fully present in the moment rather than mentally preparing answers or replies. Correspondingly, the nurse uses reflection to convey empathy. The nurse clarifies what has been heard by such comments as "Hmm" or "Tell me more." By acknowledging the patient's responses and exploring their meaning in a compassionate and supportive way, the nurse encourages the patient to explain difficult issues and concerns.[57] There may be times when the patient is silent. In this circumstance, it is appropriate for the nurse to just sit quietly, letting the patient reflect on the moment and the current situation. It is after these moments of silence that a patient may reveal sensitive information, concerns, thoughts, or past history (trauma, abuse, or illicit behaviors). It may be at a deeper level because he or she has been given the opportunity and permission to do so.

There are several strategy models for palliative nursing communication.[6] One model of listening and attending is ASK-TELL-ASK. In this model, the nurse asks a question. The patient then responds with both statements and questions. The nurse then responds to the content of the discussion. The nurse closes by asking a final question to determine patient understanding.[6] A second model is the SPIKES model. In this model, S is for listening skills, P is for patient perception of the current situation, I is for an invitation to provide information, K is for offering knowledge or the facts, E is for emotional exploration and empathy, and S is for summary.[6] Another model is SOLER, where the nurse sits Squarely opposite the patient, with an Open body posture, Leaning in to demonstrate empathy, using Eye contact as appropriate and with Relaxed positioning.[6] Finally, there is NURSE model, where the nurse Names the emotions, Understands the patients, offers Respect to the patient, provides Support, and Explores the patient's concerns through the use of I statements.[6] Any of these strategies are effective and depend on the communication style of the nurse.

Eliciting sensitive aspects of care: culture, religion, ethics

Sensitivity, another term for cultural competence, includes issues pertaining to religious, spiritual, cultural, ethnic, racial, gender,

---

Box 5.4 Useful cultural assessment questions

Where were you born?

Where were you raised?

How does this affect your about health and illness?

Are there any cultural considerations important to your care?

Are there other beliefs that are important to your healthcare?

Are you spiritual or religious?

How should spirituality or religion be addressed in your healthcare?

Are there any important rituals that are important to your healthcare?

How do you describe your medical condition/illness?

What do you know about your medical condition/illness?

What do you want to know about your medical condition/illness?

What do you fear most about your condition and its treatment?

How have you treated your medical condition/illness?

Who else, if anyone, do you want to know about your medical condition/illness?

Who else, if anyone, should we talk to about your medical condition/illness, treatment options, and the disease process?

Who is responsible for making healthcare decisions for you?

Are there other important people in your community involved in your healthcare?

Are there other people in your community whom we should include in your healthcare?

Sources: Dahlin (2010), reference 2; NCP (2013), reference 3.

---

and language issues. Communication norms differ, resulting in diverse cultural communication customs. These may include deference to healthcare providers, gender in care providers, or the appropriateness of discussion surrounding certain topics. Attending to culture is a very important aspect of communication, necessitating appreciation of verbal cues and interpretation of nonverbal cues. In many situations, beneficence takes precedence over autonomy. Disclosure and nondisclosure must be viewed within the context of the patient and the family, with understanding of, and respect for, their values and beliefs.

In order to be culturally sensitive, a nurse must be "self-aware of his or her own culture, cultural biases, and assumptions. Palliative care staff members cultivate cultural self-awareness and recognize how their own cultural values, beliefs, biases, and practices inform their perceptions of patients, families, and colleagues."[3] Understanding one's own background serves as a starting point for the nurse. This includes reflection and examination of one's ethical values and beliefs by reflecting on the following: ethnicity and its effect on health, illness, and death; religion and its role in death and dying and afterlife; and individual communication patterns.

Eliciting health information and awareness is essential to care. In some cultures there are social norms about whether or not the patient should know health information, especially if the patient is seriously ill. Therefore it is critical for the nurse to assess the patient's and family's religion and culture and how it affects healthcare. This includes how much, if any, information a patient wants to know. It also includes what and how much information is conveyed as dictated by culture and ethnicity. A patient may state she wants direct communication, or she may defer to family members who would then inform her. Next, the nurse asks the patient to identify others whom she wishes to be told about her medical issues and whom she wants to make healthcare and treatment decisions. Finally, it is important for the healthcare team to understand any religious or cultural practices that will affect health decisions. Some religions do not allow surgical removal of organs or blood transfusions; others may not allow pain medications. Box 5.4 offers questions to promote discussion of cultural and religious concerns.

If English is not the first language of the patient and family, it is obligatory to use a professional interpreter. Some hospitals offer interpreter services; some offer telephonic interpretation. Interpreters are invaluable to assist the nurse in phrasing questions and comments so as to be culturally sensitive and appropriate. Too often, family members are asked to interpret from English to another language, placing the family member in a double bind. Although they may be acting as translators, culturally, they must also act within their family roles. This is even more troublesome if children are translating for parents. Consequently, family translators may need to protect the patient from information, withhold information, or leave out pertinent facts. Therefore, it may be very unclear what the patient has actually been told.[58]

Case study: eliciting sensitive aspects of care: culture, religion, and ethics

A 32-year-old woman diagnosed with metastatic ovarian cancer has been briefly hospitalized for a blood transfusion and skin biopsies that tested positive for cancer on the dermis directly overlaying a tumor site. Upon entering the hospital room, the patient, Sue, is packing up for the drive home. Sue no longer walks without the support of her sister or husband, showers in a seated position, and is constantly accompanied by others regardless of the context. She has recently fallen and has a sprained right ankle, but has little sensation; this injury has caused profuse bruising and swelling in the area. Upon further inquiry, the nurse learns that Sue cannot lift herself up and down off of the toilet. Her chart notes that she has terminal cancer with metastases to the eye, liver, spine, shoulders, hips, femurs, and lungs. In answering questions about pain, Sue describes frequent intractable pain. She is eager to move forward and describes upcoming chemotherapy and radiation that is scheduled. Just then, Sue's husband enters the room to carry down luggage to their car.

NURSE: Sue, what is an average day like at home?

SUE: Well my sister helps me to move and take a shower. I am so weak I cannot do those things by myself. I also have pain no matter what I do. It never changes.

NURSE: Tell me more about your pain.

SUE: Often it is really bad. Medications don't seem to touch it. But I don't want to take many medications, as then I am too cloudy with my family. I also don't want to be any weaker, as my family is already helping me so much.

NURSE: That must be really hard. What medications are you taking?

SUE: Just the Percocet as the other drugs are stronger and I want to be able to take the full amount of chemotherapy.

NURSE: Tell me how the medications make you cloudy?

SUE: I feel so sleepy from them.

NURSE: What else happens?

SUE: I get worried as the pain is still there. I don't want my family to think I am so sick I need medications. Besides, the chemotherapy is soon. It will help. And I have the radiation.

NURSE: Do you think that having some equipment would help? Something like a walker or wheelchair or a shower chair?

HUSBAND WALKS IN: He scoffs and says, "Over my dead body," and quickly exits.

The husband's statement ("over my dead body") is an opening, a communication moment that can lead to reframing moments of tension and promoting understanding. Difficult conversations with patients and families coincide with transitions in care and truly require intimate exchanges between patient/family and nurse. The husband's comment can easily be ignored or avoided by the nurse, but that would neglect relational communication that can be used to present opportunities and possibilities for resilience. Instead of remaining committed to the discharge topics that she needs to address (task communication), the nurse has special access to respond to the most challenging aspects of serious and terminal illness for Sue and her husband. She may help them to accept the seriousness of the disease and its impact on quality of life for them both (relational communication) by acknowledging the husband's comment, inviting him to sit down and share in conversation about Sue's illness. Nurses are positioned to communicate either vaguely or directly, and the nurse in this interaction can rephrase the husband's comment ("So, it sounds like your concern is about the use of medical equipment in the home" or "It sounds like a walker may not be the most desirable option. What kinds of help might you need at home?"). Alternatively, his comment may indicate the need to give Sue and her husband some time to talk about decisions related to her transition home, by commenting: "I'm going to give you both some private time to talk about how best to accommodate Sue's move home."

Communication approaches

The context in which communication occurs influences the process and outcomes of interactions. Because of the rapidly changing complexity of healthcare, different methods may be utilized. Often, in-person or face-to-face meetings are helpful, as everyone is in the same room, hearing the same information. However with the changing work environment, families may not be able to meet in one place. Therefore telephone meetings may be helpful. Finally, patients and clinicians are using video technology, protected websites, and e-mails. All have benefits and burdens for the patient and family, as well as the nurse.

The timing of communication is important and may dictate the communication method. Quill and colleagues defined "urgent" situations that necessitate immediate communication[59]: (1) the patient is facing imminent death; (2) the patient is talking about wanting to die; (3) the patient or family is inquiring about hospice; (4) the patient has recently been hospitalized for severe, progressive illness; and (5) the patient is experiencing severe suffering and a short prognosis. Less urgent situations include (1) the discussion of prognosis, particularly if life expectancy is thought to be between 6 and 12 months; (2) the discussion of potential treatment options with low probability of success; and (3) the discussion of hopes and fears. More "routine" palliative communication includes circumstances when stability or recovery is predicted.[59]

Due to work commitments and personal schedules, in-person meetings may need to occur via technology. With cell phones and computers, meetings occur in novel ways and can be more inclusive. The most basic form is teleconference. A phone can be put on speaker mode to allow the family to listen and join the conversation. Missing is the nonverbal communication for either the participants in the conference room or the family member on the end of the phone. Moreover, it is important to remember that participants in the conference room need to attend to the family member who is listening on the phone. First, this requires removing extraneous background noises by closing doors to avoid overhead pages, or shutting windows to avoid street noise because these impact the ability to hear conversations. Second, the attendees need to avoid side conversations; attend to extraneous noises such as heavy breathing near the microphone and reduce the noise of clicking pens, shuffling feet, or the like. Third, there should be frequent check-ins to assure the listeners are hearing the conversation and understand what is being said, as telephone lines can be inconsistent. Finally, all participants need to identify themselves before they speak so the listener can follow who is saying what. At the end of the call, the summary is especially important to ensure everyone heard the same plan.

Other more novel meetings can occur via video on Face time, Google Chat, or Skype. This allows for full involvement by all participants because both verbal and nonverbal communication are visible. Introductions are important to allow each participant to be viewed by the person on computer or cell phone. All participants must be patient with the process. There is a delay time from when something is said on one end of the computer to when it is received on the other end. So the meeting pace may need to be slowed to accommodate this. Again, like telephones, sometimes there are bad connections, which make for static. Thus, various parts of the conversation may need to be repeated. Similar to telephone conversations, background noise should be reduced. However, overall, families appreciate the effort to be included and healthcare providers are happy to have family hear the consistent conversations.

E-mail and Web technology

Many patients request to use e-mail or social media communication, creating opportunities and challenges. It is important to set guidelines for the use of these methods of communication. These methods, if done incorrectly, cannot assure confidentiality. Any health information should be discussed through appropriate organizational guidelines and policies, which usually call for the use of institutional secure Web portals and secure correspondence. Nonetheless, only routine communication should occur this way. Expectations should be set around appropriate overall use of e-mail or phone contact. Moreover, there should be one designated person to communicate with the team in addition to the patient thereby discouraging multiple e-mails by different family members to the healthcare provider. Patients and families should be given guidelines about not using this method when the clinician is off service or on vacation.

The clinician should delineate the types of communication that are appropriate for e-mail or Web-based requests. It is important that patients understand that clinical assessment is difficult to accomplish via e-mail. Clear explanation should cover the principle that e-mail does not substitute for in-person visit and complex e-mails usually necessitate a face-to-face visit. Usual e-mail or Web-based correspondence includes nonurgent medication requests or refills, durable medical equipment requests, home services, follow-up of a stable response to a new treatment, referral information, follow-up appointments, or routine check-ins.

The response time of such communication should be considered. Patients need to be informed of expectations in response times. Because clinicians cannot monitor these sites during clinical duties, there may be a lag of several hours in response time. All health facilities have protocols for urgent and emergent issues to be attended to and any patient emergencies or urgent issues should be directed to 911 or the office triage service. All clinical assessments should occur by phone and go through the triage system.

Patient and family meetings

Patient and family meetings are a wonderful but underutilized tool. These meetings promote respectful and sensitive delivery of information in a timely, thorough, current, comprehensive, and accurate fashion. The patient may or may not attend depending on his or her condition, decision-making capacity, and preference for involvement. It can be helpful to hear consistent messages. For the family, it is a time to meet the various team members and understand their role. Family meetings help the family understand the disease process and options of care while providing reassurance that a plan is in place and everyone is working toward a consistent goal.[60] The family meeting also provides clinicians an opportunity to collaboratively formulate a plan of care that is consistent with the goals and wishes of the patient and family.

There are several types of meetings that occur within the context of palliative care: information meetings, advanced care planning meetings, bad news discussions, and code status discussions. The first meeting type a straightforward information meeting. These can occur to form a working relationship between the patient and family and the care team. These may have no particular agenda other than to convey information about the patient's current status or the nature of the illness and its symptoms. There may be no decisions to be made and no future planning. Other topics include future predictions about the course of illness and treatment options. There may be discussion of home care, symptom, management, medications, and nursing support. Box 5.5 reviews the process of a family meeting.

Before calling a family meeting, it is important to maximize the effective use of time by clarifying the goal of a meeting. For more complex or contentious families, having a meeting specifically to plan strategies to deal with a difficult family is time well spent. A meeting goal can range simply from an update of care, to more complex discussions of withdrawal of technological interventions, poor prognosis, and imminent death. Consideration should be given to the attendance of essential healthcare providers. A premeeting should be held to clarify the messages to be conveyed and determine who should lead the meeting; the leader may not necessarily be the physician. Organizational culture may dictate this.

The leader should ensure that everyone in the room is introduced and review the goal of the meeting. The nurse may facilitate the

---

Box 5.5 The family meeting

Premeeting planning

1. Ensure clinician premeeting to assure consistency of message and process.
2. Clarify goals of meeting with patient and family and staff.
3. Decide on the essential people to attend the meeting—patient, family, and healthcare providers.

The actual meeting

4. Arrange appropriate setting.
5. Introduce everyone in room and relationship to patient.
6. Review goal of meeting.
7. Elicit patient/family understanding of care to date.
8. Review of current medical condition.
9. Attend to questions.
10. Review options for care.
11. Elicit response from patient if decisional.
12. Elicit response from family in terms of what patient would choose for him or herself if he/she could.

Summary

13. Review plan. If agreement—then decision. If no agreement—what follow-up is planned?
14. Document meeting—who attended, what was discussed, and plan.

Sources: Adapted from Rabow et al. (2004), reference 61; and Dahlin (2010), reference 2.

---

initial conversation by serving as a focal point for continuity of care. The meeting may proceed as suggested under the section "Scheduled Meetings and the Role of the Nurse." This includes determining patient and family understanding of the illness, their values, preferences, and beliefs along with their informational needs for decision-making (see Box 5.5). The designated meeting leader offers a summary of the care. The next part of the meeting addresses questions and issues that require clarification. After this discussion, the leader summarizes the issues and develops a plan of care in collaboration with the patient and family. One of the most important yet often neglected tasks after the meeting is documentation. The names and titles of the people who attended, the issues discussed, and the decisions made should be recorded in the medical record.

The actual steps for a family meeting are fairly straightforward and based on common sense. There are eight steps: (1) finding an appropriately private space for the meeting; (2) introductions of all the participants at the meeting; (3) using open-ended questions to establish what the patient (and family) knows; (4) determining how the patient wishes the information to be presented; (5) presenting information in a straightforward manner, using understandable language, in small quantities and with pauses for processing and questions to assess understanding; (6) responding to emotions; (7) clarifying goals of care and treatment priorities; and (8) establishing a plan.[61]

Scheduled meetings and the role of the nurse

Scheduled meeting times are critical in allowing the patient to prepare emotionally and psychologically for any potential news. This includes allowing for the presence of the patient's support network to hear and validate information conveyed. Nurses play a vital role in these meetings because they are often responsible for organizing the meeting. Before the meeting, the nurse may assess the patient's physical, emotional, and psychological concerns to be conveyed in a meeting. This information can assist the team in planning discussion points at the scheduled meetings. After the meeting, the nurse can follow up and reinforce information communicated.

Because of their perceived formality, scheduled meetings tend to take on more importance than informal meetings. Several steps are important to their success. After introductions have been done, the goals of the meeting can be stated. Then the patient can be asked about his or her understanding of the medical condition and situation. This is followed by ascertaining the patient's worries and fears, how much information the patient wishes to know, and which other people the patient wishes to be informed concerning clinical issues or involved in his or her care.[57] A patient who is hesitant to express emotional concerns may need prompting or an invitation to speak.

The nurse may facilitate the initial conversation by serving as a reference point for the patient and family in conveying important concerns or worries from previous interactions. Often this occurs at the beginning of the meeting and personalizes the discussions to the specific needs of the patient and family. In addition, the nurse may act as a translator between the medical team and the patient, facilitating information-sharing, interpreting information and medical jargon in language the patient understands, and also ensuring that the members of the care team understand the patient's words and language. If the patient/family agrees to the plan, the meeting can end with a synopsis of the meeting and the decisions made. If the family disagrees, another meeting can be suggested. Box 5.6 offers questions to promote conversation.

Difficult or overbearing families may shift the conversation to their own needs and concerns. If overbearing or difficult patients or families obstruct meetings with anger, blame, and criticism, it is important to reinforce the goals of the meeting and to restate that the focus of care is on the patient.[62] It may also be necessary to set ground rules about appropriate behavior. After the completion of such a meeting, these family members may be offered resources and referrals for their own individual grief and coping.

Advance care planning

Advance care planning is essential to palliative care; it serves as a valuable guide to the healthcare team. The National Consensus Project for Quality Palliative Care *Clinical Practice Guidelines for Quality Palliative Care 3rd edition* describes how "person-centered goals, preference, and choices form the basis for the plan of care."[3] Advance care planning is a social process based on the ethical principle of autonomy of the patient. Advance care planning prepares for lack of capacity in decision-making and relieves the burden of decision-making on others. These comprehensive discussions promote the determination of the patient's values, goals, fears, and concerns while also developing the core topics for patient education, including the right to high-quality pain control and symptom management.

Box 5.6 Questions to address patients' and families' coping

How have you/your family coped with crises or difficult situations in the past?

Have you/your family been through something like this before?

How did you/your family react/cope?

Can you identify/anticipate any potential areas of concern for you and your family?

Have you told your family what you would want in terms of life-prolonging treatments?

Did the patient ever tell you what they wanted for themselves in terms of life-prolonging treatments?

Is there anyone you need to see? Is there anyone you think the patient would like to see?

Who is supporting you now? Is there anyone you'd like us to call?

Who could you call if things became more serious, difficult, or you needed emotional support?

Source: Revised from Dahlin (2010), reference 2.

There are three discreet elements of ACP: designation of healthcare durable power of attorney, completion of an advance directive, and out of hospital resuscitation orders. A healthcare durable power of attorney is the person whom the patient designates to make decisions if/when he or she is unable to do so.[63] This is otherwise known as the surrogate decision-maker. It is beneficial for the nurse to help describe this role as well as to educate both the patient and the surrogate decision-maker on the role and when it is invoked. Moreover, the nurse can facilitate discussion between the patient and the surrogate decision-maker about the patient's wishes. The designation of a healthcare durable power of attorney can take place on its own or within an advance directive documents such as a living will. There are several popular and easily accessible documents: Aging with Dignity Five Wishes, Making Choices (Gunderson Lutheran), and Project GRACE (Project Grace).[64,65,66]

Because the process of advanced care planning involves setting goals of therapy, developing care directives, and making decisions about specific forms of medical therapy, it is more effective if anchored in a personal experience. For instance, if a patient has had a family member or friend with chronic illness, poor health, and/or a terminal illness, they may be able reflect on the actual aspects of care. For chronically ill, debilitated, and terminally ill patients, planning topics includes decisions about life-sustaining therapies (code status), artificial feeding and hydration, and palliative and hospice care. Box 5.7 offers questions to start such conversations.

It is essential that culture, health literacy, and linguistic literacy are considered within the process of advance care planning. Discussions need to be consider and respect the education level of the patient in order for the patient to make meaningful choice.

Box 5.7 Initiating advance directive conversations

Normalizing comments/questions:

I'd like to talk with you about possible healthcare decisions in the future.

I'd like to discuss a topic I bring up with all my patients.

I often like to make sure I understand my patients' preferences and wishes for aggressive care if there were a serious change in condition.

I would like to discuss your feelings about going to the emergency room, the intensive care unit, and being on life support.

Inquiries of patient's understanding of illness:

What do you understand about your current health situation?

What do you understand from what the doctors have told you?

What more do you want to understand about the current situation?

Inquiries to elicit hopes and expectations:

What do you hope the future holds?

What do you expect in the future?

Have you ever thought about if things don't go the way you hope?

How can we help you live in the best way possible for you?

How do you wish to spend whatever time you have left?

What activities or experiences are most important for you to do to maximize the quality of your life?

Inquiries to elicit thoughts regarding cardiopulmonary resuscitation:

Have you ever thought about life support or life-prolonging treatment measures?

If you should stop breathing or your heart stops beating, would you want us to use "heroic measures" to bring you back?

Have you ever thought about if anything were to happen to you and you could not breathe on your own or your heart could not work on its own?

Have you given any thought to what kinds of treatment you would want or not want if you become unable to speak for yourself in the future?

For the family:

Did the patient or your loved one ever tell you what he or she wanted for him or herself?

Did he or she ever talk about life-prolonging therapies?

Did he or she witness other family members or friends undergoing treatment and comment on his or her own preferences for care?

Did he or she ever talk about the care of another family member and state whether they would have wanted the same type of treatment?

Source: Revised from Dahlin (2010), reference 2.

The use of interpreters is paramount to reflect the nuances of culture and language differences. In some cultures, any conversation related to death, dying, or planning at end of life, is not an appropriate conversation. In other cultures, discussions about limiting the use of life-sustaining technology is akin to hastening death. These viewpoints must be respected and supported, even if the team disagrees.

Ideally, advanced care planning and completion of advance directives should begin within preventive or primary care settings. These discussions are best completed over time, which normalizes them. This allows opportunity for reflection and discussion with family and friends about possible scenarios, which in itself may prepare the patient for the course of disease. However, if not initiated early, then discussions should occur before acute, disabling events and, hopefully, before the end stage of a terminal illness. Otherwise, they are laden with more emotional burden. Unfortunately, there are a number of reasons that these conversations do not occur, including reluctance to initiate such discussions due to time constraints, lack of comfort with such discussions, lack of skills in such communications, and fear of upsetting the patient even though she or he may wish to have the conversation.

There seems to be agreement on the importance of (1) naming a surrogate decision-maker, (2) documentation of care preferences, (3) promoting illness understanding through education, (4) willingness to discuss death and dying, and (5) completion of personal finances and business affairs. Patients differ in the extent to which they wish to participate in treatment decisions; therefore it is essential to determine this. Being provided with adequate information and direction in realistic healthcare choices is critical. Without any structure or context, the weight of these decisions can cause patients and families to feel a sense of self-blame or loss of confidence in the team. This is because the burden of stopping care is heavy and patients and family may feel this is giving up.

To promote consistency of care preferences in the community, out of hospital or community resuscitation medical order sets are appropriate. These orders usually consist of do-not-resuscitate orders because the default in our health system is full resuscitation. However, they may be known as Comfort Care Orders, Allow Natural Death Orders, POLST (Physician/Provider Orders for Life Sustaining Treatment), or MOLST (Medical Orders for Life Sustaining Treatment). As stated on the POLST website, "POLST alone is not an advanced directive; rather a set of medical orders" developed, they explain, "to improve the quality of patient care and reduce medical errors by creating a system that identifies patients' wishes regarding medical treatment and communicates and respects them by creating portable medical orders."[67]

Survival estimates affect the patient decision-making, thereby necessitating accurate prognostic information. However, there are several barriers to this. First, physicians are poor at estimating and reporting accurate survival times to patients.[68] Second, patients often receive conflicting information from various team members. Unsubstantiated information on the Internet furthers disparity in prognosis. Interviews of 56 terminally ill patients concluded that all patients wanted honesty when their physicians offered a prognosis.[69] Third, the patient's wish to hear optimistic information and the physician's reluctance to present information on disease progression may impair accurate portrayal of the patient's condition.[70] Nurses can promote a consistency in such information by their attendance when such information is delivered. Given their knowledge and working with professional colleagues, nurses may also temper the overly optimistic survival times.

A change in focus from future cure-oriented treatments to current functional status can facilitate realistic, authentic conversations. For instance, if the patient is talking about more treatment, but they are essentially bed-bound, there is opportunity to discuss the reality of actually participating in such treatment. Having the patient consider potential situations may be helpful. One such statement may be, "There may come a time when you need help breathing with a ventilator. But we may not be able to get you off the machine. What should we do then?" Such a scenario may offer understanding of the seriousness of the illness, realistic options for therapy, and potential circumstances of death. The result is that the patient may share their values and express their preferences for care. The result may be a sense of control, a sense of trust with healthcare providers, and a sense of resolution in aspects of one's life.

Advance care planning and the role of the nurse

A central communicative role of the palliative nurse is to identify opportunities to engage patients and families about ACP. Discussions of ACP are identified as essential task-focused communication to be accomplished during the first visit or to be shared during interdisciplinary team meetings when reviewing patient plans of care.[71] The goal of ACP discussions is to impart information to help the patient and family understand, requiring the use of clear explanations, a review of options, and formal clarification on the difference between hospice and palliative care.[4] Common barriers to discussions about ACP include patient-family unwillingness to listen, noncommunicative patients, nurse discomfort, and perceived physician hesitance to discuss the topic.[4] Importantly, discussions about ACP need to be reviewed during interdisciplinary team meetings to ensure that all team members are aware of the patient's preferences.[72] Nurses are encouraged to engage in relational focused communication as part of these discussions and address spiritual concerns.[73]

Case study: advanced care planning

NURSE: Have you heard of advance directives?

PATIENT: I have. Yeah, that's where I tell what I want in my healthcare.

FAMILY MEMBER: You remember. There was that guy at the senior center that came to talk about that one time.

PATIENT: Oh, that's right. That's right. Yeah.

NURSE: Well, It's basically a blanket term. There are three components to advanced directives. Number one is where you would assign someone who would speak for you in case that you cannot speak for yourself.

PATIENT: Yeah.

NURSE: Say, if you were to become very ill, in a coma, you may want to tell us whom you would like us to talk to. And then the second component is a living will, where you just state your wishes about your healthcare. Just general. Anything that you can think of. And then third would be about your heart and lungs. If your heart was to stop beating or if your lungs were to stop working, would you want to be resuscitated? Resuscitated means that your chest would be squeezed and you would likely be placed on a ventilator, which is a machine that helps you breath.

PATIENT: Oh no.

NURSE: So, there are three components. Now this is very important to start or to implement because we don't know when we're going to become ill.

FAMILY MEMBER: Do you have one?

NURSE: Yes, I do have one. I encourage all patients to have one. I think it's very important. What kinds of treatment are not acceptable to you?

Although families and patients have questions about their healthcare, many of them may not understand or be familiar with medical terms often used by nurses and other clinicians. Take the interaction above as an example in which the nurse uses lay language to explain advance care planning terms and concepts. Consider the language used versus the medical language the medical team uses:

Lay Language	Medical Language
you would assign someone	You assign a durable power of attorney
you may want to tell us	You may appoint someone
about your heart and lungs	About resuscitation
your chest would be squeezed	We would perform chest compressions

Central to educating patients and families is an awareness of the observable cues that may indicate accommodation needs. This patient does not withdraw when the topic is broached and acknowledges hearing about it previously in the presence of a family member.

Ongoing discussions of goals of care

The patient's priorities and needs shift, resulting in a changing and evolving care plan. Many palliative care specialists have emphasized the importance of systematic meetings to discuss the patient's concerns. In particular, the early introduction of such conversations in the disease process promotes better outcomes.[48,61] These outcomes include more informed choices, better palliation of symptoms, and more opportunity for resolution of important issues. Nurses may be particularly helpful in advocating for patients when they are unable to speak for themselves. The nurse may assist the surrogate decision-maker to convey the patient's wishes by inquiring more about the patient's personal history. Such questions as "Are there things that would be left undone if you were to die sooner rather than later?" stimulate thought and discussion about dying and important life closure issues such as healing relationships and completing financial transactions. However, a nurse may ask this in a different way, such as, "Are there things you need to do in case things do not go as well as we hope?" Encouraging patients to hope for the best outcome, while preparing for the possibility that treatment may not work—"hope for the best, prepare for the worst"—is helpful in guiding the patient.[74] Again, the advocacy role facilitates the provision of all essential information the patient needs to make choices. This includes managing care at home and support structures for family caregivers.

Box 5.8 Questions for discussion about ongoing care

How do you spend your days?

What is an average day like for you?

If you were not ill, how would you spend your time or how would you like to spend your time?

How has your disease interfered with your daily activities?

What practical problems has your illness created for you?

Which symptoms bother you the most?

How are things with family and friends?

Have you been feeling worried, sad, or frightened about your illness?

Do you have a preference for where you spend your time, at home, in the hospital, or at health appointments?

Source: Revised from Dahlin (2010), reference 2.

As patients decline, they may wish to defer such conversations to family or surrogates. If the surrogate decision-maker is unsure about the patient's wishes or if no advance directive is available, the nurse, by posing questions such as those recommended by Harlow in "Family Letter Writing," can be very helpful.[75] Such questions include, "What type of person was the patient?" "Did she/he ever comment on another person's situation when they were incapacitated or on life support?" "Did she/he relate those experiences to her/his own personal views of her/himself?" and "What vignettes can you recall from his/her life that illustrate his/her values?" This written letter offers a healing life review done by family members and captures the essence of the person. In addition to helping to clarify a patient's wishes, addressing these questions may also serve as a healing review of the person's life and help identify what has brought them meaning. Box 5.8 offers many questions for discussing ongoing care.

Bad-news discussions

In palliative care, bad news includes disease diagnosis, recurrence, disease progression, lack of further curative treatments, lack of any treatments to stabilize disease, transition to comfort care, and a terminal prognosis. Bad or unfavorable medical news may be defined as "any news that drastically and negatively alters the patient's view of her or his future."[18] There is no specific algorithm approach to giving bad news. Rather, it depends on the relationship with the patient and family, their understanding of the condition and its trajectory. Nurses, particularly advanced practice registered nurses, along with their physician colleagues, communicate a wide range of bad news to patients.

Nurses often convey a variety of bad news to patients and families such as cancellations or delays in treatments, confirmation of a serious or life-threatening illness, decrease in quality of life, and care setting options.[76] Nurses working in inpatient care settings, especially critical care nurses, are particularly prone to bad news disclosures as they develop relationships with patients and families in a constantly changing environment.[77] The person who delivers the bad news may depend on multiple factors: the relationship of the patient with the team, the clinician the patient most trusts and, sometimes, institutional culture or practice guidelines.

Bad news disclosures are emotionally charged events for both patient/family and nurse and require continuous assessment of patient understanding, fears, and information preferences.[78] Coyle and Sculco beautifully describe the emotional setting of giving bad news for the clinician and the patient[79]:

> Is it possible for any news, transmitted by a doctor [or nurse] to a patient, to be "good news" in the face of advancing disease that is not responsive to chemotherapy? The doctor [or nurse] is in a position of having to give information that the patient does not want to hear, and yet the patient needs to have the information in order to make necessary life decisions. Does it matter how the information is given when medical information itself can remove hope for continued existence? In a way, both parties—the doctor and the patient—are engaged in a communication dance of vulnerability. The physician is vulnerable because he/she must deliver the facts, whatever they may be, and the patient is vulnerable because he/she doesn't want to hear any more bad news.

Physicians and nurses are part of this communication dance. Patients with advanced disease generally want to have the information. Paradoxically, however, although patients may want information, they may be reluctant to initiate such a discussion.[80] Nurses may feel uncomfortable, wanting to tell patients more but disempowered to do so. Physicians may avoid telling the patient too much because they want to avoid feelings of failure.

Behaviors for effective presentation of bad news may be grouped into four domains: (1) preparation, (2) message or content delivery, (3) responding to the patient (and family), and (4) closing the encounter.[74] Essential within the preparation of giving bad news is attention to the healthcare provider's own emotional stress. There may be a range of possible feelings: guilt, lack of control, failure, loss, fear, or resentment.[46] Awareness of these feelings allows for clarity in ownership of issues and a more objective encounter. Nurses, in particular, may also need to deal with their own emotions either from a long-term relationship with the patient or family or from a connection in which there was a personality match.

Recommended steps for family meetings focus on the following: (1) ensuring privacy and adequate time, (2) assessing patients' understanding, (3) providing information about diagnosis and prognosis simply and honestly, (4) avoiding the use of euphemisms, (5) encouraging expression of their feelings, (6) being empathetic, (7) giving a broad but realistic time frame regarding prognosis, and (8) arranging review or follow-up.[61] Other points are summarized in Box 5.9.

Often in response to bad news, patients may ask difficult questions, such as, "Why me?" Rather than feeling the need to answer, one approach is to offer therapeutic presence. Acknowledgment, such as "That is a tough question," allows the nurse to comment and explore further. This can be followed up by, "Can you tell me what you are thinking right now? Or, another statement could be, "That was difficult news, how was it to hear?" By acknowledging and normalizing the patient's feelings, the nurse invites the patient to voice his or her thoughts, feelings, and concerns. By sharing the patient's distress, the nurse may reduce the patient's sense of isolation and suffering. Box 5.10 reviews nursing communication in bad-news situations.

After listening to the patient's and family members' fears and concerns, it is essential to provide accurate, hopeful information.

Box 5.9 Delivering bad news

1. Prepare for the meeting.

    Determine with the patient whom they want present.
    Determine with the team which healthcare providers should be present.

2. Create a comfortable, quiet setting with seating for all participants and free of interruptions. Obtain interpreter as needed.

3. Clarify and clearly state your and the patient's goals for the meeting.

4. Determine what the patient and family know about the patient's condition and what they have been told.

5. Provide the foundation of a brief overview of the patient's course and condition for understanding of the entire group.

6. Give a warning of the news to come
    "Unfortunately, I have some bad/difficult news to share with you." Or "I wish I had better news."
    Pause.
    Give the bad news.

7. Sit quietly and allow the patient and family to absorb the information.

    Wait for the patient to respond.
    After being silent, check in with the patient such as by saying, "I have just told you some difficult news. Do you feel comfortable sharing your thoughts about this?" This may help the patient verbalize concerns.[18]

8. Listen carefully and acknowledge the patient's and family's emotions such as by reflecting on both the meaning and the affect of their responses. Give an opportunity for questions and comments.

9. Provide a summary and give description of follow up.

Source: Revised from Dahlin (2010), reference 2.

When the patient asks whether he or she can partake in some activity that may or may not be in a realistic time frame, the nurse can respond, "I wish that were possible, but I am worried it won't happen." Or, "I hope that you can do that too, but if you can't, here is what we can do in the meantime." The issue of abandonment should be deliberately addressed. This can achieved with such words as, "I wish things were different. But no matter what, I will be there to support you in your decisions and promote your quality of life." This allays fear that even though the patient can no longer tolerate treatment, the providers will continue caring for them.

Case study: bad news

After a second brain resection, Melanie, 17, has lost substantial movement and gait control. One week after surgery, she is moved to the medical floor. This surgery and loss of movement follows an 18-month treatment process of medullablastoma. Beth, Melanie's mother, meets the nurse Clara at the hospital room door.

BETH— Please come outside so I can ask some questions about her medication. Outside the room.

BETH— Please do not tell Melanie anything about her loss of function. It will devastate her. And can we make sure no one asks her to do any movement that would highlight that?

CLARA— I will not tell her unless she brings it up. Let's see her together. Upon entering the room, they find Melanie in bed and has very low affect.

CLARA— How are you today Melanie?

MELANIE— Fine (but looks down).

CLARA— Are you having any pain?

MELANIE— No (and closes her eyes).

BETH— It doesn't appear so. Isn't that great Melanie? You will be going home soon.

CLARA— Melanie, what do you want to do today?

MELANIE— Nothing, it doesn't matter. She looks down. There is a tear in her right eye and she tries to wipe away any evidence before Beth notices.

CLARA— So let's get you washed up and think about planning for getting you home.

BETH— Well, Melanie had hoped to participate at some level in her cheerleading squad, but the recovery time necessary from this surgery will make that impossible now.

MELANIE— Mom, it doesn't matter.

BETH— The "brain surgeon" hasn't returned since I asked him about the future.

MELANIE— Mom, let it go.

Devastating news can come in many forms for patients and families, and nurses cannot expect to anticipate with accuracy what news will be considered bad. When information is bad, as interpreted by patient and family, a nurse's compassionate presence does not mean having the right answers, or all the answers, but rather just "being there" for patients. Mindful presence in bad news disclosures can attend to the spiritual, religious, and existential aspects of care. Nurses are often charged with regularly exploring and assessing patient fears, beliefs, preferences, and desires. Simply talking about these concerns is noted as very meaningful to patients and families.[81] In this occasion, the nurse's role is not to shy away from the feelings of loss between Melanie and Beth, but rather to listen without interrupting. By observing Melanie's body language (her silent tears) and Beth's nonverbal communication (lowering her voice to stress importance and privacy) are indicators that the nurse needs to attend to the content of the message. Stopping other activities to acknowledge this loss and sitting in silence with Melanie, with or without the presence of Beth, may be more therapeutic than encouraging dialogue. Additionally, the nurse should reflect on what issues are significant to the patient/family (consider if cheerleading is more important to Beth than Melanie).

Prognosis

Another common and difficult question is the patient's response to such news with the question, "How long do I have to live?" Responding to and acknowledging such a question normalizes the discussion around death and dying. The nurse may choose to answer in several ways, depending on his or her comfort in these discussions. One response is, "Are you asking for a specific timeline?" Here the nurse is trying to ascertain whether the patient is asking about dying or is thinking of a certain event that he or she wishes to live to experience. Another response is, "How long do you think you have to live?" This allows the patient to voice his or her concern about time and offer their own impression of their remaining time. The patient may say, "Not long, but I wanted to see how long you thought," comparing input from different

---

Box 5.10 Nurse communication with difficult news

Topic of bad news is directly shared with patient/family
Prognosis is explained or elaborated

OBSERVATIONS TO NOTE:
Has someone on the healthcare team told you that the patient/family has already received bad news?
What aspect of the patient's life is a priority?
Are there any indications that this patient/family doesn't understand?

QUESTIONS TO ASK:
Are there any treatments or decisions about your care that you wish you could change?
Is there a special event coming up in your life that you are worried about or looking forward to?

STATEMENTS TO MAKE:
Use a unique adjective to describe the patient/family to other team members (teams can determine the type of adjective to be used by month, e.g., colors, cars, animals)
I see a gap between what you expect from care and what we expect to see from your care.

Nonverbal compassion expressed
Substantial demonstration of closeness, touching

OBSERVATIONS TO NOTE:
Other than moments when providing care, do you touch the patient?
How do you acknowledge the patient/family, other than verbally?

QUESTIONS TO ASK:
Can I hold your hand?
May I sit here with you?

STATEMENTS TO MAKE:
Ask others not to bother the patient/family over a designated window of time.
Consider how you can adjust the environment/setting to create more intimacy and privacy for the patient/family.

Discusses team structure
Determine if patient has immediate needs for specific team members

OBSERVATIONS TO NOTE:
Does the patient/family appear uncomfortable or quiet when the team meets with the patient? Does he or she defer to a family member?
Does the patient have a special connection/relationship with one member of the team or aide staff?

QUESTIONS TO ASK:
Is there a member of the team whom you feel most comfortable with?
Our team meets to discuss your care, is there anything you would like me to tell the team for you?

STATEMENTS TO MAKE:
I'd like to introduce you to someone I work with and trust. (Always have team member known to patient introduce new team member.)
We can provide many services to you because there are several of us who are working on your care.

---

members of the team. A third response may be along the lines of, "Why are you asking that question now?", "What makes you ask that question now?, or "Why do you ask?" This invites the patient to share his or her fears and concerns about dying. The nurse may also reflect on difficult information with, "I imagine it is very frightening not knowing what will happen and when. Do you have particular fears and concerns?" Finally, if the anticipated survival time is short or the nurse is uncomfortable, he or she may reply, "What has the team told you?" In this case, the patient may state that the team has given a certain estimate of time, or the patient may be seeking validation of the prediction.

When it is appropriate to offer a timeline, it is helpful to give a range of time rather than exact times. Instead of the specific time of 2 weeks or 6 months, it is more helpful to say, "weeks to months."

This prevents the patient or family from making a calendar and ticking the days till death. If the patient surpasses the exact time, there is often anger about the countdown. However, when death is imminent, it is helpful to say "hours to days". It is also useful to explain what supports that timeline, such as significant changes, signs and symptoms of dying, or rapid disease progression. This allows the patient and family to prepare for their final time together.

Discussion of life-sustaining treatments

Often when patients are critically ill and have advanced disease, the healthcare team seeks clarification on the use or continuation of life-sustaining measures. Life-sustaining measures may include vasopressors to help the heart pump more efficiently and effectively, dialysis for kidney failure, and antibiotics for infections and artificial nutrition and hydration. "Code status" is commonly defined as the use, or limitation of use of life-sustaining therapy in the event of clinical deterioration of respiratory function and/or cardiac arrest. Major life-sustaining measures within cardiopulmonary resuscitation (CPR) include invasive ventilator support consisting of nasotracheal or endotracheal intubation, noninvasive ventilator support (CPAP, BiPAP), and defibrillation (cardiac electroshock). The use, continuation, or discontinuation of life-sustaining measures are all necessary aspects to these discussions.

Currently, when a patient in any setting experiences a cardiac arrest and/or respiratory failure, the default is full resuscitation. Thus, CPR is performed unless the patient, or the patient's surrogate, has indicated do not resuscitate (DNR) and/or not to be intubated and supported with mechanical ventilation—do not intubate (DNI). The public has little understanding of the reality of implementing CPR. Only 8% of people survive CPR.[82] These statistics decline in patients with serious life-threatening illness. Additionally, patients and families need to be informed that returning to previous function and quality of life is unlikely. Rather, if the patient survives, functional status often diminishes along with quality of life. To dispel concerns of abandonment, it is particularly important to reassure the patient, family, and surrogate that even though CPR will not be performed, all beneficial care will be actively provided. The team should offer recommendations because patients and families cannot make responsible decisions without survival rates, prognosis, and resultant quality of life from CPR.

The process is similar to other patient and family meetings. The recommended steps include (1) establishing an appropriate setting; (2) inquiring of patient and family what they understand of the patient's condition; (3) finding out what the patient expects for the future; (4) discussing resuscitation within the context of the patient's condition; (5) eliciting the patient's understanding of present condition and thoughts of the future, including the context in which resuscitation would be considered; (6) responding to concerns and emotions; and (7) developing a plan.

There are several important concepts around code status discussions. Use of medical vernacular, such as "full code" or "no code" and "Do you want everything done?" is ambiguous at best. Rather it indicates whether or not to perform a procedure, offering little insight into the patient's goals of care. Instead, code status that includes definition of quality of life, preferences, values, or beliefs guides care decisions. Box 5.11 offers some exploratory questions on quality of life.

The focus of discussion on the use of life-sustaining technology is to review the anticipated benefits and burdens of interventions. A possible statement could be, "If we did 'everything,' you still have a serious illness that is incurable. Full code will mean returning to the intensive care unit. This would cause further weakness and debility and keep you away from your family." Or another statement could be, "We know that resuscitation is not without pain from chest compressions and discomfort of ventilator tubes. You have stated you did not want to be in restrained in any way." However, the process of determining the use of life-sustaining treatment is incomplete without documentation. Both the plan and the context of the conversation must be documented in the record and accessible to other healthcare professionals.[3] Ideally, it should be accompanied by a completed state-recognized comfort care/DNR order forms.

Box 5.11 Questions to facilitate quality-of-life discussions

How is your quality of life? How would you describe quality of life?

What would not be quality of life? What would be an unacceptable life?

Is this how you thought disease-focused treatment or advanced illness would be?

What would make this time especially meaningful for you?

What makes life worth living for you?

How have your religious or spiritual beliefs been affected by your illness?

Source: Revised from Dahlin (2010), reference 2.

There are often circumstances when the patient and family convey their overwhelming sense of pressure or responsibility about the decisions they are being asked to make. When this occurs, often the responsibility of making such a decision is too great for patients and families. They may feel that by making a choice to refuse resuscitation, they are "pulling the plug." In these situations, nurses can take an active role in creating an interdisciplinary care plan as described by ANA's Position Statement *Registered Nurses' Roles and Responsibilities in Providing Expert Care and Counseling at the End of Life*. The team can offer the patient and family a plan that focuses on aggressive pain and symptom management, psychological support, and better quality of life. They can then ask for agreement from the patient and family, thereby allowing the patient and family to assent to a plan. Assent means the family agrees to the plan without having to take on the burden of choosing a specific option. Consent means the family is offered a range of options and they choose which option. By assenting, the burden of the decision is removed from the family and placed on the care team. For many families, this feels like less of a burden as the team makes the difficult decision. It may still be the same plan, but the team has allowed the patient and family to "unshoulder" the burden or weight of the decision.

Discussions of life-sustaining treatments and the role of the nurse

Nurses are heavily invested in clarification of code status. They are often the ones who find the patient with a life-threatening illness in respiratory or cardiac arrest and must initiate a code. It is not uncommon that the wish for code status clarification arises from concerned nurses who do not want to call a code because the patient is so ill and they want to avoid inflicting further suffering. Nurses fear situations in which the primary physician is unavailable and they must deal with a covering physician unfamiliar with the patient and goals of care. Therefore, most nurses want to quickly establish the code status with providers familiar with the patient's medical condition.

It is essential that nurses understand the use of life-sustaining treatments among a variety of patient populations. Explaining the benefits and risks of such treatments to patients and families requires nurses to be competent in their appropriate use.[83] Incorporating clinical ethics in decision-making about life-sustaining treatments is a key component to discussions with family.[84] There are several important communication points regarding life-sustaining measures. First and foremost is that the nurse remains present and open to the patient and family's rationale about these difficult issues. Second is that discussion with the patient and/or the patient's surrogate includes (1) perception of the benefits and burdens of life sustaining treatments and the suffering with or without these interventions; (2) any values, beliefs, and culture of the patient and family that affect the decision or need for such interventions; (3) the available data regarding the benefits and burdens of the interventions; and (4) collaborative decision-making about these interventions to meet the patient's goals.

The significant role of nurses in providing information provision and family guidance during challenging decision-making about life-sustaining measures cannot be overemphasized. When the patient is dependent on a ventilator, the nurse must assess the patient's literacy level and understanding along with any visual or auditory impairments in order to teach family members how to communicate with the patient.[85] Teaching patient and family how to use communication tools, such as picture/letter boards, to use and understand nonverbal cues (e.g., head nods, mouthing words), and to create an appropriate environment (visual and proximal positioning) to facilitate patient-family communication are the responsibility of the nurse.[86]

Because of the 24-hour presence with the patient, the nurse may be the one to whom the patient and family turn for explanations, recommendations, reassurance, validation, and support. Questions to the nurse may focus on the meaning of medical jargon such as "CPR/DNR/DNI," presser support, ventilators, and so forth. This is usually followed by patient and family questions such as, "What do you think?" or "What should I do?" The nurse must first define these terms and their intended effect. By educating the patient about the actual intervention and likely outcome, a nurse may be able to reassure the patient.[68] The nurse can offer the facts and reflect back the patient's values and preferences such as, "Mr. X, you told me you want to be comfortable and not return to the hospital. We can get support at home to keep you comfortable and aggressively treat any symptoms." Reassurance and support for the appropriateness of preferences and decisions develops from questions such as, "Do you feel I made the right decision?" or "What would you do?" They may need reassurance that the nurses will continue to provide care. The nurse may respond with, "I support your decision."

Case study: discussing life-sustaining treatments

Mrs. Hill, a 73-year-old widow, was admitted to the intensive care unit 2 weeks ago for advanced ovarian cancer and was immediately intubated. Her sons Reed and Robby (twins) and Kevin arrived from out of town to join their brother, Colton. Reed and Robby agree that ventilator withdrawal would be what their mother would want, however, Colton, who has provided the most hands-on caregiving, and Kevin adamantly believe that their mother will regain consciousness and become well enough to return home. Kevin, the oldest of the brothers, has not seen his mother in 2 years and has had little contact with his brothers. Obviously distraught, he informs the nurse, "My twin brothers have always thought I was stupid. They may be mother's favorites, but I'm going to have the last say!" Mrs. Hill remains in the intensive care unit until the family can make a decision.

To help this family come to a consensus regarding ventilator support for their mother, the nurse should be aware of the family communication patterns among Mrs. Hill's children, patterns that have long existed for this family and are now heightened by their mother's illness. Family conformity is high for the Hill family, as is evidenced by the quick attendance of all her children who have remained at her bedside, and appears to be highest for Colton, who has served as caregiver, and lowest for Kevin, who has not remained connected to the family over the last 2 years. A communication tactic that can be used during a family meeting is to ask *each member of the family* to speak about family inclusion (e.g., "who is most upset in your view?"). A more strategic approach is to incorporate a solution into the question (e.g., "how long are you willing to have your mother on life support before other options are explored?") or pose a reflexive question that invites the family to reflect on possibilities (e.g., "Did your mother ever tell you about her wishes at the end-of-life?"). While family conversation is low for the Hill family, evident by their inability to engage in debate about care options, the nurse's communication task is to help them come to consensus while relational goals include further understanding the family, their communication patterns, and how the family has coped in prior crises.

Conversations about artificial hydration and nutrition

Numerous cultures place great social and cultural importance on drinking and eating. When patients are not able to take food or fluid by mouth, artificial hydration and nutrition may be provided through the gastrointestinal tract using a nasogastric or gastric tube or may be administered intravenously. Finally, for some cultures, intravenous fluids and nutrition may be necessary to prevent any sense of hastening death. Many people believe that not eating and drinking causes great physical suffering. Artificial hydration and nutrition may alleviate any guilt for patients and family arising out of the feeling that they had not tried everything. Therefore, it is necessary to discuss the potential benefits and burdens of both instituting and withholding artificial hydration and nutrition. The rationale for and against these procedures is discussed in chapter 64, "Ethical Considerations in Palliative Care."

Conversations about the transition to palliative care or hospice

The transition in care away from curative-directed therapies is often an emotional time for patients, families, and clinicians alike. Patients may feel a sense of sadness, anger, denial, and loss of control to the disease. Families may finally come to terms with the reality of the situation or the serious nature of the illness. Physicians may feel a sense of failure for not curing the disease, and frustration with the lack of any further medical options. Nurses may feel grief from the impending termination of the patient and family relationship. The focus of care shifts from curing the disease, from physical cure to emotional and psychological healing.

A direct nursing approach is helpful, stating, "We are no longer able to cure or control your disease. We would like to optimize your quality of life, manage pain and symptoms to avoid suffering, and promote optimal functioning. We have expert nurses who care for patients with life-threatening illness, helping you avoid the hospital.

We will work with them to care for you at home." This allows the patient and family to understand they will continue to be cared for and not feel abandoned. Such discussions lend themselves to completing legal and financial business. This allows for life closure in preparation for death and legacy work. Usually, this also includes attending to psycho-emotional-spiritual work. For the family, such discussions promote preparation and planning for a home death and strategies for sustainability in caregiving.

The nurse has a central role to empower the patient at this time. This is accomplished by the continued dialogue about hopes, preferences, and quality of life. Each situation is individual and cannot be determined by an algorithm or recipe approach; personalizing the experience promotes emotional healing. Guidelines for initiating conversations during the last phase of life include (1) focusing on the patients' unique experiences of illness, (2) discussing issues of closure, (3) promoting discussions about pain and symptom management at the end of life, (3) addressing and planning for the preferred site of death and who will provide care for them, (4) facilitating home health and hospice arrangements, and (5) promoting a respectful death. Box 5.12 offers questions to open exploration of changing goals.

Nurses offer information to patients and families about resources and transitions of care. This includes hospice, home health, and other community-based healthcare resources, when such resources are consistent with the patient's and family's values, beliefs, preferences, and goals of care.[3] The nurse is then responsible for the coordination and communication of the plan. He or she promotes continuity of care and continued support in the home. The hospice, palliative, or home care nurse must educate the patient and family about necessary caregiving skills around medications, equipment, and personal care.

Box 5.12 Questions for changing goals of care

What do you understand about your disease and current condition?

What do you understand about further treatment?

What are some of the concerns you have at this time?

What, if anything, are you worried about or afraid of?

Given the severity of your illness, what is most important for you to achieve?

Have you given any thought to what kinds of treatment you would want (and not want) if you become unable to speak for yourself in the future?

We want to focus on maximal comfort and optimal functioning with as much support as possible. Is that okay?

How is your family handling your illness and its change?

How is your family coping with your changing condition?

Are there topics you need help in discussing with them?

Would it be helpful to have us talk to them with you about changes in goals?

Source: Revised from Dahlin (2010), reference 2.

Transition to death

When curing is no longer viable, there is the potential for physical comfort and psychological healing instead of cure. Simple presence, listening, and attending to the basic humanity of the dying patient may be one of the nurse's most powerful contributions. Nurses may reduce anxiety and help prepare patients and families just by describing the dying process. As appropriate, the explanation includes the actual physiological and biological process of dying in simple language. The alleviation of pain and symptoms is based on a patient's previously stated preferences regarding desired level of alertness. Often this includes discussion about the withdrawal of ineffective and/or burdensome medical treatments including preferences around artificial hydration and nutrition.

Often, a patient considers the meaning of his or her life or performs a life review. This facilitates healing in recognition of personal purpose and meaning, resolution of past conflicts, attaining forgiveness and reconciliation, and achievement of personal integration and inner peace. Additional strategies to help relieve emotional and spiritual suffering include guided imagery, music, reading, and art that focuses on healing.[87] This may all include the collaboration of social work, volunteers, and chaplain colleagues.

The nurse's therapeutic presence with the patient in his or her state of vulnerability and decline can be profound. Here, the nurse consciously and nonjudgmentally listens and bears witness to the patient, encouraging any expression of emotion, doubts, or regrets. The simple acts of visitation, presence, and attention can in itself be a potent healing affirmation—a sacramental gesture received by the dying person who may be feeling helpless, diminished, and fearful that he or she has little to offer others. The willingness to demonstrate concern to the patient far outweighs any technique or expertise in the art of listening.

During the dying process, the nurse guides the care while promoting healthy bereavement within the family. One critical nursing task is role modeling for families. Specifically, the nurse demonstrates the art of being present to the dying person. Simply encouraging the family to engage in loving, physical contact, such as holding hands, embracing, or lying next to the patient can be healing. It may help the patient in his or her transition and may help the survivors in their anticipatory grief. For families who want to be present at the time of death, explaining that patients often wait until they are alone to die may prevent the family from feeling a sense of guilt if they are not present at the time of death. Allowing the family to be with the patient after death may help the surviving family members grieve the loss of their loved one.

After death, the nurse offers continued presence, support, and information. The nurse informs them of the process of certifying death and may assist the family in informing others about the death. Awareness of anticipatory grief and bereavement guides care at this time. Bereaved families are often in most need of having someone to listen to them. Such activities, including telling the story of the loved one's illness, including details of the days and weeks around the death of their loved one, and sharing memories of the loved one, are therapeutic. The nurse may offer information for burial or funeral services as well as grief services. When the family is ready to leave their loved one, the nurse assures respect for the body and explains the process of postmortem care.

Team communication and collaboration

Collaboration within an interdisciplinary team is a vital force in working with patients with serious, life-threatening illness. Hanson and Spross describe collaboration as a "dynamic inter-personal process in which two or more individuals make a commitment to each other to interact authentically and constructively to solve problems and to learn from one another to accomplish identified goals, purposes, or outcomes. The individuals recognize and articulate the shared values that make this commitment possible."[88] Good communication ensures better collaboration, ensures comprehensive care, and assures safety and quality.[85,89] Collaboration enables the sustainability of the team.[90]

However, teams are social systems, and have their own dynamics just as a family does. In effect, the team can be a "work family." With good leadership, role delineation, and flexibility, interdisciplinary teams have the capacity to work well, creating a synergy that promotes positive outcomes.[91] If working effectively, the team identity as a palliative care team member supersedes the individual member's discipline. There are necessary qualities to promote effective collaborative teams. First, the participation of all members is essential; the degree of involvement may depend on the issues of the patient and family. Each member's role should be well defined and respected. Good communication and negotiation are necessary to delineate roles. Second, each team member should have a voice in team processes. Third, the team's mission and goals should be periodically reviewed to assure that all members are working on the same premise. Team members share information and work both independently and together to develop goals. Each team member should be committed to quality care. Fourth, each team member should understand his or her role in patient care and maintain the process of the group. Leadership is shared among team members depending on the task at hand. This means there must be respect for different styles, trust in clinical competence, and compassion for each other.[88,90] Periodic review of these guidelines will ensure the team's effectiveness and efficiency as a team.

Effective teams promote collaboration through effective team communication, team organization and coordination, and competency. This teamwork will be characterized by different environmental and organizational cultures, which dictate the nature of the teamwork as collaborative, deferential, or hierarchical. It is also variable depending on a nurse's role and level of practice. Part of teamwork is the development of working relationships and understanding differing communication styles. This necessitates:

◆ Recognition of individual team member contributions.

◆ Respect for and acknowledgment of the competence and expertise of team members.

◆ Clear definition of roles, responsibilities, and tasks.

◆ Well-defined reporting structures for both work functions and practice.

◆ Scheduled communication among team members and meeting times.

◆ Skilled leadership to manage nurses who are novices, intermediate practitioners, and experts.

◆ Evaluation processes for quality of care and team effectiveness.

◆ Psychological and spiritual support for team.

◆ Ethical and legal resources for the team.

◆ Respect for patients as individuals.

There is a negative process to teamwork as well. Barriers to effective teamwork include lack of training, hierarchical team structures, organizational rules, and reimbursement issues that cause inherent authority issues. Ineffective leadership results in lack of mission and vision. Moreover, team attitude can have an effect in care. There has been an emerging arrogance among palliative care team members that "they know best, are the most caring, effective, and ethical." This can incur negative feelings among other healthcare colleagues, who may feel they are just as caring and committed to patient care.

Poor communication results in poor care, negative outcome, conflicts, and ultimately team demoralization.[92] If roles and responsibilities have not been clearly delineated, nurses may feel restrained to broach and discuss certain topics with patients and families, defaulting to the physician, who may prefer that these discussions occur at the nursing level. Consequently, a lack of clear roles between nurse and physician can leave patients and families with no communication about their illness, treatment, or prognosis. Ongoing discussions between physician and nurse occur more as a task-focused discussion about the patient assessment and response to treatment.[84] Nurses also play an important role in mediating communication between physician and patient and family.[93]

Kane describes how stress, tension, and conflicts among team members may arise and result in bad relationships.[92] Eight problematic team behaviors include: (1) overwhelming the patient, (2) making the patient part of the team, (3) squelching of individual team members, (4) lack of accountability, (5) team process trumping client outcome, (6) orthodoxy and groupthink, (7) overemphasis on health and safety goals, and (8) squandering of resources. All of these issues can occur at various times within the palliative care team and necessitate good communication and conflict resolution. Examples of these problems include the following:

1. Overwhelming the patient—This occurs in several ways. One is overwhelming the patient with too much information. The patient and family have just heard difficult news and have yet to absorb it when palliative care or hospice enters to fix everything. Another overwhelming experience is attendance of many healthcare providers in family meetings. When the ration of healthcare professionals far outweighs the patient and family members, it is overwhelming. The patient or family may feel outnumbered and disempowered to raise individual issues or concerns.

2. Making the patient part of the team—Patients are told that they are part of the decision-making team and are asked for input. The boundaries about what decision they can or cannot make is ambiguous, especially if they disagree. Moreover as the patient declines, they may not really be able to participate in decision-making.

3. Squelching of individual team members— The team may explicitly express that everyone's input is equal when implicitly that is not the case. Nonphysician voices may be dismissed, minimized, marginalized, or trumped by physicians when there is disagreement. Or when trying to advocate a certain unpopular perspective, a team member may be discounted as being "not

really understanding the situation," "no longer objective," or "too close to the situation."

4. Lack of accountability—This is often a challenge when there are too many healthcare consultants working with the primary team. Sometimes with everyone on the palliative care team working on the same issues, no one takes responsibility for the overall care of the patient. In addition, there may be cases where a primary team is detached but asks for input from the palliative care team, but nothing is implemented. Or there may be too many consultants, and the patient receives many mixed opinions with no clear advocate.

5. Team process trumping client outcome— Healthcare providers often have certain ideas or feelings about what is right or wrong and how things are done. The challenge is to allow an open process to occur and not to limit it to one particular pathway simply because that is the way it is always done. Patients and families are unique in their needs and don't always follow algorithms.

6. Orthodoxy and groupthink—A group can become insular and not incorporate new ideas. The team becomes unable to assess itself, and obvious problems are overlooked. In end-of-life situations, this often happens in relation to the dying process. A nurse may understand that the patient is dying, but other health professionals look for a specific symptom and treat it. The team may think the nurse is "giving up," rather than admit the patient is dying.

7. Overemphasis on health and safety goals—The care plan itself takes precedence over the patient's needs or choices. This is often seen in the discharge process when the healthcare team disagrees with the patient's lifestyle choices. So the team resorts to making a plan based on their "safety agenda" rather than a patient's choice.

8. Squandering of resources—The needs of patients are missed, especially in the dying phase, resulting in implementation of high-cost interventions with low impact on the patient's overall care.

Teamwork and the role of the nurse

Among the team, nurses work the most closely with physicians, either implementing medical orders or following care plans. However, nurses and physicians differ in their communication styles. Nurses tend to be more narrative or qualitative and emphasize more process and reflection. Physicians tend to be more quantitative and want facts and numbers. Neither style is better than the other; rather both styles are essential in patient- and family-centered care. The goal of a communication interaction between the nurse and the physician dictates whether reflection or facts are needed. If the contact is about information sharing, the nurse may need to present details, short and brief. If a treatment change is warranted, the nurse provides supporting evidence. For example, if calling about pain and symptoms, the nurse should know the medications the patient is taking, when they were last taken and the patient's pain scores, and should offer a suggested plan. Or if calling about a patient's change in code status of goals of care, it is critical the nurse offer the rich narrative of the context of the conversation, so that the physician may have an effective follow-up conversation.

Quality communication between physician and nurse includes: delineating communication roles, reviewing topics to be discussed with the patient and family and by whom, fostering an active communicative role for nurses rather than blindly following physicians' requests, and limiting their own communication with others.[88] When nurses receive authorization or permission from physicians to communicate with patients and families about designated topics or participate in breaking bad news disclosures, it removes a barrier to nurse communication and promotes patient safety.[93]

Conflict resolution

Conflict is a situation in which two or more people or parties disagree. This can occur due to different perspectives of care, different goals of patient goals, different values, different ethics, or different role expectations. Task communication for teams involves gathering information from each other about clinical care of the patient and family, while relational team communication emerges from the general support team members share regarding workplace stress, coping, and burnout.

Nurses on the front line deal with conflict all the time. This may occur between a patient and a nurse, between a nurse and a doctor, between an advanced practice nurse and a registered nurse, or between two healthcare teams. Conflict is inevitable and healthy for palliative teams, secondary to different perspectives, different experience, length of time in palliative care, and the sense of urgency to alleviate symptoms. If managed well, it helps people look at different perspectives and can allow for creativity and positive movement. If dismissed or ignored, it can breed demoralization and negativity.

Nurses deal with conflict differently, depending on their level of practice, practice site, and experience. Often, nurses avoid conflict if they constantly have difficulty dealing with a team member who will not talk about disagreements. However, in palliative care, the goal should be collaboration in which all problems are discussed and mutual solutions are reached.

There are several methods to resolve conflict; negotiation, accommodation, and collaboration. What differentiates these approaches are the perceived power differences. Conflict resolution occurs through a process (Box 5.13). This involves looking at the facts of a conflict, the feelings of a conflict and the identity in the conflict.[94]

First, the nurse identifies the source of the conflict in terms of reviewing the facts of what happened and what the impact was. Second, the nurse reflects on the emotional aspect of the conflict—these are the feelings. Then the nurse addresses goal of conflict resolution in terms of what she or he hopes to accomplish as it relates to the patient and or family. Sometimes, this may be looking at the role each provider has at stake and then thinking what is best for the patient.

There are several steps in meeting with a team member about a conflict. Be curious about your colleague's perspective by learning his or her story. In doing so, the two parties share their common purposes and differing interests. Express your views, including statements of feelings, and take the time to listen. This leads to exploration of the conflict and letting each party tell his or her perspective while acknowledging feelings and each party's version of the events. Among the hardest things to learn to say are "I am sorry," "I was wrong," and "You could be right." It is not necessary for the nurse to feel pressured to agree instantly. Rather it is important to discuss the

Box 5.13 Effective conflict negotiation

I. Reflection of the conflict

A. Identify the conflict—the facts

Review -
  What happened? Objective data.
  What emotions contributed to conflict? Subjective data.
Consider -
  What impact has the situation had on you?
  How did you contribute to the problem?

B. Identify the goal of conflict resolution

Clarify -
  What do you hope to accomplish?
  What is best way to address the issue?
  What is at stake for you?

II. Negotiation of the conflict

A. Address the conflict with the other person.

Consider -
  When and how is the best way to raise the issue?
  How is the best way to achieve the purpose of resolution?

B. Identify each individual's purpose to conflict resolution—the feelings

Review -
  Where do you and the other person share purposes?
  Where do you and the other person's interests differ?

C. Explore the conflict

Discuss-
  What is the other person's perspective? Listen to other individual and explore the story.
  What are the other person's feelings? Acknowledge feelings behind story and paraphrase them.
  Does the other person understand your perspective? Ask other individual to "listen to you as you share your version of the events and your intentions."

D. Problem solve—with patient's best interest as goal

Invent options to meet each side's most important concerns and interests.
  Decide tack of resolution—avoidance, collaborate, compromise.
  Use objective criteria or palliative care standards (NCP *Clinical Practice Guidelines*) for what should happen.
  Determine approach for future communication.

Source: Revised from Dahlin (2010), reference 2.

range of the issues. Problem-solve together with the common goal of the patient's well-being and decide on a tack of resolution.

Conclusion

Communication in palliative nursing is the essential tool by which nurses deliver care. Effective communication sets the foundation on which the care plan is established and guides the care. There is the art of nursing communication based on the use of presence, listening, silence, and therapeutic presence. This is enhanced through emotional intelligence. The science of nursing communication involves skills in verbal and nonverbal communication and application of communication strategies to promote effective, quality care. Patient- and family-centered care necessitates effective nurse communication to impart communication, gather information, and provide a therapeutic presence. Communication is essential in team collaboration and resolving conflict. Nurses have a direct role in difficult conversations ranging from information sharing about diagnosis and treatment, counseling about end-of-life choices, determining values and preferences, supporting patients and families in bad news conversations, and facilitating transitions to palliative and hospice care.

References

1. Lynch M, Dahlin C, Hultman T, Coakley E. Palliative care nursing: defining the discipline? J Hosp Palliat Nurs. 2011;13(2):106–111.
2. Dahlin C. Communication in palliative care: an essential competency for nurses. In: Ferrell BR, Coyle N (eds.), Oxford Textbook of Palliative Nursing. 3rd ed. New York, NY: Oxford University Press, 2010:107–133.
3. National Consensus Project for Quality Palliative Care. Clinical Practice Guidelines for Quality Palliative Care. 3rd ed. Pittsburgh, PA: National Consensus Project; 2013.
4. Cohen A, Nirenberg A. Current practices in advance care planning: implications for oncology nurses. Clin J Oncol Nurs. 2011,15(5):547–553.
5. American Association of Colleges of Nursing. Peaceful Death: Recommended Competencies and Curricular Guidelines for End-of-Life Nursing Care. www.aacn.nche.edu/Publications/death-fin.htm. Published 1997. Accessed June 13, 2013.
6. Peereboom K, Coyle N. Facilitating goals-of-care discussions for patients with life-limiting disease: communication strategies for nurses. J Hosp Palliat Nurs. 2012;14(4):251–258.
7. American Nurses Association. Nursing: Scope and Standards of Practice. 2nd ed. Silver Spring, MD: Nursebooks.org; 2010.
8. American Nurses Association. Position Statement: Registered Nurses' Roles and Responsibilities in Providing Expert Care and Counseling at the End of Life. http://www.nursingworld.org/MainMenuCategories/EthicsStandards/Ethics-Position-Statements/etpain14426.pdf. 2010. Posted June 14, 2010. Accessed October 20, 2013.
9. American Nurses Association. Position Statement: Nursing Care and Do Not Resuscitate (DNR) and Allow Natural Death (AND) Decisions. http://www.nursingworld.org/MainMenuCategories/EthicsStandards/Ethics-Position-Statements.aspx. Posted March 12, 2012. Accessed October 20, 2013.
10. American Nurses Association and Hospice and Palliative Nurses Association. Palliative Nursing: Scope and Standards of Practice—An Essential Resource for Hospice and Palliative Nurses. 5th ed. Silver Spring, MD: American Nurses Association and Hospice and Palliative Nurses Association; 2013.
11. Hospice and Palliative Nurses Association. Competencies for the Generalist Hospice and Palliative Nurse. 2nd ed. Pittsburgh, PA: Hospice and Palliative Nurses Association; 2010.
12. Hospice and Palliative Nurses Association. 2011. Position Statement: The Nurse's Role in Advanced Care Planning. www.hpna.org/DisplayPage.aspx?Title=Position. Accessed October 20, 2013.
13. White K, Coyne P. Nurses' perceptions of educational gaps in delivering end-of-life care. Oncol Nurs Forum. 2011;38(6):711–717.
14. Degner L, Gow C. Evaluations of death education in nursing: a critical review. Cancer Nurs. 1988;11(3):151–159.

15. Mathews M, Park A. Identifying patients in financial need: cancer care providers' perceptions of barriers. Clin J Oncol Nurs. 2009;13(5)501–505.

16. Northfield S, Nabauer M. The caregiving journey for family members of relatives with cancer: how do they cope? Clin J Oncol Nurs. 2010;14(5):567–577.

17. Malloy P, Virani R, Kelly K, Munevar C. Beyond bad news: communication skills of nurses in palliative care. J Hosp Palliat Nurs. 2010;12(3):166–174.

18. Buckman R. Practical plans for difficult conversations in medicine. Baltimore, MD: Johns Hopkins University Press; 2010.

19. Ferrell BR, Coyle N. The Nature of Suffering and the Goals of Nursing. New York, New York: Oxford University Press; 2008.

20. Field D, Copp G. Communication and awareness about dying in the 1990s. Palliat Med. 1999;13(6):459–468.

21. Buckman R. Communication skills in palliative care. Neurol Clin. 2001;19(4):989–1004.

22. Cloyes K, Berry P, Reblin M, Clayton M, Ellington L. Exploring communication patterns among hospice nurses and family caregivers. J Hosp Palliat Nurs. 2012;14(6):426–437.

23. Grant M. Communication. In: Dahlin C, Lynch A (eds.), Core Curriculum for the Advanced Practice Hospice and Palliative Registerd Nurse. 2nd ed. Pittsburgh, PA: Hospice and Palliative Nurses Association, 2012:61–76.

24. Lowey S. Communication between the nurse and family caregiver in end-of-life care: a review of the literature. J Hosp Palliat Nurs. 2008;10(1):35–48.

25. Sheldon L, Hilaire D, Berry D. Provider verbal response to patient distress cure during ambulatory oncology visits. Oncol Nurs Forum. 2011;38(3):369–375.

26. Williams B, Lewis D, Burgio KL, Goode P. "Wrapped in their arms": next-of-kin's perceptions of how hospital nursing staff support family presence before, during, and after the death of a loved one. J Hosp Palliat Nurs. 2012;14(8):541–550.

27. Codier E, Munero L, Frietas E. Emotional intelligence abilities in oncology and palliative care. J Hosp Palliat Nurs. 2011;13(3):183–188.

28. Wilson S, Coenen A, Doorenbos A. Dignified dying as a nursing phenomenon in the United States. J Hosp Palliat Nurs. 2006;8:34–41.

29. Wenrich MD, Curtis JR, Shannon SE, Carline JD, Ambrozy DM, Ramsey PG. Communicating with dying patients within the spectrum of medical care from terminal diagnosis to death. Arch Intern Med 2001;161(6):868–874.

30. Martins C, Basto M. Relieving the suffering of end of life patients: a grounded theory study. J Hosp Palliat Nurs. 2011;13(3):161–171.

31. Krammer L, Hanks-Bell M J, Cappleman J. Therapeutic presence. In: Panke J, Coyne P (eds.), Conversations in Palliative Care. 3rd ed. Pittsburgh, PA: Hospice and Palliative Nurses Association, 2011:45–52.

32. Waldrop D, Meeker MA, Kerr C, Skretny J, Tangeman J, Milch R. The nature and timing of family-provider communication in late-stage cancer: a qualitative study of caregivers' experiences. J Pain Symptom Manage. 2012;43(2):182–194.

33. Hebert R, Schulz R, Copeland V, Arnold R. Preparing family caregivers for death and bereavement: insights from caregivers of terminally ill patients. J Pain Symptom Manage. 2009;37(1):3–12.

34. Dahlin C, Kelley J, Jackson V, Temel J. Early palliative care for lung cancer: improving quality of life and increasing survival. Int J Palliat Nurs. 2010;16(9):420–423.

35. Perrin K. Communicating with seriously ill and dying patients, their families and their health care providers. In: Matzo M, Sherman DW (eds.), Palliative Care Nursing: Quality Care to the End-of-Life. 3rd ed. New York, NY: Springer Publishing Company, 2010:169–185.

36. Carter N, Bryant-Lukosius D, Dicenso A, Blythe J, Neville A. The supportive care needs of men with advanced prostate cancer. Oncol Nurs Forum. 2011;38(2):189–198.

37. Pierce S. Improving end-of-life care: gathering questions from family members. Oncol Nurs Forum. 1999;34(2):5–14.

38. Dunne K. Effective communication in palliative care. Nursing Standard. 2005;20(13):57–64.

39. Ragan S. Verbal play and multiple goals in the gynaecological exam interaction. J Lang Soc. 1990(1–2);9:67–84.

40. Tracy K, Coupland N. Multiple goals in discourse: an overview of issues. J Lang Soc. 1990;9(1–2):1–12.

41. Boyd D, Merkh K, Rutledge D, Randall V. Nurses' perceptions and experiences with end-of-life communication and care. Oncol Nurs Forum. 2011;38(3):229–239.

42. Wittenberg-Lyles E, Goldsmith J, Ferrell B, Ragan S. Communication in Palliative Nursing. New York, NY: Oxford University Press; 2013.

43. Andershed B, Ternestedt BM. Being a close relative of a dying person: development of concepts, "involvement in the light and the dark." Cancer Nurs. 2000;23(2):151–159.

44. Kruijver IP, Kerkstra A, Bensing JM, van de Wiel HB. Nurse-patient communication in cancer care: A review of the literature. Cancer Nurs. 2000;23(1):20–31.

45. Ferrell BR, Virani R, Grant M. Analysis of end-of-life content in nursing textbooks. Oncol Nurs Forum. 1999;26(5):869–876.

46. Beckstrand R, Collette J, Callister L, Luthy K. Oncology nurses' obstacles and supportive behaviors in end-of-life care: providing vital family care. Oncol Nurs Forum. 2012;39(5):E398–E406.

47. Heaven C, Magure P. Communication issues. In: Lloyd-Williams M (ed.), Psychosocial Issues in Palliative Care. New York, NY: Oxford University Press; 2003:13–34.

48. Quill T E. Initiating end-of-life discussions with seriously ill patients: addressing the "elephant in the room". JAMA. 2000; 284(19):2502–2507.

49. Zanchetta M, Moura S. Self-determination and information seeking in end-stage cancer. Clin J Oncol Nurs. 2006;10(6):803–807.

50. Borrell-Carrio F, Suchman AL, Epstein RM. The biopsychosocial model 25 years later: principles, practice, and scientific inquiry. Ann Fam Med. 2004;2(6):576–582.

51. DasGupta S, Irvine C, Spiegel M. The possibilities of narrative palliative care medicine: "Giving Sorry Words." In: Gunaratnam Y, Oliviere D (eds.), Narrative Stories in Health Care: Illness, Dying and Bereavement. New York, NY: Oxford University Press; 2009.

52. Boreale K, Richardson B. Communication. In: Panke J, Coyne P (eds.), Conversations in Palliative Care. 3rd ed. Pittsburgh, PA: Hospice and Palliative Nurses Association, 2011:33–44.

53. Wood J. Relational Communication: Continuity and Change in Personal Relationships. 2nd ed. Belmont, CA: Wadsworth; 2000.

54. Wilkerson S, Mula C. Communication in care of the dying. In: Ellershaw J, Wilkerson S (eds.), Care of the Dying: A Pathway to Excellence. New York, NY: Oxford University Press, 2003.

55. Grant M, Hanson J. Families. In: Panke J, Coyne P (eds.), Conversations in Palliative Care. 3rd ed. Pittsburgh, PA: Hospice and Palliative Nurses Association, 2011:25–32.

56. Pasacreta J, Minarik P, Neil-Anderson L. Anxiety and depression. In: Ferrell BR, Coyle N (eds.), Oxford Textbook of Palliative Nursing. 3rd ed. New York, NY: Oxford University Press, 2010:425–448.

57. Neff P, Lyckholm L, Smith T. Truth or consequences: what to do when the patient doesn't want to know. J Clin Oncol. 2002;21(9):3035–3037.

58. Lapine A, Wang-Cheng R, Goldstein M, Nooney A, Lamb G, Derse A. When cultures clash: physicians, patient, and family wishes in truth disclosure for dying patients. J Palliat Med. 2001;4(4):475–480.

59. Quill TE, Arnold RM, Platt F. "I wish things were different": expressing wishes in response to loss, futility, and unrealistic hopes. Ann Intern Med. 2001;135(7):551–555.

60. Hannon B, O'Reilly V, Bennett K, Breen K, Lawlor PG. Meeting the family: measuring effectiveness of family meetings in a specialist inpatient palliative care unit. Palliat Support Care. 2012;10(1):43–49.

61. Rabow MW, Hauser JM, Adams J. Supporting family caregivers at the end of life. "They don't know what they don't know." JAMA. 2004;291(4):483–489.

62. Detmar SB, Aaronson NK, Wever LD, Muller M, Schornagel JH. How are you feeling? Who wants to know? Patients' and oncologists' preferences for discussing health-related quality-of-life issues. J Clin Oncol. 2000;18(18):3295–3301.

63. Warm E. Fast Facts # 12: Myths About Advance Care Planning. 2nd ed. EPERC Fast Facts. http://www.eperc.mcw.edu/EPERC/FastFactsIndex/ff_012. 2009. Updated March 2009. Accessed October 20, 2013.

64. Aging with Dignity. Five Wishes. http://www.agingwithdignity.org/five-wishes.php. Updated 2013. Accessed October 20, 2013.

65. Gunderson Lutheran Medical Foundation. Making Choices. http://respectingchoices.org/patient_support/making_choices_information_booklet_5562.asp. Updated 2013. Accessed October 20, 2013.

66. Project Grace. What Are Advance Directives. http://www.projectgrace.org/Advance-Directives. Updated 2012. Accessed October 19, 2013.

67. POLST. POLST: What It Is and What It Is Not. http://www.polst.org/polst-what-it-is-and-what-it-is-not/. Posted June 23 2013. Accessed October 20, 2013.

68. Christakis N A, Lamont E B. Extent and determinants of error in doctors' prognoses in terminally ill patients: prospective cohort study. BMJ. 2000;320:469–472.

69. Kutner JS, Steiner JF, Corbett KK, Jahnigen DW, Barton PL. Information needs in terminal illness. Soc Sci Med. 1999;48(10):1341–1352.

70. The AM, Hak T, Koeter G, van der Wal G. Collusion in doctor–patient communication about imminent death: an ethnographic study. BMJ. 2000;321:1376–1381.

71. Blackford J, Street AF. Facilitating advance care planning in community palliative care: conversation starters across the client journey. Int J Palliat Nurs. 2013;19(3):132–139.

72. Jeong SY, Higgins I, McMillan M. The essentials of advance care planning for end-of-life care for older people. J Clin Nurs. 2010;19(3–4):389–397.

73. Chrash M, Mulich B, Patton C. The APN role in holistic assessment and integration of spiritual assessment for advance care planning. J Am Acad Nurse Pract. 2011;23(10):530–536.

74. Back A, Arnold R, Tulsky J. Mastering Communication with Seriously Ill Patients: Balancing Honesty with Empathy and Hope. New York, NY: Cambridge University Press, 2009.

75. Last Acts. Family Letter Writing: An Interview with Navah Harlow, MA. Innovations in End-of-Life Care: An International Journal of Leaders in End-of-Life Care. http://www2.edc.org/lastacts/archives/archivesmarch99/featureinn.asp. Last update July 17, 2000. Accessed October 20, 2013.

76. McGuigan D. Communicating bad news to patients: a reflective approach. Nurs Stand. 2009;23(31):51–56; quiz 57.

77. Warnock C, Tod A, Foster J, Soreny C. Breaking bad news in inpatient clinical settings: role of the nurse. J Adv Nurs. 2010;66(7):1543–1555.

78. Stayt LC. Death, empathy and self preservation: the emotional labour of caring for families of the critically ill in adult intensive care. J Clin Nurs. 2009;18(9):1267–1275.

79. Coyle N, Sculco L. Communication and patient/physician relationship: phenomenological inquiry. J Support Oncol. 2003;1(3):206–215.

80. Hancok K, Clayton J, Parker S, et al. Truth telling in discussing prognosis in advanced life-limiting illnesses: a systematic review. Palliat Med. 2007;21:506–517.

81. Visser A, Wysmans M. Improving patient education by an in-service communication training for health care providers at a cancer ward: communication climate, patient satisfaction and the need of lasting implementation. Patient Educ Couns. 2010;78(3):402–408.

82. American Heart Association. CPR and statistics. http://www.heart.org/HEARTORG/CPRAndECC/WhatisCPR/CPRFactsandStats/CPRStatistics_UCM_307542_Article.jsp. Last update April 13, 2013. Accessed October 20, 2013.

83. Lopez RP, Amella EJ, Mitchell SL, Strumpf NE. Nurses' perspectives on feeding decisions for nursing home residents with advanced dementia. J Clin Nurs. 2010;19(5–6):632–638.

84. Blackwood B, Junk C, Lyons JD, McAuley DF, Rose L. Role responsibilities in mechanical ventilation and weaning in pediatric intensive care units: a national survey. Am J Crit Care. May 2013;22(3): 189–197.

85. Freise C, Manojlovich M. Nurse-physician relationships in ambulatory oncology settings. J Nurs Sch. 2012;44(3):258–365.

86. Grossbach I, Stranberg S, Chlan L. Promoting effective communication for patients receiving mechanical ventilation. Crit Care Nurse. 2011;31(3):46–60.

87. Fogarty LA, Curbow BA, Wingard JR, McDonnell K, Somerfield MR. Can 40 seconds of compassion reduce patient anxiety? J Clin Oncol. 1999;17(1):371–379.

88. Hanson C, Spross J. Collaboration. In: Hamric A, Spross J, Hanson C (eds.), Advanced Practice Nursing-An Integrative Approach. St. Louis, MO: Elsevier Saunders; 2009:283–314.

89. American Association of Critical Care Nurses. 2005. ACCN Standards for Establishing and Sustaining Healthy Work Environments: A Journey to Excellence. www.aacn.org/WD/HWE/Docs/HWEStandards.pdf. Accessed October 20, 2013.

90. Lindeke L, Sieckert A. Nurse-physician workplace collaboration. Online J Issues Nurs. 2005;10(1). http://www.nursingworld.org/MainMenuCategories/ANAMarketplace/ANAPeriodicals/OJIN/TableofContents/Volume102005/No1Jan05/tpc26_416011.aspx. Accessed October 20, 2013.

91. Crawford G, Price S. Team working: palliative care as a model of interdisciplinary practice. Med J Aust. 2003;Suppl 6(179):s32–s34.

92. Kane R. Avoiding the dark side of geriatric teamwork. In: Mezey MD, Cassel CK, Bottrell MM, Hyer K, Howe JL, Fuher TT (eds.), Ethical Patient Care: A Casebook for Geriatric Health Care Teams. Baltimore, MD: John Hopkins Press; 2002:187–207.

93. Manojlovich M, Antonakos CL, Ronis DL. Intensive care units, communication between nurses and physicians, and patients' outcomes. Am J Crit Care. 2009;18(1):21–30.

94. Stone D, Patton B, Heen S. Difficult Conversations: How to Discuss What Matters Most. New York, NY: Penguin Books; 1999.

SECTION II

Symptom assessment and management

CHAPTER 6

Pain assessment

Regina M. Fink, Rose A. Gates, and
Robert K. Montgomery

> Pain is such an uncomfortable feeling that even a tiny amount of it is enough to ruin every enjoyment.
>
> Will Rogers[1]

Key points

- Pain is multifactorial and affects the whole person and family caregivers.

- Multiple barriers to pain assessment exist.

- Patients or residents should be screened for pain on admission to a hospital, clinic, nursing home, hospice, or home care agency.

- If pain or discomfort is reported, a comprehensive pain assessment should be performed at regular intervals, whenever there is a change in the pain, and after any modifications in the pain management plan.

- Reassessment of pain intensity should occur within 1 hour of analgesic administration or other nonpharmacological intervention.

- The patient's self-report of pain is the gold standard, even for those patients who are nonverbal or cognitively impaired.

- Multiple pain scales are available for use in nonverbal or cognitively impaired patients or residents; these should be used in combination with clinical observation and information from healthcare professionals and family caregivers.

- Evaluate pain assessment instruments used in your care setting. Ensure evidence-based, valid and reliable, culturally sensitive tools are being used for your patient populations.

Pain is a common companion of birth, growth, death, and illness; it is intertwined intimately with the very nature of human existence. Most pain can be palliated, and patients can be relatively pain free. To successfully relieve pain and suffering, accurate, continuous pain assessment and reassessment is critical. However, evidence demonstrates that pain is undertreated in the palliative care setting, contributing significantly to patient discomfort and suffering at the end of life. Studies suggest that as many as 25% of newly diagnosed cancer patients, 60% of those undergoing treatment, and 75% of those with life-threatening illness and in the terminal phase of disease, have unrelieved pain; 33% received inadequate analgesia.[2–5] Results from a systematic review of pain prevalence in cancer patients indicate that greater than one-third of those experiencing pain report moderate to severe pain.[5] Expanding evidence suggests that among hospitalized patients, 25%–40% may suffer from uncontrolled pain within the last few days of life.[6] Kutner and colleagues[7] report that, even in the care-oriented culture of hospice, 82% of their patients in the Population-Based Palliative Care Research Network listed pain as the most bothersome symptom and required more intensive pain management during the last weeks of life, at times requiring sedation. In addition to assistance with goals of care clarification, unrelieved pain is one of the most frequent reasons for palliative care consultation.[8] Although nursing homes are increasingly becoming the most common site of death for the elderly,[9] pain relief in long-term care facilities varies widely, with 45% to 80% of residents having substantial pain with suboptimal pain management.[10–14] Pain continues to be poorly assessed with over one-third of long-term care residents having no formal or regularly scheduled pain assessment, despite implementation of the pain assessment documentation required by the Minimum Data Set (MDS) 3.0.[14]

This chapter considers various types of pain, describes barriers to optimal pain assessment, and reviews current clinical practice guidelines for the assessment of pain in the palliative care setting. A multifactorial model for pain assessment is proposed, and a variety of instruments and methods that can be used to assess pain in nonverbal and cognitively impaired patients are reviewed. Case studies are used for discussion purposes.

Types of pain

According to the International Association for the Study of Pain (IASP), pain is defined as "an unpleasant sensory or emotional experience associated with actual or potential tissue damage. The inability to communicate verbally does not negate the possibility that an individual is experiencing pain and is in need of appropriate pain-relieving treatment."[15] Pain has also been clinically defined as "whatever the experiencing person says it is, existing whenever the experiencing person says it does."[16]

Pain is commonly described in terms of categorization along a continuum of duration. Acute pain may be associated with tissue damage, inflammation, a disease process that is relatively brief, or a surgical procedure. Regardless of its intensity, acute pain is usually of brief duration: hours, days, weeks, or a few months. Acute pain serves as a warning that something is wrong and is generally viewed as a time-limited experience. In contrast, persistent or chronic pain worsens and intensifies with the passage of time, lasts for an extended period (months, years, or a lifetime), and adversely affects the patient's function or well-being. In the literature, the words "persistent" and "chronic" have often been used interchangeably to describe long-lasting pain. This newer term "persistent" is favored as it is not associated with the negative stereotype often associated with a chronic pain patient label.[11] Chronic, persistent pain has been further subclassified into chronic malignant and chronic nonmalignant pain. Cancer pain may be nociceptive or neuropathic. It may be related to primary or metastatic disease in two-thirds of patients, may be the result of treatment (surgery, chemotherapy, biotherapy, radiation therapy, or procedures), or other causes (side effects, infection).[4] Persistent pain may accompany a disease process such as human immunodeficiency virus (HIV) infection and acquired immune deficiency syndrome (AIDS), arthritis or degenerative joint disease, osteoporosis, chronic obstructive pulmonary disease, heart failure, neurological disorders (e.g., multiple sclerosis, cerebrovascular disease), fibromyalgia, sickle cell disease, cystic fibrosis, and diabetes. It may also be associated with an injury that has not resolved within an expected period of time, such as low back pain, trauma, spinal cord injury, complex regional pain syndrome (formerly known as reflex sympathetic dystrophy), postherpetic neuralgia, or phantom limb pain.

The American Geriatric Society (AGS) Panel on Persistent Pain in Older Persons[10,11] has classified persistent pain in pathophysiological terms that assist the healthcare professional to determine the cause of pain and select the appropriate pain management interventions. The four pain subcategories that have been delineated are nociceptive pain (visceral or somatic pain resulting from stimulation of pain receptors), neuropathic pain (pain caused by peripheral or central nervous system stimulation), mixed or unspecified pain (having mixed or unknown pain mechanisms), and pain due to psychological disorders.

Barriers to optimal pain assessment

Inadequate pain control is not the result of a lack of scientific information. Over the last four decades, a plethora of research has generated knowledge about pain and its management. Reports that document the inability or unwillingness of healthcare professionals to use knowledge from research and advances in technology continue to be published. The armamentarium of knowledge is available to assist professionals in the successful assessment and management of pain; the problems lie in its misuse or lack of use. Undertreatment of pain often results from clinicians' failure or inability to evaluate or appreciate the severity of the patient's problem.

Multiple barriers to the achievement of optimal pain assessment and management have been identified (Box 6.1).[17–21] The knowledge and attitudes of healthcare professionals toward pain assessment are extremely important, because these factors influence the priority placed on pain treatment.

Box 6.1 Barriers to optimal pain assessment

Healthcare professional barriers

Lack of identification of pain assessment and relief as a priority in patient care

Inadequate knowledge about how to perform a pain assessment

Perceived lack of time to conduct and document a pain assessment and reassessment

Failure to use validated pain measurement tools

Inability of clinician to empathize or establish rapport with patient

Lack of continuity of care

Lack of communication among the healthcare professional team

Prejudice and bias in dealing with patients

Failure to accept patient's/resident's pain reports

Healthcare system barriers

A system that fails to hold healthcare professionals accountable for pain assessment

Lack of criteria or availability of culturally sensitive instruments for pain assessment in healthcare settings

Lack of institutional policies for performance and documentation of pain assessment

Patient/family/societal barriers

The highly subjective and personal nature of the pain experience

Lack of patient and family awareness about the importance of speaking out about pain

Lack of patient communication with healthcare professionals about pain

- ◆ Patient reluctance to report pain
- ◆ Patient not wanting to bother staff
- ◆ Patient fears of not being believed
- ◆ Patient age-related stoicism
- ◆ Patient doesn't report pain because "nothing helps"
- ◆ Pain presence is a sign of deterioration
- ◆ Patient concern that curative therapy might be curtailed with pain and palliative care
- ◆ Lack of a common language to describe pain
- ◆ Presence of unfounded beliefs and myths about pain and its treatment

Sources: Adapted from references 17–21.

Pain assessment guidelines and standards

Recognition of the widespread inadequacy of pain assessment and management has prompted corrective efforts within many healthcare disciplines, including nursing, medicine, pharmacy, and pain management organizations. Representatives from various healthcare professional groups have convened to develop clinical practice guidelines and quality assurance standards and recommendations for the assessment and management of acute, cancer, and end-of-life pain.[4,10–12,22–30] The establishment of a formal monitoring program to evaluate the efficacy of pain assessment and interventions has been encouraged.[30] The American Pain Society (APS) Guidelines for the Management of Cancer Pain in Adults, APS Recommendations for Improving Quality of Acute and Cancer Pain Management, the APS Position Statement on Treatment of Pain at the End of Life, the Oncology Nursing Society (ONS) Position on Cancer Pain Management and ONS Putting Evidence into Practice: Pharmacologic and Nonpharmacologic Interventions for Pain, the National Comprehensive Cancer Network Adult Cancer Pain Clinical Practice Guidelines, the American Society of Pain Management Nurses (ASPMN) Position Statements on Pain Management at the End of Life and Pain Assessment in the Patient Unable to Self-Report, the Hospice and Palliative Nurses Association Position Statement on Pain Management, the American Geriatrics Society Panel on Persistent Pain in Older Persons, the American Geriatrics Society Panel on the Pharmacological Management of Persistent Pain in Older Person, the American Medical Directors Association Clinical Practice Guidelines for Pain, and an Interdisciplinary Expert Consensus Statement on Assessment of Pain in Older Persons are reflective of the national trend to assess quality of care in high-incidence patients by monitoring outcomes as well as assessing and managing pain.

Joint Commission surveyors routinely inquire about pain assessment and management practices and quality improvement activities designed to monitor pain assessment and reassessment practices, patient satisfaction, and outcomes within healthcare institutions. The Joint Commission provides standards for assessing and managing pain in hospital, ambulatory, home care, and long-term care settings, recommending that culturally sensitive, age-appropriate pain rating scales be available to assist with assessment activities. The Joint Commission launched a national campaign, the Speak Up program, to help persons with pain become better informed and more involved with their pain management plan of care.[28] Patient-centered care requires that healthcare professionals seek opportunities to empower patients and families in decision-making about their care, taking into account their personal preferences and values. Involving patients and families in the pain assessment process is integral to improving pain management with the desired outcome of decreased pain for patients.

Healthcare reform processes require that patients be discharged sooner, without adequate time to assess pain or to evaluate newly prescribed pain management regimens. Therefore, the prevalence of inadequate pain assessment and management may be even greater than reported, because more persons may be suffering silently in their homes. Healthcare professionals may not be aware of the patient's pain, have the time to communicate or understand the meaning of the pain experience for the patient, or be available due to less-than-adequate resources. With the changes in the delivery of healthcare and at times decreased continuity of care, pain assessment and management may not be a priority.

Process of pain assessment

Accurate pain assessment is the basis of pain treatment; it is a continuous process that encompasses multidimensional factors.

In formulating a pain management plan of care, an assessment is crucial to identify the pain syndrome or the cause of pain. A comprehensive assessment addresses each type of pain and includes the following: a detailed history, including an assessment of the pain intensity, its characteristics, and its effects on function, and a history of previous substance abuse; a physical examination with pertinent neurological examination, particularly if neuropathic pain is suspected; a psychosocial and cultural assessment; and an appropriate diagnostic workup to determine the cause of pain.[4] Attention should be paid to any discrepancies between patients' verbal descriptions of pain and their behavior and appearance. The physical examination should focus on an examination of the painful areas and common referred pain locations. In frail or terminally ill patients, physical examination maneuvers and diagnostic tests should be performed only if the findings will potentially change or facilitate the treatment plan. The burden and potential discomfort of any diagnostic test must be weighed against the potential benefit of the information obtained. Ongoing and subsequent evaluations are necessary to determine the effectiveness of pain-relief measures and to identify any new pain. Patients or residents should be asked whether they have pain (screened for pain) on admission to a hospital, clinic, nursing home, hospice, or home care agency. If pain or discomfort is reported, a comprehensive pain assessment should be performed at regular intervals, whenever there is a change in the pain, and after any modifications in the pain management plan. Reassessment of pain intensity should occur after each pain management intervention, once a sufficient time has elapsed for the treatment to reach peak effect (e.g., 15–30 minutes after a parenteral medication and within 1 hour of oral medication administration or other nonpharmacological intervention).[4,31] Pain reassessment is crucial because subsequent actions of the pain algorithm depend on the patient's response. The frequency of pain assessment and reassessment is determined by the patient's or resident's clinical situation. Pain assessment and reassessment should be individualized and documented so that all interdisciplinary team members involved will have an understanding of the pain problem. Information about the patient's pain can be obtained from multiple sources: verbal self-report, observations, interviews with the patient and significant others, review of medical data, and feedback from other healthcare providers.

Pain is uniquely personal and subjective. The first opportunity to understand the pain experience is at the perceptual level. Perception incorporates the patient's self-report and the results of a pain assessment accomplished by the healthcare provider. *Perception* is "the act of perceiving, to become aware directly in one's mind, through any of the senses; especially to see or hear, involving the process of achieving understanding or seeing all the way through; using insight, intuition, or knowledge gained"; *assessment* is defined as "the act of assessing, evaluating, appraising, or estimating by sitting beside another."[32] Perception is an abstract process in which the person doing the perceiving is not just a bystander but is immersed in understanding the other's situation and has the capacity for such insight. Perception is influenced by "higher-order" processes that characterize the cognitive and emotional appraisal of pain—what people feel and think about their pain and their future with the pain. Perception also includes the interpersonal framework in which the pain is experienced (with family or friends or alone), the meaning or reason for the pain, the person's coping pattern or locus of control, the presence of additional symptoms, and others' concerns (e.g., significant others' distress). Alternatively, assessment is a value judgment that occurs by observing the other's experience.

Assessment and perception of the patient's pain experience at the end of life is essential before planning interventions. However, the quality and usefulness of any assessment is only as good as the ability of the assessor to be thoroughly patient focused. This means listening empathetically, maintaining open communication, and validating and legitimizing the concerns of the patient and significant others. A clinician's understanding of the patient's pain and accompanying symptoms confirms that there is genuine personal interest in facilitating a positive pain management outcome.

Pain does not occur in isolation. Other symptoms and concerns experienced by the patient compound the suffering associated with pain. Total pain has been described as the sum of all of the following interactions: physical, psychological, social, and spiritual.[33] At times, patients describe their whole life as painful. The provision of palliative care to relieve pain and suffering is based on the conceptual model of the whole person experiencing "total pain."

It is not always necessary or relevant to assess all dimensions of pain in all patients or in every setting. At the very least, both the sensation and intensity of pain and the patient's response to pain management must be considered during an assessment. The extent of the assessment should be dictated by its purpose, the patient's condition or stage of illness, the clinical setting, feasibility, and the relevance of a particular dimension to the patient or healthcare provider. For example, a comprehensive assessment may be appropriate for a patient in the early stage of palliative care, whereas only a pain intensity score is needed when evaluating a patient's response to an increased dose of analgesic. Incorporation of the multidimensional factors described in the following section into the pain assessment will ensure a comprehensive approach to understanding the patient's pain experience.

Multifactorial model for pain assessment

Pain is a complex phenomenon involving many interrelated factors. The multifactorial pain assessment model is based on the work of a number of researchers over the last four decades.[34–38] An individual's pain is unique; it is actualized by the multidimensionality of the experience and the interaction among factors both within the individual and in interaction with others.

Melzack and Casey[34] suggested that pain is determined by the interaction of three components: the sensory/discriminative (selection and modulation of pain sensations), the motivational/affective (affective reactions to pain via the brain's reticular formation and limbic system), and the cognitive (past or present experiences of pain). Evidence presented by Ahles[35] supported the usefulness of a multidimensional model for cancer-related pain by describing the following theoretical components of the pain experience: physiological, sensory, affective, cognitive, and behavioral. McGuire[36] expanded the work of Ahles and colleagues by proposing the integration of a sociocultural dimension to the pain model. This sociocultural dimension, comprising a broad range of ethnocultural, demographic, spiritual, and social factors, influences an individual's perception of, and responses to, pain and its management. Bates[37] proposed a biocultural model, combining

Table 6.1 Multifactorial pain assessment

Factors	Question
Physiological/sensory	What is causing the patient's pain?
	How does the patient describe his/her pain?
Affective	How does the patient's emotional state affect his/her report of pain?
	How does pain influence the patient's affect or mood?
Cognitive	How do the patient's knowledge, attitudes, and beliefs affect their pain experience?
	What is the meaning of the pain to the patient?
	How does the patient's past experience with pain influence the pain?
Behavioral	How do you know the patient is in pain?
	What patient pain behaviors or nonverbal cues inform you that pain is being experienced?
	What is the patient doing to decrease his or her pain?
Sociocultural	How does the patient's sociocultural background affect the pain experience, expression, and coping?
Environmental	How does the patient's environment affect the pain experience or expression?

social learning theory and the gate control theory, as a useful framework for studying and understanding cultural influences on human pain perception, assessment, and response. She believed that different social communities (ethnic groups) have different cultural experiences, attitudes, and meanings for pain that may influence pain perception, assessment, tolerance, and neurophysiological, psychological, and behavioral responses to pain sensation. Hester[38] proposed an environmental component, referring to the setting, environmental conditions, or stimuli that affect pain assessment and management. Excessive noise, lighting, or extreme temperatures may be sources of stress for individuals in pain and may negatively affect the pain experience.

Given the complexity of the interactions among the factors, if a positive impact on the quality of life of patients is the goal of palliative care, then the multifactorial perspective provides the foundation for assessing and managing pain. Some questions that can guide a multifactorial pain assessment are reviewed in Table 6.1.

Physiological and sensory factors

The physiological and sensory factors of the pain experience explain the cause and characterize the person's pain. Over 80% of cancer patients with advanced metastatic disease suffer pain due to direct tumor involvement.[39] Patients should be asked to describe their pain, including its quality, intensity, location, temporal pattern, and aggravating and alleviating factors. Five key factors included in a basic pain assessment are outlined in Figure 6.1.[40]

In the palliative care setting, the patient's cause of pain may have already been determined. However, changes in pain location or character should not always be attributed to these pre-existing causes, but should prompt a reassessment. Treatable causes, such as infections or fractures, may be the cause of new or persistent pain.

University of Colorado Hospital
UNIVERSITY OF COLORADO HEALTH

Pain Assessment Guide
Tell Me About Your Pain

W Words to describe pain (discomfort)

Somatic	Visceral	Neuropathic
aching	crampy	numb
dull	gnawing	burning
throbbing	deep	radiating
sharp	squeezing	shooting
stabbing	pressure	electrical
sore	stretching	tingling
penetrating	bloated	pins & needles

Pain in Other Languages

Japanese - itami	Spanish - dolor	Croatian-Bosnian - bol
Chinese - tong	French - douleur	Arabic - أَلَم
Vietnamese - dau	Russian - bolno	Ethiopian - amonyal

I Intensity (0-10)

If 0 is no pain and 10 is the worst pain possible, what is your pain now?
....at rest? ..... with movement? ...
In the last 24 hours what was your least pain? ...worst? ... average?
What is your comfort-function goal?

L Location

Where is your pain?

D Duration

Is the pain constant? ...intermittent? ..... both types?

A Aggravating and Alleviating Factors

What makes the pain worse? ...better?

How does the pain affect:

activity	energy	relationships	appetite
function	sleep	mood	

Are you experiencing medication side effects?

nausea/vomiting	drowsiness	itching	urinary retention
sleepiness	constipation	confusion	dizziness

Things to Check
vital signs, response to past medication/treatment, substance abuse history, use of nonpharmacological techniques, chronic pain history

Figure 6.1 2013 Pain Assessment Guide. A pocket pain assessment guide for use at the bedside. The nurse or other healthcare professional may use this guide to help the patient identify the type and intensity of pain and to determine the best approach to pain management in the context of overall care. Source: ©2013 Regina Fink, RN, PhD, AOCN, FAAN, University of Colorado Hospital, Aurora, Colorado, used with permission (reference 40).

Words

Patients are asked to describe their pain or discomfort using words or qualifiers. Table 6.2 summarizes various pain types, word qualifiers, etiological factors, and choice of analgesia based on pain type. Identifying the qualifiers enhances understanding of the patient's pain etiology and should optimize pain treatment. Not doing so may result in an incomplete pain profile. Screening tools are available to enhance and refine neuropathic pain assessment.[41–43]

Intensity

Although an assessment of intensity captures only one aspect of the pain experience, it is the most frequently used parameter in clinical practice. Obtaining a pain intensity score will quantify how much pain a person is experiencing. Pain intensity should be evaluated not only at the present level, but also at its least, worst, average, and at rest or with movement. Patients should be asked how their pain compares with yesterday or with their worst day. They should be asked for a personal comfort-function goal describing how much pain can occur without interfering with function or quality of life or the level of pain that will enable function and comfort.[21] A review of the amount of pain experienced after analgesic or adjuvant drug administration, and/or use of nonpharmacological approaches can also add information about the patient's level of pain. Pain intensity can be measured quantitatively with the use of a visual analog scale, numeric rating scale, verbal descriptor scale, faces scale, or pain thermometer. In using these tools, patients typically are asked to rate their pain on a scale of 0 to 10: no pain = 0; mild pain is indicated by a score of 1 to 3; moderate pain, 4 to 6; and severe pain, 7 to 10.[4] No single scale is appropriate for all patients. During instrument selection, the nurse must consider the practicality, ease, and acceptability of the instrument's use by palliative care patients. (For a description of these instruments, see later discussion.) To ensure consistency, nurses and other healthcare professional staff should carefully document which scale worked best for the patient, so that all members of the healthcare team will be aware of the appropriate scale to use.

Location

The majority of persons with cancer have pain in two or more sites[4]; therefore, it is crucial to ask questions about pain location. Encourage the patient to point or place a finger on the area involved. This will provide more specific data than verbal self-report. Separate pain histories should be acquired for each major pain complaint, since their causes may differ and the treatment plan may need to be tailored to the particular pain type. For example, neuropathic pain may radiate and follow a dermatomal path; pain that is deep in the abdomen may be visceral; and when a patient points to an area that is well localized and nonradiating, the pain may be somatic, possibly indicating bone metastasis. Metastatic bone pain is one of the most common pain syndromes in cancer patients, with up to 60% of patients experiencing severe pain.[44]

Duration

Learning whether the pain is constant, intermittent, or both will guide the selection of interventions. Patients may experience "breakthrough" pain (BTP), an intermittent, transitory flare of pain, with several subtypes described—incidental, spontaneous, or end-of-dose pain.[45] This BTP may require a fast-acting opioid, whereas constant pain is usually treated with long-acting, continuous-release opioids. Patients with progressive diseases such as cancer and AIDS may experience persistent pain that has an ill-defined onset and unknown duration.

Aggravating and alleviating factors

If the patient is not receiving satisfactory pain relief, inquiring about what makes the pain worse or better—the aggravating and alleviating factors—will assist in determining which diagnostic tests need to be ordered or which nonpharmacological approaches can be incorporated into the plan of care. Pain interference with

Table 6.2 Pain descriptors

Pain type	Qualifiers	Possible etiological factors	Intervention
Neuropathic	Numb, burning, radiating, shooting, electrical, tingling, "pins and needles"	Injury to peripheral or central nervous tissue Nerve involvement by tumor (cervical, brachial, lumbosacral plexi), postherpetic or trigeminal neuralgia, diabetic neuropathies, HIV associated neuropathy (viral or antiretrovirals), chemotherapy-induced neuropathy, post-stroke pain, post-radiation plexopathies, phantom pain	Anticonvulsants, antidepressants, local anesthetics, ±opioids (e.g., tramadol, methadone), ±steroids, nerve blocks
Visceral (poorly localized)	Crampy, gnawing, deep, squeezing, pressure, stretching, bloated	Bowel obstruction, venous occlusion, ischemia, liver metastases, ascites, thrombosis, post-abdominal or post-thoracic surgery, pancreatitis	Opioids (caution must be used in the administration of opioids to patients with bowel obstruction), nonsteroidal antiinflammatory drugs (NSAIDs)
Somatic (well localized)	Aching, dull, throbbing, sore	Activation or injury of nociceptors/pain fibers in superficial cutaneous and deep musculoskeletel structures Bone or spine metastases, fractures, arthritis, osteoporosis, immobility	NSAIDs, ±opioids, steroids, muscle relaxants, bisphosphonates, radiation therapy (bone metastasis)
Psychological	All-encompassing, everywhere	Psychological disorders	Psychiatric treatments, support, nonpharmacological approaches

functional status can be measured by determining the pain's effects on activities such as activity, function (walking or repositioning in bed), energy, falling and/or staying asleep, relationships, mood, or appetite. Researchers have found that pain interference with functional status is highly correlated with pain intensity scores; for example, a pain intensity score greater than 4 has been shown to significantly interfere with daily functioning.[2] In addition, Fainsinger and colleagues found that pain intensity scores at initial assessment have been found to be significant predictors of pain management complexity and length of time to stable pain control in cancer patients.[46]

Affective factor

The affective factor includes the emotional responses associated with the pain experience and, possibly, such reactions as depression, anger, distress, anxiety, decreased ability to concentrate, mood disturbance, and loss of control. A person's feelings of distress, loss of control, or lack of involvement in the plan of care may affect outcomes of pain intensity and patient satisfaction with pain management.

Cognitive factor

The cognitive factor refers to the way pain influences the person's thought processes; the way the person views himself or herself in relation to the pain; the knowledge, attitudes, and beliefs the person has about the pain and its management; and the meaning of the pain to the individual. Past experiences with pain may influence one's beliefs about pain. Whether the patient feels that another person believes in his or her pain also contributes to the cognitive dimension. Bostrom and colleagues[47] interviewed 30 palliative care patients with cancer-related pain to examine their perceptions of the management of their pain. Patients expressed a need for open communication with healthcare professionals about their pain problem and a need for being involved in the planning of their pain treatment. Those who felt a trust in their healthcare organization, their nurse, and their doctor described an improved ability to participate in their pain management plan. Porter and colleagues examined self-efficacy for managing pain

in lung cancer patients and their caregivers and found that patients who rated their self-efficacy as high experienced lower pain levels and improved quality of life.[48] Perceived control over pain is an important aspect of the pain response. Interventions to assist patients and caregivers in becoming a part of the pain plan of care is critical.

Patients' knowledge and beliefs about pain play an obvious role in pain assessment, perception, function, and response to treatment. Patients may be reluctant to tell the nurse when they have pain; they may attempt to minimize its severity, may not know they can expect pain relief, and may be concerned about taking pain medications for fear of deleterious effects. A comprehensive approach to pain assessment includes evaluation of the patient's knowledge and beliefs about pain and its management and common misconceptions about analgesia (Box 6.2).[19,21]

Behavioral factor

Pain behaviors may be a means of expressing or coping with pain. The behavioral factor describes actions the person exhibits related to the pain, such as verbal complaints, moaning, groaning, crying, facial expressions, posturing, splinting, lying down, pacing, rocking, or suppression of the expression of pain. Other cues can include anxiety, sleeplessness, inability to concentrate, and restlessness. Unfortunately, some of these behaviors or cues may relate to causes or symptoms other than pain. For example, insomnia caused by depression may complicate the pain assessment.

Nonverbal expression of pain can complement, contradict, or replace the verbal complaint of pain. Observing a patient's behavior or nonverbal cues, understanding the meaning of the pain experience to the patient, and collaborating with family members and other healthcare professionals to determine their thoughts about the patient's pain, are all part of the pain assessment process.

The behavioral dimension also encompasses the unconscious or deliberate actions taken by the person to decrease the pain. Pain behaviors include, but are not limited to, using both over-the-counter and prescribed analgesics; seeking medical assistance; using nonpharmacological approaches and other coping

Box 6.2 Common patient concerns and misconceptions about pain and analgesia

Pain is inevitable. I just need to bear it.

If I tell about my pain it may lead to a loss of independence and more tests.

If the pain is worse, it must mean my disease (cancer) is spreading.

I had better wait to take my pain medication until I really need it or else it won't work later.

My family thinks I am getting too "spacey" on pain medication; I'd better hold back.

If it's morphine, I must be getting close to the end.

If I take pain medicine (such as opioids) regularly, I will get "hooked" or addicted.

If I take my pain medication before I hurt, I will end up taking too much. It's better to "hang in there and tough it out."

I'd rather have a good bowel movement than take pain medication and get constipated.

I don't want to bother the nurse or doctor; they're busy with other patients.

If I take too much pain medication, it will hasten my death.

Admitting I have pain is a sign of weakness.

Good patients avoid talking about pain.

Sources: Adapted from references 19, 21.

---

strategies such as removing aggravating factors (e.g., noise and light). Behaviors used to control pain in patients with advanced-stage disease include assuming special positions, immobilizing or guarding a body part, rubbing, and adjusting pressure to a body part.

Sociocultural factor

The sociocultural factor encompasses all of the demographic variables of the patient experiencing pain. The impact of these factors (e.g., age, gender, ethnicity, spirituality, marital status, social support) on pain assessment, treatment, and outcomes has been examined in the literature. Although many studies have promoted each individual dimension, few have concentrated on their highly interactive nature. Ultimately, all of these factors can influence pain assessment.

Age

Much of the pain literature has called attention to the problem of inadequate pain assessment and management in the elderly in a palliative care setting. Elderly patients suffer disproportionately from chronic painful conditions and have multiple diagnoses with complex problems and accompanying pain. Elders have physical, social, and psychological needs distinct from those of younger and middle-aged adults, and they present particular challenges for pain assessment and management. Pain assessment may be more problematic in elderly patients because their reporting of pain may differ from that of younger patients due to their increased stoicism.[19] Elderly people often present with failures in memory,

depression, and sensory impairments that may hinder history taking; they may also underreport pain because they believe pain is a part of aging. Moreover, dependent elderly people may not report pain because they do not want to bother the nurse or doctor and are concerned that they will cause more distress in their family caregivers.[19]

Multiple studies have documented the problem of inadequate pain assessment in the elderly in both hospital and long-term care settings. For example, a classic study published by Cleeland and colleagues[2] of 1308 outpatients with metastatic cancer found that those 70 years of age or older were more likely to have inadequate pain assessment and analgesia. Approximately 40% of elderly nursing home patients with cancer experience daily pain according to Bernabei, who reviewed Medicare records of more than 13,625 cancer patients aged 65 years or older discharged from hospitals to almost 1500 nursing homes in five states.[49] Pain assessment was based on patient self-report and determined by a team of nursing home personnel involved with the patients. Of the more than 4000 patients who complained of daily pain, 16% were administered a nonopioid drug, 32% were given a weak opioid, 26% received morphine, and 26% received no analgesic. As age increased, a greater proportion of patients in pain received no analgesia (21% of patients aged 65 to 74 years, 26% of those aged 75 to 84 years, and 30% of those 85 years of age and older; $P = 0.001$). Fewer than half of over 2000 elderly urban and rural nursing home residents with multiple medical problems and predictably recurrent pain were prescribed scheduled pain medication.[14] It is important to pay particular attention to pain assessment in the elderly patient, so that the chance of inadequate analgesia is decreased. Dementia, cognitive and sensory impairments, and disabilities can make pain assessment and management more difficult and will be discussed later in this chapter.

Gender

Gender differences affect sensitivity to pain, pain tolerance, pain distress, willingness to report pain, exaggeration of pain, and nonverbal expression of pain. Multiple studies have demonstrated that men show more stoicism than women, women exhibit lower pain thresholds and less tolerance to noxious stimuli than men, women become more upset when pain prevents them from doing things they enjoy, women seek care of pain sooner, and responses to analgesics and pain prevalence in various conditions may vary according to gender.[50–52] Although coping with pain and the experience of pain may be influenced by an individual's gender,[52] the reasons for these differences remain unclear or unidentified. It is important to note that gender differences in pain response are not universal and do not exert a large effect.[51] Explanations that require further investigation include molecular and genetic mechanisms, hormonal influences, as well as social, cultural, psychological, and experimental bias.[52] Nurses and other healthcare professionals need to be mindful of possible gender differences when assessing pain and planning individualized care for persons in pain. However, until there is more definitive data, men and women should receive similar pain care based on individualized assessments.

Ethnicity

The term "ethnicity" can refer to one or more of the following: (1) a common language or tradition, (2) shared origins or social background, and (3) shared culture and traditions that are passed through generations and create a sense of identity. Ethnicity may be a predictor of pain expression and response. While assessing pain, it is important to remember that certain ethnic groups and cultures have strong beliefs about expressing pain and may hesitate to complain of unrelieved pain. Bates's biocultural model proposed that culturally accepted patterns of ethnic meanings of pain may influence the neurophysiological processing of nociceptive information that is responsible for pain threshold, pain tolerance, pain behavior, and expression.[37] Thus, the manner in which a person reacts to the pain experience may be strongly related to cultural background. The biocultural model also hypothesizes that social learning from family and group membership can influence psychological and physiological processes, which in turn can affect the perception and modulation of pain. Bates stressed that all individuals, regardless of ethnicity, have basically similar neurophysiological systems of pain perception.

Ethnicity is increasingly recognized as predictive of poor pain assessment and management. There is documented variation across ethnic groups in how pain symptoms are reported and how pain is managed. Studies reveal that racial and ethnic minorities are not adequately assessed for pain and are at risk for undertreatment of pain.[53–55] Differences in cultural backgrounds between healthcare providers and patients can result in misunderstandings, mistrust, and lack of communication about pain. While the number of Latinos in the United States continues to increase, pain treatment disparities of Latinos persist with reasons including: patients' limited health literacy, language proficiency, discomfort communicating in healthcare settings, fears of addiction, prioritizing family above pain control, a belief in the role of suffering at the end-of life, and a lack of cultural understanding by providers.[53,54]

It is important for nurses to realize that racial and ethnic disparities exist in pain care and that too little is known about how culture and ethnicity affect pain responses, pain interventions, and pain measurement. Although pain assessment or pain tools may be available in languages spoken by the patients, the translations may be inadequate or may not capture cultural nuances or meanings.[56] When caring for any patient who is experiencing pain, the nurse must avoid cultural stereotyping and provide culturally sensitive assessment and educational materials, enlisting the support of an interpreter when appropriate.

Marital status and social support

The degree of family or social support in a patient's life should be assessed, because these factors may influence the expression, meaning, and perception of pain and the ability to comply with therapeutic recommendations. Few studies have examined the influence of marital status on pain experience and expression. Morgan et al.[57] studied 177 dyads (45% women, 55% men) with cancer pain and found that the quality of the couples' relationship had a positive effect on the patients' pain, quality of life, and improved strategies to manage pain. Taylor et al. studied 251 women with chronic pain due to osteoarthritis and/or fibromyalgia and found that living in a happy union or relationship may increase the capacity to cope better with pain.[58] Happily partnered patients experiencing pain show less pain-related physical disability, more adaptive and cognitive response to daily pain changes, and an increased sense of pain coping during pain episodes. While there is scant literature related to the influence of marital status and family support on a patient's pain experiences, nurses need to understand and assess the type of support patients receive from family and significant others as it may influence their expression of and coping with pain.

Spirituality

The spiritual dimension may influence the person's pain response, expression, and experience. Whereas pain refers to a physical sensation, suffering refers to the quest for meaning, purpose, and fulfillment. Unrelieved physical pain may cause emotional or spiritual suffering yet suffering may occur in the absence of pain. Many patients believe that pain and suffering are meaningful signs of the presence of a higher being and must be endured; others are outraged by the pain and suffering they must endure and demand alleviation. The nurse must verify the patients' beliefs and give them permission to verbalize their personal points of view. Assessing a patient's existential view of pain, suffering, and spiritual pain is important because it can affect the processes of healing and dying. In a study to understand the relationship among spirituality, religiosity, spiritual pain, symptom assessment, and quality of life, 100 advanced cancer patients receiving palliative care were interviewed in an outpatient oncology clinic.[59] Spiritual pain (defined as a pain deep in the person's soul/being that is not physical) was reported in 44% of patients and was significantly associated with lower self-perceived religiosity and contributed adversely to physical and emotional symptom experience, including pain. A literature review by Unruh[60] found that spiritual views can have a considerable impact on patients' understanding of pain and choices about its management. Suggestions for clinical implications include nurses' examination of their own spirituality and how that could affect their communication with patients, exploring respectful communication with patients about spirituality and its effects on pain, inclusion of spirituality in education and support programs for both patients and healthcare providers, incorporation of spiritual preferences in pain management where appropriate, and referral to pastoral care. Understanding patients' use of spiritual comfort strategies is also an area for further exploration. For additional information about spiritual assessment, please refer to chapter 32 for greater detail.

Environmental factor

The environmental factor refers to the environment in which the person receives pain management. Creating a peaceful environment free from bright lights, extreme noise, and excessive heat or cold may assist in alleviating the patient's pain. Context of care, setting, or where the patient receives care may also refer to the environmental aspect.

A multifactorial framework describing the influences of all of these factors on the assessment of pain and the pain experience is desirable to attain positive pain outcomes. The factors comprising the framework are assumed to be interactive and interrelated. Use of this framework for pain assessment has clear implications for clinical practice and research.

Quantitative assessment of pain

Although pain is a subjective, self-reported experience of the patient, the ability to quantify the intensity of pain is essential to monitoring a patient's responsiveness to analgesia.

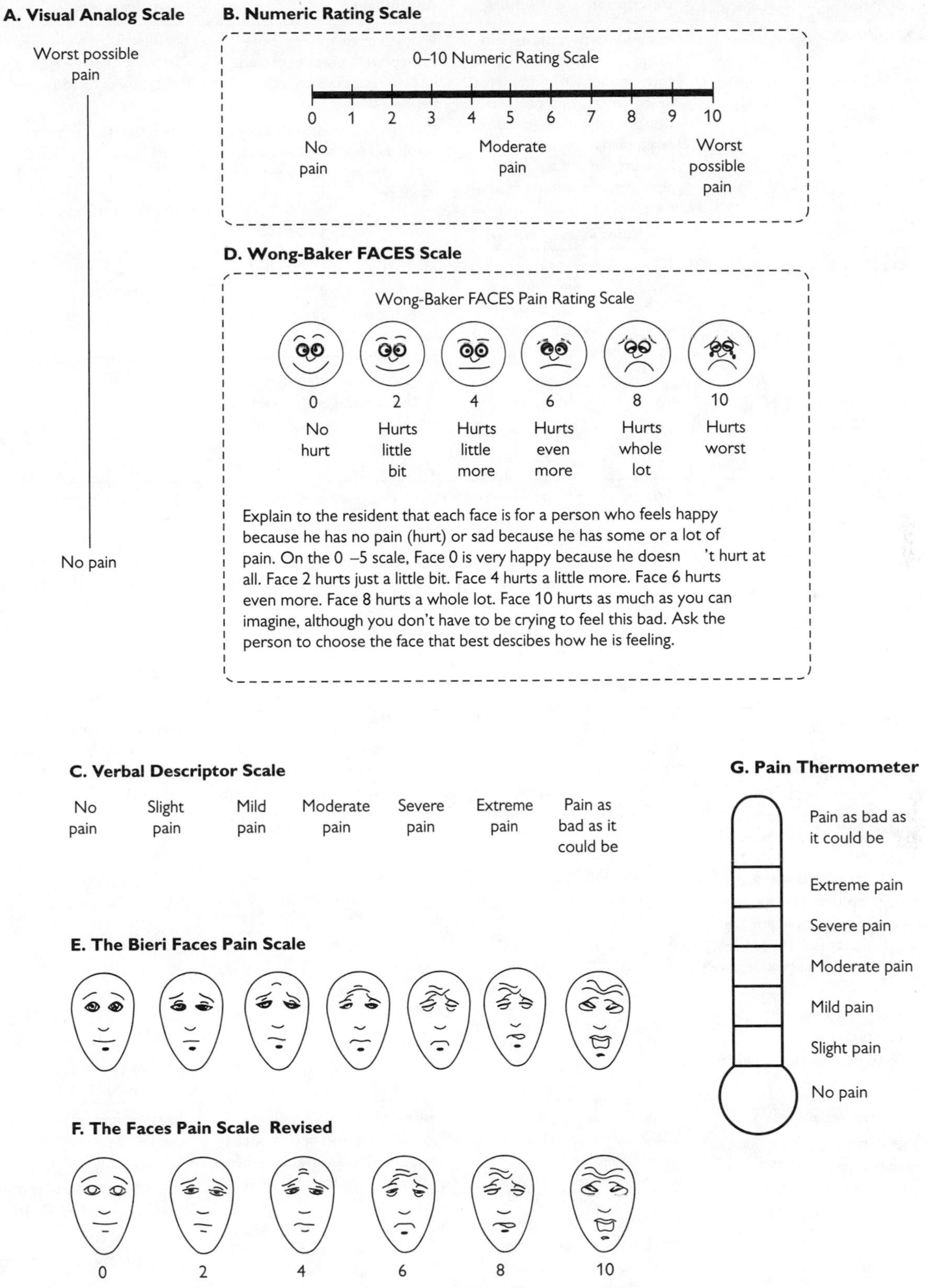

A. Visual Analog Scale

Worst possible
pain

No pain

B. Numeric Rating Scale

0–10 Numeric Rating Scale

0 1 2 3 4 5 6 7 8 9 10

No
pain

Moderate
pain

Worst
possible
pain

D. Wong-Baker FACES Scale

Wong-Baker FACES Pain Rating Scale

0	2	4	6	8	10
No hurt	Hurts little bit	Hurts little more	Hurts even more	Hurts whole lot	Hurts worst

Explain to the resident that each face is for a person who feels happy because he has no pain (hurt) or sad because he has some or a lot of pain. On the 0 –5 scale, Face 0 is very happy because he doesn   't hurt at all. Face 2 hurts just a little bit. Face 4 hurts a little more. Face 6 hurts even more. Face 8 hurts a whole lot. Face 10 hurts as much as you can imagine, although you don't have to be crying to feel this bad. Ask the person to choose the face that best descibes how he is feeling.

C. Verbal Descriptor Scale

No pain | Slight pain | Mild pain | Moderate pain | Severe pain | Extreme pain | Pain as bad as it could be

E. The Bieri Faces Pain Scale

F. The Faces Pain Scale Revised

0   2   4   6   8   10

G. Pain Thermometer

Pain as bad as it could be

Extreme pain

Severe pain

Moderate pain

Mild pain

Slight pain

No pain

Figure 6.2 Commonly used pain intensity scales. Refer to Table 6.3 for descriptions, advantages, and disadvantages. Sources: (D) From Hockenberry MJ, Wilson D: Wong's *Essentials of Pediatric Nursing*, ed. 8, St. Louis, 2009, Mosby. Used with permission. Copyright Mosby (reference 67). (F) This Faces Pain Scale-Revised has been reproduced with permission of the International Association for the Study of Pain® (IASP). Ask the patient to "point to the face that shows how much you hurt now." Score the chosen face 0, 2, 4, 6, 8, or 10 from left to right. This scale is intended to measure how the patient feels inside, not how their face looks.

Table 6.3 Pain intensity assessment scales

Scale	Description	Advantages	Disadvantages
Visual Analogue Scale (VAS) (See Figure 6.2A)	A horizontal or vertical line of 10 cm (or 100 mm) in length anchored at each end by verbal descriptors (e.g., no pain and worst possible pain). Patients are asked to make a slash mark or X on the line at the place that represents the amount of pain experienced. Often used in research studies.	Positive correlation with other self-reported measures of pain intensity and observed pain behaviors.[61] Qualities of ratio data with high number of response categories make it more sensitive to changes in pain intensity.[62]	Scoring may be more time-consuming and involve more steps. Patients may have difficulty using and understanding a VAS measure. Too abstract for many adults, and may be difficult to use with elderly, non-English-speaking, and patients with physical disability, immobility, or reduced visual acuity, which may limit their ability to place a mark on the line.[63]
Numeric Rating Scale (NRS) (See Figure 6.2B)	The number that the patient provides represents his/her pain intensity from 0 to 10 with the understanding that 0 = no pain and 10 = worst possible pain.	May be used with most children over 8 years of age.[64] Verbal administration to patients allows those by phone or who are physically and visually disabled to quantify pain intensity.[65] Ease in scoring, high compliance, high number of response categories.[65] Scores may be treated as interval data and are correlated with VAS.	Lack of research comparing sensitivity to treatments impacting pain intensity.
Verbal Descriptor Scale (VDS) (See Figure 6.2C)	Adjectives reflecting extremes of pain are ranked in order of severity. Each adjective is given a number, which constitutes the patient's pain intensity.	Short, ease of administration to patients, easily comprehended, high compliance.[61] Easy to score and analyze data on an ordinal level. Validity is established.[61]	Patients must choose one word to describe their pain intensity even if no word accurately describes it.[61] Variability in use of verbal descriptors may be associated with affective distress. Scores on VDS are considered ordinal data; however, the distances between its descriptors are not equal but categorical.[65] Less reliable among illiterate patients and persons with limited English vocabulary.[66]
FACES Scale (Wong-Baker)[67] (See Figure 6.2D) Explain to the patient or resident that each face is for a person who feels happy because he has no pain (hurt) or sad because he has some or a lot of pain. On the 0–10 scale, Face 0 is very happy because he doesn't hurt at all. Face 2 hurts just a little bit. Face 4 hurts a little more. Face 6 hurts even more. Face 8 hurts a whole lot. Face 10 hurts as much as you can imagine, although you don't have to be crying to feel this bad. Ask the person to choose the face that best describes how he is feeling. *Source:* From Hockenberry MJ, Wilson D. *Wong's Essentials of Pediatric Nursing*, ed. 8, St. Louis, 2009, Mosby. Used with permission. Copyright Mosby, reference 67.	The scale consists of six cartoon-type faces. The no pain (0) face shows a widely smiling face and the most pain (10) face shows a face with tears. The scale is treated as a Likert scale and was originally developed to measure children's pain intensity or amount of hurt. It has been used in adults.	Simplicity, ease of use, and correlation with VAS makes it a valuable option in clinical settings. Short, requires little mental energy and little explanation for use.[68]	Presence of tears on the "most pain" face may introduce cultural bias when the scale is used by adults from cultures not sanctioning crying in response to pain.[69]
Faces Pain Scale—Revised (FPS-R)[8,70,71] (See Figure 6.2F) Score the chosen face 0, 2, 4, 6, 8, or 10, counting left to right, so "0" = "no pain" and "10" = "very much pain." Do not use words like "happy" and "sad." This scale is intended to measure how children feel inside, not how their face looks. *Source:* This Faces Pain Scale-Revised has been reproduced with permission of the International Association for the Study of Pain® (IASP). Used with permission IASP, reference 71	The FACES Pain Scale Revised (FPS-R) was adapted from the FPS (seven faces) (See Figure 6.2e)[72] in order to make it compatible with a 0–10 metric scale. The FPS-R measures pain intensity consists of six oval faces ranging from a neutral face (no pain) to a grimacing, sad face without tears (worst pain).	Easy to administer. Oval-shaped faces without tears or wide smiles are more adult-like in appearance, possibly making the scale more acceptable to adults. Recommended for use in research studies on the basis of utility and psychometric features [73]	Facial expressions may be difficult to discern for patients who have visual difficulties. The FPS-R may measure other constructs (anger, distress, and impact of pain on functional status) than just pain intensity.
Pain Thermometer[74] (See Figure 6.2G)	Modified vertical verbal descriptor scale which is administered by asking the patient to point to the words that best describe his/her pain.	Increased sensitivity. Preferred for patients with moderate to severe cognitive deficits or those with difficulty with abstract thinking and verbal communication.[74]	Allow for practice time to use this tool.

Pain intensity assessment scales

The most commonly used pain intensity scales—the visual analog scale (VAS), the numeric rating scale (NRS), the verbal descriptor scale (VDS), the Wong-Baker FACES pain scale, the Faces Pain Scale-Revised (FPS-R), and the pain thermometer—are illustrated and reviewed in Table 6.3 with advantages and disadvantages delineated. These scales have been a very effective, reproducible means of measuring pain and other symptoms, and they can be universally implemented and regularly applied in many care settings. How useful these tools are in the assessment of pain in the palliative care patient is a question that still needs to be answered.

Although no one scale is appropriate or suitable for all patients, universal adoption of a 0-to-10 scale, rather than a 0-to-5 or a 0-to-100 scale, for clinical assessment of pain intensity in adult patients is recommended.[65,75] Standardization may promote collaboration and consistency in evaluation among caregivers across multiple settings (i.e., inpatient, ambulatory, home care/hospice, or long-term care environments) and would facilitate pain research across sites. Collection of comparative data would be enabled, allowing for simplification of the analytical process. Detailed explanation of how to use the pain scales is necessary before use by patients in any clinical care area.

Another concern is healthcare professionals' inconsistent use of word anchors on pain intensity scales. The intention behind the use of a word anchor to discriminate pain intensity is to provide a common endpoint; although that point may have not been reached by a patient, it would provide a place for any pain experienced to date or pain that may be experienced in the future. Some of the common endpoint word anchors that have been used are "worst possible pain," "pain as bad as it can be," "worst pain imaginable," "worst pain you have ever had," "most severe pain imaginable," and "most intense pain imaginable." Inconsistent or different word anchors may yield different pain reports. Therefore, it is important for healthcare professionals to achieve consensus about consistent use of word anchors.

Comparison of pain intensity scales

Several studies have been systematically reviewed,[26,61] and although many are limited in sample size and population, a positive correlation has been demonstrated among the VAS, VDS, NRS, Wong-Baker FACES scale, and FPS-R. Each of the commonly used pain rating scales appears to be adequately valid and reliable as a measure of pain intensity in both cancer patients and elders.

Herr and Mobily[63] studied 49 senior citizens 65 years of age with reported leg pain to determine the relationships among the various pain intensity measures, to examine the ability of patients to use the tools correctly, and to determine elder's scale preferences. The VAS consisted of 10-cm horizontal and vertical lines; the VDS had six numerically ranked choices of word descriptors, including "no pain," "mild pain," "discomforting," "distressing," "horrible," and "excruciating"; the NRS had numbers from 1 to 20; and the pain thermometer had seven choices, ranging from "no pain" to "pain as bad as it could be." The VDS was the scale preferred by most respondents. Of the two VAS scales, the vertical scale was chosen most often because the elderly subjects had a tendency to conceptualize the vertical presentation more accurately. Elderly patients may have deficits in abstract ability that make the VAS difficult to use. Increased age is associated with an increased incidence of incorrect response to the VAS.[61]

Paice and Cohen[65] used a convenience sample of 50 hospitalized adult cancer patients with pain to study their preference in using the VAS, the VDS, and the NRS. Fifty percent of the patients preferred using the NRS. Fewer patients preferred the VDS (38%), and the VAS was chosen infrequently (12%). Twenty percent of the patients were unable to complete the VAS or had difficulty in doing so. Problems included needing assistance with holding a pencil, making slash marks that were too wide or not on the line, marking the wrong end of the line, and asking to have instructions read repeatedly during the survey.

Additional problems exist with use of the VAS and may influence its reliability. Physical disability or decreased visual acuity may limit the ability of the palliative care patient to mark the appropriate spot on the line. Photocopying VAS forms may result in distortion so that the scales may not be exactly 10 cm long. When multiple horizontal scales are used to measure different aspects or dimensions (e.g., pain intensity, distress, depression), subjects tend to mark all of the scales down the middle.

The use of a faces pain scale to measure pain intensity avoids language barriers and may cross cultural differences. Several faces pain scales have been used[67,70–72] to assess pain in both pediatric and adult populations. A systematic review of commonly used faces scale for self-report of pain intensity in children recommended that the FPS-R be used in research studies[73]; however, there were no recommendations for using one faces scale over another in clinical use and there is no consensus as to the type of faces scale to use in the palliative care setting.

The literature regarding choice of scale among ethnic groups is equivocal. Jones et al.[76] asked elderly nursing home residents of various ethnicity to choose which of three pain intensity scales (NRS, VDS, and Faces Pain Scale [FPS]) they preferred to use to rate their pain. Of those able to choose, the VDS was the most commonly selected (52%); 29% chose the NRS; 19% preferred the FPS. More men than women and those residents with moderate to severe pain preferred the NRS; a higher percentage of minority (Hispanic) residents preferred the FPS. Participants clearly agreed that the FPS represented pain but also agreed that the FPS may represent other constructs, such as sadness or anger, depending how they were cued; this may suggest that the FPS may be measuring pain affect, not just intensity. Other researchers[77] found that Hispanic patients preferred the FPS-R over the Iowa Pain Thermometer (IPT) and other instruments used to measure pain intensity. In a similar study in China, the FPS-R, VAS, NRS, and a VDS were compared in postoperative patients, and researchers found that all had good reliability and validity but the FPS-R was most preferred with a low rate of error.[78]

Research[26,77] indicates that the VDS, NRS, FPS and FPS-R, and IPT are also reliable and valid in older adults with mild to moderate degrees of cognitive impairment. Ware et al. recommend consideration of the FPS-R when repeat assessments are indicated in older cognitively impaired minority adults.[77] While the FPS-R is generally favored for *both* cognitively intact and cognitively impaired older adults, it should be noted that the FPS-R may not clearly represent pain intensity only but may also represent a broader construct "pain affect."[77]

In summary, a variety of scales have been used to assess pain in varied patient populations. Each has been widely used in clinical research and practice. Little research has been done on the appropriateness of pain scales in the palliative care setting. Intellectual understanding and language skills are prerequisites for such pain assessment scales as the VAS and VDS. These scales may be too abstract or too difficult for palliative care patients. Because most dying patients are elderly, simple pain scales, such as the NRS or a faces scale, may be more advantageous.

Multidimensional pain instruments

There are several pain measurement instruments that can be used to standardize pain assessment, incorporating patient demographic factors, pain severity scales, pain descriptors, pain influence on function, and other questions related to pain. Five instruments have been considered short enough for routine clinical use; however, their utilization in seriously ill, actively dying patients needs further study.

- The *Short Form McGill Pain Questionnaire* (SF-MPQ)[79] has demonstrated reliability and validity, is available in multiple languages, and includes 15 words to describe pain. Each word or phrase is rated on a four-point intensity scale (0 = none, 1 = mild, 2 = moderate, and 3 = severe). Three pain scores are derived from the sum of the intensity rank values of the words chosen for sensory, affective, and total descriptors. Two additional pain measures are included in the SF-MPQ: the Present Pain Intensity Index (PPI) and a 10-cm VAS.

- The *Brief Pain Inventory* (BPI)[80] is a multidimensional instrument that addresses pain etiology, history, intensity, quality, location, and interference with activities. Patients are asked to rate the severity of their pain at its worst, least, average, and at present. Using a NRS (0 to 10), patients are also asked for ratings of how much their pain interferes with walking ability, mood, general activity, work, enjoyment of life, sleep, and relationships with others. The BPI also asks patients to represent the location of their pain on a drawing and asks about the cause of pain and the duration of pain relief.

- The *Memorial Pain Assessment Card* (MPAC)[81] is a simple, valid tool consisting of three VAS for pain intensity, pain relief, and mood and one VDS to describe the pain. The MPAC can be completed by patients in 20 seconds or less and can distinguish between pain intensity, relief, and psychological distress.

- The *City of Hope Patient and Family Pain Questionnaires*[82] were designed to measure the knowledge and experience of patients with persistent cancer pain and their family caregivers. The

16-item surveys use an ordinal scale format and can be administered in inpatient or outpatient settings.

- The *American Pain Society Patient Outcomes Questionnaire-Revised (APS-POQ-R)*[30] is a 23-item, 2-page patient survey designed to be used through patient-reporting or patient-interviewing methods by adult inpatients for the purposes of quality improvement. The questionnaire takes approximately 10 minutes to complete, has established reliability and validity in adult hospitalized medical-surgical patients, and measures six aspects of quality, including (1) pain severity and relief; (2) impact of pain on activity, sleep, and negative emotions; (3) side effects of treatment; (4) helpfulness of information about pain treatment; (5) ability to participate in pain treatment decisions; and (6) use of nonpharmacological strategies. Its use in a palliative care population has not been determined.

Because terminally ill patients have multiple symptoms, it is impossible to limit an assessment to only the report of pain. Complications or symptoms related to the disease process may exacerbate pain, or interventions to alleviate pain may cause side effects that result in new or worsening symptoms, such as constipation or nausea. Symptoms such as fatigue and anxiety are distressful and may affect quality of life in seriously ill cancer and noncancer patients. Therefore, pain assessment must be accompanied by assessment of other symptoms. Various surveys or questionnaires not only assess pain but also incorporate other symptoms into the assessment process. Many of these instruments are discussed in other chapters.

Pain assessment in nonverbal or cognitively impaired patients

The patient's self-report, the gold standard for pain assessment, is not always feasible in patients who cannot verbalize their pain and for patients with severe cognitive impairment (e.g., dementia and delirium). The inability to communicate by speaking, writing, or signing and cognitive impairment represent major barriers to adequate pain assessment and treatment. As noted by the IASP, "the inability to communicate verbally does not negate the possibility that an individual is experiencing pain and is in need of appropriate pain-relieving treatment."[15]

The potential for unrecognized and unrelieved pain is greater in patients who cannot verbally express their discomfort. Older, nonverbal, and cognitively impaired patients are at increased risk for pain due to underassessment and undertreatment of pain.[25,26,83,84] Patients who are nonverbal or cognitively impaired are often excluded from pain studies; thus, pain assessment and treatment in these groups are poorly understood.

The inability to communicate effectively due to impaired cognition and sensory losses is a serious problem for many patients with life-threatening illness. Cognitive failure develops in the majority of cancer patients before death, and agitated delirium is frequently observed in patients with advanced cancer. Clearly, pain assessment techniques and tools are needed that apply to patients, whether mentally incompetent or nonverbal, who communicate only through unique behavioral responses.

In addition to verbal self-reports, other ways to assess pain, such as observation of behaviors or surrogate reporting, must be utilized in persons who cannot verbally communicate their pain. It is important to remember that "No single objective assessment strategy, such as interpretation of behaviors, pathology, or estimates of pain by others, is sufficient by itself."[25] The ASPMN Position Statement on Pain Assessment in the Patient Unable to Self-Report[25] provides recommendations for assessing pain in special populations including nonverbal older adults with dementia and those who are intubated and/or unconscious. Pain assessment can be guided by the following principles and framework:

1. Use the hierarchy of pain assessment techniques[21,25,26]
   a. Obtain self-report, if possible.
   b. Search for potential causes of pain or other pathologies that could cause pain.
   c. Observe patient behaviors that are indicative of pain.
   d. Obtain proxy reporting (family members, parents, caregivers) of pain and behavior/activity changes.
   e. Attempt an analgesic trial to assess a reduction in possible pain behaviors.
2. Establish a procedure for pain assessment.
3. Use behavioral pain assessment tools, as appropriate.
4. Minimize emphasis on physiological indicators.
5. Reassess and document.

Pain behaviors

It may be more complicated to assess nonverbal cues in the palliative care setting because seriously ill patients with persistent pain, in contrast to patients with acute pain, may not demonstrate any specific behaviors indicative of pain. It is also unreasonable and even inaccurate to assess pain by reliance on involuntary physiological bodily reactions, such as increases in blood pressure, pulse, or respiratory rate and depth. Elevated vital signs may occur with sudden, severe pain, but they usually do not occur with persistent pain after the body reaches physiological equilibrium.[21] The absence of behavioral or involuntary cues does not negate the presence of pain. Assessment of behavior for signs of pain during rest and movement may provide a potentially valid and reliable alternative to verbal and physiological indices of pain. Examples of pain behaviors in cognitively impaired or nonverbal patients or residents are displayed in Table 6.4.[10,12,83]

Pain indicators in elderly demented patients identified by nursing home staff members include specific physical repetitive movements, facial expressions, vocal repetitions, physical signs of pain, and behavioral changes from the norm for that person. Observations of facial expressions may not be valid in patients with some types of dementia in which facial expressions are muted or in conditions that result in distorted facial expressions, such as Parkinson's disease or stroke.[83]

The pain experience in patients with cognitive failure

Pain behaviors in individuals with cognitive failure or dementia may be different from those of patients or residents who are cognitively intact. Patients with increased levels of cognitive impairment may report less severe pain and patients with progressive dementia may have fewer pain complaints, which may be related to a diminished capacity or difficulty in communicating pain. There is no consistent evidence to indicate that persons with dementia experience less pain sensation.[84] It has been proposed that the white matter lesions produced by vascular dementia may cause an increase in pain experience via central neuropathic pain mechanisms.[85] Instead of being less sensitive to pain, older adults with dementia may not interpret sensations as painful.[86]

Behavior or responses caused by noxious stimuli in individuals with cognitive impairment or dementia may not necessarily reflect classic or typical pain behaviors. There is considerable variability and uniqueness in behavior expressions of pain in nonverbal older adults with dementia.[83] For example, pain may be exhibited by withdrawn behavior, aggressive behavior, or verbally abusive behavior. In a study of 26 patients with painful conditions from a nursing home Alzheimer's unit, Marzinski[87] reported diverse responses to pain that were not typical of conventional pain behaviors. A patient who normally moaned and rocked became quiet and withdrawn when experiencing pain; pain in another nonverbal patient caused rapid blinking. Other patients who normally exhibited disjointed verbalizations could, when experiencing pain, give accurate descriptions of their pain.

Table 6.4 Possible pain behaviors in nonverbal and cognitively impaired patients or residents

Behavior category	Possible pain behaviors
Facial expressions	Grimace, frown, wince, sad or frightened look, wrinkled forehead, furrowed brow, closed or tightened eyelids, rapid blinking, clenched teeth or jaw
Body movements	Restless, agitated, jittery, "can't seem to sit still," fidgeting, pacing, rocking, constant or intermittent shifting of position, withdrawing
Protective mechanisms	Bracing, guarding, rubbing or massaging a body part, splinting, clutching or holding onto side rails, bed, tray table, or affected area during movement
Verbalizations	Saying common phrases such as "help me," "leave me alone," "get away from me," "don't touch me," "ouch," cursing, verbally abusive, praying out loud
Vocalizations	Sighing, moaning, groaning, crying, whining, oohing, aahing, calling out, screaming, chanting, breathing heavily
Mental status changes	Confusion, disorientation, irritability, distress, depression
Changes in activity patterns, routines, or interpersonal interactions	Decreased appetite, sleep alterations, decreased social activity participation, change in ambulation, immobilization, aggressive, combative, resisting care

Sources: Adapted from references 10, 12, 83.

Box 6.3 Assessment and treatment of pain in the nonverbal or cognitively impaired patient or resident

- Is there a reason for the patient to be experiencing pain? Review the patient's diagnoses.

- Was the patient previously treated for pain? If so, what regimen was effective (include pharmacological and nonpharmacological interventions)?

- How does the patient usually act when he/she is in pain? (Note: the nurse may need to ask family/significant others or other healthcare professionals.)

- What is the family/significant others' interpretation of the patient's behavior? Do they think the patient is in pain? Why do they feel this way?

- Try to obtain feedback from the patient, for example, ask patient to nod head, squeeze hand, move eyes up or down, raise legs, or hold up fingers to signal presence of pain.

- If appropriate, offer writing materials or pain intensity charts that patient can use or point to.

- If there is a possible reason for or sign of acute pain, treat with analgesics or other pain-relief measures.

- If a pharmacological or nonpharmacological intervention results in modifying pain behavior, continue with treatment.

- If pain behavior persists, rule out potential causes of the behavior (delirium, side effect of treatment, symptom of disease process); try appropriate intervention for behavior cause.

- Explain interventions to patient and family/significant other.

Questions in Box 6.3 can be used as a template for assessment and treatment of pain in the nonverbal or cognitively impaired patient or resident.

Instruments used to assess pain in nonverbal or cognitively impaired patients

Pain behavior scales

Assessing pain in patients/residents who are nonverbal or cognitively impaired and are unable to verbally self-report pain presents a particular challenge to clinicians. An instrument that could detect the presence of or a reduction in pain behaviors could facilitate effective pain management plans. However, because pain is not just a set of pain behaviors, the absence of certain behaviors does not necessarily mean that the patient is pain free. As evident from several excellent reviews of pain tools[25,26,83,88] many healthcare providers and researchers have attempted to develop an easy-to-use yet valid and reliable instrument for the assessment of pain in this vulnerable population. There is no one current tool based on nonverbal pain behaviors that can be recommended for general applicability in clinical practice and palliative care settings. A basic summary of instruments used to assess pain in nonverbal or cognitively impaired patients is found in Table 6.5.

Herr and colleagues[25,83] have performed an extensive and critical evaluation of many of these existing tools (conceptualization,

subject/setting, reliability and validity data based on research, administration/scoring methods, strengths/weaknesses) with the intent of providing up-to-date information to clinicians and researchers as it becomes available. These detailed reviews can be accessed at http://prc.coh.org/pain_assessment.asp.

Additionally, the Edmonton Symptom Assessment System (ESAS) is a validated tool for use in the palliative care setting. Originally tested in palliative care inpatients, 83% of symptom assessments were completed by nurses or patients' relatives.[117] The ESAS is a brief and reproducible scale consisting of separate visual analog or numeric scales that evaluate pain and eight additional symptoms (activity, nausea, depression, anxiety, drowsiness, appetite, sensation of well-being, and shortness of breath). The recently modified version, the ESAS-revised (ESAS-R), was compared to the ESAS in cognitively intact palliative care patients and it was found to be clearer in format and easier to understand with accompanying definitions describing the various symptoms, including pain.[118] On both the ESAS and ESAS-R, if patients are unable to complete the form, a space is provided for the person completing the assessment. If patients or residents are unresponsive and incapable of reporting their own pain (e.g., during the final days of life), observer judgments of pain become necessary. In this situation, the main caregiver completes the Edmonton Comfort Assessment Form (ECAF).

Proxy pain assessment in the nonverbal or cognitively impaired patient or resident

Just as the experience of pain is subjective, observing and interpreting a patient's or resident's pain is a subjective experience. Without verbal validation from the patient, the clinician must rely not only on behavioral observations but also on intuition and personal judgment. It is also particularly important to elicit the opinions of the individuals closest to the patient, which are also subjective.

Nurses and other healthcare providers reflect the difficulty of accurately assessing pain in nonverbal or cognitively impaired patients in studies that show low concurrence between patients' self-ratings of pain and clinicians' ratings.[119] Other findings are equivocal, with some studies suggesting that family caregivers or significant others accurately estimate the amount of pain cancer patients experience and others proposing that family caregivers overestimate patients' pain. Bruera and colleagues[120] studied relatives and the nurses who cared for 60 unresponsive, dying patients. Both were asked to rate a patient's discomfort level, six observed behaviors (grimacing, groaning, shouting, touching or rubbing an area, purposeless movement, labored breathing), and the suspected reason for the discomfort. Although the mean levels of perceived discomfort were similar, relatives reported significantly more observed behaviors and more often indicated pain as a reason for discomfort than did the nurse caregivers. According to Cohen-Mansfield,[121] relatives of cognitively impaired nursing home residents are better able to interpret facial expressions and other pain behaviors if they visit their loved ones at least once a week and have a close relationship. To detect pain in cognitively impaired nursing home residents, it is essential for family members and certified nursing assistants to know the resident's usual behavior and patterns to be able to detect pain.

Table 6.5 Pain assessment tools for the cognitively impaired or nonverbal patient or resident

Tool	Goal	Dimensions/parameters	Comments
Abbey Pain Scale[89]	Assess pain in late-stage demented patients in nursing homes	Vocalization Facial expression Change in body language Behavioral change Physiological change Physical change	Based on previous research this scale was developed for use with end-/late-stage dementia residents unable to express needs. Six behavioral indicators are scored with four grades of severity (0 = absent through 3 = severe) for a total possible score of 18.
Assessment of Discomfort in Dementia Protocol (ADD)[90,91]	Improve the recognition and treatment of pain and discomfort in patients with dementia who cannot report their internal states, with the added goal of decreasing inappropriate use of psychotropic medication administration	Facial expression Mood Body language Voice Behavior	Based on DS–DAT[92] items, the ADD protocol includes more overt symptoms (physical aggression, crying, calling out, resisting care, and existing behaviors). Protocol implementation when basic care interventions failed to ameliorate behavioral symptoms resulted in significant decreases in discomfort, significant increases in the use of pharmacological and nonpharmacological comfort interventions and improved behavioral symptoms.[90,91]
Certified Nurse Assistant Pain Assessment Tool (CPAT)[93]	Assess pain in patients with severe dementia by nursing assistants	Facial expression Behavior Mood Body language Activity level	Developed as a nursing assistant-administered instrument. Each of the five items is scored (0–1) for the presence or absence of pain and summed for a total score ranging from 0 to 5; higher scores require evaluation by nursing staff.
Checklist of Nonverbal Pain Indicators (CNPI)[94]	Measure pain behaviors in cognitively impaired elders	Nonverbal vocalizations Facial grimaces/winces Bracing Rubbing Restlessness Verbalizations	Rates the absence or presence of six behaviors, at rest and on movement. A summed score of the number of nonverbal pain indicators observed at rest and on movement is calculated (total possible score 0–12).
Critical Care Pain Observation Tool (CPOT)[95,96]	Assess pain in adult patients in critical care who are unable to self-report	Facial expression Body movements Compliance with the ventilator (intubated patients) or Vocalization (extubated patients) Muscle tension	Each of the four domains is scored on three behaviors from 0 to 2 for a total score ranging from 0 to 8. Presence of pain is suspected at scores above 2 or when the score increases by 2 or more.
Discomfort Behavior Scale (DBS)[97]	Identify discomfort in persons with cognitive impairment in nursing homes	Facial expression Verbalizations/vocalizations Body language Changes in activity patterns or routines Mental status changes Changes in interpersonal interactions	Does not necessarily differentiate those in pain, but identifies those with discomfort that may be due to pain or other sources. Intended to be used quarterly with information from the Minimum Data Set for nursing homes and must be computer scored.
Disability Distress Assessment Tool (DisDAT)[98]	Observe and identify discomfort in people with severely limited communication due to cognitive impairment or physical illness	Facial signs Vocal sounds Habits and mannerisms Body posture Body observation	The rater selects from a series of identical adjectives for each of the five categories to describe patient expression in both content and distressed states. There are a total of 77 descriptors of content and distressed states between the five categories. The tool loosely incorporates all six American Geriatric Society indicators of pain and is designed to identify behavior change from a content base line.

(continued)

Table 6.5 Continued

Tool	Goal	Dimensions/parameters	Comments
Discomfort Scale for Dementia of the Alzheimer Type (DS–DAT)[92]	Measure discomfort, defined as a negative state, in elders with advanced dementia who have decreased cognition and verbalization.	Noisy breathing Negative vocalizations Contented facial expression Sad facial expression Frightened facial expression Frown Relaxed body language Tense body language Fidgeting	The negative state could be pain, anguish, or suffering. Scoring is based on evaluation of frequency, intensity, and duration of the behaviors and may be cumbersome, requiring more training and education than is feasible or realistic for clinicians in hospital or long-term care settings. As the DS–DAT has been criticized for being too complex for routine nursing care, it has been revised.[99]

Doloplus-2[100,101]	Assess pain in nonverbal elders experiencing chronic, persistent pain.	Somatic reactions (5 items)
		  ♦ Somatic complaints
		  ♦ Protective body postures at rest
		  ♦ Protection of sore areas
		  ♦ Expression
		  ♦ Sleep pattern
		Psychomotor reactions (2 items)
		  ♦ Washing and/or dressing
		  ♦ Mobility
		  ♦ Psychosocial reactions (3 items)
		  ♦ Communication
		  ♦ Social life
		  ♦ Behavioral problems
			Each of the ten items is given a score (0–3) representing increased severity and summed for a total score ranging from 0 to 30. A total score of 5 or above indicates pain.

Elderly Pain Caring Assessment 2 (EPCA-2)[102]	Observe and rate the intensity of both persistent and acute pain in nonverbal communicating older adults.	Observations before caregiver intervention
		  ♦ Facial expression
		  ♦ Spontaneous posture adopted at rest
		  ♦ Movements of the patient out of bed and/or in bed
		  ♦ Interaction of all kinds with other people
		Observations during caregiver intervention
		  ♦ Anxious anticipation of caregiver intervention
		  ♦ Reactions during caregiver intervention
		  ♦ Reactions of the patient when painful parts of the body nursed
		  ♦ Complaints voiced in the course of caregiving
			Each item is rated on a 5-point scale from 0 (no pain) to 4 (intense pain). The total score is the sum of corresponding scores in the two dimensions. EPCA-2 is hypothesized to measure pain intensity through doctors', nurses', and other caregivers' proxy ratings of the presence and qualitative intensity of identified pain behaviors.

FLACC[103] FLACC-R[104]	Measure pain severity in postoperative children. Has also been tested in critically ill, cognitively impaired adults.[105]	Face Legs Activity Cry Consolability	Each of the five items is given a score (0–2) representing increased severity and summed for a total score ranging from 0 to 10. The FLACC-R can be used for all nonverbal, cognitively impaired children. Parent-identified specific descriptors and unique behaviors have been added to the FLACC to improve its reliability and validity.

(continued)

Table 6.5 Continued

Tool	Goal	Dimensions/parameters	Comments
Mobilization-Observation-Behavior-Intensity-Dementia Pain Scale-2 (MOBID-2)[106]	Observe pain behaviors and infer pain intensity at rest and with standardized guided activity in patients with severe cognitive impairment (SCI).	Facial expressions Pain noises Defensive gestures	Patient is moved through standardized guided movements of joints in hands/arms, legs and trunk; with each activity, caregiver observes for presence and intensity of pain on an 11-point NRS; caregiver assigns an independent overall pain intensity rating on an 11-point NRS. Incorporates patient self-report or expression, observation, and proxy assessment.
Multidimensional Objective Pain Assessment Tool (MOPAT)[107]	Assess acute pain in noncommunicative patients in hospice.	Behavioral indicators • Restless • Tense muscles • Frowning/grimacing • Patient sounds Physiological indicators • Blood pressure • Heart rate • Respirations • Diaphoresis	Based on previous research, this tool has a four-item behavioral dimension ranked on a 3-point scale with 0 being none and 3 severe, and a three-item physiological dimension rated as "no change from usual" or "change from usual." Both dimensions are summed for a total score of pain severity.
Non-communicative Patient's Pain Assessment Instrument (NOPPAIN)[108]	Assess pain behaviors in patients with dementia by nursing assistants.	Care conditions under which pain behaviors are observed • Bathing • Dressing • Transfers Presence/absence of pain behaviors • Pain words • Pain noises • Pain faces • Bracing • Rubbing • Restlessness Pain behavior intensity using 6-point Likert scale Pain thermometer for rating overall pain intensity	Developed as a nursing assistant–administered instrument. Pain is observed at rest and on movement while nursing assistants perform resident care. Pain behaviors are observed and pain intensity is scored using a pain thermometer.
Pain Assessment for the Dementing Elderly (PADE)[109,110]	Assess pain behaviors in patients with advanced dementia.	Physical • Facial expression • Breathing pattern • Posture Global • Proxy pain intensity Functional • Dressing • Feeding oneself • Wheelchair to bed transfers	Twenty-four items (three domains) were developed after a literature review, interviews with nursing staff, and observations of residents in a dementia unit.
Pain Assessment Tool in Confused Older Adults (PATCOA)[111]	Observe nonverbal cues to assess pain in acutely confused older adults.	Quivering Guarding Frowning Grimacing Clenching jaws	An ordinal scale includes nine items of nonverbal pain cues rated as absent or present while the patient is at rest; higher scores indicate higher pain intensity.

(continued)

Table 6.5 Continued

Tool	Goal	Dimensions/parameters	Comments
		Points to where it hurts Reluctance to move Vocalizations of moaning Sighing	
Pain Assessment in Advanced Dementia (PAINAD)[99,112]	Assess pain in patients with advanced dementia.	Breathing (independent of vocalization) Negative vocalization Facial expression Body language Consolability	Derived from the behaviors and categories of the FLACC,[103] DS-DAT,[92] and clinicians' pain descriptors of dementia. The intent is to simply measure pain using a 0–10 score (each item is scored as 0–2 and summed) in noncommunicative individuals.
Pain Assessment Behavioral Scale (PABS)[113]	Assess pain in nonverbal hospital critically ill inpatients.	Face Restlessness Muscle tone Vocalization Consolability	Each of the five items is given a score (0–2) representing increased severity and summed for a total score ranging from 0–10. The patient is observed at rest and with movement. Two scores are generated; the higher score is documented.
Pain Assessment Checklist for Seniors with Limited Ability to Communicate (PACSLAC)[114]	Assess common and subtle behaviors in seniors with advanced dementia.	Facial expressions Activity and body movements Social/personality/mood indicators Physiological indicators/eating and sleeping/vocal behaviors	Can differentiate between pain and distress; scores were positively correlated with cognitive impairment level.
Pain Behaviors for Osteoarthritis Instrument for Cognitively Impaired Elders (PBOICIE)[115]	Assess osteoarthritis (OA) pain in the knee or hip for severely cognitively impaired elders.	Distorted ambulation or gesture ◆ Excessive stiffness ◆ Shifting weight ◆ Clutching or holding area ◆ Rigid, tense body posture ◆ Massaging affected area ◆ Facial/nonaudible expressions of distress ◆ Clenching teeth	A dichotomous scale (absent or present) with scores total ranging from 0 to 6 was used; if the presence of one behavior on the PBOICIE is observed then it is indicative of the presence of pain. Limitation in practice setting based on use only in population with a specific diagnosis of OA.
Pain Assessment in Noncommunicative Elderly Persons PAINE[110,116]	Assess pain in noncommunicative elders.	Facial expressions Verbalizations Body movements Changes in activity/patterns Nurse-identified physical and vocal behaviors Visible pain cues	22 item scale with a 6-point rating scale (1 = never to 7 = several times an hour) to measure frequency of occurrence of pain behaviors.

Implications for treatment

Although pain assessment in the nonverbal or cognitively impaired patient or resident presents a challenge to clinicians, it should not pose a barrier to optimal pain management. If patients are no longer able to verbally communicate whether they are in pain or not, the best approach is to assume that their underlying disease is still painful and to continue pain interventions based on analgesic history.[27] Nonverbal patients should be empirically treated for pain if there is preexisting pain or evidence that any individual in a similar condition would experience pain. Likewise, palliative measures should be considered in nonverbal patients with behavior changes potentially related to pain.

Summary

In summary, multiple factors should be incorporated into the assessment of the pain experience. The following case examples include some of the pain assessment techniques discussed in this chapter and may prove beneficial in applying this content for nurse clinicians.

Case studies

Monica, cancer patient with pain undergoing treatment and palliative care

Monica is a 60-year-old, Caucasian woman who was diagnosed with metastatic non-small cell lung cancer after an incidental discovery of a pulmonary nodule noted on a chest X-ray following a motor vehicle accident. Her only injury after the accident was a fractured, right lower rib. Further imaging studies and biopsies showed metastasis of her lung cancer to both lobes of her liver. Brain MRI was negative. She elected to receive chemotherapy treatment with palliative intent and was agreeable to referral to a palliative care service. Prior to her diagnosis, she was in her usual good state of health with the exception of progressive fatigue and weight loss of 10 pounds over 1 year. She also had intermittent pain in her right chest which was attributed to pleurisy. She is married and worked as fourth grade school teacher until she started chemotherapy. She completed four cycles of carboplatin, paclitaxel, and bevacizumab. A restaging PET/CT at the completion of treatment revealed remission. She was unable to receive maintenance therapy with bevacizumab due to hypertension and proteinuria, but did elect to receive prophylactic whole brain radiation therapy. During treatment, Monica experienced symptoms of fatigue, nausea, memory problems, anorexia, intermittent chest pain, and depression. Seven months after completion of treatment, Monica was asymptomatic; however, imaging studies revealed new pulmonary nodules and right hilar adenopathy, suspicious for progressive disease.

Discussion Questions

1. What is the best way to assess Monica's pain?

2. After her diagnosis and initiation of treatment, was it appropriate to refer Monica for early palliative care?

3. What are the benefits of early palliative care in patients with non-small cell lung cancer?

4. List factors that could impact Monica's pain.

5. How can Monica be assisted to consider her options for further treatment or no treatment?

Lucia, patient with breast cancer cared for by hospice

Lucia is a 39-year-old Hispanic woman who underwent bilateral mastectomies with right axillary sentinel lymph node biopsy for a high-grade, triple negative, invasive ductal breast carcinoma. She declined participation in a clinical trial, but did pursue adjuvant chemotherapy and breast reconstruction. After being disease free for about 7 years, she developed lung and liver metastases. Despite palliative radiation therapy and chemotherapy, Lucia's disease continued to progress and she elected hospice care. Lucia has been depressed since her husband divorced her after discovery of her metastases because he could not deal with her illness. She has no children and lives with her supportive father. She has lost touch with her good girlfriends. She has persistent pain in her left chest related to pleural metastases and intermittent right abdominal pain related to liver metastases. She takes OxyContin 40 mg every 12 hours with hydromorphone 8 mg every 3 hours as needed for breakthrough pain. Lucia's father is concerned that she is taking too much pain medication now and that it will not work when she needs it later. She is worried that she will not have adequate pain control if she goes into a hepatic coma or is unable to talk with her providers. Her other symptoms include anxiety, peripheral neuropathy in her fingers related to chemotherapy, fatigue, dyspnea, and constipation.

Discussion Questions

1. How can Lucia be reassured that her pain will be adequately controlled when she is no longer able to verbally communicate?

2. What should Lucia's father be taught about her pain control now and when her condition declines?

3. What are appropriate assessment tools to use when and if Lucia is cognitively impaired?

4. How can Lucia's father tell if her pain is being controlled?

5. What are the cultural impacts on the assessment and management of this patient's pain?

References

1. Rogers W. Will Rogers Says. . . Favorite Quotations. Available at: http://en.www.thinkexist.com/quotes/will_rogers/. Accessed November 17, 2013.
2. Fisch MJ, Lee JW, Weiss M et al. Prospective, observational study of pain and analgesic prescribing in medical oncology outpatients with breast, colorectal, lung, or prostate cancer. J Clin Onc. 2012;30(16):1980–1988.
3. Higginson IJ, Murtaugh F. Cancer pain epidemiology: a systematic review. In Bruera ED, Portenoy RK (eds.), Cancer Pain, Assessment and Management, 2nd ed. Cambridge, UK: Cambridge University Press; 2010:37–52.
4. National Comprehensive Cancer Network (NCCN). Adult Cancer Pain: Clinical Practice Guidelines in Oncology, version 2.2013. Available at http://www.nccn.org/professionals/physician_gls/f_guidelines.asp#pain. Accessed September 11, 2013.
5. van den Beuken-van Everdingen MH, de Rijke JM, Kessels AG, Schouten HC, van Kleef M, Patijn J. Prevalence of pain in patients with cancer: a systematic review of the past 40 years. Ann Oncol. 2007;18:1437–1449.
6. Dalal S, Bruera E. Assessment and management of pain in the terminally ill. Prim Care Clin Office Pract. 2011;38:195–223.
7. Kutner JS, Bryant LL, Beaty BL, Fairclough DL. Time course and characteristics of symptom distress and quality of life at the end of life. J Pain Symptom Manage. 2007;34:227–236.
8. Kamal AH, Swetz KM, Carey EC, et al. Palliative care consultations in patients with cancer: a Mayo Clinic 5-year review. J Onc Prac. 2011;7(1):48–53.
9. Teno JM, Gozalo PL, Bynum JPW, et al. Change in end-of-life care for Medicare beneficiaries site of death, place of care, and health care transitions in 2000, 2005, and 2009. JAMA. 2013;309(5):470–477.
10. American Geriatrics Society (AGS) Panel on Persistent Pain in Older Persons. Clinical practice guideline: the management of persistent pain in older persons. J Am Geriatr Soc. 2002;50(6 Suppl):S205-S224.
11. American Geriatrics Society (AGS) Panel on the Pharmacological Management of Persistent Pain in Older Persons. Pharmacological management of persistent pain in older persons. J Am Geriatr Soc. 2009;57:1331–1346.
12. American Medical Directors Association. Pain Management in the Long-Term Care Setting: Clinical Practice Guideline. Columbia, MD: AMDA; 2012.
13. Takai Y, Yamamoto-Mitani N, Okamoto Y, Koyama K, Honda A. Literature review of pain prevalence among older residents of nursing homes. Pain Manage Nurs. 2010;11(4):209–223.
14. Hutt E, Pepper GA, Vojir C, Fink R, Jones KR. Assessing the appropriateness of pain medication prescribing practices in nursing homes. J Am Geriatr Soc. 2006;54:231–239.
15. Merskey H, Bogduk N, eds. Classification of Chronic Pain, 2nd ed. International Association for the Study of Pain, Task Force on Taxonomy. Seattle, WA: IASP Press; 1994:209–214.
16. McCaffery M. Nursing Practice Theories Related to Cognition, Bodily Pain, and Man-Environment Interactions. Los Angeles, CA: UCLA Press; 1968:95.
17. Reynolds J, Drew D, Dunwoody C. American Society of Pain Management Nursing Position Statement: Pain Management at the End of Life. Pain Manage Nurs. 2013;14(3):172–175.
18. Goldberg GR, Morrison RS. Pain management in hospitalized cancer patients: a systematic review. J Clin Oncol. 2007;25:1792–1801.

19. Jones K, Fink R, Clark L, Hutt E, Vojir CP, Mellis BK. Nursing home resident barriers to effective pain management: why nursing home residents may not seek pain medication. J Am Med Dir Assoc. 2005;6:10–17.

20. Borneman T, Koczywas M, Sun V, et al. Effectiveness of a clinical intervention to eliminate barriers to pain and fatigue management in oncology. J Palliat Med. 2011;14(2):197–205.

21. Pasero C, McCaffery M. Pain Assessment and Pharmacologic Management. St. Louis, MO: Elsevier Mosby; 2011.

22. Miaskowski C, Bair M, Chou R, et al. Principles of Analgesic Use in the Treatment of Acute and Cancer Pain, 6th ed. Chicago, IL: American Pain Society; 2008.

23. Oncology Nursing Society Position on Cancer Pain Management. 2013. Available at: http://www.ons.org/Publications/Positions/Pain/. Accessed September 16, 2013.

24. Max M, Cleary J, Ferrell BR, Foley K, Payne R, Shapiro B. Treatment of Pain at the End of Life: A Position Statement from the American Pain Society. Chicago, IL: American Pain Society; 2006.

25. Herr K, Coyne PJ, McCaffery M, Manworren R, Merkel S. Pain assessment in the patient unable to self-report: position statement with clinical practice recommendations. Pain Manage Nurs. 2011;12:230–250.

26. Hadijistavropoulos T, Herr K, Turk DC, et al. An interdisciplinary expert consensus statement on assessment of pain in older persons. Clin J Pain. 2007; 23:S1–S43.

27. Hospice and Palliative Nurses Association Position Statement on Pain Management. 2012. Available at: http://www.hpna.org/DisplayPage. aspx?Title1=Position%20Statements. Accessed October 30, 2013.

28. The Joint Commission. Speak Up: What You Should Know About Pain Management. Available at: http://www.jointcommission.org/assets/1/18/painmanagementbrochure.pdf. Accessed June 26, 2013.

29. Irwin M, Brant J, Eaton L. Putting Evidence into Practice: Pharmacologic and Nonpharmacologic Interventions for Pain. Pittsburgh, PA: Oncology Nursing Society; 2012.

30. Gordon DB, Polomano RC, Pellino TA, et al. Revised American Pain Society Patient Outcome Questionnaire (APS-POQ-R) for quality improvement of pain management in hospitalized adults: preliminary psychometric evaluation. J Pain. 2010;11(11):1172–1186.

31. Gordon DB, Rees SM, McCauland MP, et al. Improving reassessment and documentation of pain management. Jt Comm J Qual Patient Saf. 2008;34(9):509–517.

32. American Heritage Dictionary of the English Language, 5th ed. Boston, MA: Houghton Mifflin; 2012.

33. Saunders CM. The Management of Terminal Malignant Disease, 1st ed. London, England: Edward Arnold; 1978.

34. Melzack R, Casey KL. Sensory, motivational, and central control determinants of pain: a new conceptual model. In: Kenshalo D (ed.), The Skin Senses. Springfield, IL: Charles C Thomas; 1968:423–439.

35. Ahles TA, Blanchard EB, Ruckdeschel JC. The multidimensional nature of cancer-related pain. Pain. 1983;17:277–288.

36. McGuire D. Comprehensive and multidimensional assessment and measurement of pain, J Pain Symptom Manage. 1992;7:312–319.

37. Bates MS. Ethnicity and pain: a biocultural model. Soc Sci Med. 1987;24:47–50.

38. Hester NO. Assessment of acute pain. Baillieres Clin Paediatr. 1995;3:561–577.

39. Jost L, Roila F. Management of cancer pain: ESMO clinical recommendations. Ann Oncol. 2008;19:119–121.

40. Fink RM. University of Colorado Hospital, University of Colorado Health, WILDA Pain Assessment Card. Aurora, CO; 2013.

41. Haanpaa M, Attal N, Backonja M, et al. NeuPSIG guidelines on neuropathic pain assessment. Pain. 2011;152:14–27.

42. Cruccu GM, Sommer C, Anand P, et al. EFNS guidelines on neuropathic pain assessment: revised 2009. Eur J Neurol. 2010;17:1010–1018.

43. Rayment C, Hjermstad MJ, Aass N, et al. Neuropathic cancer pain: prevalence, severity, analgesics, and impact from the European Palliative Care Research Collaborative–computerised symptom assessment study. Palliat Med. 2013;27(8):714–721.

44. Jackson SY Wu, Beaton D, Smith PM, Hagen N. Patterns of pain and interference in patients with painful bone metastases: a brief pain inventory validation study. J Pain Symptom Manage. 2010;39(2):230–240.

45. Portenoy RK, Hagen NA. Breakthrough pain: definition, prevalence, and characteristics. Pain 1990;41:273–281.

46. Fainsinger RL, Fairchild A, Nekolaichuk C, Lawlor P, Lowe S, Hanson H. Is pain intensity a predictor of the complexity of cancer pain management? J Clin Oncol. 2009;27:585–590.

47. Bostrom B, Sandh M, Lundberg D, Fridlund B. Cancer-related pain in palliative care: patients' perceptions of pain management. J Adv Nurs. 2004;45:410–419.

48. Porter LS, Keefe FJ, Garst J, McBride CM, Baucom D. Self-efficacy for managing pain, symptoms, and function in patients with lung cancer and their informal caregivers. Pain. 2008;137(2):306–305.

49. Bernabei R, Gambassi G, Lapane K, et al. Management of pain in elderly patients with cancer. SAGE Study Group. JAMA. 1998;279:1877–1882.

50. Fillingim RB, King CD, Ribeiro-Dasilva MC, Rahim-Williams B, Riley JL. Sex, gender, and pain: a review of recent clinical and experimental findings. Pain. 2009;10(5):447–485.

51. Hurley RW, Adams MCB. Sex, gender, and pain: an overview of a complex field. Anesth Analg. 2009;107:309–317.

52. Chin ML, Rosequist R. Sex, gender, and pain: "Men are from Mars, women are from Venus." Anesth Analg. 2008;107:4–5.

53. Anderson KO, Green CR, Payne R. Racial and ethnic disparities in pain: causes and consequences of unequal care. J Pain. 2009;10(12):1187–1204.

54. Chiauzzi E, Black RA, Frayjo K, et al. Health care provider perceptions of pain treatment in Hispanic patients. Pain Pract. 2011;11:267–277.

55. Epps CD, Ware LJ, Packard A. Ethnic wait time differences in analgesic administration in the emergency department. Pain Manage Nurs. 2008;9(1):26–32.

56. Gélinas C, Loiselle CG, LeMay S, Ranger M, Bouchard E, McCormack D. Theoretical, psychometric, and pragmatic issues in pain measurement. Pain Manage Nurs. 2008;9:120–130.

57. Morgan MA, Small BJ, Donovan KA, Overcash J, McMillan S. Cancer patients with pain: the spouse/partner relationship and quality of life. Cancer Nurs. 2011;34(1):13–23.

58. Taylor SS, Davis MC, Zautra AJ. Relationship status and quality moderate daily pain-related changes in physical disability, affect, and cognitions in women with chronic pain. Pain. 2013;154(1):147–153.

59. Delgado-Guay M, Hui D, Parsons HA, et al. Spirituality, religiosity, and spiritual pain in advanced cancer patients. J Pain Symptom Manage. 2011;41(6):986–994.

60. Unruh AM. Spirituality, religion, and pain. Can J Nurs Res. 2007;39(2):66–86.

61. Jensen M. The validity and reliability of pain measures in adults with cancer. J Pain. 2003;4;2–21.

62. Revill SI, Robinson JO, Rosen M, Hogg MIJ. The reliability of a linear analogue for evaluating pain. Anaesthesia. 1976;31:1191–1998.

63. Herr KA, Mobily PR. Comparison of selected pain assessment tools for use with the elderly. Appl Nurs Res. 1993;6:39–49.

64. von Baeyer CL, Spagrud LJ, McCormick JC, Choo E, Neville K, Connelly MA. Three new datasets supporting use of the Numerical Rating Scale (NRS-11) for children's self-reports of pain intensity. Pain. 2009;143(3):223–227.

65. Paice JA, Cohen FL. Validity of a verbally administered numeric rating scale to measure cancer pain intensity. Cancer Nurs. 1997;20:88–93.

66. Ferraz MB, Quaresma MR, Aquino LRL, Atra E, Tugwell P, Goldsmith CH. Reliability of pain scales in the assessment of literate and illiterate patients with rheumatoid arthritis. J Rheumatol. 1990;17:1022–1024.

67. Hockenberry MJ, Wilson D. Wong's Essential of Pediatric Nursing, 8th ed. St. Louis: Mosby; 2009.

68. Stuppy DJ. The Faces Pain Scale: reliability and validity with mature adults. Appl Nurs Res. 1998;11:84–89.

69. Casas JM, Wagenheim BR, Banchero R, Mendoza-Romero J. Hispanic masculinity: myth or psychological schema meriting clinical consideration. Hisp J Behav Sci. 1994;16:315–331.

70. Hicks CL, von Baeyer CL, Spafford P, van Korlaar I, Goodenough B. The Faces Scale-Revised: toward a common metric in pediatric pain measurement. Pain. 2001;93:173–183.

71. International Association for the Study of Pain. Available at: http://www.iasp-pain.org/Content/NavigationMenu/GeneralResourceLinks/FacesPainScaleRevised/default.htm. Accessed September 27, 2013.

72. Bieri D, Reeve R, Champion GD, Addicoat L, Ziegler JB. The Faces Pain Scale for the self assessment of the severity of pain experienced by children: development, initial validation, and preliminary investigation for ratio scale properties. Pain. 1990;41:139–150.

73. Tomlinson D, von Baeyer CL, Stinson JN, Sung L. A systematic review of faces scales for the self-report of pain intensity in children. Pediatrics. 2010;126(5):e1168–e1198.

74. Herr KA, Garand L. Assessment and management of pain in older adults. Clin Geriat Med. 2001;17:457–478.

75. Dalton JA, McNaull F. A call for standardizing the clinical rating of pain intensity using a 0 to 10 rating scale. Cancer Nurs. 1998;21:46–49.

76. Jones K, Fink R, Hutt E, et al. Measuring pain intensity in nursing home residents. J Pain Symptom Manage. 2005;30:519–527.

77. Ware LJ, Epps CD, Herr K, Packard A. Evaluation of the revised faces pain scale, verbal descriptor scale, numeric rating scale, and Iowa pain thermometer in older minority adults. Pain Manage Nurs. 2006;7:117–125.

78. Li L, Liu X, Herr K. Postoperative pain intensity assessment: a comparison of four scales in Chinese adults. Pain Med. 2007;8(3):223–234.

79. Melzak R. The short-form McGill Pain Questionnaire. Pain. 1987;30:191–197.

80. Daut RL, Cleeland CS, Flanery R. Development of the Wisconsin Brief Pain Inventory to assess pain in cancer and other diseases. Pain. 1983;17:197–210.

81. Fishman B, Pasternak S, Wallenstein SL, Houde RW, Holland JC, Foley KM. The Memorial Pain Assessment Card: a valid instrument for the evaluation of cancer pain. Cancer. 1987;60:1151–1158.

82. Ferrell BR. Patient and Family Pain Questionnaires. Available at: http://prc.coh.org/res_inst.asp. Accessed June 26, 2013.

83. Herr K, Bjoro K, Decker S. Tools for assessment of pain in nonverbal older adults with dementia: a state of the science review. J Pain Symptom Manage. 2006;31:170–192.

84. Reynolds KS, Hanson LC, De Vellis RF. Disparities in pain management between cognitively intact and cognitively impaired nursing home residents. J Pain Symptom Manage. 2008;35:388–396.

85. Scherder EJA, Plooij B. Assessment and management of pain with particular emphasis on central neuropathic pain, in moderate to severe dementia. Drugs Aging. 2012;29:701–706.

86. Bjoro K, Herr K. Assessment of pain in the nonverbal or cognitively impaired older adult. Clin Geriat Med. 2008; 24:237–262.

87. Marzinski LR. The tragedy of dementia: clinically assessing pain in the confused nonverbal elderly. J Gerontol Nurs. 1991;17:25–28.

88. Hjermstad MJ, Gibbins J, Haugen DF, Caraceni A, Loge JH, Kaasa S. Pain assessment tools in palliative care: an urgent need for consensus. Palliat Med. 2008;22:895–903.

89. Abbey J, Piller N, De Bellis A, et al. The Abbey Pain Scale: a 1-minute numerical indicator for people with end-stage dementia. Int J Palliat Nurs. 2004;10:6–13.

90. Kovach CR, Weissman D, Griffie J, Matson S, Muchka S. Assessment and treatment of discomfort for people with late stage dementia. J Pain Symptom Manage. 1999;18:412–419.

91. Kovach CR, Noonan PE, Griffie J, Muchka S, Weissman DE. The Assessment of Discomfort in Dementia protocol. Pain Manage Nurs. 2002;3:16–27.

92. Hurley AC, Volicer BJ, Hanrahan PA, Houde S, Volicer L. Assessment of discomfort in advanced Alzheimer patients. Res Nurs Health. 1992;15:369–377.

93. Cervo FA, Bruckenthal P, Chen JJ, Bright-Long LE, Fields S, Zhang G, Strongwater I. Pain assessment in nursing home residents with dementia: psychometric properties and clinical utility of the CNA pain assessment tool (CPAT). J Am Med Dir Assoc. 2009;10:505–510.

94. Feldt KS. The Checklist of Nonverbal Pain Indicators (CNPI). Pain Manage Nurs. 2000;1:13–21.

95. Gélinas C, Fillion L, Puntillo KA. Item selection and content validity of the critical-care pain observation tool for nonverbal adults. J Adv Nurs. 2009;65:203–216.

96. Gélinas C. Nurses' evaluations of the feasibility and the clinical utility of the critical-care pain observation tool. Pain Manage Nurs. 2010;11:115–125.

97. Stevenson K, Brown R, Dahl J, Ward S, Brown M. The discomfort behavior scale: a measure of discomfort in the cognitively impaired based on the minimum data set 2.0. Res Nurs Health. 2006;29:576–587.

98. Regnard C, Reynolds J, Watson B, Matthews D, Gibson L, Clarke C. Understanding distress in people with severe communication difficulties: developing and assessing the Disability Distress Assessment Tool (DisDAT). J Intellect Disability Res. 2007; 51: 277–292.

99. Warden V, Hurley AC, Volicer L. Development and psychometric evaluation of the Pain Assessment in Advanced Dementia (PAINAD) scale. J Am Med Dir Assoc. 2003;9–15.

100. Wary B. Doloplus-2: a scale for pain measurement. Soins Gerontol. 1999;19:25–27.

101. Pautex S, Herrmann F, Michon A, Giannakopoulos P, Gold G. Psychometric properties of the Doloplus-2 observational pain scale and comparison to self-assessment in hospitalized elderly. Clin J Pain. 2007;23:774–779.

102. Morello R, Jean A, Alix M, et al. A scale to measure pain in non-verbally communicating older patients: the EPCA-2 study of its psychometric properties. Pain. 2007;133:87–98.

103. Merkel SI, Voepel-Lewis T, Shayevitz JR, Malviya S. The FLACC: a behavioral scale for scoring postoperative pain in young children. Pediatr Nurs. 1997;23:293–297.

104. Malviya S, Voepel-Lewis T, Burke C, Merkel S, Tait AR. The revised FLACC observational pain tool: improved reliability and validity for pain assessment in children with cognitive impairment. Paediatr Anaesth. 2006;16(3):258–265.

105. Voepel-Lewis T, Zanotti J, Dammeyer JA. Reliability and validity of the faces, legs, activity, cry, consolability behavioral tool in assessing acute pain in critically ill patients. Am J Crit Care. 2010;19(1):55–62.

106. Husebo BS, Strand LI, Moe-Nilssen R, Husebo SB, Ljunggren AE. Pain in older persons with severe dementia: psychometric properties of the Mobilization-Observation-Behaviour-Intensity-Dementia (MOBID2) Pain Scale in a clinical setting. Scan J Caring Sci. 2010;24(2):380–391.

107. McGuire DB, Reifsnyder J, Soeken K, Kaiser KS, Yeager KA. Assessing pain in nonresponsive hospice patients: development and preliminary testing of the multidimensional objective pain assessment tool (MOPAT). J Palliat Med. 2011;14:287–292.

108. Snow AL, Weber JB, O'Malley KJ, et al. NOPPAIN: a nursing assistant-administered pain assessment instrument for use in dementia. Dement Geriatr Cogn Disord. 2004;17:240–246.

109. Villanueva MR, Smith TL, Erickson JS, Lee AC, Singer C. Pain Assessment for the Dementing Elderly (PADE): reliability and validity of a new measure. J Am Med Dir Assoc. 2003;4:1–8.

110. Cohen-Manfield J, Lipson S. The utility of pain assessment for analgesic use in persons with dementia. Pain. 2008;134:16–23.

111. Decker SA, Perry AG. The development and testing of the PATCOA to assess pain in confused older adults. Pain Manage Nurs. 2003;4:77–86.

112. DeWaters T, Faut-Callahan M, McCann JJ, et al. Comparison of self-reported pain and the PAINAD scale in hospitalized cognitively impaired and intact older adults after hip fracture surgery. Orthop Nurs. 2008;27:21–28.

113. Campbell M. Psychometric Testing of a New Pain Assessment Behavior Scale (PABS). Abstract presented at the 29th Annual MNRS Research Conference, 2005.

114. Fuchs-Lacelle S, Hadjistavropoulos T. Development and preliminary validation of the Pain Assessment Checklist for Seniors with Limited Ability to Communicate (PACSLAC). Pain Manage Nurs. 2004;5:37–49.

115. Tsai PF, Beck C, Richards KC, et al. The pain behaviors for osteoarthritis instrument for cognitively impaired elders (PBOICIE). Res Gerontol Nurs. 2008;1:116–122.

116. Cohen-Mansfield J. Pain assessment in noncommunicative elderly persons—PAINE. Clin J Pain. 2006;22:569–575.

117. Bruera E, Kuehn N, Miller MJ, Selmser P, MacMillan K. The Edmonton Symptom Assessment System (ESAS): a simple method for the assessment of palliative care patients. J Palliat Care. 1991;7:6–9.

118. Watanabe SM, Nekolaichuk C, Beaumont C, Johnson L, Myers J, Strasser F. A multi-centre comparison of two numerical versions of the Edmonton Symptom Assessment System in palliative care patients J Pain Symptom Manage. 2011;41:456–468.

119. van Herk R, van Dijk M, Baar FP, et al. Assessment of pain: can caregivers or relatives rates pain in nursing home residents? J Clin Nurs. 2009;18:2478–2485.

120. Bruera E, Sweeney C, Willey J, Palmer JL, Strasses F, Strauch E. Perception of discomfort by relatives and nurses in unresponsive terminally ill patients with cancer: a prospective study. J Pain Symptom Manage. 2003;26:818–826.

121. Cohen-Mansfield J. Relatives assessment of pain in cognitively impaired nursing home residents. J Pain Symptom Manage. 2002;24:562–571.

CHAPTER 7

Pain at the end of life

Judith A. Paice

When there is pain, there are no words. All pain is the same.
Toni Morrison

Key points

♦ Pain is highly prevalent in palliative care, yet the majority of individuals can obtain good relief with available treatment options.

♦ An awareness of barriers to adequate pain care allows palliative care nurses to assess for and to plan interventions to overcome these obstacles when caring for patients. Advocacy is a critical role of the palliative care nurse.

♦ Assessment of pain, including a thorough history and comprehensive physical exam, guides the development of the pharmacological and nonpharmacological treatment plan.

♦ Pharmacological therapies include nonopioids, opioids, coanalgesics, cancer therapies, and, in some cases, interventional techniques.

♦ Intractable pain and symptoms, although not common, must be treated aggressively. In some cases, palliative sedation may be warranted.

Of the many symptoms experienced by those at the end of life, pain is one of the most common and most feared.[1] However, this fear is largely unfounded because the majority of patients with terminal illness can obtain relief. Nurses are critical members of the palliative care team, particularly in providing pain management. The nurse's role begins with assessment and continues through the development of a plan of care and its implementation. During this process, the nurse provides education and counsel to the patient, family, and other team members. Nurses also are critical for developing institutional policies and monitoring outcomes that ensure good pain management for all patients within their palliative care program. To provide optimal pain control, all healthcare professionals must understand the frequency of pain at the end of life, the barriers that prevent good management, the assessment of this syndrome, and the treatments used to provide relief. The Institute of Medicine's report *Relieving Pain in America* identified that effective pain control and alleviation of suffering results not from the clinician's intervention alone, but rather the strength of the clinician, patient, and family relationship.[2] This is a key strength of nursing at all phases of palliative care.

Prevalence of pain

The prevalence of pain in the terminally ill varies by diagnosis and other factors. Approximately one-third of persons who are actively receiving treatment for cancer and two-thirds of those with advanced malignant disease experience pain.[1,3–5] Individuals at particular risk for undertreatment include the elderly, minorities, and women.[6,7] Almost three-quarters of patients with advanced cancer admitted to the hospital experience pain at admission. In a study of cancer patients very near the end of life, pain occurred in 54% at 4 weeks and 34% at 1 week before death.[8] In other studies of patients admitted to palliative care units, pain often is the dominant symptom, along with fatigue and dyspnea. Children dying of cancer also are at risk for pain and suffering.[9]

The prevalence of pain in those with human immunodeficiency virus (HIV) disease varies widely and can have a profound negative effect on quality of life. Headache, abdominal pain, chest pain, and neuropathies are the most frequently reported types of pain. Lower CD4 cell counts and HIV-1 RNA levels are associated with higher rates of neuropathy. Numerous studies have reported undertreatment of persons with HIV disease, including those patients with a history of addictive disease.

Unfortunately, there has been little characterization of the pain prevalence and experience of patients with other life-threatening disorders. However, those working in palliative care are well aware that pain frequently accompanies many of the neuromuscular and cardiovascular disorders, such as multiple sclerosis and stroke, seen at the end of life. Furthermore, many patients in hospice and palliative care are elderly and more likely to have existing chronic pain syndromes, such as osteoarthritis or low back pain.

Additional research is needed to fully characterize the frequency of pain and the type of pain syndromes seen in patients at the end of life. This information will lead to improved detection, assessment and, ultimately, treatment. Unfortunately, pain continues to be undertreated, even when prevalence rates and syndromes are well understood. The undertreatment is largely due to barriers related to healthcare professionals, the system, and patients and their families.

Barriers to pain relief

Barriers to good pain relief are numerous and pervasive.[10] Often, because of lack of education, misconceptions, or attitudinal issues, these barriers contribute to the large numbers of patients who do not get adequate pain relief.[11] Careful examination of these barriers provides a guide for changing individual practice, as well as building an institutional plan within the palliative care program to improve pain relief (Box 7.1). Most studies address the barriers

---

Box 7.1 Barriers to cancer pain management

Problems related to healthcare professionals

Inadequate knowledge of pain management

Poor assessment of pain

Concern about regulation of controlled substances

Fear of patient addiction

Concern about side effects of analgesics

Concern about patients' becoming tolerant to analgesics

Problems related to the healthcare system

Low priority given to cancer pain treatment

Inadequate reimbursement

Restrictive regulation of controlled substances

Problems of availability of treatment or access to it

Problems related to patients

Reluctance to report pain

Concern about distracting physicians from treatment of under-lying disease

Fear that pain means disease is worse

Concern about not being a "good" patient

Reluctance to take pain medications

Fear of addiction or of being thought of as an addict

Worries about unmanageable side effects

Concern about becoming tolerant to pain medications

Source: Adapted from reference 13.

---

associated with cancer pain. Therefore, barriers facing individuals with other disorders commonly seen in palliative care are not well characterized. One might suggest that these individuals are affected to an even greater extent, as biases may be more pronounced in those with noncancer diagnoses.

Healthcare providers

Fears related to opioids held by professionals lead to underuse of these analgesics. Numerous surveys have revealed that physicians, nurses, and pharmacists express concerns about addiction, tolerance, and side effects of morphine and related compounds.[12,13] This concern has increased as rates of misuse and even deaths due to recreational opioid use have increased in the community. Inevitability of pain is also expressed, despite evidence to the contrary. Not surprisingly, lack of attention to pain and its treatment during basic education is frequently cited. Those providing care at the end of life must evaluate their own knowledge and beliefs, including cultural biases, and strive to educate themselves and colleagues.

Healthcare settings

Lack of availability of opioids is pervasive, affecting not only sparsely populated rural settings but also inner-city pharmacies

reluctant to carry these medications.[14] Pain management continues to be a low priority in some healthcare settings, reimbursement for these services is poor, and as a result some settings lack qualified professionals with expertise in pain management. All of this is complicated by the cost of analgesic therapies and other treatments.[15]

Patients and families

Understanding these barriers will lead the professional to better educate and better counsel patients and their families. Since these fears are insidious, patients and family members or support persons should be asked if they are concerned about addiction and tolerance (often described as becoming "immune" to the drug by laypersons). Studies have suggested that these fears lead to undermedication and increased intensity of pain. Concerns about being a "good" patient or belief in the inevitability of cancer pain lead patients to hesitate in reporting pain. In these studies, less educated and older patients were more likely to express these beliefs. Patients seeking active treatment may believe that admitting to pain or other symptoms may reduce their eligibility for clinical trials. Adherence to the medication regimen, complicated by a lack of understanding, can lead to unrelieved pain. Some patients and family members delay taking opioids, believing they are only for the dying.

At the end of life, patients may need to rely on family members or other support persons to dispense medications. Each person's concerns must be addressed or provision of medication may be inadequate. Studies suggest that little concordance exists between patients' and family members' beliefs regarding analgesics. The interdisciplinary team is essential, with nurses, social workers, chaplains, physicians, volunteers, and others providing exploration of the meaning of pain and possible barriers to good relief. Education, counseling, reframing, and spiritual support are imperative. Nurses are particularly well trained to offer the education and "coaching" that has been shown to provide improved relief. A randomized controlled clinical trial demonstrated that integrated video and print materials presented by oncology nurses could reduce patient barriers and improve pain control.[16] Other studies have used technologies such as Internet-based programs, telehealth, and videoconferencing to educate patients, particularly those in rural areas.[17] Overall, patient education has resulted in modest improvements in pain outcomes.[18]

Effects of unrelieved pain

Although many professionals and laypersons fear that opioid analgesics lead to shortened life, there is significant evidence to the contrary. A large cohort study revealed that individuals experiencing chronic pain had a 10-year increased mortality.[19] It is likely that inadequate pain relief hastens death by increasing physiological stress, potentially diminishing immunocompetence, decreasing mobility, worsening proclivities toward pneumonia and thromboembolism, and increasing work of breathing and myocardial oxygen requirements. For example, a large study of men with prostate cancer revealed a significant association between pain interference scores and risk of death.[20] Furthermore, pain may lead to spiritual death as the individual's quality of life is impaired. Therefore, it is the professional and ethical responsibility of clinicians to focus on, and attend to, adequate pain relief for their patients and to properly educate patients and their caregivers about all analgesic therapies, including opioids.

Assessment and common pain syndromes

Comprehensive assessment of pain is imperative. This must be conducted initially, regularly throughout the treatment, and during any changes in the patient's pain state.[13] For a complete discussion of pain assessment, see chapter 6.

Pharmacological management of pain in advanced and end-stage disease

A sound understanding of pharmacotherapy in the treatment of pain is of great importance in palliative care nursing. First, this knowledge allows the nurse to contribute to and fully understand the comprehensive plan of care. Thorough understanding also allows the nurse to recognize and assess medication-related adverse effects, to understand drug–drug and drug–disease interactions, and to educate patients and caregivers regarding appropriate medication usage. This will assure a comfortable process of dying for the well-being of the patient and for the sake of those in attendance.

This section provides an overview of the most commonly used agents and some of the newer pharmaceutical agents available in the United States for the treatment of unremitting and recurrent pain associated with advanced disease. The intent of this section is to arm the reader with a fundamental and practical understanding of the medications that are (or should be) available in most contemporary care settings, emphasizing those therapies for which there is clear and convincing evidence of efficacy. For an extensive review of mechanisms of pain and analgesia, pharmacological principles of analgesics, and more-detailed lists of all drugs used for pain control throughout the world, the reader is referred to a recent comprehensive review.[21] Since patients or family members are not always aware of the names of their medications, or they may bring pills to the hospital or clinic that are not in their original bottles, several Web-based resources provide pictures that can assist the nurse in identifying the current analgesic regimen. These can be found at http://www.drugs.com/pill_identification.html or http://www.webmd.com/pill-identification/default.htm. Some of these programs are available as applications for mobile phones and tablets.

Nonopioid analgesics

Acetaminophen

Acetaminophen has been determined to be one of the safest analgesics for long-term use in the management of mild pain or as a supplement in the management of more intense pain syndromes. It is especially useful in the management of nonspecific musculoskeletal pains or pain associated with osteoarthritis, but acetaminophen (also abbreviated as APAP and referred to as paracetamol in the rest of the world) should be considered an adjunct to any chronic pain regimen. It is often forgotten or overlooked when severe pain is being treated, so a reminder of its value as a "coanalgesic" is warranted. However, acetaminophen's limited antiinflammatory effect should be considered when selecting a nonopioid. Reduced doses or avoidance of acetaminophen is recommended in the face of renal insufficiency or liver dysfunction.[22] The Food and Drug Administration has required manufacturers of opioid/acetaminophen combination products to reduce the amount of acetaminophen to no greater than 325 mg. A complete review of both prescribed as well as over-the-counter

(OTC) medications taken by the patient is indicated. Many OTCs contain acetaminophen, and patients may not be aware of the risk of overdose. An intravenous formulation of acetaminophen is currently available, although cost issues may preclude its use in palliative care.[23]

Nonsteroidal antiinflammatory drugs

Nonsteroidal antiinflammatory drugs (NSAIDs) affect analgesia by reducing the biosynthesis of prostaglandins, thereby inhibiting the cascade of inflammatory events that cause, amplify, or maintain nociception. These agents also appear to reduce pain by influences on the peripheral or central nervous system independent of their antiinflammatory mechanism of action. This secondary mode of analgesic efficacy is poorly understood. The "classic" NSAIDs (e.g., aspirin or ibuprofen) are relatively nonselective in their inhibitory effects on the enzymes that convert arachidonic acid to prostaglandins. As a result, gastrointestinal ulceration, renal dysfunction, and impaired platelet aggregation are common.[24] The cyclooxygenase-2 (COX-2) enzymatic pathway is induced by tissue injury or other inflammation-inducing conditions. It is for this reason that there appears to be less risk of GI bleeding with use of the COX-2 selective NSAID celecoxib.[25] (Table 7.1).

Table 7.1 Acetaminophen and selected nonsteroidal antiinflammatory drugs

Drug	Dose if patient > 50 kg	Dose if patient < 50 kg
Acetaminophen[*†]	500–1000 mg q 4–6h oral; maximum 4000 mg/24 h	10–15 mg/kg q 4h (oral)
	1000 mg q 6 h IV (given over 15 minute infusion); maximum 4000 mg/24 h	15 mg/kg q 6 h; maximum 75 mg (IV)
		15–20 mg/kg q 4h (rectal)
Aspirin[*†]	4000 mg/24h maximum, given q 4–6h	10–15 mg/kg q 4h (oral)
		15–20 mg/kg q 4h (rectal)
Ibuprofen[*†]	2400 mg/24h maximum, given q 6–8h	10 mg/kg q 6–8h (oral)
Naproxen[*†]	1000 mg/24h maximum, given q 8–12h	5 mg/kg q 8h (oral/rectal)
Choline magnesium trisalicylate[*§]	2000–3000 mg/24h maximum, given q 8–12 h	25 mg/kg q 8h (oral)
Indomethacin[†]	75–150 mg/24h maximum, given q 8–12h	0.5–1 mg/kg q 8–12h (oral/rectal)
Ketorolac[‡]	30–60 mg IM/IV initially, then 15–30 mg q 6h bolus IV/IM or continuous IV/SQ infusion; short-term use only (3–5 days)	0.25–1 mg/kg q 6h short-term use only (3–5 days)
Celecoxib[§¶]	100–200 mg PO up to BID.	No data available

[*]Commercially available in a liquid form.
[†]Commercially available in a suppository form.
[‡]Potent antiinflammatory (short-term use only due to gastrointestinal side effects).
[§]Minimal platelet dysfunction.
[¶]Cyclooxygenase-2-selective nonsteroidal antiinflammatory drug.

The NSAIDs, as a class, are very useful in the treatment of many pain conditions mediated by inflammation, including those caused by cancer.[21] The NSAIDs offer the potential advantage of causing minimal nausea, constipation, sedation, or other effects on mental functioning. Therefore, depending on the cause of pain, NSAIDs may be useful for moderate to severe pain control, either alone or as an adjunct to opioid analgesic therapy.[26] The addition of NSAIDs to opioids has the benefit of potentially allowing the reduction of the opioid dose when sedation, obtundation, confusion, dizziness, or other central nervous system effects of opioid analgesic therapy alone become burdensome. As with acetaminophen, decreased renal function and liver failure are relative contraindications for NSAID use. Similarly, platelet dysfunction or other potential bleeding disorders contraindicate use of the nonselective NSAIDs due to their inhibitory effects on platelet aggregation, with resultant prolonged bleeding time. Cardiovascular risk associated with NSAIDs, including myocardial infarction and stroke, has been identified and appears to be higher in those with preexisting risk factors. Additionally, diclofenac appears to produce higher risk, while ibuprofen and naproxen are associated with lower risks of cardiovascular events.[27,28]

Opioid analgesics

As a pharmacological class, the opioid analgesics represent the most useful agents for the treatment of pain associated with advanced disease. The opioids are nonspecific insofar as they decrease pain signal transmission and perception throughout the nervous system, regardless of the pathophysiology of the pain. Moderate to severe pain is the main clinical indication for the opioid analgesics. Despite past beliefs that opioids were ineffective for neuropathic pain, these agents have been found to be useful in the treatment of this complex pain syndrome, however higher doses are usually warranted.[29] Other indications for opioid use include the treatment of dyspnea, use as an anesthetic adjunct, and as a form of prophylactic therapy in the treatment of psychological dependence to opioids (e.g., methadone maintenance for those with a history of heroin abuse).[30]

The only absolute contraindication to the use of an opioid is a history of a hypersensitivity reaction (rash, wheezing, and edema). Allergic reactions are almost exclusively limited to the morphine derivatives. In the rare event that a patient describes a true allergic reaction, one might begin therapy with a low dose of a short-acting synthetic opioid (e.g., IV fentanyl) or try an intradermal injection as a test dose. The rationale for using a synthetic opioid (preferably one without dyes or preservatives, as these can cause allergic reactions) is that the prevalence of allergic reactions is much lower. If the patient does develop a reaction, using a low dose of a short-acting opioid will produce a reduced response for a shorter period of time when compared with long-acting preparations.

Because misunderstandings lead to undertreatment, it is incumbent on all clinicians involved in the care of patients with chronic pain to clearly understand and differentiate the clinical conditions of tolerance, physical dependence, addiction, pseudoaddiction, and pseudotolerance (Box 7.2).

It is also critically important for clinicians who are involved in patient care to be aware that titration of opioid analgesics to affect pain relief is rarely associated with induced respiratory depression and iatrogenic death.[31,32] In fact, the most compelling evidence suggests that inadequate pain relief hastens death by increasing

---

Box 7.2 Definitions

Addiction:

Addiction is a primary, chronic, neurobiological disease, with genetic, psychosocial, and environmental factors influencing its development and manifestations. It is characterized by behaviors that include one or more of the following: impaired control over drug use, compulsive use, continued use despite harm, and craving.

Physical dependence:

Physical dependence is a state of adaptation that is manifested by a drug-class-specific withdrawal syndrome that can be produced by abrupt cessation, rapid dose reduction, decreasing blood level of the drug, and/or administration of an antagonist.

Tolerance:

Tolerance is a state of adaptation in which exposure to a drug induces changes that result in a diminution of one or more of the drug's effects overtime.

Pseudoaddiction:

Pseudoaddiction is the mistaken assumption of addiction in a patient who is seeking relief from pain.

Pseudotolerance:

Pseudotolerance is the misconception that the need for increasing doses of drug is due to tolerance rather than disease progression or other factors.

Source: Adapted from reference 13.

---

physiological stress, decreasing immunocompetence, diminishing mobility, increasing the potential for thromboembolism, worsening inspiration and thus placing the patient at risk for pneumonia, and increasing myocardial oxygen requirements. Furthermore, in a recent retrospective study of opioid use in a hospice setting, there was no relationship between opioid dose and survival.[33] And, finally, in a small study of opioid use for the treatment of dyspnea, there was no increased risk of respiratory depression in opioid naive patients when compared with those patients who had been receiving opioids.[34]

There is significant inter- and intraindividual variation in clinical responses to the various opioids, so in most cases a dose-titration approach should be viewed as the best means of optimizing care. This implies that close follow-up is required to determine when clinical endpoints have been reached. Furthermore, idiosyncratic responses may require trials of different agents to determine the most effective drug and route of delivery for any given patient. Box 7.3 lists more specific suggestions regarding optimal use of opioids.

Another factor that needs to be continually considered with opioid analgesics is the potential to accumulate toxic metabolites, especially in the face of decreasing drug clearance and elimination as disease progresses and organ function deteriorates. Due to its neurotoxic metabolite, normeperidine, meperidine use is specifically discouraged for chronic pain management. As well, the

Table 7.2 Approximate equianalgesic doses of most commonly used opioid analgesics*

Drug	Parenteral route	Enteral route
Morphine[†]	10 mg	30 mg
Codeine	130 mg	200 mg (not recommended)
Fentanyl[†††]	50–100 mcg	TIRF[‡]
Hydrocodone	Not available	30 mg
Hydromorphone[§]	1.5 mg	7.5 mg
Levorphanol[¶]	2 mg acute, 1 chronic	4 mg acute, 1 chronic
Methadone[¶]	See text & Table 7.3	See text & Table 7.3
Oxycodone[**]	Not available	20 mg

*Dose conversion should be closely monitored since incomplete cross-tolerance may occur. Interindividual variation in duration of analgesic effect is not uncommon, signaling the need to increase the dose or shorten the dose interval.
[†]Available in continuous- and sustained-release pills and capsules, formulated to last 12 or 24 hours. Also available in transdermal and TIRF, see package insert materials for dose recommendations. TIRF = transmucosal immediate release fentanyl.
[§]Available as a continuous-release formulation lasting 24 hours.
[¶]These drugs have long half-lives, so accumulation can occur; close monitoring during first few days of therapy is very important.
[**]Available in several continuous-release doses, formulated to last 12 hours.
[††]Fentanyl 100-mcg patch ≈ 4 mg IV morphine/h.
Sources: Adapted from references 13, 21.

mixed agonist–antagonist agents, typified by butorphanol, nalbuphine, and pentazocine, are not recommended for the treatment of chronic pain. They have limited efficacy, and their use may cause an acute abstinence syndrome in patients who are otherwise using pure agonist opioid analgesics.

Morphine

Morphine is most often considered the "gold standard" of opioid analgesics and is used as a measure for dose equivalence (Table 7.2).[13] Although some patients cannot tolerate morphine due to itching, headache, dysphoria, or other adverse effects, common initial dosing effects such as sedation and nausea often resolve within a few days. In fact, one should anticipate these adverse effects, especially constipation, nausea, and sedation, and prevent or treat appropriately (see below). Metabolites of morphine and hydromorphone, morphine-3-glucuronide (M3G) and hydromorphone-3-glucuronide (H3G), respectively, may contribute to myoclonus, seizures, and hyperalgesia (increasing pain), particularly when patients cannot clear these metabolites due to renal impairment.[35,36] However, a small study of hospice patients showed increased levels of either M3G or H3G were not correlated with the presence of myoclonus.[37] If adverse effects exceed the analgesic benefit of the drug, convert to an equianalgesic dose of a different opioid. Because cross-tolerance is incomplete, reduce the calculated dose by one-third to one-half and titrate upward based on the patient's pain intensity scores (see chapter 19 for more information on the neurotoxicity of opioids).[13]

Morphine's bitter taste may be prohibitive, especially if "immediate-release" tablets are left in the mouth to dissolve. When patients have dysphagia, several options are available. The 24-hour, long-acting morphine capsule can be broken open and the "sprinkles" placed in applesauce or other soft food. Oral morphine solution can be swallowed, or small volumes (0.5–1 mL) of a concentrated solution (e.g., 20 mg/mL) can be placed in the mouth of patients whose voluntary swallowing capabilities are more significantly limited. Transmucosal uptake of morphine is slow and unpredictable due to its hydrophilic chemical nature. In fact, most of the analgesic effect of a morphine tablet or liquid placed buccally or sublingually is due to drug trickling down the throat and the resultant absorption through the GI tract. Furthermore, again due to the hydrophilic nature of morphine, creams, gels, and patches that contain morphine do not cross the skin and therefore do not provide systemic analgesia.[38] Another useful route of administration when oral delivery is unreasonable is the rectal route.[39] Commercially prepared suppositories, compounded suppositories, or microenemas can be used to deliver the drug into the rectum or stoma. Sustained-release morphine tablets have been used rectally, with resultant delayed time to peak plasma level and approximately 90% of the bioavailability achieved by oral administration.

Fentanyl

Fentanyl is a highly lipid soluble opioid that has been administered parenterally, spinally, transdermally, transmucosally (bucal, sublingual, and nasal), and by nebulizer for the management of dyspnea.[21] Because of its potency, dosing is usually conducted in micrograms.

Transdermal fentanyl

Transdermal fentanyl, often called the fentanyl patch, is particularly useful when patients cannot swallow, do not remember to take

---

Box 7.4 Fentanyl patch instructions to patients and caregivers

1. Place patch on the upper body in a clean, dry, hairless area (clip hair, do not shave). The patch does not need to be placed over the site of pain.

2. Choose a different site when placing a new patch, then remove the old patch.

3. If a skin reaction consistently occurs despite site rotation, spray inhaled steroid (intended for inhalational use in asthma) over the area, let dry and apply patch (steroid creams prevent adherence of the patch).

4. Remove the old patch or patches and fold sticky surfaces together, and then flush down the toilet.

5. Wash hands after handling patches.

6. All unused patches (patient discontinued use or deceased) should be removed from wrappers, folded in half with sticky surfaces together, and flushed down the toilet.

Sources: Adapted from reference 21.

---

medications, or have adverse effects to other opioids (Box 7.4).[21] Two primary systems are currently available—a reservoir-based patch (i.e., Duragesic) and a matrix type patch (i.e., Mylan). These systems exhibit quite similar effects in intact skin, differences may result when exposed to heat (greater drug permeation at 72 hours in the reservoir system) or to compromised skin (greater permeation seen in the matrix patch).[40] Although the package insert states that transdermal patches should not be used in opioid-naive patients, a small study suggests that the 12-mcg/h patch can be safely used in this population.[41] Fever, diaphoresis, cachexia, morbid obesity, liver function, ascites, and the concomitant use of 3A4 inducers may have an impact on the absorption, predictability of blood levels, and clinical effects of transdermal fentanyl.[42,43] One study comparing cachectic with normal weighted patients found reduced serum fentanyl levels in those with reduced weight.[44] Despite these lower levels, clinical experience reveals that transdermal fentanyl can be effective even in those patients with few fat stores. Higher doses may be indicated. There is some suggestion that transdermal fentanyl may produce less constipation when compared with long-acting morphine.[45] At lower doses, transdermal fentanyl has limited effect on the sphincter of Oddi, suggesting that this may be a safe and effective therapy for patients with pancreatitis.[46] Further study is needed to confirm these findings.

Some patients experience decreased analgesic effects after only 48 hours of applying a new patch; this should be accommodated by determining whether a higher dose is tolerated with increased duration of effect or a more frequent (q 48 h) patch change should be scheduled. As with all long-acting preparations, breakthrough pain medications should be made available to patients using continuous-release opioids such as the fentanyl patch.

Transmucosal immediate-release fentanyl products

Several formulations of transmucosal immediate-release fentanyl (TIRF) products are available, including oral transmucosal fentanyl citrate (OTFC), bucal tablets, soluble film, and nasal spray.[47] The OTFC is composed of fentanyl on an applicator that patients rub against the oral mucosa to provide rapid absorption of the drug. Adults should start with the 200-mcg dose and monitor efficacy, advancing to higher dose units as needed. Clinicians must be aware that, unlike other breakthrough pain drugs, the around-the-clock dose of opioid does not predict the effective dose of OTFC. Patients should use OTFC over a period of 15 minutes because too-rapid use will result in more of the agent being swallowed rather than being absorbed transmucosally. Any remaining partial units should be disposed of by placing in a child-resistant temporary storage bottle provided when the drug is first dispensed. The fentanyl buccal tablet has been shown to be effective, and, when compared with OTFC, fentanyl buccal tablets produce a more rapid onset and greater extent of absorption.[48] The adverse effects are similar to those seen with other opioids, although a small percentage of patients do not tolerate the sensation of the tablet effervescing in the buccal space. For patients who cannot place the tablet buccally (between the gum and cheek pouch), sublingual (under the tongue) administration produced comparable bioequivalence. Bioadhesive films impregnated with fentanyl are an alternate to tablet formulations, providing efficacy with few adverse effects.[49] Fentanyl nasal spray has the most rapid onset of the TIRF products, with significantly improved pain intensity scores as early as 5 minutes after administration, along with minimal adverse effects.[50]

Oxycodone

Oxycodone is a synthetic opioid available in a long-acting formulation (OxyContin), as well as immediate-release tablets (alone or with acetaminophen) and liquid. It is approximately as lipid soluble as morphine but has better oral absorption. The equianalgesic ratio is approximately 20 mg oxycodone to 30 mg oral morphine. Side effects appear to be similar to those experienced with morphine; however, one study comparing these two long-acting formulations in persons with advanced cancer found that oxycodone produced less nausea and vomiting. Another study found no difference in efficacy between oxycodone and morphine at equianalgesic doses in patients with pancreatic cancer.[51] Women may have lowered serum levels of oxycodone, and CYP3A4 may alter oxycodone pharmacokinetics.[52] For example, substances that inhibit CYP3A4, such as the highly active antiretroviral agent retonavir, the antiviral voriconazole, and even grapefruit juice, have been found to increase oxycodone concentrations.[53–55] Lower doses of oxycodone may be warranted when CYP3A4 inhibitors are administered.

Methadone

Methadone has several characteristics that make it useful in the management of severe, chronic pain. The half-life of 24 to 60 hours or longer allows prolonged dosing intervals, although for pain control, every-8-hour dosing is recommended. Methadone may also bind as an antagonist to the N-methyl-D-aspartate (NMDA) receptor, believed to be of particular benefit in neuropathic pain. Additionally, methadone can be given orally, parenterally, and sublingually.[56] Furthermore, methadone is much less costly than comparable doses of proprietary continuous-release formulations, making it potentially more available for patients without sufficient financial resources for more costly drugs.

Despite these advantages, much is unknown about the appropriate dosing ratio between methadone and morphine, as well as the safest and most effective time course for conversion from another opioid to methadone[57] (Table 7.3). As a result,

Table 7.3 Selected medications that increase or decrease methadone serum levels

CYP3A4 inducers that decrease methadone	CYP3A4 inhibitors that increase methadone
Barbiturates	Cimetidine
Carbamazepine	Ciprofloxacin
Dexamethasone	Diazepam
Phenytoin	Haloperidol
Rifampin	Ketoconazole
Spironolactone	Omeprazole
	Verapamil

recommendations suggest that patients be started on no more than 30 to 40 mg of methadone per day with very slow upward titration.[58] Methadone should not be used for breakthrough pain dosing or on a prn basis.[59] Furthermore, although the long half-life is an advantage, it also increases the potential for drug accumulation before achieving steady-state blood levels, putting patients at risk for oversedation and respiratory depression. For example, it would take 12 days to reach steady state when the half-life is 60 hours. Close monitoring of these potentially adverse or even life-threatening effects is required, and most experts suggest that methadone only be prescribed by experienced clinicians.[59] Myoclonus has been reported with parenteral methadone use.[60] Finally, recent studies suggest high doses of methadone may lead to QT wave changes (also called torsade de pointes).[59,61]

Methadone is metabolized primarily by CYP3A4, but also by CYP2D6 and CYP1A2. As a result, drugs that induce CYP enzymes accelerate the metabolism of methadone, resulting in reduced serum levels of the drug. This may be demonstrated clinically by shortened analgesic periods or reduced overall pain relief. Examples of these drugs often used in palliative care include several antiretroviral agents, dexamethasone, carbamazepine, phenytoin, and barbiturates.[62] Drugs that inhibit CYP enzymes slow methadone metabolism, potentially leading to sedation and respiratory depression. These include ketoconazole, omeprazole, and serotonin-selective reuptake inhibitors (SSRIs)—antidepressants such as fluoxetine, paroxetine, and sertraline.[62]

Patients currently receiving methadone as part of a maintenance program for addictive disease will have developed cross-tolerance to the opioids and, as a result, require higher doses than naive patients. Prescribing methadone for substitution therapy in addictive disease requires a special license in the United States.

Hydromorphone

Hydromorphone (Dilaudid) is a useful alternative when synthetic opioids provide an advantage. It is available in oral tablets, liquids, suppositories, parenteral formulations, and a long-acting formulation.[63] Hydromorphone provides an advantage when inadequate pain control or intolerable side effects occur with morphine or oxycodone.[64] Parenteral hydromorphone has been shown to be a useful alternative when other opioids were ineffective; of particular benefit is the high concentration commercially available that allows lower volumes to be delivered.[65] Although

H3G may accumulate in renal disease, this metabolite is removed when patients are receiving dialysis, providing evidence for the safety of this drug in these patients.[66] This is of particular risk in persons with renal dysfunction.

Oxymorphone

Oxymorphone is a semisynthetic opioid that has been available in a parenteral formulation for almost 50 years and is now available in oral immediate-release and extended-release formulations. The safety and efficacy profile in people with cancer is similar to other opioids, such as morphine and oxycodone.[63,67] One study suggests oxymorphone extended release may produce less sedation and cognitive impairment when compared with extended release oxycodone.[68]

Other opioids

Buprenorphine, codeine, hydrocodone, levorphanol, tramadol, and tapentadol are other opioids available in the United States for treatment of pain. Their equianalgesic comparisons are included in Table 7.2. Buprenorphine, a partial agonist, is typically used as part of an opioid maintenance program instead of methadone. A 7-day buprenorphine patch approved for moderate to severe pain is now available in the United States.[69] Codeine is limited by pharmacogenetics; as a prodrug it must be broken down by the enzyme CYP2D6 to provide analgesia, yet approximately 10% of Caucasians in the United States are poor metabolizers.[70] Conversely, some patients are ultrarapid metabolizers, which can lead to overdose.[71] Hydrocodone is only available in combination products, limiting dose escalation in palliative care due to concerns regarding excess acetaminophen or other agents. Levorphanol has similarities to methadone, including a longer half-life; it is difficult to obtain in the United States.[72] Tramadol is a weak opioid and has serotonin and norepinephrine reuptake inhibition properties. It is available in immediate- and extended-release formulations. Although effective for neuropathic pain, a systematic review found insufficient data to recommend its use as an alternative to codeine for mild to moderate pain.[73] Dose escalation is limited due to potential lowering of the seizure threshold. Tapentadol is available in immediate- and extended-release formulations, and initial reports suggest it may be useful in some palliative care settings.[74]

Alternative routes of administration for opioid analgesics

Many routes of administration are available when patients can no longer swallow or when other dynamics preclude the oral route or favor other routes. These include transdermal, transmucosal, rectal, vaginal, topical, epidural, and intrathecal. In a study of cancer patients at 4 weeks, 1 week, and 24 hours before death, the oral route of opioid administration was continued in 62%, 43%, and 20% of patients, respectively. More than half of these patients required more than one route of opioid administration. As patients approached death and oral use diminished, the use of intermittent subcutaneous injections and IV or subcutaneous infusions increased.

Thus, in the palliative care setting, nonoral routes of administration must be available. Enteral feeding tubes can be used to access the gut when patients can no longer swallow. The size of the tube should be considered when placing long-acting morphine "sprinkles" to avoid obstruction of the tube. The rectum, stoma, or vagina can be used to deliver medication. Thrombocytopenia or painful lesions preclude the use of these routes. Additionally, delivering medications via these routes can be difficult for family members, especially when the patient is obtunded or unable to assist. As previously discussed, transdermal, transmucosal, or buccal fentanyl are useful alternatives to these techniques.

Parenteral administration includes subcutaneous and IV delivery (intramuscular opioid delivery is inappropriate in the palliative care setting). The IV route provides rapid drug delivery but requires vascular access, placing the patient at risk for infection and potentially complicating the care provided by family or other loved ones. Subcutaneous boluses have a slower onset and lower peak effect when compared with IV boluses. Subcutaneous infusions may include up to 10 mL/h (although most patients absorb 2 to 3 mL/h with least difficulty). Volumes greater than 10 mL/h are poorly absorbed. Hyaluronidase has been reported to speed absorption of subcutaneously administered drugs.

Intraspinal routes, including epidural or intrathecal delivery, may allow administration of drugs, such as opioids, local anesthetics, and/or α-adrenergic agonists. One randomized controlled trial demonstrated benefit for cancer patients experiencing pain.[75] However, the equipment used to deliver these medications is complex, requiring specialized knowledge for healthcare professionals and potentially greater caregiver burden. Risk of infection is also of concern. Furthermore, cost is a significant concern related to high-technology procedures.

Preventing and treating adverse effects of opioid analgesics

Constipation

Patients in palliative care frequently experience constipation, in part due to opioid therapy. Always begin a prophylactic bowel regimen when commencing opioid analgesic therapy.[76] Most clinicians recommend a laxative/softener combination, although one study found that senna alone was more effective than senna and docusate.[77,78] Avoid bulking agents (e.g., psyllium) since these tend to cause a larger, bulkier stool, increasing desiccation time in the large bowel. Furthermore, debilitated patients can rarely take in sufficient fluid to facilitate the action of bulking agents. Fluid intake should be encouraged whenever feasible. Senna tea and fruits may be of use. A novel compound, methylnaltrexone, has been shown to be effective in relieving opioid-induced constipation when given subcutaneously at doses of 0.15 mg/kg.[78,79] Lubiprostone, an oral agent that works on chloride channels in the intestine, was approved for use in opioid-induced constipation in noncancer patients.[80] For a more comprehensive review of bowel management, refer to chapter 12.

Sedation

Excessive sedation may occur with the initial doses of opioids. If sedation persists after 24 to 48 hours and other correctable causes have been identified and treated if possible, the use of psychostimulants may be beneficial. These include dextroamphetamine 2.5 to 5 mg PO q morning and midday or methylphenidate 5 to 10 mg PO q morning and 2.5 to 5 mg midday (although higher doses are frequently used). Adjust both the dose and timing to prevent nocturnal insomnia and monitor for undesirable psychotomimetic effects (such as agitation, hallucinations, and irritability). Interestingly, in one study, as-needed dosing of methylphenidate in cancer patients did not result in sleep disturbances or agitation, even though most subjects took doses in the afternoon and evening. Modafinil, an agent approved to manage narcolepsy, has been reported to relieve opioid-induced sedation with once-daily dosing. Because of the lack of data regarding these agents, selection of drug and dosing are empirical. Opioid rotation may also be warranted.

Respiratory depression

Respiratory depression is rarely a clinically significant problem for opioid-tolerant patients in pain. When respiratory depression occurs in a patient with advanced disease, the cause is usually multifactorial. Therefore, other factors beyond opioids need to be assessed, although opioids are frequently blamed for the reduced respirations. When undesired depressed consciousness occurs along with a respiratory rate less than 8/min or hypoxemia (O_2 saturation <90%) associated with opioid use, cautious and slow titration of naloxone, which reverses the effects of the opioids should be instituted. Excessive administration may cause abrupt opioid reversal with pain and autonomic crisis. Dilute 1 ampule of naloxone (0.4 mg/mL) in 10 mL of injectable saline (final concentration 40 mcg/mL) and inject 1 mL every 2 to 3 minutes while closely monitoring the level of consciousness and respiratory rate. Because the duration of effect of naloxone is approximately 30 minutes, the depressant effects of the opioid will recur at 30 minutes and persist until the plasma levels decline (often four or more hours) or until the next dose of naloxone is administered. A relatively recently identified phenomenon is the onset, or exacerbation of, sleep apnea in patients taking opioids for pain.[81] Although this has been described in nonmalignant pain populations, this may be of concern for some palliative care patients. Risk factors appear to be the use of methadone, concomitant use of benzodiazepines or other sedative agents, respiratory infections, and obesity (which is a risk factor for sleep apnea).

Nausea and vomiting

Nausea and vomiting are common with opioids due to activation of the chemoreceptor trigger zone in the medulla, vestibular sensitivity, and delayed gastric emptying, but habituation occurs in most cases within several days.[82] Assess for other treatable causes. In severe cases, or when nausea and vomiting are not self-limited, pharmacotherapy is indicated. The doses of nausea-relieving medications and antiemetics listed below are to be used initially but can be increased as required. See chapter 10 for a thorough discussion of the assessment and treatment of nausea and vomiting.

Myoclonus

Myoclonic jerking occurs more commonly with high-dose opioid therapy, although it has also been reported with lower dosing.[60] If this should develop, switch to an alternate opioid, since evidence suggests this symptom is associated with metabolite accumulation, particularly in the face of renal dysfunction. A lower relative dose of the substituted drug maybe possible, due to incomplete cross-tolerance, which might result in decreased myoclonus. Clonazepam 0.5 to 1 mg PO q 6 to 8 hours, to be increased as needed and tolerated, may be useful in treating myoclonus in patients who are still alert, able to communicate, and take oral preparations. Lorazepam can be given sublingually if the patient is unable to swallow. Otherwise, parenteral administration of a benzodiazepine is indicated if symptoms are distressing.

Pruritus

Pruritus appears to be most common with morphine, in part due to histamine release, but can occur with most opioids. Fentanyl and oxymorphone may be less likely to cause histamine release. Most antipruritus therapies cause sedation, so this side effect must be viewed by the patient as an acceptable trade-off. Antihistamines (such as diphenydramine) are the most common first-line approach to this opioid-induced symptom when treatment is indicated. Ondansetron has been reported to be effective in relieving opioid-induced pruritus, but no randomized controlled studies exist.[83] See chapter 18 for more information regarding pruritus.

Coanalgesics

A wide variety of nonopioid medications from several pharmacological classes have been demonstrated to reduce pain caused by various pathological conditions (Table 7.4). As a group, these drugs have been called analgesic "adjuvants," but this is something of a misnomer, because they often reduce pain when used alone. However, under most circumstances, when these drugs are indicated for the treatment of severe neuropathic pain or bone pain, opioid analgesics are used concomitantly to provide adequate pain relief.

Antidepressants

The mechanism of the analgesic effect of tricyclic antidepressants appears to be related to inhibition of norepinephrine and serotonin. The tricyclic antidepressants are generally believed to provide relief from neuropathic pain.[84] Side effects often limit the use of these agents in palliative care. Cardiac arrhythmias, conduction abnormalities, narrow-angle glaucoma, and clinically significant prostatic hyperplasia are relative contraindications to the tricyclic antidepressants. The delay in onset of pain relief, from days to weeks, may preclude the use of these agents for

Table 7.4 Adjuvant analgesics

Drug class	Daily adult starting dose* (Range)	Routes of administration	Adverse effects	Indications
Antidepressants	Nortriptyline 10–25 mg	PO	Anticholinergic effects	Neuropathic pain
	Desipramine 10–25 mg	PO		
	Venlafaxine 37.5 mg BID	PO	Nausea, dizziness	
	Duloxetine 30 mg	PO	Nausea	
Anticonvulsants	Clonazapam 0.5–1 mg HS, BID, or TID	PO	Sedation	Neuropathic pain
	Carbamazapine 100 mg q day or TID	PO	Sedation, Aplastic anemia (rare)	
	Gabapentin 100 mg TID	PO	Sedation, dizziness	
	Pregabalin 50 mg BID or TID		Sedation, dizziness	
Corticosteroids	Dexamethasone 2–20 mg q day; may give up to 100 mg IV bolus for pain crises	PO/IV/SQ	"Steroid psychosis," dyspepsia	Cerebral edema, spinal cord compression, bone pain, neuropathic pain, visceral pain
	Prednisone 15–30 mg TID	PO		
Local anesthetics	Mexiletine 150 mg TID	PO	Lightheadedness, arrhythmias	Neuropathic pain
	Lidocaine 1–5 mg/kg hourly	IV or SQ infusion		
N-Methyl-D-aspartate antagonists	Dextromethorphan, effective dose unknown	PO	Confusion	Neuropathic pain
	Ketamine (see Pain Crises)	IV		
Bisphosphonates	Pamidronate 60–90 mg over 2h every 2–4 wk	IV infusion	Pain flare	Osteolytic bone pain
Calcitonin	25 IU/day	SQ/nasal	Hypersensitivity reaction, nausea	Neuropathic pain, bone pain
Capsaicin	0.025–0.075%	Topical	Burning	Neuropathic pain
Baclofen	10 mg q day or TID	PO	Muscle weakness, cognitive changes	
Calcium channel blockers	Nifedipine 10 mg TID	PO	Bradycardia, hypotension	Ischemic pain, neuropathic pain, smooth muscle spasms with pain

*Pediatric doses for pain control not well established.
Source: Reference 21.

pain relief in end-of-life care. However, their sleep-enhancing and mood-elevating effects may be of benefit.[85]

Both older antidepressants and newer atypical agents have been shown to be effective in relieving neuropathic pain, although there remains little support for the analgesic effect of SSRIs.[84] Atypical antidepressants, venlafaxine and duloxetine, have been shown to reduce neuropathy associated with chemotherapy-induced neuropathy in experimental animal models and in humans.[86,87]

Anticonvulsants

The older anticonvulsants, such as carbamazepine and clonazepam, relieve pain by blocking sodium channels. Often referred to as membrane stabilizers, these compounds are very useful in the treatment of neuropathic pain, especially those with episodic, lancinating qualities. Gabapentin and pregabalin act at the alpha-2 delta subunit of the voltage-gated calcium channel.[88] Additional evidence supports the use of these agents in neuropathic pain syndromes seen in palliative care, such as thalamic pain, pain due to spinal cord injury, and cancer pain, along with restless leg syndrome. Pregabalin has undergone extensive testing in pain due to diabetic neuropathy and has been found to be effective.[88] Withdrawal from either compound should be gradual. In a study comparing amitriptyline, gabapentin, and pregabalin in cancer patients with neuropathic pain, no significant differences were found in analgesic effect, although pregabalin had a greater morphine sparing effect.[89] Other anticonvulsants have been used with success in treating neuropathies, including lamotrigine, levetiracetam, tiagabine, topiramate, and zonisamide, yet no randomized controlled clinical trials are currently available.[90]

Corticosteroids

Corticosteroids inhibit prostaglandin synthesis and reduce edema surrounding neural tissues. Dexamethasone has been found to reduce postoperative pain and nausea after mastectomy[91] and is particularly useful for relieving painful neuropathic syndromes, including plexopathies, as well as pain associated with stretching of the liver capsule due to metastases.[92] Corticosteroids are also highly effective for treating bone pain via their antiinflammatory effects and for relieving malignant intestinal obstruction. Dexamethasone produces the least amount of mineralocorticoid effect, leading to reduced potential for Cushing's syndrome. Dexamethasone is available in oral, IV, subcutaneous, and epidural formulations. The standard dose is 2 to 24 mg/day and can be administered once daily due to the long half-life of this drug. Dexamethasone doses as high as 100 mg may be given with severe pain crises. Intravenous bolus doses should be pushed slowly, to prevent uncomfortable perineal burning and itching. An additional benefit of steroid use was revealed by a recent clinical trial in cancer patients that supported the use of dexamethasone in the relief of fatigue.[93]

Local anesthetics

Local anesthetics work in a manner similar to the older anticonvulsants—by inhibiting the movement of ions across the neural membrane. They are useful for relieving neuropathic pain. Local anesthetics can be given orally, topically, intravenously, subcutaneously, or spinally. Mexiletine has been reported to be useful when anticonvulsants and other adjuvant therapies have failed. Local anesthetic gels and patches have been used to prevent the pain associated with needle stick and other minor procedures. Both gel and patch (Lidoderm) versions of lidocaine have been shown to reduce the pain of postherpetic neuropathy. Administering IV lidocaine at 1 to 5 mg/kg (maximum 500 mg) over 1 hour, followed by a continuous infusion of 1 to 2 mg/kg/h has been reported to reduce intractable neuropathic pain in patients in inpatient palliative care and home hospice settings. Epidural or intrathecal lidocaine or bupivacaine delivered with or without an opioid can reduce neuropathic pain.[94]

N-methyl-D-aspartate antagonists

Antagonists to NMDA are believed to block the binding of excitatory amino acids, such as glutamate, in the spinal cord. Ketamine, a dissociative anesthetic, is believed to relieve severe neuropathic pain by blocking NMDA receptors (see the section "Pain Crisis," below). Case reports and small studies suggest that intravenous or oral ketamine can be used in adults and children for their relief of neuropathic pain or to reduce opioid doses.[95] A Cochrane review found insufficient trials conducted to determine safety and efficacy when used in combination with morphine in cancer pain.[96,97] However, a recent systematic review concluded that although limitations in the data exist, ketamine may be an option for refractory cancer pain.[98] Routine use often is limited by cognitive changes, hallucinations, and other adverse effects, although small studies suggest that gradual upward titration may prevent these effects.[99–101] Topical ketamine, usually in combination with amitriptyline and baclofen, may be useful for neuropathic conditions due to cancer treatment.[100,102] Oral compounds containing dextromethorphan have been tested, but were found to be ineffective in relieving cancer pain.

Bisphosphonates

Bisphosphonates inhibit osteoclast-mediated bone resorption and alleviate pain related to metastatic bone disease and multiple myeloma.[103] Pamidronate disodium reduces pain, hypercalcemia, and skeletal morbidity associated with breast cancer and multiple myeloma. Dosing is generally repeated every 4 weeks, and the analgesic effects occur in 2 to 4 weeks Zoledronic acid and ibandronate have been shown to relieve pain due to metastatic bone disease.[104] Denosumab, a newer bisphosphonate, has been shown to reduce skeletal-related events associated with solid tumors, which would reduce pain associated with fractures.[105] Clodronate and sodium etidronate appear to provide little or no analgesia.

Calcitonin

Subcutaneous calcitonin may be effective in the relief of neuropathic or bone pain, although studies are inconclusive. The nasal form of this drug may be more acceptable in end-of-life care when other therapies are ineffective. Usual doses are 100 to 200 IU/day subcutaneously or nasally.

Radiation therapy and radiopharmaceuticals

Radiotherapy can be enormously beneficial in relieving pain due to bone metastases or other lesions. In many cases, single-fraction external beam therapy can be used to facilitate treatment in debilitated patients. Goals of treatment should be clearly articulated so that patients and family members understand the role of this therapy. Targeted therapies, also referred to as radiosurgery, can be effective in selected situations. Radiolabeled agents, also described as radiopharmaceuticals, such as strontium-89 and samarium-153 have been shown to be effective at reducing metastatic bone pain.[106] Thrombocytopenia and leukopenia are relative contraindications, because strontium-89 can cause thrombocytopenia in as many as 33% of those treated and leukopenia in up to 10%. Because of the delayed onset and timing of peak effect, only those patients with a projected life span of greater than 3 months should be considered for treatment. Patients should be advised that a transitory pain flare can occur after either external beam therapy or radiolabeled agents; additional analgesics should be provided in anticipation.

Chemotherapy

Palliative chemotherapy is the use of antitumor therapy to relieve symptoms associated with malignancy. Patient goals, performance status, sensitivity of the tumor, and potential toxicities must be considered. Examples of symptoms that may improve with chemotherapy include hormonal therapy in breast cancer to relieve chest wall pain due to tumor ulceration, or chemotherapy in lung cancer to relieve dyspnea. However, in a study of patients with stage IV cancers, 69% of those with lung and 81% of those with colorectal cancers did not understand the chemotherapy was not curative.[107] Clear discussions regarding the goals of therapy are warranted.

Other adjunct analgesics

Topical capsaicin is believed to relieve pain by inhibiting the release of substance P. This compound has been shown to be useful in relieving pain associated with postmastectomy syndrome, postherpetic neuralgia, and postsurgical neuropathic pain in cancer. A burning sensation experienced by patients is a common reason for discontinuing therapy. A Cochrane review of low-dose topical capsaicin found this therapy unlikely to have meaningful effect.[108] A high concentration (8%) topical capsaicin patch has been found to be effective in treating HIV-associated and other painful neuropathies.[109,110]

Patients often ask about cannabinoids for the relief of pain, particularly as many states have legalized medical marijuana. Major advances, such as the characterization of the cannabinoid receptors (CB1 and CB2) have increased our understanding of the role of these receptors in pain and have allowed the development of more selective agents that might provide analgesia without the central nervous system depressant effects seen with tetrahydrocannabinol (THC). Evidence exists for the efficacy of some of these new selective compounds in animal models of noncancer and cancer pain.[111,112] Nabiximols, an oral cannabinoid spray shown to be effective in advanced cancer pain poorly responsive to opioids, has been approved in Canada and several countries in Europe for the relief of neuropathic pain.[113] However, review of existing literature evaluating the role of cannabinoids currently approved for human use suggests that these agents are moderately effective with comparable adverse effects.[114] Questions regarding the long-term safety and regulatory implications remain.[115] Of importance to prescribers is that although a state may have legalized marijuana, it remains a federal offense.[116]

Baclofen is useful in the relief of spasm-associated pain. Doses usually begin at 10 mg/day, increasing every few days. A generalized feeling of weakness and confusion or hallucinations often occurs with doses above 60 mg/day. A small retrospective chart review of patients with neuropathic cancer pain suggested benefit from oral baclofen.[117] Intrathecal baclofen has been used to treat spasticity and resulting pain, primarily due to multiple sclerosis and spinal cord injury, although a case report describes relief from pain due to spinal cord injury and amyotrophic lateral sclerosis.[118]

Dexmedetomidine is an alpha-2 adrenergic agonist used primarily within intensive care or during invasive procedures. Early case reports suggest it may provide relief in intractable pain, although cost and hypotension may limit its use.[119]

Interventional therapies

In addition to previously discussed spinal administration of analgesics, interventional therapies to relieve pain at end of life can be beneficial, including nerve blocks, vertebroplasty, kyphoplasty, radiofrequency ablation of painful metastases, procedures to drain painful effusions, and other techniques.[120] Few of these procedures have undergone controlled clinical studies. One technique, the celiac plexus block, has been shown to be superior to morphine in patients with pain due to unresectable pancreatic cancer.[121] A relatively new approach to providing analgesia is the administration of botulinum toxin (sometimes referred to as botox). Injections of this substance into areas of muscle spasticity, tightness, and pain can result in relief. This has been used extensively in migraine treatment and chronic pain conditions and, more recently, has been used to relieve pain in people with cancer who experience radiation fibrosis, such as cervical dystonia, trigeminal nerve pain, and headache.[122]

A complete review of interventional procedures can be found in a variety of sources. Choosing one of these techniques is dependent on the availability of experts in this area who understand the special needs of palliative care patients, the patient's ability to undergo the procedure, and the patient's and family's goals of care.

Nonpharmacological therapies

Nondrug therapies, including cognitive-behavioral techniques and physical measures, can serve as adjuncts to analgesics in the palliative care setting. This is not to suggest that when these therapies work, the pain is of psychological origin. The patient's and caregivers' abilities to participate must be considered when selecting one of these therapies, including their fatigue level, interest, cognition, and other factors.[123,124]

Cognitive-behavioral therapy often includes strategies to improve coping and relaxation, such as relaxation, guided imagery, music, prayer, and reframing.[125–129] These strategies have been found to be useful in reducing anxiety and improving sleep in those with advanced disease as well as reducing endocrine symptoms in women being treated for breast cancer. Physical measures, such as massage, reflexology, heat, chiropractic, and other techniques, have also been shown to produce relaxation and relieve pain.[125,126,130,131] One study found that massage was also useful in assisting family members in their bereavement after a loved one died after receiving palliative care services.[132] More rigorous research is needed in the palliative care setting regarding nondrug therapies that might enhance pain relief.

Difficult pain syndromes

The above therapies provide relief for the majority of patients (Box 7.5). Unfortunately, complex pain syndromes may require

Box 7.5 Guidelines for pain management in palliative care

- Sustained-release formulations and around-the-clock dosing should be used for continuous pain syndromes.

- Immediate-release formulations should be made available for breakthrough pain. Each breakthrough dose is usually 10%–20% of the 24-h dose of the sustained-release formulation. Thus, as the sustained-release dose increases, so does the immediate-release dose.

- Cost, convenience, and availability of medications (and other identified issues influencing compliance) are highly practical and important matters that should be taken into account with every prescription.

- Anticipate, prevent, and treat predictable side effects and adverse drug effects.

- Titrate analgesics based on patient goals, requirements for supplemental analgesics, pain intensity, severity of undesirable or adverse drug effects, measures of functionality, sleep, emotional state, and patients'/caregivers' reports of impact of pain on quality of life.

- Monitor patient status frequently during dose titration.

- Discourage use of mixed agonist–antagonist opioids.

- Be aware of potential drug–drug and drug–disease interactions.

- Recommend expert pain management consultation if pain is not adequately relieved within a reasonable amount of time after applying standard analgesic guidelines and interventions.

- Know the qualifications, experience, skills, and availability of pain management experts (consultants) within the patient's community before they may be needed.

These basic guidelines and considerations will optimize the pharmacological management of all patients with pain, particularly those in the palliative care setting.

additional measures. These syndromes include breakthrough pain, pain crises, and pain control in the patient with a past or current history of substance abuse.

Breakthrough pain

Intermittent episodes of moderate to severe pain that occur in spite of control of baseline continuous pain are common in patients with advanced disease. Breakthrough pains are common in palliative care patients, occurring a few times a day, lasting moments to many minutes.[30] Several studies of patients with cancer and noncancer diagnoses at end of life demonstrate an average of 4–5 breakthrough episodes per day, with the majority of these episodes occurring without any warning.[133] The risk of increasing the around-the-clock or continuous-release analgesic dose to cover breakthrough pains is that of increasing undesirable side effects, especially sedation, once the more short-lived, episodic breakthrough pain has remitted. Guidelines for categorizing, assessing, and managing breakthrough pain are described below.

Incident pain

Incident pain is predictably elicited by specific activities. Use a rapid-onset, short-duration analgesic formulation in anticipation of pain-eliciting activities or events. Use the same drug that the patient is taking for baseline pain relief for incident pain whenever possible. Educate patients and family members regarding the need to administer short-acting opioids approximately 30–60 minutes prior to the activity to prevent pain.[30]

Spontaneous pain

Spontaneous pain is unpredictable and not temporally associated with any activity or event. These pains are more challenging to control. The use of adjuvants for neuropathic pains may help to diminish the frequency and severity of these types of pain (see Table 7.4). Otherwise, immediate treatment with a potent, rapid-onset opioid analgesic is indicated.

End-of-dose failure

End-of-dose failure describes pain that occurs toward the end of the usual dosing interval of a regularly scheduled analgesic. This results from declining blood levels of the around-the-clock analgesic before administration or uptake of the next scheduled dose. Appropriate questioning and use of pain diaries will assure rapid diagnosis of end-of-dose failure. Increasing the dose of around-the-clock medication or shortening the dose interval to match the onset of this type of breakthrough pain should remedy the problem. For instance, a patient who is taking continuous-release morphine every 12 hours and whose pain "breaks through" after about 8 to 10 hours is experiencing end-of-dose failure. The dosing interval should be increased to every eight hours or, if this is not reasonable, the dose should be increased by 25% to 50%.

Bone pain

Pain due to bone metastases or pathological fractures can include extremely painful breakthrough pain, often associated with movement, along with periods of somnolence when the patient is at rest.[134] As a result, malignant bone pain is highly correlated with functional impairment. Studies in the laboratory implicate sprouting of sensory neurons within bone that is driven by nerve growth factor released by tumor cells.[135] This may lead to anti-nerve growth factor (anti-NGF) directed therapies. Current treatment of bone pain includes the use of corticosteroids, bisphosphonates, radiotherapy or radionuclides if consistent with the goals of care, and long-acting opioids along with short-acting opioids for the periods of increasing pain. Vertebroplasty or kyphoplasty may stabilize the vertebrae if tumor invasion leads to instability.[120]

Pain crisis

Most nociceptive (i.e., somatic and visceral) pain is controllable with appropriately titrated analgesic therapy. Some neuropathic pains, such as invasive and compressive neuropathies, plexopathies, and myelopathies, may be poorly responsive to conventional analgesic therapies, short of inducing a nearly comatose state. Widespread bone metastases or end-stage pathological fractures may present similar challenges. When confronted by a pain crisis, the following considerations will be helpful:

- Differentiate terminal agitation or anxiety from "physically" based pain, if possible. Terminal symptoms unresponsive to rapid upward titration of an opioid may respond to benzodiazepines (e.g., lorazepam, midazolam).

♦ Make sure that drugs are getting absorbed. The only route guaranteed to be absorbed is the IV route. Although invasive routes of drug delivery are to be avoided unless necessary, if there is any question about oral or transdermal absorption of analgesics or other necessary palliative drugs, parenteral access should be established.

♦ Preterminal pain crises that respond poorly to basic approaches to analgesic therapy merit consultation with a pain management consultant as quickly as possible. Radiotherapeutic, anesthetic, or neuroablative procedures may be indicated.

Management of refractory symptoms at the end of life

Sedation at the end of life is an important option for patients at home or in hospital with intractable pain, delirium, dyspnea, or other symptoms.[136,137] The most commonly employed agents include benzodiazepines, including midazolam or lorazepam, barbiturates, and in some cases, propofol. Palliative sedation is best delivered under the guidance of experts in palliative care and is usually reserved for those patients who are expected to die within hours to days.[138] In a large review of advanced cancer patients receiving sedation, survival was no worse when compared with those not sedated.[139] Light sedation may first be attempted to allow communication with loved ones, although in some circumstances this may be insufficient to relieve the intractable symptoms. See chapter 25 for additional discussion regarding palliative sedation.

Parenteral administration of ketamine is also useful for some patients with refractory pain at the end of life. Ketamine is a potent analgesic at low doses and a dissociative anesthetic at higher doses. In particular, ketamine can be used for the management of severe neuropathic pain and can be effective as an opioid-sparing agent, allowing in some cases increased interactive capability. Adverse effects are often dose-related and include psychotomimetic effects (hallucinations, dysphoria, and nightmares) as well as excess salivation.[95] Haloperidol can be used to treat the hallucinations, and scopolamine may be needed to reduce the excess salivation seen with this drug. Ketamine is commercially available in the United States only in a parenteral formulation. If the oral route is indicated, a palatable solution can be compounded or the parenteral solution ingested, usually mixed with juice or other liquids to mask the bitter taste. Because the opioid sparing effect is so pronounced, the opioid dose should be reduced by 25% to 50% when initiating ketamine (Box 7.6). More research is needed regarding the efficacy of, and adverse effects associated with, the use of ketamine for intractable pain in the palliative care population.

Pain control in people with substance abuse disorders

The numbers of patients entering palliative care with a current or past history of substance abuse disorders are unknown, yet thought to be significant. As approximately one-third of the US population has used illicit drugs, it would logically follow that some of these individuals will require palliative care. Therefore,

---

Box 7.6 Protocol for using ketamine to treat intractable pain

1. The typical starting dose is 10–15 mg PO every 6 hours. Reversal of morphine tolerance may occur at low doses such as this, while management of neuropathic pain is likely to require higher doses.

   a. There is no commercially available oral product. The injectable product may be diluted from its standard concentration of 50 mg/mL or 100 mg/mL with cherry syrup or cola to mask the bitter taste when given orally.

   b. Consider decreasing long-acting opioid by 25%–50%.

2. Dosing may be increased *daily* by 10 mg every 6 hours until pain is relieved or side effects occur. Do not increase doses more frequently than every 24 hours.

   a. Major side effects include dizziness, a dreamlike feeling, and auditory or visual hallucinations. If intolerable side effects occur, ketamine should be decreased to the previous dose or discontinued. Resolution may not occur for 24 hours.

   b. Oral doses as high as 1000 mg per day have been reported in the neuropathic pain literature with average oral doses of 200 mg per day in divided doses required for pain relief.

3. Ketamine may be given intravenously or subcutaneously if the oral route is not available. A trial of 5–10 mg IV can also be considered, which may be repeated in 15–30 minutes.

   a. The starting infusion dose is 0.2 mg/kg/h, can increase by 0.1mg/kg/h every 6 hours, with upward titrations to 0.5 mg/kg/h or 800 mg in 24 hours.

   b. Consider decreasing long-acting opioid by 25%–50%

   c. The injectable solution is irritating and may require the subcutaneous needle to be changed daily.

Source: Thomas Palliative Care Program, Virginia Commonwealth University, Richmond, VA; with permission.

---

all clinicians must be aware of the principles and practical considerations necessary to adequately care for these individuals (see chapter 41 for a complete discussion of care for the addicted patient at the end of life).

The underlying mechanisms of addiction are complex, including the pharmacological properties of the drug, personality and psychiatric disorders, and underlying genetic factors. Caring for these patients can be extremely challenging. Thorough assessment of the pain and their addictive disease is critical. Screening tools, such as the CAGE questionnaire (i.e., Cut down, Annoying, Guilty, Eye opener), have been found to predict long-term opioid treatment in cancer patients undergoing chemoradiation for head and neck cancer.[140] The interview should begin with general questions about the use of caffeine and nicotine and gradually become more specific about illicit drug use. Patients should be informed that the information will be used to help prevent withdrawal from these drugs, as well as ensure adequate doses of medications used to relieve pain.

Patients can be categorized in the following manner: (1) individuals who used drugs or alcohol in the past but are not using them now; (2) patients in methadone maintenance programs who are not using recreational drugs or alcohol; (3) persons in methadone maintenance programs but who continue to actively use drugs or alcohol; (4) people using drugs or alcohol occasionally, usually socially; and (5) patients who are actively abusing drugs. Treatment is different for each group, and risk stratification can be useful in clinical management.

A frequent fear expressed by professionals is that they will be "duped," or lied to, about the presence of pain. One of the limitations of pain management is that pain, and all its components, cannot be proven. Therefore, expressions of pain must be believed. As with all aspects of palliative care, an interdisciplinary team approach is indicated. This may include inviting addiction counselors to interdisciplinary team meetings. Realistic goals must be established. For example, recovery from addiction is impossible if the patient does not seek this rehabilitation. The goal in that case may be to provide a structured and safe environment for patients and their support persons. Comorbid psychiatric disorders are common, particularly depression, personality disorders, and anxiety disorders. Treatment of these underlying problems may reduce relapse or aberrant behaviors and may make pain control more effective.[141]

The pharmacological principles of pain management in the person with addictive disease are not unlike those in a person without this history. Nonopioids may be used, including antidepressants, anticonvulsants, and other adjuncts. However, psychoactive drugs with no analgesic effect should be avoided in the treatment of pain. Tolerance must be considered; thus, opioid doses may require more rapid titration and may be higher than for patients without previous exposure to opioids. Requests for increasing doses may be due to psychological suffering, so this possibility must also be explored.

An additional complicating factor is that many people with addictive disease have limited psychological, social, and financial resources. Part of the reason for self-medication may be mental illness. The lack of resources makes provision of care difficult, as many of these patients may have lost their jobs and homes and have alienated friends and family members. Innovative programs offering palliative care of homeless patients living in shelters include attention to treatment of substance abuse. Other novel programs are being proposed to allow community access to palliative care patients while limiting the potential for diversion.[142]

Consistency in the treatment plan is essential. Inconsistency can increase manipulation and lead to staff frustration. Setting limits is a critical component of the care plan, and medication contracts may be indicated.[143] In fact, one primary clinician may be designated to handle the pharmacological management of pain. Prescriptions may be written for 1-week intervals if patients cannot manage an entire month's supply. Prescriptions may be delivered to one pharmacy to reduce the potential for altered prescriptions or prescriptions from multiple prescribers. Use long-acting opioids whenever possible, limiting the reliance on short-acting drugs. Some have suggested requiring patients to bring in pill bottles to all clinic visits to conduct pill counts. Checking state prescription drug monitoring program websites for information regarding medication refills can help determine whether the patient is receiving prescriptions from multiple prescribers.

Avoid bolus parenteral administration, although at the end of life, infusions can be effective and diversion limited by keeping no spare cassettes or bags in the home. Weekly team meetings provide a forum to establish the plan of care and discuss negative attitudes regarding the patient's behavior. Family meetings may be indicated, particularly if they are also experiencing addictive behaviors. Hospices and palliative care programs should have policies in place to provide guidance in the management of these patients.[144]

Withdrawal from drugs of abuse must be prevented or minimized. These may include cocaine, benzodiazepines, and even alcohol. Alcoholism in palliative care has been underdiagnosed.[145] Thus, a thorough assessment of recreational drug use, including alcohol, must be conducted. This provides evidence for adherence to the treatment plan. Urine toxicology studies may be useful. Patients in recovery may be extremely reluctant to consider opioid therapy. Patients may need reassurance that opioids can be taken for medical indications, such as cancer or other illnesses. If patients currently are treated in a methadone maintenance program, continue the methadone but add another opioid to provide pain relief. Communicate with the program to ensure the correct methadone dose. Nondrug alternatives may also be suggested.

An emerging area of interest is whether opioid therapy is beneficial in chronic pain. Several well-designed studies suggest increased rates of depression, misuse, and overdose in those with chronic nonmalignant pain.[146–150] Long-term opioid use may lead to endocrine changes in both men and women, as well as increased incidence of fractures.[151,152] Additionally, the increase in prescribing of opioids for chronic pain may be contributing to the rising death rate associated with opioid misuse.[153] Although limited data are available for those with life-threatening illnesses, as palliative care moves upstream into outpatient practices with increasing numbers of patients with chronic pain, these issues will become prominent and will require thoughtful solutions.

Case study

Mr. Hall, a patient with osteosarcoma

John Hall is a 22-year-old college student with osteosarcoma affecting the proximal end of the tibia discovered after a football injury; this is treated with neoadjuvant chemotherapy in an attempt to reduce tumor burden so that a limb-sparing procedure could be performed. He reports severe throbbing and burning pain in the affected extremity and is taking hydrocodone/acetaminophen 10 mg/325 mg 2 every 3 hours without adequate relief. Because of the frequent requests for refills, the oncology team is concerned about misuse of the drug. The palliative care team conducts a thorough pain assessment and screens for risk for opioid misuse. Except for his young age, he has no other risk factors. Due to concerns regarding acetaminophen intake, they convert his current opioids to morphine extended release 60 mg every 12 hours with immediate-release morphine 15 mg every 3 hours as needed. He is educated about safe use and storage of the medication. This regimen provides some relief; after a few days of sedation, this dissipates and he reports feeling clear. A bowel program is started using senna/docusate twice daily with regular movements.

Unfortunately, response to chemotherapy was minimal, and an amputation above the knee was performed. He describes resolving incisional pain but is experiencing distressing phantom limb sensations and difficulty sleeping. He is not scheduled for fitting of a prosthetic device until the sutures are removed; this will likely assist in reducing uncomfortable phantom sensations. For now, the team orders an older tricyclic antidepressant, nortriptyline, to be taken at night; this has been shown to reduce neuropathic sensations and enhance sedation. After a few weeks, he does well in rehabilitation, adapting to the prosthetic device, resuming college classes, and socializing with friends. The opioids and antidepressant are gradually weaned.

Within six months he notes swelling and redness at the stump; he is found to have local recurrence as well as lung nodules. Despite aggressive therapy, the disease advances. John and his family had resisted hospice involvement, hoping for a cure, but now agree the focus should be on comfort. Pain has returned, along with anxiety and sleep disorders. Pharmacological therapies, including sustained-release and immediate-release morphine and dexamethasone, are prescribed. Gabapentin is added for neuropathic pain in the leg. When he ran out of morphine earlier than expected, review of his medication intake reveals significantly increased use of immediate-release morphine at night; he admits that he wakes often and cannot fall asleep, as his mind is racing. Taking more morphine helped him fall back asleep at first but is no longer effective. Clonazepam is added at night and in reduced doses during the daytime to address anxiety. Supportive services, including social work and chaplain visits, are increased.

Many friends and family come to visit. After one busy day, John's mother realizes a bottle of immediate-release morphine is missing; this is confirmed with the hospice nurse who has kept track of his medications to ensure that he has an adequate supply. After discussion with John to determine that he has not taken additional doses, they realize that the morphine was likely stolen and that the medications have not been adequately stored. A new plan, including a locked box, is implemented.

As John declines, he becomes more sedated and unable to take oral medications. He was taking morphine ER 60 mg every 12 hours or 120 mg/24 hours. This is reduced by approximately 20% to account for incomplete cross-tolerance. A fentanyl patch 50 mcg/hour is started (this is approximately equal to oral morphine 100 mg/24 hours). High concentration liquid morphine 20 mg/mL is started at 15 mg (7.5 mL); he may have this every hour as needed. The hospice team communicates with his football coach, who brings a jersey signed by all the team members. John dies peacefully a few days later surrounded by family and friends.

John's case illustrates several important points about pain management in palliative care, particularly highlighting the need for assessment as the patient's condition changes over time.

Other Key Concepts

- Evaluate acetaminophen intake when using combination products; this can be exacerbated by use of OTC agents.

- Neuropathic pain requires multimodal therapy, including adjuvant analgesics.

- Use of alternate routes of drug delivery is common at end of life; use equianalgesic principles when converting from one opioid to another or from one route to another.

- Frequent requests for refills do not always indicate issues related to misuse; inadequate numbers of pills may be ordered and at times, pharmacies may partially fill a prescription due to drug shortages. Further investigation is warranted. Screening for risk

factors associated with substance abuse is crucial for all patients so these issues can be adequately addressed.

- Patients and caregivers need to understand that opioids are not to be used to treat sleep, anxiety, or mood disorders. Although use of opioids may initially be sedating, tolerance will develop and high doses will be needed to obtain the original effect. Careful assessment is needed and appropriate pharmacological and nonpharmacological therapies of these comorbid conditions (sleep, anxiety, and sadness/depression) are necessary.

- Safe storage principles of controlled substances should be taught and implemented in the home.

Conclusion

Pain control in the palliative care setting is feasible in the majority of patients. Understanding the barriers that limit relief will lead to improved education and other strategies to address these obstacles. Ongoing, skilled assessment captures changes in pain and other symptoms as the patient's condition evolves. Developing comfort and skill with the use of pharmacological and nonpharmacological therapies will enhance pain relief. Together, these efforts will reduce suffering, relieve pain, and enhance the quality of life of those at the end of life.

References

1. Breivik H, Cherny N, Collett B, et al. Cancer-related pain: a pan-European survey of prevalence, treatment, and patient attitudes. Ann Oncol. 2009;20(8):1420–1433.

2. Institute of Medicine. Relieving Pain in America: A Blueprint for Transforming Prevention, Care, Education, and Research. Washington, DC, The National Academies Press, 2011.

3. Bennett MI, Rayment C, Hjermstad M, Aass N, Caraceni A, Kaasa S. Prevalence and aetiology of neuropathic pain in cancer patients: a systematic review. Pain. 2012;153(2):359–365.

4. Salminen E, Clemens KE, Syrjanen K, Salmenoja H. Needs of developing the skills of palliative care at the oncology ward. an audit of symptoms among 203 consecutive cancer patients in Finland. Support Care Cancer. 2008;16(1):3–8.

5. Valeberg BT, Rustoen T, Bjordal K, Hanestad BR, Paul S, Miaskowski C. Self-reported prevalence, etiology, and characteristics of pain in oncology outpatients. Eur J Pain. 2008;12(5):582–590.

6. Deandrea S, Montanari M, Moja L, Apolone G. Prevalence of undertreatment in cancer pain. A review of published literature. Ann Oncol. 2008;19(12):1985–1991.

7. Fisch MJ, Lee JW, Weiss M, et al. Prospective, observational study of pain and analgesic prescribing in medical oncology outpatients with breast, colorectal, lung, or prostate cancer. J Clin Oncol. 2012;30(16):1980–1988.

8. Coyle N, Adelhardt J, Foley KM, Portenoy RK. Character of terminal illness in the advanced cancer patient: pain and other symptoms during the last four weeks of life. J Pain Symptom Manage. 1990;5(2):83–93.

9. Morita T, Sakaguchi Y, Hirai K, Tsuneto S, Shima Y. Desire for death and requests to hasten death of Japanese terminally ill cancer patients receiving specialized inpatient palliative care. J Pain Symptom Manage. 2004;27(1):44–52.

10. Kwon JH. Overcoming barriers in cancer pain management. J Clin Oncol. 2014;32(16):1727–1733.

11. Paice J, Von Roenn J. Under- or overtreatment of cancer pain: How to achieve proper balance. J Clin Oncol. 2014;32(16):1721–1726.

12. Breuer B, Fleishman SB, Cruciani RA, Portenoy RK. Medical oncologists' attitudes and practice in cancer pain management: a national survey. J Clin Oncol. 2011;29(36):4769–4775.

13. American Pain Society. Principles of Analgesic Use in the Treatment of Acute Pain and Cancer Pain. 6th ed. Glenview: American Pain Society; 2008.

14. Morrison RS, Wallenstein S, Natale DK, Senzel RS, Huang LL. "We don't carry that"—failure of pharmacies in predominantly nonwhite neighborhoods to stock opioid analgesics. N Engl J Med. 2000;342(14):1023–1026.

15. Pargeon KL, Hailey BJ. Barriers to effective cancer pain management: a review of the literature. J Pain Symptom Manage. 1999;18(5):358–368.

16. Thomas ML, Elliott JE, Rao SM, Fahey KF, Paul SM, Miaskowski C. A randomized, clinical trial of education or motivational-interviewing -based coaching compared to usual care to improve cancer pain management. Oncol Nurs Forum. 2012;39(1);39–49.

17. Kim HS, Shin SJ, Kim SC, An S, Rha SY, et al. Randomized controlled trial of standardized education and telemonitoring for pain in outpatients with advanced solid tumors. Support Care Cancer. 2013:21(6):1751–1759.

18. Bennett MI, Bagnall AM, Jose Closs, S. How effective are patient-based educational interventions in the management of cancer pain? Systematic review and meta-analysis. Pain 2009:143(3);192–199.

19. Torrance N, Elliott AM, Lee AJ, Smith BH. Severe chronic pain is associated with increased 10 year mortality: a cohort record linkage study. Eur J Pain. 2010;14(4):380–386.

20. Halabi S, Vogelzang NJ, Kornblith AB, et al. Pain predicts overall survival in men with metastatic castration-refractory prostate cancer. J Clin Oncol. 2008;26(15):2544–2549.

21. Paice JA, Ferrell B. The management of cancer pain. CA Cancer J Clin. 2011;61(3):157–182.

22. Chun LJ, Tong MJ, Busuttil RW, Hiatt JR. Acetaminophen hepatotoxicity and acute liver failure. J Clin Gastroenterol. 2009;43(4):342–349.

23. Ych YC, Reddy P. Clinical and economic evidence for intravenous acetaminophen. Pharmacotherapy. 2012;32(6):559–579.

24. Takeuchi K. Pathogenesis of NSAID-induced gastric damage: importance of cyclooxygenase inhibition and gastric hypermotility. World J Gastroenterol. 2012;18(18):2147–2160.

25. Cryer B, Li C, Simon LS, Singh G, Stillman MJ, Berger MF. GI-REASONS: a novel 6-month, prospective, randomized, open-label, blinded endpoint (PROBE) trial. Am J Gastroenterol. 2013;108(3):392–400.

26. Nabal M, Librada S, Redondo MJ, Pigni A, Brunelli C, Caraceni A. The role of paracetamol and nonsteroidal anti-inflammatory drugs in addition to WHO Step III opioids in the control of pain in advanced cancer: a systematic review of the literature. Palliat Med. 2012;26(4):305–312.

27. Fosbol EL, Folke F, Jacobsen S, et al. Cause-specific cardiovascular risk associated with nonsteroidal antiinflammatory drugs among healthy individuals. Circ Cardiovasc Qual Outcomes. 2010;3(4):395–405.

28. McGettigan P, Henry D. Cardiovascular risk with non-steroidal anti-inflammatory drugs: systematic review of population-based controlled observational studies. PLoS Med. 2011;8(9):e1001098.

29. Rayment C, Hjermstad MJ, Aass N, et al. Neuropathic cancer pain: prevalence, severity, analgesics and impact from the European Palliative Care Research Collaborative-Computerised Symptom Assessment study. Palliat Med. 2013;27(8):714–721.

30. Caraceni A, Hanks G, Kaasa S, et al. Use of opioid analgesics in the treatment of cancer pain: evidence-based recommendations from the EAPC. Lancet Oncol. 2012;13(2):e58–e68.

31. Sykes N, Thorns A. The use of opioids and sedatives at the end of life. Lancet Oncol. 2003;4(5):312–318.

32. Sykes N, Thorns A. Sedative use in the last week of life and the implications for end-of-life decision making. Arch Intern Med. 2003;163(3):341–344.

33. Azoulay D, Jacobs JM, Cialic R, Mor EE, Stessman J. Opioids, survival, and advanced cancer in the hospice setting. J Am Med Dir Assoc. 2011;12(2):129–134.

34. Clemens KE, Quednau I, Klaschik E. Is there a higher risk of respiratory depression in opioid-naive palliative care patients during symptomatic therapy of dyspnea with strong opioids? J Palliat Med. 2008;11(2):204–216.

35. Paramanandam G, Prommer E, Schwenke DC. Adverse effects in hospice patients with chronic kidney disease receiving hydromorphone. J Palliat Med. 2011;14(9):1029–1033.

36. King S, Forbes K, Hanks GW, Ferro CJ, Chambers EJ. A systematic review of the use of opioid medication for those with moderate to severe cancer pain and renal impairment: a European Palliative Care Research Collaborative opioid guidelines project. Palliat Med. 2011;25(5):525–552.

37. McCann S, Yaksh TL, von Gunten CF. Correlation between myoclonus and the 3-glucuronide metabolites in patients treated with morphine or hydromorphone: a pilot study. J Opioid Manag. 2010;6(2):87–94.

38. Paice JA, Von Roenn JH, Hudgins JC, Luong L, Krejcie TC, Avram MJ. Morphine bioavailability from a topical gel formulation in volunteers. J Pain Symptom Manage. 2008;35(3):314–320.

39. Ripamonti CI. Pain management. Ann Oncol. 2012;23(Suppl 10):x294–x301.

40. Prodduturi S, Sadrieh N, Wokovich AM, Doub WH, Westenberger BJ, Buhse L. Transdermal delivery of fentanyl from matrix and reservoir systems: effect of heat and compromised skin. J Pharm Sci. 2010;99(5):2357–2366.

41. Mercadante S, Porzio G, Ferrera P, Aielli F, Adile C, Ficorella C. Low doses of transdermal fentanyl in opioid-naive patients with cancer pain. Curr Med Res Opin. 2010;26(12):2765–2768.

42. Van Nimmen NF, Poels KL, Menten JJ, Godderis L, Veulemans HA. Fentanyl transdermal absorption linked to pharmacokinetic characteristics in patients undergoing palliative care. J Clin Pharmacol. 2010;50(6):667–678.

43. Kokubun H, Ebinuma K, Matoba M, Takayanagi R, Yamada Y, Yago K. Population pharmacokinetics of transdermal fentanyl in patients with cancer-related pain. J Pain Palliat Care Pharmacother. 2012;26(2):98–104.

44. Heiskanen T, Matzke S, Haakana S, Gergov M, Vuori E, Kalso E. Transdermal fentanyl in cachectic cancer patients. Pain. 2009;144(1–2):218–222.

45. Tassinari D, Sartori S, Tamburini E, et al. Transdermal fentanyl as a front-line approach to moderate-severe pain: a meta-analysis of randomized clinical trials. J Palliat Care. 2009;25(3):172–180.

46. Koo HC, Moon JH, Choi HJ, et al. Effect of transdermal fentanyl patches on the motility of the sphincter of oddi. Gut Liver. 2010;4(3):368–372.

47. Davis MP. Fentanyl for breakthrough pain: a systematic review. Expert Rev Neurother. 2011;11(8):1197–1216.

48. Darwish M, Kirby M, Robertson P, Jr., Tracewell W, Jiang JG. Absolute and relative bioavailability of fentanyl buccal tablet and oral transmucosal fentanyl citrate. J Clin Pharmacol. 2007;47(3):343–350.

49. Rauck R, North J, Gever LN, Tagarro I, Finn AL. Fentanyl buccal soluble film (FBSF) for breakthrough pain in patients with cancer: a randomized, double-blind, placebo-controlled study. Ann Oncol. 2010;21(6):1308–1314.

50. Portenoy RK, Burton AW, Gabrail N, Taylor D, Fentanyl Pectin Nasal Spray 043 Study G. A multicenter, placebo-controlled, double-blind, multiple-crossover study of Fentanyl Pectin Nasal Spray (FPNS) in the treatment of breakthrough cancer pain. Pain. 2010;151(3):617–624.

51. Mercadante S, Tirelli W, David F, et al. Morphine versus oxycodone in pancreatic cancer pain: a randomized controlled study. Clin J Pain. 2010;26(9):794–797.

52. Andreassen TN, Klepstad P, Davies A, et al. Influences on the pharmacokinetics of oxycodone: a multicentre cross-sectional study in 439 adult cancer patients. Eur J Clin Pharmacol. 2011;67(5):493–506.

53. Nieminen TH, Hagelberg NM, Saari TI, et al. Oxycodone concentrations are greatly increased by the concomitant use of ritonavir or lopinavir/ritonavir. Eur J Clin Pharmacol. 2010;66(10):977–985.

54. Nieminen TH, Hagelberg NM, Saari TI, et al. Grapefruit juice enhances the exposure to oral oxycodone. Basic Clin Pharmacol Toxicol. 2010;107(4):782–788.

55. Hagelberg NM, Nieminen TH, Saari TI, et al. Voriconazole drastically increases exposure to oral oxycodone. Eur J Clin Pharmacol. 2009;65(3):263–271.

56. Hagen NA, Moulin DE, Brasher PM, et al. A formal feasibility study of sublingual methadone for breakthrough cancer pain. Palliat Med. 2010;24(7):696–706.

57. Mercadante S, Caraceni A. Conversion ratios for opioid switching in the treatment of cancer pain: a systematic review. Palliat Med. 2011;25(5):504–515.

58. Chatham MS, Dodds Ashley ES, Svengsouk JS, Juba KM. Dose ratios between high dose oral morphine or equivalents and oral methadone. J Palliat Med. 2013;16(8):947–950.

59. Chou R, Fanciullo GJ, Fine PG, et al. Clinical guidelines for the use of chronic opioid therapy in chronic noncancer pain. J Pain. 2009;10(2):113–130.

60. Ito S, Liao S. Myoclonus associated with high-dose parenteral methadone. J Palliat Med. 2008;11(6):838–841.

61. Krantz MJ, Martin J, Stimmel B, Mehta D, Haigney MC. QTc interval screening in methadone treatment. Ann Intern Med. 2009;150(6):387–395.

62. Kapur BM, Hutson JR, Chibber T, Luk A, Selby P. Methadone: a review of drug-drug and pathophysiological interactions. Crit Review Clin Lab Sci. 2011;48(4):171–195.

63. Wallace M, Moulin DE, Rauck RL, et al. Long-term safety, tolerability, and efficacy of OROS hydromorphone in patients with chronic pain. J Opioid Manag. 2009;5(2):97–105.

64. Pigni A, Brunelli C, Caraceni A. The role of hydromorphone in cancer pain treatment: a systematic review. Palliat Med. 2011;25(5):471–477.

65. Oldenmenger WH, Lieverse PJ, Janssen PJ, Taal W, van der Rijt CC, Jager A. Efficacy of opioid rotation to continuous parenteral hydromorphone in advanced cancer patients failing on other opioids. Support Care Cancer. 2012;20(8):1639–1647.

66. Davison SN, Mayo PR. Pain management in chronic kidney disease: the pharmacokinetics and pharmacodynamics of hydromorphone and hydromorphone-3-glucuronide in hemodialysis patients. J Opioid Manag. 2008;4(6):335–336, 339–344.

67. Mayyas F, Fayers P, Kaasa S, Dale O. A systematic review of oxymorphone in the management of chronic pain. J Pain Symptom Manage. 2010;39(2):296–308.

68. Schoedel KA, McMorn S, Chakraborty B, Zerbe K, Sellers EM. Reduced cognitive and psychomotor impairment with extended-release oxymorphone versus controlled-release oxycodone. Pain Physician. 2010;13(6):561–573.

69. Al-Tawil N, Odar-Cederlof I, Berggren AC, Johnson HE, Persson J. Pharmacokinetics of transdermal buprenorphine patch in the elderly. Eur J Clin Pharmacol. 2013;69(2):143–149.

70. Prommer E. Role of codeine in palliative care. J Opioid Manag. 2011;7(5):401–406.

71. Racoosin JA, Roberson DW, Pacanowski MA, Nielsen DR. New evidence about an old drug: risk with codeine after adenotonsillectomy. N Engl J Med. 2013;368(23):2155–2157.

72. McNulty JP. Chronic pain: levorphanol, methadone, and the N-methyl-D-aspartate receptor. J Palliat Med. 2009;12(9):765–766.

73. Tassinari D, Drudi F, Rosati M, Tombesi P, Sartori S, Maltoni M. The second step of the analgesic ladder and oral tramadol in the treatment of mild to moderate cancer pain: a systematic review. Palliat Med. 2011;25(5):410–423.

74. Schwittay A, Schumann C, Litzenburger BC, Schwenke K. Tapentadol prolonged release for severe chronic pain: results of a noninterventional study involving general practitioners and internists. J Pain Palliat Care Pharmacother. 2013;9:225–234.

75. Smith TJ, Staats PS, Deer T, et al. Randomized clinical trial of an implantable drug delivery system compared with comprehensive medical management for refractory cancer pain: impact on pain, drug-related toxicity, and survival. J Clin Oncol. 2002;20(19):4040–4049.

76. Twycross R, Sykes N, Mihalyo M, Wilcock A. Stimulant laxatives and opioid-induced constipation. J Pain Symptom Manage. 2012;43(2):306–313.

77. Hawley PH, Byeon JJ. A comparison of sennosides-based bowel protocols with and without docusate in hospitalized patients with cancer. J Palliat Med. 2008;11(4):575–581.

78. Portenoy RK, Thomas J, Moehl Boatwright ML, et al. Subcutaneous methylnaltrexone for the treatment of opioid-induced constipation in patients with advanced illness: a double-blind, randomized, parallel group, dose-ranging study. J Pain Symptom Manage. 2008;35(5):458–468.

79. Thomas J, Karver S, Cooney GA, et al. Methylnaltrexone for opioid-induced constipation in advanced illness. N Engl J Med. 2008;358(22):2332–2343.

80. Gras-Miralles B, Cremonini F. A critical appraisal of lubiprostone in the treatment of chronic constipation in the elderly. Clin Interv Aging. 2013;8:191–200.

81. Webster LR, Choi Y, Desai H, Webster L, Grant BJ. Sleep-disordered breathing and chronic opioid therapy. Pain Med. 2008;9(4):425–432.

82. Smith HS, Smith JM, Seidner P. Opioid-induced nausea and vomiting. Ann Palliat Med. 2012;1(2):121–129.

83. Seccareccia D, Gebara N. Pruritus in palliative care: getting up to scratch. Can Fam Physician. 2011;57(9):1010–1013.

84. Saarto T, Wiffen PJ. Antidepressants for neuropathic pain: a Cochrane review. J Neurol, Neurosurg, Psychiatry. 2010;81(12):1372–1373.

85. Kautio AL, Haanpaa M, Saarto T, et al. Amitriptyline in the treatment of chemotherapy-induced neuropathic symptoms. J Pain Symptom Manage. 2008;35(1):31–39.

86. Smith EM, Pang H, Cirrincione C, et al. Effect of duloxetine on pain, function, and quality of life among patients with chemotherapy-induced painful peripheral neuropathy: a randomized clinical trial. JAMA. 2013;309(13):1359–1367.

87. Xiao W, Naso L, Bennett GJ, Xiao W, Naso L, Bennett GJ. Experimental studies of potential analgesics for the treatment of chemotherapy-evoked painful peripheral neuropathies. Pain Med. 2008;9(5):505–517.

88. Baron R, Brunnmuller U, Brasser M, May M, Binder A. Efficacy and safety of pregabalin in patients with diabetic peripheral neuropathy or postherpetic neuralgia: open-label, non-comparative, flexible-dose study. Eur J Pain. 2008;12(7):850–858.

89. Mishra S, Bhatnagar S, Goyal GN, Rana SP, Upadhya SP. A comparative efficacy of amitriptyline, gabapentin, and pregabalin in neuropathic cancer pain: a prospective randomized double-blind placebo-controlled study. Am J Hosp Palliat Care. 2012;29(3):177–182.

90. Goodyear-Smith F, Halliwell J. Anticonvulsants for neuropathic pain: gaps in the evidence. Clin J Pain. 2009;25(6):528–536.

91. Gomez-Hernandez J, Orozco-Alatorre AL, Dominguez-Contreras M, et al. Preoperative dexamethasone reduces postoperative pain, nausea and vomiting following mastectomy for breast cancer. BMC Cancer. 2010;10:692.

92. Paulsen O, Aass N, Kaasa S, Dale O. Do corticosteroids provide analgesic effects in cancer patients? A systematic literature review. J Pain Symptom Manage 2013;46(1):96–105.

93. Yennurajalingam S, Frisbee-Hume S, Palmer JL, et al. Reduction of cancer-related fatigue with dexamethasone: a double-blind, randomized, placebo-controlled trial in patients with advanced cancer. J Clin Oncol. 2013;31(25):3076–3082.

94. Lundborg C, Dahm P, Nitescu P, Biber B. High intrathecal bupivacaine for severe pain in the head and neck. Acta Anaesthesiol Scand. 2009;53(7):908–913.

95. Campbell-Fleming JM, Williams A. The use of ketamine as adjuvant therapy to control severe pain. Clin J Oncol Nurs. 2008;12(1):102–107.

96. Bell R, Eccleston C, Kalso E. Ketamine as an adjuvant to opioids for cancer pain. Cochrane Database Syst Rev. 2003(1):CD003351.

97. Bell RF, Eccleston C, Kalso EA. Ketamine as an adjuvant to opioids for cancer pain. Cochrane Database Syst Rev. 2012;11:CD003351.

98. Bredlau AL, Thakur R, Korones DN, Dworkin RH. Ketamine for pain in adults and children with cancer: a systematic review and synthesis of the literature. Pain Med. 2013;14(10)1505–1517.

99. Okamoto Y, Tsuneto S, Tanimukai H, et al. Can gradual dose titration of ketamine for management of neuropathic pain prevent psychotomimetic effects in patients with advanced cancer? Am J Hosp Palliat Care. 2013;30(5):450–454.

100. Uzaraga I, Gerbis B, Holwerda E, Gillis D, Wai E. Topical amitriptyline, ketamine, and lidocaine in neuropathic pain caused by radiation skin reaction: a pilot study. Support Care Cancer. 2012;20(7):1515–1524.

101. Hardy J, Quinn S, Fazekas B, et al. Randomized, double-blind, placebo-controlled study to assess the efficacy and toxicity of subcutaneous ketamine in the management of cancer pain. J Clin Oncol. 2012;30(29):3611–3617.

102. Barton DL, Wos EJ, Qin R, et al. A double-blind, placebo-controlled trial of a topical treatment for chemotherapy-induced peripheral neuropathy: NCCTG trial N06CA. Support Care Cancer. 2011;19(6):833–841.

103. Lopez-Olivo MA, Shah NA, Pratt G, Risser JM, Symanski E, Suarez-Almazor ME. Bisphosphonates in the treatment of patients with lung cancer and metastatic bone disease: a systematic review and meta-analysis. Support Care Cancer. 2012;20(11):2985–2998.

104. Clemons M, Dranitsaris G, Ooi W, Cole DE. A Phase II trial evaluating the palliative benefit of second-line oral ibandronate in breast cancer patients with either a skeletal related event (SRE) or progressive bone metastases (BM) despite standard bisphosphonate (BP) therapy. Breast Cancer Res Treat. 2008;108(1):79–85.

105. Scott LJ, Muir VJ. Denosumab: in the prevention of skeletal-related events in patients with bone metastases from solid tumours. Drugs. 2011;71(8):1059–1069.

106. Ogawa K, Washiyama K. Bone target radiotracers for palliative therapy of bone metastases. Curr Med Chem. 2012;19(20):3290–3300.

107. Weeks JC, Catalano PJ, Cronin A, et al. Patients' expectations about effects of chemotherapy for advanced cancer. N Engl J Med. 2012;367(17):1616–1625.

108. Derry S, Moore RA. Topical capsaicin (low concentration) for chronic neuropathic pain in adults. Cochrane Database Syst Rev. 2012;9:CD010111.

109. Derry S, Sven-Rice A, Cole P, Tan T, Moore RA. Topical capsaicin (high concentration) for chronic neuropathic pain in adults. Cochrane Database Syst Rev. 2013;2:CD007393.

110. Simpson DM, Brown S, Tobias J, Group N-CS. Controlled trial of high-concentration capsaicin patch for treatment of painful HIV neuropathy. Neurology. 2008;70(24):2305–2313.

111. Khasabova IA, Khasabov S, Paz J, Harding-Rose C, Simone DA, Seybold VS. Cannabinoid type-1 receptor reduces pain and neurotoxicity produced by chemotherapy. J Neurosci. 2012;32(20):7091–7101.

112. Rahn EJ, Zvonok AM, Thakur GA, Khanolkar AD, Makriyannis A, Hohmann AG. Selective activation of cannabinoid CB2 receptors suppresses neuropathic nociception induced by treatment with the chemotherapeutic agent paclitaxel in rats. J Pharmacol Exp Ther. 2008;327(2):584–591.

113. Portenoy RK, Ganae-Motan ED, Allende S, et al. Nabiximols for opioid-treated cancer patients with poorly-controlled chronic pain: a randomized, placebo-controlled, graded-dose trial. J Pain. 2012;13(5):438–449.

114. Ashton JC, Milligan ED. Cannabinoids for the treatment of neuropathic pain: clinical evidence. Curr Opin Invest Drugs. 2008;9(1):65–75.

115. Wang T, Collet JP, Shapiro S, Ware MA. Adverse effects of medical cannabinoids: a systematic review. CMAJ: Can Med Assoc J. 2008;178(13):1669–1678.

116. Bostwick JM, Reisfield GM, DuPont RL. Clinical decisions: medicinal use of marijuana. N Engl J Med. 2013;368(9):866–868.

117. Yomiya K, Matsuo N, Tomiyasu S, et al. Baclofen as an adjuvant analgesic for cancer pain. Am J Hosp Palliat Care. 2009;26(2):112–118.

118. McClelland S, 3rd, Bethoux FA, Boulis NM, et al. Intrathecal baclofen for spasticity-related pain in amyotrophic lateral sclerosis: efficacy and factors associated with pain relief. Muscle Nerve. 2008;37(3):396–398.

119. Roberts SB, Wozencraft CP, Coyne PJ, Smith TJ. Dexmedetomidine as an adjuvant analgesic for intractable cancer pain. J Palliat Med. 2011;14(3):371–373.

120. Mendoza TR, Koyyalagunta D, Burton AW, et al. Changes in pain and other symptoms in patients with painful multiple myeloma-related vertebral fracture treated with kyphoplasty or vertebroplasty. J Pain. 2012;13(6):564–570.

121. Bain E, Hugel H, Sharma M. Percutaneous cervical cordotomy for the management of pain from cancer: a prospective review of 45 cases. J Palliat Med. 2013;16(8):901–907.

122. Stubblefield MD, Levine A, Custodio CM, Fitzpatrick T. The role of botulinum toxin type A in the radiation fibrosis syndrome: a preliminary report. Arch Phys Med Rehabil. 2008;89(3):417–421.

123. Kwekkeboom KL, Abbott-Anderson K, Wanta B. Feasibility of a patient-controlled cognitive-behavioral intervention for pain, fatigue, and sleep disturbance in cancer. Oncol Nurs Forum. 2010;37(3):E151–E159.

124. Kwekkeboom KL, Cherwin CH, Lee JW, Wanta B. Mind-body treatments for the pain-fatigue-sleep disturbance symptom cluster in persons with cancer. J Pain Symptom Manage. 2010;39(1):126–138.

125. Collinge W, MacDonald G, Walton T. Massage in supportive cancer care. Semin Oncol Nurs. 2012;28(1):45–54.

126. Toth M, Marcantonio ER, Davis RB, Walton T, Kahn JR, Phillips RS. Massage therapy for patients with metastatic cancer: a pilot randomized controlled trial. J Altern Complement Med. 2013;19(7):650–656.

127. Greer JA, Traeger L, Bemis H, et al. A pilot randomized controlled trial of brief cognitive-behavioral therapy for anxiety in patients with terminal cancer. Oncologist. 2012;17(10):1337–1345.

128. Woodward SC. Cognitive-behavioral therapy for insomnia in patients with cancer. Clin J Oncol Nurs. 2011;15(4):E42–E52.

129. Balboni MJ, Babar A, Dillinger J, et al. "It depends": viewpoints of patients, physicians, and nurses on patient-practitioner prayer in the setting of advanced cancer. J Pain Symptom Manage. 2011;41(5):836–847.

130. Sharp DM, Walker MB, Chaturvedi A, et al. A randomised, controlled trial of the psychological effects of reflexology in early breast cancer. Eur J Cancer. 2010;46(2):312–322.

131. Alcantara J, Alcantara JD, Alcantara J. The chiropractic care of patients with cancer: a systematic review of the literature. Integr Cancer Ther. 2012;11(4):304–312.

132. Cronfalk BS, Ternestedt BM, Strang P. Soft tissue massage: early intervention for relatives whose family members died in palliative cancer care. J Clin Nurs. 2010;19(7–8):1040–1048.

133. Zeppetella G. Opioids for cancer breakthrough pain: a pilot study reporting patient assessment of time to meaningful pain relief. J Pain Symptom Manage. 2008;35(5):563–567.

134. Laird BJ, Walley J, Murray GD, Clausen E, Colvin LA, Fallon MT. Characterization of cancer-induced bone pain: an exploratory study. Support Care Cancer. 2011;19(9):1393–1401.

135. Bloom AP, Jimenez-Andrade JM, Taylor RN, et al. Breast cancer-induced bone remodeling, skeletal pain, and sprouting of sensory nerve fibers. J Pain. 2011;12(7):698–711.

136. Caraceni A, Zecca E, Martini C, et al. Palliative sedation at the end of life at a tertiary cancer center. Support Care Cancer. 2012;20(6):1299–1307.

137. Mercadante S, Porzio G, Valle A, et al. Palliative sedation in advanced cancer patients followed at home: a retrospective analysis. J Pain Symptom Manage. 2012;43(6):1126–1130.

138. Dean MM, Cellarius V, Henry B, Oneschuk D, Librach Canadian Society Of Palliative Care Physicians Taskforce SL. Framework for continuous palliative sedation therapy in Canada. J Palliat Med. 2012;15(8):870–879.

139. Maltoni M, Scarpi E, Rosati M, et al. Palliative sedation in end-of-life care and survival: a systematic review. J Clin Oncol. 2012;30(12):1378–1383.

140. Kwon JH, Hui D, Chisholm G, Bruera E. Predictors of long-term opioid treatment among patients who receive chemoradiation for head and neck cancer. Oncologist. 2013;18(6):768–774.

141. Perney P, Duny Y, Nalpas B, et al. Feasibility and efficacy of an addiction treatment program in patients with upper aerodigestive tract cancer. Subst Use Misuse. 2013 Aug 6. Epub ahead of print.

142. Francoeur RB. Ensuring safe access to medication for palliative care while preventing prescription drug abuse: innovations for American inner cities, rural areas, and communities overwhelmed by addiction. Risk Manag Healthc Policy. 2011;4:97–105.

143. Kircher S, Zacny J, Apfelbaum SM, et al. Understanding and treating opioid addiction in a patient with cancer pain. J Pain. 2011;12(10):1025–1031.

144. Blackhall LJ, Alfson ED, Barclay JS. Screening for substance abuse and diversion in Virginia hospices. J Palliat Med. 2013;16(3):237–242.

145. Dev R, Parsons HA, Palla S, Palmer JL, Del Fabbro E, Bruera E. Undocumented alcoholism and its correlation with tobacco and illegal drug use in advanced cancer patients. Cancer. 2011;117(19):4551–4556.

146. Sullivan MD, Edlund MJ, Fan MY, Devries A, Brennan Braden J, Martin BC. Risks for possible and probable opioid misuse among recipients of chronic opioid therapy in commercial and medicaid insurance plans: the TROUP Study. Pain. 2010;150(2):332–339.

147. Sullivan MD, Von Korff M, Banta-Green C, Merrill JO, Saunders K. Problems and concerns of patients receiving chronic opioid therapy for chronic non-cancer pain. Pain. 2010;149(2):345–353.

148. Merrill JO, Von Korff M, Banta-Green CJ, et al. Prescribed opioid difficulties, depression and opioid dose among chronic opioid therapy patients. Gen Hosp Psychiatry. 2012;34(6):581–587.

149. Dunn KM, Saunders KW, Rutter CM, et al. Opioid prescriptions for chronic pain and overdose: a cohort study. Ann Intern Med. 2010;152(2):85–92.

150. Edlund MJ, Martin BC, Devries A, Fan MY, Braden JB, Sullivan MD. Trends in use of opioids for chronic noncancer pain among individuals with mental health and substance use disorders: the TROUP study. Clin J Pain. 2010;26(1):1–8.

151. Daniell HW. Opioid endocrinopathy in women consuming prescribed sustained-action opioids for control of nonmalignant pain. J Pain. 2008;9(1):28–36.

152. Saunders KW, Dunn KM, Merrill JO, et al. Relationship of opioid use and dosage levels to fractures in older chronic pain patients. J Gen Intern Med. 2010;25(4):310–315.

153. Okie S. A flood of opioids, a rising tide of deaths. N Engl J Med. 2010;363(21):1981–1985.

CHAPTER 8

Fatigue

Edith O'Neil-Page, Paula R. Anderson, and Grace E. Dean

This is so hard. I never knew it could be like this. I have no energy. I'm not sure I can do this anymore; a part of me just wants it to be over.

Shared by a patient with prostate cancer

Key points

- Fatigue is the most common chronic symptom associated with cancer and other chronic progressive diseases.

- Ongoing research has provided lines of evidence for improved patient outcomes through both pharmacological and nonpharmacological measures.

- Thorough assessment of all patient comorbidities and symptoms is critical to accurately diagnose and treat disease-related fatigue.

- Education interventions in fatigue directed at healthcare providers, patients, and families provide an important opportunity for consistent integration of current guidelines into practice.

Chronically ill patients often do not have the energy or forethought to communicate to healthcare professionals about what may be viewed as a nonurgent symptom. They find it difficult to convey just how exhausted they feel. Fatigue is a devastating, multidimensional symptom that involves the entire person, touching every facet of daily life. It can progressively interfere with a patient's physical and social activities resulting in increased withdrawal. Fatigue is a symptom that possibly has the greatest potential to interfere with quality of life at the end of life.[1]

Definitions of fatigue

Do you have any idea how much energy it takes to breathe? That's what I want to say, when anyone asks me a question. I can't explain it; there is not enough energy to breathe. I don't have the energy. I can't look at them or speak, I can't tell them how exhausted I am. I know they want me to fight, but I can't. And, in not fighting I am failing them, again.

A patient with end-stage
chronic obstructive pulmonary disease

Fatigue is a complex phenomenon, studied by many disciplines, yet has no widely accepted definition.[2] The discipline of nursing is no exception in addressing the definition of fatigue. Within the different specialties of nursing there has been little agreement on a definition of fatigue.

Cancer-related fatigue (CRF) is "primarily a subjective, complex whole body experience"[1] and described as a lack of energy or exhaustion that interferes with normal activities and function. Fatigue is commonly associated with cancer but is not a stranger to other chronic and accelerating disease processes such as chronic obstructive pulmonary disease (COPD), irreversible cardiomyopathies, chronic renal failure (CRF), HIV/AIDS, and multiple sclerosis. The affect and or manifestation of fatigue may differ with diagnosis and treatment. In oncology, for example, patients perceive fatigue differently depending on when fatigue occurs in the disease trajectory. Often it is the recognition of fatigue symptoms that initiates diagnosis or disease discovery and medical treatment.[3] Once diagnosed, the cancer patient experiences fatigue as a side effect of treatment. And then fatigue presents across stages of disease process as a pervasive side effect of treatment and continues well into recovery. Descriptors range from a single focus of tiredness to the broad multifocal and overwhelming multidimensional syndrome.[4] In recovery, the level of energy that returns is commonly referred to as a "new normal" and becomes the reality.[1] Fatigue is often appreciated differently by those living the experience and may continue to be perceived differently throughout the course of disease or treatment. Fatigue is often identified by patients as experiential, with descriptors of how they feel as in "I feel as if I have been run over by a truck." Differentiation of the sensation of fatigue from "tiredness" or from the impact on daily life, relationships, and patients' ability to function is often very difficult for those experiencing the phenomena but also friends and family.[5] In cancer recurrence, fatigue becomes as much an enemy as the diagnosis and progression to advanced stages. Fatigue at the end of life is experienced as the end of a very long struggle, "a natural stage of the dying process and may protect against suffering."[1]

The National Comprehensive Cancer Network (NCCN) Fatigue Practice Guidelines Panel, charged with synthesizing research on fatigue to develop recommendations for care, defines fatigue as "a distressing, persistent, and subjective sense of physical, emotional, cognitive tiredness, or exhaustion related to cancer or cancer treatment, that is not proportional to recent activity and interferes with usual functioning."[6] The European Association for Palliative Care identified a working definition of fatigue as a "subjective feeling of tiredness, weakness or lack of energy."[7]

The American Cancer Society defines CRF as "feeling tired—physically, mentally, and emotionally and "having less energy to do the things you normally do or want to do."[8] This definition is similar to that of multiple sclerosis patients, who defined fatigue as one of the most frequent and most disabling symptoms—a subjective lack of physical and/or mental energy that interferes with usual and desired activities.[9] Sufferers of nonmalignant diseases such as stroke and end-stage heart failure define fatigue as being "physically tired and mentally exhausted," and perceive it as one of their worst symptoms, yet it receives little attention.[10,11] While other definitions have been proposed, the two key elements that are dominant in most definitions of fatigue are (1) a subjective perception with physical, emotional and cognitive features and (2) the interference with an ability to function.[4,5]

With children also, there is no agreed on definition of fatigue.[12] Descriptive studies of children's perceptions of fatigue are reported as a profound sense of being weak or tired and a complex changing state of exhaustion.[13] A group of adolescents with cancer expressed significantly more fatigue than their peers without chronic disease and reported more symptoms of depression associated with quality of life.[14] More recent studies of adolescents and young adults (AYAs) report significantly worse health-related quality of life (HRQOL) during treatment, with the greatest deficits in limitations to physical and emotional roles, physical and social functioning, and fatigue."[15] Several subgroups were identified in this study, which demonstrated increased vulnerability to fatigue than their counterparts.[16] Hispanic patients and those with less education or without insurance coverage appeared to be at higher risk for fatigue. Newer researchers are focusing on identifying and describing patterns or clusters of symptoms among children and adults to explore their relationships and interactions in order to more easily identify needs and assist in recovery.[13,17,18]

Prevalence

Sometimes I wonder who I am anymore; I wake up in the morning wanting to go to work. I want to be me; I want to be a wife and a mother again. I want my kitchen back, I want my house back, and I want my life back. And I can't! Not now not ever, will it be the same. It is all so different now.

A young mother with cervical cancer

Cancer-related fatigue is currently reported to be the most common symptom linked to the clinical course of cancer and other chronic diseases. Estimates of prevalence are anywhere between 50% and 90% depending on the diagnostic category, length of disease, course of treatment, complications, physical state, and a myriad of psychosocial factors.[19] Despite the significant prevalence of disabling and distressing symptoms, fatigue remains significantly under-diagnosed and undermanaged.[20] Fatigue has been indicated as the most prevalent disabling and continuous phenomenon in patients receiving various treatments for cancer.[21–23] CRF cuts across all diagnoses, ages, genders, stages of disease, and treatment modalities.[20,24] Both chemotherapy and radiation therapy result in fatigue; combined chemotherapy-radiation therapy continues to be underestimated and profoundly affects quality of life (QOL). Furthermore, "fatigue may persist for months or years" following curative treatment.[19,20]

Cancer is only one of many diseases in which fatigue is a common symptom. Prevalence rates for cancer related fatigue and other chronic diseases are identified in Box 8.1, including cardiac disease, COPD, renal disease, HIV/AIDS, and multiple sclerosis.

The prevalence of fatigue in people with HIV infection is reported as the most common complaint not associated with physiological factors. Fatigue prevalence rates for a variety of common chronic illnesses are identified in Box 8.1. Symptom prevalence in a diverse population of patients with cancer; HIV/AIDS; coronary, renal, or chronic obstructive pulmonary disease; and multiple sclerosis was reported in up to 99% of patients for all six diseases.[25–28] While symptoms rarely occur in isolation, there is growing evidence to support the occurrence of multiple symptom "clusters" along with the concept of "symptom burden."[18] The increase in symptom cluster research, particularly in the context

---

Box 8.1 Prevalence and populations at risk

Cancer

Prevalence rates of CRF vary depending on cancer type and stage, as well as the diagnostic criteria. One study indicated that over 80% of patients receiving radiotherapy experience fatigue, as did up to 90% of incurable cancer patients. Fatigue is also the most common and distressing symptom experienced by pediatric cancer patients. In some cancer survivors, fatigue persists months or even years after treatment.

Cardiac

Research suggests the widespread presence of fatigue in patients with chronic heart failure. One such study of these patients indicated that 99% of the sample reported fatigue.

COPD

Second only to breathlessness in its prevalence, fatigue is experienced by 96% of those with COPD.

Renal disease

In renal disease the prevalence of fatigue varies depending on the method of treatment employed. Of those treated by hemodialysis, 82% report fatigue, most notably physical fatigue and reduced activity.[57] Fatigue prevalence in those treated by peritoneal dialysis was greater than 88%.

HIV/AIDS

The prevalence of fatigue in HIV-positive patients, according to one study, was 69%. While fatigue was not the most common symptom in AIDS patients, it was nonetheless widespread, affecting at least 42% of patients.

Multiple sclerosis

Fatigue is the most prevalent and potentially debilitating symptom of multiple sclerosis. It is experienced by 75–95% of multiple sclerosis patients, over half of whom name fatigue as one of their most distressing symptoms. Much of the treatment for multiple-sclerosis-related fatigue involves eliminating secondary causes of fatigue (depression, sleep problems, medications) and using energy more efficiently. The USFDA has not approved any drugs to specifically treat multiple sclerosis, however, medications such as amantadine, modafinil, or methylphenidate are sometimes used.

of cancer and comorbid conditions is expanding. Sixty percent of subjects reported fatigue when cancer was a comorbid condition in rheumatoid arthritis.[18] Other studies suggest a correlation between fatigue, physical function, and systemic inflammatory response and psychological distress in advanced cancer.

The majority of fatigue research over the past two decades has been conducted in the adult population,[18] while fatigue research in children and adolescents has received less attention. As a result identification and/or assessment of fatigue prevalence is less clear in children.[30] Children may express fatigue as being tired, not sleeping well, not being able to do the things they want to do, or not being as active as before the illness and they may report playing less. Several studies investigated fatigue and its impact on academic, physical, and social functioning of children and adolescents experiencing fatigue and on QOL during and after treatment in cohorts of adolescents with cancer[16,14] and identified the need to manage fatigue to improve perception of QOL. One review of fatigue in adolescents with cancer summarized the state of evidence and designed clinical strategies for the fatigue management in this population focusing on the role of safe and feasible exercise interventions.

In a recent study on fatigue in children with advanced cancer, parents identified 18 cancer-related symptoms of concern during the last days of their children's life. The most frequently cited symptoms included changes in behavior, respiratory difficulties, pain, change in appearance, weakness and fatigue, and change in heart rate. In an earlier study, parents reported that 89% of the children suffered "a lot" or "a great deal" from at least one symptom in their last month of life.[31] The most common symptoms reported were pain, fatigue, or dyspnea. Pain and fatigue have been reported as the most frequently occurring symptoms in children who died of cancer.[32] Other studies identified symptom clusters, grouping recurring symptoms of depression and anxiety as most prevalent followed by pain, fatigue, and QOL.[16] Much work remains in the study and analysis of symptom clusters and symptom burden in children as well as adults.

Pathophysiology

It takes all of my energy just to take a shower. I can barely walk from the shower to the bed, where I allow myself to collapse for an hour before I can dredge up the energy to get dressed. And all of that for pajamas and a robe; I can't believe this is me.

A recently diagnosed, postmastectomy woman, in early chemotherapy treatment

Historical models to explain the causes of fatigue have been developed by a variety of disciplines in the basic sciences and by clinicians. Box 8.2 represents distinctive theories, models, or frameworks to explain CRF that have been reported in the literature and demonstrate the complex, multifactorial processes over time.[33]

The two most prominent constructs are the depletion hypothesis and the accumulation hypothesis. The accumulation hypothesis describes a mechanism where waste products collect and outpace the body's ability to dispose of them, resulting in fatigue. In the depletion hypothesis, essential substances integral to muscle activity are not available or have been depleted, causing fatigue and may be applied to the end-stage renal disease patients. While these models were developed with the cancer patient in mind, another model, the central peripheral model (central nervous system [CNS] control) where fatigue is controlled between

---

Box 8.2 Chronology of fatigue theories, models, and frameworks

1896

Depletion hypothesis

Muscular activity is impaired when the supply of substances such as carbohydrate, fat, protein, and adenosine triphosphate is not available to the muscle. Anemia can also be considered a depletion mechanism.

1980

Attention fatigue model[98]

The use of attention theory is linked to attentional fatigue. When increased requirements or demands for directed attention exceed available capacity, the person is at-risk for attentional fatigue.

1987

Piper's integrated fatigue model[153]

Piper suggests that fatigue mechanisms influence signs and symptoms of fatigue. Changes in biological patterns such as host factors, metabolites, energy substrates, disease and treatment, along with psychosocial patterns, impact a person's perception and lead to fatigue manifestations, which are expressed through the person's behavior.

Aistars's organizing framework

This framework is based on energy and stress theory and implicates physiological, psychological, and situational stressors as contributing to fatigue. Aistars attempts to explain the difference between tiredness and fatigue with Selye's general adaptation syndrome.

1988

Accumulation hypothesis

Accumulated waste products in the body result in fatigue.

1998

Psychobiological entropy

Activity, fatigue, symptoms, and functional status are associated based on clinical observations that persons who become less active as a result of disease- or treatment-related symptoms lose energizing metabolic resources.

Contributory theories related to fatigue

Adaptation and energy reserves

Each person has a certain amount of energy reserve for adaptation, and fatigue occurs when energy is depleted. This hypothesis incorporates ideas from the other hypotheses but focuses on the person's response to stressors.

Central nervous system control

Central control of fatigue is placed in the balance between two opposing systems: the reticular activating system and the inhibitory system, which is believed to involve the reticular formation, the cerebral cortex, and the brainstem.

Biochemical and physiochemical phenomena

Production, distribution, use, equalization, and movement of substances such as muscle proteins, glucose, electrolytes, and hormones may influence the experience of fatigue.

the reticular activating system and the inhibitory system can be applied to other fatigue-related diagnoses, such as patients with multiple sclerosis.

Causes of fatigue are associated with multifactorial issues including anemia, chemotherapy or other related treatments, and subjective experiences such as pain, depression, and anxiety.

Anemia, a deficiency of red blood cells that results in a lack of oxygen carrying hemoglobin, can result in severe fatigue and significantly impact QOL. It has a profound impact on patients, with additional complications of dyspnea, palpitations, dizziness, and decreased cognitive function.[29] These symptoms can be common in patients with advanced disease or who are receiving aggressive therapy.[30] Use of hematopoietic growth factors or erythropoietin-stimulating factors (ESAs) are known to relieve symptomology and have been utilized to alleviate some degree of fatigue. However, recent research clearly indicates an increased risk factor for thromboembolic events with use of ESAs.[34]

Some evidence suggests that dysregulation of proinflammatory cytokines may play a mechanistic role in the symptom of fatigue as a common biological mechanism.[35] In humans, proinflammatory cytokines may be released as part of the host response to infection, a tumor, tissue damage from injury, or depletion of immune cells associated with treatments. These inflammatory stimuli can signal the CNS to generate fatigue, as well as changes in sleep, appetite, reproduction, and social behavior.

Other factors thought to be of interest are "increased levels of 5H-T (serotonin)" or upregulation of receptors due to the presence of cancer or its treatment.[35]

The search for foundational causes of fatigue continues because no one theory thoroughly explains the basis for fatigue in the patient with advanced disease. The search for such a theory is complicated. Fatigue, like pain, is not only explained by physiological mechanisms, but must be understood as a multicausal, multidimensional phenomenon that includes physical, psychological, social, and spiritual aspects.

Factors influencing fatigue

> How is it that I don't seem to have the energy to exist? I just lay here, I am too tired to weep.
>
> A patient suffering from terminal cardiomyopathy

Many characteristics that may predispose patients with other advanced diseases to develop similar fatigue syndromes have not been studied comprehensively. However, the increase of fatigue prevalence has stimulated oncology research to identify and quantify patient characteristics in treatment-related fatigue for clinical identification and development of treatment modalities. Box 8.3 provides a list of factors that have been studied and are reexamined here.

Age is one factor associated with fatigue in terminal or critical illness, both in children and in the elderly. Recent literature addressing fatigue in children and adolescents with cancer compared with healthy adolescents shows that children express more fatigue than their counterparts without disease, and also reported a higher incidence of depression. And, in the same study, Hispanic groups and those with less education also experienced higher levels of fatigue.[16] Studies related to clusters of symptoms in children identify symptoms of depression and anxiety and indicate their prevalence across pediatric diseases.[17] Also, long-term survivors of childhood cancer

---

Box 8.3 Factors associated with fatigue development

Personal factors

Age (developmental stage)

Marital status (home demands, isolation)

Menopausal status

Income/insurance

Psychosocial factors

Mental and emotional state (depression, fear, anxiety, distress, conflicts)

Culture/ethnicity

Living situation

Care-related factors

Number/cohesiveness of caregivers

Responsiveness of healthcare providers

Disease-related factors

Stage and extent of disease

Comorbidities

Anemia

Pain

Dyspnea

Nutritional changes (weight loss, cachexia, electrolyte imbalance)

Continence

Sleep patterns/interruptions

Treatment-related factors

Any treatment-related effect from surgery, chemotherapy, or radiation (skin reaction, temporary altered energy level, urinary/bowel changes, pain)

Medication issues (side effects, polypharmacy, taste changes, over-the-counter medications)

Permanent physiological changes

---

experienced lower QOL than did those in the general population.[36] One study that examined the academic, physical, and social functioning of children with chronic disease demonstrated that development of preventive measures for children with chronic disease is important in maintaining maximum function.[37]

Patients with cancer, when compared with others with nonmalignant disease, express more fatigue, have worse sleep quality, more disrupted circadian rhythms, worse QOL and lower activity levels.[38] The scientific literature supports the conclusion that the advanced stage of disease compounds the level of fatigue. And, evidence demonstrates that the more advanced the cancer, the greater the occurrence of fatigue.

Early studies associated with treatment-related fatigue in cancer patients indicate that younger adult patients with cancer reported more fatigue than older patients with cancer, suggesting that fatigue may be influenced by the developmental level of the adult.[42,43] However, in more recent studies, older cancer patients aged 70–90-years-old report fatigue occurrence as a long-lasting complication of cancer treatment and may result in or accelerate functional decline. An increase in the prevalence of cancer in the elderly, compounded by the comorbidities of chronic disease and stressors associated with multiple treatments, significantly predisposes the elderly to fatigue.[39]

The most frequent and problematic issue following an acute myocardial infarction is fatigue, which is often expressed in the same terminology used by those experiencing CRF. Symptoms are similar in that they are poorly defined and often underidentified. Yet many of the experiences parallel that of patients with malignancy. Participants in one study identified interference with daily functional status and elicited symptoms related to depression.[10,40]

Similarly, patients with end-stage renal disease on chronic dialysis complain of high levels of pain and fatigue associated with other symptoms.[41] Other associated symptoms, headaches, cramps, itching, dyspnea, nausea and vomiting, and sleep disruption often identify severe fatigue and symptom distress.

In one study 100 patients with rheumatoid arthritis (RA) were asked to identify factors that contributed to their fatigue.[42] Results indicated that the rheumatoid disease process itself was the primary cause of fatigue, joint pain was specifically mentioned. Disturbed sleep was the second most frequent factor, and physical effort to accomplish daily tasks ranked third. Patients with RA indicated that they had to exert twice the effort and energy to accomplish the same amount of work. Another study of patients with RA reported that women experienced more fatigue than men; authors explained this variance as a result of female patients' higher degrees of pain and poor quality of sleep. An international study also reported the significance of depression and pain linked with fatigue for those patients undergoing treatment for rheumatoid arthritis.[42]

Many characteristics that may predispose patients with other advanced diseases to develop similar fatigue syndromes have not been studied comprehensively. However, depression and fatigue are two related concepts often linked to cancer patients.[43] Fatigue is part of the diagnostic criteria for depression and depression may develop as a result of being fatigued. While depression is reported less frequently, feelings of depression are common in patients with cancer. Research indicates that women who are fatigued score twice as high on the depression scale as those who were not fatigued and that depression is the strongest predictor of fatigue. Depression and fatigue may coexist with cancer without having a causal relationship, since each can originate from the same pathology. Fatigue in patients undergoing cancer treatment has been closely linked with other distressing symptoms, such as pain, dyspnea, anorexia, constipation, sleep disruption, depression, anxiety, and other mood states impacting patient QOL.

One study of 215 ethnic Chinese women identified associations between symptoms of fatigue, pain, anxiety, and depression, supporting the existence of symptom clusters, and the combined effect on QOL demonstrated significant implications for nursing.[44] Rather than focusing on specific individual symptoms, earlier and more thorough nursing assessment, along with identification of symptom clusters in patients, could significantly impact overall outcomes and perhaps improve outcomes. Nursing practice is called to continue exploration of symptom relationships and identify opportunities for interdisciplinary collaboration to improve

support for this and other vulnerable populations. Exploring the patient fatigue experience in cancer and other diseases furthers the identification and definition through personal description. A qualitative, longitudinal study of patients diagnosed and treated with lymphoma found that patients identified clusters of symptoms that increased over time. Subjects describe the effects as "distressing" and "cumulative," with one symptom often leading into others.[45]

The following case study reflects challenges facing nursing staff and providers to explore the broad spectrum of fatigue.

Case study

Mr. E, a 79-year-old male with recently diagnosed acute myeloid leukemia

Mr. E, is a 79-year-old male with recently diagnosed acute myeloid leukemia (AML) in June 2013. He has a long-standing history of chronic kidney disease, obstructive uropathy, with a chronic indwelling catheter, and a history of pancytopenia, with recurrent urinary tract infections (UTIs) including panresistant ESBL (Extended-Spectrum β-Lactamases)* *Escherichia coli*.

Within the past month Mr. E was hospitalized 5 days for rectal bleeding and fatigue. He was transfused with 5 units of packed red blood cells (PRBCs) and 2 units of platelets; and underwent a bone marrow biopsy, leading to a diagnosis of AML. Following the diagnosis he received chemotherapy, decitabine 20 mg/m^2 intravenously, daily for 5 days while hospitalized. During this hospitalization he was found to have a *Citrobacter freundii* UTI and was discharged on ciprofloxin.

Several days following his discharge Mr. E became severely fatigued and weak and unable to ambulate. His apartment manager called paramedics, and Mr. E. was taken to the emergency department (ED) by ambulance. He presents to the ED complaining of worsening fatigue and weakness over 1–2 weeks.

He denies experiencing fevers but complains of intermittent chills and diarrhea since discharge. He also denies bleeding from the rectum or presence of blood in the diarrhea stools and denies blood in his urine. He complains of some perianal irritation from the diarrhea, but does not experience lightheadedness, dizziness, loss of sensation, or syncope. His vital signs (VS) on admission to the ED: 102.5/100/16; 130/74; O^2 saturation of 99% on room air. He was given IV vancomycin 1 g; piperacillin/tazobactam 3.375g IV; meropenem 500 mg IV times 1 and NS 1 liter bolus times 2.

Mr. E received consults from Infectious Disease (ID) and Hematology-Oncology (Hem/Onc.), and both consultants enjoined Mr. E in a discussion of his wishes and goals of care. These discussions identified his wishes for control of pain and treatments for comfort. Mr. E was quite clear that he does not want invasive testing, CT imaging, transfer to ICU, or placement of a central line. His primary goal is "to not have pain." His orders include a DNR/DNI and continuation of IV antibiotics to continue through the completion of the current course(s)

---

* ESBLs are enzymes that mediate resistance to extended-spectrum (third-generation) cepahlosporins (e.g., ceftazidime, cefotaxime, and ceftriaoxone) and monobactams (e.g., meropenem or imipenem). The presence of ESBLs in a clinical infection can result in treatment failure with the use of any one of the listed classes of drugs. www.cdc.gov/hai/settings/lab/lab_esbl.html.

as appropriate. In his discussion with the Hem/Onc team, Mr. E emphatically stated his refusal for further inpatient treatment, aggressive management, or further invasive testing. A request was made for Palliative Care consultation.

The consult with Palliative Care revealed some deviation in assessment, in that Mr. E. stated that while he did not want any "inpatient chemotherapy" he did not want to rule out outpatient chemotherapy as a future treatment should his condition change.

Mr. E lives alone in a small apartment significantly distant from his medical support system. He does not identify any support system other than that of an apartment manager who will occasionally assist with purchase of groceries or call paramedics for help. He currently is unable to independently transfer from his bed to a chair. He wants to ambulate but states he is unable to stand even with assistance at the side of his bed. His nutritional intake is less than 30% of his recommended diet; he is able to swallow but complains of "not being hungry" and the food is just "not what he likes." He verbalizes "tiredness" and when asked to rate his fatigue or tiredness utilizing a scale from 0 to 10 he is unable to differentiate levels upon waking after being asleep or before, during, or after activity. He continually expresses his wishes to "go home to die." He is also refusing skilled nursing facility placement.

Case study assessment

When considering patient assessment for treatment-related fatigue, this case study illustrates the importance of evaluating all physical, psychosocial, and emotional contributing factors that may respond to intervention. An analysis of the patient's condition is a continuous process. Because of the high prevalence of fatigue, patients should be screened for fatigue throughout the diagnosis and illness trajectory. A focused history and physical assessment to determine causative and contributing factors are warranted across disciplines.

As this case exemplifies, fatigue can be the focal point for management of care. Mr. E's fatigue or tiredness interferes with his ability to function safely in his current home situation without support. While his fatigue is clearly consistent with his hematological disease status he is refusing further treatment and it is evident that his fatigue is also impacting his physiological, psychological, and emotional stability. Mr. E. may in fact be experiencing symptoms of loneliness, depression, and sadness accentuating his inability to receive adequate support.

Mr. E is experiencing fatigue as a result of his physiological decline and disease history along with the new cancer diagnosis and treatment which emphasizes the need for a physical/psychosocial assessment leading to an earlier interdisciplinary plan of care which includes goals of care discussion.

Physical findings indicate Mr. E is neutropenic, anemic, and thrombocytopenic. A transfusion of 2 units of PRBCs is ordered and following the transfusion a reassessment of his fatigue should be made preferably with a visual analog scale allowing him to "pick how he feels." Mr. E verbalizes emotional distress, in that he wants to go home "to die." He is currently refusing additional chemotherapy with the statement "If I had known I would feel like this. . . No, I don't want anything anymore; I just want to go home to die." His lack of mobility may be a result of his disease process, comorbidities, treatment, and confinement to bed for a period of

time. A follow-up referral to physical therapy to enable him to be out of bed safely may positively affect his psychosocial well-being, appetite, and nutrition. Referrals to social work and case management, with a goal of nursing home placement that is acceptable to him and/or a live-in caregiver with hospice support are in order. The functional goal for this patient's care is that of reducing the side effects of the disease through proper management and maximization of physical, psychosocial, and emotional needs.

Assessment of fatigue

> At first I thought, so I'll be a little tired, I can live with that; but that's not what it is really like. What is life really worth if I don't have energy to chew? Or swallow? Or move? Some days I just don't care. I have no energy to care.
>
> A patient with pancreatic cancer

Fatigue assessment of the whole person is essential—of the mind and spirit as well as the body. When assessing pain, the patient is considered the expert on his or her pain. Fatigue, like pain is also a subjective interpretation of various stimuli[4] determined by the person who is experiencing the sensation. Caregiver or staff perceptions may differ from those articulated by the person experiencing fatigue. Guidelines from the NCCN define CRF as "a persistent subjective sense of physical, emotional, and/or cognitive tiredness or exhaustion related to cancer or cancer treatment that is not proportional to recent activity that significantly interferes with usual functioning."[6]

The NCCN guidelines for CRF clearly delineate steps and processes to put the assessment and recognition of fatigue on the same level as pain and calls "to screen every patient for fatigue as a vital sign at regular intervals" using an age-related severity scale and, based on those findings, to implement a program of patient education and strategies to manage fatigue. The guidelines also include a step-by-step diagram from a "focused history" to specific interventions of nonpharmacological and pharmacological treatment from the evaluation phase through active treatment, posttreatment and the end of life.[6] Borneman et al. developed an intervention "Passport to Comfort" program to determine the effects of applying the guidelines as outlined by the NCCN. In this trial, specific patient, professional, and system barriers were identified, including a reluctance to report to professional staff because it is "inevitable, unimportant or untreatable." This study also identified the belief that patients often feel that fatigue is not "a valid" problem, and it is often the rationale for not continuing treatment. Often professionals lack the knowledge or understand of the profound effects of fatigue and tend to overlook or "assume" it is the same as all other fatigue and perceive it as normal. And finally, institutional barriers include lack of education or knowledge of the causes of fatigue, or its depth of devastation to patients.[46]

There are numerous methods of assessing and diagnosing fatigue. Recognizing the importance of CRF, the diagnosis has been proposed for inclusion in the International Classification of Diseases[47] (Box 8.4). However, some researchers suggest that the diagnostic criteria are too stringent and the strict exclusion of those with possible "mood disorders" is of concern and may underestimate fatigue occurrence.[48]

Many scales have been developed to measure fatigue in the adult with varying levels of validity and reliability. Examples of fatigue measurement tools include the Multidimensional Assessment of

Box 8.4 Proposed criteria for diagnosing cancer-related fatigue

These symptoms have been present almost every day during the same 2-week period in the past month:

Significant fatigue, diminished energy, or increased need of rest, disproportionate to any recent change in activity as well as five or more of the following:

1. Complaints of generalized weakness or limb heaviness

2. Diminished concentration or attention

3. Decreased motivation or interest in engaging in usual activities

4. Insomnia or hypersomnia

5. Sleep is unrefreshing or nonrestorative

6. Perceived need to struggle to overcome inactivity

7. Marked emotional reactivity to feeling fatigued (sadness, frustration, irritability)

8. Difficulty in completing daily tasks attributed to feeling fatigued

9. Perceived problems with short-term memory

10. Postexertional malaise lasting several hours

The symptoms cause clinically significant distress or impairment in social, occupational, or other important areas of functioning.

There is evidence from the history, physical examination, or laboratory findings that symptoms are a consequence of cancer or cancer-related therapy.

The symptoms are not primarily the consequence of comorbid psychiatric disorders, such as major depression, somatization disorder, somatoform disorder, or delirium.

Fatigue, the Symptom Distress Scale, the Fatigue Scale, the Fatigue Observation Checklist, and a Visual Analog Scale for Fatigue.[49] These scales are available for use in research and may be used in the clinical area. A comprehensive review by Piper and colleagues[50] describes the advantages and disadvantages of the single item as well as multi-item, multidimensional CRF measures currently in use. The European Association for Palliative Care compiled a list of assessment instruments that have been used in research for fatigue in the palliative care group.[7] One scale that has been used extensively in the oncology population is the Piper Fatigue Scale. This questionnaire has 22 items that measure four dimensions of fatigue: affective meaning, behavioral/severity, cognitive/mood, and sensory. This scale measures perception, performance, motivation, and change in physical and mental activities.[50]

In clinical practice, however, a verbal rating scale may be the most efficient. Fatigue severity may be quickly assessed using a "0" (no fatigue) to "10" (extreme fatigue) scale. As with the use of any measurement tool, consistency over time and a specific frame of reference are needed. During each evaluation, the same instructions must be given to the patient. For example, the patient may be asked to rate the level of fatigue for the past 24 hours.

Fatigue, as with any symptom, is not static. Changes take place daily, and sometimes hourly in the patient with an advanced illness. As such, fatigue bears repeated evaluation on the part of the

healthcare provider. One patient, noticing the dramatic change in his energy level, remarked, "Have I always been this tired?" He seemed unable to discern whether there had ever been a time when he did not feel overwhelmed by the impact of fatigue. The imperative for palliative care nursing is to consistently take the initiative and ask the patient—and then continue to ask—about fatigue, keeping in mind that the ultimate goal is the patient's comfort. An example of a thorough assessment of the symptom of fatigue is found in Box 8.4, which uses both a subjective and an objective framework to ascertain patient fatigue and possible underlying physiological events that may exacerbate the fatigue. Important areas to explore are patient and family beliefs and expectations related to the fatigue experience and awareness of changes in energy levels, exacerbation and remission of symptoms, and what improves the level of fatigue.[51]

The recognition and measurement of fatigue in children with cancer has existed for many years and became the foundation for increased studies related to QOL in children.[52,53] Research has shown that symptom clusters associated with cancer treatments of nausea, fatigue, pain, and sleeplessness are associated with QOL and depression in some children.[54] Utilization of the PedsQL Multidimensional Fatigue Scale is demonstrating reliable measurement of fatigue in children across many illnesses, cancer, sickle cell, and other chronic health conditions. Causes of CRF are often associated with chemotherapy, anemia, and psychological factors. Behaviors often identified by nursing staff and parents as fatigue are loss of appetite, lethargy, and disinterest. Management of symptoms are most often treated with nutritional support, rest, and relaxation.[55] Several promising studies show some indication that programmed physical activity may reduce symptoms and promote physical and psychological well being.[56–59]

In the adolescent patient population, the assessment of fatigue is equally challenging. One researcher used a Fatigue and Quality of Life Diary to elicit the depth of the problem for this age group across three phases of illness. Patients were evaluated while undergoing treatment, in early remission, and in the follow-up stage.[23,60] Other studies focusing on adolescents employ a variety of tools. A review by Erickson[61] indicates that often a single-item fatigue assessment is used. Although a small number of adolescents have participated, results indicate that fatigue continues to be a problem lasting well into the posttreatment phase for adolescents.

Management/treatment of fatigue

I am so exhausted; it's 2 AM and I can't sleep. My eyelids feel propped open with toothpicks and all I can do is just lie here waiting for dawn. If I could move or do something it would help but there is no strength to move, not even enough to pull the covers back. It's like being alive in a dead body.

A cancer patient while undergoing chemotherapy

Fatigue may be identified and treated in the absence of an absolute cause through recognition of contributing factors of anemia, depression, malnutrition, infection, or other comorbidities. Identifiable goals are to alleviate recognizable factors contributing to CRF and provide support systems to develop or improve patients' and families' coping mechanisms. Often the acknowledgment of the potential of CRF assists with the understanding of the phenomena. It is beneficial for family members to understand the potential exhaustion of illness and its treatment. Frequently patient and family both are under the impression that once treatment is complete, fatigue, like the disease, will "disappear."[51]

When considering palliative care, the management of fatigue is extremely challenging. By its very definition, palliative care may encompass a prolonged period prior to death, when a person is still active and physically and socially participating in life until a few weeks before death, when participatory activity may diminish considerably. With fatigue interventions, the wishes of the patient and family are paramount; management takes into consideration the extent of the disease, symptoms, whether or not palliative treatment is still in process, and the age, developmental and emotional status, and location of the patient.

Barriers to fatigue assessment as well as interventions exist and must be considered in the context of the patient, healthcare provider, and the healthcare system. Unless asked, patients may feel that their fatigue is not a paramount problem compared with other disease- and treatment-related side effects. Healthcare providers may not recognize the need to routinely assess fatigue, and even if they do recognize it they may believe that disease-related fatigue has no concrete solution potential. Current results in translational research on the implementation of a patient and staff fatigue education program using the NCCN[6] fatigue guidelines indicate a significant decrease in barriers and fatigue in the intervention sample.[62]

Interventions for fatigue have been suggested to occur at two levels: management of symptoms that contribute to fatigue, and the prevention of additional or secondary fatigue by maintaining a balance between restorative rest and restorative activity. Fatigue interventions have been grouped into two broad categories: pharmacological interventions and nonpharmacological interventions related to associated causes and symptoms. Leading physiological causes of fatigue include anemia, deconditioning, depression, dehydration, hypoxia, metabolic and endocrine disorders, insomnia, and pain. Treatment may include both pharmacological and nonpharmacological activities and may be adjusted to meet the changes in status.

Pharmacological interventions

Pharmacological approaches to treat fatigue in patients with cancer and chronic progressive diseases continue to increase and include both FDA-approved medications and complementary alternative medications. More frequently used pharmacological therapies include corticosteroids and psychostimulants and, to a lesser degree, antidepressants, tumor necrosis factor alpha, micronutrients, and various other classes of drugs.[63] Corticosteroids such as dexamethasone are commonly used to counteract fatigue, poor appetite, and nausea. However, side effects may include insomnia, mood swings, elevation of blood glucose, and increased occurrence of thrush. The psychostimulant methylphenidate shows mixed results in management, with one out of five studies reporting positive findings. It has also been shown to counteract the somnolence of opioid use, may enhance the effects of pain medication and increase patient activity level.[63] Modafinil shows a much more positive outcome in response with severe fatigue but not in mild or moderate fatigue.[6,64]

Although treatment results suggest that erythropoietin has a positive effect on fatigue, two studies terminated their drug trials early due to safety concerns over possible thromboembolic events. Later studies clearly demonstrated that while the use of ESAs reduce the need for transfusion support, the risk of thromboembolism was increased.[65] However fewer adverse events were evidenced when administration was delayed until the Hb was less than 10 g/dL.

Other drugs have been used to combat chronic disease-related fatigue. Clinical trials of tumor necrosis factor alpha (etanercept) for fatigue have had some effects in fatigue for patients experiencing ankylosing spondylitis.[66] Modafanil has been useful predominately in patients with multiple sclerosis, where some studies report clear improvement in fatigue.

The benefit of complementary alternative medicine was clearly demonstrated with a trial for treatment of CRF with the use of American ginseng 2000 mg daily with no associated toxicities.[67] Continued exploration and positive findings with multiuse drugs and alternative medicines are very encouraging for patients with chronic progressive disease and associated fatigue.

Nonpharmacological interventions

Interventions for cancer-related fatigue encompass several disciplines. Historically, nurse clinicians and researchers have been the trailblazers in assessing and managing fatigue in the clinical setting. Research has been conducted on all of the fatigue management strategies listed in Table 8.1. Included are patient and staff educational interventions; studies on disrupted sleep patterns; nutritional deficits and their effect on patient quality of life; symptom management; and physical and attentional fatigue. Sample sizes have often been small and groups homogeneous, but the studies highlight the contribution of nurse researchers.

A recent review on the effect of exercise on fatigue has been undertaken with the evaluation of 28 studies representing 2083 participants. The outcome measures were diverse and included, but were not limited to the Functional Assessment of Cancer Therapy-Fatigue (FACT-F), Profile of Mood States (POMS), Piper Fatigue Scale, the Brief Fatigue Inventory and the SF-35 vitality scale. The authors concluded that the use of exercise could be beneficial for CRF during and after cancer treatment. An additional meta-analysis by McNeely et al. of 14 studies concentrating on breast cancer patients and survivors concluded that exercise has an effect on improving QOL, fitness, and physical functioning and decreasing fatigue.[68] Several other investigators have reported the benefits of a consistent exercise regimen in breast cancer patients. Their research confirmed that exercise decreased perceptions of fatigue and increased QOL and indicated that those patients who exercised reported half the fatigue level of those who did not exercise.

In palliative care, a group exercise program was piloted for those with incurable cancer and a short life expectancy. Outcomes indicated that physical fatigue was reduced. Toward the end of life, the NCCN guidelines recommend general strategies for fatigue management that begin with energy conservation techniques, prioritizing activities, delegating, taking rest periods and using labor-saving devices. They also recommend optimizing patient activity levels with the consideration of a referral to both physical and occupational therapy. Increased caution was emphasized for those with bone metastases and immunosupression.[4]

Attentional fatigue has been noted to be disturbing and burdensome to many cancer patients.[69] Many cancer survivors continue to suffer from acute chronic and late side effects of treatment, one of the most onerous side effects is cognitive impairment. Early

Table 8.1 Nonpharmacological symptom management strategies for fatigue

Problem	Intervention	Rationale
Lack of information or lack of preparation	Explain complex nature of fatigue and importance of communication of fatigue level with healthcare providers. Explain causes of fatigue in advanced cancer and chronic progressive diseases and evaluate fatigue level with each visit. ◆ Fatigue can increase in advanced disease. ◆ Cancer cells can compete with body for essential nutrients. ◆ Palliative treatments, infection, and fever increase the body's need for energy. ◆ Anxiety, depression, and tension can contribute to fatigue. ◆ Changes in daily schedules, or interrupted sleep schedules contributes to fatigue development. Prepare patient for planned activities of daily life and daily events (eating, moving, visitors, healthcare provider appointments).	Preparatory sensory information reduces anxiety and fatigue. Realistic expectations decrease distress and fatigue.
Disrupted rest/sleep patterns	Evaluate/establish sleep routine: ◆ Usual sleep pattern, length of uninterrupted sleep, temperature in room, activity prior to sleep. ◆ Eating habits prior to sleep, medications, exercise. ◆ Establish/continue regular, routine bedtime and awakening. ◆ Obtain as long sleep sequences as possible, plan uninterrupted time. ◆ Take short rest periods/naps that do not interfere with night sleep. ◆ Use light sources to cue the body into a consistent sleep rhythm. ◆ Pharmacological management of insomnia should be used when behavioral and cognitive approaches have been exhausted.	Minimizing time in bed helps patients feel refreshed, avoids fragmented sleep, and strengthens circadian rhythm.
Deficient nutritional status	Recommend to patient: ◆ High-protein, nutrient-dense food to "make every mouthful count." ◆ Use protein supplements to augment diet. ◆ Suggest small, frequent meals. ◆ Coordinate time up in chair with meal arrival time. ◆ Socialization may increase oral intake. ◆ Encourage adequate intake of fluids, 8 glasses/day or whatever is tolerated, unless contraindicated. ◆ Consider requesting an appetite stimulant like medroxyprogesterone acetate (Megace).	Increased nutrition will raise energy level. Less energy is needed for digestion with small, frequent meals.
Multisymptom occurrence	Assess and control symptoms contributing to or coexisting with fatigue such as pain, sleeplessness, depression, nausea, diarrhea, constipation, electrolyte imbalances, dyspnea, dehydration, infection. Assess for symptoms of anemia and evaluate for the possibility of pharmacological intervention or transfusion.	Multiple distressing symptoms drain energy and will contribute to marked physical/mental fatigue.
Decreased energy reserves	Plan/schedule activities: ◆ Identify a person to be in charge (fielding questions, answering the phone, organizing meals). ◆ Adjust method/pace of care and move slowly when providing care. ◆ Prioritize and save energy for the most important events. ◆ Eliminate or postpone noncritical activities. ◆ Learn to listen to body; if fatigued, rest.	Energy conservation helps to reduce fatigue burden and efficiently use energy available. Pleasant activities may reduce/relieve mental (attentional) fatigue.

(continued)

Table 8.1 Continued

Problem	Intervention	Rationale
	Obtain physical therapy consult:	
	◆ Mild physical therapy may help joint flexibility and prevent pain.	
	◆ Engage in individually tailored, team-approved exercise/yoga program.	
	Use distraction/restoration	
	◆ Encourage activities to restore energy: spending time in natural environment, gardening, listening to music, praying, meditating, engaging in hobbies (art, reading, journaling).	
	◆ Spend time with family/friends, joining in passive activities (riding in car, watching meal preparation).	

research indicates that exercise may be an effective intervention for improving the severity of side effects of cognitive impairment, sleep problems, depression, pain, anxiety, and physical dysfunction.[70]

Nutritional consultation for patients has been shown to be key to managing the physiological deficiencies from cachexia, nausea, and anorexia. Adequate hydration and the replacement of lost electrolytes enable the fatigue-sufferer to have the best opportunity to control fatigue symptoms that are physiologically based.[71]

One of the identified barriers to fatigue management is lack of knowledge and understanding of the relationship between physical activity and inactivity as it relates to fatigue. "The Passport to Comfort" intervention was initiated through a program to translate the NCCN supportive care guidelines into practice through education over a month period.[45] In hemodialysis patients, one study explored educational intervention to promote self-management of fatigue through education. Education at all levels opens a broad category for fatigue intervention including taking advantage of every opportunity during the advanced disease course. With both patient and family education as a constant theme, every opening should be used to explain and advise of changes in disease progression, procedures, treatment, medication side effects, or scheduling. Nurse-initiated and planned educational sessions with both the patient and the patient's family may provide a forum in which to field forgotten questions, reinforce nutritional information, and together manage symptoms to improve QOL.

Sleep disruption is a common problem encountered by the patient with advanced chronic progressive disease. Sleep cycles may be negatively affected by innumerable internal and external factors.[72] The disturbances may be actual or perceived but result in daytime impairment. Common sleep disturbances include insomnia, breathing disorders, and movement disorders. Cancer-related fatigue interferes with activities of daily living, affects QOL and may be offered as a reason to discontinue treatment. Sleep disturbances are often reported together with fatigue. One study examined the relationship between fatigue and sleep parameters in women undergoing chemotherapy.[73] This study found that fatigue worsened and sleep quality remained poor throughout the course of chemotherapy, although total time of sleep increased over the course of treatment, and concludes that more studies are necessary to identify symptoms and explore further interventions. However, a study related to fatigue in multiple myloma patients indicated

that definite improvement was shown in those patients involved in an individualized exercise program.[74] Self-care practices may be important as identified by one study that evaluated self-care practices used by patients undergoing chemotherapy and radiation therapy. The self-care methods most used were management of diet and nutrition and lifestyle changes including prayer, rest, and music.[75]

Psychosocial techniques are the last broad category of fatigue intervention. A recent meta-analysis of CRF research aimed to evaluate both physical and psychosocial interventions (cognitive-behavioral therapy and counseling) as well as behavioral and alternative treatments (massage, yoga) and their effect on fatigue. The findings provide evidence that psychosocial interventions, restorative approaches, and counseling therapies have a moderate to strong effect in not only reducing fatigue but also increasing vigor and vitality.[76] Additionally, a review of 22 studies of psychosocial treatment with cancer patients reported findings that indicate psychosocial support and individualized counseling have a fatigue-reducing effect. If deemed appropriate, the patients and/or family should be encouraged to participate in disease-specific support groups. If unable to travel, there are support groups offered by telephone and/or Internet. Individual counseling by nurses, social workers, or psychologists may also help.

Fatigue-management interventions need to be considered within the cultural context of the patient and family. For some cultures, this may include only the "nuclear" family, whereas in other cultures, there are ritual or extended relatives. When information is shared and decisions are made regarding an intervention, the "family" is acknowledged formally, and care should be made inclusive of these cultural variations.

Management of, and interventions for, fatigue in pediatric oncology have mirrored intervention techniques used in adults. Taking into account the developmental stage of the pediatric patient will provide the structure needed to be effective. Children up to 13 years old with cancer consider taking a nap or sleeping, having visitors, and participating in fun activities to be fatigue-alleviating behaviors. Adolescent patients with cancer add their own perceptions of what helps their fatigue by including interventions such as going outdoors, having protracted rest time, keeping busy, taking medication for sleep, and receiving physical therapy and blood transfusions. Pediatric interdisciplinary palliative care teams are becoming more common and can provide a comprehensive range of nonpharmacological interventions for fatigue including exercise, psychosocial interventions, and complementary and alternative therapy.

As the practice guidelines and standards for fatigue management in palliative care continue to evolve, the NCCN fatigue guidelines provide a framework for adults, children, and adolescents suffering from CRF. Consolidation of the standards provides that fatigue commonly occurs with other symptoms, and all patients—regardless of age or extent of disease—should be screened, assessed, and managed according to clinical practice guidelines, by a multidisciplinary team, at regular intervals throughout the disease course. They also recommend patient, family, and healthcare provider education programs be ongoing and that fatigue management be implemented as continuous quality improvement projects. Finally, guidance is given that suggests that medical care contracts include reimbursement for fatigue and that disability insurance address coverage for long-lasting fatigue.[6]

Summary

This chapter provides an overview of fatigue as it spans the illness trajectory and end of-life experience for patients with chronic progressive disease. While fatigue is a complex phenomenon that has been widely studied, there is still no universally accepted definition. Individuals with cancer and many other chronic, progressive diseases continue to experience fatigue and the costs associated with it not only in the economic sense but also in its physical, emotional, and psychological impact on life. Many factors, including age, psychological state, social support, access to care, disease type and status, pharmaceutical issues, cognitive impairment, and comorbid conditions influence fatigue. Cancer-related fatigue is a serious problem that interferes on multiple levels with physical, psychological, emotional, social, and economic function. The need for healthcare providers to recognize and identify symptoms and explore management strategies is crucial to the lessening of human suffering. Fatigue has a myriad of causes. Fatigue assessment checklists and guidelines can be used to identify potential sources and/or antecedents for the patient's fatigue. And professional nurses are in a unique position to recognize, identify, and explore the needs of patients who may prematurely decline further treatment as a consequence of their fatigue.

Exercise constitutes a large percentage of the positive results in successfully relieving fatigue. However, as there is no instant fix for fatigue, patients may become frustrated and feel too fatigued to introduce life changes that require the habitual practice of non-pharmacological interventions such as exercise. Nurses are challenged to identify fatigue early on or anticipate the potential of various regimens of treatment and provide management education and prevent or relieve symptoms as they develop. Nurses, physicians, and caregivers are central to support, encourage, and actively engage patients in fatigue-management strategies. Referral to appropriate members of the treatment team and use of their services is always warranted.

In the last stages of life, many patients experience fatigue in the context of multiple symptoms and comorbidities. Assessment of all treatable factors known to contribute to fatigue can and will impact fatigue amelioration. As patients decline toward the end of life, fatigue may provide a comforting form of protection and insulation from suffering.

References

1. Keeney CE, Head BA. Palliative nursing care of the patient with cancer-related fatigue. J Hosp Palliat Nurs. 2011;1:270–271. doi:10.1097/NJH.0b013e318221aa36.
2. Piper BF, Cella D. Cancer-related fatigue: definitions and clinical subtypes. J Natl Compr Canc Netw. 2010;8(8):958–966.
3. Atkinson E, Miklowski M, Lopez F, Klibert D. A 23-year-old man with fever and malaise. J La State Med Soc. 2012;164(3):164–165, 167–168, 170 passim.
4. Hauser K, Rybicki L, Walsh D. What's in a name? Word descriptors of cancer-related fatigue. Palliat Med. 2010;24(7):724–730. doi:10.1177/0269216310376557.
5. Scott JA, Lasch KE, Barsevick AM. Patients' experiences with cancer-related fatigue: a review and synthesis of qualitative research. Oncol Nurs Forum. 2011;38(3):E199.
6. National Comprehensive Cancer Network. 2013. Practice Guidelines in Oncology Cancer Related Fatigue. Rockledge, Pa: National Comprehensive Cancer Network. Available at: www.nccn.org/index. asp. Accessed August 8, 2013.
7. Radbruch L, Strasser F, Elsner F, et al. Fatigue in palliative care patients: an EAPC approach. Palliat Med. 2008;22(1):13–32. doi:10.1177/0269216307085183.
8. American Cancer Society. Fatigue in People With Cancer: What is Fatigue? Available at: http://www.cancer.org/treatment/treatmentsandsideeffects/physicalsideeffects/fatigue/fatigueinpeoplewithcancer/fatigue-in-people-with-cancer-what-is-fatigue#. Accessed August 11, 2013.
9. Putzki N, Katsarava Z, Vago S, Diener HC, Limmroth V. Prevalence and severity of multiple-sclerosis-associated fatigue in treated and untreated patients. Eur Neurol. 2008;59(3–4):136–142. doi:10.1159/000111876.
10. Fredriksson-Larsson U, Alsen P, Brink E. I've lost the person I used to be: experiences of the consequences of fatigue following myocardial infarction. Int J Qual Stud Health Well-Being. 2013;8:20836.
11. Smith ORF, van den Broek KC, Renkens M, Denollet J. Comparison of fatigue levels in patients with stroke and patients with end-stage heart failure: application of the fatigue assessment scale. J Am Geriatr Soc. 2008;56(10):1915–1919. doi:10.1111/j.1532-5415.2008.01925.x.
12. Orsey AD, Wakefield DB, Cloutier MM. Physical activity (PA) and sleep among children and adolescents with cancer. Pediatr Blood Cancer. 2013;60(11):1908–1913. doi:10.1002/pbc.24641.
13. Van Cleve L, Muñoz CE, Savedra M, et al. Symptoms in children with advanced cancer: child and nurse reports. Cancer Nurs. 2012;35(2):115–125. doi:10.1097/NCC.0b013e31821aedba.
14. Daniel LC, Brumley LD, Schwartz LA. Fatigue in adolescents with cancer compared to healthy adolescents. Pediatr Blood Cancer. 2013;60(11):1902–1907. doi:10.1002/pbc.24706.
15. Ruccione K, Lu Y, Meeske K. Adolescents' psychosocial health-related quality of life within 6 months after cancer treatment completion. Cancer Nurs. 2013;36(5):E61–72. doi:10.1097/NCC.0b013e3182902119.
16. Smith AW, Bellizzi KM, Keegan THM, et al. Health-related quality of life of adolescent and young adult patients with cancer in the United States: the adolescent and young adult health outcomes and patient experience study. J Clin Oncol. 2013;31(17):2136–2145. doi:10.1200/JCO.2012.47.3173.
17. Rodgers CC, Hooke MC, Hockenberry MJ. Symptom clusters in children. Curr Opin Support Palliat Care. 2013;7(1):67–72. doi:10.1097/SPC.0b013e32835ad551.
18. Bender CM, Engberg SJ, Donovan HS, et al. Symptom clusters in adults with chronic health problems and cancer as a comorbidity. Oncol Nurs Forum. 2008;35(1):1–1. doi:10.1188/08.ONF.E1-E11.
19. Campos MPO, Hassan BJ, Riechelmann R, Del Giglio A. Cancer-related fatigue: a practical review. Ann Oncol. 2011;22(6):1273–1279. doi:10.1093/annonc/mdq458.
20. Mitchell SA. Cancer-related fatigue: state of the science. PM R. 2010;2(5):364–383. doi:10.1016/j.pmrj.2010.03.024.
21. Karthikeyan G, Jumnani D, Prabhu R, Manoor UK, Supe SS. Prevalence of fatigue among cancer patients receiving various anticancer therapies and its impact on quality of life: a cross-sectional study. Indian J Palliat Care. 2012;18(3):165–175. doi:10.4103/0973-1075.105686.

22. Barroso J, Voss JG. Fatigue in HIV and AIDS: an analysis of evidence. J Assoc Nurses AIDS Care. 2013;24(1 Suppl):S5–14. doi:10.1016/j.jana.2012.07.003.

23. Berger AM, Gerber LH, Mayer DK. Cancer-related fatigue: implications for breast cancer survivors. Cancer. 2012;118(8 Suppl):2261–2269. doi:10.1002/cncr.27475.

24. Borneman T. Assessment and management of cancer-related fatigue. J Hosp Palliat Nurs. 15(2):77–86.

25. Doyle T, Palmer S, Johnson J, et al. Association of anxiety and depression with pulmonary-specific symptoms in chronic obstructive pulmonary disease. Int J Psychiatry Med. 2013;45(2):189–202.

26. Herr JK, Salyer J, Lyon DE, Goodloe L, Schubert C, Clement DG. Heart failure symptom relationships: a systematic review. J Cardiovasc Nurs. 2013 July 8. Epub ahead of print. doi:10.1097/JCN.0b013e31829b675e.

27. Horigan AE, Schneider SM, Docherty S, Barroso J. The experience and self-management of fatigue in patients on hemodialysis. Nephrol Nurs J. 2013;40(2):113–122; quiz 123.

28. Liu Z, Yang J, Liu H, Jin Y. Factors associated with fatigue in acquired immunodeficiency syndrome patients with antiretroviral drug adverse reactions: a retrospective study. J Tradit Chin Med. 2013;33(3):316–321.

29. Oncü J, Başoğlu F, Kuran B. A comparison of impact of fatigue on cognitive, physical, and psychosocial status in patients with fibromyalgia and rheumatoid arthritis. Rheumatol Int. 2013;33:3031. doi:10.1007/s00296-013-2825-x.

30. Barsevick AM, Irwin MR, Hinds P, et al. Recommendations for high-priority research on cancer-related fatigue in children and adults. J Natl Cancer Inst. 2013; 105(19):1432–1433. doi:10.1093/jnci/djt242.

31. Pritchard M, Burghen E, Srivastava DK, et al. Cancer-related symptoms most concerning to parents during the last week and last day of their child's life. Pediatrics. 2008;121(5):1301–1309. doi:10.1542/peds.2007-2681.

32. Von Lützau P, Otto M, Hechler T, Metzing S, Wolfe J, Zernikow B. Children dying from cancer: parents' perspectives on symptoms, quality of life, characteristics of death, and end-of-life decisions. J Palliat Care. 2012;28(4):274–281.

33. Barnett ML. Fatigue. In: Otto SE, ed. Oncology Nursing, 4th ed. St. Louis: Mosby: 2001:788.

34. Horneber M, Fischer I, Dimeo F, Rüffer JU, Weis J. Cancer-related fatigue: epidemiology, pathogenesis, diagnosis, and treatment. Dtsch Ärztebl Int. 2012;109(9):161–171; quiz 172. doi:10.3238/arztebl.2012.0161.

35. Barsevick A, Frost M, Zwinderman A, Hall P, Halyard M, GENEQOL Consortium. I'm so tired: biological and genetic mechanisms of cancer-related fatigue. Qual Life Res. 2010;19(10):1419–1427. doi:10.1007/s11136-010-9757-7.

36. Kanellopoulos A, Hamre HM, Dahl AA, Fosså SD, Ruud E. Factors associated with poor quality of life in survivors of childhood acute lymphoblastic leukemia and lymphoma. Pediatr Blood Cancer. 2013;60(5):849–855. doi:10.1002/pbc.24375.

37. Pinquart M, Teubert D. Academic, physical, and social functioning of children and adolescents with chronic physical illness: a meta-analysis. J Pediatr Psychol. 2012;37(4):376–389. doi:10.1093/jpepsy/jsr106.

38. Payne JK. Altered circadian rhythms and cancer-related fatigue outcomes. Integr Cancer Ther. 2011;10(3):221–33. doi:10.1177/1534735410392581.

39. Rao AV, Cohen HJ. Fatigue in older cancer patients: etiology, assessment, and treatment. Semin Oncol. 2008;35(6):633–642. doi:10.1053/j.seminoncol.2008.08.005.

40. Alsén P, Brink E, Persson L-O. Living with incomprehensible fatigue after recent myocardial infarction. J Adv Nurs. 2008;64(5):459–468. doi:10.1111/j.1365-2648.2008.04776.x.

41. Gamondi C, Galli N, Schönholzer C, et al. Frequency and severity of pain and symptom distress among patients with chronic kidney disease receiving dialysis. Swiss Med Wkly. 2013;143:w13750. doi:10.4414/smw.2013.13750.

42. Lisitsyna TA, Veltishchev DY, Gerasimov AN, et al. [The magnitude of fatigue and its association with depression, pain, and inflammatory activity in rheumatoid arthritis]. Ter Arkhiv. 2013;85(5):8–15.

43. Butt Z, Rao AV, Lai J-S, Abernethy AP, Rosenbloom SK, Cella D. Age-associated differences in fatigue among patients with cancer. J Pain Symptom Manage. 2010;40(2):217–23. doi:10.1016/j.jpainsymman.2009.12.016.

44. So WKW, Marsh G, Ling WM, et al. The symptom cluster of fatigue, pain, anxiety, and depression and the effect on the quality of life of women receiving treatment for breast cancer: a multicenter study. Oncol Nurs Forum. 2009;36(4):E205–E214.

45. Johansson E, Wilson B, Brunton L, Tishelman C, Molassiotis A. Symptoms before, during, and 14 months after the beginning of treatment as perceived by patients with lymphoma. Oncol Nurs Forum. 2010;37(2):E105–113. doi:10.1188/10.ONF.E105-E113.

46. Borneman T, Koczywas M, Sun V, Piper BF, Uman G, Ferrell B. Reducing patient barriers to pain and fatigue management. J Pain Symptom Manage. 2010;39(3):486–501. doi:10.1016/j.jpainsymman.2009.08.007.

47. Cella D, Peterman A, Passik S, Jacobsen P, Breitbart W. Progress toward guidelines for the management of fatigue. Oncol (Williston Park). 1998;12(11A):369–377.

48. Berger AM, Lockhart K, Agrawal S. Variability of Patterns of Fatigue and Quality of Life over Time Based on Different Breast Cancer Adjuvant Chemotherapy Regimens. Oncol Nurs Forum. 2009;36(5):563–570.doi: 10. 1188/09.ONF.563-570

49. Aaronson LS, Teel CS, Cassmeyer V, et al. Defining and measuring fatigue. Image J Nurs Sch. 1999;31(1):45–50.

50. Piper BF, Borneman T, Sun VC, et al. Cancer-related fatigue: role of oncology nurses in translating National Comprehensive Cancer Network assessment guidelines into practice. Clin J Oncol Nurs. 2008;12(5 Suppl):37–47. doi:10.1188/08.CJON.S2.37-47.

51. Luthy C, Cedraschi C, Pugliesi A, et al. Patients' views about causes and preferences for the management of cancer-related fatigue-a case for non-congruence with the physicians? Support Care Cancer. 2011;19(3):363–70. doi:10.1007/s00520-010-0826-9.

52. Hockenberry MJ, Hinds PS, Barrera P, et al. Three instruments to assess fatigue in children with cancer: the child, parent and staff perspectives. J Pain Symptom Manage. 2003;25(4):319–328.

53. Varni JW, Seid M, Rode CA. The PedsQL: measurement model for the pediatric quality of life inventory. Med Care. 1999;37(2):126–139.

54. Whitsett SF, Gudmundsdottir M, Davies B, McCarthy P, Friedman D. Chemotherapy-related fatigue in childhood cancer: correlates, consequences, and coping strategies. J Pediatr Oncol Nurs. 2008;25(2):86–96. doi:10.1177/1043454208315546.

55. Yilmaz HB, Taş F, Muslu GK, Başbakkal Z, Kantar M. Health professionals' estimation of cancer-related fatigue in children. J Pediatr Oncol Nurs. 2010;27(6):330–337. doi:10.1177/1043454210377176.

56. Hooke MC, Garwick AW, Neglia JP. Assessment of physical performance using the 6-minute walk test in children receiving treatment for cancer. Cancer Nurs. 2013;36(5):E9–E16. doi:10.1097/NCC.0b013e31829f5510.

57. Baumann FT, Bloch W, Beulertz J. Clinical exercise interventions in pediatric oncology: a systematic review. Pediatr Res. 2013;74(4):366–374. doi:10.1038/pr.2013.123.

58. Chung OKJ, Li HCW, Chiu SY, Ho KYE, Lopez V. The impact of cancer and its treatment on physical activity levels and behavior in Hong Kong Chinese childhood cancer survivors. Cancer Nurs. 2013;37(3):E43–E49. doi:10.1097/NCC.0b013e3182980255.

59. Braam KI, van der Torre P, Takken T, Veening MA, van Dulmen-den Broeder E, Kaspers GJL. Physical exercise training interventions for children and young adults during and after treatment for childhood cancer. Cochrane Database Syst Rev. 2013;4:CD008796. doi:10.1002/14651858.CD008796.pub2.

60. Ream E, Gibson F, Edwards J, Seption B, Mulhall A, Richardson A. Experience of fatigue in adolescents living with cancer. Cancer Nurs. 2006;29(4):317–326.

61. Erickson JM. Fatigue in adolescents with cancer: a review of the literature. Clin J Oncol Nurs. 2004;8(2):139–145. doi:10.1188/04.CJON.139-145.

62. Ferrell BR, Koczywas M, Borneman T, Sun V, Piper BF. Barriers to pain and fatigue management in medical oncology. J Clin Oncol (Meeting Abstracts). 2008;26:9546. Available at: http://meeting.

ascopubs.org/cgi/content/abstract/26/15_suppl/9546. Accessed June 14, 2013.

63. Minton O, Stone P, Richardson A, Sharpe M, Hotopf M. Drug therapy for the management of cancer related fatigue. Cochrane Database Syst Rev. 2008;(1). doi:10.1002/14651858.CD006704.pub2.

64. Boele FW, Douw L, de Groot M, et al. The effect of modafinil on fatigue, cognitive functioning, and mood in primary brain tumor patients: a multicenter randomized controlled trial. Neuro-Oncol. 2013;15(10):1420–1428. doi:10.1093/neuonc/not102.

65. Grant MD, Piper M, Bohlius J, et al. Epoetin and Darbepoetin for Managing Anemia in Patients Undergoing Cancer Treatment: Comparative Effectiveness Update. Rockville (MD): Agency for Healthcare Research and Quality (US); 2013. Available at: http://www.ncbi.nlm.nih.gov/books/NBK143013/. Accessed August 10, 2013.

66. Hammoudeh M, Zack DJ, Li W, Stewart VM, Koenig AS. Associations between inflammation, nocturnal back pain and fatigue in ankylosing spondylitis and improvements with etanercept therapy. J Int Med Res. 2013;41(4):1150–1159. doi:10.1177/0300060513488501.

67. Barton DL, Liu H, Dakhil SR, et al. Wisconsin Ginseng (Panax quinquefolius) to improve cancer-related fatigue: a randomized, double-blind trial, N07C2. J Natl Cancer Inst. 2013;105(16):1230–1238. doi:10.1093/jnci/djt181.

68. Cramp F, Daniel J. Exercise for the management of cancer-related fatigue in adults. Cochrane Database Syst Rev. 2008;(2). doi:10.1002/14651858.CD006145.pub2.

69. Chen M-L, Miaskowski C, Liu L-N, Chen S-C. Changes in perceived attentional function in women following breast cancer surgery. Breast Cancer Res Treat. 2012;131(2):599–606. doi:10.1007/s10549-011-1760-3.

70. Mustian KM, Sprod LK, Janelsins M, Peppone LJ, Mohile S. Exercise recommendations for cancer-related fatigue, cognitive impairment, sleep problems, depression, pain, anxiety, and physical dysfunction: a review. Oncol Hematol Rev. 2012;8(2):81–88.

71. Santarpia L, Contaldo F, Pasanisi F. Nutritional screening and early treatment of malnutrition in cancer patients. J Cachexia Sarcopenia Muscle. 2011;2(1):27–35. doi:10.1007/s13539-011-0022-x.

72. Berger AM, Mitchell SA. Modifying cancer-related fatigue by optimizing sleep quality. J Natl Compr Canc Netw. 2008;6(1):3–13.

73. Liu L, Rissling M, Natarajan L, et al. The longitudinal relationship between fatigue and sleep in breast cancer patients undergoing chemotherapy. Sleep. 2012;35(2):237–245. doi:10.5665/sleep.1630.

74. Coleman EA, Goodwin JA, Coon SK, et al. Fatigue, sleep, pain, mood and performance status in patients with multiple myeloma. Cancer Nurs. 2011;34(3):219–227. doi:10.1097/NCC.0b013e3181f9904d.

75. Williams PD, Balabagno AO, Manahan L, et al. Symptom monitoring and self-care practices among Filipino cancer patients. Cancer Nurs. 2010;33(1):37–46. doi:10.1097/NCC.0b013e3181b0f2b4.

76. Kangas M, Bovbjerg DH, Montgomery GH. Cancer-related fatigue: a systematic and meta-analytic review of non-pharmacological therapies for cancer patients. Psychol Bull. 2008;134(5):700–741. doi:10.1037/a0012825.

Abbreviations

Cancer-Related Fatigue (CRF)
Complementary Alternative Medicine (CAM).
Double Blind Placebo Controlled (DBPC)
European Organization for the Research and Treatment of Cancer (EORTC)
Functional Assessment for Chronic Illness Therapy-Fatigue (FACIT-F)
Functional Assessment of Cancer Therapy-Anemia Subscale (FACT-AN)
Functional Assessment of Cancer Therapy-Fatigue Subscale (FACT-F)
Profile of Mood State Fatigue Subscale (POMS-F)
Quality of Life (QOL)
Quality of Life Scale-Core 30 Questionnaire (QLQ-C30)
Randomized Control Trial (RCT)
Visual Analog Global Scale of Fatigue (VAS-F)

CHAPTER 9

Anorexia and cachexia

Dorothy Wholihan

I knew the end was closer, once she stopped wanting to eat. I was so frustrated. I worried that the nursing home staff didn't have the time to feed her. I came at most all mealtimes, but no matter how much I coaxed, she just wasn't interested. In the last week, all she ate was bites of chocolate ice cream. I just gave her what she loved.

Husband of woman with advanced dementia

Key points

- Anorexia and cachexia are distressing symptoms of advanced illness.

- They are distinct syndromes but clinically difficult to differentiate.

- Metabolic alterations are the primary cause of anorexia/cachexia syndrome.

- Assessment and treatment of anorexia and cachexia include determining whether exogenous etiologies such as nausea and pain are involved and vigorous treatment of any such etiologies if present.

Management of anorexia/cachexia syndrome (ACS) requires a multimodal, interdisciplinary approach, utilizing pharmacological, nonpharmacological, and psychosocial interventions.

Anorexia is defined as the reduction or loss of desire to eat[1] and is a symptom that accompanies many common illnesses. In acute events, anorexia usually resolves with resolution of the illness, and any weight lost may be replaced with nutritional supplements or increased intake. Unchecked, anorexia leads to insufficient caloric intake and protein-calorie malnutrition. Weight loss from this starvation phenomenon usually involves loss of fat, rather than muscle tissue.[2] Anorexia is common among patients with advanced cancer and advanced acquired immune deficiency syndrome (AIDS) but also characterizes the clinical course of patients with other chronic progressive diseases, such as chronic obstructive pulmonary disease (COPD), congestive heart failure (CHF), and end-stage renal disease.[1]

Anorexia and cachexia are two distinct clinical syndromes, but are often intertwined in chronic progressive disease. Cachexia is a complex syndrome that usually involves anorexia along with significant weight loss, loss of muscle tissue and adipose tissue, and generalized weakness associated with increased protein catabolism and inflammatory response.[3] The word "cachexia" is derived from the Greek *kakos*, meaning bad, and *hexis*, meaning condition or appearance; throughout medical history, cachexia has been associated with the gravely ill.[4] The first clinical definition can be traced to Hippocrates earlier than 400 BC: "The flesh is consumed and becomes water. . . the abdomen fills with water, the feet and legs swell, the shoulders, clavicles, chest and thighs melt away. . . the illness is fatal."[5] It is important to differentiate the cachexia syndrome from simple anorexia or starvation. Anorexia resulting in decreased intake is usually a component of both phenomena, but cachexia can still be found in the absence of decreased appetite. Anorexia alone does not account for the magnitude of weight loss seen in diseases like cancer, and nutritional supplementation does not restore the lean body mass of cancer ACS.[4,6] Cachexia is defined as "a devastating multi-factorial syndrome combining weight loss, depletion of skeletal muscle, anorexia, asthenia, and fatigue."[4] It occurs in more than 80% of patients with cancer before death and is the main cause of death in more than 20% of such patients.[6,7] In contrast to the starvation seen in anorexia, in cachexia there is approximately equal loss of fat and muscle, significant loss of bone mineral content, and no response to nutritional supplements or increased intake.[6]

Weight loss, regardless of etiology, has a decidedly negative effect on survival, and loss of lean body mass has an especially deleterious effect.[6] Evidence-based reviews about prognosis reveal a significant correlation between anorexia/cachexia and survival in newly diagnosed cancer patients and in patients with advanced disease.[6] Weight loss is also linked to decreased survival in CHF, COPD, end-stage renal disease, and AIDS.[1,6,8–10] The term "anorexia/cachexia syndrome" (ACS) has been used mostly in reference to patients with cancer, and thus the condition is sometimes termed "cancer-related anorexia/cachexia" (C-ACS).[7] Varying terminology has been used to describe the syndrome in other disease states for instance, HIV wasting syndrome, cardiac cachexia, pulmonary cachexia syndrome, and, in patients with advanced renal disease, "malnutrition-inflammation-cachexia syndrome" (MICS).[11] Table 9.1 lists the various terms used to describe anorexia-cachexia and estimated prevalence in different disease states. The pathophysiology and clinical presentation of ACS overlap in these various diseases, even though the underlying metabolic and neurohormonal imbalances may differ. The basic issue of underlying chronic inflammation can be seen in them all.[1] For the purposes of this chapter, the term ACS shall refer to all chronic, advanced disease-related anorexia/cachexia syndromes.

The ACS of all diseases is characterized by a variety of signs and symptoms that represent interference with energy intake

Table 9.1 Anorexia/cachexia syndrome in various disease states

Disease	Terminology	Estimated prevalence: highest in advanced disease
Cancer	Cancer-related ACS	Up to 86%
CHF	Cardiac cachexia	16–36%
COPD	Pulmonary cachexia syndrome	30–70%
HIV disease	HIV wasting syndrome	10–35%
Renal disease	MIC: malnutrition-inflammation cachexia syndrome	30–60%

Sources: Adapted from Bennani-Baiti and Davis (2008), reference 6; Freeman (2009) reference 9; Watson et al. (2009), reference 12.

(decreased appetite, early satiety, taste changes, etc.) and nutritional status, that is increased metabolic rate, weight loss, hormonal alterations, muscle and adipose tissue wasting, fatigue, and decreased performance status.[1] Whatever the specific disease, the development of ACS poses a significant clinical problem. It is a grave prognostic sign but also has a detrimental effect on quality of life, as documented by studies of all the above major diagnoses. This syndrome leads to serious physical and functional deficits, and can be devastating to self-image, social and family relationships, and spiritual well-being.

Pathophysiology of anorexia/cachexia syndrome

The basic etiologies of ACS are (1) decreased food intake, (2) metabolic abnormalities, (3) the actions of proinflammatory cytokines, (4) systemic inflammation, (5) neurohormonal dysregulation, (6) tumor by-products, and (7) the catabolic state.[1,6] These result in derangement of function with negative effects on survival and quality of life. There is within some of these mechanisms a mutually reinforcing aspect; for example, anorexia leads to fatigue, fatigue increases anorexia, anorexia increases fatigue, and so on. Table 9.2 summarizes the mechanisms and effects of ACS.

Table 9.2 Mechanisms and effects of anorexia/cachexia syndrome

Mechanisms	Effect
Loss of appetite	Generalized host tissue wasting, nausea or "sick feeling," loss of socialization and pleasure at meals
Reduced voluntary motor activity (fatigue)	Skeletal muscle wasting and inanition (fatigue)
Reduced rate of muscle protein synthesis	Skeletal muscle wasting and asthenia (weakness)
Decreased immune response	Increased susceptibility to infections
Decreased response to therapy	Earlier demise and increased complications of illness

Sources: Adapted from Bennani-Baiti and Davis (2008), reference 6; Payne et al. (2012), reference 2; Dodson et al. (2011), reference 14.

The ACS is categorized as primary or secondary, depending on its etiology. Primary ACS results from endogenous metabolic abnormalities such as cytokine production, which stimulates chronic inflammation and resulting catabolism. The syndrome is called secondary if it results from exogenous etiologies, caused by symptoms that interfere with the intake or absorption of nutrients. Examples of such interfering symptoms are pain, nausea, intestinal obstruction, or psychosocial distress.[13]

Primary anorexia/cachexia syndrome

The pathogenesis of primary ACS is multifactorial, complex, and incompletely understood. Accumulating evidence suggests that chronic illness disrupts the homeostatic function of the central nervous system, leading to profound metabolic changes. Peripheral input causes the awareness of threats such as a growing tumor, or cardiac or renal failure, and this promotes a catabolic effect which results in increased energy expenditure, reduced intake, increased muscle breakdown, and loss of adipose tissue.[14]

Metabolic alterations

Metabolic alterations are common in cancer and other diseases and are thought to be due in large part to the systemic inflammatory response and stimulation of cytokine production (principally tumor necrosis factor alpha [TNF-α], prostaglandins [PG], interleukin-1 [IL-1], interleukin-6 [IL-6], interferon α [IFN-α], and interferon β [IFN-β]). Other catabolic tumor-derived factors thought to play a role in cachexia include proteolysis-inducing factor (PIF) and lipid-mobilizing factor (LMF).[14] Major metabolic alterations include glucose intolerance, insulin resistance, increased lipolysis, increased skeletal muscle catabolism, negative nitrogen balance, and, in some patients, increased basal energy expenditure.[2,14]

A number of different theories regarding the pathophysiology of ACS are under study. The maladaptive activation of oxidative processes that may be seen in chronic illness are also thought to be partially responsible for the cachexia syndrome.[12] Recent advances in genomics suggest that specific genetic polymorphisms contribute to the prominent inflammatory component of this problem.[15] The melanocortin system of the hypothalamus, which coordinates appetite and feeding, is influenced by peptide hormones such as leptin and ghrelin.[16] Disturbances in these hormonally regulated feedback loops appear to play a role in ACS. Other potential mediators of ACS include testosterone, insulin-like growth factor-1, myostatin, and adrenal hormones.[9,17] In sum, the underlying pathophysiological processes of ACS are complex and not yet fully understood. Researchers postulate that the above mechanisms play different roles of varying importance in different diseases.[3] The relative importance of these factors and the interplay among them remains unclear. However, irrespective of the underlying mechanism or specific medical illness, patients experience progressive worsening of their clinical condition, and ultimately they perish soon after the development of cachexia.[1]

Secondary anorexia/cachexia syndrome

Secondary causes of ACS include exogenous factors that can frequently lead to weight loss, anorexia, fatigue, or other symptoms associated with this wasting syndrome.

Physical symptoms

A number of physical symptoms of advanced disease may contribute to or cause anorexia, including pain, dysguesia (abnormalities in taste, especially aversion to meat), ageusia (loss of taste), hyperosmia (increased sensitivity to odor), hyposmia (decreased sensitivity to odor), anosmia (absence of sense of smell), stomatitis, dysphagia, odynophagia, dyspnea, hepatomegaly, splenomegaly, gastric compression, delayed emptying, malabsorption, intestinal obstruction, nausea, vomiting, diarrhea, constipation, inanition, asthenia, various infections (see below), and early satiety. Alcoholism or other substance dependence may also contribute to or cause anorexia. Primary or metastatic disease sites have an effect on appetite, with cancers, such as gastric and pancreatic, having direct effects on organs of alimentation.[1,2,7,13]

In general, people who are seriously ill and/or suffering distressing symptoms have poor appetites. In addition, in cancer, metabolic paraneoplastic syndromes such as hypercalcemia or hyponatremia (SIADH) may also cause anorexia or symptoms such as fatigue that contribute to anorexia. Patients with HIV disease may also develop primary muscle disease, leading to weight loss.[18] Many treatments for chronic diseases have deleterious effects on appetite or result in side effects leading to anorexia and/or weight loss.[2] Each of these should be ruled out as a contributing cause of anorexia and, if present, treated as discussed elsewhere in this book.

Treatment side effects

Many interventions used to treat advanced chronic disease have adverse effects on nutritional status. The many medications used to treat HIV/AIDS and its sequela are an excellent example. Despite the success of highly active antiretroviral therapy (or HAART) in curbing ACS in many patients, the myriad of medications involved in the prevention and treatment of AIDS complications often lead to anorexia and malabsorption themselves, and HIV wasting remains a problem for many.[18] Cytotoxic drugs can be emetogenic, cause taste changes, or cause other gastrointestinal (GI) side effects such as oral stomatitis and diarrhea.[19] Radiotherapy can also lead to significant side effects, including nausea, vomiting, diarrhea, xerostomia, and severe fatigue.[19] Among patients with advanced renal disease on dialysis, there is a high prevalence of protein-energy malnutrition.[20]

Psychological and/or spiritual distress

Psychological and spiritual distress are often overlooked causes of anorexia. The physical effects of the illness and/or treatment coupled with psychological responses (especially anxiety and depression) and spiritual distress, may result in little enthusiasm or energy for preparing or eating food. As weight is lost, and energy decreases, changes in self-image occur. Appetite and the ability to eat are key determinants of physical and psychological quality of life.[4,14,21] Cultural influences must always be considered. For many patients, the net result of ACS and weight loss constitute a negative-feedback loop of ever-increasing magnitude and suffering in multiple dimensions. Clinicians evaluating patients with anorexia are encouraged to review basic principles for the assessment and management of depression, as covered in detail in chapter 20. Treatment of underlying depression can improve appetite considerably.

Oral issues

Special attention should be directed toward the oral cavity of patients with advanced disease. The fit of dentures may change with weight loss, or already poorly fitting dentures may not be as well tolerated in advanced disease. Dental pain may be overlooked in the context of terminal illness. Oral and esophageal infections and complications increase with disease progression and immunocompromise. Xerostomia and worsening of tooth decay can occur with radiation therapy. Basic oral hygiene can often be neglected in the setting of advanced illness. Aphthous ulcers, mucositis, candidiasis, aspergillosis, herpes simplex, and bacterial infections cause oral or esophageal pain and, thus, anorexia.[22]

Assessment

Anorexia and weight loss may begin insidiously with only decreased appetite and slight weight loss, which can accompany virtually any illness. As the disease progresses and comorbid conditions increase in number and severity, anorexia and malnutrition increase, and a mutually reinforcing process may emerge. Cachexia has long been considered a part of advanced disease and end of life. However, skeletal muscle loss may be present earlier in the disease trajectory, and the early stages may be missed in patients with underlying obesity. Early identification is optimal, but further research is needed to more clearly define the benefits of early assessment and intervention on patient outcomes.[14,23]

With ACS common, and in many cases inevitable, among patients with advanced or terminal illness, identifying specific causes is an extremely challenging task. Although several international workgroups have proposed guidelines for the definition and classification of anorexia and cachexia, none as yet have been universally accepted.[3,13,24] There have been standardized tools for the general assessment of nutrition status, but none specific to ACS for palliative care.[23,25] Nevertheless, anorexia from some etiologies is treatable; hence, assessment of the possible presence of etiologies noted above is integral to quality palliative care. Assessment parameters are used according to the patient's ability to tolerate and benefit from the assessment.

Assessment parameters should include appetite, nutritional intake, and basic nutritional status.[23,25] Appetite is a component of several well-validated tools of global symptom assessment, such as the Edmonton Symptom Assessment Scale[26] or the Memorial Symptom Assessment Scale.[27] In addition, simple assessment questions about change in appetite can be transformed into a numerical assessment scale. Intake can be measured retrospectively by recall or prospectively by calorie count. Detailed exploration with appropriate physical examination can identify associated factors (i.e., dysphagia, nausea, oral issues, or pain). Open-ended questions can be helpful in eliciting specific characteristics of the eating problem.

A variety of methods can be used to assess nutritional status, from basic tools such as the Subjective Global Assessment for Nutrition (SGA) to sophisticated anthropometric and laboratory testing.[23] Common lab values may reveal decreased serum albumin, a prognostic indicator of increased morbidity and mortality, as well as changes in several electrolyte and mineral levels.[23]

Perhaps the most important component of assessment in ACS involves the patient's goals of care. Since palliative care encompasses the entire disease continuum, stage of illness and goals of

---

Box 9.1 Assessment parameters in anorexia and cachexia

The patient is likely to report anorexia and/or early satiety.

Weakness (asthenia) and fatigue are present.

Mental status declines, with decreased attention span and ability to concentrate. Depression may increase concurrently.

Inspection/observation may show progressive muscle wasting, loss of strength, and decreased fat. There often is increased total body water, and edema may thus mask some wasting.

Weight may decrease. Weight may reflect nutritional status or fluid accumulation or loss.

Increased weight in the presence of heart disease suggests heart failure.

Triceps skinfold thickness decreases with protein calorie malnutrition (PCM; skinfold thickness and midarm circumference vary with hydration status).

Midarm muscle circumference decreases with PCM.

Serum albumin concentrations decrease as nutritional status declines. Albumin has a half-life of 20 days; hence, it is less affected by current intake than other measures.

Other lab values associated with ACS include anemia, increased triglycerides, decreased nitrogen balance, and glucose intolerance.

Sources: Bennani-Baiti and Davis (2008), reference 6; Leuenberger et al. (2010), reference 23.

---

care should be clearly determined before detailed assessment and intervention are planned or initiated. It is imperative to evaluate the degree of suffering or distress experienced as a result of the ACS. A cost/benefit analysis should be undertaken to determine whether a diagnostic workup is valuable in light of the effort, cost, or discomfort it may incur. At some point in the illness, even basic assessments, such as weight, serve only to decrease the patient's quality of life. Assessment parameters are summarized in Box 9.1.

Assessment also includes a psychosocial evaluation, particularly concerning food, determining usual intake patterns, food likes and dislikes, and the meaning of food or eating to the patient and family. Too often, a family member attaches huge significance to nutritional intake and exerts pressure on the patient to increase intake: "If he would just get enough to eat." Giving sustenance is a fundamental means of caring and nurturing, and it is no surprise that the presence of devastating illness often evokes an almost primitive urge to give food. Assessment should also include an evaluation of the patient and family health literacy level, as well as their desire and preferred means of receiving health information.[24]

In some cases the patient is less troubled than the family by poor nutritional intake. Clinicians should explore the meaning of feeding in the context of the family's cultural and religious background, and help identify other ways in which the family can participate in caring for the patient.[28]

Interventions

The palliative approach to care of the patient with ACS focuses on improving patient comfort and minimizing distress caused by the anorexia and weight loss. Assisting patients and families to adapt to progressive symptoms and alleviating symptoms that may be exacerbating the problem are two foci of interventions.

Interventions may combine a variety of approaches, including treatment of secondary (exogenous) causes of anorexia, nutritional support, enteral and parenteral nutrition, pharmacological management, and psychosocial support.

(Exogenous) symptom management

The presence of symptoms that may cause or exacerbate secondary anorexia and weight loss should be evaluated and treated as possible. If anorexia is due to an identifiable problem, such as pain, nausea, fatigue, depression, or taste disorder, appropriate interventions as discussed elsewhere in this book should be instituted. The goal here is to identify and manage potentially correctible problems that contribute to low dietary intake.[8]

Nutritional support

Oral nutritional support, in an attempt to increase intake or to maximize nutritional content, may be helpful especially early in the disease process or in specific disease states. For example, there is evidence that nutritional supplementation can be effective in patients with COPD.[8] However, C-ACS studies have been disappointing. The current evidence reveals that improving the quantity and quality of nutrition does not improve lean body mass in patients with cancer.[4,6] A recent systematic review on nonpharmacological interventions found that interventions that were able to increase protein and calorie intake showed no resulting improvement in nutritional status, tumor response, survival, or quality of life.[13,17]

Helping family members understand nutritional needs and limitations in terminal situations is essential. Consultation with a nutritionist is usually warranted for the purpose of education and recommendation of appropriate supplements. General guidelines for nutritional interventions include the following[15,29,30]:

- The nutritional quality of intake should be evaluated and appropriately modified to improve the quality. Patients who are not moribund may benefit emotionally from supplementary sources of protein and calories. Clinicians should determine the meaning to the patient and family of giving, taking, and refusing food. Strong and even unconscious beliefs about food are difficult to modify, and many families require education and frequent support in the face of helplessness and frustration related to ever-diminishing intake.

- Culturally appropriate or favored foods should be encouraged. Preserving cultural or social traditions around meals may also be helpful. Families should be encouraged to share mealtime with patients or continue habits such as a glass of wine with meals, if medically appropriate.

- Small meals, on the patient's schedule and according to the taste and whims of the patient, are helpful, at least emotionally, and should be instituted early in the illness so that eating does not become burdensome.

- Foods with different tastes, textures, temperatures, seasonings, degrees of spiciness, degrees of moisture, and colors should be tried, but the family should be cautioned against overwhelming the patient with a constant parade of foods to try. Room temperature and less spicy foods are preferred by many patients.

- Different liquids should also be tried. Cold, clear liquids are usually well tolerated and enjoyed, though cultural constraints may exist. For example, patients with illnesses that are classified as "cold" by some Southeast Asians and Latinos are thought to be harmed by taking drinks or foods that are either cold in temperature or thought to have "cold" properties.

- ◆ Measures as basic as timing intake may also be instituted. Patients who experience early satiety, for example, should take the most nutritious part of the meal first. Filling fluids without nutritional value (such as carbonated soda) should be avoided at mealtime. Oral care must be considered an integral part of nutritional support. Hygiene and management of any oral pain are essential in nutritional support. Procedures, treatments, psychological upsets (negative or positive), or other stresses or activities should be limited prior to meals.

Enteral and parenteral nutrition

Enteral feeding (via nasoenteral tube, gastrostomy, or jejunostomy) may be indicated in a small subset of terminally ill patients. Many clinicians postulate that there exist certain patients with a good functional status and relevant secondary (exogenous) component to their ACS who may benefit from invasive nutritional interventions. Examples include patients with head and neck cancer with severe dysphagia who are undergoing radiation therapy, patients with slow-growing tumors causing bowel obstruction, patients undergoing certain surgeries for upper gastrointestinal tract (UGI) malignancies, or those undergoing bone marrow transplant.[15] However, the evidence remains insufficient to recommend precise guidelines for specific populations.[15] In general, guidelines recommend against enteral feedings for cancer patients undergoing routine radiotherapy, chemotherapy, or bone marrow transplantation.[31,32] Furthermore, despite the common practice of placing percutaneous endoscopic gastrostomy (PEG) tubes in patients with head and neck cancer, insufficient evidence exists that that prophylactic PEG placement improves clinical outcomes.[33] The clinical indications for enteral nutrition in noncancer diagnoses remain controversial, perhaps no more so that in the case of dementia. Although more than 30% of patients with dementia in nursing homes have PEGs, the best available data suggest that tube feeding does not improve quality of life, reduce pressure ulcer formation or healing, limit aspiration risk, enhance functional capacity, or increase survival.[33] In these patients, careful hand feeding has been recommended as an alternative. Two nonmalignant conditions warrant consideration of enteral feeding. These include patients with stroke who otherwise have good quality of life and patients with early amyotrophic lateral sclerosis (ALS).[33,34] In general, patients with poor performance status and poor prognosis are at high risk for mortality from gastrostomy.[33] In these patients, comfort feeding should be the primary focus in maintaining quality of life.

The use of parenteral nutrition in ACS has been controversial within the palliative care field, and in nearly all cases, if the patient has a functioning gut, enteral nutrition is preferred over parenteral nutrition because of the latter's very limited benefit and because the former is associated with lower cost and fewer complications.[28,32] In palliative care settings, long-term use of parenteral nutrition should be considered only if aligned with goals of care and in those with good underlying functional status, a prognosis of 2–3 months and in whom enteral feeding is not possible.[32] Systematic reviews evaluating the use of total parenteral nutrition (TPN) in cancer patients found very limited benefit and significantly more infectious, metabolic, and mechanical complications.[13] The use of parenteral nutrition should be carefully assessed on an individual basis. The choice of nutritional support depends on the cause of the malnutrition, the expected survival, goals of care and planned therapy, and patient preferences. General consensus within palliative care is that the indications for parenteral nutrition are limited and routine use should be discouraged.[13] Medical decision-making in regard to artificial nutrition can be fraught with conflict and emotional distress for families and professionals. These decisions are often emotion-based, not evidence-based. Discussions should be approached with sensitive communication skills, realistic goals, and respect for the patient's cultural background.[35,36]

Pharmacological interventions

A plethora of pharmacological studies have targeted C-ACS,[7,37] and recent work includes other chronic advanced disease.[2,8,19] The most frequently prescribed and most studied drug is megestrol acetate (MA), a synthetic progestogen agent that acts to increase appetite and weight gain. Although the mechanisms by which MA operate are not well understood, most hypotheses suggest that the medication acts on cytokines, inhibiting the TNF.[13]

A recent Cochrane review[32] reviewed trials that examined different aspects of the use of MA to stimulate appetite and weight gain. The review found that MA significantly increased both appetite and weight in cancer patients, but there was not enough evidence to make definitive conclusions about its effect on quality of life, the optimal medication dose, or the effects of MA on patients with other underlying diagnoses. Side effects of MA include hypoadrenalism, hypogonadism, and most concerning, thrombosis and deep vein thrombosis (DVT). However, the recent systematic reviews[2,38] found the rate of adverse effects to be insignificant and concluded that MA is an effective and safe medication for improving appetite and weight in cancer patients. The medication has also shown positive results in patients with COPD and AIDS.[14] The benefit of MA in other noncancer diagnoses remains unclear; more study is needed to make conclusive recommendations. In general at this time, MA is considered the best available treatment option for ACS.[38]

Glucocorticoids are widely used in the palliative care setting to address a number of symptoms, including pain, dyspnea, and nausea.[39] In cancer patients, steroids have been shown to have a limited positive effect on appetite, nutritional intake, and sense of well-being, but no demonstrable effect on weight.[39] The wide range of side effects, including adrenal suppression, hyperglycemia, and peptic ulceration, may preclude its use in some patients.

Cannabinoids have shown similar positive effects: improved appetite and mood, but without weight gain.[13] However, the central nervous system side effects also limit use of this medication. Commonly used pharmacological options with indications and notable side effects are presented in Table 9.3.

Future directions in pharmacological management target various pathways implicated in ACS. Neurohormonal manipulation, cytokine inhibition, and antiinflammatory interventions all show some promise in clinical trials.[11,31,36]

The peptide hormone ghrelin is a circulating mediator of appetite and has been implicated in ACS. Early trials that supplement

Table 9.3 Medications commonly used in anorexia/cachexia syndrome

Medication effects and common dosing	Indications	Side effects and considerations
Progestational agents esp: Megestrol acetate 160–800 mg/day	Improves appetite, weight gain, and sense of well-being	Thromboembolic events, glucocorticoid effects, GI upset, heart failure, menstrual abnormalities, tumor flare
Corticosteroids e.g.: Dexamethasone 4 mg/day	Improves appetite and sense of well-being	Immunosuppression, masks infection, HTN, myopathy, GI disturbances, dermal atrophy, increased ICP, electrolyte imbalances, avoid abrupt cessation
Cannabinoids Dronabinol 5–20 mg/day	Increases appetite and decreases anxiety	Somnolence, confusion, dysphoria, especially in elderly
Metoclopramide 10 mg before meals	Improves gastric emptying, decreases early satiety, improves appetite	Diarrhea, restlessness, fatigue, drowsiness, extrapyramidal side effects

Sources: Payne et al. (2012), reference 2; Baldwin (2011), reference 13; Lobbe (2009), reference 17; Berenstain and Ortiz (2008), reference 32.

ghrelin in various illnesses have shown short-term increases in caloric intake in patients with cancer and renal failure, and improved lean body mass and exercise capacity in those with COPD and CHF.[36,39]

Thalidomide is a controversial medication of interest to ACS researchers. Previously withdrawn from the market due to its teratogenic side effects, thalidomide is now under study in advanced disease due to its potent antiemetic and TNF inhibitor activity. Although its safety profile remains a concern, this medication may be a useful option and is under study.[31,34] Other medications under study include melanocortin (thought to decrease circulating TNF), various anabolic steroids, such as growth factor, insulinlike growth factor, and testosterone derivatives, omega-3 polyunsaturated fatty acids (as found in fish oils), the antidepressant mirtazapine, beta-adrenergic agonists, and antiinflammatory medications.[2,32–34,38,39] These agents have shown some benefit in lab and limited clinical studies. Further research is ongoing. There is also increasing evidence that given the multifactorial process involved in ACS, treatments involving combinations of agents may show promise.[38,39]

Psychosocial support

Anorexia and cachexia can have a profound impact on the quality of life of patients, not only heralding physical decline but also leading to significant emotional and social distress.[4] Weight loss negatively affects patient self-esteem but can cause even more distress and anxiety among family and partners. In a descriptive study by Reid[4] and colleagues, patients viewed wasting as a social stigma and an ominous prognostic sign. However, family held onto beliefs that weight loss was a result of decreased appetite alone. Conflict over food was a common consequence of such dissenting views. Lack of education and a strong symbolic

Box 9.2 Components of a multimodal approach to anorexia/cachexia syndrome

1. Early and ongoing determination of goals of care
2. Optimal treatment of underlying disease according to goals of care
3. Prevention, recognition, and prompt treatment of exogenous causes
4. Guidance from nutrition specialists
5. Appropriate pharmacological interventions
6. Resistance exercise as appropriate
7. Compassionate counseling to patient, family, and significant caregivers with clear consistent and empathetic dialogue

Sources: Payne et al. (2012), reference 2; Baracos (2013), reference 8; Institute for Clinical Systems Improvement (2008), reference 29; Fearon (2008), reference 38; Solheim et al. (2012), reference 39.

attachment to food increased distress.[4] Nurses can play a critical role in assessing patients and family and providing sensitive and culturally appropriate education and support.

Multimodal approach

The devastating psychosocial consequences, pathophysiological complexities, and treatment resistance of ACS lead inevitably to consideration of a multimodal approach.[2,8,32–34,38,39] A summary of what should be included in this approach is summarized in Box 9.2.

Case study

Some issues commonly associated with anorexia/cachexia syndrome

Mrs. V was an 88-year-old woman with stage 4 CHF and dementia admitted to a long-term care facility due to her elderly husband's inability to care for her at home. She was bedbound with a stage 3 sacral decubitus. Her oral intake was poor, a phenomenon that staff attributed to her symptoms of dyspnea, poor activity tolerance, and inability to self-feed due to her dementia. Low-dose morphine was initiated to treat her dyspnea, along with a bowel regimen to address chronic constipation. The patient appeared more comfortable, but she continued to grow weaker, and her general condition slowly deteriorated. The patient's daughter came from out of state and requested placement of a feeding tube, stating, "I just can't let my mother starve to death." The care team advised against PEG placement, citing most recent evidence that it would not prolong survival or improve quality of life. Additionally, the patient's husband refused PEG placement, acknowledging his wife's terminal state and their previous conversations about avoiding aggressive care at the end of her life. After a family meeting involving the medical and nursing staff, the nutritionist, and the family, all concurred with a comfort plan of care. This plan included a Do Not Hospitalize order, careful handfeeding with the patient's favorite foods, vigilant oral care, and appropriate management of her dyspnea and pain. The patient died comfortably 3 weeks later with her husband and daughter at her side.

Summary

Increasingly, ACS is recognized as a serious aspect of advanced or terminal illness and as an area requiring further research, especially with respect to (1) the pathophysiology of cachexia and (2) increasing treatment options.

The management of ACS is complicated by numerous obstacles, including lack of clear definitions and guidelines, inconsistency in assessment and management strategies, and knowledge deficits about this complex clinical syndrome in health professionals and caregiving families. The challenge is compounded by the interwoven emotional symbolism of food and nurturance. As palliative care providers, we should strive to support, understand, and translate the developing evidence that guides our care. The complex and potentially devastating impact of this problem demands a holistic response. Palliative care nurses are optimally situated to coordinate and drive the necessary multidisciplinary approach to address anorexia and cachexia in advanced, progressive disease.

Current understanding of ACS includes the following:

◆ Anorexia and cachexia are distinct syndromes but clinically difficult to differentiate.

◆ Anorexia is characterized by decreased appetite that may result from a variety of causes (including unmanaged symptoms such as nausea and pain) It results primarily in loss of fat tissue, and resultant weight loss is reversible.

◆ Cachexia is a complex metabolic syndrome thought to result from the production of proinflammatory cytokines such as TNF and interleukin 1. In cachexia, there is approximately equal loss of fat and muscle and significant loss of bone mineral content. Weight loss from cachexia does not respond to nutritional interventions.

◆ Assessment and treatment of ACS include determination of whether exogenous etiologies such as nausea or pain are involved, the vigorous treatment of any such etiologies, and nutritional and psychosocial support if indicated.

◆ Treatment of cachexia is unsatisfactory, but some temporary gains may occur with progestational agents, especially MA, and a multimodal approach such as discussed above.

References

1. Molfino A, Laviano A, Fannelli FP. Contribution of anorexia to tissue wasting in cachexia. Curr Opin Support Palliat Care. 2010;4:249–253.

2. Payne C, Wiffen PJ, Martin S. Interventions for fatigue and weight loss in adults with advanced progressive illness. Cochrane Database Syst Rev. 2012;1:1–13.

3. Blum D, Omlin A, Fearon K. Evolving classification systems for cancer cachexia: ready for clinical practice? Support Care Cancer. 2010;18:273–279.

4. Reid J, McKenna H, Fitzsimons D, McCance T. The experience of cancer cachexia: a qualitative study of advanced cancer patients and their family members. Int J Nurs Stud. 2009;46:606–616.

5. Doehner W. Cardiac cachexia in early literature: a review of research. Int J Cardiol. 2002;85:7–14.

6. Bennani-Baiti N, Davis MP. Cytokines and the cancer anorexia cachexia syndrome. Am J Hosp Palliat Care. 2008;25:407–409.

7. Baracos VE, What medications are effective in improving anorexia and weight loss in cancer? In: Goldstein N, Morrison S (eds.), Evidence-Based Practice in Palliative Medicine. Philadelphia: Elsevier Press; 2013:153–157.

8. Baracos VE. What therapeutic strategies are effective in improving anorexia weight loss in non-malignant disease? In: Goldstein N, Morrison S (eds.), Evidence-Based Practice in Palliative Medicine. Philadelphia: Elsevier Press; 2013:158–163.

9. Freeman LM. The pathophysiology of cardiac cachexia. Curr Opin Support Palliat Care. 2009;3:276–281.

10. Schols MWJ, Gosker HR. The pathophysiology of cachexia in chronic obstructive pulmonary disease. Curr Opin Support Palliat Care. 2009;3:282–287.

11. Kalantar-Zadeh K, Norris KC. Is the malnutrition-inflammation complex the secret behind greater survival of African American dialysis patients? J Amer Soc Nephrol. 2011;22:2150–2152.

12. Watson M, Lucas L, Hoy A, Wells J. Oxford Textbook of Palliative Care, 2nd ed. Oxford: Oxford University Press; 2009.

13. Baldwin C. Nutritional support for malnourished patients with cancer. Curr Opin Support Palliat Care. 2011;5:29–36.

14. Dodson S, Baracos VE, Jatoi A, Evans WJ, Cella D, Dalton JT, Steiner MS. Muscle wasting in cancer cachexia: clinical implications, diagnosis, and emerging treatment strategies. Annu Rev Med. 2011;62:265–279.

15. Kalantar-Zadeh K, Anker SD, Horwich TB, Fonarow GC. Nutritional and anti-inflammatory interventions in chronic heart failure. Am J Cardiol. 2008;101:89E–103E.

16. Ashby D, Choi P, Bloom S. Gut hormones and the treatment of disease cachexia. Proc Nutr Soc. 2008;67:263–269.

17. Lobbe VA. Nutrition in the last days of life. Curr Opin Support Palliat Care. 2009;3:195–202.

18. Thibault R. Cano N, Pichard C. Quantification of lean tissue losses during cancer and HIV infection/AIDS. Curr Opin Clin Nutr Metab Care. 2011;14:261–267.

19. Johns KKJ, Beddall MT, Corrin RC. Anabolic steroids for the treatment of weight loss in HIV infected individuals. Cochrane Database Syst Rev. 2009;4:1–63.

20. Kim JC, Kalantar-Zadeh, K. Kopple JD. Frailty and protein energy wasting in elderly patients with end stage kidney disease. J Am Soc Nephrol. 2013;24:337–351.

21. Lam H, Arnold R. Asking About Cultural Beliefs in Palliative Care: Fast Facts and Concepts. 2009; 216. Available at: http://www.eperc.mcw.edu/EPERC?FastFactsIndex/ff_216.htm. Accessed July 1, 2013.

22. Harris D, Harriman A, Cashavelly B, Maxwell C. Putting evidence into practice: evidence-based interventions for the management of oral mucositis. Clin J Onc Nurs. 2008;12:141–152.

23. Leuenberger M, Kurmann S, Stranga, Z. Nutritional screening tools in daily clinical practice: the focus on cancer. Support Care Cancer. 2010;18:S17–S27.

24. Jensen GL, Mirtallo J, Compher C, Dhaliwal R, Forbes A, Grijalba RF, et al. Adult starvation and disease-related malnutrition: A proposal for etiology based diagnosis in the clinical practice setting from the International Consensus Guideline Committee. J Parenter Enteral Nutr. 2010;34:156–159.

25. Churm D, Andrew IM, Holden K, Hildreth AJ, Hawkins C. A questionnaire study of the approach to the anorexia-cachexia syndrome in patients with cancer by staff in a district general hospital. Support Care Cancer. 2009;17:503–507.

26. Bruera, E. The Edmonton Symptom Assessment Scale: a simple method for the assessment of palliative care patients. J Palliat Care. 1991;2:6–9.

27. Chang VT, Hwang SS, Kasimis B, Thaler B. Shorter symptom assessment instruments: the Condensed Memorial Symptom Assessment Scale (CMSAS). Canc Invest. 2004;22:526–536.

28. Hopkinson JB. The emotional aspects of cancer anorexia. Curr Opin Support Palliat Care. 2010;4:254–258.

29. Institute for Clinical Systems Improvement. Clinical Practice Guideline: Palliative Care 2008. Available at:http://www.guideline.gov/summary/summary.aspx?doc_id=12618&nr=0065268&string=cachexia.

30. Lennie TA. Nutritional self-care in heart failure: state of the science. J Cardiovasc Nurs. 2008;23:197–204.

31. Good P, Cavenagh J, Mather M, Ravenscroft P. Medically assisted nutrition for palliative care in adult patients. Cochrane Database Syst Rev. 2008;(4):CD006274.

32. Reid T, Pantilat S, When should enteral feeding by percutaneous endoscopic gastrostomy tube placement be used in treatment of head and neck cancer and in patients with non-cancer conditions? In: Goldstein N, Morrison S (eds.), Evidence-Based Practice in Palliative Medicine. Philadelphia: Elsevier Press; 2013:153–157.

33. Locher JL, Bonner JA, Carroll WR. Prophylactic percutaneous endoscopic gastrostomy tube placement in treatment of head and neck cancer: a comprehensive review and call for evidence-based medicine. J Parenter Enteral Nutr. 2011;35:365–374.

34. Miller RG, Jackson CE, Kasarskis EJ. Practice parameters update: the care of the patient with amyotrophic lateral sclerosis—drug, nutritional, and respiratory therapies (an evidence-based review) Report of the Quality Standards Subcommittee of the American Academy of Neurology. Neurology. 2009;73:1218–1226.

35. McClave SA, Martindale RG, Vanek VW, et al. Guidelines for the provision and assessment of nutrition support therapy in the adult critically ill patient: Society of Critical Care Medicine (SCCM) and American Society for Parenteral and Enteral Nutrition (ASPEN). J Parenter Enteral Nutr. 2009;33:277–316.

36. Dev R, Dalal S, Bruera E. Is there a role for parenteral nutrition or hydration at the end of life? Curr Opin Support Palliat Care. 2012;6:365–370.

37. Ashby D, Choi P, Bloom S. Gut hormones and the treatment of disease cachexia. Proc Nutr Soc. 2008;67:263–269.

38. Fearon KCH. Cancer cachexia: Developing multimodal therapy for a multidimensional problem. Eur J Cancer. 2008;44:1124–1132.

39. Solheim TS, Laird BJA. Evidence base for multimodal therapy in cachexia. Curr Opin Support Palliat Care. 2012;6:424–431.

CHAPTER 10

Nausea and vomiting

Kimberly Chow, Daniel Cogan, and Sonni Mun

The nausea is like nothing I could have ever imagined. I used to drink glasses and glasses of water all the time, all of my life. I never thought the nausea could be this bad. I never thought it would be so bad that I couldn't even stand to take a sip of water.

YC, a palliative care patient (2013)

Key points

◆ Nausea and vomiting are symptoms commonly experienced in advanced disease although the majority of available research continues to be focused on the cancer population.

◆ Clear understanding of the different concepts surrounding nausea and vomiting is essential and will aid in screening, preventing, assessing, and treating symptoms as well as improve understanding of the incidence and severity of patient distress.

◆ The cause of nausea and vomiting is often multifactorial and requires a thorough assessment and understanding of the emetic pathway and neurotransmitters involved in order to aid treatment decisions.

◆ Pharmacological and nonpharmacological interventions should be used to manage the distressful symptoms of nausea and vomiting, particularly as they can both have physiological and psychological etiologies, keeping in mind goals of care at all times in order to choose appropriate interventions.

◆ Nurses play a vital role in helping patients and family members manage and cope with nausea and vomiting.

Nausea and vomiting are symptoms commonly experienced by patients with chronic and advanced disease. These highly distressing symptoms may be directly or indirectly related to disease and can have a significant impact on both the physiological and psychological well-being of patients.[1] Physiological repercussions of poorly controlled nausea and vomiting include metabolic disturbances, malnutrition, electrolyte imbalances and impairment of functional ability[2] as well as unnecessary hospitalizations, emergency room visits, and interruptions in disease-related treatment regimens.[3] Psychologically, nausea and vomiting whether experienced together or separately, can cause distress, anxiety, and fear, leading to the erosion of one's quality of life in multiple domains[2] and may also cause additional strain on caregivers.

To date, the majority of research on nausea and vomiting addresses the oncology population, focusing largely on treatment-induced nausea and vomiting in patients receiving chemotherapy for either curative or palliative purposes. For cancer patients receiving treatment, nausea, vomiting, and retching are among some of the most distressing symptoms reported. Despite advances in antiemetic therapies, nausea continues to be ranked as one of the most severe and distressing side effects of chemotherapy.[4] As the palliative care integration model has shifted to be recommended as early as diagnosis, it is important to emphasize that proper palliation of these bothersome symptoms can help patients continue on with disease-targeted therapies with the aim of disease response or control.

Advances in a variety of disease therapies have yielded extended life, and diseases previously fatal are now chronic in nature. These advances have also led to many individuals now living longer with the potential of high symptom burden.[5,6] Unfortunately, the literature on the assessment and management of nausea and vomiting in the noncancer population and in cancer patients experiencing these symptoms from causes other than chemotherapy or from terminal illness is lacking.[7,8] Given the nature of current evidence-based literature, this chapter will use advanced cancer patients as a model for assessment and treatment of nausea and vomiting, which can then be extrapolated for use in other patients with advanced nononcological diseases.

Care providers at every level must accurately understand the emetic pathway and the main neurotransmitters involved in this process in order to properly assess and manage nausea and vomiting in the palliative care population.[9] Methods for proper symptom management including screening, preventing, assessing, treating, and follow-up will be explored, and nursing interventions and patient and family education will be highlighted.

Epidemiology of nausea and vomiting in palliative care

The extent of patient suffering with any disease is largely determined by the presence and intensity of disease-related symptoms. Due to the heterogeneity of the population being assessed and treated, prevalence of nausea and vomiting in palliative care is difficult to capture; patients may have a variety of primary diseases at different stages potentially complicated by one or multiple comorbidities.[9] A strong understanding of symptom prevalence in different diseases will allow clinicians to anticipate problems for the patient, develop a well-rounded plan of care, educate clinical staff, and plan for appropriate services.[10]

Cancer population

Prevalence of nausea and vomiting in patients with advanced cancer has been reported between 21% and 68% and is described by patients as one of the most dreaded side effects of cancer treatment.[11,12,13] Research on nausea and vomiting over the past 25 years has led to steady improvements in the control of chemotherapy-induced nausea and vomiting, with the development of 5-hydroxytryptamine3 (5HT3) receptor antagonists in the 1990s being one of the most significant advances in the chemotherapy of cancer patients.[13] Despite these advances, approximately 70%–80% of patients receiving chemotherapy continue to experience nausea, vomiting, or both, and 10%–44% experience anticipatory nausea, vomiting, or both.[1,2,10] Oncology patients may experience these symptoms as a result of disease and/or treatment. The incidence, prevalence, and severity is related to the emetic potential of the chosen treatment regimen and specific patient variables,[1] with some studies suggesting that the female gender and younger age are predisposing factors for chemotherapy-induced nausea and vomiting.[12,14–17] Severity is also seen to increase as disease progresses and in some instances may be a predictor of shortened survival.[9,18]

The data on prevalence of nausea and vomiting at end-of-life in cancer patients is mixed and may be related to cancer type and whether the patient is still receiving disease-targeted therapies. Some studies show that in certain cancer populations these symptoms become more prevalent closer to death and during the last week of life, impacting physical well-being.[9,19] Meanwhile, other studies suggest that the prevalence and severity of nausea actually decreases closer to death.[5,17] In some instances nausea was reported in only 17% of cancer patients at end-of-life as compared to pain (45%) and anxiety (30%).[5,17] Decreased prevalence may be due to underreporting and lack of standardized comprehensive assessments to facilitate symptom documentation.[10]

Noncancer population

Nausea and vomiting for patients with advanced illness other than cancer has received less attention, and recent research provides conflicting information. Multiple reports suggest that nausea and vomiting are experienced by people with advanced illness, but not to the degree previously reported, and not as commonly as pain, breathlessness, or fatigue, with incidence and severity worsening over time.[8,20,21] There are also persuasive arguments that nausea is very likely to be underreported[22] and undertreated[23] especially for patients in long-term care settings. Similar to the cancer population, drawing firm conclusions regarding the epidemiology of nausea and vomiting in the noncancer advanced illness population is complicated by methodological difficulties presented by the palliative care population and the lack of standardized symptom definition and reporting.[9]

Particular populations of noncancer patients to consider are those residing in long-term care facilities. In this setting, nausea seemed to occur less frequently than pain, dyspnea, or constipation.[22] The prevalence of nausea for residents was measured to be between 1.3% and 8%,[23,24,25] with reports of moderate to severe nausea increasing to 17% during the final 2 days of life,[8] suggesting that the symptom worsens in incidence and severity as a patient nears death. Nearly one of every four deaths in

the United States occurs in a long-term care facility, with numbers expected to increase in the near future to as high as 40% in 2040 as the population ages.[22,23] Some of the challenges to appropriate symptom management in long-term care facilities are the lack of palliative care-trained staff, high staff turnover rates, and the lack of physician or midlevel provider presence. The residents at these facilities often have high rates of serious comorbid conditions including cancer, progressive neurodegenerative conditions, and other diseases that impair functional status and ability to communicate. Although research has been conducted on assessing and managing pain in hospice care in these settings, studies on nonpain symptoms such as nausea and vomiting are lacking.[22]

Studies available on noncancer patients consistently found that nausea and vomiting occur less frequently than many other measured symptoms. A systematic review examining daily symptom burden in end-stage chronic organ failure found the prevalence of nausea to range from 2% to 48%, which was less common than fatigue, dyspnea, insomnia, and pain.[7] In multiple studies using the nine-item Edmonton Symptom Assessment Scale,[8,21] nausea was the least frequently reported symptom.

Though nausea is infrequently encountered as an acute complication of dialysis administration,[26] 14.6% of patients with end-stage renal disease receiving dialysis experience nausea.[27] A longitudinal study of patients with end-stage renal disease found 59% of patients to experience nausea during the month before death,[28] again suggesting an increase in incidence as one becomes more ill.

Conceptual concerns related to nausea and vomiting

To thoroughly examine the problem of nausea and vomiting in palliative care, it is important to be clear about certain concepts. Symptoms such as nausea and vomiting are composed of subjective components and dimensions unique to each patient. Symptoms are different from signs, which are objective and can be observed by the healthcare professional.[6,29] Symptom occurrence is composed of the frequency, duration, and severity with which the symptom presents.[30] Symptom distress involves the degree or amount of physical, mental, or emotional upset and suffering experienced by an individual. This is different from symptom occurrence. Lastly, symptom experience involves the individual's perception and response to the occurrence and distress of the symptom.[6,29]

The terms "nausea" and "vomiting," often clinically associated, are in fact distinct concepts that are many times mistakenly used interchangeably or imprecisely, impacting the ability to assess and measure prevalence and burden.[6] *Nausea* is an unpleasant feeling of the need to vomit experienced in the back of the throat and epigastrium. It is a nonobservable phenomenon that may be accompanied by autonomic symptoms such as pallor, cold sweat, salivation, and tachycardia as well as some degree of anorexia or loss of appetite. The patient often times describes the sensation as feeling "queasy" or "sick to my stomach" or may have a difficult time describing the unpleasant sensations experienced.[4,6,9,18] *Vomiting* is a physical event that results in the forceful expulsion of gastric contents from the stomach and out of the mouth or nose through a complex reflex involving the gastrointestinal (GI) tract, diaphragm, and abdominal muscles. This may be described as "barfing," "upchucking," "heaving," "flipping," or "puking."[9,18] The two should always be assessed separately.

Additional terms to be familiar with when assessing for nausea and vomiting are retching, regurgitation, rumination, and dyspepsia. *Retching* is the body's attempt to vomit without the actual expulsion of material. Patients often describe this as "gagging" or "dry heaves."[4] Nausea and vomiting should not be confused with regurgitation, rumination, or dyspepsia, syndromes that cause similar sensations in the upper abdomen but require different treatment approaches.[31]

While there are multiple etiologies for nausea and vomiting in advanced cancer, chemotherapy-induced nausea and vomiting is one of the most common and can continue even near death as many patients remain on systemic therapy throughout the late stages of their disease.[32] Three distinct types of chemotherapy-induced nausea and vomiting have been described. The acute phase occurs anywhere from minutes to 1 day following chemotherapy and usually begins 4 or more hours later, while the delayed phase usually occurs 24 hours following treatment. Anticipatory nausea and vomiting differs from the other two as it is a response to conditioned stimuli developed from significant nausea and vomiting during previous chemotherapy treatments and occurs even before treatment is administered.[4,33] Because anticipatory nausea and vomiting is a learned response it is not mediated by the usual emetogenic neurotransmitters that will be reviewed, however the best approach to anticipatory emesis is the best possible prevention and control of acute and delayed emesis.[32]

Physiological mechanisms of nausea and vomiting

Understanding the pathophysiology of nausea and vomiting is important for optimal management of a palliative care patient with these symptoms. This approach allows rational selection of pharmacological therapies using an understanding of the neural mechanisms involved in nausea and vomiting.

Vomiting occurs when the vomiting center is activated by peripheral and central afferent pathways. The vomiting center is located in the medulla oblongata. Peripherally, afferent nerves from the gastrointestinal tract activate the vomiting center when there is pathology such as mucosal irritation, bowel wall invasion by neoplasm, and activation of stretch receptors. Stretching of the bowel lumen as well as the stretching of the capsule on visceral organs can activate the afferent neural circuit. The gag reflex occurs when the glossopharyngeal nerve (cranial nerve IX) is stimulated in the pharynx by coughing or other mechanical irritation.[34,35]

Central neural circuits that induce vomiting include the chemoreceptor zone and the cortex. The chemoreceptor trigger zone (CTZ) is a vascular region in the area postrema of the fourth ventricle and is outside of the blood-brain barrier.[6]

Chemical irritants (e.g., medications), electrolyte disturbances (e.g., hypercalcemia), and infections stimulate the CTZ. Vomiting that occurs when our senses of smell, taste, sight, or hearing is stimulated is cortical as well as vomiting associated with fear and anxiety. The nausea and vomiting that occurs with motion sickness and vertigo is mediated by the vestibulocochlear nerve. Increased intracranial pressure is also associated with nausea and vomiting that is prominent in the morning.[31] The neural pathway for the nausea and vomiting associated with increased intracranial pressure is less well understood than for other neural pathways to the vomiting center. Figure 10.1[6,9,31,34,35] is a conceptual illustration of the described pathways that lead to nausea and vomiting.

The various afferent pathways and the vomiting center rely on specific neurotransmitters that result in nausea and emesis when there is an appropriate stimulus. For example, enterochromaffin cells in the gut release serotonin when there is pathology such as mucosal irritation from chemotherapeutic agents. The released serotonin binds to its receptor and this afferent signal is transmitted to the vomiting center. Previously it was believed that chemotherapy caused nausea and vomiting mainly by triggering the CTZ. Now it is understood that irritation of the gut and resultant serotonin activation of the peripheral afferent pathway from the gut is an important cause along

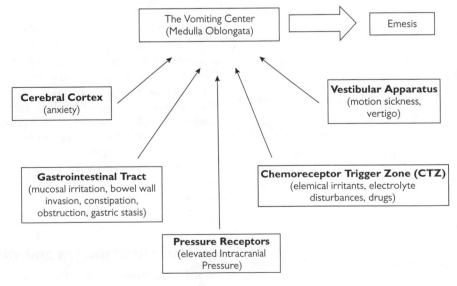

Figure 10.1 Emetic pathways.

with central afferent CTZ activation. The neurotransmitters involved in activation of the CTZ are dopamine and serotonin. The vestibular system depends on activation of histamine and acetylcholine to transmit afferent signals to the vomiting center. The vomiting center is rich in serotonin, histamine, and acetylcholine receptors.

Pharmacological therapies often target these ligand-receptor actions to prevent nausea and vomiting. Serotonin receptor antagonists such as ondansetron are particularly helpful for chemotherapy-induced nausea and vomiting because they block the activation of the gastrointestinal afferent loop to the vomiting center as well as inhibit serotonin action in the CTZ and the vomiting center. The newest pharmacological agent, aprepitant, targets another ligand-receptor pairing that was more recently discovered to be involved in vomiting. Aprepitant targets the neurokinin receptor NK1. The vomiting center is rich in NK1 receptors, and when the usual ligand, substance P, is attached to the receptor vomiting is induced.[34,36]

Causes of nausea and vomiting

There are numerous potential causes of nausea and vomiting in cancer patients with advanced disease requiring palliative care. It is helpful to have a thorough understanding of the common

---

Box 10.1 Common syndromes involving nausea and vomiting in the palliative care population

Biochemically/drug-induced

Fluid and electrolyte imbalances
(e.g., hypercalcemia, hyponatremia)

Organ failure (e.g., liver, renal)

Chemotherapy

Opioids

Antibiotics

Anticonvulsants

SSRI antidepressants

Gastric stasis

Carcinoma of stomach

Ascites

Opioid related

Anticholinergic drugs

Peptic ulcers

Gastrointestinal obstruction/irritation

Cancer related

Esophagitis

Peptic ulcers

Gastric distension or compression

Delayed gastric emptying

Bowel obstruction

Constipation

Biliary obstruction

Intra-abdominal secondaries (e.g., peritoneal disease)

Adhesions

Treatment related (e.g., chemotherapy, radiation)

Infection (e.g., cryptosporidiosis)

Medication (e.g., aspirin, NSAIDs)

Increased intracranial pressure

Cerebral edema

Intracranial tumor

Intracranial bleeding

Meningeal disease

Vestibular

Opioid induced

Cerebral secondaries

Motion sickness

Psychological

Fear

Anxiety

Anticipatory

NSAIDs = nonsteroidal anti-inflammatory drugs; SSRI = selective serotonin reuptake inhibitors

Sources: Glare et al. (2011), reference 9; Mannix (2011), reference 34; Wood et al. (2007), reference 35; National Cancer Institute (2013), reference 37.

---

causes, which can be subdivided into six clinical syndromes presented in Box 10.1.[9,34,35,37]

Although the potential causes of nausea and vomiting are extensive and the frailty of the palliative care patient often precludes invasive diagnostic testing, studies have shown that it is possible to determine the underlying cause or causes for targeted therapy.[38,39] Approach to treatment relies heavily on identifying the symptoms present, the level of patient distress, grasping the physiological mechanisms involved, and determining the underlying etiology, keeping in mind that causes are often multifactorial.[18,40–42] It is not uncommon to treat patients with advanced cancer who may have peritoneal disease causing constipation and also requiring opioids for disease-related pain. The skilled clinician will use his or her assessment to quickly identify any reasonably reversible causes that remain in line with the patient and family's goals of care.

Assessment of nausea and vomiting

Principles of emesis control for the cancer patient is first and foremost to prevent nausea and vomiting.[43] When this goal is not achieved,

- Use self-report tools rather than observational assessment whenever possible
- Check reliability and validity
- Look for clarity, precision, cultural sensitivity, and understandable wording
- Instrument should be in an easy-to-read format
- Determine and describe the symptoms and components
- Determine a time frame for recall of the symptom experienced
- Consider the purpose of the tool, the target population, and whether it is for acute, delayed, or anticipatory nausea and vomiting or for patients with advanced cancer
- Consider the ease of scoring and type of score

Source: Rhodes and McDaniel (2001), reference 6.

recommendations advocate for a structured approach to assessing and treating these symptoms.[18] Assessment is an important process and the foundation of all treatment-related decisions. It should be an ongoing process that begins with the initial patient contact.

The palliative care specialists' approach to symptom assessment and treatment requires understanding of symptom pathophysiology, which can be obtained from the patient's history, physical exam, and diagnostic test results.[41] It is rare that patients present with nausea and vomiting as a first sign of advanced cancer. Generally, patients who complain of this symptom complex have a well-documented history of their disease, including diagnosis, prior treatment, and sites of metastases. Regardless, a focused exam when a patient is complaining of nausea and vomiting is needed to narrow down the list of differential diagnoses that may include, but are not limited to: drugs, uremia, infection, anxiety, constipation, gastric irritation, and proximal gastrointestinal obstruction.[44]

History of present illness and review of systems may include pattern of symptoms, possible triggers (e.g., medications, meals, movement, position, smells), presence of epigastric pain, dysphagia, thirst (seen with hypercalcemia), hiccups (seen with uremia), heartburn, and constipation. Physical examination should include an oral assessment for thrush or mucositis and assessment of abdomen, bowel sounds, and rectum for signs of obstruction, constipation, or impaction. Laboratory studies may help rule out organ dysfunction, infection, and electrolyte imbalances; radiographic exams should only be ordered if indicated to guide treatment decisions.[44]

Information obtained by questionnaires or self-report tools such as diaries, journals, or logs is crucial for the identification and management of this symptom complex and for improving the patient's quality of life. Rhodes and McDaniel provide clear criteria when trying to choose the appropriate assessment tool for individual patients, summarized in Box 10.2.[6]

There are several measurement tools that may be used to assess one or more of the components of nausea and vomiting. Some tools provide a global measure while others measure a single component of the nausea and vomiting. Instruments may involve checklists, visual analog scales, patient interviews, or Likert scales; almost all involve self-report by the patient.[1,3,4,30,45] The most commonly used tools with reliability and validity reproducible in research studies are shown in Table 10.1.[4,6,45,46]

Nurses working in all settings and with all age ranges of patients need to use skillful observation along with effective data collection techniques for a complete and comprehensive assessment. Particularly in the long-term care population, early recognition and assessment of symptoms must be tailored to individual residents. This approach uses a combination of resident reports, caregiver reports, and direct observation, as often residents may have difficulty communicating their needs. Keep in mind, patients with different levels of cognitive impairment may still be able to make their needs known and communicate pain and other distressful symptoms. Turning to behavioral cues may also be helpful to assess discomfort.[22]

Case study

SK, a 33-year-old male with AIDS

SK is a 33-year-old male with AIDS admitted to the hospital with nausea and vomiting, severe weakness, and 10 out of 10 pain in multiple sites including his head, bones, and stomach. He has in the past refused treatment for HIV due to concerns about side effects and inability to follow up regularly for medical appointments. He recently decided to get his HIV treated because of his declining health status and fear of death. During his visit, the patient admits to past and current use of heroin and cocaine.

Table 10.1 Tools to measure nausea and vomiting

Instrument	Type	Reliability/Validity
Visual Analog Scale (VAS)	100-mm line, with anchor descriptors at each end	Reliability is a strength.
Morrow Assessment of Nausea and Emesis (MANE) Rhodes Index of Nausea and Vomiting Form 2 (INV-2)	16 item, Likert scale (onset, severity–intensity) 8 item, Likert scale	Test/retest reliability 0.61–0.78 Split-half reliability 0.83–0.99 Cronbach's alpha 0.98 Construct validity 0.87
Functional Living Index Emesis (FLIE)	18 item, Likert scale	Content and criterion validity Internal consistency

Sources: Brearley et al. (2008), reference 4; Rhodes and McDaniel (2001), reference 6; Meek et al. (2009), reference 45; Martin et al. (2003), reference 46.

Because of his past negative experiences with the medical system he is sullen and refuses many tests. His main concern is the new onset of nausea and vomiting that has been severely debilitating. He is particularly angry because he attributes the nausea and vomiting to recently starting his HIV medication, which was supposed to make him better, not worse. He also complains of pain in his head that is bandlike and constant, and says it is difficult to concentrate as a result. He has had chronic pain in his abdomen but says it has become more severe, sharper, and constant, whereas in the past it had been intermittent. He denies constipation but has had diarrhea for the last 6 months, which is less frequent. Since yesterday he has developed pain that he localizes to his bones and worse in his extremities. His main relief has been heroin or when he used his partner's hydromorphone 8 mg tabs every 2 hours. He refused blood tests and radiographic studies because of his severe discomfort. Because of his multiple severe symptoms, potential need for high opioid doses, and difficulty establishing a therapeutic relationship, a palliative care consultation was obtained.

After palliative care assessment, SK was prescribed parenteral prochlorperazine 10 mg every 6 hours around the clock for his nausea and vomiting. For his pain he was prescribed parenteral hydromorphone 4 mg every 4 hours around the clock and 2 mg every 1 hour for breakthrough pain. He stated that his goal of care was to extend his life but refused to discuss potential burdens and risks of this choice and other potential goals of care. By the second hospital day he was feeling much better and had become more engaged with the medical staff. After several more days nursing staff report that the patient violently vomits every morning and he has become more withdrawn complaining of worsening headaches. Emergent head imaging was performed and a large mass was seen. After the mass was visualized he was given dexamethasone 10 mg parenterally as an initial dose then 4 mg every 6 hours. His headache and the nausea and vomiting improved with the steroids and he also had an increase in his appetite, a welcomed side effect. He is now waiting for consultation with oncology and neurology and has agreed to ongoing palliative care involvement.

Treatment of nausea and vomiting

Management of nausea and vomiting requires a combination of both pharmacological and nonpharmacological approaches. Understanding the cause(s) of nausea and vomiting is crucial as it allows proper selection of treatment regimens. Often times the cause is multifactorial, requiring multiple interventions used concurrently. Investigations to rule out potentially reversible or treatable causes such as dehydration, electrolyte imbalances, and constipation should be considered.[33]

Pharmacological management of nausea and vomiting

In the absence of an immediately reversible cause, nausea or vomiting is palliated through the combined use of pharmacological and nonpharmacological interventions. It is essential for the nurse to know the clinical pharmacology of the large and increasing number of antiemetics available for use. This includes an understanding of nonoral routes of delivery, since patients suffering from nausea and vomiting may not be able to take oral medications reliably. Medication delivery that does not require

intravenous access is also frequently employed because patients with advanced illness may require control of severe symptoms in nonhospital settings. Similar to the management of chronic pain, patients with chronic nausea will need around-the-clock medications for baseline symptom control, supplemented with rescue dosing. The palliative care nurse will also ensure effective education of the patient and family to support symptom relief for patients outside of hospitals. Guidelines for the pharmacological treatment of this symptom rely primarily on basic pharmacology and consensus guidelines as multiple review articles have found the evidence base supporting pharmacological treatment of nausea and vomiting to be weak and suffering from a lack of strong studies.[9,47,48] Research specific to the palliative care population is particularly lacking.[43,49]

Two approaches to pharmacological treatment have been described, a mechanistic approach and an empirical approach.[9] The mechanistic approach to treatment involves the selection of medications expected to block the relevant receptors in the emetic pathway as inferred from the patient's clinical presentation. For example, a prokinetic agent such as metoclopramide is chosen when a patient's nausea is inferred to be caused by gastric stasis. Once an appropriate medication is selected, it is titrated until the symptom is relieved, maximum doses are reached, or the patient experiences dose-limiting side effects. Classes of antiemetics are listed in Box 10.3.[34] Figure 10.2[31] reviews the common dosages of drugs used for nausea and vomiting in palliative care. If the nausea is not relieved with the first agent, a second medication from another class should be added, and similarly titrated.[47] Mechanism-based treatment is limited by pharmacologic and physiologic factors. Pharmacologically, the presence of similar receptors at multiple sites of the emetic pathway and the activity of single medications at multiple receptors prevent simple targeting of treatment. Physiologically, the etiology of chronic nausea and vomiting in advanced disease is often multifactorial or not known.[31]

More commonly used to describe the initiation of antibiotic use before a definitive diagnosis is made, the empirical approach for nausea and vomiting has been described as drug selection based on prescriber preference,[9] an ad hoc approach without consideration of underlying cause,[31] or "start with one drug and, if unsuccessful, add or rotate to another."[50] Mechanistic and empirical approaches have resulted in similar response rates. Although the two methods have not been directly compared,[18] both rely on a

---

Box 10.3 Classes of antiemetics

Prokinetic agents

Dopamine receptor antagonists

Antihistaminic agents

Selective 5HT3 receptor antagonists

Corticosteroids

Benzodiazepines

Anticholinergic agents

Octreotide

Cannabinoids

Substance P antagonists (NK1 receptor antagonists)

Drug	Adults	Children
Chlorpromazine	10–25 mg every 4–6 h PO; 25–50 mg tid or qid 1M	0.5–1 mg/kg/dose lid or qid PO, IV (max 40 mg/day in children <5 years old, 75 mg/day in children 5–12 years old)[a]
Cyclizine	50–100 mg bid or lid PO; 12.5–50 mg tid or qid SC; 50–300 mg/day via CSCI	0.5–1 mg/kg tid PO/SC/IV (max 25 mg/dose in children <6 years old or 50 mg/dose in children ≥6 years) or via CSCI
Dexamethasone	Chronic nausea: 4–8 mg/day PO, SC or IV; bowel obstruction/raised intracranial pressure: up to 16 mg/day PC, SC or IV	0.1–0.2 mg/kg/dose PO/SC/IV (max 4–8 mg/dose)
Domperidone	10–20 mg tid or qid PO	0.2–0.4 mg/kg qid PO[a] (max 10-20 mg/day)[b]
Haloperidol	1.5–2.5 mg daily or bid PO; 1–2 mg bid or tid SC; 1–5 mg/day via CSCI	0.01–0.05 mg/kg/day PO/SC/IV or via CSCI (max 0.15 mg/kg/day)
Scopolamine butylbromide	80–120 mg/day via CSCI	0.5 mg/kg/dose tid or qid PO/SC/IV (max 20 mg/dose)
Scopolamine hydrobromide	0.6–2.4 mg/day via CSCI	6–10 µg/kg/dose qid PO/SC/IV (max 400 µg/dose)
Levomepromazine	6.25–25 mg bid SC; 25–50 mg/day via CSCI	0.25–1 mg/kg/dose od or bid PO/SC/IV (max 25 mg/day); 0.1–0.4 mg/kg/dose via CSCI (max 12.5–25 mg/day depending on age)[c,d]
Metoclopramide	Gastroparesis: 10 mg tid PO/SC, 30 minutes before meals and at bedtime (max 100 mg/day): partial bowel obstruction: 10 mg every 4–6 h PO; 10–20 mg every 6 h or 40–60 mg/24 h by CSCI	01–0.15 mg/kg/dose tid or qid PO/IV/SC (max 0.5 mg/ kg/day or 30 mg)
Octreotide	100 µg tid SC; 300–1200 µg/day via CSCI	1 µg/kg/dose bid or tid SC/IV (max 50 µg/dose)[a,d]
Olanzapine	2.5–10 mg/day PO	
Prochlorperazine	5–10 mg tid or qid PO; 25 mg bid or tid rectally; 5–10 mg 3–4 hourly (to a maximum of 40 mg/day) IM	0.2 mg/kg/dose bid or tid PO or slow IV (max 15 mg/dose)[a,b,d]
Promethazine	25 mg every 4–6 h (maximum 100 mg/day)	0.125–0.5 mg/kg/dose qid PO/IV[b] (max 25 mg/dose)
Ondansetron	4–8 mg od or bid PO/IV	0.15 mg/kg/dose tid PO/IV (max 8 mg/dose)
Tropisetron	5 mg od PO/IV	0.2 mg/kg od PO/IV (max 8 mg/dose)

a Not commonly used as an antiemetic in pediatric palliative care.

b If patient is <2 years old, seek advice of specialist palliative pharmacist/pediatric palliative care specialist for dosage.

c Limited availability and therefore not commonly used as antiemetic in pediatric palliative care.

d Complex dose administration/limited data available in pediatrics: seek advice of specialist palliative pharmacist/pediatric palliative care specialist.

bid = twice daily; CSCI = continuous subcutaneous infusion; IM = intramuscular: IV = intravenous; max = maximum; od = once a day; PO = oral; qid = four times a day; SC = subcutaneous; tid = three times a day

Figure 10.2 Dosages of drugs for nausea and vomiting in palliative care. Source: Glare et al. (2008), Reference 31, used with permission.

thorough understanding of the clinical pharmacology of the medications to be used.

Prokinetic agents: metoclopramide, domperidone, cisapride, erythromycin

Prokinetic agents include metoclopramide, domperidone, and cisapride. Metoclopramide is the only prokinetic medication that is currently in common use. Its use as an antiemetic is supported by small placebo-controlled trials.[18] Domperidone and cisapride are recognized as effective prokinetic medications, but neither are available for use in the United States due to QTc prolongation and risk of serious cardiac toxicity.

Prokinetic medications alleviate nausea and vomiting by stimulating motility of the upper GI tract. Four potential mechanisms for this effect have been proposed: stimulation of 5HT4 receptors in the gut wall, antagonism of 5HT3 receptors in the CTZ and gut, activation of motilin receptors, and release of the "dopaminergic brake" on gastric emptying. At higher doses metoclopramide has antiemetic activity due to dopamine (D2) receptor antagonism in the CTZ, and thus has a side-effect profile similar to antipsychotic medications, including extrapyramidal symptoms.[9] Metoclopramide's activity at the 5HT4 receptor requires acetylcholine as a mediator at the myenteric plexus, thus in theory anticholinergic medications can antagonize its effect.[18]

Metoclopramide is specifically indicated in the setting of gastric stasis, and is typically administered before meals. Higher doses are necessary to achieve central dopamine blockade in the CTZ. Reduced doses are recommended for patients with renal impairment and the elderly. Metoclopramide is contraindicated in the presence of complete bowel obstruction, GI hemorrhage, or perforation and immediately postoperatively.

The macrolide antibiotic erythromycin has also been identified as a prokinetic medication due to its motilin receptor stimulation, and it has been shown to be effective in treating diabetic gastroparesis. It is given at a dose of 250 mg orally three time daily or 250–500 mg daily intravenously. Side effects include hepatotoxicity and QTc prolongation.[9]

Dopamine receptor antagonists: butyrophenones, phenothiazines, atypical antipsychotics

There are two classes of antidopaminergic medications that are effective antiemetics: butyrophenones and phenothiazines. Though these medications are also categorized as antipsychotics, the antiemetic doses of these drugs are typically lower than the antipsychotic doses. These medications achieve their antiemetic effect through dopamine blockade in the CTZ. With the exception of haloperidol, these medications have a broad spectrum of activity, antagonizing histaminic, muscarinic, serotonergic, and/or alpha-adrenergic receptors.[9] These medications share a common side-effect and adverse-effect profile, including sedation, hypotension, anticholinergic effects, dystonias, extrapyramidal symptoms, QTc prolongation, and rarely neuroleptic malignant syndrome.[9,51] The sedating effect may be considered beneficial when caring for patients close to death. Dose reduction and caution with elderly patients is recommended for all dopamine antagonists.

Butyrophenones: haloperidol, droperidol

Droperidol and haloperidol are drugs in the butyrophenone class, acting primarily as a dopamine antagonist. They achieve their antiemetic effect by binding to the D2 receptors in the CTZ. Haloperidol is less sedating than antipsychotics of the phenothiazine class. Because of its direct antidopaminergic activity, haloperidol should not be given to patients with Parkinson's disease. Consensus-based recommendations advocate the use of haloperidol to treat nausea and vomiting caused by chemical or metabolic causes.[18,52]

There is modest evidence to support the use of haloperidol for treatment of nausea and vomiting. An uncontrolled open label study of 42 patients found haloperidol to be an effective antiemetic for patients with cancer experiencing nausea and vomiting not related to cancer treatment.[51]

Citing its effectiveness in treating nausea as well as delirium and hallucinations, researchers identified haloperidol as one of four essential drugs needed for quality care of the dying in an international survey of palliative care clinicians.[53] Separate Cochrane reviews to evaluate the use of droperidol and haloperidol to treat nausea and vomiting in the palliative care population found no randomized controlled trials of either drug for this population.[54,55] The FDA has issued black box warnings for both drugs due to concerns related to prolonged QTc.

Phenothiazines: prochlorperazine, chlorpromazine, levomepromazine

Phenothiazines possess a broader spectrum of activity compared to haloperidol, blocking histaminic, muscarinic, serotonergic, and/or alpha-adrenergic receptors in addition to dopamine blockade.[18] Their broad spectrum of activity is reflected in their numerous side effects including sedation, hypotension, anticholinergic effects, dystonias, extrapyramidal symptoms, QTc prolongation, leukopenia, and lowered seizure thresholds.[9] The availability of oral, rectal suppository, parenteral, and sustained-release formulations offers flexibility of administration in the outpatient setting, an important consideration in the palliative care population. No randomized controlled trials examining the use of levomepromazine to treat nausea and vomiting in palliative care were identified in a recent review.[56] Levomepromazine is not registered for use in the United States.

Atypical antipsychotics

Olanzapine is an atypical antipsychotic that blocks dopaminergic, serotonergic, histaminic, and muscarinic receptors. It has been used as a second-line antiemetic for patients with refractory nausea, with efficacy shown in small uncontrolled studies.[18] Olanzapine causes fewer extrapyramidal symptoms than other antipsychotics and does not usually cause QTc prolongation.[9] In a small case series, olanzapine was effective in treating nausea refractory to other treatments.[57]

Antihistaminic agents: promethazine, cyclizine, meclizine, hydroxyzine, diphenhydramine

The first generation of piperazine antihistamines have recognized antiemetic properties related to H1 receptor blockade in the vomiting center, CTZ, and vestibular nuclei.[31] Due to their action in the inner ear, antihistamines are specifically indicated for nausea and vomiting associated with movement, dizziness, or vertigo. A review of clinical evidence deemed antihistamines as a class likely to be beneficial for the treatment of nausea and vomiting in chronic diseases other than cancer.[52] Diphenhydramine is often used in combination protocols to minimize the development of extrapyramidal side effects when dopamine antagonists are used. Adverse effects include sedation, dizziness, extrapyramidal symptoms, headache, anticholinergic effects, and lowered seizure threshold.[31]

Cyclizine is an H1-antihistaminic anticholinergic medication. It achieves its antiemetic effect by decreasing excitability in the inner ear labyrinth, blocking conduction in the vestibular-cerebellar pathways, and directly inhibiting the H1 receptor in the vomiting center. It is recommended for use when nausea or vomiting is caused by elevated intracranial pressure, motion sickness, pharyngeal stimulation, or mechanical bowel obstruction, and is less sedating than promethazine.[18]

These medications also have some anticholinergic activity, which can be beneficial when treating bowel obstruction. Cyclizine has greater anticholinergic activity than promethazine, and is less sedating than scopolamine. This same anticholinergic activity may reverse the effect of prokinetic drugs such as metoclopramide.[31]

Selective 5HT3 receptor antagonists: ondansetron, granisetron, tropisetron, dolasetron, palonosetron

Serotonin antagonists achieve their antiemetic effect by antagonizing 5HT3 receptors centrally in the CTZ and vomiting center and peripherally in the gut wall. There is strong evidence to support their use in the prevention of chemotherapy-induced and radiation-induced nausea and vomiting, and their effect is enhanced by the addition of dexamethasone.[52] There is a lack of evidence to support their use outside of this indication, and consensus guidelines recommend their use for chemical causes of nausea and vomiting, vomiting refractory to dopamine antagonists, or when nausea is thought to result from massive release of serotonin from enterochromaffin cells, such as bowel obstruction and renal failure.[18,31] Due to their narrow mechanism of action compared with other antiemetics, the serotonin antagonists have a milder and more predictable side-effect profile, with constipation being the most common and significant side effect.[58]

Corticosteroids

Though the mechanism of action that produces the antiemetic effect is not well understood, there is strong evidence to support the use of corticosteroids in multidrug combination prophylactic antiemetic treatment during chemotherapy and radiation therapy.[52] It may be used to treat nausea stemming from increased intracranial pressure related to intracranial tumors,[31] hypercalcemia of malignancy, or malignant pyloric stenosis. Dexamethasone enhances the efficacy of 5HT3 receptor blockers, NK-1 blockers, and metoclopramide in the prevention of chemotherapy-induced nausea and vomiting.[18,32] In nausea and vomiting caused by bowel obstruction corticosteroids may help to resolve the obstruction.[18] Side effects are well documented, with significant adverse effects on nearly all organ systems, especially with long-term use. Short-term adverse effects include hyperglycemia, insomnia, and psychosis.

Benzodiazepines

Benzodiazepines act on the gamma-aminobutyric acid (GABA) receptors of the cerebral cortex. Lorazepam may be used alone when the intent is to treat anticipatory nausea, due to its temporary amnestic effect, or when anxiety is a contributing factor to nausea or vomiting.[9] Benzodiazepines have been shown to be effective to treat nausea in adult patients in combination with psychological techniques.[18]

Anticholinergic agents: scopolamine, atropine, hyoscamine

Scopolamine (hyoscine) is a naturally occurring muscarinic antagonist, and achieves its antiemetic effect by blocking the muscarinic receptors in the vestibular nucleus and the vomiting center. It is specifically indicated for nausea and vomiting associated with movement or dizziness[50] and with treatment of bowel obstruction if the obstruction cannot be resolved. It is commonly used in the general population to treat motion sickness. Scopolamine can cause the full range of anticholinergic side effects, including sedation, constipation, urinary retention, blurry vision, xerostomia, and delirium. Elderly patients are particularly sensitive to these side effects. In the setting of imminent death, these anticholinergic properties can be used advantageously to treat excessive respiratory secretions.

A report of three cases of cancer-related nausea and vomiting found scopolamine to be effective when selected in a mechanism-based treatment plan for nausea and vomiting, with the added benefit of being antiemetic dose sparing, since symptom control was achieved with the use of this single agent, allowing other antiemetics to be discontinued.[50]

Anticholinergic medications are available in multiple formulations, including transdermal patches, ophthalmic drops that can be administered sublingually, and intravenous and subcutaneous injections, offering flexibility of administration in nonhospital settings.

Octreotide

Octreotide acetate is a long-acting somatostatin analog that may be helpful for nausea and vomiting associated with intestinal obstruction. It is not an antiemetic per se, but is used in treatment of intestinal obstruction. Specifically, it inhibits gastric, pancreatic, and intestinal secretions and reduces gastrointestinal motility, making it useful in cases where there is high-volume emesis.[59,60]

Cannabinoids: marijuana/cannabis, nabilone, dronabinol

Marijuana is the best-known cannabinoid, dronabinol is the plant extract preparation available for prescription use. The semisynthetic agents are nabilone and levonantradol. Cannabinoids are proposed to exert an antiemetic effect by binding to specific cannabinoid receptors in the brainstem and to the opioid mu receptor.[18] In one systematic review, nabilone was found to be superior to placebo, domperidone, and prochlorperazine for management of chemotherapy-induced nausea and vomiting, but not superior to metoclopramide or chlorpromazine. Cannabinoids were not found to add to benefits of 5HT3 receptor antagonists.[48] Another systematic review found oral nabilone, oral dronabinol, and intramuscular levonantradol were more effective treatments for chemotherapy-induced nausea and vomiting than dopamine antagonists, but were associated with significantly greater side effects.[18,52]

Substance P antagonists (NK-1 receptor antagonists)

NK-1 receptor antagonists prevent the binding of substance P to NK-1 receptors. Aprepitant is an oral drug that acts as an NK-1 antagonist. It has been shown to be effective when combined with ondansetron and dexamethasone to prevent acute and delayed chemotherapy-induced nausea and vomiting.[5,49]

Combination protocols

The use of multidrug regimens for the management of chemotherapy-induced nausea and vomiting is supported by a strong base of evidence including multiple randomized controlled trials and clinical practice guidelines. Regimens are stratified based on the emetic potential of the chemotherapeutic medications used and differ based on treatment of acute or delayed emesis.[1] The reader is encouraged to refer to current guidelines from the National Comprehensive Cancer Network (NCCN),[49] the American Society of Clinical Oncology,[61] and the Multinational Association of Supportive Care in Cancer.[32] Despite the availability of effective means of controlling chemotherapy-induced nausea and vomiting, nausea as an adverse event is not reliably assessed,[62] nauseated patients often do not receive treatment,[11] and adherence to guidelines is often compromised by the omission of dexamethasone.[63]

Home hospice approach to selecting antiemetics

Routes of administration become an important consideration in the treatment of nausea and vomiting in home care and hospice. Nauseated or vomiting patients cannot take oral medications.

As opposed to hospital care, in the home it is often unrealistic to administer intravenous medications. Subcutaneous injections are far more practical to administer in the home setting, yet rely on patients or families to learn the skill of administration, which is similar in difficulty to that of insulin injection. Rectal medications are the mainstay of home antiemetic regimens, but are often not desired by patients and family caregivers. Oral dissolving tablets and intensols that can be absorbed sublingually are the best alternatives to rectal or parenteral administration of antiemetics.

To address these challenges, many hospices use topically applied gels of antiemetic medications, often in combination. Examples include ABR gel (Ativan, Benadryl, Reglan) and ABHR gel (Ativan, Benadryl, Haldol, Reglan). Early reports found these to be beneficial with minimal adverse effects.[64,65] A more recent study shows that when using these formulations, lorazepam and metoclopramide are not absorbed at all, and diphenhydramine is absorbed only in trace amounts.[66] In light of these findings, it appears that the benefit of antiemetic gels is attributable to placebo, with the lack of adverse effects due to the absence of absorption.

Nonpharmacological approach to nausea and vomiting

Despite the wide selection of pharmacological interventions with varying mechanisms of action, nausea and vomiting continues to be among some of the most distressing side effects of chemotherapy.[12] Even after treatment with antiemetics, the incidence of acute and delayed chemotherapy-induced nausea and vomiting has been reported to be greater than 50% and has the potential of interfering with the patient's willingness to undergo further disease-targeted treatment. In addition, anticipatory nausea and vomiting is difficult to control with pharmacological means.[30,67,68] Due to the high incidence of nausea and vomiting in certain disease populations, the physiological effects of uncontrolled symptoms, and the potential for negative effects on quality of life, understanding nonpharmacological approaches to symptom management and integrating them into usual care is appropriate.

Nonpharmacological management of nausea and vomiting in addition to antiemetics has been tested over many years.[69] One systematic review looking at these strategies for managing common chemotherapy adverse effects found that the majority of high-quality randomized controlled trials were focused on preventing or reducing the impact of nausea and vomiting or mucositis.[70] Treatments range from simple self-management techniques, complementary and alternative therapies, and in some instances palliative interventions to improve symptom management throughout disease treatment and at end of life. The use of certain nonpharmacological modalities has only recently been adopted into antiemetic guidelines and have been based on a lower level of evidence with uniform consensus that the interventions are appropriate.[32,43,68,69]

Self-management techniques

Self-management emphasizes patient autonomy in their own care and encourages patients and families to assume the responsibility of managing their condition.[71] Multiple self-management theories have been developed that acknowledge the complexity of living with chronic conditions and the importance of managing them in the context of one's everyday life rather than simply adhering to a series of prescribed orders.[72] There are a variety of potentially

---

Box 10.4 Self-management strategies for management of nausea and vomiting

Dietary modifications*

Eat smaller, more frequent meals
Reduce food aromas and other strong food odors
Avoid spicy, fatty, and highly salty foods
Premedicate with antiemetics prior to meals
Consume foods that minimize nausea and are "comfort foods"

Environmental modifications

Avoid the sight and smell of food when not hungry
Fresh air
Prepare small, attractive meals
Avoid strong or unpleasant odors
Minimize sights, sounds, or smells that can initiate nausea

Psychological strategies

Relaxation and meditation
Deep breathing
Distraction

*Limited evidence exist, but experts recommend the following dietary interventions in patients receiving chemotherapy to minimize nausea and vomiting

Sources: Tipton et al. (2007), reference 68; Lou et al. (2013), reference 71; Lee et al. (2010), reference 73.

---

useful self-management strategies that include psychological, cognitive, and behavioral modifications of care (Box 10.4)[68,71,73] and should take into account individual, health-status, and environmental factors when assessing for efficacy.[71] While many of these interventions are not currently backed by strong evidence, they are associated with little harm and should be considered when treating nausea and vomiting in advanced disease.

Complementary and alternative medicine

There has been growing interest in the use of complementary and alternative medicine (CAM) alongside curative and palliative treatments. This type of medicine refers to a wide variety of therapies that can be categorized into biological (e.g., nutrition supplements and herbal medicines) and nonbiological or behavioral (e.g., music therapy, mind-body therapies, massage) interventions.[74] Use has been associated with reduced therapy-related toxicity, improvement in disease-related symptoms, and improvement in quality of life.[68,70,73,74]

There is enough evidence in the literature to support the implementation of certain techniques for prevention and treatment of nausea and vomiting, however there is no convincing evidence favoring one method over another; rather, the effectiveness of these techniques appears to depend on individual preference. Randomized controlled trials are limited in number and sample size, stressing the urgent need for well-designed studies to test the effectiveness of particular complementary and alternative interventions for managing adverse effects of chemotherapy and disease-related symptoms.[70]

Patients should be educated to exercise caution before initiating certain complementary and alternative therapies due to the risk of drug interaction and adverse effects. The primary practitioner treating the patient's disease should be made aware of all conventional, complementary, or alternative modalities of treatment.

Biological therapies

Complementary and alternative biological therapies include nutritional supplements such as vitamin, minerals, enzymes, and antioxidants as well as herbal medicines. There have been few studies performed on these specific therapies in association with their effects on nausea and vomiting in advanced disease.[74]

An herbal remedy worth mentioning is ginger (zingiber officinale), which is a spice best known for its role as a flavoring agent for various foods. Ginger has actually been used in Ayurvedic and traditional Chinese medicine to treat GI symptoms such as nausea and excessive flatulence since the 16th century. Studies have suggested ginger's efficacy in treating postoperative nausea, motion sickness, and pregnancy-associated nausea and vomiting through a combination of antiinflammatory and antispasmodic activities.[75] Newer studies have demonstrated the use of ginger in acute and delayed chemotherapy-induced nausea and vomiting in both the pediatric and adult population, although findings and efficacy remain mixed.[75-77]

Reported adverse effects include grade two heartburn, bruising/flushing, and rash.[76] Potential adverse effects and herb-drug interactions must be understood before recommending ginger for symptom relief as the herb has been associated with increased risk of bleeding, hypoglycemia, and increased blood-levels of tacrolimus.[78]

Nonbiological therapies

A large body of literature exists regarding acupuncture and acupressure for nausea and vomiting in the palliative care setting as well as in the postoperative and gynecological population.[79] Behavioral treatments that have specifically been recommended in guidelines for the treatment of anticipatory nausea and vomiting include progressive muscle relaxation, systematic desensitization, and hypnosis.[32,43,68,70] More detail will be paid to these particular interventions with additional nonbiological complementary and alternative therapies listed in Table 10.2.[68,70,80–86]

Acupuncture and acupressure

Acupuncture is performed by trained specialists who insert fine, wire-thin needles into acupoints along a specific meridian on the body. Acupressure can be performed independent of a practitioner and differs from acupuncture in that it involves applying digital pressure or acustimulation bands, rather than needles, on designated points on the body. These techniques are thought to work by stimulating or easing energy flow. More specifically in regard to nausea and vomiting, both acupuncture and acupressure use the P6 acupoint, which is most commonly used to alleviate symptoms and is located on the anterior surface of the forearm, approximately three finger-widths away from the wrist crease.[68,73]

While acupuncture and acupressure have not been studied for symptom management in patients at end-of-life, benefits in the management of chemotherapy-induced nausea and vomiting has been documented since the 1980s.[69] Currently, these modalities are considered to be nonpharmacological strategies that have been evaluated as "likely to be effective" for the prevention, management, and treatment of chemotherapy-induced nausea and vomiting when used in conjunction with pharmacological interventions in mixed cancer types.[68] A review of the current available literature favors its use in the different stages of chemotherapy-induced nausea and vomiting, however some studies have shown no statistical difference when comparing acupressure to sham and control groups.[14,69,73,87] Mixed data on the effects of acupuncture and acupressure may also be due to the advances in antiemetics[14] and a stronger focus on symptom management as a part of standard care.[11,14]

Despite the suggested benefits of acupuncture and acupressure, the limited competency of practitioners to perform these nonpharmacological techniques and limited availability of such practitioners has prevented increased use.[1]

Progressive muscle relaxation

Progressive muscle relaxation allows individuals to respond to a stimulus that produces tension or anxiety by instead focusing on and isolating various muscle groups progressively up and down the body to induce relaxation.[70,88] Patients will first work with trained practitioners and may be given audiotapes for home practice.

This relaxation technique seems to have less of an effect on anticipatory nausea and vomiting versus postchemotherapy adverse effects.[88] In one study, the incidence of acute and delayed chemotherapy-induced nausea and vomiting was statistically lower for patients receiving progressive muscle relaxation during the first 4 days following treatment, although no difference in severity of symptoms between groups were found.[70]

Systematic desensitization

Commonly used to treat learning-based difficulties such as fears and phobias, systematic desensitization has proven particularly effective for treating anticipatory nausea and vomiting, as phobias may similarly develop through a learned-response or conditioning. The intervention works by teaching the patient how to counter a conditioned stimuli (e.g., entering the clinic, seeing the chemotherapy nurse) that normally elicits a maladaptive response (e.g., nausea and vomiting) with an incompatible response (e.g., muscle relaxation). Treatment has been documented as effective in over half of treated patients.[67,88]

Hypnosis

While hypnosis was the first psychological technique used to treat and control anticipatory nausea and vomiting, very few controlled studies have been performed.[67] Hypnosis is a behavioral intervention that teaches patients to focus their attention on thoughts or images unrelated to the actual source of distress, often using passive types of muscle relaxation and distraction. Similar to systematic desensitization, patients learn to invoke a physiological state incompatible with nausea and vomiting. This technique has been effective mostly with children and adolescents, as they may be more readily hypnotized. Overall, studies using hypnosis for anticipatory nausea and vomiting support the benefits of this intervention as it has no undesirable side effects and requires little training.[67,88]

Other nonpharmacological interventions

Malignant bowel obstruction is seen in approximately 3% of all advanced malignancies, particularly in the ovarian (5–42%) and

Table 10.2 Nonbiological complementary and alternative therapies

Technique	Description	Comments
Music therapy	◆ Performed by credentialed professionals ◆ Incorporated at any phase of illness ◆ Addresses multiple dimensions of QOL ◆ First introduced in hospice population in 1980s	◆ Likely to be effective ◆ Associated with significant reduction in severity and duration of CINV ◆ Perceived effects on autonomic nervous system ◆ Less time and energy to implement for patients ◆ No side effects
Aromatherapy	◆ Therapeutic use of essential oils primarily via inhalation of its vapors	◆ Oils such as peppermint and ginger have potential benefit of alleviating nausea and vomiting in postoperative and oncology patients ◆ Studies limited by design, small sample size, varied doses and methods
Massage	◆ Soft tissue manipulation using touch and movement ◆ Reduces stress and anxiety while promoting relaxation, which may lead to decreased heart rate, blood pressure, and respiratory rate	◆ Effectiveness not established ◆ Variability in episodes of CINV and retching in breast cancer patients
Exercise	◆ Any planned, structured, and repetitive bodily movement ◆ Incorporates cardiovascular, strength, and/or flexibility	◆ Effectiveness not established in a study looking at female breast cancer patients receiving chemotherapy
Cognitive distraction	◆ Studied in adults and children ◆ Learn to divert attention away from a threatening situation and toward relaxing sensations ◆ Uses videos, games, puzzles, counting objects, deep breathing	◆ No side effects ◆ Associated with decreased ANV and post chemotherapy distress

QOL = quality of life; CINV = chemotherapy-induced nausea and vomiting; ANV = anticipatory nausea and vomiting.

Sources: Tipton et al. (2007), reference 68; Lofti-Jam et al. (2008), reference 70; Karagozoglu et al. (2012), reference 80; Mahon and Mahon (2011), reference 81; Gallagher (2011), reference 82; Pawuk and Schumacher (2010), reference 83; Bourdeanu et al. (2011), reference 84; Lua and Zakaria (2012), reference 85; Sturgeon et al. (2009), reference 86.

colorectal (10–28%) cancer population with nausea, vomiting, and pain often reported.[1,9,89] Due to the potential of worsening symptom burden and impacting quality of life up until death, potential palliative interventions to treat these types of obstructions have been studied. In one review, the authors recommend that patients admitted to hospital with symptomatic malignant bowel obstruction be offered at least one of the following interventions during admission: surgery, stenting, decompression, percutaneous gastrostomy tube, nasogastric tube, or octreotide.[1]

One retrospective study looked at 94 patients with ovarian carcinoma who received percutaneous endoscopic gastrostomy (PEG) tube placement for malignant bowel obstruction over a 7-year time period. Mean age at time of placement was 56 years, and 97% had stage III or IV disease. All percutaneous endoscopic gastrostomy tubes were successfully placed using conscious sedation with 91% achieving symptomatic relief of nausea and vomiting between 0 and 3 days following placement. Median overall survival after placement was 8 weeks, and 85% of patients died either at home or under hospice care.[89] In a study looking at stage IV colorectal cancer patients, 94% of patients achieved relief of nausea and vomiting within 30 days of a palliative surgical or endoscopic procedure for malignant bowel obstruction, and median overall survival was 8.1 months.[90]

Choosing to proceed with invasive interventions should only be done if in line with the patient's treatment goals and preferences and should be reserved for those who are well enough and likely to benefit. In cases where these nonpharmacological approaches are not warranted or desired, it is important to understand the pharmacological and nonpharmacological options available to alleviate nausea, vomiting, and pain at the end of life.[9]

Nursing interventions

Palliative care is by definition active total care; thus, it is essential that nurses have a proactive attitude toward assessing and promptly relieving nausea and vomiting for patients under their care. The NCCN palliative care guidelines recommend aggressive symptom management, clarification of the intent of treatments, anticipation of the needs of patients and their families, and involvement of the caregivers in the treatment process when appropriate.[43]

As discussed in this chapter, the NCCN guidelines emphasize the need for ongoing assessment of symptoms, therapeutic interventions, and measurement of their outcomes. The palliative care nurse plays a crucial role in this aspect of care and is instrumental in promoting a collaborative approach among team members caring for their patients. Nurses in various treatment settings should be aware of the advances in the management of nausea and vomiting, changes to relevant treatment guidelines, and potential side effects of treatments being administered.[40,84]

Just as vital is the role that the patient and caregivers play in managing nausea and vomiting from disease or disease treatment. Oncology patients have reported high information needs regarding self-management of treatment adverse effects.[70] As active participants in their own care, they must be provided with the education and tools needed to confidently practice targeted symptom management and overall self-care. Personalized education plans with additional resources, including those found online,[91] can further assist patients understand how to implement the prescribed plan of care once at home. Education must include when and why to take certain antiemetics, as patients may be given multiple agents, and when to escalate symptom reporting to care providers.

For chemotherapy-induced nausea and vomiting, acute phases are usually assessed and managed in the inpatient or outpatient setting, however many patients are left to independently manage delayed nausea and vomiting, which can last up to five days post treatment. Individual characteristics may prevent patients from taking prescribed medications such as financial concerns, cost of medication, disbelief in treatment effectiveness, and perceived side effects to medication such as constipation or sedation. Likewise, certain patients may not report uncontrolled symptoms due to fear of being a "bad patient" or the perception that this is a normal part of cancer treatment.[40,68,84,91,92]

Sitting down with the patient to address their overall environment, fears, and concerns is crucial to ensure that the steps to adequately control nausea and vomiting are achieved. Referring patients to other providers and resources such as palliative care specialists, case managers, or social workers should also be considered.

Case study

Ms. SM, a 44-year-old woman with ovarian cancer

Ms. SM, a 44-year-old woman with a history of advanced ovarian cancer, is admitted to an inpatient hospice unit due to worsening nausea and vomiting, increasing abdominal distention, and escalating abdominal pain over the last 3 days. The patient has not tolerated any oral intake due to her symptoms in the last 24 hours. Vomiting occurs immediately after any oral intake now and even without oral intake she vomits greenish material several times a day. She also feels severe fatigue and admits to feeling depressed and anxious. Upon more thorough evaluation by the hospice intake nurse, the patient explains her pain is crampy and intermittent and worse when she had attempted oral intake. The abdominal pain is a 7 out of 10 most of the time but when she has spasms of pain it becomes a 10 out of 10 but the patient finds the nausea and vomiting to be the most distressing.

Previous to this acute episode, although unable to ambulate, SM was satisfied with her symptom management and quality of life. She has a teenage son and although she was honest with her son in discussing her disease stage and limited prognosis she feels her son and she herself are not ready for imminent death. She is quite upset that her son had to see her vomiting so much while at home. Medications include 100-mcg Fentanyl transdermal patch changed yesterday and concentrated oral morphine elixir for breakthrough discomfort. Because the taste and smell of the medication worsened the nausea and vomiting she has not taken breakthrough morphine in two days. She is also on four tablets of senna/docusate laxatives but has not taken either and instead used bisacodyl suppositories daily without effect. Her last bowel movement was five days ago and she normally goes every other day. Prochlorperazine suppositories have not relieved the nausea and vomiting. The patient would like treatment so that she can be well enough to go home for a few more days.

On exam she is profoundly cachectic and jaundiced appearing. She is mildly confused but can give a history. She is tachycardic, has diminished lung sounds in the bases, and on abdominal exam she is found to have a large amount of ascites. Given the goals of care patient had an abdominal X-ray, which revealed fecal impaction. She was treated with haloperidol 0.5 mg intravenous every 8 hours around-the-clock and metoclopramide 10 mg intravenous every 6 hours as needed after she was manually disimpacted. Fentanyl was continued, and she was placed on parenteral morphine 5 mg intravenous every 1 hour for breakthrough pain. She also had an ultrasound-guided paracentesis then went home in 3 days feeling much better. Before leaving she discussed with the team that she knows this is her last rally.

Her biggest fear is dying with great suffering associated with unrelenting vomiting and pain. The loss of control and her perception that she will lose her dignity from unrelenting vomiting is particularly an issue of concern to her. At this time there is a thoughtful discussion with members of the hospice team and palliative sedation was discussed and the patient expressed great satisfaction knowing that even at the very end of life she would have some control. After 2 weeks the patient is readmitted to the hospice unit, but she has declined precipitously and is vomiting bilious fluid continually. Her abdomen has become even more distended than on her prior admission. She is not able to communicate, so her 17-year-old son and her older sister are making decisions based on her wishes. The presentation is consistent with bowel obstruction related to her ovarian cancer. She is started on parental haloperidol for nausea and vomiting and her hypoactive delirium. Octreotide 100 mcg subcutaneous every 6 hours is started to help decrease her bowel secretions and vomiting, but the vomiting is unrelenting. The patient appears to be dying on this admission so she is sedated with lorazepam and dies peacefully the next night.

Conclusion

A major goal of palliative care is to improve quality of life by addressing suffering in all its dimensions. Remember that the most significant cost of inadequately controlled nausea and vomiting is patient suffering.[40] It can be difficult for nurses to meet the challenge of providing high quality palliative care when there is a limited evidence base for interventions used routinely. Multiple studies and reviews have highlighted the need for more rigorous research on the management of nausea and vomiting, particularly in patients at the end of life and within the noncancer population. Nonetheless, vigilant assessment, appropriate use and evaluation of pharmacological and nonpharmacological interventions, and appropriate patient and family education and support may avert the need for unnecessary interventions at end-of-life and allow for quality of life throughout the disease trajectory up until death and through bereavement. Nausea and vomiting profoundly affect all aspects of a person's well-being. Adequately managing these symptoms, especially at end-of-life, is essential.

References

1. Naeim A, Dy SM, Lorenz KA, Sanati H, Walling A, Asch SM. Evidence-based recommendations for cancer nausea and vomiting. J Clin Oncol. 2008;26:3903–3910.
2. Abernethy AP, Wheeler JL, Zafar SY. Detailing of gastrointestinal symptoms in cancer patients with advanced disease: new

methodologies, new insights, and a proposed approach. Curr Opin Support Palliat Care. 2009;3:41–49.

3. Kim JE, Dodd MJ, Aouizerat BE, Jahan T, Miaskowski C. A review of the prevalence and impact of multiple symptoms in oncology patients. J Pain Symptom Manage. 2009;37: 715.

4. Brearley SG, Clements CV, Molassiotis A. A review of patient self-report tools for chemotherapy-induced nausea and vomiting. Support Care Cancer. 2008;16:1213–1229.

5. van den Beuken-van Everdingen MHJ, de Rijke JM, Kessels AG, Schouten HC, van Kleef M, Patijn J. Quality of life and non-pain symptoms in patients with cancer. J Pain Symptom Manage. 2009;38: 216–233.

6. Rhodes VA, McDaniel RW. Nausea, vomiting, and retching: complex problems in palliative care. CA Cancer J Clin. 2001;51:232–248.

7. Janssen DJA, Spruit MA, Wouters EFM, Schols JMGA. Daily symptom burden in end-stage chronic organ failure: A systematic review. Palliat Med. 2008;22:938–948.

8. Brandt HE, Ooms ME, Deliens L, van der Wal G, Ribbe MW. The last two days of life of nursing home patients: a nationwide study on causes of death and burdensome symptoms in the Netherlands. Palliat Med. 2006;20:533–540.

9. Glare P, Miller J, Nikolova T, et al. Treating nausea and vomiting in palliative care: a review. Clin Interv Aging. 2011;6:243–259.

10. Teunissen SC, Wesker W, Kruitwagen C, de Haes HC, Voest EE, de Graeff A. Symptom prevalence in patients with incurable cancer: a systematic review. J Pain Symptom Manage. 2007;34:94–104.

11. Greaves J, Glare P, Kristjanson LJ, Stockler M, Tattersall MH. Undertreatment of nausea and other symptoms in hospitalized cancer patients. Support Care Cancer. 2009;17:461–464.

12. Halawi R, Aldin ES, Baydoun A, et al. Physical symptom profile for adult cancer inpatients at a Lebanese cancer unit. Eur J Intern Med. 2012;23:e185–e189.

13. Jordan K, Gralla R, Jahn F, Molassiotis A. International antiemetic guidelines on chemotherapy induced nausea and vomiting (CINV): content and implementation in daily routine practice. Eur J Pharmacol. 2014;722:197–202.

14. Lee J, Dodd M, Dibble S, Abrams D. Review of acupressure studies for chemotherapy-induced nausea and vomiting control. J Pain Symptom Manage. 2008;36(5):529–544.

15. Kirkova J, Rybicki L, Walsh D, Aktas A. Symptom prevalence in advanced cancer age, gender, and performance status interactions. Am J Hosp Palliat Care. 2012;29:139–145.

16. Yamagishi A, Morita T, Miyashita M, Kimura F. Symptom prevalence and longitudinal follow-up in cancer outpatients receiving chemotherapy. J Pain Symptom Manage. 2009;37:823–830.

17. Seow H, Barbera L, Sutradhar R, Howell D, Dudgeon D, Atzema C, Liu Y, Husain A, Sussman J, Earle C. Trajectory of performance status and symptom scores for patients with cancer during the last six months of life. J Clin Oncol. 2011;29:1151–1158.

18. Harris DG. Nausea and vomiting in advanced cancer. Br Med Bull. 2010;96:175–185.

19. Price MA, Bell ML, Sommeijer DW, et al. Physical symptoms, coping styles and quality of life in recurrent ovarian cancer: a prospective population-based study over the last year of life. Gynecol Oncol. 2013;130(1):162–168.

20. Solano JP, Gomes B, Higginson IJ. A comparison of symptom prevalence in far advanced cancer, AIDS, heart disease, chronic obstructive pulmonary disease and renal disease. J Pain Symptom Manage. 2006;31:58–69.

21. Wajnberg A, Ornstein K, Zhang M, Smith KL, Soriano T. Symptom burden in chronically ill homebound individuals. J Am Geriatr Soc. 2013;61:126–131.

22. Gonzales MJ, Widera E. Nausea and other nonpain symptoms in long-term care. Clin Geriatr Med. 2011;27:213–228.

23. Rodriguez KL, Hanlon JT, Perera S, Jaffe EJ, Sevick MA. A cross-sectional analysis of the prevalence of undertreatment of nonpain symptoms and factors associated with undertreatment in older nursing home hospice/palliative care patients. Am J Geriatr Pharmacother. 2010;8:225–232.

24. Duncan JG, Bott MJ, Thompson SA, Gajewski BJ. Symptom occurrence and associated clinical factors in nursing home residents with cancer. Res Nurs Health. 2009;32:453–464.

25. Hanson LC, Eckert JK, Dobbs D, Williams CS, Caprio AJ, Sloane PD, Zimmerman S. Symptom experience of dying long-term care residents. J Am Geriatr Soc. 2008;56:91–98.

26. Agrawal RK, Khakurel S, Hada R, Shrestha D, Baral A. Acute intradialytic complications in end stage renal disease on maintenance hemodialysis. J Nepal Med Assoc. 2012;52:118–121.

27. Gamondi C, Galli N, Schonholzer C, et al. Frequency and severity of pain and symptom distress among patients with chronic kidney disease receiving dialysis. Swiss Med Wkly. 2013;143:w13750.

28. Murtagh FE, Addington-Hall J, Edmonds P, et al. Symptoms in the month before death for stage 5 chronic kidney disease patients managed without dialysis. J Pain Symptom Manage. 2010;40:342–352.

29. Rangwala F, Zafar SY, Abernathy AP. Gastrointestinal symptoms in cancer patients with advanced disease: new methodologies, insights, and a proposed approach. Curr Opin Support Palliat Care. 2012;6(1):69–76.

30. Farrell C, Brearley SG, Pilling M, Molassiotis A. The impact of chemotherapy-related nausea on patients' nutritional status, psychological distress and quality of life. Support Care Cancer. 2013;21: 59–66.

31. Glare PA, Dunwoodie D, Clark K, et al. Treatment of nausea and vomiting in terminally ill cancer patients. Drugs. 2008;68:2575–2590.

32. Roila F, Herrstedt J, Aapro M, Gralla RJ, Einhorn LH, Ballatori E, et al. Guideline update for MASCC and ESMO in the prevention of chemotherapy- and radiotherapy-induced nausea and vomiting: results of the Perugia consensus conference. Ann Oncol. 2010;Suppl 5;v232–v243.

33. Cheung WY, Le LW, Zimmermann C. Symptom clusters in patients with advanced cancers. Support Care Cancer. 2009;17:1223–1230.

34. Mannix KA. Palliation of nausea and vomiting. In: Hanks G, Cherny N, Christakis NA (eds.), Oxford Textbook of Palliative Medicine. 4th ed. New York: Oxford University Press; 2011:801–812.

35. Wood GJ, Shega JW, Lynch B, et al. Management of intractable nausea and vomiting in patients at the end of life: "I was feeling nauseous all of the time. . . nothing was working." JAMA. 2007;298(10):1196–1207.

36. Grunberg SM, Dugan M, Muss H, et al. Effectiveness of a single-day three-drug regimen of dexamethasone, palonosetron, and aprepitant for the prevention of acute and delayed nausea and vomiting caused by moderately emetogenic chemotherapy. Support Care Cancer. 2009;17:589–594.

37. Nausea, Vomiting (emesis), Constipation, and Bowel Obstruction in Advanced Cancer. National Cancer Institute. http://www.cancer.gov/cancertopics/pdq/supportivecare/nausea/HealthProfessional/page7. Published May 2, 2013. Accessed June 2013.

38. Gordon P, LeGrand SB, Walsh D. Nausea and vomiting in advanced cancer. Eur J Pharmacol. European Journal of Pharmacology. 2014;;722:187–191.

39. Stephenson J, Davies A. An assessment of aetiology-based guidelines for the management of nausea and vomiting in patients with advanced cancer. Support Care Cancer. 2006;14:348–353.

40. Viale PH, Moore S, Grande C. Efficacy and Cost: Avoiding Undertreatment of Chemotherapy-Induced Nausea and Vomiting. Clin J Oncol Nurs. 2012;16(4):E133–E141.

41. Glare P, Pereira G, Kristjanson LJ, Stockler M, Tattersall M. Systematic review of the efficacy of antiemetics in the treatment of nausea in patients with far-advanced cancer. Support Care Cancer. 2004;2:432–440.

42. Rhondali W, Yennurajalingam S, Chisholm G, Ferrer J, Kim SH, Kang JH, Filbet M, Bruera E. Predictors of response to palliative care intervention for chronic nausea in advanced cancer outpatients. Support Care Cancer. 2013 April 16. Epub ahead of print. doi: 10.1007/s00520-013-1805-8

43. National Comprehensive Cancer Network. NCCN Clinical Practice Guidelines in Oncology: Palliative Care. Version 2.2013. http://www.

nccn.org/professionals/physician_gls/pdf/palliative.pdf. Updated June 5, 2013. Accessed June 15, 2013.

44. Shoemaker L, Estfan B, Induru R, Walsh TD. Symptom management: an important part of cancer care. Cleve Clin J Med. 2011;78(1):25–34.

45. Meek R, Kelly AM, Hu XF. Use of the visual analog scale to rate and monitor severity of nausea in the emergency department. Acad Emerg Med. 2009;16:1304–1310.

46. Martin A, Pearson J, Cai B, et al. Assessing the impact of chemotherapy-induced nausea and vomiting on patients' daily lives: a modified version of the Functional Living Index-Emesis (FLIE) with 5-day recall. Support Care Cancer. 2003;11(8):522–527.

47. Cheung WY, Zimmermann C. Pharmacologic management of cancer-related pain, dyspnea, and nausea. Semin Oncol. 2011;38:450–459.

48. Davis MP, Hallerberg G. A systematic review of the treatment of nausea and/or vomiting in cancer unrelated to chemotherapy or radiation. J Pain Symptom Manage. 2010;39(4):756–767.

49. National Comprehensive Cancer Network. NCCN Clinical Practice Guidelines in Oncology: Antiemesis. Version 1.2013. http://www.nccn.org/professionals/physician_gls/pdf/antiemesis.pdf. Updated December 06, 2012. Accessed June 20, 2013.

50. LeGrand SB, Walsh D. Scopolamine for cancer-related nausea and vomiting. J Pain Symptom Manage. 2010;40:136–141.

51. Hardy JR, O'Shea A, White C, Gilshenan K, Welch L, Douglas C. The efficacy of haloperidol in the management of nausea and vomiting in patients with cancer. J Pain Symptom Manage. 2010;40:111–116.

52. Keeley PW. Nausea and vomiting in people with cancer and other chronic diseases. Clin Evid (Online). 2009;01:2406.

53. Lindqvist O, Lundquist G, Dickman A, et al. Four essential drugs needed for quality care of the dying: a Delphi-study based international expert consensus opinion. J Palliat Med. 2013;16:38–43.

54. Dorman S, Perkins P. Droperidol for treatment of nausea and vomiting in palliative care patients. Cochrane Database Syst Rev. 2010;CD006938.

55. Perkins P, Dorman S. Haloperidol for the treatment of nausea and vomiting in palliative care patients. Cochrane Database Syst Rev. 2009;CD006271.

56. Darvill E, Dorman S, Perkins P. Levomepromazine for nausea and vomiting in palliative care. Cochrane Database Syst Rev. 2013;4:CD009420.

57. Vig S, Selbert L, Green MR. Olanzapine is effective for refractory chemotherapy-induced nausea and vomiting irrespective of chemotherapy emetogenicity. J Cancer Res Clin Oncol. 2013 Oct 31. Epub ahead of print. doi: 10.1007/s00432-013-1540-z.

58. Schwartzberg L, Barbour SY, Morrow GR, et al. Pooled analysis of phase III clinical studies of palonosetron versus ondansetron, dolasetron, and granisetron in the prevention of chemotherapy-induced nausea and vomiting (CINV). Support Care Cancer. 2013 Oct 19. Epub ahead of print. doi: 10.1007/s00520-013-1999-9.

59. Ripamonti CI. Malignant bowel obstruction: tailoring treatment to individual patients. J Support Oncol. 2008;6(3):114–115.

60. Mercadante S, Porzio G. Octreotide for malignant bowel obstruction: twenty years after. Crit Rev Oncol Hematol. 2012;83:388–392.

61. Basch E, Prestrud AA, Hesketh PJ, Kris MG, Feyer PC, Somerfield MR, et al. Antiemetics: American society of clinical oncology clinical practice guideline update. J Clin Oncol. 2011;29:4189–4198.

62. Atkinson TM, Yuelin Li Y, Coffey CW, et al. Reliability of adverse symptom event reporting by clinicians. Qual Life Res. 2012;21:1159–1164.

63. Koch S, Wein A, Siebler J, et al. Antiemetic prophylaxis and frequency of chemotherapy-induced nausea and vomiting in palliative first-line treatment of colorectal cancer patients: the Northern Bavarian IVOPAK I Project. Support Care Cancer 2013;21(9):2395–2402.

64. Weschules DJ. Tolerability of the compound ABHR in hospice patients. J Palliat Med. 2005;8:1135–1143.

65. Bleicher J, Bhaskara A, Huyck T, Constantino S, Bardia A, Loprinzi CL, Silberstein PT. Lorazepam, diphenhydramine, and haloperidol transdermal gel for rescue from chemotherapy-induced nausea/vomiting: results of two pilot trials. J Support Oncol. 2008;6:27–32.

66. Smith TJ, Ritter JK, Poklis JL, Fletcher D, Coyne PJ, Dodson P, Parker G. ABH gel is not absorbed from the skin of normal volunteers. J Pain Symptom Manage. 2012;43:961–966.

67. Roscoe JA, Morrow GR, Aapro MS, Molassiotis A, Oliver I. Anticipatory nausea and vomiting. Support Care Cancer. 2011;19:1533–1538.

68. Tipton JM, McDaniel RW, Barbour L, et al. Putting evidence into practice: evidence-based interventions to prevent, manage, and treat chemotherapy-induced nausea and vomiting. Clin J Oncol Nurs. 2007;11(1):69–78.

69. Molassiotis A, Russell W, Hughes J, et al. The effectiveness of acupressure for the control and management of chemotherapy-related acute and delayed nausea: a randomized controlled trial. J Pain Sympt Manage. 2014;47(1):12–25.

70. Lofti-Jam K, Carey M, Jefford M, et al. Non-pharmacologic strategies for managing common chemotherapy adverse effects: a systematic review. J Clin Oncol. 2008;26(34):5619–5629.

71. Lou Y, Yates P, McCarthy A, Wang HM. Self-management of chemotherapy-related nausea and vomiting: a cross-sectional survey of Chinese cancer patients. Cancer Nurs. 2013;00(0):1–13.

72. Grey M, Knafl K, McCorkle R. A framework for the study of self- and family management of chronic conditions. Nurs Outlook. 2006;54(5):278–286.

73. Lee J, Dibble S, Dodd M, Abrams D, Burns B. The relationship of chemotherapy-induced nausea to the frequency of pericardium 6 digital acupressure. Oncol Nurs Forum. 2010;37(6): E419-E425. DOI: 10.1188/10.ONF.E419-E425.

74. Oh B, Butow P, Mullan B, et al. The use and perceived benefits resulting from the use of complementary and alternative medicine by cancer patients in Australia. Asia Pac J Clin Oncol. 2010;6:342–349.

75. Hickok JT, Roscoe JA, Morrow GR, Ryan JL. A phase II/III randomized, placebo-controlled, double-blind clinical trial of ginger (zingiber officinale) for nausea caused by chemotherapy for cancer: a currently accruing URCC CCOP cancer control study. Support Cancer Ther. 2007;4(4):247–250.

76. Ryan JL, Heckler CE, Roscoe JA, et al. Ginger (zingiber officinale) reduces acute chemotherapy-induced nausea: a URCC CCOP study of 576 patients. Support Care Cancer. 2012;20:1479–1489.

77. Pillai AK, Sharma KK, Gupta YK, Bakhshi S. Anti-emetic effect of ginger powder versus placebo as an add-on therapy in children and young adults receiving high emetogenic chemotherapy. Pediatr Blood Cancer. 2011;56:234–238.

78. Memorial Sloan-Kettering Cancer Center. Integrative Medicine: Ginger. Memorial Sloan-Kettering Cancer Center. http://www.mskcc.org/cancer-care/herb/ginger. Updated October 8, 2012. Accessed June 29, 2013.

79. Cassell EJ, Rich BA. Intractable end-of-life suffering and the ethics of palliative sedation. Pain Med. 2010;11(3):435–438.

80. Karagozoglu S, Tekyasar F, Yilmaz FA. Effects of music therapy and guided visual imagery on chemotherapy-induced anxiety and nausea-vomiting. J Clin Nurs. 2012;22:39–50.

81. Mahon EM, Mahon SM. Music therapy: a valuable adjunct in the oncology setting. Clin J Oncol Nurs. 2011;15(4):353–356.

82. Gallagher LM. The role of music therapy in palliative medicine and supportive care. Semin Oncol. 2011;38(3):403–406.

83. Pawuk LG, Schumacher JE. Introducing music therapy in hospice and palliative care: an overview of one hospice's experience. Home Healthc Nurse. 2010;28(1):37–44.

84. Bourdeanu L, Twardowski P, Pal SK. Nursing considerations with pazopanib therapy: focus on metastatic renal cell carcinoma. Clin J Oncol Nurs. 2011;15(5):513–517.

85. Lua PL, Zakaria NS. A brief review of current scientific evidence involving aromatherapy use for nausea and vomiting. J Altern Complement Med. 2012;18(6):534–540.

86. Sturgeon M, Wetta-Hall R, Hart T, Good M, Dakhil S. Effects of therapeutic massage on the quality of life among patients with breast cancer during treatment. J Altern Complement Med. 2009;15(4):373–380.

87. Chao LF, Zhang AL, Liu HE, Cheng MH, Lam HB, Lo SK. The efficacy of acupoint stimulation for the management of therapy-related adverse

events in patients with breast cancer: a systematic review. Breast Cancer Res Treat. 2009;118:255–267.

88. Figueroa-Moseley C, Jean-Pierre P, Roscoe JA, et al. Behavioral interventions in treating anticipatory nausea and vomiting. J Natl Compr Canc Netw. 2007;5(1):44–50.

89. Pothuri B, Montemarano M, Gerardi M, et al. Percutaneous endoscopic gastrostomy tube placement in patients with malignant bowel obstruction due to ovarian carcinoma. Gynecol Oncol. 2005;96:330–334.

90. Dalal KM, Gollub MJ, Miner TJ, et al. Management of patients with malignant bowel obstruction and stage IV colorectal cancer. J Palliat Med. 2011;14(7):822–828.

91. Thompson N. Optimizing treatment outcomes in patients at risk for chemotherapy-induced nausea and vomiting. Clin J Oncol Nurs. 2012;16(3):309–313.

92. Hawkins B, Grunberg S. Chemotherapy-induced nausea and vomiting: challenges and opportunities for improved patient outcomes. Clin J Oncol Nurs. 2009. 13(1):54–64.

CHAPTER 11

Dysphagia, xerostomia, and hiccups

Constance M. Dahlin and Audrey Kurash Cohen

Dysphagia

Case study

RS, a patient with dementia and recurrent strokes

RS is an 87-year-old woman with a history of stroke and dementia, admitted to the hospital with mental status changes, worsening confusion, and speaking difficulty. She lives at their longtime home with her husband, who provides increasing care. Although able to ambulate, RS has become unable to perform activities of daily living such as bathing, dressing, and feeding without assistance and she had become increasingly forgetful and confused. She has been eating less food at meals, requires more assistance to eat, and has lost 20 pounds over the last year. A stroke that occurred 10 years ago impaired her right side, resulting in aphasia, affecting her ability to communicate and to swallow. The nurse focused on her swallowing difficulty because RS displayed inconsistent periods of wakefulness, drooling, and a wet cough. She requested a formal swallowing evaluation. In the meantime, both a nasogastric tube and intravenous catheter were temporarily placed to provide RS with medications and hydration.

The speech-language pathologist (SLP) completed a swallowing assessment, which demonstrated oropharyngeal dysphagia and aspiration. Given her baseline dementia, advanced age, reduced ability to self-feed, and declining swallowing ability, it was concluded that RS had an increased risk for aspiration pneumonia. The SLP recommended modifications to food texture and liquid consistencies. A family meeting was planned to discuss the best management and a plan of care that focused on quality of life.

In her advance directive, RS had clearly stated she wanted, "no extraordinary or life prolonging measures such as a breathing machine or stomach tubes." The family and team collaborated on a plan, acknowledging the inherent risks of pulmonary infection, dehydration, and malnutrition. Given the patient's stated wishes, there was unanimous agreement to forego artificial nutrition and hydration. Rather, the emphasis would be focusing on quality of life and allowing continued oral nutrition, while trying to minimize aspiration. The nasogastric tube was removed. The SLP and the nurse met with RS's husband and son to demonstrate safe feeding techniques, ways to maximize intake, and oral care prior to her discharge.

Definition

Dysphagia is defined as difficulty swallowing food or liquid. Swallowing impairments can threaten the safety and efficiency with which oral alimentation is maintained. Chronic difficulty swallowing can be both frustrating and frightening for patients. Because nutrition is compromised, generalized weakness, diminished appetite, and weight loss or malnutrition may ensue. Aspiration may also occur, causing pneumonia, fevers, malaise, shortness of breath and, rarely, death.

The psychological impact of dysphagia cannot be underestimated. Its development may be a pivotal symptom that prompts changing the goals of care to a more palliative nature.[1] Life is not compatible with absence of fluid intake. Thus, when the patient can neither drink, nor eat, nor receive artificial nutrition and hydration, death becomes more imminent.[2] The challenge in palliative care in managing dysphagia is how to ensure comfort, even at the expense of optimal nutrition and hydration.

Physiology and pathophysiology of swallowing

Normal swallowing

Understanding the physiology of normal and aberrant swallowing is critical to meeting the challenge of caring for the patient with dysphagia. Swallowing, an extremely complex physiological act, involves the passage of food or liquid from the oral cavity through the esophagus and into the stomach, where the process of digestion begins. It requires exquisite timing and coordination of more than 30 pairs of muscles under both voluntary and involuntary nervous system control.[3] Because humans swallow hundreds of times per day and are largely unaware of the activity, it is remarkable that difficulties do not occur more frequently.

The act of swallowing takes less than 20 seconds from the moment of bolus propulsion into the pharynx until the bolus reaches the stomach. For purposes of discussion, the act of swallowing is divided into three stages: the oral stage, the pharyngeal stage, and the esophageal stage (Figure 11.1). In reality, these stages occur simultaneously, with some melding and overlap of events.

The first stage of swallowing (see Figure 11.1), the oral stage, is responsible for readying the bolus (ball of food or liquid) for swallowing.[5,6] The oral cavity comprises the area extending from the lips anteriorly to the hard palate superiorly, the pharyngeal wall posteriorly, and bounded by the floor of the mouth inferiorly. The duration of the oral stage is variable, depending on the viscosity or consistency of the food bolus and individual chewing styles. Bolus preparation is under voluntary control and can be halted or changed at any point. It is during this stage that one takes pleasure

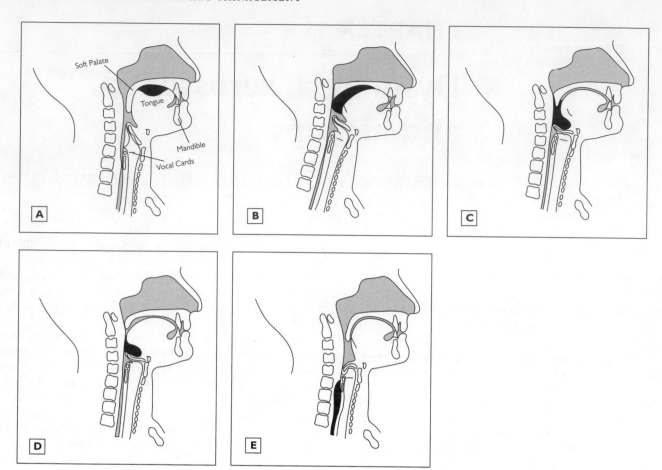

Figure 11.1 Stages of swallowing, beginning with voluntary initiation of the swallow by the tongue (A), oral transit (B), pharyngeal stage of swallowing with airway protection (C) and (D), and esophageal stage (E). Source: Logemann (1998), reference 4.

from the flavor and texture of food through the chemoreceptors of the tongue and palate.

The bolus must be partitioned and masticated into smaller portions and moistened by saliva. Sensory receptors within the oral cavity assist in mediating saliva production, as well as determining the chewing force and the configuration of the oral cavity to accommodate the bolus type and size.[3] The tongue gathers particles from the sulci of the cheek and the floor of the mouth, and prevents food from falling out of the oral cavity anteriorly, or from spilling into the pharynx posteriorly.[4] Once the bolus is formed, it is positioned on the tongue and propelled backward into the pharynx by contraction of the tongue and floor of mouth muscles. The soft palate elevates to prevent nasal regurgitation.

The second stage of swallowing, the pharyngeal stage (see Figure 11.1), lasts approximately 1 second. This stage is the most complex, requiring precise timing and coordination. The biomechanical events involved in the pharyngeal stage of swallowing are under involuntary control. They are carefully sequenced in a pattern controlled by the central swallowing center in the brainstem—the medulla. In the medulla, sensory feedback continually modulates the motor response. If this sensory feedback loop is disrupted, the onset of the pharyngeal stage of swallowing may be delayed or, in severe cases, absent.[4–6]

Anatomically, the pharyngeal stage is elicited as the posterior tongue retracts and descends, sending the bolus over the back of the tongue. The bolus is moved through the pharynx via pharyngeal muscles that progressively contract and by pressure generated from the base of the tongue contacting the pharyngeal walls. This bolus passage must be coordinated with closure of the airway and opening of the esophagus. The process of airway protection, or closure of the larynx, is quite remarkable and intricate, requiring three levels of closure to occur: epiglottic inversion at the entrance to the larynx, closure of the true vocal folds, and closure of the false vocal folds. These events occur in order to expel any material that may have entered the laryngeal vestibule, as well as prevent further material from entering.[3] During the pharyngeal stage, respiration ceases on average of 1 second for a single sip of liquid with swallowing generally occurring during expiration.

The upper esophageal sphincter (UES) separates the pharynx from the esophagus, prevents air from entering the esophagus, and prevents esophageal contents from reentering into the pharynx.[7] The opening of the UES occurs as muscles contract to pull the larynx upward and forward.[8]

The esophageal stage or final stage of swallowing (see Figure 11.1) is the longest phase and involves transport of the bolus from the upper esophageal segment, through the lower esophageal segment, and into the stomach, a distance of approximately 25 cm.[4,9] Like the pharyngeal phase of swallowing, the esophageal stage is under involuntary neuromuscular control. However, the speed of propagation of the bolus is much slower through the esophagus, with a rate of 3 to 4 cm/s compared with 12 cm/s in the pharynx.[10]

The upper portion of the esophagus consists of striated skeletal muscle, with the outer fibers arranged longitudinally and the inner fibers arranged in a circular configuration. As the bolus reaches the esophagus, the outer muscles first contract, followed by the circular fibers, which constitutes the primary peristaltic wave. The lower portions of the esophagus are composed of smooth muscle fibers. The primary peristaltic wave carries the bolus through the LES in a series of relaxation-contraction waves. A secondary peristaltic wave is generated where the striated muscle meets the smooth muscle and clears the esophagus of residue.[5,7] After passage of the bolus, the LES contracts to its resting, closed state to contain the gastric contents within the stomach.[10,11]

Pathophysiology of oropharyngeal dysphagia

Difficulty swallowing can occur during, within, or across any of the above-described stages, depending on the underlying disease. It is helpful to conceptualize the bolus transfer process according to a piston-chamber model proposed by McConnell et al.,[12] while at the same time being aware that the pressure differential that is generated in the pharynx and throughout the esophagus also works to propel the bolus.[3]

The tongue acts as the piston that creates pressure on the bolus to drive it into the esophagus. The ability of the oral cavity to fulfill its function as a closed chamber depends on the integrity of a number of muscular contractions, which form valves that open and close and are illustrated in Figure 11.2.

Bolus flow is affected by dysfunction in the chamber or the piston. If the chamber leaks, residue, regurgitation, or aspiration may occur. Inefficient bolus flow may result from weakness

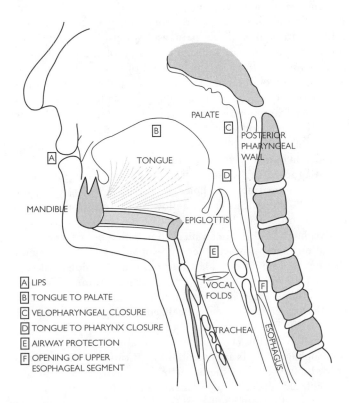

Figure 11.2 Valves of the oral cavity illustrating twin function.

PALATE

POSTERIOR PHARYNGEAL WALL

TONGUE

MANDIBLE

EPIGLOTTIS

VOCAL FOLDS

TRACHEA

ESOPHAGUS

A LIPS
B TONGUE TO PALATE
C VELOPHARYNGEAL CLOSURE
D TONGUE TO PHARYNX CLOSURE
E AIRWAY PROTECTION
F OPENING OF UPPER ESOPHAGEAL SEGMENT

in the tongue-driving force on the bolus, reduced contraction of the pharynx, or reduced excursion of the hyolaryngeal complex. This may cause loss of control over the bolus, and/or incomplete laryngeal closure, which allows the bolus to enter into the airway while it is open known as aspiration. Patients with muscle weakness due to stroke, degenerative neuromuscular disease, or neoplastic lesions involving motor and sensory function of the lips and face may experience difficulty containing the bolus in the oral cavity. Patients with severe dementia who are not aware of food in their mouth may fail to close their lips. Patients with Parkinson's disease or Amyotrophic Lateral Sclerosis (ALS) may experience lingual or facial weakness. In cases of reduced oral or lingual sensation, pocketed food may remain in the oral cavity for several hours, possibly increasing the risk of aspiration. Nasal regurgitation of liquids and particles of solids occurs when the velopharyngeal port is dysfunctional, such as in palate cancer where treatment involves resection, and in patients with progressive neuromuscular disease.

Valving of the larynx during the swallow is important for prevention of aspiration into the trachea, not only during oropharyngeal swallowing but also during periods of gastroesophageal reflux, regurgitation, or emesis. Failure of the larynx to close due to timing or muscular incompetence can result in aspiration. Reduced sensory function and weakened laryngeal musculature impair expectoration of aspirated material. Failure of the upper esophagus to open completely results in residue in the pyriform sinuses superior to the pharyngoesophageal segment and, if abundant, may spill over into the unprotected larynx and trachea.[9]

Etiology of dysphagia

Many conditions can cause dysphagia in patients receiving palliative care. In some cases, side effects of treatment such as radiation therapy or chemotherapy are the precipitating causative factors of dysphagia. In other cases, progressive disease leads to unsafe and inefficient swallowing. Understanding the physiological impact of the illness is critical in evaluation of the swallowing disorder and the method of management. Some commonly encountered etiological categories in palliative care are discussed below.

Neoplasms

Brain and central nervous system tumors

Brain tumors are classified into primary and secondary types. Primary brain tumors are a diverse group of neoplasms arising from different cells of the brain, meninges, and central nervous system (CNS). In contrast, secondary tumors originate elsewhere in the body and metastasize to the brain. There were an estimated 311,202 incidents of primary brain tumors, malignant and benign, from 2005 to 2009.[13] Although dysphagia is rarely the presenting symptom, swallowing problems can develop directly or indirectly as the tumor increases in size and compresses surrounding structures and can be present in as many as 85% of brain tumor patients in the last stages of life.[14]

Extrinsic tumors located around the brainstem, as well as those originating in the skull base, may compress or invade the lower medulla. Hence, the swallowing center may be affected, with the specific swallowing impairment dependent on which cranial nerves are disrupted. In addition to direct tumor effects, swallowing and/or inability to maintain sufficient oral nutrition may be indirectly affected by depressed levels of consciousness, reduced awareness, fatigue, depression, seizures, and sarcopenia (changes to muscle bulk and strength), as well as the need for opioids associated with tumor progression, mass effect, and associated complications, especially in high-grade gliomas.[14-17]

High-grade gliomas (glioblastomas), the most common form of malignant brain tumors, account for 16% of all primary brain tumors[13] and carry a poor prognosis. Median survival rates are 1 to 5 years with less than 5% of patients surviving 5 years post diagnosis and commonly result in seizures, altered consciousness, progressive cognitive deficits, and difficulty swallowing in the end-of-life phase.[18] These symptoms can impact the patient's ability to take oral medications in the last weeks of life, including antiseizure or glucocorticoid medications.

Head and neck cancer

It is estimated that there are 600,000 new cases of head and neck cancer around the globe each year. Oropharyngeal dysphagia is ubiquitous in patients with advanced-stage head and neck cancer.[19] Dysphagia occurs both as a direct consequence of the disease as well as an immediate or delayed consequence of the treatment. These tumors occur in a variety of sites in the oral cavity, nasal cavity, sinuses, pharynx, larynx, and upper esophagus and can affect nerve supply, muscle coordination, and strength of movements involved in swallowing. Overall, the 5-year relative survival rate for all patients with head and neck cancers is 66%[20] although this rate is rising with the increasing prevalence of HPV associated tumors, which are often quite curable.

Treatment approaches for advanced disease include surgery and chemoradiotherapy, depending on the cell type, location, tumor size, and presence of neck metastases. In extensive disease of the oral cavity or in cases of persistent or recurrent tumors, disfiguring surgical resection may be followed by reconstruction with a flap of tissue borrowed from another part of the body such as the fibula or radial forearm. Surgical resection can result in anatomical insult that interferes with the normal biomechanics of the oropharyngeal physiology, such as in the case of a glossectomy or mandibulectomy. Removal of all or a portion of the tongue will impact the ability to adequately chew, move the food around the mouth, and propel it into the pharynx.

Surgical treatment for advanced laryngeal cancer removes structures that are critical to airway protection and increase the risk for material to be misdirected into the airway and thus aspirated. Laryngectomy is seldom used as a first-line treatment for cancer of the larynx due to significant impact on patients' communication. It is used in cases of persistent or recurrent disease or may be considered an elective option for chronic, severe aspiration.

In the past two decades, "organ preservation" involving chemoradiation therapy has been the primary approach for treating cancers of the pharynx and larynx with the goal of sparing the organs involved in speech and swallowing. Unfortunately, "organ preservation" is not synonymous with "functional preservation." In spite of advances in treatment methods aimed at sparing normal tissue and targeted chemotherapy agents, patients suffer from significant treatment toxicities including pulmonary aspiration, mucositis, edema, xerostomia, and trismus (restricted jaw opening). Cranial neuropathies and fibrosis can affect airway protection, pharyngeal contraction, and bolus drive, and opening of the upper esophagus.[21,22]

Radiation effects are progressive and commonly result in chronic dysphagia and aspiration. Swallowing becomes deliberate and determined with coughing, food getting caught, and the need for large volumes of liquid intake to combat dry mouth.

Nonoral nutritional support is required in greater than 60% of patients receiving multimodality treatment, and some patients are unable to resume an oral diet once their treatment is completed.[23] A primary goal of therapy for these patients is to keep them eating.[22] Some patients manage to compensate for their dysphagia with use of a prosthetic device fitted by a prosthodontist and changes in posture or diet consistencies suggested by the SLP. Therapy to maximize jaw opening can be beneficial for patients with a condition known as trismus, the limited mobility of the mouth and jaw opening due to surgery or radiation that interferes with mastication. With local disease progression and distant metastasis, facial edema and pain increase and eating and drinking become chronically uncomfortable, effortful, and difficult.

Malignant esophageal tumors

The incidence of malignant esophageal tumors in the United States was estimated to rise to over 17,000 new cases in 2013.[24,25] Esophageal carcinoma can arise either from squamous cells of the mucosa or as adenocarcinomas of the columnar lining of Barrett's epithelium. In the last several decades adenocarcinoma has increased, and is now four to five times more prevalent in newly diagnosed cases.[26] Tumors of the squamous cell type are generally located in the upper or midesophagus, while tumors of the adenocarcinoma type are located more distally.[27]

Treatment options are more numerous and survival rates are much higher when the disease is detected early. Unfortunately, symptom presentation usually occurs late in the disease, resulting in diagnosis of advanced malignancy. Patients commonly complain of weight loss and progressive dysphagia with solid foods rather than liquids, throat pain, and vomiting. In some cases, intractable cough may indicate extension of the tumor to the mediastinum or trachea. The presence of local extension to the aorta, trachea, or other mediastinal structures eliminates the possibility of surgical resection. Symptom presentation for patients with adenocarcinoma is gastroesophageal reflux disease rather than dysphagia and weight loss.[27] Survival rates are reported to be between 10% and 20% at 5 years, and thus, palliative care is the foundation of management for this disease.[24]

If diagnosed early, esophagectomy or esophagogastrectomy may be the treatment of choice, even with a 5% mortality rate and a 64% complication rate following these procedures.[28] In cases of unresectable advanced disease, symptomatic relief of dysphagia and pain can be accomplished by external beam radiation therapy, brachytherapy, esophageal dilation, chemotherapy, placement of a plastic or wire mesh esophageal stent to open the lumen of the esophagus, or laser tumor ablation.[25] Concomitant radiation therapy and chemotherapy is more effective than radiation alone for localized esophageal cancer and is increasingly being used for palliative treatment.[29,30] Esophageal perforation during laser surgery or dilation and migration of the esophageal stents are potential complications from palliative procedures.[29] Each of these treatments is associated with considerable side effects that can make swallowing painful and difficult, including esophagitis, mucositis, xerostomia, loss of taste, and lymphedema.

Cancer, non–head and neck

Oncology patients may develop transient or persistent oropharyngeal dysphagia due to a wide range of issues including presence of tumor, radiation, cytotoxic effects of chemotherapy, cancer-related weakness and fatigue, and neurological or respiratory compromise.[17,30] One study found that of 11 non–head and neck cancer patients receiving palliative care, nine reported either dysphagic symptoms, the need to modify their food texture to softer foods, or an impact on their quality of life due to swallowing difficulties at some point in the course of their disease.[17] Of particular note, patients with intrathoracic malignancies, such as lung and mediastinal tumors that invade the left recurrent laryngeal nerve and result in laryngeal nerve palsies, may experience impaired airway protection and cough, as well as dysphagia. Alternatively, damage can occur during hilar lung tumor resection, mediastinal lymph node biopsy, and thyroidectomy. Radiation therapy to the mediastinum may cause esophagitis, which can result in odynophagia, pain on swallowing.

Chemotherapy toxicity affects the oral, pharyngeal, and/or esophageal mucosa, or may result in infection during periods of myelosuppression. This results in altered taste, pain, reduced appetite, nausea, mucosal bleeding, and formation of lesions such as herpes simplex virus or varicella zoster.[31] Cancer cachexia occurs in 50%–75% cancer patients, and results in wasting syndrome. This loss of muscle and fat either directly or indirectly as a response to the tumor leads to weakness, fatigue, and metabolic disturbances and results in poorer outcomes. Thus, the prevention of weight loss and provision of ways to maximize safety, efficiency and enjoyment of eating can improve quality of life[32] and may require an interdisciplinary team management approach.

Progressive neuromuscular diseases

Motor neuron disease

Motor neuron disease, of which the most common disease is ALS, is encountered with unfortunate regularity in patients on a palliative care service. A rapidly progressive, degenerative and terminal disease, ALS involves the motor neurons of the brain and spinal cord.[33,34] One-quarter of ALS patients initially present with swallowing difficulty, while other patients begin with distal weakness that travels proximally to involve the bulbar musculature. As the disease progresses, it encompasses upper and lower motor neurons, affecting speaking, walking, writing, and ultimately the respiratory system. Respiratory failure is the usual cause of death in patients with ALS because of weakness in diaphragmatic, laryngeal, and lingual function.[34]

Patients generally live between 3 and 5 years after diagnosis of ALS, making a coordinated and multidisciplinary team approach part of standardized treatment, essential in caring for these patients.[35] Although there is no cure for ALS, numerous pharmacological agents are being researched to treat various symptoms of the disease. Riluzole, a glutamate antagonist, is currently the only pharmacological treatment for ALS approved by the US Food and Drug Administration (FDA) and has been found to slow the progression of the disease and extend life expectancy by several months.[36–39]

As respiratory muscles weaken, breathing becomes impaired, inducing poor gas exchange and hypoventilation.[40] Typically, patients with bulbar ALS experience a reduction in tongue mobility, oral and pharyngeal muscle weakness, and fatigue with eating. They develop increasing difficulty with the ability to chew and to control material in the mouth. Nasal regurgitation of fluids and loss of control over liquids may occur, resulting in aspiration and coughing before the swallow is triggered. With disease progression, heavier foods—even pureed ones—are difficult to manipulate, resulting in significant residue in the oral cavity. Reduced pharyngeal drive also results in residue in the pharynx. Diet modifications with calorie-dense foods and postural alterations are necessary if oral intake is to continue.

Many patients reach a point where the burden of eating outweighs the pleasure; significant weight loss and frequent choking may occur. Maintenance of nutrition is further challenged by muscle atrophy and a state of hypermetabolism. Gastrostomy tube placement, if undertaken before body mass index has significantly dropped and before vital capacity drops below 50% anticipated,[38,41,42] may stabilize weight loss, prolong survival, reduce complications, and improve quality of life in some patients.

Parkinson's disease and Parkinsonian Syndromes

Parkinson's disease (PD) is a relatively common, slow progressive disease of the CNS, marked by an inability to execute learned motor skills automatically.[36] Classic motor symptoms include resting tremor, bradykinesia (slowness of movement) and rigidity, gait dysfunction, and postural instability. Nonmotor features may include autonomic disturbances, sleep problems, and cognitive dysfunction.[43] The largest etiological group is idiopathic; however, Parkinson-like symptoms may occur as a result of medications, toxins, head trauma, or degenerative conditions.[34]

Dysphagia in Parkinson's disease may occur in the oral, pharyngeal, and/or esophageal stages. It is related to changes in striated muscles under dopaminergic control and in smooth muscles under autonomic control.[34] The oral stage is associated with rigidity of the lingual musculature rather than weakness.[44] Small-amplitude, ineffective tongue-rolling movements are observed as patients attempt to propel the boluses into the pharynx. As a result, pharyngeal swallow responses are delayed, with aspiration occurring before and during the swallow. Expectoration of aspirated material may be reduced due to a weak cough because of rigidity of the laryngeal musculature. Incomplete opening of the upper esophageal sphincter and esophageal dysmotility are also commonly observed in patients with PD.[34,44] Even mild swallowing impairments may negatively affect quality of life for patients with PD and their caregivers, often adding to their perceived burden and worries.[37]

In the early stages, antiparkinsonian medications such as levodopa or dopamine agonists improve flexibility and speed during swallowing. This medical therapy does not stop progression of the disease, however, and the majority of patients with PD continue to decline.[43] In patients with dysphagia who develop severe symptoms, pharmacotherapy has a limited benefit.[45] Dysphagia and resultant pneumonia is one of the most prevalent causes of death in patients with Parkinson's disease.[34,37]

Two other progressive neuromuscular diseases include progressive supranuclear palsy (PSP) and multiple system atrophy (MSA). Progressive supranuclear palsy is often initially misdiagnosed as Parkinson's.[46] Early development of orthostasis, falls, and vertical gaze palsy are cardinal features of PSP and distinguish it from Parkinson's disease.[47–496] Patients with PSP do not respond as well as patients with Parkinson's disease to pharmacological treatment, and thus their dysphagia may be more aggressive and more life threatening.[30]

Multiple system atrophy is a progressive neurodegenerative disorder characterized by parkinsonism, ataxia, pyramidal signs such as spasticity, and autonomic failure such as urinary dysfunction and orthostatic hypotension. Generally, most patients with MSA do not respond to levodopa treatment or respond only short-term, and thus therapy is generally symptomatic.[47] Dysphagia onset occurs within 5 years after diagnosis with MSA-P (the parkinsonian subtype).[47]

Myopathies

Myopathy is a neuromuscular disorder that results in muscle weakness and can be either inherited or acquired. Some causes can be treated, such as infectious, toxic, endocrine, and alcohol related. The group of myopathies, known as muscular dystrophies, is chronic and progressive, resulting in continued muscle weakness affecting oral, pharyngeal, and esophageal muscles. Oculopharyngeal muscular dystrophy (OPMD) is an autosomal dominant muscle disorder with hallmark features of a slowly progressive ptosis and dysphagia, proximal limb and facial weakness, and abnormal gait, with onset generally occurring after age 40. The leading causes of death for patients with OPMD are recurrent aspiration pneumonia and malnutrition.[48]

Duchene's muscular dystrophy is a childhood form that generally occurs in boys before the age of 6 and results in severe dysphagia by age 12.[30] The dysphagic symptoms include reduced palatal elevation, weak pharyngeal contraction, reduced hyolaryngeal excursion, and reduced esophageal motility. Patients tend to have secretions that pool in their pharynx, aspiration, reflux, and poor gastrointestinal (GI) motility. Medical and drug treatments are ineffective in managing the disease, and thus treatment focuses on alleviation of symptoms. Surgically, there is some evidence that a myotomy (cutting of the UES) and/or upper esophageal dilation may be beneficial in cases of moderate/severe dysphagia to open the channel from the pharynx to the esophagus more readily.[49]

Multiple sclerosis

Multiple sclerosis (MS) is characterized by multifocal plaques of demyelination within the CNS. It affects approximately 400,000 people in the United States.[50] The scattered inflammatory white-matter lesions observed in the CNS result in varying combinations of motor, sensory, and cognitive deficits. It usually follows a remitting-relapsing course that within 10 years advances to the secondary progressive form.[4,34] Symptoms that affect quality of life include fatigue, spasticity, paroxysmal symptoms, pain, ataxia, bladder and bowel dysfunction, depression, cognitive problems, and dysphagia.[51] Dysphagia occurs in 34% of end-stage MS patients and appears to be related to nonambulatory patients with brainstem impairment.[52] Swallowing dysfunction depends on the location of the lesions. For instance, difficulties may arise with the feeding process as a result of hand tremors and spasticity. Alternatively, sclerosed plaques can be found in the cortex and the brainstem and can affect cranial nerves, whereby people are unable to perform certain activities.

Dementia

Dementia encompasses Alzheimer's disease, cumulative brain damage from multiple small cerebral infarcts (vascular dementia),

advanced Parkinson's or Huntington's disease, frontotemporal dementia, Lewy body disease, and brain damage from excessive and chronic alcohol. Symptoms include progressive memory loss, poor awareness, loss of language abilities, inactivity, agitation, and confusion. Dysphagia in patients with dementia is extremely prevalent, and may be as high as 93%.[30] As a result, patients with dementia frequently develop pneumonia, malnutrition, and dehydration particularly in the advanced stages of the disease.[53] Aspiration and weight loss increase mortality risk, irrespective of the dementia severity. Since early identification of dysphagia may reduce the onset and severity of these symptoms, frequent screening and monitoring of swallowing function is suggested. Swallowing and feeding problems that arise in the late stages of dementia are not reversible, although treating concomitant infections, metabolic disarray, and/or dehydration may result in improved functioning.[30,54,55]

The different types of dementia and their varying trajectories result in an unspecific dysphagia. However, common attributes include the inability to independently self-feed and inability to focus for the duration of meal times. With disease progression, patients may not engage in the task of eating and swallowing at all. They may hold food in their mouth for prolonged periods without mastication or bolus formation, especially with uniformly textured foods such as pureed items or bland foods. This often occurs when a swallowing dyspraxia (poor motor planning) of advanced dementia occurs. Decreased consciousness and sedation predispose patients to both food and liquid aspiration. Additionally, sensory impairments and lack of attention reduce the ability to control the bolus in the mouth, resulting in aspiration from premature spillage before the pharyngeal swallow has been elicited. Moreover, behaviors such as distraction or agitation may prolong the feeding time and hence reduce the amount of nutrition and hydration received. As dementia progresses, patients develop a lack of desire to eat and reduced appetite as a hallmark feature of late-stage dementia.[56]

There is growing consensus among medical care providers that a palliative care approach is appropriate in advanced and late stage dementia, particularly foregoing the use of feeding tubes. In 2013, two new position statements were published addressing the growing evidence of the burdens associated with tube feeding in patients with advanced dementia. The revised 2013 statement by American Geriatrics Society (AGS) states, "Percutaneous feeding tubes are not recommended for older adults with advanced dementia. Careful hand-feeding should be offered; for persons with advanced dementia, hand feeding is at least as good as tube-feeding for the outcomes of death, aspiration pneumonia, functional status and patient comfort. Tube feeding is associated with agitation, increased use of physical and chemical restraints, and worsening pressure ulcers."[54] A special task force from the American Academy of Hospice and Palliative Medicine (AAHPM) recommended against placing feeding tubes in patients with advanced dementia. Rather, focus should be on assisted feeding for comfort and human interaction.[57]

Medical etiologies

Systemic dysphagia

The broadest category of causes of dysphagia includes inflammatory and infectious factors, which affect oral, pharyngeal, and esophageal stages of swallowing. Autoimmune inflammatory disorders can affect swallowing in either specific organs or the immune system as a whole. This category of diseases includes polymyositis, scleroderma, inflammatory myopathy, and secondary autoimmune diseases. Sometimes, intrinsic obstruction is observed, such as in Wegener's granulomatosis. With other disorders, there is external compression, as in sarcoidosis, abnormal esophageal motility as in scleroderma, or inadequate lubrication as in Sjögren's syndrome.[30]

Poor esophageal motility restricts patients to small meals of pureed or liquid substances, resulting in long drawn out eating. Weight loss is frequent, and gastroesophageal reflux can result from poor esophageal peristalsis.[58] Immunocompromised hosts, such as patients with AIDS, patients who have undergone chemotherapy, and patients on steroid therapy, are prone to candida esophagitis. Dysphagia for solids is greater than for liquids, and patients frequently complain of food getting caught. Heartburn, nausea, and vomiting are other common complaints.[30]

General deconditioning, aging, and chronic illness

Multisystem progressive diseases, including end-stage chronic obstructive pulmonary disease (COPD), coronary artery disease, congestive heart failure (CHF), and chronic renal failure, cause insidious weakness. Weight loss in these patients is a common consequence because of reduced endurance for activities of daily living, including eating and swallowing. Body wasting, or cardiac cachexia, is a serious complication of CHF and associated with poor prognosis.[59] Patients with emphysema or COPD have difficulty coordinating swallowing and respiration, resulting in inability to tolerate the obligatory cessation of breathing required for airway protection during the swallow. General immobility impairs spontaneous pulmonary clearance, resulting in an inability to expectorate material if it is aspirated. Patients are often discouraged and depressed by their loss of independence and declining health.

Frail elders, or elderly with "failure to thrive," constitute another set of patients who may present with chronic dysphagia.[60] Aging can result in changes to the muscle bulk and strength (sarcopenia) and tissue elasticity in the tongue and pharynx, resulting in reduced ability to push the bolus through.[61] Additionally, aging affects the larynx; specifically the vocal folds may not close sufficiently or timely enough to protect the airway.[62] Sensorimotor changes may occur that impact salivary production, taste, and smell. While many of these changes occur as part of normal aging, a subset of elders progress further into a state of poor nutrition, loss of weight, poor mobility and strength, and poor emotional state. The body then becomes unable to meet the metabolic demands imposed on it. While there is some evidence that direct muscle strengthening may be effective,[63] some patients may experience irreversible declines. One theory is the reduction in functional reserve leaves older individuals highly vulnerable to insults to the swallowing system for which they are unable to compensate.[61,64]

Dysphagia may present in hospitalized medical patients who may already have cachexia, loss of muscle mass, significantly compromised pulmonary systems that impede airway protection and/or general weakness and deconditioning from a multitude of illnesses and lengthy hospital stays. In a fragile and immunocompromised condition, there is a higher risk for suffering from pulmonary infections, poor outcomes from aspiration, and fatigue, which impacts the ability to sustain appropriate nutrition. Moreover, this group of hospitalized medical patients is prone to negative outcomes from dysphagia, including increased length of hospital days and increased risk of mortality.[65] Particularly, difficulty in completing oral care due to a low level of consciousness and/or the presence of an endotracheal tube can promote colonization of oral bacteria in the hospitalized patient. If aspiration of colonized oropharyngeal contents occurs (secretions, vomitus, food/liquid mixed with colonized secretions) it can be a major contributor to aspiration pneumonia.[66]

Dysphagia as a side effect of medications

There are 160 known medications with dysphagia specified as a potential adverse effect. Any medication should be reviewed to determine if contributes to or causes dysphagia.[67] Medications may affect all stages of swallowing including lubrication of the oral cavity and pharynx, taste and smell, reduced coordination or motor function, impaired consciousness, GI dysfunction, and local mucosal toxicity.[30,67] Antipsychotic or neuroleptic medications can produce extrapyramidal motor disturbances, resulting in impaired function of the striated musculature of the oral cavity, pharynx, and esophagus. Long-term use of antipsychotics may result in tardive dyskinesia, with choreiform tongue movements affecting the coordination of swallowing. Delayed swallow initiation is a reported side effect of some neuroleptic medications. Use of antipsychotic medications within the hospital setting has been found to result in impaired swallowing function with worsening of swallowing function as dosage increases.[68]

Anticonvulsants such as phenobarbital, carbamazepine, and phenytoin may all have adverse effects and may impact CNS functioning, drowsiness, and motor incoordination.[30] Antihistamines and antidepressants may reduce taste and smell and decrease lubrication. Many of these medications can also alter GI motility, cause mucositis, or increase reflux including antipsychotics, antidepressants, and antihistamines.[67]

Role of the Speech-language pathologist in end-of-life care

Speech-language pathologists (SLP) are the expert specialists in assessment and management of communication and oropharyngeal swallowing disorders. They play a critical role as part of the multidisciplinary team for palliative care patients and can help to add comfort and maximize quality of life, as well as educate the patient and family and help prepare them to deal with the progressive symptoms of dysphagia that may accompany the disease. The SLP can use his/her knowledge to carefully explain the swallowing process and any impairments, evaluate empirical data to determine swallowing potential, prognosticate to assist in decision-making, and guide families and caregivers in safe feeding methods.[1] The SLP provides further assistance to the care team by implementing the most effective strategies to best communicate with a patient who has impaired communication ability, including speaking valves for the patient with a tracheostomy and/or assistive and augmentative communication devices. Such interventions can improve the patient's ability to participate in decision-making and in expressing their wishes, and in maintaining social connections—hallmark features of palliative care.[1,68]

A comprehensive swallow evaluation done by the SLP includes a thorough review of the patient's medical history and presenting complaint, evaluation of alertness, hemodynamic stability, and oromotor functioning, and observation of swallowing of various liquid and solid food consistencies, depending on the safety and appropriateness. An instrumental swallow evaluation (via videofluoroscopy or endoscopy) may be indicated to further delineate swallowing physiology, determine effectiveness of various swallowing strategies, and clarify or confirm aspiration risk (see below for more information). Treatment goals are individualized to the patient and may focus on improving swallow function, maximizing residual abilities, or maintaining some oral intake while ensuring safety and efficiency of nutrition. Because of their expertise in swallowing, SLPs can assist patients and families during the decision-making process of alternative hydration and nutrition with a focus on comfort, maintaining quality of life, and upholding the patient's wishes.[54]

Speech-language pathologists who care for palliative care patients must carefully weigh what will benefit the patient and what will be burdensome. They must understand the underlying disease processes while attending to the individual, spiritual, and emotional issues, and must be skilled in biomedical ethics and legal issues and highly sensitive to the psychosocial ramifications of altering oral diets.[69-71]

Assessment of dysphagia

Evaluation of dysphagia in patients receiving palliative care is best accomplished within a multidisciplinary framework. Approaching the evaluation of swallowing in the terminally ill patient demands a holistic view and reaches beyond the physiology of deglutition.[72] While aspiration of food or liquid could realistically evolve into pneumonia, paradoxically, committing a patient to nonoral feeding or non per os (NPO) is also fraught with complications. It therefore behooves caregivers to carefully consider the multiple parameters in decision-making about oral nutrition in the terminally ill patient.

For the patient with a serious and life-limiting illness, the goals of the swallowing evaluation are to: (1) identify the underlying physiological nature of the disorder, (2) determine whether any short-range interventions can alleviate the dysphagia, and (3) collaborate with the patient, family, and caregivers on the safest and most efficacious method of nutrition and hydration. Balancing the safety and health of the patient with quality of life issues is integral to the assessment. Eliciting a description of the patient's complaints about swallowing, current eating habits, appetite, and diet is critical to understanding the physiological basis of the problem and to integrating these hypotheses with attitudes and wishes about eating and not eating. Details of disease progression and prognosis, along with the accompanying emotional and psychological impact on the patient and the family and consideration of a patient's cognitive status, alertness, and ability to follow directions are also be considered when determining the aggressiveness of a swallowing work-up and its treatment. The patient with a poor appetite, fatigue, and a sense of hopelessness will understandably be less compliant and less motivated to engage in a complex treatment program. Alternatively, the patient who derives much satisfaction from eating and drinking and wishes to continue with a regular diet, will not be satisfied with significant alterations in texture and consistency.

Examination of swallowing by direct observation

Direct observation of the patient eating, drinking, or taking medications by a perceptive clinician can yield valuable information about the underlying disorder. As discussed previously, the SLP is vigilant for indications of chewing inefficiencies, aspiration, difficulties managing secretions, or obstruction.

Typically, the clinician assesses the patient's oral-motor and sensory function and cognitive communicative abilities, while observing the partaking of a variety of liquid and solid foods (e.g., semisolid, soft solid, and, where appropriate, food requiring mastication). Speech and voice are analyzed to assist in understanding the underlying physiology of the swallowing disorder. Functional airway protection is a critical predictor of safe swallowing and, thus, an important element of the swallowing evaluation although it cannot be definitively discerned from clinical observation alone. Patients who have weak voices and weak respiratory force for coughing and pulmonary clearance are at risk for pulmonary compromise.

Since aspiration may be silent in up to 40% of patients with dysphagia, (e.g., present with no overt sign or symptom that material has entered into the airway such as a cough or throat clear),[73] close attention is paid to occult signs of aspiration, including wet vocal quality or gurgliness, frequent throat clearing, delayed coughing, and oral/pharyngeal residue.[4] Silent aspiration can only be confirmed definitively with an instrumental examination. Depending on the stage of progression of the patient's illness and overall management goals, it may be prudent to identify silent aspiration with the aim of limiting progression with behavioral strategies.

Screening of swallowing function

In the last several years there has been increased awareness for the need to screen swallowing and assess risk for aspiration before giving patients anything to eat or drink, including oral medications.[74] This has been largely driven by the extensive research done on acute stroke patients and their high risk of aspiration (40–60%), the close relationship between aspiration and aspiration pneumonia, and the evidence that reveals mortality rates in acute stroke patients with pneumonia are three times higher than those without.[75] As a result, since 2005, several national regulatory and safety guidelines including the Joint Commission and American Heart Association state that all acute stroke patients should have their swallowing screened before any oral intake. Although this currently relates to acute stroke patients, there is increasing awareness of the risk of aspiration and the need to determine swallowing safety in many hospitalized patient populations.[76,77]

The swallow screening, typically done by the nurse, identifies potential aspiration risk, assists in determining whether it is safe for a patient to start eating and drinking, and helps to determine whether a patient requires a full evaluation by the SLP. It cannot, however, determine an etiology or underlying physiology of the swallowing disorder and therefore cannot determine appropriate compensatory strategies, treatment, or prognosis. Additionally, the registered dietician may identify warning signs of dysphagia during a nutrition intake and request SLP involvement. If a patient is suspected of having a swallowing disorder (see Box 11.1), a comprehensive swallow evaluation should be completed.

Box 11.1 Indications of a swallowing disorder

Reduced alertness or cognitive impairment

Coma, heavy sedation, dementia, delirium
Inattention during eating
Impulsivity with regard to eating
Playing with food

Alterations in attitudes toward eating

Refusal to eat in the presence of others
Avoidance of particular foods or fluids
Protracted meal times, incomplete meals, large amounts of fluids to flush solids
Changes in posture or head movements during eating
Laborious chewing, multiple swallows per small bites
Weight loss

Signs of oral-pharyngeal dysfunction

Dysarthria or slurred, imprecise speech
Copious secretions coating the tongue and palate
Wet voice with "gurgly" quality
Drooling or leaking from the lips
Residual food in the oral cavity after eating
Frequent throat clearing, coughing, or choking during or immediately after meals
Nasal regurgitation
Recurrent aspiration pneumonias

Signs of esophageal dysfunction

Regurgitation or emesis after swallowing
Sour taste in mouth after eating
Solids caught in the chest region
Burping during/after eating
Pain on swallowing

Specific patient complaints

Sensation of food caught in the throat
Coughing and choking while eating
Regurgitation of solids through the nose after eating or drinking
Pain on swallowing
Food or fluid noted in tracheotomy tube
Inability to manage secretions
Drooling
Shortness of breath while chewing or after meals
Difficulty initiating the swallow
Unexplained weight loss
Protracted meal times or inability to complete a meal

A word of caution is needed regarding the gag reflex and oropharyngeal swallowing. The gag reflex and the pattern of neuromuscular events comprising the swallow are very different, both in their innervation and in their execution. The gag reflex is a protective reflex that prevents noxious substances arising from the oral cavity or digestive tract from entering the airway. It is not elicited during the normal swallow, and its assessment is not clinically relevant to swallowing ability.[78] In fact, 20% to 40% of normal, healthy adults do *not* have a gag reflex.[70] In addition, the gag reflex can be extinguished or reduced by a nasogastric feeding tube, endotracheal intubation, or repeated stimulation.

Instrumental evaluation

An instrumental swallow evaluation may be indicated to further delineate swallowing physiology, locate a specific etiology that may provide valuable information for management, assess for integrity of the swallowing anatomy and mucosa, determine effectiveness of swallowing strategies, and clarify or confirm aspiration risk. Instrumental or objective evaluations may take many forms, depending on the patient complaints and likely cause.

Videofluoroscopic evaluation of swallowing

Radiographic swallowing studies are to determine the pathology of impaired swallowing.[4] The videofluoroscopic swallowing study (VFSS; commonly known as modified barium swallow study or MBS) examines oropharyngeal swallowing with the patient positioned upright while swallowing a variety of consistencies of barium-coated foods (liquids, semisolids, and solids) in controlled volumes. The study, completed by an SLP and radiology staff, is recorded digitally and the results are reviewed following the study for closer inspection of the anatomy and physiology. The goal of this study is not only to determine the presence or absence of aspiration; but also to evaluate the effectiveness of compensatory swallowing strategies that may decrease the risk of aspiration and increase swallowing efficiency. The test is noninvasive, takes little time to administer, and provides valuable information to manage the dysphagia.[4,79]

Fiberoptic endoscopic evaluation of swallowing

Using fiberoptic endoscopic evaluation of swallowing (FEES), examination of oropharyngeal swallowing can be performed at the bedside by a trained SLP. The oropharynx and larynx can be visualized transnasally while the patient is swallowing food substances dyed with food coloring. The presence of laryngeal penetration, aspiration, and pharyngeal retention can be observed; laryngeal and oropharyngeal anatomy viewed; and sensory integrity of the pharynx and larynx assessed. As with the VFSS, compensatory swallowing strategies such as postural modifications or swallowing maneuvers can be evaluated for their efficacy in the FEES. The use of the endoscope can also provide visual feedback to the patient during treatment.[80]

Barium swallow and upper GI study

In contrast to the VFSS, which focuses on the oropharyngeal mechanism, a barium swallow study and upper GI (UGI) series examines esophageal and stomach function and focuses on the anatomy of the esophagus, stomach, and duodenum. The barium swallow, completed by a radiologist, identifies mucosal and anatomical abnormalities, esophageal strictures, tumors, and esophageal motility. It has low sensitivity for diagnosing gastroesophageal reflux, which is better assessed with pH monitoring and/or manometry.[54,81] This test is conducted with the patient positioned upright and in the supine position while swallowing liquid barium or, in some cases, a barium tablet. Since the esophagus is under involuntary neural control, compensatory swallowing strategies cannot be assessed with this procedure. However, recommendations can be made for changing to liquid consistencies in a patient with an esophageal stricture.

Esophagogastroduodenoscopy

In contrast, endoscopic evaluation of the entire UGI tract, or esophagogastroduodenoscopy (EGD), is completed by a gastroenterologist and confirms the presence of strictures and mucosal anomalies, tumors, or bleeding. Endoscopy uses a thin, flexible tube (endoscope) to look at the lining of the esophagus, stomach, and upper small intestine (duodenum). The assistance of a gastroenterologist may be required in cases requiring palliative dilation of the esophagus.[30]

Esophageal manometry

This procedure measures the strength and pattern of muscle contractions in the esophagus by the use of pressure readings. Lower esophageal sphincter muscle pressure can also be taken. This test, completed by a gastroenterologist, helps determine whether there is a problem with motility of the esophagus or the function of the LES.

pH probe

An ambulatory 24-hour pH probe is a test that consists of a small tube passed through the nose into the esophagus. The tip of the tube has pH sensor that measures acid exposure in the esophagus and collects the data on a portable computer. These results are compared with "normal" acid exposure in the esophagus. This is considered the "gold standard" for determining the presence of gastroesophageal reflux disease (GERD).

Management of dysphagia

Direct swallowing intervention

Active strengthening exercises and rehabilitation aimed at restoring or improving swallowing function may be recommended by the SLP following a swallowing assessment, although consideration of overall goals of care and treatment plan should be closely aligned. Exercises may be aimed at increasing tongue strength or movement,[82] pharyngeal contraction, heightened airway and vocal fold closure, and increased opening of the UES. Like any other strengthening program, exercises are only beneficial in certain instances, such as when muscle strength is impaired and can be improved, and must be individualized to the specific dysfunction. The effectiveness and appropriateness of direct swallowing intervention in a patient with a degenerative process, or with advanced stages of disease may be questionable. Therefore, it will be necessary to discuss realistic impact and the appropriate implementation of a course of swallowing exercises. There are many causes of dysphagia other than muscle weakness, such as dementia-related cognitive impairment, that will not benefit from direct strengthening. Lastly, the overall level of endurance and cognitive ability to follow directions will also need to be considered before starting an exercise program.

Compensatory swallowing strategies

The physiological information obtained from clinical and instrumental swallowing assessment facilitates determination of intervention strategies aimed at increasing swallowing safety and efficiency. These include alterations in head and neck posture,

consistency of food, sensory awareness, and feeding behaviors. The principal advantage of these strategies is that they are simple for the patient to learn and to perform. In addition, once their effectiveness is determined, the patient can improve swallow function use during meals by utilizing these interventions. In 2008, a large, multisite, randomized clinical trial of patients with a diagnosis of dementia and/or PD was published examining the effects of three compensatory interventions to prevent aspiration of liquids, including chin-down posture, nectar-thickened liquids, and honey-thickened liquids. It demonstrated that strategies must be highly individualized, that there is no uniform effectiveness in any one of these strategies, and that effectiveness can only be determined by an objective swallowing evaluation.[83]

Postural modifications

Postural changes during swallowing often have the effect of diverting the food or liquid to prevent aspiration or obstruction but do not change the swallowing physiology.[3,4] A commonly used strategy is the chin-tuck posture. This posture has the advantage of increasing the pressure on the bolus and restricting the opening of the larynx during swallowing, thus potentially reducing the risk of laryngeal penetration and aspiration. However, in select cases, a chin tuck may exacerbate the aspiration, underscoring the need for radiographic evidence of its clinical value, if at all possible. These strategies may be used in isolation or in combination, depending on the nature of the underlying swallowing pathophysiology. Table 11.1 lists some of the postural strategies that the SLP may introduce, and their potential benefits on bolus flow.

Changes in texture, consistency, and nutritional content of food

Changes in the consistency of food and liquid necessitate emotional adjustment and support for patients because they are often unappealing. Thus, this management strategy should be reserved for patients who are unable to follow directions to use postural changes or for whom other compensatory strategies

Table 11.1 Compensatory postural changes that improve bolus flow and may reduce aspiration and residue during swallowing

Postural strategy	Rationale
Chin tuck	Closes larynx, pushes tongue closer to posterior pharyngeal wall, and promotes epiglottic deflection
Head back	Promotes bolus movement through the oral cavity with assistance of gravity
Head tilt to stronger side	Directs bolus down stronger side with assistance of gravity
Head turned to weaker side	Diverts bolus away from weaker side of pharynx, promotes opening of upper esophagus
Head tilt plus chin tuck	Directs bolus down stronger side while increasing closure of larynx
Head rotation plus chin tuck	Diverts bolus away from weaker side while facilitating closure of laryngeal vestibule and vocal folds

Source: Adapted from Logemann (1998), reference 4.

are not feasible.[4] Underlying physiological impairments, such as reduced tongue control or strength, may affect the safety of swallowing certain food consistencies. Some patients may exhibit signs of aspiration on thin liquids, but may have sufficient control to drink liquids thickened to nectarlike or honeylike consistency in small sips. Patients debilitated by chronic disease and who lack endurance to complete a meal may benefit from ground or pureed moist foods that require limited mastication. In certain circumstances, the initiation of altered food consistency is the only option to assure a patient's comfort or safe oral intake. Examples and rationale of modified diets are listed in Table 11.2.

Specialized commercial agents derived from modified food starch or gum-based (xanthan, guar, cellulose) thickeners can be used to thicken liquids. Gum-based thickeners have improved performance over starch-based in terms of stability over time and temperature.[84] Thickened liquids release the fluid in the gastrointestinal tract, do not alter the body's absorption rate of fluids, and provide water for hydration requirements.[85] Additionally, some nutritional supplement drinks are thicker liquids and calorically fortified, providing a safer alternative to more solid consistencies, while others come in a pudding format.

The patient and caregivers should understand and consider the competing benefits and risks regarding nutrition, with attention to the patient's preferences. A guiding principle for the diet of an individual with dysphagia is to ingest the maximum amount of calories for the least amount of effort. A patient with dysphagia who requires adaptations in texture and consistency, or supplemental alternative nutrition, benefits from a collaborative approach to maximize safety, health, and satisfaction with eating.[86] Nutritionists can provide individualized suggestions for calorie-dense foods or high-calorie nutritional supplements, depending on the patient's metabolic status. Food preparation in a manner that increases caloric and nutritional value, as well as maximizing hydration, is helpful. A close partnership and collaboration with the registered dietician (a specialist who performs a nutrition assessment and develops a nutrition care plan) will ensure the best outcome. Box 11.2 provides a list of cookbooks that can assist

---

Box 11.2 Cookbooks for altered food consistency diets

- *Gourmet Puree Recipes: The Ultimate Collection.* Daniel Tyler. Amazon Digital Services, 2013.

- *Soft Foods for Easier Eating.* Sandra Woodruff, MS, RD, LDN, and Leah Gilbert-Henderson, PhD, LDN. Square One Publishers, 2011.

- *Eat Well Stay Nourished: A Recipe and Resources Guide for Coping with Eating Challenges.* Compiled and edited by Nancy E. Leupold. Published by SPOHNC Support for People with Oral and Head and Neck Cancer, 2000.

- *Easy-to-Swallow, Easy-to-Chew Cookbook: Over 150 Tasty and Nutritious Recipes for People Who Have Difficulty Swallowing.* Donna Weihoffen, JoAnne Robbins, Paula Sullivan. John Wiley, 2002.

- *The Dysphagia Cookbook.* Elayne Achilles. Cumberland House Publishing, 2004.

- *I-Can't-Chew Cookbook.* J. Randy Wilson and Mark A. Piper. Hunter House, 2003.

---

patients and care providers in preparing foods and liquids that have altered textures and may be easier to swallow.

Increased sensory awareness

Sensory enhancement techniques include increasing downward pressure of a spoon against the tongue when presenting food in the mouth and presenting a sour bolus, a cold bolus, a bolus requiring chewing, or a large-volume bolus. These techniques may elicit a quicker pharyngeal swallow response while reducing the risk of aspiration. Some patients benefit from receiving food or liquid at a slower rate, while others are more efficient with larger boluses. Enhancing the bolus characteristics to include more texture can sometimes induce mastication and bolus formation more readily than a bolus that is both flavorless and homogeneous in texture. This is particularly evident in patients with advanced

---

Table 11.2 Diet modifications for patients with dysphagia

Diet	Definition	Example	Indication
Pureed diet	Blenderized food with added liquid to form smooth consistency No chewing necessary	Applesauce, yogurt, moist mashed potatoes, puddings	Significantly reduced chewing, impaired pharyngeal contraction, esophageal stricture
Mechanically altered diet	Ground, finely chopped or diced foods that easily form a cohesive bolus with minimal chewing	Pasta, soft scrambled eggs, cottage cheese, ground meats	Some limited chewing possible, but protracted
Soft, moist diet	Naturally soft foods requiring some chewing; food is cut in small pieces; serve with gravy to moisten	Soft meats, canned fruits, baked fish Avoid raw vegetables, bread, nuts, and tough meats	Reduced endurance for prolonged meal, reduced attention span, tongue/lip weakness
Liquids	Nectar consistency	Similar in viscosity to tomato juice; less thick than honey consistency	Reduced liquid bolus control, delayed swallow initiation and airway closure
	Honey consistency	Similar in viscosity to honey; available in ready-to-serve packaging or use thickening agent	Reduced oral or lingual control of liquid bolus, delayed swallow initiation and airway closure

dementia. Patient responses to these behaviors can be evaluated at the bedside, and the findings can be easily communicated to the caregivers.[4]

Pharmacological and medical management of dysphagia

There are no pharmacological agents that have been shown to directly act on oropharyngeal swallowing function. Studies on medical treatment such as hyperbaric oxygen therapy and medications that increase oxygenation or that may mediate the effects of fibrosis in head and neck cancer patients are inconclusive.[22] However, there are agents for concurrent issues, which can exacerbate an underlying mucosal problem and medications that may effectively treat GI motility, reflux, nausea and vomiting, yeast infections such as candidiasis, and sialorrhea (excess secretions).

Candida esophagitis requires oral antifungal agents such as nystatin topical. Other antifungal medications include ketoconazole, miconazole, fluconazole, and amphotericin B. Immunocompromised patients with candidiasis require potent systemic antifungal medications. Resistance can occur, however, in patients with long-term prophylaxis. Patients who fail the above regimen may be considered for antiviral agents.[87] A prokinetic agent may be prescribed for poor esophageal motility, and proton pump inhibitors or histamine-2 blockers such as ranitidine have been found to be effective in patients with GERD.[67] Botulinum toxin (Botox) can be used in the management of sialorrhea or can be injected into the LES, which can temporarily induce relaxation when LES spasm is present.[67]

Other interventions

Complementary and alternative medicine

It is estimated that nearly half of all Americans practice some form of complementary and alternative medicine (CAM) and there is an increasing rise in interest in these treatments.[88] Clinical evidence for CAM therapy for dysphagia and some of the underlying symptoms is somewhat limited for certain treatments. Acupuncture following stroke has raised much interest because dysphagia can be prevalent and debilitating in this population. However, two Cochrane reviews were unable to demonstrate clear evidence to support the use of acupuncture for dysphagia after stroke, and more large-scale trials are needed to determine its clinical efficacy.[89,90] Lastly, there are some promising results using acupuncture to treat GERD and esophageal dysmotility.[91]

Oral hygiene/oral care

The status of the oral mucosa and general oral hygiene reflect a patient's ability to manage secretions and swallowing. Oral health is often compromised in those who are critically ill, while oral hygiene can be neglected in tube-fed patients. A clean and moist oral cavity is not only for patient comfort, but also can reduce nosocomial infections and thereby reduce days in the hospital and other negative outcomes. Patients who require supplemental oxygen delivered via a nasal cannula frequently experience dryness in the oral cavity, which may further exacerbate, and in some cases even cause, difficulty swallowing. Severe illness and many medications may alter the normal oral environment, salivary production, and the growth of oral bacteria.[92] This change in oral flora increases risk of bacterial pneumonia in critically ill patients as a result of aspiration of contaminated secretions.[93] It is not uncommon to find dry secretions crusted along the tongue, palate, and pharynx in patients who have not eaten orally in some time. Dental caries and dentures that are not well cared for can also contribute to a state of poor oral hygiene as well as poor quality of life.

The American Association of Critical-Care Nurses issued a practice alert in 2006 for oral care procedures that include: frequent oral assessments, suctioning, and providing moisture to the lips and oral mucosa.[94] Other measures included the following:

- Carefully inspect and assess the condition of the entire oral cavity with the use of a flashlight prior to giving the patient food, liquids, or oral medications.

- Providing humidification via a shovel mask or face tent and consistent oral care for the hospitalized patient may help to loosen secretions, moisten the oropharyngeal mucosa, and maximize comfort. Caution should be taken when completing oral care, as dried oral secretions may loosen during trials of fluid and inadvertently obstruct the airway.

- Chlorhexidine, a broad-spectrum antibacterial agent, is highly effective in reducing the risk of nosocomial respiratory infections and ventilator-associated pneumonia in critically ill patients.[95]

Oral feeding options

Effortless, efficient, and safe swallowing are important criteria for continued oral nutrition. While there is no cure for a swallowing disorder in palliative care patient, continued oral intake may be facilitated by careful hand-feeding techniques employed by family and caregivers. These techniques will vary depending on the underlying swallowing/feeding difficulty. Hand feeding has been found to produce similar outcomes of death, aspiration pneumonia, functional status, and patient comfort for patients with dementia, as initiating tube feeding.[54] The respect for the ethical principle of patient autonomy within in a shared decision-making process is a critical. It should be accompanied by a clear understanding of the risks involved in oral intake. Specifically, families and patients should be informed about the risks and consequences of developing aspiration pneumonia and malnutrition. If the decision is to continue with oral intake, even if it impacts sufficient nutrition, the safest diet should be suggested and aspiration precautions introduced, using assessment of the swallowing problem as a guide. Family members are more likely to feed a patient a particular diet and in a particular manner if they understand the physiological and psychological reasons for the recommendation and if they have been included in the decision-making.[4]

Additional suggestions for feeding the patient with dysphagia include:

1. *Remove distractions at mealtime.* This can help patients who need to concentrate on swallowing to increase safety, in individuals who are using compensatory swallowing strategies, and for patients who easily lose their focus and need to be fed, such as patients with dementia.[96]

2. *Emphasize heightened awareness of sensory cues.* Feeding patients larger boluses and increasing downward pressure of the spoon on the tongue alert the patient that food is in the mouth. Feeding patients cold or sour boluses or foods requiring some mastication may improve oral sensation and awareness. Some patients with dementia demonstrate the most efficient swallow when offered finger foods that require chewing, allowing them greater access to the automatic motor rhythm of chewing and swallowing that is reminiscent of the patterns they have used all their lives.

3. *Provide feeding utensils.* Patients who have feeding difficulties associated with hand tremors or weakness may be aided with devices such as weighted cuffs or built-up utensils.

4. *Optimize the position of the patient.* Ensure optimal posture of the patient at meals. Sit the patient as upright as possible when eating, drinking, or taking medications. Reduce the tendency to slump forward or to the side, or head extension, which can promote an open airway and make the patient more vulnerable to aspiration.

5. *Schedule meal times.* Timing of meals to coincide with increased function, and to avoid effects from fatigue or medications may enhance swallowing efficiency and safety.

6. *Consider more frequent, smaller meals with high-calorie supplements.* Increased frequency of small meals may help patients who do not have sufficient efficiency or endurance to complete an entire meal at one time.

Medication administration

Oral medications can present enormous challenges to patients with dysphagia. One study looking at pill swallowing in patients with chronic dysphagia found that more than 60% of subjects had difficulty swallowing tablets. Some of the physiological difficulties they experienced included multiple swallows to clear the pill, residue in the pharynx after swallowing, increased time needed to swallow pills, use of liquid to assist in washing the pill down, and airway compromise.[97] Because difficulty swallowing may impact compliance with medications, finding alternative modes of presentation can be critical.

Medications deemed nonessential may be temporarily or permanently discontinued. Crushing medications or burying them whole in a semisolid food such as applesauce or ice cream creates a uniform consistency and makes swallowing easier. However, crushing, opening, or chewing a medicine can alter its pharmacological properties, render it unlicensed, and may result in a potentially toxic and lethal dose.[98] Thus, always clarify whether a medication can be altered. Patients can be offered their medications in elixir form.

Consider alternative routes for medication administration including transdermal, buccal, or rectal. Compounding, done by a pharmacist, creates a medication tailored to the specialized needs of an individual patient by producing an alternative form such as a powder, nebulized substances, liquid, lozenge, or suppository. However, compounded medications are not FDA approved, their safety and effectiveness are not verified, and most third-party payers at this time will not reimburse. Due to recent tragic events occurring as a result of nonsterile injectable medications, this practice is currently under scrutiny.

Healthcare providers and patients should refer to the FDA statement on regulation of compounded drugs found at http://www.fda.gov/Drugs/GuidanceComplianceRegulatoryInformation/PharmacyCompounding/default.htm.

Orally disintegrating medication (ODT) technology has been used to formulate medications that rapidly disintegrate in the oral cavity once placed on or under the tongue. FDA guidelines regarding ODTs can be found at http://www.fda.gov/downloads/Drugs/GuidanceComplianceRegulatoryInformation/Guidances/UCM070578.pdf. One study comparing this method of presentation with oral tablets found that dysphagic patients rated orally disintegrating medications easier to swallow.[97]

Alternative nutrition and hydration

For patients with a disease process that results in dysphagia and an inability to swallow, a decision may need to be made regarding placement of a gastrostomy or jejunostomy tubes to provide alternative hydration and nutrition (see chapter 13). Expected medical benefits often include improved nutrition and hydration, easier administration of medications, prolongation of life, prevention of aspiration, diminished pain, and facilitation of nursing home placement. Irrespective of the scenario, the following should be considered:

1. Patients and their families need to be fully informed regarding benefits and risks of nonoral and oral feeding options in order to make fully informed decisions and to incorporate patient's wishes early into the care plan.[54] For certain conditions, early placement of tube feeding may provide the patient with several more months of improved quality of life afforded by strength and endurance. Patients and families may also feel a sense of relief afforded to them because of the tube feeding itself.

2. However, a growing body of literature shows that overall there are limited medical benefits in improving survival rates, reducing aspiration risk, or improving functional status and that the expected benefits may exceed actual outcomes.[99,100]

3. The presence of a feeding tube does not inherently imply NPO, or nothing by mouth. Some patients may continue to take small amounts of food or liquid for their pleasure and comfort.

4. More creative solutions may help to ease the feeding decision. Although hand feeding is time consuming, it allows for continued intimate contact between patient and caregiver. One prominent geriatrician has proposed creating new solutions, such as Ensure lollipops or sublingual high-calorie drops.[101,102]

Sialorrhea and secretion management

Sialorrhea, or excessive salivation and drooling due to the inability to control oral secretions, is common in patients with neurological conditions such as motor neuron disease and PD, with estimates of up to 80% of patients with PD experiencing excessive salivation.[103–105] This is caused by impaired swallowing function, reduced frequency of swallowing, reduced oropharyngeal or laryngeal sensation, poor head posture, inability to close the oral cavity, and a weak cough with poor clearance of secretions. Hypersecretion may also occur in the setting of oral or dental infection, as a side effect of medication, or following extensive surgical reconstruction and repair such as in head and neck cancer.[105] Excessive salivation can be embarrassing and socially disabling, as well as contribute to skin irritation, poor oral health, dehydration, and increased risk of aspiration pneumonia.[105] In the early stages, behavioral, compensatory, and/or strengthening exercises via speech-language therapy to improve oromotor function and sensation, tongue control, self-management, and general body posture may be helpful.[106]

In more severe disease, treatment options include anticholinergic medications (glycopyrrolate, scopolamine, benzotropine); botulinum toxin; radiation therapy to the parotid and submandibular glands; and surgical resection of either the parasympathetic neural pathway or of the submandibular and salivary glands. However, each of these treatment options has significant side effects, such as thickened secretions that are more difficult to expectorate, mucus plugging, dehydration, constipation, and drowsiness[106] and may be contraindicated or poorly tolerated in various populations.[107–109]

Caregiver and family members' experience

The experience of a family member providing care for a terminally ill patient is stressful. Managing the tube feeding, care of a gastrostomy tube stoma, changing diet textures, and altering social lives due to dysphagia is a significant burden, both physical and psychological. One study that examined the experience of caring for a dysphagic relative with head and neck cancer revealed the stress of becoming a "nurse–caregiver," the sense of "living between tube feedings" and feeling tied down by it, and the distress experienced from an inability to attend important social events because of the dysphagic individual's inability to eat.[110] Partnering with the caregiver and the healthcare team's engagement with the caregiver throughout the care of the dysphagic patient at the end of- life is essential to alleviating burden and stress to the extent possible.

Dry mouth (xerostomia)

Case study

Mrs. F, a woman with multiple medical problems

Mrs. F is a 60-year-old woman with a history of worsening Hepatitis C, Hepatitis B, HIV, renal impairment, and pulmonary disease. She is on multiple medications, which results in dry mouth. She is deconditioned and requires oxygen. She frequently develops pneumonia that necessitates hospital admission. Her main complaint is dry mouth. She cannot sleep at night as her dry mouth wakes her up at night, even with gel substitute saliva. She is unable to drink as often as she would like because of the fluid restriction necessitated by her kidney disease. Moreover, she doesn't like to drink too much at one time because then she needs to use the restroom frequently. Her medication schedule was adjusted to space out the medications to prevent enhanced dry mouth. She did not want to add any other medications because she is on so many. She brushes her teeth several times a day to stimulate saliva. She is trialing a saliva substitute spray.

Definition

Xerostomia is the sensation of oral dryness, which may or may not be accompanied by decreased salivary secretions. Xerostomia is also known as salivary gland dysfunction or hyposalivation.[111] Although patients receiving palliative care commonly experience oral dryness, it is often difficult to identify the exact underlying cause and/or contributing factors.[112–115] Decreased salivary function and prolonged xerostomia cause significant oral symptoms in the mouth, including dental caries, oral pain, gum, tongue, oral mucosal irritations and lesions, mouth infections, taste changes, and bad breath.[111,115,116] In the esophageal region, problems include swallowing difficulties, along with alterations in speech formation and voice function.[115,117] Such conditions may cause physical discomfort and emotional suffering, resulting in the retreat from socializing.[113,118]

Although a serious side effect, many health professionals consider it a trivial or minimal symptom.[119] However, it has a negative impact on quality of life. Xerostomia may cause not only physical discomfort but emotional suffering and a retreat from socializing.[113,118] Social rituals, particularly meal times, offer a time to communicate, laugh or smile, and eat, all of which provide an avenue of support for patients and families coping with chronic progressive or serious life-threatening illness. Therefore, treatment not only offers the benefits of better nutrition, better sleep, and better dental health but also offers social structure to promote coping.

Incidence

In several studies, xerostomia appears to be common in 30%–50% of patients.[120] Other authors estimate that xerostomia affects 30% of palliative care patients.[114,121,122] In palliative care, xerostomia appears to be a major source of discomfort in patients with cancer. Well described in the cancer literature, it has been described in other conditions: diabetes, end-stage renal failure, end-stage cardiac disease in addition to end-stage liver disease.[121,123] In the population at large, xerostomia increases with age and with increased pharmacological treatment secondary to medical problems.

Pathophysiology

Dry mouth is rooted in reduced saliva. Saliva is produced by numerous glands in the oropharynx.[124,125] The average production of saliva in a healthy adult is 1.5 liters a day. The parotid glands, the submandibular glands, and the sublingual glands produce 90% of saliva, the other 10% produced in the oral pharynx. Parotid glands, located below and in front of each ear, produce a serous and watery saliva.[124,125,126] Therefore, damage to the parotid gland will produce a thicker saliva. Submandibular glands, located in the lower jaw, secrete mostly serous saliva with some mucinous elements.[124,126] Sublingual glands produce purely mucous saliva.[124,126] The overall viscosity of saliva is dependent on the functioning of the various glands.

Saliva is necessary to the process of oral nutrition in initiating the breakdown of food; it also facilitates chewing, swallowing, and talking. The properties of saliva allow for oral lubrication, gum and tissue repair and aid in gustation with food-bolus formation and food breakdown. Additionally, saliva breaks down bacterial substances, offering immunoprotection for oral mucosa and dental structures.[125–127] Saliva thereby inhibits dental caries and infections, while providing protection against extreme temperatures of food and drink.[124,128] In this way, it has antimicrobial properties, buffering properties, and liquid properties to help with gustation.[128]

Saliva production is regulated by the nervous system. Within 2 to 3 seconds, smell, sight, or taste of food stimulates salivary production.[126] There is a two-step process to saliva secretion: (1) production at the acinar level of the cells and (2) secretion where saliva is actually secreted into the mouth via the ducts.[100] Saliva comprises several elements. Ninety-nine percent of saliva is fluid composed of water and mucus, providing a lubricative element. The remaining 1% of saliva is solid, containing salts, proteins, minerals such as calcium bicarbonate ions, and enzymes such as pytalin, antibodies, and other antimicrobial agents.[124,126] Four general categories of xerostomia exist: (1) reduced salivary secretions, (2) buccal erosion, (3) local or systemic dehydration, and (4) other miscellaneous conditions.

Reduced salivary secretion is commonly caused by medication side effects, infections, hypothyroidism, autoimmune processes, and sarcoidosis. Oral dryness may result from oral diseases such as acute and chronic parotitis, or partial or complete salivary obstruction.[124] In cancer patients, reduced saliva production may be caused by tumor-induced salivary gland destruction or treatment. Cancer treatment including both radiation and chemotherapy affect salivary production. Radiation to the head and neck can reduce saliva production by 50% to 60% within the first week of treatment because of inflammation.[126] Chemotherapy and cytotoxic agents may also cause dry mouth, particularly in advanced disease.[126] Medications are notorious culprits of dry mouth, particularly several classifications common in of medications commonly used in palliative care: sedatives, tranquilizers, antihistamines, antiparkinsonian medications, antiseizure medications, skeletal muscle relaxants, tricyclic antidepressants, and anticholinergics.[124,126]

Buccal erosion frequently occurs in cancer and cancer treatment, particularly chemotherapy and radiation.[111] The duration of radiation and/or radiation doses affects the persistence and degree of salivary reduction.[111] In addition, buccal erosion and subsequent dry mouth is common in immune-related conditions such as Sjögren's syndrome, diabetes mellitus, HIV/AIDS, scleroderma, sarcoidosis, lupus, Alzheimer's disease, and graft versus host disease.[111,124,126]

Systemic dehydration-induced xerostomia results from a wide spectrum of conditions including debility, anorexia, vomiting, diarrhea, fever, drying oxygen therapies, mouth breathing, polyuria, diabetes, hemorrhage, and swallowing difficulties. Mental health issues may induce dry mouth including depression, coping reactions, anxiety, and depression.[116,118] Due to diurnal production, dry mouth sensations are worse at night, resulting in sleep interruptions. Over longer periods of time, lack of sleep may cause anxiety, depression, and distress as part of the stress response.[118]

The number of comorbidities with resultant complex pharmacotherapy, and not the age of the patient, increases the risk of xerostomia.[124,129,130] These same comorbidities make the management of plaque and gum difficult.[124,129,130] Patients undergoing cancer treatment or other immunosuppressive therapies may either be too immunocompromised to undergo oral surgery or treatment procedures. Thus, patients may experience simultaneous discomfort from their chronic progressive illness, or serious life-threatening illness as well as subsequent oral distress.

Assessment

As stated above, xerostomia is a dry mouth. However, it may be accompanied by other oral symptoms such as burning, smarting, and soreness of both the oral mucosa and the tongue, with or without the presence of ulcers. There may be difficulty with mastication, swallowing, and speech. Or, there may be taste alterations, difficulty with dentures, and an increase in dental caries subsequent to the lack of the protective characteristics of saliva. Common secondary concerns are nutritional issues, sleep, and rest.[131–132] Therefore, a thorough history should review these problem areas along with the subjective distress of xerostomia and current medications (Box 11.3).[124,133]

A comprehensive assessment will assist in determining etiology. Assessment should include patient rating in eight aspects of dry mouth. These areas include overall mouth and lip dryness, speech, chewing, sleeping, dry mouth with eating and swallowing, resting, and the frequency of sipping liquids for eating and during the rest of the day.[130,132,134,135] Sample questions are included in Box 11.3.

Oral examination

An intraoral examination will reveal clear indications of dry mouth: pale and dry mucosal and buccal areas, the presence of a dry and fissured tongue, a red raw tongue, the absence of salivary pooling, and the presence of oral ulcerations, gingivitis, or candidiasis.[114,126,134] Salivary glands should be noted for swelling, indicating obstruction, and dentition should be examined for caries. Extraoral examination reveals cracked lips, often with angular cheilitis (lip inflammation) or candida at the corners of the mouth.

There are several diagnostic tests for xerostomia, saliva measurement, and dry mouth evaluation. There are two standard

---

Box 11.3 Xerostomia assessment questions

Do you experience dry mouth? How frequently?
Does dry mouth bother you?
Do you have dry lips?
Do you have dry nasal passages?
Do your gums bleed when you brush your teeth?
Is your tongue red and raw?

Do you find there are times you need to drink more fluids? When?
Do you experience difficulty speaking due to a dry or sticky mouth?
Do you have difficulty chewing? What types of foods?
Do you have difficulty swallowing? Solids or liquids?

Do you need extra fluid to help you swallow food? All foods or solids or semisolids?
Do you use hard candies or gum for your dry mouth?
Do you find your sleep is disrupted dry mouth? How often do you wake up at night because of a dry mouth?
Have you experienced altered taste sensations? What types of tastes? Any types of foods?

Do you use tobacco? How often?
Do you drink alcohol? How often?
Do you drink caffeine? In what drinks? In what foods?
Are you taking any prescription medications, over-the-counter medications or preparations?

Sources: Fehrenbach (2010) reference 130; Cancer Care Ontario (2013), reference 132; Dahlin, Cohen, and Goldsmith (2010), reference 133.

bedside tests for xerostomia: the cracker biscuit test and the tongue blade test. The cracker biscuit test involves giving a patient a dry cracker or biscuit. If the patient cannot eat the cracker without extra fluids, xerostomia is present.[117] The tongue blade test is an extension of mouth inspection. After inspection is complete, the tongue blade is placed on the tongue. Since dry mouth makes for ropey, pasty saliva, the tongue blade will stick to the tongue of a patient with xerostomia. Another, more aggressive test is unstimulated or stimulated sialometric measurement of saliva.[53,131,135] This test measures the amount of saliva collected by spitting into a container, swabbing the mouth with a cotton-tipped applicator, or salivating into a test container at a set time. However, for most palliative care patients, this may be a burdensome and unnecessary test.

Documentation of the extent of xerostomia is essential. There are many rating scales specifically designed for this purpose. There are several scales suggest in Box 11.4. The American Dental Hygienists' Association documentation is the most comprehensive versus documentation based only on saliva changes as offered by the American Cancer Society or the Oncology Nursing Society.

Prevention

Prevention occurs in pretreatment considerations. The National Institute of Dental and Craniofacial Research suggests a pretreatment screening ideally four to six weeks prior to the commencement of any treatments.[138] During this screening assessment, oral examination is performed to identify potential issues, such as infection, fractured teeth or restorations, or periodontal disease that could contribute to oral complications once treatment begins. The evaluation also establishes baseline data for comparison in subsequent examinations. Should any treatment such as fillings, extractions, or periodontal surgery be necessary before treatment initiation, 2 weeks of recovery allows time for healing and reduces further complications of infection from low blood counts.

Box 11.4 Dry mouth rating scales

American Dental Hygienists Association[130]

Tissue changes (tongue and mucosal color)
Oral disease (bad breath, cavities, infection)
Saliva, glands, and function

American Cancer Society[136]

Decreased saliva
Thick saliva
No saliva

Oncology Nursing Society[137]

0 No dry mouth

1 Mild dryness, slightly thickened saliva, little change in taste

2 Moderate dryness, thick and sticky saliva, markedly altered taste

3 Complete dryness of mouth

4 Salivary necrosis

---

[138] Further education about both the importance and comfort of good oral care is essential.

Management

Much of xerostomia management focuses on interventions to alleviate rather than interventions to eradicate or prevent the symptom. The goal is to protect patients from further complications. Table 11.3 offers suggestions for pharmacological management. A stepwise approach should guide management and treatment, as suggested in Box 11.5.

Nonpharmacological interventions

Nonpharmacological interventions should be tried first. Of course preventive measures may help reduce dry mouth. Nonpharmacological use of gustatory stimulation includes a myriad of measures (see Table 11.4). All of these interventions are short term and relatively inexpensive with few adverse effects. Insurances may cover some of these costs as well except procedures. Acupuncture during and after radiation therapy for head

---

Box 11.5 Stepwise process for managing Xerostomia[133]

1. Treat underlying infections—Candidiasis should be treated using nystatin swish-and-swallow or fluconazole 150 mg PO.[139]

2. Review and alter current medications as appropriate. It is important to first evaluate the necessity of specific xerostomia-inducing drugs. There are numerous medications that list oral dryness as a side effect.[126] Specifically, anticholinergics, antihistamines, phenothiazines, antidepressants, opioids, β-blockers, diuretics, anticonvulsants, sedatives, and tobacco all may cause oral dryness.[123] Thus, patients with heart conditions, mental health issues, depression, anxiety, neurological disorders, and pain disorders may be at risk for dry mouth. If eliminating possible culprit medication is not possible, other possible strategies include decreasing the dosage to decrease dryness, or altering the schedule to assure that the peak effect of medication does not coincide with nighttime peak of decreased salivary production.

3. Stimulate salivary flow—Salivary stimulation can occur with both nonpharmacological and pharmacological interventions.

4. Replace lost secretions with saliva substitutes—Saliva substitutes are better tolerated than artificial salivas. Oral spray preparations are best tolerated.[140] Saliva substitutes are based on aqueous solution and may contain carboxymethyl cellulose or mucin from animals. Attention must be paid to any philosophical, cultural, or religious prohibitions concerning the animal ingredients of saliva substitutes.[141]

5. Protect teeth—Continue meticulous mouth care. Protect with fluoride rinses.

6. Rehydrate—Drink plenty of liquids.

7. Modify diet—Avoid mouth pain from acids or hard foods.

Table 11.3 Pharmacological interventions

Medication	Description	Dose	Side effect
Pilocarpine	◆ Nonselective muscarinic ◆ A parasympathetic agent that increases exocrine gland secretion and stimulates residual functioning tissue in damaged salivary glands. Increases saliva production.[146] ◆ New studies have shown that pilocarpine given before and during radiotherapy can reduce xerostomia.[114,115]	Dose may be given at 5 mg TID or QID depending on how well patients tolerate the medication and its side effect.	◆ Response varies with severity of xerostomia. ◆ Pilocarpine should not be used in patients with chronic obstructive pulmonary disease, asthma, bradycardia, renal or hepatic impairment, glaucoma or bowel obstruction.[146] ◆ Side effects include mild to moderate sweating, visual disturbances, nausea, rhinitis, chills, flushing, sweating, dizziness, increased urinary frequency, abdominal cramping, and asthenia.[146] ◆ Side effects can be lessened if taken with milk.[146]
Bethanechol	M-3 muscarinic relieves anticholinergic side effects of tricyclic antidepressants.		
Methacholine	A parasympathomimetic compound that increases salivation.[146]	Dose is 10 mg a day.	◆ Hypotension ◆ Short acting.[146]
Yohimbine	Blocks α-2 adrenoreceptors	Dose is 14 mg a day.	◆ Drowsiness, confusion, and atrial fibrillation, lasting up to 3 hours.[146]
Cevimeline	◆ A M-1 and M-3 muscarinic agonist. ◆ Acts to increase saliva by inhibiting acetylcholinesterase. ◆ Works on salivary glands and lacrimal glands, promoting increased salivary flow and tears in the eyes.[146]	Used in a spray or mouthwash gargle, it lasts up to 6 hours.[146]	◆ Less effect than pilocarpine.
Antifungals	◆ May be needed for oral dryness caused by oral candidial infections.	First-line treatment is nystatin (suspension or troches, depending on swallowing ability), which is inexpensive. Second treatment includes fluconazole. For fungal infections of the lips may necessitate the use of miconazole, clotrimazole, or ketonacozole.[115]	◆ Taste changes

Sources: Davies (2011), reference 111; Dahlin, Cohen, and Goldsmith (2010), reference 133.

and neck cancer has been found to prevent chronic dry mouth. A randomized controlled trial using acupuncture concurrently with radiation therapy for patients with nasopharyngeal cancer reduced the incidence and severity of xerostomia and improved quality of life,[147] while another small sample study demonstrated that 9 of 10 patients treated with acupuncture for radiation-induced dysphagia and xerostomia reported subjective improvements in swallowing, xerostomia, and pain.[148] Others have shown lasting benefits and effectiveness in other patient populations with xerostomia, such as Sjogren's syndrome, and recommend a 3- to 4-week regimen of weekly acupuncture treatments.[149]

Special considerations for older adults with impaired cognition

There are several considerations to managing xerostomia in the patient with cognitive impairment.[115] First, if a patient forgets oral care, the nurse should strategize on reminders and enlist family or other providers to assist. Second, their dentures need to be attended to and need to be thoroughly cleaned daily by brushing with appropriate cleansers. If the nurse is unable to remove or insert dentures to do oral exam due to the patient's agitation, the nurse may need to another person to do simultaneous distraction or enlist the assistance of another provider while cleaning dentures. Third, if the patient refuses oral care, the nurse needs to assess the reason for refusal and ameliorate that issue if possible. If the patient bites on a toothbrush, have several toothbrushes available to allow the patient to bite on one, while care occurs with another. Finally, if the patient has difficulty with mouthwash and toothpastes, it may be helpful for the nurse to use a suction toothbrush.

Nursing interventions

Interventions will vary from one patient to the next based on the degree of xerostomia. Strong evidence supporting the efficacy of one treatment over another has not been demonstrated. Education is indispensable in dry mouth, and nurses provide essential information about xerostomia. During palliative treatments, patients need encouragement and support in ongoing dental care. This

Table 11.4 Interventions for xerostomia management

Intervention	Role/Effect	Benefit	Comment
I. Preventative			
Oral care	◆ Reduces xerostomia severity ◆ Promotes well-being		Frequent brushing with soft brushes, water jet, denture cleaning, fluoride rinses, mouthwash, and flossing, can stimulate salivation. This can help prevent candidiasis, particularly since dentures can harbor infections.[115,138]
Lip protectants	◆ Prevents cracked lips, and use of saliva moistens lips ◆ Includes use of lip protectants such as balms, chap sticks, and other preparations		Care should be taken not to use products with alcohol, since these can be irritating. Angular chelitis at corners of the mouth need protection with the use of lanolin and KY Jelly.[115,138]
Dentifrices	◆ Cleans teeth of food and fluid debris ◆ Protects teeth from caries		Several are manufactured for patients with dry mouth that contain antimicrobial enzymes to reduce oral infections and enhance mouth wetting. Examples are Biotene, Oral Balance, and Oasis.[142]
Mouthwashes Non-alcohol containing	◆ Helps rinse debris from mouth		Includes homemade mouthwashes made from saline, sodium bicarbonate, glycerin.[138]
II. Diet modifications			
	◆ Allows patient to eat	Soft texture foods are better tolerated than rough foods. In addition, instruct patients to take fluids with all meals and snacks. The use of gravies and juices with foods can add moisture to swallowing.[112,113]	Soups, pudding, mashed potatoes, and shakes rather than foods with rough edges such as crackers or toast. Olive oil or another light oil to the gums and mucosa may help act as a lubricant.[113] Patients may sip such foods in milk, tea, or water to assist in swallowing. Education regarding the avoidance of sugars, spicy foods, sometimes salt, and dry or piquant foods is important, although preferred tastes may vary from one patient to the next. For dry mouth without oral ulcerations, provide carbonated drinks such as ginger ale, as well as cider, apple juice, or lemonade. Fresh fruits, papaya juice, or pineapple juice may help some patients refresh their mouths; however, citrus products may be too acidic and irritating for other patients.[132,133]
III. Nonpharmacological			
Peppermint water	◆ Mucous saliva	Inexpensive	Interacts with metoclopramide[117]
Vitamin C	◆ Chemical reduction ◆ Disrupts salivary mucin to reduce viscosity of saliva[143]	Inexpensive Reduces viscosity	Can irritate mouth if sores present Use in lozenges or other forms as preferred. May be irritating to the mouth, particularly if the patient has mouth sores.[104] Can erode dental enamel.
Citric acid/sweets	For mucous saliva	Inexpensive	Can irritate like vitamin C. In sweets, can cause caries. Presents in malic acid or in sweets Can cause burning[104]

Table 11.4 Continued

Chewing gum, mints	For watery saliva ♦ May create a buffer system to compensate for dietary acids.[143] ♦ Effective as salivary stimulants due to the effect on chemoreceptors and mechanical receptors.	Inexpensive	Chewing gum is more effective than mints. In particular, a low tack gum is preferable for patients with dentures.[111] Preferably, gum is sugarless, to prevent caries and infections, because an immunocompromised state promotes cavities and infections. Attention must be paid to social acceptance of gum chewing, particularly in older populations.[141] Side effect of diarrhea from sorbitol if too much gum or mints taken.[141]
Rehydration	Replenish oral hydration by sipping water, spraying water, and increasing humidity in the air.		This includes adding humidity to oxygen systems, and using vaporizers to add humidity to the dying effects of indoor heating and air conditioning. To assist in sleep, instituting these measures at night may help rest.
Saliva replacement			
Water sprays or sip	Reduces pain or decreases saliva It is usually well tolerated and easily accessible.	Inexpensive	Short acting There is no research on whether optimal relief results from either warm or cold. Thus, temperature is a personal choice.[143]
Artificial saliva	Artificial saliva contains carboxymethylcellulose or mucin; dose 2 mL every 3 to 4 hours.	Inexpensive	Those with a mucin base appear to be better tolerated than those derived from carboxymethylcellulose.[142] Both types of preparation bases are better tolerated as an oral spray than as a gel or rinse.[144]
Procedures			
Laser treatment	Stimulate saliva production	Longer lasting Expensive	Administered in an office to salivary glands.[145]
Electrostimulation	Stimulate saliva production	Longer lasting Less expensive than laser therapy	Delivered to the glands and tongue via a battery-operated process.[128]
Acupuncture	Increase production	Noninvasive Variable costs	Can be expensive. Relief may occur in a single treatment or regular weekly treatment with needle placement in the ears and finger. One study showed that 6 weeks of twice-weekly treatment increased salivation for up to 1 year. Another study used a 3-to-4 weekly regimen, with monthly maintenance visits to relieve xerostomia.[128,145]

Sources: Davies (2011) reference 111; Dahlin, Cohen, and Goldsmith (2010), reference 133.

includes the use of soft tooth brushes, wetting the brush before using, the long term need for fluoride rinses and toothpaste, and dietary restrictions of sugar to prevent further infections and caries. As a patient declines, teaching the family how to provide mouth care offers a tangible and important role in the comfort of the patient. Standardized oral care procedures and protocols vary from one institution to another. The nurse may help a family systematically try a variety of therapies from nonpharmacological to pharmacological to achieve relief. However, goals of care and medication interactions and side effects should be reviewed in the context of the patient's overall condition.

Summary

As a symptom, dry mouth may be considered inconsequential. However, it has considerable quality of life implications. To create a suitable management plan, the nurse must assess the distress from xerostomia and determine financial considerations. Patients may be responsible to pay out-of-pocket costs for nonpharmacological interventions or may have limited coverage of pharmacological agents. Oral care and education are an essential strategy and may prevent severe dry mouth. There is no strong data to support pharmacological over nonpharmacological strategies. Patients may choose nonpharmacological therapy because it is inexpensive and has fewer side effects. Families will need to help manage the symptom as the patient declines. However, continued oral care can promote dignity.

Hiccups

Case study

GS, an older male with HIV

GS is a 55-year-old male with HIV. He is an infectious disease physician who contracted HIV from a central line. He is more symptomatic and is very sick. He has been considering how long he wants to endure the disease. However, he is admitted for pneumocystis pneumonia (PCP). He develops hiccups, which affect his talking, eating, and sleep. A thorough examination is performed to determine the etiology. He is prescribed metoclopramide to decrease abdominal distention and lactulose to relieve constipation. He is treated for anxiety. An endoscopy is performed to stimulate the vagal nerve. He is then started on baclofen 10 mg TID, which reduces the hiccups. This is increased to 20 QID but then causes too much sedation and dry mouth. He is placed on chlorpromazine 15 mg BID with discussion for sedation if the hiccups persist.

Definition

Hiccup, or singultus, is defined as sudden, involuntary contractions of one or both sides of the diaphragm and intercostal muscles, terminated by an abrupt closure of the glottis, producing a characteristic sound of "hic." Hiccup occurs with a frequency of approximately 4 to 60 times per minute.[150] Prolonged hiccups result in fatigue and exhaustion from both respiratory insufficiency and sleep interferences. Anxiety, depression, and frustration result if eating and/or sleeping are routinely interrupted. Although seemingly insignificant, hiccups affect quality of life.[150]

Prevalence and impact

Hiccups, in the palliative care population, have undergone more review. However, the literature focuses on case studies rather than research into treatment. Therefore, the incidence and prevalence are not known. Estimates of prevalence of hiccups in cancer patients is about 10% to 20%.[151]

Pathophysiology

The precise pathophysiology and the physiological function of hiccups are not well understood. They are believed to be a primitive function, such as yawning or vomiting, that developed within the evolutionary process that now serves no discrete purpose.[150] However, functionally, hiccups arise from a synchronous clonic spasm or spasmodic contraction of the diaphragm and the intercostal muscles, which results in sudden inspiration and prompt closure of the glottis, causing the hiccup sounds. The anatomical cause of hiccups is thought to be bimodal, with association either with the phrenic or vagus nerve,[150] or central nervous involvement, which causes misfiring. It is hypothesized that a hiccup reflex arc is located within the phrenic nerves, the vagal nerves, and T6–T12 sympathetic fibers, as well as a possible hiccup center in either the respiratory center, the brainstem, or the cervical cord

between C3 and C5.[150] However, there does not appear to be a discrete hiccup center comparable to the chemoreceptor trigger zone for nausea.

Evidence suggests an inverse relationship between partial pressure of carbon dioxide (pCO_2) and hiccups; that is, an increased pCO_2 decreases the frequency of hiccups and a decreased pCO_2 increases frequency of hiccups.[150] Interestingly, hiccups have a minimal effect on respiration, although they cause fatigue and a sensation of inability to take deep breaths. Hiccup strength or amplitude varies within discrete hiccup episodes as well as from patient to patient. This amplitude produces the distress, as continuous strong hiccups are exhausting as a result of the energy used in hiccupping.

There are three categories of hiccups: benign, persistent, and intractable hiccups. Benign, self-limiting hiccups occur frequently; an episode can last from several minutes to 2 days. The primary etiology is gastric distention; other causes include sudden changes in temperature, alcohol ingestion, excess smoking, and psychogenic alternations. Persistent, or chronic, hiccups continue for more than 48 hours but less than 1 month. Third and last are intractable hiccups, which persist longer than 1 month.[150–152,153,154] In palliative care, the duration may not be as important as the amplitude or strength of the hiccup depending on the population. For instance, a patient with ALS or COPD may have more distress than a cardiac patient, as they are already weak and breathing is compromised.

Intractable hiccups result from more than 100 different causes ranging from metabolic disturbances to complex structural lesions of the CNS or infections.[151,150] Particular causes can be consolidated into four categories: structural, metabolic, inflammatory, and infectious disorders.[150,151] Structural conditions specifically affect or irritate the peripheral branches of the phrenic and vagus nerves, such as in abdominal or mediastinal tumors, hepatomegaly, ascites, or gastric distention, and CNS disorders. Persistent hiccups can indicate serious underlying disorders, such as thoracic aneurysm, brainstem tumors, metabolic and drug-related disorders, infectious diseases, and psychogenic disorders.[150,151] Common causes in terminal illness include neurological disorders such as stroke, brain tumors, and sepsis and metabolic imbalances; phrenic nerve irritations such as tumor compression or metastases; pericarditis, pneumonia, or pleuritis; and vagal nerve irritations such as esophagitis, gastric distention, gastritis, pancreatitis, hepatitis, and myocardial infarction.[150,151] Medications including steroids, chemotherapy, dopamine antagonists, megestrol, methyldopa, nicotine, opioids, and muscle relaxants may also cause hiccups.[151] Dexamethasone, a frequently used palliative medication, may cause hiccups.[152]

Assessment

Extensive work-up for hiccups in palliative care is impractical, uncomfortable, and reveals little to assist in determining the etiology or delineating treatment. Studies have not revealed that laboratory tests provide any useful information to determine optimal management.[153] Nonetheless, assessment should include a subjective review of the qualitative distress induced by the hiccups. For example, in a patient with an abdominal or lung tumor, hiccups can cause excruciating pain; whereas in the obtunded patient in renal failure, hiccups may cause little distress at all.

In reviewing distress, it is important to evaluate conditions caused by the hiccups. Patients may experience weight loss due to anorexia, fatigue due to the energy use from hiccups, and inability to eat from impaired swallowing; shortness of breath from inability to take deep breaths; insomnia from hiccupping all night; heartburn from acid reflux produced by hiccups; and depression resulting from all of the above, as well as the worry that hiccups are untreatable.[150] Objective assessment includes the history and duration of the current episode of hiccups, previous episodes, and interference with rest, eating, or daily routines. Inquiry into possible triggers may be helpful, including patterns during the day, and activities preceding the hiccups such as eating, drinking, or positioning. A review of recent trauma, surgery, procedures, and acute illness, as well as a medication history, is important to help focus on potential causes. There are case reports on oral and epidural steroid- and bupivacaine-induced hiccups.[153]

The presence of hiccups themselves is quite apparent. Further physical exam may not reveal much related to the hiccups themselves but rather assists in ruling out other conditions. Oral examination may reveal signs of swelling or obstruction. Observation of the patient's general appearance includes inspection for signs of a toxic or septic process. Any wounds or infections should be examined, in addition to a through respiratory examination.[116,150] More specifically, evaluation includes temporal artery tenderness, foreign bodies in the ear, infection of the throat, goiter in the neck, pneumonia or pericarditis of the chest, abdominal distention or ascites, and signs of stroke or delirium—all diagnoses that may have hiccups as part of the constellation of signs and symptoms.[116,150] Abdominal distention, hepatomegaly, should be noted.

In very rare circumstances, specific testing may be warranted to eliminate other causes. Chest X-ray may rule out pulmonary or mediastinal processes, as well as phrenic/vagal irritation from peritumor edema in the abdominal area.[150] Blood work including a complete blood count with differential electrolytes may rule out infection, as well as electrolyte imbalances and renal failure.[150] Sometimes a CT scan of the abdomen or head may be done to rule out abnormalities or a cerebral bleed.[150]

Management

The absence of larger randomized controlled studies on the nature of hiccups therapy has resulted in lack of consensus around treatment and anecdotal therapy.[153] Consequentially, treatment is based on the bias of previous success rather than a systematic, evidence-based approach. Similar to treatment of dysphagia or xerostomia, treatment for hiccups should be focused on the underlying disease. If the etiology questionably includes simple causes such as gastric distention or temperature changes, "empiric" treatment should be initiated. Both nonpharmacological and pharmacological interventions may be used.[153] Therapies include physical maneuvers, medications, and other procedures that interfere with the hiccup arc.[153] Otherwise, treatment for more complex episodes of hiccups without clear etiology will focus on various pharmacological interventions.

Nonpharmacological treatment

Nonpharmacological treatments can be divided into seven categories and are outlined in Box 11.6. The first category is simple respiratory maneuvers. These include breath holding, rebreathing in a bag, compression of the diaphragm, ice application in the

---

Box 11.6 Nonpharmacological interventions for hiccups

Respiratory measures
- Breath holding
- Rebreathing in a paper bag
- Diaphragm compression
- Ice application in mouth
- Induction of sneeze or cough with spices or inhalants

Nasal and pharyngeal stimulation
- Nose pressure
- Stimulant inhalation
- Tongue traction
- Drinking from far side of glass
- Swallowing sugar
- Eating soft bread
- Soft touch to palate with cotton-tipped applicator
- Lemon wedge with bitters

Miscellaneous vagal stimulation
- Ocular compression
- Digital rectal massage
- Carotid massage

Psychiatric treatments
- Behavioral techniques
- Distraction

Gastric distention relief
- Fasting
- Nasogastric tube to relieve abdominal distention
- Lavage
- Induction of vomiting

Phrenic nerve disruption
- Anesthetic block
- Phrenic block
- Suboccipital release gentle traction and pressure applied to the posterior neck

Miscellaneous treatments
- Bilateral radial artery compression
- Peppermint water to relax lower esophagus
- Acupuncture

Sources: Dahlin, Cohen, and Goldsmith (2010), reference 133; Calsina-Berna et al. (2012), reference 150.

---

mouth, and induction of sneeze or cough.[150] The second category is nasal and pharyngeal stimulation. These techniques use pressure on the nose, inhalation of a stimulant, traction of the tongue, drinking from the far side of a glass, swallowing sugar, eating a lemon wedge with bitters, eating soft bread, or soft touch to the palate with a cotton-tipped applicator.[150] The third category is miscellaneous vagal stimulation, including ocular compression, and carotid massage. The fourth category is psychiatric treatments, mainly behavioral therapy. The fifth category is relief of gastric distention, comprising of repositioning, fasting, a nasogastric tube to decrease distention, lavage, and induction of vomiting.[150] The sixth category is phrenic nerve disruption, such as an anesthetic injection or traditional acupuncture.[150] The seventh and final category is miscellaneous benign remedies, such as bilateral compression of radial arteries, peppermint water to relax the lower esophagus, use of distraction, or acupressure.[150]

Pharmacological treatment

Initial therapy should attempt to decrease gastric distention, the common cause in 95% of cases. Subsequent measures include hastening gastric emptying, and relaxing the diaphragm with simethicone and metoclopramide. If ineffective, second-line therapy should focus on suppression of the hiccup reflex.[150] Common pharmacological interventions, listed in Table 11.5, include the use of various classes of medications: muscle relaxants such as baclofen, midazolam, and chlordiazepoxide; anticonvulsants such as gabapentin, carbamazepine, and valproate, corticosteroids such as dexamethasone and prednisone; dopamine antagonists such as haloperidol, droperidol, and chlorpromazine; calcium channel blockers/antiarrhythmic such as nifedipine, nimodipine, nefopam, phenytoin, lidocaine, quinidine; SSRI antidepressants, specifically sertraline; and various other medications such as ketamine, tetrahydrocannabinol (THC), and methylphenidate.[150] Third-line therapy is the use of other drugs to disrupt diaphragmatic irritation or other possible causes of hiccups, which may include anesthesia and phrenic and cervical blocks.[150] However, there is little evidence as to which interventions are effective or harmful. Drugs used in the treatment of hiccups have included chlorpromazine, metoclopramide, sodium valproate, haloperidol, amitriptyline, carbamazepine, magnesium sulfate, baclofen, gabapentin, peppermint water, simethicone, benzodiazepines, and nifedipine.[150,153]

Nursing interventions

Although hiccups appear to be a simple reflex, their specific mechanism of action is unclear due to myriad etiologies. Many patients are frustrated because their discomfort and disruption were not taken seriously. The nurse can help discuss with the patient their concerns about treatment and their desire for comfort. Nursing interventions should focus on information regarding the broad range of strategies to eliminate the hiccups. Thus, the nursing role is one of advocate to promote comfort, empathetic listener, and educator.

The extent of aggressive treatment will depend on the degree of distress of the hiccups and the interference with quality of life—in particular, the extent of impact that hiccups have on the daily routine, specifically on sleep and nutrition. Information should include nonpharmacological maneuvers such as respiratory maneuvers, nasal and pharyngeal stimulation, distraction, and peppermint waters. If these measures fail to eradicate the hiccups, the nurse can discuss the range of pharmacological options and offer reassurance to continue various efforts because patients respond differently. Antacids may decrease gas, antiemetics may affect dopamine levels, and muscle relaxants may affect both gamma-aminobutyric acid channels and skeletal muscle. Separately they may be ineffective, but together they target several regions that trigger hiccups.

If all of these medications fail to induce hiccup reduction or cessation, the nurse should suggest a referral to a palliative care service,

Table 11.5 Suggested pharmacological treatment for hiccups[150]

Agent	Effect
Agents to decrease gastric distention	
Simethicone 15–30 mL PO q 4 h	Promotes emptying
Metoclopramide 10–20 mg PO/IV q 4–6 h (cannot use with peppermint water)	Promotes gastric emptying
Muscle relaxants	
Baclofen 5–20 mg PO q 6–12 h up to 15–37 mg/d	Acts at synaptic level
Midazolam 5–10 mg PO q 4 h	Reduces muscles spasm
Anticonvulsants	
Gabapentin 300–600 mg PO TID[154]	Acts on cortex area
Pregabalin 25 mg BID[155] Pregabalin is active at lower doses. Does not require a long titration (maximal doses can be reached within 1–2 weeks)	Interaction of pregabalin with the $\alpha2\delta$ subunit inhibits N- and P/Q-type voltage-sensitive Ca^{2+} channels, which control neurotransmitter release in the brain and spinal cord.
Carbamazepine 600–1200 mg PO QID-TID	Reduces muscle spasm
Valproic acid 15 mg/kg/24 hours PO divided in one or three doses. May increase by 250 mg/wk until hiccups stop	Reduces muscle spasm
Phenytoin 200 mg IV × 1, then 100 mg PO QID	Reduces muscle spasm
Antidepressants	
Amitriptyline 10–50 mg PO	Acts at central nervous system
Sertraline 50–150 mg PO QD	Acts at central nervous system
Corticosteroids	
Dexamethasone 40 mg PO QD	Reduces inflammation
Dopamine agonists	
Haloperidol 2–10 mg PO/IV/SQ q 4–12 h	Reduces muscle spasm
Chlorpromazine 5–50 mg PO/IM/IV q 4–8 h or 25–50 mg IM/IV in 1 L 0.9% normal saline	Blocks dopamine and alpha-adrenergic receptors
Calcium channel blockers	
Lidocaine 1 mg/kg loading dose followed by infusion of 2 mg/min	Blocks sodium channels
Nifedipine 10–80 mg PO QD	Causes vasodilation to suppress spasm
Other medications	
Ketamine 0.4 mg/kg	Acts on cortex and limbic system
Amitriptyline 25–90 mg PO QD	Inhibits serotonin and norepinephrine uptake

Sources: Dahlin, Cohen, and Goldsmith (2010), reference 133; Calsina-Berna et al. (2012), reference 150; Moretto et al. (2013), reference 153; Porzio et al. (2010), reference 154.

a pain service, or an anesthesia service to explore further treatment options. These services can consider possible invasive procedures such a nerve block, or infusion. However, as always, discussion with the patient should include prognosis and the benefit and burden of any procedure. If hiccups become extremely burdensome and all therapies have failed, sedation may be a consideration. Again, the nurse may act as an advocate to provide the necessary information about the implications of sedation. For further discussion of palliative sedation, the reader is referred to chapter 25.

Summary

The development of hiccups can truly affect quality of life. Though perceived as more of an annoyance rather than a symptom, hiccups can impact sleep, rest, speech, and oral nutrition. The challenge is that there is not clear evidence of one treatment over another. Quality of life and goals of care should dictate management, particularly since medications have significant side effects that may be unacceptable to the patient. Expert consensus suggests a systematic approach of nonpharmacological interventions should be initiated by pharmacological interventions. It is hoped that more research into hiccups will offer evidence-based practice.

Conclusion

Dysphagia, xerostomia, and hiccups are common problems that have not garnered much interest in research. There is more research to support evidence-based practice for dysphagia management. A multidisciplinary approach utilizing nurses, speech and language pathologists, nutritionists, dietitians, and social workers will promote successful treatment. On the other hand, xerostomia and hiccups are considered minor symptoms. Therefore, they appear to be underreported and underestimated. Nurses at the bedside, whether in a facility or at home, may be the first to identify the presence of these symptoms and understand the negative impact on quality of life. The mere act of listening to a patient's distress offers affirmation of the existence of the symptoms and validation that the symptoms will be taken seriously. Given the lack of hard evidence to manage these symptoms, the nurse must be creative in his or her approach. Working with a team can offer relief to patients and their families.

Acknowledgment

The authors would like to acknowledge and thank Tessa Goldsmith, MS, CCC-SLP, who served as the original coauthor of this chapter in the first edition and third author in the second edition, for the excellent foundation of the dysphagia portion of this chapter.

References

1. Pollens R. Role of the speech-language pathologist in palliative hospice care. J Palliat Med. 2004;7(5):694–702.
2. Schmidlin E. Artificial hydration: the role of the nurse in addressing patient and family needs. Int J Palliat Nurs. 2008;14(10):485–489.
3. Corbin-Lewis K, Liss JM, Sciortino KL. Clinical Anatomy and Physiology of the Swallow Mechanism. New York, NY: Thomson Delmar Learning; 2004.
4. Logemann JA. Evaluation and Treatment of Swallowing Disorders. Austin, TX: Pro-Ed; 1998.
5. Shaker R, Hogan WJ. Normal physiology of the aerodigestive tract and its effect on the upper gut. Am J Med. 2003;115(Suppl 3A):2S–9S.
6. Bieger D, Neuhuber W. Neural Circuits and Mediators Regulating Swallowing in the Brainstem. GI Motility online. 2006. http://www.nature.com/gimo/contents/pt1/full/gimo74.html.
7. Easterling CS. Getting acquainted with the esophagus. Perspectives on Swallowing and Swallowing Disorders (Dysphagia). 2003;12(2):3–7.
8. Kendall KA, Leonard RJ, McKenzie SW. Sequence variability during hypopharyngeal bolus transit. Dysphagia. 2003;18(2):85–91.
9. Cook IJ, Dodds WJ, Dantas RO, et al. Opening mechanisms of the human upper esophageal sphincter. Am J Physiol. 1989;257(5 Pt 1):G748–G759.
10. Mashimo H, Goyal RK. Physiology of Esophageal Motility. GI Motility online. 2006; 2013. http:www.nature.com/gimo/contents/pt1/full/gimo3.html.
11. Massey BT. Physiology of oral cavity, pharynx, and upper esophageal sphincter GI Motility online. 2006. http://www.nature.com/gimo/contents/pt1/full/gimo2.html.
12. McConnel FM, Cerenko D, Mendelsohn MS. Manofluorographic analysis of swallowing. Otolaryngol Clin North Am. 1988;21(4):625–635.
13. Dolecek TA, Propp JM, Stroup NE, Kruchko C. CBTRUS statistical report: primary brain and central nervous system tumors diagnosed in the United States in 2005–2009. Neuro Oncol. 2012;14(S 5):v1–v49.
14. Pace A, Lorenzo CD, Guariglia L, Jandolo B, Carapella CM, Pompili A. End of life issues in brain tumor patients. J Neurooncol. 2009;91(1):39.
15. Drappatz J, Schiff D, Kesari S, Norden AD, Wen PY. Medical management of brain tumor patients. Neurol Clin. 2007;25(4):1035–1071, ix.
16. Oberndorfer S, Lindeck-Pozza E, Lahrmann H, Struhal W, Hitzenberger P, Grisold W. The end-of-life hospital setting in patients with glioblastoma. J Palliat Med. 2008;11(1):26–30.
17. Roe JW, Leslie P, Drinnan MJ. Oropharyngeal dysphagia: the experience of patients with non-head and neck cancers receiving specialist palliative care. Palliat Med. 2007;21(7):567–574.
18. Sizoo EM, Braam L, Postma TJ, et al. Symptoms and problems in the end-of-life phase of high grade glioma patients. Neuro Oncol. 2010;12(11):1162–1166.
19. Mehanna H, Paleri V, West CML, Nutting C. Head and neck cancer. Part 1: epidemiology, presentation, and prevention. BMJ. 2010;341:663–666.
20. Pulte D, Brenner H. Changes in survival in head and neck cancers in the late 20th and early 21st century: a period analysis. Oncologist. 2010;15(9):994–1001.
21. Goldstein NE, Genden E, Morrison RS. Palliative care for patients with head and neck cancer: "I would like a quick return to a normal lifestyle." JAMA. 2008;299(15):1818–1825.
22. Hutcheson KA. Late radiation-associated dysphagia (RAD) in head and neck cancer patients. Perspectives on Swallowing and Swallowing Disorders (Dysphagia). 2013;22(2):61.
23. Caudell JJ, Schaner PE, Meredith RF, et al. Factors associated with long-term dysphagia after definitive radiotherapy for locally advanced head-and-neck cancer. Int J Radiat Oncol Biol Phys. 2008;72(3):410–415.
24. American Cancer Society. Esophagus Cancer: What are the Key Statistics About Esophageal Cancer? 2013. http://www.cancer.org/cancer/esophaguscancer/detailedguide/esophagus-cancer-key-statistics. Last updated January 18, 2013. Accessed June 30, 2013.
25. Freeman RK, Ascioti AJ, Mahidhara RJ. Palliative therapy for patients with unresectable esophageal carcinoma. Surg Clin N Am. 2012;92(5):1337–1351.
26. Classen M, Tytgat G, Lightdale C. Gastroenterological Endoscopy. 2nd ed. New York, NY: Thieme Medical; 2010.
27. National Cancer Institute, National Institute of Health. Esophageal Cancer. 2013. http://www.cancer.gov/cancertopics/pdq/screening/esophageal/healthprofessional/allpages#Section_22. Last update February 27, 2012. Accessed October 21, 2013.
28. Wilson JA. Management of esophageal dysphagia: the otolaryngologist's perspective updated. Perspectives on Swallowing and Swallowing Disorders (Dysphagia). 2007;16(4):7–10.

29. McLoughlin MT, Byrne MF. Endoscopic stenting: where are we now and where can we go? World J Gastroentero. 2008;14(24):3798–3803.

30. Murry T, Carrau RL. Clinical Management of Swallowing Disorders. 3rd ed. San Diego, CA: Plural; 2012.

31. Groher M, Crary M. Dysphagia: Clinical Management in Adults and Children. Maryland Heights, MO: Mosby; 2010.

32. Granda-Cameron C, DeMille D, Lynch MP, et al. An interdisciplinary approach to manage cancer cachexia. Clin J Oncol Nurs. 2010;14(1):72–80.

33. Ferguson TA, Elman LB. Clinical presentation and diagnosis of amyotrophic lateral sclerosis. NeuroRehabilitation. 2007;22(6):409–416.

34. Yorkston KM, Miller RM, Strand EA, Britton D. Management of Speech and Swallowing Disorders in Degenerative Diseases. 3rd ed. Austin, TX: Pro Ed; 2012.

35. Miller RG, Jackson CE, Kasarskis EJ, et al. Practice parameter update: the care of the patient with amyotrophic lateral sclerosis: multidisciplinary care, symptom management, and cognitive/behavioral impairment (an evidence-based review): report of the Quality Standards Subcommittee of the American Academy of Neurology. Neurology. 2009;73(15):1227–1233.

36. Elman LB, Houghton DJ, Wu GF, Hurtig HI, Markowitz CE, McCluskey L. Palliative care in amyotrophic lateral sclerosis, Parkinson's disease, and multiple sclerosis. J Palliat Med. 2007;10(2):433–457.

37. Miller N, Noble E, Jones D, Burn D. Hard to swallow: dysphagia in Parkinson's disease. Age Ageing. 2006;35(6):614–618.

38. Miller RG, Jackson CE, Kasarskis EJ, et al. Practice parameter update: the care of the patient with amyotrophic lateral sclerosis: drug, nutritional, and respiratory therapies (an evidence-based review): report of the Quality Standards Subcommittee of the American Academy of Neurology. Neurology. 2009;73(15):1218–1226.

39. Gordon PH. Amyotrophic lateral sclerosis: an update for 2013 clinical features, pathophysiology, management and therapeutic trials. Aging Dis. 2013;4(5):295–310.

40. Howard RS, Orell RW. Management of motor neurone disease. Postgrad Med J. 2002;78(926):736–741.

41. Langmore SE, Kasarskis EJ, Manca ML, Olney RK. Enteral tube feeding for amyotrophic lateral sclerosis/motor neuron disease. Cochrane Database Syst Rev. 2006;4(4):CD004030.

42. Spataro R, Ficano L, Piccoli F, LaBella V. Percutaneous endoscopic gastrostomy in amyotrophic lateral sclerosis: effect on survival. J Neurol Sci. 2011;304(1–2):44.

43. Halbig TD, Tse W, Olanow CW. Neuroprotective agents in Parkinson's disease: clinical evidence and caveats. Neurol Clin. 2004;22(3 Suppl):S1–S17.

44. Micieli G, Tosi P, Marcheselli S, Cavallini A. Autonomic dysfunction in Parkinson's disease. Neurol Sci. 2003;24(Suppl 1):S32–S34.

45. Menezes C, Melo A. Does levodopa improve swallowing dysfunction in Parkinson's patients? J Clin Pharm Ther. 2009;34(6):673–676.

46. Warren NM, Burn DJ. Progressive supranuclear palsy. Pract Neurol. 2007;7:16–23.

47. Stefanova N, Bucke P, Duerr S, Wenning G. Multiple system atrophy: an update. Lancet Neurol. 2009;8(12):1172–1178.

48. Ruegg S, Lehky Hagen M, Hohl U, et al. Oculopharyngeal muscular dystrophy—an under-diagnosed disorder? Swiss Med Wkly. 2005;135(39–40):574–586.

49. Hill M, Hughes T, Milford C. Treatment for swallowing difficulties (dysphagia) in chronic muscle disease. Cochrane Database Syst Rev. 2004(2):CD004303.

50. Hauser SG, Goodin DS. Multiple sclerosis and other demyelinating diseases. In: Longo DL, Fauci AS, Kasper DL, Hauser SL, Jameson JL, Loscalzo J (eds.), Harrison's Principles of Internal Medicine. 18th ed. New York, NY: McGraw-Hill; 2012:3395–3409.

51. Schapiro RT. Managing symptoms of multiple sclerosis. Neurol Clin. 2005;23(1):177–187, vii.

52. Calcagno P, Ruoppolo G, Grasso MG, De Vincentiis M, Paolucci S. Dysphagia in multiple sclerosis—prevalence and prognostic factors. Acta Neurol Scand. 2002;105(1):40–43.

53. Van der Steen JT, Ooms ME, Mehr DR, van der Wal G, Ribbe MW. Severe dementia and adverse outcomes of nursing home-acquired pneumonia: evidence for mediation by functional and pathophysiological decline. J Am Geriatr Soc. 2002;50(3):439–448.

54. American Geriatrics Society. Feeding Tubes in Advanced Dementia Position Statement. New York, NY: American Geriatrics Society; 2013.

55. Waters S, Sullivan P. An approach to guiding and supporting decision-making for individuals with dementia: feeding, swallowing, and nutrition considerations. Perspectives on Swallowing and Swallowing Disorders (Dysphagia) 2012; 21:105–111

56. Chen JH, Chan DC, Kiely DK, Morris JN, Mitchell SL. Terminal trajectories of functional decline in the long-term care setting. J Gerontol A Biol Sci Med Sci. 2007;62(5):531–536.

57. Fischberg D, Bull J, Casarett D, et al. Five things physicians and patients should question in hospice and palliative medicine. J Pain Symptom Manage. 2013;45(3):595–604.

58. Schechter GL. Systemic causes of dysphagia in adults. Otolaryngol Clin North Am. 1998;31(3):525–535.

59. Anker SD, Steinborn W, Strassburg S. Cardiac cachexia. Ann Med. 2004;36(7):518–529.

60. Murray J, Sullivan PA. Frail Elders and the Failure to Thrive. The ASHA Leader. October 16, 2006.

61. Sura L, Madhavan A, Carnaby G, Crary MA. Dysphagia in the elderly: management and nutritional considerations. Clin Interv Aging. 2012;7:287–298.

62. Leonard R. How Aging Affects Our Swallowing Ability. 2013; http://www.swallowingdisorderfoundation.com/how-aging-affects-our-swallowing-ability/. Last updated March 3, 2013. Accessed July 1, 2013, 2013.

63. Burkhead L, Sapienza C, Rosenbek J. Strength-training exercise in dysphagia rehabilitation: principles, procedures, and directions for future research. Dysphagia. 2007;22(3):251–265.

64. Murray J. Frailty, functional reserve, and sarcopenia in the geriatric dysphagic patient. Perspectives on Swallowing and Swallowing Disorders (Dysphagia). 2008;17(1):3.

65. Altman K, Yu G, Schaefer S. Consequence of dysphagia in the hospitalized patient: impact on prognosis and hospital resources. Arch Otolaryngol Head Neck Surg. 2010;136(8):784–789.

66. Marik PE, Kaplan D. Aspiration pneumonia and dysphagia in the elderly. Chest. 2003;124(1):328–336.

67. Carl LC, Johnson PR. Drugs and Dysphagia: How Medications Can Affect Eating and Swallowing. Austin, TX: PRO-ED, 2006.

68. Rudolph JL, Gardner KF, Gramigna GD, McGlinchey RE. Antipsychotics and oropharyngeal dysphagia in hospitalized older patients. J Clin Psychopharmacol. 2008;28(5):532–535.

69. Brady Wagner L. Dysphagia: Legal and ethical issues in caring for persons at the end of life. Perspectives on Swallowing and Swallowing Disorders (Dysphagia). 2008;17(1):27–32.

70. Davis LA. Quality of life issues related to dysphagia. Topics in Geriatric Rehabilitation. 2007;23(4):352–365.

71. Levy A, Dominguez-Gasson L, Brown E, Frederick C. Managing Dysphagia in the Adult Approaching End of Life: Technology at End of Life Questioned. The ASHA Leader. July 24, 2004.

72. Logemann J, Rademaker AW, Pauloski BR, et al. What information do clinicians use in recommending oral versus nonoral feeding in oropharyngeal dysphagic patients? Dysphagia. 2008;23(4):378–384.

73. Ramsey D, Smithard D, Kalra L. Silent aspiration: what do we know? Dysphagia. 2005;20(3):218–225.

74. Hinchey JA, Shephard T, Furie K, Smith D, Wang D, Tonn S. Formal dysphagia screening protocols prevent pneumonia. Stroke. 2005;36(9):1972–1976.

75. Sharma JC, Fletcher S, Vassallo M, Ross I. What influences outcome of stroke--pyrexia or dysphagia? Int J Clin Pract. 2001;55(1):17–20.

76. Terre R, Mearin F. Prospective evaluation of oro-pharyngeal dysphagia after severe traumatic brain injury. Brain Inj. 2007;21(13–14):1411–1417.

77. Wesling M, Brady S, Jensen M, Nickell M, Statkus D, Escobar N. Dysphagia outcomes in patients with brain tumors undergoing inpatient rehabilitation. Dysphagia. 2003;18(3):203–210.

78. Leder SB. Gag reflex and dysphagia. Head Neck. 1996;18(2):138–141.

79. Puntil Sheltman J. Fluoroscopic assessment of dysphagia: which radiological procedure is best for your patient? Perspectives on Swallowing and Swallowing Disorders (Dysphagia). 2007;16(4):11–14.

80. Leonard RJ. Endoscopy in assessing and treating dysphagia. In: R Leonard, K Kendall (eds.), Dysphagia Assessment and Treatment Planning. San Diego, CA: Plural; 2008:167–183.

81. Katz PO, Gerson LB, Vela MF. Guidelines for the diagnosis and management of gastroesophageal reflux disease. Am J Gastroenterol. 2013;108(3):308–328.

82. Robbins J, Gangnon R, Theis S, Kays S, Hewitt A, Hind J. The effects of lingual exercise on swallowing in older adults. J Am Geriatr Soc. 2005;53(9):1483.

83. Logemann JA, Gensler G, Robbins J, et al. A randomized study of three interventions for aspiration of thin liquids in patients with dementia or Parkinson's disease. JSLHR. 2008;51(1):173–183.

84. Mills RH. Dysphagia Management: Using Thickened liquids. The ASHA Leader. October 14, 2008.

85. Sharp HM, Wagner LB. Ethics, informed consent, and decisions about nonoral feeding for patients with dysphagia. Topics in Geriatric Rehabilitation. 2007;23(3):240–248.

86. Heiss CJ, Goldberg L, Dzarnoski M. Registered dietitians and speech-language pathologists: an important partnership in dysphagia management. J Am Diet Assoc. 2010;110(9):1290–1293.

87. Sullivan DJ, Moran GP, Pinjon E, et al. Comparison of the epidemiology, drug resistance mechanisms, and virulence of *Candida dubliniensis* and *Candida albicans*. FEMS Yeast Res. 2004;4(4–5):369–376.

88. Ernst E, Cohen M, Stone J. Ethical problems arising in evidence-based complementary and alternative medicine. J Med Ethics. 2004;30(2):156 159.

89. Xie Y, Wang L, He J, Wu T. Acupuncture for dysphagia in acute stroke. Cochrane Database Syst Rev. 2008;3.

90. Geeganage C, Beavan J, Ellender S, Bath PMW. Interventions for dysphagia and nutritional support in acute and subacute stroke. Cochrane Database Syst Rev. 2012;10.

91. Michelfelder A, Lee KC, Bading EM. Integrative medicine and gastrointestinal disease. Prim Care Clin Office Pract. 2010;37(2):255–267.

92. Ashford J, Skelley M. Oral care and the elderly. Perspectives on Swallowing and Swallowing Disorders (Dysphagia). 2008;17:19–26.

93. Niederman MS. American Thoracic Society: Infectious Diseases Society of America. Guidelines for the management of adults with hospital-acquired, ventilator-associated, and healthcare-associated pneumonia. Am J Respir Crit Care Med. 2005;171(4):388.

94. Ames N. Evidence to support tooth brushing in critically ill patients. Am J Crit Care. 2011;20(3):242–250.

95. Panchabhai TS, Dangayach NS, Krishnan A, Kothari VM, Karnad DR. Oropharyngeal cleansing with 0.2% chlorhexidine for prevention of nosocomial pneumonia in critically ill patients: an open-label randomized trial with 0.01% potassium permanganate as control. Chest. 2009;135(5):1150–1156.

96. Mitchell SL, Buchanan JL, Littlehale S, Hamel MB. Tube-feeding versus hand-feeding nursing home residents with advanced dementia: a cost comparison. J Am Med Dir Assoc. 2003;4(1):27–33.

97. Carnaby-Mann G, Crary M. Pill swallowing by adults with dysphagia. Arch Otolaryngol Head Neck Surg. 2005;131(11):970–975.

98. Griffith R, Tengnali C. A guideline for managing medication related dysphagia. Br J Community Nurs. 2012;12(9):426–429.

99. Cai S, Gozalo P, Mitchell S, et al. Do patients with advanced cognitive impairment admitted to hospitals with higher rates of feeding tube insertion have improved survival? J Pain Symptom Manage. 2013;45(3):524–533.

100. Hanson LC, Garrett JM, Lewis C, Phifer N, Jackman A, Carey TS. Physicians' expectations of benefit from tube feeding. J Palliat Med. 2008;11(8):1130–1134.

101. Gillick MR, Volandes AE. The standard of caring: why do we still use feeding tubes in patients with advanced dementia? J Am Med Dir Assoc. 2008;9(5):364–367.

102. Mitchell SL, Kiely DK, Miller SC, Connor SR, Spence C, Teno JM. Hospice care for patients with dementia. J Pain Symptom Manage. 2007;34(1):7–16.

103. Proulx M, de Courval FP, Wiseman MA, Panisset M. Salivary production in Parkinson's disease. Mov Disord. 2005;20(2):204–207.

104. Volonte MA, Porta M, Comi G. Clinical assessment of dysphagia in early phases of Parkinson's disease. Neurol Sci. 2002;23(Suppl 2):S121–S122.

105. Hockstein NG, Samadi DS, Gendron K, Handler SD. Sialorrhea: a management challenge. Am Fam Physician. 2004;69(11):2628–2635.

106. Walshe M, Smith M, Pennington L. Interventions for drooling in children with cerebral palsy. Cochrane Database Syst Rev. 2012(11):13–30.

107. Elman LB, Dubin RM, Kelley M, McCluskey L. Management of oropharyngeal and tracheobronchial secretions in patients with neurologic disease. J Palliat Med. 2005;8(6):1150–1159.

108. Meningaud JP, Pitak-Arnnop P, Chikhani L, Bertrand JC. Drooling of saliva: a review of the etiology and management options. Oral Surg Oral Med Oral Pathol Oral Radiol Endod. 2006;101(1):48–57.

109. Molloy L. Treatment of sialorrhoea in patients with Parkinson's disease: best current evidence. Curr Opin Neurol. 2007;20(4):493–498.

110. Penner JL, McClement S, Lobchuk M, Daeninck P. Family members' experiences caring for patients with advanced head and neck cancer receiving tube feeding: a descriptive phenomenological study. J Pain Symptom Manage. 2012;44(4):563–571.

111. Davies A, Hall S. Salivary gland dysfunction (dry mouth) in patients with cancer. Int J Palliat Nurs. 2011;17(10):477–482.

112. Kim J, Dodd M, Aouizerat B, Jahan T, Miaskowski C. A review of the prevalence and impact of multiple symptoms in oncology patients. J Pain Symptom Manage. 2009;37(4):715–736.

113. Rohr Y, Adams J, L. Y. Oral discomfort in palliative care: results of an exploratory study of the experiences of terminally ill patients. Int J Palliat Nurs. 2010;16(9):439–444.

114. Alt-Epping B, Nejad RK, Jung K, Gross U, Nauck F. Symptoms of the oral cavity and their association with local microbiological and clinical findings: a prospective survey in palliative care. Support Care Cancer. 2012;20(3):531–537.

115. Johnson V. Oral hygiene care for functionally dependent and cognitively impaired older adults. J Geron Nurs. 2012;38(11):11–19.

116. Sreebny L. Dry mouth: a common worldwide tormentor. In: Sreebny L, Vissinik A (eds.), Dry Mouth, the Malevolent Symptom: A Clinical Guide. Hoboken, NJ: Wiley; 2010:3–9.

117. Sreebny L, Valdini A. Xerostomia. Arch Intern Med. 1987;147:1333–1337.

118. Wilberg P, Hjermstad MJ, Ottesen S, Herlofson BB. Oral health is an important issue in end-of-life cancer care. Support Care Cancer. 2012;20(12):3115–3122.

119. Folke S, Fridlund B, Paulsson G. Views of xerostomia among health care professionals: a qualitative study. J Clin Nurs. 2008;18(791–798).

120. Berti-Couto Sde A, Couto-Souza PH, Jacobs R, et al. Clinical diagnosis of hyposalivation in hospitalized patients. J Appl Oral Sci. 2012;20(2):157–161.

121. Grossmann S, Teixeira R, Oliveira G, et al. Xerostomia, hyposalivation and sialadenitis in patients with chronic hepatitis C are not associated with the detection of HCV RNA in saliva or salivary glands. J Clin Pathol. 2010;63(11):1002–1007.

122. van der Putten GJ, Brand HS, Schols JM, de Baat C. The diagnostic suitability of a xerostomia questionnaire and the association between xerostomia, hyposalivation and medication use in a group of nursing home residents. Clin Oral Investig. 2011;15(2):185–192.

123. Borges BC, Fulco GM, Souza AJ, de Lima KC. Xerostomia and hyposalivation: a preliminary report of their prevalence and associated factors in Brazilian elderly diabetic patients. Oral Preven Dent. 2010;8(2):153–158.

124. de Almedia P, Gregio AMT, Machado MAN, de Lima AAS, Azevedo LR. Saliva composition and function: a comprehensive review. J Contemp Dent Pract. 2008;9(3):72–80.

125. Amerongen AV, Veerman EC, Vissinik A. Saliva: a remarkable fluid. In: Sreebny L, Vissinik A (eds.), Dry Mouth, thc Malevolent Symptom: A Clinical Guide. Hoboken, NJ: Wiley and Blackwell, 2010:10–25.

126. Porter S, Scully C, A H. An update of the etiology and management of xerostomia. Oral Surg Oral Med Oral Pathol Oral Radiol Endod. 2004;97:28–46.

127. Jensen SB, Pedersen AM, Reibel J, B N. Xerostomia and hypofunction of the salivary glands in cancer therapy. Support Care Cancer. 2003;11:207–225.

128. Bryan G, Furness S, Birchenough S, McMillan R, Worthington HV. Interventions for the management of dry mouth: nonpharmacological interventions. Cochrane Database Syst Rev. 2012(2).

129. Oregon Geriatric Education Center. Oral Health for Older Adults. http://www.ohsu.edu/xd/education/schools/school-of-nursing/about/centers/oregon-geriatric-education/upload/Oral-Health-Care.pdf. Accessed October 30, 2013.

130. Fehrenbach M. American Dental Hygienists' Assocation Hyposalivation with Xerostomia Screening Tool. Access; 2010. http://www.adha.org/resources-docs/72614_Access_Hyposalivation_Tool.pdf. Accessed October 30, 2013.

131. Wiener RC, Wu B, Crout R, et al. Hyposalivation and xerostomia in dentate older adults. J Am Dent Assoc. 2010;141(3):279–284.

132. Cancer Care Ontario, Action Cancer Ontario. Xerostomia. Symptom management guides 2013. https://www.cancercare.on.ca/toolbox/symptools/.

133. Dahlin C, Cohen A, Goldsmith, T. Dysphagia, xerostomia, and hiccups. In: BR Ferrell, N Coyle (eds.), Oxford Textbook of Palliative Nursing. New York, NY: Oxford University Press; 2010:239–267.

134. Meirovitz A, Murdoch-Kinch CA, Schipper M, Pan C, Eisbruch A. Grading xerostomia by physicians or by patients after intensity-modulated radiotherapy of head-and-neck cancer. Int J Radiat Oncol Biol Phys. 2006;66(2):445–453.

135. Thomson WM, van der Putten GJ, de Baat C, et al. Shortening the xerostomia inventory. Oral Surg Oral Med Oral Pathol Oral Radiol Endod. 2011;112(3):322–327.

136. American Cancer Society. External Radiation Side Effects Worksheet. 2013. http://www.cancer.org/acs/groups/content/@nho/documents/document/acsq-009503.pdf Accessed June 22, 2013.

137. Oncology Nursing Society. Radiation Therapy Patient Care Record. Pittsburgh: PA: Oncology Nursing Society Press, 2002.

138. National Institute of Dental and Craniofacial Research. Oral Complications of Cancer Treatment: What the Dental Team Can Do. 2011. http://www.nidcr.nih.gov/OralHealth/Topics/CancerTreatment/OralComplicationsCancerOral.htm. Last updated July 28, 2013. Accessed June 23, 2013.

139. Tagaki Y, Kimura Y, Nakamura T. Cevimeline gargle for the treatment of xerostomia in patients with Sjogren's syndrome. Ann Rheum Dis. 2004;63(6):749.

140. Mouly S, Orler JB, Tillet Y, et al. Efficacy of a new oral psychotropic drug induced xerostomia-a randomized controlled trial. J Clin Psychopharmacol. 2007;27(5):437–443.

141. Bots C, Brand H, Veerman E, et al. Chewing gum and a saliva substitute alleviate thirst and xerostomia in patients on haemodialysis. Nephrol Dial Transplant. 2005;20:578–584.

142. Furness S, Worthington HV, Bryan G, Birchenough S, McMillan R. Interventions for the management of dry mouth: topical therapies (Review). Cochrane Database Syst Rev. 2011;12.

143. Amerongen AV, Veerman EC. Current therapies for xerostomia and salivary gland hypofunction associated with cancer therapies. Support Care Cancer. 2003;11:226–231.

144. Sweeney M, Bagg J, Baxter W, Aitchison T. Clinical trial of mucin-containing oral spray for treatment of xerostomia in hospice patients. Palliat Med. 1997;11:225–232.

145. O'Sullivan EM, IJ H. Clincial effectiveness and safety of acupuncture in the treatment of irradiation induced xerostomia in patients with head and neck cancer: a systematic review. Acupunct Med. 2010;24(4):191–199.

146. Olasz L, Nyarady Z, Szentirmy M. Assessment of relieving symptoms of xerostomia with oral pilocarpine during irradiation in head-and-neck cancer patients. Cancer Detect Prev. 2000;24(Suppl 1):489.

147. Meng Z, Garcia K, Hu C, et al. Randomized controlled trial of acupuncture for prevention of radiation-induced xerostomia among patients with nashopharyngeal carcinoma. Cancer. 2012;118(13):3337–3344.

148. Lu W, Posner MR, Wayne P, Rosenthal DS, Haddad RI. Acupuncture for dysphagia after chemoradiation therapy in head and neck cancer: a case series report. Integr Cancer Ther. 2010;9(3):284–290.

149. Johnstone P, Niemtzow R, Riffenburgh R. Acupuncture for xerostomia. Cancer. 2002;94(5):1151–1156.

150. Calsina-Berna A, Garcia-Gomez G, Gonzalez-Barboteo J, Porta-Sales J. Treatment of chronic hiccups in cancer patients: a systematic review [Review]. J Palliat Med. 2012;15(10):1142–1150.

151. Woelk CJ. Managing hiccups. Can Fam Physician. 2011;57(6):672–675.

152. Kang JH, Hui D, Kim MJ, et al. Corticosteroid rotation to alleviate dexamethasone-induced hiccup: a case series at a single institution. J Pain Symptom Manage. 2012;43(3):625–630.

153. Moretto EN, Wee B, Wiffen PJ, Murchison AG. Interventions for treating persistent and intractable hiccups in adults. [Review]. Cochrane Database Syst Rev. 2013;1.

154. Porzio G, Aielli F, Verna L, Aloisi P, Galletti B, C F. Gabapentin in the treatment of hiccups in patients with advanced cancer: a 5-year experience. Clin Neuropharmacol. 2010;33(4):179–180.

155. Nicoletti F, Gradini R, Bassi PF, Rampello L. Lyrica cures the tenor. Clin Neuropharmacol. 2009;32(2):119.

CHAPTER 12

Bowel management
Constipation, diarrhea, obstruction, and ascites

Denice Caraccia Economou

With all that is going on, managing the constipation is exhausting. I was afraid of the unknown when I was first diagnosed.... now I am afraid of the pain.

JC, a 50-year-old with stage IV colon cancer

Key points

- Multiple factors contribute to constipation. Proactive management is essential for successful outcomes.

- Treating diarrhea requires a thorough assessment and therapy directed at the specific cause.

- Palliative care should allow for a thoughtful and realistic approach to management of symptoms within the goals of care.

Constipation

Functional constipation affects 30% of the general population.[1,2] The incidence may be as high as 30% to 100% in palliative care patients.[3,4] Constipation is a major problem in cancer patients, and responsible for great amounts of suffering and embarrassment.[4] The use of opioids for pain contributes to constipation, and this side effect is the principal reason for their discontinuation.[5-7] Constipation is common, yet prophylactic treatment is inconsistently begun by both physicians and nurses.[4] The costs of treating constipated patients per month is higher than treating patients without constipation, and, though this symptom can be minimized, still the problem is undermanaged.[8]

Definitions

Constipation is subjective to many patients, making assessment much more difficult. Constipation is defined as "a decrease in the frequency of passage of formed stools and characterized by stools that are hard and small and difficult to expel." Understanding the normal functioning of the bowel can provide insight into the contributing factors leading to constipation, diarrhea, and obstruction. Associated symptoms of constipation vary, but may include excessive straining, a feeling of fullness or pressure in the rectum, the sensation of incomplete emptying, abdominal distention, and cramps.[9-11] The assessment of constipation includes past history of bowel function, current physical dysfunction and the person's subjective understanding of constipation for themselves, and objective measures to document level of constipation.[10] In an effort

to establish a validated and objective way to define functional constipation and develop a scientific approach to understanding and treating functional gastrointestinal disorders (FGIDs) researchers developed the first Rome I in 1994. They have expanded their classification system with scientific evidence and continue to use scientific evidence to provide the best treatment for FGIDs. The Rome III criteria was established in 2007 and is used in many palliative care settings.[12] Patients are constipated if they experience at least two of the following symptoms: less than three stools per week; straining with at least 25% of stools; lumpy, hard stool at least 25% of the time; feeling of incomplete evacuation or sensation of blockage for at least 25% of stools; need to manually remove stool at least 25% of the time; loose stools are rarely present without the use of laxatives; or lack of sufficient criteria for irritable bowel syndrome.[9,13,14] The subjective experience of constipation may vary for different individuals, underscoring the importance of individualized patient assessment and management.[3,9,15,16]

Prevalence and impact

It is estimated that 54% of hospice patients are constipated; this maybe an underestimate, as many of those patients are on opioids and stool softeners/laxatives at baseline.[9,17] Inpatient hospitalization and ambulatory clinic visits for constipation and related side effects cost the healthcare system $235 million annually.[18,19] Constipation is considered a symptom of bowel dysfunction (BD) and opioid bowel dysfunction (OBD) relating to opioid-induced constipation. The impact of constipation on quality of life is substantial. Constipation causes social, psychological, and physical distress for patients, which additionally impacts the caregiver and healthcare staff. Failure to anticipate and manage constipation in a proactive way significantly affects the difficulty a patient will experience in attempting to relieve this problem.

Pathophysiology

Normal bowel function includes three areas of control: small intestinal motility, colon motility, and defecation. This includes the processes of secretion, absorption, transport, and storage.[6,8]

Small-intestinal activity is primarily the mixing of contents by bursts of propagated motor activity that are associated with increased gastric, pancreatic, and biliary secretion. This motor activity occurs every 90 to 120 minutes, but is altered when food is ingested. Contents are mixed to allow for digestion and absorption of nutrients. When the stomach has emptied, the small intestine returns to regular propagated motor activity.[17,20]

The colon propels contents forward through peristaltic movements. The colon movement is much slower than that of the small intestine. Contents may remain in the colon for up to 2 to 3 days, whereas small-intestinal transit is 2–4 hours. Motor activity in the large intestine occurs approximately six times per day, usually grouped in two peak bursts. The first is triggered by awakening and breakfast, and a smaller burst is triggered by the afternoon meal. Contractions are stimulated by ingestion of food, psychogenic factors, and somatic activity. Sykes[21] found that 50% of the constipated patients in a hospice setting had a transit time between 4 and 12 days.

The physiology of defecation involves coordinated interaction between the involuntary internal anal sphincter and the voluntary external anal sphincter. The residual intestinal contents distend the rectum and initiate expulsion. The longitudinal muscle of the rectum contracts, and, with the voluntary external anal sphincter relaxed, defecation can occur. Additional coordinated muscle activity also occurs and includes contraction of the diaphragm against a closed glottis, tensing of the abdominal wall, and relaxation of the pelvic floor.

The enteric nervous system plays an important role in the movement of bowel contents through the gastrointestinal (GI) tract as well. Smooth muscles in the GI tract have spontaneous electrical, rhythmic activity, resembling pacemakers in the stomach and small intestine that communicate with the remainder of the bowel. There are both submucosal and myenteric plexuses of nerves. These nerves are connected to the central nervous system through sympathetic ganglia, splanchnic nerves, and parasympathetic fibers in the vagus nerve and the presacral plexus. Opioid medications affect the myenteric plexus, which coordinates peristalsis. Therefore, peristalsis is decreased and stool transit time is decreased, leading to harder, dryer, and less frequent stools, or constipation.[19,20] Constipation therefore is related to dysfunction of either the colon or neuromuscular system.[15] Important factors that promote normal functioning of the bowel include the following:

1. *Fluid intake.* Nine liters of fluid (which includes 7 liters secreted from the salivary glands, stomach, pancreas, small bowel, and biliary system, and the average oral intake of 2 liters) are reduced to 1.5 liters by the time they reach the colon. At this point, water and electrolytes continue to be absorbed, and the end volume for waste is 150 mL.[22,23] Decreased fluid intake may make a significant difference in the development of constipation.[2]

2. *Adequate dietary fiber.* The presence of food in the stomach initiates the muscle contractions and secretions from the biliary, gastric, and pancreatic systems that lead to movement of the bowels.[17,19] The amount of dietary fiber consumed is related to stool size and consistency.[24] Smaller meal size also reduces the natural trigger for peristalsis adding to constipation.[17]

3. *Physical activity.* Colonic propulsion is related to intraluminal pressures in the colon. Lack of physical activity and reduced intraluminal pressures can significantly reduce propulsive activity.[21] Lack of mobility may also interfere with the patient's ability to sit on the toilet because of decreased muscle mass or increased fatigue.[17]

4. *Adequate time or privacy to defecate.* Changes in normal bowel routines, such as morning coffee or reading the paper, can decrease peristalsis and lead to constipation. Emotional disturbances are also known to affect gut motility.[17,18,24]

Primary, secondary, and iatrogenic constipation

Causes of constipation in cancer patients are divided into three different categories.[20,21]

1. Primary constipation is caused by reduced fluid and fiber intake, decreased activity, lack of privacy, and advanced age.

2. Secondary constipation is related to structural, metabolic, or neurological disorders. These changes may include tumor; partial intestinal obstruction; metabolic effects of hypercalcemia, hypothyroidism, hypokalemia, or hyperglycemia; spinal cord compression at the level of the cauda equina or sacral plexus; sacral nerve infiltration; and cerebral tumors.

3. Iatrogenically induced constipation is related to pharmacological interventions. Opioids are the primary medications associated with constipation. In addition, chemotherapies (vincristine, oxaliplatin, temozolomide, thalidomide), anticholinergic medications (belladonna, antihistamines), antiemetic therapy (5-HT_3 antagonists), tricyclic antidepressants (nortriptyline, amitriptyline), neuroleptics (haloperidol and chlorpromazine), antispasmodics, anticonvulsants (phenytoin and gabapentin), muscle relaxants, aluminum antacids, iron, diuretics (furosemide), and antiparkinsonian agents cause constipation.[20,21]

Constipation related to cancer and its treatment

Multiple factors associated with cancer and its treatment cause constipation. When it primarily involves the GI system or is anatomically associated with the bowel, cancer itself causes constipation. Pelvic cancers, including ovarian, cervical, and uterine cancers, are highly associated with constipation and mechanical obstruction.[24,25] Malignant ascites, spinal cord compression, and paraneoplastic autonomic neuropathy also cause constipation. Cancer-related causes include surgical interruption of the GI tract, decreased activity, reduced intake of both fluids and food, changes in personal routines associated with bowel movements, bed rest, confusion, and depression.[19–21,26]

Opioid-related constipation

Opioids affect bowel function primarily by inhibiting propulsive peristalsis through the small bowel and colon.[5,19,20] Chronic opioid use in noncancer patients causes constipation in 40% of the patients; in advanced cancer patients, 50% to 90% will develop bowel dysfunction.[5,27] Opioids bind with the receptors on the smooth muscles of the bowel, affecting the contraction of the circular and longitudinal muscle fibers that cause peristalsis or the movement of contents through the bowel.[5,27] Colonic transit time is lengthened, contributing to increased fluid and electrolyte absorption and dryer, harder stools.[2,14,20] Peristaltic changes occur 5 to 25 minutes after administration of the opioid and are dose related. Patients do not develop tolerance to the constipation side effects even with long-term use of opioids.[28] There is evidence associated with transdermal fentanyl versus morphine and methadone compared with morphine or hydromorphone use that constipation severity may differ among opioids.[29,30] The use of laxatives and stool softeners with opioids represents a rational, proactive approach to opioid-induced constipation.

Assessment of constipation

History

The measurement of constipation requires more than assessing the frequency of stools alone. Managing constipation requires a thorough history and physical examination. The lack of a universally accepted definition of constipation complicates diagnosis and management. Evidence has shown that healthcare providers cannot diagnose constipation in an objective way. Finding a tool to help establish a method to identify and stage constipation to aid in prophylactic management is essential.[3,16]

The Constipation Assessment Scale (CAS) was developed in 1989 and has been tested for validity and reliability and found to have a significant ability to differentiate the severity of constipation between moderate and severe constipation. It uses the criteria of the ROME III to define functional constipation.[13] It is a simple questionnaire that requires on average 2 minutes to complete (Table 12.1). The CAS includes eight symptoms associated with constipation: (1) abdominal distention or bloating, (2) change in amount of gas passed rectally, (3) less frequent bowel movements, (4) oozing liquid stool, (5) rectal fullness or pressure, (6) rectal pain with bowel movement, (7) small volume of stool, and (8) inability to pass stool.[18] These symptoms are rated as 0, not experienced; 1, some problem; or 2, severe problem. A score between 0 and 16 is calculated and can be used as an objective measurement of subjective symptoms for ongoing management.

Table 12.1 Constipation Assessment Scale Direction: Circle the appropriate number to indicate whether, during the past 3 days, you have had NO PROBLEM, SOME PROBLEM, or a SEVERE PROBLEM with each of the items listed.

Item	No problem	Some problem	Severe problem
1. Abdominal distention or bloating	0	1	2
2. Change in amount of gas passed rectally	0	1	2
3. Less frequent bowel movements	0	1	2
4. Oozing liquid stool	0	1	2
5. Rectal fullness or pressure	0	1	2
6. Rectal pain with bowel movement	0	1	2
7. Smaller stool size	0	1	2
8. Urge but inability to pass stool	0	1	2
Patient's Name			Date

Source: McMillan et al. (1989), reference 31. Reproduced with permission.

The CAS gives a good sense of bowel function and also outlines questions to use in taking a constipation history.[16,21,31] It is important to start by asking patients when they moved their bowels last and to follow up by asking what their normal movement pattern is. Remember, what is considered constipated for one person is not for someone else. What are the characteristics of their stools and did they note any blood or mucus? Were their bowels physically difficult to move? This is especially important if they have cancer in or near the intestines or rectal area that may contribute to physical obstruction. Ovarian cancer patients usually complain of feeling severely bloated. They may say things like "If you stick a pin in me, I know I will pop!" Evaluating the abdomen or asking patients if they feel bloated or pressure in the abdomen is important. Does the patient feel pain when moving the bowels? Is the patient oozing liquid stool? Does the patient feel that the volume of stool passed is small? Many patients may experience unexplainable nausea.

Medication- or disease-related history

The patient's medical status and anticipated disease process are important in providing insight into areas where early intervention could prevent severe constipation or even obstruction. Constipation may be anticipated with primary and secondary bowel cancer, as well as with pelvic tumors, peritoneal mesothelioma or spinal cord compression, previous bowel surgery, or a history of vinca alkaloid chemotherapy. Changes in dietary habits related to the above medications or the addition of new medications may contribute to constipation.[2,23,26] Anticholinergic medications, antihistamines, tricyclic antidepressants, aluminum antacids, and diuretics can cause constipation. Hypercalcemia, hyperglycemia, and hypokalemia contribute to constipation by slowing down motility.[32] Several factors aggravate and contribute to the experience of constipation including confusion, immobility, and dehydration.[19] Ask patients if there are things they do to aid in defecation. Sometimes physical actions the patient may use can help causes related to rectocele, or rectal ulcer.[21] Understanding the baseline status of the patient, bowel history and contributing issues like fatigue and muscle weakness must be evaluated to plan care.[32] Box 12.1 outlines causes of constipation in cancer and other palliative care patients.

Physical examination

Begin the physical examination in the mouth, to ensure that the patient is able to chew foods and that there are no lesions or tumors in the mouth that could interfere with eating. Does the patient wear dentures? Patients who wear dentures and have lost a great deal of weight may have dentures that do not fit properly, which would make eating and drinking difficult. Patients may choose to eat only what they are able to chew as a result of their dentures or other dental problems. Therefore, they may not be eating enough fiber and, thus, contributing to primary constipation.

Abdominal examination

Inspect the abdomen initially for bloating, distention, or bulges. Distention may be associated with obesity, fluid, tumor, or gas. Remember, the patient should have emptied the bladder. Auscultation is important to evaluate the presence or absence of bowel sounds. If no bowel sounds are audible initially, listen continuously for a minimum of 5 minutes. The absence of bowel sounds may indicate a paralytic ileus. If the bowel sounds are

Box 12.1 Causes of constipation in cancer/palliative care patients

Etiology

Cancer-related

Directly related to tumor site. Primary bowel cancers, secondary bowel cancers, pelvic cancers.

Hypercalcemia. Surgical interruption of bowel integrity.

Intestinal obstruction related to tumor in the bowel wall or external compression by tumor. Damage to the lumbosacral spinal cord, cauda equina, or pelvic plexus. High spinal cord transection mainly stops the motility response to food. Low spinal cord or pelvic outflow lesions produce dilation of the colon and slow transit in the descending and distal transverse colon. Surgery in the abdomen can lead to adhesion development or direct changes in the bowel.

Hypercalcemia

Cholinergic control of secretions of the intestinal epithelium is mediated by changes in intracellular calcium concentrations. Hypercalcemia causes decreased absorption, leading to constipation, whereas hypercalcemia can lead to diarrhea.

Secondary effects related to the disease

Decreased appetite, decreased fluid intake, low-fiber diet, weakness, inactivity, confusion, depression, change in normal toileting habits.

Decreased fluid and food intake leading to dehydration and weakness. Decreased intake, ineffective voluntary elimination actions, as well as decreased normal defecation reflexes. Decreased peristalsis; increased colonic transit time leads to increased absorption of fluid and electrolytes and small, hard, dry stools. Inactivity, weakness, changes in normal toileting habits, daily bowel function reflexes, and positioning affect ability to use abdominal wall musculature and relax pelvic floor for proper elimination. Psychological depression can increase constipation by slowing down motility.

Concurrent disease

Diabetes (hyperglycemia), hypothyroidism, hypokalemia, diverticular disease, hemorrhoids, colitis, chronic neurological diseases.

Electrolytes and therefore water are transported via neuronal control. Like hypercalcemia, abnormal potassium can affect water absorption and contribute to constipation. Chronic neurological diseases affect the neurological stimulation of intestinal motility.

Medication-related

Opioid medications
Anticholinergic effects (hydroscine, phenothiazines)
Tricyclic antidepressants
Antiparkinsonian drugs
Iron
Antihypertensives, antihistamines
Antacids
Diuretics
Vinca alkaloid chemotherapy

hyperactive, it could indicate diarrhea. Percussion of the bowel may result in tympany, which is related to gas in the bowel. A dull sound is heard over intestinal fluid and feces. Palpation of the abdomen should start lightly; look for muscular resistance and abdominal tenderness. This is usually associated with chronic constipation. If rebound tenderness is detected with coughing or light palpation, peritoneal inflammation should be considered. Deep palpation may reveal a "sausage-like" mass of stool in the left colon. Feeling stool in the colon indicates constipation. Although Sykes[21] points out that the distinction between tumor and stool is hard to make, recognizing the underlying anatomy is helpful in distinguishing the stool along the line of the descending colon or more proximal colon, including the cecum. A digital examination of the rectum may reveal stool or possible tumor or rectocele. If the patient is experiencing incontinence of liquid stool, obstruction must be considered. Examining for hemorrhoids, ulcerations, or rectal fissures is important, especially in the neutropenic patient. Patients with neutropenia can complain of rectal pain well before a rectal infection is obvious. Evaluating the patient for infection, ulceration, or rectal fissures is very important. Additionally, determine whether the patient has had previous intestinal surgery, alternating diarrhea and constipation, complaints of abdominal colic pain or nausea, and vomiting. Examining the stool for shape and consistency can also be useful. Stools that are hard and pelletlike suggest slow transit time, whereas stools that are ribbon-like suggest hemorrhoids. Blood or mucus in the stool suggests tumor, hemorrhoids, or possibly preexisting colitis.[21] Elderly patients may experience urinary incontinence related to fecal impaction.[1,2,5] Abdominal pain may also be related to constipation. Patients will complain of colic pain related to the effort of colonic muscle to move hard stool. The history may be complicated by known abdominal tumors. Patients in pain should still be treated with opioids as needed.

Management of constipation

Preventing constipation whenever possible is the most important management strategy. Constipation can be extremely distressing to many patients and severely affects quality of life.[19,23] The complicating factor remains the individuality of a patient's response to constipation therapy. Therefore, there is no set rule for the most effective way to manage constipation. Patients with primary bowel cancers, pelvic tumors such as ovarian or uterine cancers, or metastatic tumors that press on colon structures will experience a difficult-to-manage constipation. It is not unusual for those patients to be admitted to the hospital to manage constipation and to rule out obstruction. To minimize those admissions whenever possible, as Dame Cicely Saunders, the founder of hospice recommends, "Do not forget the bowels." Nurses are at the bedside most often and are the ones who see the cumulated number and types of medication a patient may be taking. Understanding which medications and disease processes put a patient at high risk for constipation is essential for good bowel management.

Assessing the patient's constipation as discussed earlier is the best place to start. The patient's problem list should reflect the risk for constipation and the need for aggressive constipation management. For example, diabetic patients who are taking opioids for pain are at extremely high risk for constipation.

Diabetes damages the sensory fibers that are most important for temperature and pain sensation, as well as the neuronal influence on intestinal motility.[5,21,33] In addition to assessing the extent of the patient's constipation, determining the methods the patient has used to manage the constipation in the past is essential. This can usually provide information regarding what medications the patient tolerates best and where to start with recommendations for management. According to Sykes,[2] using radiography to evaluate whether constipation has advanced to obstruction may be useful if there is indecision, but in palliative medicine, the use of X-ray procedures should be limited. He also suggests that blood work be limited to corrective studies; for example, if hypercalcemia or hyperkalemia can be reversed to improve constipation, such blood work may be useful.

Opioids in particular suppress forward peristalsis and increase sphincter tone. Opioids increase electrolyte and water absorption in both the large and small intestine; this leads to dehydration and hard, dry stools. Morphine causes insensitivity of the rectum to distention, decreasing the sensation of the need to defecate. Vinca alkaloid chemotherapy has a neurotoxic effect that causes damage to the myenteric plexus of the colon. This increases nonpropulsive contractions. Colonic transit time is increased, leading to constipation. Antidepressants slow large bowel motility. Antacids (bismuth, aluminum salts) cause hard stools.[34,35]

Improving three important primary causes of constipation is essential. Encouraging fluid intake is a priority. Increasing or decreasing fluid intake by as little as 100 mL can affect constipation.[22] Increase dietary intake as much as possible. This is a difficult intervention for many patients. Focusing on food intake for some patients can increase their anxiety and discomfort. If a patient feels that bowel movements are less frequent, think about dietary intake. The Western diet is fiber-deficient.[21,26,27] Caution is needed for patients who use bulk laxatives such as psyllium, especially if they also are taking other bowel medications. Increasing the fiber intake for patients in general may be helpful, but in palliative care, high fiber in the diet can cause more discomfort and constipation. Fiber without fluid absorbs what little liquid the patient may have available in the bowel and makes the bowels more difficult to move.[5,27,36] For example, an elderly patient who experiences reduced appetite and decreased fluid intake related to chemotherapy or disease, and whose symptoms are nausea or vomiting with reduced activity, is at extreme risk for constipation. Encouraging activity whenever possible, even in end-of-life care, can be very helpful. Increased activity helps to stimulate peristalsis and to improve mood.[2,37] Physical therapy should be used as part of a multidisciplinary bowel-management approach. Providing basic range of motion, either active or passive, can improve bowel management and patient satisfaction.[5,26]

Pharmacological management

Types of laxatives

Bulk laxatives
Laxatives can be classified by their actions. Bulk laxatives provide bulk to the intestines to increase mass, stimulating the bowel to move. Increasing dietary fiber is considered a bulk laxative. The recommended dose of bran is 8 g daily. Other bulk laxatives include psyllium, carboxymethylcellulose, and methylcellulose.[21,34] Bulk laxatives are more helpful for mild constipation. Because bulk laxatives work best when patients are able to increase their fluid intake, they may be inappropriate for end-stage patients. In palliative care, patients may not ingest enough fluid. It is recommended that the patient increase fluids by 200 to 300 mL when using bulk laxatives. Patients may have difficulty with the consistency of bulk laxatives and find this approach unacceptable. Patients using bulk laxatives without the additional fluid intake are at risk of developing a partial bowel obstruction or, if an impending one exists, may risk complete bowel obstruction. The benefits of bulk laxatives in severe constipation are questionable.

Additional complications include allergic reactions, fluid retention, and hyperglycemia.[5] Bulk laxatives produce gas as the indigestible or nonsoluble fiber breaks down or ferments. The result can be uncomfortable bloating and gas.

The recommended dosage of bulk laxatives is to start with 8 g daily, then stabilize at 3 to 4 g for maintenance. Psyllium is recommended at 2 to 4 teaspoons daily as a bulk laxative. Action may take 2 to 3 days.

Lubricant laxatives
Mineral oil can lubricate the stool surface and soften the stool by penetration, leading to an easier bowel movement. However, mineral oil can cause seepage from the rectum and perineal irritation, it can lead to malabsorption of fat-soluble vitamins (vitamins A, D, E, and K). Aspiration pneumonitis or lipoid pneumonia may occur in the frail and elderly patient. Additionally, when mineral oil is regularly given with docusate (Colace) the absorption of mineral oil increases, leading to a risk of lipoid granuloma in the intestinal wall.[38] For this reason mineral oil is rarely recommended.

Surfactant/detergent laxatives
Surfactant/detergent laxatives reduce surface tension, which increases absorption of water and fats into dry stools, leading to a softening effect. According to Larkin et al.[37] and others,[23,27] medications such as docusate exert a mucosal contact effect, which encourages secretion of water, sodium, and chloride in the jejunum and colon and decreases electrolyte and water reabsorption in the small and large intestines.[22,39] At higher doses, these laxatives may stimulate peristalsis. Docusate is used alone or in combination with laxatives such as sennosides (Peri-Colace or Senokot S).

The recommended dosage of docusate sodium is 50–500 mg daily and for docusate calcium 240 mg daily.

Castor oil also works like a detergent laxative by exerting a surface-wetting action on the stool and directly stimulates the colon, but its use in cancer-related constipation is discouraged because results are difficult to control.

Combination medications
Combination softener/laxative medications have been shown to be more effective than softeners alone at a lower total dose.[40]

The recommended dosage of senna/docusate is two tablets daily to twice a day (see flow chart in Box 12.2). Results typically occur in 6 to 12 hours. Flexibility of dosing allows individual needs to be met. Combination medications are especially recommended for opioid-related constipation. Remember as the dose of opioid increases, the dose of anticonstipation medications must also be increased.

Box 12.2 Senokot S Laxative Recommendations for Cancer-Related Constipation

Day 0

- Senokot S 2 tablets at bedtime

If no BM on day 1

- Senokot S 2 tablets BID

If no BM on day 2

- Senokot S 3 or 4 tablets BID or TID

If no BM on day 3

- Bisacodyl 2 or 3 tablets TID and/or HS
- If no BM, rule out impaction
- If impacted:
- Lubricate rectum with oil-retention enema
- Medicate with opioid and/or benzodiazepine
- Disimpact
- Give enemas until clear
- Increase daily laxative therapy per above
- If not impacted:

Give additional laxatives:

- Lactulose (45–60 mL PO)
- Magnesium citrate (8 oz)
- Bisacodyl suppository (1 PR)
- Fleet enema (1 PR)

At any step, if medication is ineffective, continue at that dose. If < 1 BM per day, increase laxative therapy per steps. If > 2 BM per day, decrease laxative therapy by 24% to 50%.

Source: Adapted from Levy (1991), reference 38.

Osmotic laxatives

Osmotic laxatives are nonabsorbable sugars that exert an osmotic effect in both the small and, to a lesser extent, large intestines. They increase fluid secretions in the small intestines by retaining fluid in the bowel lumen.[19,26,34] They have the additional effect of lowering ammonia levels. This is helpful in improving confusion, especially in hepatic failure patients. Laxatives in this category include: lactulose, magnesium citrate, magnesium hydroxide (Milk of Magnesia), polyethylene glycol (PEG 3350, MiraLax), and sodium biphosphate (Phospho-Soda). These laxatives can be effective for chronic constipation, especially when related to opioid use. Onset of action is between 2 and 48 hours.[7] Milk of Magnesia can cause severe cramping and discomfort. This medication is recommended for use only as a last resort in chronically ill patients. Opioid-related constipation requires the use of aggressive laxatives earlier rather than later to prevent severe constipation, referred to as obstipation, which leads to obstruction.

Drawbacks of agents like lactulose or sorbitol are that effectiveness is completely dose related and, for some patients, the sweet taste is intolerable. The bloating and gas associated with higher doses may be too uncomfortable or distressing to tolerate.

Lactulose or sorbitol can be put into juice or other liquid to lessen the taste. Patients may prefer hot tea or hot water to help reduce the sweet taste. Lactulose is more costly than sorbitol liquid. A study that compared the two medications found that there was no significant difference, except with regard to nausea, which increased with lactulose ($P = 0.05$).[41]

The recommended dosage of lactulose/sorbitol is 30 to 60 mL initially for severe constipation every 4 hours until a bowel movement occurs. Once that happens, calculate the amount of lactulose used to achieve that movement, and then divide in half for recommended daily maintenance dose.[5] An example would be: it took 60 mL to have a bowel movement; therefore, 30 mL daily should keep the bowels moving regularly. The recommended dosage of Milk of Magnesia is 30 mL to initiate a bowel movement. For opioid-related constipation, 15 mL of Milk of Magnesia may be added to the baseline bowel medications either daily or every other day. Magnesium citrate comes in a 10-ounce bottle. For severe constipation, it is used as a one-time initial therapy. It can be titrated up or down, depending on patient response. For patients with abdominal discomfort or pain, it is recommended that obstruction be ruled out before using this medication. If the patient were obstructed, even only partially, this would only increase the discomfort or lead to perforation.[33,37]

Polyethylene glycols (PEG 3350), (MiraLax, Movical [UK]) is used frequently and can be sprinkled over food. Recommended dose is 1 tablespoon. Evacuation can take between 2 to 4 days. If bowel obstruction is suspected, do not use.[42] Osmotic rectal compounds include glycerin suppositories and sorbitol enemas. Glycerin suppositories soften stool by osmosis and act as a lubricant.

Bowel stimulants

Bowel stimulants work directly on the colon to increase motility. These medications stimulate the myenteric plexus to induce peristalsis. They also reduce the amount of water and electrolytes in the colon. They are divided into two groups: the diphenylmethanes and the anthraquinones. The diphenylmethanes include bisacodyl and the anthraquinones are bowel stimulants that include senna and cascara. However, cascara was removed from over-the-counter medications for the treatment of constipation although it remains available as a dietary supplement. They are activated in the large intestine by bacterial degradation into the large bowel, stimulating glycosides. Bisacodyl and senna may cause cramping. This action causes a 6- to 12-hour delay when taken orally. Rectal absorption is much faster, at 15 to 60 minutes. It is recommended that bisacodyl be taken with food, milk, or antacids to avoid gastric irritation.

Recommendations for use are senna 15-mg tablets used alone or as Senokot S. Starting dose is two tablets daily (see Box 12.2). These stimulating laxatives are the most effective management for opioid-related constipation. Bisacodyl comes in 10-mg tablets or suppositories and is used daily. The suppository medication has a faster onset that is much appreciated in the uncomfortable, constipated patient. Onset of action can be within 12 hours.[19]

Rectal medications

As discussed above, bisacodyl comes in a suppository. Although the thought of rectal medications is unpleasant for many patients, suppositories' quick onset of action makes them more acceptable. Bisacodyl comes in 10 mg for adults and 5 mg as a pediatric dose.

Box 12.3 Milk and molasses enema recipe

Milk and molasses enema recipe

8 oz. warm water
3 oz. powdered milk
4.5 oz. molasses

- Put water and powdered milk in a plastic jar. Close the jar and shake until the water and milk appear to be fully mixed.

- Add molasses, and shake the jar again until the mixture appears to have an even color throughout.

- Pour mixture into enema bag. Administer enema high by gently introducing tube about 12 inches. Do not push beyond resistance. Repeat every 6 hours until good results are achieved.

Sources: Bisanz (2005), reference 24; Lowell (2003), reference 43.

Suppositories should never be used in patients with severely reduced white cell or platelet counts due to the risk of bleeding or infection.

Liquid rectal laxatives or lubricants should be used infrequently. In severely constipated patients, they may be necessary. Most commonly, saline enemas are used to loosen the stool and to stimulate rectal or distal colon peristalsis. Repeated use can cause hypocalcemia and hyperphosphatemia, so it is important to use enemas cautiously. Enemas should never be considered part of a standing bowel regimen. Onset of action can be within 30 minutes.

Oil retention enemas, however, are particularly helpful for severely constipated patients, for whom disimpaction may be necessary. They work best when used overnight, to allow softening. Overnight retention is effective only if the patient is able to retain it that long. The general rule is that the longer the enema is retained, the better the results. Bisanz[24] recommends a milk-and-molasses enema (Box 12.3) for patients with low impaction to ease stool evacuation in a nonirritating way. It is a low-volume enema of 300 mL and therefore thought to cause less cramping.

Combining an enema with an oral saline-type cathartic (lactulose, Cephulac) is helpful when a large amount of stool is present.[1,24] This may help to push the stool through the GI tract.

If disimpaction is necessary, remember that it can be extremely painful; therefore, premedicate the patient with an opioid and consider use of a benzodiazepine to reduce anxiety.[20,21,27] There are few studies outlining the efficacy of one enema over another. The reported success rates for rectal enemas within 1 hour includes phosphate enemas (100%), bisacodyl suppositories (66%), and glycerine suppositories (38%).[44] If none of the above enemas is effective, Sykes recommends rectal lavage with approximately 8 liters of warmed normal saline. It is important to remember that if a patient's constipation requires this invasive intervention, you must change the usual bowel regimen once this bowel crisis is resolved. For severe constipation associated with opioids, Levy[38] suggests four Senokot S and three Dulcolax tablets three times a day and 60 mL of lactulose every other night for a goal of a bowel movement every other day (see Box 12.2).

Recent approaches to constipation management

Peripherally acting opioid antagonists have become an effective method to manage opioid-related constipation in the palliative care setting.[45] Oral naloxone and subcutaneous methylnaltrexone have been studied and shown to improve constipation and achieve bowel movements ranging between 30 minutes and 24 hours for 50% of the patients after dosing.[8,32,46–48] Naloxone, which is an opioid antagonist, has less than 1% availability systemically when given orally, due to the first-pass effect in the liver.

The opioid antagonist methylnaltrexone (Relistor) has been used with great success toward relieving constipation in the palliative care patient.[49,50] It is administered subcutaneously and is indicated for the treatment of opioid-induced constipation in patients with advanced illness who are not responding to standard laxative/stimulant regimens. Results occurred on the average between 30 minutes and 4 hours and, unlike oral naloxone, it crosses the blood-brain barrier less readily so therefore is less likely to reverse centrally mediated analgesia.[32,40,45,51] The cost of this class of medication is a concern, although it is cheaper than a hospital admission. In a Canadian study looking at the cost benefit analysis (CBA) of methylnaltrexone and patients with terminal cancer "willingness-to-pay" showed "evidence for the adoption of methylnaltrexone treatment."[40] The key to this adoption was the 50% response rate to relief of constipation. This would account for 50% fewer interventions necessary to relieve constipation either through enemas or other factors. It would mean that at least 50% of constipated patients would find relief and experience improved quality of life. Multiple aspects need to be evaluated as to the severity of the constipation and goals for the patient, but costs for managing severely constipated palliative care patients is highest.[8]

Currently, new areas of research are examining the use of inadvertent medications whose side effects involve relief of constipation. Oral erythromycin has been shown to cause diarrhea in 50% of patients who use it as an antibiotic.[21] Currently, researchers are investigating its use to promote diarrhea. There is also interest in identifying a medication that would increase colon transit time without being antibacterial.

In 2011 Mercadante et al. aimed to evaluate the effectiveness of an oral contrast that causes diarrhea and improved symptoms of constipation. Amidotrizoane (gastrografin) is an oral contrast medium that is hyperosmolar and is used as a second-line treatment for patients who are unresponsive to common laxatives in Italy.[48] Similar to methylnaltrexone for opioid-induced constipation, this intervention leads to a bowel movement in about 45% of the advanced cancer patients who did not respond to their anticonstipation regimen.[48] The benefit of this medication is the fact that it is an oral medication and fairly inexpensive. Hydration is important for patients receiving this treatment. The cost related to this medication is its unpleasant taste and possibly intravenous fluids. More research needs to be done in this class of medications.

Many herbal medicines have laxative properties, such as mulberry and constituents of rhubarb, which are similar to senna. These herbs are being evaluated for use as laxatives. Patients have been known to develop rashes; in one patient, changes were found in warfarin (Coumadin) levels that were related to natural warfarin found in a laxative tea. Many patients prefer these options instead of pharmaceutical laxatives, but they should be cautious about where they purchase any herbal product and be alert to any unexplained side effects, as their content is unregulated.

Nursing interventions for constipation

Nurses should always be proactive in initiating laxative therapy. Bowel function requires continued evaluation to follow the trajectory of the disease and the changes that occur in normal activities that affect bowel function. Nurses should also be alert to medications that can increase the risk of constipation (see Box 12.1). Some patients, especially those on long-term opioid therapy, sometimes need at least two different regimens that can be interchanged when one or the other loses its effectiveness for a time. Like opioids, over time, a standing laxative regimen may be less effective if tolerance develops.[1,21] It is also important to be aware of medication dosing changes, as it is common to forget to increase anticonstipation therapy when there is an increase in opioid therapy. Patients generally have increased risk of constipation when opioids are increased. Positioning patients to allow gravity to assist with bowel movements is helpful. Both assistance with oral fluid intake and dietary interventions are helpful. Discuss patients' management needs as well as personal cultural perspectives and factors that may contribute to good bowel hygiene. Exercise within each patient's tolerance is recommended to aid in elimination. Fatigue, advanced disease, and decreased endurance all play a role in obstructing good bowel maintenance. The importance of effective bowel management cannot be stressed enough. It remains one of the most distressing symptoms in end-stage cancer patients.

Diarrhea

Diarrhea has been a major symptom and significant problem associated with newer chemotherapeutic and biological and radiation treatment regimens.[39,42,52] It is a main symptom of 7% to 10% of hospice admissions.[53,54] Overgrowth of GI infections such as candida can cause diarrhea as well.[21] Treating diarrhea requires a thorough assessment and therapy directed at the specific cause. Diarrhea is usually acute and short-lived, lasting only a few days, as opposed to chronic diarrhea, which lasts 3 weeks or more.[39] Diarrhea can be especially severe in human immunodeficiency virus (HIV)-infected patients.[21,54,55] Diarrhea of 500 mL/day or greater occurs in 35%–50% of bone marrow transplant patients related to radiation or graft versus host disease (GVHD).[56] Uncontrolled diarrhea leads to dehydration, fluid and electrolyte imbalance, and malnutrition.[56] Similar to constipation, this symptom can be debilitating and can severely affect quality of life.[14,33,42] Diarrhea can prevent patients from leaving their homes, increase weakness and dehydration, and contribute to feelings of lack of control and depression. Nurses play a significant role in recognizing, educating, and managing diarrhea and its manifestations.

Definitions

Diarrhea is described as an increase in stool volume and liquidity resulting in three or more bowel movements per day.[39,56] Secondary effects related to diarrhea include abdominal cramps, anxiety, lethargy, weakness, dehydration, dizziness, loss of electrolytes, skin breakdown and associated pain, dry mouth, and weight loss. Diarrhea varies among patients depending on their bowel history. Acute diarrhea occurs within 24 to 48 hours of exposure to the cause and resolves in 7 to 14 days. Chronic diarrhea usually has a late onset and lasts 2 to 3 weeks, with an unidentified cause.

Prevalence and impact

Cancer patients may have multiple causes of diarrhea. It may be due to infections or related to tumor type or its treatment. Common causes of diarrhea are chemotherapy, overuse of laxative therapy or dietary fiber. Additional causes include malabsorption disorders, motility disturbances, stress, partial bowel obstruction, enterocolic fistula, villous adenoma, endocrine-induced hypersecretion of serotonin, gastrin calcitonin, and vasoactive intestinal protein prostaglandins.[1,39] Treatment-related causes include radiation and chemotherapy, which cause overgrowth of bacteria, with endotoxin production that has a direct effect on the intestinal mucosa. Local inflammation and increased fluid and electrolyte secretion occur, resulting in interference with amino acid and electrolyte transport and a shift toward secretion by crypt cells with shortened villi.[39,53]

Chemotherapy-induced diarrhea may be related to one drug or compounded when two diarrheal instigating medications are given together, for example, fluorouracil and irinotecan.[56] Irinotecan may cause delayed diarrhea starting 6–14 days after treatment. Other fluorouracil family drugs like capecitabine or taxane drugs like docetaxel will cause diarrhea as well.[39] Newer targeted therapy drugs that can cause serious diarrhea include erlotinib and gefitinib, sorafenib, sunitinib, imatinib, and bortezomib.[39] Excessive diarrhea leads to dose interruption and severe events.[39]

Diarrhea associated with radiation can occur by the second or third week of treatment and can continue after radiation has been discontinued.[21,39,57] Radiation-induced diarrhea is related to focus of radiation and total of radiation dose. Pelvic radiation alone has been shown to cause diarrhea of any grade in up to 70% of the patients receiving it. A grade 3 or 4 diarrhea is associated with approximately 20% of those patients.[39] The risk is increased in acquired immunodeficiency syndrome (AIDS), GVHD, or HIV patients.[55] The end result could be a change in the intestinal mucosa that results in a limited ability to regenerate epithelium, which can lead to bleeding and ileus. The damaged mucosa leads to increased release of prostaglandins and malabsorption of bile salts, increasing peristaltic activity.[54,55,57]

Acute enteritis or proctitis can occur within the first 6 weeks of therapy and resolve between 2 and 6 months post treatment.[39] Patients who were treated with greater than 45 Gray (GY) may develop a chronic radiation enteritis. Physical changes secondary to the radiation may cause effects from months to years after treatment.[39]

Surgical patients who have had bowel-shortening procedures or gastrectomy related to cancer experience a "dumping syndrome," which causes severe diarrhea. This type of diarrhea is related to both osmotic and hypermotile mechanisms.[21] Patients may experience weakness, epigastric distention, and diarrhea shortly after eating.[58] The shortened bowel can result in a decreased absorption capacity and an imbalance in absorptive and secretory function of the intestine.

Pathophysiology

Diarrhea can be grouped into four types, each with a different mechanism: osmotic diarrhea, secretory diarrhea, hypermotile diarrhea, and exudative diarrhea. Cancer patients rarely exhibit only one type. Understanding the mechanism of diarrhea permits more rational treatment strategies.[39,54,56,58]

Osmotic diarrhea

Osmotic diarrhea is produced by intake of hyperosmolar preparations or nonabsorbable solutions such as enteral feeding solutions.[21,58] Enterocolic fistula can lead to both osmotic diarrhea from undigested food entering the colon and hypermotile diarrhea. Hemorrhage into the intestine can cause an osmotic-type diarrhea because intraluminal blood acts as an osmotic laxative. Osmotic diarrhea may result from insufficient lactase when dairy products are consumed.

Secretory diarrhea

Secretory diarrhea is most associated with chemotherapy and radiation therapy. The cause is related to mechanical damage to the epithelial crypt cells in the GI tract.[57] The necrosis that results, along with the inflammation and ulceration of the intestinal mucosa, leads to further damage related to exposure to bile and susceptibility to opportunistic infections, atrophy of the mucosal lining, and fibrosis. This all contributes to loss of absorption due to damaged villi, causing an increase in water, electrolytes, mucus, blood, and serum to be pulled into the intestine from immature crypt cells, and increased fluid secretion, resulting in diarrhea.[39,58-60]

Secretory diarrhea is the most difficult to control. Malignant epithelial tumors producing hormones that can cause diarrhea include metastatic carcinoid tumors, gastrinoma, and medullary thyroid cancer. The primary effect of secretory diarrhea is related to the hypersecretion stimulated by endogenous mediators that affect the intestinal transport of water and electrolytes. This results in accumulation of intestinal fluids.[39,54,55] Diarrhea associated with GVHD results from mucosal damage and can produce up to 6 to 8 liters of diarrhea in 24 hours.[57] Surgical shortening of the bowel, which reduces intestinal mucosal contact and shortens colon transit time, causing decreased reabsorption, leads to diarrhea. Active treatment requires vigorous fluid and electrolyte repletion, antidiarrheal therapy, and specific anticancer therapy.[39] Preventing diarrhea associated with chemotherapy and radiation is not always realistic, but being proactive in anticipating diarrhea and prompt management may be effective.[39,54,58] Initiation of medication with the first episode is suggested. The recommendation starts with loperamide 4 mg, then 2 to 4 mg every 2 to 4 hours (max 16 mg/24 h). If there is no response at 24 to 48 hours, then, based on grade, either increase the loperamide dose, then reevaluate in 24 hours, or start octreotide 100 to 500 mcg subcutaneously, three times a day for grades 3 to 4 diarrhea.[39] The somatostatin analog octreotide is used for grades 3 to 4 diarrhea with success. One study in patients experiencing chemotherapy-induced diarrhea unresponsive to loperamide had a 92% response to octreotide SC 500 mcg three times daily.[61] The use of sustained release octreotide (LAR) for the treatment of diarrheal syndromes, as well as treatment of malignant bowel obstruction related nausea, vomiting and pain has shown benefit.[61] The goal is to prevent high-grade diarrhea that results in dose reduction or cessation of chemotherapy regimens.[62] Cost is a major issue with this medication; dosing for only 3–7 days at $42.00–$55.00/dose could run close to $165.00/day and about $1600.00 for 10 doses or a 3-day regimen.[18,39,43,63] However, along with preventing dose reduction of chemotherapy, the potential to reduce the number of episodes of diarrhea and minimize the additional effects on psychosocial issues and quality of life may make this approach worthwhile.

Hypermotile diarrhea

Partial bowel obstruction from abdominal malignancies can cause a reflex hypermotility that may require bowel-quieting medications such as loperamide.[58] Enterocolic fistula can lead to diarrhea from irritative hypermotility and osmotic influence of undigested food entering the colon. Biliary or pancreatic obstruction can cause incomplete digestion of fat in the small intestine, resulting in interference with fat and bile salt malabsorption, leading to hypermotile diarrhea, also called steatorrhea. Malabsorption is related to pancreatic cancer, gastrectomy, ileal resection or colectomy, rectal cancer, pancreatic islet cell tumors, or carcinoid tumors. Chemotherapy-induced diarrhea is frequently seen with 5-fluorouracil or N-phosphonoacetyl-L-aspartate. High-dose cisplatin and irinotecan (Camptosar) cause severe hypermotility. Other chemotherapy drugs that cause diarrhea include cytosine arabinoside, nitrosourea, methotrexate, cyclophosphamide, doxorubicin, daunorubicin, hydroxyurea and biotherapy-2, interferon and topoisomerase inhibitors (capecitabine [5-FU prodrug]), and oxaliplatin.[39]

Exudative diarrhea

Radiation therapy of the abdomen, pelvis, or lower thoracic or lumbar spine can cause acute exudative diarrhea.[39] The inflammation caused by radiation leads to the release of prostaglandins. Treatment using aspirin or ibuprofen was shown to reduce prostaglandin release and decrease diarrhea associated with radiation therapy.[39] Bismuth subsalicylate (Pepto-Bismol) is also helpful for diarrhea caused by radiotherapy.[24]

There are multiple causes of diarrhea in palliative medicine. Concurrent diseases such as diabetes mellitus, hyperthyroidism, inflammatory bowel disease, irritable bowel syndrome, and GI infection (*Clostridium difficile*) can contribute to the development of diarrhea. Finally, the dietary influences of fruit, bran, hot spices, and alcohol, as well as over-the-counter medications, laxatives, and herbal supplements, need to be considered as sources of diarrhea.[21,39]

Assessment of diarrhea

Diarrhea assessment requires a careful history to detail the frequency and nature of the stools. The National Cancer Institute Scale of Severity of Diarrhea uses a grading system from 0 to 4. Stools are rated by (1) number of loose stools per day and (2) symptoms (Table 12.2). This scale permits an objective score to define the severity of diarrhea.

The initial goal of assessment is to identify and treat any reversible causes of diarrhea. If diarrhea occurs once or twice a day, it is probably related to anal incontinence. Large amounts of watery stools are characteristic of colonic diarrhea. Pale, fatty, malodorous stools, called steatorrhea, are indicative of malabsorption secondary to pancreatic or small-intestinal causes. If a patient who has been constipated complains of sudden diarrhea with little warning, fecal impaction with overflow is the probable cause.[21,39]

Evaluate medications that the patient may be taking now or in the recent past. Is the patient on laxatives? If the stools are associated with cramping and urgency, it may be the result of peristalsis-stimulating laxatives. If stools are associated with fecal leakage, it may be the result of overuse of stool-softening agents such as Colace.[21,39] Depending on the aggressiveness of the treatment plan, additional assessment could include stool smears for

Table 12.2 National Cancer Institute Scale of Severity of Diarrhea

	National Cancer Institute grade					
	0	1	2	3	4	5
Increased number of loose stools/day	Normal	2–3	4–6	7–9	>10	Death
Symptoms		None	Nocturnal stools and/or moderate cramping	Incontinence and/or severe cramping Interferes with normal activity	Grossly bloody diarrhea and/or need for parenteral support. Life threatening	

pus, blood, fat, ova, or parasites. Stool samples for culture and sensitivity testing may be necessary to rule out additional sources of diarrhea through *C. difficile* toxin, *Giardia lamblia*, or other types of GI infection.[56] If patients have diarrhea after 2 to 3 days of fasting, secretory diarrhea should be evaluated. Osmotic and secretory causes are considered first; if ruled out, then hypermotility is the suspected mechanism.

Multifactorial causes for diarrhea make management a challenge. Assessment is essential to rule out any causes that may be easily managed. It is essential to include a registered dietician when planning management strategies.

Management of diarrhea

A combination of supportive care and medication may be appropriate for palliative management of diarrhea. The goal of diarrhea management should focus on minimizing or eliminating the factors causing the diarrhea, providing dietary interventions, and maintaining fluid and electrolyte balance as appropriate. Quality-of-life issues include minimizing skin breakdown or infections, relieving pain associated with frequent diarrhea, and maintaining the patient's dignity.[39,56]

If the patient is dehydrated, oral fluids are recommended over the IV route.[22,39] Oral fluids should contain electrolytes and a source of glucose to facilitate active electrolyte transport (Box 12.4). Foods to be avoided in patients experiencing acute diarrhea include: spicy food, high-fat and fried foods, gas causing foods, alcohol and caffeine foods, and high-sorbitol juices. Milk and dairy products for some patients should be avoided as well.[39,56]

Box 12.4 Homemade electrolyte replacement solution for adults

Adult homemade electrolyte replacement solution

1 tsp salt	6 oz. frozen orange juice concentrate
1 tsp baking soda	6 cups water
1 tsp corn syrup	47 kcal/cup, 515 mg Na$^+$, 164 mg K$^+$

Following diarrhea, the diet should start with clear liquids, flat lemonade, ginger ale, and toast or simple carbohydrates. It is recommended that the patient avoid milk if diarrhea is related to infection due to acute lactase deficiency. Protein and fats can be added to the diet slowly as diarrhea resolves. Dietary management may help minimize amount of diarrhea.

Source: Weihofen and Marino (1998), reference 59.

Medication recommendations

There are many nonspecific diarrhea medications that should be used unless infections are suspected as the cause. If *Shigella* or *C. difficile* are responsible, nonspecific antidiarrheal medications can make the diarrhea worse.[21] Loperamide (Imodium) has become the drug of choice for the treatment of nonspecific diarrhea. It is a long-acting opioid agonist.[56] The 2-mg dose of loperamide has the same antidiarrheal action as two 5 mg tablets of diphenoxylate, or 45 mg of codeine.[20] The usual management of diarrhea begins with 4 mg of loperamide, with one capsule following each loose bowel movement. Most diarrhea is managed by loperamide 2 to 4 mg once to twice a day.[56] Diphenoxylate (Lomotil 2.5 mg with atropine 0.025 mg) is given as one or two tablets orally as needed for loose stools, maximum of eight/day. Diphenoxylate is derived from meperidine and binds to opioid receptors to reduce diarrhea. Atropine was added to this antidiarrheal to prevent abuse.[5] Diphenoxylate is not recommended for patients with advanced liver disease because it may precipitate hepatic coma in patients with cirrhosis.[56] Neither diphenoxylate nor loperamide is recommended for use in children under 12 years old.[38] Codeine as an opioid for the reduction of diarrhea can be helpful. It is also less expensive than some opioid medications. Most cancer-related diarrheas respond well to this drug. For specific mechanisms, other medications might be more beneficial. Tincture of opium works to decrease peristalsis, given at 0.6 mL every 4 to 6 hours. This is a controlled substance but may also provide some pain relief.[56] Absorbent agents such as pectin and methylcellulose may help provide bulk to increase consistency of the stools.[56]

Anticholinergic drugs such as atropine and scopolamine are useful to reduce gastric secretions and decrease peristalsis. Somatostatin analogs such as octreotide (Sandostatin) are also effective for secretory diarrhea that may result from endocrine tumors, AIDS, GVHD, or post-GI resection.[21,56,58] They may be helpful for patients who experience painful cramping.[5] Side effects of that class of drug can complicate their use; they include dry mouth, blurred vision, and urinary hesitancy.

Mucosal antiprostaglandin agents such as aspirin, indomethacin, and bismuth subsalicylate (Pepto-Bismol) are useful for diarrhea related to enterotoxic bacteria, radiotherapy, and prostaglandin-secreting tumors. Octreotide (Sandostatin) is effective for patients with AIDS, GVHD, diabetes, or GI resection.[21,54,64] Octreotide is administered subcutaneously at a dose of 50 to 200 mcg two or three times per day. Ranitidine is a useful adjuvant to octreotide for patients with Zollinger-Ellison syndrome with gastrin-induced gastric hypersecretion.[38] Side effects include nausea and pain at injection site. Patients may also experience abdominal or headache pain. Clonidine is effective at controlling watery diarrhea in patients with bronchogenic cancer. Clonidine effects an α_2-adrenergic stimulation of electrolyte absorption in the small intestine. Streptozocin is used for watery diarrhea from pancreatic islet cell cancer because it decreases intestinal secretions. Hypermotile diarrhea involves problems with fat absorption. The recommended treatment is pancreatin before meals. Pancreatin is a combination of amylase, lipase, and protease that is available for pancreatic enzyme replacement. Lactaid may also be helpful for malabsorption-related diarrhea.[56]

Nursing interventions for diarrhea

Nursing interventions should include nonpharmacological interventions focused on diet and psychosocial support (Boxes 12.5 and 12.6).

Box 12.5 Nutritional management of cancer-related diarrhea: foods and medication to avoid

Medications

Antibiotics, bulk laxatives (Metamucil, methylcellulose), magnesium-containing medications (Maalox, Mylanta), promotility agents (propulsid, metoclopramide), stool softeners/laxatives, herbal supplements (milk thistle, aloe, cayenne, saw palmetto, Siberian ginseng).

Foods

Milk and dairy products (cheese, yogurt, ice cream), caffeine-containing products (coffee, tea, cola drinks, chocolate), carbonated and high-sugar or high-sorbitol juices (prune pear, sweet cherry, peach, apple, orange juice), high-fiber/gas-causing legumes (raw vegetables, whole grain products, dried legumes, popcorn), high-fat foods (fried foods, high-fat spreads, or dressings), heavily spiced foods that taste "hot."

High risk foods—sushi, street vendors, buffets.

Sources: Adapted from Muehlbauer et al. (2009), reference 56; Engelking (2004), reference 54.

◆ Evaluate medications currently being used to identify polypharmacy, where multiple medication side effects may be contributing to the problem.

◆ Minimize or prevent diarrhea accidents in an effort to reduce patient anxiety. Anticipate obstacles between the patient and the bathroom. Assist with access plans and timing needs. Recommend commode chair at bedside to allow easiest access and prevent falls or additional problems.

◆ Protecting the bed with disposable underpads can be better accepted than diapers. It may also be better for skin integrity but requires multiple layers of disposable underpads and drawsheets for best results.

◆ Applying skin ointment protection after cleaning and drying the area is also important. Thick protectant creams that apply a barrier on the skin are most beneficial. Eucerin cream, zinc oxide, and bag balm are three that have been used anecdotally with success.

◆ The psychosocial impact of diapers can be devastating for some patients. Encourage a discussion with patient and family about patient needs, fears, and perceptions.

◆ Along with focus on diet/medications, skin integrity, and psychosocial needs, odor management must also be addressed. Perfumed air fresheners sometimes only make it worse. Concentrate on being sure the perineum or periostomy area is clean and the linens are not soiled. Also be sure that dirty linens or trash are removed from the room. Using aromatherapy such as lavender may be soothing.

◆ Remember that there may be times when adult diapers are essential and can help alleviate distress to the patient; for example, when traveling or on necessary outings. Remind families to check them frequently to prevent skin breakdown and, again, be sure there is skin barrier ointment applied before the diaper padding.

Management guidelines that may help in planning care include Oncology Nursing Society ONS Putting Evidence in Practice (PEP) diarrhea resource[65] (www.ons.org/outcomes/volume4/diarrhea/pdf/ShortCard_Diarrhea.pdf.)

Conclusion

Managing diarrhea in the cancer patient is challenging at best. The nurse's role in helping the patient and caregivers talk about this difficult symptom is essential and recognizing which patients are at highest risk is important. Understanding the sensitive aspects of bowel management in acute diarrhea patients is necessary among nurse, patient, and caregiver to allow information sharing. Palliative goals of diarrhea therapy should be to restore an optimal pattern of elimination, maintain fluid and electrolyte balance as desired, preserve nutritional status, protect skin integrity, and ensure the patient's comfort and dignity.[24,56]

Malignant obstruction

As primary tumors grow in the large intestine, they can lead to obstruction. Obstruction is related to the site and stage of disease.[60,66] Tumors in the splenic flexure obstruct 49% of the time, but those in the rectum or rectosigmoid junction only 6% of the time.[66,67] Obstruction can occur intraluminally related to primary tumors of the colon. Intramural obstruction is related to tumor in the muscular layers of the bowel wall. The bowel appears thickened, indurated, and contracted.[21,68] Extramural obstruction is related to mesenteric and omental masses and malignant adhesions. The common metastatic pattern, in relation to primary disease in the pancreas, ovaries or stomach, generally goes to the duodenum, from the colon to the jejunum and ileum, and from the prostate or bladder to the rectum.[21,66,68] Bowel obstruction in cancer patients is not always due to their tumors. Hernias, radiation-induced strictures, or adhesions may be the cause, so it is important that patients with obstructive symptoms be thoroughly evaluated to rule out a correctable cause.[21,68,69]

Definition

Experts agree there is no standard definition for malignant bowel obstruction (MBO).[67,70] A current definition uses the criteria

Box 12.6 Nursing role in the management of diarrhea

Environmental assessment

- Assess the patient's and/or caregiver's ability to manage the level of care necessary.
- Evaluate home for medical equipment that may be helpful (bedpan or commode chair).

History

- Frequency of bowel movements in last 2 wks
- Fluid intake (normal 2 quarts/day)
- Fiber intake (normal 30–40 g/day)
- Appetite and whether patient is nauseated or vomiting. Does diet include spicy foods?
- Assess for current medications the patient has taken that are associated with causing diarrhea (laxative use, chemotherapy, antibiotics, enteral nutritional supplements, nonsteroidal antiinflammatory drugs).
- Surgical history that may contribute to diarrhea (gastrectomy, pancreatectomy, bypass, or ileal resection)
- Recent radiotherapy to abdomen, pelvis, lower spine
- Cancer diagnosis associated with diarrhea includes abdominal malignancies, partial bowel obstruction; enterocolic fistulae; metastatic carcinoid tumors; gastrinomas; medullary thyroid cancer.
- Immunosuppressed, susceptible to bacterial, protozoan, and viral diseases associated with diarrhea
- Concurrent diseases associated with diarrhea: gastroenteritis, inflammatory bowel disease, irritable bowel syndrome, diabetes mellitus, lactose deficiency, hyperthyroidism

Physical assessment

- Examine perineum or ostomy site for skin breakdown, fissures, or external hemorrhoids.
- Gentle digital rectal examination for impaction
- Abdominal examination for distention of palpable stool in large bowel
- Examine stools for signs of bleeding.
- Evaluate for signs of dehydration.

Interventions

- Treatment should be related to cause (i.e., if obstruction is cause of diarrhea, giving antidiarrheal medications would be inappropriate).
- Assist with correcting any obvious factors related to assessment (e.g., decreasing nutritional supplements, changing fiber intake, holding or substituting medications associated with diarrhea).
- If bacterial causes are suspected, notify physician and culture stools as instructed. *Clostridium difficile* is most common.

- Educate patient and family on importance of cleansing the perineum gently after each stool, to prevent skin breakdown. If patient has a colostomy, stomal area must also be watched closely and surrounding skin protected. Use skin barrier such as Desitin ointment to protect the skin. Frequent sitz baths may be helpful.
- Instruct patient and family on signs and symptoms that should be reported to the nurse or physician: excessive thirst, dizziness, fever, palpitations, rectal spasms, excessive cramping, water or bloody stools.

Dietary measures

- Eat small, frequent, bland meals.
- Use Low-residue diet—potassium-rich (bananas, rice, peeled apples, dry toast).
- Avoid intake of hyperosmotic supplements (e.g., Ensure, Sustacal).
- Increase fluids in diet. Approximately 3 liters of fluid a day if possible. Drinking electrolyte fluids such as Pedialyte may be helpful.
- Homeopathic treatments for diarrhea include ginger tea, glutamine, and peeled apples.

Pharmacological management

- Opioids—codeine, paregoric, diphenoxylate, loperamide, tincture of opium
- Absorbents—pectin, aluminum hydroxide
- Adsorbents—charcoal, kaolin
- Antisecretory—aspirin, bismuth subsalicylate, prednisone, Sandostatin, ranitidine hydrochloride, indomethacin
- Anticholinergics—scopolamine, atropine sulfate, belladonna
- α_2-adrenergic agonists—clonidine

Report to nurse or physician if antidiarrheal medication seems ineffective.

Psychosocial interventions

Provide support to patient and family. Recognize negative effects of diarrhea on quality of life:

- Fatigue
- Malnutrition
- Alteration in skin integrity
- Pain and discomfort
- Sleep disturbances
- Limited ability to travel
- Compromised role within the family
- Decreased sexual activity
- Caregiver burden

Sources: Levy (1991), reference 38; Bisanz (2005), reference 24; Ripamonti, Easson, and Gerdes (2008), reference 67.

Table 12.3 Sites of intestinal obstruction and related side effects

Site	Side effects
Duodenum	Severe vomiting with large amounts of undigested food. Bowel sounds: succussion splash may be present. No pain or distention noted. Anorexia present
Small intestine	Moderate to severe vomiting; usually hyperactive bowel sounds with borborygmi; pain in upper and central abdomen, colic in nature; moderate distention. Periumbilical pain
Large intestine	Vomiting is a late side effect. Borborygmi bowel sounds, severe distention. Pain central to lower abdomen, colic in nature.

Sources: Ripamonte and Mercadante (2004), reference 44; Ripamonte (2008), reference 69.

that there is "clinical evidence of bowel obstruction, obstruction beyond the ligament of Treitz (in the setting of intra-abdominal cancer with incurable disease), or non-intra-abdominal primary cancer with clear intraperitoneal disease.[71] The significance of an agreed on definition is the ability to evaluate treatment plans for evidence-based recommendations.[67]

Clinical evidence of intestinal obstruction is occlusion of the lumen or absence of the normal propulsion that affects elimination from the GI tract.[43,72] Motility disruption, either impaired or absent, leads to a functional obstruction but without occlusion of the intestinal lumen.[67] Mechanical obstruction results in the accumulation of fluids and gas proximal to the obstruction. Distention occurs as a result of intestinal gas, ingested fluids, and digestive secretions. It becomes a self-perpetuating phenomenon as when distention increases, intestinal secretion of water and electrolytes increases. A small-bowel obstruction causes large amounts of diarrhea. The increased fluid in the bowel leads to increased peristalsis, with large quantities of bacteria growing in the intestinal fluid of the small bowel.[43,69,72]

Obstruction is related to the surrounding mesentery or bowel muscle, such as in ovarian cancer. Additional factors include multiple sites of obstruction along the intestine and constipating medications (Table 12.3), fecal impaction, fibrosis, or change in normal flora of the bowel. The goal of treatment is to prevent obstruction from happening whenever possible.

Prevalence and impact

The best treatment options for bowel obstruction in a patient with advanced cancer remain undetermined.[69] Managing MBO is dependent on the level of obstruction, disease status related to prognosis, prior treatments, and the patient's current health status.[66,68] As obstruction increases, bacteria levels increase and can lead to sepsis and associated multisystem failure and death.[72] The difficulty is knowing which patients will truly benefit from surgical intervention. The impact of obstruction on the patient and family is overwhelming. The patient and caregivers have been aggressively trying to manage the patient's constipation in an effort to prevent this very problem. Obstruction for patients means failure to manage constipation or a sign of growing disease. Interventions have been evaluated in an effort to provide noninvasive approaches for the management of bowel obstruction.[61,69,73]

Bowel obstruction can occur in between 5% and 43% of patients with advanced disease. Intestinal obstruction related to benign causes in patients with a previous malignancy can be significant: 3%–48%.[66,69,70] Patients with a history of cancer who present with symptoms of bowel obstruction should be evaluated both clinically and radiologically.[67] Each case must be evaluated individually with care decisions based on goal of treatment. Unfortunately, studies also differ in agreeing on a successful outcome. Defining success may be evaluated based on ability to resume oral intake; relief of pain, nausea, or vomiting; extended survival; or improvement in quality of life.[66,69] Further research needs to be done[68,74] to evaluate the effects of surgical intervention on quality as well as quantity of life. The effect of unrelieved intestinal obstruction on quality of life for the patient and loved ones is devastating.

Assessment and management of malignant obstruction

Patients may experience severe nausea, vomiting, and abdominal pain associated with a partial or complete bowel obstruction. In the elderly patient, fecal impaction may also cause urinary incontinence.[21] General signs and symptoms associated with different sites of obstruction are listed in Table 12.3. Providing thoughtful and supportive interventions may be more appropriate than aggressive, invasive procedures. The signs and symptoms of obstruction may be acute, with nausea, vomiting, and abdominal pain. A majority of the time, however, obstruction is a slow and insidious phenomenon, which may progress from partial to complete obstruction. Palliative care should allow for a thoughtful and realistic approach to management of obstruction within the goals of care. Radiological examination should be limited unless surgery is being considered. Treatment options start with a nonsurgical approach and emergent surgical intervention is usually not necessary unless the risk of perforation is eminent. Patients who would benefit from surgical intervention for MBO are evaluated based on age, tumor status, presence of ascites, nutritional status, previous chemotherapy or radiation treatments.[66,69,72,74] A surgical intervention would most likely not benefit a patient if they have ascites, multiple bowel obstructions, carcinomatosis, or poor overall clinical status.[66]

Surgical intervention

A percentage of cancer patients may experience nonmalignant obstruction.[68] Therefore, assuming the obstruction is related to worsening cancer may prevent the healthcare team from setting realistic treatment goals. A thorough assessment should be done, with attention to poor prognostic factors.[21,43,66] These factors historically include general medical condition or poor nutritional status, ascites, palpable abdominal masses or distant metastases, previous radiation to the abdomen or pelvis, combination chemotherapy, and multiple small-bowel obstructions.[66–69]

Helyer and Easson[68] organize criteria for surgical interventions. First are patient factors including advanced age, nutritional status, performance status, comorbidities and anticancer treatment history, psychological health, and social support. Second are factors such as disease-related etiology, tumor grade and tumor extent, and presence of ascites. Third are operative factors. Will the procedure relieve symptoms for an extended amount of time with reasonable operative morbidity? Risks and benefits of the surgery in contrast to nonsurgical options and the patient's goals of care must be balanced. The use of laparoscopic surgical techniques has brought about changes in the use of open surgical techniques in the palliative care patient.

Surgical intervention should be a decision made between patient and physician within the established goals of care. The patient's right to self-determination is essential. As a patient advocate, the nurse's role is to educate the patient and family. Helping them to understand their options, as well as considering their personal desires, is essential. Patients undergoing surgical resection for obstructing cancers of the GI tract, pancreas, or biliary tracts were found to have a 3- to 7-month survival.[58] This study pointed out the importance of nutritional status at baseline and assessment of performance status for its relationship to "reasonable quality of life."[58] The important conclusion of these studies was to leave the decision to operate with an informed patient. Mortality is possible. The need for additional surgeries remains high due to recurrence of the obstruction, wound infections, sepsis, and further obstruction.[44] Survival rates with each subsequent surgery lessen.

Improved options for management of MBO have developed as pharmacology and interventional radiology have been included in palliative care options.[67] The improvements in X-ray technologies have improved the diagnosis of the cause of the MBO to help choose more appropriate interventions especially in light of the high morbidity and mortality associated with surgery in this population.[66,68,72,74–78]

Radiological examination

Bowel obstruction may be diagnosed on the basis of a plain abdominal X-ray, but contrast may help identify the site and extent of the obstruction. Exams using CT have shown an accuracy of 94% in determining the cause of a bowel obstruction. The use of either CT or MRI to help develop a treatment plan for MBO has improved decision-making between a surgical or medical management approach.[42] Barium is not recommended because it may interfere with additional studies.[69]

Alternative interventions

Nasogastric or nasointestinal tubes have been used to decompress the bowel and/or stomach. Use of these interventions, although uncomfortable for the patient, has been suggested for symptom relief while evaluating the possibility of surgery. Venting gastrostomy or jejunostomy can be a relatively easy alternative, which is especially effective for severe nausea and vomiting. It can be placed percutaneously with sedation and local anesthesia. Patients can then be fed a liquid diet, with the tube clamped for as long as tolerated without nausea or vomiting.[67,69]

Endoscopic palliation

Laparoscopic surgical techniques have brought about new options for inoperable cancers. Gastroenterologists or interventional radiologists now have an increased role in palliating obstructions.[73] The use of enteral self-expandable metal stents (SEMS) are a permanent intervention that is performed through endoscopy to improve luminal patency and allow oral intake without surgery. The use of self-expanding metallic stents has been highly effective for MBO and, in some cases, has prevented the need for colostomy.[68,73] It is done in interventional radiology and requires close clinical observation, since perforation is a potential complication. It allows emergent relief of obstruction and may be the best option for palliative care patients with poor prognosis.[67] Putting a patient

through an X-ray of the abdomen may be helpful to confirm the presence of obstruction and the site, but determining the goals of therapy is essential.[68] When patients exhibit signs of obstruction, a physical exam may be helpful to assess the extent of the problem. Asking the patient for a bowel history, last bowel movement, and a description of consistency can be helpful. Does the patient complain of constipation? Physical examination should include gentle palpation of the abdomen for masses or distention. A careful rectal exam can identify the presence of stool in the rectum or a distended empty rectum. An empty, or "ballooned," rectum may be a symptom of high obstruction. It is also difficult to distinguish stool from malignant mass.[24,69] The ability to assess whether an impaction is low or high in the intestinal tract is important to help guide the intervention planning. As discussed above, lack of stool noted in the rectum during a digital exam is usually indicative of a high impaction. Stool has not or cannot move down into the rectum. The goal then would be to use careful assessment to be sure the obstruction is not a tumor and to concentrate on softening the stool and moving it through the GI tract. Again, using a stimulant laxative for this type of patient would result in increasing discomfort and possible rupture of the intestinal wall.[24,72] Low impactions are uncomfortable, and patients may need more comforting measures. Patients may need to lie down to decrease pressure on the rectal area and avoid drinking hot liquids or eating big meals, which may increase peristalsis and discomfort until the impaction can be cleared.[24]

Multiple types of stents are available. After evaluating 600 patients who had stent placement for malignant gastric outlet obstruction (GOO), Dormann et al. found technical success with confirmation that bowel patency occurred for 97% of patients.[78] Greater than 75% of postprocedural patients were able to tolerate a full or soft solid diet.[67] Patients were able to tolerate oral diets within 24 hours of the stent placement.[58] Complications of stent placement are divided into early or late effects. Early is related to stent misdeployment or malpositioning or perforation. Late complications include tumor growth extending through the stent into the lumen, stent migration, bleeding, or perforation.[73] The use of stents has been shown to be effective in relieving malignant bowel obstruction and, compared to surgery, is less invasive with faster resumption of oral intake and shorter hospital stays, which saved money. One study found that the cost for patients who had stent placement versus surgical interventions was $7,215 to $10,190 in US dollars.[79] For complete obstructions, especially in an emergency situation, surgery has been necessary to decompress the bowel and frequently results in a colostomy. Laparoscopy is difficult in these patients due to the acutely dilated colon and the increased risk of complications when using laparoscopic instruments on that type of tissue.[73,80] Stenting versus surgery has been found to reduce morbidity and mortality of patients who would be poor candidates for surgery. It provides a way to prevent the need for a colostomy and results in shorter hospitalizations, which reduces healthcare costs.[67,80]

Decompression tubes

Colonic decompression tubes are used to reduce acutely distended bowel to prevent perforation and prevent more invasive surgical procedures. They can be placed by endoscopy or over a guidewire. They are inexpensive and widely available and prevent surgical intervention with colostomy. Disadvantages include success being dependent on the person placing them and the risk of dislodgment of the tubes. The size of these tubes allows for bowel cleansing or stool removal. These tubes are recommended as a temporizing measure to relieve distention and hopefully allow for bowel cleaning. More research needs to be done on the success of these larger decompression tubes.[73,81]

Symptom therapy

Providing aggressive pharmacological management of the distressing symptoms associated with MBO can prevent the need for surgical intervention.[21,67] The symptoms of intestinal colic, vomiting, and diarrhea can be effectively controlled with medications for most patients. The goal of pharmacological symptom management in inoperable patients should be aimed at relieving abdominal pain and intestinal colic, to reduce vomiting and prevent the need for a nasogastric tube, relieve nausea, and allow the patient to return home optimally with hospice care.[67]

Depending on the location of the obstruction, either high or low, symptom severity can be affected. As accumulation of secretions increases, abdominal pain also increases. Distention, vomiting, and prolonged constipation occur. With high obstruction, onset of vomiting is sooner and amounts are larger. Intermittent borborygmi and visible peristalsis may occur.[40] Patients may experience colic pain on top of continuous pain from a growing mass. In chronic bowel obstruction, colic pain subsides. There are

---

Box 12.7 Obstruction management options

1. Prevent obstruction if at all possible.

2. Octreotide—0.2–0.9 mg/day IV or SQ. This may prevent complete obstruction if used early.

3. Opioids IV/SQ relieve pain.

4. Antiemetic medications—haloperidol 5–15 mg/day, metoclopromide 10 mg Q 4 h. SQ—only if no colicky pain. Prochlorperazine 25–75 mg/day rectally, chlorpromazine 50–100 mg rectally/subcutaneous Q 8 h.

5. Anticholinergics—scopolamine butybromide 40–120 mg/day, scopolamine hydrobromide 0.8–2.0 mg/day

6. Corticosteroids

7. Fluids and nutrients as tolerated

8. Laxative meds—stimulating laxatives. **Contraindicated** due to ↑ peristalsis. Stool softener meds may be helpful if there is a partial obstruction only.

9. Antidiarrheal medications—subacute obstruction or fecal fistula—codeine, loperamide, or octreotide

10. Endoscopic therapeutic devices—self-expandable metal stents (SEMS)

11. Colonic decompression tubes

12. Surgery

Sources: Adapted from Frech and Adler (2007), reference 73; Helyer and Easson (2008), reference 68; Ripamonte, Easson, and Gerdes (2008), reference 67.

---

multiple options to attempt in an effort to relieve the symptoms and obstruction of an MBO (Box 12.7).

As stated above, the goal of treatment is to prevent obstruction whenever possible. The use of subcutaneous (SQ) or intravenous (IV) analgesics, anticholinergic drugs, and antiemetic drugs can be effective for reducing the symptoms of inoperable and hard-to-manage obstruction.[21,43,71,72] Octreotide may be an option in early management to prevent partial obstructions from becoming complete.[21,43,71,72] Although octreotide is used for diarrhea because it decreases peristalsis, it also slows the irregular and ineffective peristaltic movements of obstruction, reducing the activity and balancing out the intestinal movement.[56,60,72] It reduces vomiting because it inhibits the secretion of gastrin, secretin, vasoactive intestinal peptide, pancreatic polypeptide, insulin, and glucagon. Octreotide directly blocks the secretion of gastric acid, pepsin, pancreatic enzyme, bicarbonate, intestinal epithelial electrolytes, and water.[56,60] It has been shown to be effective in 60% of patients for the control of vomiting.[21,72] Octreotide is administered by SQ infusion or SQ injection every 12 hours. A negative aspect of this drug is its cost. It is expensive and requires SQ injections or SQ or IV infusions over days to weeks. The recommended starting dose is 0.3 mg/day and may increase to 0.6 mg/day.[21,72] Hyoscine butylbromide is thought to be as effective as octreotide at reducing GI secretions and motility. Hyoscine butylbromide is less sedating, since it is thought to cross the blood-brain barrier less due to its low lipid solubility.[43] A recent study compared octreotide and scopolamine butylbromide for inoperable bowel obstruction with nasogastric tubes.[43,60] Both medications relieve colicky pain; both reduce the continuous abdominal pain and distention. Although this was a small study done over 3 days, they were able to remove the nasogastric tube in three of the seven patients on the first dose of octreotide 0.3 mg/day subcutaneously; three more patients were able to have the nasogastric tube removed when the dose was doubled to 0.6 mg/day. Scopolamine was similar in results, but the octreotide regimen was felt to be more effective overall. The negative effect is associated with the cost of the drug, a definite consideration for overall quality of life. Scopolamine is less expensive. [67,82]

Analgesic medications

Opioid medications have been used to relieve pain associated with obstruction.[21,67] Providing the opioid through SQ or IV infusion via a patient-controlled analgesic (PCA) pump is beneficial for two reasons: patients may receive improved pain relief over the oral route due to improved absorption, and by giving access to a PCA pump, patients are allowed some control over their pain management. Alternative routes of opioid administration, such as rectal or transdermal, may also be effective, but usually are inadequate if the pain is severe or unstable or there are frequent episodes of breakthrough pain.

Antiemetic medications

The goal of relief of symptoms for patients with MBO from a pharmacological approach include the use of antiemetics, antisecretory drugs, steroids, and analgesics.[21] The addition of the selective serotonin antagonists, the 5-hydroxytryptamine blockers (5-HT$_3$), has made a significant difference in the treatment of nausea, especially when combined with corticosteroids for chemotherapy-induced nausea (see also chapter 10).[83,84] Metoclopramide at 10 mg Q 4 hours SQ, has been the drug of choice for patients with incomplete bowel obstruction without colicky pain.[84] It stimulates the stomach to empty its contents into the reservoir of the bowel. Once complete obstruction is present, metoclopramide is discontinued and haloperidol or another antiemetic medication is started. Haloperidol is less sedating than other antiemetic or antihistamine medications.[84] The usual dose ranges from 5 to 15 mg/day, and at some institutions it is combined with cyclizine.[6] Corticosteroids are particularly helpful antiemetics, especially when related to chemotherapy.[84]

In practice, some recommend that morphine, haloperidol, and hyoscine butylbromide be given together by continuous SQ infusion. If pain or colic increases, the dose of morphine and hyoscine butylbromide should be increased; if emesis increases, increase the haloperidol dose.[21,67,84] Fluid and nutrient intake should be maintained as tolerated. Usually, patients whose vomiting has improved will tolerate fluids with small, low-residue meals. Dry mouth is managed with ice chips, although this has been suspected to wash out saliva that is present in the mouth. The use of artificial saliva may be more beneficial.

Corticosteroid medications

Corticosteroids have been helpful as antiemetic medications. The recommended dose of dexamethasone is between 6 and 16 mg/day; the prednisolone dose starts at 50 mg/day (injection or SQ infusion).[72] Steroids increase absorption of water and salt and reduce water and electrolytes in the intestine.

Antispasmodic medications

Colic pain results from increased peristalsis against the resistance of a mechanical obstruction. Analgesics alone may not be effective. Hyoscine butylbromide has been used to relieve spasm-like pain and to reduce emesis.[67,72] Dosing starts at 60 mg/day and increases up to 380 mg/day given by SQ infusion.[43] Side effects are related to the anticholinergic effects, including tachycardia, dry mouth, sedation, and hypotension.[72] Using methods to relieve dry mouth with sips of oral fluids, ice chips, and good mouth care is important.[72]

Laxative medications

Stimulant laxatives are contraindicated due to increased peristalsis against an obstruction. Stool-softening medications may be helpful if there is only a partial obstruction in the colon or rectum. If the obstruction is in the small bowel, laxatives will not be of benefit.[72]

Antidiarrheal management

Helping families cope with symptoms associated with obstruction is important. Historically, the management of obstruction involved aggressive surgical intervention or symptom management alone. The initial assessment should include: (1) evaluating constipation, (2) evaluating for surgery, (3) providing pain management, and (4) managing nausea with metoclopramide. If incomplete obstruction, use dexamethasone, haloperidol, dimenhydrinate, chlorpromazine, or hyoscine butylbromide.[43,60,67,72] The introduction of medications, such as octreotide, as well as newer antiemetics, has made a difference in the quality of life a patient with a malignant bowel obstruction may experience. The important thing to remember is that the treatment plan must always be in agreement with the patient's wishes and promotion of quality of life. Discussing the patient's understanding of the situation and the options available are essential to effective and thoughtful care of bowel obstruction in the palliative care patient.

Ascites

Ascites associated with malignancy results from a combination of impaired fluid efflux and increased fluid influx.[43] The effect of the accumulation of fluids leads to symptoms of abdominal distention, pain, nausea, early satiety, dyspnea, and reduced mobility.[85,86] Extreme ascites can lead to vomiting caused by external pressure on the stomach or intestines.[87] Ascites may be divided into three different types. *Central ascites* is the result of tumor-invading hepatic parenchyma, resulting in compression of the portal venous and/or the lymphatic system.[88] There is a decrease in oncotic pressure as a result of limited protein intake and the catabolic state associated with cancer. *Peripheral ascites* is related to deposits of tumor cells found on the surface of the parietal or visceral peritoneum. The result is a mechanical interference with venous and/or lymphatic drainage.[88] There is blockage at the level of the peritoneal space rather than the liver parenchyma. Macrophages increase capillary permeability and contribute to greater ascites. *Mixed-type ascites* is a combination of central and peripheral ascites. Therefore, both compression of the portal venous and lymphatic systems and tumor cells in the peritoneum are involved. Chylous malignant ascites occurs when tumor infiltration of the retroperitoneal space causes obstruction of lymph flow through the lymph nodes and/or the pancreas.[87,88] Additional sources of ascites not related to malignancy include the following:

- Preexisting advanced liver disease with portal hypertension
- Portal venous thrombosis
- Congestive heart failure
- Nephrotic syndrome
- Pancreatitis
- Tuberculosis
- Hepatic venous obstruction
- Bowel perforation

Severe ascites is associated with poor prognosis (40% 1-year survival, less than 10% 3-year survival).[88] The pathological mechanisms of malignant ascites make the prevention or reduction of abdominal fluid accumulation difficult.[88,89] Invasive management of ascites is seen as appropriate based on extent of ascites, prognosis, and etiology of disease.[90] Although survival is limited, the effects of ascites on the patient's quality of life warrant an aggressive approach.[88,89]

Tumor types most associated with ascites include ovarian, endometrial, breast, colon, gastric, and pancreatic cancers.[88,89] Less common sources of ascites include mesothelioma, non-Hodgkin's lymphoma, prostate cancer, multiple myeloma, and melanoma.[88]

Assessment of ascites

Symptoms associated with ascites

Patients complain of abdominal bloating and pain. Initially, patients complain of feeling a need for larger-waisted clothing and notice an increase in belt size or weight. They may feel nauseated and have a decreased appetite. Many patients will complain of increased symptoms of reflux or heartburn. Pronounced ascites can cause dyspnea and orthopnea due to increased pressure on the diaphragm.[87,89]

Physical examination

The physical examination may reveal abdominal or inguinal hernia, scrotal edema, and abdominal venous engorgement. Radiological findings show a hazy picture, with distended and separate loops of the bowel. There is a poor definition of the abdominal organs and loss of the psoas muscle shadows. Ultrasound and CT scans may also be used to diagnose ascites.[89]

Management of ascites

Traditionally, treatment of ascites is palliative because of poor prognosis.[12] Ovarian cancer is one of the few types where the presence of ascites does not necessarily correlate with a poor prognosis. In this case, survival rate can be improved through surgical intervention and adjuvant therapy.[89,91]

Medical therapy

Advanced liver disease is associated with central ascites. There is an increase in renal sodium and water retention. Therefore, restricting sodium intake to 100 mmol/day or less along with fluid restriction for patients with moderate to severe hyponatremia (125 mmol/L) may be beneficial. Using potassium-sparing diuretics is also important. Spironolactone (100 to 400 mg/day) is the drug of choice.[89] Furosemide is also helpful at 40 to 80 mg/day to initiate diuresis. Overdiuresis must be avoided. Overdiuresis may precipitate electrolyte imbalance, hepatic encephalopathy, and prerenal failure. The above regimen of fluid and sodium reduction and diuretics may work for mixed-type ascites, which results from compression of vessels related to tumor and peripheral tumor cells of the parietal or visceral peritoneum as well. Because mixed-type ascites is associated with chylous fluid, adding changes to the diet, such as decreased fat intake and increased medium-chain triglycerides, may be important. Chylous ascites results from tumor infiltration of the retroperitoneal space, causing obstruction of lymphatic flow.[89]

Medium-chain triglyceride oil (Lipisorb) can be used as a calorie source in these patients. Because the lymph system is bypassed, the shorter fatty acid chains are easier to digest. For patients with refractory ascites and a shortened life expectancy, paracentesis may be the most appropriate therapy.[79,90] Paracentesis is the most common and effective treatment to relieve ascites.[87,90] Patients with liver disease can tolerate the removal of up to 5 liters of ascites fluid without an effect on renal function or plasma volume.[86] Although this procedure gives temporary relief of symptoms like the treatment of MBO, palliative care decisions should be based on the goals of care and patients' quality of life. New advances in paracentesis treatment options have improved long-term use to minimize the need for frequent trips to the hospital for the procedure and repeated painful needle sticks.[89,90]

Paracentesis catheters

Peritoneovenous shunts (PVS) (Denver or LeVeen shunt) are helpful for the removal of ascites in 75% to 85% of patients.[89] These shunts are used primarily for nonmalignant ascites. The shunt removes fluid from the site, and the fluid is shunted up into the internal jugular vein.

This type of shunt has the advantage of avoiding an external drainage device and can be placed with minimal invasive techniques under conscious sedation. The disadvantages are that they have a high rate of failure related to occlusion and have been associated with pulmonary edema, thrombosis of major veins, seroma formation, leaks and disseminated intravascular coagulation (DIC).[87]

Pigtail catheter

Pigtail drainage catheters are used for percutaneous abscess drainage as well as pleural effusions and percutaneous biliary and renal drainage.[87] They are placed under ultrasound or fluoroscopic guidance and can be intermittently drained to gravity or vacuum bottles. This can be done as an outpatient procedure.[55]

Dialysis catheters

Silastic peritoneal dialysis catheters are providing effective management of malignant ascites.[87] They also can be managed at home easily and can be on gravity drainage or vacuum bottle drainage as needed.

Pleurex catheter (Denver Biomedical, Denver, Colorado)

This is a single-cuff tunneled Silastic catheter approved for the drainage of malignant plural effusions and malignant ascites. It offers a one-way valve instead of a clamp and can be managed in the home as well.[87]

The management of all of these types of catheters requires careful handling and techniques to prevent infections. Peritonitis, cellulitis, and catheter occlusion are risks.[87]

Nursing management

Ascites management involves initially understanding the mechanism, then using interventions appropriately. The reality of recurring ascites requiring repeated paracentesis is present. Acknowledging the risk/benefit ratio of repeated paracentesis is essential, especially in palliative care. The placement of an indwelling catheter can reduce the need for multiple needle sticks and improve patient quality of life.[89] Nurses need to remember good supportive care in addition to other resources. These include skin care, to help prevent breakdown, and comfort interventions, such as pillow support and loose clothing whenever possible. Educating the patient and caregivers on the rationale behind fluid and sodium restrictions when necessary can help their understanding and compliance. The cycle of a patient who feels thirsty, receives IV fluids, and has more discomfort is difficult for the patient to understand. Careful explanations about why an intervention is or is not recommended can go a long way toward improving the quality of life for these patients. Research is needed that compares interventions and helps develop guidelines to manage these many symptoms from an evidence-based position.[34]

Case study

Mrs. J, a patient with metastatic ovarian cancer

Mrs. J is a 62 year-old woman who has been experiencing escalating pain with frequent increases in her pain medication dose. The family has been focused on increased pain and extreme discomfort with moving. Increased pain medication dosing has led to more sedation but not pain relief. Mrs. J is not eating or drinking as she had been just 2 weeks ago. Mrs. J continues on anticonstipation medications as part of her basic regimen. With these other factors distracting the family and palliative care team, the patient's last bowel movement has been overlooked. As her symptoms are increasing a reassessment of constipation as a potential cause for her discomfort and a new plan of care is essential. As part of the assessment the nurse inquired about bowel history; performed an abdominal and rectal assessment; evaluated medications; and ensured that opioids being used are those that cause less constipation. In addition, the nurse helped the patient to the bathroom so that gravity might instigate a bowel movement. With a bowel movement, Mrs. J's pain improved and she was able to sit up in a chair and was better able to drink fluids and increase her eating. An additional resource would be a nutrition consult to help Mrs. J manage her diet to minimize future constipation episodes. Attention to elimination is an essential part of palliative care, especially related to opioid use.

References

1. Rao SS. Constipation: evaluation and treatment of colonic and anorectal motility disorders. Gastroenterol Clin North Am. 2007;36:687–711, x.
2. Sykes NP. The pathogenesis of constipation. J Support Oncol. 2006;4(5):213–218.
3. Clark K, Currow DC. Assessing constipation in palliative care within a gastroenterology framework. Palliat Med. 2012;26(6):834–841.
4. Andrews A, Morgan G. Constipation management in palliative care: treatments and the potential of independent nurse prescribing. Int J Palliat Nurs. 2012;18(1):17–22.
5. Twycross R, Sykes N, Mihalyo M, Wilcock A. Stimulant laxatives and opioid-induced constipation. J Pain Symptom Manage. 2012;43(2):306–313.
6. Ford AC, Brenner DM, Schoenfeld PS. Efficacy of pharmacological therapies for the treatment of opioid-induced constipation: systematic review and meta-analysis. Am J Gastroenterol. 2013;108(10):1566–1574.
7. McMillan SC, Tofthagen C, Small B, Karver S, Craig D. Trajectory of medication-induced constipation in patients with cancer. Oncol Nurs Forum. 2013;40(3):E92–E100.
8. Hjalte F, Berggren AC, Bergendahl H, Hjortsberg C. The direct and indirect costs of opioid-induced constipation. J Pain Symptom Manage. 2010;40(5):696–703.
9. Fritz D, Pitlick M. Evidence about the prevention and management of constipation: implications for comfort part 1. Home Healthc Nurse. 2012;30:533–540; quiz 540–532.
10. Clark K, Currow DC. Constipation in palliative care: what do we use as definitions and outcome measures? J Pain Symptom Manage. 2013;45(4):753–762.
11. Rhondali W, Nguyen L, Palmer L, Kang DH, Hui D, Bruera E. Self-reported constipation in patients with advanced cancer: a preliminary report. J Pain Symptom Manage. 2013;45:23–32.
12. Drossman DA. Introduction: the Rome Foundation and Rome III. Neurogastroenterol Motil. 2007;19(10):783–786.
13. Longstreth GF, Thompson WG, Chey WD, Houghton LA, Mearin F, Spiller RC. Functional bowel disorders. Gastroenterology. 2006;130(5):1480–1491.
14. Andrews A, Morgan G. Constipation in palliative care: treatment options and considerations for individual patient management. Int J Palliat Nurs. 2013;19(6):266–273.
15. Clark K, Currow DC. Assessing constipation in palliative care within a gastroenterology framework. Palliat Med. 2011;26:834–841.
16. Dal Molin A, McMillan SC, Zenerino F, et al. Validity and reliability of the Italian Constipation Assessment Scale. Int J Palliat Nurs. 2012;18(7):321–325.
17. Brown E, Henderson A, McDonagh A. Exploring the causes, assessment and management of constipation in palliative care. Int J Palliat Nurs. 2009;15(2):58–64.
18. Martin BC, Barghout V, Cerulli A. Direct medical costs of constipation in the United States. Manag Care Interface. 2006;19(12):43–49.
19. Thomas JR, Cooney GA, Slatkin NE. Palliative care and pain: new strategies for managing opioid bowel dysfunction. J Palliat Med. 2008;11(Suppl 1):S1–S19; quiz S21–12.
20. Massey RL, Haylock PJ, Curtiss C. Constipation. In: Yarbro C, Goodman M (eds.), Cancer Symptom Management. Boston: Jones and Bartlett; 2004:512–527.
21. Sykes NP. Constipation and diarrhea. In: Doyle G, Cherny N, Calman K (eds.), Oxford Textbook of Palliative Medicine. New York: Oxford University Press; 2004:483–496.
22. Bruera E, Fadul N. Constipation and diarrhea. In: Bruera I, Ripamonti C, Von Gunten C (eds.), Textbook of Palliative Medicine. New York: Oxford University Press; 2006:554–570.
23. Woolery M, Bisanz A, Lyons HF, et al. Putting evidence into practice: evidence-based interventions for the prevention and management of constipation in patients with cancer. Clin J Oncol Nurs. 2008;12:317–337.
24. Bisanz A. Bowel management in patients with cancer. In: Ajani JA (ed.), Gastrointestinal Cancer. New York: Springer; 2005:313–345.
25. Clark K, Byfieldt N, Dawe M, Currow DC. Treating constipation in palliative care: the impact of other factors aside from opioids. Am J Hosp Palliat Care. 2012;29(2):122–125.
26. Davison D. Constipation. Clin J Oncol Nurs. 2006;10(1):112–113.
27. Panchal SJ, Muller-Schwefe P, Wurzelmann JI. Opioid-induced bowel dysfunction: prevalence, pathophysiology and burden. Int J Clin Pract. 2007;61:1181–1187.
28. National Comprehensive Cancer Network (NCCN). Clinical Practice Guidelines-Constipation V2.2013. 2013. www.NCCN.org. Accessed July 1, 2013.
29. Radbruch L, Sabatowski R, Loick G, et al. Constipation and the use of laxatives: a comparison between transdermal fentanyl and oral morphine. Palliat Med. 2000;14(2):111–119.
30. Adler HF, Atkinson AJ, Ivy AC. Effect of morphine and dilaudid on the Ileum and of morphine, Dilaudid and atropine on the colon of man. Arch Intern Med. 1942;69:976–985.
31. McMillan SC, Williams FA. Validity and reliability of the Constipation Assessment Scale. Cancer Nurs. 1989;12(3):183–188.
32. Librach SL, Bouvette M, De Angelis C, et al. Consensus recommendations for the management of constipation in patients with advanced, progressive illness. J Pain Symptom Manage. 2010;40:761–773.
33. Thomas J. Opioid-induced bowel dysfunction. J Pain Symptom Manage. 2008;35:103–113.
34. Clemens KE, Faust M, Jaspers B, Mikus G. Pharmacological treatment of constipation in palliative care. Curr Opin Support Palliat Care. 2013;7(2):183–191.
35. Pitlick M, Fritz D. Evidence about the pharmacological management of constipation, part 2: Implications for palliative care. Home Healthc Nurse. 2013;31:207–218.
36. Singh B. Psyllium as therapeutic and drug delivery agent. Int J Pharm. 2007;334:1–14.
37. Larkin PJ, Sykes NP, Centeno C, et al. The management of constipation in palliative care: clinical practice recommendations. Palliat Med. 2008;22:796–807.
38. Levy MH. Constipation and diarrhea in cancer patients. Cancer Bull. 1991;43:412–422.
39. Cherny NI. Evaluation and management of treatment-related diarrhea in patients with advanced cancer: a review. J Pain Symptom Manage. 2008;36:413–423.
40. Iskedjian M, Iyer S, Librach SL, Wang M, Farah B, Berbari J. Methylnaltrexone in the treatment of opioid-induced constipation in cancer patients receiving palliative care: willingness-to-pay and cost-benefit analysis. J Pain Symptom Manage. 2011;41(1):104–115.
41. Lederle FA, Busch DL, Mattox KM, West MJ, Aske DM. Cost-effective treatment of constipation in the elderly: a randomized double-blind comparison of sorbitol and lactulose. Am J Med. 1990;89:597–601.

42. Galligan JJ, Vanner S. Basic and clinical pharmacology of new motility promoting agents. Neurogastroenterol Motil. 2005;17:643–653.

43. Lowell A. New strategies for the prevention and reduction of cancer-treatment induced diarrhea. Semin Oncol Nurs. 2003;19(Suppl 3):17–21.

44. Ripamonti C, Mercadante S. Pathophysiology and management of malignant bowel obstruction. In: Doyle G, Cherny N, Calman K (eds.), Oxford Textbook of Palliative Medicine. Oxford: Oxford University Press; 2004:496–507.

45. Becker G, Galandi D, Blum HE. Peripherally acting opioid antagonists in the treatment of opiate-related constipation: a systematic review. J Pain Symptom Manage. 2007;34(5):547–565.

46. Slatkin N, Thomas J, Lipman AG, et al. Methylnaltrexone for treatment of opioid-induced constipation in advanced illness patients. J Support Oncol. 2009;7(1):39–46.

47. Kyle G. Methylnaltrexone: a subcutaneous treatment for opioid-induced constipation in palliative care patients. Int J Palliat Nurs. 2009;15(11):533–540.

48. Mercadante S, Ferrera P, Casuccio A. Effectiveness and tolerability of amidotrizoate for the treatment of constipation resistant to laxatives in advanced cancer patients. J Pain Symptom Manage. 2011;41(2):421–425.

49. Portenoy RK, Thomas J, Moehl Boatwright ML, et al. Subcutaneous methylnaltrexone for the treatment of opioid-induced constipation in patients with advanced illness: a double-blind, randomized, parallel group, dose-ranging study. J Pain Symptom Manage. 2008;35(5):458–468.

50. Chamberlain BH, Cross K, Winston JL, et al. Methylnaltrexone treatment of opioid-induced constipation in patients with advanced illness. J Pain Symptom Manage. 2009;38(5):683–690.

51. Jones C, Goodman M, Drake R, Tookman A. Laxatives or methylnaltrexone for the management of constipation in palliative care patients (Review). Cochrane Database Syst Rev. 2011(8).

52. Stern J, Ippoliti C. Management of acute cancer treatment-induced diarrhea. Semin Oncol Nurs. 2003;19(4 Suppl 3):11–16.

53. Viele CS. Overview of chemotherapy-induced diarrhea. Semin Oncol Nurs. 2003;19(4 Suppl 3):2–5.

54. Engelking C. Diarrhea. In: Yarbro C, Goodman M (eds.), Cancer Symptom Management. Boston: Jones and Bartlett; 2003:528–557.

55. Anastasi JK, Capili B. HIV-related diarrhea and outcome measures. J Assoc Nurses AIDS Care. 2001;12(Suppl):44–50, quiz 51–44.

56. Muehlbauer PM, Thorpe D, Davis A, Drabot R, Rawlings BL, Kiker E. Putting evidence into practice: evidence-based interventions to prevent, manage, and treat chemotherapy- and radiotherapy-induced diarrhea. Clin J Oncol Nurs. 2009;13:336–341.

57. Jacobsohn DA, Vogelsang GB. Acute graft versus host disease. Orphanet J Rare Dis. 2007;2:35.

58. Gwede CK. Overview of radiation- and chemoradiation-induced diarrhea. Semin Oncol Nurs. 2003;19(4 Suppl 3):6–10.

59. Weihofen DL, Marino, C. Cancer Survival Cookbook. Los Angeles: Wiley; 1998.

60. Holt AP, Patel M, Ahmed MM. Palliation of patients with malignant gastroduodenal obstruction with self-expanding metallic stents: the treatment of choice? Gastrointest Endosc. 2004;60:1010–1017.

61. Prommer EE. Established and potential therapeutic applications of octreotide in palliative care. Support Care Cancer. 2008;16(10):1117–1123.

62. Massacesi C, Galeazzi G. Sustained release octreotide may have a role in the treatment of malignant bowel obstruction. Palliat Med. 2006;20:715–716.

63. TheGoodRx. http://www.goodrx.com/octreotide?kw=price&utm_source=bing&utm_medium=cpc&utm_term=octreotide%20cost&utm_campaign=octreotide&utm_content=Ad-Group_Price#/?filter-location=&coords=&label=octreotide&form=ampule&strength=1ml+of+500mcg%2Fml&quantity=custom&qty-custom=1. Accessed November 1, 2013.

64. Ripamonti C, Mercadante S, Groff L, Zecca E, De Conno F, Casuccio A. Role of octreotide, scopolamine butylbromide, and hydration in symptom control of patients with inoperable bowel obstruction and nasogastric tubes: a prospective randomized trial. J Pain Symptom Manage. 2000;19:23–34.

65. Oncology Nursing Society. Preventing and Treating Diarrhea related to chemotherapy and/or radiation therapy. 2011. http://www.ons.org/Research/PEP/media/ons/docs/research/outcomes/diarrhea/guidelines.pdf Accessed July 1, 2013.

66. Krouse RS. Surgical palliation of bowel obstruction. Gastroenterol Clin North Am. 2006;35:143–151.

67. Ripamonti CI, Easson AM, Gerdes H. Management of malignant bowel obstruction. Eur J Cancer. 2008;44:1105–1115.

68. Helyer L, Easson AM. Surgical approaches to malignant bowel obstruction. J Support Oncol. 2008;6(3):105–113.

69. Ripamonti CI. Malignant bowel obstruction: tailoring treatment to individual patients. J Support Oncol. 2008;6(3):114–115.

70. Krouse RS. Surgical management of malignant bowel obstruction. Surg Oncol Clin N Am. 2004;13:479–490.

71. Anthony T, Baron T, Mercadante S, et al. Report of the clinical protocol committee: development of randomized trials for malignant bowel obstruction. J Pain Symptom Manage. 2007;34:S49–S59.

72. Mercadante S, Porzio G. Octreotide for malignant bowel obstruction: twenty years after. Crit Rev Oncol Hematol. 2012;83:388–392.

73. Frech EJ, Adler DG. Endoscopic therapy for malignant bowel obstruction. J Support Oncol. 2007;5(7):303–310, 319.

74. Krouse RS. The value of a systematic approach to malignant bowel obstruction. J Support Oncol. 2008;6(3):116–117.

75. Targownik LE, Spiegel BM, Sack J, et al. Colonic stent vs. emergency surgery for management of acute left-sided malignant colonic obstruction: a decision analysis. Gastrointest Endosc. 2004;60:865–874.

76. Siddiqui A, Spechler SJ, Huerta S. Surgical bypass versus endoscopic stenting for malignant gastroduodenal obstruction: a decision analysis. Dig Dis Sci. 2007;52(1):276–281.

77. Ozkan O, Akinci D, Gocmen R, Cil B, Ozmen M, Akhan O. Percutaneous placement of peritoneal port catheter in patients with malignant ascites. Cardiovasc Intervent Radiol. 2007;30(2):232–236.

78. Dormann A, Meisner S, Verin N, Wenk Lang A. Self-expanding metal stents for gastroduodenal malignancies: systematic review of their clinical effectiveness. Endoscopy. 2004;36(6):543–550.

79. Johnsson E, Thune A, Liedman B. Palliation of malignant gastroduodenal obstruction with open surgical bypass or endoscopic stenting: clinical outcome and health economic evaluation. World J Surg. 2004;28(8):812–817.

80. Osman HS, Rashid HI, Sathananthan N, Parker MC. The cost effectiveness of self-expanding metal stents in the management of malignant left-sided large bowel obstruction. Colorectal Disease. 2000;2:233–237.

81. Rath KS, Loseth D, Muscarella P, et al. Outcomes following percutaneous upper gastrointestinal decompressive tube placement for malignant bowel obstruction in ovarian cancer. Gynecol Oncol. 2013;129:103–106.

82. Mercadante S, Ripamonti C, Casuccio A, Zecca E, Groff L. Comparison of octreotide and hyoscine butylbromide in controlling gastrointestinal symptoms due to malignant inoperable bowel obstruction. Support Care Cancer. 2000;8(3):188–191.

83. Mannix KA. Gastrointestinal symptoms-palliation of nausea and vomiting. In: Doyle G, Cherny N, Calman K (eds.), Oxford Textbook of Palliative Medicine. New York: Oxford University Press; 2004:459–468.

84. Mercadante S, Ferrera P, Villari P, Marrazzo A. Aggressive pharmacological treatment for reversing bowel obstruction. J Pain Symptom Manage. 2004;28:412–416.

85. Rosenberg S, Courtney A, Nemcek AA Jr, Omary RA. Comparison of percutaneous management techniques for recurrent malignant ascites. J Vasc Interv Radiol. 2004;15:1129–1131.

86. Becker G, Galandi D, Blum HE. Malignant ascites: systematic review and guideline for treatment. Eur J Cancer. 2006;42:589–597.

87. Rosenberg SM. Palliation of malignant ascites. Gastroenterol Clin North Am. 2006;35:189–199, xi.

88. Kichian K, Bain, VG. Jaundice, ascites, and hepatic encephalopathy. In: Doyle G, Cherny N, Calman K (eds.), Oxford Textbook of Palliative Medicine. New York: Oxford University Press; 2004:459–468.

89. Keen J. Jaundice, ascites, and encephalopathy. In: Hanks G, Cherny N, Christakis N, Fallon M, Kaasa S, Portenoy R (eds.), Oxford Textbook of Palliative Medicine. 4th ed. New York: Oxford University Press; 2010.

90. Krouse RS. The role of general surgery in the palliative care of patients with cancer. In: Hanks G, Cherny N, Christakis N, Fallon M, Kaasa S, Portenoy R (eds.), Oxford Textbook of Palliative Medicine. 4th ed. New York: Oxford University Press; 2010.

91. Numnum TM, Rocconi RP, Whitworth J, Barnes MN. The use of bevacizumab to palliate symptomatic ascites in patients with refractory ovarian carcinoma. Gynecol Oncol. 2006;102:425–428.

CHAPTER 13

Artificial nutrition and hydration

Michelle S. Gabriel and Jennifer A. Tschanz

> I don't really feel like eating or drinking. I don't really have an appetite. It's become a chore and tires me. I just don't want my family to think I am giving up hope.
>
> A patient

Key points

- For many people, food and drink are synonymous with care, comfort, and hope.

- Decreased appetite or inability to tolerate or enjoy food and fluids is often a hallmark of the terminal phase of an illness and is a source of distress for patients, family, and caregivers.

- Discussions and decisions regarding initiating or withholding artificial nutrition and hydration at the end of life are guided by goals of care, evaluation of benefits and burdens, ethical and cultural considerations, and the beliefs and wishes of the patient and family.

- Patients have the right to refuse hydration and nutrition, whether parenteral or oral.

- Nurses caring for patients and families faced with the decision to start or withhold or withdraw artificial nutrition and hydration are responsible for: promoting patient autonomy, providing education regarding benefits and burdens of interventions in order to promote informed decision-making, and delivering quality care with the rest of the care team.

Case study

Mr. C, a 76-year-old man with Alzheimer's disease and progressive dementia

Mr. C is a 76-year-old man with Alzheimer's disease and progressive dementia who has been living in a nursing home for 5 years. He is admitted to the hospital for the fourth time in 6 months for aspiration pneumonia. His daughter, who lives in the area, has noticed he has become more cachectic in the last 6 months, has a decreased appetite, and recently has needed encouragement to eat. She notes her father has become weaker and less responsive with time and believes her father is getting closer to death. His son, who lives out of state and is seeing his father for the first time in a year, would like to initiate hydration and enteral feedings via a PEG tube. He believes his father just needs a little help to get through this recent infection. Mr. C does not have an advanced directive. Both children state that in previous conversations with their father, he verbalized he "would not want to suffer when the

time comes." They are conflicted about how to proceed with their father's care. The nurse is asked to set up a family meeting with the palliative care team to determine how to proceed with his care.

Introduction

In the context of providing palliative care, decisions to initiate or withhold and withdraw the interventions of artificial nutrition and hydration (ANH) can be challenging for the patient, the family, and members of the healthcare team. In many cultures, providing food and fluids is synonymous with caring, hope, and comfort.[1] Decreased appetite or inability to tolerate or enjoy food and fluids is often a hallmark of the terminal phase of an illness. Individuals and their families may ask for ANH to address a variety of situations (e.g., fears of starvation, weight loss, and dehydration). Clinicians may recommend artificial nutrition (AN) or hydration in specific circumstances (e.g., malnutrition, dehydration, new onset of delirium). As with any palliative care intervention, the nurse needs to understand the patient's illness trajectory, and patient and family goals of care, which can be influenced by a person's culture or religion. The nurse also needs to be familiar with the current evidence for ANH for patients with advanced illness, as nurses often participate in conversations regarding treatment options and have a critical role in supporting the patient in identifying interventions that best meet their goals.

The purpose of this chapter is to serve as a resource for nurses to support their ability in caring for patients and families faced with the decision to initiate or discontinue ANH. The chapter will start with a review of the clinical indications for considering ANH followed by a discussion of the current evidence for each of these interventions to address distressing symptoms in the palliative setting. The next section will review current guidelines for ANH from various professional organizations. It will then transition into a discussion of the ethics and legal precedents surrounding the provision or discontinuation of ANH. The chapter will conclude with an overview of additional factors that affect decision-making regarding these interventions (e.g., religious beliefs and culture) and communication strategies to empower nurses to actively participate in discussions about ANH and support patients and families in this decision-making process.

Artificial nutrition

Artificial nutrition is an intervention to address malnutrition, which has been linked to poorer outcomes such as increased mortality, infections, and pressure ulcers.[2] Malnutrition occurs when the body does not get the nutrients it needs.[3] Causes of malnutrition include an inadequate diet, mechanical issues with digestion or absorption of nutrients, and specific medical conditions.[4] In patients with advanced chronic disease or terminal illness, specific causes for malnutrition may result from anorexia, cachexia, and physiological issues. Anorexia manifests with a decrease in appetite, which can lead to a loss of fat tissue. The weight loss that results can be reversible depending on the underlying causes. Many patients with advanced illness experience anorexia.[5,6] Cancer cachexia is a multifactorial syndrome in which there is loss of skeletal muscle that cannot be completely reversed by nutritional support, resulting in a negative impact on functional status.[4] Mechanical issues include malignant bowel obstruction and dysphagia.

Methods of administration

Artificial nutrition is the delivery of nutrients to an individual that bypasses the oral route. It can be administered enterally or parenterally. Methods to provide enteral nutrition, which accesses the body's gastrointestinal tract, consist of nasogastric, nasointestinal, percutaneous gastrostomy (PEG) or jejunostomy access, with PEG being the preferred method of access for long-term feeding.[7] Parenteral nutrition, which instills nutrients directly into the circulatory system, can be delivered through a peripheral vein, using peripheral parenteral nutrition (PPN) or via a central line, using total parenteral nutrition (TPN).

Benefits and burdens

While the benefits of AN are clearer in patients who are expected to recover, they are not as clear for use in patients who have advanced chronic illness or who are terminally ill. While the expected benefits include improving a patient's nutritional status to alleviate distressing symptoms resulting from malnutrition, AN in the palliative care setting does not always have a positive impact. In amyotrophic lateral sclerosis (ALS), there are guidelines recommending the use and timing of AN, since malnutrition and weight loss are prognosticators for survival.[8-10] In patients with cancers of the oropharynx or esophagus, AN may be appropriate earlier in the disease trajectory, especially when the cause of malnutrition is directly related to the inability to maintain intake due to mechanical blockages and acute treatment effects (e.g., mucositis secondary to chemoradiation).[11] Patients and families worry about anorexia, and see AN as beneficial to address both physical and psychosocial symptoms.[12,13]

A study looking at whether clinical, functional, or nutritional indices could determine whether patients would benefit from AN found that comorbidity, cognitive function, and social function could predict a patient's success with AN.[14] This same study found that predictors of the ineffectiveness of AN on clinical outcomes included severe cognitive impairment and frailty.

While there may be some benefit in certain populations with end-stage diseases, enteral and parenteral feedings are interventions with the potential for associated morbidity and increased suffering. Potential complications from the administration of AN

Table 13.1 Potential complications of enteral support

Complication	Symptom	Cause
Aspiration	Coughing	Excess residual
	Fever	Large-bore tube
Diarrhea	Watery stool	Hyperosmotic solution
		Rapid infusion
		Lactose intolerance
Constipation	Hard, infrequent stools	Inadequate fluid
		Inadequate fiber
Dumping syndrome	Dizziness	High volume
		Hyperosmotic fluids

are listed in Table 13.1. Potential additional burdens include: complications from tube placement, increased risk of infection or skin excoriation around the tube, and use of mechanical or pharmacological restraints to preserve access.[5,15]

Review of the literature

Malnutrition, anorexia, and cachexia

In many end-stage diseases, weight loss due to malnutrition, anorexia, or cachexia is a common occurrence. In cancer patients with persistent anorexia and cachexia, artificial nutrition has not been shown to reverse the weight loss.[16] In one study looking at body mass index as a specific marker of nutritional status, the provision of AN helped to stabilize the decrease for patients who were alive at the 3-month follow-up (10 out of 17 patients); however, the study did not measure quality of life (QOL) for the same population.[17] In the terminal phase of diseases, such as cancer, AN may not be metabolized in a way that would reverse the effects of malnutrition, anorexia, and cachexia, and the intervention for palliative purposes is rarely recommended.[18,19]

Dysphagia

When a patient has difficulty swallowing, AN may be considered to ensure that the patient receives adequate nutrition or to reduce the risk for aspiration pneumonia. In certain disease states, such as ALS and dementia, it is a matter of when, not if, dysphagia will occur. For ALS patients, the goal for enteral feeding is to improve the QOL and the preferred mechanism to deliver AN, if indicated, is via a PEG tube.[20] The onset of dysphagia and the resulting weight loss are indications of when to start AN in the ALS patient population.[10] Providers may consider initiating enteral feeds to reduce the risk for aspiration pneumonia due to "food going down the wrong way"; however, recent studies have shown that enteral nutrition does not reduce, and may increase, the risk for aspiration pneumonia.[15,20]

Hunger

Families often express concern about their loved one experiencing hunger, or fears about their loved one starving at end of life, yet patients will often deny sensations of hunger in the terminal phase. A study looking at the incidence of hunger in a terminally ill population found that the majority of patients (63%) denied hunger on admission, and did not report any hunger during the admission.

Of the remaining patients, only 3% (one patient) reported hunger throughout the admission; the others complained initially, but the hunger disappeared over time. All of these patients were offered food by mouth as requested, and the small amounts they tolerated satisfied their hunger; none were given AN.[6] In advanced cancer and dementia, because of the disease process, hunger is not often experienced.

Pressure ulcers

Patients who are malnourished are at increased risk for pressure ulcers, yet at the end of life, there is no evidence to support the use of AN to treat or prevent pressure ulcers.[15,21] One study showed that in patients with dementia, the use of a PEG tube to administer AN was associated with an increased risk of developing new stage 2 pressure ulcers, and a decreased likelihood of the healing of existing pressure ulcers.[22] Potential reasons for this association include the following risk factors: increased likelihood of immobility due to the use of restraints that may be used to ensure that feeding tubes are maintained and potential for diarrhea due to the composition of the enteral feeds.[22]

Survival time

There is no compelling evidence that AN increases the survival of patients with end-stage diseases.[15,20] Studies have looked at the impact of enteral feeds in the dementia population, and have found no impact on survival time.[15,23] One study found a median survival post feeding tube insertion of 165 days and a 64% mortality rate, with half of those who died doing so within the first 2 months following insertion.[24] Another study compared the impact on survival time of PEG tube insertion or the timing of the insertion and found no impact.[23] Other studies have shown an increase in survival in specific populations. One study compared survival time in dementia patients in Japan who used self-feeding oral intake versus home parenteral nutrition or PEG feeding and found that the groups who used either home parenteral nutrition or PEG feeding survived almost twice as long.[25] In this study, patients were not in the end-stage of dementia, which may explain the longer survival time. Another study looked at whether dementia was a risk factor for survival after PEG, and found no difference in survival between patients with dementia and patients without who received a PEG tube.[26] The authors did not include the stage of dementia in their analysis.

Quality of life

There have not been many studies that specifically measure QOL for patients with end-stage illness receiving AN. In a Cochrane review of enteral tube feeding in an older population with advanced dementia, there were no studies reviewed that measured QOL.[15] Another Cochrane review found two studies that demonstrated unimproved QOL in populations with either motor neuron disease or advanced cancer.[27] Patients and their families determine the impact of interventions such as AN on QOL. Some studies have shown that patients and families perceive AN to have a positive impact on reducing burden from physical and psychosocial symptoms, such as maintaining the fight against the disease, reducing anxiety due to anorexia, and alleviating symptoms.[12,13] Other studies have looked at the use of AN and the prevalence of interventions that may be thought to negatively impact QOL, such as the use of restraints. In studies looking at patients with dementia receiving tube feeds, AN has been correlated with an increased use of restraints, either physical or pharmacological.[28,29] In a study assessing family member's perceptions of the impact of a feeding tube, only 32.9% of the people who responded stated that the intervention improved the patient's QOL.[29]

Summary

Artificial nutrition has been shown to have a positive impact on survival and nutritional parameters in certain populations, such as earlier in the disease trajectories for ALS or some cancers. However, there is not enough evidence to support a specific recommendation on when or if, in a palliative care population, it is best to use AN.[27] The individual patient's condition along with the goals of care need to be considered to best determine the benefit of employing AN compared to the burdens of the intervention.

Hydration

Hydration is an intervention used to address end-of-life situations such as fluid deficits and altered mental status secondary to medication toxicities.

> Fluid deficit disorders include dehydration and volume depletion. Dehydration is intracellular water depletion with hypernatremia (hyperosmolality) and usually presents with symptoms of thirst, anorexia, nausea/vomiting, fatigue and irritability. Physical findings may include lethargy, confusion, muscle twitching and hyperreflexia. Volume depletion is the loss of intravascular water (with varying sodium levels) and presents with diminished skin turgor/capillary refill and orthostatic hypotension and dizziness.[30]

Patients with advanced illness experiencing anorexia may also experience a loss of interest in drinking.[5] During the terminal phase, fluid deficits, similar to malnutrition, may result from anorexia/early satiety, nausea/vomiting, bowel obstruction, dysphagia, and cognitive impairment.[30,31]

Some patients and families believe that decreased oral intake and the ensuing dehydration cause suffering. Patients and families are concerned dehydration may precipitate symptoms of delirium, confusion, myoclonus, somnolence, fatigue, neuromuscular irritability, restlessness, thirst, hunger, and constipation, especially in the presence of opioids, benzodiazepines, and neuroleptics.[5,31] There is limited information regarding the effects of hydration in addressing these symptoms. Many patients with advanced cancer and their caregivers perceive that hydration provides hope and comfort, improves symptoms and QOL, and fulfills a basic human need for water.[1]

When considering hydration, it is important to consider where the patient is on the disease trajectory (e.g., acutely ill or in the dying phase) to help establish goals of care. Hydration can be used for the temporary relief of symptoms of fluid loss such as nausea, vomiting, diarrhea, and fevers; to decrease fatigue; to improve mental cognition status associated with medication toxicities; and as a respect to cultural and familial beliefs.

Methods of administration

There are various alternative routes to oral administration to meet the goals of care and wishes of the patient and family. Standard methods for replacement of fluids, similar to nutrition, can be achieved by the use of enteral feeding tubes and parenteral methods, such as subcutaneous or intravenous infusion.

Intravenous access requires a competent vein. Clinicians may use permanent access devices if they have previously been placed,

Table 13.2 Potential complications of routes for artificial hydration

IV Peripheral	IV Central	SC Hypodermoclysis
Pain	Sepsis	Pain
Short duration of access	Hemothorax	Infection
Infection	Pneumothorax	Third spacing
Phlebitis	Central vein thrombosis Catheter fragment thrombosis Air embolus Brachial plexus injury Arterial laceration	Tissue sloughing Local bleeding

IV, intravenous; SC, subcutaneous.

or if ongoing hydration is anticipated. Hypodermoclysis is the subcutaneous infusion of isotonic solution. It does not require special access devices and can be used for patients who have poor venous access for intravenous placement. The absorption of the subcutaneous fluids has been found to be comparable with absorption of intravenous fluids when administered appropriately.[32] Hypodermoclysis is relatively uncommon in the United States and is more frequently used in Canada and the UK.[30] Proctoclysis is used to administer water or saline into the gastrointestinal tract via the rectum using a nasogastric tube. Researchers have found proctoclysis to be safe and economical, but there has been cultural and social reluctance to accept this mode of administration.[33]

There is no consensus regarding the volume or type of fluid replacement. Clinicians make choices based on previous experiences and knowledge of the patient's condition and wishes. Some providers allow the individual to have 1 L/day despite the fact that it may be inadequate replacement. Risks and burdens must be considered, and are listed in Table 13.2.

Benefits and burdens

The decision for hydration needs to include an evaluation of goals of care, discussion of the risks and benefits, and timely reevaluation to determine if goals or symptoms are improving or worsening. Risks for overhydration, as evidenced by worsening fluid retention, signs of increased shortness of breath, increased emotional distress or change in mental status, must be monitored. Advantages of not providing artificial hydration can include reduced urine output, leading to reduced incontinence and need for catheterization; reduction of gastrointestinal secretions, leading to decreased incidence of vomiting; and decreased respiratory tract secretions, leading to decreased cough and need for suction.[31]

Factors arguing against initiating hydration include increasing the incidence of pulmonary edema, peripheral edema, increased respiratory tract secretions, cough, and ascites.[31,34,35] Starting intravenous hydration can cause pain, be distressing, restrict mobility, hinder family contact, and increase the use of restraints.[36]

Review of the literature

Dehydration and fluid retention

Dehydration can cause unpleasant symptoms such as confusion and restlessness in nonterminally ill patients. These problems are common in the dying. There is limited research regarding the effect of hydration on alleviating dehydration at the end of life. Results can be challenging to interpret due to the ways various studies define and measure dehydration. Findings suggest that providing artificial hydration may or may not affect physical signs and symptoms of dehydration at the end of life. One study demonstrated no difference in hydration status after 7 days between advanced cancer patients who were given 1000 mL per day versus 100 mL per day. The same study also scored four dehydration symptoms (fatigue, myoclonus, sedation, and hallucinations) and noted no difference in the sum of the scores after the 7-day hydration trial.[37] A retrospective chart review study showed that artificial hydration in the last 48 hours of life had no significant impact on symptoms related to hydration status (e.g., agitation, myoclonus, urinary retention, confusion, congestive cardiac failure, respiratory tract secretions, nausea and vomiting, and ascites).[31] The finding suggests there is no benefit of hydration during the terminal phase. Information regarding details of volume or reasons for initiating hydration was not discussed.

Depending on the volume of hydration administered, hydration may increase the risk of developing fluid retention symptoms. In a study that measured the effect of hydration volume on terminally ill cancer patients with abdominal malignancies, dehydration was evaluated on the basis of physical findings that included moisture on the mucous membranes of the mouth, axillary moisture, and sunkenness of the eyes within 72 hours of death. Patients in the hydration group who received 1000 mL or more of artificial hydration per day 1 and 3 weeks before death were found to have less deterioration in dehydration symptoms than the nonhydration group who received on average less than 1000 mL of artificial hydration over the 3 weeks prior to death. However, the patients who were in the hydration group were noted to have increased symptoms of overhydration such as edema, ascites, and bronchial secretions. No difference was noted between the groups regarding pleural effusion.[35] These findings are similar to a study conducted that showed increased dehydration status in the nonhydration group who did not receive hydration and increased fluid retention symptoms of peripheral edema and ascites in the hydration group.[34] A prevalence of bronchial secretions in the last 48 hours of life was noted more in the large volume group that received more than 1000 mL hydration per day compared with those in the small volume group that received less than 1000 mL per day.[38]

A national guideline for parenteral hydration therapy was established in Japan in 2007 that encouraged respecting patient and family wishes, conducting a comprehensive assessment of patient's QOL, allowing for TPN to be administered if bowel obstruction was present, and recommending that hydration be decreased to less than 1000 mL per day if fluid retention signs were present.[39] A study to measure the efficacy of this guideline demonstrated that providing hydration to patients with advanced cancer according to the guidelines led to stable measurements in global QOL, discomfort, most physical symptoms, and fluid retention signs.[38]

Thirst and dry mouth

Thirst is thought to be a nonspecific symptom of dehydration. One study looked at interventions for thirst and dry mouth as an alternative to hydration. Researchers found that routine care, defined as offering food and fluids, administering ice chips, and providing mouth care, helped to alleviate these symptoms.[6] Dry mouth is treated with an intensive, every-2-hour schedule of mouth care, including hygiene, lip lubrication, and ice chips or popsicles. Elimination of medications that cause dry mouth, such as tricyclic antidepressants and antihistamines should be considered. Sometimes, drugs that contribute to these symptoms are being administered to palliate other symptoms, such as opioids to treat pain and anticholinergics to minimize oral secretions. Mouth breathing can also contribute to dry mouth. Candida infection, a frequent cause of dry mouth, can be treated. Agents such as pilocarpine (Salagen) can be used to increase salivation.

In one study, hydration was shown to alleviate symptoms of dry mouth in patients with advanced cancer who had a relatively longer prognosis. It was noted that dry mouth intensity decreased significantly in the group receiving a large volume of hydration (1000 mL or more per day) than those in the small volume group (less than 1000 mL per day). This same group also experienced a higher incidence of bronchial secretions.[38]

Delirium, confusion, agitation

Delirium can be caused by multiple factors including end-organ failure, dehydration, and medications. Symptoms of delirium can be distressful for patients and families.[30,37] In advanced cancer patients, no significant difference in delirium and agitation was noted between patients receiving more hydration than less hydration.[35,37]

Medications such as opioids, anticholinergics, antihistamines and corticosteroids have been known to impact delirium. If delirium is related to the accumulation of opioids, interventions to decrease or rotate opioids and to increase hydration are believed to control symptoms of hyperactive delirium, such as agitation and hallucinations of opioid-induced neurotoxicity, by assisting with the clearance of toxic opioid metabolites.[38,40]

Myoclonus

Myoclonus, or involuntary contractions of muscles, is commonly associated with chronic opioid use at the end of life. It has also been reported in cancer patients without opioid use who are experiencing decreased oral intake.[30] There is limited and mixed information regarding the effects of hydration on myoclonus depending on patient setting. Myoclonus was shown to improve in the intervention group who received 1000 mL normal saline over 4 hours for 2 days versus 100 mL.[41] However, no difference in myoclonus symptoms were noted between patients with advanced abdominal malignancies in the hydration group, who were given on average 838 to 1405 mL/day during the last 3 weeks of life, or in the nonhydration group, who received 200 mL average per day.

Survival benefit

There is limited research regarding the survival benefit of hydration. Two studies noted that hydration provided no survival benefit for terminally ill cancer patients with short prognosis.[31,37]

Quality of life

There is limited research regarding the impact of hydration on QOL in the terminally ill. Research of patients with advanced cancer shows that parenteral hydration of 1000 mL per day did not improve symptoms associated with QOL over placebo of 100 mL per day.[37] Another study showed that QOL measurements remained stable when hydration was administered according to Japanese guidelines that took into account QOL and symptoms

of fluid retention, whether patients received small (less than 1000 mL per day) or large (greater than 1000 mL per day) volumes of hydration.[38] In a study that interviewed patients with advanced cancer and their caregivers, the patients and their caregivers perceived hydration as fulfilling the basic human need for water, promoting hope and dignity and enhancing QOL.[1] Caregivers in the same study reported hydration improved pain management and the patient had more energy, better sleeping habits, an improved appetite, and a healthier physical experience. The study did not include information on volumes or duration of hydration.

Summary

Parenteral hydration has been found to be effective in temporary, short-term situations to alleviate symptoms related to dehydration and improve mental cognition. In the palliative care setting, research does not support that parenteral hydration improves signs of dehydration, survival or QOL. In the setting of delirium related to opioid toxicity, there is mixed evidence supporting hydration and possible opioid rotation to improve delirium symptoms. When deciding to initiate or stop hydration, it is important to assess goals of care, risks and benefits and the patient's preferences.

Case study

Ms. C, a 44-year-old woman with metastatic breast cancer

Ms. C is a 44-year-old woman with metastatic breast cancer to the brain who was admitted to the inpatient hospice unit because of a change in mental status. Her family did not want her young children to see her "behaving funny" at home. Providers felt that she was experiencing delirium due to a recent increase in her opioid and diuretic medications. The doctor recommended intravenous hydration through her port. After 4 days of hydration and alterations in medication doses, her cognitive status improved—she was alert and returned home.

She was hospitalized 1 month later due to mental status changes and at that time progressive disease was noted in her brain, liver, and bones. Family requested that hydration be restarted as it had worked previously. After 4 days of hydration, her cognitive status did not improve. She was noted to be less responsive to touch and painful stimuli, to have increased labored breathing and to have edema in her legs. The doctor and nurse discussed their concerns for fluid overload with the family and made recommendations to discontinue hydration treatment. Her family wished to continue her hydration in hopes of improving her condition since it previously worked.

Review of position statements and guidelines

Many professional organizations have published position statements or guidelines on the use of ANH. Common themes across these documents include:

◆ ANH is an intervention that should be evaluated by the patient, family, and care team considering, its benefits and burdens.[5,42,43]

◆ ANH is considered a medical intervention that can be refused, withheld, or withdrawn based on the patient's clinical condition and goals of care.[2,5,21,42]

◆ Decisions about ANH need to reflect the patient's and family's values, beliefs, and culture.[5,42]

Table 13.3 Disease-specific guidelines for ANH

Advanced dementia[21]	◆ Feeding tubes are not recommended. ◆ Enhance oral feedings by improving the environment and supporting patient-centered approaches.
End-stage cancer[18,19]	◆ Use of nutritional support for terminally ill cancer patients is not usually indicated.
ALS[20]	◆ Early insertion of a feeding tube is recommended if enteral feeding is determined to be an appropriate intervention.

In addition to general position statements regarding ANH, disease-specific recommendations are summarized in Table 13.3.

Decision-making and artificial nutrition and hydration

Decisions about the initiation or withholding and withdrawing of ANH are complex.[44] In addition to the review of the clinical evidence regarding the efficacy of ANH to improve symptoms and QOL, it is important to consider ethical principles and legal precedents that highlight the role nurses have in advocating for the patient as well as the responsibilities in respecting patient and family wishes. Also affecting the decision-making process are religious affiliation and cultural background, as these domains may impact a patient's and family's values toward food and fluids. Religious affiliation and cultural background equally may influence a nurse's personal comfort with the concept of ANH and its role at the end of life.

Ethical issues

Initiating or withholding or withdrawing ANH, like other medical interventions, needs to be done utilizing ethical principles. The three ethical principles that are most relevant in decision-making for ANH are autonomy, beneficence, and nonmaleficence (Table 13.4).[44] Autonomy refers to the patient or surrogate's right to

Table 13.4 Artificial nutrition and hydration: examples of nursing interventions that reflect ethical principles

Ethical principle	Nursing actions
Autonomy—respecting an individual's right to make choices regarding care	◆ Encourage a conversation that provides information on the benefits and burdens of ANH to empower the patient to make an informed decision. ◆ Focus on the patient's preferences, especially when working with family and caregivers. Ask, "Did we do everything to meet the patient's goals?" not "Did we do everything possible?"
Beneficence—"to do good"	◆ Seek to understand the patient's goals and values to understand what "good" means for them. ◆ Provide interventions that match with patient goals.
Nonmaleficence—"to do no harm"	◆ Evaluate the potential risks or burdens of ANH to minimize harm, taking into account the patient's values.

self-determination.[44] Respecting autonomy in decisions about ANH means that a patient or family has the choice to accept or refuse the intervention, based on their personal values and beliefs.[45] Beneficence means "to do good" and implies that nurses must act in the interest of the patient.[44] The nurse has a responsibility to engage the patient and family in a conversation about what "good" looks like, respecting the individual's values and goals for care. For example, a patient with end-stage cancer may be experiencing dysphagia, yet still finds enjoyment in small sips of liquid. While the risk for aspiration exists in this situation, the nurse would exhibit beneficence by supporting the intake of fluids. Nonmaleficence means "to do no harm," and can be exemplified by not administering treatments that increase the risk of suffering and have no benefit or whose benefit is less than the burden.[44]

Legal precedent

Landmark cases such as the Quinlan case, Cruzan case, Barber case, and *Vacco v. Quill* case have set the foundation for current decision-making regarding ANH within the healthcare system. Karen Ann Quinlan was 21 years old when she was deemed to be in a persistent vegetative state due to anoxic brain injury. Her father sought guardianship in order to cease "extraordinary" measures keeping her alive.[46] In this case, the court supported the standard of substituted judgment, enabling her father to speak for her as if she were able to speak for herself.[47] Nancy Cruzan was thrown from her vehicle in a car accident. Although found by the paramedics with no pulse, they were able to resuscitate her. She was in a coma for several weeks before being determined by her physicians to be in a persistent vegetative state.[48] In her case, the court supported the right to refuse treatment for competent individuals. The court also supported the need for "clear and convincing evidence" since she was incompetent and had not previously recorded her wishes. This case helped to support the federal Patient Self-Determination Act passed in 1991 in an effort to help patients document their wishes.[47] The *Vacco v. Quill* case also supported the right to refuse treatment, distinguishing respecting patient wishes from intentionally hastening death.[49] In the Barber case, the court found two physicians who had discontinued ANH to be innocent of charges of murder and conspiracy to commit murder, reinforcing the precept that ANH is considered a medical intervention and not basic care.[47]

Religious and cultural issues

To deliver patient-centered care, nurses must recognize the role that religious or spiritual beliefs and culture, including race and ethnicity, play on patient and family values of food and fluids. Understanding these factors and encouraging a dialogue about patient values will enable nurses to respect patient autonomy and engage in a dialogue on how to meet patient needs regarding nutrition and hydration to maximize beneficence ("to do good") and minimize nonmaleficence ("to do no harm"). In reviewing common beliefs of various religious traditions and cultures, it is important to remember that not everyone of a particular faith or a particular culture will have the same beliefs, and nurses should inquire as to how much influence a patient's faith or culture has on their beliefs regarding ANH.[44]

Major religions have varying beliefs specific to the use of life-sustaining therapies such as ANH. Even within religions, there can be varying opinions or interpretations of religious law to guide decisions on whether to initiate or withdraw ANH.

Table 13.5 Various religious beliefs about ANH

Religious faith	Beliefs
Buddhism[50]	◆ Belief that all beings suffer. ◆ Main focus at end of life is on spiritual comfort. ◆ Less focus on extending life through ANH and other interventions.
Catholicism[51,52]	◆ Current position (as of 2011) focuses on "life prolongation based on fundamental human dignity." ◆ Some within the church assert that ANH is not considered a medical technology, but an ordinary measure to preserve life. ◆ Others feel that ANH should be evaluated using the proportionate/disproportionate framework (ordinary versus extraordinary) on an individual basis. ◆ Catholic healthcare facilities are obligated to offer food and fluids regardless of disease state. ◆ ANH can be considered extraordinary in conditions where the underlying disease would be the cause of death, not the withholding of ANH.
Hinduism[50]	◆ Withholding or withdrawal of ANH at the very end of life is acceptable. ◆ Some Hindus fast to prepare for death.
Islam[53]	◆ The "guiding purpose of Islamic law is to protect and preserve religion, life, progeny, intellect, and wealth." ◆ Islamic rules regarding care for the terminally ill are based on the principle that one should prevent or avoid injury or harm. ◆ Islamic law permits withdrawal of ANH and allowing the disease to take its natural course. ◆ There can be various beliefs among Muslims so it is necessary to ascertain the patient's values. ◆ "Islamic law states that palliative care should not shorten a patient's life, but futile treatment is not justified." ◆ "Islamic law forbids passively or actively causing death." ◆ Nutritional support is considered basic care and not medical treatment, leading to a duty to feed patients who are no longer able to feed themselves. ◆ There is varied opinion among different Islamic communities regarding withdrawing and withholding ANH.
Judaism[50]	◆ Provision of food and fluids is considered an ordinary measure, not extraordinary. ◆ Withholding food and fluids is not consistent with Jewish law. ◆ Administration of food and fluids, even via IV or feeding tube, is not considered to be artificially administered. ◆ "The religious authorities hold that (ANH) are ordinary supportive measures rather than heroic."[54] ◆ Terminal dehydration, hospice without provision of ANH, and withdrawing or withholding ANH is not considered aligned with Jewish teaching unless there is proof of "goses" (less than 72 hours until death) and futility of intervention under any denomination of Judaism. ◆ "While the [Israeli] law respects the right of a competent dying patient to refuse nutrition and hydration, it introduces a legal requirement to persuade 'the use of oxygen, nutrition and hydration,' even by artificial means."[55]
Protestant[50]	◆ There is diversity in positions regarding ANH across denominations. ◆ A common belief is that interventions such as ANH that allow time for repentance may outweigh other burdens of treatment.

Table 13.5 summarizes beliefs by selected religious traditions specific to ANH.

In addition to religious influences, culture also affects patient and family perspectives of ANH. Studies have shown variance associated with race in the use of tube feedings, with Caucasians having lower rates than people of other cultural backgrounds.[50] In studies looking at the use of feeding tubes between white subjects compared with African-American subjects, use was consistently higher in the latter group.[56] Studies have also shown that African-Americans have a stronger preference for more intensive care.[56] One study used focus groups to look at preferences among African American and Caucasian participants, assessing for factors that might affect decisions about care at the end of life, including AN. From the qualitative data gathered in the focus groups, the researchers found more similarities than differences in how the two groups thought about food, artificial nutrition, and decision-making at the end of life.[56] The differences were not by category, but more on focus within common themes.[56]

In a study looking at what meaning Singaporean Chinese caregivers attributed to feeding, the researchers saw three major themes emerge. One theme was a sense of filial piety, where duty to one's family may motivate a push for more aggressive interventions even if the patient is at the end of life. Another theme was the link between providing nutrition and hope. A third theme was that providing food showed caring for their loved one, a theme common across many cultures.[57]

While there is not a large body of research on how differing religious and cultural backgrounds influence individual preferences for ANH, there are resources that nurses can access to learn information needed to initiate a conversation with a patient on this issue. Whether it is through position statements from religious organizations or talking to leaders within a particular faith tradition or ethnic community, nurses can seek to understand how these factors play a role in each specific situation with the patient for whom they are caring.

Engaging in conversations about artificial nutrition and hydration

Ethics, religion, and culture, factors that may influence an individual's values specific to ANH, similarly influence healthcare team members' perspectives on ANH as an intervention at the end of life. In one study, the authors found that a provider's religious beliefs or legal concerns influenced the provider's likelihood of recommending ANH as an intervention.[58] Providers may not be aware of the current evidence of ANH in affecting outcomes in the palliative care population, or as familiar with the patient's clinical course when making recommendations for ANH.[15,59] In addition to provider factors, settings of care can influence the use of ANH. In patients with dementia, studies have shown variability in the prevalence of PEG tube by state and by type of healthcare facility (i.e., acute care hospital versus long-term care facility).[29,59] It has been noted that a majority of terminally ill patients in the United States almost always receive intravenous hydration when treated in acute care facilities, but almost never in hospice settings.[30,37]

In working with palliative care and terminally ill patients, nurses play a critical role in exploring a patient's values and hopes to ensure that care related to the provision of food and fluids is patient-centered. As decisions about ANH are complex, nurses have multiple responsibilities. Nurses need to self-reflect on their own personal values, similarly influenced by religious and cultural factors as well as clinical experience. Just as continuing education and experience help nurses to develop clinical skills and understanding, further and continued ethics education may be helpful to sharpen skills in reasoning through the ANH debate to better support patients and families in the decision-making process.[60] Position statements by established professional nursing and medical organizations and outcomes of landmark legal decisions regarding ANH can provide a foundation for how nurses and the healthcare team approach conversations with the family about ANH.

One of the primary tasks of the nurse is to ensure that a patient's autonomy and dignity is respected in a way that is culturally acceptable to the patient by understanding the patient's values regarding ANH and the broader goals that the individual is hoping to achieve. This task can be accomplished by promoting early conversations regarding patient and family preferences. The focus should be on the patient as the decision-maker, even if the patient is not participating in the conversation. While open-ended questions may encourage exploration of knowledge and understanding of patient and family hopes, focused and directed questions regarding preferences may guide patients and families to more concrete goals and decisions.[61] A challenge in performing this task is when patient and family preferences conflict with a nurse's or healthcare team's preferences for treatment. The focus of discussions should be "Did we do everything to meet the patient's goals?" not "Did we do everything possible?"

Additionally, nurses can empower patients and families by educating them about the normal symptoms of the dying process

and the known benefits and burdens of ANH as an intervention to effectively treat symptoms associated with dying. In order to facilitate informed decision-making, education can focus on symptoms and progression of the normal dying process, available options for ANH, known benefits and burdens of ANH interventions, limitations of evidence supporting ANH in managing some symptoms, and alternative options to treat distressing symptoms. Patients and families should also be informed that ANH can be withheld and withdrawn. If a nurse is unable to provide appropriate information, the nurse should feel comfortable with saying "I do not know" over providing false reassurances.[61] It is recommended that the nurse seek counsel from available resources such as the clinical nurse specialist, provider, the interdisciplinary team, or the palliative care team, and then return to the patient and family with information.

Initiating and withdrawing or withholding artificial nutrition and hydration

If the decision is made to initiate ANH in a patient to meet the goals of care, the nurse has a responsibility to continually assess the patient's condition, evaluating the impact of the intervention on symptoms and the patient's responses to treatment. Artificial nutrition and hydration can be offered as a time-limited trial to determine whether the patient experiences any benefits from the intervention compared to burdens. As AN is often instituted during an acute event while in the hospital, nurses can inquire about previous medical history or expressed wishes and promote conversations that look at the bigger picture beyond the acute admission.[62] Nurses in any setting can inform patients and families early in the disease continuum of the progression of the illness, and ensure that wishes are elicited and documented by the healthcare team regarding ANH. The nurse needs to facilitate ongoing conversations about ANH to ensure that the role of this therapy continues to meet patient and family goals without excessive burden.

If the decision is made to either withdraw or withhold ANH, the nurse can provide emotional support and assurances that the patient's dignity will be respected with comfort care. If unable to support a patient or family's decision regarding ANH for religious or personal reasons, it is the responsibility of the nurse to request a change in assignment and for the healthcare system to ensure that a nurse comfortable in these situations can provide patient-centered care when ANH is being withheld or withdrawn.

Summary

The provision of food and fluids is synonymous with caring across many cultures. When a patient experiences a decreased desire to eat or drink as part of the end stage of illness, the patient along with the family may struggle and seek interventions to extend life, reduce the impact of possible symptoms such as hunger or dehydration, or fulfill a religious or cultural need at the end of life. Decisions about ANH are complex, and must be guided by the ethical principles of autonomy, beneficence, and nonmaleficence.[44,45] Nurses need to understand the factors, such as religion and culture, that influence a patient's preferences. Nurses need to provide accurate and complete information about the benefits and burdens of ANH. In doing so, nurses will ensure that decisions to initiate, withhold, or withdraw ANH will be patient-centered.

References

1. Cohen MZ, Torres-Vigil I, Burbach BE, de la Rosa A, Bruera E. The meaning of parenteral hydration to family caregivers and patients with advanced cancer receiving hospice care. J Pain Symptom Manage. 2012;43(5):855–865.

2. Sobotka L, Schneider SM, Berner YN, et al. ESPEN guidelines on parenteral nutrition: geriatrics. Clin Nutr. 2009;28(4):461–466.

3. Zieve D, Eltz DR. Malnutrition. Medline Plus website. http://www.nlm.nih.gov/medlineplus/ency/article/000404.htm. June 14, 2011. Accessed July 31, 2013.

4. Fearon K, Strasser F, Anker SD, et al. Definition and classification of cancer cachexia: an international consensus. Lancet Oncol. 2011;12(5):489–495.

5. Hospice and Palliative Nurses Association. Artificial nutrition and hydration in advanced illness. J Hosp Palliat Nurs. 2012;14(3):173–176.

6. McCann RM, Hall WJ, Groth-Juncker A. Comfort care for terminally ill patients: the appropriate use of nutrition and hydration. JAMA. 1994;272(16):1263–1266.

7. Salva A, Coll-Planas L, Bruce S, et al. Nutritional assessment of residents in long-term care facilities (LTCFs): recommendations of the task force on nutrition and ageing of the IAGG European region and the IANA. J Nutr Health Aging. 2009;13(6):475–483.

8. Oliveira AS, Pereira RD. Amyotrophic lateral sclerosis (ALS): three letters that change the people's life. For ever. Arq Neuropsiquiatr. 2009;67(3A):750–782.

9. Morassutti I, Giometto M, Baruffi C, et al. Nutritional intervention for amyotrophic lateral sclerosis. Minerva Gastroenterol Dietol. 2012;58(3)253–260.

10. Thibodeaux LS, Gutierrez A. Management of symptoms in amyotrophic lateral sclerosis. Curr Treat Options Neurol. 2008;10(2):77–85.

11. Pfister DV, Ang K, Brizel DM, et al. NCCN Clinical Practice Guidelines in Oncology (NCCN Guidelines®): Head and neck cancers (Version 2.2013). National Comprehensive Cancer Network website. http://www.nccn.org/professionals/physician_gls/pdf/head-and-neck.pdf. May 29, 2013. Accessed July 21, 2013.

12. Del Río MI, Shand B, Bonati P, et al. Hydration and nutrition at the end of life: a systematic review of emotional impact, perceptions, and decision-making among patients, family, and health care staff. Psychooncology. 2012;21(9):913–921.

13. Orrevall Y, Tishelman C, Permert J, Cederholm T. The use of artificial nutrition among cancer patients enrolled in palliative home care services. Palliat Med. 2009;23:556–564.

14. Donini LM, Savina C, Ricciardi LM, et al. Predicting the outcome of artificial nutrition by clinical and functional indices. Nutrition. 2009;25(1):11–19.

15. Sampson EL, Candy B, Jones L. Enteral tube feeding for older people with advanced dementia. Cochrane Database Syst Rev. 2009;2:CD007209. doi: 10.1002/14651858.CD007209.pub2.

16. Payne C, Wiffen PJ, Martin S. Interventions for fatigue and weight loss in adults with advanced progressive illness. Cochrane Database Syst Rev. 2012;1:CD008427. doi: 10.1002/14651858.CD008427.pub2.

17. Grilo A, Santos CA, Fonseca J. Percutaneous endoscopic gastrostomy for nutritional palliation of upper esophageal cancer unsuitable for esophageal stenting. Arq Gastroenterol. 2012;49(3):227–231.

18. August DA, Huhmann MB, American Society for Parenteral and Enteral Nutrition Board of Directors. A.S.P.E.N. clinical guidelines: nutrition support therapy during adult anticancer treatment and in hematopoietic cell transplantation. J Parenter Enteral Nutr. 2009;33(5):472–500.

19. Levy MH, Back A, Baker JN. NCCN Clinical Practice Guidelines in Oncology (NCCN Guidelines®): Palliative Care (Version 2.2013). National Comprehensive Cancer Network website. http://www.nccn.org/professionals/physician_gls/pdf/palliative.pdf. June 5, 2013. Accessed July 21, 2013.

20. Anderson PM, Abrahams S, Borasio GD, et al. EFNS guidelines on the clinical management of amyotrophic lateral sclerosis (MALS): revised report of an EFNS task force. Eur J Neurol. 2012;19(3):360–375.

21. American Geriatrics Society. Feeding tubes in advanced dementia position statement. American Geriatrics Society website. http://americangeriatrics.org/files/documents/feeding.tubes.advanced.dementia.pdf. May 2013. Accessed July 5, 2013.

22. Teno JM, Gozalo P, Mitchell SL, Kuo S, Fulton AT, Mor V. Feeding tubes and the prevention or healing of pressure ulcers. Arch Intern Med. 2012;172(9):697–701.

23. Teno JM, Gozalo PL, Mitchell SL, et al. Does feeding tube insertion and its timing improve survival? J Am Geriatr Soc. 2012;60(10):1918–1921.

24. Kuo S, Rhodes RL, Mitchell SL, Mor V, Teno JM. Natural history of feeding-tube use in nursing home residents with advanced dementia. J Am Med Dir Assoc. 2009;10(4):264–270.

25. Shintani S. Efficacy and ethics of artificial nutrition in patients with neurologic impairments in home care. J Clin Neurosci. 2013;20(2):220–223.

26. Higaki F, Yokota O, Ohishi M. Factors predictive of survival after percutaneous endoscopic gastrostomy in the elderly: is dementia really a risk factor? Am J Gastroenterol. 2008;103(4):1011–1016.

27. Good P, Cavenagh J, Mather M, Ravenscroft P. Medically assisted nutrition for palliative care in adult patients. Cochrane Database Syst Rev. 2008;4. doi: 10.1002/14651858.CD006274.pub2.

28. Di Giulio P, Toscani F, Villani D, Brunelli C, Gentile S, Spadin P. Dying with advanced dementia in long-term care geriatric institutions: a retrospective study. J Palliat Med. 2008;11(7):1023–1028.

29. Teno JM, Mitchell SL, Kuo SK, et al. Decision-making and outcomes of feeding tube insertion: a five-state study. J Am Geriatr Soc. 2011;59(5):881–886.

30. Dalal S, Del Fabbro E, Bruera E. Is there a role for hydration at the end of life? Curr Opin Support Palliat Care. 2009;3(1):72–78.

31. Krishna LK, Poulose JV, Goh C. Artificial hydration at the end of life in an oncology ward in Singapore. Indian J Palliat Care. 2010;16(3):168–173.

32. Lybarger EH. Hypodermoclysis in the home and long-term care settings. J Infus Nurs. 2009;32(1):40–44.

33. Bruera E, Pruvost M, Schoeller T, Montejo G, Watanabe S. Proctoclysis for hydration of terminally ill cancer patients. J Pain Symptom Manage. 1998;15(4):216–219.

34. Morita T, Hyodo I, Yoshimi T, et al. Association between hydration volume and symptoms in terminally ill cancer patients with abdominal malignancies. Ann Oncol. 2005;16(4):640–647.

35. Nakajima N, Hata Y, Kusumoto K. A clinical study on the influence of hydration volume on the signs of terminally ill cancer patients with abdominal malignancies. J Palliat Med. 2013;16(2):185–189.

36. Fainsinger RL, Bruera E. When to treat dehydration in a terminally ill patient? Support Care Cancer. 1997;5(3):205–211.

37. Bruera E, Hui D, Dalal S, et al. Parenteral hydration in patients with advanced cancer: a multicenter, double-blind, placebo-controlled randomized trial. J Clin Oncol. 2013;31(1):111–118.

38. Yamaguchi T, Morita T, Shinjo T, et al. Effect of parenteral hydration therapy based on the Japanese national clinical guideline on quality of life, discomfort, and symptom intensity in patients with advanced cancer. J Pain Symptom Manage. 2012;43(6):1001–1012.

39. Morita T, Bito S, Koyama H, Uchitomi Y, Adachi I. Development of a national clinical guideline for artificial hydration therapy for terminally ill patients with cancer. J Palliat Med. 2007:10(3):770–780.

40. Galanakis G, Mayo NE, Gagnon B. Assessing the role of hydration in delirium at the end of life. Current Opin Support Palliat Care. 2011;5(2):169–173.

41. Bruera E, Sala R, Rico MA, et al. Effects of parenteral hydration in terminally ill cancer patients: a preliminary study. Journal Clin Oncol. 2005:23(10):2366–2371.

42. American Academy of Hospice and Palliative Medicine. Statement on Artificial Nutrition and Hydration Near the End of Life. American Academy of Hospice and Palliative Medicine. http://www.aahpm.org/positions/default/nutrition.html. December 8, 2006. Accessed July 5, 2013.

43. American Nurses Association. Forgoing nutrition and hydration. American Nurses Association website. http://www.nursingworld.org/

MainMenuCategories/Policy-Advocacy/Positions-and-Resolutions/ANAPositionStatements/Position-Statements-Alphabetically/prtet-nutr14451.pdf. March 1, 2011. Accessed July 29, 2013.

44. Geppert CM, Andrews MR, Druyan ME. Ethical issues in artificial nutrition and hydration: a review. J Parenter Enteral Nutr. 2010;34(1):79–88.

45. Best C. Introducing enteral nutrition support: ethical considerations. Nurs Stand. 2010;24(37):41–45.

46. Karen Ann Quinlan. Wikipedia. http://en.wikipedia.org/wiki/Karen_Ann_Quinlan. June 2, 2013. Accessed July 30, 2013.

47. Nash RR. Palliative care: ethics and the law. In: AM Berger, JL Shuster Jr, JH Von Roenn (eds.), Principles and Practice of Palliative Care and Supportive Oncology. 4th ed. Philadelphia, PA: Lippincott Williams & Wilkins; 2013:748–760.

48. Cruzan v. Director, Missouri Department of Health. Wikipedia. http://en.wikipedia.org/wiki/Nancy_Cruzan. May 20, 2013. Accessed July 30, 2013.

49. Vacco v. Quill. Wikipedia. http://en.wikipedia.org/wiki/Vacco_v.Quill. January 22, 2013. Accessed July 30, 2013.

50. Heuberger RA. Artificial nutrition and hydration at the end of life. J Nutr Elder. 2010;29(4):347–385.

51. Bradley CT. Roman Catholic doctrine guiding end-of-life care: a summary of the recent discourse. J Palliat Med. 2009;12(4):373–377.

52. Brody H, Hermer LD, Scott LD, Grumbles LL, Kutac JE, McCammon SD. Artificial nutrition and hydration: the evolution of ethics, evidence, and policy. J Gen Intern Med. 2011;26(9):1053–1058.

53. Alsolamy S. Islamic views on artificial nutrition and hydration in terminally ill patients. Bioethics. 2012. doi: 10.1111/j.1467-8519.2012.01996.x.

54. Rosner F, Abramson N. Fluids and nutrition: perspectives from Jewish Law (Halachah). South Med J. 2009;102(3):248–250.

55. Ravitsky V. A Jewish perspective on the refusal of life-sustaining therapies: culture as shaping bioethical discourse. Am J Bioeth. 2009;9(4):60–62.

56. Modi S, Velde B, Gessert CE. Perspectives of community members regarding tube feeding in patients with end-stage dementia: findings from African-American and Caucasian focus groups. Omega. 2010–2011;62(1):77–91.

57. Chai HZ, Radha Krishna LK, Wong VH. Feeding: What it means to patients and caregivers and how these views influence Singaporean Chinese caregivers' decisions to continue feeding at the end of life. Am J Hosp Palliat Care. 2013 Mar 15. Epub ahead of print. http://ajh.sagepub.com/content/early/2013/03/01/1049909113480883.long. Accessed August 2, 2013.

58. Duke G, Northam S. Discrepancies among physicians regarding knowledge, attitudes, and practices in end-of-life care. J Hosp Palliat Nurs. 2009;11(1):52–59.

59. Cardin F. Special considerations for endoscopists on PEG indications in older patients. ISRN Gastroenterol. 2012;2012: 607149. doi:10.5402/2012/607149. http://www.ncbi.nlm.nih.gov/pmc/articles/PMC3512294/ Accessed July 24, 2013.

60. Monturo C, Hook K. From means to ends: artificial nutrition and hydration. Nurs Clin North Am. 2009;44(4):505–515.

61. Mahon MM. Clinical decision making in palliative care and end of life care. Nurs Clin North Am. 2010;45(3):345–362.

62. Coyne PJ, Lyckholm LJ. Artificial nutrition for cognitively impaired individuals. J Hosp Palliat Nurs. 2010;12(4):263–267.

CHAPTER 14

Dyspnea, terminal secretions, and cough

Deborah Dudgeon

It's like an elephant sitting on my chest! I can't get my breath!

A patient

I can hear her bubbly breathing from the hallway. I can't go into the room. It sounds like she's drowning!!

A family member

I'm terrified! I cough and cough and can't get any air!

A patient

Key points

- Dyspnea is a subjective experience.
- Tachypnea is not dyspnea.
- Patients can be very frightened when breathless.
- Nursing and medical interventions are helpful for patients with dyspnea.
- Death rattle is common in dying patients.
- Death rattle is very distressing for people at the bedside.
- Family members need to receive good education and reassurance about death rattle.
- Anticholinergics are the drugs of choice for death rattle.
- Chronic cough can be very debilitating.
- Massive hemoptysis is very frightening and needs to be anticipated.
- Pharmacological and nonpharmacological interventions can help patients with chronic cough.

Dyspnea

Dyspnea is a very common symptom in people with advanced disease and can severely impair their quality of life. The presence of dyspnea correlates with the probability of dying in the hospital.[1] In one international study, dyspnea prompted the use of terminal sedation in 25% to 53% of patients.[2] Management of breathlessness requires understanding and assessment of the multidimensional components of the symptom, knowledge of the pathophysiological mechanisms and clinical syndromes that are common in people with advanced disease, and knowledge of the indications and limitations of the available therapeutic approaches.

Definition

The American Thoracic Society has defined *dyspnea* as "a subjective experience of breathing discomfort that consists of qualitatively distinct sensations that vary in intensity."[3] Dyspnea, like pain, is multidimensional in nature, with not only physical elements but also affective components, which are shaped by previous experience.[4,5] A neurophysiological model provides a framework to understand the variety of mechanisms that can lead to dyspnea: receptor → afferent impulse → integration/processing in the central nervous system (CNS) → efferent impulse → dyspnea.[5] Stimulation of a number of different receptors (Figure 14.1), and the conscious perception this stimulation invokes, can alter ventilation and result in both the intensity and unpleasant sensations of breathlessness.[4,5] It is proposed that dyspnea results from a "mismatch" between the afferent information to the CNS and the outgoing motor command to the respiratory muscles. This mismatch is called "neuroventilatory dissociation" or "afferent–efferent dissociation."[4]

Prevalence and impact

The prevalence of dyspnea varies according to the stage and type of underlying disease and the methodological design of the studies.[6] A systematic review of symptom prevalence in advanced cancer, AIDS, heart disease, chronic obstructive pulmonary disease (COPD), and renal disease found the prevalence of dyspnea was 10%–70% in patients with cancer, 11%–62% with AIDS, 60%–88% with heart disease, 90%–95% with COPD, and 11%–62% with renal disease.[6] In a prospective study of 400 patients with inoperable lung cancer, the intensity of dyspnea was higher in patients closer to death, and difficulty breathing was ranked as the most distressing symptom among these patients.[7] Another study of patients with end-stage COPD found that 95% of the participants experienced extreme breathlessness and that it was

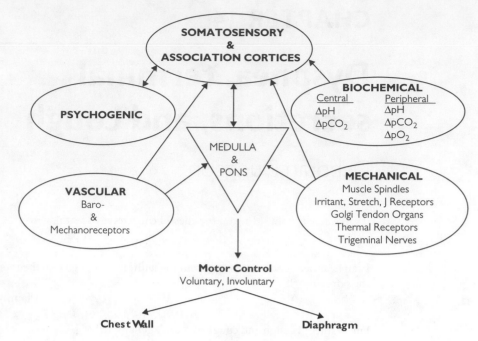

Figure 14.1 Schematic diagram of the neuroanatomical elements involved in the control of ventilation.

the most distressing and debilitating symptom.[8] Dyspnea is also quite prevalent in people with advanced congestive heart failure (CHF): 56.3% experience dyspnea, 53.4% have it "frequently" or "almost constantly," 25.9% describe it as "severe" or "very severe," and 43.1% describe the distress associated with it as "quite a bit" or "very much."[9] Likewise, dyspnea occurs in 37% of patients with cerebrovascular accident (CVA) of whom 57% were breathless for >6 months)[10]; in 47% to 50% of patients with amyotrophic lateral sclerosis (ALS); and in 70% of those with dementia.[11]

In a consecutive cohort of 5862 patients seen by a specialist palliative care service over a 4-year period, dyspnea was evaluated at every clinical encounter until death. Only 11.4% of people had "no breathlessness" recorded between referral and death. Patients with noncancer causes of breathlessness had significantly higher levels for the last 3 months of life with no significant changes. Cancer patients had significantly lower levels of breathlessness initially but the intensity worsened between 3 and 10 days before death. Despite symptomatic treatment at death, 65% of people were breathless and it was severe in 26% of the individuals.[12]

In a study of late-stage cancer patients, Roberts and associates[13] used patient self-report surveys, chart audits of patients under the care of a hospice program, and interviews of patients and nurses in a home-care hospice program to examine the occurrence of dyspnea during the last weeks of life. They found that 62% of the patients with dyspnea had been short of breath for >3 months. Various activities intensified dyspnea for these patients: climbing stairs, 95.6%; walking slowly, 47.8%; getting dressed, 52.2%; talking or eating, 56.5%; and resting, 26.1%. The patients universally responded by decreasing their activity to whatever degree would relieve their shortness of breath. Most of the patients had received no direct medical or nursing assistance with their dyspnea, leaving them to cope in isolation. Brown and colleagues[14] found that 97% of lung cancer patients studied had decreased their activities, and 80% believed they had socially isolated themselves from friends and outside contacts to cope with their dyspnea. Studies in

patients with COPD, CVA, or end-stage heart or neurological diseases have also demonstrated the presence of significant dyspnea and other symptoms, functional disability, and impaired quality of life in the last year of their lives.[8,10,11,15,16]

Patients with advanced disease typically experience chronic shortness of breath with intermittent acute episodes.[14,17] Acute attacks of breathlessness are usually accompanied by feelings of anxiety, fear, panic, and, if severe enough, a sensation of impending death.[17] Patients and family members who were participants in a qualitative study using narrative analysis consistently expressed fear of dying during a future acute episode of breathlessness, or of watching helplessly as a loved one became increasingly breathless and died before receiving any help.[18] Many dying persons are terrified of waking in the middle of the night with intense air hunger.[19] They need providers who will anticipate their fears and provide symptomatic relief of their breathlessness and anxiety as they approach death.[18,19]

Pathophysiology

Management of dyspnea requires an understanding of its multidimensional nature and the pathophysiological mechanisms that cause this distressing symptom. Exertional dyspnea in cardiopulmonary disease (Box 14.1) is caused by (1) increased ventilatory demand, (2) impaired mechanical responses, or (3) a combination of the two.[20] The effects of abnormalities of these mechanisms can also be additive.

Increased ventilatory demand

Ventilatory demand is increased because of increased physiological dead space resulting from reduction in the vascular bed (from thromboemboli, tumor emboli, vascular obstruction, radiation, chemotherapy toxicity, or concomitant emphysema); hypoxemia and severe deconditioning with early metabolic acidosis (with excessive hydrogen ion stimulation); alterations in carbon dioxide output (V_{CO_2}) or in the arterial partial pressure of carbon dioxide

Box 14.1 Pathophysiological mechanisms of dyspnea

Increased ventilatory demand

Increased physiological dead space

- Thromboemboli
- Tumor emboli
- Vascular obstruction
- Radiation therapy
- Chemotherapy
- Emphysema

Severe deconditioning

Hypoxemia

Change in Vco_2 or arterial Pco_2 set point

Psychological: anxiety, depression

Increased neural reflex activity

Impaired mechanical response/ventilatory pump impairment

Restrictive ventilatory deficit

Respiratory muscle weakness

- Cachexia
- Electrolyte imbalances
- Peripheral muscle weakness
- Neuromuscular abnormalities
- Neurohumoral
- Steroids

Pleural or parenchymal disease

Reduced chest wall compliance

Obstructive ventilatory deficit

Asthma

Chronic obstructive pulmonary disease

Tumor obstruction

Mixed obstructive/restrictive disorder (any combination of the above)

($Paco_2$) set point; and nonmetabolic sources, such as increased neural reflex activity or psychological factors such as anxiety and depression.

Impaired mechanical response/ventilatory pump impairment

Impaired mechanical responses result in restrictive ventilatory deficits due to inspiratory muscle weakness,[21] pleural or parenchymal disease, or reduced chest wall compliance; airway obstruction from coexistent asthma or COPD; or tumor obstruction. Patients may also have a mixed obstructive and restrictive disorder.

Multidimensional assessment of dyspnea

Dyspnea, like pain, is a subjective experience that may not be evident to an observer. *Tachypnea*, a rapid respiratory rate, is not dyspnea. Medical personnel must learn to ask for and accept the patient's assessments, often without measurable physical correlates. If patients say they are having discomfort with breathing, we must believe that they are dyspneic.

To determine whether dyspnea is present, it is important to ask more than the question, "Are you short of breath?" Patients often respond in the negative to this simple question because they have limited their activities so they won't become short of breath. It is therefore helpful to ask about shortness of breath in relationship to activities: "Do you get short of breath walking at the same speed as someone of your age?" "Do you have to stop to catch your breath when walking upstairs?" "Do you get short of breath when you are eating?"

Qualitative and affective aspects of dyspnea

It is now recognized that dyspnea is not a single sensation. There are at least three different "qualities" of uncomfortable breathing: "air hunger," "work," and "tightness."[22] Each of these sensations is thought to arise from a different afferent source. Air hunger arises when pulmonary ventilation is insufficient and there is a conscious perception of the urge to breath. The sense of excessive work of breathing occurs when there is an increased rate or depth, impedance to inspiration, respiratory muscle weakness, or a disadvantageous length of the respiratory muscles. Tightness is specific to bronchoconstriction. Studies show people are also able to rate the affective or unpleasant quality of breathlessness. The ratio of sensory intensity to affective rating varies among people, and to adequately characterize dyspnea it is necessary to measure both dimensions.

Clinical assessment

Clinical assessments are usually directed at determining the underlying pathophysiology, deciding appropriate treatment, and evaluating the response to therapy.

The clinical assessment of dyspnea should include a complete history of the symptom, including its temporal onset (acute or chronic); whether it is affected by positioning; its qualities, associated symptoms, precipitation, and relieving events or activities; and response to medications. A past history of smoking, underlying lung or cardiac disease, concurrent medical conditions, allergy history, and details of previous medications or treatments should be elicited.[23,24] An assessment of the impact of breathlessness on the person's quality of life, physical activities, self-care, social life, and psychological state should occur as well.

Careful physical examination focused on possible underlying causes of dyspnea should be performed. Particular attention should be directed at signs associated with certain clinical syndromes that are common causes of dyspnea. Examples are the dullness to percussion, decreased tactile fremitus, and absent breath sounds associated with a pleural effusion in a person with lung cancer; an elevated jugular venous pressure (JVP), audible third heart sound (S_3), and bilateral crackles audible on chest examination associated with CHF; and elevated JVP, distant heart sounds, and pulsus paradoxus in people with pericardial effusions.[23,24]

Gift and colleagues[25] studied the physiological factors related to dyspnea in subjects with COPD and high, medium, and low levels of breathlessness. There were no significant differences in respiratory rate, depth of respiration, or peak expiratory flow rates at the three levels of dyspnea. There was, however, a significant difference in the use of accessory muscles between patients with high and low levels of dyspnea, suggesting that this is a physical finding that reflects the intensity of dyspnea.

Diagnostic tests helpful in determining the cause of dyspnea include chest radiography; electrocardiography; pulmonary function tests; arterial blood gases; complete blood counts; serum potassium, magnesium, and phosphate levels; cardiopulmonary exercise testing; and tests specific for suspected underlying pathologies, such as an echocardiogram for suspected pericardial effusion.[23] The choice of appropriate diagnostic tests should be guided by the stage of disease, the prognosis, the risk/benefit ratios of any proposed tests or interventions, and the desires of the patient and family.

Nguyen and colleagues[26] found that the ratings of intensity of dyspnea during laboratory exercise, clinical measures of dyspnea such as the Oxygen Cost Diagram, and pulmonary function tests captured distinctly different information in patients with moderate to severe COPD. It is therefore not surprising that results of pulmonary function tests do not necessarily reflect the intensity of a person's dyspnea. Individuals with comparable degrees of functional lung impairment may also experience considerable differences in the intensity of dyspnea they perceive.[5] As mentioned earlier this may be related to the fact that the intensity:affective ratio varies between individuals.[22] Factors such as adaptation, differing physical characteristics, and psychological conditions can modulate both the quality and the intensity of the person's perception of breathlessness.

The visual analog scale (VAS) is one of the most popular techniques for measuring the perceived intensity of dyspnea. This scale is usually a 100-mm vertical or horizontal line, anchored at each end by words such as "Not at all breathless" and "Very breathless." Subjects are asked to mark the line at the point that best describes the intensity of their breathlessness. The scales can be used as an initial assessment, to monitor progress, and to evaluate effectiveness of treatment in an individual patient.[27] Numeric rating scales (NRS) are highly correlated with VAS ratings of breathlessness[28] and more repeatable measures that require a smaller sample size to detect a change in breathlessness.[28]

The modified Borg scale is a scale with nonlinear spacing of verbal descriptors of severity of breathlessness.[29] Patients are asked to pick the verbal descriptor that best describes their perceived exertion during exercise. It is usually used in conjunction with an exercise protocol with standardized power output or metabolic loads. When used in this manner, the slope of the Borg descriptors over time is very reproducible and reliable, permitting comparisons within individuals and across population groups.[30,31]

The reading numbers aloud test was designed as an objective measure of the activity-limiting effect of breathlessness in people with cancer who were breathless at very low levels of exertion.[32,33] The test involves asking subjects to read a grid of numbers as quickly and clearly as possible for 60 seconds. The number of numbers read and the number read per breath are recorded.

In a systematic review of the usefulness of different assessment tools to measure breathlessness, Bausewein and colleagues[28] concluded that no one scale accurately reflected the effects of breathlessness on the patient with advanced disease and their family. They recommended that for general clinical questions, a VAS or modified Borg scale were most useful; multidimensional tools if the focus was on quality of life; breathlessness-specific questionnaires if the focus was the sensation or functional impact of

breathlessness; and a combination of instruments or methods (qualitative and quantitative) in a research setting.

Dyspnea and psychological factors

The person's perception of the intensity of his or her breathlessness is also affected by psychological factors. Anxious, obsessive, depressed, and dependent persons appear to experience dyspnea that is disproportionately severe relative to the extent of their pulmonary disease.[5] Gift and colleagues[25] found that anxiety was higher during episodes of high or medium levels of dyspnea, compared with low levels of dyspnea. Kellner and associates[34] found in multiple-regression analyses that depression was predictive of breathlessness. Studies in cancer patients by Dudgeon and Lertzman[21,35] and others[36–38] have also shown that anxiety is significantly correlated with the intensity of dyspnea ($r = 0.3$) but explains only 9% of the variance in the intensity of breathlessness. These studies were done in people with chronic dyspnea and when the person was at rest. Carrieri-Kohlman and colleagues[39] found higher correlations between dyspnea intensity and anxiety associated with dyspnea at the end of exercise ($r = 0.49$). It is also probable that anxiety is a more prominent factor during episodes of acute shortness of breath.

Management

The optimal treatment of dyspnea is to treat reversible causes. If this is no longer possible, then both nonpharmacological and pharmacological methods are used (Box 14.2).

Pharmacological interventions
Opioids
Since the late 19th century, opioids have been used to relieve breathlessness of patients with asthma, pneumothorax, and emphysema.[40] Although most trials have demonstrated the benefit of opioids for the treatment of dyspnea,[40–50] some have been negative[51–54] or have produced undesirable side effects.[43,51]

In 2001, a systematic review examined the effectiveness of oral or injectable opioid drugs for the palliative treatment of breathlessness.[55] The authors identified 18 randomized, double-blind, controlled trials comparing the use of any opioid drug against placebo for the treatment of breathlessness in patients with any illness. In the studies involving nonnebulized routes of administration,[40,42,48,54,56–58] there was statistically strong evidence for a small effect of oral and parenteral opioids for the treatment of

---

Box 14.2 Management of dyspnea

Sit upright supported by pillows or leaning on overbed table
Fan +/– oxygen
Relaxation techniques and other appropriate nonpharmacological measures
Identify and treat underlying diagnosis (if appropriate)
Pharmacological management
Chronic
Opioids
Add phenothiazine (chlorpromazine, promethazine)
Acute
Opioids
Add anxiolytic

breathlessness.[55] Two more recent systematic reviews of the management of dyspnea in cancer patients also support the use of oral or parenteral opioids.[59,60]

In previous years, there was tremendous interest in the use of nebulized opioids for the treatment of dyspnea. Opioid receptors are present on sensory nerve endings in the airways[61]: therefore, it is hypothesized that if the receptors were interrupted directly, lower doses, with less systemic side effects, would be required to control breathlessness. The 2001 systematic review[55] identified nine randomized, double-blind, controlled trials comparing the use of nebulized opioids or placebo for the control of breathlessness.[62-70] The authors concluded that there was no evidence that nebulized opioids were more effective than nebulized saline in relieving breathlessness.[55] A double-blind, controlled, cross-over study of the effects of nebulized hydromorphone, systemic hydromorphone, and nebulized saline were compared for the relief of acute episodic dyspnea in advanced cancer patients. Over time, breathlessness decreased significantly with all treatments and there were no significant differences between the treatments.[71] Although this study did not rule out the possibility that patients' dyspnea improved because they stopped the activity that precipitated it, the results suggest that nebulized saline is an effective treatment for dyspnea. Given the results of these trials it is hard to justify the continued use of nebulized opioids alone.

Physicians have been reluctant to prescribe opioids for dyspnea since the potential for respiratory failure was recognized in the 1950s.[72] The 2001 systematic review of opioids for breathlessness identified 11 studies that contained information on blood gases or oxygen saturation after intervention with opioids.[55] Only one study reported a significant increase in the arterial partial pressure of carbon dioxide ($PaCO_2$), but it did not rise above 40 mm Hg.[56] In studies of cancer patients, morphine did not compromise respiratory function as measured by respiratory effort and oxygen saturation[41,42,73] or respiratory rate and $PaCO_2$.[41] In another study, authors found the patients' intensity of dyspnea and respiratory rates decreased significantly ($P = 0.003$) after the administration of an opioid, but there was no significant change in the transcutaneous arterial pressure of CO_2.[74] It is now thought that the development of clinically significant hypoventilation and respiratory depression from opioids depends on the rate of change of the dose, the history of previous exposure to opioids, and possibly the route of administration.[75] Early use of opioids improves quality of life and allows the use of lower doses, while tolerance to the respiratory depressant effects develops.[76] Twycross[77] suggested that early use of morphine or another opioid, rather than hastening death in dyspneic patients, might actually prolong survival by reducing physical and psychological distress and exhaustion.

Sedatives and tranquilizers
Chlorpromazine decreases breathlessness without affecting ventilation or producing sedation in healthy subjects.[78] Woodcock and colleagues[79] found that promethazine reduced dyspnea and improved exercise tolerance of patients with severe COPD. O'Neill and associates[78] did not find that promethazine improved breathlessness in healthy people, nor did Rice and coworkers[51] find that it benefited patients with stable COPD. McIver and colleagues[80] found that chlorpromazine was effective for relief of dyspnea in advanced cancer. The systematic review by Viola and colleagues

concluded that promethazine could be used orally as an alternative when systemic opioids couldn't be employed.[59]

A systematic review examined whether benzodiazepines relieved breathlessness in adults with advanced disease. Seven studies with 200 subjects with advanced cancer or COPD were included in the analysis. No significant effect of benzodiazepines for relief of breathlessness or in the percentage of breakthrough dyspnea was observed.[81]

Combinations
In a double-blind, placebo controlled, randomized trial, Light and colleagues[57] studied the effectiveness of morphine alone, morphine and promethazine, and morphine and prochlorperazine for the treatment of breathlessness in patients with COPD. The combination of morphine and promethazine significantly improved exercise tolerance without worsening dyspnea, compared with placebo, morphine alone, or the combination of morphine and prochlorperazine.[57] Ventafridda and colleagues[82] also found the combination of morphine and chlorpromazine to be effective. In a randomized, single-blinded 2-day study, dyspneic cancer patients were given subcutaneous doses of morphine routinely, every 4 hours, with breakthrough midazolam; routine midazolam with breakthrough morphine; or a routine dose of both midazolam and morphine.[83] Significant improvements in dyspnea occurred in all three arms. At 24 and 48 hours, significantly more patients who received the combined treatment of morphine and midazolam reported relief of dyspnea and had less episodes of breakthrough dyspnea with apparently no greater levels of sedation. In a subsequent study by the same group, 63 advanced cancer patients were randomized to receive oral morphine or oral midazolam in a 5-day study. The dosages of morphine and midazolam were those that improved the person's intensity of dyspnea by at least 50% as determined in a fast titration period. Dyspnea intensity decreased in both the morphine and midazolam groups on the 2nd day and was maintained or continued to drop on subsequent days. Midazolam was superior to morphine in controlling baseline and breakthrough dyspnea.[12]

Other medications
Indomethacin reduced exercise-induced breathlessness in a group of normal adults,[84] but no benefit was obtained in patients with diffuse parenchymal lung disease[85] or COPD.[86] Although inhaled bupivacaine reduced exercise-induced breathlessness in normal volunteers,[87] it failed to decrease breathlessness of patients with interstitial lung disease.[88] Inhaled lidocaine did not improve dyspnea in six cancer patients.[89] Dextromethorphan did not improve breathlessness of patients with COPD.[90] None of these medications can be recommended for the treatment of dyspnea at this time.

A review of nebulized furosemide for the management of dyspnea found encouraging results in patients with asthma, COPD, and cancer with further study recommended.[91]

Oxygen
In hypoxic patients with COPD, oxygen supplementation improves survival, pulmonary hemodynamics, exercise capacity, and neuropsychological performance.[92] Guidelines for oxygen use in this setting are shown in Box 14.3. The usefulness of oxygen to relieve breathlessness in the person with refractory dyspnea is less clear.[93] In a Cochrane review (2008) to determine whether oxygen therapy

---

Box 14.3 Guidelines for oxygen therapy

Continuous oxygen

$Pao_2 \leq 55$ mm Hg or oxygen saturation $\leq 88\%$ at rest

Pao_2 of 56 to 59 mm Hg or oxygen saturation of 89% in the presence of the following:

    Dependent edema suggesting congestive heart failure

    Cor pulmonale

    Polycythemia (hematocrit > 56%)

    Pulmonary hypertension

Noncontinuous oxygen is recommended during exercise:

$Pao_2 \leq 55$ mm Hg or oxygen saturation $\leq 88\%$ with a low level of exertion, or during sleep

Pao_2 of ≤ 55 mm Hg or oxygen saturation $\leq 88\%$ associated with pulmonary hypertension, daytime somnolence and cardiac arrhythmias

---

provided relief of dyspnea in chronic end-stage disease, Cranston and colleagues[94] identified eight cross-over studies that met their inclusion criteria. There were 144 participants (97 cancer, 35 cardiac failure, and 12 kyphoscoliosis). In the patients with cancer, the meta-analysis failed to demonstrate a significant improvement of dyspnea at rest when oxygen was compared with air inhalation, improvement in dyspnea with oxygen inhalation was independent of resting hypoxia, and there was an improvement in dyspnea with inhalation of oxygen at rest and during exercise. In cardiac failure participants, high concentration oxygen provided relief of dyspnea at 6 minutes during exercise tests, but low-flow ambulatory oxygen during a submaximal exercise test did not provide relief. In a single study of oxygen inhalation during exercise in participants with kyphoscoliosis, oxygen improved dyspnea. The authors of this systematic review stated that their outcomes were inconclusive.[94] In a subsequent randomized, double-blind, cross-over trial of the effect of oxygen versus air on the relief of dyspnea in 51 cancer patients, Philip and colleagues[95] found the mean sensation of dyspnea improved with both air and oxygen, with no significant differences in either VAS or patient preference between treatments. The 17 hypoxic patients also did not report a mean greater improvement with, or preference for, oxygen over air, despite improved oxygen saturations in all but four patients. The authors concluded that either air or oxygen via nasal prongs improved breathlessness.[95]

In a systematic review and meta-analysis comparing oxygen and air for mildly hypoxemic or nonhypoxemic people with cancer, Uronis et al. identified five randomized controlled trials with 134 patients. Oxygen did not improve dyspnea and there was a statistically significant individual preference for oxygen detected in only two of four studies.[96] In a double-blind, controlled trial, 239 nonhypoxic individuals with a life-limiting illness were randomized to receive oxygen or room air for relief of dyspnea. Participants received air or oxygen by concentrator for at least 15 hours per day for 7 days and breathlessness was measured twice a day. Compared with room air, oxygen did not provide additional benefit for relief of breathlessness.[97]

Campbell and colleagues conducted a double-blind repeated-measure study in 32 patients who were near death, with patients acting as their own controls (n-of-1 trial). Participants received medical air, oxygen, or no-flow randomly every 10 minutes via nasal cannula twice for each intervention with the Respiratory Distress Observation Scale measurement of the presence and intensity of distress at baseline and every gas or flow change. Ninety-one percent of patients tolerated the protocol with no change in respiratory comfort, and 9% required restoration of baseline oxygen. The authors concluded that oxygen was useful when the person was experiencing distress or was hypoxemic, but their findings did not support its initiation or continuation if the person was comfortable and near death.[98]

In a cohort study of 1239 patients receiving oxygen at home, 413 people had data available before and at least 1 week after the prescription of home oxygen. Approximately one-third had at least a 20% improvement in their breathlessness. It was not possible to predict the responders from demographic factors, baseline breathlessness, or underlying diagnosis.[99]

Despite the lack of clear evidence of the benefit of oxygen for terminally ill patients, some terminally ill patients report a marked improvement in both breathlessness and quality of life and as there are no predictive factors, n-of-1 therapeutic trials are warranted.

Nonpharmacological interventions

A Cochrane review by Bausewein and colleagues examined non-pharmacological interventions for breathlessness and identified 47 studies. The interventions with the highest level of evidence were all conducted in COPD patients and included neuromuscular electrical stimulation, chest wall vibration, walking aids, and breathing training.[100]

People who are short of breath often obtain relief by sitting near an open window or in front of a fan. Cold directed against the cheek[101] or through the nose[102,103] can alter ventilation patterns and reduce the perception of breathlessness, perhaps by affecting receptors in the distribution of the trigeminal nerve that are responsive to both thermal and mechanical stimuli.[101,102] Galbraith and colleagues examined the effectiveness of a hand-held fan to reduce the sensation of breathlessness in 50 patients.[104] They found that a fan directed at the face for 5 minutes significantly reduced the score on the VAS breathless scale more than if it was directed at the leg.

The Cochrane review identified 109 participants in acupuncture and 75 in acupressure studies. All participants had COPD except for one study conducted in cancer patients. They were unable to conduct a meta-analysis due to variations in the interventions, reporting of data, and timing of measurement. There were four studies of high quality, two showed significant improvement in breathlessness. The level of evidence was graded as low.[100]

Nursing interventions

Many patients obtain relief of dyspnea by leaning forward while sitting and supporting their upper arms on a table. This technique is effective in patients with emphysema,[105] probably because of an improved length-tension state of the diaphragm, which increases efficiency.[106]

Pursed-lip breathing slows the respiratory rate and increases intra-airway pressures, thus decreasing small airway collapse during periods of increased dyspnea.[107] Mueller and coworkers[45] found that pursed-lip breathing led to an increase in tidal volume and a decrease in respiratory rate at rest and during exercise in 7 of 12 COPD patients experiencing an improvement in dyspnea.

Pursed-lip breathing reduces dyspnea in about 50% of patients with COPD.[108]

Corner and colleagues[109] found that weekly sessions with a nurse research practitioner over 3 to 6 weeks, using counseling, breathing retraining, relaxation, and coping and adaptation strategies, significantly improved breathlessness and ability to perform activities of daily living compared with controls. Carrieri and Janson-Bjerklie[110] found that patients used self-taught relaxation to help control their breathlessness. Others have found that formal muscle relaxation techniques decrease anxiety and breathlessness.[111] Guided imagery[112] and therapeutic touch[113] resulted in significant improvements in quality of life and sense of well-being in patients with COPD and patients with terminal cancer, respectively, but without any significant improvement in breathlessness.

Nursing actions that intubated patients thought helpful included friendly attitude, empathy, providing physical support, staying at the bedside, reminding or allowing patients to concentrate on changing their breathing pattern, and providing information about the possible cause of the breathlessness and possible interventions.[114]

Patient and family teaching

Carrieri and Janson-Bjerklie[110] identified strategies patients used to manage acute shortness of breath. These strategies could be taught to patients and their families. Patients benefited from keeping still with positioning techniques, such as leaning forward on the edge of a chair with arms and upper body supported, and using some type of breathing strategy, such as pursed-lip or diaphragmatic breathing. Some of the patients distanced themselves from aggravating factors, and others used self-adjustment of medications. Several subjects isolated themselves from others to gain control of their breathing and diminish the social impact. Others used structured relaxation techniques, conscious attempts to calm down, and prayer and meditation. The study of Carrieri and Janson-Bjerklie[110] and another by Brown and colleagues[14] demonstrated that most subjects reported some changes in activities of living, such as changes in dressing and grooming, avoidance of bending or stooping, advanced planning or reduction in activities, staying in a good frame of mind, avoidance of being alone, and acceptance of the situation.

Patients and families should be taught about the signs and symptoms of an impending exacerbation and how to manage the situation. They should learn problem-solving techniques to prevent panic, ways of conserving energy, how to prioritize activities, use of fans, and ways to maximize the effectiveness of their medications, such as using a spacer with inhaled drugs or taking an additional dose of an inhaled beta-agonist before exercise.[115] Patients should avoid activities in which their arms are unsupported, because these activities often increase breathlessness.[111]

Patients in distress should not be left alone. Social services, nursing, and family input need to be increased as the patient's ability to care for himself or herself decreases.[116]

Case study

Mr. G, a 76-year-old man with dyspnea

Mr. G is a 76-year-old man with dyspnea. He was admitted to the hospital with worsening shortness of breath, cough, and fever and was being treated for pneumonia. He had a past history of COPD, heart disease, and a recent diagnosis of non-small-cell lung cancer. You answer his call light to find him gasping for breath and holding his chest. While getting an overbed table and pillow for him to rest on, you calmly instruct him to take slow, deep breaths and to use the breathing technique that you had previously taught him. You note that he is cyanosed and institute oxygen and fan to help relieve his breathlessness. On further questioning you ask if he has pain, whether it radiates to the jaw or arm, if this is similar to his angina or a new pain and what brought it on? The pain is in his right chest, completely unlike his angina and had awakened him from sleep. On examination you note a tachycardia, absent breath sounds in right base, with a rub, a loud pulmonary second sound, and that he has a swollen left leg. With institution of the oxygen, fan, and focused breathing, you note that he is slightly less distressed, but you ask his wife to stay with him while you prepare a dose of prn morphine. On your return 5 minutes later, Mr. G's breathing has further improved but is still a little labored, so you administer the morphine. His wife stays with him, and 15 minutes later, when you return, she has helped him back into bed, where he is resting comfortably. You explain that arrangements are underway for him to have a CT angiogram to rule out a pulmonary embolism.

Summary

Dyspnea is a very common symptom in people with advanced disease. The symptom is often unrecognized and patients, therefore, receive little assistance in managing their breathlessness. Dyspnea can have profound effects on a person's quality of life, because even the slightest exertion may precipitate breathlessness.

Terminal secretions

Noisy, rattling breathing in patients who are dying is commonly known as death rattle. This noisy, moist breathing can be very distressing for the family, other patients, visitors, and healthcare workers, because it may appear that the person is drowning in his or her own secretions.[117] Management of death rattle can present healthcare providers a tremendous challenge as they attempt to ensure a peaceful death for the patient.[118]

Definition

"Death rattle" is a term applied to describe the noise produced by the turbulent movements of secretions in the upper airways that occur with the inspiratory and expiratory phases of respiration in patients who are dying.[119]

Prevalence and impact

Death rattle occurs in 23% to 92% of patients in their last hours before death.[119-125] Studies have shown that there is an increased incidence of respiratory congestion in patients with primary lung cancer,[121,124] cerebral metastases,[124,126] pneumonia, and dysphagia,[125] with the symptom more likely to persist in cases with pulmonary pathology.[124] The incidence of death rattle increases closer to death;[124] the median time from onset of death rattle to death is 8 to 23 hours.[122–124] Most commonly, this symptom occurs when the person's general condition is very poor, and most patients have a decreased level of consciousness.[124] If the person is alert, however, the respiratory secretions can cause him or her to feel very agitated and fearful of suffocating. Despite the identification of "noisy breathing" as a problem in 39% of patients dying in a long-term care setting, 49% of them received no treatment.[127] In one study of the attitudes of palliative care nurses about the impact of death rattle, 13% thought that death rattle distressed the dying patient; 100% thought it distressed the dying person's relatives, with 52% indicating that bereaved relatives had mentioned death rattle as a source of distress; and 79% thought that death rattle distressed nurses.[118] A qualitative study involving hospice staff and volunteers found that most participants had negative feelings about hearing the sound of death rattle and thought that relatives were distressed by it as well.[128] Studies of bereaved relatives, however, found that not all were distressed by the sound, and this was, in part, determined by whether the person appeared disturbed or if they saw fluid dribbling from the person's mouth.[129,130]

Pathophysiology

The primary defense mechanism for the lower respiratory tract is the mucociliary transport system. This system is a protective device that prevents the entrance of viruses, bacteria, and other particulate matter into the body.[131–133] The surface of the respiratory tract is lined with a liquid sol phase near the epithelium and a superficial gel phase in contact with the air.[131] Ciliated epithelial cells, located at all levels of the respiratory tract except the alveoli and the nose and throat, are in constant movement to propel the mucus up the respiratory tract, to be either subconsciously swallowed or coughed out. The mucus is produced by submucosal glands, which are under neural and humoral control. The submucosal glands are under parasympathetic, sympathetic, and noncholinergic, nonadrenergic nervous control. Resting glands secrete approximately 9 mL/min, but mechanical, chemical, or pharmacological stimulation (via vagal pathways) of the airway epithelium can augment gland secretion. Surface goblet cells also produce mucus secretions, which can be increased with irritant stimuli (e.g., cigarette smoke). The secretory flow rate and amount, as well as the viscoelastic properties of the mucus, can be altered.[131]

The audible breathing of the so-called death rattle is produced when turbulent air passes over or through pooled secretions in the oropharynx or bronchi. The amount of turbulence depends on the ventilatory rate and airway resistance.[126] Mechanisms of death rattle include excessive secretion of respiratory mucus, abnormal mucus secretions inhibiting normal clearance, dysfunction of the cilia, inability to swallow, decreased cough reflex due to weakness and fatigue, and the supine, recumbent position. Factors that may contribute to respiratory congestion include infection or inflammation, pulmonary embolism producing infarction and fluid leakage from damaged cells, pulmonary edema or CHF,[133] dysphagia, and odynophagia. Although it has been suggested that a state of relative dehydration decreases the incidence of problematic bronchial secretions,[134] Ellershaw and colleagues[121] found no statistically significant difference in the incidence of death rattle in a biochemically dehydrated group of patients, compared with a group of hydrated patients.

Bennett[126] proposed two types of death rattle. Type 1 involves mainly salivary secretions, which accumulate in the last few hours of life when swallowing reflexes are inhibited. Type 2 is characterized by the accumulation of predominantly bronchial secretions over several days before death as the patient becomes too weak to cough effectively. This characterization has been empirically

supported by Morita and colleagues[124] and therefore may prove useful to determine appropriate treatment.

Assessment

Assessment of death rattle includes a focused history and physical examination to determine potentially treatable underlying causes. If the onset is sudden and is associated with acute shortness of breath and chest pain, it might suggest a pulmonary embolism or myocardial infarction. Physical findings consistent with CHF and fluid overload might support a trial of diuretic therapy; the presence of pneumonia indicates a trial of antibiotic therapy. The effectiveness of interventions should be included in the assessment. The patient's and family's understanding and emotional response to the situation should also be assessed so that appropriate interventions can be undertaken.

A recently developed and validated assessment tool, the Victoria Respiratory Congestion Scale (VRCS)[135] is clinically useful to determine the effectiveness of interventions. This instrument rates the congestion on a scale from 0 to 3, with 0 indicating no congestion heard at 12 inches from the chest; 1 indicating congestion audible only at 12 inches from the chest; 2 indicating congestion audible at foot of patient's bed; and 3 indicating congestion audible at door of patient's room. This scale has demonstrated interrater reliability ($\kappa = 0.53$, $P < 0.001$) and concurrent validity with a noise meter ($P < 0.001$). It was weakly correlated with a caregiver distress scale ($\kappa = 0.24$, $P < 0.001$).

Management

Pharmacological interventions

Primary treatment should be focused on the underlying disorder, if appropriate to the prognosis and the wishes of the patient and family. If this is not possible, then anticholinergics are the primary mode of treatment. Hyoscine hydrobromide (scopolamine), atropine sulfate, hyoscine butylbromide (Buscopan), and glycopyrrolate (Robinul) are the anticholinergic agents that are used to treat death rattle. Anticholinergic drugs can prevent vagally induced increased bronchial secretions, but they reduce basal secretions by only 39%.[131] Wee and Hillier's Cochrane review "Interventions for Noisy Breathing Near to Death" identified 32 studies, but only four were randomized-controlled, controlled before and after, or interrupted time series studies.[136] They concluded that there was no evidence that any intervention, pharmacological or nonpharmacological was superior to placebo.

In the largest trial to date, Wildiers evaluated the effectiveness of atropine, hyoscine butylbromide or hyoscine hydrobromide for treatment of death rattle in 333 participants, Death rattle decreased in 1 hour in 42%, 42%, and 37% respectively with the effect on secretions lasting up to 24 hours. A limitation of the trial was that there was no placebo arm.[137]

In a prospective comparative audit a smaller proportion of patients responded to hyoscine hydrobromide (35%) as compared with hyoscine butylbromide (54%) or glycopyrolate (46%). They reported that 54%–65% of patients had their secretions alleviated.[138]

Hyoscine hydrobromide (scopolamine) is the primary medication used for the treatment of death rattle. It inhibits the muscarinic receptors and causes anticholinergic actions such as decreased peristalsis, gastrointestinal secretions, sedation, urinary retention, and dilatation of the bronchial smooth muscle. It is administered subcutaneously, intermittently or by continuous infusion, orally, intravenously, or transdermally.[139] In one study,[140] hyoscine hydrobromide 0.4 mg subcutaneously was immediately effective and only 6% of the patients required repeated doses. In an open-label study of the treatment of death rattle, 56% of patients who received hyoscine hydrobromide had a significantly reduced noise level after 30 minutes, compared with 27% of patients who had received glycopyrrolate ($P = 0.002$).[117] In other studies, between 22% and 65% of patients did not respond to hyoscine hydrobromide, and secretions recurred from 2 to 9 hours after the injection.[120] In a retrospective study of 100 consecutive deaths in a 22-bed hospice, 27% of patients received an infusion of hyoscine hydrobromide, with 5 of 17 requiring injections despite receiving an infusion.[126]

Atropine sulfate is another anticholinergic drug that is preferred by some centers for the treatment of respiratory congestion.[133] In a study of 995 doses of atropine, congestion was decreased in 30% of patients, remained the same in 69%, and increased in 1%.[133] Atropine is the drug of choice of this group, because it results in less CNS depression, delirium, and restlessness, with more bronchodilatory effect, than hyoscine hydrobromide. There is, however, the risk of increased tachycardia with atropine sulfate when doses >1.0 mg are given. In a recent trial 137 participants were randomized to atropine or placebo. Sublingual atropine as a single dose was no more effective than placebo.[141]

Glycopyrrolate (Robinul) is also an anticholinergic agent. It has the advantages of producing less sedation and agitation because there is limited passage through the blood-brain barrier and a longer duration of action than hyoscine hydrobromide. In two studies in which its effectiveness was compared with that of hyoscine hydrobromide, glycopyrrolate was not as effective in controlling secretions.[117,120] However, others have disputed this finding and suggest it is also more cost-effective.[142] Glycopyrrolate is available in an oral form and can be useful for patients at an earlier stage of disease, when sedation is not desired.

Hyoscine butylbromide (Buscopan) is another anticholinergic drug. It is available in injection, suppository, and tablet forms.

Nonpharmacological interventions

There are times when the simple repositioning of the patient may help him or her to clear the secretions (Box 14.4). Suctioning usually is not recommended, because it can be very uncomfortable for the patient and causes significant agitation and distress. Pharmacological measures are usually effective and prevent the need for suctioning. If the patient has copious secretions that can easily be reached in the oropharynx, then suctioning may be appropriate. In a study conducted at St. Christopher's Hospice, suctioning was required in only 3 of 82 patients to control the secretions.[121] In another study, 31% of the patients required only nursing interventions with reassurance, change in position, and occasional suctioning to manage respiratory congestion in the last 48 hours of life.[140]

Patient and family teaching

The patient and the family can be very distressed by this symptom. It is important to explain the process, to help them understand why there is a buildup of secretions and that there is something that can be done to help. The Victoria Hospice group suggests using the term "respiratory congestion" as opposed to "death rattle," "suffocation," or "drowning in sputum," because these terms instill strong emotional reactions.[133] When explaining to families the changes that can occur before death, this is one of the symptoms that should be mentioned. If the person is being treated at home, the family should be instructed as to the measures available to relieve death rattle and to notify their hospice or palliative care team if it occurs, so that appropriate medications can be ordered.

Case study

Mr. P, a 56-year-old man with metastatic laryngeal cancer

Mr. P was admitted to the palliative care unit from home 4 days ago. He had a sudden deterioration in his condition and was thought to have aspiration pneumonia. He was started on antibiotics but despite this his condition worsened. When you go in to make your initial assessment you can hear gurgling with breathing from the doorway. He is restless and is pulling at the intravenous line that is running at 125 mL/h. There are audible gurgling sounds as he breathes, with diffuse crackles throughout his chest, and 3+ pitting edema of all of his limbs. His daughter, in tears, says, "It sounds like he is choking to death! Please do something!" While you help to reposition Mr. P, you explain why this is happening. You go to the desk and get an order from the doctor for some furosemide, to change the intravenous line to a saline lock, and for an "as needed" dose of hyoscine hydrobromide subcutaneously. You administer the furosemide, but there is minimal improvement; therefore, you give Mr. P an injection of hyoscine hydrobromide, and within 20 minutes he has settled.

Summary

Although death rattle is a relatively common problem in people who are close to death, very few studies have evaluated the effectiveness of treatment. Anticholinergics are the drugs of choice at this time. Death rattle can be very distressing for family members at the bedside, and they need to receive good instruction and reassurance.

Cough

Cough is a natural defense of the body to prevent entry of foreign material into the respiratory tract. In people with advanced disease, it can be very debilitating, leading to sleepless nights, fatigue, pain and, at times, pathological fractures.

Definition

Cough is an explosive expiration that can be a conscious act or a reflex response to an irritation of the tracheobronchial tree. Cough

---

Box 14.4 Management of "death rattle"
Change position
Reevaluate if receiving IV hydration
Pharmacological management
Chronic
Glycopyrrolate or hyoscine hydrobromide patch
If treatment fails: subcutaneous hyoscine hydrobromide or atropine sulfate
Acute
Subcutaneous hyoscine hydrobromide or subcutaneous atropine sulfate

lasting 8 weeks is considered chronic.[143] A *dry cough* occurs when no sputum is produced; a *productive cough* is one in which sputum is raised. *Hemoptysis* occurs when the sputum contains blood. *Massive hemoptysis* is expectoration of at least 100 to 600 mL of blood in 24 hours.[140]

Prevalence and impact

Chronic cough is a common problem; recurrent cough is reported by 3% to 40% of the population.[144] In population surveys, men report cough more frequently than women do, but women appear to have an intrinsically heightened cough response.[144] Cough is often present in people with advanced diseases such as bronchitis, CHF, uncontrolled asthma, human immunodeficiency virus infection, and various cancers. In a study of 289 patients with non-small-cell lung cancer, cough was the most common symptom (>60%) and the most severe symptom at presentation.[145] Eighty percent of the group had cough before death. Over time, cough and breathlessness were much less well controlled than the other symptoms in this group of patients.

In a study of 26 patients with lung cancer the majority had a dry, nighttime cough. The cough could be precipitated by cold, smoke, a variety of smells, lying down, physical exertion, and/or different foods. Cough was distressing and could cause pain, fractured ribs, heaving, or retching and resulted in many patients restricting their social life.[146]

In patients with lung cancer, hemoptysis is the presenting symptom 7% to 10% of the time, 20% have it at some time during their clinical course, and 3% die of massive hemoptysis.[147] The mortality rate of massive hemoptysis in patients with lung cancer can be as high as 59% to 100%.[147]

Pathophysiology

Cough is characterized by a violent expiration, with flow rates that are high enough to sheer mucus and foreign particles away from the larynx, trachea, and large bronchi. The cough reflex can be stimulated by irritant receptors in the larynx and pharynx or by pulmonary stretch receptor, irritant receptor, or C-fiber stimulation in the tracheobronchial tree.[148] There are also central and peripheral regulatory pathways that can be both excitatory and inhibitory. Supramedullary pathways are important in conscious regulation of cough, and descending inhibitory pathways are thought to modulate the cough reflex. Overstimulation, hypersensitivity, or damage to the neuronal pathways either within the airways and/or CNS may cause excessive coughting.[149] Different mechanisms are involved in isolation or together in patients with cough of various causes.[150] The vagus nerve carries sensory information from the lung that initiates the cough reflex. Infection can physically or functionally strip away epithelium, exposing sensory nerves and increasing the sensitivity of these nerves to mechanical and chemical stimuli. It is also thought that inflammation produces prostaglandins, which further increase the sensitivity of these receptors, leading to bronchial hyperreactivity and cough. When cough is associated with increased sputum production, it probably results from stimulation of the irritant receptors by the excess secretion.[148] Cough is associated with respiratory infection, bronchitis, rhinitis, postnasal drip, esophageal reflux, medications including angiotensin-converting enzyme inhibitors,[148] asthma, COPD, pulmonary fibrosis, CHF, pneumothorax, bronchiectasis, and cystic fibrosis.[151] In the

person with cancer, cough may be caused by any of these conditions; however, direct tumor effects (e.g., obstruction), indirect cancer effects (e.g., pulmonary emboli), and cancer treatment effects (e.g., radiation therapy and/or chemo or targeted therapy) could also be the cause.[149,152]

Hemoptysis can result from bleeding in the respiratory tract anywhere from the nose to the lungs. It varies from blood streaking of sputum to coughing up of massive amounts of blood. There are multiple causes of hemoptysis, but some of the more common ones are a tracheobronchial source, secondary to inflammation or tumor invasion of the airways; a pulmonary parenchymal source, such as pneumonia or abscess; a primary vascular problem, such as pulmonary embolism; a miscellaneous cause, such as a systemic coagulopathy resulting from vitamin K deficiency, thrombocytopenia, or abnormal platelet function secondary to bone marrow invasion with tumor, sepsis, or disseminated intravascular coagulation; or an iatrogenic cause, such as use of anticoagulants, nonsteroidal antiinflammatory drugs, or acetylsalicylic acid.[153]

Assessment

In assessing someone with cough, it is important to do a thorough history and physical examination. Because cough may arise from anywhere in the distribution of the vagus nerve, the full assessment of a patient with a chronic cough requires a multidisciplinary approach with cooperation between respiratory medicine, gastroenterology, and ear, nose, and throat (ENT) departments.[144] The assessment helps to determine the underlying cause and appropriate treatment of the cough. Depending on the diagnosis, the prognosis, and the patient's and family's wishes, it may be appropriate to perform diagnostic tests, including chest or sinus radiography, spirometry before and after bronchodilator and histamine challenge, and, in special circumstances in people with earlier-stage disease, upper gastrointestinal endoscopy and 24-hour esophageal pH monitoring. In patients with significant hemoptysis, bronchoscopy is usually needed to identify the source of bleeding.

In the history and physical examination, one should look for a link between cough and the associated factors listed in the previous section, timing of the start of the cough, whether the cough is productive, nocturnal or daytime, the nature of the sputum, the frequency and amount of blood, precipitating and relieving factors, associated symptoms, and the effect on quality of life.[146]

Management

It is important to base management decisions on the cause and the appropriateness of treating the underlying diagnosis, compared with simply suppressing the symptom. This decision is based on the diagnosis, prognosis, side effects, and possible benefits of the intervention and the wishes of the patient and family. Management strategies also depend on whether the cough is productive (Box 14.5) as theoretically, cough suppressants, by causing mucus retention, could be harmful in conditions with excess mucus production.[148]

Two recent reviews on management of chronic cough in patients receiving palliative care[154] and interventions for cough in cancer[155] found there was little evidence and the majority of studies were of low methodological quality to support recommendations for practice.

Box 14.5	Treatment of nonproductive cough

Nonopioid antitussive (dextromethorphan, benzonatate)
Opioids
Inhaled anesthetic (lidocaine, bupivacaine)

Pharmacological interventions

There are three broad mechanisms of sensitization to cough relevant to treatments: peripheral sensitization, central sensitization and impaired inhibition.[156]

Centrally acting antitussives

Central sensitization occurs when the central integrating neurons develop lower thresholds for activation in response to peripheral sensory stimulation. Upregulation of the N-methyl-D-asparate (NMDA) receptor is a postsynaptic mechanism that is critical to the initiation and maintenance of central sensitization.[156] Dextromethorphan, a dextro isomer of levorphanol, is a NMDA receptor antagonist that is almost equiantitussive to codeine. Dextromethorphan blocks the NMDA receptor to increase the cough threshold.[157]

There is some evidence that gabapentin, pregabalin, and baclofen may be effective for cough inhibition by working presynaptically to inhibit the release of glutamate (gabapentin, pregabalin) and inhibit voltage-gated calcium channels (baclofen, gabapentin, pregabalin).[156]

Descending inhibitory pathways

The role of inhibitory cough mechanisms has not been specifically investigated in humans but opioids are known to activate these pathways.[156]

Opioids suppress cough, but the dose needed is higher than that contained in the proprietary cough mixtures.[148] The exact mode of action is unclear, but it is thought that opioids inhibit the mu receptor peripherally in the lung; act centrally by suppressing the cough center in the medulla or the brainstem respiratory centers; or stimulate the mu receptor, thus decreasing mucus production or increasing mucus ciliary clearance.[148] Codeine is the most widely used opioid for cough; some authors claim that it has no advantages over other opioids and provides no additional benefit to patients already receiving high doses of opioids for analgesia,[157] whereas others state that the various opioids have different antitussive potencies.[147]

Peripherally acting antitussives

Demulcents are a group of compounds that form aqueous solutions and help to alleviate irritation of abraded surfaces. They are often found in over-the-counter cough syrups. Their mode of action for controlling cough is unclear, but it is thought that the sugar content encourages saliva production and swallowing, which leads to a decrease in the cough reflex; that they stimulate the sensory nerve endings in the epipharynx, and decrease the cough reflex by a "gating" process; or that demulcents may act as a protective barrier by coating the sensory receptors.[148]

Benzonatate is an antitussive that inhibits cough mainly by anesthetizing the vagal stretch receptors in the bronchi, alveoli, and pleura.[147] Other drugs that act directly on cough receptors include levodropropizine, oxalamine, and prenoxdiazine.[147]

Inhaled anticholinergic bronchodilators, either alone or in combination with β_2-adrenergic agonists, effectively decrease cough in people with asthma and in normal subjects.[158] It is thought that they decrease input from the stretch receptors, thereby decreasing the cough reflex, and change the mucociliary clearance.

The local anesthetic lidocaine is a nonselective voltage-gated sodium channel blocker that acts as a potent suppressor of irritant-induced cough and has been used as a topical anesthetic for the airway during bronchoscopy. Inhaled local anesthetics, such as lidocaine and bupivacaine, delivered by nebulizer, suppress some cases of chronic cough for as long as 9 weeks.[148,159–161] Higher doses can cause bronchoconstriction, so it is wise to observe the first treatment. Patients must also be warned not to eat or drink anything for 1 hour after the treatment or until their cough reflex returns.

The leukotriene receptor antagonists montelukast and zafirlukast may reduce cough in cough-variant asthma. Menthol is thought to work through activation of a ligand-gated ion channel on sensory afferent fibers.[156]

Productive coughs

Interventions for productive coughs include chest physiotherapy, oxygen, humidity, and suctioning. In cases of increased sputum production, expectorants, mucolytics, and agents to decrease mucus production can be employed.[147] Opioids, antihistamines, and anticholinergics decrease mucus production and thereby decrease the stimulus for cough.

Massive hemoptysis

In patients with massive hemoptysis, survival is so poor that patients may not want any kind of intervention to stop the bleeding; in such cases, maintenance of comfort alone becomes the priority. For those patients who want intervention to stop the bleeding, the initial priority is to maintain a patent airway, which usually requires endotracheal intubation. Management options include endobronchial tamponade of the segment, vasoactive drugs, iced saline lavage, neodymium/yttrium-aluminum-garnet (Nd/YAG) laser photocoagulation, electrocautery, bronchial artery embolization, and external beam or endobronchial irradiation.[147]

Nonpharmacological interventions

If cough is induced by a sensitive cough reflex, then the person should attempt to avoid the stimuli that produce this. They should stop or cut down smoking and avoid smoky rooms, cold air, exercise, and pungent chemicals. If medication is causing the cough, it should be decreased or stopped if possible. If the cause is esophageal reflux, then elevation of the head of the bed may be tried. Adequate hydration, humidification of the air, and chest physiotherapy may help patients expectorate viscid sputum.[162] Radiation therapy to enlarged nodes, endoscopically placed esophageal stents for tracheoesophageal fistulas, or injection of Teflon into a paralyzed vocal cord may improve cough.[162]

Patient and family education

Education should include practical matters such as proper use of medications, avoidance of irritants, use of humidification, and ways to improve the effectiveness of cough. One such way is called "huffing." The person lies on his or her side, supports the abdomen with a pillow, blows out sharply three times, holds the breath, and then coughs. This technique seems to improve the effectiveness of a cough and helps to expel sputum.

If the patient is having hemoptysis and massive bleeding is a possibility, it is important to educate the family about this possibility, to prepare them psychologically and develop a treatment plan. Dark towels or blankets can help to minimize the visual impact of this traumatic event. Adequate medications should be immediately available to control any anxiety or distress that might occur. Family and staff require emotional support after such an event.[163]

Case study

CB, a 75-year-old woman with metastatic colon cancer

CB is a 75-year-old woman with metastatic colon cancer to liver and lungs. She has had extensive lung metatases for over 1 year. Her main complaint is a dry nonproductive cough and mild shortness of breath on exertion. She was previously treated with chemotherapy but developed severe diarrhea and became febrile and neutropenic and nearly died. She does not want any further disease-oriented treatment. She tends to minimize her symptoms but her husband says she coughs persistently, particularly at night and both of them are unable to sleep. She has had a trial of demulcents, dextromethorphan, inhalers, and opioids for her cough, with little effect. She is afebrile and has no evidence of pneumonia on physical examination, but does have some fine crackles. You suggest a trial of nebulized preservative-free lidocaine every 6 hours. When you next see her, she reports that her cough is much better and that she and her husband have been able to get some rest.

Summary

Chronic cough can be a disabling symptom for patients. If the underlying cause is unresponsive to treatment, then suppression of the cough is the major therapeutic goal.

References

1. Edmonds P, Higginson I, Altmann D, Sen-Gupta G, McDonnell M. Is the presence of dyspnea a risk factor for morbidity in cancer patients? J Pain Symptom Manage. 2000;19:15–22.
2. Fainsinger R, Waller A, Bercovici M et al. A multicentre international study of sedation for uncontrolled symptoms in terminally ill patients. Palliat Med. 2000;14:257–265.
3. American Thoracic Society. Dyspnea. Mechanisms, assessment, and management: a consensus statement. Am J Respir Crit Care Med. 1999;159:321–340.
4. O'Donnell DE, Banzett RB, Carrieri-Kohlman V, et al. Pathophysiology of dyspnea in chronic obstructive pulmonary disease: a roundtable. Proc Am Thorac Soc. 2007;4:145–168.
5. Mahler DA. Understanding mechanisms and documenting plausibility of palliative interventions for dyspnea. Curr Opin Support Palliat Care. 2011;5:71–76.
6. Solano JP, Gomes B, Higginson IJ. A comparison of symptom prevalence in far advanced cancer, AIDS, heart disease, chronic obstructive pulmonary disease and renal disease. J Pain Symptom Manage. 2006;31:58–69.
7. Tishelman C, Petersson L-M, Degner LF, Sprangers MAG. Symptom prevalence, intensity, and distress in patients with inoperable lung cancer in relation to time of death. J Clin Oncol. 2007;25:5381–5389.
8. Skilbeck J, Mott L, Page H, Smith D, Hjelmeland-Ahmedzai S, Clark D. Palliative care in chronic obstructive airways disease: a needs assessment. Palliat Med. 1998;12:245–254.
9. Blinderman CD, Homel P, Billings JA, Portenoy RK, Tennstedt SL. Symptom distress and quality of life in patients with advanced congestive heart failure. J Pain Symptom Manage. 2008;35:594–603.
10. Addington-Hall J, Lay M, Altmann D, McCarthy M. Symptom control, communication with health professionals, and hospital care of stroke patients in the last year of life as reported by surviving family, friends and officials. Stroke. 1995;26:2242–2248.
11. Voltz R, Borasio GD. Palliative therapy in the terminal stage of neurological disease. J Neurol. 1997;244(Suppl 4):S2–S10.
12. Currow D, Smith J, Davidson PM, Newton PJ, Agar MR, Abernethy AP. Do the trajectories of dyspnea differ in prevalence and intensity by diagnosis at the end of life? A consecutive cohort study. J Pain Symptom Manage. 2010;39:680–690.
13. Roberts DK, Thorne SE, Pearson C. The experience of dyspnea in late-stage cancer: patients' and nurses' perspectives. Cancer Nurs. 1993;16:310–320.
14. Brown ML, Carrieri V, Janson-Bjerklie S, Dodd MJ. Lung cancer and dyspnea: the patient's perception. Oncol Nurs Forum. 1986;13:19–24.
15. Barnes S, Gott M, Payne S et al. Prevalence of symptoms in a community-based sample of heart failure patients. J Pain Symptom Manage. 2006;32:208–216.
16. Gore JM, Brophy CJ, Greenstone MA. How well do we care for patients with end stage chronic obstructive pulmonary disease (COPD)? A comparison of palliative care and quality of life in COPD and lung cancer. Thorax. 2000;55:1000–1006.
17. O'Driscoll M, Corner J, Bailey C. The experience of breathlessness in lung cancer. Eur J Cancer Care. 1999;8:37–43.
18. Bailey PH. Death stories: acute exacerbations of chronic obstructive pulmonary disease. Qual Health Res. 2001;11:322–338.
19. Steinhauser KE, Clipp EC, McNeilly M, Christakis NA, McIntyre LM, Tulsky JA. In search of a good death: observations of patients, families, and providers. Ann Int Med. 2000;132:825–832.
20. O'Donnell DE. Exertional breathlessness in chronic respiratory disease. In: Mahler D (ed.), Dyspnea. New York: Marcel Dekker; 1998;97–147.
21. Dudgeon D, Lertzman M. Dyspnea in the advanced cancer patient. J Pain Symptom Manage. 1998;16:212–219.
22. Lansing RW, Gracely RH, Banzett RB. The multiple dimensions of dyspnea: review and hypotheses. Respir Physiol Neurobiol. 2009;167:53–60.
23. Silvestri GA, Mahler DA. Evaluation of dyspnea in the elderly patient. Clin Chest Med. 1993;14:393–404.
24. Ferrin MS, Tino G. Acute dyspnea. AACN Clin Issues. 1997;8:398–410.
25. Gift AG, Plaut SM, Jacox A. Psychologic and physiologic factors related to dyspnea in subjects with chronic obstructive pulmonary disease. Heart Lung. 1986;15:595–601.
26. Nguyen HQ, Altinger J, Carrieri-Kohlman V, Gormley JM, Paul SM, Stulbarg MS. Factor analysis of laboratory and clinical measurement of dyspnea in patients with chronic obstructive pulmonary disease. J Pain Symptom Manage. 2003;25:118–127.
27. Gift AG. Validation of a vertical visual analogue scale as a measure of clinical dyspnea. Am Rev Respir Dis. 1986;133:A163.
28. Bausewein C, Farquhar M, Booth S, Gysels M, Higginson IJ. Measurement of breathlessness in advanced disease: a systematic review. Respir Med. 2006;101:399–410.
29. Burdon J, Juniper E, Killian K, Hargeave F, Campbell E. The perception of breathlessness. Am Rev Respir Dis. 1982;126:825–828.
30. O'Donnell DE, Lam M, Webb KA. Measurement of symptoms, lung hyperinflation, and endurance during exercise in chronic obstructive pulmonary disease. Am J Respir Crit Care Med. 1998;158:1557–1565.
31. Tattersall MHN, Boyer MJ. Management of malignant pleural effusions. Thorax. 1990;45:81–82.
32. Wilcock A, Crosby V, Clarke D, Corcoran R, Tattersfield AE. Reading numbers aloud: a measure of the limiting effect of breathlessness in patients with cancer. Thorax. 1999;54:1099–1103.
33. Neff TA, Petty TL. Tolerance and survival in severe chronic hypercapnia. Arch Intern Med. 1972;129:591–596.
34. Kellner R, Samet J, Pathak D. Dyspnea, anxiety, and depression in chronic respiratory impairment. Gen Hosp Psychiatry. 1992;14:20–28.

35. Dudgeon D, Lertzman M. Etiology of dyspnea in advanced cancer patients [abstract]. Proc Am Soc Clin Oncol. 1996;15:165.

36. Heyse-Moore LH. On Dyspnoea in Advanced Cancer. Thesis. Southampton University; 1993.

37. Dudgeon DJ, Kristjanson L, Sloan JA, Lertzman M, Clement K. Dyspnea in cancer patients: prevalence and associated factors. J Pain Symptom Manage. 2001;21:95–102.

38. Bruera E, Schmitz B, Pither J, Neumann CM, Hanson J. The frequency and correlates of dyspnea in patients with advanced cancer. J Pain Symptom Manage. 2000;19:357–362.

39. Carrieri-Kohlman V, Gormley JM, Douglas MK, Paul SM, Stulbarg MS. Differentiation between dyspnea and its affective components. West J Nurs Res. 1996;18:626–642.

40. Woodcock AA, Gross ER, Gellert A, Shah S, Johnson M, Geddes DM. Effects of dihydrocodeine, alcohol, and caffeine on breathlessness and exercise tolerance in patients with chronic obstructive lung disease and normal blood gases. N Engl J Med. 1981;305.1611–1616.

41. Bruera E, Macmillan K, Pither J, MacDonald RN. Effects of morphine on the dyspnea of terminal cancer patients. J Pain Symptom Manage. 1990;5:6:341–344.

42. Bruera E, MacEachern T, Ripamonti C, Hanson J. Subcutaneous morphine for dyspnea in cancer patients. Ann Int Med. 1993;119:906–907.

43. Cohen MH, Johnston Anderson A, Krasnow SH, et al. Continuous intravenous infusion of morphine for severe dyspnea. South Med J. 1991;84:2:229–234.

44. Light RW, Muro JR, Sato RI, Stansbury DW, Fischer CE, Brown SE. Effects of oral morphine on breathlessness and exercise tolerance in patients with chronic obstructive pulmonary disease. Am Rev Respir Dis. 1989;139:126–133.

45. Mueller RE, Petty TL, Filley GF. Ventilation and arterial blood gas changes induced by pursed lip breathing. J Appl Physiol. 1970;28:784–789.

46. Masood AR, Subhan MMF, Reed JW, Thomas SHL. Effects of inhaled nebulized morphine on ventilation and breathlessness during exercise in healthy man. Clin Sci. 1995;88:447–452.

47. Robin ED, Burke CM. Single-patient randomized clinical trial: opiates for intractable dyspnea. Chest. 1986;90:888–892.

48. Johnson MA, Woodcock AA, Geddes DM. Dihydrocodeine for breathlessness in "pink puffers." Brit Med J. 1983;286:675–677.

49. Sackner MA. Effects of hydrocodone bitartrate on breathing pattern of patients with chronic obstructive pulmonary disease and restrictive lung disease. Mt Sinai J Med. 1984;51:222–226.

50. Timmis AD, Rothman MT, Henderson MA, Geal PW, Chamberlain DA. Haemodynamic effects of intravenous morphine in patients with acute myocardial infarction complicated by severe left ventricular failure. Br Med J. 1980;280:980–982.

51. Rice KL, Kronenberg RS, Hedemark LL, Niewoehner DE. Effects of chronic administration of codeine and promethazine on breathlessness and exercise tolerance in patients with chronic airflow obstruction. Br J Dis Chest. 1987;81:287–292.

52. Eiser N, Denman WT, West C, Luce P. Oral diamorphine: lack of effect on dyspnoea and exercise tolerance in the "pink puffer" syndrome. Eur Respir J. 1991;4:926–931.

53. Boyd KJ, Kelly M. Oral morphine as symptomatic treatment of dyspnoea in patients with advanced cancer. Palliat Med. 1997;11:277–281.

54. Poole PJ, Veale AG, Black PN. The effect of sustained-release morphine on breathlessness and quality of life in severe chronic obstructive pulmonary disease. Am J Respir Crit Care Med. 1998;157:1877–1880.

55. Jennings AL, Davies A, Higgins JPT, Broadley K. Opioids for the palliation of breathlessness in terminal illness. Cochrane Database Syst Rev. 2001;4:CD002066.

56. Woodcock AA, Johnson MA, Geddes DM. Breathlessness, alcohol and opiates. N Engl J Med. 1982;306:1363–1364.

57. Light RW, Stansbury DW, Webster JS. Effect of 30 mg of Morphine alone or with promethazine or prochlorperazine on the exercise capacity of patients with COPD. Chest. 1996;109:975–981.

58. Chua TP, Harrington D, Ponikowski P, Webb-Peploe K, Poole-Wilson PA, Coats AJ. Effects of dihydrocodeine on chemosensivity and exercise tolerance in patients with chronic heart failure. J Am Coll Cardiol. 1997;29:147–152.

59. Viola R, Kiteley C, Lloyd NS, Mackay JA, Wilson J, Wong RKS. The management of dyspnea in cancer patients: a systematic review. Support Care Cancer. 2008;16:329–337.

60. Ben-Aharon I, Gafter-Gvili A, Leibovici L, Stemmer SM. Interventions for alleviating cancer-related dyspnea: a systematic review. J Clin Oncol. 2008;26:2396–2404.

61. Belvisi MG, Chung KF, Jackson DM, Barnes PJ. Opioid modulation of non-cholinergic neural bronchoconstriction in guinea-pig in-vivo. Br J Pharmacol. 1988;95:413–418.

62. Beauford W, Saylor TT, Stansbury DW, Avalos K, Light RW. Effects of nebulized morphine sulfate on the exercise tolerance of the ventilatory limited COPD patient. Chest. 1993;104:175–178.

63. Davis CL, Hodder C, Love S, Shah R, Slevin M, Wedzicha J. Effect of nebulised morphine and morphine 6-glucuronide on exercise endurance in patients with chronic obstructive pulmonary disease. Thorax. 1994;49:393P.

64. Davis CL, Penn K, A'Hern R, Daniels J, Slevin M. Single dose randomised controlled trial of nebulised morphine in patients with cancer related breathlessness [abstract]. Palliat Med. 1996;10:64–65.

65. Harris-Eze AO, Sridhar G, Clemens RE, Zintel TA, Gallagher CG, Marciniuk DD. Low-dose nebulized morphine does not improve exercise in interstitial lung disease. Am J Respir Crit Care Med. 1995;152:1940–1945.

66. Jankelson D, Hosseini K, Mather LE, Seale JP, Young IH. Lack of effect of high doses of inhaled morphine on exercise endurance in chronic obstructive pulmonary disease. Eur Respir J. 1997;10:2270–2274.

67. Leung R, Hill P, Burdon JGW. Effect of inhaled morphine on the development of breathlessness during exercise in patients with chronic lung disease. Thorax. 1996;51:596–600.

68. Masood AR, Reed JW, Thomas SHL. Lack of effect of inhaled morphine on exercise-induced breathlessness in chronic obstructive pulmonary disease. Thorax. 1995;50:629–634.

69. Noseda A, Carpiaux JP, Markstein C, Meyvaert A, de Maertelaer V. Disabling dyspnoea in patients with advanced disease: lack of effect of nebulized morphine. Eur Respir J. 1997;10:1079–1083.

70. Young IH, Daviskas E, Keena VA. Effect of low dose nebulised morphine on exercise endurance in patients with chronic lung disease. Thorax. 1989;44:387–390.

71. Charles MA, Reymond L, Israel F. Relief of incident dyspnea in palliative cancer patients: a pilot, randomized, controlled trial comparing nebulized hydromorphone, systemic hydromorphone, and nebulized saline. J Pain Symptom Manage. 2008;36:29–38.

72. Wilson RH, Hoseth W, Dempsey ME. Respiratory acidosis*: I. Effects of decreasing respiratory minute volume in patients with severe chronic pulmonary emphysema, with specific reference to oxygen, morphine and barbitures. Am J Med. 1954;17:464–470.

73. Mazzocato C, Buclin T, Rapin CH. The effects of morphine on dyspnea and ventilatory function in elderly patients with advanced cancer: a randomized double-blind controlled trial. Ann Oncol. 1999;10:1511–1514.

74. Clemens KE, Klaschik E. Symptomatic therapy of dyspnea with strong opioids and its effect on ventilation in palliative care patients. J Pain Symptom Manage. 2007;33:473–481.

75. Dudgeon D. Dyspnea, Death Rattle, and Cough. In: Ferrell BR, Coyle N (eds.), Textbook of Palliative Nursing. New York: Oxford University Press; 2001;164–174.

76. Dudgeon D. Dyspnea: Ethical concerns. Ethics in Palliative Care, Part II. J Palliat Care. 1994;10:48–51.

77. Twycross R. Morphine and dyspnoea. In: Pain Relief in Advanced Cancer. New York: Churchill Livingstone; 1994;383–399.

78. O'Neill PA, Morton PB, Stark RD. Chlorpromazine: a specific effect on breathlessness? Br J Clin Pharmacol. 1985;19:793–797.

79. Woodcock AA, Gross ER, Geddes DM. Drug treatment of breathlessness: contrasting effects of diazepam and promethazine in pink puffers. BMJ. 1981;283:343–346.

80. McIver B, Walsh D, Nelson K. The use of chlorpromazine for symptom control in dying cancer patients. J Pain Symptom Manage. 1994;9:341–345.

81. Simon S, Higginson I, Booth S, Harding R, Bausewein C. Benzodiazepines for the relief of breathlessness in advanced malignant and non-malignant diseases in adults. Cochrane Database Syst Rev. 2010;1:CD007354. doi: 10.1002/14651858.CD007354.pub2.

82. Ventafridda V, Spoldi E, De Conno F. Control of dyspnea in advanced cancer patients. Chest. 1990;98:1544–1545.

83. Navigante AH, Cerchietti LCA, Castro MA, Lutteral MA, Cabalar ME. Midazolam as adjunct therapy to morphine in the alleviation of severe dyspnea perception in patients with advanced cancer. J Pain Symptom Manage. 2006;31:38–47.

84. O'Neill PA, Stark RD, Morton PB. Do prostaglandins have a role in breathlessness? Am Rev Respir Dis. 1985;132:22–24.

85. O'Neill PA, Stretton TB, Stark RD, Ellis SH. The effect of indomethacin on breathlessness in patients with diffuse parenchymal disease of the lung. Br J Dis Chest. 1986;80:72–79.

86. Schiffman GL, Stansbury DW, Fischer CE, Sato RI, Light RW, Brown SE. Indomethacin and perception of dyspnea in chronic airflow limitation. Am Rev Respir Dis. 1988;137:1094–1098.

87. Winning AJ, Hamilton RD, Shea SA, Knott C, Guz A. The effect of airway anaesthesia on the control of breathing and the sensation of breathlessness in man. Clin Sci. 1985;68:215–225.

88. Winning AJ, Hamilton RD, Guz A. Ventilation and breathlessness on maximal exercise in patients with interstitial lung disease after local anaesthetic aerosol inhalation. Clin Sci. 1988;74:275–281.

89. Wilcock A, Corcoran R, Tattersfield AE. Safety and efficacy of nebulized lignocaine in patients with cancer and breathlessness. Palliat Med. 1994;8:35–38.

90. Giron AE, Stansbury DW, Fischer CE, Light RW. Lack of effect of dextromethorphan on breathlessness and exercise performance in patients with chronic obstructive pulmonary disease (COPD). Eur Respir J. 1991;4:532–535.

91. Newton PJ, Davidson PM, Macdonald P, Ollerton R, Krum H. Nebulized furosemide for the management of dyspnea: does the evidence support its use? J Pain Symptom Manage. 2008;36:424–441.

92. Tarpy SP, Celli BR. Long-term oxygen therapy. N Engl J Med. 1995;333:710–714.

93. Uronis H, McCrory DC, Samsa GP, Currow DC, Abernathy AP. Palliative oxygen for non-hypoxaemic chronic obstructive pulmonary disease (Protocol). Cochrane Database Syst Rev. 2008;3:1–7.

94. Cranston JM, Crockett A, Currow D. Oxygen therapy for dyspnoea in adults (Review). Cochrane Database Syst Rev. 2008;3:1–54.

95. Philip J, Gold M, Milner A, Di Iulio J, Miller B, Spruyt O. A randomized, double-blind, crossover trial of the effect of oxygen on dyspnea in patients with advanced cancer. J Pain Symptom Manage. 2006;32:541–550.

96. Uronis HAAP. Oxygen for relief of dyspnea: what is the evidence? Curr Opin Support Palliat Care. 2008;2:89–94.

97. Abernethy AP, McDonald CF, Frith PA, et al. Effect of palliative oxygen versus room air in relief of breathlessness in patients with refractory dyspnoea: a double-blind, randomised controlled trial. Lancet. 2010;376:784–793.

98. Campbell ML, Yarandi H, Dove-Medows E. Oxygen is nonbeneficial for most patients who are near death. J Pain Symptom Manage. 2013;45:517–523.

99. DC Currow, M Agar, J Smith, AP Abernethy. Does palliative home oxygen improve dyspnoea? A consecutive cohort study. Palliat Med. 2009;23:309–316.

100. Bausewein C, Booth S, Higginson GM. Non-pharmacological interventions for breathlessness in advanced stages of malignant and non-malignant diseases (Review). Cochrane Database Syst Rev. 2008;1–22.

101. Schwartzstein RM, Lahive K, Pope A, Weinberger SE, Weiss JW. Cold facial stimulation reduces breathlessness induced in normal subjects. Am Rev Respir Dis. 1987;136:58–61.

102. Burgess KR, Whitelaw WA. Effects of nasal cold receptors on pattern of breathing. J Appl Physiol. 1988;64:371–376.

103. Burgess KR, Whitelaw WA. Reducing ventilatory response to carbon dioxide by breathing cold air. Am Rev Respir Dis. 1984;129:687–690.

104. Galbraith S, Fagan P, Perkins P, Lynch A, Booth S. Does the use of a handheld fan improve chronic dyspnea? A randomized, controlled, crossover trial. J Pain Symptom Manage. 2010;39:831–838.

105. Barach AL. Chronic obstructive lung disease: postural relief of dyspnea. Arch Phys Med Rehabil. 1974;55:494–504.

106. Sharp JT, Drutz WS, Moisan T, Foster J, Machnach W. Postural relief of dyspnea in severe chronic obstructive pulmonary disease. Am Rev Respir Dis. 1980;122:201–211.

107. Thoman RL, Stoker GL, Ross JC. The efficacy of pursed-lips breathing in patients with chronic obstructive pulmonary disease. Am Rev Respir Dis. 1966;93:100–106.

108. Make B. COPD: management and rehabilitation. Am Fam Physician. 1991;43:1315–1324.

109. Corner J, Plant H, A'Hern R, Bailey C. Non-pharmacological intervention for breathlessness in lung cancer. Palliat Med. 1996; 10:299–305.

110. Carrieri VK, Janson-Bjerklie S. Strategies patients use to manage the sensation of dyspnea. West J Nurs Res. 1986;8:284–305.

111. van den Berg R. Dyspnea: perception or reality. CACCN. 1995;6:16–19.

112. Moody LE, Fraser M, Yarandi H. Effects of guided imagery in patients with chronic bronchitis and emphysema. Clin Nurs Res. 1993;2:478–486.

113. Giasson M, Bouchard L. Effect of therapeutic touch on the well-being of persons with terminal cancer. J Holist Nurs. 1998;16:383–398.

114. Shih F, Chu S. Comparisons of American-Chinese and Taiwanese patients' perceptions of dyspnea and helpful nursing actions during the intensive care unit transition from cardiac surgery. Heart Lung. 1999;28:41–54.

115. Tiep BL. Inpatient pulmonary rehabilitation: A team approach to the more fragile patient. Postgrad Med. 1989;86:141–150.

116. Grey A. The nursing management of dyspnoea in palliative care. Nurs Times. 1995;91:33–35.

117. Back IN, Jenkins K, Blower A, Beckhelling J. A study comparing hyoscine hydrobromide and glycopyrrolate in the treatment of death rattle. Palliat Med. 2001;15:329–336.

118. Watts T, Jenkins K. Palliative care nurses' feelings about death rattle. J Clin Nurs. 1999;8:615–616.

119. Wildiers H, Menten J. Death rattle: prevalence, prevention and treatment. J Pain Symptom Manage. 2002;23:310–317.

120. Hughes AC, Wilcock A, Corcoran R. Management of death rattle. J Pain Symptom Manage. 1996;12:271–272.

121. Ellershaw JE, Sutcliffe JM, Saunders CM. Dehydration and the dying patient. J Pain Symptom Manage. 1995;10:192–197.

122. Morita T, Ichiki T, Tsunoda J, Inoue S, Chihara S. A prospective study on the dying process in terminally ill cancer patients. Am J Hosp Palliat Care. 1998;15:217–222.

123. Kass RM, Ellershaw JE. Respiratory tract secretions in the dying patient: a retrospective study. J Pain Symptom Manage. 2003;26:897–902.

124. Morita T, Tsunoda J, Inoue S, Chihara S. Risk factors for death rattle in terminally ill cancer patients: a prospective exploratory study. Palliat Med. 2000;14:19–23.

125. Morita T, Hyodo I, Yoshima T et al. Incidence and underlying etiologies of bronchial secretion in terminally ill cancer patients: a multicenter, prospective, observational study. J Pain Symptom Manage. 2004;27:533–539.

126. Bennett MI. Death rattle: an audit of hyoscine (scopolamine) use and review of management. J Pain Symptom Manage. 1996;12:229–233.

127. Hall P, Schroder C, Weaver L. The last 48 hours of life in long-term care: a focused chart audit. J Am Geriatr Soc. 2002;50:501–506.

128. Wee BL, Coleman PG, Hillier R, Holgate ST. Death rattle: its impact on staff and volunteers in palliative care. Palliat Med. 2008;22:173–176.

129. Wee BL, Coleman PG, Hillier R, Holgate SH. The sound of death rattle, I: Are relatives distressed by hearing this sound? Palliat Med. 2006;20:171–175.

130. Wee BL, Coleman PG, Hillier R, Holgate SH. The sound of death rattle, II: How do relatives interpret the sound? Palliat Med. 2006;20:177–181.

131. Nadel JA. Regulation of airway secretions. Chest. 1985;87:111S–113S.

132. Kaliner M, Shelhamer H, Borson B, Nadel JA, Patow C, Marom Z. Human respiratory mucus. Am Rev Respir Dis. 1986;134:612–621.

133. Victoria Hospice Society. Medical Care of the Dying, 3rd ed. Victoria, BC: Victoria Hospice Society, 1998.

134. Andrews MR, Levine AM. Dehydration in the terminal patient: perception of hospice nurses. Am J Hosp Care. 1989;6:31–34.

135. Downing M. Victoria Respiratory Congestion Scale. Victoria, BC: Victoria Hospice. 2004.

136. Wee B, Hillier R. Interventions for noisy breathing in patient near to death. Cochrane Database Syst Rev. 2012;1:CD005177

137. Wildiers H, Dhaenekint C, Demeulenaere P, et al. Atropine, hyoscine butylbromide, or scopolamine are equally effective for the treatment of death rattle in terminal care. J Pain Symptom Manage. 2009;38:124–133.

138. Hughes A, Wilcock A, Corcoran R, Lucas V, King A. Audit of three antimuscarinic drugs for managing retained secretions. Palliat Med. 2000;14:221–222.

139. Promer E. Anticholinergics in palliative medicine: an update. Am J Hosp Palliat Care. 2012 Sep 9. Epub ahead of print.

140. Lichter I, Hunt E. The last 48 hours of life. J Palliat Care. 1990;6:7–15.

141. Heisler M, Hamilton G, Chengalaram A, Koceja T, Gerkin R. Randomized double-blind trial of sublingual atropine vs. placebo for the management of death rattle. J Pain Symptom Manage. 2013;45:14–22.

142. Murtagh FEM, Thorns A, Oliver DJ. Correspondence: hyoscine and glycopyrrolate for death rattle. Palliat Med. 2002;16:449–450.

143. Dawson HR. The use of transdermal scopolamine in the control of death rattle. J Palliat Care. 1989;5:31–33.

144. Morice AH, Kastelik JA. Cough 1: chronic cough in adults. Thorax. 2003;58:901–907.

145. Muers MF, Round CE. Palliation of symptoms in non-small cell lung cancer: a study by the Yorkshire Regional Cancer Organisation thoracic group. Thorax. 1993;48:339–343.

146. Molassiotis A, Lowe M, Ellis J et al. The experience of cough in patients diagnosed with lung cancer. Support Care Cancer. 2011;19:1997–2004.

147. Kvale PA, Simoff M, Prakash UBS. Palliative Care. Chest. 2003;123:284S–311S.

148. Fuller RW, Jackson DM. Physiology and treatment of cough. Thorax. 1990;45:425–430.

149. Harle A, Blackhall F, Smith J, Molassiotis A. Understanding cough and its managment in lung cancer. Curr Opin Support Palliat Care.2013;6:153–162.

150. Lalloo UG, Barnes PJ, Chung KF. Pathophysiology and clinical presentations of cough. J Allergy Clin Immunol. 1996;98:S91–S97.

151. Morice AH, McGarvey L, Pavord I. Recommendations for the management of cough in adults. Thorax. 2006;61:i1–i24.

152. Dudgeon D, Rosenthal S. Pathophysiology and assessment of dyspnea in the patient with cancer. In: Portenoy RK, Bruera E (eds.), Topics in Palliative Care. New York: Oxford University Press; 1999:237–254.

153. Ripamonti C, Fusco F. Respiratory problems in advanced cancer. Support Care Cancer. 2002;10:204–216.

154. Wee B, Browning J, Adams A et al. Management of chronic cough in patients receiving palliative care: review of evidence and recommendations by a task group of the Association for Palliative Medicine of Great Britain and Ireland. Palliat Med. 2012;26:780–787.

155. Molassiotis A, Bailey C, Caress A, Brunton L, Smith J. Interventions for cough in cancer (Review). Cochrane Database Syst Rev. 2010;9:1–8.

156. Young EC, Smith JA. Pharmacologic therapy for cough. Curr Opin Pharmacol. 2011;11:224–230.

157. Hagen NA. An approach to cough in cancer patients. J Pain Symptom Manage. 1991;6:257–262.

158. Lowry R, Wood A, Johnson T, Higenbottam T. Antitussive properties of inhaled bronchodilators on induced cough. Chest. 1988;93:1186–1189.

159. Louie K, Bertolino M, Fainsinger R. Management of intractable cough. J Palliat Care. 1992;8:46–48.

160. Howard P, Cayton RM, Brennan SR, Anderson PB. Lignocaine aerosol and persistent cough. Br J Dis Chest. 1977;71:19–24.

161. Sanders RV, Kirkpatrick MB. Prolonged suppression of cough after inhalation of lidocaine in a patient with sarcoid. JAMA. 1984;252:2456–2457.

162. Cowcher K, Hanks GW. Long-term management of respiratory symptoms in advanced cancer. J Pain Symptom Manage. 1990;5:320–330.

163. Dudgeon D, Rosenthal S. Pathophysiology and treatment of cough. Topics in Palliative Care. 2000;4:237–254.

CHAPTER 15

Urinary tract disorders

Mikel Gray and Terran Sims

Cancer is terrifying, but this leakage is what I find to be the most humiliating. How am I supposed to live if I am constantly wet, never sure when the leakage will occur, and never sure whether others around me know that I am wearing this diaper.

A patient

Key points

- The urinary system is frequently the cause of bothersome or deleterious symptoms that affect the patient receiving palliative care.

- A malignancy or systemic disease may affect lower urinary tract function with urinary incontinence, urinary retention, or upper urinary tract obstruction.

- Common lower urinary tract symptoms (LUTS) include urinary incontinence, daytime voiding frequency, nocturia, urgency, feelings of incomplete bladder emptying, and incomplete bladder emptying.

- Upper urinary tract symptoms include flank or abdominal pain and constitutional symptoms related to acute renal insufficiency or failure.

- Significant hematuria leading to clot formation and catheter blockage is an uncommon but significant complication of pelvic radiation therapy. Hematuria may occur months to years following radiotherapy.

- Initial treatment of hematuria includes continuous bladder irrigation to evacuate clots from the bladder vesicle until the fragile bladder wall heals. If hematuria recurs, more aggressive treatment options include intravesical alum or prostaglandins. Intravesical formalin treatments are reserved for very severe cases of blood loss.

- Overactive detrusor contractions (sometimes referred to as bladder spasms) may be associated with urinary tract infection or catheter blockage, or they may be idiopathic. Any apparent underlying cause of bladder spasms, such as a urinary tract infection, should be treated initially.

- An antimuscarinic medication should be used for long-term relief of bladder spasms. Extended-release or transdermal agents are usually preferred because of their favorable side-effect profiles and avoidance of the need for frequent dosing. However, immediate-release agents may be administered if bladder spasms prove refractory to extended-release formulations.

- Indwelling catheterization is a viable option for managing urine elimination in the patient who is near death and has urinary retention, or when pain or immobility significantly impairs the ability to urinate. A suprapubic catheter may be used as an alternative to urethral catheterization after urethral trauma or in the presence of urethral obstruction in cases of urethral injury, strictures, prostate obstruction, after gynecological surgery, or for long-term catheterization.

In many ways, the techniques used for management of urinary symptoms are similar to those used for patients in any care setting. However, in contrast to traditional interventions, the evaluation and management of urinary tract symptoms in the palliative care setting are influenced by considerations of the goals of care and proximity to death.

Urinary system disorders may be directly attributable to a malignancy, systemic disease, or a specific treatment such as radiation or chemotherapy. This chapter provides an overview of the anatomy and physiology of the urinary system, which serves as a framework for understanding of the pathophysiology of bothersome symptoms and their management. This is followed by a review of commonly encountered urinary symptoms seen in the palliative care setting, including bothersome LUTS, lower urinary tract pain, urinary stasis or retention, and hematuria.

Lower urinary tract disorders

Lower urinary tract physiology

The lower urinary tract comprises the bladder, urethra, and supportive structures within the pelvic floor (Figures 15.1 and 15.2). Together, these structures maintain *urinary continence*, which can be simply defined as control over bladder filling and storage and the act of micturition. Continence is modulated by three interrelated factors: (1) anatomical integrity of the urinary tract, (2) control of the detrusor muscle, and (3) competence of the urethral sphincter mechanism.[1,2] Each may be compromised in the patient receiving palliative care, leading to bothersome LUTS, urinary retention, or a combination of these disorders.

Anatomical integrity

From a physiological perspective, the urinary system comprises a long tube originating in the glomerulus and terminating at the urethral meatus. When contemplating urinary continence, anatomical integrity of the urinary system is often assumed, particularly because extraurethral urinary incontinence (UI) is uncommon.

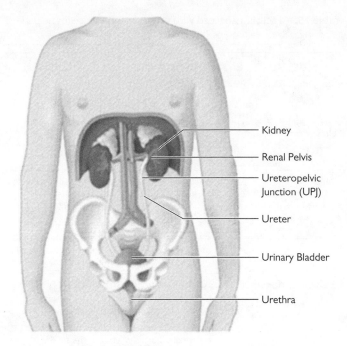

Figure 15.1 The female urinary tract.

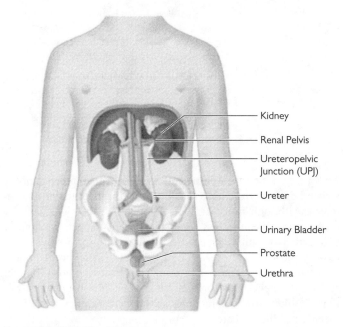

Figure 15.2 The male urinary tract.

However, anatomical integrity may be lost in the patient receiving palliative care when a fistula bypasses the urethral sphincter and opens into the vaginal vault or skin. This epithelialized tract allows continuous urinary leakage, which varies from an ongoing dribble in a patient with otherwise normal urine elimination habits to total UI characterized by failure of bladder storage.

Control of the detrusor

In addition to a structurally intact urinary system, continence requires volitional control over detrusor contractions.[1,2] Control of this smooth muscle can be conceptualized on three levels.

Multiple modulatory centers within the central nervous system modulate lower urinary tract function, ensuring low-pressure bladder filling and micturition only when the person wishes to urinate. Detrusor control is also influenced by the histological characteristics of the detrusor muscle and on a molecular level by neurotransmitters released within the neuromuscular junction.

The nervous control of the detrusor arises from multiple modulatory areas within the brain and spinal cord.[3] Bilateral modulatory centers are found in the cerebral cortex; they are involved with bladder filling and storage, and more recent evidence suggests that they play a more active role in the decision to urinate than previously thought.[4] These modulatory centers interact with neurons in the thalamus,[5] hypothalamus,[6] basal ganglia,[7] and cerebellum[8] to modulate bladder filling and voiding. Data from functional MRI and PET scans reveal that each of these areas is involved with bladder filling and/or micturition, leading to new questions and new insights into the relationships between cognition, emotional state, mood, and LUTS.[3,4] Whereas modulatory centers within the brain are essential for continence, the primary integration centers for bladder filling and micturition are found within the brainstem.[9] Specific areas within the brainstem control bladder filling and storage under the influence of higher brain regions. These areas include the periaqueductal gray matter, which is responsible for coordinating multiple groups of neurons in the brainstem; the L and M regions within the pons, which modulate bladder filling and initiate the detrusor contraction; and the pontine micturition center, which coordinates the reflexive response of the urethral sphincter mechanism. Recognition of the significance of the brainstem micturition center is particularly important when providing palliative care, because a neurological lesion above the brainstem causes urge UI with a coordinated sphincter response, whereas lesions below this center affect bladder sensations and the coordination between the detrusor and the urethral sphincter, resulting in reflex UI.

The brainstem micturition center communicates with the bladder via spinal roots in the thoracolumbar and sacral segments.[3] Neurons in the thoracolumbar spine (T10–L2) transmit sympathetic nervous impulses that promote bladder filling and storage, whereas neurons in spinal segments S2–S4 transmit parasympathetic impulses to the bladder wall, promoting micturition under the influence of the brain and brainstem. These impulses are carried through several peripheral nerve plexuses, including the pelvic and inferior hypogastric plexuses.

Histological characteristics of the detrusor also contribute to its voluntary control.[10] Unlike the visceral smooth muscle of the bowel, stomach, or ureter, the detrusor muscle bundles are innervated on an almost one-to-one basis, reflecting the critical importance of the neurological modulation described above. The smooth muscle bundles of the detrusor also lack gap junctions, observed in other visceral organs, which allow propagation of a contraction independent of nervous stimulation. These characteristics promote urinary continence because they discourage spontaneous contractions of the detrusor in response to bladder filling, as is characteristic of other visceral organs.

On a molecular level, specific chemical substances, commonly called neurotransmitters, exert local control over the detrusor muscle.[2] Several neurotransmitters are released from the axons of neurons within the bladder wall and act at specific receptors to produce smooth muscle contraction or relaxation.

Norepinephrine acts through β_3-adrenergic receptors, promoting detrusor muscle relaxation, and acetylcholine acts through muscarinic receptors, leading to detrusor contraction and micturition. Although it has long been known that the cholinergic receptors within the detrusor are muscarinic, physiological studies have identified at least five muscarinic receptor subtypes (M1 through M5) in the human body.[11] Two receptor subtypes, M2 and M3, are believed to predominate within the bladder wall and are primarily responsible for the detrusor contraction that leads to micturition.[12] Identification of these receptor subtypes is clinically relevant because it has facilitated the development of drugs that act on the bladder but produce fewer central nervous system side effects than the older (nonselective) drugs traditionally used to manage urge UI or bladder spasms.

Competence of the urethral sphincter mechanism

The urethral sphincter is a combination of compressive and tension elements that form a watertight seal against urinary leakage, even when challenged by physical exertion or sudden increases in abdominal pressure caused by coughing, laughing, or sneezing.[1,2] The soft urethral mucosa interacts with secretions produced by the urothelium (glycosaminoglycans) and the submucosal vascular cushion to ensure a watertight seal that rapidly conforms to dramatic changes in the urethral lumen such as insertion of a catheter. Whereas the elements of compression provide a watertight seal for the urethra, striated and smooth muscle within the urethral wall and within the surrounding pelvic floor are necessary when sphincter closure is challenged by physical exertion. The muscular elements of the urethral sphincter include the smooth muscle of the bladder neck and proximal urethra (including the prostatic urethra in men), the rhabdosphincter, and the periurethral striated muscles. The α_1-adrenergic receptors in the smooth muscle of the bladder neck and proximal urethra promote sphincter closure when exposed to the neurotransmitter norepinephrine.[13] Innervation of the rhabdosphincter is more complex. Acetylcholine acts on nicotinic receptors in the rhabdosphincter to stimulate muscle contraction. In addition, norepinephrine and serotonin (5HT) act on neurons within Onuf's nucleus (located at sacral spinal segments 2 through 4), modulating rhabdosphincter tone during bladder filling and storage.[14]

Pathophysiology of urinary incontinence

Urinary incontinence is defined as the uncontrolled loss of urine of sufficient magnitude to create a problem.[15] It can be divided into two types, transient (acute) and chronic, based on onset and underlying etiology.[16] Factors resulting in transient UI clearly contribute to urinary leakage, but they often arise from outside the lower urinary tract. Therefore, treatment of transient UI is typically aimed at the contributing factor, rather than the urinary system itself. Several conditions associated with transient UI are commonly encountered when caring for patients in a palliative care setting; they include delirium, urinary tract infection, adverse side effects of various drugs, restricted mobility, and severe constipation or stool impaction (Table 15.1).

Chronic UI is subdivided into types according to its presenting symptoms and underlying pathophysiology.[16] Stress UI occurs when physical stress (exertion) causes urine loss in the absence of a detrusor contraction. Two conditions lead to stress UI—urethral hypermobility (descent of the bladder base during physical

Table 15.1 Factors associated with urinary incontinence in the patient receiving palliative care

Associated factor	Effect on continence
Delirium, confusion	Reduces patient's ability to recognize and respond to cues to urinate, resulting in daytime or nighttime UI episodes.
Urinary tract infection	May exacerbate or create transient UI, especially in patients with history of UI or overactive bladder dysfunction.
Various drugs	Multiple classes of drugs predispose vulnerable patients to UI; diuretics increase urine production, potentially increasing frequency and risk for overactive detrusor contractions; antidepressants, sedatives, sleeping medications, or opioid analgesics may reduce the individual's ability to detect or respond to cues to toilet.
Excessive urine output	Polyuria associated with diabetes mellitus, diabetes insipidus, chronic venous disease, chronic heart failure, renal insufficiency, or high-volume fluid intake increases urine production, potentially increasing voiding frequency and risk for overactive detrusor contractions.
Restricted mobility	Immobility, secondary to pain as a direct result of a disease process affecting neuromuscular function, impairs the individual's ability to respond to cues to toilet and to access toilet facilities.
Constipation or stool impaction	The exact mechanism is unknown; distention of the rectal vault may reduce bladder capacity and cause functional obstruction by reflex increase in pelvic floor muscle tone, as the vault fills with stool.

activity) and intrinsic sphincter deficiency (incompetence of the striated or smooth muscle within the urethral sphincter mechanism). Although urethral hypermobility is rarely the primary cause of significant stress UI in the patient receiving palliative care, intrinsic sphincter deficiency may compromise sphincter closure and lead to severe urinary leakage. Intrinsic sphincter deficiency occurs when the nerves or muscles necessary for sphincter closure are denervated or damaged.[17] Box 15.1 lists conditions that are likely to cause intrinsic sphincter deficiency in patients receiving palliative care.

Urge UI occurs when overactive detrusor contractions produce urinary leakage (Table 15.2).[16] Urge UI is part of a larger symptom syndrome called *overactive bladder*. Overactive bladder is characterized by urgency (a sudden desire to urinate that is difficult to defer), and it is typically associated with daytime voiding frequency (more than every 2 hours) and nocturia (≥ 3 episodes per night). Reflex UI, in contrast, is caused by a neurological lesion below the brainstem micturition center.[18] It is characterized by diminished or absent sensations of bladder filling, neurogenic overactive detrusor contractions associated with urinary leakage, and a loss of coordination between the detrusor and sphincter muscles (detrusor-sphincter dyssynergia).

Functional UI occurs when long-standing deficits in mobility, dexterity, or cognition cause or contribute to urinary leakage.

Box 15.1 Causes of intrinsic sphincter deficiency in the patient receiving palliative care

Urethral surgery

Radical prostatectomy

Transurethral prostatectomy

Cryosurgery

Suburethral sling surgery for stress UI in women

Surgery indirectly affecting the urethra via local denervation

Abdominoperineal resection

Pelvic exenteration

Radical hysterectomy

Neurological lesions of the lower spine

Primary or metastatic tumors of the sacral spine

Pathological fracture of the sacral spinal column

Multiple sclerosis

Tertiary syphilis

Table 15.2 Conditions associated with detrusor overactivity in the patient receiving palliative care

Condition	Disorder
Neurological lesions above the brainstem micturition center	(Overactive bladder, with or without urge UI) Posterior fossa tumors causing intracranial pressure increased
Primary or metastatic tumors of the spinal segments	Cerebrovascular accident (stroke)
	Diseases affecting the brain, including multiple sclerosis, AIDS
Neurological lesions below the brainstem micturition center but above sacral spinal segments	Reflex UI with vesicosphincter dyssynergia
	Primary or metastatic tumors of the spinal cord
	Tumors causing spinal cord compression because of their effects on the spinal column
	Systemic diseases directly affecting the spinal cord, including advanced-stage AIDS, transverse myelitis, Guillain-Barré syndrome
Inflammation of the bladder	(Overactive bladder, with or without urge UI)
	Primary bladder tumors, including papillary tumors or carcinoma in situ
	Bladder calculi (stones)
	Radiation cystitis, including brachytherapy
	Chemotherapy-induced cystitis
Bladder outlet obstruction	(Overactive bladder usually without urge UI)
	Prostatic carcinoma
	Urethral cancers
	Pelvic tumors causing urethral compression

AIDS, acquired immunodeficiency syndrome; UI, urinary incontinence.

A variety of conditions may produce functional UI in the patient receiving palliative care. For example, neurological deficits or pain may reduce the patient's ability to reach the toilet in a timely fashion. Cognitive deficits caused by malignancies or diseases of the brain may predispose the patient to functional UI. In addition, sedative or analgesic medications may reduce awareness of bladder fullness and the need to urinate, particularly in the patient who experiences nocturia. Recently, a wound, ostomy, and continence nurse practitioner worked with the US Centers for Medicare and Medicaid Services to define an ICD-9 code for functional incontinence, which will be particularly useful for palliative care nurses providing services for this common cause of urinary leakage.[19]

Extraurethral UI occurs when a fistula creates an opening between the bladder and the vagina or skin, allowing urine to bypass the urethral sphincter. Within the context of palliative care, fistulas are usually caused by invasive pelvic or gynecological malignancies, extensive pelvic surgery, or radiation treatment.

Bladder spasm

Bladder spasms may be defined as a painful contraction of the bladder. Their pathophysiology is not well understood, but they are probably caused by an overactive detrusor contraction against a closed or partially blocked bladder outlet.[20] Patients with bladder outlet obstruction due to a urological malignancy obstructing the bladder outlet, or secondary blockage from a tumor outside the urinary tract, are at risk for bladder spasm. Foreign objects within the urinary tract, such as indwelling urinary catheters or ureteral stents, are also associated with an increased risk for bladder spasm, presumably because of their irritative effect on the urinary mucosa.[21] Instillation of potentially caustic substances into the bladder to treat significant hematuria or a urothelial tumor, or recent urological surgery also may result in bladder spasm owing to their irritative effects.[22,23]

Assessment and management of bothersome lower urinary tract symptoms

The results of a focused history, physical assessment, urinalysis, and bladder log are essential for the evaluation of UI in the patient receiving palliative care. Urine culture and sensitivity testing, blood tests, urodynamic evaluation, or imaging studies also may be completed in specific cases.

The history focuses on the duration of the problem and the probable cause of bothersome LUTS. *Transient* UI is typically characterized by a sudden occurrence of urinary leakage or an acute exacerbation of preexisting symptoms. These symptoms are typically similar to those of urge or stress UI. In contrast, chronic or established UI usually evolves over a period of time, typically months or possibly years.

The history can also be used to provide clues about the type of chronic UI. Stress UI is characterized by urine loss occurring with physical exertion or a sudden increase in abdominal pressure caused by coughing or sneezing. It occurs in the absence of a precipitous and strong urge to urinate. Approximately 36% of patients with overactive bladder syndrome experience urge UI.[24] (The diagnosis of overactive bladder is based on a combination of symptoms: diurnal voiding frequency, nocturia, and urgency with or without the symptom of urge UI).[25] A diagnosis of overactive bladder cannot be inferred from a report of the symptom of urge UI alone.

Reflex UI is suspected in the patient who experiences a paralyzing neurological lesion that affects spinal segments below the brainstem and above S2.[18] The patient frequently reports periodic urination with little or no warning and little or no associated urgency. The urinary stream may be intermittent (stuttering), and the patient may perceive a sensation of incomplete bladder emptying or report additional urinary leakage soon after completion of micturition.

Bladder spasms are diagnosed when a patient reports painful episodes localized to the suprapubic or lower abdomen.[21,26] These pains are usually characterized by a sudden onset and described as stabbing, cramping, or colicky. They are often associated with urgency and may produce bypassing of urine around an indwelling urinary catheter or urethral leakage if a suprapubic catheter is in place.

Functional UI is suspected when a general evaluation of the patient reveals significant limitations in mobility, dexterity, or cognition.[27] Continuous urinary leakage that is not associated with physical exertion raises the suspicion of extraurethral UI associated with a fistula, but it is also associated with severe stress UI caused by intrinsic sphincter deficiency. A focused physical examination provides additional evidence concerning the UI type and its severity. A general examination is used to evaluate the presence of functional UI and to determine the influence of functional limitations on other types of UI. A pelvic examination is completed to assess perineal skin integrity, to identify the presence of obvious fistulas or severe sphincter incompetence, and to evaluate local neurological function. Altered skin integrity, particularly if accompanied by a monilial rash or incontinence-associated dermatitis may occur, especially in patents with double fecal and urinary incontinence.[28] In certain cases, the source of severe leakage can be easily identified as a large fistula or severe intrinsic sphincter deficiency associated with a gaping (patulous) urethra. A local neurological examination, focusing on local sensations, pelvic floor muscle tone, and the presence of the bulbocavernosus reflex, provides clues to underlying neurological problems leading to voiding dysfunction.

A bladder log (a written record of the timing of urination, voided volume, timing of UI episodes, and fluid intake) is useful because it allows a semiquantitative analysis of the patterns of urinary elimination, UI, and associated symptoms. It can also be used to assess fluid intake or the patient's response to prompted voiding.[29] The patient is taught to record the time of voluntary urination, episodes of incontinence and associated factors (urgency, physical activity), and type and amount of fluids consumed. This record is used to determine voiding interval, frequency of UI episodes along with associated factors, and the total volume and types of fluids consumed. Recording fluid intake allows the nurse to calculate the cumulative volume of fluids consumed each day, as well as the proportion of fluids containing caffeine or alcohol—substances that exacerbate bothersome LUTS. A 3-day bladder log is strongly recommended, but valuable information can be obtained from a 1- or 2-day document if a 3-day record is not available.[30]

Urinalysis serves several useful purposes in the evaluation of the patient with UI. The presence of nitrites and leukocytes on dipstick analysis or bacteriuria and pyuria on microscopic analysis may indicate a clinically relevant urinary tract infection. Blood in the urine may coexist with a urinary tract infection, or it may indicate significant hematuria demanding prompt management (see later discussion). In the patient receiving palliative care, glucosuria may indicate poorly controlled diabetes mellitus causing osmotic diuresis and subsequent UI. In contrast, a low specific gravity may indicate diabetes mellitus or excessive fluid intake from oral or parenteral sources.

Other diagnostic tests are completed when indicated. For example, a urine culture and sensitivity analysis is obtained if the urinalysis reveals bacteriuria and pyuria, and an endoscopy is indicated if significant hematuria is present without an obvious explanation. Urodynamic testing is indicated in selected patients after transient UI is excluded and when simpler examinations have failed to establish an accurate diagnosis leading to an effective plan for management.

The management of UI is based on its type, the desires of the patient and family, and the presence of complicating factors. Transient UI is managed by addressing its underlying cause.[31] Acute delirium is managed by treating the underlying infection of disease causing the delirium, if feasible. A urinary tract infection is treated with sensitivity-driven antibiotics. Similarly, medication regimens are altered as feasible if they produce or exacerbate UI. Fecal impaction must be relieved and constipation aggressively managed. After initial disimpaction, a scheduled elimination program is frequently indicated. This program usually combines a peristaltic stimulant, such as a warm cup of coffee or tea, a mini-enema, or a suppository, and a scheduled elimination program. In addition, stool softeners or laxatives may be used if simpler programs fail to alleviate constipation. These interventions are combined with increased fluid intake as indicated and addition of fiber to the diet whenever feasible. Refer to chapter 12 for a detailed discussion of bowel elimination problems.

A number of techniques are used to manage chronic or established UI. Every patient should be counseled about lifestyle alterations that may alleviate or occasionally relieve UI and associated LUTS.[32,33] Patients are advised to avoid routinely restricting fluid intake to reduce UI, because this strategy only increases the risk of constipation and concentrates the urine, irritating the bladder wall. Instead, they should be counseled to obtain the recommended daily allowance for fluids (1.5–2.3 liters in adults; 1.2–2.3 liters in adults > 70 years of age),[34] to sip fluids throughout the day, and to avoid intake of large volumes of fluids over a brief period. Patients may also be taught to reduce or avoid bladder irritants that increase urine production or stimulate increased detrusor muscle tone, including caffeine and alcohol, depending on the goals of care and the short-term prognosis.

Containment devices may be used to provide protection while treatments designed to address underlying UI are undertaken, or they may be used for added protection if these interventions improve but fail to eradicate urine loss.[35] Women and men should be counseled about the disadvantages of using home products and feminine hygiene pads when attempting to contain urine.

Specifically, they should be counseled that home products, such as tissues or paper towels, are not designed to contain urine, and feminine hygiene products are designed to contain menstrual flow. As an alternative, patients should be advised about products specifically designed for UI, including disposable and reusable products, inserted pads, and containment briefs.

If the patient experiences primarily stress UI, the initial management is with behavioral methods, often combined with use of absorptive products. Pelvic floor muscle training is strongly recommended for mild to moderate stress UI,[36] but its applicability in the palliative care setting is limited. Instead, the patient may be taught a maneuver called the "knack." The knack describes a pelvic floor muscle contraction completed in response to physical exertion.[37] The patient is taught to identify, contract, and relax the pelvic floor muscles, typically using some form of biofeedback. Biofeedback provides sensory, audible, or palpatory cues allowing the patient to identify the pelvic floor muscles, and to differentiate contraction of these muscles from the abdominals, gluteal, or thigh muscles. Simple biofeedback maneuvers include assisting the patient to identify the pelvic floor muscles during a gentle vaginal or digital rectal examination, asking the patient to interrupt the urinary stream, or asking the patient to contract and relax while seated on a chair with a firm seat in order to maximize proprioception. After learning to identify, contract, and relax the pelvic floor muscles, the patient is taught to maximally contract (squeeze) these muscles when performing a maneuver associated with urine loss such as coughing, sneezing, walking, or bending over to don socks. This maneuver increases urethral closure and resistance to UI and relieves or prevents stress UI. It is generally preferred in the palliative care setting because it provides some relief from stress UI within a comparatively brief period of time (usually within days to a week) as compared to more formalized pelvic floor muscle training requiring 3–6 months.

Medications also may be used to treat stress UI in selected cases. Imipramine, a tricyclic antidepressant with both α-adrenergic effects that increase urethral resistance and anticholinergic actions, may be useful for patients who experience stress UI or mixed stress and urge UI symptoms.[38] Duloxetine, a norepinephrine and serotonin reuptake inhibitor, acts on neurons in Onuf's nucleus—nuclei located in spinal segments S2–4 that modulate rhabdosphincter tone in women and men—and has been found to relieve stress UI in women.[39] Duloxetine has been approved by the US Food and Drug Administration (FDA) for treatment of depression, but not stress UI, and its use for this indication is classified as off-label. Although both imipramine and duloxetine have the potential to alleviate stress UI, their benefits must be weighed carefully against the potential for adverse effects. Common side effects of imipramine include anticholinergic effects such as dry mouth, blurred vision, flushing, and heat intolerance. Imipramine also may affect the central nervous system and may be associated with short-term memory impairment, hallucinations, and nightmares. These side effects may be particularly significant in aged patients and in those with preexisting cognitive defects related to a primary tumor or disease. Common side effects of duloxetine include nausea (occurring in up to 38%), drowsiness, dry mouth, and constipation. Among patients with clinical depression, it has been associated with anxiety, agitation, anger, panic attacks, and temporary suicidal thoughts or actions.[40]

An indwelling catheter may be inserted if intrinsic sphincter deficiency and subsequent stress UI are severe. Although not usually indicated, a larger catheter size may be required to prevent urinary leakage (bypassing) around the catheter.[41] A detailed discussion of catheter management is provided later in this chapter.

Overactive bladder dysfunction, with or without urge UI, is also managed by behavioral or pharmacological modalities (or both) whenever possible.[42] Behavioral interventions include reduction or avoidance of bladder irritants such as caffeine and modification of fluid intake described previously. The patient can also be taught to identify, isolate, contract, and relax the pelvic floor muscles using principles described above. These skills are applied to a technique called *urge suppression*, which is used to inhibit specific episodes of urgency before UI occurs. When a sudden urge to urinate occurs, the patient is taught to stop, tighten the pelvic muscles in rapid succession using several "quick flick" contractions until the urge has subsided, and proceed to the bathroom at a normal pace. The patient also may be taught relaxation or other distraction techniques to cope with specific urge episodes. Behavioral methods are particularly helpful for the patient who is at risk for falling and related injuries.

Two classes of medications, antimuscarinic and β_3-adrenergic agonist medications may be used to manage overactive bladder syndrome and urge UI. Multiple agents are available. Novel agents are usually preferred because they can be taken on daily basis promoting adherence,[43] and they tend to have less pronounced adverse side effects than the older antimuscarinic agents.[42] Antimuscarinic medications block acetylcholine from binding to cholinergic receptors in the bladder wall. This increases functional bladder capacity, inhibits overactive detrusor contractions and associated incontinence episodes, and reduces voiding frequency. The principal side effect of all these agents is dry mouth, which can be severe and can interfere with appetite and mastication.[38] Other side effects include blurred vision, constipation, flushing, heat intolerance, and cognitive effects such as nightmares or altered short-term memory.

A β_3 agonist (mirabegron, Myrbetriq) has been approved by the US FDA for management of overactive bladder and urge UI.[44] This drug is the first in a new class for treating overactive bladder; it enhances the activity of the neurotransmitter norepinephrine acting at β_3 receptors within the bladder wall. Norepinephrine acts via the sympathetic nervous promote bladder filling and storage, and mirabegron has been shown to reduce detrusor overactivity,[45] voiding frequency, and number of urge UI episodes. Clinical experience is limited, but the most prevalent side effect observed during pivotal trials was hypertension observed in 5.9%; urinary tract infection, nasopharyngitis, and arrhythmia occurred in $\leq$ 4%. Table 15.3 describes pharmacological options for managing overactive bladder and urge UI and related nursing considerations.[43,44,46–49]

Although antimuscarinic medications are often viewed as an alternative to behavioral therapies, they are better viewed as complementary modalities.[50] Specifically, all patients who wish to use antimuscarinic medications for overactive bladder or urge UI should be advised to void according to a timed schedule (usually every 2 to 3 hours, depending on the urinary frequency documented on a bladder log obtained during assessment), and taught urge-suppression skills. Similarly, patients whose LUTS are not managed adequately by behavioral methods should be

Table 15.3 Pharmacological management for overactive bladder and urge urinary incontinence*

	Dosage	Nursing considerations
Antimuscarinic Drugs		
Tolterodine ER (Detrol LA)	2–4 mg daily	May be administered at night to reduce dry mouth; administration with antacid or proton pump inhibitor may reduce bioavailability of drug; does not cross blood-brain barrier as readily as oxybutynin IR; the lower (2 mg) dose is recommended for patients with impaired hepatic function.
Fesoterodine (Toviaz)	4–8 mg daily	Prodrug that is metabolized by ubiquitous esterases; metabolically active product is same as that for tolterodine; head to head trial demonstrated 8 mg dose superior to 4 mg tolterodine
Oxybutynin IR (Ditropan IR)	5 mg twice daily to three times daily	Associated with higher incidence of moderate to severe dry mouth than extended-release agents; readily crosses blood-brain barrier, potentially increasing the risk of central nervous system side effects.
Oxybutynin ER (Ditropan XL)	5–15 mg daily	Administered via osmotic releasing system; advise patient that skeleton of tablet will pass in stool 24–48 hours after ingestion; incidence and severity of dry mouth less than IR formulation; may be administered at bedtime to reduce dry mouth.
Oxybutynin TDS (Oxytrol)	3.9 mg patch twice weekly	Incidence of dry mouth not statistically different than placebo in pivotal trials; transdermal delivery systems avoids first-pass effects of oral drug formulations, increasing bioavailability of drug; local skin irritation associated with use of patch not seen with oral agents.
Oxybutynin transdermal gel (Gelnique)	Apply 1 package daily (equivalent to 10 mg daily dose)	Transdermal gel reduces likelihood of skin irritation associated with transdermal patch. Incidence of dry mouth similar to oxybutynin patch.
Solifenacin (Vesicare)	5–10 mg daily	Half-life of drug approximately 45–68 hours; may be administered at night to minimize dry mouth; use with caution in patients with impaired hepatic function
Darifenacin (Enablex)	7.5–15 mg daily	Drug has greater affinity for M3 muscarinic receptors; this receptor type is common in the bladder wall, bowel, and other peripheral organs, but absent in the central nervous system, reducing the potential for adverse central nervous system side effects; constipation rates reported in pivotal trial for this drug are higher than other drugs, possibly associated with presence of M3 receptors in bowel wall.
Trospium ER (Sactura XR)	60 mg daily	Drug is primarily excreted in urine rather than metabolized in liver, should be administered on empty stomach to maximize bioavailability; comparatively large size of trospium molecule (it is a quaternary amine) and lipophobic properties reduce likelihood drug will cross blood-brain barrier producing central nervous system side effects.
β-3 Agonist Drugs		
Mirabegron (Myrbetriq)	25–50 mg	New class of drug acts at β-3 receptors in bladder wall; avoids or reduces likelihood of specific adverse side effects of antimuscarinics such as dry mouth, flushing or blurred vision. Adverse side effects include hypertension.

* These drugs are also used for managing painful bladder spasms because of their association with detrusor overactivity.

counseled about antimuscarinic medications before placement of an indwelling catheter is considered. Nevertheless, use of a catheter is often necessary for patients managed in a palliative care setting. Traditionally, indwelling catheters have been preferred, but external collection devices often provide a viable alternative to indwelling devices in men.

Application of a condom catheter or hydrocolloid-based external collection device is indicated when urge UI is severe and refractory of other treatments.[51,52] Alternatively, an indwelling catheter may be inserted in men who are unable to wear an external device and in women. Indwelling catheterization is also indicated if urge UI is complicated by clinically relevant urinary retention or if the patient is near death and immobile. Because reflex UI is typically associated with diminished sensations of bladder filling, it is not usually responsive to behavioral treatments.[18] A minority of patients with reflex UI retain the ability to urinate spontaneously, but most cases must be managed with an alternative program. For men, an external collection device may be used to contain urine. Several devices are

available, including a hydrocolloid-based collection device.[51,52] This device attaches to the glans penis, without covering the penile shaft. Multiple condom catheters are also available. A latex-free device is typically selected, preferably with adhesive incorporated into the wall of the condom. In some patients, an α-adrenergic blocking agent such as terazosin, doxazosin, tamsulosin, or alfuzosin is administered, to minimize the obstruction caused by detrusor-sphincter dyssynergia.[53] Intermittent catheterization is encouraged whenever feasible. The patient and at least one significant other should be taught a clean intermittent catheterization technique. For the patient with reflex UI, an anticholinergic medication is usually required in addition to catheterization, to prevent UI. If intermittent catheterization is not feasible or if reflex UI develops near the end of life, an indwelling catheter may be inserted. Although the indwelling catheter is associated with serious long-term complications and is avoided in patients with spinal cord injury and a significant life expectancy, it remains a viable alternative for the patient receiving palliative care.

Functional UI is treated by minimizing barriers to toileting and the time required to prepare for urination.[54,55] Strategies designed to remove barriers to toileting are highly individualized and are best formulated with the use of a multidisciplinary team, combining nursing with medicine and physical and occupational therapy as indicated. Strategies used to maximize mobility and access to the toilet include using assistive devices such as a walker or wheelchair, widening bathroom doors, adding support bars, and providing a bedside toilet or urinal. The time required for toileting may be reduced by selected alterations in the patient's clothing, such as substituting tennis shoes with good traction for slippers or other footwear with slick soles and substituting Velcro- or elastic-banded clothing for articles with multiple buttons, zippers, or snaps.

If the patient has significant contributing cognitive disorders, functional UI is usually managed by a prompted voiding program.[56,57] Baseline evaluation includes a specialized bladder log, which is completed over a 48- to 72-hour period. The caregiver is taught to assist the patient to void on a fixed schedule, usually every 2 to 3 hours. The caregiver is taught to help the patient move to the toilet and prepare for urination; the caregiver also uses this opportunity to determine whether the pad incontinence brief reveals evidence of UI since the previous scheduled toileting. Patients who are successful, dry, and able to urinate with prompting on more than 50% of attempts completed during this trial period are considered good candidates for an ongoing prompted voiding regimen; those who are unsuccessful are considered poor candidates and are managed by alternative methods, including indwelling catheterization in highly selected cases.

Because extraurethral UI is caused by a fistulous tract and produces continuous urinary leakage, it must be managed initially by containment devices and preventive skin care. The type of containment device depends on the severity of the UI; an incontinent brief is frequently required. In some cases, the fistula may be closed by conservative (nonsurgical) means. An indwelling catheter is inserted, and the fistula is allowed to heal spontaneously.[58] This intervention is most likely to work for a traumatic (postoperative) fistula. If the fistula is a result of an invasive tumor or radiation therapy, it is not as likely to heal spontaneously. In such cases, cauterization and fibrin glue may be used to promote closure.[59] Alternatively, a suspension containing tetracycline may be prepared and used as a sclerosing agent. The adjacent skin is prepared by applying a skin protectant (such as a petrolatum, dimethicone, or zinc-oxide-based ointment) to protect it from the sclerosing agent. Approximately 5 to 10 mL of the tetracycline solution is injected into the fistula by a physician, and the lesion is monitored for signs of scarring and closure. If UI persists for 15 days or longer, the procedure may be repeated under the physician's direction. For larger fistulas or those that fail to respond to conservative measures, surgical repair is undertaken if feasible.

All patients who experience UI are at risk for developing incontinence-associated dermatitis (IAD), particularly when they also experience fecal incontinence and when urinary leakage is managed by an absorptive containment brief.[60] Skin damage is characterized by inflammation, often accompanied by erosion. Usually IAD is associated with burning and itching, and it increases the risk for pressure ulceration. Prevention focuses on a structured regimen of skin cleansing, moisturization, and application of a skin protectant.[61] An incontinence or perineal skin cleanser that contains a moisturizing agent such as an emollient or humectant may be selected, followed by application of an ointment-based skin protectant or alcohol-free liquid acrylate moisture barrier. Alternatively, these steps may be combined using a single use perineal cloth that combines a skin cleanser, moisturizer, and dimethicone-based skin protectant. Treatment of IAD begins with establishment of a structured skin cleansing regimen unless one is already in place. Often IAD is associated with cutaneous candidiasis, which may be treated by applying a thin layer of an antifungal powder covered by a skin protectant, or application of an ointment-based antifungal agent. An ointment containing as active ingredients Balsam Peru, castor oil, and trypsin also may be applied for IAD; this ointment combines active ingredients that promote wound healing with a skin protectant, shielding the skin from additional exposure to urine or stool.

Assessment and management of urinary stasis and retention

A precipitous drop or sudden cessation of urinary outflow is a serious urinary system complication that may indicate *oliguria* or *anuria* (failure of the kidneys to filter the blood and produce urine), *urinary stasis* (blockage of urine transport from the upper to lower urinary tracts), or *urinary retention* (failure of the bladder to evacuate itself of urine). The following sections review the pathophysiology and management of urinary stasis or acute postrenal failure caused by bilateral ureteral obstruction and urinary retention.

Obstruction of the upper urinary tract

Upper urinary tract stasis in the patient receiving palliative care is usually caused by obstruction of one or both ureters.[62] The obstruction is typically attributable to a primary or metastatic tumor, and most arise from the pelvic region. In men, prostatic cancer is the most common cause, whereas pelvic (cervical, uterine, and ovarian) malignancies produce most ureteral obstructions in women. In addition to malignancies, retroperitoneal fibrosis secondary to inflammation or radiation may obstruct one or both ureters. Unless promptly relieved, bilateral ureteral obstruction leads to acute renal failure with uremia and elevated serum potassium, which can cause life-threatening arrhythmias.

When a single ureter is obstructed, the bladder continues to fill with urine from the contralateral (unobstructed) kidney. In this case, urinary stasis produces symptoms of ureteral or renal colic. Left untreated, the affected kidney is prone to acute failure and infection, and it may produce systemic hypertension because of increased renin secretion.

Case study

VC, a 65-year-old patient with hematuria and percutaneous nephrostomy tube

VC is a 65-year-old female with hypertension, cardiac disease, and a new diagnosis of hydronephrosis. She has a high grade, advanced-stage invasive bladder cancer diagnosed at age 64 years. Due to her hydronephrosis she underwent placement of a right percutaneous nephrostomy tube. Her renal function improved and her pelvic pain was reduced. She then was able to begin neoadjuvant chemotherapy. The initial hope was that she would respond to chemotherapy and undergo cystectomy for bulky reduction of tumor.

However, after 4 cycles of chemotherapy she had progression of metastatic disease with new pulmonary metastasis and she was deemed no longer a cystectomy candidate. She underwent repeat transurethral resection of bladder tumor (TURBT) in hopes of identifying the ureteral orifice and internalizing the nephrostent. However, the tumor could not be completely resected nor could the nephrostomy tube be internalized. She elected to undergo permanent percutaneous nephrostomy tube status.

She began a routine of nephrostomy tube changes every 6–8 weeks. She did well for 2 months then began to experience additional problems associated with tumor progression. After extensive discussions with her care team, she decided to undergo palliative chemotherapy in hopes of reducing her tumor size and associated sequelae. When undergoing palliative chemotherapy for tumor progression, she again developed pelvic pain and severe gross hematuria resulting in anemia and requiring transfusion. While her energy level improved post transfusion, her hematuria continued. She then underwent repeat cystoscopy and bladder tumor fulguration. This stopped her hematuria. Pain relief was achieved through medication management.

After 4 more weeks, she elected to discontinue of palliative chemotherapy. She was referred to radiation oncology for painful bony metastasis. She achieved good pain relief of bony metastases. She also expressed a desire to receive hospice care at her home. Her family was close by to provide care. After several weeks she decided she wanted the percutaneous nephrostomy tube to be removed if at all possible owing to the discomfort it produced. The urine volume from the nephrostomy tube had gradually decreased to less that 30 mL daily, and a plan for removal was developed. The nephrostomy tube was capped by the angiography team, and a urine culture from the nephrostomy tube was obtained. Culture results and sensitivity-guided antimicrobials were prescribed to clear bacteria that had colonized the tube. She was observed for 1 week following occlusion of her nephrostomy tube; she remained free from pain or swelling around in the tube and experienced no fevers or chills during this period. She began sensitivity-guided oral antibiotics prior to her return for nephrostomy tube removal. She tolerated the removal well; she completed 5 days of the oral antibiotic. Drainage from the nephrostomy tube site gradually diminished, and no dressing was required after 4 days. She experienced less discomfort following nephrostomy tube removal and reported a significant improvement in sleep quality.

This case demonstrates the circuitous course that patients may experience with treatment of hydronephrosis and bladder cancer with a percutaneous nephrostomy tube. Her nephrostomy tube served a purpose for her trial of therapy in hopes of pursuing surgery. Relief of the hydronephrosis and flank pain improved her quality of life while she sought curative therapy. Her tube also temporarily improved her renal function so she was able to undergo potentially nephrotoxic chemotherapy. This diversion of the urine allowed the kidney to be saved but after diversion was not serving a curative purpose and she had disease progression, she sought removal. Removing a nephrostomy tube has potential issues. Since a percutaneous tract has formed often patients will have leakage if the tube is capped or experience sepsis or infection. The stepped approach to culture and capping the tube, along with administration of a short course of sensitivity-guided antibiotics enabled her to achieve her goal of tube removal for comfort purposes. While placement of a nephrostomy tube can relieve flank pain in some patients with upper urinary tract obstruction, the presence of a nephrostomy tube can be problematic if the kidney is no longer producing large volumes of urine at the end of life, when patients may be bed-bound or experiencing positional pain due to the presence of the tube and drainage system. Some patients' kidneys will not allow for tube removal due to the volume of urine created on a daily basis. Therefore, assessing output from the nephrostomy tube prior to attempting its removal is essential. Considering the goal of nephrostomy tube placement prior to starting the process is important in patients who may not be able to progress to a curative surgical option.

Urinary retention

Urinary retention is the inability to empty the urinary bladder despite micturition.[63] Acute urinary retention is an abrupt and complete inability to void. Patients are almost always aware of acute urinary retention because of the increasing suprapubic discomfort produced by bladder filling and distention and the associated anxiety. Chronic urinary retention occurs when the patient is partly able to empty the bladder by voiding but a significant volume of urine remains behind. Although no absolute cutoff point for chronic urinary retention can be defined, most clinicians agree that a residual volume of 200 mL or more deserves further evaluation.

Urinary retention is caused by two disorders: bladder outlet obstruction or deficient detrusor contraction strength. Bladder outlet obstruction occurs when intrinsic or extrinsic factors compress the urethral outflow tract. For the patient receiving palliative care, malignant tumors of the prostate, urethra, or bladder may produce anatomical obstruction of the urethra, whereas lesions affecting spinal segments below the brainstem micturition center but above the sacral spine cause functional obstruction associated with detrusor-sphincter dyssynergia.[64] In addition, brachytherapy may cause inflammation and congestion of the prostate, producing a combination of urinary retention and overactive bladder dysfunction.[65] In the patient receiving palliative care, deficient detrusor contraction strength usually occurs as a result of denervation or medication. Alternatively, it may result from histological damage to the detrusor muscle itself, usually caused by radiation therapy or by detrusor decompensation after prolonged obstruction. Neurological lesions commonly associated with deficient detrusor contraction strength include primary or metastatic tumors affecting the sacral spine or spinal column, multiple sclerosis lesions, tertiary syphilis, and diseases associated with peripheral polyneuropathies, such as advanced-stage diabetes mellitus or alcoholism. Poor detrusor contraction strength also may occur as a result of unavoidable denervation from large abdominopelvic surgeries, such as abdominoperineal resection or pelvic exenteration.

Assessment and management of upper tract obstruction and urinary retention

Accurate identification of the cause of a precipitous drop in urine output is essential, because the management of upper urinary tract obstruction versus urinary retention differ. Because both conditions cause a precipitous drop in urinary output, the LUTS reported by the patient may be similar. Patients usually report difficulty initiating urination and a dribbling, intermittent flow. In contrast, these conditions produce few or no bothersome symptoms in some instances. However, upper urinary tract obstruction is more likely to produce flank pain, whereas acute urinary retention is more likely to produce discomfort localized to the suprapubic area. The pain associated with upper urinary tract obstruction is usually localized to one or both flanks, although it may radiate to the abdomen and even to the labia or testes if the lower ureter is obstructed. Its intensity varies from moderate to intense. It typically is not relieved by changes in position, and the patient is often restless. The discomfort associated with acute urinary retention is typically localized to the suprapubic area or the lower back. The patient with acute urinary retention also may feel restless, although this perception is usually attributable to the growing and unfulfilled desire to urinate.

A focused physical examination assists the nurse to differentiate urinary retention from upper urinary tract obstruction. The patient with bilateral ureteral obstruction and acute renal failure may have systemic evidence of uremia, including nausea, vomiting, and hypertension. In some cases, obstruction may by complicated by pyelonephritis, causing a fever and chills. An abdominal assessment also should be performed. Physical assessment of the patient with upper urinary tract obstruction reveals a nondistended bladder, whereas the bladder is grossly distended and may extend above the umbilicus in the patient with acute urinary retention. Blood analysis reveals an elevated serum creatinine, blood urea nitrogen, and potassium in the patient with bilateral ureteral obstruction, but these values are typically normal in the patient with urinary retention or unilateral ureteral obstruction.[62] Ultrasonography of the kidneys and bladder reveals ureterohydronephrosis above the level of the obstruction or bladder distention in the patient with acute urinary retention.

In contrast to the patient with ureteral obstruction or acute urinary retention, many patients with chronic retention remain unaware of any problem, despite large residual volumes of 500 mL or more.[59] When present, LUTS vary and may include feelings of incomplete bladder emptying, a poor force of stream, or an intermittent urinary stream. Patients are most likely to complain of diurnal voiding frequency and excessive nocturia (often arising four times or more each night), but these symptoms are not unique to incomplete bladder emptying. Although acute renal failure is uncommon in the patient with chronic urinary retention, the serum creatinine concentration may be elevated, indicating renal insufficiency attributable to lower urinary tract pathology.

Obstruction of the upper urinary tract is initially managed by reversal of fluid and electrolyte imbalances and prompt drainage.[62] Urinary outflow can be reestablished by insertion of a ureteral stent (drainage tube extending from the renal pelvis to the bladder) via cystoscopy. A ureteral stent is preferred because it avoids the need for a percutaneous puncture and drainage bag. In the case of bilateral obstruction, a stent is placed in each ureter under endoscopic guidance; a single stent is placed if unilateral obstruction is diagnosed. The patient is advised that the stents will drain urine into the bladder. However, because the stents often produce bothersome LUTS, the patient is counseled to ensure adequate fluid intake while avoiding bladder irritants, including caffeine and alcohol. In certain cases, an antimuscarinic medication may be administered to reduce the irritative LUTS or bladder spasms that sometimes are associated with a ureteral stent. Alternatively, belladonna and opium (B&O) suppositories may be administered if painful ureteral spasms occur that are not responsive to antimuscarinic agents. The B&O suppositories contain 16.2 mg of belladonna (an anticholinergic agent) and 30–60 mg of opium (an opioid analgesic). One to 2 suppositories are administered once or twice daily. The suppository should be moistened prior to insertion and care taken to place it immediately beside the rectal wall rather than in a bolus of stool. Potential side effects include anticholinergic effects such as dry mouth and constipation, as well as sensitivity to light, drowsiness, and central nervous system depression owing to their opium content.

If the ureter is significantly scarred because of radiation therapy or distorted because of a bulky tumor, placement of a ureteral stent may not be feasible and a percutaneous nephrostomy tube may be required. The procedure may be done in an endoscopy suite or an interventional radiographic suite under local and systemic sedation or anesthesia. Unlike the ureteral stent that drains into the bladder, the nephrostomy tube is drained via a collection bag. The patient and family are taught to monitor urinary output from the bag and to secure the bag to the lower abdomen or leg in a manner that avoids kinking. The success of placement of a ureteral stent or nephrostomy tube is measured by the reduction in pain and in serum creatinine and potassium concentrations, indicating reversal of acute renal insufficiency.

Acute urinary retention is managed by prompt placement of an indwelling urinary catheter.[63,66] The patient is closely monitored as the bladder is initially drained, because of the very small risk of brisk diuresis associated with transient hyperkalemia, hematuria, hypotension, and pallor.[67] This risk may be further reduced by draining 500 mL, interrupted by a brief period during which the catheter is clamped (approximately 5 minutes), and followed by further drainage until the retained urine is evacuated. The catheter is left in place for up to 1 month, allowing the bladder to rest and recover from the overdistention typical of acute urinary retention. After this period, the bladder may be slowly filled with saline, preferably heated to body temperature, and the catheter removed.[68] The patient is allowed to urinate, and the voided volume is measured. This volume is compared with the volume infused, to estimate the residual volume, or a bladder ultrasound study can be completed to assess the residual volume. If the patient is able to evacuate the bladder successfully, the catheter is left out and the patient is taught to recognize and promptly manage acute urinary retention. If the patient is unable to urinate effectively, the catheter may be replaced or an intermittent catheterization program may be initiated, depending on the cause of the retention and the patient's ability to perform self-catheterization.

The patient with chronic urinary retention may be managed by behavioral techniques, intermittent catheterization, or an indwelling catheter.[63,66] Behavioral methods are preferred because they are noninvasive and not associated with any risk of adverse side effects. Scheduled toileting with double voiding may be used in the patient with low urinary residual volumes (approximately 200 to 400 mL). The patient is taught to attempt voiding every 3 hours while awake and to double void (urinate, wait for 3 to 5 minutes, and urinate again before leaving the bathroom). Higher urinary residual volumes and clinically relevant complications caused by urinary retention, including urinary tract infection or renal insufficiency, are usually managed by intermittent catheterization or an indwelling catheter.

Many factors enter into the choice between intermittent and indwelling catheterization, including the desires of the patient and family, the presence of an obstruction or low bladder wall compliance (e.g., a small or contracted bladder), and the prognosis. From a purely urological perspective, intermittent catheterization is preferable because it avoids long-term complications associated with an indwelling catheter, including chronic bacteriuria, calculi, urethral erosion, and catheter bypassing. However, an indwelling catheter may be preferable in a palliative care setting when the urethra is technically difficult to catheterize; the patient has a small capacity with low bladder wall compliance; the patient is experiencing significant pain or limited upper extremity dexterity that interferes with the ability to effectively evacuate the bladder via micturition; or UI is complicated by retention.

Managing the indwelling catheter

Although the decision to insert a catheter may be directed by a physician or nurse practitioner, decisions concerning catheter size, material of construction, and drainage bag are usually made by the nurse.[41,69,70] A relatively small catheter is typically sufficient to drain urine from the bladder. A 14- to 16-French catheter is adequate for men and a 12- to 14-French catheter is usually adequate for women. Larger catheters (18 to 20 French) are reserved for patients with significant intrinsic sphincter deficiency, hematuria, or sediment in the urine. Silastic, Teflon-coated tubes are avoided if the catheter is expected to remain in place more than 2 to 3 days. Instead, a silicone-coated, all silicone, or hydrogel-coated latex catheter is selected because of its increased comfort.[71] A hydrogel catheter coated with a silver alloy, or a silicone catheter impregnated with nitrofurazone, may be inserted when catheterization is anticipated to last for 2 weeks or less in order to reduce the risk of catheter-associated urinary tract infection.[67] However, these have not been found to provide protection when left indwelling more than 2 weeks and they are not recommended for patients managed by long-term catheters.

In men, water-soluble lubricating jelly should be injected into the urethra before catheterization and, in women the gel is liberally applied to the catheter. A lubricant containing 2% xylocaine may be used to reduce the discomfort associated with catheter insertion. The catheter is inserted to the bifurcation of the drainage port. The retention balloon is filled with 10 mL to fill the dead space in the port while ensuring proper inflation, and the inflated balloon is gently withdrawn near the bladder neck.

A drainage bag that provides adequate storage volume and reasonable concealment under clothing should be chosen. A bedside bag is preferred for bed-bound patients and for overnight use in ambulatory persons. The bedside bag should hold at least 2000 mL, should contain an antireflux valve to prevent retrograde movement of urine from bag to bladder, and should include a drainage port that is easily manipulated by the patient or care provider. In contrast, a leg bag or belly bag is preferred for ambulatory patients. It should hold at least 500 mL, should be easily concealed under clothing, and should attach to the leg or waist by elastic straps or a cloth pocket rather than latex straps, which are likely to irritate the underlying skin.

The patient is taught to keep the drainage bag level with or below the symphysis pubis. All indwelling catheters should be secured using a manufactured leg strap or adhesive backed device to reduce unintentional traction against the bladder neck or inadvertent urethral trauma.[72] Typically, the patient is encouraged to drink at least the recommended daily allowance of fluids, and to drink additional fluids if hematuria or sediment is present. However, these recommendations may be altered depending on the clinical setting and the patient's short-term prognosis. The catheter is routinely monitored for blockage caused by blood clots, sediment, or kinking of the drainage bag above the urinary bladder. The patient and family are also advised to monitor for signs and symptoms of clinically relevant infection, including fever, new hematuria, or urinary leakage around the catheter. They are also advised that bacteriuria is inevitable, even with the use of catheters containing a bacteriostatic coating, and that only clinically relevant (symptomatic) urinary tract infections should be treated.

Assessment and management of bladder spasm

Irritative LUTS, including a heightened sense of urgency and urethral discomfort, are common in patients with a long-term indwelling catheter or ureteral stent. In certain cases, these irritative symptoms are accompanied by painful bladder spasms. Bladder spasms are characterized by intermittent episodes of excruciating, painful cramping localized to the suprapubic region. They are caused by high-pressure, overactive detrusor contractions in response to a specific irritation.[62] Urine may bypass (leak around) the catheter or cause urge UI in the patient with a stent. Painful bladder spasms may be the direct result of catheter occlusion by blood clots, sediment, or kinking, or they may be associated with a needlessly large catheter, an improperly inflated retention balloon, or hypersensitivity to the presence of the catheter or stent or to principal constituents. Other risk factors include pelvic radiation therapy, chemotherapeutic agents (particularly cyclophosphamide), intravesical tumors, urinary tract infections, and bladder or lower ureteral calculus.

Bladder spasms are managed by altering modifiable factors, administering anticholinergic medications, or more invasive therapies in highly selected cases. Changing the urethral catheter may relieve bladder spasms. An indwelling catheter is usually changed every 4 weeks or more often because of the risk of blockage and encrustation with precipitated salts, hardened urethral secretions, and bacteria.

In addition to changing the catheter, the nurse should consider altering the type of catheter. For example, a catheter with a smaller French size may be inserted if the catheter is larger than 16 French, unless the patient is experiencing a buildup of sediment causing catheter blockage. Similarly, a catheter with a smaller retention balloon (5 mL) may be substituted for a catheter with a larger balloon (30 mL), to reduce irritation of the trig-one and bladder neck. Use of a catheter that is constructed of hydrophilic polymers or latex-free silicone may relieve bladder spasms and diminish irritative LUTS because of their greater biocompatibility when compared with Teflon-coated catheters.

Botulinum toxin A is a neurotoxin derived from *Clostridium botulinum*. When injected directly into the detrusor, it blocks the release of acetylcholine from the neuromuscular junction by cleaving the SNAP 25 protein needed to transport acetyl choline from nerve to muscle cell.[73] Limited evidence also suggests that the drug may reduce afferent signals from the bladder to the central nervous system, leading to reduction in perceptions of urgency.[74]

Botulinum toxin A is injected directly into the detrusor muscle under cystoscopic guidance; the duration of the effect is approximately 9 months. It is indicated for management of neurogenic detrusor overactivity associated with multiple sclerosis, spinal cord injury, and related neurological disorders. Its dual effect on detrusor overactivity and sensory urgency, combined with the durability of its effect renders it an attractive alternative for treating painful bladder spasms or refractory urge incontinence in selected cases.

Instruction about the position of the catheter, drainage tubes, and bags is reinforced; and the drainage tubes and urine are assessed for the presence of sediment or clots likely to obstruct urinary drainage. In certain cases, such as when the urethral catheter produces significant urethritis with purulent discharge from the urethra, a suprapubic indwelling catheter may be substituted for the urethral catheter. A suprapubic catheter also may be placed in patients who have a urethra that is technically difficult to catheterize, or who tend to encrust the catheter despite adequate fluid intake. Once established, these catheters are changed monthly, usually in the outpatient, home care, or hospice setting.

Patients with indwelling catheters who are prone to rapid encrustation and blockage present a particular challenge for the palliative care nurse. Options for management include frequent catheter changes (sometimes as often as one or two times per week) and irrigation of the catheter with a mildly acidic solution such as Renacidin. Irrigation may be completed once or several times weekly, and a small volume of solution is used (approximately 15 mL) to provide adequate irrigation of the catheter while avoiding irritation of the bladder epithelium.[75]

Bladder spasms also may indicate a clinically relevant urinary tract infection. The catheter change provides the best opportunity to obtain a urine specimen. This specimen should be obtained from the catheter and never from the drainage bag. Although bacteriuria is inevitable with a long-term indwelling catheter, cystitis associated with painful bladder spasms should be managed with sensitivity-guided antibiotic therapy.

The patient is taught to drink sufficient fluids to meet or exceed the recommended daily allowance of 30 mL/kg (0.5 oz/lb) whenever feasible. Reduced consumption of beverages or foods containing bladder irritants, such as caffeine or alcohol, also may alleviate bladder spasms in some cases.

If conservative measures or catheter modification fail to relieve bladder spasms, an anticholinergic medication may be administered. These medications work by inhibiting the overactive contractions that lead to painful bladder spasms.

Case study

Mr. W, a patient with bladder spasms in hospice care

Mr. W is an 81-year-old man with progressive, metastatic lung cancer with significant pain and limited mobility. He developed urinary incontinence and a silastic, 18-French indwelling urethral catheter with a 30-mL retention balloon was placed based on hospice protocol. After a week spent with the indwelling catheter, the urology team was consulted for bladder spasms and leakage of urine around the Foley catheter (catheter bypassing). During this period, he also developed IAD affecting his penis and the skin folds underneath the scrotum and on the inner thighs. The hospice nurse reported that the discomfort from his bladder spasm and skin irritation was not addressed by the opioid analgesics he was receiving for his metastatic lung cancer.

His indwelling catheter was replaced with a 16-French hydrogel-coated catheter, with a 5-mL retention balloon. A Velcro leg strap catheter securing device was placed to prevent traction of the retention balloon on the bladder neck. In addition, a skin care regimen comprising twice-daily cleansing with a disposable washcloth containing a perineal cleanser, moisturizer, and 3% dimethicone cleanser was instituted. Mr. W initially experienced relief from bladder spasm, and his IAD resolved within 7 days of beginning his skin care regimen. Unfortunately, his bladder spasms returned 2 days later, resulting in intermittent episodes of pain and catheter bypassing. In an effort to control leakage, the hospice nurses inflated the balloon to 10 and then 15 mL. However, the bladder spasms did not improve and appeared to increase, although the leakage diminished. Urology nursing was again consulted and suggested reduction in balloon inflation size, as this may have been contributing to spasms. The balloon was deflated to 5 mL and the patient started 2 mg extended release tolterodine capsules (Detrol™ LA) daily. This resulted in relief from his bladder spasms, but he reported a very dry mouth. The Detrol was discontinued, and a 3.9 mg transdermal oxybutynin patch (Oxytrol) was prescribed. This transdermal medication reduced the need for one more oral agent on a daily basis, and it did not cause the dry mouth associated with the oral antimuscarinic. After 3 days of this medication, along with adjusted and reduced balloon size, the patient's bladder spasms and leakage stopped altogether.

This case illustrates several important aspects of indwelling catheter care, management of bladder spasms, and perineal skin care in the palliative care setting. Because of his metastatic lung cancer, Mr. W was experiencing significant pain and limited ability to ambulate. A decision to insert an indwelling catheter was made when he developed urinary incontinence in order to reduce the need for him to move to a toilet, to protect his skin from the potentially damaging effect of repeated exposure to urine, and to preserve him from the indignity of repeated episodes of urinary incontinence. However, the original indwelling catheter resulted in bladder spasms and catheter bypassing. Rather than increasing the catheter and balloon size, the urology team appropriately chose to reduce the catheter size to 16 French, and to reduce the retention balloon size to 5 mL. They also elected to insert a catheter with a hydrogel coating, and to employ a leg strap securing device, in an attempt to reduce irritation and traction at the bladder neck and within the urethra. These actions resulted in relief from bladder spasm for approximately 48 hours. When the spasms recurred, the hospice nurses increased the balloon size to 15 mL, which reduced urinary leakage around the catheter. However, increasing the balloon size probably increased the irritation at the level of the bladder neck, and failed to relieve the underlying bladder spasms. Instead, the patient was managed by reducing the balloon size to a standard 5 mL, and an antimuscarinic medication was begun. This combination of interventions relieved the bladder spasms and catheter bypassing, but he experienced bothersome dry mouth. He was then switched to a transdermal oxybutynin patch, which avoids the first-pass metabolic effect associated with oral agents and is associated with a low occurrence of dry mouth. It relieved his painful bladder spasm and associated leakage without causing recurrence of his bothersome dry mouth.

Hematuria

Hematuria is defined as the presence of blood in the urine. It results from a variety of renal, urological, and systemic processes. When gross hematuria presented as an initial complaint or finding in an adult, further evaluation in one study revealed that 23% of patients had an underlying malignancy.[70,76] In the palliative care setting, hematuria may be associated with a variety of disorders, including pelvic irradiation or chemotherapy, or as the result of a major coagulation disorder or a newly diagnosed or recurring malignancy.[77]

Hematuria is divided into two subtypes according to its clinical manifestations. Microscopic hematuria is characterized by hemoglobin or myoglobin on dipstick analysis and more than 3 to 5 red blood cells (RBCs) per high-power field (hpf) under microscopic urinalysis, but the presence of blood remains invisible to the unaided eye. Macroscopic (gross) hematuria is also characterized by dipstick and microscopic evidence of RBCs in the urine, as well as a bright red or brownish discoloration that is apparent to the unaided eye.

In the context of palliative care, hematuria can also be subdivided into three categories depending on its severity.[81] Mild hematuria is microscopic or gross blood in the urine that does not produce obstructing clots or cause a clinically relevant decline in hematocrit or hemoglobin. Moderate and severe hematuria are associated with more prolonged and high-volume blood losses; hematuria is classified as moderate if less than 6 units of blood are required to replace blood lost within the urine and as severe if 6 or more units are required. Both moderate and severe hematuria may produce obstructing clots that lead to acute urinary retention or obstruction of the upper urinary tract.

Pathophysiology

Hematuria originates as a disruption of the endothelial-epithelial barrier somewhere within the urinary tract.[75] Inflammation of this barrier may lead to the production of cytokines, with subsequent damage to the basement membrane and passage of RBCs into the urinary tract. Laceration of this barrier may be caused by an invasive tumor, iatrogenic or other trauma, vascular accident, or arteriovenous malformation. Hematuria that originates within the upper urinary tract is often associated with tubulointerstitial disease or an invasive tumor, whereas hematuria originating from the lower urinary tract is typically associated with trauma, an invasive tumor, or radiation- or chemotherapy-induced cystitis.

In the patient receiving palliative care, significant hematuria most commonly occurs as the result of a hemorrhagic cystitis related to cancer, infection (viral, bacterial, fungal, or parasitic), chemical toxins (primarily from oxazaphosphorine alkylating agents), radiation, anticoagulation therapy, or an idiopathic response to anabolic steroids or another agent.[81] Radiation and chemotherapeutic agents account for most cases of moderate to severe hematuria.

Radiation cystitis is typically associated with pelvic radiotherapy for cancer of the uterus, cervix, prostate, rectum, or lower urinary tract. Most of these patients (80% to 90%) experience bothersome LUTS (diurnal voiding frequency, urgency, and dysuria) that reach their maximum intensity near the end of treatment and subside within 6 to 12 weeks after cessation of therapy. However, about 10% to 20% of patients experience clinically relevant cystitis that persists well beyond the end of treatment or occurs months or even years after radiotherapy.[78,79] In addition to bothersome LUTS, these patients experience pain and hematuria caused by mucosal edema, vascular telangiectasia, and submucosal hemorrhage. They also may experience interstitial and smooth muscle fibrosis with low bladder compliance and markedly reduced bladder capacity.[81] Severe fibrosis associated with radiotherapy can lead to moderate to severe hematuria, as well as upper urinary tract distress (ureterohydronephrosis, vesicoureteral reflux, pyelonephritis, and renal insufficiency) caused by chronically elevated intravesical pressures.

Chemotherapy-induced cystitis usually occurs after treatment with an oxazaphosphorine alkylating agent, such as cyclophosphamide or isophosphamide.[81] A urinary metabolite produced by these drugs, acrolein, is believed to be responsible. Hemorrhage usually occurs during or immediately after treatment, but delayed hemorrhage may occur in patients undergoing long-term therapy. The effects on the bladder mucosa are similar to those described for radiation cystitis.

Assessment

Because bleeding can occur at any level in the urinary tract from the glomerulus to the meatus, a careful, detailed history is needed to identify the source of the bleeding and to initiate an appropriate treatment plan.[77] The patient should be asked whether the hematuria represents a new, persistent, or recurrent problem. This distinction is often helpful, because recurrent or persistent hematuria may represent a benign predisposing condition, whereas hematuria of new or recent onset is more likely to result from conditions related to the need for palliative care. A review of prior urinalyses also may provide clues to the onset and history of microscopic hematuria in particular. The patient is queried about the relation of grossly visible hematuria to the urinary stream. Bleeding limited to initiation of the stream is often associated with a urethral source, bleeding during the entire act of voiding usually indicates a source in the bladder or upper urinary tract, and bleeding near the termination of the stream often indicates a source within the prostate or male reproductive system.

The patient with gross hematuria should also be asked about the color of the urine: a bright red hue indicates fresh blood, whereas a darker hue (often described as brownish, rust, or "Coke" colored) indicates older blood. Some patients with severe hematuria report the passage of blood clots. Clots that are particularly long and thin, resembling a shoestring or fishhook, suggest an upper urinary tract source; larger and bulkier clots suggest a lower urinary tract source.

The patient is asked about any pain related to the hematuria; this questioning should include the site and character of the pain and any radiation of pain to the flank, lower abdomen, or groin. Flank pain usually indicates upper urinary tract problems, abdominal pain radiating to the groin usually indicates lower ureteral obstruction and bleeding, and suprapubic pain suggests obstruction or infection causing hematuria.

In addition to questions about the hematuria, the nurse should ask about specific risk factors, including a history of urinary tract infections; systemic symptoms suggesting infection or renal insufficiency including fever, weight loss, rash, and recent systemic infection; any history of primary or metastatic tumors of the genitourinary system; and chemotherapy or radiation therapy of the pelvic or lower abdominal region. A focused review of medications includes all chemotherapeutic agents used currently or in the past and any current or recent administration of anticoagulant medications, including warfarin, heparin, aspirin, nonsteroidal antiinflammatory drugs, and other anticoagulant agents.

Physical examination

Physical examination also provides valuable clues to the source of hematuria. When completing this assessment, the nurse should particularly note any abdominal masses or tenderness, skin rashes, bruising, purpura (suggesting vasculitis, bleeding, or coagulation disorders), or telangiectasia (suggesting von Hippel-Lindau disease). Blood pressure should be assessed, because a new onset or rapid exacerbation of hypertension may suggest a renal source for hematuria. The lower abdomen is examined for signs of bladder distention, and a rectal assessment is completed to evaluate apparent prostatic or rectal masses or induration.

Laboratory testing

A dipstick and microscopic urinalysis is usually combined with microscopic examination when evaluating hematuria. This provides a semiquantitative assessment of the severity of hematuria (RBCs/hpf), and it excludes pseudohematuria (reddish urine caused by something other than RBCs, such as ingestion of certain drugs, vegetable dyes, or pigments).

Urinalysis provides further clues to the likely source of the bleeding.[80] Dysmorphic RBCs, cellular casts, renal tubular cells, and proteinuria indicate upper urinary tract bleeding. In contrast, hematuria from the lower urinary tract is usually associated with normal RBC morphology.

Additional evaluation is guided by clues from the history, physical examination, and urinalysis. For example, the presence of pyuria and bacteriuria suggests cystitis as the cause of hematuria and indicates the need for culture and sensitivity testing. The calcium/creatinine ratio should be assessed in a random urine sample for patients with painful macroscopic hematuria, to evaluate the risk for stone formation, particularly for individuals with hyperparathyroidism or prolonged immobility. A random urine protein/creatinine ratio and measurement of the C3 component of complement may be indicated in patients with proteinuria or casts, to evaluate for glomerulopathy or interstitial renal disease. Further studies also may be completed, to evaluate the specific cause of hematuria and implement a treatment plan.

Imaging studies

Ultrasonography is almost always indicated in the evaluation of hematuria in the patient receiving palliative care.[81] It is used to identify the size and location of cystic or solid masses that may act as the source of hematuria and to assess for obstruction, most stones, larger blood clots, and bladder-filling defects. A CTIVP, or computerized axial tomography intravenous pyelogram, or MRI urogram also may be used to image the upper and lower urinary tracts, but clinical use is limited by the risk of contrast allergy or nephropathy. Cystoscopy is performed if a bladder lesion is suspected, and ureteroscopy with retrograde pyelography may be completed if an upper urinary tract source of bleeding is suspected.

Management

The management of hematuria is guided by its severity and its source or cause. Preventive management for chemotherapy-induced hematuria begins with administration of sodium 2-mercaptoethanesulfonate (mesna) to patients receiving an alkylating agent for cancer.[81] This is given parenterally or orally, and it oxidizes to a stable, inactive form within minutes after administration. It becomes active when it is excreted into the urine, where it neutralizes acrolein (the metabolite postulated to cause chemotherapy-induced cystitis and hematuria) and slows degradation of the 4-hydroxy metabolites produced by administration of alkylating drugs. It is given with cyclophosphamide (20 mg/kg at time 0 and every 4 hours for 2 or 3 doses). When combined with vigorous hydration, it has been shown to protect the bladder from subsequent damage and hematuria. Chemotherapy guidelines have suggested oral therapy is also acceptable after initiation with a single dose in intravenous mesna.[82,83]

Mild urinary retention is managed by identifying and treating its underlying cause. For example, sensitivity-guided antibiotics are used to treat a bacterial hemorrhagic cystitis, and extracorporeal lithotripsy may be used to treat hematuria associated with a urinary stone. While the hematuria persists, the patient is encouraged to drink more than the recommended daily allowance for fluids, to prevent clot formation and urinary retention. In addition, the patient is assisted in obtaining adequate nutritional intake to replace lost blood, and iron supplementation is provided if indicated.

In contrast to mild hematuria, moderate to severe cases often lead to the formation of blood clots, causing acute urinary retention and bladder pain. In these cases, complete evacuation of clots from the bladder is required before a definitive assessment and treatment strategy are implemented.[62] A large-bore urethral catheter (24 or 26 French in the adult) is placed, and manual irrigation is performed with a Toomey syringe. The bladder is irrigated with saline until no further clots are obtained and the backflow is relatively clear.[54] A 22- or 24-French three-way indwelling catheter is then placed, to allow continuous bladder irrigation using cold or iced saline. Percutaneous insertion of a suprapubic catheter is not recommended because of limitations of size and the potential to "seed" the tract if a bladder malignancy is present.

Unsuccessful attempts to place a urethral catheter or recurrent obstruction of the irrigation catheter provide a strong indication for endoscopic evaluation. Rigid cystoscopy is preferred because it allows optimal evacuation of bladder clots and further evaluation of sites of bleeding; retrograde pyelography or ureteroscopy may also be completed if upper urinary tract clots are suspected. Based on the findings of endoscopic evaluation, sites of particularly severe bleeding are cauterized or resected.

After the initial evacuation of obstructing clots, bladder irrigations or instillations may be completed if multiple sites of bleeding are observed or if the risk of recurrence is high, as in the case of radiation- or chemotherapy-induced hematuria. Table 15.4 summarizes treatment options for moderate to severe hematuria and their route, administration, and principal nursing considerations.

Case study

VC, a 54-year-old female with bladder cancer and gross hematuria

VC is a 54-year-old female who originally presented to her provider with gross hematuria. Scans and cystoscopy led to identification of a large and unresectable bladder tumor blocking the right ureteral orifice. There was questionable spread outside the bladder wall into the perivesicle tissue. She underwent transurethral resection of the bladder (TURBT) placement of right percutaneous nephrostomy tube for right hydronephrosis. She was evaluated by cardiology and felt to be high risk for cystectomy surgery but could be optimized. Medical management of her cardiac issues was ensured and she improved from a risk perspective.

She was then treated with 4 cycles of Cisplatin Gemcitabine neoadjuvant chemotherapy in hopes of undergoing tumor resection. Unfortunately she did not tolerate full dose chemotherapy; treatment was complicated by severe neutropenia and anemia. Her scans showed some reduction in tumor size, but the remaining tumor remained visible on imaging studies. She then underwent a second attempt at bladder tumor resection and stent placement into the right ureter. Unfortunately, the right ureter could not be opened, and she was left with the percutaneous right nephrostomy.

Following this second procedure, the severity of her hematuria subsided and her anemia remained stable. Staging scans revealed a new metastatic lung lesion. She elected for a 2-week time off from chemotherapy, followed with a return visit with her team for discussion of pelvic radiation and chemotherapy consolidation.

On the day she returned for radiation consolation she reported worsening of her hematuria and exacerbation of the fatigue she elected not to communicate during her time off from chemotherapy. She was found to be hypotensive and while urine in the percutaneous nephrostomy was clear, she admitted to passing grossly visible blood and clots in her voided urine. Because of her hypotension, she was transferred to the Emergency Department for evaluation and laboratory work. Her CBC returned with hemoglobin of 3.3 and hematocrit of 11.1. She was immediately admitted to the facility's medical intensive care unit, where she received blood transfusions and stabilized. She experienced transient acute renal failure but that rapidly resolved with hydration and transfusion. After stabilization a left percutaneous nephrostomy was placed to divert urine away from the bladder. The hematuria resolved with this urinary diversion. During this hospitalization she was accepted for palliative and support care given the radiographically proven widely metastatic nature of her disease. She was also evaluated and found to be a good candidate for bladder/pelvic radiation therapy.

She was discharged home with supportive care. The following week she began palliative IMRT for bladder cancer that she tolerated well. She was able to manage the bilateral percutaneous

Table 15.4 Treatment options for hemorrhagic cystitis

Agent	Action route of administration/Dosage	Problems/Contraindications
ε-Aminocaproic acid	Acts as an inhibitor of fibrinolysis by inhibiting plasminogen activation substances 5-g loading dose orally or parenterally, followed by 1–1.25 g hourly to max of 30 g in 24 h; maximum response in 8–12 h	Potential thromboembolic complications Increased risk of clot retention Contraindicated in patients with upper urinary tract bleeding or vesicoureteral reflux Decreased blood pressure
Silver nitrate	Chemical cautery Intravesical instillation: 0.5% to 1.0% solution in sterile water instilled for 10–20 min followed by no irrigation; multiple instillations may be required Reported as 68% effective	Case report of renal failure in patient who precipitated silver salts in renal collecting system, causing functional obstruction
Alum (may use ammonium or potassium salt of aluminum)	Chemical cautery Continuous bladder irrigation: 1% solution in sterile water, pH = 4.5 (salt precipitates at pH of 7) Requires average of 21 h of treatment	Thought to not be absorbed by bladder mucosa; however, case reports of aluminum toxicity in renal failure patients
Formalin (aqueous solution of formaldehyde)	Cross-links proteins; exists as monohydrate methylene glycol and as a mixture of polymeric hydrates and polyoxyethylene glycols; rapidly "fixes" the bladder mucosa Available as 37%–40%, aqueous formaldehyde (= 100% formalin) diluted in sterile water to desired concentration (1% formalin = 0.37% formaldehyde); instillation: 50 mL for 4–10 min or endoscopic placement of 5% formalin-soaked pledgets placed onto bleeding site for 15 min and then removed	Painful, requires anesthesia Vesicoureteral reflux (relative contraindication): patients placed in Trendelenburg position with low-grade reflux, or ureteral occlusive balloons used with high-grade reflux Extravasation causes fibrosis, papillary necrosis, fistula, peritonitis
Intravesical prostaglandins	Prostaglandins (PGs) E1, E2, and F2α may be used to treat cyclophosphamide-induced hematuria; PGs are postulated to act by promoting platelet aggregation, vasoconstriction via contraction of smooth muscles of arterioles in mucosa and submucosa and a cytoprotective action influencing glycosaminoglycan function of the urothelium. PGs are introduced following introduction of a three-way indwelling catheter and evacuation of clots; PG E1,E2, F2α is introduced in a diluted aqueous solution and retained in the bladder for approximately 1 hour, dosing varies according to the individual formulations; multiple treatments are required (median 6–7 days reported in several case series). Gross hematuria resolves in approximately 50% of cases.	Bladder spasms commonly occur; nevertheless, PGs are associated with less systemic toxicity than formalin; treatment may be administered at the bedside.

Sources: References 73, 74, and 75.

nephrostomies with minimal assistance. She remained hematuria free, and her anemia improved. During radiation she had lab monitoring for cytopenias. She experienced none, and her hemoglobin was stable.

The value of percutaneous nephrostomy tubes for relief of ureteral obstruction and for hematuria due to tumor is substantial. This patient had percutaneous diversions for each reason and at the time of the diversion it provided both clinical improvement and relief of life-threatening hematuria.

Summary

Patients receiving palliative care frequently experience urinary system disorders. A malignancy or systemic disease may affect voiding function and produce UI, urinary retention, or upper urinary tract obstruction. In addition, upper acute renal insufficiency or renal failure may occur if the upper urinary tract becomes obstructed. These disorders may be directly attributable to a malignancy or systemic disease, or they may be caused by a specific treatment such as radiation, chemotherapy, or a related medication. Nursing management of patients with urinary system disorders is affected by the nature of the urological condition, the patient's general condition, and the nearness to death.

References

1. Gray ML, Moore KN. Urologic Disorders: Adult and Pediatric Care. St. Louis, MO: Mosby-Elsevier; 2009.
2. Gray ML. Physiology of voiding. In: Doughty DB (ed.), Urinary and Fecal Incontinence: Current Management Concepts. 3rd ed. St. Louis, MO: Mosby-Elsevier; 2006:21–54.
3. Griffiths D, Tadic SD. Bladder control, urgency, and urge incontinence: evidence from functional brain imaging. Neurourol Urodyn. 2008;27:466–474.
4. Hruz P, Lovblad KO, Nirkko AC, Thoeny H, El-Koussy M, Danuser H. Identification of brain structures involved in micturition with functional magnetic resonance imaging (fMRI). J Neuroradiol. 2008;35:144–149.
5. Kitta T, Kakizaki H, Furuno T, Moriya K, Tanaka H, Shiga T, Tamaki N, Yabe I, Sasaki H, Nonomura K. Brain activation during detrusor overactivity in patients with Parkinson's disease: a positron emission tomography study. J Urol. 2006;175:994–998.
6. Peterson R, Haig Y, Nakstad PH, Wyller TB. Subtypes of urinary incontinence after stroke: relation to size and location of cerebrovascular damage. Age Ageing. 2008;37(3):324–327.
7. Yamamoto T, Sakakibara R, Hashimoto K, Nakazawa K, Uchiyama T, Liu Z, et al. Striatal dopamine level increases in the urinary storage phase in cats: An in vivo microdialysis study. Neuroscience. 2005;135:299–303.
8. Morrison JF. The discovery of the pontine micturition centre by F. J. F. Barrington. Exp Physiol. 2008;93:742–745.
9. Kavia RB, Dasgupta R, Fowler CJ. Functional imaging and the central control of the bladder. J Comp Neurol. 2005;493:27–32.
10. Andersson KE, Arner A. Urinary bladder contraction and relaxation: physiology and pathophysiology. Physiol Rev. 2004;84:935–986.
11. Giglio D, Tobin G. Muscarinic receptor subtypes in the lower urinary tract. Pharmacology. 2009;83(5):259–269.
12. Anisuzzaman AS, Morishima S, Suzuki F, Tanaka T, Yoshiki H, Sathi ZS, et al. Assessment of muscarinic receptor subtypes in human and rat lower urinary tract by tissue segment binding assay. J Pharmacol Sci. 2008;106:271–279.
13. de Groat WC, Fraser MO, Yoshiyama M, Smerin S, Tai C, Chancellor MB, et al. Neural control of the urethra. Scand J Urol Nephrol Suppl. 2001;207:35–43; discussion 106–125.
14. Thor KB. Serotonin and norepinephrine involvement in efferent pathways to the urethral rhabdosphincter: implications for treating stress urinary incontinence. Urology. 2003;62(4 Suppl):3–9.
15. Abrams P, Cardozo L, Fall M, Griffiths D, Rosier P, Ulmstem U, et al. The standardization of terminology of lower urinary tract function: Report for the standardization sub-committee of the International Continence Society. Neurourol Urodyn. 2002;21:167–178.
16. Gray M. An update on the physiology of urinary continence. Continence UK. 2007;1(2):28–36.
17. McGuire EJ, English SF. Periurethral collagen injection and female sphincteric incontinence: indications, techniques and result. World J Urol. 1997;15:306–309.
18. Gray M. Pathology and management of reflex urinary incontinence/neurogenic bladder. In: Doughty DB (ed.), Urinary and Fecal Incontinence: Nursing Management. 3rd ed. St. Louis, MO: Mosby-Elsevier; 2006:105–143.
19. Hurlow J. View from here: functional urinary incontinence ICD-9. J Wound Ostomy Continence Nurs. 2009;36:79–81.
20. Gulati A, Khelemsky Y, Loh J, Puttanniah V, Malhorta V, Cubert K. The use of lumbar sympathetic blockade at L4 for management of malignancy-related bladder spasms. Pain Physician. 2011;14:305–310.
21. Wilson M. Causes and management of indwelling urinary catheter-related pain. Br J Nurs. 2008;17:232–239.
22. Chang D, Ben-Meir D, Pout K, Dewan PA. Management of postoperative bladder spasm. J Pediatr Child Health. 2005;41(1–2):56–58.
23. Hendrickson K, Gleason D, Young JM, Saltsstein D, Gershman A, Lerner A, et al. Safety and side effects of immediate instillation of apaziquone following transurethral resection in patients with non-muscle invasive bladder cancer. J Urol. 2008;180:116–120.
24. Stewart W, Herzog R, Wein A, et al. The prevalence and impact of overactive bladder in the U.S.: results from the NOBLE program. Neurourol Urodyn. 2001;20.406–408.
25. Gray M, Marx RM, Peruggio M, Patrie J, Steers WD. A model for predicting motor urge urinary incontinence. Nurs Res. 2001;50:116–122.
26. Zhang B, Gao X, Wen XQ. Abderxit. [Analysis of the causes of postoperative chest or/and abdomen colic in benign prostatic hyperplasia]. Zhong Hua Nan Ke Xue. 2005;11:288–289, 295.
27. Jirovec MM, Wells TJ. Urinary incontinence in nursing home residents with dementia: The mobility–cognition paradigm. Appl Nurs Res. 1990;3:112–117.
28. Gray M, Beeckman D, Bliss DZ, Fader M, Logan S, Junkin J, Selekof J, Doughty D, Kurz P. Incontinence-associated dermatitis: a comprehensive review and update. J Wound Ostomy Continence Nurs. 2012;39(1)61–74.
29. Robinson D, McClish DK, Wyman JF, Bump RC, Fantl JA. Comparison between urinary diaries with and without intensive patient instructions. Neurourol Urodyn. 1996;15:143–148.
30. Sampselle CM. Teaching women to use a voiding diary. Am J Nurs. 2003;103:62–64.
31. Ermer-Seltun J. Assessment and management of acute or transient urinary incontinence. In: Doughty DB (ed.), Urinary and Fecal Incontinence: Current Management Concepts. 3rd ed. St. Louis, MO: Mosby-Elsevier; 2006:55–76.
32. Tomlinson BU, Doughery MC, Pendergrast JF, Boyington AR, Coffman PA, Pickens SM. Dietary caffeine, fluid intake and urinary incontinence in older rural women. Int J Urogynecol Pelvic Floor Dysfunct. 1999;10:22–28.
33. Gray ML. Altered patterns of urinary elimination. In: Ackley BJ, Ladwig GB (eds.), Nursing Diagnosis Handbook. St. Louis, MO: Mosby; 1999:643–646.
34. Institute of Medicine. US Food and Science Board, Dietary Reference for Water and Sodium Intake. http://www.iom.edu/Global/News%20Announcements/~/media/442A08B899F44DF9AAD083D86164C75B.ashx. Accessed 6/30/2013.
35. Cottenden A, Fader M, Getliffe K, Paterson J, Szonyi G, Wilde M. Management with continence products. In: Abrams P, Cardozo L,

Khoury A, Wein A (eds.), Incontinence: Basics and Evaluation. Paris, France: Health Publications; 2005:149–254.

36. Gray M, Marx R. Results of behavioral treatment for urinary incontinence in women. Curr Opin Urol. 1998;8:279–282.

37. Miller JM, Ashton-Miller JA, Delancey JO. A pelvic muscle precontraction can reduce cough-related urine loss in selected women with mild SUI. J Am Geriatr Soc. 1998;46:870–874.

38. Ghoneim GM, Hassouna M. Alternative for the pharmacologic management of stress urinary incontinence in the elderly. J Wound Ostomy Cont Nurs. 1997;24:311–318.

39. Hunsballe JM, Djurhuus JC. Clinical options for imipramine in the management of urinary incontinence. Urol Res. 2001;29:118–125.

40. Duloxetine Side Effects. Available at: http://anxiety.emedtv.com/duloxetine/duloxetine-side-effects.html. Accessed December 26, 2008.

41. Newman DK. The indwelling urinary catheter: principles for best practice. J Wound Ostomy Continence Nurs. 2007;34:655–661.

42. Burgio KL, Locher JL, Goode PS, Hardin JM, McDowell BJ, Dombrowski M, et al. Behavioral vs. drug treatment for urge urinary incontinence in older women: a randomized controlled trial. JAMA. 1998;280:1995–2000.

43. D'Souza AO, Smith MJ, Miller LA, Doyle J, Ariely R. Persistence, adherence, and switch rates among extended release and immediate-release overactive bladder medications in a regional managed care plan. J Manag Care Pharm. 2008;14:291–301.

44. Sanford M. Mirabegron: a review of its use in patients with overactive bladder. Drugs. 2013;73:1213–1225.

45. Nitti V, Rosenberg S, Mitcheson D, et al. Urodynamic safety of the potent and selective beta3-adrenergic agonist, mirabegron, in males with lower urinary tract symptoms and bladder outlet obstruction [Abstract POD 03.05]. Urology. 2012;80(3 Suppl 1):S10.

46. Michel MC. Fesoterodine: a novel muscarinic receptor antagonist for the treatment of overactive bladder syndrome. Exp Opin Pharmacother. 2008;9:1787–1796.

47. Dmochowski RR, Sand PK, Zinner NR, Staskin DR. Trospium 60 mg once daily (QD) for overactive bladder syndrome: results from a placebo-controlled interventional study. Urology. 2008;71:449–454.

48. MacDiarmid SA. How to choose the initial drug treatment for overactive bladder. [Review]. Curr Urol Rep. 2007;8:364–369.

49. Andersson KE, Olshansky B. Treating patients with overactive bladder syndrome with antimuscarinics: heart rate considerations. BJU Int. 2007;100:1007–1014.

50. Burgio KL, Locher JL, Goode PS. Combined behavioral and drug therapy for urge incontinence in older women. J Am Geriatr Soc. 2000;48:370–374.

51. Smith DA. Devices for continence. Nurse Pract Forum. 1994;5:186–189.

52. Wells M. Managing urinary incontinence with BioDerm external continence device. Br J Nurs. 2008;17:s24–s29.

53. Nickel JC. The use of alpha1-adrenoceptor antagonists in lower urinary tract symptoms: beyond benign prostatic hyperplasia. Urology. 2003;62(Suppl 1):34–41.

54. Anson C, Gray M. Secondary urologic complications of spinal injury. Urol Nurs. 1993;13:107–112.

55. Van Gool JD, Vijverberg MA, Messer AP, Elzinga-Plomp A, De Jong TP. Functional daytime incontinence: non-pharmacologic treatment. Scand J Urol Nephrol. 1992;141:93–105.

56. Fink HA, Taylor BC, Tacklind, JW, Rutks IR, Wilt TJ. Treatment interventions in nursing home residents with urinary incontinence: a systematic review of randomized trials. Mayo Clin Proc. 2008; 83(12):1332–1343.

57. Schnelle JF, Keeler E, Hays RD, Simmons S, Ouslander JG, Siu AL. A cost and value analysis of two interventions with incontinent nursing home residents. J Am Geriatr Soc. 1995;43:1112–1117.

58. Golomb J, Ben-Chaim J, Goldwasser B, Korach J, Mashiach S. Conservative treatment of a vesicocervical fistula resulting from Shirodkar cervical cerclage. J Urol. 1993;149:833–834.

59. Tostain J. Conservative treatment of urogenital fistula following gynecological surgery: the value of fibrin glue. Acta Urol Belg. 1992;60:27–33.

60. Gray M, Bliss DZ, Doughty DB, Ermer-Seltun J, Kennedy-Evans KL, Palmer MH. Incontinence-associated dermatitis: A review. J Wound Ostomy Continence Nurs. 2007;34:45–56.

61. Gray M. Perineal skin care for the continence professional. Continence UK J. 2008;2:29–39.

62. Norman RW. Genito-urinary. In: Hanks G, Cherny NI, Christakis NA, Fallon M, Kaasa S, Portenoy RK (eds.), Oxford Textbook of Palliative Medicine. 5th ed. Edited. Oxford: Oxford University Press; 2011:667–676.

63. Gray M. Urinary retention: Management in the acute care setting. Am J Nurs. 2000;15:42–60.

64. Gray M. Functional alterations: bladder. In: Gross J, Johnson BL (eds.), Handbook of Oncology Nursing. Boston: Jones and Bartlett; 1998:557–583.

65. Blaivas JG, Weiss JP, Jones M. The pathophysiology of lower urinary tract symptoms after brachytherapy for prostate cancer. BJU Int. 2006;98:1233–1237.

66. Parker D, Callan L, Harwood J, Thompson DL, Wilde M, Gray M. Nursing interventions to reduce the risk of catheter-associated urinary tract infection. Part 1: Catheter selection. J Wound Ostomy Continence Nurs. 2009;36:23–34.

67. Willette P, Coffield S. Current trends in the management of difficult urinary catheterizations. West J Emerg Med. 2012;13(6):472–478.

68. Thees K, Dreblow L. Trial of voiding: what's the verdict? Urol Nurs. 1999;19:20–24.

69. Newman DK. The indwelling urinary catheter: principles for best practice. J Wound Ostomy Cont Nurs. 2007;34(6):655–661.

70. Tu WH, Shortliffe LV. Evaluation of asymptomatic, atraumatic hematuria in children and adults. Nat Rev Urol. 2010; 7(4):189–94.

71. Gray M. Does the construction material affect outcomes in long-term catheterization? J Wound Ostomy Cont Nurs. 2006;33:116–120.

72. Gray M. Securing the indwelling catheter. Am J Nurs. 2008; 108:44–50.

73. Tincello DG. Botulinum toxin treatment for overactive bladder and detrusor overactivity in adults. World J Urol. 2012;30:451–456.

74. Apostolodis A, Dasgupta D, Fowler CJ. Proposed mechanism for the efficacy of injected botulinum toxin in the treatment of human detrusor overactivity. Eur Urol. 2006;49:644–650.

75. Getliffe K. Managing recurrent urinary catheter blockage: problems, promises, and practicalities. J Wound Ostomy Cont Nurs. 2003;30:146–151.

76. Openbrier D. Asymptomatic hematuria. Adv Nurse Pract. 2003;11:81–88.

77. Groninger H. Phillips JM. Gross hematuria: assessment and management at end of life. J Hosp Palliat Nurs. 2012;14(3):184–188.

78. Levenbach C, Eifel PJ, Burke TW, Morris M, Gershenson DM. Hemorrhagic cystitis following radio therapy for stage Ib cancer of the cervix. Gynecol Oncol. 1994;55:206–210.

79. de la Taille A, Zerbib M. Urologic complications of radiotherapy. Ann Urol (Paris). 2003; 37(6): 345–357.

80. Glenn S, Gerber MD, Brendler CB. Evaluation of the urologic patient: history, physical examination, and urinalysis. In: Wein AJ, Kavoussi LR, Novick AC, Partin AW (eds.), Campbell-Walsh Urology. 9th ed. Elsevier: St Louis;2012;95–108.

81. Ghahstani SM, Shakhssalim N. Palliative treatment of intractable hematuria in context of advanced bladder cancer. Urology. 2009;6(3):149–156.

82. American Society of Clinical Oncology Practice Guidelines for the Use of Chemotherapy and Radiotherapy Protectans. J Clin Oncol. 1999;17:3333–3355.

83. Up to Date. Ifosamide: Pediatric drug information Lexicomp. www.Uptodate.com/contents/ifosfamide-pediatric-drug-information? Accessed July 21, 2013.

CHAPTER 16

Lymphedema management

Mei R. Fu and Bonnie B. Lasinski

With breast cancer, you go in for your treatment, once cancer is under control you are kind of done with it. With lymphedema, you will never be done with it because you are having this big arm, pain, burning, heaviness, and soreness every day. It's something that you have to live with for the rest of your life.

Mrs. S, 7 years of lymphedema

Key points

◆ Lymphedema is a syndrome of abnormal accumulation of lymph fluid and multiple symptoms that is caused by irreversible damage to and congenital malformation of the lymphatic system.

◆ There is no cure for lymphedema, and management of lymphedema requires daily self-care and changes in lifestyle.

◆ Promotion of lymph fluid flow and prevention of infection is fundamental to achieve long-term effective lymphedema management.

Nurses are the ideal resource for providing and improving quality care for patients suffering from lymphedema because they have access to large, diverse patient populations. Lymphedema or abnormal swelling is seen regularly in palliative and acute care settings. Lymphedema is often overlooked or neglected despite its capacity to cause pain, immobility, infection, skin problems, and psychosocial distress.[1,2] This chapter prepares nurses to understand, assess, and manage lymphedema in various clinical settings, including acute, outpatient, community, and palliative care.

Definitions

Lymphedema is a chronic syndrome of abnormal swelling and multiple symptoms, resulting from abnormal accumulation of protein-rich lymph fluid in the interstitial tissue spaces due to an imbalance between lymph fluid production and transport.[3,4] *Edema*, a symptom, refers to excessive accumulation of fluid within interstitial tissues and is one of the manifestations of lymphedema. Long-term, neglected edema, such as lower extremity venous insufficiency, can develop into chronic lymphedema. Discerning the difference between edema and lymphedema ensures appropriate treatment.

One or several factors can precipitate an imbalance in extracellular fluid volume. Excess fluids, proteins, immunological cells, and debris in affected tissues can produce chronic inflammation and connective tissue proliferation, including hypertrophy of adipose tissue.[5,6] Some degree of progression usually occurs and can produce subcutaneous and dermal thickening and

fibrosis.[3] Lymphedema and edema are contrasted in Table 16.1, which provides definitions, signs and symptoms, and basic pathophysiology.[7,8]

Prevalence and risk factors

The world prevalence of edema is unknown,[8] and that of lymphedema is poorly documented. According to the World Health Organization, lymphedema affects 250 million people worldwide and the global burden of lymphedema is estimated at 5.78 million disability-adjusted life years lost annually.[8] Primary lymphedema, a genetic disorder, is attributed to embryonic developmental abnormalities, which may be sporadic or part of a syndrome caused by either chromosomal abnormalities (e.g., Turner's syndrome) or inherited single-gene defects.[9,10] Primary lymphedema occurs in about one in 6000 individuals and is more common in women than men, with a 3:1 ratio.[11] The overall prevalence of primary lymphedema has been estimated as about 2%.[12]

Secondary (acquired) lymphedema results from obstruction or obliteration of lymph nodes or lymphatic vessels.[5,6,12] Cancer, trauma, surgery, severe infections, cardiac disease, poor venous function, immobility, or paralyzing diseases are major causes of secondary lymphedema.[12] In developed countries, cancer treatment is the main cause of lymphedema. Prevalence of cancer-related lymphedema has been reported in patients treated for breast cancer (5%–60%), melanoma (16%), gynecological (20%), genitourinary (10%), and head/neck cancer (4%).[13–15] Risk factors related to cancer treatment include extent of surgery, extent of lymph node resection, and radiation therapy.[16,17] In developing countries, lymphatic filariasis, a parasitic infection transmitted by mosquitoes, is the predominant worldwide cause of secondary lymphedema. Mosquitoes transmit filariasis nematodes, which embed in human lymphatics and release inflammatory substances that cause progressive lymphatic damage. It is estimated that the worldwide incidence of filariasis is 750 million.[18]

Other major factors of lymphedema risk include inflammation, infection, and higher body mass index (BMI).[18–20] Breast cancer survivors who undergo surgery and dissection of lymph nodes and vessels are known to have a compromised lymphatic system, which makes them more vulnerable to infection and

Table 16.1 Comparison of edema and lymphedema

	Edema	Lymphedema
Disorder	A symptom of various disorders	A chronic, currently incurable edema
Definition	Swelling caused by the excessive fluid in interstitial tissues—due to imbalance between capillary filtration and lymph drainage over time	Swelling (edema) caused by accumulation of lymph fluid within interstitial tissues as a result of lymphatic drainage failure, increased production of lymph fluid over time, or both
Signs and symptoms	Swelling, decreased skin mobility	Swelling, decreased skin mobility
	Tightness, tingling, or bursting	Tightness, heaviness, firmness, tingling, feeling of fullness, or bursting sensations
	Decreased strength and mobility	Decreased strength and mobility
	Discomfort (aching to severe pain)	Discomfort (aching, soreness to severe pain)
	Possible skin color change	Progressive skin changes (color, texture, tone, temperature), impairment in integrity such as blisters, weeping (lymphorrhea), hyperkeratosis, warts, papillomatosis, and elephantiasis
	Pitting scale is often used:	*Pitting scale is NOT used.*
	1+ Edema barely detectable	
	2+ Slight indentation with depression	
	3+ Deep indentation for 5–30 s with pressure	
	4+ Area 1.5–2 times greater than normal	
Pathophysiology	Capillary filtration rate exceeds fluid transport capacity	Inadequate lymph transport capacity
		Primary—Inadequately developed lymphatic pathways
	Example: Heart failure, fluid overload, and/or venous thrombosis are common causes of increased capillary pressure, leading to an increased capillary filtration rate that causes edema	*Secondary*—Damage outside lymphatic pathways (obstruction/obliteration)
		Initial sequelae of transport failure:
		Lymphatic stasis →
		Increased tissue fluid →
	Note:	Accumulated protein and cellular metabolites →
	Timely treatment of the underlying cause or causes usually reduces edema	Further increased tissue water and pressure
		Potential long-term sequelae:
	Prolonged, untreated edema can transition to lymphedema	Macrophages seek to decrease inflammation
		Increased fibroblasts and keratinocytes cause chronic inflammation
		Gradual increase in adipose tissue
		Lymphorrhea (leakage of lymph through skin)
		Gradual skin and tissue thickening and hardening progressing to hyperkeratosis, papillomatosis, and other problems
		Ever-increasing risk of infection and other complications

Sources: References 3, 4, 5, and 6.

impaired lymphatic drainage.[6] Women who had previous infections were 3.8 times more likely to develop lymphedema[14,19,20,21]; weight gain and obesity (BMI >30 kg/m^2) increase lymphedema risk. Survivors with each increase of 1 kg/m^2 in their BMI were at 1.11 greater risk for developing lymphedema.[14,16,19] Nevertheless, these risk factors only partially explain who develops lymphedema. Lymphedema can and does occur in women lacking these risk factors. It is possible that inherited genetic susceptibility may play a role in the pathogenesis of cancer-related lymphedema. Research on the effect of genetics or genetic variations on secondary lymphedema related to cancer treatment is very limited. However, mutations and genetic variations in lymphatic specific growth factors, such as vascular endothelial growth factor (VEGF-C, VEGF-D, VEGFR2, VEGFR3), are associated with hereditary lymphedema and secondary lymphedema related to breast cancer.[10,22]

Impact

Often, the most visible manifestation of lymphedema is persistent swelling.[1,2,3] However, lymphedema is much more than just swelling. Lymphedema impacts an individual's quality of life, causing physical discomfort, functional disabilities, impaired occupational roles, poor self-image, decreased self-esteem, interrupted interpersonal relationships, financial burden, and life-style changes.[1,23–25] Physically, lymphedema leads to distressing symptoms such as swelling, firmness, tightness, heaviness, pain, fatigue, numbness, and impaired limb mobility.[2,23] In addition, lymphedema predisposes individuals to skin and tissue fibrosis, cellulitis, infections, lymphadenitis, and septicemia.[20,26] Prolonged fluid stasis can lead to severe skin and tissue symptoms, sometimes referred to as elephantiasis. Symptoms include hyperkeratosis (hard, reptile-like skin), warts, and papillomas (engorged and raised lymph vessels on the skin surface).[20,26] Chronic lymphedema, over a number of years, has also been associated with the development of the rare, usually fatal cancer, lymphangiosarcoma.[26] Functionally, lymphedema makes it difficult for individuals to accomplish tasks and impairs their abilities to fulfill work that involves heavy lifting, gripping, holding, fine motor dexterity, and repetitive movement of the affected limb.[23,25] Some individuals have to give up hobbies that exacerbate their lymphedema.[27] Psychologically, individuals feel stigmatized and some experience loss of sexual attractiveness because of obvious disfigurement, which often elicits emotional distress, social anxiety, depression, and disruption of interpersonal relationships.[1] Routine check-ups for lymphedema management, long-term physical therapy, management equipment (compression garments, bandages, special lotions), and repeated cellulitis, infections, and lymphangitis create financial and economic burdens not only for survivors but also for the healthcare system.[24] Breast cancer survivors with lymphedema have significantly higher healthcare costs than those without; they spend more days annually either hospitalized or visiting physicians' offices. They also have more days absent from work, which could adversely affect employment.[24]

Anatomy, physiology, and pathophysiology

Edema

Edema is a symptom that results from an imbalance between capillary filtration and lymph drainage. Edema requires treatment of the underlying disorder that is precipitating tissue fluid excess. Precipitators can include cardiac, hepatic, renal, allergic, or hypoproteinic disease; venous obstruction; and medication complications[28] (see Table 16.1). Chronic edema can develop into secondary lymphedema with sufficient lymphatic damage, such as in chronic venous insufficiency, posttraumatic swelling from significant soft tissue injury, or fractures of the lower extremities.[29,30]

Lymphedema

A healthy lymphatic system helps regulate the tissue cellular environment, including collecting and returning plasma and proteins.[31,32] Daily, 20% to 50% of the total accumulating plasma proteins travel through 2 to 4 liters of lymph fluid in a healthy lymphatic system.[31,32] Lymphatics also remove cellular waste products, mutants, and debris; eliminate non-self-antigens; and regulate local immune defense in the process of maintaining homeostasis[31,32] (Figure 16.1). Unidirectional vessels traverse from superficial to deep lymphatics through 600 to 700 lymph nodes, carrying lymph fluid to the venous system at the right or left venous angle of the anterior chest on either side of the neck (Figure 16.2). Lymph nodes filter, concentrate, and purify lymph fluid, eliminating defective cells, toxins, and bacteria, explaining the increased risk of infection for patients with compromised lymphatics.[31,32] Lymphedema pathology signifies malfunction in any part of the process of collecting, transporting, filtering, and depositing lymph into the venous system. Lymphedema pathophysiology suggests disruption of these processes and is described in Table 16.1.

In brief, lymph fluid is transported initially from the interstitium by the initial lymphatic vessels, moving proximally through progressively larger collecting lymph vessels, filtered through lymph nodes, then drained into the two large lymph collecting ducts, and finally returned to the venous bloodstreams via the left and right subclavian veins (Figure 16.3). Damage to any structures of the lymphatic system can lead to accumulation of lymph fluid in the affected area. Further, physiological variations in each individual's lymphatic system, such as numbers or sizes of lymph nodes, make it difficult to quantify each individual's risk for lymphedema.

Secondary lymphedema from cancer treatment is caused by trauma to the lymphatic system mainly from surgery and radiotherapy.[16,17] Surgery creates disruption to the lymphatic system by directly dissecting lymph vessels and removing lymph nodes.[31] Unfortunately, lymph nodes do not regenerate once dissected.[31,32] Formation of scar tissue and tissue fibrosis from surgery create further impairment to lymph flow. The disruption or blockage of the lymphatic system reduces its ability to transport and filter the lymph, resulting in a functional overload and insufficient capability of the lymphatic system to transport the normal volume of lymph.[33] As a result, an abnormal accumulation of lymph fluid occurs, which leads to the swelling of the affected area.

Radiation exposure during radiotherapy is also traumatic to the lymphatic system. Radiation impairs the lymphatic system by causing tissue fibrosis surrounding the lymphatic vessels,[16,17] and it reduces lymphatic transport reserve by increasing long-term changes in basal lymph circulation and lymph flow in the affected area.[33] While lymphatic vessels are relatively insensitive to radiotherapy, lymph nodes are radiosensitive to conventional doses of radiotherapy.[31,32] The radiated lymph nodes respond first with lymphocyte depletion, followed by fatty replacement, then by fibrosis.[31,32] As a result, radiation hinders lymph nodes from properly filtering and transporting lymph and alters immune function. Research has not clarified the specific roles of chemotherapy in contributing to lymphedema.

In addition to the definite risk from cancer treatment, certain personal risk factors such as weight gain or obesity (BMI>30), infection, and immobility increase an individual's risk for lymphedema.[14–19] Other factors related to lifestyle have been cautioned including avoiding repetitive activity, overuse of the affected limb, lifting weighted objects, avoiding needle punctures and blood draws, and avoiding extremes of temperature and rigorous exercise, and compression garments have been recommended for air travel. However, high quality evidence to support these practices to reduce the risk of lymphedema is lacking.[13,34]

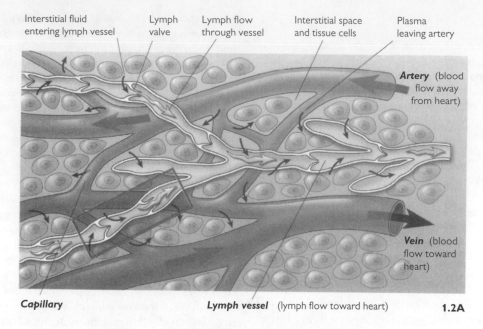

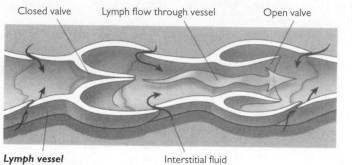

Figure 16.1 Lymphatic vessels and valves. Source: Reprinted, with permission, from the American Cancer Society. *Lymphedema: Understanding and Managing Lymphedema After Cancer Treatment.* Atlanta, GA: American Cancer Society; 2006, www.cancer.org/bookstore.

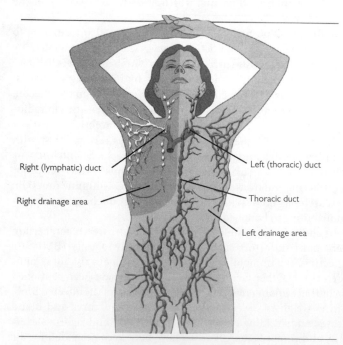

Figure 16.2 Right (lymphatic) duct, left (thoracic) duct, and drainage areas. Source: Reprinted, with permission, from the American Cancer Society. *Lymphedema: Understanding and Managing Lymphedema After Cancer Treatment.* Atlanta, GA: American Cancer Society; 2006, www.cancer.org/bookstore.

Assessment and diagnosis

Diagnosing lymphedema remains a clinical challenge. Several factors contribute to the challenge: lack of universally recognized diagnostic criteria; failure to precisely evaluate symptoms; coexisting conditions; and lack of awareness of lymphedema among healthcare professionals.[35] To ensure accurate diagnosis, it is important to conduct a careful review of the patient's health history to rule out other medical conditions that may cause similar symptoms, such as recurrent cancer, deep vein thrombosis, chronic venous insufficiency, diabetes, hypertension, and cardiac, hepatic, thyroid, and renal disease. These alternative diagnoses should be ruled out before establishing a diagnosis of lymphedema and referring the patient for lymphedema therapy. "Best practice"[35–37] components of lymphedema nursing assessment are displayed in Box 16.1.

The first assessment priority is proper diagnosis. For example, the assessment of a frail elderly woman with suspected lymphedema reveals that early symptoms of congestive heart failure are responsible for a suspected lymphedema. When the results of the physical assessment and patient history are combined with dialogue, the patient reports that she has replaced her cardiac medication with several natural supplements in order to save money and avoid "toxic drugs." Her edema resolves within several days after she resumes her cardiac medications. Some patients, especially those who are elderly, chronically ill, or significantly

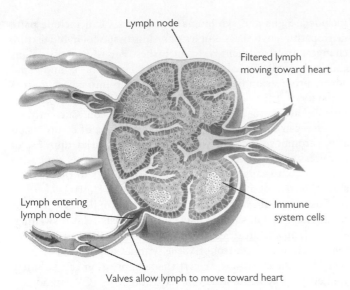

Lymph node

Filtered lymph moving toward heart

Lymph entering lymph node

Immune system cells

Valves allow lymph to move toward heart

Figure 16.3 Lymph node. Source: Reprinted, with permission, from the American Cancer Society. *Lymphedema: Understanding and Managing Lymphedema After Cancer Treatment.* Atlanta, GA: American Cancer Society; 2006, www.cancer.org/bookstore.

distressed, are not able to provide an accurate medical history. Reviewing the medical record can provide excellent assessment information. However, even the best medical record isn't always complete. Supportive dialogue with the patient can encourage them to be open and not afraid to "admit" to deviations from their recommended treatment/medication regimens, which helps the clinician to accurately assess the patient's condition and response to treatment. Asking open-ended questions such as "How do you manage taking diuretics if you have to go out of the house for extended period of time?" may elicit the fact that the patient skips

---

Box 16.1 Sequential components of lymphedema assessment

Rule out or address immediate complications (i.e., infection, thrombosis, severe pain, new or recurrent cancer, significant nonrelated disorders)

History and physical examination

Routine physical assessments: vital signs, blood pressure, height and weight, body mass index

Past and current health status, including medications and allergies (especially antibiotic allergies and history of infection, trauma, or surgery in affected area)

Current activities of daily living (job, home responsibilities, leisure activities, sleep position, activities that aggravate lymphedema)

Current psychological health, support people, view of lymphedema and health

History of lymphedema etiology, presentation, duration, and progression

Patient knowledge of and response to lymphedema, interest in assistance and goals

Third-party payer status

Quantification of lymphedema status (lymphedema signs and symptoms, volume, pain and other neurological symptoms, tissue status, range of motion of nearby joints, site-specific and overall patient function)

---

their diuretic dose on those days for fear of "wetting themselves" instead of asking the question "do you take your diuretic every day as prescribed?"

A patient health history questionnaire facilitates assessment. Useful health categories include: patient demographics; health history; etiology; signs and symptoms; complications; work and household responsibilities; support from significant others; spiritual health; and lymphedema goals.[36,38,39] Completion of the questionnaire before the initial assessment improves assessment accuracy and content and allows additional time for important nurse-patient dialogue.[38] Dialogue helps nurses to understand patients' perspective and gain essential information, including the patient's (1) view of lymphedema, (2) readiness for instruction and treatment, (3) pertinent work and lifestyle, (4) spiritual concerns, (5) illness and adjustment issues, and (6) desired goals. Often the patient's initial goal is cure, which is unattainable. In this situation, the patient needs time to understand the chronicity of lymphedema and to formulate new goals. Nurses' awareness of patient quality-of-life goals[36] fosters collaboration and management success. Instruction, support, multidisciplinary referrals, goal setting, assistance with self-care, complication avoidance, and long-term management are improved by nurses' and healthcare providers' understanding of patients' perspectives and knowledge.[36,38,39]

For example, a 58-year-old woman presents with large lower extremity primary lymphedema. She expresses a positive, easygoing life view; has a boyfriend, children, and grandchildren; cares for an elderly mother; and works full-time, 50 miles away from home. She states that her treatment goal is to "wear boots." If the nurse's goals are complete limb reduction and perfect adherence, both the nurse and the patient would be likely to experience frustration and failure. This failure *could* cause the nurse to conclude that the patient's poor outcome was caused by poor adherence. Alternatively, the nurse could collaborate with the patient on goals that are realistic to achieve given the nature of her particular condition, her life view/responsibilities, and the external factors affecting her ability to follow through with recommended compression garments, exercise, and risk-reduction strategies following treatment. Together, they can develop a workable treatment and self-care plan that would facilitate better adherence and outcome. For example, treatment goals could be to decrease fibrosis, heaviness, and swelling in her lower extremity; patient to wear compression garment daily and night compression alternative 4 of 7 nights and perform lymphedema exercises 3–5 times per week; patient to perform simple self-manual lymph drainage (MLD) in shower daily. This gives the patient some flexibility to try to fit her self-care into her busy life, affording her the self-confidence to know that she can achieve success with a modified program.

An early lymphedema diagnosis is often determined solely from a history and physical examination,[35,37] especially if conservative management is planned and symptoms are not severe. Questionable clinical symptoms or etiology may require further evaluation. Lymphoscintigraphy (isotope lymphography) can ensure definite lymphedema diagnosis.[4] Lymphography (direct), is now rarely used in lymphedema patients[35] because of its potential to cause lymphatic injury and its inability to clarify function.[32,40]

Assessment for infection, thrombosis, or cancer metastasis (Figure 16.4) is required at every patient contact.[35,40] Although later signs of infection or thrombosis are well known, awareness and careful assessment allow early diagnosis and treatment. Lymphedema progression or treatment resistance may be the earliest sign of complication or may represent a lack of response to current treatment. Changes in pain or comfort, skin (color, temperature, condition), or mobility and range of motion are other possible early signs of major complications. Most infections develop subcutaneously, beneath intact skin. Cultures are not recommended, because they rarely document a bacterial source and can further increase the risk of infection.[32] Suspected thrombosis or new or recurring cancer requires appropriate diagnostic evaluation (e.g., Doppler ultrasonography, magnetic resonance imaging, positron emission tomography, computed tomographic scanning). Venous ultrasonography is reported to be safer than venography for evaluation of suspected thrombosis in a limb with, or at high risk for, lymphedema.[41]

Figure 16.4 depicts ongoing complication assessment and decision-making. Basic treatment of complications is also

included. Signs and symptoms of metastasis can include pain, neuropathies, new masses or lesions, skin/tissue color and texture changes, and treatment-resistant rashes. For thrombosis, signs can include distended veins, venous telangiectasis, and rapid edema progression beyond the affected limb into adjacent areas of the torso.[29] Thrombosis requires anticoagulation, pain control, rest, and avoidance of use of external compression. Currently, no research clarifies the appropriate timing for use of compression after thrombosis, and the traditional 6-month delay until use of compression should be assumed.[42] Discussion of this issue with the physician is appropriate. Compression refers to the deliberate application of pressure to produce a desired clinical effect.[7] In contrast, some physicians recommend the use of limb support for several days or longer after painful thrombosis-related swelling, especially in the presence of metastatic cancer. Support signifies the retention and control of tissue without application of pressure.[7,41] Some clinicians suggest that compression can be safely applied post acute central venous thrombosis (CVT) and can

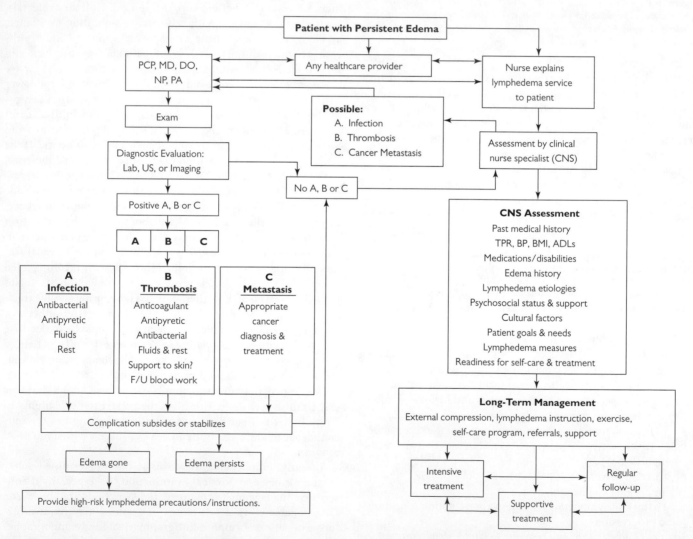

Figure 16.4 Assessment of complications in lymphedema management. ADLs, activities of daily living; BMI, body mass index; BP, blood pressure; DO, doctor of osteopathy; F/U, follow-up; MD, doctor of medicine; NP, nurse practitioner; PA, physician assistant; PCP, primary care physician; TPR, temperature, pulse, and respirations; US, ultrasonography.

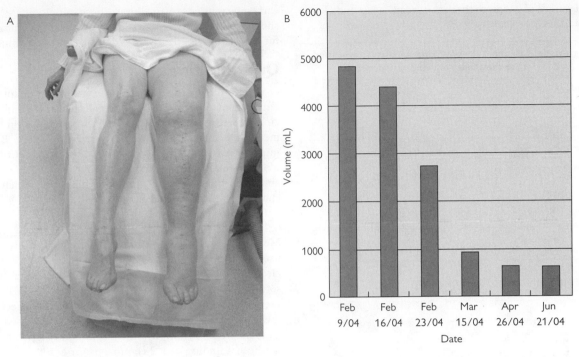

Figure 16.5 Metastatic lymphoma patient with severe deep venous thrombosis in the left leg, showing excess edema volume (mL) in the affected compared with the unaffected leg. The graph shows the improvement in the lymphedema over time.

ameliorate the exacerbation of swelling and other symptoms that occur in post thromobic symdrome.[41–42] Until research enables a practice standard, the timing of support and compression is based on clinician preference.

A diagnosis of early thrombosis was made for a 67-year-old patient with advanced metastatic lymphoma and leukemia when left leg thrombosis developed rapidly while the patient was hospitalized for a cancer complication. Thrombosis encompassed the entire leg. During anticoagulation, leg edema, pain, and signs of venous insufficiency continued to progress. Several weeks later, the patient was referred to the clinical nurse specialist for assistance. Excess edema volume in the affected leg (compared with the unaffected leg) was 94% (4816 mL). A compression garment (similar to those elastic garments used after cosmetic surgery) was provided (with physician approval) for 1 week, and 9% limb reduction was achieved. Good product tolerance was reported. A demonstration of compression legging (lower extremity, full-leg product that uses high-low foam and a spandex compression sleeve was then provided with instructions to use it as tolerated, reverting to the compression garment whenever the compression legging was removed. One week later, follow-up assessment revealed edema reduction of 43%, compared with the initial volume. Excess volume had decreased from 94% to 54% (2730 mL). The patient also agreed to referral to a lymphedema therapist to obtain daytime compression stockings and to undergo several sessions of lymphatic drainage massage. Five weeks after the initial assessment, the patient returned for follow-up wearing her new stockings, her "tight-legged" slacks, her wig, and a large smile. Pain level, skin color and condition, gait, and range of motion of the ankle, knee, and hip were significantly improved (Figure 16.5A). Edema

reduction in the lymphedema limb was 81%; excess volume was 18% (926 mL). By 4½ months following the initial assessment, edema reduction had continued. Treatment included daytime stockings and compression legging usage several nights a week. Edema reduction at this time was 87%. Excess limb volume, compared to the contralateral leg, was 12% (634 mL). Figure 16.5B displays improvement from the initial assessment through the 4-month follow-up.

Assessment of symptoms

Lymphedema symptoms, such as heaviness, tightness, firmness, pain, numbness, or impaired mobility in the affected limb, may indicate a latent stage of lymphedema in which changes cannot be detected by objective measurements.[3,43] The latent stage of lymphedema may exist months or years before overt swelling occurs. Assessing lymphedema-related symptoms plays an important role in diagnosis until objective measurements capable of detecting latent stage of lymphedema are established in at-risk individuals.[44]

Symptom assessment is essential since very often observable swelling and measurable volume changes are absent during the initial development of lymphedema.[3,4,45] Table 16.2 presents an example of a symptom checklist for breast-cancer-related lymphedema.[4] These symptoms may be the earliest indicator of increasing interstitial pressure changes associated with lymphedema.[4,45,46] As the fluid increases, the limb may become visibly swollen with an observable increase in limb size. Recent research shows that limb volume change (LVC) has significantly increased as breast cancer survivors' reports of swelling, heaviness, tenderness, firmness, tightness, and aching have increased.[46] On average, breast cancer survivors reported 4.2 symptoms for survivors

Table 16.2 Example of symptom checklist—breast cancer and lymphedema symptom experience index

The following questions are about symptoms in your affected arm, hand, breast, axilla (under arm), or chest today or in the past month.		
Have you had ___?	No	Yes
1. Limited shoulder movement		
2. Limited elbow movement		
3. Limited wrist movement		
4. Limited fingers movement		
5. Limited arm movement		
6. Hand or arm swelling		
7. Breast swelling		
8. Chest wall swelling		
9. Firmness		
10. Tightness		
11. Heaviness		
12. Toughness or thickness of skin		
13. Stiffness		
14. Tenderness		
15. Hotness/increased temperature		
16. Redness		
17. Blistering		
18. Pain/aching/soreness		
19. Numbness		
20. Burning		
21. Stabbing		
22. Tingling (pins and needles)		
23. Arm or hand fatigue		
24. Arm or hand weakness		

Source: Copyright 2006–2009 College of Nursing, New York University. Contact Mei R. Fu, PhD, RN, ACNS-BC, FAAN; Telephone: 212-998-5314; e-mail: mf67@nyu.edu

with <5.0% LVC; 5.5 symptoms for 5.0%–9.9% LVC, 7.0 symptoms for 10.0%–14.9% LVC, and 12.5 symptoms for ≥15% LVC, respectively ($p < 0.001$).[46] Most importantly, a count of lymphedema symptoms is able to differentiate healthy adults from breast cancer survivors with lymphedema and those at risk for lymphedema.[4] A diagnostic cutoff of three symptoms discriminated breast cancer survivors with lymphedema from healthy women with sensitivity of 94% and specificity of 97% (AUC [area under the curve] = 0.98). A diagnostic cutoff of nine symptoms discriminated at-risk survivors and survivors with lymphedema with sensitivity of 64% and specificity of 80% (AUC = 0.72). In the absence of objective measurements capable of detecting early development of lymphedema, count of symptoms may be a useful and cost-effective initial screening tool for detecting lymphedema.[4,45]

Because symptoms elicit tremendous distress and impair quality of life, lymphedema symptoms should warrant institution of early interventions to ameliorate those symptoms.[23,43] Symptoms should be one of the essential patient-centered clinical outcomes for evaluating the effectiveness of lymphedema treatment.

Quantification of lymphedema

A variety of measurement approaches make quantification of lymphedema a problem. Methods of measuring limb volume or circumference include sequential circumference limb measurement, water displacement, and infrared perometry.[47] Bioelectrical impedance is emerging as a possible alternative.[44] Unfortunately, lymphedema can also occur in the face, neck, shoulder, breast, abdomen, thoracic regions, and genital areas, which presents a challenge for quantification.

Sequential circumferential arm measurements

Measuring limb volume and circumference are the most widely used diagnostic methods. A flexible nonstretch tape measure for circumferences is usually used to assure consistent tension over soft tissue, muscle, and bony prominences[47] (see Figure 16.6). Measurements are done on both affected and nonaffected limbs at the hand proximal to the metacarpals, wrist, and then every 4 cm from the wrist to axilla. The most common criterion for diagnosis has been a finding of ≥ 2 centimeters or ≥ 200 mL difference in limb volume as compared with the nonaffected limb, or 10% volume difference in the affected limb. [47]

Water displacement

Although water displacement has been considered the "gold standard" for limb volume measurement and is identified as a sensitive

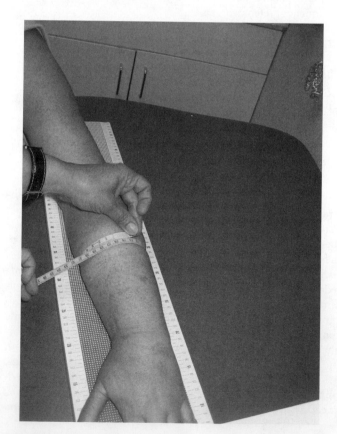

Figure 16.6 Tape measurement.

and accurate measure in the laboratory setting, water displacement is seldom used in clinical settings because of spillover and hygienic concerns. Patients submerge the affected arm in a container filled with water and the overflow of water is caught in another container and weighed. This method does not provide data about localization of the edema or shape of the extremity.[47,48] The method is contraindicated in patients with open skin lesions. Patients may find it difficult to hold the position for the time needed for the tank overflow to drain.

Infrared perometry

The perometer, an optoelectronic device developed to meet the need for a quick, hygienic, and accurate method for volume calculation, works similarly to computer-assisted tomography, but makes use of light instead of X-rays (Figure 16.7).[47–49] The volume and shape of the limb can be measured and volume changes can be calculated in seconds. Perometry and circumference are reliable measurement of limb volume change over time in individuals undergoing breast cancer treatment.

Bioelectrical impedance analysis

Bioelectrical impedance analysis (BIA) has been used for many years to detect early-onset lymphedema and to monitor results of lymphatic drainage massage in clinical settings outside the United States.[50] Bioelectrical impedance analysis measures impedance and resistance of the extracellular fluid using a single frequency below 30 kHz. The device uses the impedance ratio values between the unaffected and affected limb to calculate a *Lymphedema Index*, termed L Dex ratio. A recent published study has demonstrated that the L-Dex ratio with a cutoff point of > +7.1 can discriminate between at-risk breast cancer survivors and those with lymphedema with 80% sensitivity and 90% specificity (AUC = 0.86). In comparison, using the recommended cutoff point of L-Dex >+10 can only identity 66% of true lymphedema cases among at-risk breast cancer survivors, that is, miss 34% of true lymphedema cases (AUC = 0.81; sensitivity = 0.66 [95% CI: 0.51–0.79]). Since early treatment usually leads to better clinical outcomes, it is important to have higher sensitivity to avoid missing large numbers of true lymphedema cases. Using the diagnostic cutoff of L-Dex > +7.1, which is able to identify 80% of true lymphedema cases and 90% of nonlymphedema cases, may be an optimal choice for assessment of BIA without preoperative BIA measurement. It should be noted that there is a significant correlation between BIA and interlimb volume ratio by sequential circumferential tape measurements. Thus, objective measures of interlimb volume difference and lymph fluid change by BIA can be used to detect lymphedema objectively in clinical practice. Since there are still about 20% of true lymphedema cases missed by BIA, it is critical for clinicians to integrate other assessment methods (such as self-report, clinical observation, or perometry) to ensure the accurate detection of lymphedema.[44] The BIA technique is currently of limited use assessing individuals with bilateral swelling (Figure 16.8).

Lymphedema risk reduction

No research has demonstrated that "prevention" of lymphedema is possible. Rigid prevention measures may promote fears and frustration. The term "risk reduction" appears more accurate.[13,43] Over 50% of at-risk breast cancer survivors were found to be exceedingly worried about their risk of developing lymphedema.[13] Multiple factors may be associated with this fear of developing lymphedema among breast cancer survivors, including symptom experience, type of cancer surgery, education level, earlier experiences, or the way healthcare professionals educate and counsel individuals about risk-reducing practices.[13]

Patient education focusing on risk-reduction strategies holds great promise for reducing the risk of lymphedema. A recent study of 136 breast cancer survivors demonstrated patients who received lymphedema information reported significantly fewer symptoms and more frequent practice of risk-reduction behaviors than those who did not.[43] After controlling for confounding factors of treatment-related risk factors, patient education remains an important predictor of lymphedema outcome.[43] One essential risk-reduction behavior under patient control is maintaining ideal body weight, because excess body weight is associated with decreased lymphatic function.[16,17,19]

Infection prevention is vital for lymphedema risk reduction.[16,17,20] Infection is a significant risk factor and is the most frequent lymphedema complication.[20] Risk increases with breaches in skin integrity. Occasional drawing of blood from the limb at risk is necessary for some patients when no other reasonable option exists.[34] Patients can request an experienced phlebotomist and emphasize their increased infection risk. Subcutaneous, intramuscular, or intravenous injections in the limb at risk can cause an allergic or inflammatory response and/or infection that may compromise a weakened lymphatic system. These risks must be compared with the benefit and risk of use of a central venous catheter or suboptimal venipuncture site such as the lower extremity.[51] Diabetes potentially increases breast cancer patients' lymphedema risk when the affected limb is used for continual blood sticks or insulin injections. Patients with bilateral limb risk, especially of the upper extremities, face lifelong decisions regarding adherence to precautions.

Breast cancer disease and treatment factors are associated with increased lymphedema risk, including advanced cancer stage at diagnosis and radiation therapy to the axilla or supraclavicular area after a mastectomy. The benefits of early nursing intervention in decreasing lymphedema occurrence, severity of secondary lymphedema, and lymphedema symptoms in breast cancer survivors have been well documented.[43] Nurses can assist

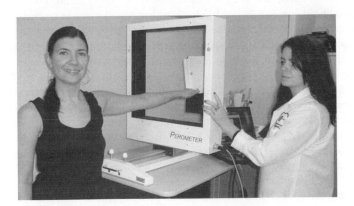

Figure 16.7 Infrared perometer measurement.

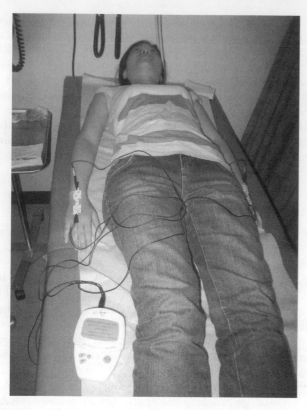

- The Imp SCA® (Impedimed, Brisbane, Australia) uses a single frequency below 30 kHz to measure impedance and resistance of the extracellular fluid.

- The device uses the impedance ratio values to calculate a *Lymphedema* Index [L-Dex], ranging from - 10 to +10.

☐ **Advantages:**
✓ Time- and cost-efficient, hygienic
✓ Easy mastery of procedure
✓ Portable
✓ Reliability is established

☐ **Limitations:**
✓ Further research is neeeded to establish validity and sensitivity of the device.

Figure 16.8 Bioelectrical impedance analysis (ImpXCA). Source: © Copyright by Mei R. Fu. All rights reserved.

high-risk patients by presenting or reinforcing prevention information and encouraging use of a well-fitted compression sleeve and gauntlet or glove at the earliest sign of edema. Emphasis on self-protection rather than rigid rules fosters patient empowerment.[34,43] For example, an empowered patient assumes responsibility for reminding staff to avoid use of the affected arm rather than expecting medical personnel to remember to do so.

In the past, breast cancer survivors were cautioned to restrict exercise as a way to reduce their risk for lymphedema. However, a growing body of evidence suggests that exercise does not necessarily increase lymphedema risk.[52] Research suggests that breast cancer survivors should be encouraged to carry out all postoperative exercises, resume normal precancer activities as tolerated, and be as fit as possible, while regularly monitoring their high-risk or affected limb.[52] In addition to the importance of physical exercise in general health, weight control, and quality of life, physical exercise can promote lymph fluid drainage through large muscle movement. Individuals should be instructed to perform physical exercise according to the general exercise guidelines[37,53]: (1) initiate exercise at lower intensity gradually increasing intensity as tolerated, monitoring the at-risk limb/s for signs and symptoms of swelling; (2) exercise to the extent that the affected body part is not fatigued; (3) modify physical exercise to reduce the risk of trauma and injury; and (4) use a compression garment during exercise if recommended by healthcare professionals with lymphedema training.

Long-term management versus treatment

Edema usually subsides with proper treatment, whereas lymphedema is a lifelong and chronic condition requiring long-term management.[27,36,54] Long-term management focuses on daily activities and strategies undertaken to decrease the swelling, relieve symptom distress, and prevent acute exacerbations and infections.[54] Components of long-term lymphedema management are listed in Box 16.2 and described throughout the chapter. Long-term management is a process of fostering optimal physical, functional, psychosocial, and spiritual wellness. Spiritual care guidelines have been gradually evolving in nursing for several decades. Spiritual care supports patients' efforts to make meaning out of illness and to redefine themselves in their new state of being. Specific spiritual interventions can include (1) support during the struggle with and exploration of life's ambiguities; (2) acknowledgment of patients' real and potential losses and victories; and (3) guidance in patients' exploration of end-of-life issues and decisions.[38,55]

Long-term management requires quantification of ongoing patient, nurse, and program outcomes.[36,54,56] Limb size or volume has been commonly used in both research and practice to evaluate treatment effectiveness. Managing limb size or volume requires patients to initiate and maintain behaviors that promote lymph drainage and reduce triggering factors leading to severe lymphedema.[27,54] Other important outcomes include pain level, skin condition, range of motion of nearby joints, affected area and overall patient function, BMI, and incidence of infection and other complications.[37,54,57] Patient's overall lymphedema-symptom experience such as psychological distress and fatigue are subjective outcomes that require supportive services. Nurses who detect distress may call on the interdisciplinary team, such as psychologists for support.[1,56]

Long-term management necessitates a multidisciplinary approach.[56,57] Nurses should assess for signs of infection, changes in limb or torso contour, and degree of swelling at each patient visit.

Box 16.2 Components of long-term lymphedema management

History, physical examination, and ongoing assessment and support
- Individualized and holistic care coordination
- Multidisciplinary referrals
- Comprehensive initial and ongoing patient instruction
- Ongoing psychosocial support
- Promotion of ongoing optimal self-care management
- Facilitation of appropriate evidence-based, individualized treatment
- Patient and practice outcome measurement
- Access and long-term follow-up and management
- Communication and collaboration with related healthcare providers

Additional inquiries need to be made as to any other symptoms patients may be experiencing because of the lymphedema. Nurses should assess self-care behaviors and encourage patients with lymphedema to wear their compression garment as prescribed. Patients with new onset or worsening lymphedema should be referred to certified lymphedema therapists for volume reduction treatment. Antibiotics may be prescribed for infections. Certified lymphedema therapists provide assessment and treatment for the swollen limb or area as well as any musculoskeletal impairment that may develop as a consequence of surgery, radiation, and or chemotherapy to treat cancer. In addition, certified lymphedema therapists also design individualized patient education about self-care practices, skin care, wear and care of compression garments, exercise and exercise progression based on individual lymphedema risk factors, and level of fitness. Certified lymphedema therapists have the expertise to recommend home and workplace modifications if needed to reduce risk for injury or overuse of the at-risk or affected limbs. Collecting and reviewing outcomes with patients over time fosters ongoing instruction, complication prevention, sustained lymphedema improvement, and patient empowerment.[27,54,57]

Case study

Ms. S, a 51-year-old female with ovarian cancer

Ms. S is a 51-year-old female who underwent a total abdominal hysterectomy and bilateral salpingo-oopherectomy in April 2008 (TAH BSO 4-08) for ovarian cancer. She received postop external beam radiation treatment to her abdomen and pelvis. Postoperatively she developed a pelvic abscess, sigmoid perforation, and an ileovaginal fistula. The fistula and perforation were repaired in December 2012, and an ileostomy was done. Ms. S stated that the swelling in her right lower extremity began after the fistula repair and ileostomy surgery 12/12. She presented for evaluation in February 2013 with genital swelling and fluid leakage from vagina as well as moderate pitting edema of her right lower extremity toes to groin with complaint of ache and heaviness 4 out of 10 (4/10). She denied swelling in her left lower extremity, which was at risk because of lymph node dissection (LND) and radiation treatment (XRT). The skin of both lower extremities was intact but taut with a slight violaceous discoloration suggestive of some venous impairment. She had chemotherapy-induced peripheral neuropathy in both feet (CIPN both feet), chronic low back pain (chronic LBP) related to herniated disc L5-S1, hypertension, adult onset diabetes

mellitus, hypothyroidism, and asthma. Patient scored herself 52% impairment on the Lower Limb Functional Index tool. She reported that her right lower extremity and pelvic area become more swollen and painful as the day progresses, limiting her ability to walk or drive any distance. Ms. S was taking ibuprofen and Percocet to control her pain and Cymbalta for depression. Pretreatment volume difference between legs was 49.7% (5288 mL). Complete decongestive therapy (CDT) 5 days per week for 4 weeks was recommended to address Ms. S's goals to decrease her pain, tightness, and edema in her right lower extremity and genital area as feasible, improve collateral lymph drainage from her lower extremities and trunk to the axillae and to increase her endurance for functional activities as tolerated. Ms. S needed to be able to walk long distances and wanted to drive with her eldest son, a high school senior, to visit colleges. At the completion of treatment she did achieve an 81% (4270 mL) reduction in volume in her right lower extremity and a reduction in the genital swelling. She was fitted with custom flat-knit chap and thigh style compression stockings Class 3 (36.1–44.5 mm Hg compression) for the right lower extremity. Pantyhose, while theoretically optimal to apply pelvic and abdominal compression, were not feasible because of abdominal discomfort, and her ileostomy appliance often leaked, causing her great distress. She was fitted with a custom thigh-length inelastic foam and fabric compression legging for night compression on her right lower extremity. She did obtain an inexpensive, ready-to-wear, lightweight microfiber panty shaper (we cut out a window for the ileostomy appliance) to provide some genital compression when she could tolerate it. Initially, post CDT treatment, she was able to walk longer distances with more comfort and she made several college visits with her eldest son and was able to take a family vacation with her husband and two sons. However, her back and abdominal pain increased and she was later admitted to the hospital with a bowel obstruction from progression of the cancer. She was able to control her swelling in the hospital with her inelastic compression legging, which she donned with nursing assistance. Although her disease progressed, she was able to obtain some relief of the pain and heaviness as well as reduce her risk for cellulitis infection in her right leg. She was happy that by treating her lymphedema, she was able to travel with her son to help him choose the college he wanted to attend the next year.

Case study

Mrs. L, an 84-year-old female with lymphedema

Mrs. L is an 84 year-old female with lymphedema in her right upper extremity (RUE) secondary to a right mastectomy and axillary lymph node dissection in 1976 to treat cancer of the right breast. She did not require chemotherapy or radiation treatment and she underwent reconstruction of the right breast with a silicone implant and reduction and lift of the left breast in 1980. Other medical diagnoses included polymyalgia rheumatica, hypertension, and diverticulitis. In 2002 with the onset of back pain it was discovered that the silicone implant was leaking and it was removed and replaced with a saline implant. In 1982 Mrs. L developed cellulitis in her right arm after sustaining scratches while cutting hedges. The infection resolved with oral antibiotics, but her RUE swelled and did not reduce after the infection cleared. In 2006, after piercing her right thenar eminence with the spoke of her umbrella, she developed a second cellulitis infection, which progressed to lymphangitis. She was hospitalized for IV antibiotics followed by a course of oral antibiotics after discharge. She was hospitalized again in September 2012, when she developed cellulitis in her RUE after cutting her right middle and ring fingers on a key ring. Since that infection, the swelling in her right forearm became more severe, interfering with fitting into blouses or jackets with long sleeves. If she wears a tight sleeve (blouse or jacket) for any period of time her right hand (which is usually not swollen) swells. Prior to the 2012 infection, Mrs. L had several courses of lymphedema treatment (variations of CDT)—some daily, some 1–2 times per week for several weeks—some with compression bandaging of her RUE, some with MLD and compression applied by a compression garment instead of bandages. She has worn a variety of compression sleeves and gauntlets and an inelastic Velcro compression armsleeve prior to the 2012 infection but following the increased swelling (that did not reduce after the infection resolved), none of these garments fit appropriately. Mrs. L reported a heaviness and tight feeling from the swelling but minimized pain per se, having adjusted with living with the swelling for so many years. The difficulty fitting into clothing and her limited ability to lift and hold her arm stable to dance (her favorite social activity) was upsetting to her.

Lymphedema assessment done on May 8, 2013 revealed severe, fibrotic, nonpitting edema of the dominant RUE from the fingers through the axilla, extending into the right posterior axilla. There was significant subcutaneous fibrosis from the right wrist through the distal aspect of the right upper arm. Initial volume difference between right and left upper extremities was 45.8 cm as measured over 8 different levels from the midhand to the axilla. Range of motion was impaired in internal rotation 0–45 degrees on the right compared with 0–60 degrees on the left, external rotation of both shoulders was 0–80 degrees, but rotations were painful. Shoulder flexion and abduction were within functional limits. Upper extremity strength was 4 out of 5. Her Quick DASH (disability arm, shoulder, and hand) score was 41%, indicating significant impairment in function because of the lymphedema. Her BMI was 23.9.

The impression was severe stage 2 breast cancer-related lymphedema (BCRL) RUE from the fingers to the axilla, extending into the right posterior axilla, with episodes of edema in the right hand. This was complicated by the patient's history of three cellulitis infections, two requiring hospitalization for IV antibiotics. The lymphedema caused significant impairment in function and quality of life for Mrs. L. A 4-week course of CDT was recommended to address the major goals of resolving/minimizing discomfort RUE; reducing risk for infection RUE; reducing edema RUE at least 10 cm; softening fibrosis RUE; preventing further skin and subcutaneous tissue changes RUE; Mrs. L to be independent in lymphedema self-care, exercises, and donning and doffing compression garments; and improving function RUE and quality of life. Mrs. L hoped to be able to fit better into her blouses and jackets and to be able to hold her RUE comfortably to dance with her partner.

Mrs. L completed 19 CDT treatments consisting of skin care, MLD directing lymph flow from her right upper extremity to her left axillary and her right inguinal lymph node regions; multilayer, short-stretch compression bandaging of her RUE from her fingers to the axilla with foam chip pads to soften fibrosis in her forearm and distal upper arm, instruction in simple self-MLD, exercises to promote lymph flow, measurement and fitting of custom seamed compression armsleeves and gloves, 25 mm Hg compression, instruction in night compression bandaging over the inelastic foam and fabric garment she had from past treatment, education in risk reduction

and resistive exercise progression. Mrs. L achieved a 21.7 cm reduction (47%) in the volume of her right upper extremity which improved to 24.3 cm (53%) at her 1-month follow-up when she reported adherence to wearing her prescribed compression garments day and night and performing her lymphatic exercises and simple self-MLD daily (30 minutes total). At her one year follow-up her reduction stabilized at 47%. Her Quick DASH score improved from 40.9% to 9.2% (a 31.7% decrease in disability). Most importantly, Mrs. L happily reported that she now fits into many blazers and blouses she had not been able to wear for several years and went dancing with her husband and friends for the first time in several years.

Edema treatment

Edema treatment focuses on detection and intervention related to the causative factor or factors. Effective treatment stabilizes the interstitial fluid volume.[8] Tissue support and/or gentle compression can be useful in relieving edema that might progress to lymphedema.

Lymphedema treatment

Lymphedema treatment refers to therapies to help reduce swelling and associated symptoms as well as maintain reductions achieved through treatment while minimizing exacerbations of swelling. Treatments include surgery, pharmacological therapy, and CDT.[37,40,54] Pharmacological therapy and surgery have limited proven effectiveness. In the past, pharmacological therapy for lymphedema has included use of coumarin (a benzopyrone) and diuretics; however, coumarin and diuretics are not recommended for the treatment of lymphedema and are proven to be ineffective.[37]

There are cases where lymphedema is combined with edema from other comorbid conditions such as heart or renal failure where diuretics are part of the medical management of these combined edemas. Patients may have heard that "diuretics are not a treatment for lymphedema" and they need to be cautioned to continue their diuretics if they have been prescribed to treat hypertension, heart or renal failure or other comorbid conditions.

Surgical treatment for lymphedema may include microsurgical lymphovenous or lympholymphatic anastomoses, debulking, and liposuction. Surgical procedures aimed at enhancing lymphatic function by removing excess fluid or tissue in the affected area have been shown to be only marginally effective.[58] Surgery does not cure lymphedema, and follow-up use of compression is necessary.[58] Surgery has provided cosmetic improvement in eyelid or genital edema.[53] Potential complications may occur with surgical management of lymphedema, such as recurrence of swelling, poor wound healing, and infection; thus surgical treatment should only be considered when other treatments fail, and with careful consideration of the benefits to risks ratio.[58]

Liposuction has been performed on patients with long-standing, breast cancer-related lymphedema.[58,59] It removes excess fat tissue and is considered only if the limb has not responded to standard conservative therapy.[58–61] Lack of response to conventional treatment results from formation of excess subcutaneous adipose tissue secondary to slow or absent lymph flow.[58–61] Liposuction has been shown to increase skin capillary blood flow without further impairing already decreased lymph transport capacity in breast cancer patients with lymphedema.[59–61] Patients are able to maintain limb reductions with concordant use of compression garments after liposuction.[37,59-61] Liposuction does not correct inadequate lymph drainage and is not indicated when pitting is present. Liposuction has also been performed on individuals with primary and secondary leg lymphedema with promising results.[37,58]

Infection prevention and treatment

Infection is the most common lymphedema complication.[20] Lymph stasis, decreased local immune response, tissue congestion, and accumulated proteins and other debris foster infection.[26] Traditional signs and symptoms (fever, malaise, lethargy, and nausea) are often present. Decades of literature support prompt oral or intravenous antibiotic therapy.[20] Because streptococci and staphylococci are frequent precipitators, antibiotics must have good skin penetration and cover normal skin flora, as well as gram-positive cocci.[62,63] Early detection and treatment of infections can help prevent the need for intravenous therapy and hospitalization.[20,62,63] Intravenous antibiotic therapy is recommended for systemic signs of infection or insufficient response to oral antibiotics.[62] Nursing activities include assisting patients in obtaining prompt antibiotic therapy, monitoring and reporting signs and symptoms, and providing instruction regarding high fluid intake, rest, elevation of the infected limb, and avoidance of strenuous activity. Garment-type compression is encouraged as soon as tolerable during infection. Wound care or infectious disease specialists can be helpful in complicated cases. Infection prophylaxis has been highly effective for patients who experience repeated serious infections or inflammatory episodes.[20,62,63] Effective edema reduction and control may also help reduce the incidence of lymphedema infection.[62]

The feet, which are especially susceptible to fungal infections in lower extremity lymphedema, can exhibit peeling, scaly skin, and toenail changes. Antifungal powders are recommended prophylactically. Antifungal creams should be used at the first sign of fungus. Diabetic-like skin care and use of cotton socks and well-fitted, breathable (leather or canvas), sturdy shoes are beneficial.[64]

Pain management

Approximately 30% to 60% of patients with lymphedema post breast cancer treatment reported pain.[46,47] Causes of pain included infection, postoperative changes in the axilla, postmastectomy pain syndrome, brachial plexopathy, various arthritic conditions, peripheral entrapment neuropathies, vascular compromise, and cancer recurrence.[64] Sudden onset of pain requires careful assessment for complications (see Figure 16.5). Use of the 0-to-10 pain scale is recommended for cancer pain assessment.[64,65] Standard pain management principles are applicable for lymphedema-related pain.

Self-care

Optimal patient self-care typically includes adherence to risk-reduction behaviors, use of compression, weight management, fitness and lymphedema exercises, optimal nutrition and hydration, healthy lifestyle practices, and seeking assistance for lymphedema-related problems.[54] Patient empowerment for optimal self-care is a great impetus to long-term management success.[27,54]

For example, one female patient with primary lymphedema attended school, worked part-time, and was a single parent of two sons. She had experienced many lymphedema treatment failures after her initial presentation of lymphedema at age 5. Treatments had been painful, distressing, and unsuccessful. Emotional scars had resulted from having legs so different from those of her friends. Five years of intermittent support and encouragement were required to achieve patient treatment readiness. Achieving a successful treatment program required another year and included surgical repair of ingrown toenails. Use of outcomes provided concrete data that fostered excellent compression adherence (daytime garment and nighttime lower leg compression). Ultimately, external compression reduced pain and fatigue sufficiently to allow 3 extra hours of activity per day. Long-term treatment success included sustained reduction of lymphedema and pain, elimination of recurrent infections, excellent compression adherence and self-care, high treatment satisfaction, and minimal need for lymphedema assistance.

Elevation

Elevation of the affected limb above the level of the heart is often recommended to reduce swelling.[3,37] Elevation promotes the drainage of lymph fluid by maximizing venous drainage and by decreasing capillary pressure and lymph production. Elevation is recommended for early-stage lymphedema of an upper limb.[3] Anecdotal evidence suggests that limb elevation when the patient is sitting or in bed may be a useful adjunct to active treatment but should not be allowed to impede function or activity.[37] Patients should be encouraged not to sleep in a chair but to go to bed at night to avoid the development of "arm chair" legs or exacerbation of lower limb lymphedema. Patient avoidance of limb dependency is also an appropriate risk-reduction strategy and may ameliorate some of the symptoms of lymphedema.

Exercise

Exercise or body movement is an integral part of lymphedema management and risk reduction. Exercise improves muscular strength, cardiovascular function, psychological well-being, and functional capacity.[52] Gentle resistance exercise stimulates muscle pumps and increases lymph flow; aerobic exercise facilitates changes in intra-abdominal pressure, which facilitates pumping of the thoracic duct.[52,53,62] A tailored exercise or body movement program that combines flexibility, resistance, and aerobic exercise may be beneficial in reducing the risk of, and controlling, lymphedema. General exercise guidelines include the following[37,52,62]:

- Start with low to moderate intensity exercise

- Walking, swimming, cycling, and low impact aerobics are recommended

- Flexibility exercises should be performed to maintain range of movement

- Appropriate warming up and cooling down phases should be implemented as part of exercise to avoid exacerbation of swelling

- Compression garments should be worn by individuals with lymphedema during exercise

Skin care

Skin care is important for lymphedema risk reduction and management, which optimizes the condition of the skin and prevents infection.[56,57,63] Diligent care is especially important for patients with lower extremity, genital, breast, head, neck, or late-stage lymphedema, additional skin alterations, or unrelated debilitating conditions. Lymphedema can cause skin dryness and irritation, which is increased with long-term use of compression products. Bland, nonscented products are recommended for daily cleansing and moisturizing.[37,63] Low pH moisturizers, which discourage infection, are recommended for advanced lymphedema, because skin and tissue changes increase infection risk. Water-based moisturizers, which are absorbed more readily, are less likely to damage compression products but are not suitable for all patients. Cotton clothing allows ventilation and is absorbent.

Advanced lymphedema can cause several skin complications, including lymphorrhea, lymphoceles, papillomas, and hyperkeratosis. Lymphorrhea is leakage of lymph fluid through the skin that occurs when skin cannot accommodate accumulated fluid. Nonadherent dressings, good skin care, and compression are used to alleviate leakage. Compression and good skin care also reduce the occurrence of lymphoceles, papillomas, and hyperkeratosis; these complications reflect skin adaptation to excess subcutaneous lymph.

Bandages

Multilayer lymphedema bandaging (MLLB) provides external compression. For some patients, MLLB may be used as part of long-term or palliative management. It uses inelastic or low-stretch bandages to produce a massaging effect and stimulate lymph flow,[37,66] and is especially important for patients with severe lymphedema, such as lymphedema complicated by morbid obesity or neglected primary lymphedema. It is also important for patients who choose self- or caregiver bandaging to enhance comfort or for nighttime compression when they wear a compression garment during the day.[37,66] Foam or other padding is often used under bandages to improve edema reduction, soften fibrosis, and restore normal limb contours. The time, effort, and dexterity required for bandaging can become burdensome and is not practical or possible for some patients, necessitating the use of an alternative compression method.[27] Multilayer lymphedema bandaging should be avoided for the following conditions: (1) severe arterial insufficiency with an ankle/brachial index (ABI) of < 0.6, although modified MLLB with reduced pressures can be used under close supervision; (2) uncontrolled heart failure; and (3) severe peripheral neuropathy.[37,66] Some components of the MLLB system can be washed and dried according to the manufacturer's instructions and reused. Over time, inelastic bandages will progressively lose their extensibility, which will increase their stiffness. Heavily soiled, cohesive, and adhesive bandages should be discarded after use.[37,66]

Compression garments

Compression garments are recommended for patients with lymphedema of the extremities.[62,66] Compression garments may be used in the initial management of patients who have mild upper or lower limb lymphedema with minor pitting, no significant tissue changes, no or minimal shape distortion, or palliative needs.[3,37,66] Proper fit of the compression garment is imperative. An ill-fitting garment can cause swelling to develop in an area proximal or distal to the end of the garment, that is, in the hand or in the anterior or posterior axillary/shoulder areas or in the toes or genital/pubic/buttock/abdominal areas. Patients must be instructed to remove their garment if this type of swelling, pain, numbness, or muscle cramps occur and consult with

their lymphedema specialist regarding revision of the garment to ensure proper fit and function. Physiological effects of compression include edema control or reduction, decreased accumulation of interstitial proteins, decreased arteriole outflow into the interstitium, improved muscle pump effect with movement and exercise of the affected area, and protection of skin. Gradient compression provides the greatest pressure distally and less pressure proximally; this is optimal for improved lymphatic transport.[37,66] Skin care, exercise or body movement, elevation and self-lymph drainage should be taught, along with self-monitoring help to relieve lymphedema symptoms in individuals receiving palliative care. Patients should be reassessed 4 to 6 weeks after initial fitting and then approximately every 3 to 6 months.[37,66]

Compression garments should be laundered every time they are worn and replaced every 3–6 months. Although some manufacturers suggest machine drying, elastic compression garments last longer if they are air-dried; patients need a minimum of 2 so that they have one to wash and one to wear. Patients need to moisturize and check their skin daily for signs of irritation/infection. A variety of helpful products exist to assist patients in applying garments, which may be an especially challenging task for elderly and disabled patients. Pain or impairment in hand dexterity or strength secondary to arthritic changes or neuropathies may limit a patient's tolerance of garments. If a compression garment causes pain, neurological symptoms, or color or temperature changes it should be removed and the patient instructed to consult with their lymphedema specialist to resolve the problem. Individuals with significant lymphedema will experience worsening of their lymphedema if they are without compression for extended periods of time. They need to know whom to contact and how to advocate for themselves to correct the problem. Readjustment and movement may remedy the problem; often, product replacement is required. Thanks to the variety of products that exist, staff and patient persistence is likely to result in good patient tolerance. Ridged rubber gloves (dishwashing gloves) facilitate application of garments and extend their longevity. Timely garment replacement (usually every 6 months) is essential for good edema control.[37,66]

Other compression products

A growing number of alternative commercial compression products have become available. Semirigid products use inelastic fabric, foam, Velcro straps, and an outer spandex compression sleeve to provide nonelastic compression designed to simulate bandaging while saving time and energy. The compression sleeve allows adjustment for limb size changes, which can be ideal for limb reduction or increase or for weight changes affecting limb size. Distinct advantages of these products include ease and speed of application, overall comfort and tolerance, and product longevity. Haslett and Aitken[67] reported that such a foam and fabric compression garment appeared to contribute to maintenance of previously achieved decongestive lymphatic therapy (DLT) reduction. Lund[68] reported that use of an inelastic Velcro closure garment provided an acceptable substitute for bandaging. Use of inelastic Velcro closure products on the lower extremities is currently contraindicated with ABI < 0.6.[37,66] Research is needed to provide insight and direction regarding the use of these promising products.

Decongestive lymphatic therapy and lymph drainage massage

Decongestive lymphatic therapy (DLT) evolved in Europe when Michael Foldi[32,54,66] combined Vodder's MLD technique with bandaging, exercises, and specialized skin care. Dr. Foldi described his four-modality lymphedema treatment as "complete decongestive therapy" (CDT). This includes MLD; multilayer, short-stretch compression bandaging; gentle exercise; meticulous skin care; education in lymphedema self-management; and elastic compression garments, and has become the standard of care for treating lymphedema.[66] Patients generally receive 2-hour treatments 5 days a week for 3 to 8 weeks and are required to make a commitment to continue performing the exercise and skin care and to wear the compression garments. Adherence to the prescribed treatment can be difficult because even the most customized garments or sleeves sometimes are uncomfortable, unsightly, and laborious to put on.[66] A constellation of complex factors (e.g., physical, financial, aesthetic, time) can influence survivors' adherence with treatment. Lymphedema is a complex condition that needs to be treated by therapists with special training and experience in this field, as outlined by the National Lymphedema Network position paper on educational training for lymphedema therapists (http://www.lymphnet.org/pdfDocs/nlntraining.pdf) and the Lymphology Association of North America (LANA) (http://www.clt-lana.org/). These multidisciplinary organizations have outlined training requirements for clinicians to gain certification in this field.

Pneumatic (mechanical) pumps—intermittent pneumatic compression devices

Mechanical pneumatic pumps use electricity to inflate a single-chamber or multichamber sleeve that produces external limb compression. A decreased tissue capillary filtration rate (documented by lymphoscintigraphy) facilitates tissue fluid reduction and, consequently, limb volume decrease.[69] Lymph formation decreases, but lymph transport, which would address lymphedema pathophysiology, is not affected. Pneumatic pumps can reduce swelling, but concern exists regarding the way in which swelling is decreased as well as the rapid displacement of fluid elsewhere in the body. In addition, the use of pumps does not eliminate the need for compression garments and may not provide more benefit than garments alone.[69] Using pumps may cause complications, including lymphatic congestion and injury proximal to the pump sleeve, increased swelling adjacent to the pump cuff in up to 18% of patients,[69,70] lack of benefit in all but stage I (reversible) lymphedema, and development of genital lymphedema in some patients with cancer-related lower extremity lymphedema.[69,70] After more than 50 years of pump use in lymphedema care and long-established Medicare reimbursement, no guidelines exist, significant complications are reported, and research has not clarified benefit.

Case study

Mr. K, a 59-year-old man with lymphedema

Mr. K, a 59-year-old airline baggage handler, was diagnosed in May 2012 with lymphedema in his RUE, right anterior and posterior axillary, and scapular areas after undergoing right axillary dissection in April 2012 to stage melanoma. The original excision of the melanoma on his right upper back was in January 2012. Mr. K was on disability from his job due to pain, limited mobility, and swelling in his RUE (self score 5-7/10). Initial evaluation revealed that Mr. K had mild to moderate mixed pitting and nonpitting edema of his RUE from the fingers through the axilla, extending into the right anterior and posterior axillary and scapular areas. The skin of his RUE was taut and shiny, and range of motion of the right shoulder was impaired as follows: shoulder flexion 0–90 degrees, abduction 0–80 degrees, and both internal and external rotation of the right shoulder 0–70 degrees. Range of motion of his left shoulder was within normal limits. Strength of the right shoulder was 3+-4/5 compared with 5/5 on the left. Initial volume difference between right and left upper extremities was 26% (692 mL). The assessment was mild to moderate stage 1/stage 2 secondary lymphedema RUE from the fingers through the axilla, extending into the right anterior and posterior axillary and scapular areas. This was combined with impairment in range of motion and strength and function of the RUE. His Quick DASH score was 100% impairment in the work module and 58.6% impairment for activities of daily living (ADLs). Mr. K completed 19 CLT treatments consisting of skin care, MLD directing lymph flow from his right upper extremity to his left axillary and right inguinal lymph node regions, short-stretch compression bandaging of his RUE from his fingers to his axilla, measurement and fitting of custom seamed compression armsleeves and gloves, 20 mm Hg compression, education in self-care, simple self-MLD, lymphatic exercises to facilitate lymph flow, active and active assistive range of motion and strengthening exercises to improve ROM and strength right shoulder, education in lymphedema risk reduction, and discussion in job modification to reduce risk for injury RUE. He achieved a 25% (180 mL) reduction in volume in his RUE. This improved to 55% (382ml) at his 1-year follow-up. He was adherent with wearing his prescribed compression garments day and night but was inconsistent with his self-MLD and exercises. His pain/discomfort reduced to 1–2/10. His Quick DASH score improved from 58.6% to 38.6%. He decided to take an early retirement from the airline and has applied for Social Security Disability. He is comfortable with that decision and is focusing on good nutrition and daily exercise at the gym, following exercise progression guidelines learned during lymphedema treatment, and monitoring his RUE for any signs of worsening lymphedema after each exercise session, which he has not experienced.

Case study

Mr. F, a 64-year-old male with swelling in the neck

Mr. F is a 64-year-old male with swelling in the neck secondary to surgery and radiation treatment to treat tongue cancer. Mr. F had surgery to remove cancerous lesions on the tongue in 2007. No lymph node dissection was done at that time. He reported that the cancer recurred in May 2012 and the new lesions were excised and he received radiation treatment to the head and neck for 6 weeks, ending September 4, 2012. He had been seen in rehab for tightness in his neck and evaluation for an appliance to help increase mouth opening. He was referred to a lymphedema therapy center in January 2013. Assessment revealed a mobile male, within ideal body weight (BMI 25.3). There was fibrotic swelling noted in the submandibular region as well as distal to that around the hyoid area. The skin of the head and neck were intact. There was significant fibrosis palpable in the mandibular and maxillary areas. The skin in the neck was discolored from the radiation treatments. Range of motion of the neck was functional, but he exhibited a forward head and round-shouldered posture in sitting. He denied difficulty chewing or swallowing but complained that he could not open his mouth fully. He reported his discomfort/tightness/pain as 3/10. He never received the mouth appliance, stating that no one contacted him after he was seen in rehab. The impression was that of mild stage 2 secondary lymphedema of the neck, and a few sessions of MLD from the neck and submandibular area to the supra- and infraclavicular and axillary lymph nodes bilaterally, and facial and postural exercises were recommended; treatment included instruction in self-MLD and risk-reduction strategies to reduce the risk for infection or worsening of the swelling. A call was placed to the rehab physician to facilitate an appointment to fit a mouth appliance.

Treatment goals were to decrease discomfort from 3/10 to 1/10, reduce risk for infection in the head and neck, minimize skin and subcutaneous tissue changes in the head and neck associated with chronic lymphedema, patient to be independent in lymphatic and postural exercises, patient to apply the principles of risk reduction to his activities of daily living. Mr. F completed 4 treatment sessions and reported reduction in discomfort from 3/10 to 1/10 and demonstrated good technique with self-MLD and facial and postural exercises. Follow-up appointment March 2013—discomfort still 1/10, skin face and neck intact but dry and peeling. Posture in sitting was improved. He was using moisturizer daily and denied any infection in the head/neck. He had received his mouth appliance and reported improvement in mouth opening. His surgeon was pleased with his progress and Mr. F was discharged with suggestion to call for follow-up if needed.

Unusual lymphedemas

Palliative care may require the management of unusual and challenging lymphedema sites, such as breast, head, neck, trunk, or genitals.[56] Manual lymph drainage, skin-softening techniques, foam chip pads, and external compression (if possible) are recommended.[2] External compression may be achieved with collars, vests, custom pants or tights, scrotal supports,[37,56] or spandex type exercise apparel. The assistance of occupational or physical therapists and a seamstress may be helpful. Nationally, instructional courses are available to provide guidance for managing these difficult lymphedemas, such as courses provided by the Lymphology Association of North America (LANA) (http://www.clt-lana.org/). Box 16.3 presents detailed information about neck lymphedema from head and neck cancer.

Conclusion

Edema is a symptom usually relieved by addressing the causative factor. Lymphedema, often labeled as edema, is a chronic disorder that requires long-term management. Although external compression is essential for effective lymphedema management, third-party payer reimbursement is inadequate and frustrating. Patients are frequently fitted with products they cannot tolerate, and many patients have not been adequately prepared for compression products and therefore discontinue use when their product does not "cure" the lymphedema. Newer inelastic compression products for night compression offer exciting product alternatives, but lack controlled research substantiation. Benefits of two commonly supported treatments, DLT and pneumatic compression pumps, have not been

---

Box 16.3 Lymphedema secondary to cancer of the head and neck

Lymphedema secondary to head and neck cancer commonly presents following surgery and radiotherapy. Lymphedema is frequently found below the chin in the anterior neck. Difficulty in swallowing and breathing are the major symptoms causing distress from neck lymphedema. Mild swelling often progresses fairly rapidly to firm, nonpitting swelling and thus may often not be recognized or treated as lymphedema.

Quantification of neck edema can be achieved by measuring from the tip of one ear lobe to the tip of the contralateral ear lobe along the line of the chin, and then measuring this distance for every 2 cm (or 4 cm) interval down to the intersection of the neck and chest. Quantifiable outcome measurement over time fosters patient participation, improved long-term outcomes, and might be beneficial as substantiation for third-party payers.

Compression supports used after cosmetic facial surgery can be useful for neck lymphedema. These products provide gentle compression to the chin using two sets of long narrow Velcro straps that extend from the chin to the top of the head and to the back of the neck. This size-adjustable "chin strap" provides gentle, size-adjustable compression to the chin and neck. Patients are encouraged to use the product continually for at least several weeks or a month to achieve optimal edema reduction. Although lifelong product use is encouraged for optimal lymph function, some patients have been able to transition to mainly nighttime product use and still maintain acceptable edema control.

Nursing interventions for head and neck lymphedema include:

- Help patients to make an informed decision in a supportive environment.
- Instruction and support in establishment of a lifelong daily self-care regimen including range-of-motion exercises, skin assessment, and application of moisturizers and early, skilled patient complication assistance and use of safe external compression. A written self-care program may foster patient self-care adherence.
- Monitor external neck compression. External neck compression must provide sufficient pressure to stimulate lymphatic function without causing skin irritation/injury or impairment of breathing, eating, or swallowing.
- Encourage the use of daily self-care using MLD and exercises for facial, neck, and postural muscles to further improve edema control and posture.
- Document patient outcomes, including interval neck circumferences, skin integrity, pain level, and neck range of motion.

---

substantiated by randomized controlled clinical trials, according to several expert literature reviews. Controlled clinical trials are essential for establishing "gold standard" treatments and should be the basis for third-party payer reimbursement. This research deficit has precluded the establishment of outcome and practice standards, allowing an "anything goes" treatment environment.

Nevertheless, over the last two decades, progress has been achieved in both lymphedema awareness and scientific research. Oncology nurses and other nurses have increasingly contributed to lymphedema management as they have improved cancer survivorship. Nursing's unique focus and scope of practice is ideally suited to chronic illness management, both at entry and advanced practice levels. To meet the physical and psychological needs of patients, nurses and other healthcare professionals must make an effort to understand the pathophysiology and chronic nature of lymphedema, as well as its physical, functional, and psychosocial impact. Armed with such information, nurses can then engage patients in supportive dialogue about risk reduction and lymphedema management.[27,54] Combined with nurses' immense and diverse patient contact, enormous potential exists for nurses to dramatically improve both edema and lymphedema management.

References

1. Fu MR, Ridner SH, Hu SH, Steward B, Cormier JN, Armer JM. Psychosocial impact of lymphedema: a systematic review of literature from 2004 to 2011. Psycho-Oncol 2013; 22(7):1466–1484. DOI: 10.1002/pon.3201. Epub 2012 Oct 9. PMID: 23044512

2. Chachaj A, Malyszczak K, Pyszel K, Lukas J, et al. Physical and psychological impairments of women with upper lymphedema following breast cancer treatment. Psycho-Oncol. 2009;19:299–305.

3. International Society of Lymphology. The diagnosis and treatment of peripheral lymphedema: consensus document of the International Society of Lymphology. Lymphology. 2003;36:84–91.

4. Fu MR, Cleland CM, Guth AA, Qiu Z, Haber J, Cartwright-Alcarese F, et al. The role of symptom report in detecting and diagnosing breast cancer-related lymphedema. Euro J Clin Med Oncol. 2013.

5. Olszewski WL. Pathophysiological aspects of lymphedema of human limb: I. Lymph protein composition. Lymphatic Res Biol. 2003;1(1):235–243.

6. Stanton AW, Modi S, Mellor RH, Levick JR, Mortimer PS. Recent advances in breast cancer-related lymphedema of the arm: lymphatic pump failure and predisposing factors. Lymphatic Res Biol. 2009;7(1):29–45.

7. Brorson H, Aberg M, Svensson H. Chronic lymphedema and adipocyte proliferation: clinical therapeutic implications. The Lymphatic Continuum. National Institutes of Health, Bethesda, USA, 2002. Lymphat Res Biol. 2003;1:88.

8. WHO: The World Health Report 2004—Changing History. Geneva: World Health Organization, 2004.

9. Ferrell R, Kimak M, Lawrence E, Finegold D. Candidate gene analysis in primary lymphedema. Lymphat Res Biol. 2008;6:69–76.

10. Ghalamkarpour A, Morlot S, Raas-Rothschild A, et al. Hereditary lymphedema type I associated with VEGFR3 mutation: the first de novo case and atypical presentation. Clin Genet. 2006;70:330–335.

11. Spiegel R, Ghalamkarpour A, Daniel-Spiegel E, Vikkula M, Shalev S. Wide clinical spectrum in a family with hereditary lymphedema type I due to a novel missense mutation in VEGFR3. J Human Genet. 2006;51:846–850.

12. Moffatt CJ, Franks PJ, Doherty D, et al. Lymphoedema: an underestimated health problem. QJM. 2003;96:731–38.

13. McLaughlin SA, Bagaria S, Gibson T, Arnold M, Diehl N, et al., Trends in risk reduction practices for the prevention of lymphedema in the first 12 months after breast cancer surgery. J Am Coll Surg. 2013;216(3):380–389.

14. Paskett ED, Naughton MJ, McCoy TP, Case LD, Abbott JM. The epidemiology of arm and hand swelling in premenopausal breast cancer survivors. Cancer Epidemiol Biomarkers Prev. 2007;16:775–782.

15. Cormier JN, Askew RL, Mungovan KS, Xing Y, Ross MI, Armer JM. Lymphedema beyond breast cancer. Cancer. 2010;116:5138–5149. doi:10.1002/cncr.25458.

16. Kwan ML, Darbinian J, Schmitz KH, Citron R, Partee P, et al. Risk factors for lymphedema in a prospective breast cancer survivorship study: the Pathways study. Arch Surg. 2010;145:1055–1063. doi: 10.1001/archsurg.2010.231.

17. Ahmed RL, Schmitz KH, Prizment AE, Folsom AR. Risk factors for lymphedema in breast cancer survivors, the Iowa Women's Health Study. Breast Cancer Res Treat. 2011;130:981–991. doi: 10.1007/s10549-011-1667-z.

18. Vaqas B, Ryan TJ. Lymphoedema: pathophysiology and management in resource-poor settings—relevance for lymphatic filariasis control programmes. Filaria J. 2003;2:4.

19. Mak SS, Yeo W, Lee YM, Mo KF, Tse KY, Tse SM, et al. Predictors of lymphedema in patients with breast cancer undergoing axillary lymph node dissection in Hong Kong. Nurs Res. 2008;57:416–425.

20. Ridner SH, Deng J, Fu MR, Radina E, Thiadens SRJ, Weiss J, et al. Symptom burden and infection occurrence among individuals with extremity lymphedema. Lymphology. 2012;45(3):113–123.

21. Angeli V, Randolph GJ. Inflammation, lymphatic function, and dendritic cell migration. Lymphatic Res Biol. 2006;4(4):217–228.

22. Newman B, Lose F, Kedda MA, Francois M, Ferguson K, Janda M, et al. Possible genetic predisposition to lymphedema after breast cancer. Lymphatic Res Biol. 2012;10(1):1–12. doi: 10.1089/lrb.2011.0024.

23. Fu MR, Rosedale M. Breast cancer survivors' experience of lymphedema related symptoms. J Pain Symptom Manage. 2009;38(6):849–859. PMID: 19819668.

24. Shih YC, Xu Y, Cormier JN, Giordano S, Ridner SH, Buchholz TA, et al. Incidence, treatment costs, and complications of lymphedema after breast cancer among women of working age: a 2-year follow-up study. J Clin Oncol. 2009;27(12):2007–2014.

25. Fu MR. Women at work with breast cancer-related lymphoedema. J Lymphedema. 2008;3:30–36.

26. Ruocco V, Schwartz RA, Ruocco E. Lymphedema: an immunologically vulnerable site for development of neoplasms. J Am Acad Dermat. 2002;47:124–127.

27. Fu MR. Breast cancer survivors' intentions of managing lymphedema. Cancer Nurs. 2005;28:446–457.

28. Firth J. Idiopathic oedema of women. In: Warrell DA, Cox TM, Firth JD (eds.), Oxford Textbook of Medicine. Oxford: Oxford University Press; 2004:1209–1210.

29. Szuba A, Razavi M, Rockson SG. Diagnosis and treatment of concomitant venous obstruction in patients with secondary lymphedema. J Vasc Interv Radiol. 2002;13:799–803.

30. Ganong WF. Dynamics of blood and lymph flow. In: Ganong WF (ed.), Review of Medical Physiology. Chicago: Lange Medical Books, McGraw-Hill Medical Publishing Division; 2001:570–571.

31. Fu MR, Ridner SH, Armer J. Pathophysiology of post-breast cancer lymphedema. Am J Nurs. 2009;109(7):48–54.

32. Foldi M, Foeldi E, Clodius L, Neu H. Complications of lymphedema. In: Foeldi M, Foeldi E, Kubik S (eds.), Textbook of Lymphology for Physicians and Lymphedema Therapists. Munich: Urban & Fischer Verlag: Elsevier GmbH; 2003:267–275, English text revised by Biotext LLC, San Francisco.

33. Perbeck L, Celebioglu F, Svensson L, Danielsson R. Lymph circulation in the breast after radiotherapy and breast conservation. Lymphology. 2006;39:33–40.

34. Cemal Y, Pusic A, Mehrara BJ. Preventative measures for lymphedema: separating fact from fiction. J Am Coll Surg. 2011; 213(4):543–551. doi: 10.1016/j.jamcollsurg.2011.07.001.

35. Fu MR, Ridner SH, Armer J. Post-breast cancer lymphedema: impact and diagnosis. Am J Nurs. 2009;109:48–54.

36. Fu MR. Post-breast cancer lymphedema and management. Recent Adv Res Updates. 2004;5:125–138.

37. Morgan PA, Moffat CJ. Lymphoedema Framework. Best Practice for the Management of Lymphoedema. International Consensus. London: MEP Ltd, 2006.

38. Parran L. Spiritual care is elemental and fundamental to the heart. ONS News. 2003;8(3):1,4,5.

39. Armer JM, Stewart BR, Wanchai A, Lasinski BB, Smith K, Cormier JN. Rehabilitation concepts among aging survivors living with and at risk for lymphedema: a framework for assessment, enhancing strengths, and minimizing vulnerability. Top Geriatric Rehabil. 2012;28(4):260–268.

40. Radina EM, Fu MR. Preparing for and coping with breast cancer-related lymphedema. In: Alberto Vannelli (ed.), Lymphedema. InTech: Open Science/Open Mind; 2012. www.intechweb.org.

41. Shrubb D, Mason W. The management of deep vein thrombosis in lymphoedema: a review. Br J Community Nurs. 2006;11:292–297.

42. Partsch H, Flour M, Smith PC. Indications for compression therapy in venous and lymphatic disease consensus based on experimental data and scientific evidence. Under the auspices of the IUP. Int Angiol. 2008;27:193–219.

43. Fu MR, Chen C, Haber J, Guth A, Axelrod D. The effect of providing information about lymphedema on the cognitive and symptom outcomes of breast cancer survivors. Ann Surg Oncol. 2010;17(7):1847–1853. Epub 2010 Feb 6. PMID: 20140528. doi 10.1245/s10434-010-0941-3

44. Fu MR, Cleland CM, Guth AA, Kayal M, Haber J, Cartwright-Alcarese F, et al. L-Dex ratio in detecting breast cancer-related lymphedema: reliability, sensitivity, and specificity. Lymphology. 2013;46(2):85–96.

45. Armer JM, Radina ME, Porock D, Culbertson SD. Predicting breast cancer-related lymphedema using self-reported symptoms. Nurs Res. 2003;52:370–379.

46. Cormier JN, Xing Y, Zaniletti I, Askew RL, Stewart BR, Armer JM. Minimal limb volume change has a significant impact on breast cancer survivors. Lymphology. 2009;42:161–175.

47. Armer JM, Stewart BR. A comparison of four diagnostic criteria for lymphedema in a post-breast cancer population. Lymphat Res Biol. 2005;3:208–217.

48. Tierney S, Aslam M, Rennie K, Grace, P. Infrared optoelectronic volumetry, the ideal way to measure limb volume. Eur J Vasc Endovasc Surg. 1996;12:412–417.

49. Petlund CF. Volumetry of limbs. In: Olszewski WI (ed.), Lymph Stasis: Pathophysiology, Diagnosis and Treatment. Boston: CRC Press; 1991:444–451.

50. Cornish BH, Chapman M, Hirst C, Mirolo B, Bunce IH, Ward LC, Thomas BJ. Early diagnosis of lymphedema using multiple frequency bioimpedance. Lymphology. 2001;34:2–11.

51. Venipuncture Policy. Penrose-St. Francis Health Services. Nursing Policy Committee, Colorado Springs, CO; 2003.

52. Kwan ML, Cohn JC, Armer JM, Stewart BR, Cormier JN. Exercise in patients with lymphedema: a systematic review of the contemporary literature. J Cancer Survivorship. 2011;5(4):320–336.

53. National Lymphedema Network (NLN). Position Paper on Lymphedema Risk Reduction Practices. Available at: http://www.lymphnet.org/lymphedemaFAQs/positionPapers.htm. Accessed July, 24 2013.

54. Ridner SH, Fu MR, Wanchai A, Stewart BR, Armer JM, Cormier JN. Self-management of lymphedema: a systematic review of literature from 2004 to 2011. Nurs Res. 2012;61(4):291–299.

55. Highfield ME. Providing spiritual care to patients with cancer. Clin J Oncol Nurs. 2000;4:115–120.

56. Beck M, Wanchai A. Stewart BR, Cormier JN, Armer JM. Palliative care for cancer-related lymphedema: a systematic review. J Palliat Med. 2012;15(7):821 827.

57. Fu MR, Ridner SH, Armer J. Post-breast cancer lymphedema: risk-reduction and management. Am J Nurs. 2009;109:34–41.

58. Cormier JN, Rourke L, Crosby M, Chang D, Armer J. The surgical treatment of lymphedema: a systematic review of the contemporary literature (2004–2010). Ann Surg Oncol. 2012;19(2);642–651.

59. Brorson H, Svensson H. Complete reduction of lymphoedema of the arm by liposuction after breast cancer. Scand J Plast Reconstr Surg Hand Surg. 1997;31:137–143.

60. Brorson H. Liposuction in arm lymphedema treatment. Scand J Surg. 2003;92:287–295.

61. Brorson H, Ohlin K, Olsson G, Langstrom G, Wiklund I, Svensson H. Quality of life following liposuction and conservative treatment of arm lymphedema. Lymphology. 2006;39(1):8–25.

62. Arsenault K, Reilly L, Wise H. Effects of complete decongestive therapy on the incidence rate of hospitalization for the management of recurrent cellulitis in adults with lymphedema. Rehabilitation Oncology. 2011;29(3):14–20.

63. Fu MR. Preventing skin breakdown in lymphoedema. Wounds International. 2010;1(4):17–19.

64. Wanchai A, Beck M, Stewart BR, Armer JM. Management of lymphedema for cancer patients with complex needs. Semin Oncol Nurs. 2013;29(1):61–65.

65. Serlin R, Mendoza T, Nakamura Y, Edwards KR, Cleeland CS. When is cancer pain mild, moderate or severe? Grading pain severity by its interference with function. Pain. 1995;61:277–284.

66. Lasinski BB, Thrift KM, Squire D, Austin MK, Wanchai A, Green JM, et al. A systematic review of the evidence for complete decongestive therapy in the treatment of lymphedema from 2004 to 2011. Physic Med Rehab. 2012;4(8):580–601.

67. Haslett ML, Aitken MJ. Evaluating the effectiveness of a compression sleeve in managing secondary lymphoedema. J Wound Care 2002;11:401–404.

68. Lund E. Exploring the use of the CircAid legging in the management of lymphoedema. Int J Palliat Nurs. 2000;6:383–391.

69. Feldman JL, Stout NL, Wanchai A, Stewart BR, Cormier JN, Armer JM. Intermittent pneumatic compression therapy: a systematic review. Lymphology. 2012;45(1):13–25.

70. Boris M, Weindorf S, Lasinski B. The risk of genital edema after external pump compression for lower limb lymphedema. Lymphology. 1998;31:15–20.

CHAPTER 17A

Skin disorders

Pressure ulcers: prevention and management

Barbara M. Bates-Jensen and Sirin Petch

It's his fourth stage 4 pressure ulcer in the last 5 years. He's had multiple surgeries and is not a candidate for any more. I just don't know what we can do for his ulcer.

A nurse caring for a patient with recurrent severe pressure ulcers

I always thought that bedsores came from neglect. I feel so guilty that I let this happen.

A patient's family member

Key points

♦ Palliative pressure ulcer care is not "lack of care"; but care focused on comfort and limiting the extent or impact of the wound.

♦ Pressure ulcer prevention for palliative care includes use of flexible repositioning schedules with attention to adequate pain relief interventions before movement and use of pressure-redistributing support surfaces for the bed and chair.

♦ Palliative care for pressure ulcers includes attention to prevention measures; obtaining and maintaining a clean wound; management of pain, exudate, and odor; and prevention of complications such as wound infection.

♦ It is essential to involve the individual, family members, and caregivers in establishing goals of care, enacting a plan of care, and defining the individual's wishes.

Palliative care for skin disorders is a broad area, encompassing prevention and care for chronic wounds such as pressure ulcers, management of malignant wounds and fistulas, and management of stomas. The goals of treatment are to reduce discomfort and pain, manage odor and drainage, and provide for optimal functional capacity. In each area, involvement of the caregiver and family in the plan of care is important. Management of skin disorders involves significant physical care as well as attention to psychological and social care. To meet the needs of the patient and family, access to the multidisciplinary care team is crucial, and consultation by an enterostomal therapy nurse; a certified wound, ostomy, and continence nurse; or a certified wound care nurse is highly desirable.

Because skin disorders are such an important issue in palliative nursing care, chapter 17 has been divided into two distinct parts. Chapter 17A addresses pressure ulcers in depth, and chapter 17B

addresses malignant wounds, fistulas, and stomas. While pressure ulcers are not the only wounds to occur at the end of life, they are the most common wound type to occur in patients receiving palliative care, accounting for 40% to 50% of wounds.[1,2] Pressure ulcer prevalence in palliative care patients in acute care settings ranges from 22%[3] to 60%[4] with acute care incidence varying from 10%[3,5] to 22%.[2] In home care, pressure ulcer prevalence in palliative care patients has been reported between 10.7%[6] and 26.9%[7] with 3-month incidence at 10%, 75% of which were stage 1 or 2 pressure ulcers.[8] In nursing homes, pressure ulcer prevalence is 9% (based on one large database study),[9] and incidence has been reported as high as 55% among terminally ill nursing home residents.[10] Studies in palliative care settings or hospice settings report prevalence rates from 17.5%[1] to 23%[11] and incidence rates at 6.5%.[11] The majority of pressure ulcers that occur in patients receiving palliative care are stage 1 or stage 2 ulcers.[2,3,5,8,10] Of interest, when patients receiving palliative care are separated by cancer versus noncancer diagnoses, those patients with noncancer diagnoses receiving palliative care have a higher incidence of pressure ulcers (50.8% versus 22.4%).[2] Pressure ulcer prevalence among cancer patients is not significantly different when compared with prevalence in noncancer patients.[12] Studies attempting to compare pressure ulcer incidence between these two groups have been inconclusive, though there is evidence that cancer patients demonstrate higher pressure ulcer risk assessment scores and increased numbers of comorbidities associated with developing pressure ulcers than noncancer patients.[11,13] Therefore, greater attention should be focused toward prevention among oncology patients. Pressure ulcers often occur in the 2 to 3 weeks prior to death and have been suggested as an indicator of failure of the skin as an organ.[14,15] This suggests that some pressure ulcers may be unavoidable in persons receiving palliative care. Contrary to many healthcare practitioner's beliefs, once a pressure ulcer develops healing is possible, with reports of wound healing in persons receiving palliative care ranging from 44% for those with cancer diagnoses to 78% for those with noncancer diagnoses.[13] Thus, the emphasis on palliative wound care does not negate the potential for wound closure and healing even in those at the end of life.

Definition

Pressure ulcers are areas of local tissue trauma that usually develop where soft tissues are compressed between bony prominences and external surfaces for prolonged periods. Mechanical injury to the skin and tissues causes hypoxia and ischemia, leading to tissue necrosis. Caring for the patient with a pressure ulcer can be frustrating for clinicians because of the chronic nature of the wound and because additional time and resources are often invested in the management of these wounds. Further, many family caregivers and healthcare providers view development of pressure ulcers as an indication of poor care or impending death. Pressure ulcers are painful, care is costly, and treatment costs increase as the severity of the wound increases. Additionally, not all pressure ulcers heal, and many heal slowly, causing a continual drain on caregivers and on financial resources. The chronic nature of a pressure ulcer challenges the healthcare provider to design more effective treatment plans.

Once a pressure ulcer develops, the usual goals are to manage the wound to support healing. However, some patients will benefit most from a palliative wound care approach. Palliative wound care goals are comfort and limiting the extent or impact of the wound, but without the intent of healing. Palliative care for chronic wounds, such as pressure ulcers, is appropriate for a wide variety of patient populations. Palliative care is often indicated for terminally ill patients, such as those with cancer or other diseases and those at the end of life. Institutionalized older adults with multiple comorbidities and older adults with severe functional decline at the end of life may also benefit from palliative care. Sometimes individuals with long-standing wounds and other life expectations benefit from a palliative care approach for a specified duration of time. For example, a wheelchair-bound young adult with a sacral pressure ulcer may make an informed choice to continue to be up in a wheelchair to attend school even though this choice severely diminishes the expectation for wound healing. The healthcare professional may decide jointly with the patient to treat the wound palliatively during this time frame.

The foundation for designing a care plan for the patient with a pressure ulcer is a comprehensive assessment. This is true even if the goals of care are palliative. Comprehensive assessment includes assessment of wound severity, wound status, and the total patient. Management of the wound is best accomplished within the context of the whole person, particularly if palliation is the outcome. Thus, including the patient, family, and significant others is essential to determine goals and develop the care plan. This is particularly true as many patients and their families are actively engaged in their healthcare and want to be involved in their own plan of care. Assessment is the first step in maintaining and evaluating a therapeutic plan of care. Without adequate baseline wound and patient assessment and valid interpretation of the assessment data, the plan of care for the wound may be inappropriate or ineffective—at the least, it may be disjointed and fragmented due to poor communication. An inadequate plan of care may lead to impaired or delayed healing, miscommunication regarding the goals of care (healing versus palliation), and complications such as infection.

Pathophysiology of pressure ulcer development

Pressure ulcers are the result of mechanical injury to the skin and underlying tissues. Traditionally, pressure (stress), shear, and friction were considered the primary external factors involved in pressure ulcer development.[16–21] More recently deformation (strain),[22–29] heat,[30] reperfusion injury,[31–33] and impaired lymphatic function[34] have been considered as additional primary forces involved in pressure damage.[35,36] Pressure is the perpendicular force or load exerted on a specific area; it causes ischemia and hypoxia of the tissues. The gravitational pull on the skeleton causes loading and deformation of the soft tissue between the bony prominence and external support surface. The mechanical physical forces of shear, which is force applied against a surface as it moves or slides in an opposite but parallel direction stretching tissues and displacing blood vessels laterally, and deformation, which stretches and pulls cells, are also key factors in pressure ulcer development. Friction, which is the resistance to motion or rubbing of one object or surface against another in a parallel direction, and moisture, which macerates tissues and increases the coefficient of friction between surfaces, are major forces in superficial damage over bony prominences, abrading the epidermal surface and increasing the risk for infection. Areas prone to these mechanical forces in the supine position are the occiput, sacrum, and heels. In the sitting position, the ischial tuberosities exert the highest pressure, and the trochanters are affected in the side-lying position.[16–21,37]

As the amount of soft tissue available for compression decreases, the pressure gradient increases. Likewise, as the tissue available for compression increases, the pressure gradient decreases. For this reason, most pressure ulcers occur over bony prominences, where there is less tissue for compression.[37] This relationship is important to understand for palliative care, because most of the likely candidates for palliative care will have experienced significant changes in nutritional status and body weight, with diminished soft tissue available for compression and a more prominent bony structure. This more prominent bony structure is more susceptible to skin breakdown from external forces, because the soft tissue that is normally used to deflect physical forces (e.g., pressure, shear) is absent. Therefore, the tissues are less tolerant of external forces, and the pressure gradient within the vascular network is altered.[37]

Alterations in the vascular network allow an increase in the interstitial fluid pressure, which exceeds the venous flow. This results in an additional increase in the pressure and impedes arteriolar circulation. The capillary vessels collapse, and thrombosis occurs. Increased capillary arteriolar pressure leads to fluid loss through the capillaries, tissue edema, and subsequent autolysis. Lymphatic flow is decreased, allowing further tissue edema and contributing to the tissue necrosis.[18,20,38–40]

Pressure, over time, occludes blood and lymphatic circulation, causing deficient tissue nutrition and buildup of waste products due to ischemia. If pressure is relieved before a critical time period is reached, a normal compensatory mechanism, reactive hyperemia, restores tissue nutrition and compensates for compromised circulation. If pressure is not relieved before the critical time period, the blood vessels collapse and thrombose, causing tissue deprivation of oxygen, nutrients, and waste removal. In the absence of oxygen, cells utilize anaerobic pathways for metabolism and produce toxic byproducts. The toxic byproducts lead to tissue acidosis, increased cell membrane permeability, edema, and, eventually, cell death.[18,38]

Tissue damage may also be caused by reperfusion and reoxygenation of the ischemic tissues or by postischemic injury.[41] Oxygen is reintroduced into tissues during reperfusion after ischemia. This triggers oxygen free radicals, known as superoxide anion, hydroxyl radicals, and hydrogen peroxide, which induce endothelial damage and decrease microvascular integrity. Ischemia and hypoxia of body tissues are produced when capillary blood flow is obstructed by localized pressure. The degree of pressure and the amount of time necessary for ulceration to occur have been a subject of study for many years. In 1930, Landis,[42] using single-capillary microinjection techniques, determined normal hydrostatic pressure to be 32 mm Hg at the arteriolar end and 15 mm Hg at the venular end. His work has served as a criterion for measuring occlusion of capillary blood flow. Generally, a range from 25 to 32 mm Hg is considered normal and is used as the marker for adequate relief of pressure on the tissues. In severely compromised patients, even this level of pressure may be too high.

During critical illness or at the end of life (the period of time when a person is living with an illness that will often worsen and may eventually cause death), the skin, as with all organs, can and often fails. This dysfunction of the skin as an organ occurs in varying degrees with resultant varying levels of injury. Dysfunction can occur at the tissue, cellular, or molecular level, all of which relate to decreased cutaneous perfusion leading to local hypoxia.[43,44] The end result is a reduced ability to use nutrients to maintain normal skin function. Thus, skin failure is a result of hypoperfusion, which creates an intense inflammatory reaction associated with severe dysfunction.[43] As the body faces critical illness, peripheral vasoconstriction may occur to shunt blood from the periphery and skin to the central vital organs. Much of the skin has collateral vascular supply, but some areas have a single vascular route. These areas include distal areas such as fingers and toes and the sacral coccygeal area, which has no direct blood flow. The decrease in blood flow to the skin also results in reduced cutaneous metabolic processes, thus minor forces can lead to major damage such as pressure ulcers. Both acute and chronic skin failure have been described.[44]

Pressure is greatest at the bony prominence and soft tissue interface and gradually lessens in a cone-shaped gradient to the periphery.[17,45,46] Therefore, although tissue damage apparent on the skin surface may be minimal, the damage to deeper structures can be severe. In addition, subcutaneous fat and muscle are more sensitive than the skin to ischemia. Muscle and fat tissues are more metabolically active and, therefore, more vulnerable to hypoxia with increased susceptibility to pressure damage. The vulnerability of muscle and fat tissues to pressure forces explains pressure ulcers, in which large areas of muscle and fat tissue are damaged, termed undermining or pocketing, yet the skin opening is relatively small.[39] In patients with severe malnutrition and weight loss, there is less tissue between the bony prominence and the surface of the skin, so the potential for large ulcers with extensive undermining or pocketing is much higher.

There is a relationship between intensity and duration of pressure in pressure ulcer development. Low pressures over a long period of time are as capable of producing tissue damage as high pressures for a shorter period.[17] Tissues can tolerate higher cyclic pressures compared with constant pressure.[47] Pressures differ in various body positions. They are highest (70 mm Hg) on the buttocks in the lying position and in the sitting position can be as high as 300 mm Hg over the ischial tuberosities.[17,37] These levels are well above the normal capillary closing pressures and are capable of causing tissue ischemia. If tissues have been compressed for prolonged periods, tissue damage will continue to occur even after the pressure is relieved.[43] This continued tissue damage relates to changes at the cellular level that lead to difficulties with restoration of perfusion (reperfusion injury). Initial skin breakdown can occur in 6 to 12 hours in healthy individuals and more quickly (less than 2 hours) in those who are debilitated.

More than 95% of all pressure ulcers develop over five classic locations: sacral/coccygeal area, greater trochanter, ischial tuberosity, heel, and lateral malleolus.[19] Correct anatomical terminology is important when identifying the true location of the pressure ulcer. For example, many clinicians often document pressure ulcers as being located on the patient's hip. The hip, or iliac crest, is actually an uncommon location for pressure ulceration. The iliac crest, located on the front of the body, is rarely subject to pressure forces. The area most clinicians are referring to is correctly termed the greater trochanter. The greater trochanter is the bony prominence located on the side of the body, just above the proximal, lateral aspect of the thigh, or "saddlebag" area. The majority of pressure ulcers occur on the lower half of the body. The location of the pressure ulcer may affect clinical interventions. For example, the patient with a pressure ulcer on the sacral/coccygeal area with concomitant urinary incontinence requires treatments that address the incontinence problem. Ulcers in the sacral/coccygeal area are also more at risk for friction and shearing damage due to the location of the wound. Figure 17A.1 shows the correct anatomical terminology for pressure ulcer locations. The most common locations for pressure ulcer development in palliative care patients are the sacral/coccygeal area and heels. Patients with contractures are at special risk for pressure ulcer development due to the internal pressure of the bony prominence and the abnormal alignment of the body and its extremities. Institutionalized older adults with severe functional decline are particularly susceptible to contractures due to immobilization for extended periods of time in conjunction with limited efforts for maintenance of range of motion. Other locations of concern are body areas under or around medical devices.[48] In the case of medical devices, individuals are at special risk due to the pressure on tissues caused by the medical device itself.[49] In many instances the medical device cannot be removed and it may not be possible to reduce the pressure on the tissues from the device.[48,49] This is particularly true if the device is applied when edema is present. One study found that patients with medical devices were 2.4 times more likely to develop a pressure ulcer.[49]

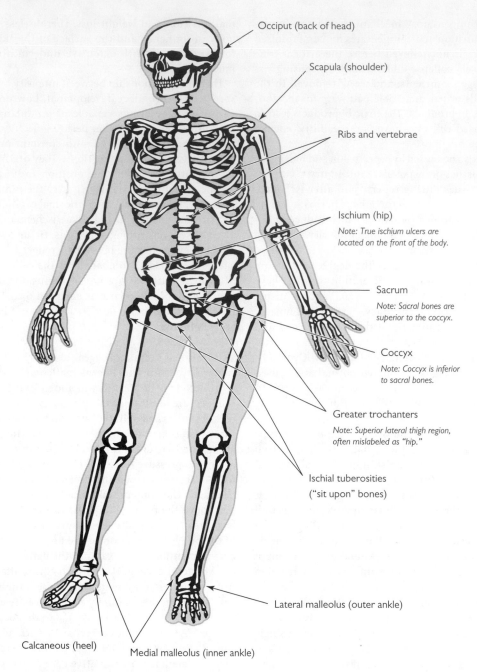

Figure 17A.1 Common anatomical locations of pressure ulcers.

Risk factors for pressure ulcers

Pressure ulcers are physical evidence of multiple causative influences. Factors that contribute to pressure ulcer development can be thought of as those that affect the pressure force over the bony prominence and those that affect the tolerance of the tissues to pressure.

Mobility, sensory loss, and activity level are related to the concept of increasing pressure. Extrinsic factors including shear, friction, and moisture, as well as intrinsic factors such as nutrition, age, and arteriolar pressure, relate to the concept of tissue tolerance.[50] Several additional areas may influence pressure ulcer development, including emotional stress, temperature, smoking, and interstitial fluid flow.[51] Given their advanced illnesses and decreased functional capacity, patients receiving palliative care exhibit most or all of the risk factors for pressure ulcer development. Characteristics of palliative care patients that predict pressure ulcers include age, immobility, and physical inactivity.[6,52,53] Caregiver frailty in conjunction with patient risk factors increases the risk for pressure ulcer development.

Immobility

Immobility, inactivity, and decreased sensory perception affect the duration and intensity of the pressure over the bony prominence. Immobility or severely restricted mobility is the most important risk factor for all populations and a necessary condition for the development of pressure ulcers. Mobility is the state of being movable. The immobile patient cannot move, or facility and ease of movement is impaired. Closely related to immobility is limited activity.

Inactivity

Activity is the production of energy or motion and implies an action. Activity is often clinically described by the ability of the individual to ambulate and move about. Those persons who are bed- or chair-bound, and thus inactive, are more at risk for pressure ulcer development.[52,54] In bed-bound individuals, ability to self-reposition is an important activity and if the individual is capable of self-movement, activity level may be less of a risk factor. A sudden change in activity level may signal significant change in health status and increased potential for pressure ulcer development.

Sensory loss

Sensory loss places patients at risk for compression of tissues and pressure ulcer development, because the normal mechanism for translating pain messages from the tissues is dysfunctional. Patients with intact nervous system pathways feel continuous local pressure, become uncomfortable, and change their position before tissue ischemia occurs. Spinal cord–injured patients have a higher incidence and prevalence of pressure ulcers.[55,56] Patients with paraplegia or quadriplegia are unable to sense increased pressure; if their body weight is not shifted, pressure ulceration develops. Likewise, patients with changes in mental status or functioning are at increased risk for pressure ulcer formation. They may not feel the discomfort from pressure, may not be alert enough to move spontaneously, may not remember to move, may be too confused to respond to commands to move, or may be physically unable to move. This risk factor is particularly evident in the palliative care population, in which individuals may use opioids and sedative drugs that inhibit spontaneous movements, may be at the end of life and not alert enough to move spontaneously, or may be physically unable to move.

Shear

Extrinsic risk factors are those forces that make the tissues less tolerant of pressure. Extrinsic forces include shear, friction, and moisture. Whereas pressure acts perpendicularly to cause ischemia, shear causes ischemia by displacing blood vessels laterally and thereby impeding blood flow to tissues.[56–58] Shear is caused by the interplay of gravity and friction. Shear is a parallel force that stretches and twists tissues and blood vessels at the bony tissue interface; as such, it affects the deep blood vessels and deeper tissue structures. The most common example of shear is seen in the bed patient who is in a semisitting position with knees flexed and supported by pillows on the bed or by head-of-bed elevation. If the patient's skeleton slides down toward the foot of the bed, the sacral skin may stay in place (with the help of friction against the bed linen). This produces stretching, pinching, and occlusion of the underlying vessels, resulting in ulcers with large areas of internal tissue damage and less damage at the skin surface.

Friction

Friction and moisture are not direct factors in pressure ulcer development, but they have been identified as contributing to the problem by reducing tolerance of tissues to pressure.[59] Friction occurs when two surfaces move across one another. Friction acts on tissue tolerance to pressure by abrading and damaging the epidermal and upper dermal layers of the skin. Additionally, friction acts with gravity to cause shear. Friction abrades the epidermis, which may lead to pressure ulcer development by increasing the skin's susceptibility to pressure injury. Pressure combined with friction produces ulcerations at lower pressures than does pressure alone.[59] Friction acts in conjunction with shear to contribute to the development of sacral/coccygeal pressure ulcers on patients in the semi-Fowler position.

Moisture

Moisture contributes to pressure ulcer development by removing oils on the skin, making it more friable, as well as interacting with body support surface friction. Constant moisture on the skin leads to maceration of the tissues. Waterlogging leads to softening of the skin's connective tissues. Macerated tissues are more prone to erosion, and once the epidermis is eroded, there is increased likelihood of further tissue breakdown. Moisture alters the resiliency of the epidermis to external forces. Both shearing force and friction increase in the presence of mild to moderate moisture. Excess moisture may be caused by wound drainage, diaphoresis, or fecal or urinary incontinence.

Incontinence

Urinary and fecal incontinence are common risk factors associated with pressure ulcer development. Incontinence contributes to pressure ulcer formation by creating excess moisture on the skin and by chemical damage to the skin. Fecal incontinence has the added detrimental effect of bacteria in the stool, which can contribute to infection as well as skin breakdown. Fecal incontinence is more significant as a risk factor for pressure ulceration because of the bacteria and enzymes in stool and their effects on the skin. Inadequately managed incontinence poses a significant risk factor for pressure ulcer development, and fecal incontinence is highly correlated with pressure ulcer development.

Nutritional risk factors

There is some disagreement concerning the major intrinsic risk factors affecting tissue tolerance to pressure. However, most studies identify nutritional status as playing a role in pressure ulcer development. Hypoalbuminemia, weight loss, cachexia, and malnutrition are commonly identified as risk factors predisposing patients to pressure ulcer development.[60–63] Low serum albumin levels are associated both with having a pressure ulcer and with developing a pressure ulcer.

Age

Age itself may be a risk factor for pressure ulcer development, with age-related changes in the skin and in wound healing increasing the risk of pressure ulcer development. The skin and support structures undergo changes in the aging process. There is a loss of muscle, a decrease in serum albumin levels, diminished inflammatory response, decreased elasticity, and reduced cohesion between dermis and epidermis. These changes combine with other changes related to aging to make the skin less tolerant of pressure forces, shear, and friction.

Medical conditions and psychological factors

Certain medical conditions or disease states are also associated with pressure ulcer development. Orthopedic injuries, altered mental status, and spinal cord injury are such conditions.[54–56,63–66] In palliative care populations, diagnoses of cancer and central nervous system disorders such as dementia are associated with higher incidence of pressure ulcer development.[2,53] Other psychological factors may affect risk for pressure ulcer development. Self-concept, depression, and chronic emotional stress have been cited as factors in pressure ulcer development.

Environmental resources

Environmental resources include socioeconomic, psychosocial, healthcare system, and therapy resources. These factors are less understood than other risk factors; however, several of them play important roles in determining risk for pressure ulcer development and course of pressure ulcer care in patients receiving palliative care. Socioeconomic resources that may influence pressure ulcer development and healing are cost of therapy, type of payor (insurance type), and access to healthcare. In palliative care, cost of therapy becomes an important issue, particularly in long-term care facilities, where financial resources are limited and cost of therapy may hinder access to treatment.

Healthcare system resources are the type of healthcare setting and the experience, education level, and discipline of healthcare professionals. Patients receiving palliative care are often in long-term care facilities and dependent on the direct-care practices of nurse aides with minimal education in healthcare, nursing, and, especially, the needs of the palliative care patient. Therapy resources include topical treatments for wounds and systemic treatments. Palliative care patients often receive concomitant therapy that impairs mobility or sensory perception (e.g., pain medication) or normal healing mechanisms (e.g., steroids, radiation therapy).

Psychosocial resources include adherence to the therapy plan, cultural values and beliefs, social support network (family and caregiver support), spiritual support, and alternative medicine use. The social support network is a key factor for palliative care. Patients receiving palliative care are often cared for in the home or in a long-term care facility. Home caregivers may be family members of the patient, often the spouse or significant other. If the patient is older and frail, it is typical to find that the caregiver is also older and frail, yet responsible for providing direct care 24 hours a day with minimal respite or support. Many times the nurse is dealing with two patients, the patient receiving palliative care and the patient's caregiver, who may also be frail and in need of services. The family member may be physically unable to reposition the patient or to provide other care services. In long-term care facilities, the problem may not be physical inability to perform the tasks but lack of staff, time, or motivation. The limited availability of nurse attendants in the long-term care facility may be such that turning and repositioning of palliative care patients are not high-priority tasks.

In summary, environmental resources are not all well defined and typically are not included in formal risk-assessment tools for development of pressure ulcers. However, the importance of environmental resources in both the development and healing of pressure ulcers is clinically relevant in palliative care.

Use of risk-assessment scales

For practitioners to intervene in a cost-effective way, a method of screening for risk factors is necessary. Several risk-assessment instruments are available to clinicians. Screening tools assist in prevention by distinguishing those persons who are at risk for pressure ulcer development from those who are not. The only purpose in identifying patients who are at risk for pressure ulcer development is to allow for appropriate use of resources for prevention. The use of a risk assessment tool allows for targeting of interventions to specific risk factors for individual patients. The risk-assessment instrument selected is based on its reliability for the intended raters, its predictive validity for the population, its sensitivity and specificity under consideration, and its ease of use including the time required for completion. The most common risk-assessment tools for adults are the Braden Scale for Predicting Pressure Sore Risk,[51] and the Norton Scale.[67] There is minimal information on the use of either instrument in palliative care patients, but both tools have been used in long-term care facilities, where many patients are assumed to be receiving palliative care. Three risk assessment tools specific to hospice patients have been developed and validated, the Hospice Pressure Ulcer Risk Assessment Scale in use in Sweden,[4] the Hunters Hill Marie Curie Center risk assessment tool,[15] and the Pressure Ulcer Scale in Oncology (PUSO),[68] the latter being a simplified adaptation of the Hunters Hill Marie Curie Center tool.

Norton Scale

The Norton tool is the oldest risk-assessment instrument. Developed in 1961, it consists of five subscales: physical condition, mental state, activity, mobility, and incontinence.[67] Each parameter is rated on a scale of 1 to 4, with the sum of the ratings for all five parameters yielding a total score ranging from 5 to 20. Lower scores indicate increased risk, with scores of 16 or lower indicating "onset of risk" and scores of 12 or lower indicating high risk for pressure ulcer formation.[69]

Braden Scale for predicting pressure sores

The Braden Scale is the most commonly used risk assessment tool in the United States. The Braden Scale was developed in 1987 and is composed of six subscales that conceptually reflect degrees of sensory perception, moisture, activity, nutrition, friction and shear, and mobility.[50,51] All subscales are rated from 1 to 4, except for friction and shear, which is rated from 1 to 3. The subscales may be summed for a total score ranging from 6 to 23.

Lower scores indicate lower function and higher risk for development of a pressure ulcer. The cutoff score for hospitalized adults is considered to be 16, with scores of 16 and lower indicating at-risk status.[51] In older patients, some have found cutoff scores of 17 or 18 to be better predictors of risk status.[15,30] Levels of risk are based on the predictive value of a positive test. Scores of 15 to 16 indicate mild risk, with a 50% to 60% chance of developing a stage 1 pressure ulcer; scores of 12 to 14 indicate moderate risk, with 65% to 90% chance of developing a stage 1 or 2 lesion; and scores lower than 12 indicate high risk, with a 90% to 100% chance of developing a stage 2 or deeper pressure ulcer.[51,70] The Braden Scale has been tested in acute care and long-term care with several levels of nurse raters and demonstrates high interrater reliability with registered nurses.

Validity has been established by expert opinion, and predictive validity has been studied in several acute care settings, with good sensitivity and specificity demonstrated.[51,70] Some have shown that Braden Scale scores are highly correlated with Karnofsky/Palliative Performance Scale (PPS) scores ($r = 0.885$; $P < 0.001$)[71]

which are prognostic performance status tools commonly used in palliative care settings.[72,73] The PPS is based on the Karnofsky performance scale, which is a tool to classify patients receiving cancer treatment according to their level of functional impairment. The PPS is scored 0 (death) to 100% (no limitation) in 10-unit increments.[72] Both the Karnofsky and PPS are scored similarly and used interchangeably in hospice settings. A score of 40% indicates that the patient spends most of his or her time in bed; a score of 30% indicates that the patient has increasing debility and requires total care. In the absence of a standardized risk assessment tool such as the Braden Scale, the PPS could be used as a proxy to determine risk for pressure ulcer development in hospice patients.[8,72] The Braden Scale is the model used in this chapter for prevention of pressure ulcers in patients requiring palliative care.

The Hospice Pressure Ulcer Risk Assessment Scale

The Hospice Pressure Ulcer Risk Assessment Scale was developed in 2003 after comparison of the Norton Scale and nine new scales derived from the Norton scale with various changes. Validity of the new scale was tested during development in 98 hospice patients. The items on the Hospice Pressure Ulcer Risk scale are physical activity, mobility, and age.[4]

Hunters Hill Marie Curie Center Risk Assessment Tool

The Hunters Hill Risk Assessment tool was developed in 2000 and is composed of seven subscales: sensation, mobility, moisture, activity in bed, nutrition/weight change, skin condition, and friction/shear.[15] Each factor is assessed on a 4-point numerical scale with 1 indicating less risk and scores of 4 indicating highest risk for that factor. Individual factor scores can be summed for a total score that ranges from 7, signifying minimal risk, to 28, demonstrating very high risk. The Hunters Hill tool was developed specifically for palliative care and validated in hospice patients using comparative analysis of the clinical judgment of experienced palliative care nurses.[15]

The Pressure Ulcer Scale in Oncology

The PUSO is an additional risk assessment tool adapted from the Hunters Hill tool for use in cancer patients.[68] The PUSO score assigns a binary value (0 or 1) to three factors—activity in bed, moisture or incontinence, and friction/shear. A score of 1 or more indicates high risk for pressure ulcer development. A prevalence survey among 582 patients comparing the PUSO scale's predictive validity to the Hunters Hill tool and the Braden scale, demonstrated a kappa value of 0.60 ($P < 0.0001$). The PUSO offers a simplified risk assessment with good sensitivity and specificity for predicting pressure ulcer development among oncology patients.

Regardless of the instrument chosen to evaluate risk status, the clinical relevance is threefold. First, assessment for risk status must occur at frequent intervals. Assessment should be performed at admission to the healthcare organization (within 24 hours), at predetermined intervals (usually weekly), and whenever a significant change occurs in the patient's general health and status. The second clinical implication is the targeting of specific prevention strategies to identified risk factors. The final clinical implication is for those patients in whom prevention is not successful. For patients with an actual pressure ulcer, the continued monitoring of risk status may prevent further tissue trauma at the wound site and development of additional wound sites.

Prevention of pressure ulcers

Prevention strategies are targeted at reducing risk factors and can be focused on eliminating specific risk factors. Early intervention for pressure ulcers is risk-factor specific and prophylactic in nature. The prevention strategies are presented here by risk factor, beginning with general information and ending with specific strategies to eliminate particular risk factors. Prevention is a key element for palliative care. If pressure ulcers can be prevented, the patient is spared tiresome, sometimes painful, and often overwhelming treatment. The Braden Scale is the basis for these prevention interventions. Prevention interventions that are appropriate to the patient's level of risk and specific to individual risk factors should be instituted. For example, the risk factor of immobility is managed very differently for the comatose patient compared with the patient with severe pain on movement with a single position of comfort, the patient with dyspnea or nausea on moving, or the patient who is still active even if bed-bound. The comatose patient requires caregiver education and caregiver-dependent repositioning. The patient with severe pain on movement requires special support surface intervention and minimal movement methods with a foam wedge. The patient who is still active but bed-bound requires self-care education and may be able to perform self-repositioning. The interventions for the risk factor of immobility and inactivity are very different for these patients.

Immobility, inactivity, and sensory loss

Patients who have impaired ability to reposition and who cannot independently change body positions must have local pressure alleviated by any of the following: passive repositioning by caregivers, pillow bridging, or pressure redistribution support surfaces for bed and chair.[54] Additional strategies include measures to increase mobility and activity and to decrease friction and shear. This is true for persons receiving palliative care until the terminal stage of the disease process. The difference for those receiving palliative care is the emphasis on providing adequate pain management as part of prevention interventions related to movement and repositioning.

Overhead bed frames with trapeze bars are helpful for patients with upper body strength and may increase mobility and independence with body repositioning. Wheelchair-bound patients with upper body strength can be taught and encouraged to do wheelchair pushups or body tilts to the side and forward leans to relieve pressure and allow for reperfusion of the tissues in the ischial tuberosity region. For patients who are weak from prolonged inactivity, providing support and assistance for reconditioning and increasing strength and endurance may help prevent further decline even among palliative care patients. Mobility plans for each patient should be individualized, with the goal of attaining the highest level of mobility and activity possible in light of the goals of overall care. Caregivers in the home are often left to fend for themselves for prevention interventions and may be frail and have health problems themselves. A repeat demonstration of a repositioning procedure can be very informative to the nurse. The nurse may need to coach, improvise, and think of creative strategies for caregivers to use in the home setting to meet the patient's needs for movement and tissue reperfusion. This is especially important for palliative care patients as caregivers may be unaware of the need for repositioning and the consequences of not repositioning even for terminally ill individuals; they may be afraid of causing pain and suffering with repositioning activities, which may make caregivers resistant to repositioning activities.

Passive repositioning by caregiver

Turning schedules or passive repositioning by caregivers is the normal intervention response for patients with immobility risk factors. Typically, turning schedules are based on time or event. Event-based schedules relate to typical events during the day (e.g., turning the patient after each meal). If time based, turning is usually done every 2–4 hours for full-body change of position and more often for small shifts in position. Full-body change of position involves turning the patient to a new lying position, such as from the right side-lying position to the left side-lying position or the supine position. If the side-lying position is used in bed, avoid direct pressure on the trochanter. To avoid placing pressure on the trochanter, the patient is placed in a 30-degree, laterally inclined side-lying position instead of the commonly used 90-degree side-lying position, which increases tissue compression over the trochanter. The 30-degree, laterally inclined side-lying position allows for distribution of pressure over a greater area. Small shifts in position involve moving the patient but keeping the same lying position, such as changing the angle of the right side-lying position or changing the position of the lower extremities in the right side-lying position. Both strategies are helpful in achieving reperfusion of compressed tissues, but only a full-body change of position completely relieves pressure.

A foam wedge is very useful in positioning for frail caregivers and for patients with severe pain on movement. The foam wedge should provide a 30-degree angle of lift when fully inserted behind the patient, usually extending from the shoulders to the hips/buttocks. Once it is in place, even the most frail of caregivers can easily pull the wedge out slightly every hour, providing for small shifts in position and tissue reperfusion. Even patients with pain on movement find the slight movement from the foam wedge tolerable. There are other techniques to make turning patients easier and less time-consuming. Turning sheets, draw sheets, and pillows are essential for passive movement of patients in bed. Turning sheets are useful in repositioning the patient to a side-lying position. Draw sheets are used for pulling patients up in bed; they help prevent dragging of the patient's skin over the bed surface. There are devices available to assist with turning and repositioning that decrease the time and physical effort required to reposition patients. One such system offloads the sacrum, includes a method of managing moisture due to incontinence, minimizes friction and shear, and assists in positioning the patient at the 30-degree angle with use of two small foam wedges. It includes a low-friction material that has one side that holds a shoulder-to-knee body pad in place under the patient and one side that is ripstop nylon that slides easily across the bed linens. The ripstop nylon decreases friction and helps the sheet move with the patient to make turning easier. Devices such as this can decrease the time and effort required to reposition a patient making it easier for caregivers to engage in repositioning activities. New pressure-mapping devices have been introduced that provide real-time monitoring of pressure magnitude, location, and duration of pressure. These devices use multiple sensors woven into a fabric sheet that provide data on interface pressure—both the magnitude of pressure at specific anatomical sites and the

duration of that pressure. The data is presented as a real-time color map of bony prominences with pressure magnitude and duration of pressure displayed. Pressure-mapping devices also can provide alarms for triggering timed repositioning episodes, pressure at an anatomical location over a predetermined threshold, and for determining accuracy of the new position in offloading a particular bony prominence. This type of technology may be helpful in providing more information on pressure magnitude and duration to clinicians and caregivers, allowing for more individualized repositioning programs.

Frequency of repositioning should be based on the individual's tissue tolerance, level of mobility and activity, medical condition, skin integrity, treatment goals, and pressure-redistribution support surface use.[54,74] Use of 4-hour repositioning schedules in conjunction with use of viscoelastic support surfaces has been shown to reduce the frequency and time to occurrence of stage 2 or greater pressure ulcers compared with standard care (no turning schedule), those on standard hospital mattresses who were turned every 2 and every 4 hours, and with persons on a viscoelastic support surface who were turned every 6 hours.[75] Further, there was no significant difference in the incidence of stage 2 or greater pressure ulcers between patients on a viscoelastic support surface who were placed in a lateral position for 2 hours and those who were allowed to remain in a lateral position for 4 hours; thus supporting use of a 4-hour repositioning frequency when used in conjunction with a viscoelastic pressure redistributing support surface.[75,76] In general, for patients on a standard hospital mattress repositioning should occur every 2 hours. Four-hour repositioning programs in conjunction with use of nonpowered viscoelastic support surfaces may be beneficial for those receiving palliative care and for whom more frequent repositioning is too painful.[77]

Similar approaches to repositioning are useful for patients in chairs. Full-body change of position involves standing the patient and then resitting the patient in a chair. Small shifts in position for those in chairs might involve changing the position of the lower extremities or inserting a small foam pillow or wedge. For the chair-bound patient, it is also helpful to use a foot stool or the foot rest in wheel chairs to help reduce the pressure on the ischial tuberosities and to distribute the pressure over a wider surface. Attention to proper alignment and posture is essential. Individuals at risk for pressure ulcer development should avoid uninterrupted sitting in chairs, and clinical practice guidelines suggest repositioning every hour.[54,74] The rationale behind the shorter time frame is the extremely high pressures generated on the ischial tuberosities in the seated position. Those patients with upper-body strength should be taught to shift weight every 15 minutes, to allow for tissue reperfusion. Use of an alarm system may be helpful in reminding patients and caregivers to shift weight. Again, pillows may be used to help position the patient in proper body alignment. Physical therapy and occupational therapy can assist in body-alignment strategies with even the most contracted patient.

In many instances, patients receiving palliative care at home spend much of their time up in recliner chairs. The ability of recliner chairs to provide a pressure-reduction support surface is not known, and individual recliner chairs probably have various levels of pressure-reducing capability. Therefore, it is still prudent to institute a repositioning schedule for those using recliner chairs. Repositioning of patients in recliner chairs is more difficult due to the physical properties of the chair and requires some creativity. The repositioning schedule should mimic the schedule for those in wheelchairs.

For patients with significant pain on movement, premedication 20 to 30 minutes before a scheduled large position change may make routine repositioning more acceptable for the patient and the family. The same is true for persons with nausea on movement—providing antiemetics prior to movement may be helpful. In those close to death, repositioning schedules may be used solely for maintaining comfort, with few or no attempts to reposition as a strategy for preventing skin problems.

Pillow bridging

Pillow bridging involves the use of pillows to position patients with minimal tissue compression. The use of pillows can help prevent pressure ulcers from occurring on the medial knees, the medial malleolus, and the heels. Pillows should be placed between the knees, between the ankles, and under the heels.

Pillow use is especially important for reducing the risk of development of heel ulcers regardless of the support surface in use.[54] The best prevention strategy for eliminating pressure ulcers on the heels is to keep the heels off the surface of the bed. Use of pillows under the lower extremities, if they remain in place, can keep the heel from making contact with the support surface of the bed. The pillows should extend and support the leg from the groin or perineal area to the ankle. Pillows help to redistribute the pressure over a larger area, thus reducing high pressure in one specific area, however it can be difficult to keep them appropriately positioned under the legs with the heels floated off the end.[78]

Some specialized heel-pressure-redistributing devices are effective in reducing pressure on heels. Look for devices that are easy to apply and remove to assure compliance. There are several considerations for choosing a heel-pressure-redistribution support surface. Use of foam wedges that span the width of the end of the bed and keep the legs cradled in place do successfully suspend the heels off the bed surface. However, these devices may limit mobility and do not address foot drop. Heel pressure redistribution boots stay in place and do address foot drop issues. Those that incorporate a brace should be properly fitted by a physical therapist for proper attention to foot drop and leg alignment. Boots without a brace may be made of foam or air cushions, fiber filled, or made of medical grade sheepskin. Those made of high specificity foam may be warm and limit ease of movement in bed because of friction, however they are relatively inexpensive. Air-filled cushions address friction and shear, they are light and do not limit bed mobility. They do require monitoring to be sure sufficient inflation is present. Fiber-filled boots can be washed, and they wick moisture and heat from the foot. Sheepskin boots may increase temperature.[78] Additional questions to address in deciding on a heel support surface include the following:

- Foot drop addressed by device?
- Moisture and temperature issues?
- Able to ambulate with device?
- Ability to remain in place?
- Shear and friction addressed?
- Bed mobility issues?
- Able to wash device?[78]

Use of donut-type or ring cushion devices is contraindicated. Donut ring cushions cause venous congestion and edema and actually increase pressure to the area of concern.[54]

Use of pressure-redistribution support surfaces

The use of support surfaces to prevent and manage pressure ulcers is important; however, regardless of the type of support surface in use with the patient, the need for scheduled repositioning continues to be an important component of the prevention program.[54,74] The support surface serves as an adjunct to strategies for positioning and careful monitoring of patients. The National Pressure Ulcer Advisory Panel (NPUAP) defines a support surface as a specialized device for pressure redistribution developed for managing tissue loads, microclimates, or other therapeutic functions.[79] Pressure-redistribution support surfaces assist in pressure ulcer risk reduction by managing tissue loading by reducing either the load or the duration of loading. The type of support surface chosen is based on a multitude of factors, including clinical condition of the patient and expected future condition of the patient, type of care setting, ease of use, maintenance, cost, characteristics of the support surface, and whether or not the patient can tolerate scheduled repositioning. The primary concern should be the therapeutic benefit associated with the surface. Support surfaces are used to redistribute pressure in bed and chairs, and over the heels as discussed above.

The NPUAP categorizes support surfaces as nonpowered and powered and describes different pressure-redistribution surfaces according to intensity of redistribution properties and physical characteristics.[79]

Nonpowered support surfaces

Pressure-redistributing devices that are nonpowered (do not use electricity or batteries) include overlays (devices placed on top of a standard mattress) and mattresses or beds composed of foam, air, or water. Generally, these devices lower tissue interface pressures but do not consistently maintain interface pressures below capillary closing pressures in all positions on all body locations. Nonpowered devices do not move; they reduce pressure by spreading the load over a larger area, and do not require electricity or a battery to function. Pressure-redistribution nonpowered support surfaces increase the body surface area that comes in contact with the support surface to decrease the interface pressure (pressure between the body and the support surface interface). Increasing the body surface area that comes in contact with the support surface is accomplished by immersion and envelopment (i.e., the body sinks into or is engulfed by the surface). Nonpowered support surfaces are indicated for patients who are at risk for pressure ulcer development, who can be turned, and who have skin breakdown involving only one sleep surface.[54] Patients with an existing pressure ulcer who are at risk for development of further skin breakdown should be managed on a nonpowered support surface.

The difficulties with foam devices include retaining moisture and heat and not reducing shear. Air and water nonpowered devices also have difficulties associated with retaining moisture and heat. Viscoelastic and elastic foam nonpowered surfaces are both types of porous materials that conform in proportion to the applied weight and assist in reducing friction and shear.

One concern when using mattress overlays (nonpowered or powered), is the "bottoming-out" phenomenon. Bottoming-out occurs when the patient's body sinks down, the support surface is compressed beyond function, and the patient's body lies directly on the hospital mattress. When bottoming-out occurs, there is no pressure reduction for the bony prominence of concern. Bottoming-out typically happens when the patient is placed on a static air mattress overlay that is not appropriately filled with air or when the patient has been on a foam mattress for extended periods. The nurse or caregiver can monitor for bottoming-out by inserting a flat, outstretched hand between the overlay and the patient's body part at risk. If the caregiver feels less than an inch of support material, the patient has bottomed-out. It is important to check for bottoming-out when the patient is in various body positions and to check at various body sites. For example, when the patient is lying supine, check the sacral/coccygeal area and the heels; and when the patient is side-lying, check the trochanter and lateral malleolus.

Powered support surfaces

Powered support surfaces more consistently *reduce* tissue interface pressures to a level below capillary closing pressure in any position and in most body locations. A simple definition of a powered support surface is one that requires a motor or pump and electricity to operate. A powered support surface may have the ability to change its load distribution properties. Powered redistribution support surfaces work by sequentially altering the parts of the body that bear load and so reduce the duration of loading on the tissues at any given anatomical location.[54,80] Examples are alternating-pressure air mattresses and overlays. Most use an electric pump alternately to inflate and deflate air cells or air columns, thus the term *alternating*-pressure air mattress. The air cells in alternating-pressure air mattresses need to be greater than 10 cm in order to be sufficiently inflated to ensure pressure relief over the deflated cells.[54] Powered support surfaces may also have difficulties with moisture retention and heat accumulation. Use of alternating-pressure powered support surfaces reduces incidence of pressure ulcers in hospitalized patients compared with standard hospital mattresses.[80–83] Alternating-pressure active support surfaces should be used for patients at higher risk of pressure ulcer development when repositioning is not possible.[54] The key to determining effectiveness is the length of time over which cycles of inflation and deflation occur. Powered devices may be preferable for palliative care patients, especially those with significant pain on movement, because they may help with tissue reperfusion when patients cannot be turned because of pain. Some patients have reported varying levels of comfort based on size of the cells in powered alternating-pressure air surfaces. When using powered devices, the caregiver must ensure that the device is functioning properly and that the patient is receiving pressure reduction.

Powered support surfaces are indicated for patients who are at high risk for pressure ulcer development and who cannot turn independently or have skin breakdown involving more than one body surface. High-end powered support surfaces include low air loss, fluidized air or high air loss, and kinetic or lateral rotation devices. These devices often assist with pain control as well as redistributing pressure.

Low air loss therapy devices use a bed frame with a series of connected air-filled pillows with surface fabrics of low-friction material. The amount of pressure in each pillow or zone can be controlled and calibrated to provide maximal pressure relief for the individual patient. These devices provide pressure redistribution in any position, and most models have built-in scales. Low air loss therapy devices that are placed on top of standard hospital mattresses may be of particular benefit for palliative care patients at home.

Fluidized air or high air loss therapy devices consist of bed frames containing silicone-coated glass beads and incorporate both air and fluid support. The beads become fluid when air is pumped through the device, making them behave like a liquid. High air loss therapy has bactericidal properties due to the alkalinity of the beads (pH 10), the temperature, and entrapment of microorganisms by the beads. High air loss therapy relieves pressure and reduces friction, shear, and moisture (due to the drying effect of the bed). These devices cause difficulties when transferring patients because of the bed frame. The increased airflow can increase evaporative fluid loss, leading to dehydration. Finally, if the patient is able to sit up, a foam wedge may be required, limiting the beneficial effects of the bed on the upper back. In palliative care cases, use of high air loss therapy is typically not indicated for pressure ulcers alone but may be indicated for patients with significant pain as well as pressure ulcers.

One additional factor to consider when choosing a support surface is the microclimate at the skin and surface interface. The microclimate is the local temperature and moisture at the body-support surface interface. Heat is a risk factor for pressure ulcer development as it contributes to superficial ulcerations. Heat accumulates at the skin surface over time. So, the longer the patient is in one position the more likely the local temperature of the skin and tissue is elevated. Controlling the microclimate can be accomplished with thermal mass, low air loss devices, and regular repositioning. Support surface coverings that wick moisture away from the body or those that have continual air flow at the skin-surface interface reduce local temperature and control the microclimate. Determining which support surface is best for a particular patient can be confusing. The primary concern must always be the effectiveness of the surface for the individual patient's needs. There are no controlled trials indicating one specific support surface is superior to another.

Seating support surfaces

Support surfaces for chairs and wheelchairs can be categorized similarly to support surfaces for beds. In general, providing adequate pressure relief for chair-bound or wheelchair-bound patients is critical. The patient at risk for pressure ulcer formation is at increased risk in the seated position because of the high pressures across the ischial tuberosities. Most pressure-redistributing devices for chairs are nonpowered overlays composed of foam, gel, air, or some a combination. Positioning of chair- or wheelchair-bound individuals must include consideration of individual anatomy and body contours, postural alignment, distribution of weight, balance, and stability in addition to pressure redistribution. The use of a chair support surface can help lessen the burden of wheelchair pushups or side leans, but does not eliminate the need for reperfusion of the tissues. This is difficult as few people can actually consistently sustain the rigor associated with maintaining a schedule of weight changes.

Reducing friction and shear

Measures to reduce friction and shear relate to passive or active movement of the patient. To reduce friction, several interventions are appropriate. Providing topical preparations to eliminate or reduce the surface tension between the skin and the bed linen or support surface assists in reducing friction-related injury. To lessen friction-induced skin breakdown, appropriate techniques must be used when moving patients so that skin is never dragged across the linens. Patients who exhibit voluntary or involuntary repetitive body movements (particularly movements of the heels or elbows) require stronger interventions. Use of a protective film such as a transparent film dressing or a skin sealant, a protective dressing such as a thin hydrocolloid, or protective padding helps to eliminate the surface contact of the area and decrease the friction between the skin and the linens. Even though heel, ankle, and elbow protectors do nothing to reduce or relieve pressure, they can be effective aids against friction.

Most shear injury can be eliminated by proper positioning, such as avoidance of the semi-Fowler position and limited use of upright positions (i.e., positions more than 30 degrees inclined). Avoidance of upright positions may prevent sliding- and shear-related injuries. Use of footboards and knee Gatch (or pillows under the lower leg) to prevent sliding and to maintain position is also helpful in reducing shear effects on the skin. Observation of the patient when sitting is also important, because the patient who slides out of the chair is at equally high risk for shear injury. Use of footstools and the foot pedals on wheelchairs, together with appropriate 90-degree flexion of the hip (which may be achieved with the use of pillows, special seat cushions, or orthotic devices) can help prevent chair sliding.

Nutrition

Nutrition is an important element in maintaining healthy skin and tissues. There is a strong relationship between nutrition and pressure ulcer development.[60] Pressure ulcer prevention methods continue to improve with increased caregiver knowledge, the implementation of repositioning schedules and higher availability of support surfaces. Subsequently, management of malnutrition plays an increasingly important role in the prevention of pressure sores.[84] One study analyzing data on pressure ulcer incidence among 746 patients in a home-care setting showed that after controlling for other risk factors such as age, immobility, support surface, and comorbidities, malnutrition was found to have the highest odds ratio of all other risk factors.[85] Severity of pressure ulceration was also significantly associated with caregiver knowledge or nutrition assessment deficit. Nutritional assessment is key in determining the appropriate interventions for the patient. A short nutritional assessment should be performed at routine intervals on all patients who are determined to be at risk for pressure ulcer formation.

The severity of pressure ulceration is correlated with severity of nutritional deficits, especially low protein intake and low serum albumin levels.[60–63,84–90] Malnutrition may be diagnosed if the serum albumin level is lower than 3.5 mg/dL, the total lymphocyte count is less than 1800 cells/mm^3, or body weight has decreased by more than 15%. Malnutrition impairs the immune system, and total lymphocyte counts are a reflection of immune competence. If the patient is diagnosed as malnourished, nutritional supplementation should be instituted to help achieve a positive nitrogen balance. Examples of oral supplements are assisted oral feedings and dietary supplements. Tube feedings have generally not been effective for patients with pressure ulcers. The goal of care is to provide approximately 30 to 35 calories per kilogram of weight per day and 1.25 to 1.5 g of protein per kilogram of weight per day.[54] It may be difficult for a palliative care patient at-risk for pressure ulcers or with a pressure ulcer to ingest enough protein and calories necessary to maintain skin and tissue health. Oral supplements can be very helpful in boosting calorie and protein intake, but they are designed only to be an adjunct to regular oral intake. Monitoring of nutritional indices is helpful to determine the effectiveness of the care plan. Serum albumin, protein markers, body weight, and nutritional assessment should be performed every 3 months to monitor for changes in nutritional status if appropriate.

In palliative care, nutrition can be a major risk factor for pressure ulcer development. Nutritional supplementation may not be possible in all cases; however, if the patient can tolerate it, supplementation should be encouraged if it is in keeping with the overall goals of care. Involvement of a dietitian during the early assessment of the patient is important to the overall success of the plan. Maintenance of adequate nutrition to prevent pressure ulcer development and to repair existing pressure ulcers in palliative care patients is fraught with differing opinions. The issue is how to balance nutritional needs for skin care without providing artificial nutrition to prolong life. One of the problems in this area is the limited research available, which leaves clinicians to rely on expert opinion and their own clinical experience. Perhaps the best advice is to look at the whole clinical picture rather than focusing only on the wound. Viewing the pressure ulcer as a part of the whole, within the contextual circumstances of the patient and the goals of care, should provide some assistance in determining how aggressive to be in providing nutrition. The overriding concern in palliative care is to provide for comfort and to minimize symptoms. If providing supplemental nutrition aids in providing comfort to the patient and is mutually agreed on by the patient, family, caregivers, and healthcare provider, then supplemental nutrition (in any form) is very appropriate for palliative wound care. If the patient's condition is such that to provide supplemental nutrition (in any form) increases discomfort and the prognosis is expected to be poor and rapid, then providing supplemental nutrition should not be a concern and is not appropriate for palliative wound care. It is important to remember that little evidence exists for either of these viewpoints, yet expert opinions on the topic abound.

Managing moisture

The preventive interventions related to moisture include general skin care, diagnosis of incontinence, and appropriate incontinence management.

General skin care

General skin care involves routine skin assessment, incontinence assessment and management, skin hygiene interventions, and measures to maintain skin health. Routine skin assessment involves observation of the patient's skin, with particular attention to bony prominences. Incontinence-associated dermatitis (IAD) or moisture-associated skin damage (MASD) is inflammation of the skin that happens when the perineal area is subject to prolonged contact with urine or stool.[91,92] Objective signs of IAD include erythema, swelling, vesiculation, oozing, crusting, and scaling, with subjective symptoms of tingling, itching, burning, and pain.[93,94] In persons with dark skin tones, IAD presents with white, dark red, purple, or yellow skin discoloration.[94,95] Incontinence-associated dermatitis is often misdiagnosed as a stage 2 pressure ulcer. The condition can occur anywhere in the perineal region, which is broadly defined as the perineum (area between the vulva or scrotum and anus), buttocks, perianal area, coccyx, and upper/inner thigh regions. The clinical presentation is variable and may be dependent on the frequency of incontinence episode, rapidity and efficacy of postepisode hygiene, and duration of incontinence.[93]

Incontinence-associated dermatitis may present with manifestations characteristic of acute episodes, or chronic skin changes suggestive of more long-standing incontinence. In acute episodes, the skin characteristics most predominant are erythema, papulovesicular reaction, frank erosions and abrasions, and, in some cases, evidence of monilial infection, due to the moist warm environment. In general, a diffuse blanchable erythema is present involving buttock areas, coccyx area, perineum, perianal area, and upper/inner thighs. The extent of the erythema varies, and the intensity of the reaction may be diminished in immunocompromised and some elderly patients. A papulovesicular rash is particularly evident in the groin and perineum areas (upper/inner thigh, vulva/scrotal area). Secondary skin changes include crusting and scaling, and are usually evident at the fringes of the reaction. Erosions and frank denudation of the skin may be more common with incontinence associated with feces. The distribution of the dermatitis differs in men and women, as might be expected. Typically, the more severe damage in male patients occurs on the posterior aspect of the penile shaft and the anterior aspect of the scrotum. More damage is seen in the lower perineal regions, such as the inner thighs and low buttocks, than in the higher perineal regions, such as the sacral/coccygeal area or groin. In women, the skin damage usually involves the vulva and groin areas, and spreads distally from those sites.

Chronic skin changes in patients with long-standing incontinence include a thickened appearance of skin where moisture is allowed to maintain skin contact, and increased evidence of scaling and crusting. The thickened appearance of the skin is due to urine or stool pooling on the skin. This skin is overhydrated and easily abraded, with minimal friction. The reaction is notable at the coccyx, scrotum, and vulva. Excoriation from patients' scratching at affected sites may also be present. In many cases of long-standing incontinence, partial-thickness ulcers are present over the sacral/coccygeal area and medial buttocks region, close to or in the gluteal fold. Although these lesions present in a typical pressure ulcer location, some characteristics of these partial-thickness ulcers differ from characteristics seen with superficial pressure-induced skin trauma. First, the lesions tend to be multiple. The lesions may or may not be directly over a bony prominence, the lesions are typically surrounded by other characteristics of IAD (e.g., diffuse blanchable erythema), they may present as copy lesions where one lesion on the buttocks mirrors a second lesion on the opposite buttock and they may present in the gluteal cleft itself.

When caring for patients who are incontinent of urine and feces, there is the challenge of preventing IAD and pressure ulceration as a result of the decreased tissue tolerance to trauma. When moisture, urine, and feces have caused maceration and overhydration of the epidermis, the skin and tissues are less tolerant of friction forces. Further moisture increases the coefficient of friction, which increases damage to the epidermis with less friction force applied.[96] Stage 2 pressure ulcers and partial-thickness skin lesions, such as abrasions, are most commonly attributed to friction and shearing forces and it is likely that incontinence plays a critical role in the development of stage 2 pressure ulcers. Reddened areas should not be massaged. Massage can further impair the perfusion to the tissues. Use moisture barrier creams/ointments to protect from moisture and apply skin emollients liberally to maintain adequate skin moisture.

Incontinence management

This discussion is meant to serve as an overview to those resources available to clinicians concerning management of incontinence. It does not include all management strategies and only briefly mentions several strategies that are most pertinent to palliative care patients at high risk of development of pressure ulcers. Management of incontinence is dependent on assessment and diagnosis of the problem.

Incontinence assessment

Assessment of incontinence should include history of the incontinence, including patterns of elimination, characteristics of the urinary stream or fecal mass, and sensation of bladder or rectal filling. The physical examination is designed to gather specific information related to bladder or rectal functioning and therefore is limited in scope. A limited neurological examination should provide data on the mental status and motivation of the patient and caregiver, specific motor skills, and condition of back and lower extremities. The genitalia and perineal skin are assessed for signs of perineal skin lesions and perineal sensation.

The environmental assessment should include inspection of the patient's home or nursing home facility to evaluate for the presence of environmental barriers to continence. A voiding/defecation diary is very helpful in planning the treatment and management of incontinence. In cognitively impaired patients, the caregiver may complete the diary, and management strategies can be identified from the baseline data.

Incontinence management strategies

Palliative care patients who are at risk for pressure ulcer development may be candidates for behavioral management strategies for incontinence. Incontinence in palliative care patients may be successfully managed with scheduled toileting. Scheduled toileting is caregiver dependent and requires a motivated caregiver to be successful. Adequate fluid intake is an important component of a scheduled toileting program.

Scheduled toileting, or habit training, is toileting at planned time intervals. The goal is to keep the patient dry by assisting him or her to void at regular intervals. There can be attempts to match the interval to the individual patient's natural voiding schedule. There is no systematic effort to motivate patients to delay voiding or to resist the urge to void. Scheduled toileting may be based on the clock (e.g., toileting every 2 hours) or on activities (e.g., toileting after meals and before transferring to bed).

Underpads and briefs may be used to protect the skin of patients who are incontinent of urine or stool. These products are designed to absorb moisture, wick the wetness away from the skin, and maintain a quick-drying interface with the skin. Studies in both infants and adults demonstrate that products that are designed to present a quick-drying surface to the skin and to absorb moisture do keep the skin drier and are associated with a lower incidence of dermatitis.[91] The critical feature is the ability to absorb moisture and present a quick-drying surface, not whether the product is disposable or reusable. Regardless of the product chosen, containment strategies imply the need for a check-and-change schedule for the incontinent patient, so that wet linens and pads may be removed in a timely manner. Underpads are not as tight or constricting as briefs. Alternating use of underpads and briefs allows the skin to dry out between wet periods, which can diminish the effects of moisture on the skin. Use of briefs when the patient is up in a chair, ambulating, or visiting and use of underpads when the patient is in bed is one suggestion for combining the strengths of both products.

External collection devices may be more effective with male patients. External catheters or condom catheters are devices applied to the shaft of the penis that direct the urine away from the body and into a collection device. Many external catheters are self-adhesive and easy to apply. For patients with a retracted penis, a special pouching system, similar to an ostomy pouch, can be used. A key concern with the use of external collection devices is routine removal of the product for inspection and hygiene of the skin.

There are special containment devices for fecal incontinence as well. There are special indwelling fecal drainage tube systems designed for prolonged use and made of soft flexible plastic can be inserted rectally and will allow management of stool of varying consistencies as well as diarrhea. These devices provide access to the bowel for colonic irrigation and permits delivery and retention of rectally administered medications. External collection devices also exist. Fecal incontinence collectors are composed of a self-adhesive skin barrier attached to a drainable pouch. Application of the device is somewhat dependent on the skill of the clinician. To facilitate success, the patient should be put on a routine for changing the pouch before leakage occurs. The skin barrier provides a physical obstacle to keep the stool away from the skin and helps to prevent dermatitis and associated skin problems. Skin barrier wafers or hydrocolloid dressings without an attached pouch can be useful in protecting the skin from feces or urine. Use of moisturizers for dry skin and use of lubricants for reduction of friction injuries are also recommended skin care strategies.[54] Moisture barriers are used to protect the skin from the effects of moisture. Although products that provide a moisture barrier are recommended, the reader is cautioned that the recommendation is derived from usual practice and clinical practice guidelines and is not research based. The success of the particular product is linked to how it is formulated and the hydrophobic properties of the product. Generally, pastes are thicker and more repellent of moisture than ointments. As a quick evaluation, one can observe the ease with which the product can be removed with water during routine cleansing: if the product comes off the skin with just routine cleansing, it probably is not an effective barrier to moisture. Mineral oil may be used for cleansing some of the heavier barrier products (e.g., zinc oxide paste) to ease removal from the skin.

Pressure ulcer assessment

The foundation for designing a palliative care plan for the patient with a pressure ulcer is a comprehensive assessment. Comprehensive assessment includes assessment of wound severity, wound status, and the total patient.

Wound severity

Assessment of wound severity refers to the use of a classification system for diagnosing the severity of tissue trauma by determining the tissue layers involved in the wound. Classification systems such as staging pressure ulcers provide communication regarding wound severity and the tissue layers involved in the injury.

Pressure ulcers are commonly classified according to grading or staging systems based on the depth of tissue destruction. The NPUAP staging classification system is most commonly used to describe depth of tissue damage.[54] Staging systems measure only one characteristic of the wound and should not be viewed as a complete assessment independent of other indicators. Staging systems are best used as a diagnostic tool for indicating wound severity. Table 17A.1 presents pressure ulcer staging criteria according to the NPUAP. Pressure-induced skin damage that manifests as purple, blue, or black areas of intact skin may represent suspected deep tissue injury (DTI). These lesions commonly occur on heels and the sacrum and signal more severe tissue damage below the skin surface. These DTI lesions

Table 17A.1 Selected characteristics for classes of support surface

Performance characteristics	Powered air fluidized	Powered low air loss	Powered alternating pressure air	Nonpowered air, water	Nonpowered foam	Standard hospital mattress
Increased support area	Yes	Yes	Yes	Yes	Yes	No
Low moisture retention	Yes	Yes	No	No	No	No
Reduced heat accumulation	Yes	Yes	No	No	No	No
Shear reduction	Yes	Yes	Yes	Yes	No	No
Pressure reduction	Yes	Yes	Yes	Yes	Yes	No
Dynamic	Yes	Yes	Yes	No	No	No
Cost per day	High	High/Moderate	Moderate	Low	Low	Low

reflect tissue damage at the bony tissue interface in the muscle tissue and may progress rapidly to large tissue defects. Pressure ulcers that occur at the end of life may present with characteristics of DTI. Persons at life's end, during an acute critical illness, or with severe trauma may experience skin failure or terminal pressure ulcers.[97,98] Skin failure is defined as an acute episode where the skin and subcutaneous tissues die (become necrotic) due to hypoperfusion that occurs concurrent with severe dysfunction or failure of other organ systems.[97] It is the hypoperfusion that creates an extreme inflammatory reaction along with severe dysfunction or failure of multiple organ systems that compromises the skin.[99] The skin, the largest organ of the body, is no different from other organs in that it also can become dysfunctional. Skin compromise, including changes related to decreased perfusion and hypoxia, can occur at the tissue, cellular, or molecular level resulting in decreased oxygen availability and reduction in nutrient use by the tissues.[97–100] These changes weaken the skin making it less tolerant of mechanical forces such as pressure, shear, and friction. Skin failure may present anywhere on the body (not just bony prominences) but often occurs over bony prominences.

One manifestation of skin failure may be a terminal pressure ulcer. One of the first clinical descriptions of terminal ulcers was by Kennedy in 1989.[101] Kennedy described a specific subgroup of pressure ulcers that some individuals developed as they were dying. They present typically over the sacrum and are shaped like a pear, butterfly, or horseshoe.[101] The ulcers are a variety of colors including red, yellow, or black; are sudden in onset; typically deteriorate rapidly; and usually indicate that death is imminent, with just over half (55.7%) dying within 6 weeks of discovery of the ulcer. Others have also reported terminal pressure ulcers occurring in the 2 weeks prior to death.[1] The Centers for Medicare and Medicaid Services (CMS) recently recognized the Kennedy ulcer as a precursor to death and part of the dying process and specifically recommends that the ulcer not be coded as a pressure ulcer once it is determined to be a Kennedy ulcer.[103]

Wound status

Pressure ulcer assessment is the base for maintaining and evaluating the therapeutic plan of care. Assessment of wound status involves evaluation of multiple wound characteristics. Initial assessment and follow-up assessments at regular intervals to monitor progress or deterioration of the sore are necessary to determine the effectiveness of the treatment plan. Adequate assessment is important even when the goal of care is comfort, not healing. The assessment data enable clinicians to communicate clearly about a patient's pressure ulcer, provide for continuity in the plan of care, and allow evaluation of treatment modalities. Assessment of wound status should be performed weekly and whenever a significant change is noted in the wound. Assessment should not be confused with monitoring of the wound at each dressing change. Monitoring of the wound can be performed by less skilled caregivers, but assessment should be performed on a routine basis by healthcare practitioners. Use of a systematic approach with a comprehensive assessment tool is helpful.

There are few tools available that encompass multiple wound characteristics to evaluate overall wound status and healing. Two available tools are the Pressure Ulcer Scale for Healing (PUSH)[104] and the Bates-Jensen Wound Assessment Tool (BWAT).[105]

The PUSH tool incorporates surface area measurements, exudate amount, and surface appearance. These wound characteristics were chosen based on principal component analysis to define the best model of healing.[104,106] The clinician measures the size of the wound, calculates the surface area (length times width), and chooses the appropriate size category on the tool (0 to 10). Exudate is evaluated as none (0), light (1), moderate (2), or heavy (3). Tissue type choices include closed (0), epithelial tissue (1), granulation tissue (2), slough (3), and necrotic tissue (4). The three subscores are then summed for a total score.[104]

The PUSH tool may offer a quick assessment to predict healing outcomes. The PUSH tool is best used as a method of prediction of wound healing. Therefore, it may not be the best tool for palliative care patients, because healing is not an expected outcome of care. Assessment of additional wound characteristics may still be needed, to develop a treatment plan for the pressure ulcer. The BWAT includes additional wound characteristics that may be helpful in designing a palliative plan of care for the wound.

The BWAT (Figure 17A.2), originally developed as the Pressure Sore Status Tool in 1990 by Bates-Jensen[105,107] and revised in 2001 and 2006, evaluates 13 wound characteristics with a numerical rating scale and rates them from best to worst possible. The BWAT is recommended as a method of assessment and monitoring of pressure ulcers and other chronic wounds. It is a pencil-and-paper instrument comprising 15 items: location, shape, size, depth, edges, undermining or pockets, necrotic tissue type, necrotic tissue amount, exudate type, exudate amount, surrounding skin color, peripheral tissue edema, peripheral tissue induration, granulation tissue, and epithelialization. Two items, location and shape, are nonscored. The remaining 13 are scored items, and each appears with characteristic descriptors rated on a scale of 1 (best for that characteristic) to 5 (worst attribute of the characteristic). It is recommended that wounds be scored initially for a baseline assessment and at regular intervals to evaluate therapy. Once a wound has been assessed for each item on the BWAT, the 13 item scores can be added to obtain a total score for the wound. The total score can then be monitored to determine "at a glance" the progress in healing or degeneration of the wound. Total scores range from 13 (skin intact but always at risk for further damage) to 65 (profound tissue degeneration). Figure 17A.2 presents the instructions for use of the BWAT.

Reliability of the tool has been evaluated in an acute care setting with enterostomal therapy (ET) nurses (nurses with additional training in wound care)[105] and in long-term care with a variety of healthcare professionals and one wound certified nurse expert.[108] Interrater reliability ranged from r = 0.915 (P = 0.0001) for the ET nurses[105] to 0.78% agreement for the variety of healthcare professionals.[108] The BWAT is widely used in a variety of healthcare settings with all chronic wounds.[109,110]

An additional benefit associated with the assignment of numeric values to items on the BWAT is that it assists in setting realistic goals, which may be beneficial in palliative care. Clinical experience shows that not all wounds heal and certainly not always in the same setting. The BWAT allows for more realistic goal setting as appropriate to the healthcare setting and the individual patient and wound. For example, the patient with a large, necrotic, full-thickness wound in acute care will probably not be in the facility long enough for the wound to heal completely. However, the tool enables clinicians to set intermediate or secondary goals,

BATES-JENSEN WOUND ASSESSMENT TOOL   NAME

Complete the rating sheet to assess wound status. Evaluate each item by picking the response that best describes the wound and entering the score in the item score column for the appropriate date. If the wound has healed/resolved, score items 1,2,3, & 4 as = 0.

Location: Anatomic site. Circle, identify right **(R)** or left **(L)** and use **"X"** to mark site on body diagrams:

_____	Sacrum & coccyx	_____	Lateral ankle
_____	Trochanter	_____	Medial ankle
_____	Ischial tuberosity	_____	Heel
_____	Buttock	_____	Other site: _____→

Shape: Overall wound pattern; assess by observing perimeter and depth.

Circle and <u>date</u> appropriate description:

_____	Irregular	_____	Linear or elongated
_____	Round/oval	_____	Bowl/boat
_____	Square/rectangle	_____	Butterfly Other Shape

Item	Assessment	Date Score	Date Score	Date Score
1. Size*	*0 = Healed, resolved wound 1 = Length × width <4 sq cm 2 = Length × width 4–<16 sq cm 3 = Length × width 16.1–<36 sq cm 4 = Length × width 36.1–<80 sq cm 5 = Length × width >80 sq cm			
2. Depth*	*0 = Healed, resolved wound 1 = Non-blanchable erythema on intact skin 2 = Partial thickness skin loss involving epidermis &/or dermis 3 = Full thickness skin loss involving damage or necrosis of subcutaneous tissue; may extend down to but not through underlying fascia; &/or mixed partial & full thickness &/or tissue layers obscured by granulation tissue 4 = Obscured by necrosis 5 = Full thickness skin loss with extensive destruction, tissue necrosis or adamage to muscle, bone or supporting structures			
3. Edges*	*0 = Healed, resolved wound 1 = Indistinct, diffuse, none clearly visible 2 = Distinct, outline clearly visible, attached, even with wound base 3 = Well-defined, not attached to wound base 4 = Well-defined, not attached to base, rolled under, thickened 5 = Well-defined, fibrotic, scarred or hyperkeratotic			
4. Under-mining*	*0 = Healed, resolved wound 1 = None present 2 = Undermining < 2 cm in any area 3 = Undermining 2–4 cm involving < 50% wound margins 4 = Undermining 2–4 cm involving > 50% wound margins 5 = Undermining > 4 cm or Tunneling in any area			
5. Necrotic Tissue Type	1 = None visible 2 = White/grey non-viable tissue &/or non-adherent yellow slough 3 = Loosely adherent yellow slough 4 = Adherent, soft, black eschar 5 = Firmly adherent, hard, black eschar			
6. Necrotic Tissue Amount	1 = None visible 2 = < 25% of wound bed covered 3 = 25% to 50% of wound covered 4 = > 50% and < 75% of wound covered 5 = 75% to 100% of wound covered			
7. Exudate	1 = None 2 = Bloody 3 = Serosanguineous: thin, watery, pale red/pink 4 = Serous: thin, watery, clear 5 = Purulent: thin or thick, opaque, tan/yellow, with or without odor			

Figure 17A.2 (Continued)

Item	Assessment	Date Score	Date Score	Date Score
8. Exudate Amount	1 = None, dry wound 2 = Scant, wound moist but no observable exudate 3 = Small 4 = Moderate 5 = Large			
9. Skin Color Sur-rounding Wound	1 = Pink or normal for ethnic group 2 = Bright red &/or blanches to touch 3 = White or grey pallor or hypopigmented 4 = Dark red or purple &/or non-blanchable 5 = Black or hyperpigmented			
10. Peripheral Tissue Edema	1 = No swelling or edema 2 = Non-pitting edema extends <4 cm around wound 3 = Non-pitting edema extends >4 cm around wound 4 = Pitting edema extends < 4 cm around wound 5 = Crepitus and/or pitting edema extends >4 cm around wound			
11. Peripheral Tissue Induration	1 = None present 2 = Induration, < 2 cm around wound 3 = Induration 2–4 cm extending < 50% around wound 4 = Induration 2–4 cm extending > 50% around wound 5 = Induration > 4 cm in any area around wound			
12. Granu-lation Tissue	1 = Skin intact or partial thickness wound 2 = Bright, beefy red; 75% to 100% of wound filled &/or tissue overgrowth 3 = Bright, beefy red; < 75% & > 25% of wound filled 4 = Pink, &/or dull, dusky red &/or fills ≤ 25% of wound 5 = No granulation tissue present			
13. Epithe-lializa-tion	1 = 100% wound covered, surface intact 2 = 75% to <100% wound covered &/or epithelial tissue extends >0.5cm into wound bed 3 = 50% to <75% wound covered &/or epithelial tissue extends to <0.5cm into wound bed 4 = 25% to < 50% wound covered 5 = < 25% wound covered			
	TOTAL SCORE			
	SIGNATURE			

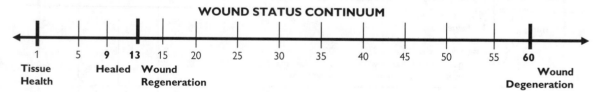

WOUND STATUS CONTINUUM

1 — Tissue Health | 5 | 9 Healed | 13 Wound Regeneration | 15 | 20 | 25 | 30 | 35 | 40 | 45 | 50 | 55 | 60 Wound Degeneration

Plot the total score on the Wound Status Continuum by putting an **"X"** on the line and the date beneath the line. Plot multiple scores with their dates to see-at-a-glance regeneration or degeneration of the wound.

© 2001 Barbara Bates-Jensen

Figure 17A.2 The Bates-Jensen Wound Assessment Tool (BWAT) for measuring pressure sore status.

such as, "Necrotic tissue in the wound will decrease in amount and type." The BWAT allows for monitoring of improvement or deterioration in individual characteristics, as well as the total score. This in turn enables assessment of the patient's response to specific treatments. For example, the characteristics of necrotic tissue type and amount may be tracked with exudate type and amount to evaluate the response to debridement or infection management. The ability to track wound symptoms such as exudate allows evaluation of interventions designed to alleviate distressing wound symptoms and as such is very useful for palliative care, wound-related complaints, and when symptoms affect the patient's quality of life.[110] In palliative care an example of a goal might be to maintain the total BWAT score between 20 and 22.

The severity of a wound, as well as overall health status of the patient, can determine the appropriate management approach for healing. Severity states are a measure of the degree of the tissue insult or wound burden on the patient and can be useful for patients with a single wound as well as for those with multiple wounds. The goals of wound care are to decrease the overall severity status and to make this decrease in a timely fashion. The BWAT can be used to identify wound severity state, and thereby guide care planning. The BWAT average total scores can be divided into four suggested severity states for the single wound:

◆ 13–20 indicate minimal severity

◆ 21–30 indicates mild severity

◆ 31–40 is moderate severity

◆ 41–65 is extreme severity

For patients with multiple wounds, the average BWAT total score should be used to determine severity state. For example, a patient with an ulcer on the heel with a BWAT score of 20 and a sacral ulcer with a BWAT score of 28 would have a BWAT severity score of 24 and would be classified in the mild severity state. An example of a treatment algorithm based on clinical practice guidelines for one wound in each of these severity states is presented below.

◆ Wounds with a BWAT total score of 13–20 are generally shallow, partial-thickness wounds. The main goals for wounds in this severity state are to prevent further damage and to provide a moist wound environment for healing.

◆ Wounds with mild severity include both partial-thickness and full-thickness clean and necrotic wounds. The goals of care for mild severity wounds are to eliminate any necrotic debris, absorb excess wound exudate, maintain a clean wound bed, and maintain a moist environment.

◆ Wounds with moderate severity scores are full-thickness clean or necrotic wounds and the goals are to obtain/maintain a clean wound bed, provide a moist environment, absorb excess exudate, prevent premature closure, and reduce wound dead space. Wounds with moderate (and some mild) severity scores have the most diverse presentations clinically, so choices regarding treatment are numerous. Treatment is often focused on debridement, absorbing exudate, eliminating dead space, and preparing a clean wound bed. The goals of care for wounds in this severity state are to obtain/maintain a clean wound bed, absorb excess exudate, eliminate dead space to prevent premature wound closure, and provide a moist wound environment.

◆ Wounds with BWAT total scores between 41 and 65 are generally deep, full-thickness wounds with more critical clinical manifestations, including undermining and significant necrosis. The goals of care for wounds in this severity state are to identify and treat infection, obtain a clean wound bed, absorb excess exudate, eliminate dead space to prevent premature wound closure, and provide a moist wound environment.

Wound characteristics

Adequate initial wound assessment should encompass a composite of wound characteristics, which forms a base for differential diagnosis, therapeutic intervention, and future reassessment comparisons.[109] The indices for wound assessment include all of the following: location, size of ulcer, depth of tissue involvement, stage or classification, condition of wound edges, presence of undermining or tunneling, necrotic tissue characteristics, exudate characteristics, surrounding tissue conditions, and wound-healing characteristics of granulation tissue and epithelialization. Wound characteristics of concern for the palliative care patient include wound edges, undermining and tunneling, necrotic tissue characteristics, exudate characteristics, and surrounding tissue conditions. These five characteristics, as well as healing attributes of granulation tissue and epithelialization, are discussed in the following sections.

Edges or margins

Wound edge, or margin, includes characteristics of distinctness, degree of attachment to the wound base, color, and thickness. In pressure ulcers, as tissues degenerate, broad and indistinct areas, in which the wound edge is diffuse and difficult to observe, become shallow lesions with edges that are more distinct, thin, and separate. As tissue trauma from pressure progresses, the reaction intensifies with a thickening and rolling inward of the epidermis, so that the edge is well defined and sharply outlines the ulcer, with little or no evidence of new tissue growth. In long-standing pressure ulcers, fibrosis and scarring result from repeated injury and repair, with the edges hyperpigmented, indurated, and firm and impairment in the migratory ability of epithelial cells.[111] Pressure ulcers in palliative care may show significant tissue damage, and the edges may indicate areas of full-thickness tissue loss with other areas of partial-thickness damage. In palliative care, pressure ulcers may be present for prolonged periods with no change in the wound; the wound edges often exhibit hemosiderin staining or hyperpigmentation in conjunction with epiboly or the rolled-under and thickened appearance.

When assessing edges, the nurse should look at the clarity and distinctness of the wound outline. With edges that are indistinct and diffuse, there are areas in which the normal tissues blend into the wound bed and the edges are not clearly visible. Edges that are even with the skin surface and the wound base are attached to the base of the wound. This means that the wound is flat, with no appreciable depth. Well-defined edges, on the other hand, are clear and distinct and can be outlined easily on a transparent piece of plastic. Edges that are not attached to the base of the wound imply a wound with some depth of tissue involvement. A crater or bowl or boat shape indicates a wound with edges that are not attached to the wound base. The wound has walls or sides. There is depth to the wound.

As the wound ages, the edges become rolled under and thickened to palpation. The edge achieves a unique hyperpigmented coloring due to hemosiderin staining. The pigment turns a gray or brown color in both dark- and light-skinned persons. Long-standing wounds may continue to thicken, with scar tissue and fibrosis developing in the wound edge, causing the edge to feel hard, rigid, and indurated. The wound edges are evaluated by visual inspection and palpation.

Undermining and tunneling

The terms *undermining* and *tunneling* refer to the loss of tissue underneath an intact skin surface. Undermining, or pocketing, usually involves a greater percentage of the wound margins and more shallow length, compared with tunneling. Undermining usually involves subcutaneous tissues and follows the fascial planes next to the wound.

Wounds with undermining have more aerobic and anaerobic bacteria than do wounds that are in the process of healing with no undermining.[112] The degree and amount of undermining indicate the severity of tissue necrosis. As subcutaneous fat degenerates, wound pockets develop. Initially, deep fascia limits the depth of pocketing, encouraging more superficial internal spread of undermining. Once the fascia is penetrated, undermining of deeper tissues may proceed rapidly.[111,112] Internal dimensions of wound undermining are commonly measured with the use of cotton-tipped applicators and gentle probing of the wound. There are also premeasured devices that can be inserted under the wound edge and advanced into the deeper tissues to aid in determination of the extent of undermining.

Undermining and wound pockets should be assessed by inserting a cotton-tipped applicator under the wound edge, advancing it as far as it will go without using undue force, raising the tip of the applicator so that it may be seen or felt on the surface of the skin, marking the surface with a pen, and measuring the distance from the mark on the skin to the edge of the wound. This process is continued all around the wound. Then the percentage of the wound involved is determined with the help of a transparent metric measuring guide with concentric circles divided into quadrants. Another noninvasive method of assessment of wound pockets is the use of ultrasound to evaluate the undermined tissues. Ultrasonography provides a visual picture of the impaired tissues and can be repeated to monitor for improvement.

Necrotic tissue type and amount

Necrotic tissue characteristics of color, consistency, adherence, and amount present in the wound must be incorporated into wound assessment. As tissues die during wound development, they change in color, consistency, and adherence to the wound bed. The level and type of tissue death influence the clinical appearance of the necrotic tissue. For example, as subcutaneous fat tissues die, a collection of stringy, yellow slough is formed. As muscle tissues degenerate, the dead tissue may be more thick or tenacious.

The characteristic "necrotic tissue type" is a qualitative variable, with most clinicians using descriptions of clinical observations of a composite of factors as a method of assessment. The characteristics of color, consistency, and adherence are most often used to describe the type of necrosis. Color varies, as necrosis worsens, from white/gray nonviable tissue, to yellow slough, and finally to black eschar. Consistency refers to the cohesiveness of the debris (i.e., thin or thick, stringy or clumpy). Consistency also varies on a continuum as the necrotic area deepens and becomes more dehydrated.

The terms *slough* and *eschar* refer to different levels of necrosis and are described according to color and consistency. A slough is described as yellow (or tan) and as thin, mucinous, or stringy, whereas eschar is described as black (or brown), and as soft or hard; eschar represents full-thickness tissue destruction. *Adherence* refers to the adhesiveness of the debris to the wound bed and the ease with which the two may be separated. Necrotic tissue tends to become more adherent to the wound bed as the level of damage increases. Clinically, eschar is more firmly adherent than is yellow slough.

Necrotic tissue is assessed for color, consistency, and adherence to the wound bed. The predominant characteristic present in the wound should be chosen for assessment. Necrotic tissue type changes as it ages in the wound, as debridement occurs, and as further tissue trauma causes increased cellular death. Slough usually is nonadherent or loosely adherent to the healthy tissues of the wound bed. By definition, nonadherent tissue appears scattered throughout the wound; it appears as if the tissue could easily be removed with gauze. Loosely adherent tissue is attached to the wound bed; it is thick and stringy and may appear as clumps of debris attached to wound tissue.

Eschar signifies deeper tissue damage

Eschar may be black, gray, or brown in color. It is usually adherent or firmly adherent to the wound tissues and may be soggy, soft or hard, or leathery in texture. A soft, soggy eschar is usually strongly attached to the base of the wound but may be lifting from (and loose from) the edges of the wound. A hard, crusty eschar is strongly attached to the base and edges of the wound. Hard eschars are often mistaken for scabs. Sometimes nonviable tissue appears before a wound is apparent. This can be seen as a white or gray area on the surface of the skin. The area usually demarcates within a day or two, when the wound appears and interrupts the skin surface.

Necrotic tissue retards wound healing because it is a medium for bacterial growth and a physical obstacle to epidermal resurfacing, wound contraction, and granulation. The greater the amount of necrotic tissue present in the wound bed, the more severe the insult to the tissue and the longer the time required to heal the wound. The amount of necrotic tissue usually affects the amount of exudate from the wound and causes wound odor, both of which are distressing to the patient and to caregivers. Because of the amount of necrotic tissue present, modifications of treatment and debridement techniques may be made. The depth of the wound cannot be assessed in the presence of necrosis that blocks visualization of the total wound.

The amount of necrotic tissue present in the wound is one of the easier characteristics to assess. The nurse visualizes the wound as a pie divided into four quadrants. The percentage of necrosis present is judged by evaluating each quadrant to determine the percent of the wound covered with necrosis. Alternatively, the length and width of the necrotic tissue may be measured to determine the surface area involved in the necrosis.

Exudate type and amount

Wound exudate (also known as wound fluid, wound drainage) is an important assessment feature, because the characteristics of the exudate help the clinician to diagnose signs of wound infection, to evaluate appropriateness of topical therapy, and to monitor wound healing. Wound infection retards wound healing, causes odor, and should be treated aggressively in most instances. Proper assessment of wound exudate is also important because it affirms the body's brief, normal inflammatory response to tissue injury. Accurate assessment and diagnosis of wound exudate and infection are critical components of effective wound management. One of the main goals of palliative wound care is to prevent infection and to control exudate, because these conditions lead to discomfort from the wound.

The healthy wound normally has some evidence of moisture on its surface. Healthy wound fluid contains enzymes and growth factors, which may play a role in promoting reepithelialization of the wound and provide needed growth factors for all phases of wound repair. The moist environment produced by wound exudate allows efficient migration of epidermal cells and prevents wound desiccation and further injury.[113]

In pressure ulcers, increased exudate is a response to the inflammatory process or infection. Increased capillary permeability causes leakage of fluids and substrates into the injured tissue. When a wound is present, tissue fluid leaks out of the open tissue. This fluid normally is serous or serosanguineous.

In the infected wound, the exudate may thicken, become purulent in nature, and continue to be present in moderate to large amounts. Examples of exudate character changes in infected wounds are the presence of *Pseudomonas*, which produces a thick, malodorously sweet-smelling, green drainage, or *Proteus* infection, which may have an ammonia-like odor. Wounds with foul-smelling drainage are generally infected or filled with necrotic debris, and healing time is prolonged as tissue destruction progresses.[111] Wounds with significant amounts of necrotic debris often have a thick, tenacious, opaque, purulent, malodorous drainage in moderate to copious amounts. True wound exudate must be differentiated from necrotic tissue that sloughs off the wound as a result of debridement efforts. Exudate from sloughing necrotic tissue is commonly attached to or connected with the necrotic debris; frequently, the only method of differentiation is adequate debridement of necrotic tissue from the wound site. Liquefied necrotic tissue occurs most often as a result of enzymatic or autolytic debridement. Often, removal of the necrotic tissue reduces the amount and changes the character of wound exudate.

Exudate should be assessed for the amount and type of drainage that occurs. The type and color of wound exudate vary depending on the degree of moisture in the wound and the organisms present. Characteristics used to examine exudate are color, consistency, adherence, distribution in the wound, and presence of odor.

Estimating the amount of exudate in the wound is difficult due to wound size variability and topical dressing types. One problem with assessment of exudate amount is the size of the wound. What might be considered a large amount of drainage for a smaller wound may be considered a small amount for a larger wound, making clinically meaningful assessment of exudate difficult.

Certain dressing types interact with or trap wound fluid to create or mimic certain characteristics of exudate, such as color and consistency of purulent drainage. For example, both hydrocolloid and alginate dressings mimic a purulent drainage on removal of the dressing. Preparation of the wound site for appropriate assessment involves removal of the wound dressing and cleansing with normal saline to remove dressing debris in the wound bed, followed by evaluation of the wound for true exudate.

Although it is not a part of exudate assessment, evaluation of the wound dressing provides the clinician with valuable data about the effectiveness of treatment. Evaluation of the percentage of the wound dressing involved with wound drainage during a specific time frame is helpful for clinical management that includes dressings beyond traditional gauze. In estimating the percentage of the dressing involved with the wound exudate, clinical judgment must be quantified by putting a number to visual assessment of the dressing. For example, the clinician might determine that 50% of the hydrocolloid dressing was involved with wound drainage over a 4-day wearing period. Based on the data, the clinician might quantify the judgment for this type of dressing, length of dressing wear time, and wound cause as being a "minimal" amount of exudate. Clinical judgment of the amount of wound drainage requires some experience with expected wound exudate output in relation to phase of wound healing and type of wound, as well as knowledge of absorptive capacity and normal wear time of topical dressings.

Certain characteristics of exudate indicate wound degeneration and infection. If signs of cellulitis (erythema or skin discoloration, edema, pain, induration, purulent drainage) are present at the wound site, the exudate amount may be copious and seropurulent or purulent in character. The amount of exudate remains high or increases, and the character may change to frank purulence, with further wound degeneration. Wound infection must be considered in these cases.

Pressure ulcers manifest with a variety of wound exudate types and amounts. In partial-thickness pressure ulcers, the wound exudate is most likely to be serous or serosanguineous in nature and to be present in minimal to moderate amounts. In clean full-thickness pressure ulcers, the wound exudate is similar, with minimal to moderate amounts of serous to serosanguineous exudate. As healing progresses in the clean full-thickness pressure ulcer, the character of the exudate changes; it may become bloody if the fragile capillary bed is disrupted, and it lessens in amount.

For full-thickness pressure ulcers with necrotic debris, wound exudate is dependent on the presence or absence of infection and the type of therapy instituted. Exudate may appear moderate to large but, in fact, is related to the amount of necrotic tissue present and to liquefaction of the debris in the wound. Typically, the necrotic full-thickness pressure ulcer manifests with serous to seropurulent wound exudate in moderate to large amounts. With appropriate treatment, the wound exudate amount may temporarily increase, as the character gradually assumes a serous nature.

Surrounding tissue condition

The tissues surrounding the wound should be assessed for color, induration, and edema. The tissues surrounding the wound are often the first indication of impending further tissue damage and are a key gauge of successful prevention strategies. Color of the surrounding skin may indicate further injury from pressure, friction, or shearing. The tissues within 4 cm of the wound edge should be assessed. Dark-skinned persons show the colors "bright red" and "dark red" as a deepening of normal skin color or a purple or black hue. As full thickness wound healing occurs in dark-skinned persons, the new skin is pink and lacks pigmentation and thus may never darken. In both light- and dark-skinned patients, new epithelium must be differentiated from tissues that are erythematous. To assess for blanchability in light-skinned patients, the nurse presses firmly on the skin with a finger, then lifts the finger and looks for "blanching," or sudden whitening, of the tissues followed by prompt return of color to the area. Nonblanchable erythema signals more severe tissue damage.

Edema in the surrounding tissues delays wound healing in the pressure ulcer. It is difficult for neoangiogenesis, or growth of new blood vessels into the wound, to occur in edematous tissues. Again, tissues within 4 cm of the wound edge are assessed. Nonpitting edema appears as skin that is shiny and taut, almost glistening. Pitting edema is identified by firmly pressing a finger down into the tissues and waiting for 5 seconds; on release of pressure, tissues fail to resume their previous position and an indentation appears. Crepitus is the accumulation of air or gas in tissues. The clinician should measure how far edema extends beyond the wound edges.

Induration is a sign of impending damage to the tissues. Along with skin-color changes, induration is an omen of further pressure-induced tissue trauma. Tissues within 4 cm of the wound edge are assessed. Induration is an abnormal firmness of tissues with margins. The nurse should palpate where the induration starts and where it ends by gently pinching the tissues. Induration results in an inability to pinch the tissues. Palpation proceeds from healthy tissue, moving toward the wound margins. It is usual to feel slight firmness at the wound edge itself. Normal tissues feel soft and spongy; induration feels hard and firm to the touch.

Granulation tissue and epithelialization

Granulation and epithelial tissues are markers of wound health. They signal the proliferative phase of wound healing and usually foretell wound closure. Granulation tissue is the growth of small blood vessels and connective tissue into the wound cavity. It is more observable in full-thickness wounds because of the tissue defect that occurs in such wounds. In partial-thickness wounds, granulation tissue may occur so quickly, and in concert with epithelialization, or skin resurfacing, that it is unobservable in most cases. The granulation tissue is healthy when it is bright, beefy red; shiny; and granular with a velvety appearance. The tissue looks "bumpy" and may bleed easily. Unhealthy granulation tissue, resulting from poor vascular supply, appears pale pink or blanched to a dull, dusky red. Usually, the first layer of granulation tissue to be laid down in the wound is pale pink and, as the granulation tissue deepens and thickens, the color becomes bright, beefy red.

The percentage of the wound that is filled with granulation tissue and the color of the tissue are characteristics indicative of the health of the wound. The clinician makes a judgment as to what percent of the wound has been filled with granulation tissue. This is much easier if there is some past history with the wound. If the wound has been monitored by the same person over multiple observations, it is simple to judge the amount of granulation tissue present. If the initial observation was done by a different observer or if the data are not available, the clinician simply must use his or her best judgment to determine the amount of tissue present.

Partial-thickness wounds heal by epidermal resurfacing and regeneration. Epithelialization occurs via lateral migration at the wound edges and the base of hair follicles as epithelial cells proliferate and resurface the wound. Full-thickness wounds heal by scar formation: The tissue defect fills with granulation tissue, the edges contract, and the wound is resurfaced by epithelialization. Therefore, epithelialization may occur throughout the wound bed in partial-thickness wounds but only from the wound edges in full-thickness wounds.

Epithelialization can be assessed by evaluating the amount of the wound that is surrounded by new tissue and the distance to which new tissue extends into the wound base. Epithelialization appears as pink or red skin. Visualization of the new epithelium takes practice. A transparent measuring guide is used to help determine the percentage of wound involvement and the distance to which the epithelial tissue extends into the wound.

Monitoring the wound

In palliative care, monitoring of the wound is important, to continue to meet the goals of comfort and reduction in wound pain and wound symptoms such as odor and exudate. Evaluation of wound characteristics at scheduled intervals allows the nurse to revise the treatment plan as appropriate and often provides an indication of the overall health of the patient. In many cases, the pressure ulcer worsens as death approaches and as the patient's condition worsens. The skin may be the first organ to actually "fail," with other systems following the downward trend. Progressive monitoring is also important to determine whether the treatment is effectively controlling odor, managing exudate, preventing infection, and minimizing pain—the goals of wound care during palliative care.

Total patient assessment

Comprehensive assessment includes assessment of the total patient as well as of wound severity and wound status. Generally, diagnosis and management of the wound are best accomplished within the context of the whole person. Comprehensive assessment includes a focused history and physical examination, attention to specific laboratory and diagnostic tests, and a pain assessment. Box 17A.1 presents an overview of assessment for the patient with a pressure ulcer.

It is important to obtain a focused history and physical examination as part of the initial assessment. The patient history determines which relevant systems reviews are needed in the physical

---

Box 17A.1 National Pressure Ulcer Advisory Panel recommended palliative care pressure ulcer guidelines

1. Assess the risk for new pressure ulcer development by using a validated risk assessment tool.

2. Reposition the individual at periodic intervals in accordance with the individual's wishes.

3. Strive to maintain adequate nutrition and hydration compatible with the individual's condition and wishes. Adequate nutrition is often not attainable if the individual is unable or refuses to eat.

4. Maintain skin integrity to the extent possible.

5. Set treatment goals that are consistent with the values and goals of the individual.

6. The goal for the palliative care individual with a pressure ulcer is often to enhance quality of life, even if the pressure ulcer cannot/does not lead to closure.

7. Assess the individual initially and whenever there is a change in factors placing the individual at risk.

8. Assess the pressure ulcer initially and weekly and document findings. Assess the pressure ulcer with each dressing change.

9. Assess the impact of the pressure ulcer on quality of life of the patient and family.

10. Manage the pressure ulcer and periwound area on a regular basis.

11. Control wound odor.

12. Assess wound pain.

13. Assess resources.

examination. The goals for treatment and the direction of care (e.g., curative with a goal of wound closure, palliative with a goal of reduced wound pain) can be determined with, at a minimum, the following patient history information: reason for admission to care facility or agency; expectations and perceptions about wound healing; psychological, social, cultural, and economic history; presence of medical comorbidities; current wound status; and previous management strategies.

The systems review portion of the patient history and physical examination provides information on comorbidities that may impair wound healing. Specific comorbidities such as diabetes,[114-118] vascular disease[119,120] and immunocompromise[121-123] have been related to impaired healing. The individual's capacity to heal may be limited by specific disease effects on tissue integrity and perfusion, patient mobility, nutrition, and risk for wound infection. Therefore, throughout the patient history, systems review, and physical examination, the clinician considers host factors that affect wound healing. Additionally, the patient's prognosis as determined by the physician should be factored into the patient's goals of wound care. For example, a patient who is receiving palliative care may have a prognosis that is 6 months or longer and the treatment chosen for the pressure ulcer may be quite different from the treatment chosen for a patient with a prognosis that is only weeks.

Specific laboratory and diagnostic tests in a comprehensive assessment include data on nutrition, glucose management, and tissue oxygenation and perfusion. Nutritional parameters typically include evaluation of serum albumin. Serum albumin is a measure of protein available for healing; a normal level is greater than 3.5 mg/dL. Clinicians should evaluate laboratory values such as arterial blood gases to assess tissue perfusion and oxygenation abilities. Review of laboratory values is prudent to determine the level of diabetic control. Normal glucose levels are 80 mg/dL. Concentrations of 180 to 250 mg/dL or higher indicate that glucose levels are out of control. The nurse should look specifically for a fasting blood glucose concentration lower than 140 mg/dL and a glycosylated hemoglobin concentration (HgbA1C) lower than 7%. The HgbA1C helps to determine the level of glucose control the patient has had over the last 2 to 3 months.

Pain is an important factor in healing, and pressure ulcers can lead to pain and disfigurement. Patients can quantify pressure ulcer pain and can differentiate pressure ulcer pain from pain due to other conditions.[124] Of those persons with pressure ulcers who are able to report pain, across nursing homes and home health and hospital settings, 87% report pain with dressing changes, 84% report pain at rest, and 42% report pain both at rest and during dressing changes.[125] Further, 18% of those persons reporting dressing change wound pain report pain at the highest level (e.g., "excruciating"). Yet, only 6% of those persons reporting pressure ulcer pain receive any medication for pain.[125] The average stage 1 and stage 2 pressure ulcer pain has been reported at 4 cm and 3.5 cm on a 10-cm visual analog scale, respectively. There is some evidence that a higher proportion of persons with stage 3 or 4 ulcers report ulcer pain compared with those persons with stage 2 ulcers and they report more severe pain than those with stage 2 pressure ulcers with a mean numerical rating scale (0–100) of 54 for stage 3/4 and 48 for stage 2.[126] Persons with chronic wounds such as pressure ulcers experience procedural and nonprocedural pain.[124] Procedural pain relates to pain associated with activities such as debridement, dressing changes, and repositioning.

Nonprocedural pain is the daily pain associated with having an open wound.

Wound pain can be assessed using numerical rating scales, the FACES scale, or a visual analog scale.[127] Patients who are nonverbal should be observed for withdrawal, grimacing, crying out, or other nonverbal signs of pain. The Pain Detection Interview (PDI) may be helpful in screening for wound pain in persons with cognitive impairment. The PDI consists of four yes/no response questions:

1. Do you have wound pain now?

2. Do you have wound pain every day?

3. Does wound pain keep you from doing the activities you enjoy?

4. Does wound pain keep you from sleeping?

An affirmative response to question 2 (wound pain every day) or affirmative responses to any two of the four questions indicate probable chronic wound pain, and the patient should have a more extensive pain assessment conducted. Pain assessments should be done before and during wound procedures, such as dressing changes or debridement, and also at times when the dressing is intact and no procedures are in progress. The patient or caregiver should be encouraged to keep a pain diary, because the data may be valuable in evaluating changes in wound pain over time. The focused history, physical examination, evaluation of laboratory and diagnostic data, pain assessment, and patient/family goals for care provide the context for the wound itself and, along with wound severity and wound status assessment, the basis for pressure ulcer treatment. Total patient assessment should also encompass evaluation of treatment appropriateness in light of the overall condition of the patient and the goals of palliative care.

Pressure ulcer management

Pressure ulcer management should be based on clinical practice guidelines. The NPUAP in conjunction with the European Pressure Ulcer Advisory Panel presented updated and pressure ulcer guidelines in 2009.[54] The revised pressure ulcer clinical practice guidelines include specific guidelines for palliative care and pain management. The general NPUAP palliative care guidelines are listed in Table 17A.2. Guidelines for palliative care include:

◆ Repositioning the individual at periodic intervals in accordance with the individual's wishes.

◆ Striving to maintain adequate nutrition and hydration compatible with the individual's condition and wishes, with the understanding that adequate nutrition is often not attainable if the individual is unable or refuses to eat.

◆ Managing the pressure ulcer and periwound skin on a routine, regular basis.

◆ Controlling wound odor

◆ Reducing wound pain

Repositioning and management of tissue loads

Repositioning and management of tissue loads refers to care related to those with pressure ulcers who are at risk for development of additional pressure ulcers. This is an important part of pressure ulcer treatment, because many individuals with a pressure ulcer are at risk for further pressure-induced tissue trauma.

Table 17A.2 Pressure ulcer staging criteria

Pressure ulcer stage	Definition and clinical description
Stage I	Intact skin with nonblanchable redness of a localized area usually over a bony prominence. Darkly pigmented skin may not have visible blanching; its color may differ from the surrounding area.
	The area may be painful, firm, soft, warmer, or cooler as compared to adjacent tissue. Stage I may be difficult to detect in individuals with dark skin tones. May indicate "at-risk" persons (a heralding sign of risk).
Stage II	Partial-thickness loss of dermis presenting as a shallow open ulcer with a red pink wound bed, without slough. May also present as an intact or open/ruptured serum-filled blister.
	Presents as a shiny or dry shallow ulcer without slough or bruising.* This stage should not be used to describe skin tears, tape burns, perineal dermatitis, maceration, or excoriation.
Stage III	Full-thickness tissue loss. Subcutaneous fat may be visible but bone, tendon, or muscle is not exposed. Slough may be present but does not obscure the depth of tissue loss. May include undermining and tunneling.
	The depth of a stage III pressure ulcer varies by anatomical location. The bridge of the nose, ear, occiput, and malleolus do not have subcutaneous tissue, and stage III ulcers can be shallow. In contrast, areas of significant adiposity can develop extremely deep stage III pressure ulcers. Bone/tendon is not visible or directly palpable.
Stage IV	Full-thickness tissue loss with exposed bone, tendon, or muscle. Slough or eschar may be present on some parts of the wound bed. Often includes undermining and tunneling.
	The depth of a stage IV pressure ulcer varies by anatomical location. The bridge of the nose, ear, occiput, and malleolus do not have subcutaneous tissue and these ulcers can be shallow. Stage IV ulcers can extend into muscle and/or supporting structures (e.g., fascia, tendon, or joint capsule) making osteomyelitis possible. Exposed bone/tendon is visible or directly palpable.
Unstageable	Full-thickness tissue loss in which the base of the ulcer is covered by slough (yellow, tan, gray, green, or brown) and/or eschar (tan, brown, or black) in the wound bed.
	Until enough slough and/or eschar is removed to expose the base of the wound, the true depth, and therefore stage, cannot be determined. Stable (dry, adherent, intact without erythema or fluctuance) eschar on the heels serves as "the body's natural (biological) cover" and should not be removed.
Suspected deep tissue injury	Purple or maroon localized area of discolored intact skin or blood-filled blister due to damage of underlying soft tissue from pressure and/or shear. The area may be preceded by tissue that is painful, firm, mushy, boggy, warmer, or cooler as compared to adjacent tissue.
	Deep tissue injury may be difficult to detect in individuals with dark skin tones. Evolution may include a thin blister over a dark wound bed. The wound may further evolve and become covered by thin eschar. Evolution may be rapid, exposing additional layers of tissue even with optimal treatment.

Source: National Pressure Ulcer Advisory Panel (2007), http://www.npuap.org/pr2.htm. Accessed December 20, 2008.

More information on support surfaces and management of tissue loads was presented in the earlier discussion of prevention of pressure ulcers. For persons who are unable or unwilling to be repositioned at regular intervals, a low air loss mattress or alternating air support surface are appropriate. Strive to reposition the individual every 4 hours on a pressure redistribution surface but use a flexible repositioning schedule that is in accordance with the individual's preferences. Avoid positioning the patient directly on the pressure ulcer unless this is the single position of comfort for the individual. For individuals with pain on movement, premedicate 20–30 minutes prior to scheduled large position changes as this may make routine repositioning more acceptable to the patient and family. However, comfort is of primary importance and may supersede prevention and wound care for those that are actively dying or have conditions causing them to have a single position of comfort. Observe individual choices after explaining the rationale for this intervention. It is important to understand that the goal of repositioning and managing tissue loads in the palliative care patient is to ease suffering and discomfort from the wound.

Nutrition and hydration support

Because many studies have linked malnutrition with pressure ulcers, adequate nutritional support is an important part of pressure ulcer management. Prevention of malnutrition reduces the patient's risk for further tissue trauma related to pressure or impaired wound healing. As noted in the discussion of prevention, maintenance of adequate nutrition in the palliative care patient may not be possible. The palliative care pressure ulcer guidelines recommend nutrition and hydration support that is consistent with the palliative care patient's condition and wishes. This includes allowing the patient to consume foods and fluids of choice and allowing the patient to direct nutritional intake. Other recommendations include consuming multiple small meals throughout the day and offering nutritional supplements. As such, nutritional supplementation should not be provided in end-of-life cases if it increases the patient's discomfort, and the decision to provide or withhold supplementation should be agreed on by the patient, family, and caregivers.[54]

Managing the ulcer and periwound skin

Direct pressure ulcer care involves adequate debridement of necrotic material, management of bacterial colonization and infection, wound cleansing, management of odor and exudate, and selection of topical dressings.

Ulcer care: debridement

Adequate debridement of necrotic tissue is necessary for wound healing. Necrotic debris in the wound bed forms an obstacle to healing and provides a medium for bacterial growth. The patient's condition and the goals of care determine the method of debridement. Conservative methods of debridement may be more appropriate for palliative care patients who may not tolerate sharp debridement procedures. If sharp debridement is tolerated, it is important that debridement should include all necrotic tissue as well as the wound edge and debridement may need to be repeated. Conservative debridement methods, including mechanical, enzymatic, biosurgical, or autolytic techniques, may be used if there is no urgent need for drainage or removal of devitalized material from the wound. In the presence of advancing cellulitis, sepsis, or large and adherent amounts of necrotic debris, sharp debridement is most beneficial in promoting comfort and reducing wound symptoms of pain, exudate, and odor and should be performed. In palliative care, debridement is still important, because the removal of nonviable material decreases wound odor and exudate. In the case of the black eschar that forms on heels, debridement is not necessary, however frequent monitoring for signs such as erythema, drainage, odor, or bogginess of the tissues is required. If signs of erythema, drainage, odor, or bogginess appear, then debridement is advised and should be considered.

Mechanical debridement includes the use of hydrotherapy, or wound irrigation. Of these methods, wound irrigation is the most favorable for wound healing and most appropriate for palliative care. It should be noted that wet-to-dry dressings are not advised because of the time and labor involved in performing the dressing technique correctly and the high potential for pain. Hydrotherapy or whirlpool treatments may be helpful for wounds with large amounts of necrotic debris adherent to healthy tissues. In these cases, hydrotherapy helps to loosen the material from the wound bed for easier removal with sharp debridement. Patients receiving palliative care may not tolerate the movement to and from the whirlpool tank much less the sharp debridement. Wound irrigation may be performed using a pulsatile lavage device or a simple catheter and syringe.

Enzymatic debridement is performed by applying a topical agent containing an enzyme that destroys necrotic tissue. Enzymatic debridement may be an appropriate method for palliative care, because the frequency of dressing changes is usually once a day and the method is easy to use in conjunction with periodic sharp debridement by a certified wound care nurse or other healthcare professional with training in sharp debridement.

Biosurgical debridement is the application of maggots (disinfected fly larvae, *Phaenicia sericata*) to the wound typically at a density of 5–8 per cm^2.[128] Comparative controlled studies evaluating the use of maggot therapy for pressure ulcer debridement compared to standard debridement therapy reported maggot therapy to be more effective for debridement and granulation tissue formation.[128,129] However, biosurgery may not be acceptable to all patients and may not be available in all areas and there no studies specific to the palliative care population.

Autolytic debridement involves the use of moisture-retentive dressings to cover the wound and allow necrotic tissue to self-digest from enzymes normally found in wound fluid or exudate.[130] Autolytic debridement may be used in conjunction with other debridement methods such as periodic sharp debridement or wound irrigation. Again, autolytic debridement may be particularly effective for palliative care. Autolytic debridement has the added benefits of decreased frequency of dressing changes (typically every 3 to 5 days) and odor containment, so the suffering associated with dressing changes is diminished.

Ulcer care: bacterial colonization and infection

Open pressure ulcers are colonized with microorganisms. In many cases, adequate debridement of necrotic debris and wound cleansing prevent the bacterial colonization from proceeding to the point of clinical infection. These two steps alone are often sufficient to prevent wound infection in pressure ulcers, because they remove the debris that supports bacterial growth.[54,130] Prevention of infection is an important goal for the palliative care patient.

Use of prolonged silver-release topical dressings or other forms of silver-impregnated dressings should be considered for pressure ulcers deemed to be high risk for microbial colonization and infection. However, they should be discontinued when microbial burden is reduced or the ulcer begins healing.[54,130] Cadexomer iodine dressings also help control wound surface microorganisms and can reduce wound exudates, but should be avoided in individuals with thyroid disease, iodine sensitivity, or large-cavity ulcers requiring frequent dressing changes.[54] These dressings are effective against a broad range of pathogens, including methicillin-resistant *Staphylococcus aureus* (MRSA). Dressings impregnated with medical-grade honey have been shown to have antibacterial, antiinflammatory, and odor-reduction properties, and can also improve healing rates.[131]

Identification of infection can be accomplished by clinical assessment. The common method of determining clinical infection is by assessing for presence of the classical clinical signs of erythema (rubor), edema (tumor), heat (calor), pain (dolor), and purulent exudate. In chronic wounds such as pressure ulcers other signs and symptoms of wound infection include: increasing wound pain, wound breakdown including pocketing or undermining development at the base of the wound, friable granulation tissue, and foul odor.[132] Among palliative care patients with poor immune defense systems, delayed healing with friable granulation tissue were the most sensitive indicators of infection, while pain, heat, and foul odor had a high specificity for determining infection.[54]

There is some evidence to suggest that nursing assessment of wound colonization may not correlate well with actual bacterial burden identified through cultures.[130] Needle aspiration or tissue biopsy are the most accurate methods of identifying invading microorganisms but these procedures are not easily accomplished in home care settings or nursing home settings.[133] Further, these procedures may increase discomfort and suffering for the palliative care patient. If cultures are deemed essential in order to meet the goals of reducing wound pain, odor, and exudate then an alternative method involves use of surface swabs. After cleansing the wound with normal saline to remove any dressing debris, the nurse swabs a 1-cm^2 area of the wound bed with the surface swab for 5 seconds, until tissue fluid is apparent on the swab, and then sends the swab directly to the laboratory. This technique may better reflect actual microorganism invasion of the wound tissues than standard swab methods do.[133] Routine swab cultures should not be used to identify infection in most pressure ulcers. Swab cultures simply reflect the contamination on the surface of the wound and may not accurately identify the organisms causing tissue infection.

Use of topical antimicrobial solutions is not indicated for clean pressure ulcers. Indeed, most topical antimicrobial solutions are toxic to the fibroblast, which is the cell responsible for wound healing and may cause a burning sensation, adding to the patient's discomfort. Topical antiseptics, such as povidone iodine, iodophor, sodium hypochlorite (Dakin's solution), hydrogen peroxide, and acetic acid, do not *significantly* reduce the number of bacteria in wound tissue; however, they do harm the healthy wound tissues.[134] As such, these substances usually have no place in the treatment of clean pressure ulcers. In wounds with necrotic debris, antiseptic/antimicrobial solutions may be used for a short course of therapy (typically 2 weeks), to assist with decreasing surface bacteria and odor reduction, and then evaluated for further use. Within the context of palliative care, if necrosis and odor persists beyond the short course period, then continuation of antimicrobial therapy is appropriate.

Ulcer care: wound cleansing

Cleansing of a wound assists healing because it removes necrotic tissue, excess wound exudate, dressing residue, and metabolic wastes from the wound bed. Wound healing is optimized and the potential for wound infection is decreased when wound cleansing is a part of the treatment plan for pressure ulcers. Wound cleansing involves the selection of a solution for cleansing and a method of delivering the solution to the wound. Routine wound cleansing should be accomplished with minimal trauma to the wound bed. Wounds should be cleansed initially and at each dressing change. Minimal force should be applied when using gauze, sponges, or cloth to clean the wound bed. Skin cleansers and antimicrobial solutions are not indicated as solutions for cleaning pressure ulcers because they destroy the healthy wound tissues and are toxic to the fibroblast cell.[54] Normal saline is the preferred solution, because it is physiological and will not harm healing tissues. Additional alternatives include potable water and surfactant wound cleansers.

When wound irrigation is used to cleanse wounds, the irrigation pressure should fall within the range of 4 to 15 pounds per square inch (psi). Higher pressures may drive bacteria deeper into wound tissues or cause additional wound trauma. A 35-mL syringe with a 19-gauge angiocatheter delivers saline at 8 psi and is an effective method for removing bacteria from the wound bed.

Ulcer care: exudate and topical dressings

In general, moisture-retentive wound dressings are the most appropriate dressing for pressure ulcers. For palliative care, they are the dressings of choice because of the decreased frequency of required changes (typically every 3 to 5 days). The goal of the wound dressing is to provide an environment that keeps the wound bed tissue moist and the surrounding intact skin dry. Use of moist wound healing dressings supports a better rate of healing than use of dry gauze dressings[54]; more importantly in palliative care, moist wound healing dressings contain odor, absorb exudate, and minimize dressing change discomfort. Clinical judgment is needed to determine the best dressing for the wound. The appropriate dressing should keep the surrounding intact skin dry while controlling wound exudate and should provide a minimal amount of pain during dressing changes.

The clinician must be aware of the absorptive capacity and pain reduction properties of the major dressing types. In general, thin film dressings have no absorptive capacity and minimize pain by covering exposed nerve endings. Thin film dressings are adherent to the skin surrounding the wound and sometimes to the

wound itself, making dressing removal more likely to be painful. Hydrocolloids, hydrogels, and foam dressings typically have a minimal to moderate absorptive capacity. Hydrocolloid dressings are occlusive and reduce pain by preventing exposure of the wound to air. They are appropriate for clean stage 2, or shallow noninfected stage 3 pressure ulcers. They have adhesive properties and can cause pain if removed improperly. Foam dressings are moderately absorptive and nonadherent, resulting in reduced pain during dressing changes. They should be considered for exudative stage 2 and shallow stage 2 pressure ulcers, and on areas or ulcers at risk for friction/shear injuries. Hydrogel dressings are cool and soothing and are particularly effective in wounds that induce a burning sensation. Hydrogel dressings also are nonadherent, reducing wound pain during dressing changes. Calcium alginates, alginate collagen dressings, and exudate-absorbing beads, flakes, pastes, or powders absorb large amounts of drainage. Dressings with a large absorptive capacity reduce pain related to maceration of surrounding tissues and to pressure caused by the excess exudate. Calcium alginates and exudate-absorbing dressings are nonadherent and are easily removed from the wound during dressing changes. Soft silicone dressings absorb minimal amounts of drainage but are nonadherent and reduce pain associated with dressing changes.

Wounds with small or minimal amounts of exudate can benefit from a variety of dressings, including hydrocolloids, hydrogels, and thin film dressings. Wounds with moderate amounts of exudate may require dressings with a higher absorptive capacity, such as hydrocolloids, foam dressings, hydrogel sheet dressings, or composite dressings (those including a combination of products, such as a thin film with a foam island in the center). Wounds with a large amount of drainage require dressings that are capable of absorbing it, such as calcium alginates, alginate collagen combinations, or specific beads, pastes, or powders designed to handle large amounts of drainage. Wounds with significant odor benefit from dressings formulated with charcoal, such as charcoal foam and dressings with a charcoal filter overlay.

If a wound shows a significant loss of tissue or if undermining or pockets are present, the wound cavities should be loosely filled with dressing to eliminate the potential for abscess formation. Eliminating the dead space helps to prevent premature wound closure with resulting abscess formation. Dressings such as calcium alginates, impregnated hydrogel gauze strips, or wound cavity fillers are useful for eliminating the dead space. Loose filling of the undermined areas also assists with exudate management, because these wounds tend to have large amounts of exudate.

Wounds in the sacral area require additional protection from stool or urine contamination. Because dressings near the anus may be difficult to maintain, the clinician must monitor dressings in this area more frequently. Some hydrocolloid dressings have been designed with specific shapes to improve their ability to stay in place over sacral/coccygeal wounds.

Control odor

Wound odor results from bacterial overgrowth and necrotic tissue. Malodorous wounds are frequently polymicrobic with both anaerobic and aerobic microorganisms present. Anaerobes release putrescine and cadaverine, both of which have been linked to ulcer smell.[135,136] The first step to controlling odor is to eliminate the cause if possible. Thus, frequent and adequate debridement of necrotic tissue is essential for odor control. Wound cleansing decreases microorganisms on the wound surface and also is helpful in reducing odor. Odor can also arise from infection. Use of topical antimicrobials including broad spectrum topical antibiotics, metronidazole, cadexomer iodine dressings, or silver-release dressings all reduce odor by reducing bacterial burden. Topical metronidazole gel (0.77–1.0%) can be applied directly to the wound once a day for a week or more often as needed to control odor.[137] If the gel is not available, metronidazole tablets can be crushed and used topically.[138] Metronidazole acts by disrupting the DNA and protein synthesis of susceptible organisms. Wound dressings with activated charcoal can be used to reduce wound odor. Activated charcoal attracts and binds wound odor molecules. Once exudate leaks through activated charcoal dressings odor control is lost, thus these dressings are typically secondary dressings. For odorous pressure ulcers not anticipated to heal, moist dressing using povidone iodine or Dakin's solution (0.25%) can help reduce odor. Use of kitty litter, vinegar, coffee beans, or candles can help control odor in the patient's room by absorbing or filtering the odor.

Reducing wound pain

Wound pain must be managed with the same attention given to choice of wound dressings. In general, pain that is moderate to severe should be managed pharmacologically. The pressure ulcer alone may not require continuous pharmacological analgesia, but medication before procedures is essential. Lower levels of pain may be manageable with appropriate wound dressing choice and topical wound analgesia. Techniques useful for wound pain associated with procedures (e.g., debridement, dressing changes) include use of distraction (e.g., talking to the patient while performing the procedure), allowing the patient to call a "time-out" during the procedure, allowing the patient to control and participate in the procedure, providing opioids and/or nonsteroidal antiinflammatory drugs or acetaminophen 30 minutes prior to procedures and afterward, and administering topical anesthetics or topical opioids using hydrogels as a transport media. The lidocaine patch 5% (Lidoderm) blocks sodium channels and has been approved for postherpetic neuralgia.[139] It is effective for chronic neuropathic pain and can be placed along the wound edge. Another option is EMLA cream (eutectic mixture of lidocaine 2.5% and prilocaine 2.5%), which reduces debridement pain scores in persons with venous leg ulcer and might have a vasoactive effect cutaneously.[140,141] Low-dose topical morphine (diamorphine in a hydrogel vehicle) can be used topically to reduce pressure ulcer pain.[142,143]

As evidenced by this discussion, attention to multiple wound characteristics helps to determine the most appropriate wound dressing. Evaluation of wound characteristics in follow-along assessments provides the basis for changes in topical dressings. For example, a wound that is heavily exudative may be treated topically with a calcium alginate dressing for several weeks; as the amount of wound exudate decreases, the wound dressing may appear dry at dressing changes. This indicates that use of a dressing with high absorptive capacity may not be needed any longer, and the wound dressing can be changed to one with minimal to moderate absorptive capacity, such as a hydrocolloid dressing. As the wound continues to heal and wound exudate becomes minimal or nonexistent, a thin film dressing may be used to provide protection from the environment.

Patient and caregiver teaching guidelines

Patient and caregiver instruction in self-care must be individualized according to specific pressure ulcer development risk factors, individual learning styles and coping mechanisms, and the ability of the patient or caregiver to perform procedures. In teaching prevention guidelines to caregivers, it is particularly important to use return demonstration to evaluate learning. Observing the caregiver perform turning maneuvers, repositioning, managing incontinence, and providing general skin care can be enlightening and provides a context in which the clinician supports and follows up education. In palliative care, it is important to include the reasons for specific actions, such as the continuation of some level of turning and repositioning to prevent further tissue damage and lessen discomfort from additional wounds. The patient and family should be informed about pressure ulcer development at the end of life, and the information should be presented so there is understanding that not all pressure ulcers are avoidable. If a pressure ulcer develops, reminding the patient and caregiver of the care that has been provided and that the pressure ulcer is not a reflection of poor care is important to help allay caregiver's guilt.

Summary

Poorly managed pressure ulcers can increase pain and suffering in those with a chronic debilitating illness. Although preventive measures in patients identified as at risk for developing such pressure ulcers can be effective, some patients do develop pressure ulcers that require expert nursing management. Expert nursing management includes instituting preventive measures to preserve intact skin, obtaining and maintaining a clean wound, management of exudate and odor, and prevention of complications such as a superimposed wound infection. Because many dying and chronically ill debilitated patients are cared for at home, educating family members about the development of pressure ulcers and involving family caregivers in the plan of care is critical. This is especially true as many caregivers view pressure ulcers as a reflection of poor care, and, in reality, pressure ulcer development in persons at the end of life or in persons with certain comorbidities may be unavoidable even with the best care.

References

1. Tippett AW. Wounds at the end of life. Wounds. 2005;17(4):91–98.
2. Maida V, Corbo M, Dolzhykov M, Ennis M, Irani S, Trozzolo L. Wounds in advanced illness: a prevalence and incidence study based on a prospective case series. Int Wound J. 2008;5(2):305–314.
3. Galvin J. An audit of pressure ulcer incidence in a palliative care setting. Int J Palliat Nurs. 2002;8(5):214–220.
4. Henoch I, Gustafsson M. Pressure ulcers in palliative care: development of a hospice pressure ulcer risk assessment scale. Int J Palliat Nurs. 2003;9(11):474–484.
5. Bonaldi A, Parazzini F, Corli O, Lodetti L. Palliative care at home in Milan. Eur J Palliat Care. 2009;16(1):40–42.
6. Brink P, Smith TF, Linkewich B. Factors associated with pressure ulcers in palliative home care. J Palliat Med. 2006;9(6):1369–1375.
7. Reifsnyder J, Hoplamazian LM, Maxwell T. Preventing and treating pressure ulcers in hospice patients. Caring. 2004;30:30–37.
8. Reifsnyder J, Magee H. Development of pressure ulcers in patients receiving home hospice care. Wounds. 2005;17(4):74–79.
9. Thein H-H, Gomes T, Krahn MD, Wodchis WP. Health status utilities and the impact of pressure ulcers in long term care residents in Ontario. Qual Life Res. 2010;19(1):81–89.

10. Kayser-Jones J, Kris AE, Lim K, et al. Pressure ulcers among terminally ill nursing home residents. Res Gerontol Nurs. 2008;1(1): 14–24.

11. Hendrichova I, Castellie M, Mastroianni C, Piredda M, Mirabella F, Surdo L, et al. Pressure ulcers in cancer palliative care patients. Palliat Med. 2010;24(7) 669–673.

12. Masaki F, Riko K, Seiji H, Shuhei Y, Aya Y. Evaluation of pressure ulcers in 202 patients with cancer. Wounds. 2007;19(1):13–19.

13. McNees P, Meneses KD. Pressure ulcers and other chronic wounds in patients with and patients without cancer: a retrospective, comparative analysis of healing patterns. Ostomy Wound Manage. 2007;53(2):70–78.

14. Brown G. Long-term outcomes of full-thickness pressure ulcers: healing and mortality. Ostomy Wound Manage. 2003;49(10):42–50.

15. Chaplin J. Pressure sore risk assessment in palliative care. J Tissue Viability. 2000;10(1):27–31.

16. Daniel RK, Priest DL, Wheatley DC. Etiologic factors in pressure sores: an experimental model. Arch Phys Med Rehabil. 1981;62:492–498.

17. Kosiak M. Etiology and pathology of ischemic ulcers. Arch Phys Med Rehabil. 1959;40:62–69.

18. Reuler JB, Cooney TG. The pressure sore: pathophysiology and principles of management. Ann Intern Med. 1981;94:661.

19. Seiler WD, Stahelin HB. Recent findings on decubitus ulcer pathology: implications for care. Geriatrics. 1986;41:47–60.

20. Witkowski JA, Parish LC. Histopathology of the decubitus ulcer. J Am Acad Dermatol. 1982;6:1014–1021.

21. Berlowitz DR, Brienza DM. Are all pressure ulcers the result of deep tissue injury? A review of the literature. Ostomy Wound Manage. 2007;53(10):34–38.

22. Farid KJ. Applying observations from forensic science to understanding the development of pressure ulcers. Ostomy Wound Manage. 2007;53(4):26–28, 30, 32 passim.

23. Gefen A. Reswick and Rogers pressure-time curve for pressure ulcer risk. Part 2. Nurs Stand. 2009;23(46):40–44.

24. Stekelenburg A, Gawlitta D, Bader DL, Oomens CW. Deep tissue injury: how deep is our understanding? Arch Phys Med Rehabil. 2008;89(7):1410–1413.

25. Stekelenburg A, Strijkers GJ, Parusel H, Bader DL, Nicolay K, Oomens CW. Role of ischemia and deformation in the onset of compression-induced deep tissue injury: MRI-based studies in a rat model. J Applied Physiology. 2007;102(5):2002–2011.

26. Peeters EA, Oomens CW, Bouten CV, Bader DL, Baaijens FP. Mechanical and failure properties of single attached cells under compression. J Biomechanics. 2005;38(8):1685–1693.

27. Gefen A, van Nierop B, Bader DL, Oomens CW. Strain-time cell-death threshold for skeletal muscle in a tissue-engineered model system for deep tissue injury. J Biomechanics. 2008;41(9):2003–2012.

28. Linder-Ganz E, Yarnitzky G, Yizhar Z, Siev-Ner I, Gefen A. Real-time finite element monitoring of sub-dermal tissue stresses in individuals with spinal cord injury: toward prevention of pressure ulcers. Ann Biomed Eng. 2009;37(2):387–400.

29. Linder-Ganz E, Gefen A. The effects of pressure and shear on capillary closure in the microstructure of skeletal muscles. Ann Biomed Eng. 2007;35(12):2095–107.

30. Iaizzo PA. Temperature modulation of pressure ulcer formation: using a swine model. Wounds. 2004;16:336–343.

31. Salcido R, Donofrio JC, Fisher SB, et al. Histopathology of pressure ulcers as a result of sequential computer-controlled pressure sessions in a fuzzy rat model. Adv Wound Care. 1994;7:23–28.

32. Peirce SM, Skalak TC, Rodeheaver GT. Ischemia-reperfusion injury in chronic pressure ulcer formation: a skin model in the rat. Wound Rep Reg. 2000;8:68–76.

33. Houwing R, Overgoor M, Kon M, et al. Pressure-induced skin lesions in pigs: reperfusion injury and the effects of vitamin E. J Wound Care. 2000;9:36–40.

34. Miller GE, Seale J. Lymphatic clearance during compressive loading. Lymphology. 1981;14:161–166.

35. Gefen A. Risk factors for a pressure-related deep tissue injury: a theoretical model. Med Bio Eng Comput. 2007;45:563–573.

36. Shabshin N, Zoizner G, Herman A, Ougortsin V, Gefen A. Use of weight-bearing MRI for evaluating wheelchair cushions based on internal soft-tissue deformations under ischial tuberosities. J Rehabil Res Dev. 2010;47(1):31–42.

37. Lindan O, Greenway RM, Piazza JM. Pressure distributor on the surface of the human body. Arch Phys Med Rehabil. 1965;46:378.

38. Scales JT. Pressure on the patient. In: Kenedi RM, Cowden JM (eds.), Bedsore Biomechanics. London: University Park Press; 1976.

39. Parish LC, Witkowski JA, Crissey JT. The Decubitus Ulcer. New York: Masson; 1983.

40. Slater H. Pressure Ulcers in the Elderly. Pittsburgh, PA: Synapse; 1985.

41. Parish LC, Witkowski JA, Crissey JT. The Decubitus Ulcer in Clinical Practice. Berlin: Springer; 1997.

42. Landis EM. Micro-injection studies of capillary blood pressure in human skin. Heart. 1930;15:209.

43. Witkowski JA, Parish LC. The decubitus ulcer: skin failure and destructive behavior. Int J Dermatol. 2000;39(12):894–896.

44. Langemo DK, Brown G. Skin fails too: acute, chronic and end-stage skin failure. Adv Skin Wound Care. 2006;19(4):206–211.

45. Husain T. An experimental study of some pressure effects on tissues, with reference to the bedsore problem. J Pathol Bacteriol. 1953;66:347–358.

46. Salcido R, Donofrio JC, Fisher SB, LeGrand EK, Dickey K, Carney JM, et al. Histopathology of decubitus ulcers as a result of sequential pressure sessions in a computer-controlled fuzzy rat model. Adv Wound Care. 1994;7(5):40.

47. Kosiak M, Kubicek WG, Olsen ME. Evaluation of pressure as a factor in the production of ischial ulcers. Arch Phys Med Rehabil. 1958;39:623.

48. Black JM, Edsberg LE, Baharestani MM, Langemo D, Goldberg M, McNichol L, et al., National Pressure Ulcer Advisory Panel. Pressure ulcers: avoidable or unavoidable? Results of the national pressure ulcer advisory panel consensus conference. Ostomy Wound Manage. 2011;57(2):24–37.

49. Black JM, Cuddigan JE, Walko MA, Didier LA, Lander MJ, Kelpe MR. Medical device related pressure ulcers in hospitalized patients. Int Wound J. 2010;7(5):358–365.

50. Braden BJ, Bergstrom N. A conceptual schema for the study of etiology of pressure sores. Rehabil Nurs. 1987;12:8–12.

51. Bergstrom N, Demuth PJ, Braden BJ. A clinical trial of the Braden Scale for Predicting Pressure Sore Risk. Nurs Clin North Am. 1987;22:417–428.

52. Franks PJ, Winterberg H, Moffat CJ. Health-related quality of life and pressure ulceration assessment in patients treated in the community. Wound Rep Reg. 2002;10(3):133–140.

53. Allman RM, Goode PS, Patrick MM, Burst N, Bartolucci AA. Pressure ulcer risk factors among hospitalized patients with activity limitations. JAMA. 1995;273:865–870.

54. National Pressure Ulcer Advisory Panel and European Pressure Ulcer Advisory Panel. Prevention and Treatment of Pressure Ulcers: Clinical Practice Guideline. Washington, DC: National Pressure Ulcer Advisory Panel; 2009.

55. Curry K, Casady L. The relationship between extended periods of immobility and decubitus ulcer formation in the acutely spinal cord injured individual. J Neurosci Nurs. 1992;24:185–189.

56. Hammond MC, Bozzacco VA, Stiens SA, Buhrer R, Lyman P. Pressure ulcer incidence on a spinal cord injury unit. Adv Wound Care. 1994;7:57–60.

57. Reichel SM. Shearing force as a factor in decubitus ulcers in paraplegics. JAMA. 1958;166:762–763.

58. Bennett L, Kavner D, Lee BY, Trainor FS, Lewis JM. Skin stress and blood flow in sitting paraplegic patients. Arch Phys Med Rehabil. 1969;65:186–190.

59. Dinsdale SM. Decubitus ulcers: role of pressure and friction in causation. Arch Phys Med Rehabil. 1974;55:147–152.

60. Pinchcovsky-Devin G, Kaminsky MV Jr. Correlation of pressure sores and nutritional status. J Am Geriatr Soc. 1986;34:435–440.

61. Iizaka S, Okuwa M, Sugama J, Sanada H. The impact of malnutrition and nutrition-related factors on the development and severity of pressure ulcers in older patients receiving home care. Clin Nutr. 2009;29(1), 47–53.

62. Bobel LM. Nutritional implications in the patient with pressure sores. Nurs Clin North Am. 1987;22:379–390.

63. Allman RM, Laprade CA, Noel LB, Walker JM, Moorer CA, Dear MR, et al. Pressure sores among hospitalized patients. Ann Intern Med. 1986;105:337–342.

64. Lindholm, C Sterner E, Romanelli M. et al. Hip fracture and pressure ulcers—the Pan European Pressure Ulcer Study—intrinsic and extrinsic risk factors. Int Wound J. 2008;5:315–328.

65. Baumgarten M, Margolis D, Orwig D, et al. Pressure ulcers in elderly patients with hip fracture across the continuum of care. J Am Geriatr Soc. 2009;57:863–870.

66. Campbell K, Woodbury G, Labate T, LeMesurier A, Houghton P. Heel ulcer incidence following orthopedic surgery: a prospective observational study. Ostomy Wound Manage. 2010;56(8):24–31.

67. Norton D, McLaren R, Exton-Smith NA. An Investigation of Geriatric Nursing Problems in Hospitals. London: National Corporation for the Care of Old People; 1962.

68. Fromantin I, Falcou MC, Baffie A, Petot C, Mazerat R, Jaouen C, et al. Inception and validation of a pressure ulcer risk scale in oncology. J Wound Care. 2011;20(7), 328–334.

69. Norton D. Calculating the risk: Reflections on the Norton scale. Decubitus. 1989;2:24–31.

70. Braden B, Bergstrom N. Clinical utility of the Braden scale for predicting pressure sore risk. Decubitus. 1989;2:44–51.

71. Maida V, Lau F, Downing M, Yang J. Correlation between Braden Scale and Palliative Performance Scale in advanced illness. Int Wound J. 2008;5(4):585–590.

72. Morita T, Tsunoda J, Inoue S, Chihara S. Validity of the palliative performance scale from a survival perspective. J Pain Symptom Manage. 1999;18(1):2–3.

73. Virik K, Glare P. Validation of the palliative performance scale for inpatients admitted to a palliative care unit in Sydney, Australia. J Pain Symptom Manage. 2002;23(6):455–457.

74. Stechmiller JK, Cowan L, Whitney JD, et al. Guidelines for the prevention of pressure ulcers. Wound Rep Reg. 2008;16:151 168.

75. Defloor T, De Bacquer D, Grypdonck MH. The effect of various combinations of turning and pressure reducing devices on the incidence of pressure ulcers. Int J Nurs Stud. 2005;42(1):37–46.

76. Vanderwee K, Grypdonck MHF, De Bacquer D, Defloor T. Effectiveness of turning with unequal time intervals on the incidence of pressure ulcer lesions. J Adv Nurs. 2006;57(1):59–68.

77. Langemo DK, Black J, National Pressure Ulcer Advisory Panel. Pressure Ulcers in Individuals Receiving Palliative Care: A National Pressure Ulcer Advisory Panel White Paper [White Paper]. Retrieved from http://www.npuap.org/resources/white-papers/.

78. Junkin J, Gray M. Are pressure redistribution surfaces or heel protection devices effective for preventing heel pressure ulcers? J Wound Ostomy Continence Nurs. 2009;36(6):602–608.

79. National Pressure Ulcer Advisory Panel Support Surface Standards Initiative. Terms and definitions related to support surfaces. Washington, DC:National Pressure Ulcer Advisory Panel; 2007.

80. Cullum N, McInnes E, Bell-Syer SE, Legood R. Support surfaces for pressure ulcer prevention. Cochrane Database Syst Rev. 2004;(3):CD001735.

81. McInnes E, Bell-Syer SE, Dumville JC, Legood R, Cullum N. Support surfaces for pressure ulcer prevention. Cochrane Database Syst Rev. 2008;8(4):CD001735.

82. Vanderwee K, Grypdonck MH, Defloor T. Effectiveness of an alternating pressure air mattress for the prevention of pressure ulcers. Age Ageing. 2005;34(3):261–267.

83. Nixon J, Cranny G, Iglesias C, Nelson EA, Hawkins K, Phillips A, et al. Randomised, controlled trial of alternating pressure mattresses compared with alternating pressure overlays for the prevention of pressure ulcers: PRESSURE (pressure relieving support surfaces) trial. BMJ. 2006;332 (7555);1413.

84. Langer G, Schloemer G, Knerr A, Kuss O, Behrens J. Nutritional interventions for preventing and treating pressure ulcers. Cochrane Database Syst Rev. 2003;(4):CD003216.

85. Stratton RJ, Ek AC, Engfer M, et al. Enteral nutritional support in prevention and treatment of pressure ulcers: a systematic review and meta-analysis. Ageing Res Rev. 2005;4(3):422–450.

86. Bourdel-Marchasson I, Barateau M, Rondeau V, Dequae-Merchadou L, et al. A multi-center trial of the effects of oral nutritional supplementation in critically ill older inpatients. GAGE Group. Groupe Aquitain Geriatrique d'Evaluation. Nutrition. 2000;16(1):1–5.

87. Hartgrink HH, Wille J, Konig P, et al. Pressure sores and tube feeding in patients with a fracture of the hip: a randomized clinical trial. Clin Nutrition. 1998;17(6):287–292.

88. Houwing RH, Rozendaal M, Wouters-Wesseling W, et al, A randomized, double-blind assessment of the effect of nutritional supplementation on the prevention of pressure ulcers in hip-fracture patients. Clin Nutrition. 2003;22(4):401–405.

89. Chernoff RS, Milton KY, Lipschitz DA. The effect of very high-protein liquid formula on decubitus ulcers healing in long-term tube fed institutionalized patients. J Am Diet Assoc. 1990;90:A–130.

90. Breslow RA, Hallfrisch J, Guy DG, et al. The importance of dietary protein in healing pressure ulcers. J Am Geriatr Soc. 1993;41(4): 357–362.

91. Zimmerer RE, Lawson KD, Calvert CJ. The effects of wearing diapers on skin. Pediatr Dermatol. 1986;3:95–101.

92. Willis I. The effects of prolonged water exposure on human skin. J Invest Dermatol. 1973;60:166–171.

93. Gray M, Bliss DZ, Doughty DB, Emer-Seltun J, Kennedy-Evans KL, Palmer MH. Incontinence-associated dermatitis: a consensus. J Wound Ostomy Continence Nurs. 2007;34:45–54.

94. Gray M. Incontinence-related skin damage: essential knowledge. Ostomy Wound Manage. 2007;53(12):28–32.

95. Schnelle JF, Adamson GM, Cruise PA, et al. Skin disorders and moisture in incontinent nursing home residents: intervention implications. J Am Geriatr Soc. 1997;45(10):1182–1188.

96. Dinsdale JM. Decubitus ulcers: role of pressure and friction in causation. Arch Phys Med Rehabil. 1974;55:147–153.

97. Langemo DK, Brown G. Skin fails too: acute, chronic, and end-stage skin failure. Adv Skin Wound Care. 2006;19(4):206–211.

98. Sibbald RG, Krasner DL, Lutz JB, et al. The SCALE Expert Panel: Skin Changes At Life's End. Final Consensus Document. October 1, 2009.

99. Witkowski JA, Parish LC. Skin failure and the pressure ulcer. Decubitus. 1993;6(5):4.

100. Witkowski JA, Parish LC. The decubitus ulcer: skin failure and destructive behavior. Int J Dermatol. 2000;39(12):894–896.

101. Kennedy KL. The prevalence of pressure ulcers in an intermediate care facility. Decubitus. 1989;2(2):44–45.

102. Hanson D, Langemo DK, Olson B, et al. The prevalence and incidence of pressure ulcers in the hospice setting: analysis of two methodologies. Am J Hosp Palliat Care. 1991;8(5):18–22.

103. Levine J. CMS recognizes the Kennedy Terminal Ulcer in long-term care hospitals. 2013. http://www.jeffreymlevinemd.com/unavoidable-kennedy-ulcer-in-long-term-care-hospitals/. Last accessed July 10, 2013.

104. Thomas DR, Rodeheaver GT, Bartolucci AA, Franz RA, Sussman C, Ferrell BA, et al. Pressure Ulcer Scale for Healing: derivation and validation of the PUSH tool. Adv Wound Care. 1997;10:96–101.

105. Bates-Jensen BM, Vredevoe DL, Brecht ML. Validity and reliability of the Pressure Sore Status Tool. Decubitus. 1992;5:20–28.

106. Stotts NA, Rodeheaver GT, Thomas DR, Frantz RA, Bartolucci AA, Sussman CA, et al. An instrument to measure healing in pressure ulcers: development and validation of the Pressure Ulcer Scale for Healing (PUSH). J Gerontol A Biol Sci Med Sci. 2001;56(12):M795–M799.

107. Bates-Jensen B. New pressure ulcer status tool. Decubitus. 1990;3:14–15.

108. Bates-Jensen BM, McNees P. Toward an intelligent wound assessment system. Ostomy Wound Manage. 1995;41(Suppl 7A):80–87.

109. Bates-Jensen B. The Pressure Sore Status Tool: an outcome measure for pressure sores. Top Geriatr Rehabil. 1994;9:17–34.

110. Bates-Jensen BM. The Pressure Sore Status Tool a few thousand assessments later. Adv Wound Care. 1997;10:65–73.

111. Seiler WD, Stahelin HB. Identification of factors that impair wound healing: a possible approach to wound healing research. Wounds. 1995;6:101–106.

112. Sapico FL, Ginunas VJ, Thornhill-Hoynes M, Canawati HN, Capen DA, Klen NE, et al. Quantitative microbiology of pressure sores in different stages of healing. Diagn Microbiol Infect Dis. 1986;5:31–38.

113. Winter GD. Formation of the scab and the rate of reepithelialization of superficial wounds in the skin of the young domestic pig. Nature. 1965;193:293–294.

114. De Laat EH, Scholte OP, Reimer WH, van Achterberg T. Pressure ulcers: diagnostics and interventions aimed at wound-related complaints: a review of the literature. J Clin Nurs. 2005;14(4):464–472.

115. Bagdade JD, Root RK, Bulger RJ. Impaired leukocyte function in patients with poorly controlled diabetes. Diabetes. 1974;23:9–15.

116. Pecoraro RE, Ahroni JH, Boyko EJ, Stensel VL. Chronology and determinants of tissue repair in diabetic lower extremity ulcers. Diabetes. 1991;40:1305–1313.

117. Goodson WH 3rd, Hunt TK. Studies of wound healing in experimental diabetes mellitus. J Surg Res. 1977;22:221–227.

118. Yue DK, McLennan S, Marsh M, Mai YW, Spaliviero J, Delbridge L, et al. Effects of experimental diabetes, uremia, and malnutrition on wound healing. Diabetes. 1987;36:295–299.

119. Coleridge Smith PD, Thomas P, Scurr JH, Dormandy JA. Causes of venous ulceration: a new hypothesis. BMJ. 1998;296:1726–1727.

120. Falanga V. Growth factors and wound healing. Dermatol Clin. 1993;11:667–674.

121. Barbul A, Lazarou SA, Efron DT, Wasserkrug HL, Efron G. Arginine enhances wound healing and lymphocyte immune responses in humans. Surgery. 1990;108:331–336.

122. Kagan RJ, Bratescu A, Jonasson O, Matsuda T, Teodorescu M. The relationship between the percentage of circulating B cells, corticosteroid levels, and other immunologic parameters in thermally injured patients. J Trauma. 1989;29:208–213.

123. Mosiello GC, Tufaro A, Kerstein M. Wound healing and complications in the immunosuppressed patient. Wounds. 1994;6:83–87.

124. Dallam L, Smyth C, Jackson BS, et al. Pressure ulcer pain: assessment and quantification. J Wound Ostomy Continence Nurs. 1995;22(5):211–215;discussion 217–218.

125. Szor JK, Bourguignon C. Description of pressure ulcer pain at rest and at dressing change. J Wound Ostomy Continence Nurs. 1999;26(3):115–120.

126. Roth RS, Lowery JC, Hamill JB. Assessing persistent pain and its relation to affective distress, depressive symptoms, and pain catastrophizing in patients with chronic wounds: a pilot study. Am J Phys Med Rehabil. 2004;83(11):827–834.

127. Freeman K, Smyth C, Dallam L, Jackson B. Pain measurement scales: a comparison of the visual analogue and faces rating scales in measuring pressure ulcer pain. J Wound Ostomy Continence Nurs. 2001;28(6):290–296.

128. Sherman RA. Maggot versus conservative debridement therapy for the treatment of pressure ulcers. Wound Repair Regen. 2002;10(4):208–214.

129. Steenvoorde P, Jacobi CE, Oskam J. Maggot debridement therapy: free-range or contained? An in-vivo study. Adv Skin Wound Care. 2005;18(8):430–435.

130. Miller CN, Carville K, Newall N, Kapp S, Lewin G, Karimi L, et al. Assessing bacterial burden in wounds: comparing clinical observation and wound swabs. Int Wound J. 2011;8(1):45–57.

131. Gunes UY, Eser I. Effectiveness of a honey dressing for healing pressure ulcers. Ostomy Wound Manage. 2007;34(2):184–190.

132. Gardner SE, Frantz RA, Doebbeling BN. The validity of the clinical signs and symptoms used to identify localized chronic wound infection. Wound Repair Regen. 2001;9(3):178–186.

133. Stotts NA. Determination of bacterial burden in wounds. Adv Wound Care. 1995;8(4):suppl 46–52.

134. Sibbald RG, Orsted HL, Coutts PM, Keast DH. Best practice recommendations for preparing the wound bed. Update 2006. Wound Care Canada. 2006;4(1):15–29.

135. Holloway S. Recognizing and treating the causes of chronic malodor wounds. Professional Nurse. 2004;19(7):380–384.

136. Kalinski C, Schnepf M, Laboy D, Hernandez L, Nusbaum J, McGrinder B, et al. Effectiveness of a topical formulation containing metronidazole for wound odor and exudate control. Wounds. 2005;17(4):74–79.

137. Paul JC, Pieper BA. Topical metronidazole for the treatment of wound odor: a review of the literature. Ostomy Wound Manage. 2008:54(3):18–27.

138. McDonald A, Lesage P. Palliative management of pressure ulcers and malignant wounds in patients with advanced illness. J Palliat Med. 2006;9(2):285–295.

139. Argoff CE. New Analgesics for neuropathic pain: the lidocaine patch. Clin J Pain. 2000;16(2 Suppl):S62–S66.

140. Briggs M, Nelson EA. Topical agents or dressings for pain in venous leg ulcers. Cochrane Database Syst Rev. 2003;(1):CD001177.

141. Hafner HM, Thomma SR, Eichner M, Steins A, Junger M. The influence of EMLA cream on cutaneous microcirculation. Clin Hemorrheol Microcirc. 2003;28:121–128.

142. Zeppetella G, Paul J, Ribeiro M. Analgesic efficacy of morphine applied topically to painful ulcers. J Pain Symptom Manage. 2003;25:555–558.

143. Flock P. Pilot study to determine the effectiveness of diamorphine gel to control pressure ulcer pain. J Pain Symptom Manage. 2003;25:547–554.

CHAPTER 17B

Skin disorders
Malignant wounds, fistulas, and stomas

Susie Seaman and Barbara M. Bates-Jensen

The drainage and odor are so bad, I am embarrassed to go out in public, and I feel like my family does not want to be around me because of it....I don't want to be around me either.

A palliative care patient

I feel so helpless. I don't know how to help her, and I feel nauseated whenever I see or smell her wound.

A loved one

Key points

- Management of drainage, odor, bleeding, and pain are key components of palliative care for malignant wounds.
- Palliative cares for the person with an ostomy is focused on maintenance of an efficient management plan and provision for optimal functional capacity.
- It is essential to involve caregivers and family members in the plan of care.

Malignant wounds

Definition

Malignant wounds, also known in the literature as fungating tumors, tumor necrosis, ulcerative malignant wounds, or fungating malignant wounds, present both a physical and an emotional challenge for the patient, caregiver, and clinician. These wounds are frequently associated with pain, odor, bleeding, and an unsightly appearance. They may be a blow to self-esteem and may cause social isolation just when the patient needs more time with loved ones. The goals in the care of patients with malignant wounds include managing wound exudate, odor, bleeding, and pain; preventing infection; and promoting the emotional welfare of the patient and family.

Malignant cutaneous lesions occur in up to 5% of patients with cancer and 10% of patients with metastatic disease. To date, the largest study examining the incidence of cutaneous involvement of internal malignancies was performed by Lookingbill and colleagues,[1] who retrospectively reviewed data accumulated over a 10-year period from the tumor registry at Hershey Medical Center in Pennsylvania. Of 7316 patients, 367 (5.0%) had cutaneous malignancies. Of these, 38 patients had lesions as a result of direct local invasion, 337 had metastatic lesions, and 8 had both. A secondary analysis from the same registry found that 420 patients (10.4%) of 4020 with metastatic disease had cutaneous involvement.[2] In women, the most common origins of metastasis were breast carcinoma (70.7%) and melanoma (12.0%). In men, melanoma (32.3%), lung carcinoma (11.8%), and colorectal cancer (11.0%) accounted for the most common primary tumors. In a 10-year retrospective review of 677 patients with lung cancer, Ambrogi et al.[3] found that 26 (3.8%) patients had cutaneous metastasis. Mueller et al.[4] performed a meta-analysis of eight studies examining cutaneous metastasis of internal malignancies. Out of 81,618 primary visceral cancers, they identified 2369 (2.9%) cases of metastasis to the skin. Wong et al.[5] found that in 401 patients with skin metastasis cared for over a 25-year period at a single cancer center, the primary tumor sites, starting with the most common, were breast (32.7%), bronchus and lung (13.2%), skin (melanoma; 9.5%), lymph nodes (7.5%), mouth/pharynx/larynx (6.2%), blood and bone marrow (5.5%), and colorectal (4.2%). Although breast, lung, gastrointestinal tract, and melanoma account for the majority of cutaneous metastases, these lesions may arise from any type of malignant tumor.[6–9] In some cases, the tumor of origin may not be identified.[10]

Pathophysiology of malignant wounds

Malignant wounds may occur from infiltration of the skin by local invasion of a primary tumor or by metastasis from another site.[6,11] Local invasion may initially manifest as inflammation with induration, redness, heat, tenderness, or some combination of these features. The skin may have a peau d'orange appearance and may be fixed to underlying tissue. As the tumor spreads and further tissue destruction occurs, the skin eventually ulcerates.

The presentation may differ in metastatic cutaneous infiltration. Tumor cells detach from the primary site and travel via blood or lymphatic vessels, or tissue planes, to distant organs, including the skin.[8,12,13] In general, cutaneous metastasis occurs in the region of the primary tumor, most commonly on the chest, head, neck, abdomen, and groin.[6,8,9,13] These lesions may initially manifest as an erythematous rash or plaque, known as carcinoma erysipelatoides, which is due to the presence of malignant cells in the dermal lymphatics.[8] More commonly, they present as well-demarcated, painless nodules ranging in size from a few millimeters to several centimeters. Their consistency may vary from firm to rubbery. Pigmentation changes may be noted over the lesions, from deep red to brown-black. Both locally invasive and metastatic lesions may initially be misdiagnosed as rashes, plaques, cellulitis, epidermal cysts, lipomas, or other benign conditions. However, unlike many benign skin problems, these lesions will not resolve and over time may ulcerate, fungate, drain, and become very painful.

As these malignant lesions extend, changes in vascular and lymphatic flow lead to edema, exudate, and tissue necrosis.[14] The resulting lesion may be fungating, in which the tumor mass extends above the skin surface with a fungus or cauliflower-like appearance, or it may be erosive and ulcerative.[15,16] The wound bed may be pale to pink with very friable tissue, completely necrotic, or a combination of both. The surrounding skin may be erythematous, fragile, and exceedingly tender to touch. The skin may also be macerated in the presence of excessive wound exudate. The presence of necrotic tissue is an ideal culture medium for bacterial colonization, which may result in significant malodor.[17,18] The degree of pain experienced by the patient depends on wound location, depth of tissue invasion and damage, nerve involvement, and the patient's previous experience with pain and analgesia.[15]

Assessment of malignant wounds

Ongoing comprehensive assessment of the patient and malignant wound facilitates formulation of an appropriate treatment plan, allows for adjustment of the treatment plan as findings change, and promotes recognition of wound complications. Specifically, wound location, size, appearance, exudate, odor, and condition of the surrounding skin guides local therapy. Associated symptoms should be noted so that appropriate measures can be taken to provide comfort. The potential for serious complications such as hemorrhage, vessel compression or obstruction, or airway obstruction should be noted so that the caregiver can be educated regarding their palliative management. Table 17B.1 presents highlights for the assessment of malignant wounds and associated rationale.

Malignant wounds may change over time based on the aggressiveness of the cancer and whether the patient is undergoing palliative surgery, chemotherapy, or radiation. Although palliative treatment may result in regression or even disappearance of the cutaneous lesion, it may recur. Ongoing assessment allows the clinician to tailor the local wound management based on the current needs of the patient and wound.

Part of holistic assessment includes evaluation of how the patient and significant others are coping with the malignant wound and the cancer diagnosis.[19,20] How the wound affects daily life and relationships, and the availability and use of social support networks in the community should be examined.

Table 17B.1 Assessment of malignant wounds

Assessment	Rationale
Wound location	
Is mobility impaired?	Consider occupational therapy referral to facilitate activities of daily living
Located near wrinkled or flat skin?	Affects dressing selection Affects dressing fixation
Able to hide from public view?	Affects psychological coping
Wound appearance	
Size: length, width, depth, undermining, deep structure exposure	Affects dressing selection, provides information on deterioration or response to palliative treatment
Fungating or ulcerative	Affects dressing selection and fixation
Percentage of viable vs. necrotic tissue	Need for cleansing/debridement
Tissue friability and bleeding	Need for nonadherent dressings and other measures to control bleeding
Presence of odor	Need for odor-reducing strategies
Presence of fistula	Possible need for pouching
Exudate amount	Affects dressing selection
Wound colonized or clinically infected	Need for local vs. systemic care
Surrounding skin	
Erythematous	Infection or tumor extension
Fragile or denuded	Impacts dressing type and fixation
Nodular	Tumor extension/metastasis
Macerated	Need for improved exudate management
Radiation-related skin damage	Need for topical care of skin, affects dressing fixation
Symptoms	
Deep pain: aching, stabbing, continuous	Need to adjust systemic analgesia
Superficial pain: burning, stinging, may be associated only with dressing changes	Need for topical analgesia and rapid-onset, short-acting analgesics
Pruritus	Related to dressings? If not, may need systemic antipruritic medications
Potential for serious complications	
Lesion is near major blood vessels: potential for hemorrhage	Need for education of patient/family about palliative management of severe bleeding
Lesion is near major blood vessels: potential for vessel compression/obstruction	Need for education of patient/family about palliative management of severe swelling and pain, possible tissue necrosis
Lesion is near airway: potential for obstruction	Need for education of patient/family about palliative management of airway obstruction

Management of malignant wounds

The goals of care for patients with malignant wounds include control of infection and odor, management of exudate, prevention and control of bleeding, and management of pain.[11,14,15,21–24] In determining the appropriate treatment regimen, the abilities of the caregiver must also be considered. There is limited published information on treatment effectiveness, which reflects the absence of evidence-based care in this area and the significant need for further research and dissemination of findings.[25] Many articles regarding malignant wounds are based on expert opinion and the personal experience of practitioners knowledgeable in palliative and hospice care. Although research-based treatment is the gold standard of care, anecdotal reports on successful treatment of these challenging wounds are helpful to nurses striving to provide the best care for their patients.

Infection and odor control

Control of infection and odor is achieved by controlling local bacterial colonization with wound cleansing, wound debridement, and use of local antimicrobial agents.[26] Because malignant wounds are frequently associated with necrotic tissue and odor, wound cleansing is essential to remove necrotic debris, decrease bacterial counts, and thus reduce odor. If the lesion is not very friable, the patient may be able to shower. This not only provides for local cleansing but also gives the added psychological benefit of helping the patient to feel clean. The patient should be instructed to allow the shower water to hit the skin above the wound and then run over the wound. If there is friable tissue (i.e., tissue that bleeds easily with minimal trauma) or the patient is not able to shower, the nurse or caregiver should gently irrigate the wound with normal saline or a commercial wound cleanser. Skin/incontinence cleansers, which contain mild soaps and antibacterial ingredients used in bathing, can be very effective at controlling local bacterial colonization and odor. As long as they do not cause burning, they may be sprayed directly on the wound. If pain and burning occur with use of skin cleansers in the wound, they should be used only on the surrounding skin. Topical antimicrobial agents such as hydrogen peroxide, sodium hypochorite (Dakin's solution), and povidone iodine are recommended by some authors,[27] however their use should be weighed against the potential negative effects of local pain, skin irritation, wound desiccation with subsequent pain and bleeding on dressing removal, and unpleasant odor associated with Dakin's and povidone iodine. Newer antimicrobial wound cleansers containing polyhexamethylene biguanide (PHMB) may help decrease bacterial colonization while minimizing toxicity to healthy cells.[28,29] Gauze soaked with a PHMB cleanser can be applied to the wound for 15 minutes prior to new dressing application for optimal decolonization.

The necrotic tissue in malignant wounds is typically moist yellow slough. Occasionally, in the absence of exudate, there may be dry black eschar, but this is less common. Debridement is best done with the use of autolytic and/or gentle mechanical methods, as opposed to wet-to-dry dressings, which are traumatic and can cause significant bleeding and pain upon removal. Autolytic debridement, which is the natural breakdown of necrotic tissue by enzymes and white cells present in wound fluid, can be achieved with the use of dressings that support a moist wound environment,[30] but odor may be increased under occlusion and/or with the use of hydrogels. Local debridement may be performed by very gently scrubbing the necrotic areas with gauze saturated with skin or wound cleanser. Low-pressure irrigation with normal saline using a 35-mL syringe and a 19-gauge needle can be used to remove loose necrotic tissue and decrease bacterial counts. Care should be taken to avoid causing pain with either procedure. In addition, careful sharp debridement by clinicians trained in this procedure can be performed to remove loose necrotic tissue. Penetration of viable tissue should be avoided, because bleeding may be difficult to control. If necrotic tissue in the wound is extensive, surgical debridement may be indicated to promote infection control, odor reduction, and exudate management, if compatible with the palliative goals of care for the patient.

Local colonization and odor can be reduced with the use of topical antibacterial preparations. Odor is by far the most difficult management aspect of treating malignant wounds and is frequently the most distressing complaint that affected patients have. The literature supports use of topical metronidazole, which has a wide range of activity against anaerobic bacteria, to control wound odor.[31–38]

Topical therapy is available by crushing metronidazole tablets in sterile water and creating either a 0.5% solution (5 mg/mL) or a 1% solution (10 mg/mL).[31,32] This may be used as a wound irrigant, or gauze may be saturated with the solution and packed into wound cavities. Care must be taken not to allow the gauze packing to desiccate, because dressing adherence may lead to bleeding and pain.

An easy, effective alternative to metronidazole solution is metronidazole 0.75% gel, which is applied in a thin layer to the entire wound. Poteete[38] evaluated the use of metronidazole 0.75% gel in the treatment of 13 patients with malodorous wounds. Metronidazole gel was applied to the wounds daily and covered with either saline-moistened or hydrogel-saturated gauze. At the end of the 9-day observation period, no odor was detected in any wound after the dressings were removed. Finlay et al.[33] prospectively studied subjective odor and pain, appearance, and bacteriological response in 47 patients with malodorous wounds treated with daily application of metronidazole 0.75% gel. Ninety-five percent of the patients reported decreased odor at 14 days. Anaerobic colonization was discovered in 53% of patients and eliminated in 84% of these cases after treatment. Patients reported decreased pain at day 7, and both discharge and cellulitis were significantly decreased by day 14. Bale et al.[34] conducted a randomized controlled trial of the daily application of topical metronidazole gel versus placebo gel in the treatment of 41 patients with malodorous wounds, including venous, arterial, and pressure ulcers, and other types of wounds. Based of subjective ratings of odor by the patient at start of therapy and days 1, 3, and 7, metronidazole gel eliminated odor faster than placebo gel. Interestingly, whereas all the patients treated with metronidazole gel noted odor elimination, 76% of placebo gel–treated patients also noted odor elimination by the end of the study. The authors speculated that this good result in the placebo group may have been from daily wound attention and care. Kalinski et al.[35] conducted a prospective, uncontrolled trial of metronidazole 0.75% gel in 16 patients with malodorous, malignant fungating wounds. Metronidazole gel was applied to the wounds once or twice daily and covered with a nonadherent contact layer and a secondary gauze dressing. Using a subjective odor rating scale of 0–10, complete odor elimination was noted at day 1 in 10 patients, and significant improvement (> 3 units of improvement on rating scale) was noted in the other six patients. No adverse effects were seen with this regimen. Although metronidazole gel is now available generically, it may still be costly for some patients, depending on insurance coverage, or may not be available in developing countries. In these cases, making a solution from crushed tablets as mentioned previously may be the best option. Choice of dressing over metronidazole gel should be based on the amount of exudate. In low exudate wounds in which dressing adherence is a concern, the gel should be covered with a nonadherent contact layer, and then absorbent dressings such as gauze or ABD pads should be applied. In more heavily draining wounds, a nonadherent contact layer may not be necessary, and the absorbent dressings can be applied directly to the wound. For optimum odor control, dressings should be changed daily, and more often for high levels of exudate that soak through the bandage. In the United States, use of metronidazole gel is considered off-label use, but with significant support for its use in the literature, it can be considered an appropriate choice in the standard care of patients with malodorous malignant wounds.[36] Systemic use of metronidazole should only be used in patients with invasive infection, not those with local bacterial colonization.

Another topical antimicrobial agent is Iodosorb gel (Smith & Nephew), 0.9% cadexomer iodine, which is iodine complexed in a starch copolymer. This product contains slow-release iodine and has been shown to decrease bacterial counts in wounds without cytotoxicity.[39,40] Cadexomer iodine is available in a 40-g tube and is applied to the wound in a 1/8-inch layer. An advantage of this product is exudate absorption: each gram absorbs 6 mL of fluid. Disadvantages include cost (comparable to metronidazole 0.75% gel) and possible burning on application.

A PHMB-based gel is available for odor reduction. Prontosan gel (B. Braun) contains PHMB, to provide bacterial control, and betaine, a surfactant that softens and facilitates debridement of necrotic debris. It is applied in a 3- to 5-mm layer over the wound and covered with secondary dressings similar to what are used over metronidazole gel. It can also be applied to gauze packing for wounds with depth.

There are dressings that may also help decrease bacterial colonization and odor in malignant wounds.[41] Charcoal dressings, which absorb and trap odor, are available as either primary or secondary bandages. Some products trap odor under the bandage, requiring application of a perfect seal around the dressing for effectiveness. This can be a disadvantage in that adhesive will have to be applied to fragile surrounding skin. Some charcoal products are complexed with absorptive ingredients such as alginates or hydrocolloids, which help to trap the odor in the dressings. Because these dressings vary in their application and performance, package inserts should be reviewed before use.

Any dressing that decreases bacterial counts in a wound has the potential to decrease odor. Silver has broad-spectrum activity against microorganisms found in wounds.[42] Silver-based dressings are available in multiple different types including alginates, hydrocolloids, hydrogels, hydrofibers, foams, contact layers, and mesh gauze. Dressing type is chosen based on exudate level; for example, a silver-based alginate or hydrofiber might be used on a high exudating wound, whereas a silver-based contact layer and/or a silver-based hydrogel may be used on a low draining wound. Medical grade honey-based dressings and gels may also decrease wound odor as honey is naturally antibacterial.[41,43,44]

Lund-Nielsen et al.[45] compared the use of honey-coated bandages with silver coated bandages in the treatment of 69 subjects with malignant wounds. Subjects were randomized to receive either treatment, and dressing effects on wound size, cleanliness, malodor, exudate, and pain were assessed. After 4 weeks of treatment, no differences were noted between the groups regarding outcomes, but when the data was pooled for all 69 subjects, there were significant decreases in subject-rated visual analog scale scores for malodor ($P = 0.007$) and exudate level ($P < 0.0001$) from study start to study end. Although a meta-analysis by Lo et al.[46] concluded that silver dressings improve healing and reduce odor, pain, and exudate in nonmalignant chronic wounds, Cochrane reviews of the use of topical silver for both prevention and treatment of wound infections have concluded insufficient evidence to provide recommendations for practice.[47,48] A Cochrane review of honey used as a topical treatment for acute and chronic wounds resulted in the same conclusion.[49] Further research is needed on these treatments for firm conclusions to be made regarding their efficacy.

Less conventional methods of odor management are also available. Environmental deodorizers such as cat litter or charcoal briquettes can be placed under the bed to help reduce room odor for patients at home.[11] Use of peppermint oil or other aromatherapy products, applied below the nostril or near the bed may help mask the odor. Odor-eliminating room sprays are more effective than room deodorant sprays and can be used before and after wound care to reduce the odor associated with wound exposure.

Although local colonization is treated with topical cleansing, debridement, and antibacterial agents, clinical infection, as evidenced by erythema, induration, increased pain and exudate, leukocytosis, and fever, should be treated with systemic antibiotics. Cultures should be used to identify infecting organisms once the wound is diagnosed with an infection based on clinical signs; cultures should not be taken routinely to diagnose infection. Because of the local inflammatory effects of the tumor, wounds may have many of the same signs as infection, so the clinician must be discriminating in differentiating between the two. A complete blood count, assessing the white cell count and differential, may be helpful in guiding assessment and therapy. It is crucial to avoid treating patients with oral antibiotics if they are only colonized and not infected, to prevent side effects and emergence of resistant organisms.

Management of exudate

Because of the inflammation and edema commonly associated with malignant wounds, there tends to be significant exudate. Dressings should be chosen to conceal and collect exudate and odor. This is essential because a patient who experiences unexpected drainage on clothing or bedding may suffer significant feelings of distress and loss of control. Specialty dressings, such as foams, alginates, or starch copolymers, are notably more expensive than gauze pads or cotton-based absorbent pads. However, if such dressings reduce the overall cost by reducing the need for frequent dressing changes, they may be cost-effective. Table 17B.2 summarizes dressing considerations with malignant wounds. Nonadherent dressings are best utilized as the primary contact layer, because they minimize the trauma to the wound associated with dressing changes. Seaman[23] suggests using nonadherent contact layers, such as Vaseline gauze, for the primary dressing on the wound bed, and covering these with soft, absorbent dressings,

Table 17B.2 Dressing choices for malignant wounds

Type of wound and goals of care	Dressing choice
Low exudate	
Maintain moist environment Prevent dressing adherence and bleeding	Nonadherent contact layers ◆ Adaptic (Systagenix) ◆ Adaptic Touch (Systagenix) ◆ Conformant 2 (Smith & Nephew) ◆ Dermanet (DeRoyal) ◆ Mepitel One (Mölnlycke) ◆ Mepilex Transfer (Mölnlycke) ◆ Petrolatum gauze (numerous manufacturers) ◆ Restore Contact Layer (Hollister) ◆ Tegaderm Contact (3M Health Care) Amorphous hydrogels Sheet hydrogels Hydrocolloids: contraindicated with fragile surrounding skin, may increase odor Semipermeable films: contraindicated with fragile surrounding skin
High exudate	
Absorb and contain exudate Prevent dressing adherence in areas of lesion with decreased exudate	Alginates Foams Starch copolymers Gauze Soft cotton pads Menstrual pads (excessive exudate)
Malodorous wounds	
Wound cleansing (see text) Reduce or eliminate odor	Charcoal dressings Topical metronidazole (see text) Iodosorb Gel (Healthpoint): iodine-based, may cause burning Prontosan Gel (B. Braun) Honey-based dressings Silver-based dressings

such as gauze and ABD pads, for secondary dressings to contain drainage. The entire dressing should be changed once a day; the secondary dressing should be changed twice a day if drainage strikes through to the outside of the bandage. When applied over metronidazole gel, this dressing regimen is both clinically and cost effective. Many active patients may prefer to use menstrual pads as the secondary dressing, not only because of their excellent absorption, but also because the plastic backing blocks exudate and protects clothing. For patients with highly exudating wounds in which frequent bandage changes are required, an ostomy pouch may be used to contain the drainage. An appliance with a spout, such as urostomy pouch or wound management pouch, is applied to completely enclose the wound, and is changed twice a week. These devices are odor-proof as long as the seal is maintained; however, pouch deodorants may be used to decrease odor that will be noticed when the device is emptied. Partnering with a Certified

Wound, Ostomy, and Continence Nurse (CWOCN) when deciding whether to pouch a malignant wound is recommended.

Protection of the surrounding skin is another goal of exudate management. The skin around the malignant wound may be fragile secondary to previous radiation therapy, inflammation due to tumor extension, repeated use of adhesive dressings, and/or maceration. Although adhesive dressings may assist with drainage and odor control, their potential to strip the epidermis upon removal may outweigh their benefit. Using flat ostomy skin barriers on the skin surrounding the wound and then taping the dressings to the skin barriers is one method of protecting against excess drainage and skin stripping due to tape removal. The ostomy barriers are changed every 5 to 7 days. Another method of protecting the surrounding skin is to use a barrier ointment or skin sealant on the skin surrounding the ulcer. These barriers protect the fragile tissue from maceration and the irritating effects of the drainage on the skin. Avoid excessive use of skin barrier ointments though; they can actually cause or increase maceration if too much is used. Dressings can then be held in place with tape affixed to the skin barrier placed on healthy skin, flexible netting, tube dressings, sports bras, panties, briefs, snug tank tops, or tube tops. New silicone-based adhesive tapes may also be effective at keeping dressings in place while allowing for atraumatic removal.

Controlling bleeding

The viable tissue in a malignant wound may be very friable, bleeding with even minimal manipulation. Prevention is the best therapy for controlling bleeding. Prevention involves use of a gentle hand in dressing removal and thoughtful attention to the use of nonadherent dressings or moist wound dressings. On wounds with a low amount of exudate, the use of hydrogel sheets, or amorphous hydrogels under a nonadherent contact layer, may keep the wound moist and prevent dressing adherence. Even highly exudating wounds may require a nonadherent contact layer to allow for atraumatic dressing removal. If dressings adhere to the wound on attempted removal, they should be soaked away with normal saline to lessen the trauma to the wound bed. If bleeding does occur, the first intervention should be direct pressure applied for 10 to 15 minutes. Local ice packs may also assist in controlling bleeding. If pressure alone is ineffective, several other options exist.[50-52] Application of an alginate dressing or sucralfate paste (1 g sucralfate tablet crushed in 5 mL water-soluble gel) may stop mild bleeding. Gauze soaked with 1:1000 epinephrine applied to the wound may control bleeding, but can lead to local tissue necrosis. Other local vasoconstrictive agents may be used, including topical cocaine or oxymetazoline spray.[51] Small bleeding points can be controlled with silver nitrate sticks. As an alternative, use of topical, absorbable hemostatic agents made from gelatin, collagen, and/or oxidized regenerated cellulose (e.g., Gelfoam, Surgicel, Promogran) may be appropriate, but are costly. Moh's Paste, a chemical fixative applied topically to the wound, has been shown to be successful at controlling bleeding in gynecological and breast cancer tumors.[53,54] Caution must be used to avoid excessive tissue damage, periwound dermatitis, and pain associated with this treatment. More aggressive therapy may be necessary in cases of significant bleeding,[50] including transcatheter embolization of the arteries feeding the tumor[55,56] intra-arterial infusion chemotherapy, and/or radiotherapy[57,58] or surgery if compatible with palliative care goals of the patient. Oral fibrinolytic inhibitors, such as tranexamic acid or a minocaproic acid, have been used in the palliative management of cancer-associated bleeding[59] and have been used topically in patients with hemophilia.[60] If terminal hemorrhage is expected to occur, crisis medications such as midazolam should be kept ready at the bedside for immediate use if needed.[52] Clinicians should not hesitate to consider any of these options if they will improve the quality of life in patients with malignant wounds.

Pain management

Several types of pain are associated with tumor malignant wounds: deep pain, neuropathic pain, and superficial pain related to procedures.[15] Deep pain should be managed by premedication before dressing changes. Opioids for preprocedural medication may be needed, and rapid-onset, short-acting analgesics may be especially useful for those already receiving other long-acting opioid medication. For management of superficial pain related to procedures, topical lidocaine or benzocaine may be helpful.[61] These local analgesics may be applied to the wound immediately after dressing removal, with wound care delayed until adequate local anesthesia is obtained. Ice packs used before or after wound care may also be helpful to reduce pain.

Another option for topical analgesia is the use of topical opioids, which bind to peripheral opioid receptors.[61-64] Back and Finlay[65] reported on the use of diamorphine 10 mg added to an amorphous hydrogel and applied to the wounds of three patients on a daily basis. Two of the patients had painful pressure ulcers, and the third had a painful malignant ulcer. All three were receiving systemic opioid therapy. The patients noted improved pain control on the first day of treatment. Zeppetella et al.[66] demonstrated efficacy of topically applied morphine sulfate 10 mg/mL in 8 g amorphous hydrogel in the treatment of five hospice patients with painful pressure ulcers. The results of this pilot study were later validated in a larger randomized controlled study.[67] Sixteen hospice inpatients with painful pressure or malignant wounds were randomized to receive topical morphine as described above or placebo (water for injection 1 mL in 8 g amorphous hydrogel) to their wounds. After 2 days of treatment, patients entered a 2-day washout period and then were crossed over to the opposite group for two more days. Patients assigned a numerical rating score to the analgesia that they obtained in each 2-day period, the lower score indicating better pain relief. Topically applied morphine provided significantly lower scores compared to pretreatment and placebo ($P < 0.001$) and was well tolerated. Topical opioids may be a viable adjunct to systemic analgesia in the care of patients with malignant wounds.

Adjunctive therapies

Palliative care of the patient with a malignant wound may include surgical debulking of fungating masses and/or resection of new nodules, or chemotherapy, radiotherapy, hyperthermia, and/or radiofrequency ablation for tumor shrinkage and pain control.[50,68-70] Electrochemotherapy, a treatment in which the application of electric pulses to tumors facilitates penetration of topical chemotherapy, has been shown to have high efficacy at reducing or eliminating cutaneous tumors, while having minimal side effects.[71-73] Topical chemotherapy regimens can also help to shrink the tumor and thus ease local care.[74] Although these interventions will not cure patients of their advanced cancers, they may extend life, ease pain and bleeding, and improve quality of life. Patients with malignant wounds should be referred for these treatments if compatible with the palliative goals of care.

Promotion of patient and caregiver welfare through education

Dealing with a cancer diagnosis is traumatic enough without the added physical and psychological burden of a malignant wound.[75] Lo et al.[76] interviewed 10 patients with malignant fungating wounds to examine how this condition affected their lives. Central issues that negatively affected quality of life were pain, social isolation secondary to exudate and odor, and ignorance of both patients and healthcare providers regarding appropriate wound care. Piggin and Jones[77] interviewed five women with malignant fungating wounds to gain an understanding of their lived experiences. Four central themes were found: the wound was the "worst part" of having cancer, there was "an overwhelming sense of vulnerability of living within a body that cannot be trusted," they experienced "a changing relationship with family and friends" that was mainly related to unrelenting malodor and an unsightly wound, and had "a loss of identity while striving to be normal, yet feeling different." Probst et al.[78] conducted a similar study of nine women with malignant fungating wounds secondary to breast cancer. Key findings included the difficulty in dealing with the unpredictability of the wound, including odor, exudate, bleeding, and pain, and the embarrassment of having the wound, especially around family and when out in public. Similar findings have been published by other authors.[79–80] Lo et al.[81] measured quality of life in 70 subjects with malignant fungating wounds using the McGill Quality of Life (QOL) Questionnaire. Subjects had low QOL scores with their age, frequency of dressing change, pain, comfort of wound dressing, wound pain, bleeding and malodor negatively correlating with QOL at a statistically significant level. Probst et al.[78] examined the caregiver experience of tending to loved ones with these wounds. Caregivers described "shock, disgust and nausea" when providing local care and highlighted their isolation and lack of knowledge in how to care for their loved ones. The main conclusions of these studies are that the key to improving quality of life for these patients is access to a wound care team or specialist who educates patients and caregivers on how to care for the wound with appropriate dressings and how to control exudate and odor. Education must also focus on the psychosocial aspects of having a malignant wound. As noted, patients may experience grief, anxiety, embarrassment, and stigma and may withdraw from loved ones.[19] Caregivers may experience feelings of helplessness and fear about caring for the patient. The nurse can facilitate a trusting relationship with the patient and caregivers by reviewing the goals of care and by openly discussing issues that the patient may not have talked about with other providers. For example, it is helpful to acknowledge odor openly and then discuss how the odor will be managed. Attention to the cosmetic appearance of the wound with the dressing in place can assist the patient in dealing with body image disturbances. Use of soft flexible dressings that can fill a defect and protect clothing may help to restore symmetry and provide security for the patient.

Assisting the patient and the caregiver to cope with the distressing symptoms of the malignant wound such that odor and bleeding is managed, exudate is contained, and pain is alleviated will improve the quality of life for these patients and contribute to the goal of satisfactory psychological well-being. Education must include realistic goals for the wound. In these patients, the goal of complete wound healing is seldom achievable; however, quality of life can be maintained even as the wound degenerates. Continual education and reevaluation of the effectiveness of the treatment plan are essential to maintaining quality of life for those suffering from a malignant wound.

Fistulas

Definition

A fistula is an abnormal passage or opening between two or more body organs or spaces. The most frequently involved organs are the skin and either the bladder or the digestive tract, although fistulas can occur between many other body organs and/or spaces. Often, the organs involved and the location of the fistula in difficult anatomical areas or open abdominal wounds influence management

methods and complicate care. For example, fistulas involving the small bowel and the vaginal vault and those involving the esophagus and skin create extreme challenges in care related to both the location and the organs involved in the fistula. Although spontaneous closure occurs in at least 50% of all enteric or small-bowel fistulas, the time required to achieve closure is 4 to 7 weeks, so long-term treatment plans are required for all patients with fistulas. Ninety percent of those fistulas that close spontaneously do so within the 4- to 7-week time frame.[82] Therefore, if the fistula has not spontaneously closed with adequate medical treatment within 7 weeks, the goal of care may change to palliation, particularly if chances of closure are limited by other factors. Factors that inhibit fistula closure include complete disruption of bowel continuity, distal obstruction, presence of a foreign body in the fistula tract, an epithelium-lined tract contiguous with the skin, presence of cancer, previous radiation, and Crohn's disease. The presence of any of these factors can be deleterious for spontaneous closure of a fistula. The goals of management for fistula care involve containment of effluent, management of odor, comfort, and protection of the surrounding skin and tissues.

Pathophysiology of fistula development

In cancer care, those with gastrointestinal cancers and those who have received irradiation to pelvic organs are at highest risk for fistula development. Fistula development occurs in 1% of patients with advanced malignancy.[82] In most cases of advanced malignancy, the fistula develops in relation to either obstruction from the malignancy or irradiation side effects. Radiation therapy damages the vasculature and underlying structures. In cancer-related fistula development, management is almost always palliative. However, fistula development is not limited to patients with cancer.

In addition to cancer and radiation therapy, postsurgical adhesions, inflammatory bowel disease (Crohn's disease), and small-bowel obstruction place an individual at high risk for fistula development. The number one cause of fistula development is postsurgical adhesions. Adhesions are scar tissues that cause fistula development by providing an obstructive process within the normal passageway. Enterocutaneous fistulas also arise as complications in 0.8%–2% of abdominal operations.[83] The incidence of fistula development as a result of abdominal surgery has declined due to techniques of modern wound management using plastic barriers to protect exposed viscera and topical negative pressure on the soft tissues in open abdominal wounds.[83–86] Further, the use of biological dressings like human acellular dermal matrix and fibrin glue to help seal the orifice of acute fistula has helped support early fistula closure.[87–89] Unfortunately, once an enterocutaneous fistula develops, mortality remains 10%–30%.[83] Those with inflammatory bowel disease—Crohn's disease in particular—are prone to fistula development by virtue of the effects of the disease process on the bowel itself. Crohn's disease often involves the perianal area, with fissures and fistulas being common findings. Because Crohn's disease is a transmural disease, involving all layers of the bowel wall, patients are prone to fistula development. Crohn's disease can occur anywhere along the entire gastrointestinal tract, and there is no known cure. Initially, the disease is managed medically with steroids, immunotherapy, and metronidazole for perianal disease. If medical management fails, the patient may be treated with surgical creation of a colostomy, to remove the portion of bowel affected by the disease. In later stages of disease, if medical and surgical management have failed, multiple fistulas may present clinically, and the goal for care becomes living with the fistulas and palliation of symptoms.

Other factors contributing to fistula development include the presence of a foreign body next to a suture line, tension on a suture line, improper suturing technique, distal obstruction, hematoma/abscess formation, tumor or additional disease in anastomotic sites, and inadequate blood supply. Each of these can contribute to fistula formation by promoting an abnormal passage between two body organs. Typically, the contributing factor provides a tract for easier evacuation of stool or urine along the tract rather than through the normal route. Such is the case with a foreign body next to the suture line and with hematoma or abscess formation. In some cases, the normal passageway is blocked, as with tumor growth or obstructive processes. Finally, in many cases, the pathology relates to inadequate tissue perfusion, as with tension on the suture line, improper suturing, and inadequate blood supply.

Fistula assessment

Assessment of the fistula involves assessment of the source, surrounding skin, output, and fluid and electrolyte status. Evaluation of the fistula source may involve diagnostic tests such as radiographs to determine the exact structures involved in the fistula tract. Assessment of the fistula source involves evaluation of fistula output, or effluent, for odor, color, consistency, pH, and amount. These characteristics provide clues to the origin of the output. Fistulas with highly odorous output are likely to originate in the colon or may be related to cancerous lesions. Fistula output with less odor may have a small-bowel origin. The color of fistula output also provides clues to the source: clear or white output is typical of esophageal fistulas, green output is usual of fistulas originating from the gastric area, and light brown or tan output may indicate small-bowel sources. Small-bowel output is typically thin and watery to thick and pasty in consistency, whereas colonic fistulas have output with a pasty to a soft consistency. The volume of output is often an indication of the source. For small-bowel fistulas, output is typically high, with volumes ranging from 500 to 3000 mL over 24 hours, for low-output and high-output fistulas, respectively. Esophageal fistula output may be as high as 1000 mL over 24 hours. Fistulas can be classified according to output, with those producing less than 500 mL over 24 hours classified as low output and those producing greater volumes classified as high output.[82]

The anatomical orifice location, proximity of the orifice to bony prominences, the regularity and stability of the surrounding skin, the number of fistula openings, and the level at which the fistula orifice exits onto the skin influence treatment options. Fistulas may be classified according to the organs involved and the location of the opening of the fistula orifice. Fistulas with openings from one internal body organ to another (e.g., from small bowel to bladder, from bladder to vagina) are internal fistulas; those with cutaneous involvement (e.g., small bowel to skin) are external fistulas.[82]

The location of the fistula often impedes containment of output. Skin integrity should be assessed for erythema, ulceration, maceration, or denudation from fistula output. Typically, the more caustic the fistula output, the more impaired the surrounding

skin integrity. Multiple fistula tracts may also impede containment efforts.

Assessment of fluid and electrolyte balance is essential because of the risk of imbalance in both. In particular, the patient with a small-bowel fistula is at high risk for fluid volume deficit or dehydration and metabolic acidosis due to the loss of large volumes of alkaline small-bowel contents. Significant losses of sodium and potassium are common with small-bowel fistulas. Laboratory values should be monitored frequently. Evaluation for signs of fluid volume deficit is also recommended.

Fistula management

Wherever anatomically possible, the fistula should be managed with an ostomy pouching technique. The surrounding skin should be cleansed with warm water without soap or antiseptics; skin barrier paste should then be used to fill uneven skin surfaces, so that a flat surface is created to apply the pouch. Pediatric pouches are often smaller and more flexible and may be useful for hard-to-pouch areas where flexibility is needed, such as the neck for esophageal fistulas. The type of pouch should be chosen based on the output of the fistula. For example, if the fistula output is watery and thin, a pouch with a narrow spigot or tube for closure is chosen; in contrast, a fistula with a thick, pasty output would be better managed with a pouch with an open end and a closure clamp. Pouches must be emptied frequently, at least when one-third to one-half full. There are several wound drainage pouching systems on the market that allow for visualization and direct access to the fistula through a valve or door that can be opened and closed. These wound management pouches are available in large sizes and often work well for abdominal fistulas. Pouching of the fistula allows for odor control (many fistulas are quite malodorous), containment of output, and protection of the surrounding skin from damage. Gauze dressings with or without charcoal filters may be used if the output from the fistula is less than 250 mL over 24 hours and is not severely offensive in odor. Colostomy caps (small, closed-end pouches) can be useful for low-output fistulas that continue to be odorous.

There are specific pouching techniques that are useful in complex fistula management, including troughing, saddlebagging, and bridging. These techniques are particularly helpful when dealing with fistulas that occur in wounds, most commonly the small-bowel fistula that develops in the open abdominal wound. Troughing is useful for fistulas that occur in the posterior aspect of large abdominal wounds.[90] The skin surrounding the wound and fistula should be lined with a skin barrier wafer and the edge nearest the wound sealed with skin barrier paste. Then, thin film dressings are applied over the top or anterior aspect of the wound, down to the fistula orifice and the posterior aspect of the wound. Finally, a cut-to-fit ostomy pouch is used to pouch the opening in the thin film dressing at the fistula orifice. Wound exudate drains from the anterior portion of the wound (under the thin film dressing) to the posterior portion of the wound and out into the ostomy pouch, along with fistula output. The trough technique does not prevent fistula output from contaminating the wound site.

The bridging technique prevents fistula output from contaminating the wound site and allows for a unique wound dressing to be applied to the wound site. Bridging is appropriate for fistulas that occur in the posterior aspect of large abdominal wounds, where it is important to contain fistula output away from the wound site. Using small pieces of skin barrier wafers, the clinician builds a "bridge" by consecutively layering the skin barriers together until the skin barrier has the appearance of a wedge or bridge and is the same height as the depth of the wound.[82] With the use of a skin barrier paste, the skin barrier wedge is adhered to the wound bed (it does not harm the healthy tissues of the wound bed), next to the fistula opening. An ostomy pouch is then cut to fit the fistula opening, using the wedge or bridge as a portion of intact surrounding skin to adhere the pouch.[82] The anterior aspect of the wound may then be dressed with the dressing of choice.

Saddlebagging is used for multiple fistulas, if it is important to keep the output from each fistula separated and the fistula orifices are close together. Two cut-to-fit ostomy pouches (or more for more fistulas) are used. The fistula openings are cut on the back of the pouch, off-center, or as far to the side as possible, and the second pouch is cut to fit the next fistula, off-center, or as far to the other side as possible. The skin is cleansed with warm water, and skin barrier paste is applied around the orifices. Ostomy pouches are applied and, where they contact each other (down the middle), they are affixed or adhered to each other in a "saddlebag" fashion. Multiple fistulas can also be managed with one ostomy pouching system that accommodates the multiple openings. Consultation with an enterostomal therapy (ET) nurse or ostomy nurse is extremely advantageous in these cases.

Another method of managing fistulas is by a closed suction wound drainage system. Jeter and colleagues[91] described the use of a Jackson-Pratt drain and continuous low suction in fistula management. After the wound is cleansed with normal saline, the fenestrated Jackson-Pratt drain is placed in the wound, on top of a moistened gauze that has been opened up to line the wound bed (primary contact layer); a second fluffed wet gauze is placed over the drain, and the surrounding skin is prepared with a skin sealant. Next, the entire site is covered with a thin film dressing, which is crimped around the tube of the drain where it exits the wound. The tube exit site is filled with skin barrier paste, and the drain is connected to low continuous wall suction; the connection site may need to be adjusted and may require use of a small "Christmas tree" connector or device and tape to secure it. Jeter and colleagues[91] advised changing the system every 3 to 5 days. Others have used a similar setup for pharyngocutaneous fistulas.[92]

Negative pressure wound therapy (NPWT) devices present an easier method of closed suction and have also been used for fistula management.[83-85] In certain circumstances, NPWT may help to promote healing in wounds with an enteric fistula. Candidates must have a fistula that has been examined/explored, and the fistula opening must be readily visualized and accessible. The patient must be receiving nothing by mouth, on total parenteral nutrition with fistula effluent that is thin to viscous. In most cases, fistulas managed by NPWT occur in open abdominal wounds and use of NPWT assists with both fistula closure and wound healing.[83-85] Use of NPWT in open abdominal wounds with fistula formation should be used with caution, as there have been reports of new fistula formation after wound closure and an associated high mortality rate in these cases.

Pouches to contain the fistula output usually assist in containing odor as well. If odor continues to be problematic with an intact pouching system, internal body deodorants such as bismuth subgallate, charcoal compositions, or peppermint oil may be helpful.[93] Taking care to change the pouch in a well-ventilated room also helps with odor. If odor is caused by anaerobic bacteria, use of 400 mg metronidazole orally three times a day may be helpful. Management of high-output fistulas may be improved with administration of octreotide 300 mcg subcutaneously over 24 hours.[82]

Nutrition management and fluid and electrolyte maintenance are essential for adequate fistula care. Fluid and nutritional requirements may be greatly increased with fistulas, and there are difficulties with fistulas that involve the gastrointestinal system. As a general guideline, the intestinal system should be used whenever possible for nutritional support. If nutrition can bypass the fistula site, absorption and tolerance are better with use of the intestinal tract. For small-bowel fistulas, bypass of the fistula orifice is not always feasible. If the small-bowel fistula is located distally, enough of the intestinal tract may be available to adequately absorb nutrients before the fistula orifice is reached. If the fistula is located more proximally, there may not be enough intestinal tract available for nutrient absorption ahead of the fistula orifice. Many of these patients must be given intravenous hyperalimentation during the early stages of fistula management. The specific goals of fluid and electrolyte and nutritional support for fistula management must be discussed with the patient and family in view of the palliative nature of the overall care plan.

Patient and caregiver education

Patient and caregiver teaching first involves adequate assessment of the self-care ability of the patient and of the caregiver's abilities. The patient and caregiver must be taught the management method for the fistula, including pouching techniques, how to empty the pouch, odor control methods, and strategies for increasing fluid and nutritional intake. Many of the pouching techniques used to manage fistulas are complicated and may require continual surveillance by an expert such as an ET nurse or ostomy nurse.

Palliative Stoma Care

The significance of palliative care for an individual with a stoma is to improve well-being during this critical time and to attain the best quality of life possible. In regard to the stoma, palliative care and is achieved by restoring the most efficient management plan and providing optimal functional capacity. It is essential to involve the family in the plan of care and to provide care to the extent of the patient's wishes.

Management of the ostomy includes physical care as well as psychological and social care. To meet the needs of the patient and family, access to the multidisciplinary care team is crucial. This team may include the ET nurse, physicians such as the surgeon and oncologist, a nutritionist, and social service personnel. The urinary or fecal stoma can be managed (by the ET nurse) to incorporate the needs and goals of both the patient and the caregiver and to provide the highest quality of life possible.

Pathophysiology

A stoma is an artificial opening in the abdominal wall that is surgically created to allow urine or stool to be eliminated by an alternative route. The most common indications for the creation of a stoma are as follows:

1. Cancers that interfere with the normal function of the urinary or gastrointestinal system

2. Inflammatory bowel diseases such as Crohn's or ulcerative colitis

3. Congenital diseases such as Hirschsprung's disease or familial adenomatous polyposis

4. Trauma

In planning the care of an individual with a stoma, it is necessary to understand the type of ostomy that was created, including the contents that will be eliminated.

Types of diversion

The three types of diversion created with a stoma as the outlet for urine or stool are the ileoconduit (urinary output), the ileostomy (fecal output), and the colostomy (fecal output). Construction of any of these diversions requires the person to wear an external appliance to collect the output.

Ileoconduit

Since the early 1950s, the Bricker ileoconduit has been the primary method for diverting urinary flow in the absence of bladder function. This procedure involves isolation of a section of the terminal ileum. The proximal end is closed, and the distal end is brought out through an opening in the abdominal wall at a site selected before surgery. The ileal segment is sutured to the skin, creating a stoma. The ureters are implanted into the ileal segment, urine flows into the conduit, and peristalsis propels the urine out through the stoma. An external appliance is worn to collect the urine; it is emptied when the pouch is one-third to one-half full, or approximately every 4 hours.

Ileostomy

The ileostomy is created to divert stool away from the large intestine, typically using the terminal ileum. The stoma is created by bringing the distal end of the ileum through an opening surgically created in the abdominal wall and suturing it to the skin. The output is usually a soft, unformed to semiformed stool. Approximately 600 to 800 mL/day is eliminated. An external appliance is worn to collect the fecal material; it is emptied when the bag is one-third to one-half full, usually four to six times per day.

An ileostomy may be temporary or permanent. A temporary ileostomy usually is created when the colon needs time to heal or rest, such as after colon surgery or a colon obstruction. A permanent ileostomy is necessary if the entire colon, rectum, and anus has been surgically removed, such as in colorectal cancer or Crohn's disease.[93]

Colostomy

The colostomy is created proximal to the affected segment of the colon or rectum. A colostomy may be temporary or permanent. There are three sections of the colon: the ascending, transverse, and descending colon. The section of colon used to create the stoma determines in part the location and the consistency of output, which may affect the nutritional and hydration status of the individual at critical times. The ascending colon stoma usually is created on the right midquadrant of the abdomen, and the output is a semiformed stool. The transverse stoma is created in the upper quadrants and is the largest stoma created; the output is usually a semiformed to formed stool. The descending colon stoma most closely mirrors the activity of normal bowel function; it usually is located in the lower left quadrant.

The stoma is created by bringing the distal end of the colon through an opening surgically created in the abdominal wall and suturing it to the skin. An external appliance is worn to collect the fecal material; it is emptied when the bag is one-third to one-half full, usually one or two times per day. A second option for management is irrigation, to regulate the bowel. The patient is taught to instill 600 to 1000 mL of lukewarm tap water through the stoma, using a cone-shaped irrigation apparatus. This creates bowel distention, stimulating peristaltic activity and therefore elimination within 30 to 45 minutes. Repetition of this process over time induces bowel dependence on the stimulus, reducing the spillage of stool between irrigations. The elimination process after initial evacuation is suppressed for 24 to 48 hours.[94,95]

Assessment

Stoma characteristics

Viability of the stoma is assessed by its color. This should be checked regularly, especially in the early postoperative period. Normal color of the stoma is deep pink to deep red. The intestinal stomal tissue can be compared with the mucosal lining of the mouth. The stoma may bleed when rubbed because of the capillaries at the surface. Bleeding that occurs spontaneously or excessively from stoma trauma can usually be managed by the application of pressure. Bleeding that persists or that originates from the bowel requires prompt investigation, with the management plan based on the cause of the bleeding and the overall status of the individual.[94,95]

A stoma with a dusky appearance ranging from purple to black, or a necrotic appearance, indicates impairment of circulation and should be reported to the surgeon. A necrotic stoma may develop from abdominal distention that causes tension on the mesentery, from twisting of the intestine at the time of surgery, or from arterial or venous insufficiency. Necrotic tissue below the level of the fascia indicates infarction and potential intra-abdominal urine or stool leakage. Prompt recognition and surgical reexploration are necessary.

Stoma edema is normal in the early postoperative period as a result of surgical manipulation. This should not interfere with stoma functioning, but a larger opening will need to be cut in the appliance to prevent pressure or constriction of the stoma. Most stomas decrease by 4 to 6 weeks after surgery, with minor changes over 1 year. Teaching the individual to continue to measure the stoma with each change of appliance should alleviate the problem of wearing an appliance with an aperture too large for the stoma. The stoma needs only a space one-eighth of an inch in diameter to allow for expansion during peristalsis.

Stoma herniation occurs when the bowel moves through the muscle defect created at the time of stoma formation and into the subcutaneous tissue. The hernia usually reduces spontaneously when the patient lies in a supine position, as a result of decreased intra-abdominal pressure. Problems associated with the formation of a peristomal hernia are increased difficulty with ostomy pouch adherence and possible bowel strangulation and obstruction. The peristomal hernia may be managed conservatively with the use of a peristomal hernia belt to maintain a reduction of the hernia. The belt is an abdominal binder with an opening to allow for the stoma and pouch. The belt is applied with the patient in a supine position, while the hernia is reduced, creating an external pressure that maintains the bowel in a reduced position. Aggressive treatment includes surgical intervention for correction of the peristomal hernia. However, this is usually reserved for emergency situations, such as obstruction or strangulation of the bowel. Colostomy patients who irrigate should be taught to irrigate with the hernia in a reduced position, to prevent perforation of the bowel.

Stoma prolapse occurs as a result of a weakened abdominal wall caused by abdominal distention, formation of a loop stoma, or a large aperture in the abdominal wall. The prolapse is a telescoping of the intestine through the stoma. Stoma prolapse may be managed by conservative or surgical intervention. Surgical intervention is required if there is bowel ischemia, bowel obstruction, or prolapse of excessive length and unreducible segment of bowel. Conservative management includes reducing the stoma while in a supine position to decrease the intra-abdominal pressure, then applying continuous gentle pressure at the distal portion of the prolapse until the stoma returns to skin level. If the stoma is edematous, cold soaks or a hypertonic solution such as salt or sugar is applied to reduce the edema before stoma reduction is attempted. Once the stoma is reduced, a support binder is applied to prevent recurrence. In most cases, it is necessary to alter the pouching system by including a two-piece appliance and cutting the barrier size opening larger to accommodate changes in stoma size.

Retraction of the stoma below skin level can occur in the early postoperative period due to tension on the bowel or mesentery or related to breakdown at the mucocutaneous junction. Late retraction usually occurs as a result of tension on the bowel from abdominal distention, most likely as a result of intraperitoneal tumor growth or ascites. Stomal retraction is managed by modification of the pouching system—for example, by using a convex appliance to accommodate changes in skin contour. Stomas that retract below the fascia level require prompt surgical intervention.

Stenosis of the stoma can occur at the skin level or at the level of the fascia. Stenosis that interferes with normal bowel elimination requires intervention. Signs and symptoms of stenosis include change in bowel habits (e.g., decreased output, thin-caliber stools), abdominal cramping, abdominal distention, flank pain from urinary stomas, and nausea or vomiting. The stenotic area may be managed conservatively by dilatation or may require surgical intervention by local excision or laparotomy.[94,95] Many of the stoma problems discussed can occur from simple stretching and displacement of normal organs due to bulky tumors, as might occur in the end stages of some disease states.

Peristomal skin problems

Peristomal skin complications commonly include mechanical breakdown, chemical breakdown, rash, and allergic reaction. Mechanical breakdown is caused by trauma to the epidermal skin layer. This is most often related to frequent appliance changes that cause shearing or tearing to the epidermal skin. The result is denuded skin or erythematous, raw, moist, and painful skin. The use of pectin-based powder with or without a light coating of skin sealant aids in healing and protecting the skin from further damage, while allowing appliance adherence.

Chemical breakdown is caused by prolonged contact of urine or fecal effluent with the peristomal skin. Inappropriate use of adhesive skin solvents may also result in skin breakdown. The result of chemical breakdown is denudation of the peristomal skin that has been exposed to the caustic effects of the stool, urine, or adhesive solvents. Prompt recognition and management are essential. Modification of the pouching system, such as using a convex wafer instead of a flat wafer or adding protective skin products such as

a paste (or both), can be used to correct the underlying problem. Instructing patients and caregivers to thoroughly cleanse the skin with plain water after using the skin solvent can eliminate the problem of denuded skin. Treatment of denuded skin is the same as described previously.

A peristomal fungal rash can occur as a result of excessive moisture or antibiotic administration that results in overgrowth of yeast in the bowel or, at the skin level, due to perspiration under a pouch or leakage of urine or stool under the barrier. The rash is characterized as having a macular, red border with a moist, red to yellow center; it is usually pruritic. Application of antifungal powder, such as nystatin powder, to the affected areas usually produces a prompt response. Blotting the powder with skin preparation or sealant may allow the pouching system to adhere more effectively.

Allergic reactions are most often caused by the barrier and tape used for the pouching system. Erythematous vesicles and pruritus characterize the area involved. Management includes removal of the offending agent. The distribution of the reaction can usually aid in defining the allergen. It may be necessary to perform skin testing if the causative agent is not clear. Patients with sensitive skin and those who use multiple products may respond to simple pouching techniques such as using water to clean the skin, patting the skin dry, and applying the wafer and pouch without the use of skin preparations. Changing to products from a different manufacturer may also eliminate the allergen. A nonadhesive pouching system may be used temporarily for patients with severe blistering and hypersensitivity, to allow healing and prevent further peristomal skin damage. Patients with severe blistering and pruritus may also require temporary use of systemic or topical antihistamines or corticosteriods.[94,95]

Principles and products for pouching a stoma

The continuous outflow of urine or stool from the stoma requires the individual to wear an external appliance at all times. Ideally, the stoma protrudes one-half to three-fourths of an inch above the skin surface, to allow the urine or stool to drain efficiently into a pouch.[95] The objective of stoma management is to protect the peristomal skin, contain output, and control odor.

The skin around the stoma should be cleaned and thoroughly dried before the appliance is positioned over the stoma. An effective pouch should adhere for at least 3 days, although this is not always possible. If no leakage occurs, the same pouch may remain adhered to the skin for up to 10 days. It should then be changed for hygienic reasons and to observe the peristomal area. Today, there is an ever-changing supply of new appliances. Materials and design are being updated rapidly to provide the consumer with the best protection and easiest care.[96] Factors to consider when choosing a pouch include the consistency and type of effluent, the contour of the abdomen, the size and shape of the stoma, and the extent of protrusion, as a well as patient preferences.

Pouching systems are available as one-piece or two-piece systems. The one-piece system is constructed with the odor-proof pouch joined to a barrier ring that adheres to the skin. The barrier can be precut to the size of the stoma, or it can be customized with a cut-to-fit barrier. A two-piece system usually consists of an individual barrier with a flange ring and an odor-proof pouch, which attach (snap) together by matching the ring size of the barrier and pouch. The pouch barrier may be flat or convex and is chosen based on the contour of the abdomen and the extent of stoma protrusion. The colostomy pouch maybe closed-ended or open-ended with a clip for closure. Some individuals choose to

Table 17B.3 Pouch options

Type	Barrier	Odor-proof pouch
1 piece	Flat	Open end with clip (ileostomy with colostomy)
2-piece	Convex	Closed end (colostomy)
	Cut-to-fit precut	Spout opening (urostomy)

clean the pouch daily. The pouch of the one-piece system can be cleaned by instilling water into the pouch (with a syringe or turkey baster) and rinsing while preventing the water from reaching the stoma area. The pouch of the two-piece system can be cleaned daily by detaching and washing it in the sink with soap and water and drying it before reattaching it to the barrier.

The urinary pouch has a spout opening to allow for controlled emptying of the pouch. This end may also be attached to a bedside bag or bottle to collect urine. It typically holds up to 2000 mL of urine. The urinary system can be easily disassembled and cleaned with soap and water. After cleaning, a vinegar-and-water solution should be rinsed through the tubing and bag/bottle to prevent urine crystallization.

Skin barriers, skin sealants, powders such as Stomahesive powder or karaya powder, and pastes such as Stomahesive paste or karaya paste are available to protect the peristomal skin from the caustic affects of urine or stool. These products may also be used to aid in the healing of peristomal skin problems.

Belts and binders are available to assist in maintaining pouch adherence and for management of certain stoma problems.[95] Table 17B.3 presents an overview of pouching options for patients with fecal or urinary diversions.

Interventions

Prevention of complications

Stoma surgery performed as a palliative measure is not intended to provide a cure but, rather, to alleviate difficulties such as obstruction, pain, or severe incontinence. Unfortunately, at a difficult time in patients' and families' lives, the created stoma disrupts normal physical appearance, normal elimination of urine or stool, and control of elimination with, in some cases, loss of body parts and/or sexual function. The patient then has to learn to care for the stoma or allow someone else to care for them. Physically and psychologically, the patient has to come to terms with the presence of the stoma, its function, and care. This takes time and energy to cope emotionally, physically, and socially.[94,97]

Educating the patient and family regarding management issues related to ostomy care and palliation could assist in the physical and psychological adaptation to the ostomy. Additional therapies that may be required for treatment of the underlying disease or a new disease process, such as progressed or recurrent cancer, may affect the activity of the stoma or the peristomal skin. Additional therapies may include chemotherapy, radiation therapy, or analgesics for pain management.

Chemotherapy and radiation therapy may affect a fecal stoma by causing diarrhea. Associated symptoms include abdominal discomfort, larger quantities of loose or liquid stool produced per day, and potential dehydration and loss of appetite with prolonged diarrhea. The ostomy bag requires more frequent emptying, and the ostomy pouch seal needs to be monitored more closely for leakage. In addition, radiation therapy that includes the stoma in the radiation field can cause peristomal skin irritation, particularly redness and maceration. The effects on the peristomal skin may be exacerbated by leakage of urine or stool, as described earlier.[94]

Analgesic use may result in constipation and ultimately bowel obstruction. It is necessary to coadminister stool softeners or laxatives for the prevention of constipation. Irrigation of the colostomy may also assist in treating constipation. The patient and family need to be instructed regarding these measures so that they can be used to treat and prevent constipation. The patient and family need to be aware that adequate pain relief and prevention of constipation can be achieved.[94,97]

Patients may become very tired or may experience anxiety, nausea, or pain as a result of their condition and palliative management. Patients often want to remain as independent as possible but may allow assistance from family and staff. For example, the patient may want to perform the actual pouch change but allow someone else to gather and prepare the supplies. This allows for conservation of energy during part of the task to be accomplished. The patient may also choose the time of day to perform such tasks—when he or she has the most energy and maximal pain and nausea control.[96]

Nutrition and hydration

Anorexia and dehydration can be major problems for the patient with advancing disease or disease-related treatments such as chemotherapy and radiation therapy. Compromised ingestion, digestion, and absorption can have major influences on nutritional and hydration status.

Anorexia is the loss of appetite resulting from changes in gastrointestinal function, including changes in taste, changes in metabolism, psychological behaviors, and the effects of disease and treatment. Decreased oral intake and changes in metabolism, including decreased protein and fat metabolism, increased energy expenditure, and increased carbohydrate consumption, result in loss of muscle mass, loss of fat stores, and fatigue, leading to weight loss and malnutrition.[98]

Managing the underlying cause of poor nutritional and hydration status, such as controlling the cancer or disease, treating an infection, or slowing down the high-volume ileostomy output, can improve the nutritional state. However, despite effective treatment, other assistance may be necessary, such as small and more frequent meals, nutritional liquid supplements, appetite stimulants (e.g., megestrol acetate), corticosteroids, and parenteral or enteral support.[99] Foods and drinks need to be appealing to the patient. Strong odors and large-portion meals may result in appetite suppression. Promoting comfort before meals may also increase appetite; this may include administering antiemetics or analgesics, oral care, or resting for 30 minutes before mealtime.[99]

Management issues

Controlling odor, reducing gas, and preventing or managing diarrhea or constipation are management issues related to patients with a colostomy. Odor can be controlled by ensuring that the pouch seal is tight, that odor-proof pouches are used, and that a clean pouch opening is maintained. In addition, deodorants such as bismuth subgallate or chlorophyllin copper complex may be taken orally. Gas can be reduced by decreasing intake of gas-producing foods such as broccoli, cabbage, beans, and beer. Peppermint or chamomile tea may be effective in gas reduction.[94,97]

Diarrhea can be managed as in a patient with an intact rectum and anus. Diarrhea may be a result of viral illness or use of a chemotherapeutic agent. Management includes increased fluid intake, a low-fiber and low-fat diet, and administration of antidiarrhea medications such as loperamide (Imodium), bismuth subsalicylate (Pepto-Bismol), or diphenoxylate plus atropine (Lomotil) by prescription.[95,100] If the patient irrigates, it is necessary to hold irrigation until formed stools return. Constipation more commonly occurs in patients with advanced malignancies due to the affects of analgesic use, reduced activity level, and reduced dietary fiber intake. Management of constipation includes administration of laxatives such as milk of magnesia, mineral oil, or lactulose and initiation of a plan for prevention of constipation with use of stool softeners and laxatives as needed. Cleansing irrigation may be necessary for patients who normally do not irrigate. Cleansing irrigation is performed as described previously for individuals with a colostomy who irrigate for control of bowel movements.[95]

Skin protection, fluid and electrolyte maintenance, prevention of blockage, and modification of medications are management issues related to an ileostomy. Because of the high-volume liquid or loose stools, protecting the skin from this effluent is critical. Leakage of effluent can cause chemical skin breakdown and pain from the irritated skin. The ET nurse can work with the patient and family to determine the cause of the effluent leak. It may be necessary to modify the pouching system, to ensure a proper fit. The peristomal skin may need to be treated with a powder or skin sealant, or both, to aid in healing. The transit time of food and wastes through the gastrointestinal system and out through the ileostomy is rapid and potentially contributes to dehydration and fluid and electrolyte imbalance. Ensuring adequate fluid and electrolyte intake is essential and may be accomplished by ingestion of sports drinks or nutrition shakes. Patients with an ileostomy are instructed to include fiber in their diet, to bulk stools and promote absorption of nutrition and medications.

Food blockage occurs when undigested food particles or medications partially or completely obstruct the stoma outlet at the fascia level. It is necessary to instruct the patient and family about the signs of a blockage, including malodorous, high-volume liquid output or no output accompanied by abdominal cramping, distention, and/or nausea and vomiting. These symptoms should be reported as soon as they occur. Blockage is resolved by lavage or mini-irrigation performed by the physician or ET nurse. A catheter is gently inserted into the stoma until the blockage is reached, 30 to 60 mL of normal saline is instilled, and the catheter is removed to allow for the return. This process is repeated until the blockage has resolved. Patient teaching should be reinforced regarding the need to chew food well before swallowing, to prevent food blockage. Timed-release tablets and enteric-coated medications should be avoided because of inadequate or unpredictable absorption. Medications often come in various forms, including liquid, noncoated, patch, rectal suppository, and subcutaneous or intravenous administration. Choosing the most appropriate route that provides the greatest efficacy for the individual is essential. For example, a transdermal patch may be used for analgesia instead of a timed-release pain tablet. For patients who have an intact rectum that is no longer in continuity with the proximal bowel, rectal administration of medications is effective.[95]

Management issues for an individual with an ileoconduit include prevention of a urinary tract infection, stone formation, peristomal skin protection, and odor control. Each of these issues is preventable by the maintenance of dilute and acidic urine through adequate fluid intake (1800 to 2400 mL/day). Vitamin C (500 to 1000 mg/day) and citrus fruits and drinks may assist in accomplishing acidic urine. Alkaline urine can cause encrustations on the stoma and peristomal skin damage with prolonged exposure. Acetic acid soaks may be applied three or four times per day to treat the encrustations until they dissolve. Adjustments in the pouching system may be necessary to prevent leakage of urine onto the skin, and the temporary addition of powder, paste, skin sealant, or some combination of these products may be needed to aid healing of the affected skin.[95]

Case study

Wound care in a woman with breast cancer and a fungating ulcerative lesion of her chest

A 64-year-old woman was referred to the wound clinic for assessment and management of wounds on the left anterior chest wall, shoulder, upper arm, and upper abdomen. She had a history of a left modified radical mastectomy for breast cancer, followed by local radiation therapy and chemotherapy 6 years prior. About 2 years prior to being referred to the wound clinic, she developed painless nodules on the left anterior chest. Biopsy revealed a local recurrence of breast cancer. She was started on a course of chemotherapy, but despite this, the lesions spread to her upper abdomen and left shoulder and upper arm. The left anterior chest wall eventually ulcerated and drained. Her main complaints to the nurse practitioner (NP) were exudate that leaked through her clothing during the day and her nightgown at night, and odor. She said that she had stopped meeting her girlfriends for their weekly lunch because of her embarrassment over this. She shared that she was quite disgusted by the lesions and was very afraid to touch them, so she would just lightly dab them with water to clean them and would cover the chest wounds with gauze in her bra, and tape gauze over the lesions on her abdomen. The nodules on the shoulder and upper arm were not draining, and she questioned whether or not she could have these surgically removed.

Assessment revealed a 12 × 8 cm irregularly shaped ulcerative lesion on the left chest wall with fungating tissue along the wound edges that was mildly friable. There was a moderate amount of serous exudate from this wound and mild to moderate odor. Surrounding skin was thin, mildly erythematous, and fragile. There were multiple nodules, some of which were coalesced, on her upper abdomen. Some had dry crust on their surface, but no apparent exudate. There were a few isolated, nondraining nodules on her left shoulder and upper arm.

She had continuous aching, vise-like pain in the left chest wall, which she rated a 5–8 on a scale of 0–10. She only used acetaminophen for this, strongly refusing to take narcotics, stating that she did not want to get "hooked on drugs." Her husband, who accompanied her, was very concerned about his wife's uncontrolled pain, and he stated that he was available to help in any way that he could.

Goals of care included exudate and odor control, and pain management. A long discussion about palliative goals of care was undertaken. The nurse practitioner concentrated on what could be done (exudate, odor, pain control) versus what could not be offered (permanent cure). The hope for quality of life with return to her social activities (which the patient stated she desired) was promoted. The patient's fears about touching the wound were also explored. With the NP's confidence that the patient could learn how to take care of the wound, she agreed to try. The patient was instructed regarding daily care:

1. Spray wound/incontinence cleanser on ulcerative wound and on surrounding skin.

2. Stand in shower and allow water to hit the skin above the wound and rinse over it.

3. Pat area dry with clean towel or paper towels or gauze.

4. Apply thin coat (the thinness of a dime) of metronidazole gel to the ulcerative wound on the chest.

5. Cover wound edges with petrolatum-impregnated contact layer (Adaptic)

6. Cover wound area with two large ABD pads and secure with boy's-size tank top (this ended up being more comfortable than the bra). Small squares of paper tape were applied to a few areas of the ABD pad that contacted healthy skin.

7. Cover crusted abdominal lesions with ABD pad to protect from friction from clothing, and secure with paper tape.

8. No dressings were needed on the shoulder nodules, and the patient preferred not to cover them with dressings. If she had preferred coverage, soft gauze or an ABD pad could have been used.

The NP, patient, and husband had a long philosophical discussion about use of narcotics for pain management. The benefits of adequate pain management were discussed including the ability to enjoy activities, sleep better, and generally feel better. Misconceptions about opiate addiction versus dependence were cleared up and the patient agreed to try some hydrocodone with acetaminophen, 5/500, 1–2 tabs every 4 hours as needed for pain.

The NP believed that it was entirely reasonable for the patient to have the discreet nodules on the left shoulder and upper arm removed. The patient was instructed that they might or might not return. She was referred back to her surgeon, who removed them, sutured the skin together, and she healed uneventfully.

The patient returned to the wound clinic 2 weeks later for a recheck. She was in better spirits and reported a complete cessation in the odor, good control of exudate, and much better pain control. She actually had plans to meet her friends for lunch, and because she was still concerned about exudate leakage, it was suggested that she use unscented menstrual pads over the chest wound instead of the ABD pads. She was grateful that the NP had "nagged" her about the pain management and acknowledged that she was sleeping better and feeling more rested. She appeared to have more hope that she could have some good quality of life.

She was seen every month thereafter. At one point, her odor was so well controlled that she stopped the metronidazole gel and just used the skin cleanser with daily showers. This resulted in satisfactory odor control. She eventually started long-acting morphine for pain, and this led to a significant improvement in overall comfort.

The ulcer on the chest eventually eroded so that a rib was exposed. Six months after treatment started in the wound clinic, she had an episode of significant bleeding from the wound, which could not be stopped. She was sent to interventional radiology and underwent successful intra-arterial embolization of the artery feeding the tumor in her chest wall. At her next wound clinic visit, she was very afraid of further bleeding, and did complain of mild

oozing from the wound edges. She and her husband were reassured and given written and verbal instructions regarding a stepwise approach for local control of bleeding:

1. Rest in a reclined position with the chest elevated.

2. Apply local pressure with water-moistened gauze for 10–15 minutes.

3. If still bleeding, apply collagen/oxidized regenerated cellulose dressing (Promogran) to the area and hold pressure for 15 minutes.

4. If still bleeding, apply ice packs for 15–20 minutes.

5. May spot-treat bleeding areas with silver nitrate (the husband was competent to do this).

6. Contact wound clinic if these measures fail.

7. For severe bleeding, go to ER (this was compatible with the patient's wishes as she still wanted aggressive care).

Thereafter, the patient had mild episodes of bleeding but reported that she and her husband felt confident in their ability to control this with the instructions provided.

Although she did slow down in her remaining months, she remained fairly active until a week before her death, which occurred 11 months after first being seen at the wound clinic. She finally accepted hospice, and was able to die at home with her loved ones at her side. Her husband later called the NP and thanked her for helping them to cope with the wounds, stating that just knowing how to take care of them and what to expect had decreased their stress significantly and helped his wife have some quality and happiness in her last year of life.

Summary

Skin disorders are both emotionally and physically challenging for patients and caregivers. Cutaneous symptoms may be the result of disease progression (e.g., malignant wounds, fistula development), complications associated with end-stage disease or the end of life (e.g., pressure ulcers), or simple changes in function of urinary or fecal diversions. All cutaneous symptoms require attention to basic care issues, creativity in management strategies, and thoughtful attention to the psychosocial implications of cutaneous manifestations. Palliative care intervention strategies for skin disorders reflect an approach similar to those for nonpalliative care. Although the goals of care do not include curing the condition, they always include alleviating the distressing symptomology and improving quality of life. The most distressing symptoms associated with skin disorders are odor, exudate, and pain. The importance of attention to skin disorders for palliative care is related to the major effect of these conditions on the quality of life and general psychological well-being of the patient.

References

1. Lookingbill DP, Spangler N, Sexton FM. Skin involvement as the presenting sign of internal carcinoma. J Am Acad Dermatol. 1990;22:19–26.

2. Lookingbill DP, Spangler N, Helm KF. Cutaneous metastases in patients with metastatic carcinoma: a retrospective study of 4020 patients. J Am Acad Dermatol. 1993;29:228–236.

3. Ambrogi V, Nofroni I, Tonini G, Mineo TC. Skin metastasis in lung cancer: analysis of a 10-year experience. Oncol Rep. 2001;8:57–61.

4. Mueller TJ, Wu H, Greenberg RE, et al. Cutaneous metastases from genitourinary malignancies. Urology. 2004;63:1021–1026.

5. Wong CY, Helm MA, Helm TN, Zeitouni N. Patterns of skin metastases: a review of 25 years, experience at a single cancer center. Int J Dermatol. 2014;53(1):56–60.

6. El Khoury J, Khalifeh I, Kibbi AG, Abbas O. Cutaneous metastasis: clinicopathological study of 72 patients from a tertiary care center in Lebanon. 2014 53(2):147–58.

7. Nashan D, Meiss F, Braun-Falco M, Reichenberger S. Cutaneous metastases from internal malignancies. Dermatol Ther. 2010;23:567–580.

8. Alcarez I, Cerroni L, Rütten A, Kutzner H, Requena L. Cutaneous metastases from internal malignancies: a clinicopathologic and immunohistochemical review. Am J Dermatopathol. 2012;34:347–393.

9. Flores-Fernandez A. Cutaneous metastases: a study of 78 biopsies from 69 patients. Am J Dermatopathol. 2010;32:222–239.

10. Carroll MC, Fleming M, Chitambar CR, Neuburg M. Diagnosis, workup, and prognosis of cutaneous metastases of unknown primary origin. Dermatol Surg. 2002;28:533–535.

11. Bergstrom KJ. Assessment and management of fungating wounds. J Wound Ostomy Continence Nurs. 2011;38:31–37.

12. De Giorgi V, Grazzini M, Alfaioli B, et al. Cutaneous manifestations of breast carcinoma. Dermatol Ther. 2010;23:581–589.

13. Hu SC, Chen GS, Lu YW, Wu CS, Lan CC. Cutaneous metastases from different internal malignancies: a clinical and prognostic appraisal. J Eur Acad Dermatol Venereol. 2008;22:735–740.

14. Grocott P, Cowley S. The palliative management of fungating malignant wounds: generalising from multiple-case study data using a system of reasoning. Int J Nurs Stud. 2001;38:533–545.

15. Naylor W. Assessment and management of pain in fungating wounds. Br J Nurs. 2001;10(22 Suppl):S33–S36, S38, S40.

16. Nashan D, Müller ML, Braun-Falco M, et al. Cutaneous metastasis of visceral tumors: a review. J Cancer Res Clin Oncol. 2009;135:1–14.

17. Bowler PG, Davies BJ, Jones SA. Microbial involvement in chronic wound malodour. J Wound Care. 1999;8:216–218.

18. Grocott P, Gethin G, Probst S. Malignant wound management in advanced illness: new insights. Curr Opin Support Palliat Care. 2013;7:101–105.

19. Piggin C. Malodorous fungating wounds: Uncertain concepts underlying the management of social isolation. Int J Palliat Nurs. 2003;9:216–221.

20. Alexander S. Malignant fungating wounds: epidemiology, aetiology, presentation and assessment. J Wound Care. 2009;18:273–280.

21. Chrisman CA. Care of chronic wounds in palliative care and end-of-life patients. Int Wound J. 2010;7:214–235.

22. Lazalle-Ali C. Psychological and physical care of malodorous fungating wounds. Br J Nurs. 2007;16(15):S16–S24.

23. Seaman S. Management of malignant fungating wounds in advanced cancer. Semin Oncol Nurs. 2006;22:185–193.

24. Hawthorn M. Caring for a patient with a fungating malignant lesion in a hospice setting: reflecting on practice. Int J Palliat Nurs. 2010;16:70–76.

25. Adderly U, Smith R. Topical agents and dressings for fungating wounds. Cochrane Database Syst Rev. 2007;(2):CD003948.

26. Wilkins RG, Unverdorben M. Wound cleaning and wound healing: a concise review. Adv Skin Wound Care. 2013;26:160–163.

27. Alvarez OM, Kalinski C, Nusbaum J, et al. Incorporating wound healing strategies to improve palliation in patients with chronic wounds. J Palliat Med. 2007;10:1161–1189.

28. Hübner NO, Kramer A. Review on the efficacy, safety and clinical applications of polihexanide, a modern wound antiseptic. Skin Pharmacol Physiol. 2010;23(suppl 1):17–27.

29. Butcher M. PHMB: an effective antimicrobial in wound bioburden management. Br J Nurs. 2012;21(12):S16, S18–S21.

30. Powers JG, Morton LM, Phillips TJ. Dressings for chronic wounds. Dermatol Ther. 2013;26:197–206.

31. Whedon MA. Practice corner: what methods do you use to manage tumor-associated wounds? Oncol Nurs Forum. 1995;22: 987–990.

32. Gomolin IH, Brandt JL. Topical metronidazole therapy for pressure sores of geriatric patients. J Am Geriatr Soc. 1983;31:710–712.

33. Finlay IG, Bowszyc J, Ramlau C, Gwiezdzinski Z. The effect of topical 0.75% metronidazole gel on malodorous cutaneous ulcers. J Pain Symptom Manage. 1996;11:158–162.

34. Bale S, Tebble N, Price P. A topical metronidazole gel used to treat malodorous wounds. Br J Nurs. 2004;13(11):S4–S11.

35. Kalinski C, Schnepf M, Laboy D, et al. Effectiveness of a topical formulation containing metronidazole for wound odor and exudate control. Wounds. 2005;17(4):84–90.

36. Paul JC, Pieper BA. Topical metronidazole for the treatment of wound odor: a review of the literature. Ostomy Wound Manage. 2008;54(3):18–27.

37. da Costa Santos CM, de Mattos Pimenta CA, Nobre MR. A systematic review of topical treatments to control the odor of malignant fungating wounds. J Pain Symptom Manage.2010;39:1065–1076.

38. Potcctc V. Case study: eliminating odors from wounds. Decubitus. 1993;6(4):43–46.

39. Danielsen L, Cherry GW, Harding K, Rollman O. Cadexomer iodine in ulcers colonised by Pseudomonas aeruginosa. J Wound Care. 1997;6:169.

40. Schwartz JA, Lantis JC, Gendics C, Fuller AM, Payne W, Ochs D. A prospective, non comparative, multicenter study to investigate the effect of cadexomer iodine on bioburden load and other wound characteristics in diabetic foot ulcers. Int Wound J. 2012;10:193–199.

41. Hampton S. Malodorous fungating wounds: how dressings alleviate symptoms. Br J Community Nurs. 2008;13(6):S31–S32, S34, S36, S38.

42. Lo SF, Hayter M, Chang CJ, Hu WY, Lee LL. A systematic review of silver-releasing dressings in the management of infected chronic wounds. J Clin Nurs 2008;17:1973–1985.

43. Acton C, Dunwoody G. The use of medical grade honey in clinical practice. Br J Nurs. 2008;17:S38–S44.

44. Belcher J. A review of medical-grade honey in wound care. Br J Nurs. 2012;21:S4–S9.

45. Lund-Nielsen B, Adamsen L, Kolmos HJ, Rorth M, Tolver A, Gottrup F. The effect of honey-coated bandages compared with silver-coated bandages on treatment of malignant wounds—a randomized study. Wound Rep Reg. 2011;19:664–670.

46. Lo SF, Chang CJ, Hu WY, Hayter M, Chang YT. The effectiveness of silver-releasing dressings in the management of non-healing chronic wounds: a meta-analysis. J Clin Nurs. 2009;18:716–728.

47. Storm-Versloot MN, Vos CG, Ubbink DT, Vermeulen H. Topical silver for preventing wound infection. Cochrane Database Syst Rev. 2010;(3):CD006478.

48. Vermeulen H, van Hattem JM, Storm-Versloot MN, Ubbink DT. Topical silver for treating infected wounds. Cochrane Database Syst Rev. 2007;(1):CD005486.

49. Jull AB, Walker N, Deshpande S. Honey as a topical treatment for wounds. Cochrane Database Syst Rev. 2013;(2):CD005083.

50. Pereira J, Phan T. Management of bleeding in patients with advanced cancer. Oncologist. 2004;9:561–570.

51. Recka K, Montagnini M, Vitale CA. Management of bleeding associated with malignant wounds. J Palliat Med. 2012;15:952–954.

52. Harris DG, Noble SIR. Management of terminal hemorrhage in patients with advanced cancer: a systematic literature review. J Pain Symptom Manage. 2009;38:913–927.

53. Kakimoto M, Tokita H, Okamura T, Yoshino K. A chemical hemostatic technique for bleeding from malignant wounds. J Palliat Med. 2010;13:11–13.

54. Yanazume Y, Douzono H, Yanazume S, et al. Clinical usefulness of Moh's Paste for genital bleeding from the uterine cervix or vaginal stump in gynecologic cancer. J Palliat Med. 2013;16:193–197.

55. Rzewnicki I, Kordecki K, Lukasiewicz A, et al. Palliative embolization of hemorrhages in extensive head and neck tumors. Pol J Radiol. 2012;77(4):17–21.

56. Moriarty JM, Xing M, Loh CT. Particle embolization to control life-threatening hemorrhage from a fungating locally advanced breast carcinoma: a case report. J Med Case Rep. 2012;6:186–191.

57. Murakami M, Kuroda Y, Sano A, et al. Validity of local treatment including intraarterial infusion chemotherapy and radiotherapy for fungating adenocarcinoma of the breast: case report of more than 8-year survival. Am J Clin Oncol. 2001;24:388–391.

58. Huang SF, Wu RC, Chang JT, et al. Intractable bleeding from solitary mandibular metastasis of hepatocellular carcinoma. World J Gastroenterol. 2007;13:4526–4528.

59. Dean A, Tuffin P. Fibrinolytic inhibitors for cancer-associated bleeding. J Pain Symptom Manage. 1997;13(1):20–24.

60. Coetzee MJ. The use of topical crushed tranexamic acid tablets to control bleeding after dental surgery and from skin ulcers in haemophilia. Hemophilia. 2007;12:443–444.

61. Sawynok J. Topical and peripherally acting analgesics. Pharmacol Rev. 2003;55:1–20.

62. Parley P. Should topical opioid analgesics be regarded as effective and safe when applied to chronic cutaneous lesions? J Pharm Pharmacol. 2011;63:747–756.

63. LeBon B, Zeppetella G, Higginson IJ. Effectiveness of topical administration of opioids in palliative care; a systematic review. J Pain Symptom Manage. 2009;37:913–917.

64. Zeppetella G, Poraio G, Aielli F. Opioids applied topically to painful cutaneous malignant ulcers in a palliative care setting. J Opioid Manage. 2007;3(3):161–166.

65. Back IN, Finlay I. Analgesic effect of topical opioids on painful skin ulcers. J Pain Symptom Manage. 1995;10:493.

66. Zeppetella G, Paul J, Ribeiro M. Analgesic efficacy of morphine applied topically to painful ulcers. J Pain Symptom Manage. 2003; 25:555–558.

67. Zeppetella G, Ribeiro MD. Morphine in intrasite gel applied topically to painful ulcers. J Pain Symptom Manage. 2005;29:118–119.

68. vanSonnenberg E, Shankar S, Parker L, et al. Palliative radiofrequency ablation of a fungating symptomatic breast lesion. AJR Am J Roentgenol. 2005;184:S126–S128.

69. Marchal F, Brunaud L, Baxin C, et al. Radiofrequency ablation in palliative supportive care: early clinical experience. Oncol Rep. 2006;15:495–499.

70. Zagar TM, Higgins KA, Miles EF, et al. Durable palliation of breast cancer chest wall recurrence with radiation therapy, hyperthermia, and chemotherapy. Radiother Oncol. 2010;97:535–540.

71. Matthiessen LW, Johannesen HH, Hendel HW, Moss T, Kamby C Gehl J. Electrochemotherapy for large cutaneous recurrence of breast cancer: a phase II clinical trial. Acta Oncologica. 2012;51:713–721.

72. Sersa G, Cufer T, Paulin SM, Cemazar M, Snoj M. Electrochemotherapy of chest wall breast cancer recurrence. Cancer Treat Rev. 2012;38:379–386.

73. Benevento R, Santoriello A, Perna G, Canonico S. Electrochemotherapy of cutaneous metastases from breast cancer in elderly patients: a preliminary report. BMC Surgery. 2012;12(suppl 1):S6–S8.

74. Leonard R, Hardy J, van Tienhoven G, et al. Randomized, double-blind, placebo-controlled, multicenter trial of 6% miltefosine solution, a topical chemotherapy in cutaneous metastases from breast cancer. J Clin Oncol. 2001;19:4150–4159.

75. Goode ML. Psychological needs of patients when dressing a fungating wound: a literature review. J Wound Care. 2004;13:380–382.

76. Lo S, Hu W, Hayter M, Chang S, Hsu M, Wu L. Experiences of living with a malignant fungating wound: a qualitative study. J Clin Nurs. 2008;17:2699–2708.

77. Piggin C, Jones V. Malignant fungating wounds: an analysis of the lived experience. J Wound Care. 2009;18:57–64.

78. Probst S, Arber A, Faithfull S. Malignant fungating wounds—the meaning of living in an unbounded body. Eur J Oncol Nurs. 2013;17:38–45.

79. Alexander SJ. An intense and unforgettable experience: the lived experience of malignant wounds from the perspectives of patients, caregivers and nurses. Int Wound J. 2010;7:456–465.

80. Gibson S, Green J. Review of patients' experiences with fungating wounds and associated quality of life. J Wound Care. 2013;22:265–275.

81. Lo SF, Hayter M, Hu WY, Tai CY, Hsu MY, Li, YF. Symptom burden and quality of life in patients with malignant wounds. J Adv Nurs. 2012;68:1312–1321.

82. Bryant RA. Management of drain sites and fistula. In: Bryant RA (ed.), Acute and Chronic Wounds: Nursing Management. St. Louis: Mosby Year Book; 1992:248–287.

83. Wainstein DE, Fernandez E, Gonzalez D, Chara O, Berkowski D. Treatment of high-output enterocutaneous fistulas with a vacuum-compaction device: a ten-year experience. World J Surg. 2008;32(3):430–435.

84. Becker HP, Willms A, Schwab R. Small bowel fistulas and the open abdomen. Scand J Surg. 2007;96(4):263–271.

85. Goverman J, Yelon JA, Platz JJ, Singson RC, Turcinovic M. The "Fistula VAC," a technique for management of enterocutaneous fistulae arising within the open abdomen: report of 5 cases. J Trauma. 2006;60(2):428–431; discussion 431.

86. Girard S, Sideman M, Spain DA. A novel approach to the problem of intestinal fistulization arising in patients managed with open peritoneal cavities. Am J Surg. 2002;184(2):166–167.

87. Jamshidi R, Schecter WP. Biological dressings for the management of enteric fistulas in the open abdomen: a preliminary report. Arch Surg. 2007;142(8):793–796.

88. Evenson AR, Fischer JE. Current management of enterocutaneous fistula. J Gastrointest Surg. 2006;10(3):455–464.

89. Dearlove JL. Skin care management of gastrointestinal fistulas. Surg Clin North Am. 1996;76(5):1095–1109.

90. Wiltshire BL. Challenging enterocutaneous fistula: a case presentation. J Wound Ostomy Continence Nurs. 1996;23:297–301.

91. Jeter KF, Tintle TE, Chariker M. Managing draining wounds and fistula: new and established methods. In: Krasner D (ed.), Chronic Wound Care. King of Prussia, PA: Health Management Publications; 1990:240–246.

92. Harris A, Komray RR. Cost-effective management of pharyngocutaneous fistulas following laryngectomy. Ostomy Wound Manage. 1993;39:36–44.

93. McKenzie J, Gallacher M. A sweet smelling success. Nurs Times. 1989;85:48–49.

94. Doughty D. Principles of fistula and stoma management. In: Berger A, Portenoy R, Weissman D (eds.), Principles and Practice of Supportive Oncology. New York: Lippincott-Raven; 1998:285–294.

95. Erwin-Toth P, Doughty DB. Principles and procedures of stomal management. In: Hampton BG, Bryant RA (eds.), Ostomies and Continent Diversions: Nursing Management. Philadelphia: Mosby Year Book; 1992:29–94.

96. Dodd M. Self-care and patient/family teaching. In: Yarbro C, Frogge M, Goodman M (eds.), Cancer Symptom Management. Boston: Jones and Bartlett; 1999:20–32.

97. Breckman B. Rehabilitation in palliative care: stoma management. In: Doyle D, Hanks G, MacDonald N (eds.), Oxford Textbook of Palliative Medicine. New York: Oxford University Press; 1998:543–549.

98. Tait N. Anorexia–cachexia syndrome. In: Yarbro C, Frogge M, Goodman M (eds.), Cancer Symptom Management. Boston: Jones and Bartlett; 1999:183–208.

99. Bruera E. ABC of palliative care: Anorexia, cachexia, and nutrition. BMJ. 1997;315:1219–1222.

100. Martz C. Diarrhea. In: Yarbro C, Frogge M, Goodman M (eds.), Cancer Symptom Management. Boston: Jones and Bartlett; 1999:522–545.

CHAPTER 18

Pruritis, fever, and sweats

Philip J. Larkin

The itch drove me crazy. It seemed to be worse at night, particularly in my arms and legs. Nothing helped. The tablets really didn't do anything for me. My skin was sore from scratching and I would find blood on the bedsheets. It made me really miserable.

Mary, a 60-year-old woman with end-stage renal disease

Key points

- Pruritus, fever, and sweats are complex and debilitating symptoms.
- The patient's experience warrants a nursing response to care of the body.
- Comfort remains the key priority.

Responding effectively to distressing symptoms is one core task of palliative care nursing.[1] Clear links are evident between philosophical constructs of nursing and modern concepts of palliative care, for example, hope, dignity, comfort, and empathy.[2,3] This chapter offers a clear example of the way in which good nursing care complements a biomedical approach to palliative management. Pruritus, fevers, and sweats (including hot flashes) are a range of complex and often interrelated symptoms that, although not as evident as pain or constipation in the palliative care population, can be equally debilitating and distressing. From a nursing perspective, the patient's experience of these symptoms warrants a nursing response to care of the body. Efforts should be directed simultaneously toward both professional, objective management of symptoms and effective response to subjective patient experience. At its best, attention to the suffering and discomfort caused by these symptoms demonstrates what nursing intervention can truly contribute to palliative management in terms of focus toward quality of life.

In this chapter, although each of these symptoms will be addressed separately for clarity of explication, patients may experience them in combination. For example, fever and sweating are frequently linked, and treating the former may well relieve both symptoms. A structured response to assessment and treatment has mutual benefits to symptom management, regardless of the root cause. This is important in a palliative care context, since the most appropriate response may be to manage the impact of the symptom rather than attempting to investigate or treat the underlying cause. This said, the shift in palliative care from a cancer-oriented practice to one that now considers a wider range of chronic and nonmalignant disease within its spectrum means that the extent to which clinical intervention to relieve the problem is deemed appropriate may vary. As is often the case in palliative care, the requirement to balance benefit over burden means that the implications of practice need to be considered. For example, treating fever with antibiotics can bring both benefit and burden to patients at end-of-life. This debate will be examined in the context of appropriate nursing responses and the use of measures beyond the biomedical framework to alleviate the discomfort imposed by these symptoms. A case history will be used to focus the discussion around each symptom and its appropriate medical management. This will be followed by a review of the nursing response and care of the patient.

Pruritus

Case study

The impact of itch on a patient's quality of life

Mary was a 60-year-old woman with stage 5 chronic kidney disease (CKD) managed by the Renal Unit in her district hospital, supported by the palliative care team. In discussion with Mary, a decision had been taken to manage her care without dialysis. At review, among a range of symptoms, including edema, breathlessness, and nausea and vomiting, she complained of a generalized itch, which she rated at 6/10 on a linear scale of 0 = no discomfort to 10 = worst discomfort possible, notably worse at night. Itch prevented sleep, and she was unable to tolerate bedding on her body. Nursing records noted that Mary's skin had been broken by constant scratching, particularly around her lower abdomen and arms. Even when sleep occurred with night sedation, Mary would be restless in bed and scratching, which left her exhausted and frustrated.

Mary was frail with clear evidence of clinical deterioration. A histamine antagonist had been prescribed with limited effect but was supported by a nursing management regimen of skin cleansing, moisturizing, and cool bathing in the early evening, which Mary appreciated. A short course of topical corticosteroids was prescribed for areas of persistent itch across her abdomen and front of her legs and arms, but again with limited benefit. A bout of persistent nausea and vomiting associated with uremia warranted the use of a 5-HT3 antagonist, ondansatron. This was not only successful in the relief of vomiting, but also appeared to have a positive effect on the pruritus. A shift in rating scale from 8/10 to 4/10 was noted once ondansatron therapy commenced. A proposal to consider a low dose of Sertraline was under review when Mary's clinical condition worsened. Her last days were managed through consultation with the palliative care team and she died peacefully 72 hours later.

Interpreting pruritus

Pruritus has been defined as "an unpleasant sensation that elicits either a conscious or reflex desire to scratch.[4] A recent Cochrane systematic review of pharmacological interventions for pruritus in palliative care patients describes it as a pathological condition exhibited by an intense sensation of itch that triggers scratching to alleviate discomfort.[5] It is seen across both malignant and nonmalignant disease, notably in hematological cancers, cancers of the biliary tract, and hepatic and uremic disease (as in the case of Mary).[6–9] Pruritus has received increasing research interest in terms of its neurological basis, differentiation of typology, and responses to treatment.[9–12] However, it remains poorly defined and understood, particularly within a palliative care context. The Cochrane review cited above[5] reviewed 40 studies, of which only one related specifically to pruritus in patients receiving palliative care, and ideal interventions for the management of itch in this population are lacking. The evidence to explain the neurophysiology of pruritus remains weak, and therefore management is challenging, with a need for care to be targeted to individual variation. Pruritus should not be considered simply a skin disorder, but rather a systemic problem for which there are multiple causes.[13,14] Four descriptive categories have been noted, which highlight the challenge in diagnosis and management.[11] These are described as *prurioreceptive* (within the skin), *neuropathic* (damage to the afferent pathway), *neurogenic* (cerebrally induced), and *pyschogenic* (related to psychiatric disorder). As in many palliative care clinical situations, it is difficult to isolate these entirely and some degree of overlap is likely. Why scratching relieves an itch is not fully understood, but it has been postulated from the Melzak-Wall "gate theory" that scratching stimulates the large C fibers to open the "gate" and thereby inhibit the itch stimulus in the dorsal horn of the spinal cord.[15] However, where the physiological response is altered due to disease or damage, it may initiate a cycle of itching, localized histamine release, exacerbation of the itch, and further scratching, so that the symptom is unrelieved. The psychological element as both cause and consequence of pruritus should not be discounted, particularly if the patient is anxious or fearful. There would appear to be some physiological synchronicity between pruritus and pain, given the fact that similar chemical messengers excite the unmyelinated C fibers. It may be that a specific subset of these fibers responds particularly to pruritus-inducing stimuli and mediators such as histamine and prostaglandins.[16] The ability to trace the neurological pathways of histamine through the dorsal horn and into the thalamus and sensorimotor cortex would appear to confirm this as the primary mediator of itch.[17] However, other peripheral mediators have been identified, including serotonin, prostaglandin, and dopamine.[16]

Contemporary review of the neurophysiology of itch would support the view that similarities exist but would also indicate increasing understanding of the differences in neuronal pathways between pain and itch.[10] Mary's expression of the severity and impact of this symptom would not be uncommon. Sleep deprivation and broken skin from scratching are noted phenomena, and the impact of chronic unrelieved pruritus has been equated to the debilitation associated with chronic pain.[12] Its subjective nature makes it both unrelenting and unpredictable, and although scratching behavior is observable and measurable, the burden experienced by the patient is not conducive to measurement.

Nursing assessment and differential diagnosis

In considering the categories of pruritus noted above,[11] it is important to remember that it may be both localized and generalized. There is a distinction between primary or idiopathic pruritus (where no cause can be determined) and secondary pruritus (related to systemic or localized disease), and decisions on the extent of investigation of the systemic problem need to be considered.[16] General skin disorders such as eczema, psoriasis, or infestation should be ruled out, or treated as necessary, before attributing the problem to an internal cause. However, systemic etiology may be present in up to 40% of all cases.[4] Therefore, in cases of nonspecific generalized pruritus, it is important to monitor for the development of systemic disease over time. Table 18.1 lists some of the key causes of pruritus based on Bernhard's classification[17] with a specific focus on those causes seen in palliative care practice.

In Mary's case, it is important to quantify the level of discomfort imposed by itch. A thorough clinical assessment reflective of any systemic disease should include a consideration of the factors identified in Box 18.1. If appropriate in the context of palliative stage of disease, laboratory blood tests may be useful in diagnosis. At the least, a complete blood count including urea and creatinine should be considered, as well as tests to rule out endocrine or metabolic dysfunction (for example, serum glucose, thyroxine, and bilirubin levels). The patient should also be questioned sensitively about his or her personal hygiene regimen and use of specific deodorants, lotions, and bath products. Associations with food, weather, and exposure to new environments (e.g., pets, new bedding or clothes) should also be explored. In Mary's case from a nursing perspective, the presence of edema, which is not uncommon in renal disease, is an additional factor that may challenge skin integrity or lead to fluid loss and risk of infection, which need to be managed.

Pruritus and opioids

Given the link between the physiological mechanisms of pain and pruritus, it is important here to make specific mention of the relationship of opioids and itch. It is known from animal studies that generalized pruritus is a side effect of morphine, particularly when administered centrally. A reaction to morphine salts has been suggested as one reason for morphine-induced pruritus.[17] The degranulation of mast cells by opiates stimulates histamine release, and this is considered the most likely causative factor for generalized pruritus in opioid-dependent patients. There is also evidence that naltrexone is beneficial in the management of pruritus where the cause is cholestatic or uremic in origin. A reported case history of nine patients with chronic liver disease has suggested that the slow and careful intravenous administration of naloxone followed by oral naltrexone therapy can be beneficial, without risk of the opioid withdrawal phenomena commonly associated with opioid antagonists.[18] Conversely, the evidence derived from the Cochrane review[5] suggests caution is advised in its use in palliative care populations because of the perceived risk to analgesia. The complexity here is that one treatment possibility for pruritus may inhibit treatment for another, equally important symptom, pain. Therefore, careful monitoring of outcome and response is essential.

Medical management of pruritus

Due to the breadth of possible causes for pruritus, management needs to balance the response between intervention, patient

Table 18.1 Key causes of pruritus

Bernhard's classification	Overall problem	Clinical presentation
Dermatological	Generalized skin problems	Psoriasis, eczema, urticaria, scabies, pediculosis, xerosis (dry skin)
		Contact dermatitis, atopic dermatitis, allergy (e.g., nickel, bathing products)
	Medication (including hypersensitivity)	Opioids, amphetamines, acetylsalisylic acid, quinidine
	Blood dyscrasias (including hematological malignancy)	Iron deficiency anemia
		Polycythemia rubravera
		Leukemias
		Lymphomas
		Hodgkin's disease
Systemic	Organ failure	Liver failure (malignant cholestasis, primary biliary cirrhosis, hepatitis)
		Renal failure (uremia, postdialysis dermatosis)
	Endocrine and metabolic dysfunction	Diabetes mellitus
		Hyperthyroidism/hypothyroidism
		Hyperparathyroidism/hypoparathyroidism
		Zinc deficiency
	Connective tissue disorder	Systemic lupus erythematosus
		Chronic graft versus host disease
Neuropathic/Neurogenic (including neuroanatomical and neurochemical disorders)	Chronic and potentially life-limiting disease	Neuroendocrine tumors
		Paraneoplastic tumors
		Multiple sclerosis
		Stroke
		Brain injury
		Post herpes zoster infection
		Syphilis

perception of the problem, and clinical status. Centrally acting antihistamine preparations can be effective but sedating and are therefore best administered at night. Since the symptom may be exacerbated at night as Mary experienced, the sedative effect may not be a problem and might even assist the patient in getting to sleep. However, in terms of life quality, oversedation would not be an appropriate palliative care response and so would need careful monitoring and the evidence for the use of antihistamine preparations is limited.[12]

There is a wide array of medications that have been efficacious in the treatment of pruritus. The potential use of the antibiotic rifampicin has been noted in the literature. Particularly where pruritus is considered opioid-induced and not responsive to

Box 18.1 Clinical assessment of pruritus

Specific questions which may form part of a clinical assessment would include:

- Can a location for itch be specified?
- Is there presence or absence of rash?
- Is there evidence of a fungal or parasitic infection?
- Is there evidence of broken or dry skin?
- Is there bleeding or seepage of serous fluid?

antihistamine therapy, rifampicin has been shown to achieve a rapid resolution of the symptom.[5]

As seen in this case, another medication that has been demonstrated as beneficial in the treatment of pruritus is ondansatron, commonly used in the treatment of chemotherapy-induced nausea and vomiting. As a 5-HT3 serotonin antagonist, ondansatron has shown a dramatic effect in reducing itch following intravenous infusion and regular oral administration in patients with malignant cholestasis and has also been noted as effective in other patient populations.[19] Other potential choices of treatment would include topical treatments, local anesthetics and antidepressants such as mirtazapine, which has antiserotonergic effects at the 5-HT2 and 5-HT3 receptors, and offers benefits similar to those of ondansatron. Gabapentin has also been utilized to good effect, as has buprenorphine.[20–22]

Topical and systemic corticosteroids have a place in treatment, although their use may be limited because of potential side effects. Paroxetine has also been considered most effective with stronger supporting evidence for its use.[5] However, it is important to note that most of the evidence available on the treatment of pruritus is limited to clinical reports, case histories, and small-scale studies. This has been supported in the findings of the recent Cochrane review, where the quality of studies was variable, with high levels of bias reported in some studies.[8] Further research trials are needed to identify best treatment options. In the palliative context, particularly where there may be multiorgan failure, systemic treatment choices may be very limited,[4] particularly if opiate use for optimal pain control is not stabilized. Therefore, a program of nursing management is an essential component of the approach to care.

Nursing management

Regardless of cause, the patient complaint focuses on the skin, and nursing management should endeavor to provide the highest standard of skin care to supplement medical intervention. Although topical treatment alone may have minimal benefit, it may contribute to relieving the patient's discomfort. Skin cleansing is important, along with the prevention of xerosis (dry skin), which may exacerbate the pruritus. Bathing may assist hydration in the short term, but the essential need is to keep the skin moist. Emollient oils should be added to the bath near the end, as doing so at the beginning may have a drying effect. A "soak and seal" method that involves bathing, patting (not rubbing) the skin dry, and then adding an occlusive cream or moisturizer may be beneficial. The choice of skin cleanser and moisturizer should ideally be pH neutral and free from fragrance and alcohol. Soap and talcum powder should be avoided due to their drying properties. The water content of the product should be relatively low, since it may evaporate quickly.[16]

Frequent application of moisturizer and the use of soft, cool clothing, preferably cotton, should be encouraged.[16] Topical antihistamine preparations, such as an oil-based calamine lotion, may soothe excoriated and scratched skin. Cool packs, cool oatmeal baths, and loose, light bedding can be beneficial, particularly when settling the patient for sleep. An ambient room temperature (cooler rather than warmer) may be relaxing, although this is less easy to regulate if the patient is hospitalized. The patient should be advised to keep nails short, and to rub or pat rather than scratch, if at all possible. A physical examination for damage to skin or evidence of a secondary infection should be carried out regularly, and any damage or infection treated accordingly. One recently reported therapy is the "wet pajama treatment," where topical lotions are applied and then nightclothes are soaked and worn to keep the skin moist.[12] Although its benefit in a palliative care patient may be very limited, it highlights the need to seek innovative measures to relieve this distressing symptom.

Fever

Case study

Management of fever in relation to a patient's goals of care

Thomas, a 58-year-old man with advanced non-small-cell lung cancer (NSCLC) was admitted to the local district hospital at the request of his general practitioner (GP). He presented with a history of fatigue, anorexia, fever, and chills in the week prior to the GP review. On admission he appeared flushed, diaphoretic, dyspneic, and mildly confused, possibly due to dehydration. Baseline measurements indicated a body temperature of 39.6°C (103.28°F) although his family reported that this had exceeded 40.2 °C (104.36 °F) at home, which prompted the GP visit. Although his oxygen saturation level was below 90%, a subsequent chest examination and X-ray were unremarkable. Blood bacterial cultures were undertaken and Thomas commenced on a broad spectrum antibiotic therapy three times daily, as well as an antipyretic

comfort program by nursing staff with particular emphasis on increased oral fluid intake and skin care. Results of the blood culture were inconclusive as to causative organism. Thomas's condition was unresolved, and he "spiked" a further temperature of 40.1°C (104.18 °F) despite antipyretic measures. Following discussion with Thomas and his family, a short trial of intravenous antibiotics was prescribed, which was considered appropriate since Thomas was otherwise clinically stable. Following 3 days of intravenous antibiotics, later converted to oral therapy, Thomas was discharged home, where his family cared for him until his death 4 months later.

Interpreting fever

Fever is defined as a rise in body temperature exceeding 38°C (100.4°F) from the norm (37°± 1°C) (98.78°F).[23] However, the degree to which a rise in temperature denotes "fever" varies widely in the literature.[24] Raised body temperature and fever occur as a response to an elevation in a thermal set-point regulated by the anterior hypothalamus.[16] Pathogens (viruses, bacteria, or fungi) may break down to release both exogenous and endogenous pyrogens. The most commonly noted endogenous pyrogens are interleukin-1 (IL-1), interleukin-6 (IL-6), tumor necrosis factor (TNFα), and interferon (INF).[25] The neurophysiological mechanism by which the thermal set-point is raised remains unclear, although cytokines and prostaglandins are considered influential. Once the thermal set-point is raised, the hypothalamus continues to regulate body temperature, albeit around a higher set-point.

Table 18.2 outlines the many and varied causes of fever, most of which have direct relevance for palliative care patients. Notably, patients with advanced dementia may have fever as a common

Table 18.2 Key causes of fever

Causative factors	Causative agent
Infection	Bacteria, fungi, viruses, parasites, tuberculosis, hepatitis, endocarditis, contaminated food, HIV-AIDS
Inflammation	Trauma, surgery, splenectomy heat, ulcerative colitis, pulmonary embolism, radiation, gastrointestinal bleeding
Cancer treatment	Chemotherapeutic agents, blood products, immunosuppression, neutropenia, external devices for venous access, catheters
Tumors	Hodgkin's and non-Hodgkin's lymphoma, leukemia, carcinoma of the liver, lung and genitourinary systems, adrenal cancer, Ewing's sarcoma, renal disease, tumors affecting the thermoregulatory system of the brain
Autoimmune disease	Rheumatoid arthritis, connective tissue disorder, anaphylaxis, polymyalgia
Neurological disorder	Spinal/brain injury or infection, stroke
Environmental	Allergens
Other	Constipation, dehydration, medication

symptom of their end-of-life stage of illness. Further, older people may exhibit an altered febrile response, which makes the assessment of body temperature a limited diagnostic tool.[25]

The particular problems of fever in hematological conditions as part of a spectrum of symptoms (fever, infection, anemia, and bleeding) has prompted a call for greater integration with palliative care services.[26]

The presentation of fever often manifests in three stages.[16] These have been described as chill, fever, and flush.[25] In the chill phase, the body attempts to respond to the raised thermal set-point by vasoconstriction of the skin to prevent heat loss and muscle contraction to generate heat. This results in shivering and, in marked cases, rigors. The second phase is dominated by a sensation of warmth, flushed skin, lethargy, weakness, and possibly dehydration, delirium, and/or seizure. This occurs as the core body temperature rises to the new set-point. During fever, the basal metabolic rate is increased to meet new tissue and oxygenation requirements by up to 13% per 1°C increase.[16] In the third and final phase, the core temperature attempts to normalize with the new set-point through vasodilatation and sweating (diaphoresis). For the palliative care population, and particularly those with a cancer diagnosis that has led to episodes of neutropenia, infection and fever are not uncommon. As the patient becomes increasingly immunosuppressed, attack by pyrogens may lead to overwhelming sepsis and death if left untreated.[16] Recent review of approaches to febrile neutropenia (FN) would argue that risk stratification tools such as the MASCC Index (assessing high or low complication risk to determine treatment options) should be utilized.[27,28] In Thomas's case, it may have been an option to treat at home if the risk of hospitalization was perceived to be greater in terms of sepsis. Although there are challenges in terms of the sensitivity of risk stratification tools, there is evidence that outpatient treatment even with intravenous therapy and early discharge in cases of hospitalization lead to higher health outcomes.[29,30] As always in palliative care, the justification for aggressive intervention needs to be considered in relation to the patient's overall health status. The use of blood transfusions in palliative care is a debate in itself, but the risk of hemolytic reaction and associated fever is possible. Therefore, for many reasons, its benefit should be carefully evaluated. Given that bacterial infection can account for up to 90% of fevers,[16] anything that might introduce infection through damaged skin integrity (such as venous access and urinary catheters) also warrants judicious use and scrupulous aseptic practice. Medications may also trigger a febrile response, most commonly penicillins, cephalosporins, antifungals (e.g., amphotericin) and, of course, chemotherapy agents (e.g., bleomycin).[24,30] A recent case study has also shown that PCP (pneumocystis pneumonae), commonly associated with HIV/AIDS, is increasingly prevalent in non-HIV+ populations and often overlooked in terms of a causative factor, even though it has a noted prevalence in the cancer population.[31]

Nursing assessment and differential diagnosis

The differential diagnosis of fever will determine realistic goals and the most appropriate plan of care. Understanding the experience from the perspective of the patient is critically important.[32] Clearly, a thorough physical examination and recent history are essential. Box 18.2 identifies common diagnostic questions relevant to and inclusive of clinical examination. The list is not intended to be

---

Box 18.2 Clinical assessment of fever

Is there evidence suggestive of a respiratory tract infection?
Is there evidence suggestive of a urinary infection?
How long has the patient been febrile?
What is the pattern of the fever (day or night, number of peaks of temperature over 24 hours)?
What medication or treatment is in progress or recently completed?
Has there been a recent blood transfusion?
Have there been any recent invasive procedures?
Have blood tests been obtained?
Is there evidence of damage to the skin integument?
Are there any venous access devices or catheters?

---

exhaustive, but rather to guide a holistic assessment in the context of increasing frailty and the likelihood of impending death.

Medical management of fever

In the palliative context, the degree to which fever is treated aggressively raises the debate about burden over benefit—life quality versus the risk of prolonged dying. Clearly, as in Thomas's case, antibiotics can be beneficial and therefore have a place in palliative care practice. In one recent study, both physicians and family members rated antibiotics highly in terms of treatment options for their patient/relative, second only to opiates, and more highly than intravenous nutrition.[33] The challenge for palliative care is to decide how far to treat and when "enough is enough." This is a necessary discussion if the aim is to prevent undue suffering and to ensure patient and family involvement in decision-making, which should be a priority for practice.

The complexity of the decision whether or not to use antibiotics is evidenced by the diversity of opinion within the literature as to their value and efficacy. Whatever decision is made regarding antibiotics, it is important that a plan of care includes decisions on the conditions that would herald cessation of treatment. For Thomas, the decision to proceed to intravenous antibiotics was clearly the right action. It would seem that there is something of a general consensus that antibiotic use in the terminal phase is inappropriate. However, even if the patient's status is deemed "palliative," debate may arise about where active treatment ends and palliative care begins. A good principle on which to base the decision to treat actively is the degree of symptom burden to the patient, regardless of the clinical presentation.[25]

Acetaminophen has the benefit of offering relatively rapid response to pyrexia and is available in a variety of forms—tablet, suspension, or suppository. An intravenous route has been approved in the United States for treating mild to moderate pain and fever. Aspirin, if tolerated, may also be effective. Corticosteroids also hold antipyretic properties, although their benefit needs to be weighed against the possible side effects.[16] Unless antipyretic medication is prescribed and administered regularly and not on a "PRN" basis, it may induce fluctuating patterns of fever and sweating. More intensive management may be required depending on the cause of the fever. Fever related to tumor may be responsive to radiation, if the patient's condition is stable enough for treatment. Further, neuroleptic agents such as chlorpromazine may be beneficial where the fever is centrally mediated.[16]

Nursing management of fever

Using Thomas's case as an example, comfort should be the key priority in the palliative approach. It is important to obtain a balance between "cooling" and "cold," the latter of which may only exacerbate the discomfort caused by shivering and heat-generation. Bathing with tepid water, drying off gently and using light bedding may add to comfort, but cold packs and ice should be avoided. Cool fluids should be encouraged, and attention to mouth and skin care is imperative, particularly in cases where there is a risk of dehydration. Thomas's fatigue and lethargy placed him at risk of decubitus ulcer formation, so an air mattress was used to good effect. A fan should be used to cool the ambient air and not be focused directly on the patient. Attention to these details in the evening may help to promote sleep. Accurate and methodical recording and interpretation of temperature may help in deciding clinical care planning as well as the timing and spacing of comfort care. Such review revealed a moderate elevation to Thomas's temperature that within a few hours progressed to an overall degeneration in his condition and a decision to treat the infection more aggressively. The outcome of discharge home supported the clinical decisions made at this time.

Sweats and hot flashes

Case study

Sweats with both disease-related and emotions-related components

Catherine was a 48-year-old single woman with advanced breast cancer, previously treated with surgery, chemotherapy, radiotherapy, and hormone therapy (tamoxifen). She had evidence of metastatic spread of her disease and had been admitted to the palliative care unit for management of increasing unresolved pain, unresponsive to opiates. During her first night, Catherine experienced a drenching sweat that occurred without warning and required a full change of clothes and bed linen. She reported that this had happened on two other occasions at home. She also reported that she had experienced hot flashes during the day, which had led to profuse sweating and palpitations. She experienced a similar sweat on the second night, at which point opioids were considered a causative factor and therefore reduced slightly, with minimal effect. Although sweating was presumed to be hormone-related, Catherine found some relief from the symptom through aromatherapy and relaxation sessions offered by the Complementary and Supportive Care Team. The introduction of gabapentin to assist in pain management also appeared to have a positive effect on the episodes of sweating. On discharge, nursing records indicated that no further episodes of sweating at night occurred following treatment with gabapentin and complementary support sessions were established.

Interpreting Sweats

Although sweats are considered one of the major problems experienced by patients,[34] research evidence for the management and treatment of sweats remains sparse. Night sweats have been identified as a significant problem for up to 48% of advanced cancer patients, and a specific association has been noted in patients who present with anorexia-cachexia as part of their advanced disease.[35]

Evidently, there is a strong link between fever and sweating, although there is a distinction between the thermal diaphoresis described in the previous section, and controlled by the hypothalamus, and emotional sweating that is controlled by the limbic system.[16] Age, gender, ambient temperature, and exercise are all known to influence the amount of sweating that takes place, and that is usually greater from palms of the hands and soles of the feet.[16]

Hot flashes are reported in up to 75% of menopausal women and described as a sensation of heat, associated with flushing, palpitations, and anxiety.[36] Completely unpredictable, hot flashes interfere greatly with life quality and in particular, sleep. It is common in breast cancer due to estrogen deprivation and noted in up to 70% of breast cancer patients on tamoxifen therapy. Although the pathophysiology is not well understood, it is known that as estrogen levels fall, a subsequent rise in hypothalamic serotonin receptors increases body temperature and may narrow the thermoregulatory zone. Hence, the person finds they may more easily "tip" outside the normal zone into overheating or cold. What is also known is that the degree of decline in estrogen levels, rather than the absolute level of estrogen would be an important indicator.[36] Specifically, hormone treatment as prescribed to Catherine is known to influence hyperhidrosis through estrogen withdrawal.[16,25] The problem is also seen in men with prostate cancer.[37]

Beyond breast and prostate cancer, sweating is noted in a variety of illnesses, including malignancy. Hyperhidrosis (excessive sweating) may be directly related to disease or indeed, may have no evident cause. In each case, it can be localized or generalized.[25] This may present as "night sweats" as described above.[35] Table 18.3 presents key causes of sweating.

Nursing assessment and differential diagnosis

Box 18.3 identifies some key questions that may be helpful when ascertaining the impact of the problem on the life quality of the patient.

Medical management of sweats

Unfortunately, drug therapy options for the management of sweating are relatively limited and there is very little evidence beyond case reports and pilot trials to support the use of any specific treatment. Medications that work as antispasmodics and anticholinergics have also demonstrated some benefit.[16,25] One small-scale study has indicated benefit in the use of the cannabinoid nabilone for persistent night sweats.[35]

There is a growing body of research looking at options for the management of hot flashes and in a number of small studies

Table 18.3 Key causes of sweating

Endocrine disorders	Estrogen deficiency, hyperthyroidism, hypoglycemia
Malignancy	Lymphoma, breast cancer, prostate cancer, neuroendocrine tumors
Chronic infection	Tuberculosis, lupus
Medication (including withdrawal from)	Opioids, barbiturates, estrogen-depriving agents (e.g., tamoxifen)
Emotion	Stress, anxiety, fear

Box 18.3 Questions for clinical assessment

How often do you find yourself sweating?
How would you describe these sweats?
Are they a particular problem at night?
Do you have any other problems when you sweat?
(nausea, vomiting, feeling faint, anxious or fearful)
Have you changed any medication recently?
Is your sweating all over your body, or confined to certain parts?
Have you identified anything that seems to make your sweating better or worse?
How much of a problem is this sweating for you?

---

in relation to the use of progestational agents (such as megestrolacetate), clonidine, SSRIs and gabapentin have been proposed.[38-41] This may explain the benefit that Catherine received in relation to her sweating when the latter medication was introduced for her pain management. However, there is contrasting evidence in relation to the use and efficacy of hormone replacement therapy (HRT—a standard treatment offered to healthy menopausal women) and therefore, in addition to the progestational agents it is not recommended for women with a history of breast cancer.

Given the link to "menopausal" symptoms, a number of nonpharmacological preparations have been proposed, including evening primrose oil, phytoestrogens, and herbs.[25] Although there is weak evidence for the use of complementary and supportive therapies, there is some suggestion that relaxation techniques to address the emotional component of the symptom may be beneficial.[36,42-44] One recent review of the management of hot flashes would suggest greater evidence for the use of cognitive-behavioral therapy (CBT) and yoga as of benefit. However, the evidence remains weak, and the discomfort associated with this symptom indicates the need for sensitive and responsive nursing care.

Nursing management of sweats

It is argued that the ethics of care begin with that which is most basic, and the care for the body is an example of that basic—but notably not simple—care. Since the burden of sweats on the patient's quality of life would appear to be great, nursing care must include an approach that addresses the immediate discomfort and anxiety. Patients should be advised to have extra changes of nightwear (or day clothes if the symptoms are not restricted to the night) and additional bedding should be available. Just as in the fever type response, the patient may feel cold following diaphoresis, and so should be kept comfortable in an ambient temperature while washing and changing. Similar to the treatment of fever, cool (but not cold) fluids should be encouraged to avoid dehydration, since the occurrence of multiple sweats in one night is not uncommon.[16] Avoiding hot and spicy foods, encouraging loose clothing, and keeping the room cool may also assist in maintaining comfort.[36] Anecdotal reports suggest reducing alcohol and red wine intake in particular as beneficial.

Patients may fear that their sweating indicates a deterioration or recurrence of disease. Night sweats may indicate this in the case of lymphoma.[16] The patient may be embarrassed by the symptom and withdraw from social events. Gentle discussion about the problem and reassurance that efforts are being made to find a solution may ease distress. Careful observation of factors relating to the sweats (time, duration, extent, patient response) may indicate a possible treatment pathway. Referral for complementary and supportive therapy should always be considered for the practical and emotional benefit it can bring.

Conclusions

Perhaps of all symptoms that palliative care patients endure, those of pruritus, fever, and sweats most remind nurses of their fundamental grounding in caring for others. The care given to patients with these symptoms is reflective of skills learned and nurtured throughout the nursing career, and then specifically honed to meet end-of-life needs. Comfort remains the key priority, particularly where drug therapy may have limited effect. The "benefit-burden calculus"[33] should be uppermost in the mind with respect to the goals of treatment. As the clinical team member with closest proximity to the patient, the nurse may need to voice his or her concerns, and the concerns of others, where an intervention appears to be unwarranted or even futile.

The attention to detail required in order to address these symptoms highlights the importance to palliative nursing of those philosophical constructs noted at the beginning of this chapter—hope, dignity, comfort, and empathy.

References

1. Payne S, Seymour J, Ingleton C, eds. Palliative Care Nursing Principles and Evidence for Practice. Berkshire: McGraw-Hill Open University Press; 2004:3.
2. Penz K. Theories of hope: are they relevant for palliative care nurses and their practice? Int J Palliat Nurs. 2008;14:408–412.
3. Currow DC, Ward AM, Plummer JL, Bruera E, Abernathy AP. Comfort in the last 2 weeks of life: relationship to accessing palliative care services. Support Care Cancer. 2008;16:1255–1263.
4. Summey BT. Pruritus. In: Walsh D, Caraceni AT, Fainsinger R, et al. (eds.), Palliative Medicine. Philadelphia PA: Saunders Elsevier; 2008:910–913.
5. Xander C, Meerpohl JJ, Galandi D, Buroh S, Schwarzer G, Antes G, Becker G. Pharmacological interventions for pruritus in adult palliative care patients. Cochrane Database Syst Rev. 2013(6): CD008320. doi: 10.1002/14651858.CD008320.pub2.
6. Chaing HC, Huang V, Cornelius LA. Cancer and itch. Sem Cutaneous Med Surg. 2011;30 (2):107–112.
7. Metz M, Ständer S. Chronic pruritus—pathogenesis, clinical aspects and treatment. J Eur Acad Dermatol Venereol. 2010;24:1249–1260.
8. Wang H, Yosipovitch G. New insights into the pathophysiology and treatment of chronic itch in patients with end-stage renal disease, chronic liver disease, and lymphoma. Int J Dermatol. 2010;49: 1–11.
9. Weisshaar E, Dalgard F. Epidemiology of itch: adding the burden of skin morbidity. Acta Derm Venereol. 2009;89:339–350.
10. Dhand A, Aminoff MJ. The neurology of itch. Brain. Brain 2014;137(2):313–322.
11. Seccareccia D, Gebara N. Pruritus in palliative care. Can Fam Physician. 2011;57:1010–1013.
12. Yosipovitch G, Barnard JD. Chronic pruritus. N Engl J Med. 2013;368: 1625–1634
13. Noble H, Meyer J, Bridges J, Johnson B, Kelly D. Exploring symptoms in patients managed without dialysis: a qualitative research study. J Renal Care. 2010;36(1):9–15.
14. Misery L, Ständer S. Pruritus. London: Springer; 2010.

15. Ständer S, Weisshaar E, Luger TA. Neurophysiological and neurochemical basis of modern pruritus treatment. Exp Dermatol. 2008;17(3):161–169.

16. Rhiner M, Slatkin NE. Pruritus, fever and sweats. In: Ferrell B, Coyle N (eds.), Textbook of Palliative Nursing (2nd ed). Oxford: Oxford University Press; 2004:345–363.

17. Bernhard JD. Itch and pruritus: what are they, and how should itches be classified? Dermatol Ther. 2005;18:288–291.

18. Jones EA, Zylicz Z. Treatment of pruritus caused by cholestasis with opioid antagonists. J Palliat Med. 2005;6:1290–1294.

19. Manenti L, Tansinda P, Vaglio A. Uraemic pruritus: clinical characteristics, pathophysiology and treatment. Drugs. 2009;69(3):251–263.

20. Anand S. Gabapentin for pruritus in palliative care. Am J Hosp Palliat Care. 2013;30:192–196.

21. Rayner H, Baharani J, Smith S, Suresh V, Dasgupta I. Uraemic pruritus: relief of itching by gabapentin and pregabalin. Nephron Clin Pract. 2012;122:75–79.

22. Elmariah SB, Lerner EA. Topical therapies for pruritus. Sem Cutan Med Surg. 2011;30(2): 118–126.

23. Cleary JF. Fever and sweats. In: Berger AM, Portenoy RK, Weissman DE (eds.), Principles and Practice of Palliative Care and Supportive Oncology. 2nd ed. Philadelphia: Williams and Wilkins; 2002:154–167.

24. Mackowiak PA. Fever: Basic Mechanisms and Management. 2nd ed. Philadelphia: Lippincott-Raven; 1997.

25. Bobb B, Lyckholm L, Coyne P. Fever and sweats. In: Walsh D, Caraceni AT, Fainsinger R, et al. (eds.), Palliative Medicine. Philadelphia: Saunders Elsevier; 2008:890–893.

26. Hung Y-S, Wu J-H, Chang H, Wang P-N, Kao C-Y, Wang H-M, et al. Characteristics of patients with hematological malignancies who received palliative care consultation services in a medical center. Am J Hosp Palliat Care. 2013 Jan 8. Epub ahead of print. doi: 101177/1049909112471423.

27. deNaurois J, Novitzky-Basso I, Gill MJ, Marti FM, Cullen MH, Roila F. Management of febrile neutropenia: ESMO clinical practice guidelines. Ann Oncol. 2010;21(Suppl 5): v252–v256.

28. Pascoe J. Developments in the management of febrile neutropaenia. Br J Cancer. 2011;105:597–598.

29. Carmona-Bayonas A, Gomez J, Gonzalez-Billalabeitia E, Canteras M, Navarrete A, Gonzalvez MI, et al. Prognostic evaluation of febrile neutropaenia in apparently stable adult cancer patients. Br J Cancer. 2011;105:612–617.

30. Cheng S, Teuffel O, Ethier MC, Diorio C, Martino J, Mayo C, et al. Health-related quality of life anticipated with different management strategies for paediatric febrile neutropaenia. Br J Cancer. 2011;105:606–611.

31. El Ghoul R, Eckardt SM, Muckopadhyay S, Ashton BW. Fever and dyspnea in a 61 year old woman with metastatic breast cancer. Chest. 2009;136:634–638.

32. Ames NJ, Peng C, Power JH, Kline Leidy N, Miller Davies C Rosenberg A et al. Beyond Fever Patient Fever Symptom Experience Journal of Pain and Symptom Management. 2013. Downloaded 28th June 2013 at http://dx.doi/10.1016/jpainsymman 2013.01.012

33. Oh DY, Kim JE, Lee CH, et al. Discrepancies among patients, family members and physicians in Korea in terms of values regarding the withholding of treatment form patients with terminal malignancies. Cancer. 2004;100:1961–1966.

34. De Lima L. The IAHPC list of essential medicines in palliative care. Palliat Med. 2006;20:647–651.

35. Maida V. Nabilone for the treatment of paraneoplastic night sweats. J Palliat Med. 2008;11(6):929–934.

36. Morrow PKH, Mattair DN, Hortobagyi GN. Hot flashes: a review of pathophysiology and treatment modalities. Oncologist. 2011;16:1658–1664.

37. Loprinzi CL, Dueck AC, Khoyratty BS, et al. A phase III randomized, double-blind, placebo—controlled trial of gabapentin in the management of hot flashes in men (N00CB). Ann Oncol. 2009;20:542–549.

38. Pandya KJ, Morrow GR, Roscoe JA, et al. Gabapentin for hot flashes in 420 women with breast cancer: a randomised double-blind placebo-controlled trial. Lancet. 2005;366:818–824.

39. Loprinzi CL, Barton DL, Sloan JA, et al. Mayo Clinic and North Central Cancer Treatment Group hot flash studies: a 20-year experience. Menopause. 2008;15:655–660.

40. Bordeleau L, Pritchard KI, Loprinzi CL, et al. Multicenter, randomized, cross-over clinical trial of venlafaxine versus gabapentin for the management of hot flashes in breast cancer survivors. J Clin Oncol. 2010;28:5147–5152.

41. Tremblay A, Sheeran L, Aranda SK. Psycho-educational interventions to alleviate hot flashes: a systematic review. Menopause. 2008;15:193–202.

42. Casey Lefkowits C, Arnold RM. Hot flashes in palliative care. Part 1 §261. J Palliat Med. 2013;16(1):100–101.

43. Casey Lefkowits C, Arnold RM Hot flashes in palliative care. Part 2 §262. J Palliat Med. 2013;16(1):101–102.

44. Casey Lefkowits C, Arnold RM Hot Flashes in Palliative Care Part 3 §263. J Palliat Med. 2013;16(2):203–204.

CHAPTER 19

Neurological disorders

Margaret A. Schwartz

It looked so uncomfortable—his arm would start first, then his face and leg, then his whole body. When he woke up from the seizures, he was groggy. Usually he'd have sore muscles for a few days. It was hard to watch.

A mother describing her son's seizures

The palliative care nurse is likely to encounter a patient with advanced neurological disorder or with a medical condition with neurological complications. It behooves the palliative care nurse to prepare for the variety of symptoms and diagnoses that he or she will clinically encounter. This chapter aims to lead the palliative care nurse to the appropriate, evidence-based interventions for the patient with neurological disturbances. We will address broad symptom categories as well as common neurological diseases with heavy symptom burden deserving of special attention.

Abnormal movements

The human body is capable of a broad variety of involuntary and abnormal movements—shivering, tremor, seizures, fasciculations, myoclonus, and chorea to name a few. See Table 19.1 for definitions of the abnormal movements most frequently encountered. Although it is beyond the scope of this chapter to delve into all of the possibilities, we will review those most relevant to the practice of the palliative care nurse.

Seizures

Seizures are defined as electrical discharges of the cerebral cortex with resulting changes in the functions of the central nervous system. For an aberrant electrical phenomenon to propagate and result in a seizure, three physiological conditions must exist: neurons capable of undergoing excitation, capacity for spread of the electrical phenomenon to surrounding neurons, and diminished ability of GABA-ergic neurons to suppress excitatory events. Any condition that disturbs the normal environment of the central nervous system can result in a seizure. Thus, any given patient has the capacity to experience a seizure. There are a number of conditions that increase the risk of an epileptic event. Most common are acute metabolic derangements, medications and substances, space-occupying lesions of the brain, ischemic events, and infection (see Tables 19.2 and 19.3). It is important to note that a single seizure does not constitute epilepsy.

Witnessing a seizure can be a traumatic event for caregivers and providers. Additionally, the emotional burden for patients with seizures is great. The impact of seizures on health is enormous—an estimated 50 million people worldwide have epilepsy. The incidence of a single unprovoked seizure event is estimated to be between 23 and 61 per 100,000 person-years.[1] Research on patients with epilepsy and their caregivers reveals persistent societal and individual stigma associated with this disorder and the resulting seizures.[2] Patients with new-onset seizures or uncontrolled epilepsy are at higher risk of impaired sleep, mood disorder, pain, and psychological distress.[3,4] Unchecked, seizures can result in significant morbidity—delirium, physical injury, aspiration, rhabdomyolysis and renal injury, pain, temporary paralysis, and loss of function. Among oncology patients there are a number of factors increasing the risk for seizures. Brain metastases, chemotherapy, and radiation, as well as metabolic and endocrinological changes in the patient with cancer increase the risk for seizures. In patients with primary brain tumors, the burden of seizures is staggering. Estimates of seizures in this group are as high as 80%. The financial, emotional, and social burden of seizures is also an important consideration. There are many interventions available to the palliative care nurse to reduce the impact of seizures.

The palliative care nurse begins with a careful history and physical exam. Any new physical findings may suggest an underlying physiological change that has lowered the seizure threshold. The patient with recent medication changes requires careful review—medication changes are frequently at play in the patient with new-onset seizure. In patients with primary brain tumors or intracranial metastatic disease, seizures are generally a result of edema and blood-brain barrier disturbance, mass effect, and cortical involvement. Additionally, the patient entering inpatient or hospice care with a history of substance abuse is at elevated risk for seizures if the patient is newly abstinent from alcohol, benzodiazepines, opioids, or illicit substances. Of special interest to the palliative care nurse is the patient with undiagnosed substance abuse entering into a hospice or palliative program.[5] If no source is immediately identified, radiographic or metabolic evaluation may be indicated if it is within the goals of care.

Family and patient teaching are important to dispel fear and to maximize patient comfort. Education goals focus on safety during seizures, postictal care, medications, eliminating the cause of the seizure when feasible and when to contact the provider. Safety during a seizure focuses on minimizing injury—falls and physical trauma during clonic movements as well as minimizing the length of seizure if possible. Padding the patient's surroundings (bed rails) is traditionally done in patients with refractory seizures.

Table 19.1 Commonly encountered neurological definitions

Agraphia	Inability to write. Of note, agraphia rarely occurs in isolation.
Akathisia	A sensation of restlessness, often accompanied by a compulsion to move the effected limbs. Most commonly found in patients with Parkinson's disease, dementia, and those receiving neuroleptics.
Alexia	Inability to read.
Aphasia	Impaired verbal or written communication because of an acquired insult to the brain.
	Expressive aphasia is an impairment in the ability to generate spoken language (also known as anterior/nonfluent/Broca's/motor aphasia).
	Receptive aphasia is difficulty or inability to understand spoken word (also known as posterior/fluent/ Wernicke's/sensory aphasia).
	Global aphasia is the inability to speak and understand spoken words. Patients with global aphasia can neither read nor write.
Asterixis	Also known as "flapping tremor," asterixis is commonly encountered in patients with metabolic and toxic encephalopathy (most notably in ammonia-retention). It is characterized by irregular lapses of a sustained posture, often followed by an overcorrection. It is also observed in neck and arms of the drowsy person.
Ataxia	Lack of coordination of voluntary movements.
Athetosis	Involuntary and abnormal slow, complex writhing movements. Most commonly involves fingers, hands, toes, and feet. Encountered in various forms with encephalitis, hepatic encephalopathy, Parkinson's disease, Huntington's disease, and cerebral palsy.
Chorea	Arrhythmic movements characterized by a writhing, rapid, and jerky quality. The movements are purposeless and involuntary. Often accompanied by a general state of hypotonia—the limbs hang slack. The major distinguishing feature of Huntington's disease.
Clonus	Rhythmic contraction and relaxation of antagonistic muscle groups.
Corticospinal tracts	The neurons connecting the cortex of the brain (gray matter) with the lower motor neurons in the ventral horn of the spinal cord.
Dysarthria	Impaired speech output due to oral, lingual, or pharyngeal motor impairment.
Dyskinesia	A wide-encompassing term meaning abnormal movement. Movements can be intermittent or persistent. In tardive dyskinesia, the movements are slow, rhythmic, and automatic.
Dysmetria	Ataxia with overshoot or undershoot of movement, dysmetria results from difficulty processing or perceiving the position of the body in relation to its surroundings.
Dsyphagia	Impaired ability to swallow in a coordinated and timely fashion.
Dystonia	A unilateral movement defined by involuntary muscle contraction of both the agonist and antagonist muscles. The result is the limb held in a twisted, distorted posture. Can affect a limb, the head and neck, the face, or the spinal muscles.
Fasciculation	A small, localized pattern of muscle contraction and relaxation, often observable through the skin. Commonly noted in the eyelid of healthy individuals, it can also be seen in ALS, progressive spinal muscle atrophy, or in states causing nerve fiber irritability (dehydration, muscular exhaustion, metabolic imbalance).
Lower motor neuron	The neurons that connect the upper motor neurons to the muscle fibers. Lower motor neurons originate in the ventral horn of the spinal cord or in the brainstem motor nerve nucleii and terminate on the neuromuscular plate of effector muscles.
Myoclonus	Rapid and irregular shocklike contractions of a group of muscles. The most commonly experienced myoclonic events are hiccups and "sleep starts." Palliative care nurses are likely to encounter opioid-induced myoclonus.
Myokymia	The irregular firing of several motor units, seen as a rippling of the skin.
Nystagmus	Involuntary jerking movement of the eyes in either a lateral or vertical direction.
Opsoclonus	Involuntary and irregular multidirectional movement of the eyes.
Seizures	Aberrant electrical activity of a part or the entire cortex of the brain, resulting in altered neurological functions.
Tardive dyskinesia	A specific dyskinesia characterized by repetitive and stereotyped movements often of the face, mouth, and tongue. It is most commonly an effect of antipsychotic medications.
Tremor	Rhythmic contraction of a muscle or group of muscles in opposing directions.
Upper motor neuron	The motor neurons originating in the motor cortex of the brain or brainstem and carrying synapses down to the lower motor neurons. Upper motor neurons do not directly contact the target muscle.

Table 19.2 Common conditions resulting in seizures

Metabolic changes	Electrolyte imbalances
	Thyrotoxic storm
	Uremia
	Hypertensive encephalopathy
	Hypertension of pregnancy (eclampsia and preclampsia)
	Fever
	Dehydration and overhydration
	Hyperventilation
Medication-related, illicit substance-related	Missed doses/withdrawal
	New medications
	Metabolite accumulation
Intracranial tumors	Metastatic tumors
	Primary central nervous system tumors
Ischemia	Stroke
	Diffuse cerebral hypoxia
Infections	Encephalitis
	Meningitis
	Intracranial abscess
	Parasitic lesions
Paraneoplastic syndromes	NMDA-receptor encephalitis
Trauma-related	Subdural hematoma
	Subarachnoid hemorrhage
	Intraventricular hemorrhage
	Trauma-induced gliosis
	Post-traumatic epilepsy
Vascular lesions	Atreovenous malformation
	Intracranial aneurysm
	Subdural hemorrhage or fluid collection
	Epidural hemorrhage
	Subarachnoid hemorrhage
Idiopathic or congenital disorders	Birth injury
	Congenital malformation
	Enzyme deficiencies
	Lysosomal storage disorders
	Channelopathies

Although a prudent intervention, no data exists to support this long-standing nursing intervention. See Box 19.1 for seizure first-aid and safety suggestions. Placing objects in the mouth and restraining the patient are absolutely contraindicated. Patients should not be given food or liquid until they have fully recovered consciousness. Should the patient fail to regain full consciousness between seizures or continue to seize after several minutes—a condition known as status epilepticus—urgent action is required. Status epilepticus is treated as a serious and life-threatening situation requiring immediate administration of medication to break the seizures. If the seizure occurs in the home, emergency medical services may be appropriate if consistent with the goals of care. Of note, there remain several states in the United States that require providers to report seizure events to the Department of Motor

Vehicles. Certainly, patients with seizures should abstain from driving until cleared by a neurologist.

Of utmost importance for patient comfort and safety is to stop the seizure as it happens. Seizure-ablative medications may be limited by the specific patient situation. The patient receiving hospice at home will likely be best served by administration of rapid-acting benzodiazepines. Orally administered concentrated lorazepam drops are readily available from the hospice pharmacy. Other choices include rectal diazepam gel, nasal lorazepam gel, or clonazepam wafers applied to the buccal surface. In the patient with intravenous access, slow intravenous push administration is generally the preferred choice.

Several issues require specific attention in the palliative care setting. In a patient with a reversible condition, antiepileptic drugs (AEDs) may not be required. Patients with epilepsy or significant risk for ongoing seizures will require careful consideration for AED choice. If the patient with metastatic or primary brain tumors has never experienced a seizure, the current recommendation is not to prophylactically administer anticonvulsants.[6] For a brief overview of factors to be considered when introducing AEDs, see Box 19.2. Notably, several choices have arisen in recent years for the patient with medically refractory seizures. A restrictive diet inducing a ketogenic state has been studied for decades for medically refractory childhood epilepsy with some success. Surgical options include resection of the seizure focus or lesion as well as vagal nerve stimulator placement. Careful consideration must be given to the life expectancy and appropriateness of the patient for such procedures and interventions.

Myoclonus

Emily W was dying of end-stage renal carcinoma. After nephrectomy and several rounds of treatments, the cancer returned in her bones. She enrolled in hospice care at home. Emily developed progressive somnolence and diminishing urine output but continued to moan in pain. The hospice team increased her morphine but after 3 days, Emily's husband called the hospice nurse to report a distressing development. "Emily's body is twitching all over. There's no pattern to the twitches except that it worsens when we turn her."

Myoclonus is a series of brief muscular contractions. The contractions are irregular in both the amplitude of contraction and rhythm, and it denotes a disturbance of the central nervous system. There are a wide variety of myoclonic syndromes. In the palliative care setting, the nurse is most likely to encounter diffuse myoclonus rather than myoclonus simplex or segmental myoclonus. See Table 19.4 for other causes of myoclonus. Diffuse myoclonus is characterized by random jerks, widespread throughout the body. It can be either a passing or persistent phenomenon. Myoclonus has gained increasing awareness in the palliative care setting as it can lead to increased pain, fatigue, and other distressing symptoms. Intervention begins with recognizing the causative factors. The palliative care nurse is most likely to encounter diffuse myoclonus from acquired neurological disease or metabolite accumulation. Several other causes of myoclonus are known: epileptic, hereditary, and essential causes and immune and toxic disorders. Myoclonus also results from forms of degenerative neurological disorders.

The palliative care nurse begins with careful examination and review of medications. An interview of the patient and

Table 19.3 Seizure definitions

Simple focal (partial) seizure	The uncontrolled electrical activity in a simple partial seizure is limited to a small area of the cortex. The resulting seizure is not accompanied by loss of consciousness. Symptoms include shaking of a single area of the body. Less commonly, simple partial seizures can result in abnormal sensations of the affected limb or in abnormal sensations such as auditory, visual, or gustatory changes. Rarely, simple partial seizures can result in behavioral and emotional changes.
Complex focal (partial) seizure	Affecting a larger area of the brain, complex partial seizures result in impairments in the ability of the person to interact with his of her surroundings. They often start with a blank look or staring spell and progress to stereotyped, repetitive movements. Also termed "psychomotor seizures."
Generalized seizure	The most common and obvious of the seizures. Generalized seizures involve the entire cortex of the brain. The typical generalized seizure begins with limb stiffening (tonic posturing) and a period of apnea or hypoventilation. This gives way to clonic movements (jerking of the limbs and/or head as muscles contract and relax together). During the clonic phase, breathing returns, although it is often irregular.
Absence seizure	A generalized seizure in which the patient abruptly ceases activity and stares blankly. The patient is unable to interact with his or her environment during the seizure. As soon as the seizure is finished, the patient returns to the activity preceding the ictal event.
Atonic seizure	Atonic (drop-attack/astatic/akinetic) seizures are generalized seizures resulting in an abrupt loss of postural tone. Loss of tone can vary from head drooping to full collapse.
Aura	In epilepsy, an aura is the initial phase of a focal seizure. It is generally experienced as a motor, sensory, autonomic, or psychic event. For some patients, the aura alone constitutes the seizure.
Epilepsy	A syndrome of repeated seizures
Febrile seizure	A seizure occurring in infants and children (ages 6 months to 5 years) in the setting of a temperature usually above 38° C. Febrile seizures are usually a single generalized motor seizure as the patient's temperature peaks. Be certain to distinguish between febrile seizures and complicated febrile seizures, the latter occurring repeatedly during a febrile illness.
Ictal	Latin for "stroke," ictal has come to mean the height of a seizure or migraine.
Psychogenic nonepileptic seizures	Also called "pseudoseizures," these are events characterized by changes in neurological function in the absence of electroencephalographic changes indicating abnormal electrical activity of the cortex.
Status epilepticus	A cluster of seizures without return to full neurological baseline between events or a single, ongoing seizure lasting more than a few minutes. Considered a medical emergency, status epilepticus carries an elevated risk of brain damage, hypoxia, and death.

family may illicit a recent change. Emily's urine output diminished, indicating renal impairment. Renal impairment is associated with opioid-induced myoclonus (OIM). The patient or family will describe nonrhythmic jerking movements. Stimulation of the patient or tapping on the muscles may bring on or worsen myoclonus. Hyperalgesia and hallucinations in

---

Box 19.1 Seizure safety

Seizure first aid

- prevent injury by moving furniture or hard objects out of the way
- refrain from putting anything in the mouth of the patient
- place a pillow or soft item under the patient's head
- loosen tight clothing around the neck

After-seizure care

- avoid situations dangerous to the epileptic (open flame, unaccompanied boating/swimming/tub-bathing)
- avoid seizure triggers (sleep deprivation, blood sugar lows, alcohol consumption, excess caffeine intake)

---

the setting of myoclonus raise the suspicion of OIM and should trigger an evaluation of pain medications. In the patient with opsoclonus-myoclonus syndrome, the myoclonus is typically diffuse or focal with titubation (rhythmic tremoring of the head or trunk). Ataxia and other cerebellar symptoms may also be apparent. The diagnosis of opsoclonus-myoclonus is based on clinical, serological, and radiographic testing. In the palliative care setting, the goals of care are always considered when deciding whether to conduct this testing.

Elimination of the causative factor, if possible, is most likely to induce remission of the myoclonus. In the patient on opioid medications, opioid rotation is indicated. The precise mechanisms behind OIM are unknown. The leading theorized mechanism points to accumulation of neuroexcitatory metabolites, particularly hydromorphone-3-glucuronide and morphine-3-glucuronide in the setting of impaired kidney function.[7–12] Although higher doses of opioids are more commonly implicated in OIM, it can occur in patients with relatively low doses and preserved renal function.[13,14] Opioids implicated in OIM in the literature include morphine, hydromorphone, fentanyl, methadone, and meperidine.[15–19] If OIM is suspected, opioid rotation, addition of a benzodiazepine such as clonazepam or midazolam, and a trial of adjuvant medications are indicated.[20,21]

Box 19.2 Special considerations when introducing an antiepileptic drug

- Drug interactions are common with AEDs, especially older generation medications that induce the cytochrome P450 hepatic enzymes.

- Many AEDs can alter mood and are used as psychotropic medications.

- carefully review comorbidities; for example, phenytoin can cause osteoporosis, topiramate can induce weight loss in the patient with limited life expectancy. Impaired level of consciousness or diminished ability to swallow makes most oral AEDs poor choices—consider scheduled benzodiazepines.

- Most AEDs do not require drug-level monitoring.

- Dexamethasone is neither an antiepileptic medication nor a seizure-ablating drug.

- Phenytoin increases metabolism of corticosteroids, and corticosteroids can alter the metabolism of phenytoin—consider a different AED.

- consultation with a neurologist may be warranted

Table 19.4 Etiologies of Myoclonus

Drug-related	Opioid-induced myoclonus (OIM)
	Lithium toxicity
	Haloperidol
	Phenothiazines
	Cyclosporine
	Beta-lactam antibiotics
	Antidepressants
Metabolic disorders	Hepatic encephalopathy
	Nicotinic acid deficiency
	Uremia
	Storage diseases
Inflammatory disorders	Thyroiditis
Infectious diseases	Whipple disease of the central nervous system
	Tetanus
	Herpes zoster myelitis
Central nervous system disorders	Hypoxic brain injury
	Multiple sclerosis
	Paraneoplastic syndromes
	AIDS dementia complex
	Viral encephalitis
	Advanced dementias
	Cerebellar degenerative conditions
	Basal ganglia degenerative conditions
	Creutzfeldt-Jakob disease
	Parkinson's disease
	Subacute sclerosis panencephalitis
	Myoclonic epilepsy syndromes

Treatment of non-OIM myoclonus includes eliminating causative conditions. Few medications have been found to ease myoclonus. Anticonvulsants can be helpful in chronic myoclonus, although typically multidrug therapy is needed. Clonazepam is the most frequently used and most effective agent. Other drugs have been tried, including valproic acid, levetiracetam, zonisamide, acetazolamide, and sodium oxybate, although strong data for each of these medications is lacking.[22] Several non-AEDs have been tried for myoclonus, including baclofen and dantrolene, also with varying success.

Nursing-specific care for myoclonus is multifaceted. Safety takes priority. Padded side rails and helmets may be necessary. For patients with severe myoclonus, ambulation may not be possible. Physical or occupational therapy assessment will determine whether durable medical equipment, assistive devices, or a gait belt are needed. Offer strategies for safe patient transfers to families and caregivers. As with all palliative care measures, assessment for pain is necessary. During opioid rotation the risk for discomfort is high because of variability in cross-tolerance. Myoclonus is fatiguing. Teaching patients and family members energy conservation is important. Myoclonus increases caloric expenditure, and in the medically frail patient nutritional supplementation or counseling may prevent weight loss. Provide a low level of stimulation (low light, minimizing noise).

Spasticity

Jamie P. was 14 when his dirt bike flipped. He fractured C4 in the accident and sustained a complete spinal cord injury. After spinal shock resolved, Jamie was left with severe spasticity below the level of injury. When Jamie yawns, coughs, or sneezes his entire body is consumed with a tremendous spasm. Jamie, now 28 years old, came to the emergency room last week reporting an increase in spasticity: "every time I get spasms this bad it means I've got a bladder infection."

Spasticity is increased muscle tone to the extreme. It results from denervation of muscles or from demyelination of neurons in the central nervous system—typically because of a lesion of the upper motor neuron (UMN). Spasticity occurs in many neurological conditions. It is commonly encountered with spinal cord injury, multiple sclerosis (MS), cerebral palsy, stroke, brain or head trauma, amyotrophic lateral sclerosis (ALS), hereditary spastic paraplegias, and metabolic diseases.

The most sensitive indicator of an UMN lesion is a positive Babinski sign. It is elicited by firmly stroking the lateral plantar surface of the foot. A positive Babinski sign is extension of the large toe accompanied by fanning and extension of the other toes during and immediately after the stimulus. The Babinski sign mimics the physiological reflex observed in infancy. Spasticity shows a predilection for antigravity muscles: brachialis, brachioradialis, biceps, pectoralis, anterior deltoid, and the flexor carpi muscles of the arms as well as the hip flexors, gastrocnemius, hamstrings, and popliteus muscles of the legs. Other physical exam signs include hyperreflexia of the deep tendon reflexes, clonus, muscle spasms, and scissoring of extremities. Spasticity can occur in any muscle or muscle group. One notable example is the spasticity and dystonia of cranial nerves in bulbar or pseudobulbar palsy.

Spasticity can be uncomfortable and painful. It can also severely limit functional abilities and thus requires considered treatment. The palliative care nurse will consider whether the condition is established spasticity with worsening, as with our example of Jamie P. In this situation, the nurse will seek secondary causes—infection, constipation, pain, or autonomic dysreflexia. If the spasticity is new, further investigation is required. In a patient with MS, the primary concern is for disease progression. It is imperative to balance spasticity with the functional abilities of the patient. For example, the patient with spastic cerebral palsy must preserve some muscle tone in order to ambulate.

Many treatments are available for spasticity. Research into the neurochemical changes of spasticity has demonstrated that glutamic acid is the primary neurotransmitter of the corticospinal tracts. Baclofen, a gamma-aminobutyric acid derivative, is the mainstay treatment. Other commonly used oral antispasmodics include dantroline, diazepam, and tizanidine for a desired effect of diminished force of contraction. Spasticity is one of the few generally agreed on medical uses for marijuana.[23,24] See Table 19.5 for a summary of oral antispasmodic medications. Phenol and botulinum toxin are injected for patients with persistent spasticity and torticollis. Surgical interventions are also available for the patient with medically intractable spasticity. Intrathecal administration of baclofen has become a mainstay of treatment for patients with persistent spasticity with significant side effects from oral baclofen.[25,26] These interventions must be carefully weighed,

Table 19.5 Medications used to treat spasticity

Drug name	Mechanism of action	Most common use	Common side effects
Baclofen	Inhibition of synaptic reflexes at the spinal cord level	Spasticity Hiccups	Central nervous system (CNS) depression, weakness, hypotension, gastrointestinal (GI) disturbance, polyuria
Carisoprodol	Unknown	Spasticity Muscle pain due to injury Adjunctive to opioids—use carefully in combination any CNS depressant, especially synthetic opioids	CNS depression, idiosyncratic reactions of weakness and euphoria, seizures
Chlorzoxazone	Reduces polysynaptic reflexes	Muscle spasm and pain	Withdrawal if abruptly discontinued, CNS depression, paradoxical stimulation, GI disturbance, rash, hepatotoxicity, hypersensitivity reaction
Cyclobenzaprine	Unknown	Spasticity	CNS depression, dry mouth, dizziness, agitation
Dantrolene	Local action on the excitation-contraction units of the muscle	Spasticity Malignant hyperthermia Serotonin syndrome "Ecstasy" intoxication	CNS depression, hallucinations, hepatotoxic effects, GI disturbance
Diazepam	Reduced neuronal excitability via enhanced GABA-ergic inhibition	Agitation Alcohol detoxification Anticonvulsant Anxiolysis Spasticity Sedation	CNS depression Anterograde amnesia Psychiatric disturbance Seizures if acutely withdrawn Abuse
Gabapentin	Reduced neuronal excitability via enhanced GABA-ergic inhibition	Anticonvulsant Neuropathic pain Spasticity	CNS depression, dizziness, weight gain, fatigue, peripheral edema, risk of suicidality
Orphenadrine	Anticholinergic	Low back pain, sciatica Adjuvant treatment of neuropathic pain and spasticity	CNS depression, dry mouth, dizziness, restlessness, insomnia, constipation, urine retention, orthostasis, euphoria
Metaxalone	Unknown	Muscle pain due to spasticity	CNS depression, rash, GI disturbance, leukopenia, hemolytic anemia, hepatotoxicity
Methocarbamol	Unknown	Spasticity Tetanus	CNS depression, seizures, bradycardia, syncope, hypotension, rash, GI disturbance, leukopenia, vision changes, hypersensitivity reactions
Tizanidine	Reduced neuronal excitability via alpha-2 adrenergic agonist	Spasticity Chronic headache Migraine	CNS depression, hepatotoxicity, sweating, GI disturbance, dry mouth, constipation, urine retention

particularly for the palliative care patient who may have limited life expectancy.

Nursing care for spasticity focuses on comfort and maximizing function. Physical and occupational therapy consultation are invaluable for prescribed stretching regimens and to determine appropriate durable medical equipment. Patient and family education are important to set realistic goals. Education also focuses on factors that worsen spasticity, prevention of pressure ulcers and contractures, fatigue, and psychosocial concerns. Early education is crucial to prevent complications. Appropriate medication use and indications for their use is also taught. Repositioning, application of heat, and strategies to improve functional abilities are helpful.

Headaches

Tracey W. was 13 when she had her first migraine. She noticed vision changes followed by a severe one-sided headache. As she grew, Tracey's migraines increased in frequency and intensity. She cannot work and experiences vomiting on a weekly basis secondary to her migraines. During a recent visit to her neurologist, Tracey reported, "I'm not sure I can ever get pregnant. How could I parent a child when I can't get off the couch?"

Tracey W. elegantly illustrates the degree of debilitation that can result from headaches and migraines. Headaches are a common ailment—an estimated 78% of Americans will experience a tension-type headache in their lifetime and 16% will suffer a migraine.[27] Quality-of-life studies demonstrated that the impact of migraines on an individual is striking—in one study 59% of migraine sufferers reported missing a family or social activity as a result of a migrainous event.[28]

A wide variety of conditions can trigger headaches and migraines. Common conditions encountered in the palliative setting include intracranial tumors, vascular disorders, infection, and head trauma. A selection of etiologies is found in Table 19.6. Of certain importance to the palliative care nurse is the medication overuse headache (MOH, also known as rebound headache), in which attempt at withdrawal from certain substances leads to onset of headache. The typical scenario encountered in MOH is a patient using acetaminophen, NSAIDs, or combination migraine preparation. Other identified substances include caffeine, triptans, antidepressants, cocaine, estrogen, marijuana, and opioids.[29] The headache typically resolves in the absence of the offending substance after a period of days to weeks. In some cases, gradual reduction of dose may be a safer option, particularly if the substance has the potential for an acute withdrawal syndrome, as with opioids.

As with all neurological changes in the palliative setting, the nurse begins with an assessment. The pain and its accompanying characteristics (intensity, location, quality, exacerbating/alleviating factors, response to previous therapies, related symptoms) can guide care. The typical tension-type headache is bilateral and characterized by a sensation of constant pressure. Episodic-type headache is thought to transform into tension-type headache with constant pericranial muscle tension.[30] The pain can range from mild to moderate, and in extreme cases can be severe. Conversely, migrainous events are commonly unilateral. The pain can be pulsatile in nature

Table 19.6 Causes of head pain

Headache syndromes	Cluster headache
	Tension-type headache
	Withdrawal/medication overuse headache
Migraine syndromes	Migraine with or without aura
Cranial and intracranial lesions	Metastatic brain tumors
	Primary brain tumors
	Skull base tumors
	Leptomeningeal metastases
General medical diseases and conditions	Fasting state/hunger
	Eyestrain
	Stress
	Muscle strain/tension, prolonged sitting, poor posture
	Sleep deprivation
	Stroke
	Vascular disorders
	Multiple sclerosis
	Increased intracranial pressure
	Sinus infection
	Temporal arteritis
	Varied infections, both systemic and CNS
Head trauma	Trigeminal neuralgia
Atypical pain syndromes	Postherpetic neuralgia

and is often associated with phonophobia, photophobia, and nausea/vomiting. Sleep alleviates the migraine and physical activity aggravates it. A significant number of migraineurs will experience an aura of transient sensory (usually visual), language, or motor disturbance. Focal deficits indicate either a complex migraine, or more seriously, a new intracranial lesion. The "thunderclap" headache of subarachnoid hemorrhage is a sudden-onset and very severe headache often accompanied by profuse vomiting and mental status changes. A headache accompanied by nuchal rigidity, vomiting, and photophobia suggests irritation of the meninges and warrants emergent evaluation. The typical headache of a patient with intracranial metastasis is dull, poorly localized, and of moderate intensity. Some patients will have ipsilateral pain to the metastatic lesion. Signs of increased intracranial pressure include an increase in pain intensity when lying down, coughing, or sneezing as well as nausea, vomiting, mental status changes, and pupillary changes. In some situations of headache, radiographic evaluation will be appropriate. Cerebrospinal fluid sampling via lumbar puncture may also be warranted.

Physical assessment includes palpation over the area of pain. Careful neurological examination may elicit deficits—skull base metastases will commonly compress an isolated cranial nerve. Leptomeningeal metastases will commonly result in multiple cranial or spinal neuropathies as well as headache.

Treatment is dictated by the classification of headache or migraine as well as by the etiology. In the case of Tracey W., she was surprised to realize the frequency with which she was using a combination medication (acetaminophen/caffeine/aspirin)—as often as 20 doses per month. When the medication was eliminated and a prophylactic migraine medication was initiated, Tracey W. found her migraine frequency reduced to once per month. After journaling her sleep pattern and food intake, Tracey W. was able to identify red wine and oversleeping as triggers.

The patient with an isolated skull base metastasis may find symptom stabilization and pain relief with palliative radiation or chemotherapy. Dexamethasone is commonly used in the palliative care setting because of its oral and parental formulations, lower mineralocorticoid effects, and ease of dosing.[31]

Nursing interventions also include patient and family education. It is distressing to care for a loved one with severe, persistent headaches. Caregivers may express feelings of impotence to change the symptoms as well as loss and sadness in the setting of progressive neurological deficits. Patients and family members benefit from education regarding pain management measures and medications. In the event of neurological deficits, education about safety measures is important. Other nonpharmacological interventions can be useful—ice and heat, reduced light/sound exposure, meditation and distraction, physical activity or rest, and positioning. Commonly, head-of-bed elevation is useful in the setting of increased intracranial pressure.

Impaired communication

Pete U. is 82 years old. He suffered a left-hemisphere stroke last year and now struggles to make himself understood. He has expressive aphasia. Pete's daughter finds herself sad, angry, and frustrated that she cannot understand her father: "I just want to hear my dad's voice again—it would do me a world of good to just hear him tell me what flavor ice cream he wants!"

Communication is arguably at the heart of the human existence. Impaired communication is distressing to both the patient and their caregivers. Impairments in communication from neurological disorders can take the form of aphasia, mutism, deafness, agraphia, alexia, or dysarthria. Additionally, several conditions can impede the patient's ability to express wishes—the ventilator-dependent patient is one such example. The patient with a massive brainstem injury from a basilar artery occlusion is "locked-in" and has retained cognitive abilities but lost all control of his body save for voluntary eye movement.

Any number of disorders can result in impaired communication. Aphasia is caused by any disease disturbing the cortex of the brain responsible for language production or reception. Traditional neurological teaching identifies the key cortical areas as Broca's area, Wernicke's area, and the supplemental motor area. Functional hemisphere dominance determines the localization of language in the right or left cerebral hemisphere. For most people, language production and comprehension occur in the left hemisphere.

Nursing care for the patient with disorders of speech or language focuses on strategizing alternative means of communication and maximizing functional ability for speech. As the case study illustrates, impaired communication is highly distressing and frustrating for patients and caregivers alike. If the patient is capable of cognition, the nurse identifies alternative communication

> **Box 19.3** Key points for optimizing communication
>
> ◆ Provide the optimal setting for communication: ensure the patient has glasses on and hearing aids in if appropriate, and adequate lighting.
>
> ◆ Avoid correcting grammatical mistakes or speaking for the patient.
>
> ◆ Do not raise the volume of your voice unless the patient is hearing impaired.
>
> ◆ Use facial expression to emphasize spoken communication.
>
> ◆ Face the patient directly while communicating.
>
> ◆ If the patient has other neurological impairment, such as a visual field cut, compensate by standing on the patient's best side.
>
> ◆ Simplify the message.
>
> ◆ Allow adequate time for cognitive processing and response.

strategies regardless of the patient's prognosis and the setting of care. Intensive care nurses and home hospice nurses alike can use communication boards, yes/no questions, and written instructions. Several key points are important for the patient with aphasia (Box 19.3).

Speech-language pathology consultation can be immensely helpful to clarify the specific communication deficiencies. Speech pathologists are a wonderful resource to the palliative care nurse for strategizing alternative communication methods. One particularly fascinating communication strategy for the patient with expressive aphasia is to use song rather than spoken word to communicate. Patients with nonfluent aphasia may be able to put words to familiar melody in order to communicate. A technique known as melodic intonation therapy has been developed for patient with left-hemisphere lesions to increase length of spoken phrases.[32] Music therapy has a potential role as well for the patient with communication difficulty.

Neurological diseases

A number of neurological diseases result in devastating symptom clusters and require increasingly complex nursing care. Many of these diseases are progressive neurological degenerative disorders such as ALS, MS, and Parkinson's disease (PD). This section will address the palliative care needs of these patients

Amyotrophic lateral sclerosis

Amyotrophic lateral sclerosis (ALS, also known as Lou Gehrig's disease) is a devastating progressive neurological condition characterized by progressive muscle wasting from denervation (amyotrophy) with hyperreflexia. Amyotrophic lateral sclerosis is the most common of all motor neuron diseases. It results from the destruction of both upper and lower motor neurons. There are both familial and sporadic cases of ALS, with familial cases accounting for approximately 10% to 20% of total cases.[33] The mechanism of neuron destruction is a defect in the degradation of misfolded proteins. The resulting accumulation and clumping of nonfunctional proteins results in neuronal death.[34] The end result of the disease process is paralysis and respiratory failure.

Jack P. was a police officer. One day Jack stepped out of the squad car and had difficulty picking up his left foot to walk: "I thought my foot was asleep from sitting in traffic. I didn't pay attention to it until it didn't go away." Jack's internist was immediately suspicious of a serious problem when she noticed Jack's calf muscle quivering. After meeting with a neurologist, Jack was diagnosed with ALS. "I don't want to suffocate to death—that will be my fate with this disease. I know who Lou Gehrig was and how he died." Jack inquired of his treatment team if they would assist him "to make the end easier when the time came."

Jack's story highlights the fears and psychological distress that underlies a diagnosis with a progressive and devastating neurological disorder. Table 19.7 highlights the typical symptom clusters of ALS.

The treatment team is prepared to address a number of symptoms as well as the emotional impact of the disease. Goals-of-care discussions are important early in the disease trajectory. Median life expectancy is under 5 years,[35] although life expectancy is considerably shorter if the patient declines artificial nutritional or respiratory support. Riluzole is the only therapy demonstrated to extend survival and time to tracheostomy.[36] Gastrointestinal distress and liver enzyme elevation can occur with riluzole treatment. Nursing interventions for the patient with ALS focus on the impact on quality of life, symptom palliation, and functional ability as well as end-of-life planning and support.

The ALS patient requires an extensive team. Neurologists, pulmonologists, speech pathologists, physical and occupational therapists, nurses (see Table 19.8), and social workers will all play a role. Functional assessment and physical/occupational therapy needs are immediate; patients may require assistive devices at diagnosis. Therapy services have been shown to maintain endurance and strength, promoting functional independence, and limit complications and pain.[37] Formal speech-language pathology and nutrition assessment is needed for swallowing evaluation and feeding strategies. The patient with ALS is at high risk for malnutrition from dysphagia, depression, cognitive impairment, difficulty with self-feeding and meal preparation, hypermetabolism, anxiety, respiratory insufficiency, and fatigue with meals[38]—some of these problems can be managed with speech pathology and dietary intervention. Early intervention to maximize nutrition and feeding is shown to extend survival and improve quality of life.[39,40] Augmentative communication strategies will become key as paralysis progresses. Patients with ALS have increasingly accepted alternative communication strategies as compared with previous years.[42] Both low-tech strategies such as alphabet boards and high-tech solutions like speech-generating devices can be helpful. Sialorrhea is a common and uncomfortable symptom of ALS. Unilateral radiotherapy to the salivary or parotid gland and botulinum toxin injection are effective interventions.[43–45]

The terminal phase of ALS is marked by significant challenges, and symptoms are best managed by a hospice team. The dying phase of ALS is often marked by pain, psychological distress, episodes of choking and loss of respiratory capacity, diminishing communicative ability, and increasing physical dependency. Sadly, symptoms from disease progression are commonly inadequately

Table 19.7 Symptoms common to the patient with amyotrophic lateral sclerosis

Bulbar-onset	Limb-onset
Dysphagia	Muscle weakness
Dysarthria	Hyperreflexia
Sialorrhea	Fasciculations

controlled.[40] A remarkable responsibility thus falls to the family and caregivers. Should the patient opt for long-term ventilatory support (LTVS) or noninvasive ventilation (NIV), the family and caregivers will require considerable teaching—from managing the tracheostomy wound to airway suctioning and maintaining equipment. Palliative sedation may be useful in select patients with ALS who decline or terminate mechanical ventilation.[46]

The wish to hasten death is expressed not uncommonly in a patient with a terminal illness. The palliative care nurse must be prepared for assessment, intervention, and thoughtful discussion of these issues. Suicidality and depression are associated with poorer quality of life in patients with ALS.[47] A single review of cases in The Netherlands revealed that 20% of patients with ALS chose euthanasia or physician-assisted suicide.[48] Depression and hopelessness require urgent attention. Pseudobulbar affect (PBA) is common in patients with ALS. It is characterized by uncontrolled expression of emotion that does not correlate to the underlying mood. Frequently the emotion expressed is inappropriate to the situation. Pseudobulbar affect has also been called emotional incontinence. Importantly, the phenomenon of PBA is not isolated to ALS. It has been described in other neurological disorders—MS, traumatic brain injury, Alzheimer's disease and PD. Coadministration of dextromethorphan 20 mg with quinidine 10 mg (the latter to slow the metabolism of the first) has been found effective at treating PBA.[49] A combination pill was approved by the US FDA in 2010 under the trade name Nuedexta.

Parkinson's disease

Angelique O. was 58 years old. She worked as a postal carrier and was nearing retirement. Angelique's children noticed a change in Angelique's walking when they gathered for the holidays. At her children's urging, Angelique finally saw her provider when she fell and broke her nose several months later. The general practitioner noticed that Angelique's fingers tremored during the visit, prompting a referral to neurology. The neurologist determined that Angelique was suffering from PD and started her on ropinirole.

Parkinson's disease is the second most common neurological degenerative disorder. Related conditions include multiple system atrophy and progressive supranuclear palsy. The defining characteristics of PD are tremor, postural instability, bradykinesia, and rigidity of the extremities or trunk. It is important to distinguish PD from parkinsonism. Parkinsonism is an umbrella term indicating that the patient has symptoms of PD that may not originate from loss of dopaminergic neurons in the substantia nigra.

As with ALS, care for the patient with PD requires a team of healthcare providers. The palliative care nurse will be initially focused on maximizing functional ability and diminishing falls. Medication education, home safety, physical and occupational

Table 19.8 Nursing management of amyotrophic lateral sclerosis

Airway and secretions	
Sialorrhea	◆ Excessive saliva in the oral cavity ◆ Anticholinergics, use with care due to risk of mucous plugging, orthostasis, confusion, sedation ◆ Glycopyrrolate, amitriptyline, atropine, benztropine mesylate, trihexypenidyl, hyoscyamine, transdermal scopolamine (Miller et al.[43]) ◆ Radiation to salivary gland (Stalpers and Moser[44]) ◆ Botulinum toxin to parotid gland (Scott et al.[45])
Mucous pooling	◆ Suction ◆ Cough-assist device ◆ Guaifenesin ◆ Beta blockers
Airway	◆ Early discussion of goals of care and patient preferences ◆ Noninvasive ventilation (NIV) such as positive-pressure ventilation with CPAP, biPAP ◆ Tracheostomy with or without long-term mechanical ventilation (LTMV) ◆ Oxygen support ◆ Positioning
Communication impairment	◆ Speech-language pathologist evaluation ◆ Alphabet boards, picture board, yes/no board ◆ Electronic equipment if appropriate
Pseudobulbar affect (PBA)	◆ Not a mood disorder, but a separate mood disorder may underlie the PBA ◆ SSRIs ◆ TCAs ◆ Dextromethorphan/quinidine (Brooks et al.[49])
Falls, loss of mobility	◆ Early physical and occupational therapy referral ◆ Home nursing referral ◆ Durable medical equipment ◆ Assistive devices ◆ Stretching, range of motion ◆ Positioning, exercises ◆ Anticipating toileting needs ◆ Energy-sparing strategies
Spasticity, cramps, ALS-specific pain	◆ Pain is common in ALS ◆ Opioids ◆ Nonopioids ◆ Balancing opioids with concerns for tenuous respiratory status and patient preferences
Mood disorder, anxiety	◆ Strategies for managing requests for euthanasia/assisted suicide ◆ Increased risk for suicide, suicidal ideation ◆ Treat underlying depression, anxiety
Nutrition	◆ Changes in food and liquid consistency ◆ Smaller, more frequent meals ◆ Ensuring solid foods are soft and moist ◆ Using straws, chin-tuck maneuver if appropriate ◆ Gastrostomy tube if consistent with patient's preferences
Cognitive changes	◆ Frontotemporal dementia, although an unusual presentation, can occur in ALS patients ◆ Managing dementia behaviors
Terminal phase of ALS	◆ Early discussion with patients and caregivers about when to refer to hospice ◆ Highly aggressive symptom management ◆ Palliative sedation has been explored for patients with ALS[46]

therapy, and establishing a routine of exercise and rest are important goals of nursing care. Interestingly, dance therapy and Tai-Chi have been found to improve objective measures of gait and balance for PD.[50–55] As PD and the dopaminomimetic therapies can result in a degree of autonomic instability, the nurse will evaluate for hypotensive episodes and gastrointestinal dysmotility. The speech therapist also has a role in the evaluation of the patient with PD—dysphagia, impaired communication, drooling, and aspiration are common. Fluctuating energy expenditure, medication-food interactions, impaired gastrointestinal motility, and fluid balance leaves patients with PD at risk of nutritional deficiencies. As a result, the nutritionist has a role across the disease trajectory for the patient with PD.[56] One key point for the nurse is the potential for diminished drug absorption when PD medications are taken with protein-rich meals. The psychosocial needs of the patient with PD and the family must be addressed. The nurse assesses for depression, anxiety, and caregiver distress. Grief, feelings of loss, and uncertainty of the future are common. Financial concerns and social isolation should also be addressed. A summary of available medical treatments can be found in Box 19.4. The medication regimens for PD can be complex, and doses are terrifically time-sensitive due to the rapid onset/offset of activity of most levodopa-containing medications. For a select group of patients, surgical intervention has a role. Currently available surgical interventions include deep brain stimulator placement and ablative surgical techniques such as thalamotomy and pallidotomy.

The terminal phase of PD is typically heralded by progressive loss of mobility, worsening dysphagia, and aspiration. Parkinson's-associated dementia can occur as well. The palliative care nurse will expand the goals of nursing intervention to include continence care, preserving patient preferences, managing medication effects, and patient/family education about symptoms at the end of life (Table 19.9).

Huntington's disease

Tracy P. was a young nurse when she pursued genetic testing for Huntington's disease (HD). Tracy's father and uncle both died in their 40s from the disease. Tracy's testing was positive. Tracy's mother and best friend were present when the neurologist and geneticist delivered this news. Mrs. P. stated, "I knew that one of my kids would die of this awful disease. I had prepared myself for that after my husband died, but that doesn't make this easier to bear. I am going to bury my baby girl." Although she was asymptomatic of HD, Tracy knew what the future held for her. Tracy decided that she would neither marry nor have children.

Huntington's disease is characterized by a classical triad—dementia, choreoathetosis, and autosomal dominant inheritance. It is a devastating disease with all-encompassing effects on the patient and family. Indeed, the family is often familiar with the disease—typically a family will have affected members across several generations. Huntington's disease is caused by the accumulation of the huntingtin protein and the resulting destruction of many brain structures, particularly the cerebral cortex and basal ganglia. Repetition of the trinucleic acid CAG encodes for huntingtin on the short arm of chromosome 4. The disease is diagnosed when the number of repeats exceeds 35. Patients are typically diagnosed in the third through the fifth decades of life, although juvenile-onset HD is well established. In the case of Tracy P., she was found to have 52 repeats of CAG. As her case

Box 19.4 Medications commonly used for movement disorders in Parkinson's disease

Levodopa and levodopa-modifying drugs

Levodopa (l-dopa), levodopa/carbidopa (LC), and levodopa/benserazide (LB)

- Mechanism of action: levodopa is the metabolic precursor to dopamine, carbidopa and benserazide increase the availability of levodopa in the central nervous system
- Dosing schedule: to prevent the "on/off" effects of levodopa treatment in some patients, tightly follow the prescribed schedule
- Rationale: increases survival and quality of life
- Adverse effects: nausea and vomiting, psychosis, compulsive behaviors
- Bioavailability of LC and LB when taken with protein-rich meals is reduced

Catechol-O-methyl transferase inhibitors (COMT inhibitors)

- Mechanism of action: decreases metabolism of l-dopa
- Increase the half-life of l-dopa, LC, and LB, simultaneously increasing efficacy of doses
- Available as entacapone and tolcapone
- Leads to longer "on" periods and shorter "off" periods
- Notably does not decrease the dyskinesia effects of l-dopa

Monoamine oxidase inhibitors

- Dopamine metabolizer
- Can reduce the needed dose of l-dopa by 30%–40%

Dopamine angonists

- Often used for initial treatment
- Lower risk of causing dyskinesia
- Available in extended-release formulations
- Shortened "off" time compared with l-dopa
- Risk of compulsive behaviors such as gambling, hypersexual behavior, and eating disorders
- Available in oral formulations, continuous subcutaneous infusion, or as a continuous duodenal infusion via portable minipump
- Apomorphine injection for sudden "off" periods

illustrates, identification of the causative gene has allowed recent generations to make informed life decisions. There is also a psychological burden of knowing that one will die of a devastating neurological disease. The ideal setting for the HD patient is in a multidisciplinary clinic that includes nurses with palliative care training. Affected patients ultimately require care with all personal needs.

Palliative care nursing for the patient with HD ideally begins with early identification. There is currently no cure for HD. Symptoms

Table 19.9 Nursing care in Parkinson's disease

Fatigue, falls, loss of independence	◆ Referral for physical, occupational therapy ◆ Dance therapy ◆ Tai-Chi to improve balance ◆ Home modifications ◆ Home nursing evaluation ◆ Durable medical equipment ◆ Evaluate for hypotensive episodes
Communication and swallowing disorders	◆ Impaired facial expression ("masked face") further impairs functioning ◆ Assess for pseudobulbar affect (PBA) if expressed mood and affect are dyscongruent

must be treated carefully. The most outwardly obvious symptom is the movement disorder. Notably, the chorea may not be bothersome to the patient and should be treated only if it is functionally impairing to the patient. Treating the chorea must be done carefully and ideally with the assistance of a skilled neurologist. Dopamine-blocking agents and dopamine-depleting agents are both used.

Psychiatric disorders in HD are common and highly disabling. The cognitive dysfunction is progressive, but the psychiatric symptoms are typically static. Cognitive dysfunction typically precedes the onset of motor symptoms and evolves into full dementia. In the case of Tracy P., she opted for semiannual neurocognitive evaluation to ensure her patients' safety: "I'd hate to think that someday I'll cause one of my patients harm because I forget a medicine or mis-dose a drug. My neurologist is certain that we'll catch any problem when it's still subtle." The neurocognitive effects of HD are characterized by bradyphrenia, poor spatial memory, diminished working memory, impaired capacity for planning, poor judgment, and decreased mental flexibility. No agent has been found to be effective at delaying the cognitive decline of HD—ACH-ase inhibitors such as donepezil are ineffective.[57] Rivastigmine was studied in a small open-label study with modest improvements in motor function and cognitive impairment but has yet to be replicated in a large phase III trial.[58] Psychiatric disturbances range from emotional lability and behavior disorder to major mood disorder, suicidality, or homicidality. Tracy P. required three psychiatric hospitalizations during the course of her disease, each time for careful titration of medications when she became depressed, delusional, and suicidal.

As HD progresses, end-stage symptoms emerge (Table 19.10). Chorea progresses until the patient is unable to be still for more than a few moments at a time. Eventually, chorea gives way to a hypokinetic, abulic state and then to a vegetative state. Muscles become rigid. Patients may experience tremor, bradykinesia, and dysphagia. Many patients will be placed in residential facilities by this stage. Nursing care involves safety assessment, positioning, and feeding assistance. Patients commonly suffer pain from falls, injuries, and hyperkinetic movements. The palliative care nurse facilitates occupational and physical therapy referrals when necessary. Speech therapy and dietician assistance are also commonly required. Food and drink consistency may be modified, and

Table 19.10 Symptomatic treatment of Huntington's disease

Chorea	◆ Treat carefully and only if distressing to the patient/functionally impairing ◆ Halperidol 2–10 mg/day ◆ Olanzapine has been found to reduce chorea, stabilize mood, and augment antidepressants; may also improve ambulation ◆ Tetrabenzapine improves motor function/suppresses chorea; monitor closely for parkinsonism, mood disorder, suicidality, sedation, akathisia
Parkinsonism of HD	◆ Treated with standard PD therapy ◆ Poor candidates for neurosurgical interventions ◆ Often characterized by rigidity in the terminal stages of disease
Bruxism	◆ Separate from the effects of neuroleptics ◆ Well managed with botulinum toxin
Dystonia	◆ May be painful ◆ Functionally impairing ◆ No specific treatment has been evaluated in trials
Aggressive behavior, mood disorder	◆ Antidepressants ◆ Antipsychotics ◆ Propranolol ◆ Mood stabilizers ◆ Buspirone ◆ Suicidal and homicidal assessment
Sleep-wake cycle disruption	◆ Significant circadian rhythm disturbance ◆ Insomnia is not the dominant feature ◆ Although efficacy is not established, scheduled hypnotics are reported in the literature ◆ Nursing interventions for sleep-wake cycle disturbances[61]

dietary modifications can slow the weight loss. One fascinating feature of HD is weight loss in the setting of preserved appetite.

Certainly the most difficult task is supporting the patient and family through the inevitable decline. Emotional support and evaluation for mood disorder will be ongoing tasks for the nurse. Family and caregiver education will focus on the disease process, and the risk for potentially affected family members. Early discussions about end-of-life preferences are also important. Because of the financial burden of care, the nurse will also facilitate conversation about financial planning. Tracy P. eventually passed away at age 39 in the same nursing facility specializing in HD that cared for her father and uncle.

Multiple sclerosis

Multiple sclerosis is a neuroimmunological disease with widely varying clinical courses. Multiple sclerosis is typically diagnosed in young to middle adulthood. It is more commonly found in people of northern European decent and those living farther from the Equator. Prevalence is estimated at 5 to 200 per 100,000 persons.

Chad T. was a 41-year-old father of two. While working out one morning, Chad felt that his left side "didn't feel right." He saw his internist the following week and was sent for an MRI of the brain and spine. Three white matter lesions were identified. Chad experienced a period of disease stability for 4 years, followed by two relapses within a 3-month period. He developed more lesions on MRI scan. Chad opted for immunomodulatory therapy under the direction of a neurologist.

Multiple sclerosis symptom clusters have been well described in the literature. Although no cure exists for MS at the present, much can be done to alleviate the symptom burden. Cognitive dysfunction is seen in severe disease. Patients describe disabling fatigue, functional impairments, bowel and bladder dysfunction, and sexual dysfunction, among others (Table 19.11).

Managing disability is at the heart of nursing interventions for the patient with MS. Mobility and activities of daily living typically decline as the disease progresses. Early and scheduled physical and occupational therapy assessments are wise. Home and workplace modifications can preserve the patient's functional independence. As with most incurable diseases, emotional support is frequently necessary. Multiple sclerosis is traditionally a disease of young adults—it strikes at a time when the patient may be contemplating marriage and pregnancy. The risk for depression is high. Referral to the MS Society can be helpful for patients—both peer support and case management services are available.

Myasthenia gravis

Myasthenia gravis (MG) is a life-threatening neuroimmunological disease. The disease stems from the destruction of acetylcholine receptors at the neuromuscular junction. The common presentation is a patient with fluctuating weakness of the muscles, especially the muscles innervated by brainstem motor neurons. Weakness can be induced with repetitive movement and strength is restored with rest. Strength is characteristically restored dramatically with anticholinesterase drugs.

Table 19.11 Managing symptoms of multiple sclerosis

Fatigue	Neurostimulants
	Amantadine
	Regular exercise
	Planned rest breaks, energy-sparing techniques
Cognitive dysfunction	Neuropsychological assessment
Neurogenic bladder: urinary frequency, urgency, bladder spasticity, incomplete emptying	Urinary retention:
	♦ Bethanechol
	♦ Intermittent catheterization
	♦ Monitor and treat high postvoid residual volumes to reduce risk of urinary tract infection
	Frequency and urgency:
	♦ Propantheline, oxybutynin
Sexual dysfunction	Men: PDE-5 inhibitors
Pain	Pain assessment
	Traditional methods of pain control can be effective, especially neuroleptics, gabapentin, tricyclic antidepressants
Tremor	Severe postural tremor can respond to isoniazide with pyridoxine[62]
	Carbamazepine
	Clonazepam
	Limb weights of small poundage applied to the wrists
Neurogenic bowel	Prescribed bowel program of:
	♦ Scheduled toileting (especially after eating or exercising)
	♦ Stool softeners, laxatives, suppositories, enemas if needed
	♦ Digital rectal stimulation if needed
Mood disorder	Aggressive management of depression
	Referral for neuropsychological testing

Table 19.12 Symptoms of intracranial lesion by location

Structure	Normal function	Altered function in the presence of tumor
Frontal lobe	Personality Voluntary skeletal movements Fine repetitive motor movements Eye movements	Personality change or disinhibition Altered responses to stimuli, emotional lability Difficulty with speaking, chewing, or facial expressions Uncoordinated swallowing, or movement of hands, arms, torso, pelvis, legs, and feet
Parietal lobe	Sensory processing: tactile, visual, gustatory, olfactory, auditory, body position	Trouble integrating language, vision, and tactile stimuli Loss of sense of body positioning or vibratory sense Difficulty with verbal and nonverbal memory Paresthesias Loss of tactile discrimination Inability to write or do math calculations
Occipital lobe	Interpretation of visual input	Difficulty naming visual images and words Difficulty reading and writing, identifying colors Inability to identify if an object is moving
Temporal lobe	Auditory perception and interpretation	*Right lobe:* Difficulty hearing, understanding, organizing, and concentrating on what is seen or heard Inability to recognize musical tones and nonspeech information such as illustrations Olfactory or gustatory hallucinations Vertigo, unsteadiness, or tinnitus *Left lobe:* Difficulty hearing and with understanding, organizing, and concentrating on what is seen or heard Inability to recognize spoken words Vertigo, unsteadiness, or tinnitus
Cerebellum	Processing of sensory information from eyes, ears, and tactile and musculoskeletal receptors Refining motor activity into coordinated movement	Frequent loss of balance, unstable posture or gait Uncoordinated movement of extremities Alterations of some reflexive movements Nystagmus, muscle tremors, or ataxia
Brainstem and cranial nerves (CN)	*Brainstem:* Gateway from cerebrum and cerebellum to spinal cord. Maintains consciousness, cardiovascular and respiratory functioning Relays motor and sensory information *Cranial nerves:* Nuclei of cranial nerves III-XII arise within the brainstem structures	CN I: loss of smell (anosmia) CN II: vision compromise, visual field defect CN III: loss of pupillary constriction and ability to raise eyelid, extraocular movements, diplopia CN IV: loss of inferior/medial eye movement CN V: inability to clench jaw and chew, numbness of mouth and nose, numbness of face, loss of corneal reflex CN VI: inability to abduct the eye CN VII: facial paralysis, taste disturbance, salivary and lacrimal dysfunction CN VIII: loss of hearing, disequilibrium CN IX: swallowing difficulty, taste disturbance CN X: loss of ear sensation, GI disturbance, voice hoarseness CN XI: difficulty turning head and shrugging shoulders CN XII: difficulty swallowing and articulating lingual sounds

Madeline V. presented with shortness of breath to the emergency room. The ER physician noted Madeline's eyes were droopy and ordered a urine toxicology screen and a neurology consult. The toxicology screen was negative, but the neurologist admitted Madeline to the intensive care unit. Her bedside respiratory function tests on arrival to the intensive care unit revealed that Madeline was suffering from dramatically reduced inspiratory capacity. Before the afternoon was out, Madeline was intubated and on mechanical ventilation for respiratory failure.

Myasthenia gravis was once a fatal disease shortly after diagnosis. Discovery of anticholinesterase inhibiting medications has allowed many patients with MG to pursue full lives. Although there is no cure for MG, many with MG enjoy a full life. Treatment is initiated with thymectomy—hyperplastic thymus tissue is found in 70% of newly diagnosed patients with MG.[59] Anticholinesterase medications and immunomodulation are the backbone of therapy. Symptom control focuses on managing and preventing acute MG crisis. During crisis, palliative management focuses on symptoms of dyspnea and anxiety. In the long-term care of patients with MG, careful discussions about intubation and the possibility of prolonged mechanical ventilation are warranted. Some patients will ultimately require tracheostomy.

Intracranial lesions

Intracranial tumors encompass both primary and metastatic tumors and may involve cerebrospinal fluid, bony structures of the skull and skull base, dura, and cranial nerves. Cancers that commonly metastasize to the central nervous system are lung, melanoma, renal cell carcinoma, breast, and colorectal. The most common primary central nervous system tumors include meningioma, the gliomas, embryonal tumors such as medulloblastoma, and primary central nervous system lymphoma.[60] The palliative care goals will be different for the patient with widely metastatic cancer, newly diagnosed intracranial metastases but stable system disease, and the patient with primary central nervous system tumors. A thoughtful discussion with the oncologist can be immensely helpful for the nurse in any of these settings. Symptoms of intracranial lesions vary widely by location of tumor (Table 19.12). Notably, patients with intracranial lesions can be asymptomatic.

Symptoms from central nervous system tumors result from edema, infiltration of normal brain by tumors, and mass effect—displacement of normal brain structures. The concern in cases of large lesions or significant edema is for brain herniation. Herniation involves displacement of a piece of brain tissue under a rigid structure such as the foramen magnum, tentorium, or falx cerebrii. There are six distinct herniation syndromes: uncal (transtentorial), central, cingulate (subfalcine), transcalvarial, upward cerebellar, and tonsillar (downward cerebellar). In the uncal herniation, most common herniation syndrome, the medial temporal gyrus compresses the brainstem and nearby cranial nerves. This scenario is typically heralded by an ipsilateral third cranial nerve palsy (the pupil fails to constrict when stimulated with light and the eye deviates inferiorly and laterally). Treatment for the palliative care patient typically incorporates high-potency corticosteroids. Corticosteroids restore the blood-brain barrier by reducing the permeability of vascular endothelial cells and thus reducing intracranial pressure. Steroids can alleviate headache and pain from metastases. The nurse will also avoid hypotonic intravenous solutions (this includes all dextrose-containing IV solutions except D5 0.9% NS). In emergency and intensive care situations, hypertonic intravenous solutions such as mannitol and 3% saline are used. This intervention is for short-term situations only as the brain gradually increases osmolality. Controlled hyperventilation is also used in these scenarios, although it is typically reserved for aggressive last-ditch efforts. In scenarios where it is consistent with goals of care, neurosurgical intervention may be appropriate. For the patient with impending herniation, removal of a portion of the skull (craniectomy) and lobectomy may be performed. Some

patients may benefit from removal of the lesion—this applies to patients with most primary central nervous system tumors and to some patients with metastatic disease.

Seizures are not uncommon with intracranial tumors. Typically, seizures from primary brain tumors are focal in onset and can have localizing significance. Seizures from all intracranial tumors are usually well managed with AEDs. Seizures also tend to respond well to lesionectomy. Patients with seizures from primary central nervous system tumors will usually experience improved seizure control with tumor treatment. Patients with known intracranial tumors who have not experienced a seizure do not require prophylactic treatment with AEDs.[6]

Conclusion

Arguably, the role of the palliative care nurse is first to alleviate suffering and second to advocate for the patient's choices. The task of assisting the patient to identify his or her healthcare choices in the face of a devastating and often terminal neurological illness is no easy one. Several other themes emerge—advocating for early therapy referral, pain control, bowel and bladder care, preserving functional abilities, maintaining patients' independence, and providing education about medications and disease processes.

Additional resources

Seizures

Care of the Patient with Seizures. 2nd ed. American Association of Neuroscience Nurses Clinical Practice Guideline Series. 2007. www.aann.org/pdf/cpg/aannseizures.pdf.

General resources

DeAngelis L, Posner J. Neurologic Complications of Cancer. 2nd ed. New York: Oxford University Press; 2009.

Spasticity

NINDS Spasticity Information Page
http://www.ninds.nih.gov/disorders/spasticity/spasticity.htm
NINDS Motor Neuron Fact Sheet
http://www.ninds.nih.gov/disorders/motor_neuron_diseases/
    detail_motor_neuron_diseases.htm

Headache and migraine

International Headache Society. Headache Classifications. 2nd ed.
http://www.ihs-headache.org/upload/ct_clas/ihc_II_main_no_
    print.pdf.
Kelman L. The triggers or precipitants of the acute migraine attack. Cephalalgia. 2007;27:394–402. doi: 10.1111/j.1468-2982 .2007.01303.x.

Aphasia

American Speech-Language-Hearing Association
http://www.asha.org/public/speech/disorders/aphasia.htm
National Aphasia Association
http://aphasia.org/
Aphasia Hope Foundation
http://www.aphasiahope.org/
Academy of Neurologic Communication Disorders Science
http://www.ancds.org/

Amyotrophic lateral sclerosis

ALS Foundation Guide to Nursing Care for Patients with ALS
http://www.alsa.org/als-care/resources/publications-videos/fact-sheets/nursing-management-in-als.html

Mitsumoto H, Rabkin JG. Palliative care for patients with amyotrophic lateral sclerosis: "Prepare for the worst and hope for the best." JAMA. 2007;298(2):207–216.

Torres AL. The management of respiratory insufficiency in patients with ALS. Home healthcare nurse. 2012;30(3):186–194. doi: 10.1097/NHH.0b013e318246d45a.

McCluskey L. Amyotrophic lateral sclerosis: ethical issues from diagnosis to end of life. Neurorehabilitation [serial online]. 2007;22(6):463–472.

Parkinson's disease

Johnson ML. Parkinson's disease: speech and swallowing. National Parkinson Foundation. http://www3.parkinson.org/site/DocServer/Speech___Swallowing.pdf?docID=193&JServSessionIdr004=2u6sv9pks2.app337a.

National Parkinson Foundation
www.parkinson.org

Intracranial lesions

AANN Guide to Care of the Patient After Craniotomy

References

1. Hauser WA, Beghi E. First seizure definitions and worldwide incidence and mortality. Epilepsia. 2008;49(s1):8–12.
2. Westphal-Guitti AC, Alonso NB, Migliorini RC, et al. Quality of life and burden in caregivers of patients with epilepsy. J Neurosci Nurs. 2007;39(6):354–360.
3. Wheless JW. Intractable epilepsy: a survey of patients and caregivers. Epilepsy Behav. 2006;8(4):756–764.
4. Loring DW, Meador KJ, Lee GP. Determinants of quality of life in epilepsy. Epilepsy Behav. 2004;5(6):976–980.
5. Dev R, Parsons HA, Palla S, Palmer JL, Del Fabbro E, Bruera E. Undocumented alcoholism and its correlation with tobacco and illegal drug use in advanced cancer patients. Cancer. 2011;117(19):4551–4556.
6. Glantz MJ, Cole BF, Forsyth PA, Recht LD, Wen PY, Chamberlain MC, Grossman SA, Cairncross JG. Practice parameter: anticonvulsant prophylaxis in patients with newly diagnosed brain tumors. Neurology. 2000;54:1886–1893.
7. Wright AW, Mather LE, Smith MT. Hydromorphine-3-glucuronide: a more potent neuro-excitant than its structural analogue, morphine-3-glucuronide. Life Sci. 2001;69:409–420.
8. Gretton SK, Ross JR, Rutter D, Sato H, Droney JM, Welsh KI, Joel S, Riley J. Plasma morphine and metabolite concentrations are associated with clinical effects of morphine in cancer patients. J Pain Symptom Manage. 2013;45(4):670–680.
9. Hemstapat K, Monteith GR, Smith D, Smith MT. Morphine-3-glucuronide's neuro-excitatory effects are mediated via indirect activation of N-methyl-D-aspartic acid receptors: mechanistic studies in embryonic cultured hippocampal neurones. Anesth Analg. 2003;97:494–505.
10. Smith MT. Neuroexcitatory effects of morphine and hydromorphone: evidence implicating the 3-glucuronide metabolites. Clin Exp Pharmacol Physiol. 2000;27:524–528.
11. Mercadante S. Pathophysiology and treatment of opioid-related myoclonus in cancer patients. Pain. 1998;74:5–9.
12. Portenoy RK, Khan E, Layman M, Lapin J, Malkin MG, Foley KM, et al. Chronic morphine therapy for cancer pain: plasma and cerebrospinal fluid morphine and morphine-6-glucuronide concentrations. Neurology. 1991;41:1457–1461.
13. Lee MA, Leng ME, Tiernan EJ. Retrospective study of the use of hydromorphone in palliative care patients with normal and abnormal urea and creatinine. Palliat Med. 2001;15:26–34.
14. Klepstad P, Borchgrevink PC, Dale O, Zahlsen K, Aamo T, Fayers P, et al. Routine drug monitoring of serum concentrations of morphine, morphine-3-glucuronide and morphine-6-glucuroide do not predict clinical observations in cancer patients. Palliat Med. 2003;17:679–687.
15. Essandoh S, Sakae M, Miller J, Glare PA. A cautionary tale from critical care: resolution of myoclonus after fentanyl rotation to hydromorphone. J Pain Symptom Manage. 2010;40(5):e4–e6.
16. Ito S, Liao S. Myoclonus associated with high-dose parenteral methadone. J Palliat Med. 2008;11(6):838–841.
17. Patel S, Roshan VR, Lee KC, Cheung RJ. A myoclonic reaction with low-dose hydromorphone. Ann Pharmacother. 2006;40(11):2068–2070.
18. Sarhill N, Davis MP, Walsh D, Nouneh C. Methadone-induced myoclonus in advanced cancer. Am J Hosp Palliat Care. 2001;18(1):51–53.
19. Kaiko RF, Foley KM, Grabinski PY, Heidrich G, Rogers AG, Inturrisi CE, Reidenberg MM. Central nervous system excitatory effects of meperidine in cancer patients. Ann Neurol. 1983;13(2):180–185.
20. Cherny N, Ripamonti C, Pereira J, Davis C, Fallon M, McQuay H, et al.; Expert Working Group of the European Association of Palliative Care Network. Strategies to manage the adverse effects of oral morphine: an evidence-based report. J Clin Oncol. 20011;19(9):2542–2554.
21. Parsons HA, de la Cruz M, El Osta B, Li Z, Calderon B, Palmer JL, Bruera E. Methadone initiation and rotation in the outpatient setting for patients with cancer pain. Cancer. 2010;116(2):520–528.
22. Stone P, Minton O. European Palliative Care Research collaborative pain guidelines. Central side-effects management: what is the evidence to support best practice in the management of sedation, cognitive impairment and myoclonus? Palliat Med. 2011;25(5):431–441.
23. Corey-Bloom J, Wolfson T, Gamst A, Jin S, Marcotte TD, Bentley H, Gouaux B. Smoked cannabis for spasticity in multiple sclerosis: a randomized placebo-controlled trial. CMAJ: Can Med Assoc J. 2012;184(10):1143–1150.
24. Collin C, Davies P, Mutiboko IK, Ratcliffe S; Sativex Spasticity in MS Study Group. Randomized controlled trial of cannabis-based medicine in spasticity caused by multiple sclerosis. Eur J Neurol. 2007;14(3):290–296.
25. Guillaume D, Van Havenbergh A, Vloeberghs M, Vidal J, Roeste G. A clinical study of intrathecal baclofen using a programmable pump for intractable spasticity. Arch Phys Med Rehabil. 2005;86:2165–2171.
26. Staal C, Arends A, Ho S. A self-report of quality of life of patients receiving intrathecal baclofen therapy. Rehabil Nurs. 2003;28(5):159–163.
27. Rasmussen BK, Jensen R, Schroll M, Olesen J. Epidemiology of headache in a general population—a prevalence study. J Clin Epidemiol. 1991;44:1147–1157.
28. Lipton RB, Stewart WF, Diamond S, et al. Prevalence and burden of migraine in the United States: data from the American Migraine Study II. Headache. 2001;41(7):646–657.
29. Rapaport AM. Medication overuse headache: awareness, detection and treatment. CNS Drugs. 2008;22(12):995–1004.
30. Ashina S, Bendtsen L, Ashina M. Pathophysiology of tension-type headache. Curr Pain Headache Rep. 2005;9(6):415–422.
31. El Kamar FG, Posner JB. Brain metastases. Semin Neurol. 2004;24(4):347–362.
32. Norton A, Zipse L, Marchina S, Schlaug G. Melodic intonation therapy: shared insights on how it is done and why it might help. Ann NY Acad Sci. 2009;1169:431–436. doi: 10.1111/j.1749-6632.2009.04859.x.
33. Chio A, Calvo A, Moglia C, Mazzini L, Mora G; ParALS Study Group. Phenotypic heterogeneity of amyotrophic lateral sclerosis: a population based study. J Neurol Neurosurg Psychiatry. 2011;82(7):740–746. doi: 10.1136/jnnp.2010.235952

34. Fecto F, Siddique T. UBQLN2/P62 cellular recycling pathways in amyotrophic lateral sclerosis and frontotemporal dementia. Muscle Nerve. 2012;45(2):157–162. doi: 10.1002/mus.23278.

35. Turner MR, Parton MJ, Shaw CE, Leigh PN, Al-Chalabi A. Prolonged survival in motor neuron disease: a descriptive study of the King's database 1990–2002. J Neurol Neurosurg Psychiatry. 2003;74(7):995–997. doi: 10.1136/jnnp.74.7.995

36. Bensimon G, Lacomblez L, Delumeau JC, Bejuit R, Truffinet P, Meininger V. A study of riluzole in the treatment of advanced stage or elderly patients with amyotrophic lateral sclerosis. J Neurol. 2002;249(5):609–615.

37. Lewis, M, Rushanan S. The role of physical therapy and occupational therapy in the treatment of amyotrophic lateral sclerosis. NeuroRehabilitation. 2007;22(6):451–461.

38. Greenwood DI. Nutrition management of amyotrophic lateral sclerosis. Nutr Clin Pract. 2013;28(3):392–399.

39. Park JH, Seong-Woong K. Percutaneous radiologic gastrostomy in patients with amyotrophic lateral sclerosis on noninvasive ventilation. Arch Phys Med Rehabil. 2009;90:1026–1029.

40. Mitsumoto H, Rabkin JG. Palliative care for patients with amyotrophic lateral sclerosis: "Prepare for the worst and hope for the best." JAMA. 2007;298(2):207–215.

41. Ball L, Beukelman D, Pattee G. Augmentative and alternative communication acceptance by persons with amyotrophic lateral sclerosis. Augment Altern Commun. 2004;20(2):113–123.

42. Miller RG, Rosenberg JA, Gelinas DF, et al. Practice parameter: the care of the patient with amyotrophic lateral sclerosis (an evidence-based review). Neurology. 1999;52:1311–1323.

43. Kasarskis EJ, Hodskins J, St Clair WH. Unilateral parotid electron beam radiotherapy as palliative treatment for sialorrhea in amyotrophic lateral sclerosis. J Neurol Sci. 2011;308:155–157.

44. Stalpers LJA, Moser EC. Results of radiotherapy for drooling in amyotrophic lateral sclerosis. J Otolaryngol. 2001;30:242–245.

45. Scott KR, Kothari MJ, Simmons Z, et al. Parotid gland injections of botulinum toxin a are effective in amyotrophic lateral sclerosis. J Clin Dis. 2005;7(2):62–65.

46. Berger JT. Preemptive use of palliative sedation and amyotrophic lateral sclerosis. J Pain Symptom Manage. 2012;43(4):802–805.

47. Ganzini L, Johnston WS, Silveria MJ. The final month of life in patients with ALS. Neurology. 2002;59:428–431.

48. Veldink JH, Wokke JH, van der Wal G, Vianney de Jong JM, van den Berg LH. Euthanasia and physician-assisted suicide among patients with amyotrophic lateral sclerosis in the Netherlands. N Engl J Med. 2002; 346:1638–1644.

49. Brooks BR, Thisted RA, Appel SH, Bradley WG, Olney RK, Berg JE, et al.; AVP-923 ALS Study Group. Treatment of pseudobulbar affect in ALS with dextromethorphan/quinidine: a randomized trial. Neurology. 2004;63(8):1364–1370.

50. Hackney ME, Earhart GM. Effects of dance on gait and balance in Parkinson's disease: a comparison of partnered and nonpartnered dance movement. Neurorehabil Neural Repair. 2010;24(4):384–392.

51. Duncan RP, Earhart GM. Randomized controlled trial of community-based dancing to modify disease progression in Parkinson's disease. Neurorehabil Neural Repair. 2012;26(2):132–143.

52. Klein PJ, Rivers I. Taiji for individuals with Parkinson's disease and their support partners: a program evaluation. J Neurol Phys Ther. 2006;30(1):22–27.

53. Li F, Harmer P, Fisher JK, Xu J, Fitzgerald K, Vongjaturapat N. Tai Chi-based exercise for older adults with Parkinson's disease: a pilot-program evaluation. J Aging Phys Act. 2007;15(2):139–151.

54. Hackney ME, Earhart GM. Tai chi improves balance and mobility in people with Parkinson disease. Gait Posture. 2008;28(3):456–460. doi: 10.1016/j.gaitpost.2008.02.005.

55. Li F, Harmer P, Fitzgerald K, Eckstrom E, Stock R, Galver J, et al. Tai chi and postural stability in patients with Parkinson's disease. NEJM. 2012;366(6):511–519. doi: 10.1056/NEJMoa1107911.

56. Barichella M, Cereda E, Pezzoli G. Major nutritional issues in the management of Parkinson's disease. Mov Disord. 2009;24(13):1881–1892. doi: 10.1002/mds.22705.

57. Cubo E, Shannon KM, Tracy D, Jaglin JA, Bernard BA, Wuu J, et al. Effect of donepezil on motor and cognitive function in Huntington disease. Neurology. 2006;67(7):1268–1271.

58. DeTommaso M, et al. Two years' follow-up of rivastigmine treatment in Huntington disease. Clin Neuropharmacol. 2007;30:43–46.

59. Mao ZF, Xue-An M, Qin C, Lai Y-R, Hacket ML. Incidence of thymoma in myasthenia gravis: a systematic review. J Clin Neurol. 2012;8(3):161–169.

60. CBTUS (Central Brain Tumor Registry of the United States) 2012. CBTRUS Statistical Report: Primary Brain and Central Nervous System Tumors Diagnosed in the United States in 2004–2008 (March 13, 2012 revision). Central Brain Tumor Registry of the United States, Hinsdale, IL.

61. Song Y, Dowling GA, Wallhagen MI, Lee KA, Strawbridge WJ. Sleep in older adults with Alzheimer's disease. J Neurosci Nurs. 2010; 42(4): 190–198.

62. Hallett M, Lindsey JW, Adelstein BD, Riley PO. Controlled trial of isoniazid therapy for severe postural cerebellar tumor in multiple sclerosis. Neurology. 1985; 35(9): 1347–1377.

CHAPTER 20

Anxiety and depression

Jeannie V. Pasacreta, Pamela A. Minarik,
Leslie Nield-Anderson, and Judith A. Paice

I cannot live like this—I am no good to anyone and am a burden to everyone.

Palliative care patient

Key points

- The psychosocial issues in persons facing life-threatening illness are influenced by individual, sociocultural, medical, and family factors.

- Emotional turmoil may occur at times of transition in the disease course.

- Anxiety and depression are common symptoms in individuals facing chronic or life-threatening illness but should not be regarded as an inevitable consequence of advanced disease.

- These symptoms warrant evaluation and appropriate use of pharmacological and psychosocial interventions.

This chapter provides information regarding the assessment and treatment of anxiety and depression among individuals faced with chronic or life-threatening illness, and delineates psychosocial interventions that are effective at minimizing these troubling symptoms. Practical guidelines regarding patient management and identification of patients who may require formal psychiatric consultation, are offered.

Case study

Ms. Johnson, a patient with depression

Ms. Johnson, a 50-year-old woman with advanced lung cancer told the oncology nurse during chemotherapy infusion that she did not want to go on with therapy any longer, despite the fact that she denied adverse effects. When asked to explain her decision, the patient stated, "It is hopeless—why bother?" In further discussion with the nurse she described lifelong anxiety, which had worsened to the point that she could not sleep during the night due to intrusive thoughts of death. She felt guilty that she might have contributed to the development of cancer through a long history of smoking. She was also depressed and withdrawn, not wanting to see her adult children or other family members. The anxiety and hopelessness together were overwhelming, and she could not focus on anything else.

Changes in healthcare that have accentuated psychiatric symptoms

Changes in healthcare delivery and rapid scientific gains are simultaneously increasing the number of individuals receiving or in need of palliative care at any given time, the longevity and course of chronic diseases, and the prevalence and intensity of the psychological symptoms that accompany them.[1,2] Furthermore, psychological distress is experienced within an increasingly complex, fragmented, and impersonal healthcare system that tends to intensify these symptoms. Despite these realities, psychological symptoms receive minimal attention, and healthcare providers often lack the needed education and support regarding assessment, treatment, and referral of these common problems.

Advances in science and technology have moved the crisis of a life-threatening medical diagnosis to the prediagnostic period, extending life expectancy and the number of treatment courses delivered over a lifetime. Individuals are being diagnosed earlier and living longer, with increasing opportunities to experience simultaneous, interrelated psychosocial and medical comorbidity. The human genome project has, theoretically and in some cases, practically, moved the psychosocial implications of chronic disease into the prediagnostic period. Concurrent treatment discoveries have increased quantity of life, albeit with ill-defined consequences to quality of life.[2,3] For example, an individual who learns of an inherited predisposition to cancer at age 25, is diagnosed at age 50, and receives intermittent treatment until death at age 79, incurs innumerable insults to her mental health and psychological well-being.

Soaring medical costs, managed-care arrangements, and the stigma associated with mental illness, have simultaneously placed a low priority on the recognition and treatment of psychosocial distress within our healthcare system. There is abundant documentation that psychiatric morbidity, particularly depression and anxiety, enhances vulnerability and creates formidable barriers to integrated healthcare.[3] Psychological factors have long been implicated as barriers to disease prevention, early diagnosis, and comprehensive treatment.[3,4] Lack of assessment and treatment of the common psychiatric sequelae to chronic disease have been linked to such problems as treatment-resistant depression and anxiety, family dysfunction, lack of compliance with prevention and treatment recommendations, potentiation of physical symptoms, and suicide, to name just a few.[3-6] These issues create long-term problems that drive up healthcare expenses and diminish access, quality, and efficiency of care. In healthcare settings, physical problems assume priority in the growing competition for scarce resources. Clinicians confronted with ambiguous symptoms are likely to interpret them within diagnostic paradigms most consistent to their specialty and theoretical orientation. As a consequence, the psychological symptoms that accompany life-threatening conditions may be interpreted and treated inappropriately, rendering care that is not comprehensive or cost effective.

We are at a critical juncture in the evolution of healthcare in this country. Systems are being overwhelmed by serious, often preventable, diseases that are not being treated comprehensively after diagnosis. Furthermore, in spite of cutting-edge therapies, a significant number of individuals experience unfavorable outcomes. As budget constraints limit the use of psychiatric specialists, these issues have intensified, and the importance of educating "front-line" health providers to recognize and address psychiatric morbidity is compelling. In a healthcare system focused largely on pathogenesis, cure, and cost, psychological symptoms are all too often unrecognized and untreated in clinical settings, despite their insidious harm to patients As psychiatric consultation-liaison nurses, who work primarily in nonpsychiatric settings, the authors have been consistently struck by the limited knowledge of nursing and medical staff regarding key signs and symptoms that characterize depression and anxiety in the medically ill. Often, young patients with particularly poor prognoses, who elicit anxiety and sadness from staff, are referred for psychiatric evaluation, while their objectively depressed or anxious counterparts are not.

In dealing with depressed and/or anxious patients referred for evaluation, the decision to intervene with psychotherapy or pharmacological agents may be based largely on the philosophy, educational background, and past experience of individual clinicians. Not uncommonly, a diagnosis of clinical anxiety or depression is ruled out if the symptoms seem reactive and "appropriate" to the situation, or are viewed as organic in nature. Patients who exhibit depressive or anxious symptoms not considered severe enough to classify for "psychiatric" status are frequently not offered psychotherapeutic services, and the natural history of their symptoms is rarely monitored over time. The lack of attention to assessment and treatment of depression and anxiety among the medically ill may, for example, lead to ongoing dysphoria, family conflict, noncompliance with treatment, increased length of hospitalization, persistent worry, and suicidal ideation. Because depression and anxiety are common among individuals with chronic illness, recognition and management of these symptoms is extremely important, particularly because they are often responsive to treatment. Patients, family, and professional caregivers need to be informed of the factors that affect psychological adjustment, the wide range of psychological responses that accompany chronic and progressive disease, and the efficacy of various modes of intervention.

The clinical course of chronic illness

Acute stress is a common response to the diagnosis of a life-threatening illness, and resurfaces at transitional points in the disease process (beginning treatment, recurrence, treatment failure, disease progression).[7] The response is characterized by shock, disbelief, anxiety, depression, sleep and appetite disturbance, and difficulty performing activities of daily living. Under favorable circumstances, these psychological symptoms should resolve within a short period.[7,8] The time period is variable, but consensus is that once the crisis has passed, and the individual knows what to expect in terms of a treatment plan, psychological symptoms diminish.[7,9] Patients who are diagnosed with late-stage disease, or have aggressive illnesses with no hope for cure, are often most vulnerable to psychological distress—particularly anxiety, depression, family problems, and physical discomfort.

Diagnostic phase

The period from time of diagnosis through initiation of a treatment plan is characterized by medical evaluation, the development of new relationships with unfamiliar medical personnel, and the need to integrate a barrage of information that, at best, is frightening and confusing. Patients and families frequently experience a heightened sense of responsibility, worry, and isolation during this period. They are particularly anxious and fearful when receiving initial information regarding diagnosis and treatment. Consequently, care should be taken by professionals to repeat information over several sessions and to inquire about patients' and families' understanding of the facts and treatment options. Weissman and colleagues described the first 100 days following a cancer diagnosis as the period of "existential plight."[8] Psychological distress varied according to patient diagnosis. Individuals with late-stage lung cancer were more distressed than individuals with early-stage disease, supporting the need for palliative care services directed toward psychological symptoms.

During the diagnostic period, patient concerns commonly focus on existential issues of life and death, rather than on concerns related to health, work, finances, religion, self, or relationships with family and friends. While it is unusual to observe extreme and sustained emotional reactions as the first response to diagnosis, it is important to assess the nature of early reactions because they are often predictive of later adaptation.[10,11] Early assessment by clinicians can help to identify individuals at risk for later adjustment problems or psychiatric disorders, and in the greatest need of ongoing psychosocial support.[7,12]

The initial response to diagnosis may be profoundly influenced by a person's prior association with a particular disease.[13] Those with memories of close relatives with the same illness often demonstrate heightened distress, particularly if the relative died or had negative treatment experiences. During the diagnostic period, patients may search for explanations or causes for their disease and may struggle to give personal meaning to their experience. Since many clinicians are guarded about disclosing information until a firm diagnosis is established, patients may develop highly personal explanations that can be inaccurate and provoke intensely negative emotions. Ongoing involvement and accurate information will minimize uncertainty and the development of maladaptive coping strategies based on erroneous beliefs.

While the literature substantiates the devastating emotional impact of a life-threatening chronic illness, it also well documents that many individuals cope effectively. Positive coping strategies, such as taking action and finding favorable characteristics in the situation, have been reported to be effective.[14] Contrary to the beliefs of many clinicians, denial also has been found to assist patients in coping effectively,[15] unless sustained and used excessively to a point that it interferes with appropriate treatment. Healthcare practitioners play an important role in monitoring and supporting the patient's and family's psychosocial adjustment. With an awareness of the unique meaning the individual associates with the diagnosis, it is critical that practitioners keep patients informed and involved in their care. Even though patients may not be offered hope for cure, other hopes and goals to be achieved can be offered. Assisting the patient and family in maintaining comfort and control helps to facilitate adaptation and improved quality of life.

Recurrence and progressive disease

Development of a recurrence after a disease-free interval can be especially devastating for patients and those close to them. The point of recurrence often signals a shift into a period of disease progression, and is clearly a time when palliative care services aimed at alleviating psychological symptoms are indicated. The medical workup may be difficult and anxiety-provoking[16]; psychosocial problems experienced at the time of diagnosis frequently resurface, often with greater intensity.[17,18] Shock and depression are not uncommon after relapse, and require individuals and their families to reevaluate the future. This period is a difficult one, during which patients may also experience pessimism, renewed preoccupation with death and dying, and feelings of helplessness and disenchantment with the medical system. Patients tend to be more guarded and cautious at this time and feel as if they are in limbo.[18] Silverfarb and colleagues[18] examined emotional distress in a cross-sectional study of 146 women with breast cancer at three points in the clinical course (diagnosis, recurrence, stage-of-disease progression). The point of recurrence was found to be the most distressing time, with an increase in depression, anxiety, and suicidal ideation. As a disease progresses, the person frequently reports an upsetting scenario that includes frequent pain, disability, increased dependence on others, and diminished functional ability, which then potentiates psychological symptoms.[19] Investigators studying quality of life in cancer patients have demonstrated a clear relationship between an individual's perception of quality of life and the presence of discomfort.[20] As uncomfortable symptoms increase, perceived quality of life diminishes. Thus, an important goal in the psychosocial treatment of patients with advanced chronic illness focuses on symptom control.

An issue that repeatedly surfaces among patients, family members, and professional care providers deals with the use of aggressive treatment protocols in the presence of progressive disease. Often, patients and families request to participate in experimental protocols even when there is little likelihood of extending survival. Controversy continues about the efficacy of such therapies, and the role health professionals can play in facilitating patients' choices about participating. These issues become even more important because changes in the healthcare system may limit payment for costly and highly technical treatments, such as hematopoietic stem cell transplants. It is essential for healthcare professionals to establish structured dialogue with patients, family members, and care providers regarding treatment goals and expectations. Despite the existence of progressive illness, certain individuals may respond to investigational treatment with increased hope. Efforts to separate and clarify values, thoughts, and emotional reactions of care providers, patients, and families to these delicate issues, are important if individualized care with attention to psychological symptoms is to be provided. Use of resources such as psychiatric consultation-liaison nurses, psychiatrists, psychologists, social workers, and chaplains can be invaluable in assisting patients, family members, and staff to grapple with these issues in a meaningful and productive manner.

Terminal disease and dying

Once the terminal period has begun, it is usually not the fact of dying but the quality of dying that is the overwhelming issue confronting the patient and family.[21,22] Continued palliative care into the terminal stage of cancer relieves physical and psychological symptoms, promotes comfort, and increases well-being. Patients and families who have received such services along the illness trajectory have been found to be more open and accepting of palliative efforts in the final stage of life.

Patients living in the final phase of any advanced chronic illness experience fears and anxiety related to uncertain future events, such as unrelieved pain, separation from loved ones, burden on family, and loss of control. Psychological distress is more likely in persons confronting diminished life span, physical debilitation associated with functional limitation, and/or symptoms associated with toxic therapies.[20,23] Therapeutic interventions should be directed toward increasing patients' sense of control and self-efficacy within the context of functional decline and increased dependence. In addition, if patients so desire, it is often therapeutic to let them know that there is help available to discuss the existential concerns that often accompany terminal illness. Personal values and beliefs, socioeconomic and cultural background, and religious belief systems influence patients' expectations about quality of life and palliative care. Cultural affiliation can have a significant influence on perception of pain. Awareness of the family system's cultural, religious, ethnic, and socioeconomic background is important to the understanding of their beliefs, attitudes, practices, and behaviors related to illness and death.[24] Cultural patterns play a significant role in determining how individuals and families cope with illness and death.[25,26]

Delirium, depression, suicidal ideation, and severe anxiety are among the most common psychiatric complications encountered in terminally ill cancer patients.[27] When severe, these problems require urgent and aggressive assessment and treatment by psychiatric personnel, who can initiate pharmacological and psychotherapeutic treatment strategies. Psychiatric emergencies require the same rapid intervention as distressing physical symptoms and medical crises. In spite of the seemingly overwhelming nature of psychosocial responses along the chronic illness trajectory, most patients do indeed cope effectively. Periods of intense emotions, such as anxiety and depression, are not necessarily the same as maladaptive coping.

Factors that affect psychological adjustment

Psychological responses to chronic illness vary widely and are influenced by many individual factors. A review of the literature points to key factors that may impact psychological adjustment

Table 20.1 Common medical conditions associated with anxiety and depression

Anxiety	Depression
◆ Endocrine disorders: hyperthyroidism and hypothyroidism, hyperglycemia and hypoglycemia, Cushing's disease, carcinoid syndrome, pheochromocytoma	◆ Cardiovascular: cardiovascular disease, congestive heart failure, myocardial infarct, cardiac arrhythmias
	◆ Central nervous system: cerebrovascular accident, cerebral anoxia, Huntington's disease, subdural hematoma, Alzheimer's disease, human immunodeficiency virus (HIV) infection, dementia, carotid stenosis, temporal lobe epilepsy, multiple sclerosis, postconcussion syndrome, myasthenia gravis, narcolepsy, subarachnoid hemorrhage
◆ Cardiovascular conditions: myocardial infarction, paroxysmal atrial tachycardia, angina pectoris, congestive heart failure, mitral valve prolapse, hypovolemia	
◆ Metabolic conditions: hyperkalemia, hypercalcemia, hypoglycemia, hyperthermia, anemia, hyponatremia	
◆ Respiratory conditions: asthma, chronic obstructive pulmonary disease, pneumonia, pulmonary edema, pulmonary embolus, respiratory dependence, hypoxia	◆ Autoimmune: rheumatoid arthritis, polyarteritis nodosa ◆ Endocrine: hyperparathyroidism, hypothyroidism, diabetes mellitus, Cushing's disease, Addison's disease
◆ Neoplasms: islet cell adenomas, pheochromocytoma	◆ Other: alcoholism, anemia, systemic lupus erythematosus, Epstein-Barr virus, hepatitis, malignancies, pulmonary insufficiency, pancreatic or liver disease, syphilis, encephalitis, malnutrition
◆ Neurological conditions: akathisia, encephalopathy, seizure disorder, vertigo, mass lesion, postconcussion syndrome	

Sources: Fernandez et al. (1995), reference 28; Kurlowicz (1994), reference 29; Wise and Taylor (1990), reference 19.

and the occurrence and expression of anxiety and depression. Three of the most important factors are previous coping strategies and emotional stability, social support, and symptom distress. In addition, there are common medical conditions, treatments, and substances that may cause or intensify symptoms of anxiety and depression (Tables 20.1 and 20.2).

Previous coping strategies and emotional stability

One of the most important predictors of psychological adjustment to chronic illness is the emotional stability and coping strategies used by the person prior to diagnosis.[30] Individuals with a history of poor psychological adjustment and of clinically significant anxiety or depression, are at highest risk for emotional decompensation[31] and should be monitored closely throughout all phases of treatment. This is particularly true for people with a history of major psychiatric syndromes and/or psychiatric hospitalization.[32]

Social support

Social support consistently has been found to influence a person's psychosocial adjustment to chronic illness.[33] The ability and availability of significant others in dealing with diagnosis and treatment can significantly affect the patient's view of him- or herself, and potentially the patient's survival.[34] Individuals diagnosed with all types of life-threatening chronic disorders experience a heightened need for interpersonal support. Individuals who are able to maintain close connections with family and friends during the course of illness are more likely to cope effectively with

the disease than those who are not able to maintain such relationships.[35] This is especially true during the palliative care period.

Symptom distress

The effects of treatment for a variety of chronic diseases, as well as the impact of progressive illness, can inflict transient and/or permanent physical changes, physical symptom distress, and functional impairments in patients. It is a well-known clinical observation supported by research[36] that excessive psychological distress can exacerbate the side effects of cancer-treatment agents. Conversely, treatment side effects can have a dramatic impact on the psychological profiles of patients.[37] The potential for psychological distress, particularly anxiety and depression, appears to increase in patients with advanced illness,[38–41] especially when cure is not viable and palliation of symptoms is the issue. In a study that elicited information from oncology nurses regarding psychiatric symptoms present in their patients, almost twice as many patients with metastatic disease were reported to be depressed, in contrast to those with localized cancers.[42] Investigators studying quality of life in cancer patients have demonstrated a clear relationship between an individual's perception of quality of life, and the presence of discomfort.[20] As uncomfortable symptoms increase, perceived quality of life diminishes and psychiatric symptoms often worsen. The presence of increased physical discomfort, combined with a lack of control and predictability regarding the occurrence of symptoms, amplifies anxiety, depression, and organic mental symptoms in patients with advanced disease.

Table 20.2 Common medications and substances associated with anxiety and depression

Anxiety	Depression
Alcohol and nicotine withdrawal	Antihypertensives
Stimulants, including caffeine	Analgesics
Thyroid replacement	Antiparkinsonian agents
Neuroleptics	Hypoglycemic agents
Corticosteroids	Steroids
Sedative-hypnotic withdrawal or paradoxical reaction	Chemotherapeutic agents
Bronchodilators and decongestants	Estrogen and progesterone
Cocaine	Antimicrobials
Epinephrine	L-dopa
Benzodiazepines and their withdrawal	Benzodiazepines
Digitalis toxicity	Barbiturates
Cannabis	Alcohol
Antihypertensives	Phenothiazines
Antihistamines	Amphetamines
Antiparkinsonian medications	Lithium carbonate
Oral contraceptives	Heavy metals
Anticholinergics	Cimetidine
Anesthetics and analgesics	Antibiotics
Toxins	
Antidepressants	

Sources: Fernandez et al. (1995), reference 28; Kurlowicz (1994), reference 29; Wise and Taylor (1990), reference 19.

Differentiating psychiatric complications from expected psychological responses

Differentiating between symptoms related to a medical illness and symptoms related to an underlying psychiatric disorder is particularly challenging to healthcare practitioners. Anxiety and depression are normal responses to life events and illness, and occur throughout the palliative care trajectory. It is the intensity, duration, and extent to which symptomatology affects functioning that distinguishes an anxiety or depressive disorder from symptoms that individuals generally experience in the progression of an illness. Symptoms following stressful events in a person's life (employment difficulties, retirement, death of a family member, loss of a job, diagnosis of a medical illness/life-threatening illness) are expected to dissipate as an individual copes, with reassurance and validation from family and friends, and adapts to the situation. When responses predominantly include excessive nervousness, worry, and fear, diagnosis of an adjustment disorder with anxiety is applied. If an individual responds with tearfulness and feelings of hopelessness, he or she is characterized as experiencing an adjustment disorder with depressed mood. An adjustment disorder with mixed anxiety and depressed mood is characterized by a combination of both anxiety and depression.[43]

Referrals from primary care providers for psychiatric assistance with psychopharmacological treatment are indicated when symptoms continue, intensify, or disrupt an individual's life beyond a 6-month period, or when symptoms do not respond to conventional reassurance and validation by the primary care provider, and support from an individual's social network. Most patients develop transient psychological symptoms that are responsive to support, reassurance, and information about what to expect regarding a disease course and its treatment. There are some individuals, however, who require more aggressive psychotherapeutic intervention, such as pharmacotherapy and ongoing psychotherapy.

Guidelines can help clinicians identify patients who exhibit behavior that suggests the presence of a psychiatric syndrome. If the patient's problems become so severe that supportive measures are insufficient to control emotional distress, referral to a psychiatric clinician is indicated. Factors that may predict major psychiatric problems along the chronic illness trajectory include past psychiatric hospitalization; history of significant depression, manic-depressive illness, schizophrenia, organic mental conditions, or personality disorders; lack of social support; inadequate control of physical discomfort; history of or current alcohol and/or drug abuse; and currently prescribed psychotropic medication.

The need for psychiatric referral among patients receiving psychotropic medication deserves specific mention because it is often overlooked in clinical practice. Standard therapies used to treat major chronic diseases, such as surgery and chemotherapy, and/or disease progression itself can significantly change dosage requirements for medications used to treat major psychiatric syndromes such as anxiety, depression, and bipolar disorder. For example, dosage requirements for lithium carbonate, commonly used to treat the manic episodes associated with bipolar disorder and the depressive episodes associated with recurrent depressive disorder, can change significantly over the course of treatment for a number of chronic diseases. Therapeutic blood levels of lithium are closely tied to sodium and water balance. Additionally, lithium has a narrow therapeutic window, and life-threatening toxicity can develop rapidly. Treatment side effects such as diarrhea, fever, vomiting, and resulting dehydration warrant scrupulous monitoring of dosage and side effects.

Careful monitoring is also indicated during pre- and postoperative periods. Another common problem among patients treated with psychotropic medication is that medications may be discontinued at specific points in the treatment process, such as the time of surgery, and not restarted. This may produce an avoidable recurrence of emotionally disabling psychiatric symptoms, when the stress of a life-threatening chronic disease and its treatment is burden enough.

For some patients, psychological distress does not subside with the usual supportive interventions. Unfortunately, clinically relevant and severe psychiatric syndromes may go unrecognized by nonpsychiatric care providers.[43,44] Particularly, as a chronic illness progresses, anxiety and depression can occur in greater numbers of patients and with greater intensity.[45] One of the reasons that it may be difficult to detect serious anxiety and depression in patients is that several of the diagnostic criteria used to evaluate their presence, such as lack of appetite, insomnia, decreased sexual interest, psychomotor agitation, and diminished energy, may overlap with usual disease and treatment effects.[46]

Additionally, healthcare providers may confuse their own fears about chronic illness with the emotional reactions of their patients (e.g., "I too would be extremely depressed if I were in a similar situation").

The coexisting nature of psychiatric and medical symptoms

Depression and anxiety are appropriate to the stress of having a serious illness, and the boundary between normal and abnormal symptoms is often unclear. Even when diagnostic criteria are met for a major depressive episode or anxiety disorder, there is disagreement regarding the need for psychiatric treatment, as psychiatric symptoms may improve on initiation of medical treatment. A major source of diagnostic confusion is the overlap of somatic symptoms associated with several chronic illnesses and their treatments, and those pathognomonic to depression and anxiety themselves (e.g., fatigue, loss of appetite, weakness, weight loss, restlessness, agitation). Separating out whether a symptom is due to depression, anxiety, the medical illness and its treatment, or a combination of factors, is often exceedingly difficult.

Figure 20.1 diagrams the overlap between the symptoms of a chronic medical condition and/or its treatment effects, and the

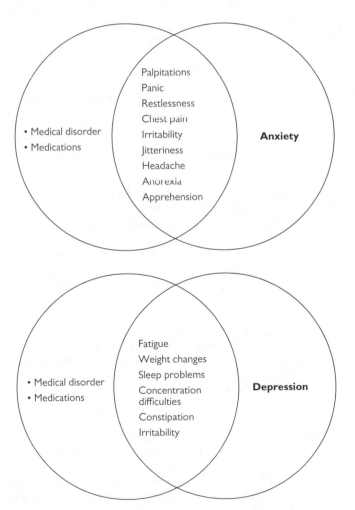

Figure 20.1 Symptoms of depression and anxiety with medical etiologies.
Source: Adapted from Derogatis et al. (1989), reference 39.

clinical manifestations of anxiety or depression. The symptoms of anxiety or depression may be intrinsic to the medical disorder or induced by certain treatment agents. Symptoms may cease when the medical disorder is treated or the medication is discontinued or decreased. Whether the psychiatric symptoms have a primary psychiatric etiology, occur following the medical diagnosis, or receive equal causal contributions from medical and psychiatric sources, neurovegetative symptoms are not reliable assessment parameters and treatment may be delayed or never started.

Anxiety or depression with a medical or pharmacological etiology

During progressive or active treatment phases of a chronic disease, symptoms of anxiety or depression may recur at various intervals relative to a specific causative agent, the stress associated with the illness, or a combination of those and other factors. Diagnostic data from earlier points, both before the onset of the current illness and at various points along the illness course, are important and should routinely be incorporated into the plan of care. As psychiatric symptoms become more prevalent within the context of the lengthening chronic illness trajectory, attention to the collection of this diagnostic information is an intrinsic aspect of quality comprehensive care. Physical and medication history, mental status, psychosocial and psychiatric histories (see Box 20.1 for screening instruments), electrocardiogram, comprehensive laboratory tests including toxicology screening, and relevant family information regarding available support systems, changes in lifestyle and functioning, all will promote accurate assessment and close monitoring throughout the palliative care trajectory. This information will assist the healthcare team in determining the etiology of anxiety and depressive symptoms and to treat and monitor them appropriately.

Some patients may have a primary psychiatric disorder that precedes the diagnosis of their chronic medical condition. This situation is encountered in primary care and chronic illness treatment settings. During the diagnostic phase, fear and anxiety are expected reactions to the diagnosis of a life-threatening or potentially life-threatening disease. Heightened apprehension coincides with the anticipated course of treatment, uncertainty, and concerns about the potential impact on lifestyle. These initial responses usually resolve in a few weeks with the support of family and friends, use of personal resources, provision of professional care, and maintenance of hope.[28,47] Lingering reports of feeling weak, dizzy, worried, or tense, and of difficulty concentrating, are often confusing to providers and may suggest an anxiety disorder. When anxiety is accurately diagnosed and treated, somatic

Box 20.1 Brief screening measures used in nonpsychiatric settings for cognitive functioning, anxiety, and depression

Folstein Mini-Mental Exam
Beck Depression Inventory
Center for Epidemiological Studies of Depression Scale
Geriatric Depression Scale
Hospital Anxiety and Depression Scale
Zung Self-Rating Depression Scale
Zung Self-Rating Anxiety Scale
PHQ9

complaints may diminish. If symptoms are not correctly identified and treated, suffering can become needlessly prolonged.[41,43]

Depression occurs frequently during the recurrence and progressive disease phase. An illness course marked with recurrences engenders anxiety and fear with each relapse, as well as feelings of desperation. Individuals experiencing depression do not always present with a dysphoric affect or report distressing feelings of hopelessness and helplessness.[48] Instead, they may present with somatic complaints such as dizziness, headaches, excessive fatigue, sleep disturbances, or irritability. Disturbances in appetite, sleep, energy, and concentration are hallmark symptoms of depression. However, in the medically ill, these symptoms are frequently caused by the medical illness.[49] Symptoms such as fearfulness, depressed appearance, social withdrawal, brooding, self-pity, pessimism, a sense of punishment, and mood that cannot be changed (e.g., cannot be cheered up, not smiling, does not respond to good news) are considered to be more reliable. It has been recommended that assessment of these affective symptoms provides more accurate diagnostic information for depression in medically ill patients than neurovegetative symptoms commonly used in healthy individuals.[49–52] Boxes 20.2 and 20.3 list general criteria to diagnose an anxiety and depressive disorder in the medically ill.[43,51,52] Whenever symptoms are unremitting, or intensify and do not respond to conventional professional and family support, psychiatric evaluations for psychopharmacological and psychotherapeutic interventions are warranted.

Untreated or undertreated psychiatric disorders can be profoundly disabling and, as such, can precipitate or exacerbate the physical manifestations of chronic disease. The degree of anxiety and depression experienced by an individual at any given point is influenced by the degree to which individuals and their families have been prepared for what to expect. These considerations include: physical and psychological manifestations of the illness; speed and extent of physical deterioration expected, including the likelihood of pain and other symptoms; available treatment options; and the individual's history of psychiatric illness.[42]

Box 20.2 Symptoms indicating an anxiety disorder in the medically ill in the absence of physiological course

Chronic apprehension, worry, inability to relax not related to illness or treatment
Difficulty concentrating
Irritability or outbursts of anger
Difficulty falling asleep or staying asleep not explained by illness or treatment
Trembling or shaking not explained by illness or treatment
Exaggerated startle response
Perspiring for no apparent reason
Chest pain or tightness in the chest
Fear of places, events, certain activities
Unrealistic fear of dying
Fear of "going crazy"
Recurrent and persistent ideas, thoughts, or impulses
Repetitive behaviors to prevent discomfort

Sources: Barraclough (1997), reference 47; Fernandez et al. (1995), reference 28.

Box 20.3 Symptoms indicating a depressive disorder in the medically ill in the absence of physiological course

Enduring depressed or sad mood, tearful
Marked disinterest or lack of pleasure in social activities, family, and friends not explained by pain or fatigue
Feelings of worthlessness and hopelessness
Excessive enduring guilt that illness is a punishment
Significant weight loss or gain not explained by dieting, illness, or treatments
Hopelessness about the future
Enduring fatigue
Increase or decrease in sleep not explained by illness or treatment
Recurring thoughts of death or suicidal thoughts or acts
Diminished ability to think and make decisions

Sources: Cassem (1995), reference 45; Cavanaugh (1995), reference 46; Kurlowicz (1994), reference 29.

Anxiety and depression typically accompany difficult decisions regarding both the addition of comfort measures and the withdrawal of diagnostic procedures and aggressive medical treatments. Distress regarding separation from family and friends, worries about burdening caregivers, feeling overwhelmed with end-of-life decisions, and living in existential uncertainty are just a few of the issues that individuals and families confront during terminal phases of illness. Severe distress, thoughts of suicide, panic, and/or questions about assisted suicide may occur. Such responses require immediate attention and intervention. Suicide and assisted suicide are discussed at a later point in this chapter.

Anxiety or depression precipitated by a medical disorder

In many cases, an anxiety or depressive disorder occurs secondary to the diagnosis of a chronic medical condition.[53] The stress of the medical illness itself typically induces anxiety or depression. Often these symptoms diminish when treatment is explained and initiated and hope is offered. When a patient with a chronic illness experiences increasing physical dependence on others, prolonged pain, progressive loss of function, and/or immobility, anxiety and depression can become severe and prolonged. Disease progression may affect body image, self-esteem, social relationships, employment, and family roles. The extent and speed at which disabling aspects of a chronic illness occur can impact an individual's ability to react and to integrate the changes and, subsequently, to develop adjustment skills. The development of adaptive coping mechanisms is influenced by many factors, particularly the patient's premorbid coping strategies and the availability of outside support.

Within the context of a chronic medical condition, anxiety and depression often occur simultaneously. In general, anxiety precedes depression, and depression is more likely to persevere in individuals who also have an anxiety disorder. When anxiety and depression coexist, assessment and treatment may be more challenging, underscoring the need for an aggressive, ongoing approach to assessment and treatment.

A common but erroneous assumption by clinicians is that the psychological distress that accompanies a medical condition, even when it is severe and unremitting, is natural, expected, and does not require or respond to treatment. This is thought to be particularly true when hope for a cure is unrealistic or the prognosis is grave. This attitude leads to underrecognition and undertreatment of high levels of suffering. Receiving a life-threatening medical diagnosis and undergoing invasive treatment are potent catalysts for an acute stress response that is not typically expected, planned for, or routinely addressed in healthcare settings. Providers' dominant concerns are usually centered around treatment options, the pursuit of a cure or life-prolongation, improving prognosis, and relieving physical discomfort. Providers may also be desensitized to the intrusiveness of medical protocols and treatment environments. Most patients are not comfortable with, and are not encouraged to express to professional or family care providers, their feelings of helplessness, dependency, or fear. In fact, they frequently avoid such discussions in an attempt to decrease burden on others.

Untreated psychological symptoms can lead to a posttraumatic stress disorder (PTSD). Posttraumatic stress disorders, typically induced by exposure to extreme stress and/or trauma, are increasingly being linked in the literature to medical treatment situations. Providers are apt to confuse PTSD symptoms such as avoidance and withdrawal as nonpathological responses, for example, acceptance adjustment. It is common for providers to hear "I do not remember anything about the hospitalization; it is a blur. I feel like I was in a daze ... ask my wife/husband ... my memory isn't so great." In the treatment of PTSD, psychopharmacological agents alone are inadequate and must be accompanied by aggressive psychotherapeutic interventions, education, and support. Posttraumatic stress disorder is best treated by a professional skilled in treating this disorder. Routine psychiatric assessment and the availability of prompt treatment across the palliative care trajectory is needed to reduce the prevalence and morbidity of PTSDs that occur in response to medical diagnosis and treatment.[37]

Assessment and screening considerations

Assessment of anxiety

The experience of anxiety is virtually universal, especially when a person has a serious chronic illness. Anxiety is a vague, subjective feeling of apprehension, tension, insecurity, and uneasiness, usually without a known, specific cause identifiable by the individual. Normally, anxiety serves as an alerting response resulting from a real or perceived threat to a person's biological, psychological, or social integrity, including self-esteem, identity, or status. This alert occurs in response to actual happenings, or to thoughts about happenings in the past, present, or future. The greater the perceived threat, the greater the anxiety response.[26] A wide variety of signs and symptoms accompany anxiety along the continuum of mild, moderate, severe, and panic levels. Anxiety responses can be adaptive, and anxiety can be a powerful motivating force for productive problem-solving. Talking, crying, sleeping, exercising, deep breathing, imagery, and relaxation techniques are adaptive anxiety-relief strategies. Responses to anxiety also can be maladaptive and may indicate psychiatric disorder, but not all distressing symptoms of anxiety indicate a psychiatric disorder.

Box 20.2 lists anxiety symptoms that indicate a psychiatric disorder and call for psychiatric assessment and treatment. Skill in early recognition of anxiety is important so that care providers can intervene to alleviate symptoms, prevent escalation and loss of control, and enable adjustment and coping. Anxiety is interpersonally contagious. As a result, therapeutic effectiveness can be severely compromised when care providers fail to recognize and manage their own anxiety.

Assessment of depression

Underrecognized and undertreated, depression has the potential to decrease immune response, decrease survival time, impair ability to adhere to treatment, and impair quality of life.[54] The assessment of depression in any setting depends on the provider's awareness of its potential to occur. In addition, providers must be cognizant of the risk factors associated with depression as well as its key signs, symptoms, and historical aspects. In addition to medical comorbidity, risk factors that favor the development of a depressive disorder include prior episodes of depression, family history of depression, prior suicide attempts, female gender, age under 40 years, postpartum period, lack of social support, stressful life events, personal history of sexual abuse, and current substance abuse.[55–57] The experience of chronic and progressive disease may increase dependence, helplessness, and uncertainty, and generate a negative, self-critical view. Cognitive distortions can easily develop, leading to interpretation of benign events as negative or catastrophic. Motivation to participate in care may be diminished, leading to withdrawal. Patients may see themselves as worthless and burdensome to family and friends. Family members may find themselves immobilized, impatient, or angry about the patient's lack of communication, cooperation, or motivation.[57]

Cultural considerations

Culture can be a powerful influence on the occurrence and presentation of psychiatric morbidity. In some cultures, anxiety and depression may be expressed through somatic symptoms rather than affective/behavioral symptoms such as guilt or sadness. Complaints of "nerves" and headaches (in Latino and Mediterranean cultures); of weakness, tiredness, or "imbalance" (in Chinese or Asian cultures); of problems of the "heart" (in Middle Eastern cultures); or of being "heartbroken" (among the Hopi) may be depressive equivalents. Cultures may differ in judgments about the seriousness of dysphoria; for example, irritability may be a greater concern than sadness or withdrawal. Experiences distinctive to certain cultures, such as fear of being hexed, or vivid feelings of being visited by those who have died, must be differentiated from actual hallucinations or delusions that may be part of a major depressive episode with psychotic features. However, a symptom should not be dismissed because it is seen as characteristic of a particular culture (see Box 20.3).[43,49,50,52]

Conceptual and diagnostic considerations

The conceptualization of psychological distress is varied. Depression in particular has a variety of meanings, and has been used to describe a broad spectrum of human emotions and behaviors ranging from expected, transient, and nonclinical sadness following upsetting life events, to the clinically relevant extremes of suicidality and major depressive disorder. Depression is common among people with chronic illness. The term *depressive syndromes* refers to a specific constellation of symptoms that comprise a discrete psychiatric disorder. Examples are: major depression, dysthymia, organic affective disorder, and adjustment disorder with depressed features. Depressive symptoms describe varying degrees of depressed feelings not necessarily associated with psychiatric illness. Five major theoretical viewpoints have been used to understand and treat depression. In the psychoanalytic view, depression represents the introjection of hostility subsequent to the loss of an ambivalently loved object.[58] Cognitive views emphasize the mediating role that distorted and negative thinking plays in determining mood and behavior.[59] In the sociological view, depression is a social phenomenon in which a breakdown of self-esteem involves the loss of possessions such as status, roles and relationships, and life meaning.[60] Cultural and societal factors, including illness, increase vulnerability to depression. The biological view of depression emphasizes genetic vulnerability and biochemical alterations in neurotransmitters.[61] In studies of medically ill patients, depression is often equated with a crisis response, in which demands on the individual exceed the ability to respond.[62]

Conceptual viewpoints are important to the extent that they influence the understanding and subsequent treatment of the psychiatric symptoms experienced by patients with chronic physical illness. Diverse conceptualizations do not diminish the ability to plan and deliver effective care, and most often simply offer complementary ideas concerning the etiological significance of symptoms. In many healthcare settings, nurses have the most patient contact and are likely to talk with individuals about their physical and emotional problems and thus to detect psychiatric symptoms and syndromes. Specific screening instruments, such as those listed in Box 20.1, may be used for assessment. In addition, direct questioning and clinical observation of mood, behavior, and thinking can be carried out concomitant with physical care. Questions related to mood may include the following: How have your spirits been lately? How would you describe your mood now? Have you felt sad or blue? Questions about behavior relate to sleeping patterns, appetite, activity level, and changes in energy: How are you sleeping lately? How much energy do you have now compared with 1 month or 6 months ago? Have you experienced recent changes in your appetite? Have you lost or gained weight? What do you usually do to cope with stress (talk to someone? go to a movie? work? exercise? drugs? alcohol?)? Questions related to cognition are as follows: What do you see in your future? What are the biggest problems facing you now? Are you as interested as usual in your family and friends, work, hobbies, and so forth? Have you felt satisfied with yourself and with your life? Can you concentrate as well as you usually can? Do you have family or close friends readily available to help you? Do you feel able to call on them? As noted previously, disturbances in appetite, sleep, energy, and concentration may be caused by the illness and not necessarily indicative of depression.

Screening for anxiety and depression

In chronic illness settings, the need for routine psychiatric screening has been well documented for identifying patients at high risk for psychiatric morbidity, as well as to identify those who can benefit from early-intervention programs. Patients may require different interventions based on their placement on the distress continuum. Researchers[63] concluded that newly diagnosed patients who are highly distressed can benefit from evaluation and treatment for psychiatric consequences of illness, and that adaptation to the disease can be improved through the use of psychosocial interventions and close monitoring.

A number of tools have been developed to screen for psychological distress but have not been consistently incorporated into clinical care.[64,65] One tool that is easy to administer, reliable, and palatable to patients is the Distress Thermometer. This tool, developed by a team led by Dr. Jimmie Holland at Memorial Sloan Kettering Cancer Center, is similar to pain measurement scales that ask patients to rate their pain on a scale from 0 to 10, and consists of two cards. The first card is a picture of a thermometer, and the patient is asked to mark his or her level of distress. A rating of 5 or above indicates that a patient has symptoms indicating a need to be evaluated by a mental health professional and potential referral for services. The patient is then handed a second card and asked to identify which items from a six-item problem list relate to the patient's distress; that is, illness-related, family, emotional, practical, financial, or spiritual. This tool is part of the National Comprehensive Cancer Network (NCCN) distress-management practice guidelines in oncology. This interdisciplinary workgroup chose the term "distress management" because it was "more acceptable and less stigmatizing than psychiatric, psychosocial or emotional," and could be defined and measured by self-report.[66]

Again, striving for simplicity and clinical utility, Harvey Chochinov and colleagues compared the performance of four brief screening measures for depression in the terminally ill.[51] They found that asking the question "Are you depressed?" was reliable and valid for diagnosing depression and was extraordinarily useful in care of the terminally ill. Both the NCCN practice guidelines for distress management and the simple three-word screening sentence for depression can easily be incorporated into daily clinical practice.

Addressing deficits in case-finding strategies

Individuals are living longer with chronic illnesses, within the context of aggressive, physically and psychologically debilitating treatments. These trends promise to continue, and further study is needed to identify effective approaches to treatment. Available data clearly support a policy of routine psychological assessment in chronic-illness settings. Additional studies are needed to support intervention development that, at a minimum, will likely lead to improved quality of life for patients and cost savings at the systems level. In clinical settings, detection and case identification are particularly difficult. As mentioned, this is due to several factors, including: the high prevalence of clinically significant "subsyndromal" psychiatric symptoms in medically ill samples (symptoms not severe enough, or of sufficient duration, to be classified as a psychiatric disorder), and the overlapping nature of physical and neurovegetative symptoms such as fatigue, changes in appetite, sleep, and sex drive. Different clinical sites have their own unique limitations, including lack of knowledge, comfort, or time by health professionals to assess patients for these symptoms. Consequently, recognition of significant psychological distress (psychiatric morbidity) is seriously impeded in clinical settings.

Clinicians need to be trained to recognize the prognostic importance of comorbid medical illness and psychiatric symptoms, and to understand how the subtleties of case identification can affect treatment planning. The range in severity of psychiatric symptoms, and the often rapid change in both psychiatric and physical symptoms across the treatment trajectory, create both a great variance and the need to observe and record the dynamic interchange between physical and psychological phenomena over a small time span. The difficulties in case identification discussed may be highlighted by the severity of physical symptoms and the low prevalence of prior mood disorder. The presence of acute physical illnesses places the individual under severe physiological, psychological, and psychosocial stress. In addition, patients are often removed from their usual social support systems to receive treatment, and are exposed to psychosocial stressors unique to the treatment setting (e.g., dependency on hospital staff, unfamiliar and sometimes painful diagnostic and therapeutic procedures, altered eating, bathing, and sleep routines, and uncertain prognosis). Symptom assessments must strike a balance between overly inclusive (e.g., mistakenly treating the fatigue of cancer treatment as depression) and overly exclusive (e.g., erroneously dismissing the patient's mood symptoms as "understandable"). Case identification is a crucial first step. The approach to identifying psychiatric symptoms potentially confounded by medical illnesses must be defined explicitly. Choice of an inclusive approach avoids premature exclusion of relevant phenomena. The use of similar screening instruments across clinical sites would greatly facilitate comparisons of information and standardization of assessment and case-finding guidelines.

Suicide

Suicide is the ninth leading cause of death in the United States. Five percent of suicides occur in patients with chronic medical illnesses, with spinal cord injuries, multiple sclerosis, cancer, and human immunodeficiency virus disease.[67] Because of underreporting, statistics underestimate the magnitude of suicide; intentional overdoses by the terminally ill and intentional car accidents are rarely labeled as suicides. The strongest suicide predictor is the presence of a psychiatric illness, especially depression and alcohol abuse, although a chronic deteriorating medical illness with perceived poor health, recent diagnosis of a life-threatening illness, and recent conflict or loss of a significant relationship also are considered to be predictive.[67] Being male, over age 45 years, and living alone and lacking a social support system are risk factors.[68] Hopelessness was found to be more important than depression as a clinical marker of suicidal ideation in the terminally ill.[67] Individuals with progressive chronic illness, particularly during the terminal stages, are at increased risk for suicide.[67] Other cancer-related risk factors include oral, pharyngeal, or lung cancer; poor prognosis; confusion and delirium; inadequately controlled pain; and the presence of deficits, such as loss of mobility, loss of bowel or bladder control, amputation, sensory loss, inability to eat or swallow, and exhaustion.[67,69] The highest-risk patients are those with severe and rapidly progressive disease producing rapid functional decline, intractable pain, and/or history of depression, suicide attempts, or substance abuse.[67–69]

Physician-assisted suicide

Whereas suicide is the intentional ending of one's own life, physician-assisted suicide (PAS) refers to a physician acting to aid a person in the ending of his or her life.[70] Public demand for PAS has been fueled by burdensome, exhausting, and expensive dying in acute care settings.[71] It is highly controversial; the American Medical Association, the American Nurses Association, and the National Hospice and Palliative Care Organization have taken positions against it. Implications for healthcare providers include the following: to be knowledgeable about the legal and moral/ethical aspects of PAS; to do a personal evaluation and prepare responses for situations with patients where the topic may arise; to improve education about pain management, symptom control, and related issues in the care of dying and seriously ill patients; to conduct rigorous research on the attitudes and practices of healthcare professionals with respect to assisted suicide; and to develop effective mechanisms to address conflicts.[72]

There is an ongoing debate about the legalization of PAS. Oregon was the first state in the United States where the majority of voters approved legalization of PAS. However some fear that providing adequate pain relief might be seen as hastening the patient's death rather than controlling pain at end-of-life. Events in Oregon highlight care as a priority and increase the understanding about the distinction between assisting suicide and honoring patient preferences for limiting life-sustaining treatment. Patient concerns most often related to desire to hasten death are: unrelieved pain, poorly managed symptoms, depression, worries about loss of control, being a burden, being dependent on others for personal care, and loss of dignity.[72]

Assessment of suicide risk

Assessment and treatment of depression, often overlooked in chronic-illness treatment settings, is a key suicide-prevention strategy. In addition, managing symptoms, communicating, and helping patients to maintain a sense of control are vitally important prevention strategies. An assessment of depression should always include direct questions about suicidal thinking, plans or attempts, despair or hopelessness, distress from poorly managed symptoms, and personal or family history of suicidal ideation, plans, or attempts.[73] When any indicator of suicide risk is recognized, there should be a thorough evaluation of risk factors, clues, suicidal ideation, level of depression, hopelessness and despair, and symptom distress, in order to estimate individual lethality. The rationality of the suicidal request or intent must also be evaluated. The nurse should interview the patient and family members to find out why the patient is thinking about suicide now.[73] Find out what method the patient is considering, and whether the means are available. Ask the patient what has prevented suicide before, and if he or she wants help or hopes someone else will decide.[74] Most people are relieved to be asked about suicidal thoughts because it opens communication. Initial and periodic evaluation of suicidal potential is necessary for patients with a history, thoughts, or risk factors of suicide.

Recognition of clues

Suicidal persons usually give verbal and/or behavioral clues, such as isolated or withdrawn behavior, or death wishes or death themes in art, writing, play, or conversation. Clues may be subtle or obvious; for example, joking about suicide, asking questions concerning death (e.g., "How many of these pills would it take to kill someone?"), comments with a theme of giving up, or statements that indicate hopelessness or helplessness. Keys to determining lethality are suicide plan, method, intended outcome (e.g., death or rescue), and availability of resources and ability to communicate.[73,74] Lethal means include guns, knives, jumping from heights, drowning, or carbon monoxide poisoning. Other potentially lethal means include hanging or strangulation (using strong pieces of twine, rope, electric cords, sheets), taking high doses of aspirin or Tylenol, being in a car crash, or undergoing exposure to extreme cold. Low to moderately lethal methods are wrist cutting and mild aspirin overdose.

Suicide interventions

Severely depressed and/or potentially suicidal patients must be identified as soon as possible to ensure a safe environment and appropriate treatment. Prompt action should be taken including provision of safety, supervision, and initiation of psychiatric evaluation. A patient with an immediate, lethal, and precise suicide plan needs strict safety precautions such as hospitalization and continuous or close supervision. The low-risk patient should not be underestimated. If circumstances change, risk could change. In all cases, notify the primary provider, and document the patient's behavior and verbatim statements, suicide assessment, and rationale for decisions, as well as the time and date the provider was notified.[73,74] If the provider is not responsive to the report of the patient's suicidal ideation, it is important to maintain observation and to pursue psychiatric consultation. The motivation for suicide can be reduced through palliative care interventions such as improved pain and symptom management; referral and treatment for depression or other psychiatric disorders; discussion of alternative interventions to improve quality of life; referral to spiritual, social, and psychiatric resources; and education and accurate facts about options for terminal care or end-of-life decision-making. Openness to talking about suffering, distress, death preferences, and decision-making in a sensitive and understanding manner, and advocacy to aid communication with others, are helpful for patients and their families.

Management of anxiety and depression

Psychosocial interventions can exert an important effect on the overall adjustment of patients and their families to chronic illness and treatment. Several studies document the beneficial effect of counseling on anxiety, feelings of personal control, depression, and generalized psychological distress.[75] Increased length of survival from time of diagnosis has highlighted the need for psychopharmacological, psychotherapeutic, and behaviorally oriented interventions to reduce anxiety and depression and to improve quality of life for patients diagnosed with a chronic illness.

Pharmacological interventions

Pharmacotherapy, as an adjunct to one or more of the psychotherapies, can be an important aid in bringing psychological symptoms under control.

Pharmacological management of anxiety

The prevalence of anxiety in medical illness is relatively high. As described in Figure 20.1, a variety of disorders have anxiety as a prominent symptom of the clinical presentation (see Tables 20.1 and 20.2), and many commonly used medications are associated with anxiety as a side effect. Studies have shown a high prevalence in cardiovascular, pulmonary, cerebrovascular, and

gastrointestinal diseases, as well as cancer and diabetes. In addition, patients with a history of anxiety disorders have increased rates of diabetes, heart disease, arthritis, and physical handicaps compared with the general population. Pain, metabolic abnormalities, hypoxia, and drug withdrawal states can present as anxiety. Before instituting pharmacological treatment, any patient with acute or chronic symptoms of anxiety should be thoroughly evaluated, including a review of medications to assess the contribution of medical condition and/or medication-related etiologies for their complaints.

The following brief review of pharmacological treatment must be supplemented with other references concerning assessment, intervention, evaluation, and patient education. Benzodiazepines are the most frequently used medications for anxiety in both medical and psychiatric settings. When longer-acting benzodiazepines, such as diazepam, are used in the elderly or in the presence of liver disease, dosages should be decreased and dosing intervals increased. They may suppress respiratory drive. Consultation-liaison services often use lorazepam in medically ill patients because its elimination half-life is relatively unaffected by liver disease, age, or concurrent use of selective serotonin reuptake inhibitors (SSRIs) or nefazodone. Drawbacks include amnestic episodes, and interdose anxiety caused by its short half-life. The latter can be remedied by more frequent dosing. If medically ill patients need a longer-acting benzodiazepine for panic disorder or generalized anxiety disorder, clonazepam is often used because it is not affected by concurrent use of SSRIs. Clonazepam may accumulate and result in oversedation and ataxia in the elderly; therefore, low doses are used. Temazepam is useful as a sedative-hypnotic. Buspirone, used primarily for generalized anxiety disorder, is preferable for anxiety in the medically ill because of its lack of sedation, lack of negative effects on cognition, insignificant effect of age on elimination half-life, and limited effect of liver disease on half-life. Buspirone has almost no clinically significant interactions with drugs commonly used in general medicine. It may stimulate the respiratory drive, which makes it useful in patients with pulmonary disease or sleep apnea.

Cyclic antidepressants are well established as anxiolytic agents, which are particularly effective in the treatment of panic disorder and in generalized anxiety disorder. If these drugs are used for anxiety in depressed medically ill patients, or used because of their sedating properties in patients with major depression or panic disorder, the side effects must be carefully considered. Potentially deleterious side effects in the medically ill are sedative, anticholinergic, orthostatic hypotensive, and quinidine-like. Liver disease and renal disease may affect metabolism and excretion of the drug and, therefore, require careful dosage titration.[76] Other drugs that may be used for anxiety include the β-adrenergic blocking agents, antihistamines, monoamine oxidase inhibitors, and neuroleptics. Beta-adrenergic blocking agents may be used for milder forms of generalized anxiety, but there are cautions and contraindications in the presence of pulmonary disease, diabetes, and congestive heart failure. Antihistamines are sometimes used, although the effects are largely nonspecific and sedative. Side effects, such as sedation and dizziness, can be significant for medically ill patients. Monoamine oxidase inhibitors are rarely used in the medically ill because of the precautions that must be taken to prevent drug interactions. Neuroleptics, such as haloperidol in low doses, are used for anxiety associated with severe behavioral agitation or psychotic symptoms.[76] When anxiety develops in the context of the terminal stages of cancer, it is often secondary to hypoxia and/or an untreated pain syndrome. Intravenous opiates, and oxygen if hypoxia is present, are usually an effective palliative treatment. Anxiolytics are most effective when doses are scheduled; if given on an as-needed basis, anxiety may increase in patients already frightened and anxious. Anxiolytic medications help patients gain control over agonizing anxiety. Use of these medications may also assist the patient in psychotherapy, which can help control symptoms. All pharmacological treatments must be monitored for effectiveness and side effects. The effects of benzodiazepines are felt within hours, with a full response in days. Buspirone has no immediate effect, with a full response after 2 to 4 weeks. The sedating effects of benzodiazepines are associated with impaired motor performance and cognition. Benzodiazepines have dependence and abuse potential and the possibility of withdrawal symptoms when discontinued.

Pharmacological management of depression

Patients with chronic illness commonly exhibit transient depressive symptoms at various points in the disease trajectory, particularly during the palliative care period when a hope for cure is no longer possible. As explained previously, depressive symptoms can be caused by the medical disorder itself, associated with medications used for treatment or symptom management, or caused or worsened by the stress related to coping with illness. Depression can also predate and recur with the medical illness. To further complicate matters, individuals with medical illness are often older, with potentially greater risk of adverse effects from both psychotropic and nonpsychotropic medications. Medical illnesses and the medications required to treat or manage symptoms may impose significantly modified prescribing regimens on the use of antidepressants. Therefore, it is necessary to evaluate the possible role of existing medical conditions and medications that could cause the depressive symptoms. Other general guidelines include: (1) use the medication with the least potential for drug–drug interactions and for adverse effects based on the patient's drug regimen and physiological vulnerabilities, and the greatest potential for improving the primary symptoms of the depression; (2) begin with low dosage, increase slowly, and establish the lowest effective dosage; and (3) reassess dosage requirements regularly.[76,77]

In the past, antidepressant drug selection was limited by the nearly sole availability of tricyclic antidepressants; but new drugs, such as the SSRIs, bupropion, and venlafaxine, have vastly simplified pharmacological treatment of depression in the medically ill.[78–80] No one medication is clearly more effective than another. The SSRIs have fewer long-term side effects than the tricyclic antidepressants and, in general, are the first line of pharmacological antidepressant treatment unless specific side-effect profiles associated with other classes of drugs are desired.

Psychostimulants, such as methylphenidate, have been useful in the treatment of depression in medically ill patients.[81–83] Advantages include rapid onset of action and rapid clearance if side effects occur. They can also counteract opioid-induced sedation and improve pain control through a positive action on mood.[83] Common side effects of psychostimulants include insomnia, anorexia, tachycardia, and hypertension, although incremental dosage increases allow adequate monitoring of therapeutic

---

Box 20.4 Selected medications commonly used for the treatment of anxiety in the medically ill

Benzodiazepines

Diazepam (Valium and others)
Alprazolam (Xanax)
Clonazepam (Klonopin)
Lorazepam (Ativan and others)
Oxazepam (Serax and others)

Azapirones

Buspirone (Buspar)

Cyclic antidepressants

Nortriptyline (Pamelor and others)

Other antidepressents

Fluoxetine (Prozac), an SSRI
Sertraline (Zoloft), an SSRI
Paroxetine (Paxil), an SSRI
Citalopram (Celexa) an SSRI
Escitalopram (Lexapro) an SSRI
Duloxetine (Cymbalta) an SNRI
Venlafaxine (Effexor), an SNRI
Mirtazapine (Remeron)

Other medications selectively used for their anxiolytic effects

β-Adrenergic blocking agents, such as propranolol
Neuroleptics (antipsychotics), such as olanzapine (Zyprexa), Quetiapine (Seroquel)

Source: References 76 and 77.

---

versus side effects. In medically ill patients, a 1- to 2-month trial can provide remission from depression even after discontinuation of the drug. Different studies have shown a 48% to 80% improvement in depressive symptoms, and this class of medication is often quite effective but underutilized in medical settings (Box 20.4).

Certain medications and treatment agents can produce severe depressive states. As reiterated throughout this chapter, a diagnosis of major depression in medically ill patients relies heavily on the presence of affective symptoms such as hopelessness, crying spells, guilt, preoccupation with death and/or suicide, diminished self-worth, and loss of pleasure in most activities, for example, being with friends and loved ones. The neurovegetative symptoms that usually characterize depression in physically healthy individuals are not good predictors of depression in the medically ill, because disease and treatment can also produce these symptoms. A combination of psychotherapy and antidepressant medication will often prove useful in treating major depression in medically ill patients. Peak dosages of antidepressants, regardless of drug class, are usually substantially lower than those tolerated by physically healthy individuals. Antidepressant medications may take 2 to 6 weeks to produce their desired effects. Patients may need ongoing support, reassurance, and monitoring before experiencing the antidepressant effects of medication. It is essential that patients are monitored closely by a consistent provider during the initiation and modification of psychopharmacological regimens. Patient education is essential in this area to decrease the possibility of nonadherence to the medication regimen.

Psychotherapeutic modalities

Psychosocial interventions are defined as systematic efforts applied to influence coping behavior through educational or psychotherapeutic means.[18] The goals of such interventions are to improve morale, self-esteem, coping ability, sense of control, and problem-solving abilities, and to decrease emotional distress. The educational approach is directive, using problem-solving and cognitive methods. It is important that the educational approach both clarify medical information that may be missed due to fear and anxiety, or misconceptions and/or misinformation regarding illness and treatment, and normalize emotional reactions throughout the illness trajectory. The psychotherapeutic approach uses psychodynamic and exploratory methods to help the individual understand aspects of the medical condition such as emotional responses and personal meaning of the disease. Psychotherapeutic interventions, as opposed to educational interventions, should be delivered by professionals with special training in both mental health and specific interventional modalities as applied to patients with chronic medical illnesses and palliative care needs. Psychotherapy with a patient who has cancer should maintain a primary focus on the illness and its implications, using a brief therapy and crisis-intervention model. Expression of fears and concerns that may be too painful to reveal to family and friends is encouraged. Normalizing emotional distress, providing realistic reassurance and support, and bolstering existing strengths and coping skills are essential components of the therapeutic process. Gathering information about previous associations with the medical condition experienced through close relationships can also be instrumental in clarifying patients' fears and concerns and establishing boundaries for and differences from the current situation.

Depending on the nature of the problem, the treatment modality may take the form of individual psychotherapy, support groups, family and marital therapy, or behaviorally oriented therapy such as progressive muscle relaxation and guided imagery.[84–86] A primary role for clinicians is to facilitate a positive adjustment in patients under their care. Periodic emotional distress and coping problems can be expected during the palliative care trajectory and monitored routinely. Emotional display is not the same as maladaptive coping. Understanding an individual's unique circumstances can assist nurses in supporting the constructive coping abilities that seem to work best for a particular patient.

Psychotherapeutic interventions targeted to symptoms of anxiety

Anxiety responses can be thought of as occurring along a continuum, from mild to moderate to severe to panic. Lazarus and Folkman's[87] differentiation of problem-focused coping and emotion-focused coping provides a framework for intervention strategies matched to the continuum of responses (Table 20.3). As a person moves along the continuum to moderate, severe, and panic levels of anxiety, the problem causing the distress recedes from view and distress itself becomes the focus of attention. Both preventive and treatment strategies can be used with patients and family members in a variety of settings. Before assuming that

Table 20.3 Hierarchy of anxiety interventions

Anxiety level	Interventions
Level 1	*Prevention strategies*
Mild to moderate	Provide concrete objective information.
	Ensure stressful-event warning.
	Increase opportunities for control.
	Increase patient and family participation in care activities.
	Acknowledge fears.
	Explore near-miss events, past and/or present.
	Control symptoms.
	Structure uncertainty.
	Limit sensory deprivation and isolation.
	Encourage hope.
Level 2	*Treatment strategies*
Moderate to severe	Use presence of support person as "emotional anchor."
	Support expression of feelings, doubts, and fears.
	Explore near-miss events, past and/or present.
	Provide accurate information for realistic restructuring of fearful ideas.
	Teach anxiety-reduction strategies, such as focusing, breathing, relaxation, and imagery techniques.
	Use massage, touch, and physical exercise.
	Control symptoms.
	Use antianxiety medications.
	Delay procedures to promote patient control and readiness.
	Consult psychiatric experts.
Level 3	*Treatment strategies*
Panic	Stay with the patient.
	Maintain calm environment and reduce stimulation.
	Use antianxiety medications and monitor carefully.
	Control symptoms.
	Use focusing and breathing techniques.
	Use demonstration in addition to verbal direction.
	Repeat realistic reassurances.
	Communicate with repetition and simplicity.
	Consult psychiatric experts.

Sources: Minarik (1996), reference 30; Lazarus & Folkman, 1984; reference 87.

anxiety has a psychological basis, consider the models of interaction and review the patient's history for recent changes in medical condition and/or medications. Asking whether the patient was taking medications for "nerves," depression, or insomnia will help to determine whether drugs were inappropriately discontinued, or whether anxiety symptoms predated the current illness. In addition, ask about over-the-counter medications, illegal drugs, alcohol intake, and smoking history. Documentation and communication of findings are essential to enhance teamwork among providers.

Frequently, patients can identify the factors causing their anxiety, as well as coping skills effective in the past, and when they do, their discomfort decreases. Anxiety may be greatly reduced by initiating a discussion of concerns that are painful, frightening, or shameful, such as being dependent or accepting help. Use open-ended questions, reflection, clarification, and/or empathic remarks, such as "You're afraid of being a burden?" to help the patient to identify previously effective coping strategies and to integrate them with new ones. Use statements such as "What has helped you get through difficult times like this before?" "How can we help you use those strategies now?" or "How about talking about some new strategies that may work now?" Encourage the patient to identify supportive individuals who can either help emotionally or with tasks.

Preventive strategies

Preventive strategies can help to maintain a useful level of anxiety, one that enhances rather than interferes with problem solving (see Table 20.3). Effective preventive strategies that can be used by all providers involved with the patient follow:

1. *Provide concrete, objective information.* Fear of the unknown, lack of recent prior experience, or misinterpretations about an illness, procedure, test, or medication, especially when coupled with a tendency to focus on emotional aspects of experiences, may be a source of anxiety. Help patients and families know what to expect, and focus attention by realistically describing the potentially threatening experience with concrete objective information.[88] Describe both the typical subjective (e.g., sensations and temporal features) and objective (e.g., timing, nature of environment) features of stressful healthcare events, using concrete terminology. Avoid qualitative adjectives, such as "terrible." Also known as mental rehearsal and stress inoculation, concrete information increases the patient's understanding of the situation, allows for preparation under less emergent and more supportive conditions, and facilitates coping. Encourage the patient to ask questions, and then match the detail of the preparatory information to the request. Since anxiety hinders retention, use of understandable terms and repetition is helpful. Too much information at once may increase anxiety.

2. *Ensure stressful event warning before the event.* For example, a person may experience magnetic resonance imaging as entrapping or traumatic, or the placement of a central line as painful and threatening. Giving time to anticipate and mentally rehearse coping with the experience helps the person to maintain a sense of control and endure the procedure.

3. *Increase opportunities for control.* Illness can seriously disrupt a person's sense of control and increase anxiety. Help the patient to make distinctions between what is controllable, partially controllable, or not controllable. Focus on what is controllable or partially controllable and create decision-making and choice opportunities that fit the patient's knowledge. Ask patients to make choices about scheduling the day of the visit and the readiness for, and timing of, procedures and interventions.

4. *Increase patient and family participation in care.* Participation in care helps directly in coping and can be taught to both the patient and family members. Participation may reduce helplessness and increase a sense of control. Patients and family members may vary in their interest in participating, and in their ability to do so. Often, female family members are more likely to be caregivers. Other factors influencing the ability to participate include family roles such as spouse, parent, and sibling; quality of relationships; presence or absence of conflicts; and other commitments, such as work or other family roles. Cultures also vary in expectations and the duty or obligation to caregiving based on gender or family position. Participation may also help with the resolution of ineffective denial when a person's condition is deteriorating. Family members who are caring for a person may recognize and adjust to the deterioration.

5. *Encourage self-monitoring and the use of a stress diary.* Self-monitoring of stress is a cognitive-behavioral intervention. Ask the patient to record the situations, thoughts, and feelings that elicit stress and anxiety. The patient may record incidences of treatment-related stress, illness-related stress, or other, unrelated anxiety-provoking situations. Not only does this intervention provide assessment information, it also enhances collaboration with the patient and helps the patient understand the relationship between situations, thoughts, and feelings.

6. *Acknowledge fears.* Encourage and listen to the expression of feelings. Avoid denying the existence of problems or reassuring anxious people that "everything will be fine." Structure your availability. Refrain from avoiding anxious persons or their fears. Avoidance is likely to increase vulnerability, isolation, helplessness, and anxiety. Early structured intervention is more economical of time and more effective.

7. *Explore near-miss events.* Past or current exposure to a near-miss event is a potent generator of extreme stress and anxiety, with heightened vigilance. A near miss is a harrowing experience that overwhelms the ability to cope. It may be a one-time experience, such as a person's own near-death experience, the cardiac arrest of another person in similar circumstances, or something faced repeatedly, such as daily painful skin and wound care. Near misses should be explored, fears acknowledged and realistically evaluated in view of the person's situation, and help given in developing coping strategies.

8. *Manage symptoms.* Managing symptoms such as pain, dyspnea, and fatigue is an essential part of promoting self-control. Symptoms such as pain signal threat, and may lead to worries about the meaning of the symptom and whether necessary treatments will be worse or more frightening. Ensure pain control, especially before painful or frightening procedures. Severe anxiety may increase the perception of pain and increase the requirement for analgesia. Symptom management reduces distress and allows for rest.

9. *Structure uncertainty.* Even when there are many unknowns, the period of uncertainty can be framed with expected events, procedures, updates, and meetings with providers.

10. *Reduce sensory deprivation.* Sensory deprivation and isolation can heighten attention to various signals in the environment. Without the means for the patient to accurately interpret the signals, to be reassured, and to feel in control, the signals take on frightening meanings, such as abandonment and helplessness. Feeling isolated and helpless increases the sense of vulnerability and danger.

11. *Build hope.* Provide information about possible satisfactory outcomes and means to achieve them. Hope also may be built around coping ability, sustaining relationships, revising goals such as pain-free or peaceful death, and determination to endure. Many additional suggestions are provided in this text.

Treatment strategies

When it is evident that the person's anxiety level has escalated to the point of interfering with problem solving or comfort, the following strategies may be helpful.[26,89]

1. *Presence of supportive persons.* Familiar and supportive people, a family member, friend, or staff member can act as an "emotional anchor." Family and friends may need coaching to enable them to help in the situation without their own anxiety increasing.

2. *Expression of feelings, doubts, and fears.* Verbalizing feelings provides the opportunity to correct or restructure unrealistic misconceptions and automatic anxiety-provoking thoughts. Accurate information allows restructuring of perceptions and lends predictability to the situation. Aggressive confrontation of unrealistic perceptions may reinforce them, and is to be avoided.

3. *Use of antianxiety medications.* If medications are used, they should be given concurrently with other interventions and monitored. Use caution to avoid delirium from toxicity, especially in the older person.

4. *Promoting patient control and readiness.* If a patient is very frightened of a particular procedure, allow time for the patient to regain enough composure to make the decision to proceed. Forging ahead when a patient is panicked may appear to save time in the immediate situation, but it will increase the patient's sense of vulnerability and helplessness, possibly adding time over the long term.

5. *Management of panic.* When anxiety reaches panic, use presence and acknowledgment: "I know you are frightened. I'll stay with you." Communicate with repetition and simplicity. Guide the person to a smaller, quieter area away from other people and use quiet reassurance. Maintain a calm manner and reduce all environmental stimulation. Help the patient to focus on a single object (see below), and guide the patient in recognizing the physical features of the object while breathing rhythmically. Consider using prescribed anxiolytic medication.

6. *Massage, touch, and physical exercise.* For those who respond well to touch, massage releases muscle tension and may elicit emotional release. Physical exercise is a constructive way of releasing energy when direct problem solving is impossible or ineffective, because it reduces muscle tension and other physiological effects of anxiety.

7. *Relaxation techniques.* Relaxation techniques are likely to be effective for patients with mild to moderate anxiety who are able to concentrate and who desire to use them. Some techniques require learning and/or regular practice for effectiveness. Environmental awareness is reduced by focusing inward, with deliberate concentration on breathing, a sound, or an image, and suggestions of muscle relaxation. Progressive relaxation and autogenic relaxation are commonly used techniques, which require approximately 15 minutes. Relaxation and guided imagery scripts are readily available for use by clinicians.

8. *Breathing techniques.* Simple and easy to learn, breathing exercises emphasize slow, rhythmic, controlled breathing patterns that relax and distract the patient while slowing the heart rate, thus decreasing anxiety. Ask the patient to notice his or her normal breathing. Then ask the patient to take a few slow, deep abdominal breaths and to think "relax" or "I am calm" with each exhalation. Encourage practice during the day. Some patients are helped by seeing photographs and drawings of lungs and breathing to visualize their actions.

9. *Focusing techniques.* Useful for patients with episodes of severe-to-panic levels of anxiety, focusing repeatedly on one person or object in the room helps the patient to disengage from all other stimuli and promotes control. A combination of focusing, with demonstration and coaching of slow, rhythmic breathing (using a calm, low-pitched voice) is helpful. These techniques enhance the patient's self-control, which is desirable when the stress reaction is excessive and the stressful event cannot be changed or avoided. Both focusing and deep-breathing techniques can be used without prior practice and during extreme stress.

10. *Music therapy.* Soothing music or environmental sounds reduce anxiety by providing a tranquil environment and prompting recall of pleasant memories, which interrupt the stress response through distraction or direct sympathetic nervous system action.[88] Music most helpful for relaxation is primarily of string composition, low-pitched, with a simple and direct musical rhythm and a tempo of approximately 60 beats per minute, although music with flute, a cappella voice, and synthesizer is also effective.

11. *Imagery and visualization techniques.* Imagery inhibits anxiety by invoking a calm, peaceful mental image, including memories, dreams, fantasies, and visions. Guided imagery is the deliberate, goal-directed use of the natural capacities of the imagination. Using all the senses, imagery serves as a bridge for connecting body, mind, and spirit. Imagery, especially when combined with relaxation, promotes coping with illness by anxiety reduction, enhanced self-control, feeling expression, symptom relief, healing promotion, and dealing with role changes. Regular practice of imagery enhances success. Guided imagery for pain or anxiety reduction should not be attempted the first time during periods of extreme stress. Imagery in conversation is subtle and spontaneous. Often, without being aware of it, healthcare providers' questions and statements to patients include imagery. Easily combined with routine activities, the deliberate use of conversational imagery involves listening to and positively using the language, beliefs, and metaphors of the patient. Be aware of descriptors used for the effects of medications or treatments, because they affect the patient's attitude and response. Healthcare providers can enhance hope and self-control if they give empowering, healing messages that emphasize how the treatment will help.

Psychotherapeutic interventions targeted to symptoms of depression

Depression is inadequately treated in palliative care, although many patients experience depressive symptoms. Goals for the depressed patient are (1) to ensure a safe environment, (2) to assist the patient in reducing depressive symptoms and maladaptive coping responses, (3) to restore or increase the patient's functional level, (4) to improve quality of life if possible, and (5) to prevent future relapse and recurrence of depression.

Table 20.4 Nonpharmacological interventions for treatment of depression

Cognitive interventions	Behavioral interventions
Review and reinforce realistic ideas and expectations.	Provide directed activities.
Help the patient test the accuracy of self-defeating assumptions.	Develop a hierarchy of behaviors with the patient and use a graded task assignment.
Help the patient identify and test negative automatic thoughts.	
Review and reinforce patient's strengths.	Develop structured daily activity schedules.
Set realistic, achievable goals.	Encourage the at-home use of a diary or journal to monitor automatic thoughts, behaviors, and emotions; review this with the patient.
Explain all actions and plans, seek feedback and participation in decision-making.	
Provide choices (e.g., about the timing of an activity).	Use systematic application of reinforcement.
Teach thought stopping or thought interruption to halt negative or self-defeating thoughts.	Encourage self-monitoring of predetermined behaviors, such as sleep pattern, diet, and physical exercises.
Encourage exploration of feelings only for a specific purpose and only if the patient is not ruminating (e.g., constant repeating of failures or problems).	Focus on goal attainment and preparation for future adaptive coping.
Direct the patient to activities with gentle reminders to focus as a way to discourage rumination.	Specific Behavioral Strategies
	Observe the patient's self-care patterns, then negotiate with the patient to develop a structured, daily schedule.
Listen and take appropriate action on physical complaints, then redirect and assist the patient to accomplish activities.	Develop realistic daily self-care goals with the patient to increase sense of control.
Avoid denying the patient's sadness or depressed feelings or reason to feel that way.	Upgrade the goals gradually to provide increased opportunity for positive reinforcement and goal attainment.
Avoid chastising the patient for feeling sad.	
	Use a chart for monitoring daily progress; gold stars may be used as reinforcement; a visible chart facilitates communication, consistency among caregivers, and meaningful reinforcement (i.e., praise and positive attention from others).
Interpersonal Interventions	
Educate the patient about the physical and biochemical causes of depression and the good prognosis.	
Enhance social skills through modeling, role-playing, rehearsal, feedback, and reinforcement.	Provide sufficient time and repetitive reassurance ("You can do it") to encourage patients to accomplish self-care actions.
Build rapport with frequent, short visits.	
Engage in normal social conversation with the patient as often as possible.	Positively reinforce even small achievements.
Give consistent attention, even when the patient is uncommunicative, to show that the patient is worthwhile.	Provide physical assistance with self-care activities, especially those related to appearance and hygiene, that the patient is unable to do.
Direct comments and questions to the patient rather than to significant others.	
Allow adequate time for the patient to prepare a response.	Adjust physical assistance, verbal direction, reminders, and teaching to the actual needs and abilities of the patient; and avoid increasing unnecessary dependence by overdoing.
Mobilize family and social support systems.	
Encourage the patient to maintain open communication and share feelings with significant others.	Teach deep breathing or relaxation techniques for anxiety management.
Supportively involve family and friends and teach them how to help.	
Avoid sharing with the patient your personal reactions to the patient's dependent behavior.	Complementary Therapies
	Guided imagery and visualization

(continued)

Table 20.4 Continued

Cognitive interventions	Behavioral interventions
Avoid medical jargon, advice giving, sharing personal experiences, or making value judgments.	Art and music therapies
	Humor
Avoid false reassurance.	Aerobic exercise
	Phototherapy
	Aromatherapy and massage

Source: Minarik (1996), reference 30.

Crisis intervention

Crisis intervention is appropriate treatment for a grief-and-loss reaction and when a patient feels overwhelmed. Effective strategies also include providing guidance on current problems, reinforcing coping resources and strengths, and enhancing social supports.

Cognitive interventions

Cognitive interventions (Table 20.4) are based on a view of depression as the result of faulty thinking. A person's reaction depends on how that person perceives and interprets the situation of chronic illness. Patterns of thinking associated with depression include self-condemnation, leading to feelings of inadequacy and guilt; hopelessness, which is often combined with helplessness; and self-pity, which comes from magnification or catastrophizing about one's problems. Cognitive approaches involve clarification of misconceptions and modification of faulty assumptions by identifying and correcting distorted, negative, and catastrophic thinking. Cognitive approaches are effective in treating forms of depression. Therapy is usually brief, with the primary goal of reversing and decreasing the likelihood of recurrence of the symptoms of depression by modifying cognitions. It requires effort on the part of the patient. The effect is more powerful if homework and practice are included. Cognitive restructuring is one of the strategies used in cognitive therapy. In this strategy, patients are aided in identifying and evaluating maladaptive attitudes, thoughts, and beliefs by self-monitoring and recording their automatic thoughts when they feel depressed. The patient is then helped to replace self-defeating patterns of thinking with more constructive patterns. For example, "The treatment is not working. I can't cope; nothing works for me," could be replaced with a rational response such as "I can cope. I have learned how to help myself and I can do it." New self-statements and their associated feeling responses can also be written on the self-monitoring form. Over time, the patient learns to modify thinking, and learns a method for combating other automatic thoughts.

Imagery rehearsal is a useful strategy for helping patients to cope with situations in which they usually become depressed. The first step is to anticipate events that could be problematic, such as a magnetic resonance procedure. The patient is helped to develop constructive self-statements; then, imagery is used to provide an opportunity for the patient to mentally rehearse how to think, act, and feel in the situation. The combination of imagery with cognitive restructuring increases the effectiveness.

Interpersonal interventions

Interpersonal interventions (see Table 20.4) focus on improved self-esteem, the development of effective social skills, and dealing with interpersonal and relationship difficulties. Interpersonal difficulties that could be a focus include role disruptions or transitions, social isolation, delayed grief reaction, family conflict, or role enactment. Psychotherapies include individual, group, and support groups led by a trained professional. Patient-led support groups or self-help groups are effective for the general chronic illness population, but are less able to address the needs of depressed persons.

Behavioral interventions

Behavioral interventions (see Table 20.4) are based on a functional analysis of behavior and on social learning theory. These interventions are often used in combination with cognitive interventions, such as self-monitoring and imagery rehearsal. The key to the behavioral approach is to avoid reinforcement of dependent or negative behaviors. Instead, provide a contingency relationship between positive reinforcement and independent behavior and positive interactions with the environment. This approach suggests that, by altering behavior, subsequent thoughts and feelings are positively influenced. It is helpful to structure this approach using the following self-care functional areas: behavior related to breathing, eating, and drinking; elimination patterns; personal hygiene behavior; rest and activity patterns; and patterns of solitude and social interaction. The aim is to maintain involvement in activities associated with positive moods and, if possible, to avoid situations that trigger depression. This approach has been effective at helping family members of terminally ill patients see and accept functional decline.

Alternative and complementary therapies

Complementary therapies may help reduce mild depressive symptoms, or they may be used as an adjunct to other therapies for more severe depressive symptoms. Strategies described for anxiety, such as guided imagery and visualization, the use of drawings or photographs, and music therapy, also may be used for depression. Art therapy for creative self-expression, use of humor and laughter, aerobic exercise, and aromatherapy massage have been helpful for mild depressive symptoms. Phototherapy, which is exposure to bright, wide-spectrum light, has shown promise in patients with cancer.[90] See chapter 26, "Complementary and Alternative Therapies in Palliative Care," for a more in-depth review.

Conclusion

The psychosocial issues in persons facing life-threatening illness are influenced by individual, sociocultural, medical, and family factors. Most patients receiving palliative treatment, and their families, experience expected periods of emotional turmoil that occur at transition points, as is seen, for example, along the clinical course of cancer. Some patients experience anxiety and depressive disorders. This chapter has described the spectrum of anxiety and depressive symptoms during the palliative care trajectory; models useful for understanding the interaction of psychiatric and medical symptoms and for designing appropriate treatments; guidelines for referral to trained psychiatric clinicians; and a range of treatments for anxiety and depression. Supportive psychotherapeutic measures, such as those described in this chapter, should be used routinely because they minimize distress, and enhance feelings of control and mastery over self and environment. Assessment and treatment of psychosocial problems, including physical symptoms, psychological distress, caregiver burden, and psychiatric disorders, can enhance quality of life throughout the palliative care trajectory.

References

1. Zabora J, Brintzenhofeszoc K, Curbow B, Hooker C, Piantadosi S. The prevalence of psychological distress by cancer site. Psychooncology. 2001;10:19.
2. Kirkova J, Walsh D, Rybicki L, et al. Symptom severity and distress in advanced cancer. Palliat Med. 2010;24:330–339.
3. Hsu T, Ennis M, Hood N, Graham M, Goodwin PJ. Quality of life in long-term breast cancer survivors. J Clin Oncol. 2013;31(28):3540 3548.
4. Syrjala KL, Chapko MK, Vitaliano PP, et al. Recovery after allogenic marrow transplantation: a prospective study of predictors of long-term physical and psychosocial functioning. Bone Marrow Transplant. 1993;11:319.
5. Tschuschke V, Hertenstein B, Arnold R, et al. Associations between coping and survival time of adult leukemia patients receiving allogeneic bone marrow transplantation: results of a prospective study. J Psychosom Res. 2001;50:277.
6. Steinhauser KE, Christakis NA, Clipp EC, et al. Factors considered important at the end of life by patients, family, physicians, and other care providers. JAMA. 2000;284:2476.
7. Holland JC, Alici Y. Management of distress in cancer patients. J Support Oncol. 2010;8(1):4–12.
8. Weissman A, Worden JW. The existential plight in cancer: significance of the first 100 days. Int J Psychiatry Med. 1976;7:1.
9. Walker J, Holm Hansen C, Martin P, et al. Prevalence of depression in adults with cancer: a systematic review. Ann Oncol. 2013;24(4): 895–900.
10. Graydon JE. Factors that predict patients' functioning following treatment for cancer. Int J Nurs Stud 1988;25:117–124.
11. Richardson JL, Zamegar Z, Bisno B, Levine A. Psychosocial status at initiation of cancer treatment and survival. J Psychosom Res. 1990;34:189.
12. Vickberg SMJ, Duhamel KN, Smith MY, et al. Global meaning and psychological adjustment among survivors of bone marrow transplant. Psychooncology. 2001;10:29.
13. van Laarhoven HW, Schilderman J, Bleijenberg G, et al. Coping, quality of life, depression, and hopelessness in cancer patients in a curative and palliative, end-of-life care setting. Cancer Nurs. 2011;34(4):302–314.
14. Watson M, Greer S, Blake S, Sharpnell K. Reaction to a diagnosis of breast cancer: relationship between denial, delay, and rates of psychological morbidity. Cancer. 1984;53: 2008–2012.
15. Molassiotis A, Van Den Akker OBA, Milligan DW, Goldman JM. Symptom distress, coping style and biological variables as predictors of survival after bone marrow transplantation. J Psychosomatic Res. 1997;42:275.
16. Bope E. Follow-up of the cancer patient: surveillance for metastasis. Prim Care. 1987;14:391–401.
17. Savard J, Ivers H. The evolution of fear of cancer recurrence during the cancer care trajectory and its relationship with cancer characteristics. J Psychosom Res. 2013;74(4):354–360.
18. Silverfarb PM, Maurer LH, Crouthamel CS. Psychosocial aspects of neoplastic disease: I. Functional status of breast cancer patients during different treatment regimens. Am J Psychiatry. 1980;137:450–455.
19. Wise MG, Taylor SE. Anxiety and mood disorders in medically ill patients. J Clin Psychiatry. 1990;51(Suppl 1):27–32.
20. Breitbart W. Identifying patients at risk for and treatment of major psychiatric complications of cancer. Support Care Cancer. 1995;3:45–60.
21. Greer JA, Jackson VA, Meier DE, Temel JS. Early integration of palliative care services with standard oncology care for patients with advanced cancer. CA Cancer J Clin. 2013;63(5):349–363.
22. Steinhauser KE, Christakis NA, Clipp EC, et al. Factors considered important at the end of life by patients, family, physicians, and other care providers. JAMA. 2000;284:2476.
23. Emanuel EJ, Emanuel LL. The promise of a good death. Lancet. 1998;351:21.
24. Puchalski CM. Spirituality in the cancer trajectory. Ann Oncol. 2012;23(Suppl 3):49–55.
25. Wright AA, Stieglitz H, Kupersztoch YM, et al. United States acculturation and cancer patients' end-of-life care. PLoS One. 2013;8(3):e58663.
26. Tang ST, McCorkle R. Determinants of place of death for terminal cancer patients. Cancer Invest. 2001;19:165.
27. Roth AJ, Breitbart W. Psychiatric emergencies in terminally ill cancer patients. Hematol Oncol Clin North Am. 1996;10:235–259.
28. Fernandez R, Levy JK, Lachar BL, Small GW. The management of depression and anxiety in the elderly. J Clin Psychiatry. 1995;56(Suppl 2):20–29.
29. Kurlowicz LH. Depression in hospitalized medically ill elders: evolution of the concept. Arch Psychiatric Nurs. 1994;7:124–136.
30. Minarik P. Psychosocial intervention with ineffective coping responses to physical illness: depression-related. In: Barry PD (ed.), Psychosocial Nursing: Care of Physically Ill Patients and Their Families. New York: Lippincott-Raven; 1996:323–339.
31. Levenson J, Lesko LM. Psychiatric aspects of adult leukemia. Semin Oncol Nurs. 1990;6:76–83.
32. Pasacreta JV, Pickett M. Psychosocial aspects of palliative care. Semin Oncol Nurs. 1998;14:110–120.
33. Bloom JR. Social support, accommodation to stress and adjustment to breast cancer. Soc Sci Med. 1982;16:1329–1338.
34. Molassiotis A, Van Den Akker OBA, Boughton BJ. Perceived social support, family environment and psychosocial recovery in bone marrow transplant long-term survivors. Soc Sci Med. 1997;44:317.
35. Andrykowski MA, Brady MJ, Henslee-Downey PJ. Psychosocial factors predictive of survival after allogenic bone marrow transplantation for leukemia. Psychosom Med. 1994;56:432.
36. Molassiotis A, Van Den Akker OBA, Milligan DW, Goldman JM. Symptom distress, coping style and biological variables as predictors of survival after bone marrow transplantation. J Psychosom Res. 1997;42:275.
37. Seitz DC, Besier T, Debatin KM, et al. Posttraumatic stress, depression and anxiety among adult long-term survivors of cancer in adolescence. Eur J Cancer. 2010;46(9):1596–1606.
38. Fitch MI. Screening for distress: a role for oncology nursing. Curr Opin Oncol. 2011;23(4):331–337.
39. Derogatis LR, Morrow GR, Petting J, et al. The prevalence of psychiatric disorders among cancer patients. JAMA. 1983;249:751–757.
40. Massie MJ, Gagnon P, Holland JC. Depression and suicide in patients with cancer. J Pain Symptom Manage. 1994;9:325–340.

41. Pasacreta JV, Massie MJ. Psychiatric complications in patients with cancer. Oncol Nurs Forum. 1990;17:19–24.

42. Pasacreta JV, Massie MJ. Nurses' reports of psychiatric complications in patients with cancer. Oncol Nurs Forum. 1990;3:347–353.

43. Pasacreta JV, McCorkle R. Psychosocial aspects of cancer. In: McCorkle R, Grant M, Stromborg MF, Baird S (eds.), Cancer Nursing: A Comprehensive Textbook. 2nd ed. Philadelphia: Saunders; 1991:1074–1090.

44. McDaniel JS, Messelman DL, Porter MR, Reed DA, Nemeroff CB. Depression in patients with cancer: diagnosis, biology and treatment. Arch Gen Psychiatry. 1995;52:89–99.

45. Cassem EH. Depressive disorders in the medically ill. Psychosomatics. 1995;36:S2–S10.

46. Cavanaugh S. Depression in the medically ill. Psychosomatics. 1995;36:48–59.

47. Barraclough J. ABC of palliative care: depression, anxiety, and confusion. BMJ. 1997;315:1365–1368.

48. Morse JM, Doberneck B. Delineating the concept of hope. Image J Nurs Scholarsh. 1995;27:277–285.

49. Loge JH, Abrahamsen AF, Ekeberg O, Kaasa S. Fatigue and psychiatric morbidity among Hodgkin's disease survivors. J Pain Symptom Manage. 2000;19:91.

50. McCoy, D.M. Treatment considerations for depression in patients with significant medical comorbidity. J Fam Pract. 1996;43(Suppl):S35–S44.

51. Chochinov HM, McClement SE, Hack TF, et al. Health care provider communication: an empirical model of therapeutic effectiveness. Cancer. 2013;119(9):1706–1713.

52. Rustad JK, David D, Currier MB. Cancer and post-traumatic stress disorder: diagnosis, pathogenesis, and treatment considerations. Palliat Support Care. 2012;10:213–223.

53. Mitchell AJ, Ferguson DW, Gill J, Paul J, Symonds P. Depression and anxiety in long-term cancer survivors compared with spouses and healthy controls: a systematic review and meta-analysis. Lancet Oncol. 2013;14(8):721–732.

54. Lutgendorf SK, Sood AK. Biobehavioral factors and cancer progression: physiological pathways and mechanisms. Psychosom Med. 2011;73(9):724–730.

55. Sarna L, McCorkle R. Living with lung cancer: a prototype to describe the burden of care for patient, family and caregivers. Cancer Pract. 1996;4:245–251.

56. McCorkle R, Yost LS, Jespon C, et al. A cancer experience: relationship of patient psychosocial responses to caregiver burden overtime. Psychooncology. 1993;2:21.

57. Robinson LA, Berman JS, Neimeyer RA. Psychotherapy for the treatment of depression: a comprehensive review of controlled outcome research. Psychol Bull. 1990;108:30–49.

58. Beck AT, Rush AJ, Shaw BF, et al. Cognitive Therapy of Depression. A Treatment Manual. New York: Guilford Press; 1979.

59. Beck AT. Cognitive therapy: a 30-year retrospective. Am Psychol. 1991;46:368–375.

60. Johnson J, Weissman MM, Klerman GL. Service utilization and social morbidity associated with depressive symptoms in the community. JAMA. 1992;267:1478–1483.

61. Koenig HG, George LK, Peterson BL, Pieper CF. Depression in medically ill hospitalized older adults: prevalence characteristics, and course of symptoms according to six diagnostic schemes. Am J Psychiatry. 1997;154:1376–1383.

62. Kissane DW. The relief of existential suffering. Arch Intern Med. 2012;172:1501–1505.

63. DiMatteo MR, Lepper HS, Croghan TW. Depression is a risk factor for noncompliance with medical treatment: metaanalysis of the effects of anxiety and depression on patient adherence. Arch Intern Med. 2000;160:2101–2107.

64. Barg F, Cooley M, Pasacreta JV, Senay B, McCorkle R. Development of a self-administered psychosocial cancer screening tool. Cancer Pract. 1994;2:288–296.

65. Roth AJ, Kornblith AB, Batel-Copel L, Holland J. Rapid screening for psychologic distress in men with prostate carcinoma. Cancer. 1998;82:1904–1908.

66. Pasacreta JV, McCorkle R, Jacobsen P, Lundberg J, Holland JC. Distress management training for oncology nurses: description of an innovative and timely new program. Cancer Nurs. 2008;31: 485–490.

67. Anguiano L, Mayer DK, Piven ML, Rosenstein D. A literature review of suicide in cancer patients. Cancer Nurs. 2012;35(4):E14–E26.

68. Misono S, Weiss NS, Fann JR, Redman M, Yueh B. Incidence of suicide in persons with cancer. J Clin Oncol. 2008;26(29):4731–4738.

69. Urban D, Rao A, Bressel M, Neiger D, Solomon B, Mileshkin L. Suicide in lung cancer: who is at risk? Chest. 2013;144(4):1245–1252.

70. Steck N, Egger M, Maessen M, Reisch T, Zwahlen M. Euthanasia and assisted suicide in selected European countries and US states: systematic literature review. Med Care. 2013;51(10):938–944.

71. St John PD, Man-Son-Hing M. Physician-assisted suicide: the physician as an unwitting accomplice. J Palliat Care. 1999;15:56–58.

72. Hendry M, Pasterfield D, Lewis R, Carter B, Hodgson D, Wilkinson C. Why do we want the right to die? A systematic review of the international literature on the views of patients, carers and the public on assisted dying. Palliat Med. 2013;27(1):13–26.

73. Cooke L, Gotto J, Mayorga L, Grant M, Lynn R. What do I say? Suicide assessment and management. Clin J Oncol Nurs. 2013;17(1):E1–E7.

74. Qill TE. Suicidal thoughts and actions in cancer patients: the time for exploration is now. J Clin Oncol. 2008;10:4705–4707.

75. Stuber ML, Reed GM. "Never been done before": consultative issues in innovative therapies. Gen Hosp Psychiatry. 1991;13:337.

76. Snyderman D, Wynn D. Depression in cancer patients. Prim Care. 2009; 36:703–719.

77. Koenig HG, Breitner JCS. Use of antidepressants in medically ill older patients. Psychosomatics. 1990;31:22–32.

78. Frank L, Revicki DA, Sorensen SV, Shih YC. The economics of selective serotonin reuptake inhibitors in depression: a critical review. CNS Drugs. 2001;15:59–83.

79. Katzelnick DJ, Kobak KA, Jefferson JW. Prescribing pattern of antidepressant medications for depression in a HMO. Formulary. 1996;31:374–388.

80. Shuster JL, Stern TA, Greenberg DB. Pros and cons of fluoxetine for the depressed cancer patient. Oncology. 2002;11:45–55.

81. Prommer E. Methylphenidate: established and expanding roles in symptom management. Am J Hosp Palliat Care. 2012;29(6):483–490.

82. Vigano A, Watanabe S, Bruera E. Methylphenidate for the management of somatization in terminal cancer patients. J Pain Symptom Manage. 1995;10:167–170.

83. Woods SW, Tesar GE, Murray GB. Psychostimulant treatment of depressive disorders secondary to medical illness. J Clin Psychiatry. 1996;47:12–15.

84. Anderson CM, Griffin S, Rossi A. A comparative study of the impact of education vs process groups for families of patients with affective disorders. Fam Process. 1986;25:185–204.

85. Gallagher DE, Thompson LW. Treatment of major depressive disorder in older adult outpatients with brief psychotherapies. Psychother Theory Res Practice. 1982;19:482–490.

86. Persons JB, Burns DD, Perloff JM. Predictors of dropout and outcome in cognitive therapy for depression in a private practice setting. Cognit Ther Res. 1998;12:557–574.

87. Lazarus RS, Folkman S. Stress, Appraisal and Coping. New York: Springer; 1984.

88. Archie P, Bruera E, Cohen L. Music-based interventions in palliative cancer care: a review of quantitative studies and neurobiological literature. Support Care Cancer. 2013;21(9):2609–2624.

89. Beliles K, Stoudemire A. Psychopharmacologic treatment of depression in the medically ill. Psychosomatics. 1998;39: S2–S19.

90. Leavitt M, Minarik PA. The agitated, hypervigilant response. In: Rigel B, Ehrenreich D (eds.), Psychological Aspects of Critical Care Nursing. Rockville, MD: Aspen; 1989:49–65.

CHAPTER 21

Delirium, confusion, agitation, and restlessness

Debra E. Heidrich and Nancy K. English

> You said you wouldn't let them take me. I won't go! Please don't let them hurt me; I will be good.
>
> SC, a patient experiencing delirium

Key points

◆ Delirium, confusion, and agitation are common symptoms in the palliative care setting and are extremely distressing to both patient and family.

◆ Identifying patients at risk of developing these symptoms can lead to early recognition and prompt treatment.

◆ The etiology of these symptoms is frequently multifactorial; some causes are reversible and others not.

◆ The bedside nurse and advanced practice palliative care nurse are central to the assessment and management of patients experiencing delirium.

◆ Patient and family education regarding the reasons for these mental changes and how they will be managed is essential.

Case study

Mrs. Rice, a patient with delirium

Mrs. Rice is a 78-year-old widow with advanced stage COPD and moderate dementia. She lives with her adult daughter, Darlene, and Darlene's husband. Mrs. Rice has been hospitalized three times over the past 6 months with exacerbation of her COPD and pneumonia and required intubation and mechanical ventilation on her last admission. She is now admitted to the hospital in acute respiratory distress, requiring noninvasive ventilator support with a bilevel positive airway pressure (BiPAP) machine. The palliative care team has been consulted to discuss goals of care and to assist with symptom management.

Darlene reports that she noticed Mrs. Rice's cough was more productive than usual a couple of days ago, but Mrs. Rice did not report any change in her breathing and she did not have a fever. At about 3 AM, Darlene heard her mother calling for help. Mrs. Rice was struggling to breathe and looked frightened. Darlene called 911. When the paramedics arrived, Mrs. Rice became combative and begged Darlene to not let them "take her away." The paramedics reported they had to restrain Mrs. Rice during transport as she kept pulling off the oxygen mask and tried to hit the paramedic when he was putting the mask back on her. A chest X-ray showed bilateral

pneumonia. On admission she was oriented to person only. Her respiratory status continued to deteriorate, and she continued to be very agitated. BiPAP was initiated and she had to be restrained to prevent her from pulling off the BiPAP mask. When Darlene arrived in the emergency department (ED), Mrs. Rice told her, "They're trying to kill me! Get me out of here." Darlene and the staff worked to calm Mrs. Rice, with little effect. She was given lorazepam 0.5 mg IV. She became even more agitated. Two additional doses of lorazepam were given. Mrs. Rice slept after the third dose for about 1 hour, during which time she was transferred to a medical unit. When she woke, she again tried to pull of the BiPAP mask. When assessed by the nursing staff, Mrs. Rice appears fearful and tries to pull away. She sometimes refuses to answer questions. She called her daughter by name this morning; this afternoon she is calling her "mom."

Darlene states, "I know everyone thinks she's just a crazy old lady, but she never acts like this." Mrs. Rice was diagnosed with Alzheimer's dementia about 1 year ago. She is usually oriented to person, place, and time of year, although she often forgets what day of the week it is; she recognizes family and friends, but often can't remember the names of her grandchildren that she doesn't see regularly. And, she's usually very "mild-mannered" and cooperative. If she is "noncompliant" in any way, it is usually just that she forgets to do things. Darlene is both frightened and embarrassed by her mother's behavior.

Introduction

Delirium is a common neuropsychiatric disorder seen in all healthcare settings, and is frequently underdiagnosed, misdiagnosed, and poorly managed. Often, patients are labeled as "confused" and no further evaluation is performed to determine the cause of this confusion. This is particularly an issue with the elderly, whose confusion is often dismissed as dementia and for those with terminal illness, whose confusion may be accepted as part of disease progression. Patients at highest risk for delirium include those who are elderly, in intensive care units, or postoperative, as well as those with advanced illnesses. This syndrome is associated with significant morbidity and mortality, leading to increased length of hospital and nursing home stays, and risk of earlier death. The experience of delirium is frightening to both patients and their significant others; it impairs quality of living—and quality of dying. Prompt recognition and treatment are essential to improve patient outcomes, especially in the final stages of an illness. This chapter will discuss the prevalence of delirium, its associated symptoms, factors that contribute to delirium, assessment for delirium, interventions to prevent or lessen the severity of delirium, and important patient/family teaching points.

Incidence, prevalence, and outcomes

Delirium is considered the most common and serious cognitive disorder in hospitals and in the palliative care setting.[1-3] Reported incidence and prevalence rates vary depending on population being studied, criteria used to identify delirium, and setting. The majority of studies focus on the elderly population and the intensive care unit setting. Delirium is reported to be found in 0.5% to 10% of community-based elders, 8.9% to 47% of institutionalized elders, 14% to 56% of hospitalized elderly, 45% of elderly after general anesthesia, 60% to 80% of mechanically ventilated adult patients in intensive care units, 26% to 62% of palliative care admissions, and 58.8% to 88% of persons in the weeks or hours preceding death.[1-10] However, the true incidence of delirium is unknown because it often goes undetected or misdiagnosed. In a retrospective review of 319 patient care notes in three palliative care centers in the United Kingdom, Hey and colleagues found a documented diagnosis of delirium in 0% to 8.4% of charts, but when descriptions in the chart suggestive of delirium were taken into account the prevalence was estimated at 35.7% to 39.2%.[11] A systematic review of the literature in 2008 revealed that nurse recognition of delirium ranged from 26% to 83%.[12] Factors that contribute to a missed diagnosis include the following[12-16]:

- History of a past psychiatric diagnosis or cognitive disorder, such as dementia, to which the symptoms may be attributed

- Acceptance of confusion is an expected consequence of old age and dying

- The presence of pain

- Transient and fluctuating nature of symptoms

- Imprecise and overlapping use of terminology, such as delirium, acute confusion, and terminal restlessness

- Inconsistencies in use of and types of assessment tools used to diagnose delirium

Delirium is associated with adverse physical, cognitive, and psychological outcomes. It is associated with short- and long-term decline in cognitive functioning and increases in falls, length of hospital stays, need for institutionalized care after hospitalization, and mortality.[3,6-8,17-19]

While not everyone remembers their experience of delirium, those who do report having distressing feelings during the experience, including fear, anxiety, and feeling threatened.[20-24] Visual hallucinations of people or animals in the room intertwine with the people who are actually present, to create a confusing and frightening experience. Misinterpretations of real sensory experiences also lead to fear, anxiety, or the sense of being trapped in the experience, as illustrated by the quote at the beginning of this chapter. Procedures like injections may be interpreted as attempts to do harm, and interventions to reorient or reassure delirious patients

may be met with suspicion and the fear that everyone is lying to them.[20] Feeling threatened, the delirious patient may try to escape from the experience, leading to wandering behavior and falls as well as aggression toward caregivers. After the episode of delirium, persons report feeling humiliated and ashamed of their behavior while delirious. They also report a fear of experiencing delirium again in the future and may exhibit signs of posttraumatic stress disorder.[21,23,25] Caregivers also experience distress related to delirium. Family members recall more symptoms of delirium than both the patient and the bedside nurse and are more distressed by the experience.[22,23,26,27] Family members know the patient's baseline cognitive status and spend more time at the beside, so it is not surprising that they witness and, therefore, recall more delirium symptoms. Agitation and delusions/hallucinations are particularly distressing to both family members and nurses.[22,28] Interventions to decrease the incidence of delirium and prompt treatment of delirium symptoms may help decrease caregiver distress. And, providing information about delirium and support throughout this difficult time may reduce both acute and long-term distress in family members.[23,29]

Restlessness or agitation at the end of life, sometimes called "terminal restlessness" or "terminal delirium," has been viewed as an expected part of the dying process.[1,30-33] However, descriptions of terminal restlessness overlap considerably with the defining characteristics of delirium. It is likely that what is labeled terminal restlessness is actually delirium.[1,3,30,33] Importantly, delirium is potentially reversible in some persons, even at the end of life. Two frequently cited studies from 2000 report that up to 50% of delirium episodes in the palliative care setting are reversible.[10,34] Leonard and colleagues followed 121 persons diagnosed with delirium in an inpatient palliative care unit; 27% recovered from delirium before death[30]—fewer than the 50% reported by others, but still significant. Those with reversible delirium tend to be of younger age, have less severe cognitive disturbance, and absence of organ failure as a cause of delirium.[30,35] Given this potential for reversibility, a thorough evaluation of treatable causes of delirium is required, followed by appropriate interventions based on the patient's overall condition and the goals of care.

In addition to the negative physical and psychological impacts of this syndrome, there is a significant financial burden, in part due to the increased length of stays in hospital and increased use of long-term care facilities associated with delirium. A study examining 1-year healthcare costs associated with delirium in the elderly estimated the total cost attributable to delirium to be $16,303 to $64,421 per patient, implying that the national burden of delirium on the healthcare systems ranges from $38 billion to $152 billion each year.[36] Zaubler and colleagues implemented a multicomponent delirium intervention program for patients over the age of 70 admitted to a general medical floor at a community hospital and showed a 40% reduction in the incidence of delirium, resulting in an annual cost savings of $1.1 million for that facility alone.[8] A comprehensive plan that includes prevention, assessment and early detection, and appropriate intervention has the potential to save lives, improve quality of life, and significantly decrease costs.

Definition and key features of delirium

Understanding the many symptoms, syndromes, and diagnoses associated with cognitive changes in persons with an advanced illness can be difficult at best. Terms such as "confusion," "acute confusion," "delirium," and "terminal restlessness" are often used to describe changes in mental status without clear definitions or use of standard psychiatric classifications. The use of imprecise terminology can lead to mislabeling of behaviors, miscommunication among healthcare professionals, and misdiagnoses of cognitive changes. Therefore, the potential for the mismanagement of any cognitive change is extremely high.

The fifth edition of the *Diagnostic and Statistical Manual of Mental Disorders* (DSM-5) criteria for delirium are listed in Box 21.1.[37] Key features are that the disturbances develop over a short period of time, tend to fluctuate in severity during the course of a day, and represent a change from baseline.[37,38] There are no diagnostic tests for delirium; the diagnosis is primarily clinical, based on careful observation and awareness of the criteria.[17] Because the presentation of symptoms can sometimes be subtle, and symptoms fluctuate throughout the day, nurses, who have more frequent and continuous contact with patients, are key to the early recognition of delirium. However, without education about delirium and use of tools to assist in identifying it, nurses often miss the diagnosis.[11,12,14,15] Vasilevskis and colleagues showed that with education and integration of delirium assessment into routine documentation in an ICU, bedside nurse measurements of delirium were valid, reliable, and sustainable over time.[39]

Disturbance in attention refers to a reduced ability to direct, focus, sustain, and shift attention. In delirium, the disturbed attention is combined with a *disturbance in awareness*, defined as having a reduced orientation to the environment. Previous versions of the DSM used "disturbances in consciousness" as a criterion for delirium. However, there is no consensus on what is meant by the term "consciousness"; awareness and attention are included in the DSM-5 as these are operational terms to describe consciousness and can be assessed with bedside tests in the clinical setting.[38] Patients may be hypoalert, slow to respond, unable to maintain eye contact, or may fall asleep between stimuli, requiring an increased amount of stimuli (touch, calling name) to elicit a response. Conversely, patients may be hyperalert, overreact to stimuli, startle easily, rapidly change from one topic to another in conversation, and exhibit signs of agitation.[17,40] In the early stage of delirium, the abnormalities in attention and awareness may be subtle and easily overlooked.[40]

Changes in cognition in delirium include memory deficit, disorientation, language disturbances, and perceptual disturbances.[17,38,40] Disruptions in orientation usually manifest as disorientation to time or place, with time disorientation being the first to be affected. Short-term memory deficits are the most evident memory impairments. Patients may not remember conversations, television shows, or verbal instructions. For example, the person experiencing cognitive changes may remember the nurse visiting, but not anything the nurse said or did. Language disturbances include incoherent or jumbled speech, use of repetitive phrases, abnormally long pauses in the conversation, or difficulty with finding the proper words to convey a message.[17,40] Perceptual disturbances are no longer considered essential to the diagnosis of delirium.[1] When they are present, these disturbances may include misinterpretations, illusions, or hallucinations. Visual misperceptions and hallucinations are most common, but auditory, tactile, gustatory, and olfactory misperceptions or hallucinations can also occur. Aggressive or combative behavior may occur if the patient misperceives caregivers' actions as intent to harm.

Development over a short time and fluctuation during the course of the day are important considerations in both identifying delirium and in differentiating it from dementia. In dementia, short-term memory problems occur progressively over months versus over hours or days with delirium. Importantly, persons with dementia are at high risk of developing delirium.[4,6,7] Obtaining a history of memory issues from the family is vital to establishing the patient's baseline, as it is the change from the baseline that indicates delirium in persons with and without dementia. Because the symptoms fluctuate, assessment throughout the course of the day is essential to identify delirium. Family member reports of subtle changes in attention, cognition, or sleep pattern disturbances are indicators that a more thorough assessment is needed.[27,29,41,42]

Additional clinical features of delirium that are not included in the diagnostic criteria but are frequently present include sleep-wake cycle disruption (73% of cases), hallucinations or perceptual distortions (50%), delusional or fixed false beliefs (30%), and mood lability.[35,41] Some of these features help in differentiating delirium from dementia, as persons with dementia do not typically have delusions or hallucinations. Sleep-wake cycle disruptions are more pronounced in persons with delirium and are of new onset. "Sundowning," or increased confusion and agitation at night, should be viewed as a potential sign of delirium unless this behavior has been present for weeks to months in the person with dementia.

Subtypes of delirium

There are three clinical subtypes of delirium based on arousal disturbance and psychomotor behavior: hyperactive, hypoactive, and mixed.[1,17,38,43–45] Box 21.2 outlines the characteristics of the subtype categories. There are some variations in the definitions of these subtypes from one author to another, but in general hyperactive delirium is associated with hypervigilance, restlessness, and agitation; the hypoactive subtype is characterized by confusion and somnolence; and the mixed subtype has alternating features of hyperactive and hypoactive delirium. Although psychotic features, such as delusions or hallucinations, are most often associated with hyperactive delirium, these symptoms are present in many patients with hypoactive delirium.[44,45] Some patients, may

---

Box 21.1 Diagnostic criteria for delirium

A. Disturbance in attention and awareness

B. The disturbance develops over a short period of time and tends to fluctuate in severity during the course of the day.

C. Disturbance in cognition

D. The disturbances in criteria A and C are not explained by another preexisting, established, or evolving neurocognitive disorder and do not occur in the context of a severely reduced level of arousal, such as coma.

E. History, physical examination, or laboratory findings indicate that the disturbance is caused by a medical condition, substance intoxication or withdrawal, or exposure to a toxin, or is because of multiple etiologies.

Source: Adapted from American Psychiatric Association (2013), reference 37.

Box 21.2 Motor subtypes of delirium

Hyperactive subtype if definite evidence in the previous 24 hours of at least two of the following*:

1. Increased quantity of motor activity, e.g., pacing, fidgeting, general overactivity

2. Loss of control of activity, e.g., unable to remain still when required

3. Restlessness, e.g., complains of mental restlessness or appears agitated

4. Wandering, e.g., moving around without clear direction or purpose

Hypoactive subtype if definite evidence in the previous 24 hours of two or more of the following**:

1. Decreased amount of activity, e.g., sits still with few spontaneous movements

2. Decreased speed of actions, e.g., slow movements, including walking

3. Reduced awareness of surroundings, e.g., passive attitude to surroundings

4. Decreased amount of speech, e.g., doesn't answer questions or answers are restricted to a minimum

5. Decreased speed of speech, e.g., long pauses or slowed pace of speech

6. Listlessness, e.g., slow or reduced response to environment

7. Reduced alertness/withdrawal, e.g., detached or lacking awareness of surroundings

*The symptoms must be a deviation from predelirious baseline.

**Where at least one of either decreased amount of activity or speed of actions is present.

Mixed motor subtype if evidence of both hyperactive and hypoactive subtype in the previous 24 hours.

No motor subtype if evidence of neither hyperactive or hypoactive subtype in the previous 24 hours.

Source: Adapted from Meagher et al. (2008), reference 43.

---

not exhibit enough symptoms to identify a subtype.[35,43,44] One study in an inpatient palliative care unit showed that the few subjects (6 of 100) whose delirium fit no subtype had fewer symptoms, were more likely to recover from the delirium, and were more likely to survive greater than 1 month than any other subtype.[35] In this study, delirium assessments were done twice weekly. Given the fluctuating nature of delirium, it is not clear whether these subjects may have exhibited symptoms at times that would have placed them in one of the defined categories.

Subsyndromal delirium is described by some as occurring in those persons who have some symptoms associated with delirium, but are not symptomatic enough to fit the criteria for the diagnosis of delirium. The DSM-5 does not include subsyndromal delirium as a category because it is not clear that this distinction is clinically practical given the fluctuating course of delirium.[38] Persons who

exhibit these more subtle symptoms are certainly at risk of developing the diagnosable syndrome of delirium. Clinicians need to intervene to eliminate as many factors that contribute to delirium as possible, and they need to monitor these patients routinely for progression to delirium.

Hyperactive delirium is identified more often in the clinical setting than the other subtypes because the symptoms of hypervigilance, restlessness, and agitation attract caregiver attention. However, the hypoactive and mixed forms appears to be more prevalent.[2,17,35,40,46] The hypoactive form of delirium is likely underdiagnosed as symptoms are less noticeable, or may be misdiagnosed as depression or fatigue.[1,2,7,15,17,40,46,47]

An interesting area of study is determining whether the subtype of delirium exhibited by a patient can be associated with its underlying causes and, therefore, assist in identifying reversible causes. Some studies suggest that delirium associated with metabolic factors, organ failure, and older age is hypoactive while delirium associated with substance withdrawal or intoxication is hyperactive.[44,48,49] Other studies, however, show no association between subtype and etiology.[35,50,51] Variations in the population being studied, assessment tools, and definitions of subtypes account for some inconsistencies in the conclusions of these studies. Until more data are available, no assumptions as to underlying cause can be made solely on subtype of delirium.

Many studies have looked at outcomes related to subtype of delirium and show inconsistent findings.[1,17,30,35,44,45,50,52] Again, a lack of consistency in definitions and clinical criteria to identify subtypes may account for some of the variation seen in outcome studies. In some settings, patients with hyperactive delirium did worse; in other studies those with hypoactive delirium had poorer outcomes. In a review of these studies, Meagher concluded that the evidence suggests that persons with hypoactive delirium appear to have a worse prognosis.[44] A study of 100 consecutive cases of diagnosed delirium in patients admitted to a palliative care unit supports the conclusion that those with hypoactive delirium have worse outcomes.[35]

Delirium in the final days of life and deathbed phenomena

Most patients who exhibit signs of the dying process, experience symptoms consistent with delirium.[31–33,53] In a retrospective review, Chirco, Dunn, and Robinson found delirium usually occurs 24 to 48 hours prior to death, with subtle signs being evident approximately 7 days before death.[31] Delirium around the time of death is sometimes referred to as terminal restlessness, terminal delirium, terminal agitation, preterminal restlessness, preterminal delirium, or terminal psychosis. To avoid confusion, the qualifiers "terminal" and "preterminal" should be avoided and standardized assessment tools should be used to diagnose delirium throughout the course of illness, including in the final phase of life.

While delirium may be very frequent at the end of life, restless behaviors in the dying patient should not be accepted as simply "part of the dying process"; reversal of delirium maybe possible even in very advanced stages of illness.[30,34,35,53] Keep in mind that the studies that show up to 49% of terminally ill patients may have reversible delirium included all patients admitted during the data collection period.[30,34,35] One can speculate that if only patients who exhibit objective signs of the dying process are included, far fewer cases of documented delirium would be reversible. An evaluation to determine reversibility of a delirium is essential to facilitate a conscious, comfortable death whenever possible.

As death draws near, patients' may experience apparitions of "helpers" or family members who have died and now appear to the patient as "guides" in the transition from life to death. Deathbed visions (DBVs) have been defined as "spiritual, mystical or unexplainable experience[s] or coincidental occurrence[s] that take place in the arena of death."[54] Patients have reported seeing angels, religious figures, spiritual guides and deceased loved ones.[54–56] It has been reported that 10% of patients are aware and conscious prior to death. Of these, approximately 50% to 60% are reported to have experienced a DBV.[57] Fenwick and colleagues in the United Kingdom decided to demystify this phenomenon and record the frequency of end-of-life experiences, including DBVs, by interviewing 38 caregivers about their personal observations of dying patients in nursing and palliative care centers. Sixty-two percent of the caregivers reported that patients or their relatives spoke of DBVs and that it brought comfort to both the patient and the family. The caregivers described DBVs and end-of-life experiences as "intense, subjective experience[s] that held a profound personal meaning for the dying patient."[56]

Hospice nurses Callanan and Kelly refer to these kind of phenomena as "nearing death awareness" and define this concept as a special knowledge about the process of dying that may reveal what dying is like, or what is needed to die peacefully.[58] Themes of nearing death awareness include describing a place, talking to or being in the presence of someone who is not alive, knowledge of when death will occur, choosing the time of death, needing reconciliation, preparing for travel or change, being held back, and symbolic dreams.

Deathbed phenomena may be differentiated from delirium-related hallucinations or misperceptions by observing verbal and nonverbal behaviors. Persons experiencing DBVs tend to be calm or questioning but not fearful of the visions, are able to focus their attention on the vision and describe the experience coherently to others, may converse with the person(s) in the vision, and are comforted and consoled by this experience.

Pathophysiology and etiology of delirium

The pathophysiology of delirium is not clearly understood. Disturbances in cerebral oxygenation or blood flow, neurotransmitters, cytokine production, and plasma esterase activity have all been identified as potential contributing factors. Diminished blood flow and decreased oxygenation are seen with aging, hypotension, hypoxia, cirrhosis, and sepsis,[59–63] and may explain the long-term cognitive changes seen with prolonged delirium.[64,65] Acetylcholine deficiency, gamma-aminobutyric acid (GABA) deficiency, and dopamine excess are three of several neurotransmitter disturbances associated with delirium; neurotransmitter changes help to explain delirium associated with the use of medications such as anticholinergics and benzodiazepines, withdrawal from opioids and alcohol, organ system failure, sleep deprivation, and insults to the brain, such as ischemia.[44,62,66–71] Elevated levels of various cytokines have been shown in patients with delirium associated with sepsis and severe physical stresses such as hip fracture and surgery.[64,72–77] A decrease in the activity of plasma esterases, important drug metabolizing enzymes,

has been found in delirium and explains, in part, the mechanism behind medication-induced delirium.[71] These various theories to explain delirium are complementary; it is likely an interconnection of several pathological mechanisms that leads to delirium.[44,62,71]

Delirium usually develops due to the interrelationship between patient vulnerability (predisposing factors) and noxious insults (precipitating factors).[78–80] Table 21.1 identifies some of the common predisposing and precipitating factors for delirium. While a single precipitating factor in the predisposed patient may be enough to lead to delirium (for example, a single

Table 21.1 Predisposing and precipitating factors for delirium

Predisposing factors	Precipitating factors
Demographic characteristics	*Drugs*
Age of 65 years or older	Sedative hypnotics
Male sex	Narcotics
Cognitive status	Anticholinergic drugs
Dementia	Treatment with multiple drugs
Cognitive impairment	Alcohol or drug withdrawal
History of delirium	*Primary neurological diseases*
Depression	Stroke, particularly nondominant hemispheric
Functional status	Intracranial bleeding
Functional dependence	Meningitis or encephalitis
Immobility	*Intercurrent illnesses*
Low level of activity	Infections
History of falls	Iatrogenic complications
Sensory impairment	Severe acute illness
Visual impairment	Hypoxia
Hearing impairment	Shock
Decreased oral intake	Fever or hypothermia
Dehydration	Anemia
Malnutrition	Dehydration
Drugs	Poor nutritional status
Treatment with multiple psychoactive drugs	Low serum albumin level
Treatment with many drugs	Metabolic derangements (e.g., electrolyte, glucose, acid–base)
Alcohol abuse	*Surgery*
Coexisting medical conditions	Orthopedic surgery
Severe illness	Cardiac surgery
Multiple coexisting conditions	Prolonged cardiopulmonary bypass
Chronic renal or hepatic disease	Noncardiac surgery
History of stroke	*Environmental*
Neurological disease	Admission to an intensive care unit
Metabolic derangements	Use of physical restraints
Fracture or trauma	Use of bladder catheter
Terminal illness	Use of multiple procedures
Infection with human immunodeficiency virus	Pain
	Emotional stress
	Prolonged sleep deprivation

Source: Adapted from Inouye (2006), reference 71.

dose of an anticholinergic medication in a patient with dementia), there are often multiple factors involved in the development of delirium. Addressing only a single factor likely will not aid in improving delirium; an approach that addresses as many predisposing and precipitating factors as possible is needed for resolution.[78]

Cognitive impairment and dementia are the leading predisposing factors for delirium,[3,7,78,81-83] and persons with dementia are vulnerable to delirium at lower levels of medical acuity than nondemented persons.[4,6,81,84,85] One study showed that persons with dementia had poorer functional and nutritional status than those in the same age group who did not have dementia.[86] As both poor functional status and malnutrition are additional predisposing factors for delirium (see Table 21.1), this higher risk of delirium with dementia is not surprising. There likely are other factors (e.g., changes in levels of neurotransmitters and cerebral blood flow) in persons with dementia that also contribute to this increased vulnerability. Nurses must be aware of the increased risk of delirium in patients with dementia, carefully assess for signs of delirium, and work to eliminate or decrease precipitating factors that can be controlled. Too often, changes in behavior are dismissed as signs of the individual's dementia instead of being identified as signs of delirium. Table 21.2 identifies the factors that help in differentiating dementia from delirium. Knowledge of the patient's baseline cognitive status is critical for identifying recent changes in cognition and attention.

Several studies have identified key factors that increase the risk of delirium in subsets of populations. Despite an incidence rate of 40% to 80% in persons with cancer, delirium is rarely appreciated as a source of symptom distress in oncology settings.[1,40,48,89] Table 21.3 outlines the cancer-specific considerations as they relate to the risk factors for delirium, illustrating that persons with cancer have many predisposing risk factors and are exposed to multiple precipitating factors for delirium. Studies of patients undergoing surgery showed that preoperative cognitive deficits, preexisting depression, and impaired vision are common predisposing factors for delirium and that duration of surgery, prolonged intubation, surgery type, and elevated inflammatory markers are frequent precipitating factors for postoperative delirium.[84,90-92] In the hospice and palliative care setting, poor sleep quality, uncontrolled pain, multiple medications (including high dose opioids), dehydration, infection, dementia, and organ failure are associated with delirium.[30,33,41,93-96] Inouye and colleagues identified five risk factors for persistent delirium in the elderly at discharge from the hospital: dementia, vision impairment, functional impairment, high comorbidity, and use of physical restraints during delirium.[97] These studies reinforce the increased vulnerability of persons with underlying dementia or cognitive impairments and demonstrate the multiple precipitating factors common in many care settings.

Assessment

Comprehensive and ongoing assessment is necessary to identify patients at risk for delirium and for early detection of delirium. During routine assessments, nurses frequently observe behavior

Table 21.2 Differentiating delirium from dementia

	Delirium	Dementia
Onset	Acute or subacute, occurs over a short period of time (hours–days).	Insidious, often slow and progressive
Course	Fluctuates over the course of the day, worsens at night. Resolves over days to weeks	Stable over the course of the day; is progressive
Duration	If reversible, short term	Chronic and nonreversible
Consciousness	Impaired and can fluctuate rapidly. Clouded, with a reduced awareness of the environment	Clear and alert until the later stages. May become delirious, which will interfere
Cognitive defects	Impaired short-term memory, poor attention span	Poor short-term memory; attention span less affected until later stage
Attention	Reduced ability to focus, sustain, or shift attention	Relatively unaffected in the earlier stages
Orientation	Disoriented to time and place	Intact until months or years with the later stages. May have anomia (difficulty recognizing common objects) or agnosia (difficulty recognizing familiar people)
Delusions	Common, fleeting, usually transient and poorly organized	Often absent
Hallucinations	Common and usually visual, tactile, and olfactory	Often absent
Speech	Often uncharacteristic, loud, rapid, or slow (hypoactive)	Difficulty in finding words and articulating thoughts; aphasia
Affect	Mood lability	Mood lability
Sleep-wake cycle	Disturbed; may be reversed	Can be fragmented
Psychomotor activity	Increased, reduced, or unpredictable; variable depending on hyper/hypo-delirium	Can be normal; may exhibit apraxia

Sources: Adapted from Arnold (2005), reference 87; Milisen et al. (2006), reference 88.

Table 21.3 Cancer-specific risk factors for delirium

Type of physiological risk factor	Cancer-specific considerations
Nutritional deficiencies B vitamins Vitamin C Hypoproteinemia	◆ Symptom distress: nausea, emesis, mucositis, diarrhea, pain, and anorexia or cachexia syndrome ◆ Surgical alteration of the head and neck region or gastrointestinal tract ◆ Nonoral feeding routes: gastrostomy feeding tube and use of total parenteral nutrition
Cardiovascular abnormalities Decreased cardiac output states: myocardial infarction, dysrythmias, congestive heart failure, and cardiogenic shock Alterations in peripheral vascular resistance: increased and decreased states Vascular occlusion: emboli and disseminated intravascular coagulopathy	◆ Septic shock syndrome ◆ Hypercoagulopathy and hyperviscosity ◆ Anthracycline-related cardiomyopathy ◆ Central-line occlusion ◆ Thrombi associated with immobility and paraneoplastic syndromes ◆ Disseminated intravascular coagulopathy
Cerebral disease Vascular insufficiency: transient ischemic attacks, cerebral vascular accidents, and thrombosis Central nervous system infection: acute or chronic meningitis, brain abscess, and neurosyphylis Trauma: subdural hematoma, contusion, concussion, and intracranial hemorrhage	◆ Intracerebral bleed caused by thrombocytopenia ◆ Meningeal carcinomatosis ◆ Central nervous system edema secondary to brain malignancy or whole-brain radiation therapy ◆ Fall risk ◆ Malignancy: primary or metastatic involving brain and cranial irradiation
Endocrine disturbance Hypothyroidism Diabetes mellitus Hypercalcemia Hyponatremia Hypopituitarism	◆ Mantle field radiation therapy ◆ Steroid induced ◆ Related to bone metastases ◆ Syndrome of inappropriate antidiuretic hormone, rigorous hydration, and dehydration ◆ Brain tumor in or adjacent to pituitary gland
Temperature regulation fluctuation Hypothermia Hyperthermia	◆ Absence of customary warm clothes ◆ Fever
Pulmonary abnormalities Inadequate gas-exchange states: pulmonary disease and alveolar hypoventilation Infection: pneumonia	◆ Hypoxemia ◆ Anemia ◆ Lung metastases ◆ Bleomycin-induced pulmonary fibrosis ◆ Radiotherapy to chest ◆ Chest tubes ◆ Neutropenia and immobility
Systemic infective process (acute or chronic) Viral Fungal Bacterial: endocarditis, pyelonephritis, and cystitis	◆ Prominence of neutropenia ◆ Steroids ◆ Hypogammaglobunemia
Metabolic disturbance Electrolyte abnormalities: hypercalcemia, hypo- and hypernatremia, hypo- and hyperkalemia, hypo- and hypercalcemia, and hyperphosphatemia Acidosis and alkalosis Hypo- and hyperglycemia Acute and chronic renal failure Volume depletion: hemorrhage, inadequate fluid intake, diuretics, and diarrhea Hepatic failure	◆ Syndrome of inappropriate antidiuretic hormone ◆ Bone metastases ◆ Diabetes secondary to steroids ◆ Renal malignancy ◆ Dehydration and diarrhea secondary to pelvic radiotherapy or chemotherapy ◆ Liver primary or metastases with ascites or encephalopathy ◆ Tumor lysis syndrome

(continued)

Table 21.3 Continued

Type of physiological risk factor	Cancer-specific considerations
Drug intoxication (therapeutic or substance abuse)	
Misuse of prescribed medications Side effects of therapeutic medications Drug-drug interactions Drug and herb interactions Improper use of over-the-counter medications Alcohol intoxication or withdrawal	◆ Polypharmacy with drugs having anticholinergic or central nervous system effects ◆ Inadequate knowledge about geriatric-specific pharmacokinetic considerations in dosing ◆ Self-medication with over-the-counter or herbal remedies in the absence of healthcare professional awareness ◆ Alcohol withdrawal perioperatively in patients with head and neck cancer

Source: Boyle (2006), reference 89 (used with permission).

changes that are signs of delirium, but often do not "put the pieces together" to recognize this syndrome. Standardized assessment tools for delirium administered by healthcare providers trained in using these tools improves the identification of delirium in the clinical setting.[3,11,12,15,39,98] Assessment tools include those designed to screen for delirium symptoms, those designed to make a formal diagnosis of delirium, and those designed to rate the severity of delirium.

The Mini-Mental State Examination (MMSE) is a 20-item screening tool that provides a clinical evaluation of cognitive function but is not specifically designed to assess for delirium and does not differentiate between dementia and delirium.[99,100,101] It assesses orientation, attention, recall, and language function. The MMSE is widely used in practice and research, and data support the scoring system to identify the severity of cognitive impairment. The length of this examination and the writing and drawing

questions included in it may be cumbersome and difficult to perform in a palliative care population.[101] Fayers and colleagues reported that a subset of four items from the MMSE is adequate to screen for delirium and cognitive impairment: current year, date, backward spelling, and copy a design.[101] Additional research would be required to support the validity of using only these four items for screening. Whether using the full MMSE or a modification, it may be best to view it as a predictive instrument that directs the clinician to use a delirium assessment instrument for additional information.

Table 21.4 provides an overview of the instruments used to assess delirium. These instruments are reviewed because they distinguish delirium from dementia and assess at least several of the multiple features of delirium. While all of these instruments require further study to determine application across varied settings and among different patient populations, the following have

Table 21.4 Overview of delirium assessment tools

	MDAS	DRS	CAM	NCS	BCS	DOS	Nu-DESC
DSM-IV criterion							
Acute onset		X	X			X	X
Fluctuating nature		X	X			X	X
Physical disorder		X	X				
Consciousness	X		X		X	X	X
Attention/concentration	X		X	X	X	X	
Thinking	X	X	X	X	X	X	X
Disorientation	X		X	X		X	X
Memory	X	X	X	X	X	X	
Perception	X	X	X			X	X
Purpose							
Screening/diagnosis		X	X	X	X	X	X
Symptom severity	X	X					
Number of items	10	10	9	9	2	13	5
Time to complete (minutes)	10	Not specified	<5	10	<2	5	1

MDAS, Memorial Delirium Assessment Scale; DRS, Delirium Rating Scale; CAM, Confusion Assessment Method; NCS, NEECHAM Confusion Scale; BCS, Bedside Confusion Scale; DOS, Delirium Observation Scale; Nu-DESC, Nursing Delirium Screening Scale.

shown good reliability and validity in identifying delirium in selected populations.[102,103]

- The Memorial Delirium Assessment Scale (MDAS) is a 10-item tool based on the DSM-IV criteria (which are consistent with the DSM-5 criteria) designed to quantify the severity of delirium.[103–105] It takes about 10 minutes to administer. The MDAS requires minimal training for use and is appropriate for both clinical practice and research.

- The Delirium Rating Scale (DRS) is a 10-item scale, and the Delirium Rating Scale—Revised-98 (DRS-R98) is a 16-item scale. Both are intended to be used by clinicians with psychiatric training. It looks at symptoms over a 24-hour period and may be used to assess severity of delirium.[103,106,107]

- The Confusion Assessment Method (CAM) is based on the DSM–IV criteria for delirium and is designed for use by a trained interviewer to assess cognitive functioning in elderly patients on a daily scheduled basis.[108] The CAM and the CAM-ICU (revised for use in the intensive care unit setting) have been evaluated in a number of studies and show good reliability and validity.[9,49,102,109–112] A related tool, the Family Confusion Assessment Method (FAM-CAM), is designed to get family caregiver assessments and has been shown to correlate with a formal CAM evaluation.[113]

- Nurses designed the NEECHAM Confusion Scale (NCS) for rapid and unobtrusive assessment and monitoring of acute confusion in hospitalized elderly.[102,114] It contains nine scaled items divided into three subscales and takes about 10 minutes to complete. The NCS has been studied in many populations, including nonintubated patients in intensive care units.[115]

- The Bedside Confusion Scale (BCS) consists of observation of the level of consciousness and timed recitation of the months of the year in reverse order starting with December, and is designed for use in the palliative care setting.[113,116] It requires minimal training and only about 2 minutes to complete. The BCS was found to correlate with the CAM, but it is subject to bias or inappropriate interpretation, and has a limited capacity to assess the multiple cognitive domains influenced by delirium.[117]

- The Delirium Observation Screening Scale (DOSS) is based on the DSM-IV criteria and is designed to assist nurses in the early recognition of delirium during routine care.[102,118] The original version of the scale has 25 items. After studies on geriatric and hip fracture patients, the scale was reduced to 13 items that can be rated as present or absent in less than 5 minutes.[118]

- The Nursing Delirium Screening Scale (Nu-DESC) is an observational 5-item instrument designed to be completed in about 1 minute at the bedside.[119] It has been shown to have validity and sensitivity comparable to the MDAS in oncology populations and is a sensitive test in the recovery room to detect delirium.[119,120]

Given the fluctuating nature of delirium, every-shift assessment in hospital and nursing home settings, using a simple screening tool such as the CAM, BCS, DOSS, or Nu-DESC is appropriate, especially for high-risk populations. There are no published recommendations on the frequency with which delirium assessment tools should be used in outpatient and home care settings.

Too-frequent evaluation for delirium in persons at low risk is burdensome to both the patient and the clinician. It makes sense to complete a baseline evaluation on all patients, and then base the frequency of follow-up assessments on the number of risk factors present for delirium. Simply asking the family, "Do you think [the patient] has been more confused lately?" may serve as a clinical screening tool to determine which patients require a more thorough evaluation.[42]

Management of delirium

Optimal care of the person at risk for, or experiencing, delirium requires application of evidence-based practice guidelines by an interdisciplinary team that includes both palliative care bedside nurses and advanced practice nurses (APNs). The plan of care must align with the patient and family goals of care. Creation of the plan of care is initiated by the palliative care nurse with the guidance of the palliative care team. The plan should be both proactive, to prevent delirium when possible, and focused on alleviation of suffering for both patient and family. The following management guidelines address interventions appropriate for all types of delirium that commonly occur in patients with serious medical conditions: hyperactive, hypoactive, and mixed-type, as well as irreversible delirium that may occur at the end of life. Deathbed phenomena are discussed as a separate syndrome.

Evidenced-based guidelines focus on primary prevention by implementing risk prevention measures, using reliable and valid delirium screening and assessment tools, and addressing contributing factors for delirium for all patients with serious or advanced medical conditions. Figure 21.1 illustrates a suggested care pathway.

Care of patients at risk for delirium

The correlation between the number of risk factors and the incidence of delirium suggests that a proactive plan of care may reduce the severity of a delirious episode or possibly prevent an acute delirious episode. Five risk factors in the elderly hospitalized patient are predictive of delirium: physical restraints, malnutrition, three medications recently added, indwelling urinary catheter, and any recent medical event such as admission to an emergency room.[79,121] McCusker and colleagues demonstrated that an absence of reading glasses and not having access to a glass of water was associated with increased delirium score, while having reading glasses and presence of a family member decreased delirium scores.[85] The Hospital Elder Life Program (HELP), developed by Inouye and colleagues, has been shown to decrease the incidence of delirium in the hospitalized elderly in a cost-effective manner and serves as a model for incorporating specific nonpharmacological interventions in the care planning process.[8,122,123] To do this, HELP encourages engaging patients in meaningful conversation, providing frequent orientation cues, socialization, and daily exercise. Attention is also given to promoting sleep using methods such as back rubs, warm drinks, and relaxation tapes.

The American College of Critical Care Medicine published revised guidelines for the management of pain, agitation, and delirium in the intensive care unit setting in 2013.[9,124] These guidelines, often referred to as the "PAD bundle," emphasize (1) frequent reorientation and assuring access to eyeglasses and hearing aids, if needed, (2) maintaining patients' sleep-wake

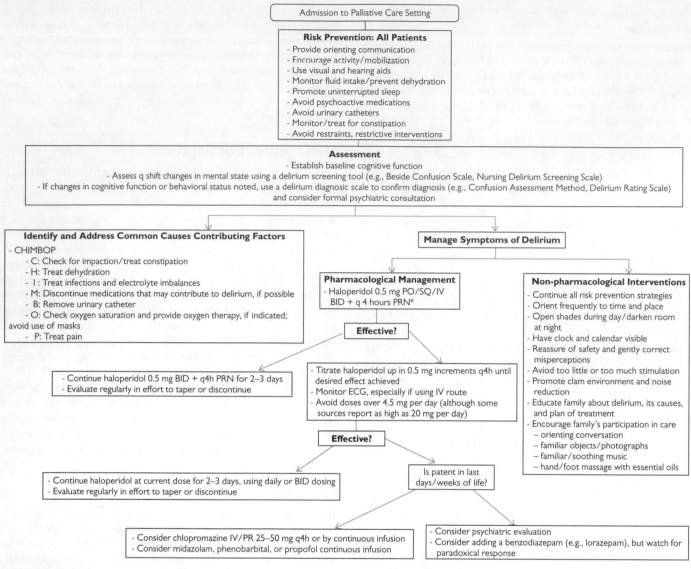

Figure 21.1 Delirium algorithm. Sources: Adapted from Inouye (2006), reference 71; Irwin et al. (2013), reference 53.

cycles by minimizing environmental and procedural disturbances at night, and (3) advancing patients' mobility during the day as tolerated, with the goal of getting patients out of bed each day, even when they are intubated and mechanically ventilated.[124]

Based on the impact of the HELP model of care for hospitalized elderly and the PAD bundle in the ICU, the palliative nursing plan of care includes frequent orientation, normalizing sleep routines, mobilizing the patient, engaging the patient in mentally stimulating activities, maintaining consistent/familiar caregivers, ensuring use of eyeglasses and hearing aids, monitoring fluid and food intake, and monitoring bowel function.[8,53,85,122,124,125] Evaluation of and interventions to improve sleep quality cannot be overemphasized as this is both a contributing factor for delirium and one of the earliest signs of a developing delirium.[30,41,93] Nurses are key to advocating for the least invasive and least restrictive

interventions, for example, avoiding urinary catheters, intravenous lines, and use of restraints whenever possible.

Despite an excellent plan of care that eliminates or minimizes risk factors, delirium may not be preventable in the final stages of life.[10,30,35] A study incorporating a multicomponent prevention intervention at two inpatient palliative care centers was ineffective in reducing the incidence or severity of delirium among cancer patients receiving end-of-life care.[10] There are several potential reasons this prevention program did not show the anticipated benefits, including that the prevention program used was not as comprehensive as the HELP program (in order to minimize burden for both the family and the bedside nurses) and that the population included only patients with advanced cancer, that is, patients in whom the underlying causes of delirium may not be reversible.[10] The benefits and burdens of interventions must be evaluated in all settings and care taken to assure that the plan of care is congruent with the patient and family goals of care throughout the illness trajectory.

This proactive prevention and mitigation approach requires that nurses have a thorough knowledge of the patient's primary diagnosis, comorbidities, symptoms, prior activity, cognitive status, nutritional status, and prognosis. The physical examination rules out infectious, metabolic, endocrine, cardiovascular, and cerebrovascular disease that could contribute to delirium.[46,126] This information along with identifying medications that could contribute to delirium alerts the palliative care team to patients who are at high risk for delirious episodes.[33,46,96,127]

A review of the patient's medications is an essential component of delirium risk assessment. Sedative hypnotics, opioids, medications with anticholinergic effects, benzodiazepines, and the use of multiple medications are all potential precipitating factors for delirium.[33,95,96,127] With the help of an interdisciplinary review, the medication profile can be streamlined.

Because delirium is frequently undiagnosed in the clinical setting,[11,15,127] evidenced-based guidelines focus on screening all patients with serious or advanced medical conditions to identification delirium on admission and at early onset. The BCS, the Nu-DESC, or asking the family if the patient has been confused lately (all described in the section on assessment tools) can be added to routine patient assessments. In the home, the FAM-CAM is a helpful tool to document changes in the patient's behavior.[128] Prior to initiating any delirium screening assessment, however, it is important to establish a baseline by questioning the patient and family caregivers about the patient's preadmission cognitive and emotional status, sleep-wake patterns, and daily care routines. When screening indicates changes associated with delirium, a diagnostic tool, for example, the CAM or DRS, can be administered by the nurse and reported to the interdisciplinary team for further evaluation and intervention.

Because delirium is a medical diagnosis, concern is sometimes raised that bedside nurses are functioning outside their scope of practice by diagnosing delirium. Multiple studies support that the use of tools like the CAM are within the scope of the practice of the bedside nurse. Using this, or a similar tool, nurses can report the patient's score on the CAM and the formal diagnosis can be made by the physician or APN.

Management of acute delirium

When delirium is present, a detailed workup is essential to identify the underlying cause, when possible. Laboratory examinations include complete blood count, blood urea nitrogen and creatinine levels, liver function, and thyroid function. If an infectious process is suspected, urine culture, chest X-ray, or, possibly, arterial blood gases are evaluated. Serum vitamin B_{12} and folate levels may reveal nutritional imbalances. Brain imaging and scans could be of value when other more common causes have been ruled out, as several advanced illness pathologies may extend to the brain, for example, cancer and acquired immune deficiency syndrome (AIDS), causing an acute delirium.[46,53] All laboratory and imaging tests are initiated only after consideration of what impact the information will have on the plan of care and whether the tests are consistent with patient/family goals.[53] For example, if brain metastasis is suspected and the patient would not be a candidate for, or does not want, additional treatment, a brain scan would not be appropriate.

The acronym CHIMBOP can assist the nurse to rule out seven common causes of delirium.[117] While this tool does not address all of the potentially reversible causes of delirium, it provides a framework for nurses to begin searching for the etiologies of the delirium.

- ◆ C = Constipation—check for impaction; obtain order for and administer bowel stimulants and stool softeners.
- ◆ H = Hypovolemia, hypoglycemia—encourage oral intake or provide parenteral fluids; treat hypoglycemia.
- ◆ I = Infection—evaluate for signs and symptoms of infection; contact the physician or APN to determine whether antiinfective medications are appropriate at this time.
- ◆ M = Medications—review the patient's medications for those known to contribute to delirium; discuss minimizing or discontinuing medications, as possible, with the physician, APN, and pharmacist.
- ◆ B = Bladder catheter, bladder outlet obstruction—avoid the use of or remove urinary catheters; check for bladder distension and insert catheter (straight or indwelling) only if required.
- ◆ O = Oxygen deficiency—check oxygen saturation or signs of hypoxia and administer oxygen as indicated.
- ◆ P = Pain—evaluate for and treat pain.

While dehydration is a documented contributing factor for delirium, artificial hydration is not necessarily helpful. Two studies demonstrated that administration of a liter of fluid a day to persons with advanced cancer did not decrease the incidence of delirium, and did not improve symptoms, quality of life, or survival.[128,129] A thorough evaluation of the patient's overall condition is necessary to determine whether a trial of artificial hydration is indicated. And, careful monitoring is required to assure the patient does not experience any uncomfortable symptoms associated with overhydration if artificial hydration is initiated.

Additional measures include providing a safe, quiet, and comforting environment for the patient. If the patient is in an area of high activity, either in the home or hospital, moving the patient to a quiet location may help. Eliminate extraneous noises such as televisions and intercoms that may stimulate the overtaxed brain. And, involve the family.[26,85] The voice of a family member or significant other or the touch of their hand can communicate understanding and reassurance to the patient.[58,130]

Physical restraints should be avoided whenever possible. The use of physical restraints is a recognized independent risk factor for delirium and for its persistence at discharge.[97] Restraints should be used only when a patient poses a clear risk of harm to self or others. A better way to ensure patient safety is to arrange for one-on-one observation of the patient. Not only does one-on-one observation promote safety but the presence of a trusted person may also reduce the patient's anxiety and provide orientation cues. This person becomes part of the treatment plan for delirium.

An acute phase of delirium can last for hours or days. Following resolution of the acute phase of delirium, the nurse should continue assessments and delirium screenings as the patient remains at high risk for a reoccurrence of delirium.[46] In the elderly a syndrome referred to as "persistent delirium" may continue in the posthospital period for as long 6 months.[46]

In the postdelirium state, it is important to debrief the patient about what they remember. As mentioned previously, patients may recall distressing images or feel embarrassed about their behavior. Debriefing the experience can help the patient and caregivers to normalize the event and reduce any stigma that the patient may feel about being out of control and seemingly unaware of their behavior.

Management of delirium at the end of life

When delirium is present in the final hours and days of life, every effort needs to be made to address the presenting symptoms and ensure patient safety. Further invasive testing and examinations may increase the distress and are not recommended. Often this is a time where the search for any underlying cause is limited to only the most common causes of delirium (see CHIMBOP above). Pharmacological interventions are used as discussed in the following section.

Management of deathbed phenomena

As discussed above, deathbed phenomena are usually not distressing to patients. Therefore, a nonpharmacological approach may be the most beneficial. Yet, these behaviors may create some concern on the part of the caregivers who wonder how to respond to the patient who is seeing and speaking to someone who is not visible to others.

The palliative care team can guide caregivers in listening carefully to the patient's words as they describe their visions. Often a theme emerges in phases such as "please open the door," "I will be home soon," or "I will catch the next train." The nurse can normalize the event by explaining that these experiences are common and that they indicate the patient is preparing for death. And the nurse can teach the family responses that may be helpful, such as "The door is open, you can go on when you are ready"; "We will miss you, but you can go when it's time"; "They are waiting and will be happy to see you"; or, "It is OK to catch the next train." The nurse and spiritual caregivers reframe the experience as a sacred passage for the patient, where family and loved ones are offered a time to say good-bye.

Pharmacological management of delirium

Nonpharmacological approaches and interventions to treat or lessen risk factors causing delirium are the first-line treatments for this syndrome.[1,46,53,78] No medications have been approved by the US Food and Drug Administration (FDA) for the treatment of delirium, but when pharmacological agents are required, antipsychotic agents are the medications of choice.[1,32,40,53,131–133] However, the use of antipsychotics for the treatment of delirium is not without controversy. Some clinicians feel that pharmacological management should be used only for those who have severe agitation that interferes with medical treatments, or in patients that pose a danger to themselves.[3,78] This approach means that those with hypoactive delirium rarely receive antipsychotics. Others suggest that pharmacological interventions should be considered in all patients with delirium, especially those who have agitation, paranoia, hallucination, or altered sensorium, because of the distressing nature of these symptoms.[1,45,53,123,124] Additional support for using antipsychotics for more than the severely agitated is that these medications have been shown to improve both arousal

disturbance and impaired cognitive functioning in patients with hypoactive delirium.[42,134] And current evidence does not indicate a difference in response rates between clinical subtypes of delirium.[133] Clinicians who choose to take a "wait-and-see" approach before using antipsychotics for the delirious patient who is not agitated or having distressing hallucinations should be prepared to act quickly, as the hypoactive, somnolent patient can become agitated very quickly.[1] What is clear from the literature is that there is a wide range of prescribing patterns in the use of antipsychotics to manage delirium.[33,135] Table 21.5 provides an overview of the more common medications used to treat delirium.

Haloperidol is the most widely studied and used antipsychotic for delirium.[3,9,46,53,78,131,133,136] After review of the literature, Jackson and Lipman concluded that there is not enough evidence to draw any conclusions about the role of pharmacology in terminally ill patients with delirium but that perhaps haloperidol is the most suitable drug therapy for delirium treatment near the end of life.[65] Haloperidol has fewer anticholinergic side effects, is less sedating, and has fewer active metabolites than other typical antipsychotics. There are little data to support the optimal dose or route of administration of haloperidol for delirium, and little is known about the optimal duration of treatment. Typical starting doses are 1 to 2 mg (oral, intramuscularly, intravenously, subcutaneously) for mild agitation, 5 mg for moderate agitation, and 7.5 to 10 mg for severe agitation.[3,124] In the elderly, lower doses, for example, 0.25 to 0.5 mg may be sufficient.[46,124] Doses are repeated every 30 minutes until the patient is calm but arouses to normal voice.[53,124] When symptoms are controlled, the total dose given in the last 24 hours is given once per day or divided for twice-daily administration. Doses above 20 mg per day are not recommended,[1] but doses as high as 250 mg in 24 hours have been used.[1,53] A systematic review of the literature concluded that doses greater than 4.5 mg per day were associated with more adverse side effects than the atypical antipsychotics.[131] Generally, after 2 to 3 days with no evidence of delirium, the medication can be weaned while evaluating for return of symptoms.[124] Ideally, during this time other interventions to address the underlying cause(s) of delirium are also used. Long-term use of antipsychotics for persistent delirium has not been studied and increases the risk of adverse events and increases costs.[138]

Haloperidol can be given by the oral, sublingual, rectal, subcutaneous, intramuscular, or intravenous routes. Parenteral doses are approximately twice as potent as oral doses.[1] The oral route is associated with more frequent extrapyramidal side effects than the intravenous route, but the intravenous route is not without problems.[131,136] Haloperidol can prolong the QTc interval and has been associated with torsades de pointes (TdP), especially when given intravenously or in higher doses than recommended. In 2007, the FDA issued an alert warning that cases of sudden death, TdP, and QTc prolongation have been reported even in the absence of predisposing factors; this warning included a reminder that haloperidol is not approved for intravenous administration, and recommended ECG monitoring if it is given intravenously.[139] Monitoring of QTc intervals is recommended before long-term, high-dose antipsychotic therapy, and there is some support for not initiating treatment with haloperidol administration if the QTc interval is greater than 450 ms.[124] However, two published studies, one of 326 elderly patients with delirium and one evaluating safety reports from 1972 to 2010, found no association between

Table 21.5 Pharmacological treatment of delirium

Class & drug	Starting dose & titration	Usual daily dose	Comments
Typical Antipsychotic			
◆ Haloperidol	0.5–2 mg PO/SL/SQ/IM/IV every 30 minutes until settled, then up to 20 mg daily given in one or two divided doses, based on dose needed to settle	1–5 mg over 24 hours	◆ Most commonly used and studied medication for delirium ◆ EPS, especially if dose is > 4.5 mg PO per day ◆ Monitor QTc interval ◆ Due to long half-life may be able to dose once daily after effective dose established
◆ Chlorpromazine	25–50 mg PO/SL/PR/IM/SQ/IV every 1 h until settled, then 25 mg–100 mg 6–8 h ATC or PRN, based on dose needed to settle	PO: 50 mg tid SQ: 5–50 mg/h	◆ Useful if a more sedating agent is desired ◆ Higher risk of anticholinergic side effects than with haloperidol ◆ Monitor blood pressure for orthostatic hypotension ◆ If using IV route, give by slow push or infusion over 10–15 minutes
Atypical Antipsychotic			**Class characteristics:** ◆ EPS equivalent to or slightly less than those of haloperidol ◆ Prolonged QTc interval ◆ More expensive than typical antipsychotics
◆ Olanzapine	2.5–5 mg PO daily, may increase to 10 mg daily	5 mg bid	◆ Available in orally disintegrating tablets
◆ Risperidone	0.25–0.5 mg PO twice daily and PRN; may increase by 0.5 mg every other day	1 mg bid	◆ Available in orally disintegrating tablets ◆ Monitor blood pressure for orthostatic hypotension
◆ Quetiapine	12.5–25 mg PO twice daily; may give 12.5 in morning and 25 mg at night, increasing as necessary	50 mg bid	◆ Most sedating of this class ◆ Preferred agent in patients with Parkinson's disease ◆ Monitor blood pressure for orthostatic hypotension
Benzodiazepine			
◆ Lorazepam	0.5–1mg PO/IV every 4 h PRN		◆ Often worsens delirium ◆ Sedating, but can see paradoxical excitation ◆ Medication of choice in patients with delirium associated with sedative or alcohol withdrawal or those with neuroleptic malignant syndrome ◆ Second-line agent for delirium in patients with Parkinson's disease

PO, oral; SL, sublingual; PR, rectal; SQ, subcutaneous; IV, intravenous; ATC, around the clock; PRN, as needed; EPS, extrapyramidal symptoms.

Sources: Irwin et al. (2013), reference 53; Breitbart and Alici (2008), reference 32; Mittal et al. (2011), reference 46; Weckmann and Morrison (2013), reference 136; Twycross and Wilcock (2008), reference 137.

use of intravenous haloperidol and increased mortality.[140,141] Weckmann and Morrison, in their review of the evidence, concluded that the choice to obtain an ECG should be based on the patient's overall condition, prognosis, expected mortality, distress level, and goals of care and that the benefits of treating delirium outweigh the risks.[124]

Chlorpromazine is another typical antipsychotic that may be used to treat delirium. Doses of 25 mg to 50 mg by the oral, sublingual or parenteral route maybe used.[53] Chlorpromazine is associated with more anticholinergic side effects, orthostatic hypotension, and sedation than haloperidol. Therefore, it is usually used only when the additional sedation will be of benefit and haloperidol has not been completely effective.

The newer, atypical antipsychotics have the advantage of fewer extrapyramidal side effects, and less effect on QTc interval.[53,131] None of these medications are FDA approved for the treatment of delirium, and all of them are more expensive than haloperidol. With the exception of olanzapine, these drugs do not come in a parenteral form. Studies support that haloperidol, risperidone, olanzapine, and quetiapine are equally effective in treating delirium with few adverse events.[131,142–144] Starting doses are outlined in Table 21.5. First-generation antipsychotics (i.e., haloperidol or chlorpromazine) are considered first-line therapy, unless the patient has Parkinson's disease, where quetiapine is recommended.[137]

Several studies evaluating the effectiveness of prophylactic antipsychotics in persons at high risk for delirium, that is, postoperative elderly patients and the intensive care unit setting, have shown a reduction in delirium incidence in subjects who received perioperative antipsychotics.[145–148] Surgery and intensive care unit stays are acute, time-limited events that increase the risk of delirium, providing a more clear rationale for time-limited prophylaxis with antipsychotic medications. The multiple factors contributing to delirium in persons with advanced progressive illnesses are often chronic and cumulative. At this time, the only potential rationale for pharmacological prophylaxis of delirium in the palliative care setting might be for patients who will be exposed to the additional risks of surgery and acute care.

Cholinesterase inhibitors have been studied for the treatment of delirium based on the understanding that disruption of the cholinergic system may be one of the underlying mechanisms of this syndrome. However, there is currently no evidence from controlled trials that the cholinesterase inhibitors are effective in the treatment of delirium.[149]

Benzodiazepines are not recommended as the first-line treatment of delirium, except for delirium associated with alcohol or sedative-hypnotic drug withdrawal.[32,131,132] This class of medications tends to cause oversedation and exacerbate confusion, potentially making delirium worse.[150] If haloperidol does not control the agitation of delirium, the clinician may consider switching to chlorpromazine or adding a benzodiazepine, most frequently, lorazepam.[32,53,124] The patient must be monitored careful to assure the addition of the benzodiazepine does not make the delirium worse. Irwin suggests that if paradoxical agitation occurs with lorazepam, rapid titration of lorazepam to higher doses will usually overcome this reaction and palliate symptoms.[53] Some clinicians will avoid benzodiazepines and treat this as a refractory delirium.

Refractory delirium is often cited as an indication for palliative sedation. Mercandante and colleagues reported that delirium alone (53.1%) or in combination with other symptoms (an additional 16.3%) was the most frequent indicator for palliative sedation in patients with advanced cancer followed at home.[151] Caraceni and colleagues followed patients seen by an inpatient palliative care service over a 5-year period and reported that of the 83 patients who required palliative sedation for symptom control, delirium was the indicator 31% of the time.[152] Midazolam, pentobarbital, phenobarbital, and propofol have been used for palliative sedation for delirium.[53,124,153] See chapter 25 for a discussion of palliative sedation.

Family/caregiver education and support

Family/caregiver education about delirium and its associated risk factors is essential because caregiver assistance is needed to maintain daily routines, decrease risk factors that precipitate delirium, and identify early signs and symptoms of delirium.[23,29,53,154] Watching a loved-one spiral into confusion and paranoia is overwhelming to caregivers. Caregivers require education and support to respond to their dying loved-one's agitation or sudden withdrawal into silence.[35,155] Psychosocial and spiritual care are essential components of the continuum of support for the caregivers' journey with illness and death.

A simple inquiry from the nurse to the caregiver, "tell me what this is like for you," provides the opportunity for caregivers to express their needs for support as well as the anguish over seeing

a loved one decline physically and mentally. In one study, families described witnessing their loved-one's confusion as "extreme suffering," and reported feeling helpless and overwhelmed.[27]

The goals of caregiver education depend on where the patient resides (home, residential, or acute care) and the stage of their chronic/terminal illness (beginning, middle, end). Consideration is given to caregivers' ethnicity and level of education and the resources available in the care setting. Education can be directed toward understanding delirium and its possible causes, ways to communicate with the patient (including while ventilated), orientation methods, and how to comfort the patient with touch, familiar sounds, and other sensory aids. Nurses can facilitate referrals to chaplains and social workers who may be available to offer additional support. Written information is helpful for reinforcing education. As an example, a "Quick Information Sheet" about delirium is available in English and Spanish from the Hospice and Palliative Nurses Association.[156]

Intensive or acute care settings

As discussed above, admission to an intensive care setting increases the risk of delirium in older adults, especially those with cognitive deficits. On admission to an acute care setting, the palliative care team can collaborate with hospital staff to educate family and caregivers on ways to help the patient adapt to the acute care setting. The family should be encouraged to let the staff know if the patient "just isn't him- or herself, today." When patients are in an intensive care unit, written material for family members may include scripts and suggestions of things to say to the patient during visits. Modeling possible conversations that may occur between the caregiver and the patient can help caregivers know what to say. For example, "[Patient name], it is [family member's name] I am here with you. It is Wednesday and it is summertime. You are in the intensive care unit at [hospital name]. [Nurse's name] is your nurse. She is taking good care of you when I am not here. You are safe and no one will hurt you." Such scripts can be followed by a short explanation of why simple communication is important during every visit in an acute care setting. The explanation could be as simple as "even though your family member is on a breathing machine and sedated, familiar voices can help him/her feel safe and less anxious."

The touch of a familiar hand can have a profound impact on a patient who is confused and fearful. Reassure caregivers that their presence is an important component of their loved one's care. Caregivers may need assistance in pulling chairs close to the bedside so that they can be near and touch their loved one.

Early and timely involvement of the palliative care team can assist in discharge planning and education of families concerning the possibilities of reoccurring delirium as well as how to prevent delirium and monitor for early signs of a potential delirium after discharge. Proactive caregiver education may serve to prevent a delirious episode and readmission into acute care.

Home care setting

In home care settings, caregivers can assist in early identification of changes in the patient's behavior that may alert the nurse to the onset of delirium. It is not uncommon for patients with advanced diseases to experience a change in sleep patterns, feel anxious or irritable, or forget the days of the week, all of which can be early signs of a delirious episode. The caregiver can be empowered through learning to observe and record specific changes in behavior through the use of a delirium assessment tool. The FAM-CAM, described earlier, provides caregivers with an easy and reliable tool to record behavioral changes.[157] Caregivers are not expected to diagnose delirium but rather to keep a consistent record of behaviors. Offering caregivers this opportunity to be involved may help reduce their anxiety about caregiving while alerting the palliative care team of changes forewarning delirium in the patient.

When appropriate, engage the patient in self-reporting about feelings of agitation or confusion or experiences of seeing things or hearing voices, explaining that these are common experiences among other patients with similar problems. Patients often refrain from telling healthcare professionals or even family members that they are seeing things or hearing voices because of the fear of being labeled "crazy." Frequent questioning of the patient by the healthcare professional can serve to normalize such changes in cognition for both the patient and the caregivers and can therefore make honest communication more comfortable for them.

In acute delirious episodes at home, help the family understand that the radio or television should be avoided, as they may increase the patient's confusion. Families can be reminded about the importance of touch and that something as simple as a hand massage can comfort the patient and let them know that love and care is present. The familiar smells of cooking and sounds of home also serve to reassure the patient.

Delirium at the end of life

When delirium occurs in the final days or hours of life, the goals of education and support will change because delirium often cannot be resolved at this time. Review the signs of approaching death with the caregivers. This conversation will require extraordinary sensitivity and can be aided with the help of a chaplain. Time is of the essence as caregivers are prepared and supported to express their farewells. Explain the administration and intended outcome of medications used to treat delirium. If the patient experiences refractory delirium and palliative sedation is considered, the palliative care team must review with the family their goals of care, the pros and cons of palliative sedation, and the medications that would be used (see chapter 25). The palliative care team reinforces that the intent of palliative sedation is not to hasten death, but to relieve the extreme suffering of the patient.

Death bed phenomena

Twenty percent of patients will experience DBVs. Often, these can be reassuring to caregivers and some have postulated that they are helpful in bereavement.[56] The palliative care team may assist in normalizing these events by informing the family and caregivers that such events are often helpful and that the patient's seemingly confused communication need not cause alarm. The following scenario helps illustrate how the nurse may support the family: A wife tells the hospice nurse that her husband is talking to his dead sister and is asking her to forgive him. The wife shares that her husband seems afraid and that she has reminded him several times that his sister died in 1985. The wife thinks it is odd because he was always fighting with his sister and she died rather suddenly before their arguments were resolved. The hospice nurse speaks with the patient and tells him to feel free to ask his sister again to forgive him. He calms down, and his wife follows the nurses lead and says, "I know Ellen forgives you. All you have to do is ask her and she will

welcome you." Soon, he becomes calm and smiles and mumbles in conversation with his "sister." He died peacefully 2 days later.

This is a spiritual time where families/caregivers can be coached to surround their dying loved-one with love and to acknowledge his/her otherworldly visions. This exercise can transform the pain of loss into an experience of death as a magnificent spiritual event. Deathbed visions can provide the opportunity for the palliative care team to model a fearless approach to dying while facilitating a peaceful transition.

Case study (continued)

Given Mrs. Rice's change from baseline, the nurse uses the CAM to evaluate for delirium. Mrs. Rice fits the diagnostic criteria for delirium as the mental status change had an acute onset and fluctuates in severity, she is easily distracted when trying to assess her, her answers to questions are often incoherent, she has misperceptions that people are trying to harm her, and she is hyperalert. These mental status changes are interfering with appropriate treatment of her medical condition and they are causing distress to both her and her daughter. The nurse reports the findings from the CAM to the APN, who confirms the diagnosis of delirium after a review of the record and assessing the patient. The APN and bedside nurse sit with Darlene to explain the syndrome of delirium. They tell her that it is common in patients that have as many risk factors as her mother, that it is usually treatable by eliminating as many risk factors as possible in addition to treating the infection and breathing problems. They list the following as likely contributing factors for Mrs. Rice's delirium: age, dementia, advanced illness, infection, low oxygen, new medications (especially the lorazepam), being restrained (wrist restraints when Darlene is not present to prevent Mrs. Rice from taking off the mask, and restricted by the medical interventions, i.e., BiPAP and intravenous lines), and being in an unfamiliar environment.

A multicomponent plan of care is developed to address the delirium, including providing frequent orientation cues, avoiding restraints, having a family member present as often as possible or using a sitter if the family is unable to be present, keeping staff members as consistent as possible, making sure Mrs. Rice has her eyeglasses on when she is awake, getting her up to a chair during the day, assuring toileting needs (bowel and bladder) are addressed, and promoting uninterrupted sleep at night. The APN also discusses the use of short-term antipsychotic medications to treat the disorganized thinking, frightening misperceptions, and agitation. The lorazepam will be stopped and the APN will review the rest of Mrs. Rice's medications with the pharmacist to evaluate if others can be eliminated.

Mrs. Rice is started on haloperidol 1 mg IV to be given now, and the nurse may give 0.5 mg IV every 30 minutes, as needed, for agitation over the next two hours, at which time the APN will check back to see how Mrs. Rice is doing. When the APN calls 2 hours after the initial dose of haloperidol, she learns that Mrs. Rice was given one additional dose of haloperidol. Mrs. Rice is sleeping intermittently, is easily arousable, is more cooperative with her mask and treatments, and no longer appears fearful.

The next day, Mrs. Rice is able to transition to a high-flow nasal cannula, which is much more comfortable for her than the BiPAP. She is oriented to person and place, correctly identifies the family members present in the room, and participates in conversations. Darlene reports that the patient's memory seems about normal for her. The APN discusses with Darlene the importance of maintaining the plan of care both here at the hospital and upon discharge because Mrs. Rice will be at risk for future episodes of delirium. The haloperidol will be continued at the current dose for another 24 hours, then switched to 1 mg oral daily for two days, then discontinued, as long as Mrs. Rice shows no signs of relapsing delirium

It appears the acute medical problems are being well managed, but the underlying COPD will continue to progress. The palliative care team arranges a meeting with Mrs. Rice and Darlene to discuss goals of care now, and for future exacerbations.

References

1. Breitbart W, Chochinov HM, Passik SD. Psychiatric symptoms in palliative care. In: Hanks G, Cherny N, Christakis NA, Fallon M, Kaasa S, Portenoy RK (eds.), Oxford Textbook of Palliative Medicine (4th ed). Oxford: Oxford University Press; 2010:1451–1482.

2. Cerejeira, J, Mukaetova-Ladinska, EB. A clinical update on delirium: from early recognition to effective management. Nurs Res Pract. 2011; Article ID 875196, published online June 16, 2011. doi: 10.1155/2011/875196.

3. Hosie A, Davidson PM, Agar M, Sanderson CR, Phillips J. Delirium prevalence, incidence, and implications for screening in specialist palliative care inpatient settings: a systematic review. Palliat Med. 2012;27:486–498.

4. Mathillas J, Olofsson B, Lovheim H, Gustafson Y. Thirty-day prevalence of delirium among very old people: a population-based study of very old people living at home and in institutions. Arch Gerontol Geriatr. 2013;57:298–304.

5. Neufeld KJ, Leoutsakos JM, Sieber FE, Wanamaker BL, et al. Outcomes of early delirium diagnosis after general anesthesia in the elderly. Anesth Analg. 2013;117:471–478.

6. Fick DM, Steis MR, Waller JL, Inouye S. Delirium superimposed on dementia is associated with prolonged length of stay and poor outcomes in hospitalized older adults. J Hosp Med. 2013;8:500–505.

7. Wand AP, Thoo W, Ting V, Baker J, Sciuriaga H, Hunt GE. Identification and rates of delirium in elderly medical inpatients from diverse language groups. Geriatr Nurs. 2013;34:355–360.

8. Zaubler TS, Murphy K, Rizzuto L, Santos R, et al. Quality improvement and cost savings with multicomponent delirium interventions: a replication of the Hospital Elder Life Program in a community hospital. Psychosomatics. 2013;54:219–226.

9. Barr J, Fraser GL, Puntillo K, Ely EW, et al. Clinical practice guidelines for the management of pain, agitation, and delirium in adult patients in the intensive care unit. Crit Care Med. 2013;41:263–306.

10. Gagnon P, Allard P, Gagnon B, Merett C, Tardif F. Delirium prevention in terminal cancer: assessment of a multicomponent intervention. Psychooncology. 2012;21:187–194.

11. Hey J, Hosker C, Ward J, Kite S, Speechley H. Delirium in palliative care: detection, documentation and management in three settings. Palliat Support Care. 2013; 21:1–5.

12. Steis M, Fick D. Are nurses recognizing delirium?: A systematic review. J Gerontol Nurs. 2008;34:40–48.

13. Kishi Y, Kato M, Okuyama T, et al. Delirium: patient characteristics that predict a missed diagnosis at psychiatric consultation. Gen Hosp Psychiatry. 2007;29:442–445.

14. Fick D, Hodo D, Lawrence F, et al. Recognizing delirium superimposed on dementia: assessing nurses' knowledge using case vignettes. J Gerontol Nurs. 2007;33:40–49.

15. Flagg B, McDowell S, Mwose JM, Buelow JM. Nursing identification of delirium. Clin Nurse Spec. 2010;24:260–266.

16. Moyer DD. Terminal delirium in geriatric patients with cancer at end of life. Am J Hosp Palliat Care. 2011;28:44–51.

17. Neufeld KJ, Thomas C. Delirium: definition, epidemiology, and diagnosis. J Clin Neurophysiol. 2013;30:438–442.

18. DeCrane S, Culp KR, Wakefield B. Twelve-month fall outcomes among delirium subtypes. J Healthc Qual. 2012;34(6):13–20.

19. Witlox J, Eurelings LS, deJonghe JF, Kalisvaart KJ, Eikenlenboom P, vanGool WA. Delirium in elderly patients and the risk of postdischarge mortality, institutionalization, and dementia: a meta-analysis. JAMA. 2010;304:443–451.

20. O'Malley G, Leonard M, Meagher D, et al. The delirium experience: A review. J Psychosom Res 2008;65:223–228.

21. DiMartini A, Dew MA, Kormos R, McCurry K, Fontes P. Posttraumatic stress disorder caused by hallucinations and delusions experienced in delirium. Psychosomatics. 2007;48:436–439.

22. Bruera E, Bush SH, Willey J, Paraskevopoulos T, et al. Impact of delirium and recall on the level of distress in patients with advanced cancer and their family caregivers. Cancer. 2009;115:2004–2012.

23. Partridge JS, Martin FC, Harari D, Dhesi JK. The delirium experience: what is the effect on patients, relatives and staff and what can be done to modify this? Int J Geriatr Psychiatry. 2013;28:804–812.

24. Grover S, Shah R. Distress due to delirium experience. Gen Hosp Psychiatry. 2011;33:637–639.

25. Davydow DS. Symptoms of depression and anxiety after delirium. Psychosomatics. 2009;50:309–316.

26. Namba M, Morita T, Imura C, et al. Terminal delirium: families' experience. Palliat Med. 2007;21:587–594.

27. Szarpa KL, Kerr CW, Wright ST, Luczkiewicz DL, Hang PC, Ball LS. The prodrome to delirium. J Hosp Palliat Nurs. 2013;15:332–337.

28. McDonnell S, Timmins F. A quantitative exploration of the subjective burden experienced by nurses when caring for patients with delirium. J Clin Nurs. 2012;21:2488–2498.

29. Otani H, Morita T, Uno S, Yamamoto R, et al. Usefulness of the leaflet-based intervention for family members of terminally ill cancer patients with delirium. J Palliat Med. 2013;16:419–422.

30. Leonard M, Raju B, Conroy M, Donnelly S, Trazepacz PT, Saunders J, Meagher D. Reversibility of delirium in terminally ill patients and predictors of mortality. Palliat Med. 2008;22:848–854.

31. Chirco N, Dunn KS, Robinson SG. The trajectory of terminal delirium at the end of life. J Hosp Palliat Nurs. 2011;13:411–418.

32. Breitbart W, Alici Y. Agitation and delirium at the end of life: "We couldn't manage him." JAMA. 2008;300:2898–2910.

33. White C, McCann M, Jackson N. First do no harm … terminal restlessness or drug-induced delirium. J Palliat Med. 2007;10:345–351.

34. Lawlor P, Gagnon B, Mancini I, et al. Occurrence, causes, and outcomes of delirium in patients with advanced cancer: a prospective study. Arch Intern Med. 2000;160:786–794.

35. Meagher DJ, Leonard M, Donnelly S, Conroy M, Adamis D, Trazepacz PT. A longitudinal study of motor subtypes in delirium: relationship with other phenomenology, etiology, medication exposure and prognosis. J Psychosom Res. 2011;71:395–403.

36. Leslie D, Marcantonio E, Zhang Y, et al. One-year health costs associated with delirium in the elderly population. Arch Intern Med. 2008;168:27–32.

37. American Psychiatric Association. Diagnostic and Statistical Manual of Mental Disorders: DSM-5. Arlington, VA: American Psychiatric Association; 2013.

38. Blazer DG, vanNieuwenhuizen AO. Evidence for the diagnostic criteria of delirium. Curr Opin Psychiatry. 2012;25:239–243.

39. Vasilevskis EE, Morandi A, Boehm L, Pandharipande PP, Girard TD, et al. Delirium and sedation recognition using validated instruments: reliability of bedside intensive care unit nursing assessments from 2007 to 2010. J Am Geriatr Soc. 2011;55(Suppl 2):S249–S255.

40. Kang JH, Shin SH, Bruera E. Comprehensive approached to managing delirium in patients with advanced cancer. Cancer Treat Rev. 2013;39:105–112.

41. Kerr CW, Donnelly JP, Wright ST, Luczkiewicz DL, et al. Progression of delirium in advanced illness: a multivariate model of caregiver and clinician perspective. J Palliat Med. 2013;16:768–773.

42. Sands MB, Dantoc BP, Hartshorn A, Ryan CJ, Lujic S. Single question in delirium (SQiD): testing its efficacy against psychiatrist interview,

the Confusion Assessment Method, and the Memorial Delirium Assessment Scale. Palliat Med. 2010;24:561–565.

43. Meagher DJ, Moran M, Raju B, Gibbons D, et al. A new data-based motor subtype schema for delirium. J Neuropsychiatry Clin Neurosci. 2008;20:185–93.

44. Meagher D. Motor subtypes of delirium: past, present, and future. Int Rev Psychiatry 2009;21:59–73.

45. Stagno D, Gibson C, Breitbart W. The delirium subtypes: A review of prevalence, phenomenology, pathophysiology, and treatment response. Palliat Support Care. 2004;2:171–179.

46. Mittal V, Muralee S, Williamson D, McEnerney N. Thomas J, Cash M, Rajesh R. Review: Delirium in the elderly: a comprehensive review. Am J Alzheimers Dis Other Demen. 2011;26:97–109.

47. Marchington KL, Carrier L, Lawlor PG. Delirium masquerading as depression. Palliat Support Care. 2012;10:59–62.

48. Morita T, Tei Y, Tsunoda J, Inoue M, Chihara S. Underlying pathologies and their associations with clinical features in terminal delirium of cancer patients. J Pain Symptom Manage. 2001;22:997–1006.

49. Peterson JF, Pun BT, Dittus RS, Thomason JW, Jackson JC, Shintani AK, Ely EW. Delirium and its motoric subtypes: a study of 614 critically ill patients. J Am Geriatr Soc. 2006;54:479–484.

50. Sagawa R, Akechi T, Okuyama T, Uchida M, Furukawa TA. Etiologies of delirium and their relationship to reversibility and motor subtype in cancer patients. Jpn J Clin Oncol. 2009;39:175–182.

51. Slor CJ, Adamis D, Jansen RW, Meagher DJ, Witlox J, Houdijk AP, et al. Delirium motor subtypes in elderly hip fracture patients: risk factors, outcomes and longitudinal stability. J Psychosom Res. 2013;74:444–449.

52. Siddiqi N, House A, Holmes J. Occurrence and outcome of delirium in medical in-patients: a systematic literature review. Age Ageing. 2006;35:350–364.

53. Irwin S, Pirreilo RD, Hirst JM, Buckholz GT, Ferris FD. Clarifying delirium management: practical, evidenced-based, expert recommendations for clinical practice. J Palliat Med. 2013;16:423–435.

54. Curtis L. 2012. Deathbed visions: social workers' experiences, perspectives, therapeutic responses, and direction for practice. Paper 17. http://sophia.stkate.edu/cgi/viewcontent.cgi?article=1016&context=msw_papers. Accessed December 8, 2013.

55. Brayne S, Lovelace H, Fenwick P. End-of-life experiences and the dying process in a Gloucestershire nursing home as reported by nurses and care assistants. Am J Hosp Palliat Care. 2008;25:195–206.

56. Fenwick P, Lovelace H, Brayne S. Comfort for the dying: five year retrospective and one year prospective studies of end of life experiences. Arch Gerontol Geriatr. 2010;51:173–179.

57. Mazzarino-Willett A. Deathbed phenomena: its role in peaceful death and terminal restlessness. Am J Hosp Palliat Care. 2010; 27:127–133.

58. Callanan C, Kelley P. Final Gifts. New York: Poseidon Press; 1992:67–71.

59. Yokota H, Ogawa S, Kurokawa A, et al. Regional cerebral blood flow in delirium patients. Psychiatry Clin Neurosci 2003;57:337–339.

60. Fong T, Bogardus S, Daftary A, et al. Cerebral perfusion changes in older delirious patients using 99mTc HMPAO SPECT. J Gerontol A Biol Sci. 2006;61:1294–1299.

61. Gottesman R, Hillis A, Grega M, et al. Early postoperative cognitive dysfunction and blood pressure during coronary artery bypass graft operation. Arch Neurol. 2007;64:1111–1114.

62. Maldonado J. Pathoetiological model of delirium: a comprehensive understanding of the neurobiology of delirium and an evidence-based approach to prevention and treatment. Crit Care Clin. 2008;24:789–856.

63. Dam G, Keiding S, Munk OL, Ott P, et al. Hepatic encephalopathy is associated with decreased cerebral oxygen metabolism and blood flow, not increased ammonia uptake. Hepatology. 2013;57:258–265.

64. Gunther M, Jackson J, Ely E. Loss of IQ in the ICU: brain injury without the insult. Med Hypotheses. 2007;69:1179–1182.

65. Jackson J, Gordon S, Hart R, et al. The association between delirium and cognitive decline: a review of the empirical literature. Neuropsychol Rev. 2004;14:87–98.

66. Gunther M, Morandi A, Ely E. Pathophysiology of delirium in the intensive care unit. Crit Care Clin. 2008;24:45–65.

67. Hshieh T, Fong T, Marcantonio E, et al. Cholinergic deficiency hypothesis in delirium: a synthesis of current evidence. J Gerontol A Biol Sci Med Sci. 2008;63:764–772.

68. Trzepacz P. Is there a common neural pathway in delirium? Focus on acetylcholine and dopamine. Semin Clin Neuropsychiatry. 2000;5;132–148.

69. Kreek M, Zhou Y, Butelman E, et al. Opiate and cocaine addiction: from bench to clinic and back to the bench. Curr Opin Pharmacol. 2009;9:74–80.

70. Segal M, Avital A, Rusakov A, et al. Serum creatine kinase activity differentiates alcohol syndromes of dependence, withdrawal and delirium tremens. Eur Neuropsychopharmacol. 2009;19:92–96.

71. Inouye S. Delirium in older persons. N Engl J Med. 2006;354:1157–1165.

72. Pfister D, Siegemund M, Dell-Kuster S, et al. Cerebral perfusion in sepsis associated delirium. Crit Care. 2008;12:R63. http://ccforum.com/content/12/3/R63. Accessed December 3, 2013.

73. Siami S, Annane D, Sharshar T. The encephalopathy in sepsis. Crit Care Clin. 2008;24:67–82.

74. deRooij S, vanMunster B, Korevaar J, et al. Cytokines and acute phase response in delirium. J Psychosom Res. 2007;62:521–525.

75. vanMunster B, Korevaar J, Zwinderman A, et al. Time-course of cytokines during delirium in elderly patients with hip fractures. J Am Geriatr Soc. 2008;56:1704–1709.

76. Beloosesky Y, Hendel D, Weiss A, et al. Cytokines and C-reactive protein production in hip-fracture-operated elderly patients. J Gerontal A Biol Sci Med Sci. 2007;62:420–426.

77. Van Gool WA, van de Beek D, Eikelenboom P. Systemic infection and delirium: when cytokines and acetylcholine collide. Lancet. 2010;375:773–775.

78. Fearing M, Inouye S. Delirium. In: Blazer D, Steffens D (eds.), The American Psychiatric Publishing Textbook of Geriatric Psychiatry (4th ed). Washington, DC: American Psychiatric Publishing; 2009:229–241.

79. Inouye S, Charpentier P. Precipitating factors for delirium in hospitalized elderly persons: predictive model and interrelationship with baseline vulnerability. JAMA. 1996;20:852–858.

80. Inouye S. Current concepts: delirium in older persons. N Engl J Med. 2006;354:1157–1165.

81. Margiotta A, Bianchetti A, Ranieri P, et al. Clinical characteristics and risk factors of delirium in demented and not demented elderly medical inpatients. J Nutr Health Aging. 2006;10:535–539.

82. Cole M. Delirium in elderly patients. Am J Geriatr Psychiatry. 2004;12:7–21.

83. Meagher DJ, Leonard M, Donnelly S, Conroy M, Saunders J, Trzepacz, PT. A comparison of neuropsychiatric and cognitive profiles in delirium, dementia, comorbid delirium-dementia and cognitively intact controls. J Neurol Neurosurg Psychiatry. 2010;81:876–881.

84. Hamann J, Bickel H, Schwaibold H, et al. Postoperative acute confusional state in typical urologic population: incidence, risk factors, and strategies for prevention. Urology. 2005;65:449–453.

85. McCusker J, Cole MG, Voyer P, Vu M, et al. Environmental factors predict the severity of delirium symptoms in long-term care residents with and without delirium. J Am Geriatr Soc. 2013;61:502–511.

86. Zekry D, Herrmann F, Grandjean R, et al. Demented versus non-demented very old inpatients: the same comorbidities but poorer functional and nutritional status. Age Ageing. 2008;37:83–89.

87. Arnold E. Sorting out the 3 D's: Delirium, dementia, depression: learn how to sift through overlapping signs and symptoms so you can help an older patient's quality of life. Holist Nurs Pract. 2005;19:99–104.

88. Milisen K, Braes T, Fick D, et al. Cognitive assessment and differentiating the 3 Ds (dementia, depression, delirium). Nurs Clin North Am. 2006;41:1–22.

89. Boyle D. Delirium in older adults with cancer: implications for practice and research. Oncol Nurs Forum. 2006;33:61–78.

90. Guenther U, Theuerkauf N, Frommann I, et al. Predisposing and precipitating factors of delirium after cardiac surgery: a prospective observational cohort study. Ann Surg. 2013;257:1160–1167.

91. Lin Y, Chen J, Wang Z. Meta-analysis of factors which influence delirium following cardiac surgery. J Card Surg. 2012;27:481–492.

92. Zhang Z, Pan L, Deng H, Ni H, Xu X. Prediction of delirium in critically ill patients with elevated C-reactive protein. J Crit Care. 2014;29:88–92.

93. Slatore CG, Goy ER, O'Hearn DJ, Boudreau EA, O'Malley JP, Peters D, Ganzini L. Sleep quality and its association with delirium among veterans enrolled in hospice. Am J Geriatr Psychiatry. 2012;20:317–326.

94. Meier DE. Less is more: pain as a cause of agitated delirium. Arch Intern Med. 2012;172:1130.

95. Oosten AW, Oldenmenger WH, van Zuylen C, Schmitz PIM, et al. Higher doses of opioids in patients who need palliative sedation prior to death: cause or consequence? Eur J Cancer. 2011;47:2341–2346.

96. Clegg A, Young JB. Which medications to avoid in people at risk of delirium: a systematic review. Age Ageing. 2011;40:23–29.

97. Inouye S, Zhang Y, Jones R, et al. Risk factors for delirium at discharge: development and validation of a predictive model. Arch Intern Med. 2007;167:1406–1413.

98. Akechi T, Ishiguro C. Okuyama T, Endo C, Sagawa R, Uchida M, Furukawa TA. Delirium training for nurses. Psychosomatics. 2010;51:106–111.

99. Folstein M, Folstein S, McHugh P. Mini-mental state: a practical method for grading the cognitive state of patients for the clinician. J Psychiatr Res. 1975;12:189–198.

100. Hjermstad M, Loge J, Kaasa S. Methods for assessment of cognitive failure and delirium in palliative care patients: implications for practice and research. Palliat Med. 2004;18:494–506.

101. Fayers P, Hjernstad M, Ranhoff A, et al. Which mini-mental state exam items can be used to screen for delirium and cognitive impairment? J Pain Symptom Manage. 2005;30:41–50.

102. Schuurmans M, Deschamps P, Markham S, et al. The measurement of delirium: Review of scales. Res Theory Nurs Pract 2003;17:207–224.

103. Wong CL, Holroyd-Leduc J, Simel DL, Straus SE. Does this patient have delirium?: Value of bedside instruments. JAMA. 2010;304:779–786.

104. Breitbart W, Rosenfeld B, Roth A, et al. The Memorial Delirium Assessment Scale. J Pain Symptom Manage. 1997;13:128–137.

105. Bosisio M, Caraceni A, Grassi L, et al. Phenomenology of delirium in cancer patients as described by the Memorial Delirium Assessment scale (MDAS) and the Delirium Rating Scale (DRS). Psychosomatics. 2006;47:471–478.

106. Trzepacz P. The Delirium Rating Scale: Its use in consultation liaison research. Psychosomatics. 1999;40:193–204.

107. Trzepacz P, Mittal D, Tores R, et al. Validation of the Delirium Rating Scale-revised-98: comparison with the delirium rating scale and the cognitive test for delirium. J Neuropsychiatry Clin Neurosci. 2001;13:229–242.

108. Inouye S. The Confusion Assessment Method (CAM): Training Manual and Coding Guide. New Haven: Yale University School of Medicine, 2003. Available at: http://elderlifeprogram.org/pdf/TheConfusionAssessmentMethodTrainingManual.pdf. Accessed November 29, 2013.

109. Lemiengre J, Nelis T, Joosten E, et al. Detection of delirium by beside nurses using the confusion assessment method. J Am Geriatr Soc. 2006;54:685–689.

110. Waszynski C, Petrovic K. Nurses' evaluation of the Confusion Assessment Method: a pilot study. J Gerontol Nurs. 2008;34:49–56.

111. Morandi A, McCurley J, Vasilevskis EE, Fick DM. Tools to detect delirium superimposed on dementia: a systematic review. J Am Geriatr Soc. 2012;60:2005–2013.

112. Guenther U, Popp J, Koecher L, Muders T, Wrigge H, Ely EW, Putensen C. Validity and reliability of the CAM-ICU flowsheet to diagnose delirium in surgical ICU patients. J Crit Care. 2010;25:144–151.

113. Sarhill N, Walsh D, Nelson K, et al. Assessment of delirium in advanced cancer: the use of the bedside confusion scale. Am J Hosp Palliat Care. 2001;18:335–341.

114. Neelon V, Champagne M, Carlson J, et al. The NEECHAM Confusion Scale: Construction, validation, and clinical testing. Nurs Res. 1996;45:324–330.

115. Matarese M, Generoso S. Ivziku D, Pedone C, DeMarinis MG. Delirium in older patients: a diagnostic study of NEECHAM confusion scale in surgical intensive care unit. J Clin Nurs. 2013;22:2849–2857.

116. Stillman M, Rybicki L. The bedside confusion scale: development of a portable bedside test for confusion and its application to the palliative medicine population. J Palliat Med. 2000;3:449–456.

117. Zama I, Maynard W, Davis M. Clocking delirium: the value of the clock drawing test with case illustrations. Am J Hosp Palliat Care. 2008;25:385–388.

118. Schuurmans M, Shortridge-Baggett L, Duursma S. The Delirium Observation Screening Scale: a screening instrument for delirium. Res Theory Nurs Pract. 2003;17:31–50.

119. Gaudreau J, Gagnon P, Harel F, et al. Fast, systematic, and continuous delirium assessment in hospitalized patients: the nursing delirium screening scale. J Pain Symptom Manage. 2005;29:368–375.

120. Radtke R, Franck M, Schneider M, et al. Comparison of three scores for delirium in the recovery room. Br J Anaesth. 2008;101:338–343.

121. Pisani, MA, Murphy T, VanNess PH, Araujo KLB, Inouye SK. Characteristics associated with delirium in older patients in a medical intensive care unit. Arch Intern Med. 2007;167:1629–1634.

122. Inouye S, Bogardus S, Charpentier P, et al. A multicomponent intervention to prevent delirium in hospitalized older patients. N Engl J Med. 1999;340:669–676.

123. Inouye S. The Hospital Elder Life Program (HELP). 2007. http://www.hospitalelderlifeprogram.org. Accessed December 2, 2013.

124. Barr J, Pandharipande PP. The pain, agitation, and delirium care bundle: synergistic benefits of implementing the 2013 pain, agitation, and delirium guidelines in an integrated and interdisciplinary fashion. Crit Care Med. 2013;41:S99-S115.

125. Gagnon P, Allard P, Gagnon B, Merett C, Tardif F. Delirium prevention in terminal cancer: assessment of a multicomponent intervention. Psychooncology. 2012;21:187–194.

126. Yennurajalingam S, Bruera E, eds. Oxford American of Hospice Palliative Medicine. New York: Oxford University Press; 2011.

127. Popeo DM. Delirium in older adults. Mt Sinai J Med. 2011;78:571–582.

128. Bruera E, Hui D, Dalal S, Torres-Vigil I, et al. Parenteral hydration in patients with advanced cancer: a multicenter, double-blind, placebo-controlled randomized trial. J Clin Oncol. 2013; 31:111–118.

129. Nakajima N, Hata Y, Kusumoto K. A clinical study on the influence of hydration volume on the signs of terminally ill cancer patients with abdominal malignancies. J Palliat Med. 2013;16:185–189.

130. White J, Hammond L. Delirium assessment tool for end of life: CHIMBOP. J Palliat Med. 2008;11:1069.

131. Lonergan E, Britton AM, Luxenberg J. Antipsychotics for delirium. Cochrane Database Syst Rev. 2007(2): CD005594. doi: 10.1002/14651858.CD005594.pub2.

132. Hatta K, Kishi Y, Wada K, Odawara T, et al. Antipsychotics for delirium in the general hospital setting in consecutive 2453 inpatients: a prospective observational study. Int J Geriatr Psychiatry. 2013. Published online in Wiley Online Library: http://onlinelibrary.wiley.com/doi/10.1002/gps.3999/pdf. Accessed November 23, 2013.

133. Meagher DJ, McLoughlin L, Leonard M, Hannon N, Dunne C, O'Regan N. What do we really know about the treatment of delirium with antipsychotics?: Ten key issues for delirium pharmacotherapy. Am J Geriatr Psychiatry. 2013;21:1223–1238.

134. Hanson E, Healey K, Wolf D, Kohler C. Assessment of pharmacotherapy for negative symptoms of schizophrenia. Curr Psychiatry Rep. 2010;12:563–571.

135. Tropea J, Slee J, Holmes A, et al. Use of antipsychotic medications for the management of delirium: an audit of current practice in the acute care setting. Int Psychogeriatr. 2008;5:1–8.

136. Weckmann MT, Morrison RS. What pharmacological treatments are effective for delirium? In: Goldstein NE, Morrison RS (eds.), Evidence-Based Practice of Palliative Medicine. Philadelphia: Elsevier; 2013:205–210.

137. Twycross R, Wilcock A., eds. Hospice and Palliative Care Formulary USA. 2nd ed. Nottingham UK: Palliativedrugs.com Ltd, 2008.

138. Jasiak KD, Meddleton EA, Camamo JM, Erstad BL, Snyder LS, Huckleberry YC. Evaluation of discontinuation of atypical antipsychotics prescribed for ICU delirium. J Pharm Pract. 2013;26:253–256.

139. US Food and Drug Administration. 2007. Information for Healthcare Professionals: Haloperidol (marketed as Haldol, Haldol Decanoate and Haldol Lactate). Available at: http://www.fda.gov/Drugs/Drug Safety/PostmarketDrugSafetyInformationforPatientsandProviders/DrugSafetyInformationforHeathcareProfessionals/ucm085203.htm. Accessed December 3, 2013.

140. Elie M, Boss K, Cole MG, McCusker J, Belzile E, Ciampi A. A retrospective, exploratory, secondary analysis of the association between antipsychotic use and mortality in elderly patients with delirium. Int Psychogeriatr. 2009;21:588–592.

141. Meyer-Massetti C, Vaerini S, Ratz Bravo AE, Meier CR, Guglielmo BJ. Comparative safety of antipsychotics in the WHO pharmacovigilance database: the haloperidol case. Int J Clin Pharm. 2011;33:806–814.

142. Yoon H, Park K, Choi W, Choi S, Park J, Kim J, Seok J. Efficacy and safety of haloperidol versus atypical antipsychotic medications in the treatment of delirium. BMC Psychiatry. 2013;13:240.

143. Hawkins SB, Bucklin M, Muzyk A. Quetiapine for the treatment of delirium. J Hosp Med. 2013;8:215–220.

144. Maneeton B, Maneeton N. Srisurapanont M. Chittawatanarat K. Quetiapine versus haloperidol in the treatment of delirium: a double-blind, randomized, controlled trial. Drug Des Devel Ther. 2013;7:657–667.

145. Teslyar P, Stock VM, Wilk CM, Camsari U, Ehrenreich MJ, Himelhoch S. Prophylaxis with antipsychotic medication reduces the risk of post-operative delirium in elderly patients: a meta-analysis. Psychosomatics. 2013;54:124–131.

146. Wang W, Li H, Wang D, Zhu X, et al. Haloperidol prophylaxis decreases delirium incidence in elderly patients after noncardiac surgery: a randomized controlled trial. Crit Care Med. 2012;40:731–739.

147. Larsen KA, Kelly SE, Stern TA, Bode RH Jr, et al. Administration of olanzapine to prevent postoperative delirium in elderly joint-replacement patients: a randomized, controlled trial. Psychosomatics. 2010;51:409–418.

148. van den Boogaard M, Schoonhoven L, van Achterberg T, van der Hoeven JG, Pickkers P. Haloperidol prophylaxis in critically ill patients with high risk for delirium. Crit Care. 2013;17:R9. Available at http://ccforum.com/content/17/1/R9. Accessed December 3, 2013.

149. Overshott R, Karim S, Burns A. Cholinesterase inhibitors for delirium. Cochrane Database Syst Rev. 2008;(1): CD005317. doi: 10.1002/14651858.CD005317.pub2.

150. Breitbart W, Marotta R, Platt M, et al. A double-blind trial of haloperidol, chlorpromazine, and lorazepam in the treatment of delirium in hospitalized AIDS patients. Am J Psychiatry. 1996;153:231–237.

151. Mercandante S, Porzio G, Valle A, Fusco F, Aielli F, Adile C, et al. Palliative sedation in advanced cancer patients followed at home: a retrospective analysis. J Pain Symptom Manage. 2012, 43:1126–1130.

152. Caraceni A, Zecca E, Martini C, Gorni G, Campa T, Brunelli C, et al. Palliative sedation at the end of life at a tertiary cancer center. Support Care Cancer. 2012;20:1299–1307.

153. Kerr CW, Luczkiewicz DL, Holahan T, Milch R, Hang PC. The use of pentobarbital in cases of severe delirium: a case series. Am J Hospice Palliat Care., 2014;34:105–108.

154. Rosenbloom-Brunton DA, Henneman EA, Inouye SK. Feasibility of family participation in a delirium prevention program for hospitalized older adults. J Gerontol Nurs. 2010;36:22–33.

155. Morita T, Akechi T, Ikenaga M, et al. Terminal delirium: recommendations from bereaved families' experiences. J Pain Symptom Manage. 2007;34(6):579–589.

156. Hospice and Palliative Nurses Association. Quick Reference Sheet: Delirium in Hospice And Palliative Patients. Revised July 2013. Available at http://www.hpna.org/DisplayPage.aspx?Title=Quick%20 Information%20Sheet. Accessed December 3, 2013.

157. Steis MR, Evans L, Hirschman KB, et al. Screening for delirium using family caregivers: convergent validity of the Family Confusion Assessment Method and Interviewer-Rated Confusion Assessment Method. J Am Geriatr Soc. 2012; 60(11):2121–2126.

CHAPTER 22

Insomnia

Laura Bourdeanu, Marjorie J. Hein,
and Ellen A. Liu

> He would lie in the bed and finally, with daylight, he would go to sleep. After all, he said to himself, it is probably only insomnia. Many must have it.
>
> Ernest Hemingway

Key points

• Insomnia is a symptom characterized as inconsistent or ineffective sleep patterns that can significantly impact a person's quality of life.

• There remains a lack of knowledge specifically related to assessing and managing insomnia in cancer patients. Many pharmacological and nonpharmacological therapies are available that can be helpful.

• All nurses in all settings can play an important role in advancing the knowledge and skills related to addressing insomnia.

Insomnia is a prevalent health complaint, with an estimated 6%–10% of Americans suffering from insomnia on a regular basis each year.[1] Insomnia is predominant among the elderly, those with chronic medical illness, and those with anxiety or depressive disorders.[2] Unchecked, insomnia can lead to various adverse sequelae in psychiatric, neurocognitive, and medical domains, as well as significant reduction in quality of life.[3,4] In addition, insomnia can lead to daytime dysfunction, such as daytime sleepiness, irritability, depressive or anxious mood, and accidents.[5]

Sleep is a "highly structured and well-organized activity following a circadian periodicity that is regulated by the interplay of internal biological processes and environmental factors."[6] According to the International Classification of Sleep Disorders and DSM-IV, insomnia is a "heterogeneous complaint that may involve difficulties falling asleep, difficulty maintaining sleep with more than 30 minutes of nocturnal awakenings, early-morning awaking with inability to resume sleep, or a complaint of nonrestorative sleep with corresponding sleep efficiency less than 85%."[7,8]

In patients with cancer, insomnia is reported to be a common problem. The prevalence of insomnia and associated symptoms in cancer patients, either newly diagnosed or recently treated, was reported to be 23%–61%. However, insomnia was still present in 23%–44% of patients 2–5 years after treatment.[9,10] The causes for insomnia in patients with cancer may be related to psychological factors (anxiety or depression), pain, treatment-related toxicity, or other comorbid medical conditions. Further, insomnia was linked with increased rates of depression, decreased quality of life, and increased fatigue in other patient populations.[2]

Though it is a common symptom noted by cancer patients, especially those undergoing aggressive forms of treatment, research regarding insomnia in cancer patients is scarce. This chapter will apply as a model for assessment and treatment of insomnia to cancer patients; however, these principles can also be considered for patients without cancer.

Case study

EH, 29-year-old Hispanic male. Diagnosis: recurrent germ cell tumor

Prior to his diagnosis of recurrent cancer, EH was an active musician and performer. He was also involved in a serious relationship, engaged to be married, and was one of the breadwinners in his family. When EH began experiencing inguinal pain and persistent left scapular pain, he decided to seek medical attention. Ultimately, radiographic scans and blood tests confirmed his diagnosis of recurrent metastatic germ cell tumor, which spread to his lungs and inguinal nodes. Not only did he recur, requiring chemotherapy and possible stem cell transplantation, but he suffered from persistent pain, which inhibited his quality of life. From the time of his diagnosis of recurrent cancer and his chronic pain syndrome, EH suffered from persistent insomnia, despite the fact he was on higher doses of narcotics, which brought along the expected sedative side effects. He was subsequently referred to a palliative program, which included a thorough evaluation of his medications, his current lifestyle, and his sleep patterns. Though there are many modalities that will be described later in this chapter, the most effective regimen for him involved the use of pharmacological agents. With patient education provided on managing his pain, maintaining his daily exercise and eating routines, and optimizing his time awake, EH was able to maintain 7–8 hours of restful sleep by using a nonbenzodiazepine drug: Zolpidem.

Factors related to insomnia

Insomnia is among the most prevalent, distressing, and undermanaged symptoms experienced by patients with cancer. Insomnia is associated with adverse outcomes and should be proactively targeted for intervention. A. J. Spielman, in the late 1980s, created a model of insomnia in terms of predisposing, precipitating, and perpetuating factors. In the context of precipitating factors such as psychosocial, medical or psychiatric, the genetic and neurobiological factors can determine a person's risk for insomnia. The process of sleep and wakefulness is active and tightly regulated and differs among individuals who have different susceptibilities to exogenous influence.[11]

Often, sleep disturbances are associated with situational stresses such as illness, aging, and drug treatments.[2] However, in patients with cancer, the physical illness, pain, hospitalization, and cancer treatment drugs, along with the psychological impact of the disease, may disrupt sleeping patterns of the individual. A history of poor sleep patterns will adversely affect the individual's daytime mood and performance. Among the general population, an individual with complaints of persistent insomnia has been associated with an increased risk of developing anxiety or depression. Complaints of sleep disturbances and a pattern of sleep-wake cycle reversals may be an early sign of a developing delirium.[12]

Paraneoplastic syndromes may exacerbate sleep disturbances if they are associated with increased steroid production and if the patient has symptoms associated with tumor invasion such as draining lesions, gastrointestinal and genitourinary changes, pain, fever, cough, dyspnea, pruritus, and fatigue. Moreover, medications used by patients to control symptoms of the disease, or side effects of treatment, may cause insomnia. For example, medications such as vitamins, corticosteroids, neuroleptics for nausea and vomiting, and sympathomimetics to relieve dyspnea may negatively impact sleep patterns. Frequently, hospitalized patients are likely to have their sleep interrupted by treatment schedules, routine hospital procedures, and other patients sharing the room. All of these factors may either singularly or collectively alter the sleep-wake cycle. Other considerations influencing the sleep-wake cycles of patients with cancer include age, comfort, pain, and anxiety; environmental noise; and temperature.[10]

There are four major categories of sleep disorders according to the Sleep Disorders Classification Committee of the American Academy of Sleep Medicine:

1. Disorders of initiating and maintaining sleep (insomnias)

2. Disorders of the sleep-wake cycle

3. Dysfunctions associated with sleep, sleep stages, or partial arousals (parasomnias)

4. Disorders of excessive somnolence[13]

In the DSM-IV-TR (*Diagnostic and Statistical Manual of Mental Disorders*, fourth edition text revision), sleep disorders are organized into four major categories according to the etiology of the sleep disorder[7]:

1. *Primary sleep disorders* consist of all etiologies other than those listed below. Primary sleep disorders are assumed to develop from endogenous abnormalities in sleep-wake patterns, accompanied by conditioning factors.

   a. *Dyssomnias* are abnormalities in the amount, quality, or timing of sleep.

   b. *Parasomnias* are abnormal behavioral or physiological events.

2. *Sleep disorder related to another mental disorder* resulting from a diagnosable mental disorder, usually mood or anxiety disorder, but severe enough to receive clinical attention.

3. *Sleep disorder due to a general medical condition* resulting from the effects of a physiological medical condition.

4. *Substance-induced sleep disorder* resulting from concurrent use or a recent discontinuation of a drug.[7]

Insomnia may also be caused by medications commonly used in the treatment of cancer. The sustained use of central nervous system (CNS) stimulants such as amphetamines, psychostimulants used to treat attention deficit disorders (e.g., methylphenidate), caffeine, and diet pills (including some dietary supplements that promote weight loss and appetite suppression); sedatives and hypnotics (e.g., glutethimide, benzodiazepines, pentobarbital, chloral hydrate, secobarbital sodium, and amobarbital sodium); cancer chemotherapeutic agents (especially antimetabolites); anticonvulsants (e.g., phenytoin); adrenocorticotropin; oral contraceptives; monoamine oxidase inhibitors; methyldopa; propranolol; atenolol; alcohol; and thyroid preparations can cause insomnia. In addition, withdrawal from CNS depressants (e.g., barbiturates, opioids, glutethimide, chloral hydrate, methaqualone, ethchlorvynol [no longer sold in the United States], alcohol, and over-the-counter and prescription antihistamine sedatives), benzodiazepines, major tranquilizers, tricyclic and monoamine oxidase inhibitor antidepressants, and illicit drugs (e.g., marijuana, cocaine, phencyclidine) can cause insomnia.[1]

Hypnotics that are commonly prescribed to patients with cancer can interfere with rapid eye movement (REM) sleep, resulting in irritability, apathy, and decreased mental alertness. An abrupt withdrawal of hypnotics and sedatives may cause nervousness, jitteriness, seizures, and REM rebound, which is a "marked increase in REM sleep with increased frequency and intensity of dreaming, including nightmares."[14] The increased physiological arousal that occurs during REM rebound may be dangerous for patients with peptic ulcers or a history of cardiovascular problems.

Pathophysiology

Normal sleep consists of two phases: REM sleep and non-rapid eye movement (NREM) sleep.[15] The brain is active during REM sleep or dream sleep; NREM sleep is the quiet or restful phase of sleep. Non-rapid eye movement sleep is divided into four stages of progressively deepening sleep based on electroencephalogram findings.[15,16] Sleep occurs in stages of a repeated pattern, or cycle, of NREM followed by REM, in which each cycle lasts approximately 90–120 minutes. The cycle is repeated four to five times during a 7- to 8-hour sleep period.[17,18]

A biological clock, or circadian rhythm, dictates the sleep-wake cycle. A disruption in an individual's sleep pattern may disturb the circadian rhythm and impair the sleep cycle.[18] Responses to exogenous influences such as caffeine, light, and stress have been indicated in recent studies to be influenced by genetic factors. An example in one study found that differences in the adenosine 2A receptor gene (ADORA2) determine the differential sensitivity to caffeine's effect on sleep. The ADORA2A c. 1083T>C genotype determines how closely the caffeine-induced changes in brain electrical activity (increased beta activity) during sleep resemble the alterations observed in patients with insomnia.[19] A mutated clocked gene has been found to cause hyperactivity, decreased sleep, lowered depression-like behavior, lowered anxiety, and increased reward-oriented behavior.[20] A patient with a history of chronic insomnia may have a mutation in the gene (GABAa beta3) that is believed to affect an individual's ability to handle stress or make them more susceptible to depression.[21]

Patients with chronic insomnia (in clinical trials) were noted to have increased brain arousal.[22] Demonstrations of fast-frequency activity during NREM sleep, an EEG sign of hyperarousal, and evidence of reduced deactivation in key sleep-wake regions during NREM sleep, were noted in patients with chronic primary insomnia. Also, patients with insomnia were noted to have higher day and night body temperatures, urinary cortisol, adrenaline secretion, and adrenocorticotropic hormone (ACTH), than patients with normal sleep. Evidence demonstrated that sleep deprivation was not a factor in the differences found between individuals with insomnia and normal sleepers. Studies have indicated that only a small percentage of patients with medical and psychiatric conditions develop insomnia, which suggests that some patients have an inherent susceptibility (whether psychosocial, medical, or psychiatric) to develop insomnia in the context of a stressful event.[21]

Perpetuating factors

Cognitive and behavioral mechanisms perpetuate insomnia, regardless of how insomnia is triggered. Patients have misconceptions about what are normal sleep requirements, and then develop excessive worry about not having adequate sleep. This often causes the patient to become obsessive about sleep. The patient develops a dysfunctional belief, often worsening the disruptive sleep behavior—for example taking daytime naps or "sleeping in late"—which in turn reduces the natural homeostatic drive to sleep at a normal bedtime.[21]

Patients develop a conditioned arousal to stimuli that would normally be associated with sleep (i.e., heightened anxiety and ruminations about going to sleep once they are in the bedroom). The patient then develops a cycle in which the more they strive to sleep, the more agitated they become, and the less they are able to fall asleep. Also, the patient may have ruminative thoughts or clock-watching behavior as they try to fall asleep in the bedroom. Therefore, conditioned environmental stimuli cause insomnia to develop from the continued association of sleeplessness with situations and behaviors that are typically related to sleep.[21]

In addition, prescription drug use, somatic disorders, neurological decline, reduced exposure to outdoor light, polyphasic sleep-wake patterns, and lack of physical activity perpetuate the greater prevalence of insomnia in elderly individuals.[23]

Treatment

Insomnia in cancer patients may be due to a variety of disease-related factors, cancer treatment, or psychological factors. The initial strategy to treat insomnia in cancer patients is to address the underlying physical and psychological factors contributing to the sleep disturbance. If the precipitating factors are not fully manageable, then pharmacological or behavioral interventions, or both, should be used to treat both acute and chronic insomnia. Pharmacological interventions are more commonly used in cancer patients who seek help for their insomnia; however, long-term pharmacotherapy is not desirable.[13] Hence, the treatment for insomnia in cancer patients must be multimodal and should include both pharmacological and nonpharmacological interventions.

Pharmacological interventions

Pharmacological interventions, particularly hypnotics, have historically played a prominent role in the management of insomnia in cancer patients, despite the lack of controlled trials. Pharmacological agents approved by the US Food and Drug Administration (FDA) for the treatment of insomnia include benzodiazepine gamma-aminobutyric acid (GABA$_A$) agonists, non-benzodiazepine GABA$_A$ agonists, melatonin-receptor agonists, and histamine-receptor antagonists (Table 22.1).[2]

Benzodiazepine receptor agonists

Benzodiazepines are still frequently used in the management of insomnia because of their undisputed efficacy and relative safety compared to other agents such as barbiturates. Benzodiazepines facilitate the GABA-mediated inhibition of cell firing by occupying the subunits of the GABA receptor complex present throughout the brain, including the ventral lateral preoptic area that controls sleep. The sleep architecture is altered by suppressing sleep stages 3 and 4 and prolonging sleep stages 1 and 2, thereby increasing total sleep time.[24] Although benzodiazepines are effective agents, they have several unwanted side effects, such as daytime drowsiness, dizziness or light-headedness, cognitive impairments, motor incoordination, tolerance, dependence, rebound insomnia, and daytime anxiety.[24]

Nonbenzodiazepine receptor agonists

Nonbenzodiazepines are the most widely used medications because they can induce sleep with fewer side effects than benzodiazepines. Nonbenzodiazepines inhibit neuronal firing by binding selectively to the alpha-1 subunit of the omega-1 receptor of the GABA receptor complex. Although both nonbenzodiazepines and benzodiazepines exert their effect on the GABA receptor complex, nonbenzodiazepines do not disturb the architecture of sleep. Nonbenzodiazepines have fewer residual side effects, including a lower risk for abuse and dependence, less psychomotor impairment, amnesia, and daytime somnolence.[25]

Melatonin-receptor agonists

Melatonin-receptor agonists are an emerging class of drugs that can be used to treat insomnia. Melatonin-receptor agonists bind to the MT1 and MT2 receptors in the suprachiasmatic nucleus. These receptors are thought to be involved in the maintenance of the circadian rhythm underlying the normal sleep-wake cycle. Melatonin-receptor agonists have the advantage of having minimal side effects and no potential for abuse or dependence.[26] Presently, the only melatonin-receptor agonist approved for the treatment of insomnia by the FDA is ramelteon (Rozerem).

Histamine-receptor antagonists

Histamine receptor antagonists, such as doxepin, are tricyclic antidepressants that are used for improving sleep-maintenance insomnia. Doxepin, the only FDA-approved drug in this class, has affinity for the H1 histaminic receptor, which produces sedating effects. Doxepin does not produce residual effects in part because of the rise of histamines in the morning that override the sedative effects of doxepin. Doxepin in low doses ($\leq$ 6 mg) has been shown to improve wake after sleep onset, total sleep time, and sleep

Table 22.1 Pharmacological agents approved by the US Food and Drug Administration for the treatment of insomnia

Drugs	Name	Dose	Contraindications
Benzodiazepine receptor agonists	Clonazepam	>0.5 mg	Hypersensitivity, liver disease, acute open-angle glaucoma
	Lorazepam	≥0.5mg	Hypersensitivity, acute narrow-angle glaucoma, sleep apnea syndrome, severe respiratory insufficiency, given intra-arterially
	Oxazepam	≥10mg	Hypersensitivity, psychoses
	Estazolam	≥1mg	Pregnancy, with ketoconazole and itraconazole
	Flurazepam	≥15mg	Hypersensitivity
	Temazepam	≥7.5mg	Pregnancy
	Triazolam	≥0.125mg	Hypersensitivity, pregnancy, with ketoconazole, itraconazole, and nefazodone, medications that significantly impair the oxidative metabolism mediated by cytochrome P450 3A (CYP 3A)
	Quazepam	≥7.5mg	Hypersensitivity, sleep apnea, or with pulmonary insufficiency
Nonbenzodiazepine receptor agonists	Zaleplon	≥5mg	Hypersensitivity
	Zolpidem	≥5mg	Hypersensitivity
	Zolipdem (extended release)	≥6.25mg	Hypersensitivity
	Eszopiclone	≥2mg	Hypersensitivity
Melatonin receptor agonists	Ramelteon	≥8mg	Hypersensitivity, with fluvoxamine
Histamine receptor antagonists	Doxepin	≥6mg	Hypersensitivity, glaucoma or a tendency to urinary retention

efficiency. Currently it is not known whether tolerance develops with long-term use.[27]

Others

Other classes of drugs have been used to treat insomnia in cancer patients, including antidepressants, antihistamines, atypical antipsychotic agents, and neuroleptics. Antidepressants are increasingly used for the management of insomnia. Specifically, tricyclic antidepressants such as amitriptyline or doxepin, trazodone, and mirtazapine, may provide sedation in patients who are not depressed, as well as those who are depressed. Antihistamines such as diphenhydramine and hydroxyzine are used for their sedative properties as well as for their anticholinergic properties to treat insomnia and help relieve nausea and vomiting. However, these are not indicated in patients over the age of 60, as this population is sensitive to the negative cognitive effects of these drugs and to their anticholinergic effects. Atypical antipsychotics such as denzapine have been used for their sedating effects and their ability to improve appetite and relieve opioid-induced nausea. Neuroleptics, such as thioridazine, have been found to promote sleep, especially in patients with insomnia associated with organic mental syndrome and delirium.[2]

Nonpharmacological interventions

Several nonpharmacological interventions have been used for the treatment of insomnia in healthy patients, but more intervention studies are needed to address insomnia in patients with cancer. Currently, there are four categories of nonpharmacological interventions for insomnia: cognitive-behavioral therapies (CBTs), complementary therapies (CTs), psychoeducation and information, and exercise.

Cognitive-behavioral therapies

Cognitive-behavioral therapies involve a variety of behavioral and psychological treatments aimed at changing negative thought processes, attitudes, and behaviors related to a person's ability to fall asleep, stay asleep, get enough sleep, and function during the day. These include, but are not limited to, sleep education, cognitive control, psychotherapy, sleep restriction, remaining passively awake, stimulus control therapy, sleep hygiene, relaxation training, and biofeedback. Cognitive-behavioral therapies that have been tested in patients with cancer include stimulus control, sleep restriction, relaxation therapy, sleep hygiene, profile-tailored CBT, and cognitive restructuring strategies. These therapies have been shown to produce significant improvement in sleep quality, longer duration of sleep, and higher sleep efficiency.[28,29]

Complementary therapies

Complementary therapies are interventions that are not considered to be part of conventional medicine. In patients with cancer, several complimentary therapies have been tested: aromatherapy, expressive therapy, expressive writing, healing, autogenic training, massage, muscle relaxation, mindfulness-based stress reduction, and yoga. These therapies have resulted in improvement in sleep quality, duration, and efficiency; use of fewer medications; and less daytime dysfunction.[29]

Herbal therapies

Several herbal supplements are currently being used for managing insomnia, especially chamomile, hops, lavender, passionflower, wild lettuce, California poppy, kava kava, St. John's Wort, lemon balm, and melatonin. However, over-the-counter supplements are not regulated by the FDA, therefore they do not have to undergo rigorous clinical trials to determine efficacy and side effects of taking these compounds. In addition, the studies hitherto investigating the benefits of herbal therapies for managing insomnia have inconclusive or contradictory results.[30]

Psychoeducation

Psychoeducation includes the use of structured education provided to patients with specific information regarding treatments and side effects. Two studies evaluated the effect of psychoeducation on the severity of the side effects from radiation and chemotherapy.[31-33] Kim and colleagues[33] found that educational information tapes increased sleep duration in men receiving radiation for localized prostate cancer. Williams and Schreier[32] found no change in sleep disturbances after using informational audiotapes in women with breast cancer undergoing chemotherapy. The results suggest that patients who receive more detailed, user-friendly information about their treatment may benefit from this form of assistance for their insomnia. Further studies are necessary to explore the benefit of psychoeducation in insomnia in patients with cancer and other diseases.

Exercise interventions

Exercise interventions involve any planned, structured, and repetitive bodily movement that is performed for the purpose of conditioning any part of the body, improving health, or maintaining fitness. Several studies that evaluated the efficacy of exercise intervention for the treatment of insomnia in patients with cancer reported less difficulty sleeping and improved sleep patterns and quality.[34,35]

Nursing interventions

One of the key components of oncology nurses' and palliative care nurses' scope of practice is symptom management. These nurses are often the first-line providers and thus are responsible for understanding the consequences of insomnia on quality of life, and for recognizing the relationships between patient insomnia and disease-related treatments (Box 22.1). Nurses are often in a position to influence decisions regarding interventions to promote optimal sleep, both pharmacological and nonpharmacological. Educational programs for nurses that offer information about insomnia and interventions are therefore important and should be introduced at the graduate and undergraduate level.[36]

Box 22.1 Potential consequences of insomnia in the context of cancer

Psychological and behavioral consequences

Fatigue
Cognitive impairments (e.g., memory, concentration)
Mood disturbances and psychiatric disorders

Psychological and health consequences

Health problems and physical symptoms (e.g., pain)
Longevity
Immunosuppression

Source: Data from Savard and Morin (2001), reference 6.

Conclusion

Insomnia remains a common and distressing complaint in patients with cancer, in cancer survivors, and in those with chronic debilitating diseases. Insomnia has been linked to psychological and/or physiological malfunction. The importance of healthy sleep in patients who are chronically ill cannot be overestimated.

Effective management of insomnia begins with a thorough assessment that includes the exploration of predisposing factors such as insomnia prior to diagnosis, usual sleep patterns, emotional status, exercise and activity level, and other disease-related symptoms and medications. Tools such as the Clinical Sleep Assessment for Adults and Children may be used to screen for insomnia.[37] Typically, insomnia is treated with hypnotic drugs; however, more recent findings support the use of cognitive-behavioral therapies, complementary therapies, psychoeducation and information, and exercise to treat insomnia.

The challenge for palliative care nurses is to adequately provide patients with education regarding healthy sleep patterns. Nurses need to acquire a better understanding of the multidimensionality of sleep and to be aware that patients may not relate their symptoms to sleep issues. Unfortunately, insomnia in patients with cancer and other debilitating chronic diseases has only recently received attention from cancer researchers. Studies aimed to determine the etiology of insomnia in this population, and the appropriate treatment, is much needed.

References

1. Morin CM, Benca R. Chronic insomnia. Lancet. 2012;379(9821): 1129–1141.
2. Deak MC, Winkelman JW. Insomnia. Neurol Clin. 2012;30:1045–1066.
3. Orzeł-Gryglewska J. Consequences of sleep deprivation. Int J Occup Med Env Health. 2010;23(1):95–114.
4. Gomes AA, Tavares J de AM. Sleep and academic performance in undergraduates: a multi-measure, multi-predictor approach. Chronobiol Int. 2011;28(9):786–801.
5. Léger D, Partinen M, Hirshkowitz M, Chokroverty S, Touchette E, Hedner J; Equinox (Evaluation of daytime Quality Impairment by Nocturnal awakenings in Outpatients eXperience) Survey Investigator Group. Daytime consequences of insomnia symptoms among outpatients in primary care practice: EQUINOX international survey. Sleep Med. 2010;11(10):999–1009.
6. Savard J, Morin CM. Insomnia in the context of cancer: a review of a neglected problem. J Clin Oncol. 2001;19(895–908).
7. American Psychiatric Association. Diagnostic and Statistical Manual of Mental Disorders. 4th ed. Washington, DC: American Psychiatric Association; 2000.
8. American Sleep Disorders Association. The International Classification of Sleep Disorders: Diagnostic and Coding Manual. Rochester, MN: American Sleep Disorders Association; 1997.
9. Savard J, Villa J, Ivers H, Simard S, Morin CM. Prevalence, natural course, and risk factors of insomnia comorbid with cancer over a 2-month period. J Clin Oncol. 2009;27(31):5233–5239.
10. Price MA, Zachariae R, Butow PN, deFazio A, Chauhan D, Espie CA, Friedlander M Australian Ovarian Cancer Study Group; Australian Ovarian Cancer Study—Quality of Life Study Investigators. Prevalence and predictors of insomnia in women with invasive ovarian cancer: anxiety a major factor. Eur J Cancer. 2009;45(18):3262–3270.
11. Spielman AJ. Assessment of insomnia. Clin Psychol Rev. 1986;6(1):11–25.
12. Cerejeira J M-LE. A Clinical update on delirium: from early recognition to effective management. Nurs Res Pract. 2011; Epub 2011 June 6.
13. Schutte-Rodin S, Broch L, Buysse D, Dorsey C, Sateia M. Clinical guideline for the evaluation and management of chronic insomnia in adults. J Clin Sleep Med. 2008;4(5):487–504.

14. Edinger JD, Wohlgemuth WK, Radtke RA, Coffman CJ, Carney CE. Dose-response effects of cognitive–behavioral insomnia therapy: a randomized clinical trial. Sleep. 2007;30(2):203–212.

15. Colrain IM. Sleep and the brain. Neuropsychol Rev. 2011;21:1–4.

16. Rosipal R, Lewandowski A, Dorffner G. In search of objective components for sleep quality indexing in normal sleep. Biol Psychol. 2013;S0301–0511(13):144–146.

17. Kim J, Tofade TS, Peckman H. Caring for the elderly in an inpatient setting: managing insomnia and polypharmacy. J Pharm Pract. 2009;22(5):494–506.

18. McNamara P, Johnson P, McLaren D, Harris E, Beauharnais C, Auerbach S. REM and NREM sleep mentation. Int Rev Neurobiol. 2010;92:69–86.

19. Kripke DF, Shadan FF, Dawson A, Cronin JW, Jamil SM, Grizas AP, et al. Genotyping sleep disorders patients. Psychiatry Investig. 2010;7(1):36–42.

20. Schutte-Rodin S, Broch L, Buysse D, Dorsey C, Sateia M. Clinical guideline for the evaluation and management of chronic insomnia in adults. J Clin Sleep Med. 2008;4(5):487–504.

21. NCI. Sleep Disorders. US National Institutes in Health. 2009. Available at: http://www.cancer.gov/cancertopics/pdq/supportivecare/sleepdisorders/HealthProfessional. Accessed June 1, 2013.

22. Riemanna D, Spiegelhalder K, Feige B, Voderholzer U, Berger M, Perlis M, et al. The hyperarousal model of insomnia: a review of the concept and its evidence. Sleep Med Rev. 2010;14(1):19–31.

23. Roth T, Roehrs T, Pies R. Insomnia: pathophysiology and implications for treatment. Sleep Med Rev. 2007;11:71–79.

24. Roehrs T, Roth T. Insomnia pharmacotherapy. Neurotherapeutics. 2012;9:728–738.

25. Nutt DJ, Stahl SM. Searching for perfect sleep: the continuing evolution of GABAA receptor modulators as hypnotics. J Psycopharmacol. 2010;24(11):1601–1612.

26. Pandi-Perumal SR, Spence DW, Verster JC, Srinivasan V, Brown GM, Cardinali DP, et al. Pharmacotherapy of insomnia with ramelteon: safety, efficacy and clinical applications. J Cent Nerv Syst Dis. 2011;3:51–65.

27. Roth T, Rogowski R, Hull S, Schwartz H, Koshorek G, Corser B, et al. Efficacy and safety of doxepin 1 mg, 3 mg, and 6 mg in adults with primary insomnia. Sleep. 2007;30(11):1555–1561.

28. Garland SN, Carlson LE, Antle MC, Samuels C, Campbell T. I-CAN SLEEP: Rationale and design of a non-inferiority RCT of mindfulness-based stress reduction and cognitive behavioral therapy for the treatment of Insomnia in CANcer survivors. Contemp ClinTrials. 2011;32(5):747–754.

29. Sarris J, Byrne GJ. A systematic review of insomnia and complementary medicine. Sleep Med Rev. 2011;15(2):99–106.

30. Sarris J, Byrne GJ. A systematic review of insomnia and complementary medicine. Sleep Medicine Reviews. 2011;115(2):99–106.

31. Erickson J, Berger, AM. Sleep-wake disturbances. Clin J Oncol Nurs. 2011;15(2):123–127.

32. Williams SA, Schreier AM. The role of education in managing fatigue, anxiety, and sleep disorders in women undergoing chemotherapy for breast cancer. Appl Nurs Res. 2005;18:138–147.

33. Kim Y, Roscoe JA, Morrow GR. The effects of information and negative affect on severity of side effects from radiation therapy for prostate cancer. Support Care Cancer. 2002;10:416–421.

34. Tang M, Liou T, Lin C. Improving sleep quality for cancer patients: benefits of a home-based exercise intervention. Support Care Cancer. 2010;18(10):1329–1339.

35. Payne JK, Held J, Thorpe J, Shaw H. Effect of exercise on biomarkers, fatigue, sleep disturbances, and depressive symptoms in older women with breast cancer receiving hormonal therapy. Oncol Nurs Forum. 2008;35(4):635–642.

36. Berger AM. Update on the state of the science: sleep-wake disturbances in adult patients with cancer. Oncol Nurs Forum. 2009;36(4):E165–E177.

37. Buysse DJ, Hall ML, Strollo PJ, Kamarck TW, Owens J, Lee L, et al. Relationships between the Pittsburgh Sleep Quality Index (PSQI), Epworth Sleepiness Scale (ESS), and clinical/poly somnographic measures in a community sample. J Clin Sleep Med. 2008;4(6):563–571.

CHAPTER 23

Sexuality

Marianne Matzo

I think it might have to do with your own attitude about it, too. Because I remember, gosh, I think it was maybe a day or two after my surgery; and I still had tube drains hooked up and all that stuff, and I was like, this is how I'm going to make my statement to my husband, that I'm not going to let cancer take us over. I actually made the moves on him. And he was totally shocked. You know? He wasn't expecting anything for a really long time. And I'll tell you from my experience, that empowered me so much. It's kind of like, "Ha! Cancer. You're not taking this." And, so in a way, you know I have to say I wasn't really exactly wanting it, you know I wasn't in the mood or anything. But this was more of a conscious decision that I was looking cancer in the eye and saying, "You're not doing this."

A 52-year-old woman with ovarian cancer

Key points

◆ Sexuality is an integral part of the human experience.

◆ Healthcare providers often overlook the sexual needs of those receiving palliative care.

◆ Communication, privacy, and practical solutions to physical changes may have a positive impact on sexual health for the palliative care patient.

Terminal advanced illness and end-of-life care can interfere with sexual health and physical sexual functioning in many ways. These include: physiological changes; tissue damage; other organic manifestations of the disease; attempts to palliate the symptoms of advancing disease, such as fatigue, pain, nausea, and vomiting; and psychological sequelae such as anxiety, depression, and body-image changes. The complexities of human sexuality are broad, especially for people coping with life-threatening illness and those who are facing the end of their lives.

The sexual health model[1] (Figure 23.1) reflects these complexities by identifying ten broad components posited to be essential domains of healthy human sexuality: talking about sex; culture and sexual identity; sexual anatomy and functioning; sexual healthcare and safer sex; overcoming challenges to sexual health; body image; masturbation/fantasy; positive sexuality, intimacy and relationships; and spirituality and values.[1] A patient's experiences, symptoms, and concerns throughout the course of his or her illness are dynamic and complex, and are represented in the model as potentially impacting sexual health and, ultimately, quality of life. This chapter is organized according to each component of the sexual health model.[1]

Talking about sex

A cornerstone of the sexual health model is the ability to talk comfortably and explicitly about sexuality, especially one's own sexual values, preferences, attractions, history, and behaviors.[1] This communication is necessary for one to effectively express needs to a partner, and to discuss with a healthcare provider the alterations in sexual health that have resulted from illness. This is a valuable skill that must be learned and practiced.

An Institute of Medicine[2] report that addresses cancer care for the whole patient states that, in order to ensure appropriate psychosocial health, healthcare practitioners should facilitate effective communication. One study of an oncology population documented that 28% of the patients indicated their physicians do not pay attention to anything other than their medical needs.[3] Psychological distress that patients or their partners experience during diagnosis and treatment of malignancy can impair a healthy sexual response cycle.[4]

Culture and sexual identity

Culture influences one's sexuality and sense of sexual self. It is important that individuals examine the impact of their particular cultural heritage on their sexual identities, attitudes, behaviors, and health.[1] The cultural meaning of sexual behaviors needs to be taken into account, because that meaning may impact a person's willingness or interest in maintaining sexual intimacy while receiving palliative care.

The patient and family are at the center of palliative care. A patient's desire or interest in maintaining physical sexual relations is highly variable. Some may find expression of physical love an important aspect of their life right up to death, while others may relinquish their "sexual being" early in the end-of-life trajectory. Each individual's identity is influenced, in part, by his or her sexual identity. Roles between spouses or sexual partners are additionally defined by the sexual intimacy between them.

Sexual integrity can be both altered and compromised during the course of an incurable disease, deleteriously affecting both the

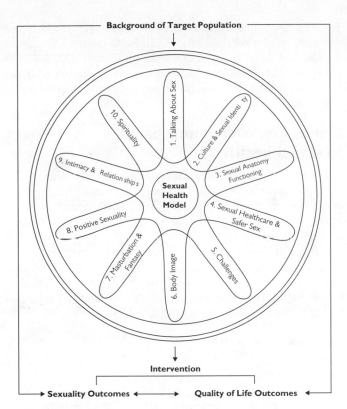

Figure 23.1 Sexual Health Model. Source: Robinson et al. (2007), reference 1. Used with permission.

identity and the role fulfillment of the affected person. Healthcare providers should not make assumptions about the level of interest or capacity a couple has for physical intimacy. Sexuality goes far beyond "sexual intercourse." Sexuality may encompass physical touch of any kind, as well as experiences of warmth, tenderness, and the expression of love.

The importance of physical intimacy vacillates throughout a relationship, and may be diminished or rekindled by a superimposed illness. Long-term palliative care providers may see sexual desire and expression ebb and flow between couples throughout the course of care. The patient may view sexual expression as an affirmation of life, a part of being human, a means to maintain role relationships, or the expression of passion in and for life itself.

There exists tremendous diversity of cultural, religious, and spiritual beliefs in relation to sexual intimacy and death. Culture often guides interactions between people, and even the mores within sexual interactions. Culturally competent healthcare providers should take into consideration the effect of culture on sexual expression. For example, do both members of the couple possess the same cultural identity? If not, are their identities similar with respect to beliefs about intimacy? What are the couple's health, illness, and sexual beliefs and practices? What are their customs and beliefs about intimacy, illness, and death? Issues such as personal space, eye contact, touch, and permissible topics to discuss with healthcare providers and/or members of the opposite sex may influence one's ability to intercede within the realm of intimate relations.

A cultural assessment is vital to determining whether these factors are an issue. Variations in sexual orientation must also be considered within the area of cultural competence. The beliefs, actions, and normative actions of homosexual and bisexual couples are important considerations when providing palliative care to a couple with alternate sexual expression.[5–7] Gay and lesbian couples may be offended by the assumption that they are heterosexual.[8]

Sexual anatomy and functioning

Sexual health assumes a basic knowledge, understanding, and acceptance of one's sexual anatomy, sexual response, and sexual functioning, as well as freedom from sexual dysfunction and other sexual problems.[1] Physical sexual expression is a basic aspect of human life, seen by many as fundamental to "being human." It is a complex phenomenon that basically comprises the greatest intimacy between two humans. The ability to give and to receive physical love is very important for many individuals, throughout the trajectory of an incurable illness.[9,10] The ability to maintain close sexual relations can be viewed as maintaining an essential part of one's "self."

Sexuality can affirm love, relieve stress and anxiety, and distract one from the emotional and physical sequelae of a life-threatening chronic illness. Sexual expression can foster hope and accentuate spirituality. Healthcare providers in all clinical settings where palliative care is provided can be pivotal in facilitating the expression of sexuality in the terminal stages of life. Holistic palliative care throughout the trajectory of an illness should include the promotion of sexual expression and assistance in preventing or minimizing the negative effects of disease progression on a couple's intimacy. Sexual partners' caring can comfortably include sexual expression if both parties are interested and able.

Sexual healthcare and safer sex

As a component of the sexual health model, physical health includes, but is not limited to, practicing safer sex behaviors, knowing one's body, obtaining regular exams, and responding to physical changes with appropriate medical interventions.[1] The promotion or restoration of sexual health begins with a sexual assessment. Interventions to address alterations in sexual health cannot be adequately planned without thorough assessment.

Assessment should include the patient as well as his or her partner. Securing permission to include the sexual partner is necessary. For the nurse to perform this assessment, she or he must be comfortable with the topic of sexuality. Comfort with one's own sexuality conveys comfort to others. Additionally, the nurse's values, beliefs, and attitudes regarding sexuality greatly influence the capacity to discuss these issues in a nonjudgmental way.[11]

Perceived insufficient knowledge on the part of the healthcare provider is often an obstacle to frank sexual discussions. Additional sexual education and consistent assessment and counseling approaches will allay this discomfort. Education can be gained informally via discussions with colleagues and through consultation with experts in the area of human sexuality. Formal training is gained through inservice education offerings, workshops, and sexual-attitude reassessment programs. Knowledge can also be fostered by keeping abreast of new developments within the field by attending conferences, and reviewing journals and professional information via the Internet.[12]

Assessment of sexuality begins with a sexual history and is then supplemented by data regarding the patient and partner's physical health as it influences intimacy, psychological sequelae of the chronic illness, sociocultural influences, and possible environmental issues.[13] Sexual health varies from person to person, so it is essential to determine whether the couple is satisfied with their current level of sexual functioning.[14] Celibacy, for example, may have been present in the relationship for years. However, the trajectory of palliative care may have forced celibacy on an otherwise sexually active couple.[15] Determining the couple's need for interventions and assistance in this area is vital to determining appropriate interventions. The healthcare provider has many interventions available to prevent or minimize the untoward effects that palliative care may impose on sexual health.[13]

Obtaining a sexual history and performing a subsequent sexual assessment can be augmented using several communication techniques: assuring privacy and confidentiality; allowing for ample, uninterrupted time; and maintaining a nonjudgmental attitude. Addressing the topic of sexuality early in the relationship with a palliative care patient legitimizes the issue of intimacy.[16] It delivers the message that this is an appropriate topic for concern within the professional relationship, and is often met with relief on the part of the patient and couple. Often, sexuality concerns are present but unvoiced.[4]

Incorporating several techniques of therapeutic communication enhances the interview. These techniques include asking open-ended questions ("Some people who have an incurable illness are frustrated by their lack of private time with their spouse/sexual partner. How is this experience for you?"); using questions that refer to frequency as opposed to occurrence ("How often do you have intimate relations with your wife/husband/partner?" as opposed to "Do you have intimate relations with your wife/husband/partner?"); and "unloading" the question ("Some couples enjoy oral sex on a regular basis, while others seldom or never have oral sex. How often do you engage in oral sex?"). This last technique legitimizes the activity and allows the patient to feel safe in responding to the question in a variety of ways.[13]

Gender and age may also play a part in the patient's comfort with sexual discussions. An adolescent boy may feel more comfortable discussing sexual concerns with a male healthcare provider, whereas an elder woman may prefer to discuss sexual issues with a woman closer to her own age. Assessment of these factors may include statements like the following: "Many young men have questions about sexuality and the effect their illness may have on sexual functioning. This is something we can discuss or, if you'd be more comfortable, I could have one of the male nurses talk to you about this. Which would you prefer?"[13]

If the sexual history reveals a specific sexual problem, a more in-depth assessment is warranted. This would include the onset and course of the problem, the patient's or couple's thoughts about what caused the problem, any solutions that have been attempted, and potential solutions and their acceptability to the patient/couple. For example, use of a vibrator in the case of male impotence may be entirely acceptable to some couples but abhorrent to others. Determining what is and is not acceptable regarding potential solutions is part of the logical next step in sexual assessment.

Finally, documentation in the patient's chart should reflect the findings of the sexual assessment. Many institutions have a section for sexual assessment embedded within their intake form.

This can be completed, and more thorough notes added to the narrative section on the chart. Findings, suggestions for remediation, and desired outcomes should be documented. This will prevent duplication of efforts, enhance communication within the healthcare team, and support continuity of care within the realm of sexual health.

Challenges: overcoming barriers to sexual health

Challenges to sexual health include previous sexual history, developmental issues, privacy, and physical symptoms or side effects of symptom management.[7] Previous sexual history such as sexual abuse, substance abuse, compulsive sexual behavior, sex work, harassment, and discrimination are critical in any discussion of sexual health. This is particularly true in the context of interventions for cultural and sexual minorities, many of whom are disproportionately affected by these issues.[1] It is not uncommon to see our patients only as they present to us, without full appreciation of their previous life histories.

Developmental issues

There are a number of developmental issues that may play a part in the patient's ability to maintain intimacy during palliative care.[17] Often, healthcare providers assume sexual abstinence in the elderly and, to some degree, in adolescents and unmarried young adults.[18] However, intimacy may be a vital part of these individuals' lives.[19]

Chronological age may or may not be a determinant of sexual activity.[20] For underage patients, parental influence may interfere with the ability to express physical love. Likewise, older adults may be inhibited by perceived societal values and judgments about their sexuality.[19–25] Maintaining an open, nonjudgmental approach to patients of all ages, sexual orientations, and marital status when assessing sexual health may foster trust and facilitate communication.

Privacy

One of the main external challenges to maintaining intimate relations during palliative care is the lack of privacy. In the acute care setting, privacy is often difficult to achieve. However, this obstacle can be removed or minimized by recognizing the need for intimacy and making arrangements to ensure quiet, uninterrupted time for couples. Private rooms are, of course, ideal. However, if this is not possible, arranging for roommates and visitors to leave for periods of time is necessary. A sign could be posted on the door that alerts healthcare providers, staff, and visitors that privacy is required. Finally, many rooms in the acute care setting have windows as opposed to walls, requiring the use of blinds and/or curtains to assure privacy. The nurse should offer such strategies rather than expecting patients to request privacy.

Similar issues may arise in the long-term care environment.[23] If privacy is a scarce commodity, assisting couples to maintain desired intimate relations is crucial in providing holistic care. Nurses in long-term care settings can initiate strategies to offer privacy. Such privacy may be more important than in acute care settings because the stay in long-term care is usually quite extended.[26] In both the acute care and long-term care settings, nurses can play a vital role in setting policy to facilitate the expression of intimacy and the maintenance of sexual health.

Home care may present an array of different obstacles for maintaining intimate relations, such as the ongoing presence of a healthcare provider other than the sexual partner. The home setting is often interrupted by professional visits as well as visits from family, friends, and clergy, which may be unplanned or unannounced. The telephone itself may be an unwelcome interruption. Often, when receiving home hospice care, the patient may have been moved from a more private bedroom setting to a more convenient central location, such as a den or family room, to aid caregiving and to enable the patient to maintain an integral role in family life. However, this move does not provide the privacy usually sought for intimate activity. There may not be a door to close; proximity of the patient's bed to the main rooms of the house may inhibit a couple's intimate activities, and they may need to schedule private time together. Necessary steps to maintain sexual relations include scheduling "rest periods" when one will not be disturbed; turning the ringer of the phone off; asking healthcare providers, friends, and clergy to call before visiting; and having family members respect periods of uninterrupted time.

Fatigue

Fatigue may be secondary to many factors. In chapter 8, the etiology and management of fatigue are thoroughly addressed. Fatigue may render a patient unable to perform sexually. If fatigue is identified as a factor in the patient's ability to initiate or maintain sexual arousal, several strategies may be suggested to diminish these untoward effects.[27] Minimizing exertion during intimate relations may be necessary. Providing time for rest before and after sexual relations is often a sufficient strategy to overcome the detrimental effects of fatigue. Likewise, avoiding the stress of a heavy meal, alcohol consumption, or extremes in temperature may be helpful. Experimenting with positions that require minimal patient exertion (male-patient, female astride; female-patient, male astride) is often helpful. Finally, timing should be taken into consideration. Sexual activity in the morning upon awakening may be preferable over relations at the end of a long day. Planning for intimate time may replace spontaneity, but this can be a beneficial tradeoff.

Pain

Sexual health can be impaired by the presence of pain, as well as the use of pain medication (especially opiates), which can interfere with sexual arousal.[28] In chapters 6 and 7, the issues of pain assessment and management are comprehensively discussed. The goal of pain therapy is to alleviate or minimize discomfort; however, attaining that goal may result in an alteration in sexual responsiveness (i.e., libido or erectile function). Temporarily adjusting pain medications, or experimenting with complementary methods of pain management, should be explored. For example, using relaxation techniques and/or romantic music may decrease discomfort through distraction and relaxation, while enhancing sexual interest.

Physical sexual activity itself can be viewed as a form of distraction and subsequent relaxation. The couple should be encouraged to explore positions that offer the most comfort. Traditional positions may be abandoned for more comfortable ones, such as sitting in a chair or taking a side-lying position. Pillows can be used to support painful limbs or to maintain certain positions. A warm bath or shower before sexual activity may help pain relief and be seen as preparatory to intimate relations. Massage can be used as both an arousal technique and a therapeutic strategy for minimizing discomfort. Finally, suggesting the exploration of alternate ways of expressing tenderness and sexual gratification may be necessary if the couple's traditional intimacy repertoire is not feasible due to discomfort.

Nausea and vomiting

Nausea and vomiting are common during the palliative care trajectory and negatively impact sexual health. Chapter 10 discusses the etiology and treatment of these symptoms. There are many medications that suppress nausea; however, they may interfere with sexual functioning due to their sedative effects. If the patient complains of sexual difficulties secondary to treatment for nausea and vomiting, assess which antiemetics are prescribed and try another medication and/or use alternate nonpharmacological methods to control nausea and vomiting. As with fatigue, timing may be an important consideration for intimate relations. If the patient/couple notes that nausea is more prevalent during a certain time of the day, planning for intimacy at alternate times may circumvent this problem.[27]

Neutropenia and thrombocytopenia

Neutropenia and thrombocytopenia, per se, do not necessarily interfere with intimacy, but they do pose some potential problems. Sexual intimacy during neutropenic phases may jeopardize the compromised patient, because severe neutropenia predisposes the patient to infections. Close physical contact may be inadvisable if the sexual partner has a communicable disease, such as an upper respiratory infection or influenza. Specific sexual practices, such as anal intercourse, are prohibited during neutropenic states due to the likelihood of subsequent infection. The absolute neutrophil count, if available, is a good indicator of neutropenic status and associated risk for infection. Patient and partner education about the risks associated with neutropenia is essential.

Thrombocytopenia and the associated risk of bleeding, bruising, or hemorrhage should be considered when counseling a couple about intimacy issues. Again, anal intercourse is contraindicated due to risk for bleeding. Likewise, vigorous genital intercourse may cause vaginal bleeding. Indeed, even forceful or energetic hugging, massage, or kissing may cause bruising or bleeding. Preventative suggestions might include such strategies as gentle lovemaking, with minimal pressure on the thrombocytopenic patient, or having the patient assume the dominant position to control force and pressure.

Dyspnea

Dyspnea is an extremely distressing occurrence in the end-of-life trajectory. In chapter 14, the management of this symptom is reviewed. Dyspnea, or even the fear of initiating dyspnea, can impair sexual functioning.[29] General strategies can be employed to minimize dyspnea during sexual play. These can include using a waterbed to accentuate physical movements, raising the dyspneic patient's head and shoulders to facilitate oxygenation, using supplementary oxygen and/or inhalers before and during sexual activity, performing pulmonary hygiene measures before intimacy, encouraging slower movements to conserve energy, and modifying sexual activity to allow for enjoyment and respiratory comfort.[30,31]

Neuropathies

Neuropathies can be a result of disease progression or complication of prior treatment. Neurological disturbances are discussed in depth in chapter 19. Neuropathies can manifest as pain, paresthesia, and/or weakness. Depending on the location and severity of the neuropathy, sexual functioning can be altered or completely suppressed. Management or diminution of the neuropathy may or may not be feasible. If not, creative ways to evade the negative sequelae of this occurrence are necessary. Such strategies might include creative positioning, use of pillows to support affected body parts, or alternate ways of expressing physical love. The distraction of physical sexual expression may temporarily minimize the perception of the neuropathy.

Mobility and range of motion

Mobility issues and compromised range of motion may interfere with sexual expression. Similar to issues related to fatigue, a decrease in mobility can inhibit a couple's customary means of expressing physical love.[32] A compromise in range of motion can result in a similar dilemma. For example, a female patient may no longer be able to position herself in such a way as to allow penile penetration from above due to hip or back restrictions. Likewise, a male patient may have knee or back restrictions that make it impossible for him to be astride his partner. Regardless of the exact nature of the range-of-motion/mobility concern, several suggestions can be offered. Antiinflammatory medication before sexual activity, experimenting with alternate positions, employing relaxation techniques before sexual play, massage, warm baths, and exploring alternative methods of expressing physical intimacy should be encouraged.[33]

Erectile dysfunction

Erectile dysfunction can be caused by physiological, psychological, and emotional factors.[34] These factors include vascular, endocrine, and neurological causes; chronic diseases, such as renal failure[35] and diabetes; and iatrogenic factors, such as surgery and medications. Surgical severing of the small nerve branches essential for erection is often a side-effect of radical pelvic surgery, radical prostatectomy, and aortoiliac surgery.[6] Vascular and neurological causes may not be reversible, although endocrine causes may be minimized. For example, the use of estrogen in advanced prostate cancer may be terminated in palliative care, which may result in the return of erectile function.

Many medications decrease desire and erectile capacity in men. The most common offenders are antihypertensives, antidepressants, antihistamines, antispasmodics, sedatives or tranquilizers, barbiturates, sex hormone preparations, opioids, and psychoactive drugs.[36] Often, these medications cannot be discontinued to permit the return of erectile function; for those patients, penile implants may be an option.[37]

The use of sildenafil (Viagra), vardenafil HCl (Levitra), tadalafil (Cialis), and yohimbine (Yohimbine) have not been researched with patients receiving palliative care. These medications are classified as selective enzyme inhibitors. They relax smooth muscle, increase blood flow, and facilitate erection.[38] If a vascular component is part of the underlying erectile dysfunction, the use of one of these medications may correct the problem.[39] Contraindications such as underlying heart disease and other current medications should be taken into consideration.[40] Otherwise, if acceptable to the couple, digital or oral stimulation of the female partner or use of a vibrator can be suggested.[41]

Dyspareunia

Dyspareunia, like erectile dysfunction, can be caused by physiological, psychological, and emotional factors. These factors include vascular, endocrine, and neurological causes as well as iatrogenic factors such as surgery and medications.[42] Vascular and neurological causes may not be reversible; endocrine causes may be minimized. For example, the use of estrogen replacement therapy (ERT), vaginal estrogen creams (estrogen replacement is contraindicated for women with hormone receptor-positive tumors), or water-soluble lubricants may be helpful in diminishing vaginal dryness, which can cause painful intercourse. Gynecological surgery and pelvic irradiation may result in physiological changes that prevent comfortable intercourse.[43]

Postirradiation changes, such as vaginal shortening, thickening, and narrowing, may result in severe dyspareunia.[44] For women, as with male patients, many medications decrease desire and function. These drugs include antihypertensives, antidepressants, antihistamines, antispasmodics, sedatives or tranquilizers, barbiturates, sex hormone preparations, opioids, and psychoactive drugs. Often, these medications cannot be discontinued in order to facilitate the return of sexual health. For those patients, digital or oral stimulation of the male partner may be suggested, if acceptable. Additionally, intrathigh and intramammary penetration may be suggested to women who find vaginal intercourse too painful. See Table 23.1 for an overview of dyspareunia management.

Anxiety and depression

Anxiety and depression related to the incurable and terminal aspects of the disease may interfere with sexual desire and response.[45] As two of the most common affective disorders during end-of-life care, they are thoroughly discussed in chapter 20. Both anxiety and depression have profound effects on sexual functioning. Decreases in sexual desire, libido, and activity are common sequelae of these affective disorders. However, some interventions, especially pharmacological management, can further compromise sexual functioning.

A thorough assessment of the patient's psychological state and an evaluation of the medications currently prescribed for this condition may reveal the source of the problem. Anxiolytics and antidepressants are often prescribed for these conditions and have the potential for interfering with sexual functioning. Patients may choose symptom management and sacrifice sexual function. However, relaxation techniques, imagery, and biofeedback may lower anxiety to a tolerable level. Additionally, the release of sexual tension may itself resolve anxiety.

If desire is maintained and function alone is compromised for male patients, the couple may explore alternate ways of pleasing each other. For female patients, use of water-soluble lubricants can offset the interference with arousal, if interest remains intact. Open communication between the partners and with the healthcare provider allows for frank discussions and the presentation of possible alternatives to expressing physical affection.

Table 23.1 Management of vaginal dryness and dyspareunia

Assess	Comments/considerations	HCP management
General history		
Location, onset, intensity of pain	Location may indicate nature of problem (details below).	Give patient the booklet: "A–Z Guide for Sexual Health" (mmatzo@ouhsc.edu).
Trend (same or worse over time)	If onset after surgery, may be related to scarring or neuropathic in nature. Pain may increase over time if pelvic muscles involved.	
Resources couple has already utilized Other comorbidities: Sjogren's syndrome, MS, diabetes, etc.	Diabetics are more prone to yeast infections, as well as decreased lubrication, orgasmic function, and cervical pain.	
General vaginal pain		
Bacterial/fungal infections	Diabetics are more prone to yeast infections, as well as decreased lubrication, orgasmic function, and cervical pain. (Patients with MS often experience painful intercourse, decreased lubrication, and decreased sensation).	Treat infection with antibiotics/antifungals.
Assess dryness/atrophy of tissue	If patient unable to localize pain, also consider all causes below. (Patients with MS often experience painful intercourse, decreased lubrication, and decreased sensation).	Adjust medications that may affect lubrication (e.g., antihistamines/anticholinergics). Educate patient on promoting healthy vaginal environment: Encourage use of pH-balanced moisturizers, Kegel exercises. Prescribe vaginal dilator and/or vacuum (Eros). As appropriate, give patient information about moisturizer/lubricant, Kegel exercises, dilator, or Eros vacuum. Consider temporary localized estradiol therapy—may be discontinued once lubrication restored with regular stimulation.
Vulvar pain		
Assess for vulvar vestibular syndrome by sensory mapping with cotton-tipped applicator	Many women with vestibular pain will also have levator spasm.	5% topical lidocaine ointment twice daily by applicator, or overnight by a cotton ball. Tricyclic antidepressants or anticonvulsants for neuropathic component. If levator muscles involved, refer to PT specializing in pelvic floor physiotherapy. Give patient information about pelvic pain and include a list of physical therapists, e.g., http://www.pelvicpainhelp.com/symptoms/levator-ani-syndrome/.
Vaginal vestibule		
Evaluate control of bulbocavernosus muscles		Refer to sexual therapist (or family therapist if relational origin). See Table 23.3, "Management of Psychosocial Issues Contributing to Sexual Problems."
Assess for vaginismus	Primary vaginismus will often have psychosocial components (see negative thoughts/feelings about sex). Secondary vaginismus is reactive to a disease process (i.e., vulvar vestibular syndrome) or relationship issues after a period of successful relations. Levator pain and/or spasm also commonly occur with involuntary contraction of introital muscles.	Patient may benefit from referral for physical therapist specializing in pelvic floor physiotherapy. Give patient information about pelvic pain and include a list of women's health physical therapists.
Mid-vaginal pain		
Assess levator muscle tension	Levator spasms can develop as protective response to pelvic pain and may continue well after original stimulus resolved, continuing the pain cycle.	Refer to physical therapist specializing in pelvic floor physiotherapy. Give patient information about pelvic pain and include a list of women's health physical therapists, e.g., http://www.pelvicpainhelp.com/symptoms/levator-ani-syndrome/.

(Continued)

Table 23.1 (Continued)

Assess	Comments/considerations	HCP management
Deep vaginal pain		
◆ Assess cervix for neuropathic pain by palpating with cotton-tipped applicator ◆ Rectovaginal exam	Pain will be focal, often elicited by palpitation of only one quadrant of cervix. Pain can be related to scarring from hysterectomy, repeated trauma, etc.	5% topical lidocaine ointment twice daily by applicator, or overnight by a cotton ball. Tricyclic antidepressants or anticonvulsants for neuropathic component of pain.
Other causes		
◆ Bladder disease ◆ Gastrointestinal (GI) illnesses ◆ Adnexal pathology ◆ Sensitivity of abdominal wall ◆ Pelvic floor or hip muscle pain ◆ Other inflammatory or visceral disorders ◆ Postoperative (especially some pelvic support surgeries)	GI illnesses such as Crohn's disease and irritable bowel syndrome can cause visceral hyperalgia. Areas of abdominal point tenderness should be evaluated with/without patient raising head off table (rectus abdominus flexion). If equal or increased with abdominal flexion, then myofascial structures of abdominal wall may be involved in pain generation.	Suspected GI/GU causes: Refer to GI/GU specialist. Musculoskeletal pain: Give patient information about pelvic pain and include a list of women's health physical therapists, e.g., http://www.pelvicpainhelp.com/symptoms/levator-ani-syndrome/.
Psychosocial factors		
◆ Relationship issues ◆ Depression, fear, or stress ◆ Past abuse	Anxiety is an independent predictor of dyspareunia, aside from structural factors. Vaginismus is often attributed to difficulties with upbringing or discomfort with sexuality in general.	See Table 23.3, "Management of Psychosocial Issues Contributing to Sexual Problems," for specific referrals.

Body image

In a culture with so many sexual images focused on a type of physical beauty unattainable for many, body image is an important aspect of sexual health. Challenging one, narrow standard of beauty and encouraging self-acceptance is relevant to all populations, and should be carried out in a culturally sensitive manner.[1] An incurable illness and concomitant end-of-life care can alter one's physical appearance. Additionally, past treatments for disease often irrevocably alter body appearance and function. Issues such as alopecia, weight loss, cachexia, the presence of a stoma, or amputation of a body part, to name a few, can result in feelings of sexual inadequacy and/or disinterest.[46,47]

End-of-life care can focus on the identification and remediation of issues related to body image changes. Although an altered appearance may be permanent, counseling and behavior modification, as well as specific suggestions to minimize or mask these appearances, can improve body image to a level compatible with positive sexual health. The use of a wig, scarf, or headbands can mask alopecia. Some patients, rather than try to conceal hair loss, choose to emphasize it by shaving their heads. Weight loss and cachexia can be masked through clothing and the creative use of padding.

The presence of an ostomy can significantly alter body image and negatively affect sexual functioning.[48,49] Specific interventions for minimizing the effect that the presence of an ostomy has on sexual functioning depend, in part, on the particular type of ostomy. Some patients are continent, while others need an appliance attached at all times.

If the patient has a continent ostomy, timing sexual activity can allow for removal of the appliance and covering the stoma. If the ostomy appliance cannot be safely removed, the patient should be taught to empty the appliance before intimate relations and to use a cover or body stocking to conceal the appliance. Alternate positions may also be considered, and in the event of a leak, sexual activity can continue in the shower. The United Ostomy Association (http://www.uoa.org) publishes four patient information booklets on sexuality and the ostomate.

Masturbation and fantasy

The topics of masturbation and fantasy are saddled with a myriad of historical myths associated with sin, illness, and immaturity that would need to be confronted in order to normalize masturbation. Encouraging masturbation as a normal adjunct to partnered sex can decrease the pressures on people to engage in penetrative sex with their partners more frequently than they have desire and arousal for.[1]

Positive sexuality

Some patients may view sexual expression as an essential aspect of their being, while others may see it as ancillary or unimportant. Some may have an established sexual partner; some may lose a partner through separation, divorce, or death; others may begin a relationship during the course of their illness trajectory. Some patients may have several sexual partners; some couples may be gay or lesbian; others, without a sexual partner, may gain pleasure by erotic thoughts and masturbation. All of these scenarios are within the realm of the palliative care provider's patient base. Understanding the various forms of sexual expression and pleasure is paramount in providing comprehensive care.

Intimacy and relationships

Intimacy is a universal need that people try to meet through their relationships.[1] A sexual partner's interest and ability to maintain sexual relations throughout the palliative care trajectory can also be affected by many variables. Sexual expression may be impeded by the partner's mood state (anxiety, depression, grief, or guilt), exhaustion from caregiving and assuming multiple family roles, and misconceptions about sexual appropriateness during palliative care. Anxiety and depression have profound effects on sexual functioning. Decreases in libido and sexual activity can result from depressive and anxious states[50,51] (Table 23.2).

Table 23.2 Management of loss of libido

Assess	Comments/considerations	HCP management
Psychosocial factors[1,2]		
◆ Relationship issues ◆ Depression, fear, or stress ◆ Past abuse ◆ Poor body image	Referral to mental health professional or social services (See Table 23.3, "Management of Psychosocial Issues Contributing to Sexual Problems").	
Medications that can impact desire		

◆ Antidepressants (especially SSRIs)
◆ Antihypertensives/cardiovascular
◆ H2 blockers
	Some substitutions may be possible within same drug class that have less of an impact on sexual functioning.	For antidepressants[3-8]
		1. Adjust current antidepressant dosing
		2. Alter timing of dose (so decreased serum levels when most likely to be sexually active)
		3. 2-day "drug holidays" (effective for sertraline and paroxitine)
		4. Substitution with another medication:
		  a. Minimal to no sexual dysfunction: bupropion, maritazapine
		  b. Low risk of sexual dysfunction: fluvoxamine, citalopram, venlafaxine

Unfavorable experiences due to pain		
See Table 23.3, "Management of Psychosocial Issues Contributing to Sexual Problems."		**Cancer-related pain**: NCCN Clinical Guideline: Adult Cancer Pain
	Vaginismus can result from dyspareunia, contributing to pain cycle and fear of sexual intimacy.	**Dyspareunia:** See Table 23.1, "Management of Vaginal Dryness and Dyspareunia." **Vaginismus**: May need referral to mental health professional, especially if patient experienced prolonged dyspareunia or contributing psychosocial factors.[9]
Fatigue: NCCN clinical guideline: cancer treatment-related fatigue: MS 8–13[10]		

◆ Cancer-related fatigue is a distressing persistent, subjective sense of physical, emotional, and/or cognitive tiredness or exhaustion related to cancer or cancer treatment that is not proportional to recent activity and interferes with usual functioning.
 	
Fatigue continued...
	Fatigue can be a result of inactivity. Some patients may benefit by gradually increasing their daily exercise.
	Psychosocial issues may contribute to fatigue. Patients should be counseled about coping and educated on how to deal with anxiety and depression, which are commonly associated with fatigue.
	Poor nutrition may contribute to fatigue.
	Consider psychostimulants to combat fatigue.
		Nonpharmacological interventions: (MS-8–M-11)
		1. Activity enhancement and physically based therapies:
		  Give the patient the hand out "Physical Activity and the Cancer Patient"
		2. Psychosocial interventions:
		  Refer to counselor
		3. Nutritional consultation:
		  Refer active patients (in treatment) to a nutritionist. Include with the referral a patient assessment form that the patient can bring with her on her first visit with the dietician.
		Pharmacological interventions: (M-12–M-13)
		1. Amphetamine psychostimulant
		  Methylphenidate
		  Only beneficial in severe fatigue or and/or advanced disease
		2. Nonamphetamine psychostimulant
		  Modfinil
		3. For anemia
		  Erythropoietin

(Continued)

Table 23.2 (Continued)

Assess	Comments/considerations	HCP management
Hormones		
Hormone levels ◆ Cortisol ◆ Free testosterone (or FTI/FAI)	High cortisol levels can compete with androgenic hormones. Decreased androgen levels with surgical menopause can be significant factor in hypoactive sexual desire disorder (HSDD). Supplementation is controversial, but increasing evidence supports safety and efficacy of transdermal medications. Consider supplementation if free testosterone levels for women: Under 50: <25 ng/dL or 1.5 pg/mL Over 50: <20 ng/dL or <1.0 ng/mL	**High cortisol levels**: Encourage stress-reducing activities. Consider mental health referral for patients experiencing psychosocial situations contributing to stress. (See Table 23.3, "Management of Psychosocial Issues Contributing to Sexual Problems.") **Low testosterone**: No FDA-approved testosterone products for treating HSDD in women, but numerous preparations commonly prescribed off-label.[11] Transdermal matrix (Intrinsa) shown to be effective at 150–300 mcg/d, with no increase in breast cancer risk. Monitor serum FT for therapeutic effectiveness.

A partner may feel that the patient is "too ill" to engage in sexual activity. In turn, the partner may feel remorse or guilt for even thinking about their loved one in a sexual capacity during this time. Partners may fear that they may injure their loved one during sexual activity due to the loved one's perceived or actual weakened state or appearance. The partner may have difficulty adjusting to the altered physical appearance of the patient (cachexia, alopecia, stomatitis, pallor, amputation, etc.). The role of caregiver may seem incompatible with that of sexual partner.

As the ill partner's health deteriorates, the well partner may assume caretaking roles that may seem incompatible with those of a lover. The myriad of responsibilities sequentially assumed by the well partner may leave him or her exhausted, which can interfere with sexual health and impede sexual performance. The partner may harbor misconceptions about sexual relations with a terminally ill partner, including diminishing the patient's waning energy reserves or causing the illness to progress more rapidly.

Spirituality and values

Sexual health assumes congruence between one's ethical, spiritual, and moral beliefs and one's sexual behaviors and values. In this context, spirituality may or may not include identification with formal religions, but it addresses moral and ethical concerns. Exposure to multiple cultural traditions (e.g., Native American storytelling, African-American church activism, etc.) is important, especially in those traditions that have a positive and life-affirming view of sexuality.[1]

Individual, family, and cultural factors influence the development of healthy sexuality in adolescents. One factor that is less often considered, but may play a role, is religion/spirituality. Attitudes or beliefs about having sex before marriage, decisions about the timing of coital debut, or contraceptive practices may be shaped by their religious/spiritual belief system, or the cultural/religious context in which they were raised.[52] These values may influence the decisions that an adolescent with a life-limiting disease may make regarding sexual experiences that they choose to engage in before they die.

Case study

A patient with end-stage ovarian cancer

"I think that I prefer that at least I have information, so the more information I have at least I feel like I'm in control of at least

reading the information, so the more information I have the more I'll be, if it's online, or if it's a speaker, or whatever, books. I just remember getting all the information I could, however, information about intimacy was very limited out there. You know, could you have sex, could you not? What was viable, what wasn't, after surgery. Frankly, no one ever talked to me about that if you want to know the truth. Anything that I did find, I pursued it and looked for it, because it was a bullet point, or two or three in a brochure that was given to me by a nurse or a doctor or whoever. That's all I got, was a couple of bullet points, and that's really not enough."

Interventions

The specific sexual needs and concerns of the patient and couple determine the approach and type of intervention. The intervention can address current needs, or focus on potential future needs in the form of anticipatory guidance. False assumptions about intimacy during palliative care can be addressed, and anticipatory guidance regarding what to expect as a result of advancing disease and palliative treatment is included in this discussion.

Specific suggestions should go beyond limited information, and be explicit, to help the patient and their partner attain a mutually stated goal. Specific suggestions usually pertain to communication, symptom management, and alternate physical expression. Open communication between the couple and their healthcare practitioner regarding sexual health is essential for successful symptom management. Candid discussions regarding their emotional responses to this phase of their relationship, their fears and concerns, and their hopes and desires are included in these interactions.

Symptom management is essential to optimizing sexual expression (Table 23.3). Alternate expressions of physical intimacy may be necessary if sexual disruption is due to organic changes. If intercourse is difficult, painful, or impossible, the couple may be counseled regarding how to expand their sexual repertoire. A thorough discussion of the couple's values, attitudes, and preferences should be done before suggesting alternatives. Using language that is understandable to the patient/partner is essential. However, the use of slang or street language may be uncomfortable to the healthcare practitioner—defining terms early in the discussion will alleviate this potential problem.

Table 23.3 Management of psychosocial issues contributing to sexual problems

Assess	Comments/considerations	HCP management
Body image	NCCN Guideline for Distress: DIS-6; MS-8,9*	
Fertility	Premenopausal women	Encourage patient to attend an infertility support group.
		Give patient information about fertility, e.g., http://www.fertilehope. org/; http://www.cancer.org/treatment/ treatmentsandsideeffects/physicalsideeffects/ fertilityandcancerwhataremyoptions/ fertility-and-cancer-toc.
◆ Loss of womanhood ◆ Hair loss ◆ Scars	Express concern of self-image	Refer for counseling. Encourage patient to attend a support group.
Colostomy		Encourage patient to attend an ostomy support group. Give patient the booklet "Intimacy After Ostomy Surgery" (http://www.ostomy.org/ostomy_info/ pubs/uoaa_sexuality_en.pdf) with the list of support groups attached.
Emotional	NCCN Guideline for Distress: DIS-6; MS-2,8,9*	
Anxiety	Symptoms: Loss of appetite, sleep, or concentration;	Prescribe medications (anxiolytic, antidepressant).
Fear	Preoccupied with thoughts of illness/death; Sadness at loss of health;	Suggest integrative therapies—i.e., yoga, exercise, mediation, walking club, laughter club, etc.
Depression	Anger, feeling out of control.	Encourage patient to attend a support group.
	If managing symptoms with medication, consider impact on sexual function.	Refer for counseling.
Spiritual	NCCN Guideline for Distress: DIS-19,20; MS-9*	
◆ Spiritual conflict ◆ Grief/guilt ◆ Hopelessness	Most cancer patients have spiritual needs, but only a slight majority felt it was appropriate to ask about these needs. Cancer patients can experience an existential crisis.	Refer to chaplain.
Practical concerns	(NCCN Guideline for Distress: DIS-18; MS-9 *)	
◆ Finances ◆ Housing ◆ Transportation ◆ Isolation	Ask if the patient's concrete needs are met. Ask the patient about her living/support situation	Refer to Social Work Services.
Cultural/language issues	Does the patient have a language barrier?	Ask patient to bring a translator to clinic visits or provide one if needed. Spanish-speaking cancer support groups are available throughout the country.
Psychosocial	NCCN Guideline for Distress: DIS-6; MS-3*	
◆ Adjustment to illness ◆ Family conflicts ◆ Social isolation	Functional changes affecting quality-of-life issues. Help with coping or communication skills or with difficulties in decision-making.	Refer to Social Work Services.
Domestic abuse/neglect	Signs of possible abuse or neglect:** Failure to keep appointments, secrecy, discomfort when interviewed about relationship, partner will not leave patient alone with medical staff, unexplained/multiple injuries, chronic pain without apparent etiology, high number of STIs, pregnancies, miscarriages, and abortions.	
◆ Advanced directives ◆ End-of-life issues		

(Continued)

Table 23.2 (Continued)

Assess	Comments/considerations	HCP management
Relationships	NCCN Guideline for Distress: DIS-19; MS-3,9*	
Partner	Communication with partner about sexual health or needs.	Refer to AASECT sexual therapist.
		Give patient information about sexual therapists in your area.
		Refer for counseling.
		Give patient information about marriage counseling.
Family	Children of patients with difficulties coping.	Give patient information on support groups for children in your area.

There are many ways of giving and receiving sexual pleasure; genital intercourse is only one way of expressing physical love. The nurse can encourage the couple to expand their sexual expression to include hugging, massage, fondling, caressing, cuddling, kissing, hand-holding, and masturbation, either mutually or singularly. Sexual gratification may be derived from manual, oral, and digital stimulation. Intrathigh, anal, and intramammary intercourse are also options if the female partner is unable to continue vaginal penetration.

Summary

Incurable illness and end-of-life care may compromise a couple's intimacy. To prevent or minimize this, healthcare practitioners should assume a leading role in the assessment and remediation of potential or identified alterations in sexual functioning. Not all couples will be concerned about their sexual health at this point of their life together. However, if sexual health is desired, all attempts should be made to facilitate this important aspect of life. People may find that being physically close to the one they love is life-affirming and comforting.

As patients draw close to the end of life, their needs, hopes, and concerns remain intact as in any other stage of their life. Assessment of sexual health should occur for all patients to determine if these needs and hopes include maintenance of their sexual health. The healthcare practitioner's offer of information and support can make a significant difference in a couple's ability to adjust to the changes in sexual health during end-of-life care. The realm of sexual health and intimacy during end-of-life care remains an area in which further research is warranted. Incorporating intimacy research into end-of-life care research is a natural and much-needed area of inquiry.

References

1. Robinson BBE, Bockting WO, Simon Rosser BR, Miner M, Coleman E. The sexual health model: application of a sexological approach to HIV prevention. Health Educ Res. 2002;17(1):43–57.
2. Institute of Medicine. Cancer Care for the Whole Patient: Meeting Psychosocial Health Needs. Washington, DC: The National Academies Press, 2007.
3. Young P. Caring for the whole patient: the Institute of Medicine proposes a new standard of care. Community Oncol. 2007;4(12):748–751.
4. Krychman ML, Pereira L, Carter J, Amsterdam A. Sexual oncology: sexual health issues in women with cancer. Oncology. 2006;71(1–2):18–25.
5. Alfano CM, Rowland JH. Recovery issues in cancer survivorship: a new challenge for supportive care. Cancer J. 2006;12(5):432–443.
6. Galbraith ME, Crighton F. Alterations of sexual function in men with cancer. Sem Oncol Nurs. 2008;24(2):102–114.
7. Shell JA. Sexual issues in the palliative care population. Sem Oncol Nurs. 2008;24(2):131–134.
8. Dibble SL, Eliason MJ, Christiansen MAD. Chronic illness care for lesbian, gay, and bisexual individuals. Nurs Clin North Am. 2007;42(4):655–674.
9. Hordern AJ, Currow DC. A patient-centered approach to sexuality in the face of life-limiting illness. Med J Aust. 2003;179(6 Suppl):S8–S11.
10. Rice A. Sexuality in cancer and palliative care 1: Effects of disease and treatment. Int J Palliat Nurs. 2000;6(8):392–397.
11. Krebs LU. Sexual assessment: research and clinical. Nurs Clin North Am. 2007;42(4):515–529.
12. Hordern A, Street A. Communicating about patient sexuality and intimacy after cancer: mismatched expectations and unmet needs. Med J Aust. 2007;186(5):224–227.
13. Sadovsky R, Nusbaum M. Sexual health inquiry and support is a primary care priority. J Sex Med. 2006;3(1):3–11.
14. Higgins A, Barker P, Begley CM. Sexuality: the challenge to espoused holistic care. Int J Nurs Pract. 2006;12(6):345–351.
15. Sanders S, Pedro LW, Bantum EO, Galbraith ME. Couples surviving prostate cancer: long-term intimacy needs and concerns following treatment. Clin J Oncol Nurs. 2006;(4):503–508, 21–23.
16. Huber C, Ramnarace T, McCaffrey R. Sexuality and intimacy issues facing women with breast cancer. Oncol Nurs Forum. 2006;33(6):1163–1167.
17. Stausmire JM. Sexuality at the end of life. Am J Hosp Palliat Care. 2004;21(1):33–39.
18. Stroberg P, Hedelin H, Bergstrom AB. Is Sex only for the healthy and wealthy? J Sex Med. 2007;4(1):176–182.
19. Hurd Clarke L. Older women and sexuality: experiences in marital relationships across the life course. Can J Aging. 2006;25(2):129–140.
20. Lindau ST, Schumm LP, Laumann EO, Levinson W, O'Muircheartaigh CA, Waite LJ. A study of sexuality and health among older adults in the United States. N Engl J Med. 2007;357:762–774.
21. Lesser J, Hughes S, Kumar S. Sexual dysfunction in the older woman: complex medical, psychiatric illnesses should be considered in evaluation and management. Psychiatric Consultant. 2005;60(8):18–22.
22. Loehr J, Verma S, Seguin V. Issues of sexuality in older women. J Women's Health. 1997;6(4):451–457.
23. Malatesta VJ. Sexual problems, women and aging: an overview. J Women Aging. 2007;19(1–2):139–154.
24. Scott LD. Sexuality and older women. exploring issues while promoting health. AWHONN Lifelines. 2002;6(6):520–525.
25. Robinson JG, Molzahn AE. Sexuality and quality of life. J Gerontol Nurs. 2007;33(3):19–29.
26. Everett B. Supporting sexual activity in long-term care. Nurs Ethics. 2008;15(1):87–96.
27. Stead ML. Sexual function after treatment for gynecological malignancy. Curr Opin Oncol. 2004;16:492–495.

28. Abs R, Verhelst J, Maeyaert J, et al. Endocrine consequences of long-term intrathecal administration of opioids. Endocrinol Metab. 2000;85(6):2215–2222.

29. Vincent EE, Singh SJ. Review article: addressing the sexual health of patients with COPD: the needs of the patient and implications for health care professionals. Chron Respir Dis. 2007;4(2):111–115.

30. Hardin S. Cardiac disease and sexuality: implications for research and practice. Nurs Clin North Am. 2007;42(4):593–603.

31. Goodell TT. Sexuality in chronic lung disease. Nurs Clin North Am. 2007;42(4):631–638.

32. Newman AM. Arthritis and sexuality. Nurs Clin North Am. 2007;42(4):621–630.

33. Kautz DD. Hope for love: practical advice for intimacy and sex after stroke. . . including commentary by Secrest. J Rehabil Nurs. 2007;32(3):95–103, 32.

34. Resendes LA, McCorkle R. Spousal responses to prostate cancer: an integrative review. Informa Healthc. 2006;24:192–198.

35. Katz A. What have my kidneys got to do with my sex life?: The impact of late-stage chronic kidney disease on sexual function. Am J Nurs. 2006;106(9):81–83.

36. Karadeniz T, Topsakal M, Aydogmus A, et al. Erectile dysfunction under age 40: etiology and role of contributing factors. Sci World J. 2004;4(Suppl 1):171–174.

37. Mulcahy JJ, Wilson SK. Current use of penile implants in erectile dysfunction. Curr Urol Rep. 2006;7(6):485–489.

38. Ali ST. Effectiveness of sildenafil citrate (Viagra) and tadalafil (Cialis) on sexual responses in Saudi men with erectile dysfunction in routine clinical practice. Pak J Biol Sci. 2008;21(3):275–281.

39. Hartmann U, Burkart M. Erectile dysfunctions in patient–physician communication: optimized strategies for addressing sexual issues and the benefit of using a patient questionnaire. J Sex Med. 2007;4(1):38–46.

40. Ezzell A, Baum N. When Viagra doesn't work: treating erectile dysfunction. Diabetes Self Manag. 2008;25(2):29–30.

41. Bruner DW, Calvano T. The sexual impact of cancer and cancer treatments in men. Nurs Clin North Am. 2007;42(4):555–580.

42. Stead ML. Sexual function after treatment for gynecological malignancy. Curr Opin Oncol. 2004;16(5):492–495.

43. Carmack Taylor CL, Basen-Engquist K, Shinn EH, et al. Predictors of sexual functioning in ovarian cancer patients. J Clin Oncol. 2004;22(5):881–889.

44. Yamamoto R, Okamoto K, Ebina Y, Shirato H, Sakuragi N, Fujimoto S. Prevention of vaginal shortening following radical hysterectomy. BJOG-Int J Obstet Gy. 2000;107(7):841–845.

45. Brandberg Y, Sandelin K, Erikson S, et al. Psychological reactions, quality of life, and body image after bilateral prophylactic mastectomy in women at high risk for breast cancer: a prospective 1-year follow-up study.[see comment]. J Clin Oncol. 2008;26(24):3943–3949.

46. Alfano CM, Rowland JH. Recovery issues in cancer survivorship: a new challenge for supportive care. Cancer J. 2006;12(5):432–443.

47. Hinsley R. "The reflections you get": an exploration of body image and cachexia. Int J Palliat Nurs. 2007;13(2):84–89.

48. Penson RT, Gallagher J, Gioiella ME, et al. Sexuality and cancer: conversation comfort zone. Oncologist. 2000;5(4):336–344.

49. Kilic E, Taycan O, Belli AK, et al. [The effect of permanent ostomy on body image, self-esteem, marital adjustment, and sexual functioning]. Turk Psikiyatri Dergisi. 2007;18(4):302–310.

50. Barton-Burke M, Gustason CJ. Sexuality in women with cancer. Nurs Clin North Am. 2007;42(4):531–554.

51. Stead ML, Brown JM, Fallowfield L, Selby P. Communication about sexual problems and sexual concerns in ovarian cancer: a qualitative study. West J Med. 2002;176(1):18–19.

52. Cotton S, Berry D. Religiosity, spirituality, and adolescent sexuality. Adoles Med. 2007;18(3):471–483.

CHAPTER 24

Urgent syndromes at the end of life

Barton T. Bobb

Thank goodness for the palliative care team here that knows how to treat my pain. It was rough without the usual medications.

Frank, a patient who has metastatic renal cell carcinoma and paraplegia from malignant spinal cord compression. He has severe chronic pain that was controlled on a complex regimen established by his palliative care team, but this regimen was changed at another facility.

Key points

- ◆ Superior vena cava obstruction
- ◆ Pleural effusion
- ◆ Pericardial effusion
- ◆ Hemoptysis
- ◆ Spinal cord compression
- ◆ Hypercalcemia

Hallmarks of palliative care are skilled assessment and rapid evaluation and management of symptoms that impact negatively on patient and family quality of life. This chapter addresses select syndromes that unless recognized and treated promptly will cause unnecessary suffering for the patient and family.

Superior vena cava obstruction

Case study

Mrs. S, a patient with non-Hodgkin's lymphoma

Mrs. S is a 64-year-old housewife with recurrent non-Hodgkin's lymphoma currently receiving active treatment. She calls her oncologist's office complaining of worsening shortness of breath over the past week. She tells the nurse about this and when asked about any other symptoms, she reports, "Maybe a slight cough and I have noticed some new swelling, especially in my face. What do you think caused this?"

Key points

- ◆ Superior vena cava obstruction can cause distressing symptoms that are amenable to palliation.
- ◆ The common presenting symptoms are dyspnea, facial swelling, and feeling of fullness in the head.
- ◆ The patient's swollen and distorted facial features can be highly upsetting to the patient and family.
- ◆ The diagnosis of vena cava syndrome can usually be made on clinical grounds.

Definition

Superior vena cava obstruction (SVCO) is a disorder produced by obstruction of blood flow in the superior vena cava (SVC), which results in impairment of blood flow through the superior vena cava into the right atrium. Severity of the syndrome depends on rapidity of onset, location of the obstruction, and whether or not the obstruction is partial or complete. Obstruction may occur acutely or gradually, and symptoms may be severe and debilitating.[1,2]

Epidemiology

The patient most likely to experience SVCO is a 50- to 70-year-old man with a primary or metastatic tumor of the mediastinum. More than 90% of SVCO cases have been due to cancer, most commonly, endobronchial tumors.[2] More recent research indicates that the percentage of SVCO cases due to nonmalignant causes, primarily due to the higher use of intravascular devices, has probably risen.[3] In the majority of patients, the presence of SVCO is not a poor prognostic indicator of survival.[4] The prognosis of patients with SVCO strongly correlates with the prognosis of underlying disease.

Two types of obstruction may cause SVCO: (1) intrinsic obstruction, and (2) extrinsic obstruction.[1] Intrinsic obstruction is usually caused by primary tracheal malignancies that invade the airway epithelium, that is, squamous cell carcinoma and adenoid cystic carcinoma, as well as other benign and malignant tumors. Extrinsic obstruction occurs when airways are surrounded and compressed by external tumors or enlarged lymph nodes, that is, lymphoma, and locally advanced thyroid, lung, or esophageal cancers. Obstruction may be caused by a tumor arising in the right main or upper-lobe bronchus or by large-volume lymphadenopathy in the right paratracheal or precarinal lymph node chains.[5] A classification scale has been proposed that would rate the severity of SVCO on a scale of 0–5 (0 is asymptomatic, and 5 is fatal, but grades 0–2 have an estimated combined incidence of 85%).[6]

Thrombosis of the SVC is also associated with insertion of indwelling catheters and central-venous access devices, which are thought to damage the intima of vessels. Both adults and children may experience thrombosis of the SVC. More than compression or tumor, thrombosis is likely to cause acute and complete obstruction of the SVC.[7] Cancer patients are also at greater risk of experiencing hypercoagulopathies, which increase the risk of experiencing thrombosis and SVCO. Other less common nonmalignant causes associated with SVCO are mediastinal fibrosis from histoplasmosis and iatrogenic complications from cardiovascular surgery.[7,8]

Pathophysiology

The SVC is located in the rigid thoracic cavity and is surrounded by a number of structures, including the sternum, trachea, right bronchus, aorta, pulmonary artery, and several lymph node chains. There is little room for structures to move or expand within this cavity, thus the SVC is vulnerable to any space-occupying lesion in its vicinity. Venous drainage from the head, neck, upper extremities, and upper thorax collects in the SVC on its way to the right atrium. The SVC has a thin wall, and normally blood flows through the vessel under low pressure. When the vessel is compressed, blood flow is slowed, fluid pressure is increased, and occlusion may occur.[9]

The severity of symptoms related to SVCO can increase based on how quickly the obstruction develops and its location, especially if the obstruction occurs below the azygous vein.[10] The presence of collateral circulation, tumor growth rate, and extent and location of the blockage are all factors in determining how rapidly SVCO develops.[11]

Signs and symptoms

The onset of symptoms is often insidious. Patients may report subtle signs that include venous engorgement in the morning hours after awakening from sleep, difficulty removing rings from fingers, and an increase in symptoms when bending forward or stooping, all of which may not be noticed initially.[1,9] The most common symptoms/physical findings are facial/neck swelling (82%) followed by arm swelling (68%), dyspnea (66%), cough (50%), and dilated chest veins (38%).[10]

In severe or rapid cases, where collateral circulation has not yet made accommodation for increased blood flow, symptoms may be immediately life threatening. Patients may experience orthopnea, stridor, respiratory distress, headache, visual disturbances, dizziness, syncope, lethargy, and irritability. As the condition further progresses, significant mental status changes occur, including stupor, coma, seizures, and, ultimately, death.[10]

Diagnostic procedures

Plain chest X-ray films are the least invasive diagnostic modality.[7] Computed tomography (CT) is the most widely available and used modality to elucidate the location, extent of obstruction or stenosis, presence and extent of thrombus formation, and status of collateral circulation.[10] It can be performed unless the patient is so debilitated that no further treatment is indicated or desired by the patient.[12] Magnetic resonance imaging (MRI) is another diagnostic tool that can confirm the diagnosis of SVC[12] and distinguish between tumor mass or thrombosis.

Palliation of symptoms

The effectiveness of palliation of symptoms of SVCO in patients who have persistent or recurrent small-cell lung cancer (SCLC)

has been reviewed.[4] Chemotherapy or mediastinal radiation therapy were found to be very effective as initial treatment for patients who have SCLC and SVCO at first presentation, as well as in those with recurrent or persistent disease. It was recommended that radiation therapy be used in those patients who have been previously treated with chemotherapy. However, due to side effects, large fractions should be avoided.[4] When comparing the treatment modalities used to treat SVCO, including chemotherapy alone, chemotherapy and radiation therapy, and radiation therapy alone, none has proved superior.[5] Adverse prognostic indicators are dysphagia, hoarseness, and stridor.

Superior vena cava stenting

Current American College of Chest Physicians (ACCP) guidelines state that lung cancer patients with symptomatic SVCO can be treated with a combination of chemotherapy, radiation therapy, and/or insertion of an SVC stent.[13] Patients with severe symptoms are often best treated initially by SVC stenting, especially if a tissue diagnosis has not been made yet. However, the decision should be made on a case-by-case basis, as many patients with lung cancer respond very quickly to radiation or chemotherapy.[1] Although there are no controlled studies comparing radiation therapy with SVC stenting, several reviews and nonrandomized studies indicate that this procedure can relieve edema, promote improved superficial collateral vein drainage, and improve neurological impairment. It can also relieve dyspnea, provide greater relief of obstruction, create few or minor complications,[1,6,14] and allow for the full use of chemotherapy and radiation therapy,[10] thus providing more rapid relief in a higher proportion of patients.[5] Complications associated with SVC stenting procedures include bleeding due to anticoagulation, arrhythmia, septic episodes, thrombosis, fibrosis, and migration of the stent.

Thrombolytic therapies

Thrombolytic therapy has often been successful in the lysing of SVC thrombi.[15] Another alternative, percutaneous angioplasty with or without thrombolytics, may open SVC obstructions. Documented thrombi may be treated with tissue plasminogen activators (TPAs).

Drug therapy

Steroids have been one of the standard therapies for treatment of SVCO, in spite of the lack of research-based evidence to support their use. Prednisone and methylprednisolone have both been used to reduce inflammation in the treatment of SVCO, but the typical regimen is generally 4 mg of dexamethasone every 6 hours.[2]

Diuretics, such as furosemide, may be given to promote diuresis, thus decreasing venous return to the heart, which reduces pressure in the SVC. However, caution must be exercised to avoid dehydration.[16]

Nursing management

The primary nursing goals are to identify patients at risk for developing SVC syndrome, to recognize the syndrome if it does occur, and to relieve dyspnea and other symptoms. Reduction of anxiety is another important nursing goal. The patient and family may experience significant distress not only because of physical symptoms experienced, but also because of an altered physical appearance, including a ruddy, swollen, distorted face and neck.

The nurse monitors the patient for side effects of treatment and provides symptom management. For example, if the patient is receiving radiation therapy, be alert for signs of dyspnea (which may indicate presence of tracheal edema), pneumonitis, dysphagia, pharyngitis, esophagitis, leukopenia, anemia, skin changes, and fatigue. If the patient is receiving chemotherapy, be alert for signs of stomatitis, nausea and vomiting, fatigue, leukopenia, anemia, and thrombocytopenia. If the patient is receiving steroid therapy, educate the patient and family about the potential for developing proximal muscle weakness, mood swings, insomnia, oral candida, and hyperglycemia. Aspects of palliative nursing care that are always of primary importance are: early recognition and management of symptoms, educating the patient and family about these symptoms and what to report, and providing reassurance that these symptoms, if they occur, will be controlled.

Pleural effusion

Case study

Mrs. G, a patient with breast cancer

Mrs. G is a 53-year-old former lawyer who was diagnosed with metastatic breast cancer over a year ago. She has metastases to her bones, lungs, and liver, and her disease has progressed more rapidly in the past 2 months in spite of treatment. She has received surgery, radiation, and multiple regimens of chemotherapy. Over the past week, she has been experiencing worsening dyspnea and some pleuritic chest pain. "It was barely noticeable at first, but I now get pretty short-winded just going downstairs in our house." She is advised by her oncologist's office to go to the emergency room, where she is found to have some decreased breath sounds at the bases and some dullness to percussion on exam.

Key points

◆ The treatment of pleural effusion is palliative and symptomatic.

◆ The treatment approach depends on clinical circumstances, the patient's general condition, and nearness to death.

◆ Preemptive pain management is a critical nursing function when patients undergo invasive procedures.

Definition

Pleural effusion is defined as a disparity between secretion and absorption of fluid in the pleural space secondary to increased secretion, impaired absorption, or both, resulting in excessive fluid collection.[17]

Epidemiology

More than 150,000 pleural effusions (PEs) are diagnosed each year in the United States.[17] Parapneumonic disease is the most common cause of pleural effusions, followed by malignant disease. Breast, ovarian, and lung cancer plus lymphomas account for over 75% of all malignant pleural effusions (MPEs),[18] followed by ovarian cancer and gastric cancer, in order of descending frequency.[19] Almost half of patients with metastatic disease will experience a pleural effusion sometime during the course of their disease.[20]

Pleural effusions occur in 7% to 27% of hospitalized human immunodeficiency virus (HIV) patients.[21] The three leading causes of PE in those with HIV disease are parapneumonic infection, pulmonary Kaposi's sarcoma (KS), and tuberculosis.[22] The overall mortality rate associated with PE in HIV patients is 10% to 40%.[22] Unfortunately, the presence of MPE is usually associated with widespread disease and poor clinical prognosis, particularly in those with malignancy or AIDS. The overall mean survival for cancer patients who have MPE is 4 to 12 months.[18] Lung cancer patients usually die within 2 to 3 months, breast cancer patients within 7 to 15 months, and ovarian cancer patients within 9 months.[23] The mean survival period of those with pulmonary KS and MPE is 2 to 10 months; for those who have lymphoma and MPE, it is about 9 months.[24] Nearly all patients who have MPE are appropriate candidates for hospice care.[23]

Pathophysiology

Each lung is covered with a serous membrane called the *pleura*. A closed cavity is located between the pleura and the surface of each lung, called the pleural cavity. Under normal circumstances, it is bathed with 10 to 120 mL of almost protein-free fluid that continuously flows across the pleural membrane. The fluid moves from the systemic circulation into the pleural cavity and then into the pulmonary circulation.[25] Osmotic and hydrostatic pressure act to ensure that equilibrium is maintained between absorption and production of fluid in the pleural space. When this equilibrium is disturbed, fluid can accumulate in the pleural cavity.[26]

A number of factors may disturb this equilibrium: (1) metastatic implants or inflammations that cause increased hydrostatic pressure in pulmonary circulation; (2) inflammatory processes that increase capillary permeability and increase oncotic fluid pressure in the pleural space; (3) hypoalbuminemia that decreases systemic oncotic pressure; (4) tumor obstruction or lung damage that creates increased negative intrapleural pressure; (5) impaired absorption of lymph when channels are blocked by tumor; and (6) increased vascular permeability caused by growth factors expressed by tumor cells.[27] Patients with large PEs have demonstrated left-ventricular diastolic collapse and cardiac tamponade, which resolve with thoracentesis.[28]

Diagnostic procedures

A chest X-ray will usually establish the presence of the PE, and should also differentiate the presence of free versus loculated pleural fluid.[29] Computed tomography can show pleural or lung masses, adenopathy, pulmonary abnormalities such as infiltrates or atelectasis, or distant disease.[30] Chest ultrasonography may differentiate between pleural fluid and pleural-thickening disease.[31]

In some cases, once evidence of the effusion has been established and obvious nonmalignant causes have been ruled out, a diagnostic thoracentesis may be helpful in establishing the diagnosis. Sonographic guidance can avoid problems associated with performing "blind" thoracentesis.[17]

Signs and symptoms

Dyspnea is the most common symptom of PE and occurs in about 75% of patients.[17,19,20] Its onset may be insidious or abrupt, and depends on how rapidly the fluid accumulates.[23] It is almost always related to collapse of the lung from the increase of pleural fluid pressure on the lung.[27]

The patient's inability to expand the lung leads initially to complaints of exertional dyspnea. As the effusion increases in volume, resting dyspnea, orthopnea, and tachypnea develop. The patient may complain of a dry, nonproductive cough, and an aching pain or heaviness in the chest. Pain is often described as dull or pleuritic in character.[32] Generalized systemic symptoms associated with advanced disease may also be present: malaise, anorexia, and fatigue.[18,31]

Physical examination reveals the presence of dullness to percussion of the affected hemithorax, decreased breath sounds, egophony, decreased vocal fremitus, whispered pectoriloquy, and decreased or no diaphragmatic excursion.[33] A large effusion may cause mediastinal shift to the side of the effusion; tracheal deviation may be present. Cyanosis and plethora, a ruddy facial complexion that occurs with partial caval obstruction, may also be present.[34]

Medical and nursing management

Overall medical management of MPE depends on multiple factors, including the history of the primary tumor, prior patient history and response to therapy, extent of disease and overall medical condition, goals of care, and severity of symptom distress. In some cases, systemic therapy, hormonal therapy, or mediastinal radiation therapy may provide control of PEs.[30] Symptomatic management of symptoms with pharmacotherapy includes the use of opioids to manage both pain and dyspnea and anxiolytics to control concomitant anxiety.[17]

If the patient is to have a chest tube placed, or other invasive procedures to drain the fluid or to prevent fluid reaccumulation, the nurse must aggressively manage the patient's pain and anxiety. Educating the patient about what to expect, being present during the procedure, and medicating the patient preemptively are important aspects of palliative nursing care. Use of patient-controlled analgesia (PCA) for pain management is appropriate. Unfortunately, pain assessment and management is frequently not recognized as a priority when patients undergo these procedures.

Thoracentesis alone

Thoracentesis has been shown to relieve dyspnea associated with large PEs.[30] When thoracentesis is undertaken, relief of symptoms may rapidly occur, but fluid reaccumulates quickly, usually within 3 to 4 days, and in 97% of patients within 30 days.[35] The decision to perform repeated thoracenteses should be tempered by the knowledge that risks include empyema, pneumothorax, unexpandable lung from inadequate drainage and/or loculated fluid, and the possibility of increasing malnutrition as a result of the removal of large amounts of protein-rich effusion fluid.[27]

Repeated thoracenteses rarely provide lasting control of MPEs.[35] There are no studies that compare repeated thoracenteses to other management approaches.[2] Instead of a second thoracentesis, a thoracostomy with pleurodesis should be considered.[23] It can be used to reduce adhesions and draw off fluid.

Tube thoracostomy and pleurodesis

Palliative treatment, especially for those with a life expectancy of months rather than weeks, is best accomplished by performing closed-tube thoracoscopy, using imaging guidance with smaller bore tubes.[23] The goal of this therapy is to drain the pleural cavity completely, expand the lung fully, and then instill the chemical agent into the pleural cavity. However, if there is a large effusion, only 1000 mL to 1500 mL should be drained initially.[23] Too-rapid drainage of a large volume of fluid can cause reexpansion pulmonary edema, and some patients have developed large

hydropneumothoraces following rapid evacuation of fluid.[23] The thoracoscopy tube should then be clamped for 30 to 60 minutes. Approximately 1000 mL can be drained every hour until the chest is completely empty, but a slow rate of drainage is recommended.[30] The chest tube is then connected to a closed-drainage device. To prevent reexpansion pulmonary edema, water-seal drainage alone and intermittent tube clamping should be used to allow fluid to drain slowly.

Complications of chest tube placement include bleeding and development of pneumothorax, which occurs when fluid is rapidly removed in patients who have an underlying noncompliant lung. Patients who have chest tubes inserted should receive intrapleural bupivacaine or epidural and intravenous (IV) conscious sedation, as the procedure can be moderately to severely painful.[36]

Pleurodesis

Chest radiography is used to monitor the position of the tube after thoracostomy is completed. It is thought that tube irritation of the pleural cavity may encourage loculations, which can lessen the effectiveness of potential sclerosing agents.[27] If the lung fails to expand and there is no evidence of obstruction or noncompliant lung, additional chest tube placement may be considered. Fibrinolysis with urokinase or streptokinase may improve drainage in those cases where fluid is still present or is thick or gelatinous.[37] Intrapleural instillation of urokinase 100,000 units in 100-mL 0.9% saline can be attempted, and the chest tube clamped for 6 hours, with suction then being resumed for 24 hours. Once the pleural fluid has been drained and the lung is fully expanded, pleurodesis may be initiated. This can usually take place the day after chest tube insertion.[20,38]

The purpose of pleurodesis is to administer agents that cause inflammation and subsequent fibrosis into the pleural cavity to produce long-term adhesion of the visceral and parietal pleural surfaces. The goal of this procedure, which can be painful, is to prevent reaccumulation of pleural fluid.[19] Various sclerosing agents are used to treat MPE. They include bleomycin, doxycycline, and sterilized asbestos-free talc. There is some research indicating that talc should be the agent of choice based on its success rate in preventing recurrence, and overall effectiveness.[18]

Pleuroperitoneal shunt

This procedure is useful for patients who have refractory MPE despite sclerotherapy.[39] Two catheters are connected by a pump to a chamber between the pleural cavity and the peritoneal cavity. Manually pushing the pumping chamber moves fluid from the pleural cavity to the peritoneal cavity. Releasing the compression moves the fluid from the pleural cavity into the chamber.

The major advantage of this device is that it can be used on an outpatient basis and allows the patient to remain at home. Its disadvantages include obstruction risk, infection, and tumor seeding; general anesthesia is needed for placement, and the device requires motivation and ability on the part of the patient to operate it. Most patients with advanced disease are unable to physically overcome the positive peritoneal pressure required to pump the device. Pumping is required hundreds of times a day, and therefore this device is not likely to be useful in those who are close to death.[40]

Pleurectomy

Surgical stripping of the parietal pleura, with or without lung decortication (if the underlying lung is trapped), is more than

90% effective, but it has a high complication rate and should be reserved for only those who have a reasonable life expectancy and physical reserve to withstand surgery.[17] Video-assisted thoracoscopy (VATS) and pleurectomy have been performed successfully, but this intervention is probably not an appropriate choice in the palliative care patient at the end of life.

Indwelling pleural catheters

Indwelling pleural catheters can be placed under local anesthesia.[18] Those who meet criteria for ambulatory therapy—that is, those with symptomatic, unilateral effusions, and who have a reasonable performance status—may benefit from this therapy. It has been suggested that tunneled pleural catheters may permit long-term drainage and control of MPE in 80% to 90% of patients.[20] These catheters can be used to treat trapped lungs and large locules. Spontaneous pleurodesis eventually occurred in over 40% of catheter insertions (103 out of 240) in one study.[41]

Small-bore tubes attached to gravity drainage bags or vacuum drainage have been reported to be successful on an outpatient basis.[23] Rare complications include tumor seeding, obstruction, infection, cellulitis of tract site, and pain during drainage. If spontaneous pleurodesis does not occur, then continuing drainage may present management challenges. This treatment offers the potential for better quality of life and reduction in overall healthcare costs.

Subcutaneous access ports

In this procedure a fenestrated catheter is placed in the pleural cavity. It can be accessed for repeated drainage without risk of pneumothorax or hemothorax.[23] Complications include occlusion, kinking, and wound infection.

Nursing management

Dyspnea and anxiety are primary symptoms experienced by the patient who has a PE. When invasive diagnostic procedures are being considered, these choices should be guided by the stage of disease, prognosis, the risk/benefit ratio of tests or interventions, pain-management considerations, and the desires of the patient and family.[42] The nurse can educate the patient and family about each procedure, including its purpose, how it is carried out, how pain will be addressed, and possible side effects or complications that may occur. This not only allows for informed consent but also may help to reduce anxiety and thus decrease dyspnea.[42]

A variety of nonpharmacological techniques can relieve the patient's dyspnea and pain, and can be used in combination with opioids and anxiolytics, as well as concurrently with medical treatment. These approaches include positioning the patient to comfort, using relaxation techniques, and providing oxygenation as appropriate.[42] Aggressive pain assessment and monitoring are particularly important for patients who receive invasive procedures.

Pericardial effusion

Case study

Mr. D, a patient with non-small-cell lung cancer

Mr. D, a 48-year-old carpenter, has widespread metastatic non-small-cell lung cancer. He is receiving palliative chemotherapy, but he has decided that the overall goal of his treatment is to focus on quality over quantity of life. He has recently started complaining of slight dyspnea on exertion and has therefore made an appointment to see his oncology nurse practitioner. He tells her, "I just can't quite catch my breath right when I walk around for a while." On exam, his lungs are clear to auscultation and percussion, but his heart sounds seem to be a little muffled.

Key points

- Malignant pericardial effusions occur in less than 5% of patients with cancer, but the incidence may be nearer to 20% in patients with lung cancer.

- Effusions usually develop in patients with advanced disease and are usually a poor prognostic sign.

- The clinical features depend on the volume of pericardial fluid, the rate of accumulation of fluid, and the underlying cardiac function.

- Dyspnea is the most common presenting symptom.

Definition

A pericardial effusion is defined as an abnormal accumulation of fluid or tumor in the pericardial sac.[43] Pericardial effusions can lead to life-threatening sequelae. They can be caused by malignancies and their treatment and by nonmalignant conditions. Pericardial effusions can lead to cardiac tamponade, which, if not treated, will cause cardiovascular collapse and death.[43]

Epidemiology

Malignant disease is the most common cause of pericardial effusions.[44] Pericardial effusion is most commonly associated with lung and breast cancer, leukemia, and lymphoma.[44] Twenty-five percent to 50% of all patients who require surgical pericardial drainage have malignant pericardial involvement.[44] Metastatic spread or local extension from esophageal tumors and from sarcomas, melanomas, and liver, gastric, and pancreatic cancers can also occur.[45] Many pericardial effusions are asymptomatic and are discovered only on autopsy.[46] Up to 40% of cancer patients who have a symptomatic pericardial effusion will have a benign cause of the effusion.[27] Nonmalignant causes of pericardial effusions include pericarditis, congestive heart failure, uremia, myocardial infarction, and autoimmune disease, such as systemic lupus erythematosus. Other causes are infections, fungi, viruses, tuberculosis, hypothyroidism, renal and hepatic failure, hypoalbuminemia, chest trauma, aneurysm, and complications of angiographic and central venous catheter procedures.[47]

A treatment-related cause of pericardial effusion is radiation therapy to the mediastinal area of more than 4000 cGy, which can lead to pericarditis and possible cardiac tamponade.[45] The anthracycline-based chemotherapies, such as doxorubicin, can also cause pericardial effusions.[48]

Pathophysiology

The heart is covered by a thin sac called the pericardium. There are usually 15 to 50 mL of fluid between the pericardium and the heart itself.[27] Pericardial fluid originates in lymphatic channels surrounding the heart and is reabsorbed and drained by the lymph system into the mediastinum and into the right side of the heart.[11] This fluid minimizes friction, provides a barrier against inflammation, supports the chambers of the heart, and maintains the heart's position in the chest against accelerational and gravitational forces.[49] A pericardial effusion occurs when there is excessive fluid in this space. This fluid causes increased pressure to build in the pericardial sac, and the heart cannot fill or pump adequately. A pericardial effusion refers to the increased fluid or tumor in the pericardial sac. Cardiac tamponade is the physiological hemodynamic response of the heart to the effusion.[43]

Malignancies can cause effusions in the pericardial space by: (1) blocking lymph and blood drainage and preventing their resorption, (2) producing excess fluid in the space, (3) bleeding into the space, and (4) growing tumor into the space. The pericardial sac can hold up to approximately 2000 mL of fluid before the heart begins to decompensate.[43] Thus, volume of fluid and distensibility will affect the impact of effusion on intrapericardial pressure.

Cardiac tamponade occurs when the heart cannot beat effectively because of excess pressure being exerted on its muscle.[45,47] As the pressure of fluid in the pericardial sac increases, the heart chambers are compressed. First, the right side of the heart, including the right atrium and right ventricle, is compressed. Less blood volume returns to the right side of the heart, thus increasing venous pressure. As the ventricles are further compressed, the heart cannot fill adequately, which leads to decreased stroke volume and cardiac output, and poor perfusion throughout the body. The body attempts to compensate by activating the adrenergic nervous system to keep the heart stimulated and its chambers filled with circulating blood volume. Heart rate increases, veins constrict, and the kidneys increase sodium and fluid retention. The heart ultimately is overwhelmed due to increased fluid, decreased filling, and decreased cardiac output, which leads to hypotension and circulatory collapse.[9,49]

Pericardial effusion can develop gradually over a period of weeks or months. The pericardium becomes more compliant, stretching to accommodate as much as 2 liters or more of fluid, with minimal effect on pericardial pressure. This is known as the "stress relaxation" phenomenon. Unfortunately, patients with chronic pericardial effusions may not exhibit physical signs of cardiac tamponade until compression of the heart and surrounding structures occurs, leading to sudden, life-threatening cardiac decompensation.[50]

Signs and symptoms

Pericardial tamponade that results from metastatic disease has a gradual onset that may be chronic and insidious.[9,50] Vague symptoms may be reported. Early in the decompensation process it may be difficult to differentiate symptoms of cardiac dysfunction from the effects seen in advancing cancer. The severity of symptoms is related to volume of the effusion, rate of accumulation, and the patient's underlying cardiac function.[45] Generally, rapid accumulation of fluid is associated with more severe cardiac tamponade. The most powerful predictor of the development of cardiac tamponade is the size of the pericardial effusion.[45]

Dyspnea is the most common presenting symptom.[43] The patient may complain of the inability to catch his or her breath, which progresses from dyspnea on exertion to dyspnea at rest. In advanced stages, the individual may be able to speak only one word at a time. Chest heaviness, cough, and weakness are also symptoms.[27] Pressure on adjacent structures, that is, the esophagus, trachea, and lung may increase.[51]

Tachycardia occurs as a response to decrease in cardiac output. A narrowing pulse pressure (difference between systolic and diastolic blood pressure) may be seen when blood backs up in the venous system, causing the systolic blood pressure to decrease and the diastolic blood pressure to increase.[51] Compression of the mediastinal nerves may lead to cough, dysphagia, hoarseness, or hiccups.[11] Increased venous pressure in the chest may lead to gastrointestinal (GI) complaints, such as nausea.[52,53] Retrosternal chest pain that increases when the patient is supine and decreases when he is leaning forward may occur, but is often not present.[49,51] Engorged neck veins, hepatomegaly, edema, and increased diastolic blood pressure are late signs of effusion. Anxiety, confusion, restlessness, dizziness, lightheadedness, and agitation related to hypoxemia may be present as the process progresses.[9,45,49] Poor cardiac output will lead to complaints of fatigue and weakness.

As the effusion increases and the heart begins to fail, symptoms worsen and dyspnea and orthopnea progress. Increasing venous congestion leads to peripheral edema. As cerebral perfusion worsens and hypoxemia increases, confusion increases. Patients with chronic symptomatic pericardial effusions will often exhibit tachycardia, jugular venous distension, hepatomegaly, and peripheral edema.[51]

When examining the patient, one should listen for early signs of cardiac tamponade: (1) muffled heart sounds and perhaps a positional pericardial friction rub and weak apical pulse, (2) presence of a compensatory tachycardia, (3) abdominal venous congestion and possible peripheral edema, and (4) a fever.[49,51] The signs and symptoms of pericardial effusion and cardiac tamponade may be mistaken for those of other pulmonary complications or PEs. Many cancer patients have both pleural and pericardial effusions.[49] Unfortunately, symptoms of cardiac tamponade may be the first indication of the presence of pericardial effusion.

The triad of hypotension, increased jugular venous pressure, and quiet heart sounds that are diagnostic for pericardial effusion occurs in less than a third of patients.[54] If clear lung fields are present, this can help the clinician differentiate between pericardial effusion and congestive heart failure.[54] Pulsus paradoxus is a cardinal sign of cardiac tamponade. It occurs in 77% of those with acute tamponade and in only about 30% of those with chronic pericardial effusion.[50,54] However, its absence does not rule out pericardial effusion. Pulsus paradoxus is a fall in systolic blood pressure of greater than 10 mmHg with inspiration. Normally, blood pressure lowers on inspiration, but when the heart is compressed it receives even less blood flow. The resulting lowered volume and output result in a greater decrease in blood pressure.[49,55] Late in the process of deterioration, diaphoresis and cyanosis are also present. The patient develops increasing ascites, hepatomegaly, peripheral edema, and central venous pressure. Decreased renal flow progresses to anuria. Further impairment in tissue perfusion leads to loss of consciousness, obtundation, coma, and death.[9,45,49]

Diagnostic procedures

Initially, a standard chest X-ray is likely to show a change in the size or contour of the heart and clear lung fields.[27] A PE may be evident in up to 70% of patients. Chest X-ray can also demonstrate mediastinal widening or hilar adenopathy. This diagnostic tool is cost-effective, minimally invasive, readily available, and may detect tamponade before the patient becomes symptomatic.

However, when used alone, it is not specific enough to diagnose pericardial effusions and does not indicate the level of heart decompensation.[52] Two-dimensional echocardiogram (2D echo) is the most sensitive and precise test to determine if pericardial effusion or cardiac tamponade is present.[43] It can be used at the bedside and is noninvasive.

Some cancer patients may have both pericardial effusions and PEs.[49] Pleural effusions can mimic the signs and symptoms of pericardial tamponade, causing symptoms of dyspnea and respiratory distress. Chest X-ray may hide or mimic the presence of pericardial tamponade, so depending on the goals of care, a 2D-echo should be performed to differentiate between these phenomena and to detect decompensation of the heart.

Other tests, including MRI and CT, can be used to detect effusions, pericardial masses and thickening, and cardiac tamponade. However, these tests do not indicate how well the heart is functioning, and they have limited use due to safety and comfort concerns in very ill patients.[51] If echocardiography (ECG) is not available, a cardiac catheterization, which will detect depressed cardiac output and pressure levels in all four chambers of the heart, may be considered on a case-by-case basis.[51]

Medical and nursing management

Options for medical management include pericardiocentesis with or without catheter drainage, pericardial sclerosis, percutaneous balloon pericardiotomy, pericardiectomy, pericardioperitoneal shunt, tunneled pericardial catheters, radiation therapy and chemotherapy, and aggressive symptom management without invasive procedures.

Pericardiocentesis

The most simple, safe, and effective (97%) treatment is ECG-guided pericardiocentesis, with a procedural morbidity of 2% to 4% and mortality of 0%.[56] Since more than 50% of pericardial effusions reoccur, it is recommended that a 60-cm pigtail catheter (6 to 8 French) be threaded over the needle to allow for drainage of fluid over time.[51,56] The procedure can be performed emergently at the bedside, blindly or with ECG guidance, but it should not be attempted in this manner except in extreme emergencies.[57] Adverse complications of the blind procedure include myocardial laceration, myocardial "stunning," arrhythmias, pneumothorax, abscess, and infection.[58] The failure rate of this procedure is 10% to 20% because of posterior pericardial loculation or catheter obstruction.

Pericardial sclerosis

Patients who experience pericardial tamponade face a 50% rate of recurrence when the underlying disease is not effectively treatable.[51] Pericardial sclerosis should be considered in those patients whose disease is not being actively or effectively treated. Pericardial sclerosis is defined as the instilling of chemicals through an indwelling catheter into the pericardial sac for the purpose of causing inflammation and fibrosis, to prevent further fluid reaccumulation. Doxycycline and bleomycin are the most common drugs instilled into the pericardial space.[55] Twenty-two patients were treated with bleomycin in one study, 95% of them successfully.[59] A common side effect of sclerosing therapy is severe retrosternal chest pain, especially with talc administration, and sometimes with bleomycin therapy.[55] A preemptive pain

management plan is essential for the well-being of the patient. Arrhythmias, catheter occlusion, and transient fever of up to 38°C without associated bacteremia are also associated complications, primarily of talc and bleomycin therapy.[50] While sclerosing therapy may initially be "successful," that is, with evidence of disappearance of effusion or absence of tamponade symptoms for more than 30 days, multiple instillations may be necessary for true success.[51] The use of thiotepa has been recommended for pericardial instillation because it can be instilled into the drained space, is not associated with severe pain, and is reasonably effective.[55] A major complication is pericardial constriction. A serious discussion of risks, benefits, side effects of the therapy, and its impact on quality of life should take place in the context of end-of-life decision-making.

Percutaneous balloon pericardiotomy

This is a safe, nonsurgical method that can be used to relieve the symptoms of chronic recurrent pericardial effusions.[51] It is performed in a cardiac catheterization lab under fluoroscopic guidance using IV conscious sedation and local anesthesia. A guidewire is inserted into the pericardial space, and a small pigtail catheter is inserted over the wire. The wire is removed and some pericardial fluid is withdrawn. Next, the pigtail catheter is removed and replaced with a balloon-dilating catheter that is advanced into the pericardial space and inflated. A pericardial drainage catheter is left in place and is removed when there is less than 100 mL of drainage daily.[60] Patients have reported experiencing severe pain during and after this procedure. A plan for aggressive pain management must be in place before this procedure and rapidly implemented if pain occurs.

Fever and pneumothorax are the most common complications.[60] Pleural effusion has also been associated with the procedure. It is suggested that percutaneous balloon pericardiotomy can be used in place of surgical drainage in patients with malignancy and a short life expectancy.[61]

Surgical pericardiectomy

Another option is to surgically create a pericardial "window" (partial pericardiectomy), a small opening in the pericardium and suture it to the lung. This allows pericardial fluid to drain out of the pericardial cavity, especially loculated effusions.[55] One study observed a 6.4% morbidity and 2.1% mortality rate after pericardial window surgery as the definitive method of treatment for malignant pericardial effusion.[62] When other procedures fail and the patient is expected to have long-term survival and good quality of life, partial or complete pericardiectomy may be considered.[51]

Video-assisted thoracoscopic surgery

Video-assisted thoracoscopic surgery (VATS), a minimally invasive procedure, can be used to manage chronic pericardial effusions. In this case, a thoracoscope is introduced into the left or right chest and a pericardial window is performed under thoracoscopic vision.[62] The pleura and pericardium can be visualized, tissue diagnosis can be obtained, and loculated effusions can be drained.[63] It has a 100% long-term success rate, and there is no significant morbidity or mortality associated with its use.[51]

Radiation therapy and chemotherapy

In some cases, radiation therapy can be used to treat chronic effusions after the pericardial effusion has been drained[51] and when tamponade is not present. It can be effective in radiosensitive tumors such as leukemias and lymphomas but is less so in solid tumors.[50] Systemic chemotherapy can be considered if the malignancy is chemotherapy sensitive.[63]

Chronic pericardial effusions and their management can be challenging. Treatment of symptomatic chronic pericardial effusions will depend on patient prognosis, extent of symptoms, presence of concurrent medical conditions, and general condition. In many cases, treatment may be planned and carried out in a less urgent manner, keeping in mind the long-term benefits and side effects of interventions. Optimal treatment should focus on relieving symptoms caused by pressure on adjacent structures, and in the case of underlying malignancy the first priority should be the promotion of comfort. When choosing a plan, the ability to treat the underlying cause, the long-term prognosis, and patient comfort should be of greatest importance.[51]

Nursing management

The priority goals in managing this condition are to provide comfort, to promote pain relief, and to reduce anxiety. The nurse should know both early and late signs of cardiac tamponade. Early recognition of these signs and their implications is most important because early intervention may prevent life-threatening sequelae.[9]

Aggressive symptom management includes the administration of opioids and anxiolytics to reduce pain and anxiety. If invasive cardiac procedures are carried out in an emergency at the bedside, the nurse should be present to provide support to the patient and family, to control pain and anxiety, and to monitor vital signs as indicated.[9]

Hemoptysis

Case study

Mrs. H, a patient with small-cell lung cancer

Mrs. H, a 53-year-old mother of three adult children, was diagnosed with small-cell lung cancer six months ago. She is undergoing aggressive radiation therapy and chemotherapy. About a week ago, she started noticing some slight bleeding in her sputum as she coughs. She decides to see her oncologist as the bleeding gets worse over time. Her oncologist orders a CT scan and she asks her oncologist, "So what does this potentially mean for me and the future? What can we do to treat this bleeding? When should I talk to my family about this?"

Key points

◆ Hemoptysis occurs commonly in patients with advanced cancer and is most commonly due to malignant infiltration or infection.

◆ Hemoptysis should be distinguished from gastrointestinal and nasopharyngeal bleeding.

◆ Hemoptysis frequently provokes considerable anxiety.

◆ Massive hemoptysis, while rare, is a life-threatening crisis for patient, family, and staff. Massive hemoptysis occurs in fewer than 5% of cases, but the mortality rate is 85% if surgery is not feasible.

◆ Skilled palliative nursing intervention includes provision of 24-hour psychological support and guidance.

Definition

Hemoptysis is defined as blood that is expectorated from the lower respiratory tract. Hemoptysis can be classified according to the amount of blood expectorated: (1) mild—less than 15 to 20 mL in a 24-hour period, (2) moderate—greater than 15 to 20 mL but less than 200 mL in a 24-hour period, and (3) massive—greater than 200 mL to 600 mL in a 24-hour period.[64] The primary risk to the patient is asphyxiation from blood-clot formation obstructing the airway, rather than from exsanguination. Massive hemoptysis carries a high mortality rate if not treated.

Epidemiology

Tuberculosis is the most common worldwide cause of hemoptysis.[65] The most common causes of hemoptysis in the United States are bronchitis, bronchiectasis, and bronchogenic carcinoma.[65] Other nonmalignant causes of hemoptysis are lung abscess, sarcoidosis, mycobacterium invasion, emphysema, fungal diseases, and AIDS. There is no underlying cause found in 15% to 30% of hemoptic episodes.[65]

Metastatic lung disease caused by other primary tumors is associated with nonfatal hemoptysis.[66] Tumors in the trachea usually cause obstructive symptoms rather than massive bleeding.[67] Massive hemoptysis occurs in fewer than 5% of cases, but the mortality rate is 85% if surgery is not feasible.[68,69] Bleeding occurs most often from proximal endobronchial tumors that are not amenable to surgical intervention. Prognosis is usually grim in the case of end-stage lung disease and in the setting of massive hemoptysis.

Pathophysiology

Each lung is supplied with blood by way of two circulatory systems. Pulmonary circulation delivers blood under low pressure from the right ventricle to the alveolar capillaries, where oxygen and carbon dioxide are exchanged. Bronchial circulation arises from the systemic circulation that branches off the aorta, which delivers blood to the lungs under high pressure. These systems anastomose in precapillary pulmonary arterioles and pulmonary veins.[66]

The bronchial venous system returns blood to the heart by two pathways: (1) blood is returned to the right atrium by way of the azygous, hemiazygous, or intercostal veins, and (2) blood is returned to the left ventricle by way of the pulmonary veins. The second pathway carries the bulk of bronchial venous return to the heart.[66]

In the setting of inflammation, tumor, or infection, the bronchial vasculature develops new vascularization pathways. Bronchial blood flow increases as the result of increases in both size and number of these collateral vessels. When these vessels are damaged by inflammation, malignancy, or other injury, blood flow is increased and this raises pulmonary vascular pressure. Hemoptysis occurs in the setting of multiple collateral vessels, high vascular pressure, and damaged, enlarged, and diseased airways.[66,70]

In patients who have HIV disease, bacterial pneumonia and infections cause 63% of episodes of hemoptysis. Kaposi's sarcoma causes 10% of episodes, and pulmonary embolism causes 4% of episodes.[71] Patients on anticoagulant or thrombolytic therapy may also experience hemoptysis.[69]

Diagnostic procedures

Flexible fiberoptic bronchoscopy is initially the quickest and surest way to visualize the source of bleeding in the upper lung lobes and to localize it in the lower respiratory tract.[65] This procedure can be done at the bedside without putting the patient under general anesthesia, and it can also visualize distal airways.[66] If there is brisk bleeding, the rigid bronchoscope can suction more efficiently, remove clots and foreign bodies, allow for better airway control, and be used to obtain material for diagnostic purposes.[72] In some cases, bronchoscopy may locate the area of bleeding but not the direct source of bleeding. In this case, the segment of affected tissue may be purposely suctioned until it collapses.[21] Bronchoscopy should not be undertaken if there is evidence of pulmonary embolism, pneumonia, or bronchitis, or when the patient's condition is so poor or unstable that no further intervention would be undertaken no matter what the results.[70]

If treatment is to be initiated, the combination of bronchoscopy and high-resolution CT can identify the cause of hemoptysis in 81% of patients. It is also quick, noninvasive, and less costly than other modalities.[65] If pulmonary embolism is suspected and therapy is to be initiated, a ventilation-perfusion scan may be warranted.[73]

Signs and symptoms

Respiratory complaints that raise suspicion of bleeding into the lungs may include cough, dyspnea, wheezing, chest pain, sputum expectoration, and systemic clues, such as fever, night sweats, and weight loss. Clues to nasopharyngeal bleeding as the possible source include frequent nosebleeds, throat pain, tongue or mouth lesions, dysphonia, and hoarseness.[74] Clues to GI bleeding as the possible source include the presence of dyspepsia, heartburn, and/or dysphagia. Coffee-grounds-colored vomitus and blood in vomitus does not rule out hemoptysis, because blood from respiratory sources can be swallowed. Patients and family members should be asked to describe the color of blood, and should be asked about any changes in color and pattern of bleeding in vomitus and stool.[74]

During an active bleeding episode, a focused examination should be performed as quickly as possible. If possible, the nasopharynx, larynx, and upper airways should be thoroughly visually examined to rule out an upper airway source of bleeding.[65,72,74] If bleeding is brisk and views are obstructed, examination may best be accomplished with bronchoscopy. The patient may be coughing or vomiting blood, and may be short of breath. If possible, sputum, blood, and vomitus should be examined.[65,70] Some patients may not yet have a diagnosis of malignancy. In these cases one should note clubbing of fingernails and presence of cervical or supraclavicular adenopathy. This may indicate the presence of a malignancy.[74]

Massive bleeding may take place in the lung without the presence of hemoptysis, so listening to lung sounds is very important. Auscultation of the lungs may reveal localized wheezing, an indication of possible airway obstruction.[74] Fine diffuse rales and asymmetric chest excursion may indicate the presence of an infectious or consolidative process.[74] If petechiae and ecchymosis are present, then there should be strong suspicion that a bleeding diathesis is present.[74]

Medical and nursing management

If the episode of bleeding is severe and the goal is active treatment or prolongation of life, then the primary focus is to maintain an adequate airway. This will usually require endotracheal intubation, which may have to be performed immediately at the bedside, and oxygenation. If bleeding can be localized and controlled quickly, a short period of intubation may be considered if it will allow for improved quality of life.[66]

Specific methods of treatment include radiation therapy, laser coagulation therapy, bronchial arterial embolization, endobronchial balloon tamponade, epinephrine injection, iced saline lavage, and, in very rare cases, surgical resection. One case study describes the use of a self-expanding endobronchial stent to successfully stop hemoptysis.[75]

Radiation therapy

External-beam radiation therapy can stop hemoptysis in more than 80% of cases, especially in those patients who have unresectable lung cancers.[76] The goal is to provide therapy in the shortest time period possible, at the lowest dose to achieve symptom control while minimizing side effects. Complications of therapy are radiation fibrosis, and, unfortunately, massive hemoptysis.[77]

Endobronchial brachytherapy has been effective in some patients who have failed previous external-beam radiation attempts.[78] Brachytherapy and bronchoscopy laser therapy have also resulted in resolution of hemoptysis. Results have not been as favorable in patients who have failed previous external-beam radiation therapy, or when combined with laser therapy.[79] Side effects associated with brachytherapy, particularly high-dose brachytherapy, include mucositis, fistula formation, and fatal hemoptysis.[80] The benefits of this treatment should be carefully weighed against potential side effects and their impact on quality of life, particularly in those patients who have short-term prognoses.

Endobronchial tamponade

In this procedure, flexible bronchoscopy is used to find the bleeding site after the site has been lavaged with iced saline. A balloon catheter attached to the tip of the bronchoscope is placed on the site and is then inflated and left on the bleeding site for 24 to 48 hours.[81] In the case of life-threatening hemoptysis, a rigid bronchoscope should be used. This is not a uniformly successful procedure, and should be considered a temporizing measure only.[65] A different approach to endobronchial tamponade that was recently used involved the placement of two self-expanding bronchial stents that stopped the bleeding permanently and allowed the patient to be extubated and continue treatment.[82]

Laser coagulation therapy

In the case of obstructing tracheal tumors, Nd-YAG photocoagulation may control bleeding from endobronchial lesions, and it has a response rate of 60%.[83] Anecdotal reports of the effectiveness of electrocautery to control hemoptysis have been reported; argon plasma coagulation has led to resolution of hemoptysis for at least a 3-month follow-up. However, highly vascular tumors are at risk for bleeding when exposed to laser therapy.[82]

Bronchial arterial embolization

When an endoscopically visualized lung cancer is the source of bleeding, bronchial artery embolization is effective as a palliative intervention. It stops bleeding in 77% to 93% of cases.[72] Bronchial artery embolization, preceded by bronchoscopy, involves injecting a variety of agents angiographically into the bronchial artery to stop blood flow.[70,84] Thirty percent of patients will rebleed within the first or later months, and repeated embolizations may be required.[84]

There are major risks associated with this procedure, including transverse myelitis, paraplegia, ischemic colitis, severe pneumonia, esophagobronchial fistula formation, and temporary severe retrosternal pain.[85] Superselective catheterization now reduces the chance of inadvertently catheterizing the spinal cord branch of the bronchial artery, which has led to spinal cord paraplegia in the past.[86] The risks of rebleeding and the prospect of having repeated embolizations should be carefully reviewed and discussed with the patient and family before carrying out this therapy.

Endobronchial epinephrine injections

A 1:10,000 epinephrine solution may be instilled on visualized lesions to constrict veins and reduce bleeding. Vasopressin and chlorpromazine have also been used in this procedure, which is performed in patients who are not candidates for surgery and when bronchial artery embolization is not available.[65,72]

Iced saline lavage

Iced saline solution lavage has been used as a temporary nonstandard measure to provide improved visualization and localization of the bleeding site. It does not appear to improve outcomes.[63,72]

Surgery

In rare cases, some patients who continue to have life-threatening hemorrhage after receiving other therapies may be considered as candidates for surgical intervention. Only those whose life expectancy, condition, ability to tolerate major surgery, and ability to maintain an airway should be considered. It is important to remember that most lung cancers are well advanced at diagnosis and that undertaking this procedure may not meet quality of life goals for those with short-term prognoses.[63]

Palliative care

When a decision has been made to forego aggressive treatment measures, then promotion of comfort for the patient is the primary goal. Death from massive hemoptysis is usually rapid, occurring within minutes. However, even when the family has been carefully "prepared" for this possibility and coached in a step-by-step manner in what to do, family members inevitably remain unprepared and distraught if a massive hemorrhage does occur, especially in the home without medical personnel around. Preemptive planning includes anxiolytics and opioids readily available in the home, a 24-hour palliative care number to call for immediate guidance and support, and dark-colored towels to reduce the visibility of blood and thus make it less overwhelming.

Spinal cord compression

Case study

Mr. P, a patient with prostate cancer

Mr. P is a 78-year-old man diagnosed with metastatic prostate cancer over a year ago. It has gradually progressed, and he has developed bony metastases, including his spine. He is followed in a palliative care clinic for ongoing pain management of his back pain which had been well controlled on low-dose opioids. Over the past few days, however, his pain has been getting worse, and he has made an appointment to be seen in palliative care clinic today. He tells the clinic nurse, "I've been having a lot more pain in my back recently, especially when I'm lying down, and I'm no longer able to stay comfortable. I kind of feel like my legs are a little weak, too."

Key points

- Pain is the primary presenting symptom of spinal cord compression. It may be present long before neurological dysfunction occurs.
- The pain is classically worse when lying flat and improved when upright.
- In a patient with cancer, increasing back pain that is worse when lying flat and improved when standing is presumed to be cord compression until proven otherwise.
- Early detection and treatment may prevent permanent loss of function. It is therefore considered a medical emergency.
- The use of steroids and radiation therapy in patients with far advanced cancer can decrease the pain and usually preserve function. Steroids alone can usually decrease pain and preserve function in those who are close to death and do not want to undergo radiation therapy, even in truncated form.

Definition

Spinal cord compression (SCC) is compression of the thecal sac at the level of the spinal cord or cauda equina. Spinal cord injury may cause progressive and irreversible neurological damage and requires immediate intervention to prevent disability. Spinal cord compression in the presence of malignancy often carries a poor prognosis, with a median life expectancy of 3 to 6 months.[2,87] Prognostic factors for longer survival include: only one site of cord compression, ability to ambulate pre and post treatment, bone metastases only, and tumor that is responsive to radiation.[87]

Epidemiology

Compression of the spinal cord and cauda equina is a major cause of morbidity in patients with cancer. It occurs in approximately 5% to 10% of patients with malignant disease,[88,89] and is most commonly associated with metastatic disease from tumors of the breast, lung, and prostate. Less than 50% of patients will regain functional losses due to SCC.[10,89–91]

Compression of the spine in 85% to 90% of cases is caused by direct hematological extension of solid tumor cells into a vertebral body.[92] A less common pathway is by direct extension of tumor from adjacent tissue through the intervertebral foramina. Tumor cells can also enter the epidural space directly by circulating in the cerebral spinal fluid (CSF). Paraneoplastic syndromes, leptomeningeal disease, and toxicity of chemotherapy drugs can cause spinal cord syndromes.[93]

Nonmalignant causes of SCC include benign tumors, degenerative, inflammatory, and infectious diseases that affect the spinal column, and from trauma, herniated disks, osteoporosis, or other structural diseases.[93]

Pathophysiology

There are 26 vertebrae in the vertebral column: 7 cervical, 12 thoracic, 5 lumbar, 1 sacral, and 1 coccygeal. Inside this flexible protective vertebral column is the spinal cord, which is an elongated mass of nervous tissue covered and protected by membranes called *meninges*. The outermost layer is the dura mater, the middle layer is the arachnoid membrane, and the innermost layer closest to the spinal cord is the pia mater. The epidural space is located between the outer layer of the dura mater and the vertebral column.[91]

The spinal cord begins where it is attached to the medulla oblongata in the brain and descends through the foramen magnum of the skull until it ends at the level of the first lumbar vertebra. Lumbar and sacral nerve roots then descend below the distal tip of the vertebral column, and spread to the lumbar and sacral areas. These long nerve roots resemble a horse's tail that is called the *cauda equina*. Thirty-one pairs of spinal nerves exit from the spinal cord.[91] Transmission of nerve impulses travels the length of the spinal cord to and from the brain in ascending and descending tracts. Impulses from the spinal cord to the brain travel through the anterior spinothalamic tracts, and impulses from the brain to the spinal cord travel through the lateral corticospinal tracts. Injury to these nerves, or to the cord itself, can result in sensory-motor and autonomic impairment.[91]

Eighty-five percent of SCCs are extradural in nature.[9,89,94] That is, they originate outside the cord itself. Extradural metastatic tumors may be osteolytic, where lesions invade the marrow of the vertebrae and cause absorption of bone tissue, which leads to bone destruction. They may also be osteoblastic, where lesions invade the bone marrow and cause bone development, tumor invasion, and collapse of the vertebral body, which then pushes tumor or bone fragments into the spinal cord.[94] Neurological deficits caused by SCC include direct compression on the cord or cauda equina, vascular supply interruption, or pathological fracture, causing vertebral collapse. When nerve tissue dies, neurological regeneration is not always possible. Function may be quickly and irreversibly lost.

Diagnostic procedures

Plain spinal X-rays are an excellent screening tool and can determine the presence of tumor and the stability of the spine.[93] They can identify lytic or blastic lesions in up to 85% of vertebral lesions. However, false negatives can occur due to poor visualization, mild pathology, or poor interpretation.[92] More than 50% collapse and pedicle erosion must be present before X-ray can detect SCC.[95] Epidural spread of tumor through the foramina might not always be visualized using plain X-rays. A bone scan may detect vertebral abnormalities when plain films are negative.[96]

The imaging choice for emergent SCC is MRI.[95] It is noninvasive and does not require injection with contrast material. It has an advantage over CT because it can image the entire spine, thus detecting multiple areas of compression.[88,93] Decisions about diagnostic testing will be tempered by a number of factors, including the potential for treatment, prognosis, patient's condition, and the patient's and/or family's wishes for treatment.

Signs and symptoms

The presence of increasing back pain, worse on lying flat and improved on standing, with or without signs of bowel and bladder impairment, in a patient with a history of cancer, should be presumed to be SCC until proven otherwise. Neurological function before initiation of therapy is the single most important prognostic factor in SCC.[43] Misdiagnosis of SCC has been attributed to poor history, inadequate examination, and insufficient diagnostic evaluation.[97] Patients who have only localized back pain and a normal neurological examination may have more than 75% of the spinal cord compressed. Upper motor neuron weakness may occur above the L1 vertebral body in 75% of patients with SCC at diagnosis. Sensory changes occur in about half of patients at presentation. Sensory change without pain complaint is extremely rare.

A thorough history should pay special attention to the onset of pain, its location, its intensity, duration, quality, and what activities increase or decrease the pain.[94,98] A history of sensory or motor weakness and autonomic dysfunction should be evaluated and should include onset and degree of weakness; heaviness or stiffness of limbs; difficulty walking; numbness in arms, hands, fingers, toes, and trunk; and change in temperature or touch. Specific questions about bowel, bladder, and sexual function should be asked directly, because patients may not volunteer these symptoms, such as difficulty in passing urine or stool, incontinence of bowel or bladder, loss of sphincter control, and ability to obtain and maintain an erection. Constipation usually precedes urinary retention or incontinence.[94]

Physical examination includes observation of the spine, muscles, extremities and skin, and palpation and gentle percussion of vertebrae. Spinal manipulation to elicit pain responses should be carried out cautiously because it may cause muscle spasm or further injury.[93] Mental status, cranial nerves, motor function, reflexes, sensation, coordination, strength, and gait should be evaluated (where appropriate to the patient's status and closeness to death). Focused examination may include performing straight leg raises until the patient feels pain, then dorsiflexing the foot. If this action increases pain down the back of the leg, this suggests that nerve root compression is present. Testing of reflexes will indicate the presence and impact of nerve root compression on motor ability. Cord compression may cause hyperactive deep-tendon reflexes, while nerve-root compression may cause decreased deep-tendon reflexes. A positive Babinski sign and sustained ankle clonus indicate motor involvement.[94]

Sensory function should be tested by assessing pain (sharp, dull), temperature (hot, cold), touch (light), vibration (tuning fork test), and position senses (fingers and toes). Examination may reveal a demarcated area of sensory loss and brisk or absent reflexes.[94] The mapping of positive sensation can be used to pinpoint the level of SCC, usually one or two levels below the site of compression.[94] Bladder percussion and digital rectal examination will elicit retention and laxity of sphincter control, a late sign of SCC.

Pain may be reported for weeks to months before any obvious neurological dysfunction.[86] Pain may be local initially (in the central back, for example), then progress to a radicular pattern that follows a particular dermatome.[90,93] Local pain may be caused by stretching of bone periosteum by tumor or vertebral collapse and is usually described by the patient as constant, dull, aching, and progressive in nature. Radicular pain is caused by pressure of tumor along the length of the nerve root.[91] The patient who reports radicular pain will describe it as shooting, burning, or shocklike in nature and will state that it is worsened by movement, coughing, sneezing, straining, neck flexion, or by lying down.

A classic sign of cord compression is if pain is relieved by sitting up or standing and is worsened by lying flat. Also, if pain increases at night when the patient is lying down to sleep, one should be suspicious of SCC rather than degenerative or disk disease.[88] Radicular pain is present in 90% of lumbosacral SCC, 79% in cervical SCC, and in 55% of thoracic SCC.[99] Radicular pain is typically bilateral in thoracic lesions, and is often described as a tight band around the chest or abdomen, but it may also be experienced in only part of one dermatome.[86,92] Nonradicular referred pain may also be associated with vague paresthesias and point tenderness.[86,92] Vigilance is called for when these radicular symptoms occur: (1) shoulder tip pain from C7/T1 metastases; (2) anterior or abdominal, flank, or hip pain from T12–L2 metastases; or (3) lateral or anterior rib pain from thoracic metastases.[93]

The sequence of neurological symptoms usually progresses in the following manner: first there is pain, then motor weakness that progresses to sensory loss, then motor loss, and finally, autonomic dysfunction.[9] The patient will initially complain of heaviness or stiffness in the extremities, loss of coordination, and ataxia.[100] Sensory complaints include paresthesias and numbness, and loss of heat sensation. Dysfunction begins in the toes and ascends in a stocking-like pattern to the level of the lesion.[86] Loss of proprioception, deep pressure, and vibration are late signs of sensory loss.[91] When the cauda equina is affected, sensory loss is bilateral; the dermatome that follows the perianal area, posterior thigh, and lateral aspect of the leg is involved. Late signs of SCC are motor loss and paralysis. Loss of sphincter control is associated with poor return to functionality.[91]

Medical and nursing management

The focus of management of SCC should be the relief of pain and preservation or restoration of neurological function. Rapid intervention is required to prevent permanent loss of function and concomitant quality of life. The patient status (e.g., goals of care and closeness to death), rate of neurological impairment, and prior radiation therapy experience are other factors to consider.[94]Corticosteroids, surgical decompression, radiation therapy, and adjuvant chemotherapy or hormonal therapy are the standard treatments for SCC.[91]

Corticosteroids

Corticosteroids decrease vasogenic edema and inflammation and thus relieve pain and neurological symptoms, and may have some oncolytic effect on tumor.[98] Dexamethasone is the preferred corticosteroid because it is less likely to promote systemic edema caused by other steroids, or to cause cognitive and behavioral dysfunction, and it improves overall outcomes after specific therapy.[86]

There has been controversy about dosage and scheduling of dexamethasone therapy in the management of SCC.[87,88] In animal studies, neurological status has improved more rapidly with high-dose steroid therapy.[92] A recent Cochrane review examining interventions for metastatic extradural SCC was, however, unable to demonstrate any evidence-based differences in benefit from high-dose versus low-dose corticosteroids. The review did however, conclude that the incidence of adverse side effects was greater with high-dose compared with low-dose steroid therapy.[101] One suggested approach would be to administer high-dose therapy for patients who are no longer ambulatory or have rapidly increasing motor deficits and low-dose therapy for those patients who can walk and do not have significant/worsening motor deficits.[87]

Currently, high-dose therapy regimens recommend administering a 100-mg IV bolus of dexamethasone, followed by 24 mg dexamethasone orally QID for 3 days, then tapering the dose over 10 days. High-dose therapy may increase analgesia but, as mentioned, can also increase side effects that are significant.

These include GI bleeding, hyperglycemia, depression and psychosis, myopathy, osteoporosis, and acute adrenal insufficiency with abrupt withdrawal.[102] A low-dose dexamethasone regimen recommends administering a 10-mg IV bolus of dexamethasone, followed by 4 mg IV QID for 3 days, then tapering the dose over 14 days.[86] Rapid IV push of corticosteroids causes severe burning pain in the perineum, and the patient needs to be warned that this will occur but does not signify that anything is wrong. Corticosteroids are metabolized by the cytochrome P-450 system, and there are implications for interactions with other medications, particularly anticonvulsants.

Decompressive surgery

The goals of surgery are to decompress neural structures, resect tumor if possible, establish local disease control, achieve spinal stability, restore the ability to ambulate, treat pain, and improve quality of life. Surgery for SCC has been used to (1) establish a diagnosis when tissue is required for histological analysis; (2) halt rapidly deteriorating function; (3) achieve cure for primary malignancy; (4) treat those with previously irradiated radio-resistant tumor and who have continuing symptomatic progressive loss of function; (5) rule out infection or hematoma; (6) alleviate respiratory paralysis caused by high cervical spinal cord lesions; and (7) decompress and stabilize spine structure.[94,103] Benefits and burden of surgery to the patient in a palliative care setting must be carefully weighed so that the patient and family can make an informed decision.

Radiation therapy

Fractionated external-beam radiation therapy (XRT) to the spine is given to inhibit tumor growth, restore and preserve neurological function, treat pain, and improve quality of life.[9] It has been the primary treatment for SCC.[86] The standard treatment regimen is 30 Gy over the course of 10 fractions, but hypofractionation (e.g., 8 Gy once or 4 Gy over 5 fractions) maybe used in patients with limited expected survival.[76] Only symptomatic sections of the spine are treated. Seventy percent of patients who are ambulatory at the start of treatment will retain their ability to walk. Thirty-five percent of paraparetic patients will regain their ability to walk, while only 5% of completely paraplegic patients will do so.[104] Primary side effects of radiation therapy include skin alterations, including erythema, dry or moist desquamation, and pigmentation changes, and generalized fatigue.

Nursing management

The goal of nursing management is to identify patients at high risk for cord compression, to educate the patient and family regarding signs and symptoms to report, to detect early signs of SCC, and to work as a member of the palliative care team in managing symptoms. In those patients who have far advanced disease, palliative care efforts focus on promoting comfort, relieving pain, and providing family support.

Hypercalcemia

Case study

Mrs. R, a patient with multiple myeloma

Mrs. R is a 56-year-old teacher with advanced multiple myeloma. She is continuing to receive treatment for her disease and requires opioid therapy to manage her chronic back pain due to spine lesions. She is still teaching, but she has been feeling more fatigued lately and has also been having a new problem with constipation. In addition to these symptoms, she tells her oncologist during a routine visit that she also just doesn't feel "quite as sharp" mentally as she usually does.

Key points

- Hypercalcemia occurs in 8% to 10% of patients with cancer, with an incidence of 40% in patients with breast cancer and multiple myeloma.

- Common presenting signs are fatigue, lethargy, nausea, polyuria, and confusion.

- The combination of nausea and polyuria can lead to dehydration and worsening of hypercalcemia.

- Severity of symptoms depends on the level of free ionized calcium and the speed with which the level rises.

- The serum calcium level is adjusted according to the serum albumin in patients with significant hypoalbuminemia.

- All patients with hypercalcemia who are symptomatic warrant a trial of therapy.

- Control of hypercalcemia will not affect prognosis but may greatly improve symptoms and quality of life in these patients.

Definition

Hypercalcemia is an excessive amount of ionized calcium in the blood.[105,106] If hypercalcemia is left untreated, the patient may experience irreversible renal damage, coma, or death. Mortality from untreated hypercalcemia approaches 50%.

Epidemiology

About 10% to 20% of cancer patients will develop hypercalcemia at some time during their illness.[105,107] Carcinomas of the breast and lung, multiple myeloma, and squamous cell carcinomas of the head, neck, and esophagus are the most common malignancies associated with hypercalcemia. Incidence ranges from 30% to 40% for breast cancer with bone metastases, 20% to 40% for multiple myeloma, 12.5% to 35% for the squamous cell lung carcinomas, and 2.9% to 25% for head and neck malignancies.[105] Hypercalcemia is rare in prostate cancer, GI cancers, and cancers of the biliary tract.[105]

Primary hyperparathyroidism as a cause of hypercalcemia is more common in the ambulatory and asymptomatic population.[108,109] Other conditions associated with hypercalcemia include lithium therapy, Addison's disease, Paget's disease, granulomatous disease, vitamin D intoxication, hyperthyroidism, vitamin A intoxication, and aluminum intoxication.[106,110]

Pathophysiology

Calcium helps the body to maintain its acid-base balance, maintain permeability of cell membranes, promote coagulation, and maintain proper nerve and muscle function.[111] Under normal circumstances, bone resorption and bone formation are in a steady state and are regulated by three hormones—parathyroid hormone (PTH), calcitriol (1,25 dihydroxyvitamin D, a metabolite of vitamin D), and calcitonin.[106] These hormones act at bone sites, in the intestine, and in the kidney. Parathyroid hormone directly

increases resorption of calcium from the bone and calcium resorption in the renal tubule. Calcitriol stimulates absorption of calcium in the intestine. It enhances bone resorption and increases renal resorption. Calcitonin is excreted by the thyroid gland and inhibits bone resorption and increases excretion of calcium.

Bone undergoes constant remodeling in the human body. Osteoblasts form bone and osteoclasts resorb bone. About 99% of the body's calcium is found in bone. The remaining 1% circulates in the blood or is found inside cells. Half of plasma calcium is bound to either protein (albumin) or to other ions, such as phosphate, carbonate, or citrate. The remaining calcium circulates as free ions. Since free calcium is biologically active, its level is maintained in a narrow range in the normal physiological state.

Hypercalcemia in malignant disease is primarily due to increased mobilization of calcium from bone. Increased renal tubular calcium resorption is also a factor in hypercalcemia of malignancy. There are three major mechanisms that contribute to the development of malignant hypercalcemia.[107] First, higher levels of PTHrP (parathyroid hormone-related protein) are found in hypercalcemic patients who have solid tumors, particularly squamous cell carcinomas. The presence of elevated PTHrP levels is associated with more advanced cancer, a worse prognosis, and a poor response to bisphosphonate therapy. Approximately 80% of cases of malignant hypercalcemia are related to the presence of this protein.

Second, osteolysis of bone is caused by the release of tumor and other cell mediators. When this mechanism is operating, hypercalcemia occurs late in disease and is usually associated with extensive osteolytic bone metastases. Third, the increased production of calcitriol by lymphoma tumor cells, for example, leads to increased resorption of calcium in the gut. Hypercalcemia induced by calcitriol usually responds to corticosteroid therapy.

The kidney normally adapts to disturbances in calcium homeostasis. However, in the presence of malignancy, patients may experience treatment or disease-related side effects including vomiting, mucositis, anorexia, dysphagia, and fever, all of which can lead to volume depletion.[105] This imbalance signals the kidney to reabsorb sodium to correct extracellular volume depletion. Calcium and sodium resorption are closely linked in the body; when sodium is resorbed, calcium is also resorbed. As calcium ions are resorbed in the kidney, the tubules lose their ability to concentrate urine, leading to high-output polyuria and further dehydration. Poor renal perfusion, reduced glomerular filtration, and compromised excretion of calcium lead to a further increase of calcium in the blood. Ultimately, renal failure will occur.

A high calcium level can alter the patient's mental status significantly, which, in turn, can greatly affect the patient's ability to drink fluids. Cellular dehydration and resulting hypotension are exacerbated by decreased proximal renal tubule reabsorption of sodium, magnesium, and potassium. Bone loss due to immobilization, lack of physical exercise, inappropriate use of thiazide diuretics, poor diet, and general physiological wasting will also increase the amount of free calcium ions in the circulation, further increasing calcium levels.

Diagnostic tests and procedures

The ionized calcium concentration is the most important laboratory test to use in the diagnostic workup for hypercalcemia. It is the most accurate indicator of the level of calcium in the blood. (There is only a fair correlation between the total serum calcium level and ionized calcium.) When ionized calcium cannot be used as a diagnostic tool, the total serum calcium value may be used, but it must be corrected for serum albumin. A rule of thumb is to add 0.8 for each 1 g/dL the albumin has dropped below the normal range (3.7 to 5 g/dL).[105,106]

Signs and symptoms

Symptoms of hypercalcemia, their severity, and how quickly they appear will vary from patient to patient. The extent of metastatic bone disease is not associated with hypercalcemia levels.[108] It is important to remember that patients, especially the elderly and the debilitated,[105,108,110] may experience severe symptoms even when serum calcium is not extremely elevated.[105] Symptoms of hypercalcemia, such as vomiting, nausea, anorexia, weakness, constipation, and impaired mental status, may be mistakenly attributed to the disease or effects of treatment. Factors that will influence patients' response to hypercalcemia include age,[110] performance status, renal or hepatic failure, and sites of metastatic disease.

Patients with a corrected serum calcium level less than 12 mg/dL who are asymptomatic can be considered to have mild hypercalcemia. Patients who have a serum calcium level between 12 and 14 mg/dL should be closely monitored and may require urgent intervention, depending on goals of care in the palliative setting. Those patients with a calcium level greater than 14 mg/dL will require urgent treatment, again depending on goals of care in the palliative setting.[107]

The patient may complain of numerous symptoms that can mimic symptoms of advanced malignancy.[105] These include GI symptoms of nausea, vomiting, anorexia, constipation, obstipation and even complete ileus. Polydipsia and polyuria may also be present. Muscle weakness, fatigue, and difficulty climbing stairs or getting out of a car, are musculoskeletal symptoms that can progress to profound weakness, hypotonia, and fracture. Neuropsychological symptoms can begin with confusion, personality change, restlessness, and mood alterations, and can progress to slurred speech, psychotic behavior, stupor, and coma. These are also symptoms that must be evaluated. The patient may also complain of bone pain, although the precise mechanism of bone-pain hypercalcemia is unknown.

Early signs of delirium in the hypercalcemic patient are associated with multiple factors that include electrolyte imbalance, metabolic disturbance, and renal failure, among others. If recognized early, treatment of the condition can alleviate and possibly reverse the symptoms.[112] Management of confusion includes both pharmacotherapy and a reassuring and calm environment.

Medical and nursing management

Regardless of the goals of care, active treatment goals are to promote alleviation of distressing symptoms. All patients with hypercalcemia who are symptomatic warrant a trial of therapy. When the goal is to reverse the hypercalcemia, this is accomplished by replenishing depleted intravascular volume, promoting diuresis of calcium, shutting down osteoclast activity in the bone, inhibiting renal tubular reabsorption of calcium, and promoting patient mobilization to the extent it is possible.[106,107] See Table 24.1 for a list of commonly used treatments for hypercalcemia.

Hydration

Hydration is the first step in treatment. The purpose of hydration is to increase urinary calcium excretion, which improves renal

Table 24.1 Common treatments for hypercalcemia in palliative care

Treatment	Mechanism of action
Biphosphonates (pamidronate and zoledronate most frequently)	Inhibit osteoclast activity
Hydration with IV fluids	Increase urinary calcium excretion and improve kidney function
Calcitonin	Inhibits calcium resorption
Gallium nitrate and plicamycin	Mechanisms of action unknown
Dialysis	Dialyze excess calcium out

function.[107] One to 2 liters of isotonic saline is administered over 1 to 4 hours, and the patient's fluid intake and urinary output are closely monitored. The rate of fluid administration depends on the clinical estimate of the extent of hydration, patient's cardiovascular function, and renal excretion capacity.[107]

Electrolytes and other laboratory values are closely monitored in appropriate patients. These include serum calcium (ionized or corrected), potassium, magnesium, and other electrolytes and albumin and bicarbonate levels. Renal function tests, including BUN and creatinine, are monitored. In rare cases, dialysis may be considered. In most patients, cardiac effects of hypercalcemia are minimal and outcomes are not usually affected, so cardiac monitoring is not usually necessary.

Bisphosphonate therapy

Most hypercalcemic patients are treated with bisphosphonate therapy. It is an effective therapy for a number of cancers.[113,114] Bisphosphonate therapy inhibits bone resorption by osteoclasts, thus reducing the amount of calcium released into the bloodstream. Several IV bisphosphonates and aminobisphosphonates are available for use in patients.[115] Pamidronate, etidronate, risedronate sodium, ibandronate, and zoledronate are available in the United States.[116]

Pamidronate has been the most frequently used bisphosphonate, but zoledronate is becoming more widely used in the outpatient setting due to its much more rapid infusion time (30 minutes versus 2–6 hours for pamidronate). Pamidronate is usually given as 60 mg to 90 mg IV approximately every 3 to 4 weeks. In general, there is a 60% response to a 60-mg dose and a 100% response to a 90-mg dose.[109] Zoledronate, usually given as 4 mg IV, has been shown to have a higher rate and duration of control of hypercalcemia compared to pamidronate.[117] Pamidronate, and especially zoledronate, can cause renal toxicity (thus making evaluation and continued monitoring of kidney function essential prior to/during administration). Biphosphonates can cause osteonecrosis of the jaw, especially in patients with myeloma who have been treated with pamidronate and zoledronate for a long period of time and patients with dental problems.[117]

Since hypercalcemia tends to recur, pamidronate or zoledronate must be given approximately every 4 weeks. Immediate side effects of pamidronate therapy include low-grade fever appearing within 48 hours of treatment, redness, induration, and swelling at the site of catheter. Hypomagnesia and hypocalcemia may also occur. Rapid administration of IV bisphosphonates can cause significant pain, and this practice should be avoided. Subcutaneous administration of clodronate has been found to be an efficient treatment for malignant hypercalcemia.[118] This route may be particularly useful in hospital, home, and hospice settings and spares the patient discomfort and the costs associated with transportation and IV administration in the hospital environment.

Calcitonin

Calcitonin inhibits resorption of calcium and can rapidly restore normocalcemia, often within 2 to 4 hours of administration. It is much less effective than pamidronate. Its role in managing hypercalcemia is limited to short-term use, usually of only 2 to 3 days' duration. Side effects are usually mild and include nausea and vomiting, skin rashes, and flushing. Calcitonin can be an alternative for treatment in patients with kidney failure (where pamidronate and zoledronate are contraindicated).[117]

Gallium nitrate and plicamycin

Gallium nitrate is an effective bone resorptive agent. Its mechanism of action is unknown.[119] Its main disadvantages are that it has potential to cause nephrotoxicity, and it must be given as a continuous IV infusion over 5 days.[106] Plicamycin is an antitumor antibiotic.[120] Its mechanism is unknown. It has a hypocalcemic effect that occurs within 48 hours of administration and that lasts for 3 to 7 days, but it exhibits marrow, hepatic, and renal toxicities.[106] Individual response variations make this drug unpredictable, and it must be administered repeatedly.

Corticosteroids

Corticosteroids have a limited role in the treatment of hypercalcemia.[107]

Dialysis

The use of dialysis has been reserved for those patients who have severe hypercalcemia, renal failure, or congestive heart failure and cannot be given saline hydration.[121] The decision to offer this therapy is made on a case-by-case basis, but, in general, dialysis is not offered in the palliative care arena.

Palliative nursing care

Hypercalcemia can cause significantly painful and distressing symptoms, including bone pain, agitation and confusion, severe constipation, and delirium. Treatment of hypercalcemia can reduce pain and other symptoms, improve quality of life, and reduce hospitalizations. At the end of life, the promotion of comfort and management of symptoms are the primary goals of palliative nursing care. If hypercalcemia cannot be reversed, or the patient decides that the burden of interventions is greater than the benefit, the patient should be given the option of discontinuing such treatment. Ongoing management of symptoms, including sedation if desired, must be guaranteed to the patient and their family.

Conclusion

This chapter addressed a group of syndromes, which, unless recognized and treated promptly, will cause unnecessary suffering for the patient and family. Emphasis has been given to the epidemiology and basic pathophysiology of each syndrome, as well as diagnostic assessment. Providing this information, although by necessity limited in detail, enables the palliative care nurse to explain to the patient and/or family why particular symptoms are occurring and why a particular management approach is being suggested. Treatment advice and decisions are always couched within the framework of these questions: "Is the underlying cause reversible or not?", "What is the benefit/ burden ratio of the treatment and how does that fit with the patient's values and goals?", "What is the likely outcome if the syndrome is not treated?", "How will resultant symptoms be managed?", "Is palliative sedation available to a patient at end of life if desired?", and "Will the site of care impact on treatment decisions?"

Acknowledgment

The author wishes to thank Ashby Watson for her outstanding first version (in the second edition) of this chapter that made the task of updating it for future editions so much easier. Unfortunately, she could not be reached to obtain her feedback and retain her as first author.

References

1. Wilson LD, Detterbeck FC, Yahalom J. Superior vena cava syndrome with malignant causes. N Engl J Med. 2007;356:1862–1869.
2. Walji N, Chan AK, Peake DR. Common acute oncological emergencies: diagnosis, investigation and management. Postgrad Med J. 2008;84:418–427.
3. Rice TW, Rodriguez RM, Light RW. The superior vena cava syndrome: clinical characteristics and evolving etiology. Medicine. 2006;85:3742.
4. Chan RH, Dar AR, Yu E, et al. Superior vena cava obstruction in small-cell lung cancer. Int J Radiat Oncol Biol Phys. 1997;38:513–520.
5. Rowell NP, Gleeson FV. Steroids, radiotherapy, chemotherapy and stents for superior vena caval obstruction in carcinoma of the bronchus: a systematic review. Clin Oncol. 2002;14:338–351.
6. Yu JB, Wilson LD, Detterbeck FC. Superior vena cava syndrome—a proposed classification system and algorithm for management. J Thorac Oncol. 2008;3:811–814.
7. Yaholom J. Superior vena cava syndrome. In: Devita VT, Hellman S, Rosenberg SA (eds.), Cancer: Principles and Practice of Oncology. 9th ed. Philadelphia: Lippincott Williams & Wilkins; 2011:2123–2130.
8. Nickloes T. Superior Vena Cava Syndrome. Available at: http://emedicine.medscape.com/article/460865-overview. Accessed June 30, 2013.
9. Flounders JA. Oncology emergency modules: spinal cord compression. Oncol Nurs Forum. 2003;30:E17–E23.
10. Wan JF, Bezjak A. Superior vena cava syndrome. Emerg Med Clin N Am. 2009:243–255.
11. Uaje C, Kathsen K, Parish L. Oncology emergencies. Crit Care Nurs Q. 1996;18:26–34.
12. Silvestri GA, Tanoue LT, Margolis ML. The noninvasive staging of non-small cell lung cancer: the guidelines. Chest. 2003;123:147S–156S.
13. Detterbeck FC, Lewis SZ, Diekemper R, et al. Executive summary: diagnosis and management of lung cancer, 3rd ed: American College of Chest Physicians Evidence-Based Clinical Practice Guidelines. Chest. 2013;143(5 suppl):7S–37S.
14. Hague J, Tippett R. Endovascular techniques in palliative care. Clin Oncol. 2010;22:771–780.
15. Gauden SJ. Superior vena cava syndrome induced by bronchogenic carcinoma: is this anoncological emergency? Australas Radiol. 1993;37:363–366.
16. National Cancer Institute (NCI). Cancer Information Service: Physicians Desk Query Supportive Care Guideline: Superior Vena Cava Syndrome. Available at: http:// http://www.cancer.gov/cancertopics/pdq/supportivecare/cardiopulmonary/HealthProfessional/page5. Accessed June 30, 2013.
17. Neragi-Miandoab S. Malignant pleural effusion, current and evolving approaches for its diagnosis and management. Lung Cancer. 2006;54:1–9.

18. Heffner JE, Klein JS. Recent advances in the diagnosis and management of malignant pleural effusion. Mayo Clin Proc. 2008;83:235–250.

19. Sahn SA. Malignancy metastatic to the pleura. Clin Chest Med. 1998;19:351–361.

20. Pollak JS. Malignant pleural effusions: treatment with tunneled long-term drainage catheters. Curr Opin Pulm Med. 2002;8:302–307.

21. Afessa B. Pleural effusions and pneumothoraces in AIDS. Curr Opin Pulm Med. 2001;7:202–209.

22. Soubani AO, Michelson MK, Karnik A. Pleural fluid findings in patients with the acquired immunodeficiency syndrome: correlation with concomitant pulmonary disease. South Med J. 1999;92:400–403.

23. American Society of Clinical Oncology (ASCO). Optimizing Cancer Care—The Importance of Symptom Management, Vol. 2: Malignant Pleural Effusions. ASCO Curriculum 2001. Dubuque, IA: Kendall/Hunt; 2001:1–27.

24. Gill PS, Akil B, Colletti P, Rarick M, Loweiro C, Bernstein-Singer M. Pulmonary Kaposi's sarcoma: clinical findings and results of therapy. Am J Med. 1989;87:57–61.

25. Milne ENC, Pistolesi M. Pleural effusions: normal physiology, pathophysiology, and diagnosis. In: Patterson S, ed. Reading the Chest Radiograph: A Physiologic Approach. St. Louis: Mosby; 1993:120–163.

26. Shamji F, Deslauriers J. Surgeon's view: is palliative resection of lung cancer ever justified? Thoracic Surg Clin. 2013;23:383–399.

27. Ruckdeschel JC, Robinson LA. Management of pleural and pericardial effusions. In: Berger AM, Portenoy RK, Weissman DE (eds.), Principles and Practice of Palliative Care and Supportive Oncology. 2nd ed. Philadelphia: Lippincott Williams & Wilkins; 2002:389–412.

28. Kaplan LM, Epstein SK, Schwartz SL, et al. Clinical, echocardiographic, and hemodynamic evidence of cardiac tamponade caused by large pleural effusions. Am J Resp Crit Care Med. 1995;151:904–908.

29. Woodring JH, Loh FK, Kryscio RJ. Mediastinal hemorrhage: an evaluation of radiographic manifestations. Radiology. 1984;23:393–397.

30. Nemchek AA. Management of malignant pleural effusions. J Vasc Interv Radiol. 1998;9:115–120.

31. Bartter T, Santarelli R, Akers S, et al. The evaluation of pleural effusion. Chest. 1994;106:1209–1214.

32. Nally AT. Critical care of the patient with lung cancer. AACN Clin Issues: Adv Practice Acute Crit Care. 1996;7:79–94.

33. Chernecky C, Shelton B. Pulmonary complications in patients with cancer: diagnostic and treatment information for the noncritical care nurse. Am J Nurs. 2001;101:24A, 24E, 24G–24H.

34. Ruckdeschel JC. Management of malignant pleural effusion: an overview. Semin Oncol. 1988;15:24–28.

35. Beyea, A, Winzelberg, G, Stafford, RE. To drain or not to drain: an evidence-based approach to palliative procedures for the management of malignant pleural effusions. J Pain Symptom Manage. 2012;44:301–306.

36. Gaeta RR, Marcario A, Brodsky JB, et al. Pain outcomes after thoracotomy: lumbar epidural hydromorphone versus intrapleural bupivacaine. J Cardiothorac Vasc Anesth. 1995;9:534–537.

37. Robinson LA, Mouton AL, Fleming WH, et al. Intrapleural doxycycline control of malignant pleural effusions. Am Thorac Surg. 1993;55:1115–1122.

38. Gilkeson RC, Silverman P, Haaga JR. Using urokinase to treat malignant pleural effusions. Am J Roent. 1999;173:781–783.

39. Sherman S, Raviskrishnan KP, Patel AS. Optimum anesthesia with intrapleural lidocaine during chemical pleurodesis with tetracycline. Chest. 1988;94:533–536.

40. Leslie WK, Kinasewitz GT. Clinical characteristics of the patient with nonspecific pleuritis. Chest. 1988;94:603–608.

41. Tremblay A, Michaud G. Single-center experience with 250 tunnelled pleural catheter insertions for malignant pleural effusion. Chest. 2006;129:362–368.

42. Dudgeon DJ, Lertzman M, Askew GR. Physiological changes and clinical correlates of dyspnea in cancer outpatients. J Pain Symptom Manage. 2001;21:373–379.

43. McCurdy MT, Shanholtz CB. Oncologic emergencies. Crit Care Med. 2012;40:2012–2222.

44. Weinberg BA, Conces DJ Jr, Waller BF. Cardiac manifestations of noncardiac tumors. Part 1: Direct effects. Clin Cardiol. 1989;12:289–296.

45. Knoop T, Willenberg K. Cardiac tamponade. Semin Oncol Nurs. 1999;15:168–175.

46. National Hospital Discharge Summary: Annual Survey 1993. US Department of Health and Human Services, Public Health Service. Centers for Disease Control and Prevention, National Center for Health Statistics. Hyattsville, MD, 1993, DHHS Publication No. (PHS) 93–1775.

47. Bullock B. Altered cardiac function. In: Bullock B, Henze R (eds.), Focus on Pathophysiology. Philadelphia: Lippincott Williams & Wilkins; 2000:455–502.

48. Smeltzer S, Bare B. Oncology: nursing the patient with cancer. In: Smeltzer S, Bare B (eds.), Brunner and Suddarth's Textbook of Medical-Surgical Nursing. 8th ed. Philadelphia: Lippincott-Raven; 1996:309–316.

49. Beauchamp K. Pericardial tamponade: an oncologic emergency. Clin J Oncol Nurs. 1998;2:85–95.

50. Press OW, Livingston R. Management of malignant pericardial effusion and tamponade. JAMA. 1987;8:1088–1092.

51. Stouffer GA, Sheahan RG, Lenihan DJ, et al. Diagnosis and management of chronic pericardial effusions. Am J Med Sci. 2001;322:79–87.

52. Mangan C. Malignant pericardial effusions: pathophysiology and clinical correlates. Oncol Nurs Forum. 1992;19:1215–1223.

53. Nguyen DM, Schrump DS. Malignant pleural and pericardial effusions. In: DeVita V, Hellman S, Rosenberg S (eds.), Cancer Principles and Practice of Oncology. 7th ed. Philadelphia: Lippincott Williams & Wilkins; 2005:2381–2392.

54. Gueberman B, Fowler N, Engel P. Cardiac tamponade in medical patients. Circulation. 1987;64:633–640.

55. Keefe D. Cardiovascular emergencies in the cancer patient. Semin Oncol. 2000;27:244–255.

56. Kopecky SL, Callahan JA, Tajik AJ, Seward JB. Percutaneous pericardial catheter drainage: report of 42 consecutive cases. Am J Cardiol. 1986:7:633–635.

57. Chong HH, Plotnick GD. Pericardial effusion and tamponade: evaluation, imaging, modalities, and management. Compr Ther. 1995;21:378–385.

58. Shepherd F. Malignant pericardial effusion. Curr Opin Oncol. 1997;9:170–174.

59. Maruyama R, Yokohama H, Seto T, et al. Catheter drainage followed by the instillation of bleomycin to manage malignant pericardial effusion in non-small cell lung cancer: a multi-institutional phase II trial. J Thorac Oncol. 2007;2:65–68.

60. Ziskind AA, Pearce AC, Lemmon CC, et al. Percutaneous balloon pericardiotomy for the treatment of cardiac tamponade and large pericardial effusions: descriptions of technique and report of the first 50 cases. J Am Coll Cardiol. 1993;21:1–5.

61. Jackson G, Keane D, Mishra B. Percutaneous balloon pericardiotomy in the management of recurrent malignant pericardial effusions. Br Heart J. 1992;68:613–615.

62. Gross JL, Younes RN, Deheinzelin D, et al. Surgical management of symptomatic management of pericardial effusion in the patient with solid malignancies. Ann Surg Oncol. 2006;13:1732–1738.

63. Gompelmann, D, Eberhardt, R, Herth, FJ. Advanced malignant lung disease: what the specialist can offer. Respiration. 2011;82:111–123.

64. Lewis MM, Read CA. Hemoptysis. Part 1: Identifying the cause. J Resp Dis. 2000;21:335–341.

65. Corder R. Hemoptysis. Emerg Med Clin N Am. 2003;21:421–435.

66. Lipchik RJ. Hemoptysis. In: Berger AM, Portenoy RK, Weissman DE (eds.), Principles and Practice of Palliative Care and Supportive Oncology. 2nd ed. Philadelphia: Lippincott Williams & Wilkins; 2002:372–377.

67. Rizzi A, Rocco G, Robustellini M, et al. Results of surgical management of tuberculosis: experience in 206 patients undergoing operation. Ann Thorac Surg. 1995;59:896–900.

68. Chan C, Elazar-Popovic E, Farver C, et al. Endobronchial involvement in uncommon diseases. J Bronch. 1996;3:53–63.

69. Levine MN, Raskob G, Landefeld S, et al. Hemorrhagic complications of anticoagulant treatment. Chest. 1995;108:276S–290S.

70. Corey R, Hla KM. Major and massive hemoptysis: reassessment of conservative management. Am J Med Sci. 1987;294:301–309.

71. Luce K, O'Donnell EE, Morton AR. A combination of calcitonin and bisphosphonate for the emergency treatment of severe tumor-induced hypercalcemia. Calcif Tissue Int. 1993;52:70–71.

72. Lewis MM, Read CA. Hemoptysis. Part 2: Treatment options. J Resp Dis. 2000;21:392–394.

73. Saltzman HA, Alavi A, Greespan RH. Value of the ventilation/perfusion scan in acute pulmonary embolism: results of the prospective investigation of pulmonary embolism diagnosis. JAMA. 1990;263:2753–2759.

74. Colice GL. Hemoptysis: three questions that can direct management. Postgrad Med. 1996;100:227–236.

75. Chung H, Park M, Kim DH, Jeon GS. Endobronchial stent insertion to manage hemoptysis caused by lung cancer. J Korean Med Sci. 2010;25:1253–1255.

76. Kwok Y, DeYoung C, Garofalo M, et al. Radiation oncology emergencies. Hematol Oncol Clin North Am. 2006;20:505–522.

77. Makker HK, Barnes PC. Fatal hemoptysis from the pulmonary artery as a late complication of pulmonary irradiation. Thorax. 1991;46:609–610.

78. Villaneuva AG, Lo TCM, Beamis JF. Endobronchial brachytherapy. Clin Chest Med. 1995;16:445–454.

79. Sutedgja G, Baris G, Schaake-Koning C, et al. High dose rates brachytherapy in patients with local recurrences after radiotherapy of non-small cell lung cancer. Int J Radiat Oncol Biol Phys. 1992;24:551–553.

80. Hatlevoll R, Karlsen KO, Skovlund E. Endobronchial radiotherapy for malignant bronchial obstruction or recurrence. Acta Oncol. 1999;38:999–1004.

81. Aurora R, Milite F, Vander Els N. Respiratory emergencies. Semin Oncol. 2000;27:256–269.

82. Brandes JC, Schmidt E, Yung R. Occlusive endobrachial stent placement as a novel management approach to massive hemoptysis from lung cancer. J Thorac Oncol. 2008;3:1071–1072.

83. Schray MF, McDougall JC, Martinez A, et al. Management of malignant airway compromise with laser and low dose brachytherapy: the Mayo Clinic experience. Chest. 1988;93:264–269.

84. Adelman M, Haponik E, Bleeker E, et al. Cryptogenic hemoptysis. Ann Intern Med. 1985;102:829–834.

85. Brinson G, Noone P, Mauro M, et al. Bronchial artery embolization for the treatment of hemoptysis in patients with cystic fibrosis. Am J Resp Crit Care Med. 1998;157:1951–1958.

86. Hirscherg B, Biran I, Glazer M, et al. Hemoptysis: etiology, evaluation, and outcome in a tertiary referral hospital. Chest. 1997;112:440–444.

87. Cole JS, Patchell RA. Metastatic epidural spinal cord compression. Lancet Neurol 2008;7:459–466.

88. Quinn J, DeAngelis L. Neurologic emergencies in the cancer patient. Semin Oncol. 2000;27:311–321.

89. Byrne TN. Metastatic epidural spinal cord compression. In: Black P, Loeffler J (eds.), Cancer of the Nervous System. London: Blackwell Scientific; 1997:664–673.

90. Byrne TN. Spinal cord compression from epidural metastases. N Engl J Med. 1992;327:614–619.

91. Wilkes G. Neurological disturbances. In: Yarbro C, Frogge M, Goodman M (eds.), Cancer Symptom Management. 2nd ed. Boston: Jones and Bartlett; 1999:344–381.

92. Posner J. Neurologic Complications of Cancer. Philadelphia: F.A. Davis; 1995:111–142.

93. Weinstein SM. Management of spinal cord and cauda equina compression. In: Berger AM, Portenoy RK, Weissman DE (eds.), Principles and Practice of Palliative Care and Supportive Oncology. 2nd ed. Philadelphia: Lippincott Williams & Wilkins; 2002:532–543.

94. Bucholtz J. Metastatic epidural spinal cord compression. Semin Oncol Nurs. 1999;15:150–159.

95. Hewitt DJ, Foley KM. Neuroimaging of pain. In: Greenberg JO (ed.), Neuroimaging. New York: McGraw-Hill; 1995:41.

96. Algra PR, Bloem JL, Tissing H. Detection of vertebral body metastases: comparison between MR imaging and bone scintigraphy. Radiographics. 1991;11:219–232.

97. Burger EL, Lindeque BG. Sacral and non-spinal tumors presenting as a backache: a retrospective study of 17 patients. Acta Orthoped Scand. 1994;65:344–346.

98. Abrahm JL. Management of pain and spinal cord compression in patients with advanced cancer. Ann Intern Med. 1999;131:37–46.

99. Gilbert RW, Kim JH, Posner JB. Epidural spinal cord compression from metastatic tumor: diagnosis and treatment. Ann Neurol. 1978;3:40–51.

100. Hainline B, Tuzynski MH, Posner JB. Ataxia in epidural spinal cord compression. Neurol. 1992;42:2193–2195.

101. George R, Jeba J, Ramkumar G, et al. Interventions for the treatment of metastatic extradural spinal cord compression in adults. Cochrane Database Syst Rev. 2008;(4):CD006716. doi:10.1002/14651858. CD006716.pub2.

102. Leppert, W, Buss, T. The role of corticosteroids in the treatment of pain in cancer patients. Curr Pain Headache Rep. 2012;16:307–313.

103. Akram H, Allibone J. Spinal surgery for palliation in malignant spinal cord compression. Clin Oncol. 2010;22:792–800.

104. Sitton E. Nursing implications of radiation therapy. In: Itano J, Toaka K (eds.), Core Curriculum for Oncology Nursing. 3rd ed. Philadelphia: W.B. Saunders; 1998:616–629.

105. Clayton K. Cancer-related hypercalcemia: how to spot it, how to manage it. Am J Nurs.1997;97:42–48.

106. Morton AR, Ritch PS. Hypercalcemia. In: Berger AM, Portenoy RK, Weissman DE (eds.), Principles and Practice of Palliative Care and Supportive Oncology. 2nd ed. Philadelphia: Lippincott Williams & Wilkins; 2002:493–507.

107. Warrell RP. Metabolic emergencies. In: Devita VT, Hellman S, Rosenberg SA (eds.), Cancer Principles and Practice of Oncology. 6th ed. Philadelphia: Lippincott Williams & Wilkins; 2001:2633–2645.

108. Ralston SH. Pathogenesis and management of cancer-associated hypercalcemia. In: Rubens RD, Fogelman I (eds.), Bone Metastases: Diagnosis and Treatment. New York: Springer Verlag; 1991:149–169.

109. Nussbaum SR. Pathophysiology and management of severe hypercalcemia. Endocrinol Metab Clin North Am. 1993;2:343–362.

110. Kovacs CS, MacDonald SM, Chik CL, et al. Hypercalcemia of malignancy in the palliative care patient: a treatment strategy. J Pain Symptom Manage. 1995;10:224–232.

111. King PA. Oncologic emergencies: assessment, identification, and interventions in the emergency department. J Emerg Nurs. 1995;21:213–218.

112. Kuebler KK. Palliative nursing care for the patient experiencing end-stage renal failure. Urol Nurs. 2001;21:167–168, 171–178.

113. Wong MHF, Stockler MR, Pavlakis N. Bone agents for breast cancer. Cochrane Database Syst Rev 2012, Issue 2. Art. No.: CD003474. Available at: http:// http://summaries.cochrane.org/CD003474/bone-agents-for-breast-cancer. Accessed June 30, 2013.

114. Wong RKS, Wiffen PJ. Bisphosphonates for the relief of pain secondary to bone metastases. Cochrane Database Syst Rev 2002, Issue 2. Art. No.: CD002068, Available at: http://www.cochrane.org/reviews/en/ab002068.htm. Accessed June 30, 2013.

115. Gallacher SJ, Ralston SH, Fraser WD. A comparison of low versus high dose pamidronate in cancer-associated hypercalcemia. Bone Miner. 1991;15:249–256.

116. Major P, Lortholary A, Hon J, et al. Zoledronic acid is more effective than pamidronate for hypercalcemia of malignancy. Evid Based Oncol. 2001;2:159–162.

117. Lumachi F, Brunello A, Roma A, Basso U. Medical treatment of malignancy-associated hypercalcemia. Curr Med Chem. 2008;15:415–421.

118. Roemer-Becuwe C, Vigano A, Romano F, et al. Safety of subcutaneous clodronate and efficacy in hypercalcemia of malignancy: a novel route of administration. J Pain Symptom Manage. 2003;26:843–848.

119. Leyland-Jones B. Treatment of cancer-related hypercalcemia: the role of gallium nitrate. Semin Oncol. 2003;30(2 suppl 5):13–19.

120. Mundy GR. Mechanisms of bone metastasis. Cancer. 1997;80: 1546–1556.

121. Leehey DJ, Ing TS. Correction of hypercalcemia and hypophosphatemia by hemodialysis using a conventional, calcium-containing dialysis solution enriched with phosphorus. Am J Kidney Dis. 1997;29:288–290.

CHAPTER 25

Sedation for refractory symptoms

Patti Knight, Laura A. Espinosa,
and Bonnie Freeman

> I can't bear the thought of my dad dying like this; he is such a good man.
> Daughter watching her father suffer with bone pain while dying of cancer

Key points

- Palliative sedation is sedation used to control refractory and intolerable symptoms at the end of life when control of these symptoms is not possible and the person remains awake and alert.

- Proportionality is a concept that implies that a patient's consciousness is reduced just enough to relieve refractory symptoms.

- Determining refractoriness of symptoms and closeness to death can be difficult and requires assessment by a skilled practitioner.

- Clear communication with significant others, precise documentation, and informed consent are necessary.

Palliative care providers are faced with the challenge of managing a multitude of complex symptoms in terminally ill patients. Although many of these symptoms respond to skilled palliative management, others can remain refractory to treatment. Suffering at the end of life involves physical, psychological, social, and spiritual distress. In most situations, multidisciplinary palliative interventions provide effective comfort, but in some instances suffering becomes refractory and intolerable.[1–3]

This chapter explores the use of palliative sedation in the hospital setting. It presents case studies involving palliative sedation, discusses several definitions of palliative sedation, frequency of palliative sedation, reasons for palliative sedation, medications used, guidelines for nursing care, time-to-death issues, ethical considerations, informed consent, and the role of the nurse-caregiver.

The following case provides an example of a clinical situation in which decisions regarding sedation were required.

Case study 1

Mr. C, a 63-year-old man with bladder cancer

Mr. C is a 63-year-old man with a 3-month-old diagnosis of bladder cancer that metastasized to his ribs, spine, pelvis, right clavicle, and right femur and humerus. He was admitted to the acute palliative unit by his primary oncologist for management of uncontrolled pain, depressed mood, and difficulty coping with the cancer diagnosis. His primary oncologist is offering palliative treatment, but is not ruling out curative therapy if Mr. C's overwhelming symptom burden is brought under control. Mr. C, who is divorced, is accompanied by his two children and three siblings. While his family is supportive, they are also having difficulty coping with the cancer diagnosis and with watching their loved one suffer uncontrolled pain. Mr. C was initially started on a hydromorphone infusion (patient-controlled analgesia) for immediate pain relief. Palliative radiation therapy for the tumor in his femur was also started. Adopting a multidisciplinary approach, the primary oncologist asked a psychiatrist to assess Mr. C's depressed mood, an orthopedic surgeon to assess options for femur stabilization, and an anesthesia pain specialist to evaluate the feasibility of a nerve block or other interventions to provide added pain relief. Shortly after admission, Mr. C's femur fractured upon transfer to radiation therapy. Consultants from the orthopedic and pain services felt he was not a candidate for surgery for multiple reasons, including coagulopathies related to his renal cancer. The psychiatrist who evaluated Mr. C diagnosed an adjustment disorder stemming from the stress associated with his cancer diagnosis, and multiple family issues that required immediate attention. The patient and family's distress were compounded by his escalating pain and his dependency and need for daily care. His pain was initially managed by escalating his hydromorphone dose and adding steroids to his regimen. With increasing doses of hydromorphone and the addition of steroids, he developed a delirium. Haloperidol was added to his regimen and he was rotated to methadone. The patient's sensorium cleared, his pain remained difficult to control while he remained awake and alert, and he stated that he did not want further cancer-focused treatment. He acknowledged that his death was near and that he wanted to be sedated in his dying.

Definitions

From terminal sedation to palliative sedation

Numerous efforts have been made to standardize a definition for terminal sedation (this phrase was first used by Enck after a reviewing

Box 25.1 Palliative sedation definitions

Existential suffering (sometimes referred to as **terminal anguish**): Refractory psychological symptoms.

Imminent death: Death that is expected to occur within hours to days based on the person's condition, disease progression, and symptom constellation.

Intent: The purpose or state of mind at the time of an action. Intent of the patient/proxy and healthcare provider is a critical issue in ethical decision-making regarding palliative sedation. Relief of suffering, not hastening or causing death, is the intent of palliative sedation.[1,16]

Palliative sedation: The monitored use of medications intended to provide relief of refractory symptoms by inducing varying degrees of unconsciousness, but not death, in terminally ill patients.[17–20]

Refractory symptom: A symptom that cannot be adequately controlled in a tolerable time frame despite the aggressive use of usual therapies and that seems unlikely to be adequately controlled by further invasive or noninvasive therapies without excessive or intolerable acute or chronic side effects.

series of cases where physical symptoms were treated with sedation at the end of life),[4] and to separate sedation at the end of life from sedation used in other medical settings.[5–10] Terms used for sedation at end of life include "palliative sedation," "terminal sedation," "total sedation," "sedation for intractable symptoms," and "sedation for distress in the imminently dying." Palliative sedation has been termed "slow euthanasia."[11,12] This is not a widely accepted definition of palliative sedation, as the intent of sedation at end of life is to relieve suffering and not to hasten death. In this chapter the term "palliative sedation" will be used for sedation at the end of life. It is defined as the monitored use of medications to induce sedation as a means to control refractory and unendurable symptoms near the end of life.[13,14] The intent is to control symptoms, not hasten death. The acceptance of the term "palliative sedation" over "terminal sedation" has evolved to emphasize the difference between management of refractory symptoms at end of life, and euthanasia.[15] Box 25.1 lists common terms used in relation to palliative sedation.

The goal of palliative sedation is the relief of suffering and includes the concept of proportionality. Proportionality, in this setting, implies that the patient's consciousness is reduced just enough to relieve refractory suffering.[21] Depending on the patient's situation, the level of sedation that is required may be light or deep. The endpoint that is sought is the relief of suffering. This range in the depth of sedation is based on the "intentional administration of sedative drugs in dosages and combinations as required to reduce the consciousness of a terminally ill patient as much as necessary to relieve one or more refractory symptoms."[21–23] This definition reflects proportionality and clearly separates out palliative sedation at end of life from euthanasia.[24–26]

Frequency of palliative sedation

Because the definition of palliative sedation is so varied, it is difficult to determine how often palliative sedation at end of life occurs in practice. Estimates range from 10% to 52%, varying by definition and practice sites.[1,6,14,27–29]

Reasons for palliative sedation

Deep sedation is a usual and accepted standard of practice prior to surgery or an extremely painful or highly distressing procedure. However, sedation at end of life does not have the same level of acceptance.[11,30–32] Common symptoms at the end of life include pain, dyspnea, delirium, nausea, and vomiting, as well as feelings of hopelessness, remorse, anxiety, and loss of meaning. Palliative sedation is most commonly used and accepted for the relief of refractory physical symptoms.[1,33] Claessens and colleagues, in a literature review of palliative sedation, found that the majority of practitioners listed physical symptoms as the reasons for sedation at end of life, with a smaller number indicating existential suffering as the reason for sedation. The most common physical symptoms were listed as delirium, dyspnea, and pain. The nonphysical symptoms were feelings of meaninglessness, being a burden, dependency, death anxiety, and wishing to control the timing and manner of death.[22]

Fainsinger and associates, in a multicenter international study, found that 1% to 4% of terminally ill patients needed sedation for pain, 0% to 6% for nausea and vomiting, 0% to 13% for dyspnea, and 9% to 23% for delirium.[34] Multiple physical and psychological symptoms are common. Chater and colleagues surveyed a number of palliative care experts and asked a series of questions regarding symptoms and palliative sedation in their patients. These clinical experts reported that half of their patients had more than one symptom and that 34% received sedation for nonphysical symptoms such as anguish, fear, panic, anxiety, terror, and emotional, spiritual, or psychological distress.[21,33,35–37]

Various factors that may affect varying standards of practice for palliative sedation include the physician's philosophy of what constitutes a "good death," personal and/or professional experiences, religious beliefs, and level of fatigue or burnout.[34,37,38] Although there is no consensus on the use of palliative sedation for existential suffering, literature suggests that its use in these circumstances may be increasing.[28,34,36,39] Ganzini and colleagues reviewed Oregon physicians' perceptions of reasons for patients request for a hastened death and found avoidance of dependency on others and wanting to control the timing and manner of their death frequently cited.[40–42]

Medications and monitoring

Drugs most commonly used for palliative sedation outside the ICU setting are benzodiazepines, neuroleptics, barbiturates, and anesthetics.[6,43] Midazolam is the most commonly used of these drugs.[9] The drug and route chosen vary based on the route available, location of the patient, and cost, as well as the preference of the provider.[44] Usually in inpatient settings the medications are given intravenously or subcutaneously and continuously. In general, the chosen medication is started at a low dose and titrated upward rapidly until the symptom is controlled and the patient does not evidence signs of distress. Classes of medications used and routes of administration are presented in Table 25.1. Dose ranges are highly variable and determined by the patient's weight, renal and hepatic function, state of hydration, concurrent medication use, and other variables. The right dose is the dose that results in the patient resting comfortably without showing evidence of distress. It is recommended that doses be started low and titrated at approximately 30% an hour until sedation is achieved and the desired

Table 25.1 Medications used for palliative sedation

Medication	Dose and route	Comments
Benzodiazepines/midazolam	Loading dose of 0.5–5.0 mg, followed by 0.5–10 mg/h continuously infused IV or SQ	Monitor for paradoxical agitation with all benzodiazepines
Lorazepam	0.5–5.0 mg every 1–2 h PO, SL, or IV	—
Neuroleptics/haloperidol	Loading dose of 0.5–5.0 mg PO, SL, SC, or IV, followed by an IV bolus of 1–5 mg every 4 h or 1–5 mg/h continuously infused IV or SQ	Monitor for extrapyramidal side effects
Chlorpromazine	12.5–25.0 mg every 2–4 h PO, PR, or IV	More sedating than haloperidol
Barbiturates/pentobarbital	60–200 mg PR every 4–8 h; loading dose of 2–3 mg/kg bolus IV, followed by 1–2 mg/kg/h continuously infused IV	Do not mix with other drugs when given IV
Phenobarbital	Loading dose of 200 mg, followed by 0.5 mg/kg/h continuously injected SQ or IV	—
Anesthetics/propofol	Begin with 2.5–5.0 µg/kg/min and titrate to desired effect every 10 min by increments of 10–20 mg/h	—

IV, intravenously; SQ, subcutaneously; PO, per os; SL, sublingually; PR, per rectum.

Source: Lynch (2003), reference 71.

Richmond Agitation–Sedation Scale (RASS) level is reached.[45,46] The type of medication that can be administered by nurses may be influenced by state regulatory rules. The drugs used for refractory symptoms and terminal weaning in the ICU include opiates, benzodiazepines, neuroleptics, and anesthetics.[47] These drugs can be continually infused and titrated until the patient appears comfortable. Morphine or other opioids are used to provide analgesia and reduce dyspnea. Propofol is a general anesthetic but can be used at sedative doses for ICU patients. Propofol is a good drug of choice because of its rapid onset and rapid offset. Haloperidol is used in the treatment of delirium and can be combined with opiates and sedative agents to manage acute agitation or to protect against delirium in vulnerable patients.[47] The drugs of choice for deep sedation are usually classified as anesthesia medications, and therefore can only be used in monitored settings.

Assessment tools to measure sedation and agitation

Assessment tools to measure sedation and agitation are important in assessing and managing levels of consciousness in patients undergoing palliative sedation.[48] The RASS has demonstrated validity and reliability in medical and surgical, ventilated and nonventilated patients, and in sedated and nonsedated adult ICU patients. The RASS assessment scale is also being used in some palliative care units to assess and monitor patients undergoing mild or intermediate sedation.[46,49]

Guidelines for palliative sedation

Institutional guidelines are important for palliative sedation so that there is a consistent standard of care and essential education for all involved practitioners.[6,9,16,20,29,37] Box 25.2 is a sample checklist for palliative sedation and Table 25.2 is a sample checklist for palliative sedation in an ICU setting. Four factors need to be present for a patient to be considered for palliative sedation. First, the patient is terminally ill; second, the patient has severe symptoms that are refractory to treatment and intolerable to the patient, and a palliative care expert agrees that the symptoms are intractable; third, a DNR order is in effect; and fourth, death is

imminent (within hours to days), although this can be challenging to determine.[6] If the first three conditions exist, sedation may be appropriate for a patient in severe distress who has been unresponsive to skilled palliative interventions.[50] Ethics consultations or patient advocate services have been found to be useful if there is conflict about goals of care and appropriate care of someone near to death, especially in the ICU setting.[51]

Palliative sedation checklist

A major role of the palliative care team is to assist families in making the transition in treatment goals from cure to comfort. Refractory symptoms and the distress they cause can create a very difficult and abrupt need for this transition phase. Use of the interdisciplinary team to both plan for treatment options and participate in family meetings is critical to the success of the team. The social worker plays an important role in assessing caregiver stress and family dynamics, and coordinating family meetings. The chaplain and other psychosocial professionals provide spiritual assistance and counseling and support the decision-makers through anticipatory and actual grief. The nurse is a consistent presence and skilled resource to the patient and family.[43]

Nursing care: back to basics

Communication

An important role of the nurse in the end-of-life process is to facilitate communication and establish trust between the patient, family members,[53–55] and healthcare providers. Communication is vital to developing a relationship of trust and avoiding conflict during any illness, but it becomes even more important when dealing with end-of-life issues. The team has to build a trusting relationship with patients and families as they make difficult decisions together. If the patient or family members do not trust the healthcare team, conflict is likely. Communication includes (1) being honest and truthful; (2) letting the patient and family members know they will not be abandoned; (3) including

Box 25.2 Palliative sedation checklist

Part A. Background

- Confirm patient has
  - Irreversible advanced disease.
  - Apparent imminent death within hours, days, or weeks.
  - A "do not attempt resuscitation" order.
- Confirm that symptoms are refractory to other therapies that are acceptable to the patient and have a reasonable/practical potential to achieve comfort goals.
- Consider obtaining a peer consultation to confirm that the patient is near death with refractory symptoms.
- Complete informed consent process for palliative sedation.
- Discontinue interventions not focused on comfort.
  - Discontinue routine laboratory and imaging studies.
  - Review medications, limit to those for comfort, and adjust for ease of administration (timing and route).
  - Discontinue unnecessary cardiopulmonary and vital sign monitoring.
  - Review the role of cardiac support devices (e.g., pacemaker) and disable functioning implanted defibrillators.
    - Develop a plan for the use or withdrawal of nutrition and hydration during palliative sedation.
    - Identify a location and an environment acceptable for providing palliative sedation.
    - Use providers familiar with palliative sedation and the use of sedatives.

Part B. Treatment/care of the patient

- Institute and maintain aspiration precautions.
- Provide mouth care and eye protection.
- Use oxygen only for comfort, not to maintain a specific blood oxygen saturation.
- Provide medications primarily by IV or SQ route.
- Maintain bowel, bladder, and pressure point care.
- Continue, do not taper, routine opioids.
- Provide sedating medication.
  - Titrate to symptom control not level of consciousness, using frequent reevaluation.
  - Limit vital sign monitoring to temperature and respiratory rate for dyspnea.
- Choose sedating medication based on provider experience, route available, and patient location.

Home initial dosing (choose one):

- Chlorpromazine, 25 mg suppository or 12.5 mg IV infusion every 4–6 h
- Midazolam, 0.4 mg/h by continuous IV or SQ infusion
- Lorazepam, 0.5–2.0 mg IV sublingually every 4–6 h

Hospital initial dosing (choose one):

- Chlorpromazine, 12.5–25.0 mg every 4–6 h
- Midazolam, 0.4 mg/h by continuous IV or SQ infusion
- Amobarbital or thiopental, 20 mg/h by continuous IV infusion
- Propofol, 2.5 mg/kg/min by continuous IV infusion

Source: Lynch (2003), reference 71.

Table 25.2 Checklist for intensive care unit personnel end-of-life criterion

Assessment	MET	NOT MET
1. Determine that primary physician, critical care physician, family, and possibly patient are in agreement with discontinuation of life-sustaining treatment.	——	——
2. Assist family in preparation or fulfillment of familial or religious predeath rituals.	——	——
3. Place "do not resuscitate" orders on chart.	——	——
4. Provide a calm, quiet, restful atmosphere free of medical devices and technology for the patient and family, including dimming the lights in the room.	——	——
5. Turn off arrhythmia detection and turn off or decrease all auditory alarms at bedside and central station.	——	——
6. Remove all monitoring equipment from patient and patient's room except for the electrocardiograph (ECG).	——	——
7. Remove all devices unless the removal of the device would create discomfort for the patient (e.g., sequential compression device, nasogastric tube).	——	——
8. Remove or discontinue treatments that do not provide comfort to the patient.	——	——
9. Obtain orders to discontinue test and laboratory studies.	——	——
10. Liberalize visitation.	——	——
11. Notify chaplain and social worker of end-of-life care; obtain grief packet from chaplain.	——	——
12. Determine that family participants in the end-of-life process are present, if appropriate; place sufficient chairs in the patient's room for family members.	——	——
13 Maintain the patient's personal comfort and dignity with attention to hygiene, hairstyle, and providing moisturizers for lips and eyes.	——	——
14. Frequent assessment of the patient's condition assists in titrating medications per end-of-life protocol and level of patient discomfort.	——	——
15. Document the patient's signs and symptoms that indicate discomfort, including but not limited to the following:	——	——

Agitated behavior	Grimacing
Altered cognition	Increased work of breathing
Anxiety	Irritation
Autonomic hyperactivity	Moaning
Confusion	Pain
Coughing	Perspiration
Dyspnea	Tachypnea
Restlessness	Tension
Self-report of symptoms	Trembling
Splinting	
Stiffness	
Tachycardia	

16. Remain at bedside to

    a. assess patient for comfort/discomfort.

    b. promptly administer sedation, analgesics.

    c. provide emotional support to patient and family.

    d. ask patient/family if additional comfort measures are needed.

Assessment	MET	NOT MET
17. Obtain physician orders for additional or alterations in pain and sedation medications if the end-of-life protocol medications are ineffective in controlling the patient's discomfort.	——	——
18. Support and educate the patient's family regarding interpretation of the clinical signs and symptoms the patient may experience during the end of life.	——	——
19. Assess the family's need to be alone with the patient during and after the death process.	——	——
20. Assess the family to determine the amount of support they require during the end-of-life process.	——	——

(continued)

Table 25.2 Continued

Assessment	MET	NOT MET
21. Assist the family in meeting its needs and the patient's needs for communication, final expressions of love, and concern (e.g., holding a hand, talking with the patient, remembering past events).	—	—
22. Discuss signs of death and how the physician will pronounce the patient; the family will be asked to leave the room while the physician examines the patient.	—	—
23. Notify intensive care unit physician to pronounce patient. An ECG strip of a straight line or asystole is not needed to document patient death.	—	—
24. Notify primary care physician.	—	—
25. Assist family with decisions regarding need for autopsy.	—	—
26. Notify clinical nurse specialist Monday through Friday before 3 PM to complete death paperwork.	—	—
27. Notify in-house administrator after 3 PM and on weekends to complete death paperwork.	—	—
28. Notify chaplain, if chaplain not present.	—	—
29. If the patient is to have an autopsy, leave all tubes in place; if no autopsy, remove all tubes (IV lines may be clamped instead of removed).	—	—
30. Permit family visitation after the patient has been cleaned and tubes removed.	—	—
31. Prepare patient for the morgue, shroud, etc.	—	—

MET, indicates that the individual is prepared, follows suggested steps in appropriate sequence, and demonstrates minimal safe practice; NOT MET, indicates that the individual is unprepared, needs repeated assistance or suggestions in order to proceed, and or omits necessary steps.

Source: M.D. Anderson Cancer Center, Houston, Texas. Reprinted with permission.

the patient and family in care decisions; (4) helping the patient and family explore all options; (5) asking the patient and family to clearly define what they need from the team; (6) working to ensure that the entire team knows and understands the plan; and, most important, (7) practicing active listening when talking to the patient and family members.[56,57] In a qualitative study examining nurses' perceptions of palliative sedation, two factors made nurses more comfortable with their role in the dying process. The first was how well the nurse knew the patient as a person, and the second was the interdisciplinary team collaboration.[58]

When the decision is made to use palliative sedation, caring and thoughtful communication make a tremendous difference in the family's experience with the death of their loved one. The patient and/or family healthcare agent are central in this decision, and need ongoing reassurance that the decision made is the right one. They may need frequent confirmation that the person is dying of their disease, and that the intent of the sedation is to ensure a peaceful death but not to hasten death. The concept of "presence" with the patient and family during the death vigil is difficult to quantify, but critical during periods of extreme distress.[59] Untreated symptoms cause families and staff to be traumatized by a "horrible death" (Table 25.3) The family may fear that this "final event" will be equally traumatic. They don't want their loved one to suffer any more. They need constant explanations and reassurance about what to expect, what is happening, and the opportunity to express their grief.

Physical care

As the patient becomes more sedated, protective reflexes decrease. The ability to clear secretions decreases. This can be anticipated, and appropriate medication should be given proactively. Suctioning is kept to a minimum and only done if absolutely necessary. The blink reflex also decreases and eyes can become dry, requiring frequent eye drops (artificial tears).

Bowel and bladder management should be carefully monitored to maintain comfort. A urinary catheter is often appropriate to minimize the need for frequent changing and cleaning. Allowing the family to decide what basic comfort care they want provided to their loved one at end of life allows the family some sense of control in an uncontrollable situation. Some family members may want to assist in the care of their loved one, and helping with bathing, brushing the hair, and applying a lubricant to the lips can be quite meaningful to some family members. Other family members may prefer not to help with physical care and they should be reassured that their presence alone, even if in spirit only, is equally important.[43]

Time to death
Palliative sedation

One of the concerns many people have with palliative sedation is that it might hasten death. Part of this concern stems from the difficulty in predicting the time of death. Several studies using different methodologies have examined effects of sedation on survival rates.[50,60–62] The mean time-to-death in a large four-country study ranged from 1.9 to 3.2 days,[34] and the median time to death in a Taiwanese study was 5 days.[63] A study of patients in Japanese hospices indicated that sedating medications did not shorten life span.[60] However, because of ethical considerations none of these studies were controlled trials, so it is not possible to determine whether sedation may or may not result in hastening death. In situations of unbearable distress, sedation remains an appropriate option to relieve suffering.[64]

Ethical considerations concerning palliative sedation

Palliative sedation is a medical therapy for the imminently dying when pain and suffering are intolerable, and other interventions have proved inadequate. Intent is the critical issue, and separates palliative sedation at the end of life from assisted dying and

Table 25.3 Management of distressing physical symptoms

Symptom	Considerations before defining a symptom as refractory
Agitation and confusion	Discontinue all nonessential medications.
	Change required medications to ones less likely to cause delirium.
	Check for bladder distention and rectal impaction.
	Evaluate for undiagnosed or undertreated pain.
	Review role of hydration therapy.
	Consider evaluation and therapy for potentially reversible processes, such as hypoxia, hyponatremia, and hypercalcemia.
Pain	Maximize opioid, nonopioid, and adjuvant analgesics including agent, route, and schedule.
	Consider other therapies, including invasive/neurosurgical procedures, environmental changes, wound care, physical therapy, and psychotherapy.
	Anticipate and aggressively manage analgesic side effects.
Shortness of breath	Provide oxygen therapy.
	Maximize opioid and anxiolytic therapy.
	Review the role of temporizing therapy, including thoracentesis, stents, and respiratory therapy.
Muscle twitching	Differentiate from seizure activity.
	Remember the use of opioid rotation, clonidine, and benzodiazepines if muscle twitching is caused by high-dose opioids.

Source: Cowan and Palmer (2002), reference 6.

euthanasia. With sedation the intent is to produce somnolence and relieve suffering, not hasten death. In assisted dying—where the intent is to produce death to relieve suffering—the agent is the patient. In euthanasia—the intent is to produce death to relieve suffering—the agent is another. The ethical and legal principles that apply to palliative sedation are patient autonomy (patient's choice), beneficence (do good), nonmaleficence (do no harm), and the principle of double effect.[6,17-21,65] The reader is referred to chapter 64 for a more in-depth discussion on ethical principles and issues in palliative care and end-of-life care.

In 1997, the US Supreme Court ruled unanimously that "there is no constitutional right to physician-assisted suicide" but "terminal sedation is intended for symptom relief and not assisted suicide. ... and is appropriate in the aggressive practice of palliative care."[66-68] The American Nurses Association and the Oncology Nursing Society have position papers opposed to physician-assisted suicide.[69,70] Although neither of the position papers addresses the exact issue of palliative sedation, both support the risk of hastening death through treatments aimed at alleviating suffering or controlling symptoms as ethically and legally acceptable. The Hospice and Palliative Nurses Association has issued a position paper in support of palliative sedation.[17] The use of palliative sedation for existential suffering remains controversial.[35,36]

Informed consent

Informed consent is always a process. A patient's symptoms may have been difficult to control over time and may have escalated as the patient's disease has progressed. Patients (or their agents when they cannot speak for themselves) must always be involved in these decisions. Palliative sedation involves an important trade-off between symptom control and alertness, and different patients will weigh this differently. The need for sedation may be a palliative care emergency to relieve distress, and consent would be similar to obtaining consent in any other emergency situation. A family meeting to discuss the situation would then follow.

A family meeting includes a well-planned, compassionate, and clear discussion with the patient and family about the patient's goals and values in the setting of end-of-life care. The bedside nurse is an important participant in these meetings to provide insight into the care and support needed by the family. It is important to plan these meetings carefully if at all possible, to ensure that the appropriate family members are present. Allowing the designated decision-maker to invite significant people to the planned meeting allows key participants to hear the information at the same time. A religious or spiritual representative can be helpful at these meetings, if the family so desires.

The primary physician usually begins the family meeting with a brief, clear report on the current condition of the patient. Supporting documentation of the current condition, such as recent laboratory data or other diagnostic test results, may be helpful to some families. The patient and or family should be provided all the time necessary to raise concerns, clarify information, and have their questions answered.[54,55] The same questions may be raised time and time again to different team members and need to be answered with consistent information to reduce uncertainty. Next, the treatment options should be discussed. When discussing terminal sedation options, it is important to assess the patient's and family's cultural and religious beliefs and concerns. Documentation in the chart should include the parties present, the reason for sedation (symptom distress), and the primary goal (patient comfort), as well as patient terminal status, notation of any professional consultations, documentation that the patient is near death and has refractory symptoms, planned discontinuance of treatments not focused on comfort, plan regarding hydration and nutrition, and anticipated risks or burdens of sedation.[52]

Either at the end of the family meeting, or the next day in nonemergency cases, some institutions require that an informed consent document be signed by the patient, family, or healthcare agent. Because it usually is not possible to communicate verbally with the sedated patient, it is important to make sure that the patient and family are given time to talk with each other and say their goodbyes, if that is possible, prior to proceeding with sedation. A well-planned family meeting decreases miscommunication and supports the family during a difficult decision-making time by allowing all pertinent parties to hear the same information at the same time. The decision for palliative sedation or terminal wean is a patient/agent/family decision (whoever is the decision-maker) with guidance from the palliative care team.

The nurse caregiver

In a literature review examining the experience of nurses caring for terminally ill patients in ICU settings, several barriers related to provision of terminal care were identified. These included: (1) lack of involvement in the plan of care and comfort; (2) disagreement among physicians and other healthcare team members; (3) inadequacy of pain relief; (4) unrealistic expectations of families; (5) personal difficulty coping; (6) lack of experience and education; (7) staffing levels; and (8) environmental circumstances.[71] In a Japanese study of 2607 nurses involved in palliative sedation, 37% reported they wanted to leave their current jobs because of the burden of palliative sedation; 12% reported that their involvement in palliative sedation made them feel helpless; and 11% would avoid a patient who is being treated with palliative sedation if possible. This study concluded that a significant number of nurses felt serious emotional burdens related to palliative sedation.[72]

Nurses who work with patients requiring palliative sedation are at increased risk of burnout if not intimately involved with the team decision-making process. In addition, if left out of decision-making processes such as the team planning and family conferences, they are denied the information needed for effective counseling at the patient's bedside. A formal and informal support system for nurses as well as education in end-of-life care, spiritual support, and individual support are essential.[72]

An interdisciplinary team meeting after the death of the patient can function as both a learning experience and a debriefing session. Working in an environment that recognizes the need for support and education of staff, and one that recognizes the importance of mentors and advanced practice nurses, allows nurses to face these challenges as they arise.

Conclusion

Although nurses and other healthcare practitioners may disagree about what a "good death" is, there is general agreement about what is a "bad death." Palliative sedation is a necessary option for a small number of patients with refractory and intolerable symptoms and suffering at end of life. These options are part of the spectrum of palliative care and are ethically and legally supported. However, the ability to determine refractoriness of symptoms can be complicated and is largely dependent on the skills of the practitioner and the tools available to manage complex symptoms. Nurses have a central role in ensuring that a dying patient undergoing palliative sedation

has his or her symptoms well controlled, and that the family members are well supported. Education of palliative care nurses in these areas is essential.

References

1. Breura E. Palliative sedation: when and how? J Clin Oncol. 2012;30(12): 1258–1259.
2. Sanft T, Hauser J, Rosielle D, et al. Physical pain and emotional suffering: the case for palliative sedation. J Pain. 2009;10(3):238–242
3. Elsayem A, Curry E III, Boohene J, et al. Use of palliative sedation for intractable symptoms in the palliative care unit of a comprehensive cancer center. Support Care Cancer. 2009;17:53–59.
4. Enck RE. Drug-induced terminal sedation for symptom control. Am J Hosp Palliat Care. 1991;84:332–337.
5. Beel AC, Hawranik PG, McClement S, Daeninck P. Palliative sedation: Nurses' perceptions. Int J Palliat Nurs. 2006;12(11):510–518.
6. Cowan JD, Palmer TW. Practical guide to palliative sedation. Curr Oncol Rep. 2002;4:242–249.
7. Chater S, Viola R, Paterson J, Jarvis V. Sedation for intractable distress in the dying: a survey of experts. Palliat Med. 1998;12:255–269.
8. Cherny NI, Portenoy RK. Sedation in the management of refractory symptoms: guidelines for evaluation and treatment. J Palliat Care. 1994;10:31–38.
9. De Graeff A, Dean M. Palliative sedation therapy in the last weeks of life: a literature review and recommendations for standards. J Palliat Med. 2007;10(1):67–87.
10. Mercandante S, Intravaia G, Villari P, et al. Controlled sedation for refractory symptoms in dying patients. J Pain Symptom Manage. 2009;37:771–779.
11. Billings JA, Block SD. Slow euthanasia. J Palliat Care. 1996;12:21–30.
12. Claessens P, Menten J, Schotsmans P, Broeckaert B. Palliative sedation, not slow euthanasia: a prospective, longitudinal study of sedation in Flemish Palliative Care Units. J Pain Symptom Manage. 2011; 41: 14–24
13. Davis MP. Does palliative sedation always relieve symptoms? J Palliat Med. 2009;12:875–877
14. Hasselaar JC, Verhagen SC, Vissers KC. When cancer symptoms cannot be controlled: the role of palliative sedation. Curr Opin Support Palliat Care. 2009;3:14–23.
15. Koh YH, Lee OK, Wu HY. "Palliative" and not "terminal" sedation. J Pain Symptom Manage. 2009;37:e6–e8.
16. Berger JT. Rethinking guidelines for the use of palliative sedation. Hastings Cent Rep. 2010;40(3):32–38.
17. Hospice and Palliative Nurses Association. Position Statement: Palliative Sedation. Pittsburgh, PA: HPNA; 2011. Available at: www.hpna.org/DispalyPage.aspx?Title=Position%20Statements. Accessed December 20, 2013.
18. Kirk TW, Mahon MM. National Hospice and Palliative Care Organization (NHPCO) position statement and commentary on the use of palliative sedation in imminently dying terminally ill patients. J Pain Symptom Manage. 2010;39(5):914–923.
19. American Medical Association Report of the Council of Ethical and Judicial Affairs. Sedation to Unconsciousness at End of Life. CEJA Report 5-A-08. Available at www.ama-assn.org/resources/doc/code-medical-ethics/2201A.pdf. Accessed December 20, 2013.
20. Cherny NI, Radbruch L. European Association for Palliative Care (EAPC-recommended framework for the use of sedation in palliative care. Palliative Med. 2009;23:581–593.
21. Sulmasy D, Coyle N. Palliative sedation. In Doka KJ, Tucci AS, Corr CA, Jennings B (eds.), End-of-Life Ethics: A Case Study Approach. Washington, DC: Hospice Foundation of America; 2012:109–125.
22. Claessens P, Menten J, Schotsmans P, Broeckaert B. Palliative sedation: a review of the research literature. J Pain Symptom Manage. 2008;36(3):310–333.
23. Sulmasy DP, Curlin F, Brungardt CS, Cavanaugh T. Justifying different levels of palliative sedation. Ann Intern Med. 2010;152:332–333.

24. Broeckart B. Palliative sedation, physician assisted death and euthanasia: "same, same, different"? Am J Bioeth. 2011;11:62–64.

25. Carvalho TB, Rady MY, Verheijde JL, Robert JS. Continuous deep sedation in end of life care: disentangling palliation from physician assisted death. Am J Bioeth. 2011;11:60–62.

26. Lipuma SH. The lacking of moral equivalency for continuous sedation and PAS. Am J Bioeth. 2011;11(6):48–49.

27. Wein S. Sedation in the imminently dying patient. Oncology. 2000;14: 585–601.

28. Cherny N. Sedation for the care of patients with advanced cancer. Nat Clin Pract Oncol. 2006;3(9):492–500.

29. Rousseau P. Existential suffering and palliative sedation: a brief commentary with a proposal for clinical guidelines. Am J Hosp Palliat Care. 2001;18:151–153.

30. Morita T, Tsuneto S, Shima Y. Proposed definitions of sedation for symptom relief: a systematic literature review and a proposal of operation criteria. J Pain Symptom Manage. 2002;24:447–453.

31. Hallenbeck JL. Terminal sedation: ethical implications in different situations. J Palliat Med. 2000;3:313–320.

32. Hauser K, Walsh D. Palliative sedation: welcome guidance on a controversial issue. Palliative Med. 2009;23:577–579.

33. Rich BA. Terminal suffering and the ethics of palliative sedation. Camb Q Healthc Ethics. 2012;21:30–39.

34. Fainsinger RL, Waller A, Bercovici M, Bengtson K, Landman W, Hosking M, et al. A multicentre international study of sedation for uncontrolled symptoms in terminally ill patients. Palliat Med. 2000;14:257–265.

35. Bruce A, Boston P. Relieving existential suffering through palliative sedation: discussion of an uneasy practice. J Adv Nurs. 2011;67:2732–2740.

36. Schuman-Olivier Z, Brendel DH, Forstein M, Price BH. The use of palliative sedation for existential distress: a psychiatric perspective. Harv Rev Psychiatry. 2008;16:339–351.

37. Patel B, Gorawarta-Bhat R, Levine S, Shega JW. Nurses' attitudes and experiences surrounding palliative sedation: components for developing policy for nursing professionals. J Palliat Med. 2012;15:432–437.

38. Feen E. Continuous deep sedation: consistent with physician's role as healer. Am J Bioeth. 2011;11:49–51.

39. Raus K, Sterckx S, Mortier F. Is continuous sedation at the end of life an ethically preferable alternative to physician assisted suicide? Am J Bioeth. 2011;11:32–40.

40. Aungst H. "Death with dignity": the first decade of Oregon's physician-assisted death act. Geriatrics. 2008;63:20–24.

41. Hedberg K, Hopkins D, Leman R, Kohn M. The 10-year experience of Oregon's Death with Dignity Act: 1998–2007. J Clin Ethics. 2009;20(2):124–132

42. Ganzini L, Dobscha SK, Heintz RT, Press N. Oregon physicians' perceptions of patients who request assisted suicide and their families. J Palliat Med. 2003:6:381–390.

43. Lynch M. Care of the actively dying patient. In: Dahlin CM, Lynch MT (eds.), Core Curriculum for the Advanced Practice Nurse. 2nd ed. Pittsburgh, PA: Hospice and Palliative Nurses Association; 2013:573–574.

44. Alonso-Babarro A, Varela-Cerdeira M, Torres-Vigil I, Rodriquez-Barrientos R, Bruera E. At home palliative sedation for end-of-life cancer patients. Palliat Med. 2010;24(5):486–492.

45. Sessler CN, Jo Grap M, Ramsay MA. Evaluating and monitoring analgesia and sedation in the intensive care unit. Crit Care. 2008;12(Suppl 3):15.

46. Arenalo JJ, Brinkkemper T, van der Heide A, et al. Palliative sedation: reliability and validity of sedation scales. J Pain Symptom Manage. 2012 44(5):704–714

47. Troug RD, Campbell M, Curtis JR, Hass CE, Luce J, Rubenfeld GD, et al. Recommendations for end-of-life care in the intensive care unit: a consensus statement by the American College of Critical Care Medicine. Crit Care Med. 2008;36:953–963.

48. Claessens P, Menten J, Schotsmans P, Broeckaert B. Level of consciousness in dying patients: the role of palliative sedation: a longitudinal prospective study. Am J Hosp Palliat Care. 2012;29:195–200.

49. Benitez-Rosario M, Castillo-Padros M, Garrido-Bernet B, Ascanio-Leon B. Quality of care in palliative sedation: audit and compliance monitoring of a clinical protocol. J Pain Symptom Manage. 2012;44:532–541.

50. Rietjens JA, van Zuylen L, van Veluiw H, et al. Palliative sedation in a specialized unit for acute palliative care in a cancer hospital: comparing patients dying with and without palliative sedation. J Pain Symptom Manage. 2008;36:228–234.

51. Wiegand DL, Russo MM. Ethical considerations. In: Dahlin CM, Lynch MT (eds.), Core Curriculum for the Advanced Practice Nurse. 2nd ed. Pittsburgh, PA: Hospice and Palliative Nurses Association; 2013:52–53.

52. Lynch M. Palliative sedation. Clin J Oncol Nurs. 2003;7:653–667.

53. Van Doorin S, van Veluiw HT, van Zuylen L, et al. Exploration of concerns of relatives during continuous palliative sedation of their family members with cancer. J Pain Symptom Manage. 2009;38:452–459.

54. Bruinsma SM, Rietjens JAC, Seymour JE, Rotterdam EMC, van der Heide A. The experience of relatives with the practice of palliative sedation: a systematic review. J Pain Symptom Manage. 2012;44(3):431–445.

55. Bruinsma S, Rietjens J, van der Heide A. Palliative sedation: a focus group study on the experience of relatives. J Palliat Med. 2012;16(4): 349–355.

56. Dahlin CM. Communication in palliative care: an essential component for nurses, In: Ferrell BR, Coyle N (eds.), Oxford Textbook of Palliative Nursing. Oxford: Oxford University Press; 2010:107–133.

57. Peereboom K, Coyle N. Facilitating goals of care discussions for patients with life limiting disease: communication strategies for nurses. J Hosp Palliat Nurs. 2012;14(4):251–258.

58. Beel A, McClement S, Harlos M. Palliative sedation therapy: a review of definitions and usage. Int J Palliat Nurs. 2002;8:190–199.

59. Pitorak EF. Care at the time of death: how nurses can make the last hours of life a richer, more comfortable experience. Am J Nurs. 2003;103:42–53.

60. Morita T, Tsunoda J, Inoue S, Chihara S. Effects of high-dose opioids and sedatives on survival in terminally ill cancer patients. J Pain Symptom Manage. 2001;21:282–289.

61. Maltoni M, Scarpi E, Rosati M, et al. Palliative sedation in end-of-life care and survival: a systematic review. J Clin Oncol. 2012;30:1378–1383.

62. Maltoni M, Pittureri C, Scarpi E, et al. Palliative sedation therapy does not hasten death: results from a prospective multicenter study. Ann Oncol. 2009;20(7):1163–1169.

63. Chiu TY, Hu WY, Lue BH, Cheng SY, Chen CY. Sedation for refractory symptoms of terminal cancer patients in Taiwan. J Pain Symptom Manage. 2001;21:467–472.

64. Seale C. Continuous deep sedation in medical practice: a descriptive study. J Pain Symptom Manage. 2010;39:44–53.

65. National Ethics Committee of the Veterans Health Administration. The Ethics of Palliative Sedation. Washington, DC: Department for Veterans Affairs: National Center of Ethics in Health Care; 2008.

66. Orentlicher D. The Supreme Court and physician-assisted suicide: rejecting assisted suicide but embracing euthanasia. N Engl J Med. 1997;337: 1236–1239.

67. Burt RA. The Supreme Court speaks: not assisted suicide but a constitutional right to palliative care. N Engl J Med. 1997;337:1234–1236.

68. Vacco v Quill, 521 U.S. 793, 1997.

69. American Nurses Association. Code of Ethics for Nurses with Interpretive Statements. Washington, DC: American Nurses Association, 2001. Position Statement on Euthanasia, Assisted Suicide and Aid in Dying—approved 04/20/13.

70. Oncology Nursing Society. Position Statement on the Nurse's Responsibility to the Patient Requesting Assisted Suicide, revised 1/2013. Available at http://www.ons.org/about-ons/ons-position-statements/ethics-and-human-rights/nurses-responsibility-patients-requesting Accessed August 8, 2014

71. Espinosa L, Young E, Walsh T. Barriers to ICU nurses providing terminal care: an integrated literature review. Crit Care Nurse. 2008;31:83–93.

72. Morita T, Miyashita M, Kimura R, Adachi I, Shima Y. Emotional burden of nurses in palliative sedation therapy. Palliat Med. 2004;18:550–557.

CHAPTER 26

Complementary and alternative therapies in palliative care

Kate Kravits

My husband is a changed man. I think he was lost and now he has found himself again.
Wife of patient SC receiving nurse-led hypnosis

Key points

- Complementary therapies can improve quality of life in patients with cancer and those who are cancer survivors.

- Complementary therapies reduce physical, psychosocial, and spiritual symptoms and the suffering with which they are associated.

- Complementary therapies offer the patient an opportunity to develop enhanced feelings of self-efficacy.

- Nurses empower patients and families by providing education and guidance in the safe utilization of complementary therapies.

Introduction to complementary and alternative therapies

There is worldwide use of complementary and alternative medicine (CAM) by cancer patients.[1] Patients elect to use CAM therapies for many reasons, such as a desire to improve their health and well-being (Box 26.1).[2] It is common for physicians and nurses who provide care for cancer patients to have limited or no knowledge of these therapies or their benefits and risks.[3] Many CAM therapies do not have established safety and efficacy. In the absence of informed dialogue with their physicians and nurses, patients seek information about these therapies from sources that may or may not be reliable. It is difficult for most people to distinguish between reputable treatments and promotions of unproven therapies pushed by vested interests. Understanding CAM is complicated because of its unfamiliar terminology, large numbers of available therapies, the abundance of controversial anecdotal stories, and the lack of well-designed research studies. It is confusing for patients, families, doctors, and nurses to navigate the abundance of information and to determine the most effective and safest choices.

Complementary medicine has become an important aspect of palliative and supportive cancer care.[4] Palliative care has a broad mission of reducing suffering by providing symptom relief in a patient-focused, systems-oriented manner. It is holistic in its approach and strives to address needs originating in all the domains of experience: physical, cultural, psychological, social, spiritual, legal, and ethical.[5] Patient interest in CAM therapies and the palliative care mission of reducing suffering compel oncologists and nurses to develop their knowledge and competence in complementary and alternative therapies.

The focus in this chapter is on evidence-based complementary therapies. Alternative therapies will be discussed in a limited manner in order to provide a context for understanding the range of CAM therapies that are used by patients. Cancer is used as a model of a chronic progressive disease that illuminates opportunities for the use of CAM therapies.

Patients are more likely to use complementary therapies outside of the influence of a provider.[6] The independent use of evidence-based complementary therapies by patients often promotes feelings of self-efficacy with hopeful and positive attitudes arising from these feelings. Patients can participate in their care by knowing that they have options to promote comfort and quality of life. It is the role of nurses to educate themselves, their patients, and patients' families and to assist in responsible decision-making related to the use of evidence-based complementary therapies.

The goals of this chapter are (1) to define terms related to CAM; (2) to list, define, and describe the benefits and risks of the most common CAM therapies; (3) to emphasize the most beneficial, evidenced-based complementary therapies along with the supportive research; and (4) to describe the role of the nurse as educator, researcher, and clinical practitioner in the CAM setting. Patients look to their nurses to guide them to make informed and safe complementary therapy choices. Nurses can bring hope and a sense of empowerment to their patients and families by teaching, supporting, and encouraging the use of safe complementary therapies when indicated.

Box 26.1 Reasons for use of complementary and alternative medicine

Poor prognosis
Focus of care is comfort not cure
Desire to be more active in one's own healthcare
Reduce side effects of treatment
Reduce side effects of the disease
Desire to cover all the options
Suggestions by family/friends/society to try CAM
Philosophical or cultural orientation
Less expensive than conventional medicine
Easier access to health food store than physician
Dissatisfaction with or loss of trust in conventional medicine
Desire to treat the disease in a "natural" way
Hope of altering the disease progression
Decrease the feelings of helplessness and hopelessness
Improve the immune system
Improve overall health
Improve the quality of one's life

Table 26.1 Evidence-based complementary medicine therapies for symptom control and quality of life

Physical	Cognitive
Acupuncture	Art therapy
Acupressure	Biofeedback
Aromatherapy	Creative visualization
Chiropractic medicine	Focused breathing
Exercise	Guided imagery
Massage	Hypnosis
Nutrition	Meditation
Polarity	Music therapy
Qigong	Progressive muscle relaxation
Reflexology	
Reiki	
Shiatsu	
Therapeutic touch	
Yoga	

Definitions

The National Center for Complementary and Alternative Medicine defines CAM as "a group of diverse medical and health care systems, practices, therapies, and products that are not presently considered to be part of conventional medicine".[7] Complementary and alternative medicine therapies range along a continuum of safety and efficacy. Safety and efficacy must be established for CAM therapies just as it is for standard medical therapies in order for clinicians to be able to ethically recommend their use.[8] The list of what is considered to be CAM changes continually, as therapies that are proven to be safe and effective are adopted into conventional healthcare.

Although they are grouped together, complementary and alternative therapies are very different. Complementary therapies are used as adjuncts to and integrated with conventional care for the purpose of reducing suffering through symptom management[2] (Table 26.1). In research conducted by Hunt and colleagues (2010), it was found that CAM was more likely to be used by people with disturbed mood (anxiety and depression), perceptions of lack of social support, females, and those having a higher income level.[9]

In contrast, alternative therapies are used in place of surgery, chemotherapy, and radiation therapies. They are invasive, biologically active, and unproven, and are promoted as viable cures and alternatives to be used in place of mainstream cancer treatments.[10] Some examples of alternative therapies are Laetrile, dietary cancer cures, oxygen therapy, and biomagnetics. There is not a single alternative intervention (as opposed to mainstream therapies) that has been demonstrated to constitute an effective cure for cancer. The purveyors of alternative therapies can misguide, raise false hopes, and financially exploit patients, and these treatments may be associated with significant risks. They may prevent patients from seeking known, helpful medical oncological interventions.[10]

Integrative healthcare is defined by Deng and colleagues (2010) "as prospective, relationship-based, patient-centered, comprehensive, and holistic healthcare that focuses on patients' priorities for well-being, as well as preventing, managing, rehabilitating, and palliating diseases and injuries".[4] Integrative oncology medicine promotes the use of evidence-based complementary therapies along with mainstream cancer treatments. An example of an integrative oncology program is found at a major comprehensive cancer center, Memorial Sloan-Kettering Cancer Center (MSKCC) in New York City. Complementary therapy practitioners of massage, reflexology, Reiki, meditation, acupuncture, art therapy, and music therapy work with inpatients who have been self-referred or referred by doctors, nurses, or other hospital professionals. Outpatients are offered these same therapies along with nutritional counseling, yoga, Tai chi, Qigong, and other exercise classes.

History

The history of medicine is filled with descriptions of persons using herbs, potions, and physical and spiritual manipulations to heal the sick. Traditional medicine came into being in the United States in the late 1890s, when physicians began to develop the science of medicine, with a focus on cure. Anything other than the allopathic physician using science-based diagnosis and prescribing tested medicines began to be considered quackery. Recently, however, there has been a resurgence of interest in the use of herbal and other CAM therapies that fall outside mainstream medicine. People are living longer with chronic diseases, cancer being one of them. Patients look to CAM therapies to help with quality of life, to allow them to participate in their own self-care, and to provide a glimmer of hope.[2] The increasing use of CAM by Americans prompted the United States Congress to establish in 1992 the Office of Alternative Medicine (OAM) as part of the National Institutes of Health (NIH). In 1998, the name was changed to the National Center for Complementary and Alternative Medicine (NCCAM) and a larger budget was assigned. The mission of NCCAM is to explore complementary and alternative healing practices in the context of rigorous science, to train CAM researchers, and to inform the public and health professionals about the results of CAM research studies.

Prevalence

General population

The use of CAM by the general population in the United States is common and widespread. In a national health interview survey conducted by the Centers for Disease Control and Prevention (CDC) in 2007, use of CAM therapies among US adults was 38% when prayer was excluded.[2] Although some publications cite prayer as a CAM therapy, it is excluded from further discussion as a CAM therapy in this chapter. Other findings of the CDC study were that women are more likely than men to use CAM, black adults were less likely than white or Asian adults to use CAM, persons with higher education were more likely than those with lower education to use CAM, and those who have been diagnosed with multiple comorbid conditions or had 10 or more visits to the doctor in the past year were more likely to use CAM.[2]

Rural population

There are reported differences in the use of CAM therapies by urban and rural populations. The use of CAM in rural settings is reported to range from 40% to 70%.[11] Predictors of CAM use by rural populations are largely consistent with that found for urban populations with some additions. Unmarried women and older individuals have higher rates of use in rural settings than in urban settings and those older individuals are using CAM as part of a comprehensive process to manage their healthcare needs.[11] Circumstances that seem to support the use of CAM therapies by rural residents include lack of healthcare services and dissatisfaction with healthcare providers.[11] Additional research is required in order to understand the needs and opportunities for care of this diverse and underserved population.

Pediatric population

The 2007 National Health Interview Survey reports on the use of CAM therapies by adults and children. The results of this survey indicate that 12% of children use some form of CAM therapy with 23.9% using CAM therapies if their parents are using them as well.[2] This study also reported that the most commonly used therapies by children were biologically based therapies (such as nutritional supplements), mind-body therapies (such as breathing), and body-based therapies (such as chiropractic care).[2] Caucasian children were more likely to use CAM therapies than either African-American or Hispanic children.[2] While other studies produced different findings, the 2007 National Health Interview Survey reports that those families who were unable to afford conventional care were more likely to use CAM therapies.[2]

Culture and ethnicity

There appears to be a relationship between ethnicity and CAM use. The 2007 National Health Interview Survey reports that 50.3% of American Indians/Alaska Natives had used CAM therapies within the last 12 months as compared to 43.1% of white adults, 39.9% of Asian adults, and 25.5% of African-American adults. Variations in use of CAM therapies by Hispanic populations were reported as Mexican adults 18.2%, Puerto Rican 29.7%, Mexican

American 27.4%, Dominican 28.2%, and South American 23.4%.[2] Acculturation is an understudied but important aspect of cultural and ethnic use of CAM therapies. In a study by Lee and colleagues, results suggest that the longer Mexican and Asian immigrants are in the United States and the more active they are in the dominant culture, the more likely they are to use CAM therapies at rates approaching the national levels.[12] These studies suggest that culture can influence CAM choices and should be considered when caring for patients.

Elderly

Older adults are challenged by the physical consequences of the aging of their bodies. The United States, as well as many other countries around the world, is experiencing an aging population. It is important to understand how older adults use all of the types of healthcare resources available to them. Recent studies indicate that older adults use CAM therapies to manage their healthcare issues.[2] The results of a systematic review reported by Harris, Cooper, Relton, and Thomas (2012) suggest that the rate of use of CAM therapies by older adults ranges from 41% to 63%.[13] There are indications in the literature that CAM use may remain stable with age. However, there is great variability in study design, making it difficult to assess the rate of CAM use by older individuals.[14] Rural populations that have been studied have offered more consistent data, indicating that in rural areas older patients have higher rates of use of CAM therapies.[11] Accessibility to healthcare resources may influence the use of CAM by older rural patients.[11] CAM therapies commonly used by older patients are folk medicine/home remedies and vitamin/mineral supplements.[11]

Cost

Most insurance companies do not reimburse for CAM. In the United States in 2007, it is estimated that individuals spent between $36 billion and $47 billion on CAM therapies. Of this amount, between $12 billion and $20 billion were paid out-of-pocket, with $5 billion spent on herbal products alone.[15] The cost of CAM may prevent many patients from receiving these therapies. There is movement within the US Congress to begin to acknowledge the value of these therapies and to reimburse for them. It is suggested that patients check with their insurance companies to see whether use of CAM can be reimbursed.

Cancer population

Among cancer patients, rates of CAM use are usually higher than in the general urban population. Oh and colleagues report that 65% of cancer patients use at least one form of complementary therapy.[16] A study of early stage breast cancer patients by Wyatt, Sikorskii, Willis, and An (2010) reported that 56.8% of these women used some form of CAM with the most frequently used being biologically based therapies.[17]

Improved cancer therapies are resulting in a growing population of cancer survivors in the United States. A cancer survivor may be defined as "an individual from the time of a cancer diagnosis through the remaining years of his or her life."[18] Many survivors experience ongoing cancer treatment-related symptoms even after treatment has been completed in the context of limited healthcare resources available to respond to those unmet needs.[18] Gansler and colleagues reported that cancer survivors use CAM therapies for several reasons including those framed as enhancing "locus of control," reducing stress, and reducing risk of cancer recurrence.[19] The most commonly used therapies by this group excluding prayer were relaxation (44%), spiritual healing (42%), and nutritional supplements (40%).[19]

The prevalence of CAM among cancer patients varies and is influenced by cancer site, stage, and treatment goals.[1] In one systematic review and meta-analysis, pooled prevalences of CAM use in North America ranged from 35% to 56%.[1] Factors that influence CAM use are more advanced stage at diagnosis and cancer site.[19] Data indicates that breast and ovarian patients are most likely to use CAM and melanoma and kidney cancer were least likely.[19] New use of CAM after surgery in patients with early-stage breast cancer (57%) was thought to be a marker for greater psychosocial distress and worse quality of life.[17] It was suggested that physicians take note of such usage and evaluate patients for quality of life with special attention to anxiety, depression, and physical symptoms.

Case study

SC, a 60-year-old man undergoing treatment for a blood dyscrasia

SC is an outgoing and active professional. He was recently diagnosed with a blood dyscrasia and is participating in a clinical trial of a pharmaceutical agent. SC has a history of depression and anxiety and is on bupropion and alprazolam. He is experiencing anxiety, emotional distress, and insomnia secondary to increased stress due health concerns. Both he and his wife have recently lost their jobs. SC has a history of addiction and has 27 years of sobriety.

Hypnosis experience #1

SC has experienced hypnosis previously and found it useful. SC was referred by his physician to a clinical hypnotherapist working at a comprehensive cancer center for his anxiety, emotional distress, and insomnia. His goals for the use of hypnosis are to reduce his anxiety, reduce his fear of leaving his home, and to assist him in regulating his emotional distress.

After identifying SC's preferred imagery, the hypnotherapist provided a 20-minute hypnotic experience. SC responded well to requests for psychomotor signaling and was able to embrace the suggestions. Reversal of hypnosis occurred without event. He reported satisfaction with the experience.

Hypnosis experience #2

SC reported that the effects of the suggestions persisted for approximately 5 days and then he began to experience increasing difficulty with the anxiety and emotional distress. He reported that he is on methadone for pain and one of his concerns is that he will become addicted to the medication. Time was taken to explain the differences between habituation and addiction and to create a strategy for monitoring his relationship to the pharmaceuticals being used to treat him. A 20-minute hypnosis intervention was delivered with additional suggestions related to managing his anxiety and emotional distress. Suggestions related to increasing his awareness of the medications and reinforcing his ability to use them appropriately were provided. A CD will be given to him at his next visit to bridge the time between sessions and increase his successful management of the anxiety and emotional distress.

Hypnosis experience #3

Both the patient and wife came to session reporting that the patient was better this week than for many weeks previously. The patient continues to describe his anxiety as a 7 out 10, but he is able to successfully regulate his anxiety and relax. He was given the CD to use at bedtime nightly and anytime he has difficulty downregulating his anxiety. He received a 20-minute hypnosis session. Reversal of the hypnosis occurred without incident. The patient reported feeling well after the session. He will return in 1 week and if the changes remain consistent will consider extending the time between visits.

Hypnosis experience #4

SC returns to clinic after having some changes in his health status. He has taken the suggestions offered in the last hypnosis session and is actively applying them to managing his anxiety and emotional distress. He reports listening to the CD only one time, but states he will listen more regularly. SC received a 20-minute hypnosis experience. All previous suggestions were reinforced. The reversal occurred easily and he reports feeling satisfied with the experience. He will return in 2.5 weeks and the outcomes of these sessions will be reviewed.

Hypnosis experience #5

SC returns to clinic reporting that he has not had any panic attacks during the last 3 weeks. He finds that under stress he is able to emotionally regulate and minimize anxiety. He is using the CD regularly and will continue to use it. No further visits are scheduled due to the resolution of his primary complaint.

Overview of complementary and alternative therapies

The National Center for Complementary and Alternative Medicine has grouped CAM therapies into five major domains: (1) alternative medical systems (traditional Chinese medicine, ayurveda, homeopathic medicine, naturopathic medicine, Native American medicine, and Tibetan medicine); (2) mind-body interventions (meditation, focused breathing, progressive muscle relaxation, guided imagery, creative visualization, hypnosis, biofeedback, music therapy, and art therapy); (3) biologically based therapies, nutrition, and special diets (e.g., macrobiotics, megavitamin and orthomolecular therapies, metabolic therapies, individual biological therapies such as shark cartilage) and herbal medicine; (4) manipulative and body-based methods (massage, aromatherapy, reflexology, acupressure, Shiatsu, polarity, chiropractic medicine, yoga, and exercise); and (5) energy therapies (Reiki, Qi gong, and therapeutic touch). The currently popular therapies are discussed in the following sections. Many of these methods are not proven, whereas others have been documented as helpful complementary therapies.

Counseling, group therapy, prayer, and spirituality, which we already know to be very helpful to cancer patients, are not included in this chapter because many view them as part of mainstream therapies.

Alternative medical systems

Instead of disease-oriented therapies, ancient systems of healing were based on attributing health, illness, and death to an invisible energy or life force, and the suggestion of an interaction between the human body, humankind, the spirit world, and the universe. In the earliest of times, there seemed to be a link between religion, magic, and medicine. This is in contrast to modern Western medicine, which is focused on the cause and curing of the disease. These alternative medicine systems are briefly discussed in this chapter because they are followed by many people today. The best known examples of alternative medical systems are traditional Chinese medicine (TCM), India's ayurvedic medicine, homeopathic medicine, naturopathic medicine, Native American medicine, and Tibetan medicine. Ancient healing systems tend to remain unchanged, unlike modern medicine, which keeps growing and expanding on a regular basis. A common feature across alternative medical systems is an emphasis on working with internal natural forces to achieve a harmonic state of mind and body, which can promote a sense of well-being and comfort. This idea, although outmoded and unscientific, has great appeal for many in the general public and especially for cancer patients dealing with advanced disease.

Traditional Chinese medicine

The cornerstone concept in Chinese medicine is *qi* (life force), which is energy that flows through the body along pathways known as meridians. Traditional Chinese medicine views people as ecosystems in miniature.[20] Any imbalance or disruption in the circulation of chi or qi (pronounced "chee") is thought to result in illness. Restoration of one's health is therefore dependent on returning the balance and flow of the life force. A TCM diagnosis is based on examination of the person's complexion, tongue, radial pulse, and detection of scents in bodily materials. Treatment is geared toward correcting imbalances or disruptions of the qi, primarily with herbal formulas and acupuncture.[20]

Acupuncture is one of the best known forms of CAM. It is one component of TCM. It is based on the belief that qi, the life force, flows through the human body in vertical energy channels known as meridians. There are 12 main meridians, which are believed to be dotted with acupoints that correspond to every body part and organ. To restore the balance and flow of qi, very fine disposable needles are inserted into the acupoints just under the skin. Other stimuli can be used along with acupuncture, such as heat (moxibustion), suction (cupping), external pressure (acupressure), and electrical currents (electroacupuncture). The biological basis of qi or meridians has not been found, but is thought that acupuncture needling releases endorphins and other neurotransmitters in the brain.[6] There is good evidence in the oncology literature that acupuncture helps control pain and nausea and vomiting. There is current research on its possible effectiveness for fatigue and dyspnea. Risks associated with acupuncture include mild discomfort or, occasionally, a drop of blood and/or a small bruise at the site of the insertion, but they can include more serious problems, such as an infection or (in the most extreme case) a pneumothorax, which is rare, and depends on the training and experience of the acupuncturist.

Ayurveda

The term *ayurveda* comes from Sanskrit words *ayur* (life) and *veda* (knowledge) and the practice is about 5000 years old. Ayurvedic medicine is based on the idea that illness is the absence of physical, emotional, and spiritual harmony.[6] Many of the basic principles are similar to those of Chinese medicine. Ayurveda is a natural system of medicine that uses diet, herbs, cleansing and purification practices, meditation, yoga, astrology, and gemstones to bring about healing. It sees causation of disease as an accumulation of toxins in the body and an imbalance of emotions. It prescribes individualized diets, regular detoxification, cleansing from all orifices, meditation, and yoga as some of the therapies. There is no scientific evidence that ayurvedic healing techniques cure illness.

Homeopathic medicine

Homeopathy is a medical system that was devised by Samuel Hahnemann 200 years ago, when the causes of diseases, such as bacteria and viruses, were unknown, and little was understood about the workings of the bodily organs. The thinking was that symptoms of ill health represent expressions of disharmony within the person, and attempts of the body to heal itself and return to a state of balance. It is the person, not the disease, who needs treatment. The treatment of disease is based on the principle, "Like cures like." Homeopathic medicines are made by taking original substances from plants, animals, and minerals, and highly diluting them. It is believed that the body's own healing ability is stimulated by these medicines. Homeopathic medicines are sold over the counter without prescription. They are so diluted that they are thought to have no side effects, and at the same time to be ineffectual for medical conditions, including cancer-related conditions.

Naturopathic medicine

Naturopathy is more of a philosophical approach to health than a particular form of therapy. It is an alternative medical system that attempts to cure disease by harnessing the body's own natural healing powers, and restoring good health and preventing disease. Rejecting synthetic drugs and invasive procedures, it stresses the restorative powers of nature, the search for the underlying causes of disease, and the treatment of the whole person. It takes very seriously the motto, "First, do no harm." Naturopathic medicine began as a quasi-spiritual "back to nature" movement in the 19th century. European founders advocated exposure to air, water, and sunlight as the best therapy for all ailments and recommended such spa treatments as hot mineral baths as virtual cure-alls. This system relies on natural healing approaches such as herbs, nutrition, and movement or manipulation of the body. Most naturopathic remedies are considered harmless by conventional practitioners.[6]

Traditional healing systems of American Indians/Alaska Natives

It is difficult to characterize a traditional healing system of American Indian/Alaska Native (AI/AN) peoples, as there are 564 federally recognized tribes speaking over 270 different languages.[21] American Indian/Alaska Native traditional healing methods are rooted in the culture of the people. Traditional healing methods are themselves an expression of cultural identity.[22]

Despite the diversity of tribal beliefs, shared concepts that influence health behaviors can be identified. A significant belief that underlies many traditional healing systems is that all things are interconnected and composed of a spiritual essence.[23] Spirituality is a critical component of most AI/AN traditional healing methods. Therefore, traditional healing is an expression of a cultural identity that is informed by a rich tradition of spirituality.[22]

Wellness is another important concept in AI/AN traditional healing systems. Wellness is an expression of balance and harmony in individual, family, and community systems. Many traditional healing methods focus on restoring balance and harmony to one or more of these elements.[22] Concepts of illness and its causes vary among tribal groups. However, beliefs in the spiritual reality of life often serve to provide a framework for understanding illness. Even seemingly accidental causes of injury may be viewed as having occurred to someone who may be living out of balance and harmony with traditional ways of being, as defined by the group's spiritual belief systems. Therefore, illness is often attributed to the violation of spiritual norms.[22]

Healing is often viewed by American Indians/Alaska Natives as the restoration of harmony and balance. Healing may be facilitated by traditional healers, who may be called many things and take many forms depending on the native group. Rituals, herbs, and purification processes are used by traditional healers to restore balance and harmony in a manner consistent with the values and beliefs of their people. Traditional healers are considered respected leaders within and outside of their communities.[22]

It is common for AI/AN to incorporate multiple healing systems into their lives. Both traditional healing systems and the biomedicine of European-American society may be employed. Contributions to European-American biomedicine have been made by the traditional healing systems of AI/AN. The most important evidence of Native American influence on traditional American medicine is the fact that >200 indigenous medicines used by one or more tribes have been listed in the pharmacopeia of the United States of America.[24]

Tibetan medicine

Tibetan medicine views the human body as an ecological system, a microcosm directly related to the macrocosm of the world. It attempts to investigate the root causes of illness. The belief is that all of the material that makes up our universe is based on the qualities of five basic elements (earth, water, fire, wind, and space). It is understood through experience that natural environmental forces can influence the functioning of the human organism. The Tibetan doctor bases his practice of diagnosis on his own spiritual practice, intellectual training, and intuition. The Tibetan medical diagnosis is a result of the patient interview, observation of the urine, taking of the 12 pulses, looking at the sclera and surface of the tongue, and feeling for sensitivity on certain parts of the body. The treatment is similar to that used in Chinese medicine.

Mind-body interventions

Mind-body therapies (MBT) are defined by the NCCAM as "a variety of techniques designed to enhance the mind's ability to affect bodily function and symptoms."[7] There is a long history of the use of interventions currently categorized as MBTs such as distraction, breathing, relaxation, imagery, and hypnosis.[6] Frequently used outside of formal Western medical contexts, they have become accepted as useful by the public at large. One study indicates that as of 2002 approximately 17% of the adult US population used some type of MBT, and when including prayer as an MBT, 53% of the population use or have used some form of MBT. The National Health Interview Survey conducted in 2007 reports that the use of deep breathing, meditation, and yoga increased from 2002 to 2007.[2]

According to one study, MBTs are used by 17% of the public.[25] Reasons cited for the use of MBTs include pain syndromes, anxiety/depression, insomnia, irritable bowel syndrome, hypertension, and irregular heart beats.[25] The majority of MBTs are used as self-guided therapies by lay users. Only 12% of the users were shown to seek care from healthcare and/or MBT providers.[26] One reason cited in the literature for the prevalence of self-guided MBTs over practitioner-guided therapies is availability of healthcare providers who have received training in and are competent to provide MBTs.[26]

The ability to influence health with the mind is an extremely appealing concept for many individuals. One of the benefits of self-guided MBTs is the ability to support and affirm feelings of self-efficacy. Since there is emerging evidence of the effectiveness of meditation, guided imagery, hypnosis, progressive muscle relaxation, biofeedback, and yoga for stress reduction and as adjunct therapies for the management of pain, nausea and vomiting, fatigue, anxiety, and disease-related distress, it is important for nurses and other healthcare providers to be well educated about these therapies. While the evidence supports the ability of these therapies to control stress, to reduce selected symptoms, and to improve the response to cardiac rehabilitation, there are no reliable, well-controlled studies to support the idea that these therapies can cure disease.[6]

Meditation

Meditation is the intentional self-regulation of attention. It enhances concentration and awareness as the individual focuses systematically and intentionally on particular aspects of inner or outer experience. It allows one to stay present in the moment and without judgment.[27] Historically, most meditation practices were developed within a spiritual or religious context with the goal of spiritual growth, personal transformation, or transcendental experience.[27]

There are two categories of meditation: concentration and mindfulness. Concentrative methods cultivate one-point of attention and start with mantras (sounds, words, or phrases repeated), as in transcendental meditation (TM). Mindfulness-based stress reduction (MBSR) practices start with the observation, without judgment, of thoughts, emotions, and sensations as they arise in the field of awareness. "Meditation can help individuals connect with what is deepest and most nourishing in themselves, and to mobilize the full range of inner and outer resources available to them."[27] Meditation has been helpful for terminally ill cancer patients. It has shown to be helpful in the relief of physical and emotional pain when integrated into a palliative care program. Many dying cancer patients discover that the calmness and quiet of meditation promotes a profound feeling of acceptance, well-being, and inner peace.[27] Walking meditation is appealing to those that cannot sit still. The focus might be on taking one step at a time, smelling the fresh air, taking in one breath at a time, or listening to the birds as one walks.

Relaxation techniques

Relaxation techniques are those simple techniques that, when learned by the patient, can promote relaxation. They include progressive muscle relaxation (contracting and relaxing muscle groups one at a time from head to toe), passive progressive muscle relaxation (no contraction of muscles, but focusing in the mind on sequentially relaxing groups of muscles), focused breathing (counting of breaths as one exhales, which can be used by itself or as an introduction to guided imagery).[28] Relaxation is safe and is tolerated by most cancer patients.[29,30] Due to the fatigue that is often associated with cancer, it may be useful to determine the functional status of a patient before beginning relaxation training.[31] There is evidence to support the use of relaxation training for pain, anxiety, distress, insomnia, and fatigue.[6,32–36]

Guided imagery

Imagery is the formation of mental images. Guided imagery is the intentional formation of mental images in response to verbal suggestion for the purpose of achieving a specific therapeutic result.[37] Imagery is a natural phenomenon in our lives that occurs all day long. For example, when we wake in the morning we might imagine our day, where we will be going, what we will wear, what we will eat, and so forth. This is a form of self-guided visualization and imagery. Some investigators categorize guided imagery and hypnosis as part of the same continuum of experience, with imagery playing a particular role in inducing a state of relaxation necessary for therapeutic intervention. Guided imagery and hypnosis are not the same.[38]

In 2010 Lai and colleagues conducted a pilot study exploring the efficacy of guided imagery in the management of cancer-related dyspnea. Fifty-three patients were recruited for this single-group study. A combined intervention was employed combining music and guided imagery. The results indicated an improvement in the dyspnea. However, due to the design of the study it is impossible to know whether the music or the guided imagery produced the positive effect.[39]

There are minimal risks associated with guided imagery. Due to the requirement for focused attention, it is contraindicated in patients with severe cognitive impairments and/or thought disorders. It is important that those providing guided imagery be well trained and conform to the ethical standards of practice of their profession.

Hypnosis

As the technology for understanding the mechanisms underlying the experience known as hypnosis becomes more advanced, more precise and accurate definitions of the phenomenon are created. Hypnosis is defined by Kihlstrom (2013) as "a social interaction in which one person, designated the subject, responds to suggestions offered by another person, designated the hypnotist, for imaginative experiences involving alterations in conscious perception and memory, and the voluntary control of action."[40] Activation of the anterior cingulate cortex, the thalamus, and the anterior basal ganglia, along with alterations in the orbital frontal cortex, support the state of hypnosis.[41] One study using fMRI has identified the neural processes underlying the mechanism for hypnotic pain reduction. This study determined that the hypnotic state prevents nociceptive inputs from reaching the cortical structures.[42] These findings support the concept that there are specific neural processes underlying hypnosis that are responsible for its clinical affect. Hypnosis does not have the same mechanism of action as distraction, but has similar mechanisms to meditation.[41]

The data supports the efficacy of hypnosis for the management of cancer symptoms (pain, nausea and vomiting, fatigue, anxiety, and distress) and the promotion of positive surgical outcomes (decreased pain, nausea and vomiting, medication usage, recovery time, and anxiety).[43–51] Hypnosis may be practiced as a facilitated experience or a self-guided experience. It is not uncommon for practitioners of hypnosis to begin with a facilitated experience that transitions to a self-guided practice through the use of supportive tools such as audiotapes/CDs.

The hypnotic state is achieved by using a variety of strategies to induce a state of profound relaxation and focused attention, including deep breathing, relaxation, and imagery. The process of inducing the hypnotic state is known as the induction. Once a sufficient state of relaxation and focused concentration is achieved, suggestions may be used to achieve therapeutic goals. These suggestions, identified as therapeutic suggestion, are suggestions for behaving, thinking, and/or feeling in a particular way with a specific outcome in mind (i.e., pain reduction). The suggestion may be direct or indirect depending on the needs of the client and the skills and preferences of the provider.[52]

Minimal risks are associated with hypnosis. Due to the requirement for focused attention, it is contraindicated in patients with severe cognitive impairments and/or thought disorders. It is recommended that only those individuals with licensure in a healthcare profession, and who have received formal training in hypnosis, be allowed to provide this service.

Biofeedback

Biofeedback is an increasingly popular technique for the management of symptoms associated with several medical conditions. It is defined as "a self-regulation technique through which patients learn to voluntarily control what were once thought to be involuntary body processes. This intervention requires specialized equipment to convert physiological signals into meaningful visual and auditory cues, as well as a trained biofeedback practitioner to guide the therapy."[53] Patients are guided through relaxation and imagery exercises and are instructed to alter their physiological processes using as a guide the provided biofeedback (typically visual or auditory data).

Biofeedback has been shown to have established efficacy for the management of female urinary incontinence, anxiety, pain, constipation, and headache.[53]

Music therapy

Music therapy in the palliative care setting is a useful therapy for which there is preliminary evidence.[54] Music can facilitate the participation of the patient with family and hospital staff. Music therapists apply psychotherapeutic skills in the setting of music as they care for patients with advanced cancer. Music therapy interventions consist of use of precomposed songs (reflecting messages or feelings that are foremost in the patient's thoughts), improvisation (offering opportunities for spontaneous expression and discovery), chanting and toning (use of vocalization to promote attentiveness and relaxation), imagery (exploration of images and feelings that arise in the music), music listening techniques (which facilitate reminiscence and build self-esteem through reflection on accomplishments), and taping of the music session as a gift for the family.[54] Music therapy may help to facilitate a life review for the patient. While evidence is building for the efficacy and safety of music therapy, there are too few well-designed randomized controlled trials to say definitively that music therapy is efficacious.[54]

Art therapy

Art therapy is a form of psychotherapy. Art therapy focuses on assisting patients to express, explore, and transform sensations, emotions, and thoughts connected with physical and psychological suffering by representing them as visual imagery.[55] In art therapy, the art therapist and the art materials (e.g., paper, colored markers, oil pastels, cut-up images from magazines) help patients get in touch with their feelings, their fears, and their hopes, and put them out onto the paper, thus helping patients process their experience of illness. It can easily be accommodated to hospitalized inpatients as well as to outpatient art groups or individuals. Art therapy can assist patients with advanced-stage cancer in the management of pain, fatigue, and stress.[56] Art images can serve to help the dying patient with issues of anger, bereavement, and loss. The art therapist may help dying patients find "personal symbols" to express something so powerful and so mysterious as the end of life.[56] Slayton, D'Archer, and Kaplan (2010) conducted a systematic review of the literature and found that, while there was a small number of studies supporting the effectiveness of art therapy, there was a need for additional well-designed trials before there would be sufficient evidence to assert that art therapy is efficacious.[57]

Biologically based therapies

Alternative diets have an ancient history, both medical and cultural, of plants and herbs as the first medicines. The example of vitamin C curing scurvy reinforces the idea of foods being medicines and curing illness. Some of the ancient medicine systems are still being practiced today; for example, ayurveda uses special diets, herbs, and cleansings to treat illness and promote health.

Today's food pyramid recommends fiber, grains, fruits and vegetables, and less protein, meat, and dairy products than was emphasized in earlier US Department of Agriculture government guidelines. It emphasizes balance. Changes in guidelines are based on carefully controlled scientific studies. Many alternative and fad diets, herbs, and supplements are either not scientifically validated or are marketed despite having been found worthless or harmful.

Nutrition

Some alternative practitioners believe that dietary treatments can prevent cancer or even go a step further to believe that foods or vitamins can cure cancer. The American Cancer Society Guidelines on Nutrition form the basis for a healthful diet that emphasizes vegetables, fruits, legumes, and whole grains; low-fat or nonfat dairy products; and limited amounts of red meat (lean preferred). Special dietary problems should be discussed with the doctor and an oncology-registered dietitian. It should be emphasized to the patient and family that the doctor should be informed before the patient takes any vitamin, mineral, or herb.

Special diets
Macrobiotics
The philosophy of the macrobiotic diet is curing through diet. It was developed in the 1930s by a Japanese philosopher, George Ohsawa. Originally, the diet consisted of brown rice with very little liquid. It was nutritionally deficient. Today it consists of 50% to 60% whole grains, 25% to 30% vegetables, and the remainder beans, seaweeds, and soups. Soybean foods are encouraged, and a small amount of fish is allowed. In-season foods are preferred. Proponents of this diet believe that it cures cancer. There is no evidence that the macrobiotic diet is beneficial for cancer patients.

Megavitamin and orthomolecular therapy
Some alternative practitioners believe that huge doses of vitamins can cure cancer. Linus Pauling coined the term "orthomolecular," meaning large quantities of minerals and other nutrients. Side effects are associated with the use of huge doses of vitamins and minerals.[58] A nutritionally healthy diet is recommended for overall good health. Some people have special needs and may require supplements. Patients should not attempt to treat themselves with megadoses of vitamins or minerals, but should seek professional attention for nutritional advice.

Metabolic therapies
Metabolic therapies are based on the theory that disease is caused by the accumulation of toxic substances in the body. The goal of treatment is to eliminate the toxins. Metabolic therapies usually include a special diet; high-dose vitamins, minerals, or other dietary supplements; and detoxification with coffee enemas or irrigation of the colon. Colon detoxification is not used in mainstream medicine, and there are no data to support the claims that dried food and toxins remain stuck in the walls of the colon. The development of metabolic therapy is attributed to Max Gerson, a physician who emigrated from Germany in 1936. Today, cancer is the most common illness treated with metabolic therapies. Research does not substantiate the beliefs and practices of metabolic therapies, and patients may lose valuable time during which they could be receiving treatments with proven benefits.

Individual biological therapy
Advocates of shark and bovine cartilage therapy claim that it can reduce tumor size, slow or stop the growth of cancer, and help reverse bone diseases such as osteoporosis. More importantly, shark and bovine cartilage are thought to play a role in angiogenesis, which involves halting the blood supply to cancer cells. There is no firm evidence that cartilage treatment is effective against cancer.

Herbal medicine
Herbs have been used as medicines going back to ancient times. Belief in the magic of herbs for the treatment of cancer exists today, especially in the face of advanced cancer and few or no other curative options. There is a romance about herbs, in that they are natural and come from the earth and therefore must be pure, safe, and harmless. A major concern exists that patients are using herbs indiscriminately on a routine basis without knowledge that these herbs interact with drugs, can interfere with the efficacy of anticancer drugs, and can cause death. They can cause medical problems such as allergic reactions, toxic reactions, adverse effects, drug interactions, and drug contamination.[59] There is a lack of knowledge that most herbal remedies have not been tested in carefully designed clinical studies.[59] Currently, some herbal remedies are being studied for their ability to induce or extend a cancer remission.

An important aspect of cancer care is to recognize that herbs can be toxic to cancer patients and should be discussed with the doctor and other qualified practitioners. The MSKCC advises patients to avoid taking any herbs for 2 weeks before any cancer therapy and to refrain from using supplements while in the hospital. Some herbs, such as St. John's Wort, may interfere with the effectiveness of chemotherapy.[60] Garlic may alter clotting times in a surgical candidate. Dong qui may make the skin more sensitive to burns during radiation. The active ingredients in many herbs are not known. In the United States, herbal and other dietary supplements are not regulated by the US Food and Drug Administration (FDA) as drugs. This means that they do not have to meet the same standards as drugs and over-the-counter medications for proof of safety and effectiveness. Identifying the active ingredients and understanding how they affect the body are important areas of research being done by NCCAM. Differences have been found in some cases between what is listed on the label and what is in the bottle, and some contaminants have been identified as heavy metals, microorganisms, or unspecified prescription drugs and adulterants. Standardization and authentication of herbs is important. An excellent resource to obtain information about herbs can be found in a resource book by Cassileth and Lucarelli on herb-drug interactions and at http://www.mskcc.org/cancer-care/integrative-medicine/about-herbs-botanicals-other-products.[61] As the prevalence of herbal remedy use grows, equipping nurses and doctors with information and vocabulary will help them discuss these remedies with patients and offer patients information about proper precautions. Patients should be encouraged to talk to their doctors and nurses about the herbs they are taking. It is important to listen with patience and then to respond without judgment. This approach promotes open, ongoing communication between the patient and the doctor or nurse.

Manipulative and body-based methods

Touch is the first sense to develop, and it is our primary way of experiencing the world, starting at infancy up until the moment of the last breath.[62] It is critical to growth and development. Infants, the elderly, the ill, and animals that do not receive regular touch fail to thrive and eventually die. In ancient times, the "laying on of hands" was an early practice of healing by touch. Medicine consisted of touch before the advent of pharmaceutical therapies. Today drugs, technology, paperwork, and heavy patient loads keep the doctor and nurse from the bedside. Patients comment, "I don't get touched very much anymore. If I do, it is a medical touch and it can hurt. My family and friends don't seem to touch either, maybe out of fear." Touch is a healing agent, but is underutilized by healing practitioners. Touch is our most social sense and implies a communication between two people. Cultural differences in touching are essential to keep in mind so as to always be respectful.

Massage

Massage therapy is one of the oldest healthcare practices in use. Chinese medical texts referred to it more than 4000 years ago. It is one of the most widely accepted forms of complementary therapies today. Massage employs the manual techniques of rubbing, stroking, tapping, or kneading the body's soft tissues to influence the whole person and to promote well-being and relaxation.[63] Massage is contraindicated under some circumstances: over metastatic bones (for risk of bone fracture or breakage), if the platelet count is <35,000 to 40,000/mm^3 (for risk of bruising), over sites of blood clots (for risk of promoting movement of a thrombus in the circulation), and over surgical sites or rashes. Medical massage for the cancer patient, and especially for the end-stage cancer patient, uses light pressure. Deep tissue massage is not appropriate and is potentially harmful.

The benefits of massage are many and include improving circulation, relaxing muscles and nerve tissue, releasing tension, reducing pain, decreasing anxiety and depression, energizing, and promoting an overall sense of well-being. Listing and colleagues (2010) conducted a randomized controlled trial that demonstrated a reduction in cortisol and perceived stress in those participants receiving the massage intervention.[64] While evidence is building to support the use of massage for symptom relief, additional randomized controlled trials are needed.

Aromatherapy

Aromatherapy is the controlled use of plant essences for therapeutic purposes. Essential oils are the aromatic essences of plants in the form of oil or resin, which have been extracted in a highly concentrated solution.[65] Aromatherapy is often combined with a touch therapy such as massage. There are very few studies evaluating the efficacy of aromatherapy as a single intervention. Ndao and colleagues (2012) conducted a study of children and adolescents who received inhaled aromatherapy at the time of their stem cell infusion. This was a double-blind, randomized controlled study with 37 participants in the intervention arm. No benefits were found to the use of the aromatherapy. While this study was underpowered to detect a change, the results are essentially consistent with the few well-designed studies evaluating the effects of aromatherapy. At this time, there is insufficient evidence to support the efficacy of aromatherapy or to evaluate its safety. Due to the paucity of evidence, it would be inappropriate for healthcare providers to recommend this therapy.

Reflexology

Reflexology is an ancient intervention that developed from TCM and ayurvedic health practices.[66] It is based on the assumption that the body contains energy flowing through it that may be accessed by placing pressure on specific areas of the foot that correspond to internal organs.[66] Reflexology is generally used to reduce stress, to promote relaxation and sleep, to improve circulation, to energize, to diminish symptoms of pain, anxiety, nausea, and peripheral neuropathy, and to promote an overall sense of well-being. In a systematic review conducted by Ernst (2011) the results of 23 randomized controlled trials were evaluated. The majority of the included studies did not show benefit. Due to the limited number of well-designed studies and the inconclusive results of the research, there is insufficient evidence to support the use of reflexology. Until there is more convincing evidence, reflexology should not be recommended by healthcare providers.

Acupressure

Acupressure is the pressing of a specific acupuncture point to relieve pain and stress in a particular area or part of the body. More than 300 acupoints dot the lengths of the hypothesized meridians (channels) that run vertically head to toe. Acupressure promotes relaxation and comfort. Zick and colleagues (2011) conducted a trial of a 12-week acupressure intervention. Self-report measures for fatigue showed clinically relevant improvement in the treatment group.[67] It should be done to the tolerance of the patient. It need not be painful. It should not be applied near areas of fractures or broken bones, or near blood clots, wounds, sores, or bruises.

Yoga

Yoga is the Sanskrit word for union or oneness. It is a centuries-old Eastern philosophy, science, and art form that can be used as a tool to achieve inner peace and freedom. Through mental (meditation) and physical (movement and simple poses with deep breathing) techniques, pathways lead into the yoga state of oneness.[68] Yoga helps align the body, promotes relaxation, and reduces fatigue. There are different types of yoga: hatha yoga (physical posturing), pranayama (yoga breathing), mantra yoga (sacred sound symbols in the sound of a chant designed to awaken the left hemisphere of the brain to rational thinking and clarity), and yantra yoga (visualizing symbols and energy patterns).[28] In a systematic review conducted by Ross and Thomas (2010), it was found that yoga was better than exercise on all measures other than fitness.[69]

Exercise

Patients with cancer often experience lack of energy and loss of physical performance and strength. Exercise being evaluated for symptom relief with cancer patients is identified as aerobic, resistance training and combined aerobic and resistance training. Segal and colleagues (2009) conducted a randomized controlled trial of combined aerobic exercise and resistance training. A statistically significant decrease in fatigue scores was achieved. However, there was a death on the study secondary to occult coronary artery disease in a participant.[70] This study offers some compelling evidence for the use of exercise and provides cautionary evidence supporting the evaluation of fitness prior to exercise.

Energy therapies

NCCAM has classified Reiki, Qi gong, and therapeutic touch as biofield therapies. Biofield therapies are defined as those therapies intended to affect energies that purportedly surround and interpenetrate the human body. They are thought to be able to rebalance the biofield. Some believe that these therapies can remove the subtle causes of illness and enhance overall resilience. The existence of such fields has not yet been scientifically proven.

Reiki

Reiki is a vibrational or subtle energy most commonly facilitated by light touch. *Rei* means universal or highest energy, and *ki* means subtle energy. Reiki therapy is thought to balance the biofield and to strengthen the body to heal itself. Reiki is offered to a fully clothed individual and involves placement of hands on the head and front and back; it may include placement of hands on the site of discomfort, if desired. The gentle touch is described as soothing by patients and is reported to promote deep relaxation. It is estimated that 1.2 million adults and 161,000 children in the United States have received at least one session of Reiki and that 15% of US hospitals offer Reiki as a service.[2] Despite the public and institutional use of Reiki, the evidence supporting its efficacy remains in the early stages of development.

Coakley and Barron (2012) conducted a review of the literature exploring the efficacy of Reiki. The results of the review identified several well-designed studies with findings supporting the use of Reiki.[71] The majority of these studies were quite small and therefore underpowered to detect effect and ungeneralizable. Bowden, Goddard, and Gruzelier (2010, 2011) have conducted an original randomized controlled single-blind trial of Reiki followed by a replication of the same study with a different cohort of participants. In the original trial, well-being and salivary cortisol were measured, and in the second, mood and well-being were assessed. Both trials were relatively small with 35 and 40 participants respectively. In the original trial, some improvement in perceptions of well-being was noted, but did not reach significance nor were there significant changes in salivary cortisol. In the second study, improvement in mood was noted, but did not reach statistically significant levels.[72,73] Both of these studies were underpowered to detect effect. Further research

using larger numbers of participants is required to understand the role of this therapy.

Qi gong

Qi gong is a component of TCM that combines movement, meditation, and regulation of breathing to enhance the flow of qi (vital energy) in the body.[28] Very few well-designed studies have studied the efficacy of Qi gong. Oh and colleagues (2011) conducted a randomized, controlled trial evaluating the effect of Qi gong on cognitive function and quality of life and c-reactive protein. The results of their study supported improved quality of life and cognitive functioning in association with Qi gong.[16] Additional research is urgently needed.

Therapeutic touch

Therapeutic touch, as described by Dolores Kreiger, is "the conscious, intentional act of directing universal energy with the intent to help and heal."[74] Therapeutic touch embraces the belief that humans have energy systems that radiate a few inches beyond the body.[75] It is believed that healing is promoted when the body's energies are in balance. The hands are usually passed over the patient without touching the patient so that the practitioner can detect energy imbalances and facilitate rebalancing. Coakley and Duffy (2010) conducted a randomized, controlled between-subjects interventional study using a psychoneuroimmunology framework.[75] Pain and cortisol levels were measured. Natural killer cell (NKC) levels were drawn before and immediately after the intervention. Participants in the intervention arm showed lower pain and cortisol levels and higher NKC levels than the controls. Another randomized, three-group experimental study conducted by Aghabati, Mohammadi, and Esmaiel (2008) demonstrated lower postintervention pain and fatigue scores than either the usual care group or the placebo group.[76] Well-designed studies are increasing the data supporting the efficacy of therapeutic touch. More research needs to be done.

Polarity therapy

Polarity views good health as a balance among internal energies, such as earth, air, fire, water, and space. When these energies are blocked due to stress or other factors, physical and emotional problems follow. The therapist provides a series of gentle stretching, light rocking, and holding of pressure points until the body's energy is brought into balance. Mustian and colleagues (2011) conducted a small, pilot, randomized, controlled trial of polarity therapy with radiation therapy patients. A small positive effect was detected, which is consistent with other studies evaluating this modality.[77] The evidence is in the early stage of development and additional research is needed.

Pretherapy nursing assessment

The nurse needs to assess the patient first, before any therapy is given or ordered.

Current medical history

The practitioner should determine the diagnosis, extent of disease, location of tumors, sites of metastatic disease, medications, CAM therapies (including vitamins, supplements, and herbs), site of blood clots, surgical site, site of radiation, and blood counts. He or she should determine which positions are most comfortable for the patient. All information must be obtained from the chart, doctor, or patient and family before doing a touch therapy.

Symptoms

Ask patients what symptoms they are currently experiencing. Ask patients to rate their symptoms on a scale of 0 to 10 as an estimate of their level of distress. This is necessary to select the most appropriate and the most effective CAM therapy. If the patient has pain, medicate first, before therapy is provided; the patient is much more likely to enjoy it. Have patients rate their individual symptoms after the chosen therapy, to make clear to the patient and medical staff the benefit of the therapy.

Religious/cultural background

What is the patient's cultural background? What therapies were used at home? Are there any cultural taboos? For example, it is not acceptable for a Hasidic Jewish man to be touched by a woman. It is important that the patient's cultural beliefs be respected and incorporated into the plan of care as long as there is no evidence-based reason to exclude them.

Previous use

What do the patients know about these therapies? Have they had previous experiences? Were they positive or negative experiences? Do they have any fears or reticence?

Patient's requests

Who is asking for these therapies? Is it the patient or the family? What would the patient like to try?

Remember:

◆ Do not massage on bones where there is metastatic disease, because bones are at risk for fracture or breakage; if the platelet count is <35,000 to 40,000/mm^3, because there is risk for bruising; on a site of current radiation, due to increased fragility of the skin; or where there are blood clots, due to the risk of setting a clot free to travel.[78]

◆ There is no deep tissue massage given especially in a patient with advanced disease. Gentle light massage is most appropriate.

Symptom management with evidence-based complementary therapies

Complementary therapies for control of pain

Pain is a common symptom experienced by the patient with advanced-stage cancer. Cancer pain can be very difficult to manage. Peripheral neuropathy is a common problem for cancer patients receiving certain chemotherapies and for those with diabetes. It is a difficult problem to treat, and its severity and recovery can vary with each patient. It can be so severe that the oncologist may have to stop the chemotherapy. It may be described by patients as numbness, tingling, or burning. Cisplatin is known to induce sensory peripheral neuropathy, and paclitaxel causes sensory and motor neuropathy. Neurological toxicity eventually decreases the patient's ability to perform physical functions necessary for activities of daily living, and thus can interfere with quality of life. Traditional pharmaceutical-based therapies in combination with evidenced-based complementary therapies have been shown to have a positive effect. The following adjuvant

complementary therapies can provide much-needed extra help for pain control: acupuncture, massage, hypnosis, relaxation, guided imagery, music therapy, and transcutaneous electrical nerve stimulation.[79] They can be chosen based on the nurse's assessment and the patient's wishes. Control of pain is a well-known use of acupuncture. Randomized trials support the use of acupuncture for acute and chronic cancer pain, nausea and vomiting, dyspnea, and xerostomia.[6,66,80] It is safe when performed by a qualified practitioner.[6]

Massage therapy can provide immediate pain relief and a sense of well-being in cancer patients experiencing pain.[78] Relaxation and imagery can provide some pain relief.[6,32–36,78] Hypnosis has established efficacy and safety and is able to modulate pain when provided by a clinical hypnotherapist well versed in the pathophysiology of pain.[49–51]

Music therapists provide services to treat pain. Music increases the patient's comfort, is soothing, and creates a safe environment to ease the dying process.[6] While Reiki is widely used and safe, only preliminary evidence supports its use for pain management.[71]

Complementary therapies for control of nausea and vomiting

Nausea and vomiting can greatly compromise patients' quality of life. The causes may be multiple, including a reaction to medications (chemotherapy, antibiotics, opiates), bad taste in the mouth, or bowel obstruction. Nausea and vomiting can be so severe that patients would rather discontinue their chemotherapy, or wish to die. Acupuncture, relaxation techniques, acupressure, massage, music, imagery, hypnosis, art therapy, and meditation are effective therapies for nausea and vomiting and can be used alongside pharmacotherapy.[81]

Complementary therapies for control of anxiety

People with cancer often live with anxiety. Common causes of anxiety in cancer patients are situational anxiety, previous history of anxiety, poorly controlled pain, abnormal metabolic states (e.g., hypoxia, sepsis, delirium), and side effects of medications (e.g., corticosteroids, neuroleptics.[82] The complementary therapies for which there is substantial evidence of safety and efficacy are meditation, relaxation, hypnosis, guided imagery, music therapy, and exercise.[6]

Complementary therapies for control of depression

The National Comprehensive Cancer Network, in their guidelines of 2011, chose to focus on the patient's distress management. They recognized that distress extends along a continuum, ranging from feelings of vulnerability, sadness, and fear to disabling conditions such as clinical depression, anxiety, panic, isolation, and existential or spiritual crisis.[83] There is evidence supporting the use of psychotherapy, art therapy, massage, exercise, yoga, meditation, relaxation, and guided imagery with depression.[6]

Complementary therapies for control of insomnia

Insomnia is a common problem in cancer. The contributing factors, especially for advanced cancer, are hypoxia, pain, anxiety, delirium, medications, or withdrawal from medications. The causes need to be treated, but, in addition, therapies that promote stress reduction and relaxation can be considered. There is convincing evidence to support the use of progressive muscle relaxation, guided imagery, meditation, and hypnosis in the treatment of insomnia.[6,84]

Complementary therapies for control of fatigue

Fatigue is a common symptom among patients with cancer. The National Comprehensive Cancer Network defines fatigue as "a distressing, persistent, subjective sense of physical, emotional, and/or cognitive tiredness or exhaustion related to cancer and cancer treatment that is not related to recent activity and that interferes with usual functioning."[85] There are some nonpharmacological interventions for cancer-related fatigue such as exercise, yoga, hypnosis, mindfulness-based stress reduction, relation training and controlled breathing.[86] Of these, exercise and yoga have the strongest evidence supporting an effect in treating cancer-related fatigue.[6]

Complementary therapies for control of dyspnea

Breathlessness is an extremely distressing and frightening symptom that can completely dominate a patient's life. It can cause physical disability, high anxiety, dependence, and loss of self-esteem. Nonpharmacological therapies recommended for use with dyspnea include hypnosis, self-hypnosis, guided imagery, relaxation, controlled breathing, music therapy, and acupuncture.[87]

Summary

It is a privilege to work with patients who have advanced debilitating illness and are in their last days of life. Gone are the days when a patient or a family might be told, "There is nothing more we can do." There remain many treatment options, including complementary therapies that patients can choose and receive as a part of palliative care.

Nurses can educate patients and families about the safe choices of evidence-based complementary therapies that can affect their quality of life. But first, they need to educate themselves about CAM—what these therapies are, what their specific benefits and risks are, and which ones are safe—before guiding patients. Nurses want to be respectful of the patient's desire to seek out CAM in the setting of advanced disease. Nurses must listen to the patient and then give suggestions of effective complementary therapies for comfort. Palliative care nurses are exposed to an abnormal amount of suffering and death and need to take care of themselves in order to give to others. Use of complementary therapies for themselves will benefit all.

Nurses can help patients live their lives to the last with hope. One patient said, "I didn't mind returning to the hospital, because I knew Integrative Medicine would be there for me." Another inpatient reported, after her reflexology session, "You have made me want to stay alive longer, I feel so good."

References

1. Horneber M, Bueschel G, Dennert G, et al. How many cancer patients use complementary and alternative medicine: a systematic review and metaanalysis. Integr Cancer Ther. 2012;11(3):187–203.
2. Barnes PM, Bloom B, Nahin RL. Complementary and alternative medicine use among adults and children: United States, 2007. National Health Statistics Reports. 2008(12):1–23.
3. Yildirim Y, Parlar S, Eyigor S, et al. An analysis of nursing and medical students' attitudes towards and knowledge of complementary and alternative medicine (CAM). J Clin Nurs. 2010;19(7–8):1157–1166.
4. Deng G, Weber W, Sood A, Kemper KJ. Research on integrative healthcare: context and priorities. Explore. 2010;6(3):143–158.
5. Institute for Clinical Systems Improvement (ICSI). Health care guideline: palliative care. In: (ICSI) IfcI, ed. Bloomington (MN) 2011 www.icsi.org.
6. Deng GE, Frenkel M, Cohen L, et al. Evidence-based clinical practice guidelines for integrative oncology: complementary therapies and botanicals. Journal of the Society for Integrative Oncology. 2009;7(3):85–120.
7. National Center for Complementary and Alternative Medicine. 2013. What Is CAM? http://nccam.nih.gov/health/whatiscam.
8. Cassileth B, Gubili J. Integrative oncology: complementary therapies in cancer care. In: Ettinger DS (ed.), Supportive Care in Cancer Therapy. New Jersey: Humana Press; 2009:269–277.
9. Hunt KJ, Coelho HF, Wider B, et al. Complementary and alternative medicine use in England: results from a national survey. Int J Clin Pract. 2010;64(11):1496–1502.
10. Ernst E. Complementary and alternative medicine: between evidence and absurdity. Perspectives in Biology and Medicine. 2009;52(2):289–303.
11. Wardie J, Lui CW, Adams J. Complementary and alternative medicine in rural communities: current research and future directions. Journal of Rural Health. 2012;28(1):101–112.
12. Lee JH, Goldstein MS, Brown ER, Ballard-Barbash R. How does acculturation affect the use of complementary and alternative medicine providers among Mexican-Americans and Asian-Americans? Journal of Immigrant and Minority Health/Center for Minority Public Health. 2010;12(3):302–309.
13. Harris PE, Cooper KL, Relton C, Thomas KJ. Prevalence of complementary and alternative medicine (CAM) use by the general population: a systematic review and update. Int J Clin Pract. 2012;66(10):924–939.
14. Bishop FL, Lewith GT. Who uses CAM?: A narrative review of demographic characteristics and health factors associated with CAM Use. eCAM. 2010;7(1):11–28.
15. Nahin RL. Costs of Complementary and Alternative Medicine (CAM) and Frequency of Visits to CAM Practitioners. Google eBook, Diane Publishing; 2010.
16. Oh B, Butow P, Mullan B, et al. A critical review of the effects of medical qigong on quality of life, immune function, and survival in cancer patients. Integr Cancer Ther. Jun 2012;11(2):101–110.
17. Wyatt G, Sikorskii A, Wills CE, Su H. Complementary and alternative medicine use, spending, and quality of life in early stage breast cancer. Nursing Research. 2010;59(1):58–66.
18. Bell RM. A review of complementary and alternative medicine practices among cancer survivors. Clin J Oncol Nurs. 2010;14(3):365–370.
19. Gansler T, Kaw C, Crammer C, Smith T. A population-based study of prevalence of complementary methods use by cancer survivors: a report from the American Cancer Society's studies of cancer survivors. Cancer. 2008;113(5):1048–1057.
20. Cassileth BR, Deng G. Complementary and alternative therapies for cancer. Oncologist. 2004;9(1):80–89.
21. Fixico D. Bureau of Indian Affairs. Santa Barbara, CA: ABC-CLIO; 2012.
22. Johnston S. Native American traditional and alternative medicine. Annals of the American Academy of Political and Social Sciences. 2002;583:195–213.
23. Unger JB, Soto C, Thomas N. Translation of health programs for American Indians in the United States. Evaluation for Health Professions. 2008;31(2):124–144.
24. Vogel V. American Indian Medicine. Norman: University of Oklahoma Press; 1970.
25. Bertisch SM, Wee CC, Phillips RS, McCarthy EP. Alternative mind-body therapies used by adults with medical conditions. J Psychosom Res. 2009;66(6):511–519.
26. Fouladbakhsh JM, Stommel M. Gender, symptom experience, and use of complementary and alternative medicine practices among

cancer survivors in the U.S. cancer population. Oncol Nurs Forum. 2010;37(1):E7–E15.

27. Kabat-Zinn J, Massion A, Hebert J, Rosenbaum E. Meditation. In: Holland JC (ed.), Psycho-oncology. Oxford: Oxford University Press; 1998:767–779.

28. Elkins G, Fisher W, Johnson A. Mind-body therapies in integrative oncology. Current Treatment Options in Oncology. 2010;11(3–4):128–140.

29. Demiralp M, Oflaz F, Komurcu S. Effects of relaxation training on sleep quality and fatigue in patients with breast cancer undergoing adjuvant chemotherapy. J Clin Nurs. 2010;19(7–8):1073–1083.

30. Adamsen L, Stage M, Laursen J, Rorth M, Quist M. Exercise and relaxation intervention for patients with advanced lung cancer: a qualitative feasibility study. Scan J Med Sci Sports. 2012;22(6):804–815.

31. Kondo Y, Koitabashi K, Kaneko Y. Experiences of difficulty that patients with cancer faced in the learning process of progressive muscle relaxation. Japan Journal of Nursing Science. 2009;6(2):123–132.

32. Kwekkeboom KL, Wanta B, Bumpus M. Individual difference variables and the effects of progressive muscle relaxation and analgesic imagery interventions on cancer pain. J Pain Symptom Manage. 2008;36(6):604–615.

33. Lolak S, Connors GL, Sheridan MJ, Wise TN. Effects of progressive muscle relaxation training on anxiety and depression in patients enrolled in an outpatient pulmonary rehabilitation program. Psychother Psychosom. 2008;77(2):119–125.

34. Rabin C, Pinto B, Dunsiger S, Nash J, Trask P. Exercise and relaxation intervention for breast cancer survivors: feasibility, acceptability and effects. Psycho-Oncol. 2009;18(3):258–266.

35. Yang XL, Li HH, Hong MH, Kao HS. The effects of Chinese calligraphy handwriting and relaxation training in Chinese nasopharyngeal carcinoma patients: a randomized controlled trial. Int J Nurs Stud. 2010;47(5):550–559.

36. Chan AS, Cheung MC, Sze SL, Leung WW, Shi D. Shaolin dan tian breathing fosters relaxed and attentive mind: a randomized controlled neuro-electrophysiological study. eCAM. 2011;2011:180704.

37. King K. A review of the effects of guided imagery on cancer patients with pain. Com Health Pra Rev. 2010;15(2):98–107.

38. Green JP, Barabasz AF, Barrett D, Montgomery GH. Forging ahead: the 2003 APA Division 30 definition of hypnosis. International Journal of Clinical and Experimental Hypnosis. Jul 2005;53(3):259–264.

39. Lai WS, Chao CS, Yang WP, Chen CH. Efficacy of guided imagery with theta music for advanced cancer patients with dyspnea: a pilot study. Bio Res Nurs. 2010;12(2):188–197.

40. Kihlstrom JF. Neuro-hypnotism: prospects for hypnosis and neuroscience. Cortex. 2013;49(2):365–374.

41. Taylor AG, Goehler LE, Galper DI, Innes KE, Bourguignon C. Top-down and bottom-up mechanisms in mind-body medicine: development of an integrative framework for psychophysiological research. Journal of Science and Healing. 2010;6(1):29–41.

42. Schulz-Stubner S, Krings T, Meister IG, Rex S, Thron A, Rossaint R. Clinical hypnosis modulates functional magnetic resonance imaging signal intensities and pain perception in a thermal stimulation paradigm. Regional Anesthesia and Pain Medicine. 2004;29(6):549–556.

43. Richardson J, Smith JE, McCall G, Richardson A, Pilkington K, Kirsch I. Hypnosis for nausea and vomiting in cancer chemotherapy: a systematic review of the research evidence. European Journal of Cancer Care. 2007;16(5):402–412.

44. Lang EV, Benotsch EG, Fick LJ, et al. Adjunctive non-pharmacological analgesia for invasive medical procedures: a randomized trial. Lancet. 2000;355(9214):1486–1490.

45. Lang EV, Berbaum KS, Faintuch S, et al. Adjunctive self-hypnotic relaxation for outpatient medical procedures: a prospective randomized trial with women undergoing large core breast biopsy. Pain. 2006;126(1–3):155–164.

46. Neron S, Stephenson R. Effectiveness of hypnotherapy with cancer patients' trajectory: emesis, acute pain, and analgesia and anxiolysis in procedures. International Journal of Clinical and Experimental Hypnosis. 2007;55(3):336–354.

47. Elkins G, Jensen MP, Patterson DR. Hypnotherapy for the management of chronic pain. International Journal of Clinical and Experimental Hypnosis. 2007;55(3):275–287.

48. Schnur JB, Kafer I, Marcus C, Montgomery GH. Hypnosis to manage distress related to medical procedures: a meta-analysis. Contemp Hyp. 2008;25(3–4):114–128.

49. Jensen MP, Sherlin LH, Hakimian S, Fregni F. Neuromodulatory approaches for chronic pain management: research findings and clinical implications. J Neurother. 2009;13(4):196–213.

50. Mendoza ME, Capafons A. Efficacy of clinical hypnosis: a summary of its empirical evidence. Papeles del Psicologo. 2009;30(2):98–116.

51. Montgomery GH, Hallquist MN, Schnur JB, David D, Silverstein JH, Bovbjerg DH. Mediators of a brief hypnosis intervention to control side effects in breast surgery patients: response expectancies and emotional distress. Journal of Consulting and Clinical Psychology. 2010;78(1):80–88.

52. Rossi EL, Rossi KL. What is a suggestion?: The neuroscience of implicit processing heuristics in therapeutic hypnosis and psychotherapy. American Journal of Clinical Hypnosis. 2007;49(4):267–281.

53. Frank DL, Khorshid L, Kiffer JF, Moravec CS, McKee MG. Biofeedback in medicine: who, when, why and how? Men Health Fam Med. 2010;7(2):85–91.

54. Bradt J, Dileo C. Music therapy for end-of-life care. Editorial Group: Cochrane Pain, Palliative and Supportive Care Group. 2010(1):CD007169.

55. Magill L, Luzzatto P. Music therapy and art therapy. In: Berger A, Portenoy R, Weissman D (eds.), Principles and Practice of Palliative Care and Supportive Oncology. 2nd ed. Philadelphia: Lippincott Williams & Wilkins; 2002:993–1005.

56. Luzzatto P, Gabriel B. Art therapy. In: Holland J (ed.), Psychooncology. Oxford: Oxford University Press; 1998:743–757.

57. Slayton S, D'Archer J, Kaplan F. Outcome studies on the efficacy of art therapy: a review of findings. Art Therapy: Journal of the American Art Therapy Association. 2010;27(3):108–118.

58. Cassileth B. The Alternative Medicine Handbook: The Complete Reference Guide to Alternative and Complementary Therapies. New York: Norton; 1998.

59. Jordan SA, Cunningham DG, Marles RJ. Assessment of herbal medicinal products: challenges, and opportunities to increase the knowledge base for safety assessment. Toxicology and Applied Pharmacology. 2010;243(2):198–216.

60. He SM, Yang AK, Li XT, Du YM, Zhou SF. Effects of herbal products on the metabolism and transport of anticancer agents. Expert Opinion on Drug Metabolism and Toxicology. 2010;6(10):1195–1213.

61. Cassileth B, Lucarelli C. Herb-Drug Interactions in Oncology. Hamilton, Ontario: Decker; 2003.

62. Anderson JG, Taylor AG. Effects of healing touch in clinical practice: a systematic review of randomized clinical trials. J Holistic Nurs. 2011;29(3):221–228.

63. Wilkinson S, Barnes K, Storey L. Massage for symptom relief in patients with cancer: systematic review. J Adv Nurs. 2008;63(5):430–439.

64. Listing M, Krohn M, Liezmann C, et al. The efficacy of classical massage on stress perception and cortisol following primary treatment of breast cancer. Archives of Women's Mental Health. 2010;13(2):165–173.

65. Ndao DH, Ladas EJ, Cheng B, et al. Inhalation aromatherapy in children and adolescents undergoing stem cell infusion: results of a placebo-controlled double-blind trial. Psycho-Oncology. 2012;21(3):247–254.

66. Ernst E. Acupuncture for hot flashes, vasomotor symptoms, breathlessness, xerostomia, chemotherapy-induced leucopenia and for alleviating the adverse effects of conventional breast cancer therapies. 2011. http://ws.cam-cancer.org/CAM-Summaries/Alternative-Medical-Systems/Acupuntrue-for-other-cancer-related-complaints

67. Zick SM, Alrawi S, Merel G, et al. Relaxation acupressure reduces persistent cancer-related fatigue. eCAM. 2011;2011.

68. Galantino ML, Greene L, Archetto B, et al. A qualitative exploration of the impact of yoga on breast cancer survivors with aromatase inhibitor-associated arthralgias. Explore. 2012;8(1):40–47.

69. Ross A, Thomas S. The health benefits of yoga and exercise: a review of comparison studies. J Alt Com Med. 2010;16(1):3–12.

70. Segal RJ, Reid RD, Courneya KS, et al. Randomized controlled trial of resistance or aerobic exercise in men receiving radiation therapy for prostate cancer. J Clin Oncol. 2009;27(3):344–351.

71. Coakley AB, Barron AM. Energy therapies in oncology nursing. Semin Oncol Nurs. 2012;28(1):55–63.

72. Bowden D, Goddard L, Gruzelier J. A randomized controlled single-blind trial of the effects of Reiki and positive imagery on well-being and salivary cortisol. Brain Research Bulletin. 2010;81(1): 66–72.

73. Bowden D, Goddard L, Gruzelier J. A randomized controlled single-blind trial of the efficacy of Reiki at benefitting mood and well-being. eCAM. 2011;2011:381862.

74. Krieger D. The Therapeutic Touch: How to Use Your Hands to Help or to Heal. Englewood Cliffs, NJ: Prentice Hall; 1979.

75. Coakley AB, Duffy ME. The effect of therapeutic touch on postoperative patients. J Holistic Nurs. 2010;28(3):193–200.

76. Aghabati N, Mohammadi E, Pour Esmaiel Z. The effect of therapeutic touch on pain and fatigue of cancer patients undergoing chemotherapy. eCAM. 2010;7(3):375–381.

77. Mustian KM, Roscoe JA, Palesh OG, et al. Polarity therapy for cancer-related fatigue in patients with breast cancer receiving radiation therapy: a randomized controlled pilot study. Integr Can Ther. 2011;10(1):27–37.

78. Collinge W, MacDonald G, Walton T. Massage in supportive cancer care. Semin Oncol Nurs. 2012;28(1):45–54.

79. Mansky PJ, Wallerstedt DB. Complementary medicine in palliative care and cancer symptom management. Cancer J. 2006;12(5): 425–431.

80. Cassileth BR, Keefe FJ. Integrative and behavioral approaches to the treatment of cancer-related neuropathic pain. Oncologist. 2010;15(Suppl 2):19–23.

81. Roscoe JA, Morrow GR, Aapro MS, Molassiotis A, Olver I. Anticipatory nausea and vomiting. Support Care Cancer. 2011;19(10): 1533–1538.

82. Pasacreta J, Minarik PA. Anxiety and depression. In: Ferrell B, Coyle N (eds.), Palliative Nursing. New York: Oxford University Press; 2010:425–448.

83. National Comprehensive Cancer Network. 2011. Distress Management. NCCN Clinical Practice Guidelines in Oncology (NCCN Guidelines). 2011;1.2011.

84. Ebben MR, Spielman AJ. Non-pharmacological treatments for insomnia. J Behav Med. 2009;32(3):244–254.

85. National Comprehensive Cancer Network. Cancer-Related Fatigue. NCCN clinical Practice Guidelines in Oncology (NCCN Guidelines):pp. FT-5-7; MS-8; MS-10; MS-11; MS-14. 2011;1.2011.

86. Sood A, Barton D. Complementary and Alternative Treatments for the Management of Cancer-Related Fatigue. New York: Springer; 2010.

87. Bausewein C, Booth S, Gysels M, Higginson I. Non-pharmacological interventions for breathlessness in advanced stages of malignant and non-malignant diseases. Cochrane Database Syst Rev. 2008(2): CD005623.

CHAPTER 27

Withdrawal of life-sustaining therapies
Mechanical ventilation, dialysis, and cardiac devices

Margaret L. Campbell and Linda M. Gorman

> When the time comes … I want natural, no machines.
> Patient

Key points

- Any form of life-sustaining therapy or treatment can be withheld or withdrawn.
- Distress can be anticipated and treated during withdrawal of life supports.
- Death follows life support withdrawal along varying trajectories characteristic of the organ or organs in failure.

Mechanical ventilation

Case study

Lula Belle, a 73-year-old nursing home resident, developed acute respiratory distress presumed secondary to pneumonia. She was transferred to a hospital, intubated in the Emergency Department and admitted to the Medical Intensive Care Unit (MICU). Lula Belle had a history of advanced-stage Alzheimer's dementia that left her bed-bound, incontinent, largely nonverbal, and with recent feeding difficulties.

Her children were surprised to find her in the MICU with mechanical ventilation because they had completed do not resuscitate (DNR) paperwork at the nursing home prior to this acute complication. In the context of terminal-stage dementia, Lula Belle's children requested a change in treatment goals to comfort measures only and withdrawal of mechanical ventilation; the MICU team agreed with this request.

After the family had assembled at the hospital a private waiting area was made available for those who did not want to be at the bedside during ventilator withdrawal. A nurse's aide stocked the room with ice water, juice, cups and tissues. Chaplain support was offered and declined.

Lula Belle was conscious but severely cognitively impaired. The Respiratory Distress Observation Scale (RDOS) was used to evaluate her respiratory comfort during ventilator withdrawal; low RDOS scores are indicative of comfort. A cuff-leak test was done that suggested extubation could be accomplished with a low risk of postextubation stridor. She was premedicated with morphine 5 mg as an intravenous bolus, given her ability to experience distress and the probability of dyspnea as ventilation was withdrawn. A rapid terminal wean was done by discontinuing positive end-expiratory pressure, followed by a stepwise reduction in oxygen, with subsequent stepwise reduction in ventilation. Lula Belle was assessed with RDOS after each ventilator change. When distress was apparent, a bolus of morphine 5 mg was given.

After 15 minutes of rapid weaning and one morphine bolus, the ventilator was turned off. The endotracheal tube was removed, and her face and mouth were cleaned. She had received 10 mg of intravenous morphine so respiratory comfort was maintained with the initiation of a continuous infusion at 5 mg/h.

The family from the waiting room joined the family at the bedside. Lula Belle showed signs of imminent death so the family was encouraged to stay; Lula Belle died 3 hours after the ventilator was withdrawn and remained comfortable throughout.

Benefits and burdens of mechanical ventilation

Mechanical ventilation (MV) has been used for decades to support breathing when patients experienced acute or chronic respiratory failure. Mechanical ventilation is of benefit when the patient, for a number of reasons, cannot maintain normal ventilation as evidenced by increasing carbon dioxide and respiratory acidosis; invasive and noninvasive modalities are employed. Invasive MV is accomplished after the establishment of an artificial airway such as an endotracheal tube or tracheostomy. Noninvasive MV is applied over the nose or nose and mouth via a tight-fitting face mask.

Invasive MV is employed after cardiopulmonary arrest, during general anesthesia, to treat respiratory failure that is not responsive to noninvasive ventilation or for patients who are ventilator dependent. Endotracheal intubation is used for periods of less than

2 weeks of ventilation; continued ventilation after 2 weeks is supported by tracheostomy. When respiratory failure occurs during an exacerbation of chronic pulmonary disease noninvasive ventilation is often useful as a first response.[1] Patients with obstructive sleep apnea, chronic obstructive pulmonary disease (COPD), and amyotrophic lateral sclerosis (ALS) often use noninvasive ventilation at night or when breathing is difficult during the day.

Patients often experience discomfort during MV. With noninvasive modalities the tight-fitting mask may produce generalized pressure-associated discomfort, feelings of suffocation, and pressure lesions on the bridge of the nose. Endotracheal intubation causes gagging, coughing, and drooling, and leaves the patient unable to verbalize because the tube passes through the vocal cords. In many cases of endotracheal intubation and some cases of noninvasive ventilation the patient requires mechanical restraints or sedation to maintain the integrity of the life-saving treatment and to ensure ventilator synchrony.

Ventilator-dependent patients experience fewer burdens because they are routinely ventilated through a tracheostomy. Nonetheless, chronic ventilator dependence limits patient mobility and contributes to the development of immobility complications such as pressure ulcers, deep venous thrombosis, and pneumonia.

Ventilator withdrawal is considered as a treatment option when the treatment is more burdensome than beneficial, such as when the patient has a terminal illness or is unconscious or when the patient makes an informed, capable decision to cease treatment because her/his quality of life is poor.[2] In critical care units (adult, pediatric, and neonatal), ventilator withdrawal is usually undertaken because the patient is not expected to survive and/or to regain functional consciousness. Clinical standards, policies, and procedures about foregoing life-sustaining therapy, including MV, are in wide use and reflect broad agreement about the underlying principles regarding these decisions.[3]

Although withdrawal of ventilation occurs on a frequent basis across settings of care, there is little empiric evidence to guide the process. A review of the evidence to guide a ventilator withdrawal process demonstrated that small samples and largely retrospective chart reviews characterize the body of evidence about processes for ventilator withdrawal.[2] The cited research is not conclusive to make recommendations in all cases of ventilator withdrawal. However, a number of suggested processes may be useful in this clinical context, along with a team approach to the procedure and patient care to address anticipated symptoms.

Patients are ventilated because of respiratory failure and an inability to exchange respiratory gases without mechanical support. Dyspnea arises from increased inspiratory effort, hypercarbia, and/or hypoxemia; dyspnea is anticipated during and after ventilator withdrawal. Prevention and alleviation of dyspnea or respiratory distress becomes the focus of care during ventilator withdrawal. Some patients, if awake, may experience fear or anxiety before or during ventilator withdrawal, which will require attention if present. Adult patients may experience barotrauma to the trachea from the pressure in the cuff, leading to laryngeal edema or spasm after extubation with development of postextubation stridor.

Ventilator withdrawal processes

Advance preparation

The Centers for Medicare and Medicaid Services has enacted guidelines for consistent processes around organ donation.[4]

Hospital staff must notify their state Organ Procurement Organization (OPO) when decisions about ventilator withdrawal are being considered. The OPO will collaborate with the hospital staff to identify whether the patient is a donor candidate for donation after cardiac death and to seek consent from the next of kin. This evaluation by the OPO must be completed before ventilation is withdrawn.

Timing to conduct the withdrawal process is generally negotiated with the patient's family and the healthcare team. This timing will depend on which team members will be present, including support personnel, such as a chaplain. The time needs to be communicated to all clinical team members, and ideally the assigned nurse should have a reduced assignment to be able to spend 1:1 time with the patient and family.

Not all family members want to be present at the bedside during withdrawal. Another room nearby can be arranged with adequate seating, tissues, water, and access to a telephone. Religious observances or family-specific rituals need to be accommodated and completed before beginning the withdrawal process. Patient and/or family questions about what to expect can be addressed before beginning the process.[5] When ventilation is withdrawn from a small child, infant, or neonate it is customary for a parent to hold the child on his/her lap during the process.

Neuromuscular blocking agents (NMBA) are being used with less frequency in the ICU, however, when in use it is impossible to assess the patient's comfort. Thus, the NMBA should be discontinued with evidence of patient neuromuscular recovery before ventilator withdrawal is undertaken. In some cases the duration of action of these agents is prolonged, such as when the patient has liver or renal failure and impaired clearance. Therefore, although controversial, withdrawal can proceed with careful attention to ensuring patient comfort if an unacceptable delay in withdrawing MV occurs because of protracted effects of NMBA.[6]

Measuring distress

Dyspnea, also known as breathlessness, is a nociceptive phenomenon defined as "a subjective experience of breathing discomfort that consists of qualitatively distinct sensations that vary in intensity. The experience derives from interactions among multiple physiological, psychological, social and environmental factors, and may induce secondary physiological and behavioral responses."[7] Dyspnea can be perceived and verified only by the person experiencing it. Many patients who are undergoing ventilator withdrawal are cognitively impaired or unconscious as a result of underlying neurological lesions or hemodynamic, metabolic, or respiratory dysfunction that produce cognitive impairment or unconsciousness. Respiratory distress is an observable (behavioral) corollary to dyspnea; the physical and emotional suffering that results from the experience of asphyxiation is characterized by behaviors that can be observed and measured.[8]

Most patients undergoing ventilator withdrawal will be unable to provide a self-report about any dyspnea experienced, particularly patients who are unconscious, severely cognitively impaired, or infants and neonates. Attempts to elicit a self-report should be made if the patient is conscious. Skill is required to detect nuances of behaviors particularly when the patient is unable to validate the nurse's assessment. Initiation and escalation of sedatives and opioids should be guided by patient behaviors.

The RDOS is suitable for assessing the adult patient during the withdrawal of mechanical ventilation; reliability and validity have been established.[9] This eight-variable categorical scale is the only known tool for assessing respiratory distress when the patient cannot self-report dyspnea as typifies most patients undergoing ventilator withdrawal. Infants and neonates often display nasal flaring, grunting at end-expiration, and sternal retraction.[10] Brain-dead patients by definition will not show distress, cough, gag, or breathe during or following ventilator withdrawal, and sedation or analgesia is not indicated.

Premedication for anticipated distress

As is the standard with pain management, opioids should be initiated to signs of distress and the advice to "start low and titrate slowly" is sage. For the opioid-naïve adult an initial bolus of 3 or 5 mg of morphine is recommended. Pediatric dosing is usually initiated at 0.1 to 0.2 mg/kg.[11] Anticipatory premedication is a sound practice if distress is already evident and if distress can be anticipated. There is no justification for medicating a brain-dead patient, and one could argue that the patient in coma with only minimal brainstem function is also unlikely to experience distress. Doses that correspond to customary dosing for the treatment of dyspnea should guide dosing during ventilator withdrawal. Documentation of the signs of distress and rationale for dose escalation is important to ensure continuity across professional caregivers and to prevent overmedication and the appearance of hastening death. At the conclusion of the process a continuous infusion may be initiated to maintain patient comfort; an infusion rate equivalent to 50% of total amount of bolus medication is recommended. Thus, if the patient received three boluses at 5 mg (15 mg) the infusion would start at a rate of 7.5 mg/h.

Weaning method

Terminal extubation is characterized by ceasing ventilatory support and removing the endotracheal tube in one step. Terminal weaning is a process of stepwise, gradual reductions in oxygen and ventilation, terminating with placement of a t-piece or with extubation. There are no known investigations comparing one method to another.[2]

With no comparative evidence to support one method over another it is difficult to make a recommendation. Rapid terminal weaning may afford the clinician with the most control because it allows for careful, sequential adjustments to the ventilator with precise titration of medications to ensure patient comfort. Continuous patient monitoring with readily accessible opioids and sedatives will afford the patient and family with comfort regardless of method employed.

Extubation considerations

Patients who are ventilator-dependent are generally ventilated through a tracheostomy tube. After ventilator withdrawal a tracheostomy mask with humidified room air or low-flow oxygen can be placed. Patients experiencing acute respiratory failure are ventilated through a nasal or oral endotracheal tube. Adult tubes have a cuff to maintain tube placement and occlude the trachea to prevent air leaking and loss of tidal volume; neonatal tubes are cuffless.

Removal of the endotracheal tube should be performed whenever possible because of patient comfort and the aesthetic appearance of the patient. However, in some cases airway compromise can be anticipated, such as when the patient has a swollen, protuberant tongue, or has no gag or cough reflexes. In cases of airway compromise the disconcerting noises may be more distressing to the attendant family than the presence of the tube. Medication with dexamethasone may reduce airway edema permitting extubation when patients are at high risk for postextubation laryngeal edema, but dosing would need to start 12 hours before withdrawal if the timing permits. A cuff-leak test entails measuring the volume of air loss when the endotracheal tube cuff is deflated prior to extubation. Air loss of less than 140 cc predicts postextubation stridor.[12] Aerosolized racemic epinephrine is a useful intervention to reduce stridor after extubation.[13] Family counseling about usual noises that can be expected and cause no distress should be done prior to extubation.

Oxygen

A growing body of evidence suggests that oxygen is a useful palliative intervention to treat dyspnea when the patient is experiencing distress and is hypoxemic but offers no benefit when the patient has normal oxygenation.[14,15] Further, when patients are near death and in no distress, oxygen is not necessary.[16] Thus, the patient can be cared for without oxygen following ventilator withdrawal unless there are signs of respiratory distress and hypoxemia. Nasal cannula is better tolerated than a face mask if oxygen is initiated.

Dialysis discontinuation

Case study

Mildred Jones is an 85-year-old woman with end-stage renal disease related to a long history of heart failure; she has been on hemodialysis for 2 months. She also has advanced-stage Alzheimer's disease. She lives in a dementia unit at an assisted living facility, from which she is taken to dialysis 3 times a week by dialysis unit–arranged van. The facility staff saw no signs of patient suffering prior to starting dialysis. Initially her dialysis was uneventful but recently staff has noted that the patient has become increasingly agitated when the van driver arrives. She tells the staff she doesn't want to go and to leave her alone. One of the patient's daughters has started coming to the assisted living to coax her mother into going to dialysis. The patient is unable to verbalize why she doesn't want to go to dialysis. The facility staff notes that the patient is becoming more agitated, restless, with some itching and vomiting. She is unable to respond when asked about pain or other discomforts. The dialysis team is unsure how to proceed with the patient refusing to go to dialysis. She has missed 2 treatments.

The nephrologist arranges a family meeting with the patient and her 2 daughters to discuss how to improve the patient's comfort and address the treatment goals. A local outpatient palliative care team will also participate. At the meeting the patient is mute and gives no indication of being able to participate. One of the daughters presents her mother's advance directive and reports that she is the patient-appointed surrogate. The advance directive indicates the patient's wish is to be allowed to die if she is terminally ill.

Both daughters express surprise at the extent of uncomfortable symptoms since starting dialysis; both thought the dialysis would treat all of these. Neither remembers any previous discussion about the option to not begin or to discontinue dialysis. After discussion about the burdens and benefits of dialysis, the patient's goals expressed in the past, and the current prognosis for her dementia, the daughters both agree that the patient should not be "forced" to go to dialysis. This would create more suffering and they realize their mother would never want the daughters to be put in this situation of prolonging her life with this poor quality. The daughters request that the patient not be transferred to the hospital but try to manage her care as an outpatient.

The decision is made to implement an improved symptom management plan recommended by Palliative Care and continue to offer dialysis to the patient. Mildred continues to refuse dialysis over the next 2 days. She becomes increasingly agitated each time it is offered. The daughters do not want her sedated to perform it, so the decision is made to discontinue dialysis.

Mildred is placed on hospice care. She spends the next 7 days with family and staff around her at the assisted living facility. She has been restless, so hydromorphone is administered as a trial to determine if her restlessness is due to pain. She also receives some lorazepam for anxiety, haloperidol for nausea/vomiting and emollient lotions for itching. She dies 11 days after her last dialysis with her family around her.

Benefits and burdens of dialysis

Dialysis was introduced as a treatment for end-stage renal disease (ESRD) in 1962. In the early years the number of patients receiving dialysis was limited by the small number of dialysis machines available, and only individuals younger than 40 years of age, family breadwinners, and those without severe medical problems like diabetes were considered.[17] In 1973, Medicare established universal entitlement for chronic dialysis; currently over 300,000 Americans receive dialysis.[18] Also referred to as CKD stage 5, ESRD is defined as a glomerular filtration rate of less than 15 mL/min (normal is greater than 90 mL/min). The most common causes include diabetes mellitus, heart failure, hypertension, and glomerulonephritis. Acute renal failure, also known as acute kidney injury (AKI) as well as acute renal injury (ARI), is commonly seen in the critically ill who suffer from dehydration, sepsis, hypotension, and/or trauma; AKI may lead to dialysis.

In the last 10 years the dialysis population has changed. The current dialysis population is older with more comorbidities, higher symptom burden, and a higher mortality rate than previous populations. More than 75% of hemodialysis patients are over 65 years old.[19] Patients older than 80 years now constitute the fastest-growing segment of this population and have a 46% mortality rate in the first year of dialysis.[20] The cause of this change in population is multifactorial and may be due to advances in life-prolonging therapies, nephrologists' focus on "life-saving" approaches, and reports that nephrologists are increasingly being expected to dialyze patients who they believe may receive little benefit from this therapy.[21] This population will not be candidates for transplant, so they will remain on dialysis until they die or until it is discontinued. As expected, elderly patients tend to have high symptom burden, higher rates of rehospitalization within 30 days of discharge, and frequent ICU admissions as well as higher use of more intensive procedures than younger patients.[18] They also may have slower progression of renal disease, so this should also be taken into consideration before rushing to start dialysis.[22]

Box 27.1 The Renal Physicians Association Guidelines on Initiation and Withdrawal from Dialysis

1. Develop a physician-patient relationship for shared decision-making

2. Fully inform ARI, stage 4 and 5 CKD, and ESRD patients about their dialysis, prognosis, and all treatment options

3. Give all patients with ARI, stage 5 CKD, or ESRD an estimate of prognosis specific to their overall condition

4. Institute advance care planning

5. If appropriate, forgo (withhold initiating or withdraw ongoing) dialysis for patients with AKI, CKD, or ESRD in certain well-defined situations

6. Consider forgoing dialysis for AKI, CKD, or ESRD patients who have a very poor prognosis or for whom dialysis cannot be provided safely as in advanced dementia or unstable hypotension.

7. Consider a time-limited trial of dialysis for patients requiring dialysis but who have an uncertain prognosis, or for whom a consensus cannot be reached about providing dialysis

8. Establish a systematic, due process approach for conflict resolution if there is disagreement about what decision should be made with regard to dialysis

9. To improve patient-centered outcomes, offer palliative care services and interventions to all AKI, CKD, and ESRD patient who suffer from burdens of their disease

10. Use a systematic approach to communicate about diagnosis, prognosis, treatment options, and goals of care

Source: Renal Physician's Association (2010), reference 24. Reproduced with permission.

A decision to stop dialysis is a frequent occurrence, especially in a frail elderly population. The nephrology community has been moving to address improved quality of life and incorporating advances from the palliative care field. Renal and palliative care experts recommend incorporating a discussion about discontinuing dialysis in the informed consent process for dialysis routinely with this population[22] and revisiting it regularly as the patient declines.[23] National initiatives including the Renal Physicians Association Clinical Practice Guidelines are addressing the growing needs of this older, sicker population.[24] See Box 27.1. Using well-established ethical principles and processes, the ethical framework of shared decision-making as covered in these guidelines gives support to the nephrologist to address the appropriate use of dialysis.[25]

Symptoms of uremia are usually controlled quickly with dialysis; paradoxically, dialysis produces one of the highest symptom burdens as well as hospitalization rates of any chronic illness population.[26,27] Jablonski found patients experience an average of six uncomfortable symptoms while on dialysis.[28] Davison and Jhangri found a mean of seven symptoms, and over 50% of patients had chronic pain.[29] Other discomforts with dialysis include fatigue, pruritus, constipation, anorexia, anxiety, and sleep disturbances.

The frail elderly with multiple comorbidities receiving dialysis are particularly vulnerable to a high symptom burden.[30,31] Therefore, although life may be prolonged with dialytic management of uremia, this population's quality of life will often not improve. Thus, a trial of dialysis may be offered in some cases to elderly patients to see if dialysis will improve symptoms, although this will require a vascular access. Germain and colleagues have noted that a time-limited trial of dialysis is appropriate only if there is a reasonable chance it will provide a net benefit to the patient and achieve the patient's and/or family's goals.[21] Some investigators are finding that patients had poor self-reported knowledge of options in stage 5 CKD and 61% regretted their decision to start dialysis.[32] Wachterman and colleagues found that dialysis patients tended to be more optimistic about prognosis than their nephrologists, indicating that these patients had not been given accurate information or had not absorbed this information.[33]

In response to the aging population and trends of dialyzing older and sicker patients, interest is growing in nondialytic medical therapy for ESRD. Conservative management of uremia without dialysis is now being offered more frequently in the presence of advanced age and comorbidities.[21,34] Conservative treatment is associated with a high symptom burden, thus concomitant palliative care is indicated.[35]

Discontinuing dialysis

Dialysis was rarely withdrawn in the initial years of this treatment option unless there was loss of vascular access that made dialysis impossible.[17] Today 20%–25% of patients receiving dialysis have it discontinued each year.[24] Stopping dialysis remains the second leading condition prior to death in this population.[18] Mailloux notes that withholding dialysis probably occurs even more frequently than commonly thought given the frequency of it being offered or doctors feeling obligated to offer it as a trial in very ill patients.[36] Stopping dialysis should be considered when the burdens of dialysis outweigh the benefits and/or dialysis is no longer serving to substantially prolong life or is only prolonging death.

The most common reason for stopping dialysis is unacceptable quality of life. Specific causes include pain, burden of multiple symptoms, acute complications such as infection, technical problems with dialysis, dementia, stroke, and cancer.[37] Additionally, some patients become too unstable to complete the dialysis session. Peritoneal dialysis patients may be too sick to carry out exchanges and need to obtain vascular access for hemodialysis. Inserting new access lines may cause the patient to consider discontinuing dialysis.

Addressing symptom burden, including psychological symptoms, is an important consideration before making the decision to discontinue dialysis. Patients on dialysis often struggle with depression, changes in body image, sexual dysfunction, loss of control, irritability, and dependency issues along with the physical symptoms. These can all contribute to a patient's consideration of stopping dialysis. When discontinuation is being considered, addressing symptom burden is key prior to stopping it.[37] A thorough assessment and interventions to address all these issues should be part of any treatment plan when discontinuing dialysis is being considered. See Box 27.2 for guidelines on this decision. Shared decision-making with the patient/family/nephrologist discussing the burdens, benefits, possible reversible factors, goals, and outcomes need to be part of the treatment plan when considering the option of discontinuing dialysis. If the patient cannot

---

Box 27.2 Guidelines for making dialysis discontinuation decisions

- Identify patients who may benefit from discontinuation including those patients with poor prognosis, poor quality of life, pain that is poorly responsive to treatment, progressive untreatable disease, and technically difficult dialysis.
- Address patient's decision-making capacity.
  - Discuss goals with patient/family.
  - Discuss quality of life.
  - Discuss possible symptoms and their palliation.
- Identify possible reversible causes.
- Clarify that dialysis discontinuation is an option, as part of a review of treatment modalities, when educating patients who are new to dialysis.
  - Provide reassurance of a peaceful death.
  - Allow time for discussion.
- Make the recommendation to stop dialysis and request patient/family assent.

Sources: References 36, 37.

---

make his/her own decisions, surrogate decision-makers must be driven by the patient's values.

When patients make their own decisions, stopping dialysis can be a freeing, almost euphoric experience.[38] The patient often has a few days before uremic symptoms begin; this time can include eating favorite, formerly forbidden foods and opportunities to say good-bye to loved ones. This allows a patient to maintain some sense of control over his/her life and the dying process. Choosing the date of the last dialysis, where he/she wants to be for the last days, choosing what foods to eat, all can enhance a sense of control. Family members may struggle with accepting the patient's choice. Loved ones need to be prepared that the patient may become cognitively impaired suddenly as the creatinine rises.

When the patient is unable to participate in decision-making because of dementia, delirium, or critical illness, families and/or surrogates often struggle with making this literally life-and-death decision. But if the patient's suffering with dialysis has been evident, it can be easier for them to make the decision to stop. Another key factor for surrogates is the patient's inability to return to an acceptable quality of life.

Treating symptoms after discontinuation

Death after discontinuation of dialysis generally occurs in 8–12 days, though patients with many comorbidities may die sooner, and patients who make urine generally live longer. Nearly all patients discontinuing dialysis die within 1 month.[39] Death is generally caused by accumulation of toxins including potassium as well as other factors due to comorbidities.[40] Patients may have a few days of relative comfort with sudden onset of symptoms. Last days and hours are characterized by hypersomnolence followed by coma. A peaceful death can be achieved with palliative care management of symptoms. Cohen and colleagues found that the majority of families whose loved ones died after withdrawal of dialysis rated the death as good to very good.[41]

The most frequent symptoms after discontinuation include pain, delirium, dyspnea, nausea, and itching. Frequent pain assessment and aggressive analgesia is important, as symptoms can develop quickly. Though uremia itself is painless, patients may experience pain from their general medical condition.[39] Morphine should be avoided due to its metabolite morphine-3-glucuronide, which increases in kidney failure putting the patient at risk for myoclonus, seizures, and hyperalgesia. Fentanyl and methadone are better choices. Hydromorphone and oxycodone can be used but with caution. Hydromorphone does have a metabolite that can accumulate, and oxycodone has not been well studied in this population.[21,39,42–45] Myoclonus can be treated with benzodiazepines if it occurs. As the patient becomes obtunded near death, swallowing a pill may become difficult and liquid opioids may be selected. Methadone can be given as an elixir into the sublingual or buccal space, where it will gradually trickle into the pharynx and be swallowed.

Delirium, confusion, and somnolence are expected as part of the uremic syndrome. A more severe form of delirium called uremic encephalopathy occurs infrequently. It is characterized by extreme agitation and hallucinations. Haloperidol, clonazepam, or lorazepam are useful if the patient becomes agitated and doses are not dependent on renal function.

Dyspnea can occur from fluid retention and pleural effusion. Anticholinergics to reduce oral secretions, opioids for dyspnea, and low-flow oxygen may be helpful. Stopping hydration and artificial nutrition will minimize fluid retention. Pulmonary edema is a palliative care emergency that may arise from volume overload. Diuresis is not possible, but systemic vasodilation may provide relief; nitroglycerin paste every 6 hours is recommended. Ultrafiltration through the dialysis access, if patent, and if the patient is still in the hospital, will also relieve volume overload.[40]

Nausea may be an effect of uremia as well as delayed gastric emptying that is common in ESRD; haloperidol is a useful antiemetic in this context. The liberty to eat previously forbidden foods may contribute to the onset of nausea and vomiting, and the patient will need to be counseled about moderation.

Itching referred to as uremic pruritus is another effect of uremia and responds well to benzodiazepines and diphenhydramine, along with lanolin-based or capsaicin creams.[46] Principles for treating uremic symptoms follow in Box 27.3. Symptom management strategies need to be in place when dialysis is stopped, as the time frame to death is brief and symptoms can intensify quickly.

Role of palliative care and hospice

Dialysis centers are encouraged to develop a palliative care approach to address their patients' needs, which may include advance care planning for timing of discontinuation of dialysis and location of death. Cohen, Davison, and Moss,[21] leaders in nephrology, recommend that palliative care should be offered to all patients with ESRD who experience burdens of their disease regardless of whether they start or refuse dialysis therapy and whether they continue or withdraw from dialysis therapy. Palliative care consultation is especially important with complex pain and symptom management.[23]

Hospice care can also be appropriate both for dialysis patients with comorbidities and patients who are considering discontinuing dialysis; however, hospice has historically been underutilized

---

Box 27.3 Treatment principles when discontinuing dialysis

- Avoid volume overload including hydration and artificial nutrition.
- Utilize symptom management medications not metabolized via the kidneys.
- Discontinue all non-symptom-management medications to reduce risk of toxicities.
- Involve a pharmacist consultation early to ensure no medications given are metabolized via kidneys.
- Anticipate common symptoms and have appropriate medications available as symptoms can occur suddenly.
- Prepare patient and family for what to expect, especially addressing common unfounded fears of drowning in fluid.

Sources: References 39, 42.

---

in this population.[19,39] The percentage of dying ESRD patients who receive hospice is significantly less than other diagnoses.[19] See Box 27.4 for a list of barriers to hospice utilization. Hospice care is appropriate for patients when dialysis is stopped. Making a referral to hospice early in the discussion period about stopping dialysis may increase access earlier. Hospice can help these patients remain at home after dialysis is stopped and manage symptoms effectively. Patients may also qualify for hospice while continuing on dialysis due to their poor prognosis and comorbidities in some cases when they have a second terminal diagnosis in addition to ESRD such as heart failure.[21,47] These patients can

---

Box 27.4 Barriers to use of hospice in end-stage renal disease

- Financial disincentives and confusion about coverage and eligibility
- Hospice agencies and local dialysis centers often do not have relationships.
- Hospice agencies' concern about reimbursement when the patient is still on dialysis
- Nephrology professionals not addressing end-of-life issues with patients
- Dialysis staff often have inaccurate information about hospice care.
- Patients/families with lack of awareness of life-limiting nature of ESRD
- Hospice not offered when dialysis is being discontinued due to brief life expectancy
- Nephrologists often driven by "life-saving" culture
- Lack of good prognostic models for patients remaining on dialysis or receiving non dialysis medical management of renal failure who also may qualify for hospice

Sources: References 19, 21, 39

benefit from improved symptom management and ongoing discussion about goals.

Deactivation of cardiac implantable devices

Case study

Peter Rupersburg enjoyed 5 years of increased survival with his implantable cardioverter defibrillator (ICD), which had been inserted when ventricular arrhythmias were previously diagnosed. He had experienced rare activations of his device over the ensuing years. Meanwhile, this 72-year-old man developed Alzheimer's type dementia, which had progressed to an advanced stage. He was hospitalized with pneumonia, and during a discussion about hospice enrollment his wife asked about deactivation of the ICD. She was worried that ICD firing would interfere with a natural dying trajectory. A cardiology consult led to ICD deactivation. Subsequently, Peter was discharged home to the care of his family with a home hospice referral.

Benefits and burdens of cardiac assist devices

Implantable cardioverter defibrillators, pacemakers, ventricular assist devices (VADs) and even a totally artificial replacement heart used for many patients with advanced cardiac disease, represent advanced life-sustaining technology. The number of adult patients with implantable cardiac devices is rising sharply, making it among the most common cardiovascular device used in contemporary clinical practice.[48] Because these devices reduce the incidence of sudden death, patients with implantable defibrillators are more likely to die of other nonarrhythmic causes such as cancer, lung disease, advanced dementia, and congestive heart failure.[49,50]

Discussions for deactivation of cardiac devices

Prior to insertion of an ICD/pacemaker/VAD a general discussion should occur with the patient/and family regarding the possibility that the device may be deactivated at a future point in time if therapy is ineffective, no longer needed, or not desired. During the informed consent process information is provided to the patient about the device, indications, how it works, the expected benefits, the risks, required follow-up, device maintenance (e.g., battery changes) and the possibility that the device may be deactivated in the future. A statement such as the following introduces the topic: "A time may come in the future when the device may not work as we had anticipated, or you may decide that you no longer want it. If that time comes we will talk about deactivating the device." When having end-of-life "discussions with patients and their families facing the last chapter, it is easier if they have heard previously of the potential circumstances for turning the defibrillation off."[51]

Grassman reported, "We had a patient who went home with hospice care. The ICD was never turned off. As a result, the wife told us that the patient died in her arms while the defibrillator jolted him 33 times before the battery ran down."[52] Thus, not addressing deactivation of the ICD can cause not only unnecessary suffering for the patient but also distress for the patient's family. Even when death is expected and discussions have occurred regarding resuscitation and other end-of-life care, the topic of deactivating the ICD is not routinely discussed.[53,54]

Deactivation procedures

Pacemakers

A pacemaker is intended to correct an abnormal heart rate or rhythm. Some patients are only mildly reliant on the device; others are total dependent to the extent that if the pacemaker is deactivated discomfort secondary to complete heart block or bradycardia can occur. Sudden death at the time of disabling the pacemaker is unlikely, unless the patient is pacemaker-dependent.

Trained personnel should interrogate the pacemaker with the pacemaker programmer. Prepare the patient and family for a rapid death after deactivation if the patient is pacemaker-dependent. Adjust the pacemaker settings (e.g., rate and output) so pacing does not occur, this can be done gradually or all at once. The patient can be premedicated with an anxiolytic or sedative if desired, particularly if a relatively sudden death can be anticipated and the patient is capable of experiencing distress.

Implantable cardioverter defibrillators

Defibrillators are intended only to convert a lethal ventricular arrhythmia. Deactivation of an ICD will not degrade quality of life or create discomfort. Conversely, as illustrated previously, ICD firing while the patient is dying can be distressing to both the patient and family.

Deactivation should be done by trained personnel using the programmer for either device. A pacemaker magnet can be placed over the ICD generator, palpable under the skin, to deactivate when an ICD programmer is unavailable. However, it will not deactivate the backup pacing function of the ICD; this can only be done by an ICD programmer. The funeral director will need to be informed about the presence of the device, or any other implanted metallic device especially with a battery, if cremation is planned.

Ventricular assist devices

Ventricular assist devices are mechanical pumps surgically implanted to improve the performance of the damaged left (LVAD), right (RVAD), or both (BiVAD) ventricles. These VADs can be used short-term as a bridge to recovery or transplantation, or as destination therapy, that is an alternative to transplantation. Short-term support is indicated for patients who develop cardiogenic shock in which recovery is anticipated with devices outside the body attached to large consoles. The average duration of VAD support for these critically ill patients is a week, but the units are capable of providing support for up to a month. Prolonged support is associated with coagulopathy, thrombocytopenia, thromboembolism, and hemolysis. When VADs are inserted as destination therapy, it is expected that the patient will need the VAD the rest of his/her life, thus, the VAD is considered a final treatment. Technological advances have made VADs compact and portable, allowing freedom for patients to be discharged home from the hospital, with high-level home health follow-up. Initial clinical trials of older pulsatile flow VADs showed a 52% 1-year survival[55]; more recent studies of continuous flow pumps demonstrated a 73% 1-year survival.[56]

Trained personnel should stop the VAD after patient and family preparation and silencing the device alarms. The patient may experience distress from heart failure and may benefit from premedication with a diuretic and an anxiolytic. After deactivation the patient will require close monitoring and symptomatic treatment of heart failure until death occurs.

Summary

Withdrawal of mechanical ventilation, discontinuation of dialysis, and deactivation of cardiac devices are procedures that occur with relative frequency. The benefits of these therapies, when initiated are to replace failing organs, extend life, and improve quality of life by relieving symptom distress associated with organ failure. When the burdens exceed the benefits, or when the patient is near death or unresponsive, decisions may be made to cease these therapies.

In some cases, such as ICD deactivation, no distress is anticipated. In others, such as discontinuing dialysis or withdrawing MV, measures to palliate anticipated distress must be applied. A peaceful death after cessation of life-prolonging therapies can be provided.

References

1. Azoulay E, Kouatchet A, Jaber S, et al. Noninvasive mechanical ventilation in patients having declined tracheal intubation. Intensive Care Med. 2013;39:292–301.
2. Campbell ML. How to withdraw mechanical ventilation: a systematic review of the literature. AACN Adv Crit Care. 2007;18:397–403; quiz 344–345.
3. National Consensus Project for Quality Palliative Care. Clinical Practice Guidelines for Quality Palliative Care. 3rd ed. 2013.
4. Hospital Conditions of Participation About Organ/Tissue Donation. http://www.cms.gov/manuals/downloads/som107ap_a_hospitals.pdf. Accessed November 1, 2013.
5. Wiegand DL, Grant MS, Cheon J, Gergis MA. Family-centered end-of-life care in the ICU. J Gerontol Nurs. 2013;39:60–68.
6. Truog RD, Campbell ML, Curtis JR, et al. Recommendations for end-of-life care in the intensive care unit: a consensus statement by the American College [corrected] of Critical Care Medicine. Crit Care Med. 2008;36:953–963.
7. Parshall MB, Schwartzstein RM, Adams L, et al. An official American Thoracic Society statement: update on the mechanisms, assessment, and management of dyspnea. Am J Respir Crit Care Med. 2012;185:435–452.
8. Campbell ML. Fear and pulmonary stress behaviors to an asphyxial threat across cognitive states. Res Nurs Health. 2007;30:572–583.
9. Campbell ML, Templin T, Walch J. A respiratory distress observation scale for patients unable to self-report dyspnea. J Palliat Med. 2010;13:285–290.
10. Catlin A, Carter B. Creation of a neonatal end-of-life palliative care protocol. J Perinatol. 2002;22:184–195.
11. Zernikow B, Michel E, Craig F, Anderson BJ. Pediatric palliative care: use of opioids for the management of pain. Paediatric Drugs. 2009;11:129–151.
12. Chung YH, Chao TY, Chiu CT, Lin MC. The cuff-leak test is a simple tool to verify severe laryngeal edema in patients undergoing long-term mechanical ventilation. Crit Care Med. 2006;34:409–414.
13. Sinha A, Jayashree M, Singhi S. Aerosolized L-epinephrine vs budesonide for post extubation stridor: a randomized controlled trial. Indian Pediatrics. 2010;47:317–322.
14. Abernethy AP, McDonald CF, Frith PA, et al. Effect of palliative oxygen versus room air in relief of breathlessness in patients with refractory dyspnoea: a double-blind, randomised controlled trial. Lancet. 2010;376:784–793.
15. Uronis H, McCrory DC, Samsa G, Currow D, Abernethy A. Symptomatic oxygen for non-hypoxaemic chronic obstructive pulmonary disease. Cochrane Database Syst Rev. 2011;6:CD006429.
16. Campbell ML, Yarandi H, Dove-Medows E. Oxygen is nonbeneficial for most patients who are near death. J Pain Symptom Manage. 2013;45:517–523.
17. Germain MJ, Cohen LM, Davison SN. Withholding and withdrawal from dialysis: what we know about how our patients die. Semin Dial. 2007;20:195–199.
18. U.S. Renal Data System, USRDS 2013 Annual Data Report: Atlas of Chronic Kidney Disease and End-Stage Renal Disease in the United States, National Institutes of Health, National Institute of Diabetes and Digestive and Kidney Diseases, Bethesda, MD, http://www.usrds.org/adr.aspx
19. Cohen LM, Ruthazer R, Germain MJ. Increasing hospice services for elderly patients maintained with hemodialysis. J Palliat Med. 2010;13:847–854.
20. Kurella M, Covinsky KE, Collins AJ, Chertow GM. Octogenarians and nonagenarians starting dialysis in the United States. Ann Intern Med. 2007;146:177–183.
21. Germain MJ, Davison SN, Moss AH. When enough is enough: the nephrologist's responsibility in ordering dialysis treatments. Amer J Kidney Dis. 2011;58:135–143.
22. Schmidt RJ. Informing our elders about dialysis: is an age-attuned approach warranted? CJASN. 2012;7:185–191.
23. Schmidt RJ, Moss AH. Dying on dialysis: the case for a dignified withdrawal. CJASN. 2014:9:174–180.
24. Renal Physicians Association. Shared Decision-Making in the Appropriate Initiation of and Withdrawal from Dialysis: Clinical Practice Guidelines. 2nd ed. Rockville, MD: Renal Physicians Association; 2010.
25. Moss AH. To dialyze or not: the patient with metastatic cancer and AKI in the intensive care unit. CJASN. 2012;7:1507–1512.
26. Germain MJ, Cohen LM. Maintaining quality of life at the end of life in the end-stage renal disease population. Adv Chronic Kidney Dis. 2008;15:133–139.
27. Germain MJ, Kurella Tamura M, Davison SN. Palliative care in CKD: the earlier the better. Amer J Kidney Dis. 2011;57:378–380.
28. Jablonski A. Level of symptom relief and the need for palliative care in the hemodialysis population. J Hosp Palliat Nurs. 2007;9:50–60.
29. Davison SN, Jhangri GS. Impact of pain and symptom burden on the health-related quality of life of hemodialysis patients. J Pain Symptom Manage. 2010;39:477–485.
30. Wong SP, Kreuter W, O'Hare AM. Treatment intensity at the end of life in older adults receiving long-term dialysis. Arch Intern Med. 2012;172:661–663; discussion 3–4.
31. Yong DS, Kwok AO, Wong DM, Suen MH, Chen WT, Tse DM. Symptom burden and quality of life in end-stage renal disease: a study of 179 patients on dialysis and palliative care. Palliat Med. 2009;23:111–119.
32. Davison SN. End-of-life care preferences and needs: perceptions of patients with chronic kidney disease. CJASN 2010;5:195–204.
33. Wachterman MW, Marcantonio ER, Davis RB, Cohen RA, Waikar SS. Relationship between the prognostic expectations of seriously ill patients undergoing hemodialysis and their nephrologists. JAMA Int Med. 2013;27:1–8.
34. Murtagh FE, Addington-Hall J, Edmonds P, et al. Symptoms in the month before death for stage 5 chronic kidney disease patients managed without dialysis. J Pain Symptom Manage. 2010;40:342–352.
35. O'Connor NR, Kumar P. Conservative management of end-stage renal disease without dialysis: a systematic review. J Palliat Med. 2012;15:228–235.
36. Mailloux L. Initiation, withdrawal and withholding dialysis. In: Chambers E, Brown E, Germain MJ (eds.), Supportive care of the renal patient. Oxford, England: Oxford University Press; 2010:231–240.
37. Davison SN, Rosielle DA. Withdrawal of dialysis: decision making #207. J Palliat Med. 2012;15:1270–1271.
38. Cohen LM, Germain MJ, Poppel DM. Practical considerations in dialysis withdrawal: "to have that option is a blessing." JAMA. 2003;289:2113–2119.
39. Moss AH. Kidney failure. In: Emmanuel L, Librach S (eds.), Palliative Care: Core Skills and Clinical Competencies. Philadelphia: Saunders Elsevier; 2011:405–420.

40. Farrington K, Chambers E. Death and end of life care. In: Chambers E, Brown E, Germain MJ (eds.), Supportive Care of the Renal Patient. Oxford, England: Oxford University Press; 2010:281–292.

41. Cohen LM, Poppel DM, Cohn GM, Reiter GS. A very good death: measuring quality of dying in end-stage renal disease. J Palliat Med. 2001;4:167–172.

42. Davison SN, Rosielle DA. Clinical care following withdrawal of dialysis #208. J Palliat Med. 2012;15:1271–1272.

43. Mid-Atlantic Renal Coalition and the Kidney End of Life Coalition. Clinical Algorithm and Preferred Medications to Treat Pain in Dialysis Patients. Richmond, VA: Author; 2009.

44. Paramanandam G, Prommer E, Schwenke DC. Adverse effects in hospice patients with chronic kidney disease receiving hydromorphone. J Palliat Med. 2011;14:1029–1033.

45. Russon L, Mooney A. Palliative and end-of-life care in advanced renal failure. Clin Med. 2010;10:279–281.

46. Gorman L. Pruritus in end stage renal disease. In: Campbell ML, ed. Case Studies in Palliative and End of Life Care. Ames, IA: Wiley-Blackwell; 2012:183–189.

47. Trivedi DD. Palliative dialysis in end-stage renal disease. Am J Hosp Palliat Care. 2011;28:539–542.

48. Go AS, Mozaffarian D, Roger VL, et al. Executive summary: heart disease and stroke statistics—2013 update: a report from the American Heart Association. Circulation. 2013;127:143–152.

49. Bramstedt KA. Elective inactivation of total artificial heart technology in non-futile situations: inpatients, outpatients and research participants. Death Stud. 2004;28:423–433.

50. Lipman HI. Deactivation of advanced lifesaving technologies. Am J Geriatr Cardiol. 2007;16:109–111.

51. Blumer J, Wolber T, Hellermann J, et al. Predictors of appropriate implantable cardioverter-defibrillator therapy during long-term follow-up of patients with coronary artery disease. Int Heart J. 2009;50:313–321.

52. Grassman D. EOL considerations in defibrillator deactivation. Am J Hosp Palliat Care. 2005;22:179; author reply, 80.

53. Goldstein NE, Mehta D, Teitelbaum E, Bradley EH, Morrison RS. "It's like crossing a bridge": Complexities preventing physicians from discussing deactivation of implantable defibrillators at the end of life. J Gen Intern Med. 2008;23(Suppl 1):2–6.

54. Hauptman PJ, Swindle J, Hussain Z, Biener L, Burroughs TE. Physician attitudes toward end-stage heart failure: a national survey. Am J Med. 2008;121:127–135.

55. Rose EA, Gelijns AC, Moskowitz AJ, et al. Long-term use of a left ventricular assist device for end-stage heart failure. N Engl J Med. 2001;345: 1435–1443.

56. Park SJ, Milano CA, Tatooles AJ, et al. Outcomes in advanced heart failure patients with left ventricular assist devices for destination therapy. Circulation Heart Failure. 2012;5:241–248.

SECTION III

Psychosocial support

CHAPTER 28

The meaning of hope in the dying

Valerie T. Cotter and Anessa M. Foxwell

Hope is a powerful influence in our lives. Hope is potentially everywhere, including the bedside of someone who is dying. When mobilized effectively, robust hope is precious; when left untended, effete hope can send us in perilous directions.[1]

Key points

- Hope is a key factor in coping with and finding meaning in the experience of life-threatening illness.

- People with life-threatening illness and their families do not invariably lose hope; in fact, hope can increase at the end of life.

- Nurses can implement evidence-based practices to foster and sustain hope for patients and families at the end of life.

- Nurses need to understand and respect individual variations in hope processes to provide sensitive, effective care to patients and their families at the end of life.

Hope has long been recognized as fundamental to the human experience. Many authors have contemplated hope, extolling it as a virtue and an energy that brings life and joy.[2-4] Fromm[2] called hope "a psychic commitment to life and growth." Some authors assert that life without hope is impossible.[4]

Despite its positive connotations, hope is intimately bound with loss and suffering. As the French philosopher Gabriel Marcel[3] observed, "Hope is situated within the framework of the trial." It is this paradox that manifests itself so fully at the end of life.

Indeed, the critical role that hope plays in human life takes on special meaning as death nears. The ability to hope often is challenged, and it can elude patients and families during terminal illness. Hope for a cure is almost certainly destroyed, and even a prolonged reprieve from death is unlikely. Many patients and families experience multiple losses as they continue an illness trajectory that is marked by increasing disability and pain.

Even when hope appears to be strong within the dying person or the family, it can be problematic if hopefulness is perceived to be based on unrealistic ideas about the future.[5,6] Tension grows within relationships as people become absorbed in a struggle between competing versions of reality. Important issues may be left unresolved as individuals continue to deny the reality of impending death.

Despite these somber realities and the inevitable suffering, many people do maintain hope as they die, and families recover and find hope even within the experience of loss. How can this be? Part of the reason lies in the nature of hope itself—its resiliency and capacity to coexist with suffering. As witnesses to suffering and hope, palliative care nurses must understand these complexities and be confident and sensitive in their efforts to address hope and hopelessness in the people for whom they care.

To assist palliative care nurses, this chapter explores the many dimensions of hope and identifies its possible influence on health and quality of life. Nursing assessment and strategies to foster hope are described. In addition, specific issues such as "unrealistic hopefulness" and cultural considerations in the expression and maintenance of hope are discussed. The goals of the chapter are to provide the reader with an understanding about this complex but vital phenomenon; to offer guidance in the clinical application of this concept to palliative nursing care; and to explore some of the controversies about hope that challenge clinicians.

Definitions and dimensions of hope

Hope is an important concept for many disciplines, including philosophy, theology, psychology, nursing, and medicine. A classic nursing theory of hope, developed by Karin Dufault[7] is particularly notable in its comprehensiveness. Dufault[7] described hope as "a multidimensional, dynamic life force characterized by a confident yet uncertain expectation of achieving a future good which, to the hoping person, is realistically possible and personally significant." Dufault also theorized that hope has two interrelated spheres: particularized and generalized. *Particularized hope* is centered and dependent on specific, valued goals or hope objects. An example is the hope of a terminally ill patient to live long enough to celebrate a particular holiday or event. In contrast, *generalized hope* is a broader, nonspecific sense of a more positive future that is not directly related to a particular goal or desire. Dufault likened this sphere to an umbrella that creates a diffuse, positive glow on life.

Dufault postulated six dimensions of hope: affective, spiritual, relational, cognitive, behavioral, and contextual. The *affective* dimension of hope encompasses a myriad of emotions.

Of course, hope is accompanied by many positive feelings, including joy, confidence, strength, and excitement. The full experience of hope, however, also includes uncertainty, fear, anger, suffering, and, sometimes, despair.[8-11] The philosopher Gabriel Marcel, for example, argued that in its fullest sense hope could only follow an experience of suffering or trial.[3] Marcel's thesis is corroborated by the experiences described by people with cancer who see their disease as "a wake-up call" that has opened their eyes to a greater appreciation for life and an opportunity for self-growth—in other words, an event that has forced them to confront their mortality while also inspiring hope.[12] The *spiritual* dimension is a central component of hope.[12-15] Hopefulness is associated with spiritual well-being,[13,16,17] and qualitative studies have shown that spirituality and spiritual practices provide a context in which to define hope and articulate hope-fostering activities.[7,18] These activities include religious beliefs and rituals but extend to broader conceptualizations of spirituality that encompass meaning and purpose in life, self-transcendence, and connectedness with a deity or other life-force.[14,19] Although spirituality is almost always viewed as a hope-fostering influence, serious illness and suffering can challenge one's belief and trust in a benevolent deity or be viewed as punishment from God; either interpretation of suffering can result in hopelessness.[20]

Relationships with significant others are another important dimension of hope. Interconnectedness with others is cited as a source of hope in virtually every study, and physical and psychological isolation from others is a frequent threat to hope.[12,21,22] Hope levels are positively associated with social support.[23,24] In addition to family members and friends, nurses offer patients a unique and independent source of support for hope.[25,26] Harris et al.[21] reported that HIV peer-counseling relationships inspired hope in both the counseling recipients and their counselors. Despite being vital sources of hope, other people can threaten a patient's hope by distancing themselves from the patient, showing disrespect, discounting the patient's experiences, disclosing negative information, or withholding information.[20,22]

The *cognitive* dimension of hope encompasses many intellectual strategies, particularly those involving specific goals that require planning and effort to attain. Identifying goals can motivate and energize people, thereby increasing hope.[21,27] When identifying goals, people assess what they desire and value within a context of what is realistically possible.[28] They appraise the resources necessary to accomplish their goals against the resources that are available to them. They then take action to secure the resources or meet the goals, and they decide on a reasonable time frame in which to accomplish the goals.[29] Active involvement in one's situation and attainment of goals increases the sense of personal control and self-efficacy, which, in turn, increases hope.[28] If a person repeatedly fails to attain valued goals, hopelessness and negative emotions, such as anxiety, depression, or anger can result.[27]

The *behavioral*, goal-focused thoughts and activities that foster hope are similar to the problem-focused coping strategies originally described by Lazarus and Folkman.[30] This similarity is not surprising, because hope is strongly associated with coping.[31] Hope has been identified as a foundation or mediator for successful coping, a method of coping, and an outcome of successful coping.[31,32] Many strategies that people use to maintain hope have been previously identified as coping methods, and models of maintaining hope overlap substantially with models of coping.[5,31] Strategies to maintain hope include problem-focused coping methods (e.g., setting goals, actively managing symptoms, getting one's affairs in order) and emotion-focused strategies (e.g., using distraction techniques, appraising the illness in nonthreatening ways).[5,31,33]

Contextual dimensions of hope are the life circumstances and abilities that influence hope—for example, physical health, financial stability, and functional and cognitive abilities. Common threats to hope include acute, chronic, and terminal illness; cognitive decline; fatigue; pain; and impaired functional status.[31,34] These factors, particularly physical illness and impairment, do not inevitably decrease hope if people are able to overcome the threat through cognitive, spiritual, relational, or other strategies.

Influence of hope and hopelessness on adaptation to illness

Hope influences health and adaptation to illness. Empirical evidence indicates that diminished hope is associated with poorer quality of life[32] persistence of suicidal ideation,[35] and higher incidence of suicide.[36] Hopelessness also increases the likelihood that people will consider physician-assisted death as an option for themselves.[37] Hopelessness is significant in the etiology and maintenance of depression.[36]

In addition to its influence on psychological states and behaviors, there is some evidence to suggest that hope affects physical states as well. Researchers have found associations between hopelessness and early markers of endothelial dysfunction, a precursor to atherosclerosis.[38] Rawdin and colleagues[34] reported that hope was associated with the psychosocial elements of the pain experience.

Variations in hope among different populations

The preceding description of hope is derived from studies involving diverse populations, including children and older adults. In addition, research has been conducted in inpatient, outpatient, and community settings with well persons and those with a variety of chronic and life-threatening illnesses. The experiences of families also have been described. Over these diverse populations and settings, many core concepts have been identified that transcend specific groups. However, some subtle but important differences exist. For this reason, hopefulness in selected populations is addressed in the following sections.

Hope in children and their parents

A few investigators have examined hope in children and their parents. Kylma and Juvakka[39] studied hope in parents of adolescents with cancer. The findings suggested that hope appears to be central to parents who have a child with cancer. Their hope reflected an orientation toward life and the future, trust, connection with others, and wishes. Factors endangering parental hope were related to the adolescent's cancer and deteriorating health status, negative aspects in care received, poor parental resources, tightened economic situation, and other people's negative reactions. Hope-engendering factors were related to the adolescent's constructive personality, positive consequences from the adolescent's cancer, the adolescent's improving health status, good care, gradual ability to continue life, good parental resources, other people's positive reactions, having faith, and having family pets.

Salmon and colleagues[40] explored how hope arose in interactions between oncologists and parents of children aged one to twelve years with acute lymphoblastic leukemia. The investigators found an interpersonal basis of hope (e.g., most parents linked their ability to hope to "having faith in" the oncologist and consistently valued oncologists' explicit positivity) and a psychological basis of hope (e.g., focusing on short-term events associated with treatment and avoiding information about the longer term).

In another study, Mack and colleagues[41] surveyed parents of children with cancer and the children's physicians to evaluate relationships between parental recall of prognostic disclosure by the physician and possible outcomes, including hope, trust, and emotional distress. Nearly half of parents reported that physician communication always made them feel hopeful. Parents were more likely to report communication-related hope when they also recalled increased prognostic disclosure.

Hope and older adults

Numerous studies have examined hope in ill and healthy older adults.[42-44] Findings from these studies suggest that certain hope-related themes and factors take on special significance for this age group. For example in a recent metasynthesis of qualitative research, hope was described as an important psychological resource that helped older adults deal with chronic illness.[43] Older adults used two interrelated processes to help deal with their experience: (1) transcendence, a process of reaching inwardly and outwardly, and finding meaning and purpose, and (2) positive reappraisal, a recognition and acknowledgment that their situation had changed and they could see positive possibilities for the future. Although chronic illness that impairs physical functioning is linked with decreased hope, diagnosis of a life-threatening disease, such as cancer, is not associated with low levels of hope.[45] This finding may reflect an attitude among older adults that the quality of life that remains matters more than the quantity.

Hirsch and colleagues[42] studied older adults recruited from primary care settings. They found that functional impairment was associated with increased depressive symptoms and individuals with higher levels of hope experienced fewer depressive symptoms. Also, the ability to generate goals and resources to accomplish goals contributed to higher levels of hope.

Among younger European American adults, hope tends to be tied to being productive; personal and professional achievements figure prominently in one's ability to nurture and maintain hope. In contrast, older adults are more likely to focus on spirituality, relationships, leaving a legacy focused on others, and other factors that are not linked with accomplishment.[46] Hope-fostering activities include reminiscing, controlling symptoms, spirituality, and connecting with others.

Hope from the family caregiver's perspective

Family caregivers are an integral component in palliative care. Patients and families influence each other's hope, and nursing interventions must focus on both groups. Often, the physical and psychological demands placed on family caregivers are great, as are threats to hope.[33,47,48] Threats to hope in caregivers include isolation from support networks, questioning of one's spiritual beliefs; concurrent losses, including loss of significant others, health, and income; and inability to control the patient's symptoms. Holtslander and Duggleby[49] reported that difficulties in communicating with healthcare providers, feelings of depersonalization, and receipt of "too many negative messages" also eroded caregivers' hope. Other studies found that hope played a significant role in family caregivers' perception of increased strain and overall quality of life.[50,51]

Strategies to maintain hope in family caregivers are similar to those found in patients, with a few differences. Spending time with others in the support network was very important for caregivers. In addition, being able to reprioritize demands helped caregivers conserve much-needed energy. Obtaining respite from the caregiving role also promoted hope.[49]

Case study

Mr. R, a patient with recently diagnosed metastatic cancer

Mr. R, a 64-year-old married man and retired auditor, was recently diagnosed with metastatic non-small-cell lung cancer. Nine months prior Mr. R began experiencing right shoulder pain while playing golf. He sought treatment from multiple providers including an internist, an orthopedist, three different pain specialists, a physical therapist, a chiropractor and an acupuncturist. Most of these practitioners believed Mr. R to be suffering from a torn rotator cuff, until a neurologist evaluating him for right-hand weakness ordered an MRI and found a right apical lung mass. When Mr. R retired from a demanding job last year, he and his wife moved into a retirement community complete with amenities including a golf course. Mr. R promised his wife he would spend more time with their grandchildren and quit smoking as his daily stress diminished. The couple enjoyed their time together until Mr. R's undiagnosed pain and many appointments added frustration and heartache.

After finally meeting with an oncologist and receiving a definitive diagnosis Mr. R began palliative radiation to right clavicle metastases. A week later Mr. R's mobility and pain improved. As his primary caregiver, Mrs. R's hope developed as she had answers and a treatment plan. Mrs. R contacted the American Cancer Society and inquired about nearby caregiver support groups. The couple completed their advance directives together and are now working on updating financial and other paperwork. Mrs. R admits feeling overwhelmed at times by the process to get their affairs in order and with keeping up with housework. Mrs. R is grateful to be living in a very supportive retirement community, where one neighbor cooks a weekly meal for them and another knitted Mr. R a prayer shawl. Mr. and Mrs. R's hope is influenced by the possibility of a cure and the drive to remain strong for their children and grandchildren. Mrs. R finds comfort and solace in the community pool, swimming as a cathartic outlet.

Hope in terminally ill patients: is hope compatible with death?

Research demonstrates that many people are able to maintain hope during acute and chronic illness. Hope also can thrive during the terminal phase of an illness, despite the realization that no cure is possible. In qualitative studies, hope was essential to human existence, as integral to life, even when dying.[52,53]

Although hope levels may not decrease, the nature of hope often is altered through the dying process. Other changes in hope at the end of life include an increased focus on relationships and

> **Box 28.1** Sources of hope/hope-fostering strategies in terminally ill adults
>
> ◆ Love of family and friends
>
> ◆ Spirituality/having faith
>
> ◆ Setting goals and maintaining independence
>
> ◆ Positive relationships with professional carers
>
> ◆ Humor
>
> ◆ Personal characteristics
>
> ◆ Uplifting memories
>
> *Source:* Adapted from Buckley and Herth (2004), reference 54

trusting in others, as well as a desire to leave a legacy and to be well remembered.[7,33,46] Spirituality also increases in importance for some patients during the terminal phases of illness.[33] People also adopt specific strategies to foster hope at the end of life.[53,54] Many of these approaches are summarized in Box 28.1.

Although hope tends to change in people with terminal illness, maintaining a delicate balance between acceptance of death and hope for a cure often remains an important task up until the time of death, even when people acknowledge that cure is virtually impossible.[33,54] The dying person also needs to envision future moments of happiness, fulfillment, and connection.[52,53]

Case study

Mr. S, a case of hope transformed

Mr. S, a 62-year-old Jamaican man was diagnosed with gastric cancer 5 months ago and has now been admitted to the hospital with increasing abdominal distention and worsening pain at the J-tube site. Just a week prior to his admission, Mr. S had an appointment with his oncologist, during which he was told that imaging revealed progression of his disease and palliative chemotherapy was recommended. Mr. S refused chemotherapy; he was worried that his body could not handle further treatment and he would instead pursue herbal remedies. Mr. S also told his oncologist that perhaps the scans are evidence that his cancer is "breaking up" and he was hopeful that with prayer a miracle would happen.

Upon admission to the hospital, the primary team felt that Mr. S was in denial and/or did not understand the gravity of his circumstances. Thus, the primary team consulted the Palliative Care Service to help determine goals of care. Mr. S was followed by the interdisciplinary palliative care team including a spiritual care provider who was essential in uncovering his hopes for the future. Three years ago Mr. S battled colon cancer and has been in remission since a surgical resection. Spirituality has guided Mr. S throughout his life, and God, as "the ultimate physician and healer," continued to provide Mr. S with hope. Mr. S prayed and hoped that his cancer was breaking up because he did not feel as though his work was done. Mr. S looked to his four daughters for support and lived with two of them.

Mr. S hoped that he would return to Jamaica to see the birth of his first grandchild in the upcoming month. Mr. S continued to work toward achieving these goals while his symptoms worsened and he eventually transitioned to inpatient hospice care. During his last weeks, Mr. S spent time with his family, shared prayers with trusted chaplains, and filmed a legacy video for his unborn grandson. Although an ultimate hope for a miracle remained, Mr. S acquired new hopes at the end of his life through reflection that led to great comfort and peace for his family.

Multicultural views of hope

Over the past three decades, understanding of the clinical phenomenon of hope has increased dramatically through theoretical discourse and empirical investigation. Although knowledge regarding the components, processes, and outcomes of hope has grown dramatically, progress in multicultural research on hope has been limited. The samples in many studies that examine hope or hopelessness are ethnically homogeneous,[34,46,55] or their ethnic composition is unknown.[32,50] The studies that do include ethnically diverse samples are small,[56,57] precluding any comparisons or generalization of findings.

Several excellent European studies have contributed greatly to the general understanding of hope.[9,10,29,40] However, many of these investigations use frameworks and instruments developed by US researchers whose work is founded on homogeneous samples. Moreover, it may be that hopefulness for Europeans is more similar to that of middle-class Americans than it is different.[33]

Farone and colleagues[58] examined the associations among locus of control, negative affect, hope, and self-reported health in 109 older Mexican American women with cancer. They found that hope and internal locus of control both showed significant associations with better health outcomes. Although these findings are similar to those for white, non-Hispanic samples, the authors cautioned that they were unable to explore the characteristics of control that may be unique to Latina populations. They recommended that future research include attribution of control based on religious beliefs and the concept of *fatalismo* (fatalism).

Despite the growing body of research in diverse samples, existing research may not adequately reflect the experience of hope for people from non-European cultures. Several known cultural differences could certainly limit the applicability of current conceptualizations of hope, especially within the palliative care context. Three issues that theoretically could have a major impact on multicultural views of hope are time orientation, truth-telling, and one's beliefs about control.

Time orientation is identified as a cultural phenomenon that varies among cultural groups. Some cultural groups, usually highly individualistic ones, are future oriented. Within these groups, people prefer to look ahead, make short- and long-term plans, and organize their schedules to meet goals.[59] Because hope is defined as being future-oriented, with hopeful people more likely to identify and take action to meet goals, members of these future-oriented cultures may possibly appear more hopeful than people who are predominantly present-focused. On the other hand, people who are more focused on the present may be better able to sustain hope at the end of life, when the ability to create long-range goals is hindered by the uncertainty surrounding a terminal diagnosis. Additional research is needed to clarify these relationships.

The value for truth-telling in Western healthcare systems also may affect hope. Current ethical and legal standards require full disclosure of all relevant healthcare information to patients.[60] Informed consent and patient autonomy in medical decision-making, two eminent values in American healthcare, are impossible without this disclosure.[60] Although few would advocate lying to patients, truth-telling is not universally viewed as helpful or desirable.[61,62] In some cultures, it is believed that patients should be protected from burdensome information that could threaten hope. Truthful, but blunt, communication may also be seen as rude and disrespectful in some cultures, and the feeling of being devalued and disrespected has a negative impact on hope. In addition to the threats to hope that frank discussion is believed to engender, people who prefer nondisclosure of threatening information may be seen as attempting to cling to unrealistic hopes by refusing to listen to discouraging facts about their condition.

A third cultural concept that may affect hope is one's feeling of being in control. As described earlier, control is a core attribute in many conceptualizations of hope. Although control can be relinquished to others, including healthcare providers or a transcendent power, personal control often is central to the hoping process. In Euro-American cultures, applying one's will and energy to alter the course of an illness or to direct the dying process seems natural and desirable. Advance directives are one culturally sanctioned way in which members of these societies exert control over the dying process.[63] However, this desire for and belief in personal control is not a common feature in many other cultures. In cultures where death is viewed as part of the inherent harmony of living and dying, attempts to exert any influence over the dying process may seem unnatural or inappropriate.[63] People from diverse cultures who take a more passive role in their healthcare, or who do not espouse a desire to control their illness or the dying process, may be viewed as less hopeful than people who manifest a "fighting spirit" and active stance.

More research is needed to test theories of hope in multicultural groups, both to ensure the appropriate application of current conceptualizations to diverse cultural groups, and to develop new theories that are relevant for these groups. Until this work is done, palliative care clinicians must be cautious in applying current hope theories, and sensitive to the possible variations in diverse populations.

Models of maintaining hope for people with life-threatening illnesses

Many investigators have identified factors that foster hope, and strategies that enable people to sustain hope despite life-threatening or chronic illness. Although there is considerable concordance across these studies regarding many of the major themes, various models emphasize different styles and strategies that demonstrate the diversity in hope-fostering approaches.

As described previously, many people with terminal illness turn to activities and coping strategies that cultivate generalized hope rather than an emphasis on achievement and control. These strategies reflect a sense of peace and acceptance of death, and center on "being" rather than "doing." These strategies are described in Box 28.1.

In contrast, Olsson and colleagues found that patients preserved their hope using two goal-oriented or problem solving processes: (1) maintaining life, and (2) preparing for death. The patients tried to maintain life in several ways by keeping up with their day-to-day tasks and hobbies; communicating with others about practical matters and emotional feelings; involving other people such as family, friends, or professionals; and actively searching elsewhere for something to give them hope. To prepare for death, patients took responsibility for planning their own funeral and other practical matters, and arranged things so that family would have less of a burden. People use multiple strategies that allow them to confront and to avoid the negative aspects of illness and death. Although the strategies used to manage the threat of death often seem to predominate, these activities occur within a background of recognition and acknowledgment of the possibility of death. This process of negotiating between acknowledgment and management of these fears has been identified in other studies of people with life-threatening illnesses.[8]

Although some people continue to search for a cure after receiving a terminal diagnosis, hoping for a cure can coexist with awareness of death and engagement with life's activities.[53] Most people eventually accept their prognosis and mourn the loss of their original goals. At this point, they need to develop and pursue alternative goals that are possible in light of their diminished physical function, end-of-life symptoms, and loss of energy.

These different approaches for maintaining hope are important to describe and understand because they assist the palliative care nurse in designing effective strategies to foster hope. They increase clinicians' awareness regarding the various ways that people respond to chronic and terminal illness, and guide clinicians in their interactions with patients and families to sustain hope. They also help palliative care providers understand difficult or troubling responses, such as unrealistic hopefulness.

The issue of "unrealistic" hopefulness

Reality surveillance is a feature of many conceptualizations of hope. Often, clinicians, researchers, and theorists believe that mentally healthy people should choose and work toward realistic goals. In these frameworks, adhering to unrealistic hopes or denying reality is a sign of maladaptive cognitions that could lead to negative health outcomes. Therefore, denial and unrealistic hopes and ideas are discouraged and treated as pathological.[5,6]

Clinical examples of unrealistic hopes that cause consternation are numerous and diverse. For instance, one patient with advanced cancer might hope that his persistent severe sciatica is from exercise and overuse rather than spinal metastases. The nurse working with this patient may continually contradict his theory, asserting that his denial of the probable malignant cause of the pain will delay effective treatment. Another patient might insist that a new cure for her illness is imminent, causing distress for the nurse, who believes that the patient's unrealistic hopes will hinder acceptance of and preparation for death.

Despite these concerns, however, some investigators argue that the nurses' fears maybe unfounded. This perspective is based on more recent studies, which have led researchers to question the view that denial and unrealistic hopes are maladaptive. Instead, they argue that to believe these patients' professions of hope are unrealistic is to challenge or negate the legitimacy of the dominant depiction of the promise and potential cure provided by medical science.[52,53] Eliott and Olver[52] suggest that clinicians should not be concerned whether hope is real or unreal, true or false, present or not, rather they should view hope as an attempt to articulate, share, and value with others those things that connect the patient to what give their lives meaning, and ultimately, to life.[52(p. 148)]

In addition to promoting positive outcomes, "unrealistic" hopes need to be assessed within the context of uncertainty. For instance, people frequently respond to dire prognostic news with the observation that they can always "beat the odds." Given that no one can predict the future with absolute certainty, it is impossible to predict which individuals with a 2% chance of remission or recovery will actually be cured. So, if a person hopes for something in the future that appears highly unlikely, can it be known for certain that it will not occur? Patients and families often need to focus on this uncertainty to sustain hope.[8] Research supports the idea that patients' and families' hopes and goals are effective coping strategies, even when the likelihood of obtaining them seems remote.[51,53]

Olsman and colleagues[64] conducted an interpretative synthesis of the literature showing that nurses and physicians could take three perspectives on hope of palliative care patients: (1) realistic perspective, (2) functional perspective, and (3) narrative perspective. Hope is viewed from a realistic perspective when hope is truthful and focused on adjusting hope to the truth. From a functional perspective, hope helps patients cope with treatments or face uncertainty. Nurses who take a narrative perspective focus on meaning that is valuable to patients. They also suggested that clinicians can take more than one perspective at the same time.

Assessing hope

As in all nursing care, thorough assessment of physical and psychosocial factors must precede thoughtful planning and implementation of therapeutic strategies. Therefore, consistent and comprehensive evaluations of hope should be included in the palliative nursing assessment. Some conceptual elements of hope, such as those focusing on meaning and purpose in life, are included in a spiritual assessment. Rarely, however, are comprehensive guides to assessing hope included in standardized nursing assessment forms.

The guidelines produced by Farran, Wilken, and Popovich[65] for the clinical assessment of hope appropriately use the acronym HOPE to designate the major areas of evaluation: The areas are health, others, purpose in life, and engaging process. The term "engaging process" refers to identifying goals, taking actions to achieve goals, sense of control over one's situation, and identifying hope-inspiring factors in one's past, present, and future. In Table 28.1, this framework has been adapted and applied to terminally ill patients. It includes examples of questions and probes that can be used to assess hope.

Table 28.1 Guidelines for the clinical assessment of hope in palliative care

Interview question/probe	Rationale
Health (and symptom management)	
1. Tell me about your illness. What is your understanding of the probable course of your illness?	Explore the person's perceptions of seriousness of his or her illness, and possible trajectories
2. How hopeful are you right now, and how does your illness affect your sense of hope?	Determine the person's general sense of hope and the effect of the terminal illness on hope
3. How well are you able to control the symptoms of your illness? How do these symptoms affect your hope?	Uncontrolled end-of-life symptoms have been found to negatively influence hope
Others	
1. Who provides you with emotional, physical, and spiritual support?	Identify people in the environment who provide support and enhance hope
2. Whom are you most likely to confide in when you have a problem or concern?	Identify others in whom the person has trust
3. What kinds of difficulty experiences have you and your family/partner/support network had to deal with in the past? How did you manage those experiences?	Explore experiences of coping with stressful situations
4. What kinds of things do family, support people, and healthcare providers do that make you more hopeful? Less hopeful?	Identify specific behaviors that affect hope and recognize that other people can also decrease hope
Purpose in life	
1. What gives you hope?	Identify relationships, beliefs, and activities that provide a sense of purpose and contribute positively to hope
2. What helps you make sense of your situation right now?	Identify the ways in which the person makes meaning of difficult situations.
3. Do you have spiritual or religious practices or support people who help you? If "yes," what are these practices and who are these people?	Identify if and how spirituality acts as a source of hope
4. Has your illness caused you to question your spiritual beliefs? If "yes," how?	Terminal illness can threaten the person's basic beliefs and test one's faith
5. How can we help you maintain these practices and personal connections with spiritual support people?	Identify ways in which clinicians and others can support spiritual practices that enhance hope

(continued)

Table 28.1 Continued

Interview question/probe	Rationale
Goals	
1. Right now, what are your major goals?	Identify major goals and priorities
	Examine whether these goals are congruent with the views of others
2. What do you see are the chances that you will meet these goals?	Explore how realistic the person thinks the goals are; if the goals are not perceived as being attainable, assess the impact on hope
3. What actions can you take to meet these goals?	Identify specific actions the person can take to meet the goals
4. What actions have you already taken to meet these goals?	Identify how active the person has been in attaining the goals
5. What resources do you have for meeting these goals?	Determine other resources to which the person has access for the purpose of attaining goals
Sense of control	
1. Do you feel that you have much control over your current situation?	Determine whether the person feels any ability to control or change the situation
	Explore whether the person wants to have more control
2. Are there others that you feel have some control over your current situation? If "yes," who are they, and in what ways do they have control?	Determine whether the person feels as though trusted others (e.g., healthcare providers, family, deity) can control or change the situation
Sources of hope over time	
1. In the past, what or who has made you hopeful?	Identify sources of hope from the person's past that may continue to provide hope during the terminal phase
2. Right now who and what provides you with hope?	Identify current sources of hope
3. What do you hope for in the future?	Assess generalized and specific hopes for the future

Sources: Adapted from Farran, Wilken, and Popovich[65]; Farran, Herth, and Popovich.[68]

Like pain, hope is a subjective experience, and assessment should focus on self-report. However, behavioral cues can also provide information regarding a person's state of hope or hopelessness. Hopelessness is a central feature of depression; therefore, behaviors such as social withdrawal, flat affect, alcohol and substance abuse, insomnia, and passivity may indicate hopelessness.

As discussed earlier, the patient's terminal illness affects the hope of family caregivers, who, in turn, influence the hope of the patients. Therefore, the hope of the patient's family caregivers and other significant support people also should be assessed.

Over the past decades, researchers from several disciplines have developed instruments to measure hope and hopelessness. The theoretical and empirical literature documents the comprehensiveness and face validity of these tools. Advances in psychometric theory and methods have allowed the evaluation of multiple dimensions of validity and reliability. The development and use of well-designed and well-tested tools has contributed greatly to the science of hope. Although a thorough discussion of these measures is beyond the scope of this chapter, Table 28.2 provides a brief description of several widely used and tested instruments.

Nursing interventions to maintain hope at end of life

Clinicians, theorists, and researchers recognize that nurses play an important role in instilling, maintaining, and restoring hope in people for whom they care. Researchers have identified many ways in which nurses assist patients and families to sustain hope in the face of life-threatening illness. Box 28.2 provides a summary of nursing approaches to instill hope. A brief perusal of this table reveals an important point about these strategies: For the most part, nursing care to maintain patients' and families' hope fundamentally is about providing excellent physical, psychosocial, and spiritual palliative care. There are few unique interventions to maintain hope, and yet there is much nurses can do. Because hope is inextricably connected to virtually all facets of the illness experience—including physical pain, coping, anxiety, and spirituality—improvement or deterioration in one area has repercussions in other areas. Attending to these relationships reminds clinicians that virtually every action they take can influence hope, negatively or positively.

Another vital observation about hope-inspiring strategies is that many approaches begin with the patient and family. The experience of hope is a personal one, defined and determined by the hoping person. Although others greatly influence that experience, ultimately the meanings and effects of words and actions are determined by the person experiencing hope or hopelessness. Many approaches used by people with life-threatening illness to maintain hope are strategies initiated with little influence from others. For example, some people pray; others distract themselves with television watching, conversation, or other activities; and many patients use cognitive strategies, such as minimizing negative thoughts, identifying personal strengths, and focusing on the positive. For many patients and families, careful observation and active support of an individual's established strategies to maintain hope will be most successful.

Family caregivers and other support people should be included in these approaches. Ample evidence demonstrates that patients

Table 28.2 Descriptions of selected instruments to measure hope and hopelessness

Instrument name	Brief description
Beck Hopelessness Scale	◆ 20-item, true-false format ◆ Based on Stotland's definition of hopelessness: system of negative expectancies concerning oneself and one's future ◆ Developed to assess psychopathological levels of hopelessness; correlates highly with attempted and actual suicide
Herth Hope Index	◆ 12-item, 4-point Likert scale; total score is sum of all items; range of scores 12–48 ◆ Designed for well and ill populations ◆ Assesses three overlapping dimensions: (1) cognitive-temporal, (2) affective-behavioral, (3) affiliative-behavioral ◆ Spanish, Thai, Chinese, Swedish translations available
Hopefulness Scale for Adolescents (Hinds)	◆ 24-item visual analog scale ◆ Assesses the degree of the adolescent's positive future orientation ◆ Assesses only the relational and rational thought processes of hope ◆ Tested in several populations of adolescents: well, substance abusers, adolescents with emotional and mental problems, cancer patients
Miller Hope Scale	◆ 40-item scale, 5-point Likert scale ◆ Assesses 10 elements: (1) mutuality/affiliation, (2) avoidance of absolutizing, (3) sense of the possible, (4) psychological well-being and coping, (5) achieving goals, (6) purpose and meaning in life, (7) reality surveillance-optimism, (8) mental and physical activation, (9) anticipation, (10) freedom ◆ Chinese and Swedish versions
Snyder Hope Scale	◆ 12-item, 4-point Likert scale ◆ Based on Stotland's definition of hope; focus is on goals identification and achievement ◆ Tested in healthy adults, and adults with psychiatric illness ◆ Also has developed tool to measure hope in children

and people within their support systems reciprocally influence one another's hope. In addition, family and significant others are always incorporated into the palliative care plan and considered part of the unit of care. Maintenance of hope also is a goal after death, in that hope-restoring and -maintaining strategies must be an integral part of bereavement counseling.[66,67]

Specific interventions

The framework for the following discussion is adapted from Farran, Herth, and Popovich,[68] who articulated four central attributes of hope: experiential, spiritual/transcendent, relational, and rational thought. These areas encompass the major themes found in the literature, and although they are not mutually exclusive, they provide a useful organizing device. This section also includes a brief discussion of ways in which nurses need to explore and understand their own hopes and values in order to provide palliative care that fosters hope in others.

Experiential process interventions

The experiential process of hope involves the acknowledgment and acceptance of suffering while at the same time using the imagination to move beyond the suffering and find hope.[15] Included in these types of strategies are methods to decrease physical suffering and cognitive strategies aimed at managing the threat of the terminal illness.

Uncontrolled symptoms, such as pain, fatigue, dyspnea, and anxiety, cause suffering and challenge the hopefulness of patients and caregivers. Timely and adept symptom prevention and management is central to maintaining hope. In home-care settings, teaching patients and families the knowledge and skills to manage symptoms confidently and competently also is essential.

Other ways to help people find hope in suffering is to provide them a cognitive reprieve from their situation. One powerful strategy to achieve this temporary suspension is through humor. Humor helps put things in perspective and frees the self, at least momentarily, from the onerous burden of illness and suffering. Making light of a grim situation brings a sense of control over one's response to the situation, even when one has little influence over it. Of course, the use of humor with patients and families requires sensitivity as well as a sense of timing. The nurse should take cues from the patient and family, observe how they use humor to dispel stress, and let them take the lead in joking about threatening information and events. In general, humor should be focused on oneself or on events outside the immediate concerns of the patient and family.

Other ways to move people cognitively beyond their suffering is to assist them in identifying and enjoying that which is joyful in life. Engagement in aesthetic experiences, such as watching movies or listening to music that is uplifting, can enable people to transcend their suffering. Sharing one's own hope-inspiring stories also can help.

Another strategy is to support people in their own positive self-talk. Often people naturally cope with stress by comparing themselves with people they perceive to be less fortunate or by identifying attributes of personal strength that help them find hope.[21,54] For example, an elderly, married woman with advanced breast cancer may comment that, despite the seriousness of her disease, she feels luckier than another woman with the same disease who is younger or without social support. By comparing

---

Box 28.2 Nursing actions to foster hope

Experiential processes

♦ Prevent and manage end-of-life symptoms

♦ Use lightheartedness and humor appropriately

♦ Encourage the patient and family to transcend their current situation

♦ Encourage aesthetic experiences

♦ Encourage engagement in creative and joyous endeavors

♦ Suggest literature, movies, and art that are uplifting and highlight the joy in life

♦ Encourage reminiscing

♦ Assist patient and family to focus on present and past joys

♦ Share positive, hope-inspiring stories

♦ Support patient and family in positive self-talk

Spiritual/transcendent processes

♦ Facilitate participation in religious rituals and spiritual practices

♦ Make necessary referrals to clergy and other spiritual support people

♦ Assist the patient and family in finding meaning in the current situation

♦ Assist the patient/family to keep a journal

♦ Suggest literature, movies, and art that explore the meaning of suffering

Relational processes

♦ Minimize patient and family isolation

♦ Establish and maintain an open relationship

♦ Affirm patients' and families' sense of self-worth

♦ Recognize and reinforce the reciprocal nature of hopefulness between patient and support system

♦ Provide time for relationships (especially important in institutional settings)

♦ Foster attachment ideation by assisting the patient to identify significant others and then to reflect on personal characteristics and experiences that endear the significant other to the patient

♦ Communicate one's own sense of hopefulness

Rational thought processes

♦ Assist patient and family to establish, obtain, and revise goals without imposing one's own agenda

♦ Assist in identifying available and needed resources to meet goals

♦ Assist in procuring needed resources; assist with breaking larger goals into smaller steps to increase feelings of success

♦ Provide accurate information regarding patient's condition and treatment in a skillful and sensitive manner

♦ Help patient and family identify past successes

♦ Increase patients' and families' sense of control when possible

---

herself with less fortunate others, she can take solace in recognizing that "things could be worse." Similarly, a person can maintain hope by focusing on particular talents or previous accomplishments that indicate an ability to cope with illness. People may also cite their high level of motivation as a reason to feel hopeful about the future. Acknowledgment and validation of these attributes supports hope and affirms self-worth for patients and families.

Spiritual process interventions

Several specific strategies can foster hope while incorporating spirituality. These strategies include providing opportunities for the expression of spiritual beliefs and arranging for involvement in religious rituals and spiritual practices.

Assisting patients and families to explore and make meaning of their trials and suffering is another useful approach. Encouraging patients and families to keep a journal of thoughts and feelings can help people in this process. Suggesting books, films, or art that focuses on religious or existential understanding and transcendence of suffering is another effective way to help people make sense of illness and death.

Palliative care nurses also should assess for signs of spiritual distress and make appropriate referrals to spiritual care providers and other professionals with expertise in counseling during spiritual and existential crises.

Relational process interventions

To maximize hope, nurses should establish and maintain an open relationship with patients and members of their support network, taking the time to learn what their priorities and needs are and then addressing those needs in timely, effective ways. Demonstrating respect and interest and being available to listen and be with people—that is, affirming each person's worth—is essential.

Fostering and sustaining connectedness among the patient, family, and friends can be accomplished by providing time for uninterrupted interactions, which is especially important in institutional settings. Nurses can increase hope by enlisting help from others to help achieve goals. For example, recruiting friends or arranging for a volunteer to transport an ill person to purchase a gift for a grandchild can cultivate hope for everyone involved. It is important to help others realize how vital they are in sustaining a person's hope.

Rational thought process interventions

The rational thought process is the dimension of hope that specifically focuses on goals, resources, personal control and self-efficacy, and action. Interventions related to this dimension include assisting patients and families in devising and attaining goals. Providing accurate and timely information about the patient's condition and treatment helps patients and families decide which goals are achievable. At times, gentle assistance with monitoring and acknowledging negative possibilities helps the patient and family to choose realistic goals. Helping to identify and procure the resources necessary to meet goals also is important.

Often, major goals need to be broken into smaller, shorter-term achievements. For example, a patient with painful, metastatic lung cancer might want to attend a family event that is two weeks away. The successful achievement of this goal depends on many factors, including adequate pain control, transportation, and ability to transfer to and from a wheelchair. By breaking the larger goal into several smaller ones, the person is able to identify all the necessary steps and resources. Supporting patients and families to identify those areas of life and death in which they do have real influence can increase self-esteem and self-efficacy, thereby instilling hope. It also helps to review their previous successes in attaining important goals.

This domain also includes ways in which clinicians balance the need to communicate "bad news" while sustaining patients' and families' hope. The difficulties inherent in delivering negative information to patients and families does not release us from our duty to communicate openly and honestly; however, it does require that palliative care nurses and other clinicians communicate skillfully in ways that assist patients and families to sustain hope. There are many articles describing empirically derived methods for delivering bad news sensitively and communicating in ways that maintain hope.[56,69] More information about communication can be found in chapter 5.

Programs to enhance hopefulness

In addition to discrete actions that individual nurses take to foster hope, several investigators have developed and tested programs to enhance hope in people with life-threatening illness.

Duggleby and colleagues[26] evaluated the effectiveness of the Living with Hope Program (LWHP), a brief intervention designed for older adults with advanced cancer receiving home-based palliative care services. Grounded in their earlier research,[46] the LWHP is a 1-week intervention consisting of a visit from a trained assistant, a copy of the film "Living with Hope," and a choice of one of three hope-focused activities. The investigators found that compared to the control group, LWHP participants reported greater hope and existential quality of life 1 week following the intervention. The LWHP also has been pilot-tested in a sample of 10 family caregivers, and results suggest that the program may increase hope and quality of life in this group.[70]

Rustoen and colleagues[29] studied the effects of a professional-led group intervention on hope and psychological distress in a community-based sample of cancer patients. The intervention consisted of eight 2-hour sessions focused on belief in oneself and in one's ability, emotional reactions, relationships with others, active involvement, spiritual beliefs and values, and acknowledgment that there is a future. The results showed increased hope levels and decreased psychological distress immediately following the intervention, however it was not sustained at the 3- and 12-month assessments. The investigators suggested that like other cognitive-behavioral interventions, additional "booster sessions" would have been helpful.

Ensuring the self-knowledge necessary to provide palliative care

Providing holistic palliative care requires a broad range of skills. Astute management of physical symptoms and a solid command of technical skills must be matched with an ability to provide psychosocial and spiritual care for patients and families at a time of great vulnerability. To nurture these latter skills, nurses should continually reflect on and evaluate their own hopes, beliefs, and biases and identify how these factors influence their care. In an intriguing study, investigators examined the relationship between nurses' hope and their comfort in caring for and communicating with dying children and their families. They found that, after controlling for number of years in nursing, nurses' hope and hours of palliative care education both were significantly associated with comfort in caring for dying children and their families.[71] These findings underscore the importance of education and self-reflection in delivering compassionate, skilled palliative care. In providing high-quality care, nurses also should evaluate how they are affected by patients' and families' responses and strategies to maintain hope. For example, does it anger or frustrate the nurse that the patient seems to refuse to acknowledge that his or her disease is incurable? Is this anger communicated nonverbally or verbally to the patient or family? In addition to self-reflection, it is important for palliative care nurses to remain hopeful while working with dying patients by engaging in self-care activities.

Summary

Hope is central to the human experience of living and dying, and it is integrally entwined with spiritual and psychosocial well-being. Although terminal illness can challenge and even temporarily diminish hope, the dying process does not inevitably bring despair. The human spirit, manifesting its creativity and resiliency, can forge new and deeper hopes at the end of life. Palliative care nurses play important roles in supporting patients and families with this process by providing expert physical, psychosocial, and spiritual care. Sensitive, skillful attention to maintaining hope can enhance quality of life and contribute significantly to a "good death" as defined by the patient and family. Fostering hope is a primary means by which palliative care nurses accompany patients and families on the journey through terminal illness.

References

1. Feudtner C. Hope and the prospect of healing at the end of life. J Alter Complement Med. 2005;11(1):S23–S30.
2. Fromm E. The Revolution of Hope. New York: Bantam Books; 1968.
3. Marcel G. Homo Viator: Introduction to a Metaphysic of Hope. New York: Harper and Row; 1962.
4. Menninger K. Hope. Bull Menninger Clin. 1987;51(5):447–462.
5. Ersek M. Examining the process and dilemmas of reality negotiation. Image J Nurs Sch. 1992;24(1):19–25.
6. Snyder CR, Rand KL. The case against false hope. Am Psychol. 2003;58(10):820–822; authors' reply 823–824.
7. Dufault K, Martocchio B. Hope: its spheres and dimensions. Nurs Clin North Am. 1985;20:379–391.
8. De Graves S, Aranda S. Living with hope and fear: the uncertainty of childhood cancer after relapse. Cancer Nurs.2008;31(4):292–301.
9. Kylma J, Vehvilainen-Julkunen K, Lahdevirta J. Dynamically fluctuating hope, despair and hopelessness along the HIV/AIDS continuum as described by caregivers in voluntary organizations in Finland. Issues Ment Health Nurs. 2001;22(4):353–377.
10. Kylma J, Vehvilainen-Julkunen K, Lahdevirta J. Hope, despair and hopelessness in living with HIV/AIDS: a grounded theory study. J Adv Nurs. 2001;33(6):764–775.
11. Morse JM, Penrod J. Linking concepts of enduring, uncertainty, suffering, and hope. Image J Nurs Sch. 1999;31(2):145–150.
12. Cutcliffe J, Herth K. The concept of hope in nursing 2: hope and mental health nursing. Br J Nurs. 2002;11(13):885–889.
13. Gibson LM. Inter-relationships among sense of coherence, hope, and spiritual perspective (inner resources) of African-American and European-American breast cancer survivors. Appl Nurs Res. 2003;16(4):236–244.

14. Haase JE, Britt T, Coward DD, Leidy NK, Penn PE. Simultaneous concept analysis of spiritual perspective, hope, acceptance and self-transcendence. Image J Nurs Sch. 1992;24(2):141–147.

15. Herth KA. The relationship between level of hope and level of coping response and other variables in patients with cancer. Oncol Nurs Forum.1989;16(1):67–72.

16. Carson V, Soeken KL, Shanty J, Terry L. Hope and spiritual well-being: essentials for living with AIDS. Perspect Psychiatr Care. 1990;26(2):28–34.

17. Fehring RJ, Miller JF, Shaw C. Spiritual well-being, religiosity, hope, depression, and other mood states in elderly people coping with cancer. Oncol Nurs Forum. 1997;24(4):663–671.

18. Duggleby W, Wright K. Transforming hope: how elderly palliative patients live with hope. Can J Nurs Res. 2005;37(2):70–84.

19. Fanos JH, Gelinas DF, Foster RS, Postone N, Miller RG. Hope in palliative care: from narcissism to self-transcendence in amytrophic lateral sclerosis J Palliat Med. 2008;11(3):470–475.

20. Borneman T, Brown-Saltzman, K. Meaning in illness. In: Ferrell B, Coyle N (eds.), Textbook of Palliative Nursing. New York: Oxford University Press; 2010:673–683.

21. Harris GE, Larsen D. HIV peer counseling and the development of hope: perspectives from peer counselors and peer counseling recipients. AIDS Patient Care STDS. 2007;21(11):843–860.

22. Kavradim ST, Ozer ZC, Bozcuk H. Hope in people with cancer: a multivariate analysis from Turkey. J Adv Nurs. 2013;69(5):1183–1196.

23. Mattioli JL, Repinski R, Chappy SL. The meaning of hope and social support in patients receiving chemotherapy. Oncol Nurs Forum. 2008;35(5):822–829.

24. Cotter VT. Hope in early-stage dementia: a concept analysis. Holist Nurs Pract. –2009;23(5):297–301.

25. Reinke LF, Shannon SE, Engelberg RA, Young JP, Curtis JR. Supporting hope and prognostic information: nurses' perspectives on their role when patients have life-limiting prognoses. J Pain Symptom Manage. 2010;39(6):982–992.

26. Duggleby WD, Degner L, Williams A, et al. Living with hope: initial evaluation of a psychosocial hope intervention for older palliative home care patients. J Pain Symptom Manage. 2007;33(3):247–257.

27. Weis RS, et al. A meta-analysis of hope enhancement strategies in clinical and community settings. Psychol Well Being. 2011;1(5):1–16.

28. Kylma J, Duggleby W, Cooper D, Molander G. Hope in palliative care: an integrative review. Palliat Support Care. 2009;7(3):365–377.

29. Rustoen T, Cooper BA, Miaskowski C. A longitudinal study of the effects of a hope intervention on levels of hope and psychological distress in a community-based sample of oncology patients. Eur J Oncol Nurs. 2011;15(4):351–357.

30. Lazarus RS, Folkman S. Stress, Appraisal, and Coping. New York: Springer; 1984.

31. Folkman S. Stress, coping, and hope. Psycho-Oncol. 2010;19(9):901–908.

32. Rustoen T, Cooper BA, Miaskowski C. The importance of hope as a mediator of psychological distress and life satisfaction in a community sample of cancer patients. Cancer Nurs. 2010;33(4):258–267.

33. Olsson L, Ostlund G, Strang P, Jeppsson Grassman E, Friedrichsen M. Maintaining hope when close to death: insight from cancer patients in palliative home care. Int J Palliat Nurs. 2010;16(12):607–612.

34. Rawdin B, Evans C, Rabow MW. The relationships among hope, pain, psychological distress, and spiritual well-being in oncology outpatients. J Palliat Med. 2013;16(2):167–172.

35. Zhang Y, Law CK, Yip PSF. Psychological factors associated with the incidence and persistence of suicidal ideation. J Affect Disord. 2011;133(3):584–590.

36. Joiner TE, Jr., Brown JS, Wingate LR. The psychology and neurobiology of suicidal behavior. Annu Rev Psychol. 2005;56:287–314.

37. Dees MK, Vernooij-Dassen MJ, Dekkers WJ, Vissers KC, van Weel C. "Unbearable suffering": a qualitative study on the perspectives of patients who request assistance in dying. J Med Ethics. 2011;37(12):727–734.

38. Phuong Do D, Dowd JB, Ranjit N, House JS, Kaplan GA. Hopelessness, depression, and early markers of endothelial dysfunction in U.S. adults. Psychosom Med. 2010;72(7):613–619.

39. Kylma J, Juvakka T. Hope in parents of adolescents with cancer: factors endangering and engendering parental hope. Eur J Oncol Nurs. 2007;11(3):262–271.

40. Salmon P, Hill J, Ward J, Gravenhorst K, Eden T, Young B. Faith and protection: the construction of hope by parents of children with leukemia and their oncologists. Oncologist. 2012;17(3):398–404.

41. Mack JW, Wolfe J, Cook EF, Grier HE, Cleary PD, Weeks JC. Hope and prognostic disclosure. J Clin Oncol. 2007;25(35):5636–5642.

42. Hirsch JK, Sirois FM, Lyness JM. Functional impairment and depressive symptoms in older adults: mitigating effects of hope. Br J Health Psychol. 2011;16(4):744–760.

43. Duggleby W, Hicks D, Nekolaichuk C, Holtslander L, Williams A, Chambers T, et al. Hope, older adults, and chronic illness: a metasynthesis of qualitative research. J Adv Nurs. 2012;68(6):1211–1223.

44. Moore SL. The experience of hope and aging: a hermeneutic photography study. J Gerontol Nurs. 2012;38(10):28–36.

45. Esbensen BA, Swane CE, Hallberg IR, Thome B. Being given a cancer diagnosis in old age: a phenomenological study. Int J Nurs Stud. 2008;45(3):393–405.

46. Duggleby W, Wright K. Transforming hope: how elderly palliative patients live with hope. Can J Nurs Res. 2005;37(2):70–84.

47. Duggleby W, Williams A, Wright K, Bollinger S. Renewing everyday hope: the hope experience of family caregivers of persons with dementia. Issues Ment Health Nurs. 2009;30(8):514–521.

48. Holtslander LF, Duggleby WD. The hope experience of older bereaved women who cared for a spouse with terminal cancer. Qual Health Res. 2009;19(3):388–400.

49. Holtslander LF, Duggleby W, Williams AM, Wright KE. The experience of hope for informal caregivers of palliative patients. J Palliat Care. 2005;21(4):285–291.

50. Lohne V, Miaskowski C, Rustoen T. The relationship between hope and caregiver strain in family caregivers of patients with advanced cancer. Cancer Nurs. 2012;35(2):99–105.

51. Duggleby WD, Swindle J, Peacock S, Ghosh S. A mixed methods study of hope, transitions, and quality of life in family caregivers of persons with Alzheimer's disease. BMC Geriatrics. 2011;11:88.

52. Eliott JA, Olver IN. Hope and hoping in the talk of dying cancer patients. Soc Sci Med. 2007;64(1):138–149.

53. Eliott JA, Olver IN. Hope, life, and death: a qualitative analysis of dying cancer patients' talk about hope. Death Stud. 2009;33(7):609–638.

54. Buckley J, Herth K. Fostering hope in terminally ill patients. Nurs Stand. 2004;19(10):33–41.

55. Shinn EH, Taylor CL, Kilgore K, et al. Associations with worry about dying and hopelessness in ambulatory ovarian cancer patients. Palliat Support Care. 2009;7(3):299–306.

56. Curtis JR, Engelberg R, Young JP, et al. An approach to understanding the interaction of hope and desire for explicit prognostic information among individuals with severe chronic obstructive pulmonary disease or advanced cancer. J Palliat Med. 2008;11(4):610–620.

57. Berendes D, Keefe FJ, Somers TJ, Kothadia SM, Porter LS, Cheavens JS. Hope in the context of lung cancer: relationships of hope to symptoms and psychological distress. J Pain Symptom Manage. 2010;40(2):174–182.

58. Farone DW, Fitzpatrick TR, Bushfield SY. Hope, locus of control, and quality of health among elder latina cancer survivors. Soc Work Health Care. 2008;46(2):51–70.

59. Purnell LD. The Purnell Model for cultural competence. In: Purnell LD (ed.), Transcultural Health Care: A Culturally Competent Approach. 4th ed. Philadelphia: F.A. Davis; 2013:15–44.

60. Beauchamp TL, Childress JF. Principles of Biomedical Ethics. 7th ed. New York: Oxford University Press; 2013.

61. Oliffe J, Thorne S, Hislop TG, Armstrong EA. "Truth telling" and cultural assumptions in an era of informed consent. Fam Community Health. 2007;30(1):5–15.

62. Shaw S. Exploring the concepts behind truth-telling in palliative care. Int J Palliat Nurs. 2008;14(7):356–359.

63. Giger JN, Davidhizar RE, Fordham P. Multi-cultural and multi-ethnic considerations and advanced directives: developing cultural competency. J Cult Divers. 2006;13(1):3–9.

64. Olsman E, Leget C, Onwuteaka-Philipsen B, Willems D. Should palliative care patients' hope be truthful, helpful or valuable?: An interpretative synthesis of literature describing healthcare professionals' perspectives on hope of palliative care patients. Palliative Med. 2013;0(0):1–12.

65. Farran CJ, Wilken C, Popovich JM. Clinical assessment of hope. Issues Ment Health Nurs. 1992;13(2):129–138.

66. Holtslander L, Duggleby W. An inner struggle for hope: insights from the diaries of bereaved family caregivers. Int J Palliat Nurs. 2008;14(10):478–484.

67. Holtslander LF. Caring for bereaved family caregivers: analyzing the context of care. Clin J Oncol Nurs. 2008;12(3):501–506.

68. Farran CJ, Herth KA, Popovich JM. Hope and Hopelessness: Critical Clinical Constructs. Thousand Oaks, CA: Sage; 1995.

69. Robinson CA. "Our best hope is a cure": Hope in the context of advance care planning. Palliat Support Care. 2012:1–8.

70. Duggleby W, Wright K, Williams A, Degner L, Cammer A, Holtslander L. Developing a living with hope program for caregivers of family members with advanced cancer. J Palliat Care. 2007;23(1):24–31.

71. Feudtner C, Santucci G, Feinstein JA, Snyder CR, Rourke MT, Kang TI. Hopeful thinking and level of comfort regarding providing pediatric palliative care: a survey of hospital nurses. Pediatrics. 2007;119(1):e186–e192.

CHAPTER 29

Bereavement

Inge B. Corless

It's before and after—life before the death of your loved one and then after when nothing is ever the same. But how could that be? That's not to say that there are not some happy times, but it's not the same. Your loved one is no longer physically present.

Key points

- Bereavement is the state of having lost a significant other.
- "Loss" is a generic term indicating the absence of a current or future possession or relationship.
- Grief is the emotional response to loss.
- Mourning encompasses the death rituals engaged in by the bereaved.

On December 20, 2008, a young woman, a wife and mother, died after a lengthy illness. She had a two year, apparently illness-free, period that was punctuated by metastases to liver and lung. That is not the important part of her story, although it accounts for her demise. The important part of her story is how beloved she was not only by her immediate and extended family, but by the community of those she had met throughout her life and the community in which she lived. The vivid grief expressed by those in attendance at her funeral is in sharp contrast to the more restrained expression of grief typical at white Anglo-Saxon funerals. Not that all in attendance were Caucasian—the mourners at this funeral represented multiple ethnic groups. Those who were most expressive in their grief were those who, culturally, would have been expected to a stiff upper lip. Would such a response have occurred had the deceased lived her four score years and ten? How do we account for this response to bereavement? In the following pages we will examine some of the factors that might help us understand this expression of grief.

Bereavement takes many forms. It is influenced first and foremost by culture. In Victorian times, bereaved women in the northeastern United States wore black for a year and used black-edged stationery, while men wore a black armband for a matter of days before resuming their regular activities. Bereavement is also influenced by religious practice, the nature of the relationship with the deceased, the age of the deceased, and the manner of death. In this chapter, the impact of social and cultural forces on the form of bereavement is examined.

Changes have occurred in what is considered "appropriate" to the expression of grief. The wearing of black by a widow ("widow's weeds") for the remainder of her life, and the presumption that grief will be "resolved" within a year, are no longer societal or professional expectations. There are other expectations, however, that color the expressions of bereavement, loss, mourning, and grief. Given that greater emphasis is placed on the discussion of bereavement and grief, it behooves us to define these terms and examine their related elements.

A matter of definition

Bereavement

With the pronouncement of death, those who have the closest blood or legal connections to the deceased are considered *bereaved*. Bereavement confers a special status on the individual, entailing both obligations and special rights. The obligations concern disposition of the body and any attendant ceremonies, as well as disposal of the worldly goods of the deceased, unless indicated otherwise in a legal document such as a last will and testament. The rights include dispensation from worldly activities such as work and, to a lesser degree, family roles for a variable period of time. Before an expanded discussion of bereavement is undertaken, it is important to distinguish the concept of bereavement from such related terms as loss, mourning, and grief.

Loss

"Loss" is a generic term that signifies absence of an object, position, ability, or attribute. More recently it also has been applied to the death of an animal or person. Absence or loss of the same entity has different implications depending on the strength of the relationship to the owner. For example, loss of a dog with which there was an indifferent relationship results in less emotional disruption for the owner than the loss of a dog that was cherished. The term often is applied to the death of an individual, and it is the bereaved person who is considered to have experienced a loss.

A loss occurs, and its meaning is determined by the person who sustained the loss. The attributes of loss can be formulated as follows:

1. Loss signifies the absence of a relationship or possession.
2. Each loss is valued differently and ranges from no or little value to great value.
3. The meaning of the loss is determined primarily by the individual sustaining it.

This suggests that it is wiser not to make assumptions about loss, but to query further as to its meaning to the individual. This is all the more relevant in instances of ambiguous loss. Lee and Whiting[1] employ the theory of ambiguous loss to discuss the situation of foster children, whose caregivers may be physically present but psychologically absent, physically absent but psychologically present, or in transient relationships. Feelings of confusion, hopelessness, and ambivalence may accompany ambiguous loss.[1(p. 418)] Mourning and grief under these circumstances may not receive the recognition that is warranted.

Mourning

Mourning has been described in various ways. Kagawa-Singer[2] described mourning as "the social customs and cultural practices that follow a death." This definition highlights the external manifestations of the process of separation from the deceased and the ultimate reintegration of the bereaved into the family and, to varying degrees, society. Durkheim, one of the founders of sociology, stated that "mourning is not a natural movement of private feelings wounded by a cruel loss; it is a duty imposed by the group."[3(p. 443)] This duty is participation in the customary rituals appropriate to membership in a given group. These rituals and behaviors acknowledge that a loss has occurred for the individual and the group, and that the individual and the group are adjusting their relationships so as to move forward without the presence of the deceased individual.

DeSpelder and Strickland highlighted an important distinction pertinent to mourning. They stated, "The term mourning refers not so much to the reaction to loss but rather to the process by which a bereaved person integrates the loss into his ongoing life."[4(p. 336)] They continue by observing that the "process is determined at least partly by social and cultural norms for expressing grief."[4(p. 336)] An outward acknowledgment of loss consists of participation in various death and bereavement rituals. As noted, these vary by religious and cultural traditions as well as by personal preferences. In South Africa, a Zulu wife is expected to engage in mourning (ukuzila) for one year as a sign of respect.[5]

Whereas ancestor worship is important to varying degrees in Asia, Latin cultures believe in the relationship between life and death, a relationship reflected in practices such as the tradition of bringing food to the cemetery and remaining there all night for the Day of the Dead. "These practices have many functions, including signifying respect for the deceased and providing a mechanism for the expression of feelings by the bereaved. A similar relationship is observed in Africa, where "the living and the dead together constitute the social world."[6(p. 341)]

Mourning is also expressed in the symbolism entailed in funerals and burials. Burial grounds contain the expressions of what was considered appropriate in each time period for the memorialization of the deceased. These memorials may be above or below ground, in cemeteries or memorial parks, as part of individual graves or mausoleums, or various permutations. The availability of space for burials influences the manner in which burials and memorials are constructed. Bachelor examines the various reasons for the visit to cemeteries by mourners including: to fulfill obligations, to help achieve independence from the deceased; and to seek solace.[7(p. 408)]

Grief

Grief has been defined as "a reaction to loss—we can experience grief obviously when someone we're attached to dies, but we can also experience it when we lose any significant form of attachment."[8] And, as we saw in the opening paragraph of this chapter, grief can vary in the manner in which it is expressed. There are numerous definitions of grief, and these are illustrative of variations on a theme. The process of grief has been studied and reformulated, phases identified, types proposed (anticipatory, complicated, disenfranchised), and expressions of grief described.

Given that nurses work largely with individuals and families, but in some cases also with communities, several sections of this chapter focus on grief as it relates to these different entities. However, even in those sections that putatively deal with associated topics, the subject of grief is related and may be interwoven. With these preliminary definitions as a basis, bereavement, grief, and mourning can now be addressed in greater depth.

The process of bereavement

The process and meaning of bereavement vary depending on a number of factors, including age, gender, ethnicity, cultural background, education, and socioeconomic status. For African-American widows, storytelling was the means by which the bereavement experience was described.[9] The themes identified in a study of these widows included awareness of death, caregiving, getting through, moving on, changing feelings, and financial security. These themes describe well the concerns of bereavement.

The impact of grief affects the health outcomes of bereavement, notably the physical and mental health of the bereaved. These outcomes have been examined by Stroebe, Schut, and Stroebe.[10] In a review of the literature, they found that there is an increase in mortality from a variety of causes for the bereaved, including changes in personal habits and social activities, and psychological distress; that psychological distress can take the form of grief or depression.

The distinction between grief and depression in the bereaved is an important one.[11] As Middleton and associates[12] concluded, "The bereaved can experience considerable pain and yet be coping adaptively, and they can fulfill many depressive criteria yet at the same time be experiencing phenomena that are not depressive in nature (p. 452)." Even in individuals with a history of "sadness or irritability" before bereavement, although they may have more intense expressions of grief, the rate of recovery is the same as for those without such a history.[13] Other authors are not as sanguine, and caution that a past history of subsyndromal symptomatic depressions are "frequently seen complications of bereavement that may be chronic and often are associated with substantial morbidity."[14] These debates have taken on new relevance given the publication of the *Diagnostic and Statistical Manual of Mental Disorders*, 5th edition (DSM-5), as shall be discussed later in this chapter.

Rubin and Schecter conceptualized bereavement-related grief into the two-track model of bereavement as a means of understanding and addressing the bereavement process and its outcome. Track 1 addresses biopsychological functioning and is concerned with two questions: "1. Where are the difficulties in biopsychological functioning? 2. Where are the strengths and growth manifest?"[15] Track 2 examines the relationship to the deceased and focuses on two questions: "1. What is the state of the desire to reconnect with the deceased affectively and cognitively? 2. What is the nature of the ongoing relationship to the deceased? Is the death story integrated?"[15] In essence, bereavement involves adjusting to a world without the physical, psychological, and social presence of the deceased.

Prebereavement mental distress such as depression and anxiety, as well as a high level of perceived burden with lack of support, was predictive of a poor bereavement outcome.[16] Boelen and coworkers[17] pointed out that traumatic grief is distinct from bereavement-related depression and anxiety. Identifying these differences clinically is essential for appropriate treatment. Bereavement becomes complicated (in the literature and in life) when adjustment is impeded, as in posttraumatic stress disorder. Whether such bereavement occurs as a result of vehicular accident, war, or natural disaster, the suddenness or overwhelming nature of the event dislodges the sense that all is well with the world. The sense of disequilibrium is amplified when bereavement is the result of suicide. Such a death is accompanied by an overwhelming sense of guilt and the sense of abandonment and rejection.[18] Even in instances in which an elective medical procedure such as abortion occurs, the emotional response may not become evident until many years later.

Death before its time, as in children and young and middle-aged adults, not only affects the bereaved directly, but also affects the social roles of the survivors that require readjustment. The idea that parental outcomes are worse when a child's death is by suicide was not confirmed empirically, however. Another myth is that divorce is more common among bereaved couples than in the general population. The empirical evidence is insufficient either to substantiate or disconfirm this assumption. The issues occasioned by the death of a child with intellectual disabilities have much in common with disenfranchised grief.[19] Studies have underscored the need for postbereavement support in such cases.[19,20] Disenfranchised grief is compounded by stigma for children with a father on death row, who must contend first with the loss of having an incarcerated parent and then with his death by execution.[21] More will be said about disenfranchised grief shortly.

The hesitancy of children to exhibit their own sadness so as not to upset their parents requires that professionals encourage parents to give their children permission to be sad when that is how they feel. By taking care of their parents, children may not receive the attention they require. In a study that sought to identify those factors that helped or hindered adolescent sibling bereavement, a youngster stated: "What helped me the most was my mother, who was totally honest with me from the time Sarah got sick through her death. My mother took the time to listen to how I felt as well as understand and hug me."[22] Adolescents whose parents died of cancer have been noted to be more likely to engage in self-injury with a range in prevalence of from 6% to 40%.[23] The importance of support for children and adolescents cannot be overstated.

Situations where individuals are expected to "get on with it" may pose difficulties for those who are bereaved. Individuals such as university faculty members who have demanding work responsibilities may not receive the support required as a result of the need to remain productive.[24] Work factors may be compounded by the personality of the bereaved. Personality correlates were found to influence bereavement narratives, with those testing high in conscientiousness providing brief, factual narratives, those high in neuroticism being self-focused, and those high in extraversion giving narratives associated with social reasons.[25]

Cognitive processing and finding meaning can be helpful to a variety of clients. However, older persons have been noted to be more reluctant to express their feelings.[26] Nurses can be helpful to these clients by encouraging them to express their feelings and being available when needed. Routine bereavement care can be helpful in identifying people at risk for complicated grieving. For individuals who are unable to avail themselves of face-to-face support groups whether for reasons of time, distance, or responsibilities, an Internet support group may be an option. Pector[27] provides a host of such resources. Given that the best therapy is prevention, palliative care teams who identify caregivers at risk for bereavement maladjustment can intervene early to prevent long-term difficulties.

Aside from such proactive approaches for all bereaved persons, Sheldon[28] reported the following predisposing factors for a poor bereavement outcome: ambivalent or dependent relationship; multiple prior bereavements; previous mental illness, especially depression; and low self-esteem. At the time of death: sudden and unexpected death, untimely death of a young person, preparation for the death, stigmatized deaths (e.g., AIDS, suicide, culpable death), sex of the bereaved person (e.g., elderly male widower), caring for the deceased person for >6 months, and inability to carry out valued religious rituals.[28] Boyle, Feng, and Raab[29] reaffirm that widowhood increases the risk of death regardless of the type of death of the spouse, noting that the risk of mortality is increased 10%–40% for the surviving spouse.

Penultimately, after the death, such factors as level of perceived social support, hardiness, lack of opportunities for new interests, and stress from other life crises—as well as dysfunctional behaviors and attitudes appearing early in the bereavement period, consumption of alcohol and drugs, smoking, morbid guilt, and the professional caregiver's gut feeling that this patient will not do well—are predictive of poor outcomes.[28,29] Knowledge of and alertness to such predisposing factors are useful for the provision of help, both lay and professional, early in the course of the bereavement so as to prevent further debilitating events. In addition to social support, healthcare policy can have a profound effect on the experience of bereavement as part of the context in which care is provided.[30]

The nature of grief

Rando[31] observed that, although he was not the first person to examine the effects of bereavement, Freud is taken as an important point of departure. The observation that grief is a normal process and that "a lost love object is never totally relinquished" are congruent with current thinking. The notion that one needs to totally "let go" of the beloved, ascribed to Freud on the basis of some of his work, has influenced professionals to the current day.

The initiation of the modern study of death and dying, however, especially in America, is often attributed to Erich Lindemann, a physician at the Massachusetts General Hospital, who responded to the survivors of a fire in Boston's Coconut Grove nightclub. Five hundred persons died as a result of the fire, which took place on Thanksgiving eve, 1942. Lindemann, a psychiatrist, was interested at the time in the emotional reaction of patients to body disfigurement and plastic surgery.[32] With this medical interest, "Lindemann was struck by the similarity of responses between his patients' reactions to facial disfigurement or loss of a body part and the reactions of the survivors of the fire."[32(p. 105)]

This observation led Lindemann to a study of 101 patients including (1) psychoneurotic patients who lost a relative during the course of treatment, (2) relatives of patients who died in the hospital, (3) bereaved disaster victims (Coconut Grove fire) and their close relatives, and (4) relatives of members of the armed forces.[33] Based on the study of these patients, he determined the five indicators that are "pathognomonic for grief"[33]: (1) sensations of somatic distress, such as tightness in the throat, choking, and shortness of breath; (2) intense preoccupation with the image of the deceased; (3) strong feelings of guilt; (4) a loss of warmth toward others with a tendency to respond with irritability and anger; and (5) disoriented behavior patterns. Lindemann coined the term "grief work" to describe the process by which individuals attempt to adjust to their loss.[32]

Various theorists have developed a series of stages and phases of grief work. The most well known of these to the general public are the stages formulated by Elizabeth Kübler-Ross. Proposed for those facing a death, these stages have also been applied to those experiencing a loss. Kübler-Ross[34] identified five stages: denial and isolation, anger, bargaining, depression, and acceptance. The commonality among all theorists of the stages of grief is that the individual moves through (1) notification and shock, (2) experience of the loss emotionally and cognitively, and (3) reintegration. Based on these stages, Corr and Doka[35] proposed the following tasks:

1. To share acknowledgment of the reality of death

2. To share in the process of working through the pain of grief

3. To reorganize the family system

4. To restructure the family's relationship with the deceased and to reinvest in other relationships and life pursuits

With regard to the last task, some dispute has arisen concerning the degree to which separation from the deceased must occur. Klass and associates[36] made the compelling argument that such bonds continue. They averred that "survivors hold the deceased in loving memory for long periods, often forever," and that maintaining an inner representation of the deceased is normal rather than abnormal. Winston's study of African-American grandmothers demonstrated that they maintained strong bonds with the deceased.[37]

The second area of dissension is the expectation that intense grief must be resolved within 2 weeks. More will be said about the changes in the time frame for the so-called bereavement exclusion for a diagnosis of major depressive disorder later in the chapter.

A third area of discussion concerns whether the concept of recovery, or some other term, best connotes what occurs after coming to terms with a death and getting on with one's life.[38,39] It has been suggested that recovery is a term more appropriate to an illness, and that death is a normal process of life. Balk,[40] however, argues for a term that incorporates the potential for transformative growth.

A fourth area of debate is the issue of the medicalization of the grief process. Given that death is a normal part of the cycle of living, grief too is considered a normal process. As shall be observed in the following sections of this chapter, grief, although considered normal, may also become "complicated." As such, interventions may be needed. A medical diagnosis provides legitimacy to those engaged in the treatment encounter, including funding for those who are engaged in providing treatment.

A fifth area of vigorous discussion concerns the efficacy of grief counseling. Larson and Hoyt[41] provide a compelling argument that the basis of the pessimistic view of the value of grief counseling is unfounded. The question of continuing bonds and the length of the grief process are addressed again at the close of this chapter. Readers are invited to consider all of these questions in light of their own experiences and readings of the literature. In this next section, types of grief are examined.

Types of grief

The types of grief examined in this section are not exhaustive of all types of grief, but rather encompass the major categories. Different terms such as "common grief" and "chronic grief" may be used for some of these same phenomena.

Anticipatory grief

Anticipatory grief shares similarities with other forms of grief. It is also different. The onset may be associated with the receipt of bad news. Anticipatory grief must be distinguished from the concept of forewarning. An example of forewarning is learning of a terminal diagnosis. Anticipatory grief is an unconscious process, whereas forewarning is a conscious process. With forewarning of a terminal diagnosis, the question is, "What if we do?" With a death, that question becomes, "What if we had done?" With the former question, there is the potential for hope; with the latter query, there may be guilt.

Even with forewarning, preparation for loss may not occur, given that this may be perceived to be a betrayal of the terminally ill person. There also have been instances of family members unconsciously preparing for the death of an individual and going through the grieving process, only to have that person recover to find no place in the lives of his or her loved ones. This is an example of anticipatory grief.

The question of the utility of forewarning is one of how this time is used. If it is used to make some preparation for role change, such as becoming familiar with the intricacies of the role the terminally ill person plays in the family (e.g., mastering a checking account or other financial responsibilities of the family), such time may be used to the benefit of all concerned. On the other hand, anticipatory grieving resulting in reinvestment of emotional energy before the death of the terminally ill person is detrimental to the relationship.

Byrne and Raphael[42] found that "widowers who were unable to anticipate their wife's death, even when their wife had suffered a long final illness, had a more severe bereavement reaction." (The term "anticipate" is used by Byrne and Raphael in the sense of forewarning.) Family members and friends are "warned" when their loved one is diagnosed with certain disease entities such as cancer with metastases. If the primary problem is Alzheimer's disease, there may be a long decline in which, ultimately, familiar figures are no longer recognized. In either situation, the death of the ill person may be experienced both with sadness and with a sense of relief that the caregiving burden is no more. The price of that relief is that the patient is no more.

The sense of relief experienced by caregivers is often a source of guilt feelings about wishing the patient dead. It is important to clarify for the family member or significant other that feelings of relief in being freed of the caregiver burden are not equivalent to wishing someone dead. A woman who experienced relief from not having to care for her bulky husband was assisted to examine this distinction, and consequently was able to grieve uncomplicated by feelings of guilt. Further, persons who have cared for a dying person may experience a sense of accomplishment, knowing that they have done everything they could for their loved one.

Duke,[43] in a qualitative study that enlarged the understanding of the status changes of widowhood, interviewed five spouses in the second year of their bereavement. Although the findings may have been biased by the distortion of hindsight, they provide much food for thought. The research identified four areas of change: role change from spouse to caregiver during the illness, followed by loss of those roles in bereavement and needing to be cared for; relationship changes from being with spouse to being alone; coping changes from being in suspense to being in turmoil; and the change from experiencing and gathering memories to remembering and constructing memories.[43] It is interesting that these findings reflect the general changes that occur over a terminal illness and not the experience of anticipatory grief. Anticipatory grief, as noted previously, is unconscious preparation for status change and not a conscious, deliberative process. It should be noted here that the term "premature grief" has also been given to this process.[44] In the following section, anticipatory grief is contrasted with what is termed "uncomplicated grief."

Uncomplicated grief

Worthington[45] depicted a linear model of uncomplicated grief based on adjustment. In this model, an individual in a normal emotional state experiences a loss that causes a reaction and an emotional low; subsequently, the individual begins a recovery to his or her former state. This process of recovery is occasioned by brief periods of relapse, but not to the depths experienced previously. Ultimately, the individual moves to adjustment to the loss. Although this description simplifies the turmoil that may be experienced, discussion of expressions of grief later in this chapter capture the physical, psychological, behavioral, and social upset that characterizes even uncomplicated grief.

Niemeyer[46] offered a new perspective by focusing on meaning reconstruction. He developed a set of propositions to capture adaptation to loss:

1. Death as an event can validate or invalidate the constructions that form the basis on which we live, or it may stand as a novel experience for which we have no constructions.

2. Grief is a personal process, one that is idiosyncratic, intimate, and inextricable from our sense of who we are.

3. Grieving is something we do, not something that is done to us.

4. Grieving is the act of affirming or reconstructing a personal world of meaning that has been challenged by loss.

5. Feelings have functions and should be understood as signals of the state of our meaning-making efforts.

6. We construct and reconstruct our identities as survivors of loss in negotiations with others.

Niemeyer[46] viewed meaning reconstruction as the central process of grief. The inability to make meaning may lead to complications.

Complicated grief

In her discussion of complicated mourning, Rando[31] made observations applicable to complicated grief. She observed that, after a suitable length of time, the mourner is attempting to "deny, repress, or avoid aspects of the loss, its pain, and its implications and … to hold onto, and avoid relinquishing, the lost loved one. These attempts, or some variants thereof, cause the complications in mourning." These complications have also been noted to occur pre-death in the caregivers of cancer patients.[47]

Researchers have identified the diagnostic criteria for complicated grief disorder. These criteria include "the current experience (>1 year after a loss) of intensive intrusive thoughts, pangs of severe emotion, distressing yearnings, feeling excessively alone and empty, excessively avoiding tasks reminiscent of the deceased, unusual sleep disturbances, and maladaptive levels of loss of interest in personal activities."[48(p904)] Other researchers have underscored the need for the specification of complicated grief as a unique disorder, and have developed an inventory of complicated grief to measure maladaptive symptoms of loss.[49] The Inventory of Complicated Grief is composed of 19 items with responses ranging from "Never" to "Rarely," "Sometimes," "Often," and "Always." Examples of items include, "I think about this person so much that it's hard for me to do the things I usually do"; "Ever since she (or he) died it is hard for me to trust people"; "I feel that it is unfair that I should live when this person died"; and "I feel lonely a great deal of the time ever since she (or he) died."[49] This inventory may be helpful to healthcare practitioners because it differentiates between complicated grief and depression.[49] Finally, it is the severity of symptomatology and the duration that distinguishes abnormal and complicated responses to bereavement.[50] Ruminative coping as an avoidance of grief work as been proposed as a variant of complicated chronic grief.[51]

The Inventory of Complicated Grief was used by Ott[51] with 112 bereaved participants in a study in which those identified as experiencing complicated grief were compared with those who were not. Those with complicated grief both identified more additional life stressors and felt they had less social support than the other bereaved individuals in the study. Lack of preparation for the death of a loved one has also been associated with complicated grief and depression.[53] The perspective of complicated grief as a stress response syndrome has been explicated by Shear and colleagues.[54] It is important to observe that the characteristics of complicated grief have not been found to vary by race or by the violence of the loss.[55,56]

It should be noted that there is some concern among professionals that what is a normal process is being medicalized by healthcare practitioners. Complicated grief, however, may require professional intervention.[41,57] Approaches to therapy have included cognitive-behavioral therapy, presented face-to-face as well as over the Internet, and supportive counseling.[57–59] More is said about this later in the chapter. Bearing this in mind, disenfranchised grief poses different but potentially related problems.

Disenfranchised grief

Doka[60] defined disenfranchised grief as "grief that results when a person experiences a significant loss and that the resultant grief is not openly acknowledged, socially validated or publicly mourned. In short, although the individual is experiencing a grief reaction, there is no social recognition that the person has a right to grieve or a claim on social sympathy or support." Those who are grieving the loss of relationships that may not be publicly acknowledged—for example, with a mistress or with a family conceived outside a legally recognized union, or in some cases with stepfamilies, colleagues, or friends—are not accorded the deference and support usually afforded the bereaved. Further nonsanctioned relationships, either heterosexual or homosexual, may result in the exclusion of individuals not legitimated by blood or legal union. Individuals in homosexual relationships of long standing who care for their partners throughout their last illness, may find themselves barred both from the funeral and from the home that was shared.[61] A recent study underscores the finding of less social support for the bereaved spouses of same-sex couples.[62] For some time, infection with HIV was hidden from the community, thereby depriving both the infected and their caregivers of support. The AIDS quilt has done much to provide a public mourning ritual, but has not alleviated the disenfranchised status of homosexual or lesbian partners. The result is what has been termed "modulated mourning."[61] This response to stigmatization constrains the public display of mourning by the griever. In this situation, the griever is not recognized.[63] The griever with intellectual disabilities may also not be recognized. McEvoy and colleagues[64] examined the degree to which the person with intellectual disabilities comprehends the finality, universality, and inevitability of death. While they conclude that there is only a partial understanding of death by their sample of individuals with intellectual disabilities, some of the responses could easily have been uttered by those without such disabilities. As with any bereaved person, the most helpful approach is an individualized one.

There are other instances in which a loss has not been legitimized. Loss resulting from miscarriage or abortion has only recently been recognized. In Japan, a "cemetery" is devoted to letters written by families each year telling miscarried or aborted children about the important events that occurred in the family that year, and also expressing continued grief at their loss. Grieving in secret is a burden that makes the process more difficult to complete. Disenfranchised grief may also be a harbinger of unresolved grief.

Unresolved grief

Unresolved grief is a failure to accomplish the necessary grief work. According to Rando, a variety of factors may give rise to unresolved grief, including guilt, loss of an extension of the self, reawakening of an old loss, multiple loss, inadequate ego development, and idiosyncratic resistance to mourning.[65(pp. 64–65)] In addition to these psychological factors, such social factors as social negation of a loss, socially unspeakable loss, social isolation and/or geographic distance from social support, assumption of the role of the strong one, and uncertainty over the loss (e.g., a disappearance at sea) may be implicated in unresolved grief.[65(pp. 66–67)] By helping significant others express their feelings and complete their business before the death of a loved one, unresolved grief and the accompanying manifestations can be prevented to some extent.

Eakes and coworkers[66] questioned whether "closure" is a necessary outcome. They explored the concept of "chronic sorrow" in bereaved individuals who experienced episodic bouts of sadness related to specific incidents or significant dates. These authors suggested the fruitfulness of maintaining an open-ended model of grief. With this in mind, grief is always unresolved to some degree; this is not considered pathological but rather an acknowledgment of a death. This model is now known as the theory of chronic sorrow.[67]

Expressions of grief

Symptoms of grief

In some of the earlier sections of this chapter, various manifestations of grief were mentioned. In this section, expressions of grief that are within the range considered normal in this society are described. It is important to note that what is considered appropriate in one group may be considered deviant or even pathological in another. It bears repeating that the manifestations of grief and bereavement are influenced by culture.[68]

The perception of the manifestations of grief is also framed by professionals. For example, intense grieving beyond 2 weeks is considered in need of psychiatric intervention in the current *Diagnostic and Statistical Manual of Mental Disorders,* 5th edition.[69] In previous versions of the manual, grief was not mentioned or grief was considered an exclusion for a diagnosis of major depressive disorder if bereavement occurred within a year and subsequently 2 months and now, in the current edition of the manual, 2 weeks. This has been a source of considerable debate with professionals in the field of death and dying decrying such as approach as ill-advised and inappropriate. To quote from a letter from these experts "Death is a life-altering event, but grief is not a pathological condition."[70] That is not to say that there are no physical, cognitive, and emotional responses to the death of a loved one. Balk and colleagues state, "We are concerned that for reasons of economic profit and clinical efficiency, people will often be prematurely diagnosed with depression and put on medication, rather than offered person-to-person counseling. Clinicians report anecdotally that this practice already occurs."[71(p. 208)] Wakefield warns against pathologizing grief when he states that the "grief process is less a step-wise preset series of events that lead to full resolution of pain, as classically portrayed, and more an individually constructed compromise between a degree of pain that never fully resolves and the need to compartmentalize that pain to move on with one's life."[72(p. 509)] Wakefield concurs with Bowlby that "normal grief can be a very lengthy process."[72]

In Table 29.1, physical, cognitive, emotional, and behavioral symptoms of grief are presented. Table 29.1 is not exhaustive of all of the potential symptoms, but rather is illustrative of the expressions and manifestations of grief. What distinguishes so-called normal grief is that it is usually self-limited. Although manifestations of grief at 1, 3, and 15 months after the death are not the same in intensity, a recent paper may change our assumptions about grief. The widows in the study by Kowalski and Bondmass,[73] while experiencing a decline in symptomatology, also continued experiencing symptoms for up to 5 years—the limit of the bereavement experience of the research participants.

A potentially useful bereavement assessment tool links the questions to be asked to the needs in the Maslow hierarchy, thereby attempting to assess the level of need.[74] The five questions address physiological, safety, belongingness, esteem, and self-actualization needs. The author provides no clinical or research data on

Table 29.1 Manifestations of grief

Physical	Cognitive	Emotional	Behavioral
Headaches	Sense of depersonalization	Anger	Impaired work performance
Dizziness	Inability to concentrate	Guilt	Crying
Exhaustion	Sense of disbelief and confusion	Anxiety	Withdrawal
Muscular aches	Idealization of the deceased	Sense of helplessness	Avoiding reminders of the deceased
Sexual impotency	Search for meaning of life and death	Sadness	Seeking or carrying reminders of the deceased
Loss of appetite	Dreams of the deceased	Shock	
Insomnia	Preoccupation with image of deceased	Yearning	Overreactivity
Feelings of tightness or hollowness	Fleeting visual, tactile, olfactory, auditory hallucinatory experiences	Numbness	Changed relationships
		Self-blame	
Breathlessness		Relief	
Tremors			
Shakes			
Oversensitivity to noise			

Source: Adapted from Doka.[76]

the use of the hierarchy. Nonetheless, this approach merits further investigation. Requiring further discussion are the outward manifestations that are the expressions of mourning.

Mourning

O'Gorman contrasted death rituals in England with those in Ireland. She recalled the "Protestant hushed respectfulness which had somehow infiltrated and taken over a Catholic community."[75(p. 1133)] The body was taken from the home by the funeral director. Children continued with school and stayed with relatives; they were shielded from the death. By way of contrast, in an Irish wake, "The body, laid out by a member of the family in order to receive a 'special blessing,' would be in the parlour of a country house surrounded by flowers from the garden and lighted candles."[75(p. 1133)] The children, along with the adult members of the family, viewed the corpse. "When visitors had paid their last respects they would join the crowd in the kitchen, who would then spend all night recounting stories associated with the dead person."[75(p. 1133)] O'Gorman noted the plentiful availability of alcohol and stated, "by the end of the night, to the uninitiated the event would appear to be more like a party than a melancholy event."[75(p. 1133)] Although O'Gorman initially found this distasteful, she "now believes that rituals like the Irish wake celebrate death as a happy occasion and bestow grace upon those leaving life and upon a community of those who mourn them."[75(p. 1133)]

The Irish wake, like the reception held in a church basement, hall, restaurant, or private home, serves not only for the expression of condolences but also as an opportunity to reinforce the connections of the community. Anyone familiar with such events knows that a variety of social and business arrangements are made by mourners both within and outside the immediate family. And although some gatherings are more reserved and others lustier, giving the deceased a good send off ("good" being defined by the group) is central to each. The good send-off is part of the function of the funeral as a piacular rite—that is, as a means of atoning for the sins of the mortal being, and as preparation for life in the afterworld.[76] Fulton[76] noted two other functions of funerals, namely integration and separation. The former concerns the living; the latter refers to separation from the loved one as a mortal person. The value of the Irish wake, which in the United States may look more like the Protestant burial O'Gorman[75] describes, is the time spent together sharing stories and feelings.

In the United States, funeral services are held not only in religious establishments such as churches or synagogues, but also in funeral homes. These services, frequently under the aegis of a clergyperson, may also be conducted by a staff member of the funeral home. More recently these services have also taken on the earmarks of a memorial service, accompanied by pictures of the deceased and the bereaved and remarks by selected close family members and friends of the deceased.

In the Irish wake as practiced in Ireland, one is not alone with one's feelings but in the company of others who are devoting the time to mourning (integration). This devotion of time to mourning is also found in the Jewish religion, where the bereaved "sit Shiva," usually for 7 days.[77] In Judaism, the assumption is that the bereaved are to focus on their loss and the grieving of that loss. They are to pay no attention to worldly considerations. This period of time of exemption from customary roles may facilitate the process. Certainly having a "minion," in which 10 men and women (10 men for Orthodox Jews) say prayers each evening, reinforces the reality of the death and the separation. For the Orthodox, the mourning period is 1 year.

A very different pattern is practiced by the Hopi in Arizona. The Hopi have a brief ceremony with the purpose of completing the funeral as quickly as possible so as to get back to customary activities.[77] The fear of death and the dead, and of spirits, induces distancing by the Hopi from nonliving phenomena. Strobe and Stroebe[77] contrasted Shinto and Buddhist mourners in Japan with the Hopi. Both Shinto and Buddhist mourners practice ancestor worship; as a result, the bereaved can keep contact with the deceased, who become ancestors. Speaking to ancestors as well as offering food is accepted practice. In contrast to this Japanese practice, what occurs in the United States is that those bereaved who speak with a deceased person do so quietly, hiding the fact from others, believing others will consider it suspect or pathological. It is, however, a common occurrence. As mentioned previously, bringing food to the ancestor, or (e.g., to celebrate the Day of the Dead) to the cemetery, is part of the mourning practice in Hispanic and many other societies.

Practices, however, change with time, although one can often find the imprint of earlier rituals. The practice of saving a lock of hair or the footprint of a deceased newborn may have evolved from the practice in Victorian times of using hair for mourning brooches and lockets. As a salesperson of these items commented, "They liked to be reminded of their dead in those days. Now it's out of sight, out of mind."[78] But not quite. Virtual or online memorials take the form of personal Web pages in a study by Mitchell and colleagues, who suggest that "virtual memorials blur the boundaries between the living and the dead."[79(p. 426)] They posit, "Virtual memorials may even imply a kind of ethereal techno-presence whereby the ideal of heaven is being reconfigured as technologically mediated space/time: a digital set of pearly gates."[79(p. 428)] These mourning practices of virtual memorials provide continuing bonds with the deceased and offer a clue to the answer to the question posed for the last section of this chapter: When is it over? Before addressing this question, another needs to be raised, and that is the question of support.

A question of support

A question regarding support is the contribution of formal support as an addition to the support of the social network. Diamond and colleagues[80] demonstrate the utility of such outside support particularly for those not wanting to burden family and friends.

Formal support

Many of the mourning practices noted previously provide support by the community to the bereaved (Table 29.2). Formal support in the Jewish tradition is exemplified by the practice of attending a minion for the deceased person. The minion expresses support for the living. It is formal in that it is prescribed behavior on the part of observant Jews and incorporates a prayer service.

Other examples of formal support include support groups such as the widow-to-widow program and the Compassionate Friends for families of deceased children. The assumption underlying the widow-to-widow program is that grief and mourning are not in and of themselves pathological, and that laypersons can be helpful to one another. The widow-to-widow program provides a formal mechanism for sharing one's emotions and experience with individuals who have had a similar experience. The Widowed Persons Service offers support for men and women via self-help support groups and a variety of educational and social activities. The Compassionate Friends, also a self-help organization, seeks to help parents and siblings after the death of a child. Other support groups may or may not have the input of a professional to run the group. Being in such a group, one doesn't have to explain oneself. The other participants have "gone through something so close, it's quite scary."[18(p. 9)]

Formal programs for children's bereavement support include peer support programs and art therapy programs. Institutions with bereavement programs, whether for children or adults, often send cards at the time of a patient's death, on the birthday of the deceased, and at 3, 6, 12, and 24 months after the death. Pamphlets with information about grief, a bibliography of appropriate readings, and contact numbers of support groups are also helpful. Family bereavement programs have been found to lead to improved parenting, coping, and caregiver mental health. The provision of bereavement follow-up to parents who have experienced the loss of a child or a pregnancy loss is helpful to the parents and also has implications for the support of the nurses and others who deliver this service.[81]

Attention to staff bereavement support has been given by institutional trauma programs, in emergency departments, and in critical care departments.[82] Brosche[83] provides a description of a grief team within a healthcare system. Keene, Hutton, Hall, and Rushton[84] outline a format for bereavement debriefing. This attention to the grief of healthcare providers empowers those involved to express their grief rather than to suppress it. All of these programs, whether for healthcare providers or family and significant others, maintain contact with the bereaved so as to provide

Table 29.2 Bereavement practices

Lay	Professional
1. Friendly visiting	1. Clergy visiting
2. Provision of meals	2. Clergy counseling
3. Informal support by previously bereaved	3. Nurse, MD, psychologist, social worker, psychiatrist counseling
4. Lay support groups	4. Professionally led support groups
5. Participation in cultural and religious rituals	5. Organization of memorial services by hospice and palliative care organizations
6. A friendly listener	6. A thoughtful listener
7. Involvement in a cause-related group	7. Referral to individuals with similar cause-related concerns
8. Exercise	8. Referral to a health club
9. Joining a new group	9. Referral to a bereavement program

support and make referrals to pastoral care personnel and other professionals as needed.

A variety of approaches have been used in working with the bereaved. Indeed, the combination of "religious psychotherapy" and a cognitive-behavioral approach was observed to be helpful to highly religious bereaved persons.[85] Religious psychotherapy for a group of Malays who adhered to the religion of Islam consisted of discussion and reading of verses of the Koran and Hadith, the encouragement of prayers, and a total of 12 to 16 psychotherapy sessions.[85] Targeting of the follow-up approach to the characteristics of the population eschews the notion that "one size fits all."

A bereavement support group intervention was demonstrated to have a significant impact on the grief of homosexual men who were or were not seropositive for the human immunodeficiency virus (HIV-1).[86] The need for support was found to be all the more necessary for bereaved women living with HIV who "may be at increased risk for bereavement complicated with psychiatric morbidity and thoughts of suicide."[87(p. 225)] The risk reduction effects of a community bereavement support program for HIV-positive individuals was demonstrated by a community support program in Ontario, Canada.[88] These outcomes have implications for the approaches nurses use with other bereaved clients.

Support groups may be open ended (i.e., without a set number of sessions), or they may be closed and limited to a particular set of individuals. Support groups with a set number of sessions have a beginning and end and are therefore more likely to be closed to new members until a new set of sessions begins. Open ended groups have members who stay for varying lengths of time and may or may not have a topic for each session. Lev and McCorkle[89] cited the finding that short-term programs of two to seven sessions, or meeting as needed, were the most effective.

Other formal support entails working with a therapist or other healthcare provider (bereavement counseling). For those who were bereaved as a result of a suicide, the 6- to 8-week programs run by the Lifeline Community Care Group Brisbane helped to normalize the suicide bereavement experience.[18] Cloyes and colleagues[90] caution that the style of the interaction whether directive or facilitative has an impact on the opportunity for expression by the family caregiver. Arnold[91] suggested that the nurse should follow a process to assess the meaning of loss, the nature of the relationship, expressions and manifestations of grief, previous experience with grief, support systems, ability to maintain attachments, and progression of grief. Further, Arnold underscored the importance of viewing grief as a healing process (Box 29.1). She gave the following example of a patient situation and two different approaches to diagnosis:[91]

A newly widowed woman feels awkward about maintaining social relationships with a group of married couples with whom she had participated with her husband.

◆ Grief as a pathological diagnosis: social isolation.
◆ Grief as a healthy diagnosis: redefinition of social support.[91]

In addition to conventional talking therapy, such techniques as letter writing, empty chair, guided imagery, and journal writing can be used (Table 29.3). In letter writing, the empty chair technique, and guided imagery, the bereaved are

Box 29.1 Assessment of grief

The bereaved often are weary from caring for the deceased. During this period they may not have looked after themselves. An assessment should include:

1. A general health checkup and assessment of somatic symptoms
2. A dental visit
3. An eye checkup as appropriate
4. Nutritional evaluation
5. Sleep assessment
6. Examination of ability to maintain work and family roles
7. Determination of whether there are major changes in presentation of self
8. Assessment of changes resulting from the death and the difficulties with these changes
9. Assessment of social networks

The healthcare worker needs to bear in mind that there is no magic formula for grieving. The key question is whether the bereaved is able to function effectively. Cues to the need for assistance include:

1. Clinical depression
2. Prolonged deep grief
3. Extreme grief reaction
4. Self-destructive behavior
5. Increased use of alcohol and/or drugs
6. Preoccupation with the deceased to the exclusion of others
7. Perceived lack of social support

encouraged to express feelings about the past or about what life is like without the deceased. These techniques can be helpful as the "wish I had said" becomes said. A journal is also a vehicle for recording ongoing feelings of the lived experience of bereavement.

It must be emphasized that grief is not pathology. It is a normal process that is expressed in individual ways. The techniques in Table 29.3 may prove helpful to the individual who is experiencing guilt about things not said or done. This list is not exhaustive, merely illustrative.

Another part of bereavement counseling is the instillation or reemergence of hope. As Cutcliffe[92] concluded, "There are many theories of bereavement counseling, with commonalities between these theories. Whilst the theories indicate implicitly the re-emergence of hope in the bereft individual as a result of the counseling, they do not make specific reference to how this inspiration occurs." Cutcliffe saw the clear need to understand this process.

In her exposition of the concept "hope," Stephenson[93] noted the association made by Frankl[94] between hope and meaning. Stephenson stated, "Frankl equated hope with having found meaning in life, and lack of hope as [having] no meaning in life."[93]

Table 29.3 Counseling interventions

1. Letter writing	The bereaved writes a letter to the deceased expressing the thoughts and feelings that may or may not have been expressed.
2. Empty chair	The bereaved sits across from an empty chair on which the deceased is imagined to be sitting. The bereaved is encouraged to express his or her feelings.
3. Empty chair with picture	A picture of the deceased is placed on the chair to facilitate the expressions of feelings by the bereaved.
4. Therapist assumes role of the deceased	In this intervention, the therapist helps the bereaved to explore his or her feelings toward the deceased by participating in a role play.
5. Guided imagery	This intervention demands a higher level of skill than, for example, letter writing. Guided imagery can be used to explore situations that require verbalization by the bereaved to achieve completion. Imagery can also be used to recreate situations of dissension with the goal of achieving greater understanding for the bereaved.
6. Journal writing	This technique provides an ongoing vehicle for exploring past situations and current feelings. It is a helpful intervention to many.
7. Drawing pictures	For the artistically and not so artistically inclined, drawing pictures and explaining their content is another vehicle for discussing feelings and concerns.
8. Analysis of role changes	Helping the bereaved obtain help with the changes secondary to the death, such as with balancing a checkbook or securing reliable help with various home needs; assists with some of the secondary losses with the death of a loved one.
9. Listening	The bereaved has the need to tell his or her story. Respectful listening and concern for the bereaved is a powerful intervention that is much appreciated.
10. Venting anger	The professional can suggest the following: ♦ Banging a pillow on the mattress. If combined with screaming, it is the best to do with the windows closed and no one in the home. ♦ Screaming—at home or parked in a car in an isolated spot with the windows closed. ♦ Crying—at home, followed by a warm bath and cup of tea or warm milk.
11. Normality barometer	Assuring the bereaved that the distress experienced is normal is very helpful to the bereaved.

Meaning-making appears key to the emergence of hope, and hope has been associated with coping.

In hospice programs, healthcare providers encourage dying persons and their families to have hope for each day. This compression of one's vision to the here and now may also be useful for the person who is grieving the loss of a loved one. Hope for the future and a personal future is the process that Cutcliffe[92] wished to elucidate. It may be a process that is predicated on hope for each day and having found meaning for the past.

Sikkema and colleagues[87] compared the effectiveness of individual and group approaches by evaluating individual psychotherapy and psychiatric services-on-demand with a support group format. The strategies employed in dealing with grief included establishing a sense of control and predictability, anger expression and management, resolution of guilt, promotion of self-mastery through empowerment, and development of new relationships. Those assigned to individual therapy may or may not have taken advantage of the option. It is proposed that future research examine three groups: those receiving individual counseling, those receiving group therapy, and those assigned no specific intervention but given information about various options for counseling and support in a pamphlet.

A therapist provides a vehicle for ongoing discussion of the loss that informal caregivers may be unable to provide. A support group of bereaved individuals, or periodic contact by an institutional bereavement service, may also prove useful. What is helpful depends on the individual and his or her needs and also on the informal support that is available.

Informal support

Informal support that is perceived as supportive and helpful can assist the bereaved to come to terms with life after the death of the beloved. Strategies evaluated as being helpful included "presence ('being there'), expressing the willingness to listen, and expressing care and concern, whereas the least positively evaluated strategies included giving advice, and minimization of other's feelings."[95(p. 419)] Whether the bereaved is isolated, or is part of a family or social group, is of tremendous import to the physical, psychological, and social welfare of the individual. Community in a psychosocial sense and a continuing role in the group are key factors in adjustment.

In societies where the widow has no role without her husband, she is figuratively if not literally disposed of in one way or another. It is for this reason that the woman who is the first in her group to experience widowhood has a much more difficult social experience than a woman who is in a social group where several women have become widows. In the former there is no reference group; in the latter there is.

The presence of family and friends takes on added significance after the initial weeks following the funeral. In those initial weeks, friendly visiting occurs with provision of a variety of types of foods considered appropriate in the group. After the initial period, friendly visiting is likely to decrease, and bereaved individuals may find themselves alone or the objects of financial predators. The counsel by the healthcare provider, or by family and friends, not to make life-altering decisions (e.g., moving) at this time unless absolutely necessary continues to be valuable advice. On the other hand, the comment that "time makes it easier" is a half-truth that is not perceived as helpful by the bereaved.[96]

What is helpful to the bereaved is listening to music enjoyed by both the deceased and the bereaved[97] and being listened to by an interested person. Having family members with whom to grieve has been shown to be significant to the process of grief processing, and may enhance family bonding.[96] Quinton disliked the term "counseling" in that it implies the availability of a person with good counsel to confer. What Quinton considered important was "lots of listening to what the victim wants to off-load."[98(p. 32)] She observed, "The turning point for me was realizing that I had a right to feel sad, and to grieve and to feel miserable for as long as I felt the need."[98(p. 32)] By owning the grieving process, Quinton provided herself with the most important support for her recovery from a devastating experience—her mother's murder in a massacre by the Irish Republican Army in 1987. The lesson is applicable, however, to any bereaved person regardless of whether the death was traumatic or anticipated. Quinton's turning point is another clue to answering the question of the last section of this chapter: When is it over?

When is it over?

To use the colloquial phrase, it's not over until it's over. What does this mean? As long as life and memory persist, the deceased individual remains part of the consciousness of family and friends. When is the grieving over? Unfortunately, there is no easy answer, and the only reasonable response is "It depends." Lindemann's concept of grief work,[32,33] mentioned earlier in this chapter, is applicable. Sooner or later that work needs to be accomplished. Delay protracts the time when accommodation is made. And grief work is never over, in the sense that there will be moments in years to come when an occasion or an object revives feelings of loss. The difference is that the pain is not the same acute pain as that experienced when the loss initially occurred. How one arrives at the point of accommodation is a process termed "letting go."

Letting go

The term "letting go" refers to acknowledgment of the loss of future togetherness—physical, psychological, and social. There is no longer a "we," only an "I" or a "we" without the deceased. Family members speak of events such as the first time a flower or bush blooms, major holidays, birthdays, anniversaries, and special shared times. Corless[99] quoted Jacqueline Kennedy, who spoke about "last year" (meaning 1962–1963) as the last time that her husband, John Kennedy, experienced a specific occasion:

> On so many days—his birthday, an anniversary, watching his children running to the sea—I have thought, "but this day last year was his last to see that." He was so full of love and life on all those days. He seems so vulnerable now, when you think that each one was a last time.

Mrs. Kennedy also wrote about the process of accommodation, although she didn't call it that:[61]

> Soon the final day will come around again—as inexorably as it did last year. But expected this time. It will find some of us different people than we were a year ago. Learning to accept what was unthinkable when he was alive changes you.

Finally, she addressed an essential truth of bereavement:

> I don't think there is any consolation. What was lost cannot be replaced.[99]

Letting go encompasses recognizing the uniqueness of the individual. It also entails finding meaning in the relationship and experience. It does not require cutting oneself off from memories of the deceased. It does require accommodating to the loss and to the continuing bonds with the deceased.

Continuing bonds

Klass and associates[36] contributed to the reformulation of thinking on the nature of accommodating to loss. Although theorists postulated that the grief process should be completed in 1 year, with one's emotional energies once again invested in the living, the experience of the bereaved suggested otherwise. Bereaved persons visit the grave for periodic discussions with the deceased. They gaze at a picture and seek advice on various matters. They maintain the presence of the deceased in their lives in a variety of different ways—some shared and some solitary. Such behavior is not pathological.

It is a common expectation that teachers in the educational system will have an influence on their students. The students progress and may or may not have continuing contact with those educators. Given that assumption about education, how could we not expect to feel the continuing influence and memory of those informal teachers in our lives, our deceased family members and friends? Integration of those influences strengthens the individual at any point in his or her life.

A Turkish expression in the presence of death is, "May you live."[100] That indeed is the challenge of bereavement.

References

1. Lee RA, Whiting JB. Foster children's expressions of ambiguous loss. Am J Fam Ther. 2007;35:117–128. doi: 10, 1080/ 0192618060/057499.
2. Kagawa-Singer M. The cultural context of death rituals and mourning practices. Oncol Nurs Forum. 1998;25:1752.
3. Durkheim E. The Elementary Forms of Religious Life. New York: Collier; 1961.
4. DeSpelder LA, Strickland AL. The Last Dance. 9th ed. Mountain View, CA: Mayfield; 2011:207.
5. Kotze E. "Women. … mourn and men carry on": African women storying mourning practices: a South African example. Death Stud. 2012;36:742–766.
6. Lee R, Vaughn M. Death and dying in the history of South Africa since 1800. JAH. 2008;49:341–359.
7. Bachelor P. Practical bereavement. Health Soc Rev. 2007;16: 405–414.
8. Yalom V. 2010. Kenneth Doka on Grief Counseling and Psychotherapy. http://www.psychotherapy.net/interview/grief-counseling-doka.
9. Rodgers L. Meaning of bereavement among older African-American widows. Geriatr Nurs. 2004;25:10–16.
10. Stroebe M, Schut H, Stroebe W. Health outcomes of bereavement. Lancet. 2007;370:1960–1973.
11. Zisook S, Kendler KS. Is bereavement-related depression different then non-bereavement-related depression? Psychol Med. 2007;37:779–794.
12. Middleton W, Franzp MD, Raphael B, Franzp MD, Burnett P, Martinek N. Psychological distress and bereavement. J Nerv Ment Dis. 1997;185:452.
13. Hays JC, Kasl S, Jacobs S. Past personal history of dysphoria, social support, and psychological distress following conjugal bereavement. J Am Geriatr Soc. 1994;42:712–718.
14. Zisook S, Shuchter SR, Sledge PA, Paulus M, Judd LL. The spectrum of depressive phenomena after spousal bereavement. J Clin Psychiatry. 1994;55(Suppl):35.

15 Rubin SS, Malkinson R, Witztum E. Working with the Bereaved: Multiple Lenses on Loss and Mourning. New York: Routledge Taylor & Francis Group; 2012.

16. Schulz R, Herbert R, Boerner K. Bereavement after caregiving. Geriatrics. 2008;63:20–22.

17. Boelen PA, van den Bout J, de Keijser J. Traumatic grief as a disorder distinct from bereavement-related depression and anxiety: a replication study with bereaved mental health care patients. Am J Psychiatry. 2003;160:1339–1341.

18. Groos AD, Shakespeare-Finch J. Positive experiences for participants in suicide bereavement groups: a grounded theory model. Death Stud. 2013;37:1–24.

19. Todd S. Silenced grief: living with the death of a child with intellectual disabilities. J Intellect Disabil Res. 2007;51:637–648.

20. Reilly DE, Hastings RP, Vaughan FL, Huws JC. Parental bereavement and the loss of a child with intellectual disabilities: a review of the literature. Intellect Dev Disabil. 2008;46:27–43.

21. Beck E, Jones SJ. Children of the condemned: grieving the loss of a father to death row. Omega. 2008;56:191–215.

22. Hogan NS, DeSantis L. Things that help and hinder adolescent sibling bereavement. West J Nurs Res. 1994;16:137.

23. Grenklo TB, Kreicbergs U, Hauksdottir A, Valdimarsdottir UA. Nyberg T, Steineck G, et al. Self-injury in teenagers who lost a parent to cancer: a nationwide, population-based, long-term follow-up. JAMA Pediatr. 2013;167:133–140. doi:10.1001/jamapediatrics.2013.430

24. Fitzpatrick, TR. Bereavement among faculty members in a university setting. Soc Work Health Care. 2007;45:83–109.

25. Baddeley JL, Singer JA. Telling losses: personality correlates and functions of bereavement narratives. J Res Pers. 2008;42:421–438.

26. Anderson KL, Dimond MF. The experience of bereavement in older adults. J Adv Nurs. 1995;22:308–315.

27. Pector EA. Sharing losses online: do Internet groups benefit the bereaved? ICEA Journal. 2012;27:19–25.

28. Sheldon F. ABC of palliative care: bereavement. BMJ. 1998;316:456.

29. Boyle PJ, Feng Z, Raab GM. Does widowhood increase mortality risk?: Testing for selection effects by comparing causes of spousal death. Epidemiology. 2011;22:1–5. doi:10.1097/EDE.06013e3181fdcc0b.

30. Holtslander LF. Caring for bereaved family caregivers: analyzing the context of care. Clin J Onc Nurs. 2008;510–506.

31. Rando TA. Grief and mourning: accommodating to loss. In: Wass H, Neimeyer RA (eds.), Dying: Facing the Facts. Philadelphia: Taylor and Francis; 1995:211–241.

32. Fulton R, Bendikson R. Introduction: grief and the process of mourning. In: Fulton R, Bendicksen R (eds.), Death and Identity. 3rd ed. Philadelphia: Charles Press; 1994:105–109.

33. Lindemann E. Symptomatology and management of acute grief. Am J Psychiatry. (Sesquicentennial Suppl) 1994;151(6):156.

34. Kübler-Ross E. On Death and Dying. New York: Macmillan, 1969.

35. Corr CA, Doka KJ. Current models of death, dying and bereavement. Crit Care Nurs Clin North Am. 1994;6:545–552.

36. Klass D, Silverman P, Nickman S. Continuing Bonds. Philadelphia: Taylor and Francis; 1996.

37. Winston CA. African American grandmothers parenting AIDS orphans: concomitant grief and loss. Am J Orthopsychiatry. 2003;73:91–100.

38. Shapiro ER. Whose recovery of what?: Relationships and environments promoting grief and growth. Death Stud. 2008;32(1):40–58.

39. Rosenblatt PC. Recovery following bereavement: metaphor, phenomenology, and Culture. Death Stud. 2008;32(1):6–16.

40. Balk DE. A modest proposal about bereavement and recovery. Death Stud. 2008;32(1):84–93.

41. Larson DG, Hoyt WT. What has become of grief counseling?: An evaluation of the empirical foundations of the new pessimism. Prof Psychol Res Pract. 2007;38:347–355.

42. Byrne GJA, Raphael B. A longitudinal study of bereavement phenomena in recently widowed elderly men. Psychol Med. 1994;23:411–421.

43. Duke S. An exploration of anticipatory grief: the lived experience of people during their spouses' terminal illness and in bereavement. J Adv Nurs. 1998;28:829–839.

44. Grassi L. Bereavement in families with relatives dying of cancer. Curr Opin Support Palliat Care. 2007;1(1):43–49.

45. Worthington RC. Models of linear and cyclical grief: different approaches to different experiences. Clin Pediatr. 1994;33(5):297–300.

46. Neimeyer RA. Meaning reconstruction and the experience of chronic loss. In: Doka KJ, Davidson J (eds.), Living with Grief: When Illness Is Prolonged. Philadelphia: Taylor and Francis; 1997:159–176.

47. Tomarken A, Holland J, Schachter S, et al. Factors of complicated grief pre-death in caregivers of cancer patients. Psycho-Oncol. 2008;17:105–111.

48. Horowitz MJ, Siegel B, Holen A, Bonanno GA, Milbrath C, Stinson CH. Diagnostoc criteria for complicated grief disorder. Am J Psychiatry. 1997;154:904–910.

49. Prigerson HG, Maciejewski PK, Reynolds CF III, et al. Inventory of complicated grief: a scale to measure maladaptive symptoms of loss. Psychiatry Res. 1995;59:65–79.

50. Boelen PA, van den Bout J. Complicated grief and uncomplicated grief are distinguishable constructs. Psychiatry Res. 2008;157:311–314.

51. Stroebe M, Boelen PA, van den Hout M, Stroebe W, Salemink E, van den Bout J. Ruminative coping as avoidance: a reinterpretation of its function in adjustment to bereavement. Eur Arch Psychiatry Clin Neurosci. 2007;257:462–472.

52. Ott CH. The impact of complicated grief on mental and physical health at various points in the bereavement process. Death Stud. 2003;27:249–272.

53. Loke AY, Li Q, Man LS. Preparing family members for the death of their loved one with cancer. J Hosp Palliat Nurs. 2013;15:E1–E11.

54. Shear K, Monk T, Houck P, et al. An attachment-based model of complicated grief including the role of avoidance. Eur Arch Psychiatry Clin Neurosci. 2007;257:453–461.

55. Cruz M, Scott J, Houck P, Reynolds CF, Frank E, Shear MK. Clinical presentation and treatment outcome of African Americans with complicated grief. Psychiatr Serv. 2007;58:700–702.

56. Boelen PA, van den Bout J. Examination of proposed criteria for complicated grief in people confronted with violent or nonviolent loss. Death Stud. 2007;31:155–164.

57. Shear MK, Simon N, Wall M, et al. Complicated grief and related bereavement issues for DSM-5. Depress Anxiety. 2011;28:103–117.

58. Boelen PA, de Keijser J, van den Hout M, van den Bout J. Treatment of complicated grief: a comparison between cognitive-behavioral therapy and supportive counseling. J Counsel Clin Psychol. 2007;75:277–284.

59. Wagner B, Maercker A. A 1.5-year follow-up of an Internet based intervention for complicated grief. J Trauma Stress. 2007;20:625–629.

60. Doka K. Disenfranchised grief in historical and cultural perspective. In: Stroebe M, Hansson RO, Schenk H, Stroebe W, van den Blink E (eds.), Handbook of Bereavement Research and Practice: Advances in Theory and Intervention. Washington, DC: American Psychological Association; 2008:223–240.

61. Corless IB. Modulated mourning: The grief and mourning of those infected and affected by HIV/AIDS. In: Doka KJ, Davidson J (eds.), Living with Grief: When Illness Is Prolonged. Philadelphia: Taylor and Francis; 1997:108–118.

62. Boswell C. A phenomenological study of the experience of grief resulting from spousal bereavement in heterosexual and homosexual men and women. A dissertation presented to the Faculty of the College of Education University of Houston. 2007.

63. Gataric G, Kinsel B, Currie BG, Lawhorne LW. Reflections on the under-researched topic of grief in persons with dementia: a report from a symposium on grief and dementia. Am J Hosp Palliat Care. 2010;27:567–574. doi:10.1177/1049909110371315.

64. McEvoy J, MacHale R, Tierney E. Concept of death and perceptions of bereavement in adults with intellectual disabilities. J Intellect Disabil Res. 2012; 56;191–203.

65. Rando TA. Grief, Dying and Death: Clinical Interventions for Caregivers. Champaign, IL: Research Press Company, 1984.

66. Eakes GG, Burke ML, Hainsworth MA. Chronic sorrow: the experiences of bereaved individuals. Illness Crisis Loss. 1999;7:172–182.

67. Eakes GG, Burke ML, Hainsworth MA. Theory of chronic sorrow. In: Masters K. (ed.), Nursing Theories: A Framework for Professional Practice. Sudbury, MA: Jones and Bartlett Learning, 2010:349–361.

68. HardyBougere M. Cultural manifestations of grief and bereavement: a clinical perspective. J Cult Divers. 2008;15:66–69.

69. American Psychiatric Association. Diagnostic and Statistical Manual of Mental Disorders. 5th ed. Arlington, VA: American Psychiatric Publishing: 2013.

70. Attig T, Corless IB, Gilbert, KR, Larson DG, McKissock M, Roth D, Schuurman D, et al. When does a broken heart become a mental disorder? The Dougy Center The National Center for Grieving Children and Families. http://www.dougy.org.

71. Balk DE, Noppe I, Sandler I, Werth J. Bereavement and depression: possible changes to the diagnostic and statistical manual of mental disorders: a report from the scientific advisory committee of the Association for Death Education and Counseling. Omega. 2011:63:199–220.

72. Wakefield JC. Should prolonged grief be reclassified as a mental disorder in DSM-5?: Reconsidering the empirical and conceptual arguments for complicated grief disorder. J Nerv Ment Dis. 2012:200:499–511. doi:10.1097/nmd.06013e3182482155.

73. Kowalski SD, Bondmass MD. Physiological and psychological symptoms of grief in widows. Res Nurs Health. 2008;31:23–30.

74. Love AW. Progress in understanding grief, complicated grief, and caring for the bereaved. Contemp Nurse. 2007;27:73–83.

75. O'Gorman SM. Death and dying in contemporary society: an evaluation of current attitudes and the rituals associated with death and dying and their relevance to recent understandings of health and healing. J Adv Nurs. 1998;2:1127–1135.

76. Fulton R. The funeral in contemporary society. In Fulton R, Bendiksen R (eds.), Death and Identity. 3rd ed. Philadelphia: Charles Press; 1994:288–312.

77. Stroebe W, Stroebe MS. Is grief universal?: Cultural variations in the emotional reaction to loss. In Fulton R, Bendiksen R (eds.), Death and Identity. 3rd ed. Philadelphia: Charles Press; 1994:177–207.

78. Byatt AS. Possession: A Romance. New York: Vintage Books, 1990:6.

79. Mitchell LM, Stephenson PH, Cadell S, Macdonald, ME. Death and grief on-line: virtual memorialization and changing concepts of childhood death and parental bereavement on the Internet. Health Soc Rev. 2012; 21(4):413–431.

80. Diamond H, Llewelyn S, Relf M, Bruce C. Helpful aspects of bereavement support for adults following an expected death: volunteers' and bereaved people's perspectives. Death Stud. 2012;36:541–564.

81. MacConnell G, Aston M, Randel P, Zwaagstra N. Nurses' experiences providing bereavement follow-up: an exploratory study using feminist poststructuralism. J Clin Nurs. 2012; 22:1094–1102. doi: 10.1111/j.1 365-2702.2012.04272.x.

82. LeBrocq P, Charles A, Chan T, Buchanan M. Establishing a bereavement program: caring for bereaved families and staff in the emergency department. Accid Emerg Nurs. 2003;11:85–90.

83. Brosche TA. A grief team within a healthcare system. Dimens Crit Care Nurs. 2007;26:21–28.

84. Keene EA, Hutton N, Hall B, Ruchton C. Bereavement debriefing sessions: an intervention to support health care professionals in managing their grief after the death of a patient. Pediatr Nurs. 2010; 36:185–189.

85. Azhar MZ, Varma SL. Religious psychotherapy as management of bereavement. Acta Psychiatr Scand. 1995;91:233–235.

86. Goodkin K, Blaney NT, Feaster DJ, Baldewicz T, Burkhalter JE, Leeds B. A randomized controlled clinical trial of a bereavement support group intervention in human immunodeficiency virus type 1-seropositive and -seronegative homosexual men. Arch Gen Psychiatry. 1999;56:52–59.

87. Sikkema KJ, Hansen NB, Kochman A, Tate DC, Difranceisco W. Outcomes from a randomized controlled trial of a group intervention for HIV positive men and women coping with AIDS-related loss and bereavement. Death Stud. 2004;28:187–209.

88. Leaver CA, Perreault Y, Demetrakopoulos A; AIDs Bereavement Project of Ontarios' Survive and Thrive Working Group. Understanding AIDS-related bereavement and multiple loss among long-term survivors of HIV in Ontario. Can J Hum Sex. 2008:17:37–52.

89. Lev EL, McCorkle R. Loss, grief and bereavement in family members of cancer patients. Semin Oncol Nurs. 1998;4:145–151.

90. Cloyes KG, Berry PH, Reblin M, Clayton M, Ellington L. Exploring communication patterns among hospice nurses and family caregivers. J Hosp Palliat Nurs. 2012;14:426–437. doi:10.1097/ NJH.06013e318251598b.

91. Arnold J. Rethinking: nursing implications for health promotion. Home Healthc Nurse. 1996;14:779–780.

92. Cutcliffe JR. Hope, counselling, and complicated bereavement reactions. J Adv Nurs. 1998;28:760.

93. Stephenson C. The concept of hope revisited for nursing. J Adv Nurs. 1991;16:1456–1461.

94. Frankl V. Man's Search for Meaning: An Introduction to Logotherapy. New York: Simon and Schuster, 1959.

95. Rack JJ, Burleson BR, Bodie GD, Holmstrom AJ, Servaty-Seib H. Bereaved adults' evaluations of grief management messages: effects of message person centeredness, recipient individual differences, and contextual factors. Death Stud. 2008;32:399–427.

96. Pressman DL, Bonanno GA. With whom do we grieve?: Social and cultural determinants of grief processing in the United States and China. J Soc Pers Relat. 2007;24:729–746.

97. O'Callaghan CC, McDermott F, Hudson P, Zalcberg JR. Sound continuous bonds with the deceased: the relevance of music including preloss music therapy, for eight bereaved caregivers. Death Studies. 2013;37(2):101–125. doi: 10.1080/07481187.2011.617488.

98. Quinton A. Permission to mourn. Nurs Times. 1994;90:31–32.

99. Corless IB. And when famous people die. In: Corless IB, Germino BA, Pittman MA (eds.), A Challenge for Living: Dying, Death, and Bereavement. Boston: Jones & Bartlett; 1995:398.

100. [Commentary by newscaster on Turkish earthquake.] ABC News, 1999.

CHAPTER 30

Supporting families in palliative care

Rose Steele and Betty Davies

We try to spend as much time together as possible, but that's not realistic either, because there are times when I want to get out and play squash or racquetball with my friends, or get out into the yard. So I'm torn ... I want to be upstairs with her, but I realize I have a need too, that I can't be there all the time. It's the same for my boys—they have their lives too. And for her too—she wants us with her and she wants to be alone. It's a real tug of war, adjusting all the time to things slipping away.

Husband of a 64-year-old woman with cancer

Key points

♦ Family-centered care is a basic tenet of palliative care philosophy, which recognizes that terminally ill patients exist within the family system. The patient's illness affects the whole family, and, in turn, the family's responses affect the patient. Supporting families in palliative care means that nurses must plan their care with an understanding not only of the individual patient's needs but also of the family system within which the patient functions.

♦ Therapeutic nurse-patient and nurse-family relationships are central to family-centered palliative care.

♦ Families with a member who requires palliative care are in transition. Families have described this as a "transition of fading away," characterized by seven dimensions that help nurses to understand families' experiences and to support them.

♦ Level of family functioning also plays a role in family experience, and serves to guide nursing interventions for families with varying levels of functioning.

Family-centered palliative care

Recognizing the importance of a family focus necessitates clearly defining what is meant by "family." Most often, families in palliative care do consist of patients, their spouses, and their children. But in today's world of divorce and remarriage,[1] step-relatives must also enter into the family portrait. In other instances, people unrelated by blood or marriage may function as family.[2] Therefore, the definition of family must be expanded. The family is a group of individuals inextricably linked in ways that are constantly interactive and mutually reinforcing. Family can mean direct blood relatives, relationships through an emotional commitment, or the group or person with which an individual feels most connected.[3] Moreover, family in its fullest sense embraces all generations—past, present, future; those living, those dead, and those yet to be born. Shadows of the past and dreams of the future also contribute to the understanding of families.

Palliative care programs are based on the principle that the family is the unit of care. In practice, however, the family is often viewed as a group of individuals who can either prove helpful or resist efforts to deliver care. Nurses and other health professionals must strive to understand the meaning of the palliative experience to the family.[4] The best outcomes may be achieved if appropriate interventions are also directed at the family members both individually and as a group.[5] If quality care is to be provided, nurses need to understand how all family members perceive their experience, how the relationships fit together, and that a multitude of factors combine to make families what they are. In the past 5–10 years research has gone beyond focusing on the needs of dying patients for comfort and palliation, to addressing issues relevant to other family members. Much of this research has focused on the family's perceptions of their needs[6–9]; experiences and challenges faced[6–12]; adaptation and coping skills required for home care[6,11,13–16]; the supportiveness of nursing behaviors[17] or physician behaviors;[18] and satisfaction with care.[19] Though research used to focus primarily on families of patients with cancer, the current trend in palliative care extends the focus to other life-threatening illnesses. Reports for other diagnostic populations, such as Parkinson's disease,[20] cardiac disease,[21] motor neurone disease,[22] dementia,[23] and neurodegenerative diseases,[7] as well as simply advanced age[24] are becoming more available. Regardless of disease condition, findings make it clear that family members look to health professionals to provide quality care to the patient. Family members also expect health professionals to meet their own needs for information, emotional support, and assistance with care.[18] But recent research suggests that the most effective way to support family caregivers may be to help them be successful in their caregiving role rather than to focus on personal needs.[12]

Much of the research that purports to address the impact of cancer on the family is based on the perceptions of individuals—either the patient or adult family members (usually the spouse). As well, many of the studies were conducted retrospectively, that is, after the patient's death. But even studies conducted during the palliative period frequently exclude the patient—the one who is at the center of the palliative care situation. Examining the palliative experience of the family unit has been very limited.

As a basis for offering optimal support to families in palliative care, this chapter focuses on describing the findings of a research program that prospectively examined the experiences of such families.[25] The research evolved from nurses' concerns about how to provide family-centered palliative care. Nurses in a regional cancer center constantly had to attend to the needs of not only patients but also patients' families, particularly as they moved back and forth between hospital and home. In searching the literature for guidelines about family-centered care, they found that many articles were about the needs of patients and family members, about levels of family members' satisfaction with care, and about family members' perceptions of nurses, but nothing really described the families' experiences as they coped with the terminal illness of a beloved family member. Research involving families included patients with advanced cancer, their spouses, and at least one of their adult children (>18 years of age). Since the completion of the original research, families with AIDS, Alzheimer's disease, and cardiac disease have provided anecdotal validation of the findings for their experiences. In addition, families of children with progressive, life-threatening illness have provided similar validation. Therefore, it seems that the conceptualization has relevance for a wide range of families in palliative care. The findings from this research program form the basis for the description that follows; references to additional research studies are also included to supplement and emphasize the ongoing development of knowledge in the field of family-centered end-of-life care.

The transition of fading away

The common view is that transitions are initiated by changes, by the start of something new. However, as Bridges[26] suggested, most transitions actually begin with endings. This is true for families living with serious illness in a loved one. The nurses' research findings generated a theoretical scheme that conceptualized families' experiences as a transition—a transition that families themselves labeled as "fading away." The transition of fading away for families facing terminal illness began with the ending of life as they knew it. They came to realize that the ill family member was no longer living with cancer but was now dying from cancer.

Despite the fact that family members had been told about the seriousness of the prognosis, often since the time of diagnosis, and had experienced the usual ups and downs associated with the illness trajectory, for many the "gut" realization that the patient's death was inevitable occurred suddenly: "It struck me hard—it hit me like a bolt. Dad is not going to get better!" The awareness was triggered when family members saw, with "new eyes," a change in the patient's body or physical capacity, such as the patient's weight loss, extreme weakness, lack of mobility, or diminished mental capacity. Realizing that the patient would not recover, family members began the transition of fading away. As one patient

commented, "My body has shrunk so much—the other day, I tried on my favorite old blue dress and I could see then how much weight I have lost. I feel like a skeleton with skin! I am getting weaker. . . . I just can't eat much now, I don't want to. I can see that I am fading. . . . I am definitely fading away."

The transition of fading away is characterized by seven dimensions: redefining, burdening, struggling with paradox, contending with change, searching for meaning, living day by day, and preparing for death. The dimensions do not occur in linear fashion; rather, they are interrelated and inextricably linked to one another. Redefining, however, plays a central role. All family members experience these dimensions, although patients, spouses, and children experience each dimension somewhat differently.

Redefining

Redefining involves a shift from "what used to be" to "what is now." It demands adjustment in how individuals see themselves and each other. Patients maintained their usual patterns for as long as possible, and then began to implement feasible alternatives once they realized that their capacities were seriously changing. Joe, a truck driver, altered his identity over time: "I just can't do what I used to. I finally had to accept the fact that the seizures made it unsafe for me to drive." Joe requested to help out at his company's distribution desk. When he could no longer concentrate on keeping the orders straight, Joe offered to assist with supervising the light loading. One day, Joe was acutely aware he didn't have the energy to even sit and watch the others: "I couldn't do it anymore," Joe sighed. "I had reached the end of my work life and the beginning of the end of my life." Another patient, Cora, lamented that she used to drive to her son's home to babysit her toddler-aged grandchildren; then her son dropped the children off at her house to conserve the energy it took for her to travel; and now, her son has made other child care arrangements. He brings the children for only short visits because of her extreme fatigue.

Both Joe and Cora, like the other patients, accepted their limitations with much sadness and a sense of great loss. Their focus narrowed, and they began to pay attention to details of everyday life that they had previously ignored or overlooked. Joe commented, "When I first was at home, I wanted to keep in touch with the guys at the depot; I wanted to know what was going on. Now, I get a lot of good just watching the grandkids out there playing in the yard."

Patients were eager to reinforce that they were still the same on the inside, although they acknowledged the drastic changes in their physical appearance. They often became more spiritual in their orientation to life and nature. As Joe said, "I always liked being outside—was never much of an office-type person. But, now, it seems I like it even more. That part of me hasn't changed even though it's hard for some of the fellas (at work) to recognize me now." When patients were able to redefine themselves as Joe did, they made the best of their situation, differentiating what parts of them were still intact. Joe continued, "Yeah, I like just being outside, or watching the kids. And, you know, they still come to their Grandpa when their toy trucks break down—I can pretty much always fix 'em." Similarly, Cora commented: "At least, I can still make cookies for when my family comes, although I don't make them from scratch anymore." Patients shared their changing perceptions with family members and others, who then were able to offer understanding and support.

Patients who were unable to redefine themselves in this way attempted to maintain their regular patterns despite the obvious changes in their capacity to do so. They ended up frustrated, angry, and feeling worthless. These reactions distanced them from others, resulting in the patients feeling alone and, sometimes, abandoned. Ralph, for example, was an educational administrator. Despite his deteriorating health, he insisted that he was managing without difficulty. "Nothing's wrong with me, really. ... We are being accredited this year. There's a lot to do to get ready for that." Ralph insisted on going into the office each day to prepare the necessary reports. His increasing confusion and inability to concentrate made his reports inaccurate and inadequate, but Ralph refused to acknowledge his limitations or delegate the work. Instead, his colleagues had to work overtime to correct Ralph's work after he left the office. According to Ralph's wife, anger and frustration were commonplace among his colleagues, but they were reluctant to discuss the issue with Ralph. Instead, they avoided conversations with Ralph, and he complained to his wife about his colleagues' lack of interest in the project.

For the most part, spouses took the patient's physical changes in stride. They attributed the changes to the disease, not to the patient personally, and as a result, they were able to empathize with the patient. Patients' redefining focused on themselves, the changes in their physical status and intrapersonal aspects; spouses' redefining centered on their relationship with the patient. Spouses did their best to "continue on as normal," primarily for the sake of the patient. In doing so, they considered alternatives and reorganized their priorities.

Wittenberg and colleagues[4] described the "reciprocity of suffering" that family members experience, which results from the physical and emotional distress that is rooted in their anguish of dealing with the impending death of the loved one, and in their attempt to fill new roles as caregivers. The degree to which family members experienced this phenomenon varied according to patients' redefining. When patients were able to redefine themselves, spouses had an easier time. Such patients accepted spouses' offers of support; patients and spouses were able to talk about the changes that were occurring. Spouses felt satisfied in the care that they provided. But when patients were less able to redefine, then spouses' offers of support were rejected or unappreciated. For example, Ralph's wife worried about his work pattern and its impact on his colleagues. She encouraged him to cut back, but Ralph only ignored her pleas and implied that she didn't understand how important this accreditation was to the future of his school. Even when Ralph was no longer able to go to the office, he continued to work from home, frequently phoning his colleagues to supervise their progress on the report. His wife lamented, "For an educated man, he doesn't know much. I guess it's too late to teach an old dog new tricks."

In such situations, spouses avoided talking about or doing anything that reminded the patient of the changes he or she was experiencing but not acknowledging. The relationship between the spouse and patient suffered. Rather than feeling satisfied with their care, spouses were frustrated and angry, although often they remained silent and simply "endured" the situation. The ill person contributed significantly to the caregiver's ability to cope. Indeed, the ill person was not simply a passive recipient of care but had an impact on the experience of the caregiving spouse. Similarly, in their study of factors that influence family caregiving, Stajduhar and colleagues[27] found that the ill person contributed significantly to the capacity of the spouse to continue to provide care despite their experience of overwhelming emotional and physical strain. Caregivers drew strength from the dying person when the ill person accepted the impending death, had an understanding of the caregivers' needs, and had attitudes, values, and beliefs that sustained their caregivers.

Adult children also redefined the ill family member; they redefined their ill parent from someone who was strong and competent to someone who was increasingly frail. Children felt vulnerable in ways they had not previously experienced. Most often, children perceived that the changes in their ill parent were the result of disease and not intentional: "It's not my father doing this consciously." Younger adult children were particularly sensitive to keeping the situation private, claiming they wanted to protect the dignity of the patient, but seemed to want to protect their own sense of propriety. For example, one young woman in her early twenties was "devastated" when her father's urinary bag dragged behind him as he left the living room where she and her friends were visiting. It was difficult for some young adults to accept such manifestations of their parent's illness. Adolescents in particular had a difficult time redefining the situation. They preferred to continue on as if nothing was wrong and to shield themselves against any information that would force them to see the situation realistically.

When the ill parent was able to redefine to a greater degree, then children were better able to appreciate that death is part of life. They recognized their own susceptibility and vowed to take better care of their own health; older children with families of their own committed to spending more quality time with their children. Joe talked, although indirectly, with his son about the situation: "I won't be here forever to fix the kids' toys." Together, Joe and his son reminisced about how Joe had always been available to his son and grandchildren as "Mr. Fix-it." Joe's son valued his dad's active participation in his life and promised to be the same kind of father to his own sons. In contrast, when the ill parent was unable to redefine, then children tended to ignore the present. They attempted to recreate the past to construct happy memories they never had. In doing so, they often neglected their own families. Ralph's daughter described her dad as a "workaholic." Feeling as if she had never had enough time with her dad, she began visiting her parents daily, with suggestions of places she could take him. He only became annoyed with her unfamiliar, constant presence: "It's okay she comes over every day, but enough is enough."

The extent to which spouses and adult children commented on the important contribution made by the dying family member is a provocative finding that underscores the importance of relationships among and between family members in facilitating their coping with the situation of terminal illness.

Burdening

Feeling as if they are a burden for their family is common among patients.[28] If patients see themselves as purposeless, dependent, and immobile, they have a greater sense of burdening their loved ones. The more realistically patients redefined themselves as their capacities diminished, the more accurate they were in their perceptions of burdening. They acknowledged other family members' efforts, appreciated those efforts, and encouraged family members to rest and take time to care for themselves. Patients who were less able to redefine themselves did not see that they were burdening other family members in any way. They denied or minimized the strain on others. As Ralph said during the last week of his life, "I can't do much, but I am fine really. Not much has changed. It's a burden on my wife, but not much. It might be some extra work.... She was a nursing aide, so she is used to this kind of work."

Most spouses acknowledged the "extra load" of caring for their dying partner, but indicated that they did not regard the situation as a "burden." They agreed that it's "just something you do for the one you love." Spouses did not focus on their own difficulties; they managed to put aside their own distress so that it would not have a negative impact on their loved one. They sometimes shared stories of loneliness and helplessness, but also stories of deepening respect and love for their partner. Again, spouses of patients who were able to redefine were energized by the patient's acknowledgment of their efforts and were inspired to continue on. Spouses of patients who were not able to redefine felt unappreciated, exhausted, and confessed to "waiting for the patient to die."

The literature provides a comprehensive description of the multidimensional nature of the burden experienced by family caregivers, but little attention has been given to the burdening felt by patients or adult children specifically. Caregiver burden, usually by spouses, has been described in terms of physical burden, which includes fatigue and physical exhaustion, sleeplessness, and deterioration of health.[4,10–16] Social burden encompasses limited time for self and social stress related to isolation.[10–14] Regardless of the type of burden, however, most caregivers, including the ones in the fading away studies, expressed much satisfaction with their caregiving.[4,14] Despite feeling burdened, most caregivers would repeat the experience: "Yes, it was difficult and exhausting, and there were days I didn't think I could manage one more minute. But, if I had to do it over again, I would. I have no regrets for what I am doing."

Children, too, experienced burdening, but the source stemmed from the extra responsibilities involved in helping to care for a dying parent, superimposed on their work responsibilities, career development, and their own families. As a result, adult children of all ages felt a mixture of satisfaction and exhaustion. Their sense of burdening was also influenced by the ill parent's redefining—if the ill parent acknowledged their efforts, they were more likely to feel satisfaction. However, children's sense of burdening was also influenced by the state of health of the well parent. If that parent also was ill or debilitated, the burden on children was compounded. If children were able to prioritize their responsibilities so that they could pay attention to their own needs as well as helping both their parents, they felt less burdened. Children seemed less likely than their well parents to perceive caregiving as something they themselves would do. Of course, they did not have the life experience of a long-term relationship that motivated the spouses to care for their partners.

Finding effective ways to support family caregivers is critical, because an increase in the proportion of elderly people in the population means growing numbers of people with chronic, life-threatening, or serious illness require care. The responsibility for the care of such individuals is increasingly being placed on families. Respite care is often suggested as a strategy for relieving burden in family caregivers.[6,20] Respite and other resources or services should be offered to families, but each family must decide what will actually be helpful for them. For some families, inpatient respite services during the last year of life may help relieve their burden, while other caregivers may experience feelings of guilt and increased stress because of worrying about the quality of care provided.[29] Caregivers may be supported in their role simply by knowing there are other resources and support readily available, even if they do not make use of them.[6]

Another potential factor influencing the success of respite care may be the dynamics within the family, in particular between the patient and family caregivers. Respite must be assessed in conjunction with the role of redefining in burdening. Support for this suggestion comes from a study of the experiences of caregivers,[27] which showed that support from informal and professional caregivers was not sufficient to balance the stresses of caregiving and the missing element may be internal to the family. These findings encourage greater exploration into respite care and its meaning to caregivers. Family members may value cognitive breaks during which they can remain within the caregiving environment, but physical separation from the caregiving environment may be valuable only if it contributes in some meaningful way to the caregiving.

Struggling with paradox

Struggling with paradox stems from the fact that the patient is both living and dying. For patients, the struggle focuses on wanting to believe they will survive and knowing that they will not. On "good days," patients felt optimistic about the outcome; on other days, they succumbed to the inevitability of their approaching demise. Often, patients did not want to "give up" but at the same time were "tired of fighting." They wanted to "continue on" for the sake of their families but also wanted "it to end soon" so their families could "get on with their lives." Patients coped by hoping for miracles, fighting for the sake of their families, and focusing on the good days. As Joe said, "I like to think about the times when things are pretty good. I enjoy those days. But, on the bad days, when I'm tired, or when the pain gets the best of me, then I just wonder if it wouldn't be best to just quit. But you never know— maybe I'll be the one in a million who makes it at the last minute." He then added wryly, "Hmmm, big chance of that."

Spouses struggled with a paradox of their own: they wanted to care for and spend time with the patient, and they also wanted a "normal" life. They coped by juggling their time as best they could, and usually put their own life on hold. Spouses who tended to their own needs usually were less exhausted and reported fewer health problems than spouses who neglected their own needs. For years, Joe and his wife had been square dancers. They hadn't been dancing together for many months when his wife resumed going to "dance night as a sub" or to prepare the evening's refreshments. "Sometimes, I feel guilty for going and leaving Joe at home, but I know I need a break. When I did miss dance night, I could see I was getting really bitchy—I need to get out for a breather so I don't suffocate Joe."

Children struggled with hanging on and letting go to a greater extent than their parents. They wanted to spend time with their ill parent and also to "get on with their own lives." Feeling the pressure of dual loyalties (to their parents and to their own young families), the demands of both compounded the struggle that children faced.

Contending with change

Those facing terminal illness in a family member experience changes in every realm of daily life—relationships, roles, socialization, and work patterns. The focus of the changes differed among family members. Patients faced changes in their relationships with everyone they knew. They realized that the greatest change of their life was underway, and that life as they knew it would soon be gone. They tended to break down tasks into manageable pieces, and increasingly they focused inward. The greatest change that spouses faced was in their relationship with the patient. They coped by attempting to keep everything as normal as possible. Children contended with changes that were more all-encompassing. They could not withdraw as their ill parent did, nor could they prioritize their lives to the degree that their well parent could. They easily become exhausted. As Joe's son explained, "It's a real challenge coming by this often—I try to come twice a week and then bring the kids on the weekends. But I just got a promotion at work this year, so that's extra work too. Seems like I don't see my wife much—but she's a real trooper. Her dad died last year so she knows what it's like."

Searching for meaning

Searching for meaning has to do with seeking answers to help in understanding the situation.[30] Patients tended to journey inward, reflect on spiritual aspects, deepen their most important connections, and become closer to nature: "The spiritual thing has always been at the back of my mind, but it's developing more. ... When you're sick like that, your attitude changes toward life. You come not to be afraid of death."

Spouses concentrated on their relationship with the patient. Some searched for meaning through personal growth, whereas others searched for meaning by simply tolerating the situation. Some focused on spiritual growth, and others adhered rigidly to their religion with little, if any, sense of inner growth or insight. Joe's wife commented, "Joe and I are closer than ever now. We don't like this business, but we have learned to love each other even more than when we were younger—sickness is a hard lesson that way." In contrast, Ralph's wife said with resignation, "He's so stubborn—always has been. I sometimes wonder why I stayed. But, here I am." Spouses and patients may attribute different meanings to other aspects of their experience as well. For example, when seeing their loved one in pain, many spouses felt helpless and fearful. Once the pain was controlled, they felt peaceful and relaxed and interpreted this as an indication that the couple would return to their old routines. The meaning attributed to the patient's experience also influences spousal bereavement. For example, spouses who witnessed distressing sights and sounds as the patient was dying experienced posttraumatic stress and much distress after the death.[31]

Children tended to reflect on and reevaluate all aspects of their lives: "It puts in perspective how important some of our goals are. ... Having financial independence and being able to retire at a decent age. ... Those things are important, but not at the expense of sacrificing today."

Living day to day

Not all families reached the point of living day to day. If patients were able to find some meaning in their experience, then they were better able to adopt an attitude of living each day. Their attitude was characterized by "making the most of it." As one patient described it, "There's not much point in going over things in the past; not much point in projecting yourself too far into the future either. It's the current time that counts." Patients who were unable to find much meaning in their experience, or who didn't search for meaning, focused more on "getting through it." As Ralph said with determination, "Sure, I am getting weaker. I know I am sick. ... But I will get through this!"

Spouses who searched for meaning focused on "making the best of it" while making every effort to enjoy the time they had left with their partner. Other spouses simply endured the situation without paying much attention to philosophizing about the experience. Children often had difficulty concentrating on living day to day, because they were unable to defer their obligations and therefore were constantly worrying about what else needed to be done. However, some children were still able to convey an attitude of "Live for today, today—worry about tomorrow, tomorrow."

Preparing for death

Preparing for death involved concrete actions that would have benefit in the future, after the patient died. Patients had their family's needs uppermost in their minds and worked hard to teach or guide family members with regard to various tasks and activities that the patient would no longer be around to do. Patients were committed to leaving legacies for their loved ones, not only as a means of being remembered but also as a way of comforting loved ones in their grief. Joe spent time "jotting down a few Mr. Fix-it pointers" for his wife and son. Ralph's energy was consumed by focusing on the work he still had to do, so he was unable to consider what he might do for his wife and daughter.

Spouses concentrated on meeting the patient's wishes. Whatever the patient wanted, spouses would try to do. They attended to practical details and anticipated their future in practical ways. Children offered considerable help to their parents with legal and financial matters. They also prepared their own children for what was to come. A central aspect was reassuring the dying parent that they would take care of the surviving parent. Children also prepared for the death by envisioning their future without their parent: "I think about it sometimes ... about how my children will never have a grandfather. It makes me so sad. That's why the photos we have been taking are so important to me. ... They will show our children who their grandfather was."

Palliative care for diagnoses other than cancer

Traditionally, palliative care practice and discussions have focused on families of cancer patients. At the same time, care of the patient with cardiac disease, for example, has traditionally focused on restoring health and enabling a return to normal life. So, the idea of providing a patient with aggressive versus palliative treatment has, until recently, not been a well-discussed issue in the treatment of the patient with heart disease. For most patients with heart disease, and particularly for those with heart failure, the decline in functional status is slower than for patients diagnosed with cancer.[21] However, if palliative care is considered only after disease-related care fails or becomes too burdensome, the opportunity for patients to achieve symptom relief, and for patients and family members to engage in the process of fading away, may be lost. Consequently, following a model of care wherein issues of treatment and end-of-life care are discussed early and throughout the illness trajectory facilitates patient and family coping, and enables nurses to optimally support families.

Varying disease trajectories for other conditions,[32,33] such as dementia, also influence the nature of support that nurses provide patients and families. For example, the support needed by families of dementia patients often occurs within a context where the life-limiting nature of the condition is not initially recognized by families. In dementia care, there may be significantly more need to form support groups for families, offer respite care, educate families, and try to relieve families' feeling of guilt.[34]

Family involvement according to location of care

Over the past century, nursing homes and hospitals increasingly have become the site of death. A landmark national study evaluated the US dying experience at home and in institutional settings.[35] Family members of 1578 deceased individuals were asked via telephone survey about the patient's experience at the last place of care at which the patient spent >48 hours. Results showed that two-thirds (67.2%) of patients were last cared for in an institution; little has changed in the intervening years. Family members reported greater satisfaction with patient's symptom management, and with emotional support for both the patient and family, if they received care at home with hospice services. Families have greater opportunities for involvement in the care if home care is possible. Family involvement in hospital care also makes for better outcomes.[36] Nurses, therefore, must consider how best to include families in the care of their dying loved ones, regardless of the location of care.

Large variations exist in the provision of home-based palliative and terminal care across the United States, although the development of hospice home services has enabled increasing numbers of seriously ill patients to experience care at home. However, dying at home can present special challenges for family members.[37] Lack of support and lack of confidence have been found to be determinants contributing to hospital admissions and the breakdown of informal caregiving for people with a life-threatening illness. A lack of support from the healthcare system is given as the reason many caregivers have to admit their loved one to the hospital.[12] They also report that fragmentation of services and lack of forward planning jeopardizes the success of home care.[12]

Moreover, the decision for home care has a profound effect on family members.[15,16] Many caregivers believe that providing home care for their loved one is the only option.[12] Some make uninformed decisions, giving little consideration to the implications of their decision. Such decisions are often made early in the patient's disease trajectory or when the patient was imminently dying, and may be influenced by the unrealistic portrayal in the media about dying at home. The patient's needs and wishes often drive decisions, with caregivers paying little attention to their own needs.[12] Negotiated decisions for home care typically occur if caregivers and patients are able to talk openly about dying, and have done so throughout the disease trajectory. For some families, a home death can bring additional burdens, worries, and responsibilities,[37] so it is important that open discussion be facilitated.

Family members' decisions are often influenced by three major factors: making promises to care for the loved one at home, the desire to maintain as much as possible a "normal" life for the patient and themselves, and negative experiences with institutional care. Of interest, family members tend not to think of themselves as the target of professional interventions. They may be reluctant to ask for help or to let their needs be known. Consequently, when working with caregiving families, healthcare providers can mediate discussions with the aim of coming to a mutually acceptable decision about home care. Such discussions could facilitate the sharing of perspectives, to allow for decisions that would work well for all concerned. Ideally, such discussions should begin early in the disease trajectory. Importantly, ongoing attention should be paid to improving hospital end-of-life care so that families feel they have a meaningful alternative to home care.

Clinicians must recognize the emotional impact of providing palliative care at home, and must be sensitive to the sometimes overwhelming task that caregiving imposes on family caregivers. Care must be provided within the team context that is the standard of care in palliative care[38] so that families can benefit from a whole set of services needed to support death at home; availability and access to the professional is important. Further, clinicians must work with the dying patients, with family caregivers, and with each other as equal partners in the caregiving process.

Clinicians must be available to families, offering anticipatory guidance and support throughout the caregiving experience. Healthcare professionals must assist family members as they traverse the maze of treatment and care decisions, ranging from whether to give particular "as needed" medications, or what food to make for the patient to eat, to whether or not to seek hospice care, to sign "do-not-resuscitate" documents, or to terminate treatment. It is critical that palliative care professionals continually engage with caregivers in forward planning, interpretation, and monitoring of the inevitable decline and dying process of the ill person, so as to facilitate the feeling in caregivers that they are secure and supported in their physically and emotionally exhausting work. Families need to know whom to call and when, and how to reach them.

Some simple guidelines for families can serve to encourage their coping. For example, caregivers should be told to keep a small notebook handy for jotting down questions and answers. The pages may be divided in half lengthwise, using the column on the left for questions and the other column for answers. Or, the left-sided page may be used for questions and the opposite page for the answers. They should be advised to have the notebook with them whenever they talk with a member of the palliative care team. Family members should be reassured that nothing is trivial. All questions are important, and all observations are valuable. They should be encouraged to say when they do not understand something, and to ask for information to be repeated as necessary. Palliative care professionals can help by spelling words that family members do not understand or by jotting down explanations. They should reassure family members that asking for help is not a sign of failure, but rather a sign of good common sense. Following such simple guidelines helps keep families from feeling overwhelmed. And, if they do feel "out of control," such guidelines, simple as they may seem, give family members some concrete action they can take to help with whatever the situation may be.

Clinicians must also remember that their own attitudes are critical; if families feel they are a "nuisance" to healthcare providers, they tend to be more anxious and to shy away from asking for help. Furthermore, clinicians are in ideal positions to advocate with politicians and policy makers to expand resources for home-based palliative care programs so that families can adequately and humanely be supported in their caregiving work.

Caregiving at a distance

About 89% of all informal caregivers are related to the care recipient,[39] but not all caregiving is provided by family members who live with, or are geographically close to, the patient. Distant caregiving, the provision of instrumental and/or emotional support to an ill loved one who lives a long distance from the caregiver, is prevalent in today's changing society. Adult children often live far from their parents and find themselves caregiving from a distance. Millions of Americans are distant caregivers and the number is only expected to increase as baby boomers and their parents age.[40] An estimated 15% of caregivers live an hour or more from their loved one.[39] These adult children are dealing with the added challenges and stressors associated with living at a distance, such as lack of nearby family support. There is some indication that stress related to the distant caregiving is quite common in caregivers.[41] Otherwise, little is known about their experiences, yet most interventions have been designed to support local caregivers. Clinicians must remember that interventions to decrease caregiver burden and improve caregiver well-being may not be as applicable to distant caregivers, who may need extra flexibility and accommodations, such as increased telephone communication, in order to meet their needs.

Advance care planning

Whether care is provided in hospital or by families in the home or at a distance, patients at the end of life may not be able to make decisions about their own care. Family members, therefore, are often asked to make those decisions on the patient's behalf, yet they may not know explicitly what the patient would want. Advance care planning is a process that allows the patient's preferences to be made known to the family and to healthcare professionals. It involves discussions between the patient and his or her family and friends, as well as written instructions in the event that a patient can no longer express his or her choices verbally. Advance care planning is best begun while family members are healthy but when someone is ill, then as early as possible in the illness experience and revisited as needed because preferences can change over time.[42,43] However, even in the less than 30% of cases when an adult has an advance directive, it may be neither specific enough nor available when needed.[44] Clinicians should ask if advance directives are available and they might invite family discussion regardless of whether or not such directives are in place. It is important for clinicians to be familiar with a patient's advance directive and to advocate for the patient if needed. Information about advance directives is available from the American Cancer Society.[45]

Guidelines for nursing interventions

Respect for persons requires that clinicians understand diversity and are able to manage issues that may arise when caring for people with varied backgrounds. The cultural and spiritual backgrounds of families, as well as those of the clinician, need to be taken into account because cultural or spiritual beliefs may be important in assisting families to cope.[46–48] All nursing interventions should be provided with respect to an individual's background. However, despite differences across cultures, it is important to remember that similarities exist in regard to basic needs for support, dignity, and connections with others.[49] At the same, a single approach toward everyone from a particular faith group or culture is inappropriate because there may be a great deal of diversity within faiths or cultures.

Much of the nursing literature, which provides guidelines for nursing care, addresses the importance of four major interventions that have relevance for all members of the palliative care team:

1. *Maintain hope* in patients and their family members. As families pass through the illness trajectory, the nature of their hope changes from hope for cure, to hope for remission, to hope for comfort, to hope for a good death. Offering hope during fading away can be as simple as reassuring families that everything will be done to ensure the patient's comfort. Talking about the past also can help some families by reaffirming the good times spent together and the ongoing connections that will continue among family members. Referring to the future beyond the immediate suffering and emotional pain can also sustain hope. For example, when adult children reassure the ill parent that they will care for the other parent, the patient is hopeful that the surviving spouse will be all right.

2. *Involve families* in all aspects of care. Include them in decision-making, and encourage active participation in the physical care of the patient. This is their life—they have the right to control it as they will. Involvement is especially important for children when a family member is very ill. The more children are involved in care during the terminal phase, and in the activities that follow the death, the better able they are to cope with bereavement.[50]

3. *Offer information.* Tell families about what is happening in straightforward terms and about what they can expect to happen, particularly about the patient's condition and the process their loved one is to undergo. Doing so also provides families with a sense of control. Initiate the discussion of relevant issues that family members themselves may hesitate to mention. For example, the nurse might say, "Many family members feel as if they are being pulled in two or more directions when a loved one is very ill. They want to spend as much time as possible with the patient, but they also feel the pull of their own daily lives, careers, or families. How does this fit with your experience?"

4. *Communicate openly.* Open and honest communication with nurses and other health professionals is frequently the most important need of families. They need to be informed; they need opportunities to ask questions and to have their questions answered in terms that they can comprehend. Open communication among team members is basic to open communication with the families.

It is not an easy task for families to give up their comfortable and established views of themselves as death approaches. The challenge for members of the healthcare team is to help family members anticipate what lies ahead, without violating their need to relinquish old orientations and hopes at a pace they can handle. These four broad interventions assist healthcare providers in providing good palliative care; the following guidelines offer further direction. They are derived from the direct accounts of patients, spouses, and children about the strategies they used to cope with the dimensions of fading away.

Redefining

Supporting patients and other family members with redefining requires that healthcare providers appreciate how difficult it is for family members to relinquish familiar perceptions of themselves and adopt unfamiliar, unwelcome, and unasked-for changes to their self-perceptions. Disengagement from former perceptions and the adoption of new orientations occur over time. Nurses and other care providers are challenged to help family members anticipate and prepare for what lies ahead, while not pushing them at a pace that threatens their sense of integrity. Each family member redefines at his or her own pace; interventions must be tailored according to the individual needs of each. At the same time, healthcare providers must support the family as a unit by reassuring family members that their varying coping responses and strategies are to be expected.

Provide opportunities for patients to talk about the losses incurred due to the illness, the enforced changes, the adaptations they have made, and their feelings associated with these changes. Reinforce their normal patterns of living as long as possible and as appropriate. When they can no longer function as they once did, focus on what patients still can do, reinforcing those aspects of self that remain intact. Acknowledge that roles and responsibilities may be expressed in new and different ways, and suggest new activities appropriate to the patient's interest and current capabilities.

There is some evidence that families who can find positive aspects in caregiving and recognize that what they are doing has value may report improved well-being, better coping, and less traumatic grief. Acknowledge the positive aspects, such as a family member's feeling of satisfaction, greater appreciation of life, or newly uncovered sense of personal ability to foster the positives and strengths within the caregiving experience.

The focus with spouses and children centers on explaining how the disease or treatment contributes to changes in the patient physically, psychologically, and socially. Provide opportunities for spouses to talk about how changes in the patient affect their marital relationship. Help children appreciate their parent from another perspective, such as in recalling favorite memories or identifying the legacies left. Discuss how they can face their own vulnerability by channeling concerns into positive steps for self-care. Reinforce the spouse's and children's usual patterns of living for as long as possible and as appropriate; when former patterns are no longer feasible, help them to consider adjustments or alternatives.

Provide opportunities for spouses to discuss how they may reorganize priorities in order to be with and care for the patient to the degree they desire. Consider resources that enable the spouse to do this, such as the assistance of volunteers, home support services, or additional nursing services. Teach caregiving techniques if the spouse shows interest. With the children, discuss the degree to which they want to be open or private about the patient's illness with those outside the family. Acknowledge that family members will vary in their ability to assimilate changes in the patient and in their family life.

Burdening

Palliative care professionals can help patients find ways to relieve their sense of burden, and can provide patients with opportunities to talk about their fears and concerns and to consider with whom they want to share their worries. In this way, patients may alleviate their concern for putting excessive demands on family members. Explain the importance of a break for family members, and suggest that patients accept assistance from a volunteer or home-support services at those times to relieve family members from worry. Explain that when patients affirm family members for their efforts, this contributes to family members feeling appreciated and reduces their sense of burden.

Nurses and all members of the interdisciplinary team can assist spouses with burdening by supporting the spouse's reassurances to the patient that he or she is not a burden. Acknowledge spouses' efforts when they put their own needs on hold to care for the patient; help them to appreciate the importance of taking care of themselves as a legitimate way of sustaining the energy they need for the patient. Talk with spouses about how they might take time out, and consider the various resources they might use. Acknowledge the negative feelings spouses may have about how long they can continue; do not negate their positive desire to help.

For children, acknowledge the reorganization and the considerable adjustment in their daily routines. Explain that ambivalent feelings are common—the positive feelings associated with helping, and the negative feelings associated with less time spent on careers and their own families. Acknowledge that communicating regularly with their parents by telephoning or visiting often is part of the "work" of caring; the extra effort involved should not be underestimated. Encourage children to take time out for themselves, and support them in their desire to maintain involvement in their typical lives.

Struggling with paradox

Facing the usual business of living and directly dealing with dying is a considerable challenge for all members of the family. The care provider's challenge is to appreciate that it is not possible to alleviate completely the family's psychosocial and spiritual pain. Team members must face their own comfort level in working with families who are facing paradoxical situations and the associated ambivalent feelings. Like family members, nurses, social workers, physicians, and all team members may also sometimes want to avoid the distress of struggling with paradox. They may feel unprepared to handle conversations in which no simple solution exists, and strong feelings abound.

Care providers can support patients and other family members by providing opportunities for all family members to ventilate their frustrations and not minimizing their pain and anguish. On the good days, rejoice with them. Listen to their expressions of ambivalence, and be prepared for the ups and downs and changes of opinion that are sure to occur. Reassure them that their ambivalence is a common response. Encourage "time out" as a way to replenish depleted energy.

Contending with change

Palliative care team members must realize that not all families communicate openly or work easily together in solving problems. Nurses in particular can support patients and family members to contend with change by creating an environment in which families explore and manage their own concerns and feelings according to their particular coping style. Providing information so that families can explore various alternatives helps them to determine what adjustments they can make. Make information available not only verbally but also in writing. Or, tape-record informative discussions so that families can revisit what they have been told.

Rituals can be helpful during periods of terminal illness. A family ritual is a behavior or action that reflects some symbolic meaning for all members of the family and is part of their collective experience. A ritual does not have to be religious in nature. Rituals may already exist, or they can be newly created to assist the family in contending with change. For example, the writing of an "ethical will," whereby one passes on wisdom to others or elaborates on his or her hopes for their loved ones' future, can help ill family members communicate what they might not be able to verbalize to their loved ones. Developing new rituals can help with the changes in everyday life; for example, one woman had always been the sounding board for her children on their return from school. It was a pattern that continued as her children entered the work force. Cancer of the trachea prevented her participation in the same way. Instead, she requested her young adult children to sit by her side, hold her hand, and recount their days. Instead of words, the mother responded with varying hand squeezes to let them know she was listening. The altered daily ritual served both mother and children in adapting to the changes in their lives.

Searching for meaning

Palliative care professionals help families search for meaning by enabling them to tell their personal stories and make sense of them. It is essential that team members appreciate the value of storytelling—when a family talks about its current situation and recollections of the past, it is not just idle chatter. It is a vital part of making sense of the situation and coping with it. Professional team members must appreciate that much of the search for meaning involves examining spiritual dimensions, belief systems, values, and relationships within and outside the family. Nurses can be supportive by suggesting approaches for personal reflection, such as journal writing or writing letters.

Living day to day

In living day to day, families make subtle shifts in their orientation to living with a dying family member. They move from thinking that there is no future to making the most of the time they have left. This is a good time to review the resources available to the family, to ensure that they are using all possible sources of assistance so that their time together is optimally spent.

Preparing for death

In helping families prepare for death, nurses in particular must be comfortable talking about the inevitability of death, describing the dying process, and helping families make plans for wills and funerals. It is important not to push or force such issues; it is equally important not to avoid them because of the nurse's personal discomfort with dying and death. Encourage such discussions among family members while acknowledging how difficult they can be. Affirm them for their courage to face these difficult issues. Encourage patients to attend to practical details, such as finalizing a will and distributing possessions. Encourage them to do "last things," such as participating in a special holiday celebration.

Provide information to spouses and children about the dying process. If the plan is for death at home, provide information about what procedures will need to be followed and the resources that are available. Provide opportunities for family members to express their concerns and ask questions. Encourage them to reminisce with the patient as a way of saying "good-bye," and acknowledge the bittersweet quality of such remembrances. Provide information to the adult children about how they can help their own children with the impending death.

The foregoing guidelines are intended to assist nurses and all members of the palliative care team in their care of individual family members. The guidelines are summarized in Box 30.1. In addition, family-centered care also means focusing on the family as a unit. Healthcare providers must appreciate that the family as a whole has a life of its own that is distinct, but always connected to the individuals who are part of it. Both levels of care are important.[17] The families in the "fading away" study also provided insights about how family functioning plays a role in coping with terminal illness in a family member.

Family functioning and fading away

Families experienced the transition of fading away with greater or lesser difficulty, depending on their level of functioning according to eight dimensions: integrating the past, dealing with feelings, solving problems, utilizing resources, considering others, portraying family identity, fulfilling roles, and tolerating differences. These dimensions occurred along a continuum of functionality; family interactions tended to vary along this continuum rather than being positive or negative, good or bad.

Some families acknowledged the pain of past experience with illness, loss, and other adversity, and integrated previous learning into how they were managing their current situation. These families expressed a range of feelings, from happiness and satisfaction, through uncertainty and dread, to sadness and sorrow. Family members acknowledged their vulnerabilities and their ambivalent feelings. All topics were open for discussion. There were no clearcut rights and wrongs, and no absolute answers to the family's problems. They applied a flexible approach to problem-solving and openly exchanged all information. They engaged in mutual decision-making, considering each member's point of view and feelings. Each family member was permitted to voice both positive and negative opinions in the process of making decisions. They agreed on the characteristics of their family and allowed individual variation within the family. They allocated household and patient care responsibilities in a flexible way. These families were often amenable to outside intervention and were comfortable in seeking and using external resources. Such families were often appealing to palliative care nurses and other personnel, because they openly discussed their situation, shared their concerns, and accepted help willingly.

Redefining

Ensure effective symptom management, because this allows patients and family members to focus outside the illness.

Appreciate that relinquishing old and comfortable views of themselves occurs over time and does not necessarily occur simultaneously with physical changes in the patient.

Explain the importance of respite as a strategy for renewing energy for dealing with the situation.

Tailor interventions according to the various abilities of family members to assimilate the changes.

Contending with change

Reassure family members that a range of responses and coping strategies is to be expected within and among family members.

Create an environment in which family members can explore and manage their own concerns and feelings. Encourage dialogue about family members' beliefs, feelings, hopes, fears, and dilemmas so they can determine their own course of action.

Provide opportunities for patients to talk about the illness, the enforced changes in their lives, and the ways in which they have adapted; for spouses to talk about how changes in the patient affect their marital relationship; and for children to talk about their own feelings of vulnerability and the degree to which they want to be open or private about the situation.

Recognize that families communicate in well-entrenched patterns and their ability to communicate openly and honestly differs.

Normalize the experience of family members and explain that such feelings do not negate the positive feelings of concern and affection.

Reinforce normal patterns of living for as long as possible and as appropriate. When patterns are no longer viable, consider adjustments or alternatives.

Provide information so families can explore the available resources, their options, and the pros and cons of the various options. Provide information in writing as well as verbally.

Focus on the patient's attributes that remain intact, and acknowledge that roles and responsibilities may be expressed differently. Consider adjustments or alternatives when former patterns are no longer feasible.

Explain the wide-ranging nature of the changes that occur within the patient's immediate and extended family.

Searching for meaning

Help spouses consider how they might reorganize priorities and consider resources to help them do this.

Appreciate that the search for meaning involves examination of the self, of relationships with other family members, and of spiritual aspects. Help children appreciate their parent from another perspective, such as in recalling favorite stories or identifying legacies left.

Realize that talking about the current situation and their recollections of past illness and losses is part of making sense of the situation.

Burdening

Provide opportunities for patients to talk about fears and anxieties about dying and death, and to consider with whom to share their concerns.

Encourage life reviews and reminiscing. Listen to the life stories that family members tell.

Help patients stay involved for as long as possible as a way of sustaining self-esteem and a sense of control.

Suggest approaches for self-examination such as journal writing, and approaches for facilitating interactions between family members such as writing letters.

Assist family members to take on tasks appropriate to their comfort level and skill and share tasks among themselves.

Living day to day

Support family members' reassurances to patient that he or she is not a burden. Explain that when patients reaffirm family members for their efforts, this contributes to their feeling appreciated and lessens the potential for feeling burdened.

Listen carefully for the subtle shifts in orientation to living with a dying relative and gauge family members' readiness for a new orientation.

Ensure effective control of symptoms so that the patient can make the most of the time available. Assess the need for aids.

Explain the importance of breaks for family members. Encourage others to take over for patients on a regular basis so family members can take a break without minimizing their losses and concerns, affirm their ability to appreciate and make the most of the time left.

Acknowledge the reorganization of priorities and the considerable adjustment in family routines and extra demands placed on family members. Acknowledge the "work" of caring for all family members.

Review resources that would free family members to spend more time with the patient.

(continued)

Box 30.1 Continued

Preparing for death

Assess your own comfort level in talking about the inevitability of death, describing the dying process, and helping families make plans for wills and funerals.

Realize that family members will vary in their ability to assimilate the changes and that a range of reactions and coping strategies is normal.

Provide information about the dying process.

Struggling with paradox

Discuss patients' preferences about the circumstances of their death. Encourage patients to discuss these issues with their family. Acknowledge how difficult such discussions can be

Appreciate that you, as a nurse, cannot completely alleviate the psychosocial-spiritual pain inherent in the family's struggle.

Assess your own comfort level in working with people facing paradoxical situations and ambivalent feelings.

Encourage patients to do important "last things," such as completing a project as a legacy for their family.

Provide opportunities for family members to mourn the loss of their hopes and plans. Do not minimize these losses; help them modify their previous hopes and plans and consider new ones.

Provide opportunities for spouses and children to express their concerns about their future without the patient. Provide them with opportunities to reminisce about their life together. Acknowledge such remembrances will have a bittersweet quality.

Listen to their expressions of ambivalence, and be prepared for the ups and downs of opinions.

Source: Davies et al. (1995), reference 25.

Other families were more challenging for palliative care professionals. These were families who hung on to negative past experiences and continued to dwell on the painful feelings associated with past events. They appeared to avoid the feelings of turmoil and ambivalence, shielding themselves from the pain, often indicating that they did not usually express their feelings. These families approached problems by focusing more on why the problem occurred and who was at fault, rather than generating potential solutions. They often were unable to communicate their needs or expectations to each other or to healthcare professionals, and were angry when their wishes were not fulfilled. They expressed discrepant views only in individual interviews, not when all members were present, and tended not to tolerate differences. Varying approaches by healthcare workers were not generally well tolerated, either. These families did not adapt easily to new roles, nor did they welcome outside assistance. Such families showed little concern for others. They used few resources, because family members were often unable or reluctant to seek help from others. Such families often presented a challenge for nursing care. Nurses must realize that expecting such families to "pull together" to cope with the stresses of palliative care is unrealistic. It is essential not to judge these families, but rather to appreciate that the family is coping as best it can under very difficult circumstances. These families need support and affirmation of their existing coping strategies, not judgmental criticisms.

Palliative care clinicians are encouraged to complete assessments of level of family system functioning early in their encounters with families.[51] This is the best time to begin to develop an understanding of the family as a whole, as a basis for the services to be offered. In fact, the value of focusing on patterns of family functioning has been demonstrated by a clinical approach that screens for families, rather than individuals, at high risk. Assessment of family functioning provides a basis for effective interactions to ensure a family-focused approach in palliative care. The eight dimensions of family functioning provide a guideline for assessment. Table 30.1 summarizes these dimensions and gives examples of the range of behaviors evident in each dimension. The table summarizes those behaviors that on one end of the continuum are more helpful, and on the other end are less helpful to families facing the transition of fading away.

Understanding the concept of family functioning enhances the nurse's ability to assess the unique characteristics of each family. An assessment of family functioning enables the nurse to interact appropriately with the family and help them solve problems more effectively (Table 30.2). For example, in families where communication is open and shared among all members, the nurse can be confident that communication with one family member will be accurately passed on to other members. In families where communication is not as open, the nurse must take extra time to share the information with all members. Or, in families who dwell on their negative past experiences with the healthcare system, nurses must realize that establishing trust is likely to require extra effort and time. Families who are open to outside intervention are more likely to benefit from resource referrals; other families may need more encouragement and time to open their doors to external assistance.

Nurses, and all palliative care providers, must remember that each family is unique and comes with its own life story and circumstances; listening to the story is central to understanding the family. There may be threads of commonality, but there will not be duplicate experiences. Nurses must assist family members to recognize the essential role they are playing in the experience, and to acknowledge their contributions. Most importantly, nurses must realize that each family is doing the best it can. Nurses must sensitively, creatively, and patiently support families as they encounter one of the greatest challenges families must face—the transition of fading away.

Table 30.1 Dimensions of family functioning: examples of the range of behaviors

More helpful	Less helpful
Integrating the past	
Describe the painful experiences as they relate to present experience	Describe past experiences repeatedly
Describe positive and negative feelings concerning the past	Dwell on painful feelings associated with past experiences
Incorporate learning from the past into subsequent experiences	Do not integrate learning from the past to the current situation
Reminisce about pleasurable experiences in the past	Focus on trying to "fix" the past to create happy memories that are absent from their family life
Dealing with feelings	
Express a range of feelings including vulnerability, fear, and uncertainty	Express predominantly negative feelings, such as anger, hurt, bitterness, and fear
Acknowledge paradoxical feelings	Acknowledge little uncertainty or few paradoxical feelings
Solving problems	
Identify problems as they occur	Focus more on fault finding than on finding solutions
Reach consensus about a problem and possible courses of action	Dwell on the emotions associated with the problem
Consider multiple options	Unable to clearly communicate needs and expectations
Open to suggestions	Feel powerless about influencing the care they are receiving
Approach problems as a team rather than as individuals	Display exaggerated response to unexpected events
	Withhold information from or inaccurately share information with other family members
Utilizing resources	
Utilize a wide range of resources	Utilize few resources
Open to accepting support	Reluctant to seek help or accept offers of help
Open to suggestions regarding resources	Receive help mostly from formal sources rather than from informal support networks
Take the initiative in procuring additional resources	Avoid seeking or exploring additional resources on their own
Express satisfaction with results obtained	Express dissatisfaction with help received
Describe the involvement of many friends, acquaintances, and support persons	Describe fewer friends and acquaintances who offer help
Considering others	
Acknowledge multidimensional effects of situation on other family members	Focus concern on own emotional needs
Express concern for well-being of other family members	Fail to acknowledge or minimize extra tasks taken on by others
Focus concern on patient's well-being	Focus on own self
Appreciate individualized attention from healthcare professionals, but do not express strong need for such attention	Display inordinate need for individualized attention
Direct concerns about how other family members are managing rather than about themselves	Focus concerns on themselves
Identify characteristic coping styles of family unit and of individual members	Describe own characteristic coping styles rather than the characteristic way the family as a unit coped
Demonstrate warmth and caring toward other family members	Allow one member to dominate group interaction
Consider present situation as potential opportunity for family's growth and development	Lack comfort with expressing true feelings in the family group
Value contributions of all family members	Feign group consensus where none exists
Describe a history of closeness among family members	Describe few family interactions prior to illness
Fulfilling roles	
Demonstrate flexibility in adapting to role changes	Demonstrate rigidity in adapting to role changes and responsibilities
Share extra responsibilities willingly	Demonstrate less sharing of responsibilities created by extra demands of patient care

(continued)

Table 30.1 Continued

More helpful	Less helpful
Adjust priorities to incorporate extra demands of patient care and express satisfaction with this decision	Refer to caregiving as a duty or obligation
Enlist assistance as needed and entrust responsibilities to others	Criticize or mistrust caregiving provided by others
Tolerating differences	
Allow differing opinions and beliefs within the family	Display intolerance for differing opinions or approaches of caregiving
Tolerate different views from people outside the family	Demonstrate critical views of friends who fail to respond as expected
Willing to examine own belief and value systems	Adhere rigidly to belief and value systems

Source: Davies et al. (1994), reference 52.

Table 30.2 Family functioning: guidelines for interventions in palliative care

Assessing family functioning	Solving problems
Use dimensions of family functioning to assess families. For example: Do members focus their concern on the patient's well-being and recognize the effect of the situation on other family members, or do family members focus their concerns on their own individual needs and minimize how others might be affected? Putting your assessment of all the dimensions together will help you determine to what degree you are dealing with a more cohesive family unit or a more loosely coupled group of individuals, and hence what approaches are most appropriate.	*Use your assessment of family functioning to guide your approaches.* For example, in families where there is little consensus about the problems, rigidity in beliefs, and inflexibility in roles and relationships, the common rule of thumb—offering families various options so they may choose those that suit them best—tends to be less successful. For these families, carefully consider which resource provides the best possible fit for that particular family. Offer resources slowly, perhaps one at a time. Focus considerable attention on the degree of disruption associated with the introduction of the resource, and prepare the family for the change that ensues. Otherwise, the family may reject the resource as unsuitable and perceive the experience as yet another example of failure of the healthcare system to meet their needs.
Be prepared to collect information over time and from different family members. Some family members may not be willing to reveal their true feelings until they have developed trust. Others may be reluctant to share differing viewpoints in the presence of one another. In some families, certain individuals take on the role of spokesperson for the family. Assessing whether everyone in the family shares the viewpoints of the spokesperson, or whether different family members have divergent opinions but are reluctant to share them, is a critical part of the assessment.	*Be aware of the limitations of family conferences and be prepared to follow up.* Family conferences work well for more cohesive family units. However, where more disparity exists among the members, they may not follow through with the decisions made, even though consensus was apparently achieved. Though not voicing their disagreement, some family members may not be committed to the solution put forward and may disregard the agreed-on plan. The nurse needs to follow up to ensure that any trouble spots are addressed.
Listen to the family's story and use clinical judgment to determine where intervention is required. Part of understanding a family is listening to their story. In some families, the stories tend to be repeated and the feelings associated with them resurface. Talking about the past is a way of being for some families. It is important that the nurse determine whether family members are repeatedly telling their story because they want to be better understood or because they want help to change the way their family deals with the situation. Most often the stories are retold simply because family members want the nurse to understand them and their situation better, not because they are looking for help to change the way their family functions.	*Be prepared to repeat information.* In less-cohesive families, do not assume that information will be accurately and openly shared with other family members. You may have to repeat information several times to different family members and repeat answers to the same questions from various family members.
	Evaluate the appropriateness of support groups. Support groups can be a valuable resource. They help by providing people with the opportunity to hear the perspectives of others in similar situations. However, some family members need more individualized attention than a support group provides. They do not benefit from hearing how others have experienced the situation and dealt with the problems. They need one-to-one interaction focused on themselves with someone with whom they have developed trust.
	Adjust care to the level of family functioning. Some families are more overwhelmed by the palliative care experience than others. Understanding family functioning can help nurses appreciate that expectations for some families to "pull together" to cope with the stress of palliative care may be unrealistic. Nurses need to adjust their care according to the family's way of functioning and be prepared for the fact that working with some families is more demanding and the outcomes achieved are less optimal.

Source: Davies et al. (1995), reference 25.

References

1. US Census Bureau. America's Families and Living Arrangements: 2011. Family Status and Household Relationship of People 15 Years and Over, by Marital Status, Age, and Sex: 2011 (Table A2). Retrieved from http://www.census.gov/population/www/socdemo/hh-fam/cps2011.html.

2. Panke JT, Ferrell BR. The family perspective. In: Hanks G, Cherny N, Christakis NA, Fallon M, Kaasa S, Portenoy RK (eds.), Oxford Textbook of Palliative Medicine. 4th ed. Oxford: Oxford University Press; 2010:1437–1444.

3. Field MJ, Cassell CK, eds. Approaching Death: Improving Care at the End of Life. Washington, DC: National Academy Press; 1997.

4. Wittenberg-Lyles E, Demiris G, Oliver DP, Burt S. Reciprocal suffering: caregiver concerns during hospice care. J Pain Symptom Manage. 2011;41(2):383–393.

5. Northouse LL, Katapodi MC, Song L, Zhang L, Mood DW. Interventions with family caregivers of cancer patients: meta-analysis of randomized trials. CA Cancer J Clin. 2010;60:317–339.

6. Stajduhar KI, Martin WL, Barwich D, Fyles G. Factors influencing family caregivers' ability to cope with providing end-of-life cancer care at home. Canc Nurs. 2008;31:77–85.

7. Aoun S, McGonigley R, Abernethy A, Currow DC. Caregivers of people with neurodegenerative diseases: profile and unmet needs from a population-based survey in South Australia. J Palliat Med. 2010;13(6):653–661.

8. Milberg A, Olsson EC, Jakobsson M, Olsson M, Friedrichsen M. Family members' perceived needs for bereavement follow-up. J Pain Symptom Manage. 2008;35(1):58–69.

9. Milberg A, Strang P. Protection against perceptions of powerlessness and helplessness during palliative care: the family members' perspective. Palliat Support Care. 2011;9(3):251–262.

10. Corà A, Partinico M, Munafò M, Palomba D. Health risk factors in caregivers of terminal cancer patients: a pilot study. Cancer Nurs. 2012;35(1):38–47.

11. Kenny P, Hall J, Zapart S, Davis PR. Informal care and home-based palliative care: the health-related quality of life of carers. J Pain Symptom Manage. 2010;40(1):35–48.

12. Robinson CA, Pesut B, Bottorff JL. Supporting rural family palliative caregivers. J Fam Nurs. 2012;18(4):467–490.

13. Funk L, Stajduhar KI, Toye C, Aoun S, Grande GE, Todd CJ. Part 2: Home-based family caregiving at the end of life: a comprehensive review of published qualitative research (1998–2008). Palliat Med. 2010;24(6):507–607.

14. Grande G, Stajduhar K, Aoun S, et al. Supporting lay carers in end of life care: current gaps and future priorities. Palliat Med. 2009;23(4):339–344.

15. Stajduhar K, Funk L, Jakobsson E, Ohlen J. A critical analysis of health promotion and 'empowerment' in the context of palliative family care-giving. Nurs Inquiry. 2010;17(3):221–230.

16. Stajduhar K, Funk L, Toye C, Grande GE, Soun S, Todd CJ. Part 1: Home based family caregiving at the end of life: a comprehensive review of published quantitative research (1998–2008). Palliat Med. 2010;24(6):573–593.

17. Benzein EG, Saveman B. Health-promoting conversations about hope and suffering with couples in palliative care. Int J Palliat Nurs. 2008;14:439–445.

18. Fine E, Reid MC, Shengelia R, Adelman RD. Directly observed patient-physician discussions in palliative and end-of-life care: a systematic review of the literature. J Palliat Med. 2010;13(5):595–603.

19. Rhodes RL, Mitchell SL, Miller SC, Connor SR, Teno JM. Bereaved family members' evaluation of hospice care: what factors influence overall satisfaction with care? J Pain Symptom Manage. 2008;35:365–371.

20. Hasson F, Kernohan WG, McLaughlin M, Waldron M, McLaughlin D, Chambers H, et al. An exploration into the palliative and end-of-life experiences of carers of people with Parkinson's disease. Palliat Med. 2010;24(7):731–736.

21. Saunders MM. Factors associated with caregiver burden in heart failure family caregivers. West J Nurs Res. 2008;30(8):943–959.

22. Aoun SM, Connors SL, Priddis L, Breen LJ, Colyer S. Motor neurone disease family carers' experiences of caring, palliative care and bereavement: an exploratory qualitative study. Palliat Med. 2012;26(6):842–850.

23. Hennings J, Froggatt K, Keady J. Approaching the end of life and dying with dementia in care homes: the accounts of family carers. Rev Clin Geront. 2010;20:114–127.

24. World Health Organization. Palliative Care for Older People: Better Practices. Author 2011. Retrieved from http://www.euro.who.int/__data/assets/pdf_file/0017/143153/e95052.pdf.

25. Davies B, Chekryn Reimer J, Brown P, Martens N. Fading Away: The Experience of Transition in Families with Terminal Illness. Amityville, NY: Baywood; 1995.

26. Bridges W. Transitions: Making Sense of Life's Changes. Reading, MA: Addison-Wesley; 1980.

27. Stajduhar KI, Martin WL, Barwich D, Fyles G. Factors influencing family caregivers' ability to cope with providing end-of-life cancer care at home. Cancer Nurs. 2008;31(1):77–85.

28. Fitzsimons D, Mullan D, Wilson JS, et al. The challenge of patients' unmet palliative care needs in the final stages of chronic illness. Palliat Med. 2007;21(4):313–322.

29. Wolkowski A, Carr SM, Clarke CL. What does respite care mean for palliative care service users and carers? Messages from a conceptual mapping. Int J Palliat Nurs. 2010;16(8):388–392.

30. Hexem KR, Mollen CJ, Carroll K, Lanctot DA, Feudtner C. How parents of children receiving pediatric palliative care use religion, spirituality, or life philosophy in tough times. J Palliat Med. 2011;14(1): 39–44.

31. Sanderson C, Lobb EA, Mowll J, Butow PN, McGowan N, Price MA. Signs of post-traumatic stress disorder in caregivers following an expected death: a qualitative study. Palliat Med. 2013;27(7): 625–631.

32. Murray SA, Kendall M, Boyd K, Sheikh A. Illness trajectories and palliative care. BMJ. 2005;330(7498):1007–1011.

33. Murray SA, Sheikh A. Care for all at the end of life. BMJ. 2008;336(7650): 958–959.

34. van der Steen JT, Radbruch L, Hertogh CM, de Boer ME, Hughes JC, Larkin P, et al. White paper defining optimal palliative care in older people with dementia: a Delphi study and recommendations from the European Association for Palliative Care. Palliat Med. 2013 July 4. Epub online before print.

35. Teno JM, Clarridge BR, Casey V, et al. Family perspectives on end-of-life care at the last place of death. JAMA. 2004;291:88–93.

36. Spichiger E. Family experiences of hospital end-of-life care in Switzerland: an interpretive phenomenological study. Int J Palliat Nurs. 2009;15(7):332–337.

37. Stajduhar K. Burdens of family caregiving at the end of life. Clin Invest Med. 2013;36(3):E121–E126.

38. Klarare A, Hagelin CL, Fürst CJ, Fossum B. Team interactions in specialized palliative care teams: a qualitative study. J Palliat Med. 2013;16(9):1062–1069.

39. National Alliance for Caregiving, in collaboration with AARP. 2009. Caregiving in the U.S. A Focused Look at Those Caring for the 50+. Retrieved from http://assets.aarp.org/rgcenter/il/caregiving_09.pdf.

40. National Institute on Aging. So Far Away: 20 Questions and Answers About Long-Distance Caregiving. NIH Publication No. 10-5496. Bethesda MD: National Institutes of Health, 2011. Retrieved from http://www.nia.nih.gov/sites/default/files/so_far_away_twenty_questions_about_long-distance_caregiving.pdf.

41. Alzheimer's Association. 2013. Alzheimer's Disease Facts and Figures. Retrieved from http://www.alz.org/alzheimers_disease_facts_and_figures.asp.

42. Robinson CA. Advance care planning: re-visioning our ethical approach. Can J Nurs Res. 2011;43(2):18–37.

43. Robinson CA. "Our best hope is a cure." Hope in the context of advance care planning. Palliat Support Care. 2012;10:75–82.

44. Dunn PM, Tolle SW, Moss AH, Black JS. The POLST paradigm: respecting the wishes of patients and families. Ann Long-Term Care. 2007;15(9):33–40.

45. American Cancer Society. 2011. Advance Directives. Retrieved from http://www.cancer.org/acs/groups/cid/documents/webcontent/002016-pdf.pdf.

46. Yeh P-M, Bull M. Influences of spiritual well-being and coping on mental health of family caregivers for elders. Res Gerontol Nurs. 2009;2(3):173–181.

47 Ferrell B, Otis-Green S, Economou D. Spirituality in cancer care at the end of life. Cancer J. 2013;19(5):431–437.

48. Donovan R, Williams A, Stajduhar K, Brazil K, Marshall D. The influence of culture on home-based family caregiving at end-of-life: a case study of Dutch reformed family care givers in Ontario, Canada. Soc Sci Med. 2011;72(3):338–346.

49. Kongsuwan W, Chaipetch O, Matchim Y. Thai Buddhist families' perspective of a peaceful death. Nurs Crit Care. 2012;17(3):151–159.

50. Davies B. Environmental factors affecting sibling bereavement. In: Davies B. Shadows in the Sun: Experiences of Sibling Bereavement in Childhood. Philadelphia: Brunner/Mazel; 1999:123–148.

51. Steele R, Robinson C, Hansen L, Widger, K. Families and palliative/end-of-life care. In: Kaakinen J, Gedalfy-Duff V, Coehlo D, Hanson S (eds.), Family Health Care Nursing: Theory, Practice and Research. 4th ed. Philadelphia: Davis; 2010:273–306.

52. Davies B, Reimer J, Martens N. Family functioning and its implications for palliative care. J Palliat Care. 1994;10:35–36.

CHAPTER 31

Planning for the actual death

Patricia Berry and Julie Griffie

I had known Jim from my church and community for almost half of my lifetime. We met when we were both newly married and just starting down the road of life. He was brilliant, a shining star in the crowd. With a loving wife of 30+ years, he had nurtured many students, but never had the joy of being a biological father. Instead, he nurtured everyone around him. About three years ago, he suddenly appeared in our clinic. Suddenly, he was "our patient," with stage III lung cancer. He analyzed and plotted out each step of his treatment plan, and was able to successfully stay "on top" (control) of his cancer for 2 years.

When headaches started, he had a positive neuro workup, was scanned and started on radiation therapy along with a different chemotherapy. And then, one bright Monday morning, his wife arrived to tell us that Jim had experienced a seizure, and had been admitted through the ER the previous night. A neurooncologist had seen him and there was a plan for placement of an Ommaya reservoir. We had all walked this path before with other patients, and were in need of a plan for how we would assure that both our friend and his wife truly understood risks and benefits of these next steps. No one wanted to see Jim, not be able to "be Jim." It was time for us to seriously nurture Jim and his wife more aggressively, as we helped them prepare for Jim's death.

Key points

- The care of patients and families near to death and afterward is an important nursing function—arguably one of the most important things nurses do. At the end of life, there are often no dress rehearsals; nurses and other healthcare professionals often only have one chance to "get it right."

- Assessment and aggressive management of symptoms must remain a priority, especially as death approaches.

- As the dying person nears death, the goals of care inevitably change in rhythm with patient and family needs and wishes. The nurse is key in picking up the rhythm of the situation and considering the perspectives and needs of everyone involved, assuring the best experience possible for everyone involved.

- Care of the body after death, including normalizing and interpreting postmortem changes, honoring rituals and individual requests, is critically important in communicating to family members and close others that the person who died was indeed important and valued.

Issues and needs at the time of death are exceedingly important and, at the same time, exceptionally personal. While the physiology of dying is often the same for most expected deaths, the psychological, spiritual, cultural, and family issues are as unique and varied as the patients and families themselves. As death nears, the goals of care must be discussed and appropriately redefined. Some treatments may be discontinued, and symptoms may intensify, subside, or even appear anew. Physiological changes as death approaches must also be defined, normalized, explained, and interpreted to the patient whenever possible, as well as to the patient's family, close others, and caregivers. The nurse occupies a key position in assisting patients' family members at the time of death by supporting and/or suggesting death rituals, caring for the body after death, and facilitating early grief work. In past literature, most of the focus on death and dying has been on the dying process in general, making the need for a chapter focused specifically on the actual death—and the time right before and after—even more important.

Terminally ill persons are cared for in a variety of settings, including home settings with hospice care or traditional home care, hospice residential facilities, nursing homes, assisted living facilities, hospitals, intensive care units, prisons, and group homes. Deaths in intensive care settings may present special challenges, such as restrictive visiting hours and lack of space and less privacy for families—shortcomings that can be addressed by thoughtful and creative nursing care. Likewise, death in a nursing home setting may also offer unique challenges. Regardless of the setting, anticipating and managing pain and symptoms can minimize distress and maximize quality of life. Families can be supported in a way that optimizes use of valuable time and lessens distress during the bereavement period. Like it or not, health professionals only have one chance to "get it right" when caring for dying persons and their families as death nears. In other words, there is no dress rehearsal for the time surrounding death; careful, thoughtful, extensive planning ensures the least stressful and best possible outcome for all involved.

The patient's family is especially important as death nears. Family members may become full- or part-time caregivers; daughters and sons may find themselves in a position to "parent" their parents; and family issues, long forgotten or ignored, may surface. Although "family" is often thought of in traditional terms, a family may take on several forms and configurations. For the purposes of this chapter, the definition of family recognizes that many patients have nontraditional families and may be cared for by a large extended entity, such as a church community, a group of supportive friends, or the staff of a healthcare facility. Family is defined broadly to include not only persons bound by biology or legal ties but also those whom the patient defines or who define themselves as "close others" or who function for the patient as a family member would, including nurturance, intimacy, and economic, social, and psychological support in times of need; support in illness (including dealing with those outside the family); and companionship.

The occurrence of symptoms at end-of-life is temporal in nature; that is, there is a constellation of symptoms common throughout the course of end-stage disease, and symptoms that appear during the period immediately preceding death, most often 2–3 days prior. As death nears, symptoms can escalate and new ones appear. While there is much known about the assessment and management of symptoms as death nears, most research demonstrates that many people experience a death with symptoms not well controlled. It is estimated that up to 52% of patients have refractory symptoms at the very end of life that at times require palliative sedation.[1] In a recent systematic review of signs of impending death and symptoms in the last 2 weeks of life, a total of 43 unique symptoms were identified, with dyspnea (56.7%), pain (52.4%), noisy breathing/respiratory congestion (51.4%), and confusion (50.1%) as the most common.[2] Within a few days of death, many patients experience a higher frequency of noisy and moist breathing, urinary incontinence and retention, restlessness, agitation, delirium, and nausea and vomiting.[3–5] Symptoms that occur with less frequency include sweating and myoclonus, with myoclonus sometimes occurring as a reversible toxic effect of morphine, especially in older patients and those with renal impairment.[2,6] In most studies, symptoms requiring maximum diligence in assessment, prevention, and aggressive treatment during the final day or two before death are respiratory tract secretions/moist breathing, pain, dyspnea, and agitated delirium, which is very common.[2,7–8] For some patients, the pathway to death is characterized by progressive sleepiness leading to coma and death. For others, the pathway to death is marked by increasing symptoms, including restlessness, confusion, hallucinations, sometimes seizure activity, and then coma and death.[9] Assessment and intervention is focused on identifying those persons who are on the more difficult pathway and aggressively treating their symptoms to assure a peaceful death. Persons with cognitive impairment and the inability to self-report or communicate require specific attention to symptoms, especially as death nears. In any case, the nurse plays a key role in assessing and anticipating symptoms, acting promptly to assure, if at all possible, that symptoms are aggressively prevented and managed before they become severe. The nurse also has an important role in educating family members and other caregivers about the assessment, treatment, and ongoing evaluation of these symptoms.

Regardless of individual patient and family needs, attitudes, and "unfinished business," the nurse's professional approach and demeanor at the time near death is crucial and worthy of close attention. Patients experience total and profound dependency at this stage of their illness. Families are often called on to assume total caregiving duties, often disrupting their own responsibilities for home, children, and career. Although there maybe similarities, patients and families experience this time through the unique lens of their own perspective, and form their own unique meaning.

Some authors suggest theories and guidelines as the bases for establishing and maintaining meaningful, helpful, and therapeutic relationships with patients or clients and their families. One example is Carl Rogers's theory of helping relationships, in which he proposed that the characteristics of a helping relationship are empathy, unconditional positive regard, and genuineness.[10] These characteristics, defined later as part of the nurse's approach to patients and families, are essential in facilitating care at the end of life. To this may be added "attention to detail," because this additional characteristic is widely accepted as essential for individualized, patient- and family-centered quality palliative care.[11–12] Readers are urged to consider the following characteristics as they reflect on their own practice, as these characteristics can serve as a powerful foundation for facilitating and providing supportive relationships:

- Empathy: the ability to put oneself in the other person's place, trying to understand the patient or client from his or her own frame of reference; it also requires the deliberate setting aside of one's own frame of reference and bias.

- Unconditional positive regard: a warm feeling toward others, with a nonjudgmental acceptance of all they reveal themselves to be; the ability to convey a sense of respect and esteem at a time and place in which it is particularly important to do so.

- Genuineness: the ability to convey trustworthiness and openness that is real rather than a professional facade; also the ability to admit that one has limitations, makes mistakes, and does not have all the answers.

- Attention to detail: the learned and practiced ability to think critically about a situation and not make assumptions. The nurse, for example, discusses challenging patient and family concerns with colleagues and other members of the interdisciplinary team. The nurse considers every "what if" before making a decision and, in particular, before making any judgment. Finally, the nurse is constantly aware of how his or her actions, attitudes, and words may be interpreted—or misinterpreted—by others.

The events and interactions—positive as well as negative—at the bedside of a dying person set the tone for the patient's care and form lasting memories for family members. The time of death and the care received by both the individual who has died, and the family members who are present, are predominant aspects of the survivors' memories of this momentous event. Approaching patients and families with a genuine openness characterized by empathy and positive regard eases the way in making this difficult time meaningful, individualized, and deeply profound.

This chapter discusses some key issues surrounding the death itself, including advance planning and the evolving and ever-changing choices and goals of care, the changing focus of care as death nears, common signs and symptoms of nearing death and their management, and care of the patient and family at time of death. It concludes with two case examples illustrating the chapter's content.

Advance planning: evolving choices and goals of care

Healthcare choices related to wellness are generally viewed as clearcut or easy. We have an infection, we seek treatment, and the problem resolves. Throughout most of the life span, medical treatment choices are obvious. As wellness moves along the healthcare continuum to illness, choices become less clear and consequences of choices have a significantly greater impact.

Many end-of-life illnesses manifest with well-known and well-documented natural courses. Providing the patient and family with information on the natural course of the disease at appropriate intervals is a critical function of healthcare providers such as nurses. Providing an opening for discussion, such as, "Would you like to talk about the future?" "Do you have any concerns that I can help you address?" or "It seems you are not as active as you were before," may allow a much-needed discussion of fears and concerns about impending death. Family members may request information that patients do not wish to know at certain points in time. With the patient's permission, discussions with the family may occur in the patient's absence. Family members may also need coaching to initiate end-of-life discussions with the patient. End-of-life goal setting is greatly enhanced when the patient is aware of the support of family.

End-of-life care issues should always be discussed with patients and family members. The patient who is capable of participating in and making decisions is always the acknowledged decision maker. The involvement of family ensures maximal consensus for patient support as decisions are actually implemented. Decisions for patients who lack decision-making capacity should be made by a consensus approach, using family conference methodology. If documents such as a durable power of attorney for healthcare or a living will are available, they can be used as a guide for examining wishes that influence decision-making and goal setting. The decision maker, usually the person named as healthcare power of attorney (HCPOA), or the patient's primary family members, should be clearly identified. This approach is also useful with patients who are able to make their own decisions and, of course, should always include the patient as a participant.

To facilitate decision-making, convening a family conference that involves the decision makers (decisional patient, family members, and the HCPOA), the patient's physician or provider, nurse, chaplain, and social worker is ideal. A history of how the patient's healthcare status evolved from diagnosis to the present is reviewed. The family is presented with the natural course of the disease. Choices on how care may proceed, including prognostic estimations and the benefits and burdens of treatments are reviewed. Guidance or support for those choices is provided based on existing data and clinical experience with the particular disease in relation to the current status of the patient. If no consensus for the needed decisions occurs, decision-making is postponed. Third-party support by a trusted individual or consultant may then be enlisted. Decisions by patients and families cross the spectrum of care range from continuing treatment for the actual disease, such as undergoing chemotherapy or renal dialysis or utilization of medications, to initiating cardiopulmonary resuscitation (CPR). The healthcare provider may work with the patient and family, making care decisions for specific treatments and timing treatment discontinuance within a clear and logical framework. A goal-setting discussion may determine a patient's personal framework for care, such as:

◆ Treatment and enrollment in any clinical studies for which I am eligible.

◆ Treatment as long as statistically there is a greater than 50% chance of response.

◆ Full treatment as long as I am ambulatory and able to come to the clinic or office.

◆ Treatment only of "fixable" conditions such as infections or blood glucose levels.

◆ Treatment only for controlling symptomatic aspects of disease.

Once a goals of care framework has been established with the patient, the appropriateness of interventions such as CPR, renal dialysis, or intravenous antibiotics is clear. For instance, if the patient states a desire for renal dialysis as long as transportation to the clinic is possible without the use of an ambulance, the endpoint of dialysis treatment is quite clear. At this point, the futility of CPR would also be apparent. Allowing a patient to determine when the treatment is a burden that is unjustified by his or her value system, and communicating this determination to family and caregivers, is perhaps the most pivotal point in management of the patient's care. Box 31.1 suggests a format for an effective and comprehensive family conference.

Changing the focus of care as death nears

As death nears the rhythm of care changes; visiting hours in an institutional setting are relaxed, the routines of care, for example taking vital signs, tracking intake and output, and daily weights seem less important, and treatments automatically associated with caring for any patient are considered in the context of benefit and burden. Here we focus on some of these routines and treatments, recognizing the nurse again plays a key role in explaining and normalizing the shifts in the rhythm of care to the patient and family. The nurse also plays an important role in advocating on behalf of the patient, interpreting the goals of care to colleagues and assuring that the care delivered is consistent with the goals and preferences of the patient and/or family.

Vital signs

As nurses, we derive a good deal of security in performing the ritual of measurement of vital signs, one of the hallmarks of nursing care. When death is approaching, we need to question the rationale for measuring and recording vital signs. Are interventions going to change if it is discovered that the patient has experienced a drop in blood pressure? If the plan of care no longer involves intervening in changes in blood pressure and pulse rate, the measurements should cease. The time spent taking vital signs can then be redirected to assessment of patient comfort and provision of family support. Changes in respiratory rate are visually noted and do not require routine monitoring of rates, unless symptom management issues develop that could be more accurately assessed by measurement of vital signs. The measurement of body temperature using a noninvasive route should continue on a regular basis until death, if the patient appears uncomfortable, allowing for the detection and management of fever, a frequent symptom that can cause distress and may require management.

Fever often suggests infection. As death approaches, goal setting should include a discussion of the benefits and burdens of treating an infection. Indications for treatment of infection are based on the degree of distress and patient discomfort.[14] Pharmacological

Box 31.1 Moderating an end-of-life family conference

   I. Why: Clarify goals in your own mind.

  II. Where: Provide comfort, privacy, circular seating.

III. Who: Include legal decision maker/healthcare power of attorney; family members; social support; key healthcare professionals, patient if capable to participate.

IV. How:

    A. Introduction

      1. Introduce self and others.

      2. Review meeting goals: State meeting goals and specific decisions.

      3. Establish ground rules: Each person will have a chance to ask questions and express views; no interruptions; identify legal decision maker, and describe importance of supportive decision-making.

      4. If new to patient/family, spend some time getting to know the patient as a person as well as the family.

    B. Determine what the patient/family knows.

    C. Review medical status.

      1. Review current status, plan, and prognosis.

      2. Ask each family member in turn for any questions about current status, plan, and prognosis.

      3. Defer discussion of decision until the next step.

      4. Respond to emotions.

    D. Family discussion with decisional patient

      1. Ask patient, "What decision(s) are you considering?"

      2. Ask each family member, "Do you have questions or concerns about the treatment plan? How can you support the patient?"

    E. Family discussion with nondecisional patient

      1. Ask each family member in turn, "What do you believe the patient would choose if he (or she) could speak for himself (or herself)?"

      2. Ask each family member, "What do you think should be done?"

      3. Leave room to let family discuss alone.

      4. If there is consensus, go to V; if no consensus, go to F.

    F. When there is no consensus:

      1. Restate goal: "What would the patient say if he or she could speak?"

      2. Use time as ally: Schedule a follow-up conference the next day.

      3. Try further discussion: "What values is your decision based on? How will the decision affect you and other family members?"

      4. Identify legal decision-maker.

      5. Identify resources: minister/priest; other physicians; ethics committee.

 V. Wrap-up

    A. Summarize consensus, decisions, and plan.

    B. Caution against unexpected outcomes.

    C. Identify family spokesperson for ongoing communication.

    D. Document in the chart who was present, what decisions were made, follow-up plan.

    E. Approach discontinuation of treatment as an interdisciplinary team, not just as a nursing function.

    F. Continuity: Maintain contact with family and medical team; schedule follow-up meetings as needed.

Box 31.1 Continued

VI. Family dynamics and decisions

    A. Family structure: Respect the family hierarchy whenever possible.

    B. Established patterns of family interaction will continue.

    C. Unresolved conflicts between family members may be evident.

    D. Past problems with authority figures, doctors, and hospitals affect the process; ask specifically about bad experiences in the past.

    E. Family grieving and decision-making may include

        1. Denial: false hopes.

        2. Guilt: fear of letting go.

        3. Depression: passivity and inability to decide; or anger and irritability.

Source: Adapted from Ambuel and Weissman (2009), reference 13.

---

management of fever includes antipyretics, including acetaminophen, and nonsteroidal antiinflammatory drugs. In some cases, treatment of an infection with an antibiotic may increase patient comfort. Ice packs, alcohol baths, and cooling blankets should be used cautiously, because they often cause more distress than the fever itself.[14]

Fever may also suggest dehydration. As with the management of fever, interventions are guided by the degree of distress and patient discomfort. The appropriateness of beginning medically administered hydration for the treatment of fever is based on individual patient assessment, the estimated prognosis, and the goals of care.

Finally, fever may suggest that death is imminent as many people develop a central fever, that is, they are cool to the touch but have an increased temperature. In this case, as with all interventions as death nears, treat for patient comfort.

Cardiopulmonary resuscitation

Patients and family members may need to discuss, if they haven't already, the issue of the futility of CPR when death is expected from a terminal illness. Developed in the 1960s as a method of restarting the heart in the event of sudden, unexpected clinical death, CPR was originally intended for circumstances in which death was unexpected or accidental. It is not indicated in certain situations, such as cases of terminal irreversible illness where death is not unexpected; resuscitation in these circumstances may represent an active violation of a person's wish to die with dignity.

Over the years, predictors of the success of CPR have become apparent, along with the predictors of the burden of CPR. In general, a poor outcome of CPR is predicted in patients with advanced terminal illnesses, patients with dementia, and patients with poor functional status who depend on others for meeting their basic care needs. Poor outcomes or physical problems resulting from CPR include fractured ribs, punctured lung, brain damage if anoxia has occurred for too long, and permanent unconsciousness or persistent vegetative state.[15–16] Most importantly, the use of CPR negates the possibility of a peaceful death. This is considered the gravest of poor outcomes.

Medically-administered fluids

The issue of medically administered or "artificial" hydration is emotional for many patients and families because of the role that giving and consuming fluids plays in our culture. When patients are not able to take fluids, concerns may surface among caregivers. A decision must be reached regarding the appropriate use of fluids within the context of the patient's framework of goals. Beginning artificial hydration is a relatively easy task, but the decision to stop is generally much more problematic given its emotional implications. Ethical, moral, and most religious viewpoints state that there is no difference between withholding and withdrawing a treatment such as artificial hydration. However, the emotional response attached to withdrawing a treatment adds a world of difference to the decision to suspend. It is therefore much less burdensome to not begin treatment, if this decision is acceptable in light of the specific patient circumstances.[17]

Most patients and families are aware that, without fluids, death will occur quickly. The literature suggests that fluids should not be routinely administered to dying patients, nor automatically withheld from them. Instead, the decision should be based on careful, individual assessment. Zerwekh,[18] in a classic article, suggested consideration of the following questions when the choice to initiate or continue hydration is evaluated. These questions remain relevant to this important issue:

◆ Is the patient's well-being enhanced by the overall effect of hydration?

◆ Which current symptoms are being relieved by medically administered hydration?

◆ Are other end-of-life symptoms being aggravated by the fluids?

◆ Does hydration improve the patient's level of consciousness? If so, is this within the patient's goals and wishes for end-of-life care?

◆ Does hydration appear to prolong the patient's survival? If so, is this within the patient's goals and wishes for end-of-life care?

◆ What is the effect of the infusion technology on the patient's well-being, mobility, and ability to interact and be with family?

◆ What is the burden of the infusion technology on the family in terms of caregiver stress, finance? Is it justified by benefit to the patient?

Research suggests that, although some dying patients may actually benefit from dehydration, others may experience increased discomfort such as confusion, agitated delirium, or opioid metabolite toxicity that can be mitigated by hydration.[19] In any case, the uniqueness of the individual situation, the goals of care, the benefits and burdens of the proposed treatment, and the comfort of the patient must always be considered.[20]

Terminal dehydration refers to the process in which the dying patient's condition naturally results in a decrease in fluid intake. A gradual withdrawal from activities of daily living may occur as symptoms such as dysphagia, nausea, and fatigue become more obvious. Families commonly ask whether the patient will be thirsty as fluid intake decreases. The arguments are complex, but several studies have demonstrated that, although patients reported thirst, there was no correlation between thirst and hydration, resulting in the assumption that artificial hydration to relieve symptoms may be futile.[19] Medically, hydration has the potential to cause fluid accumulation, resulting in distressful symptoms such as edema, ascites, nausea and vomiting, and pulmonary congestion.

There is no evidence that rehydration actually prolongs life.[19] Healthcare providers need to assist patients and family members to refocus on the natural course of the disease and the notion that the patient's death will be caused by the disease, not by dehydration, which is a natural occurrence in advanced illness and dying. Nurses may then assist families in dealing with symptoms caused by dehydration.

Dry mouth, a consistently reported distressing symptom of dehydration, can be relieved with sips of beverages, ice chips, or hard candies. Another simple comfort measure for dry mouth is spraying normal saline into the mouth with a spray bottle or atomizer. (Normal saline is made by mixing one teaspoon of table salt in a quart of water.) Meticulous mouth care must be administered to keep the patient's mouth clean. Family members can be instructed to anticipate this need. The nurse can facilitate this care by ensuring that the necessary provisions are on hand to assist the patient.

Medications

Medications unrelated to the terminal diagnosis are generally continued as long as their administration is not burdensome. When swallowing pills becomes too difficult, the medication may be offered in a liquid or other form if available, considering patient and family comfort. Continuing medications, however, may be seen by some patients and families as a way of normalizing daily activities and therefore should be supported. Considerable tact, kindness, and knowledge of the patient and family are needed in assisting them to make decisions about discontinuing medications.

Medications that do not contribute to daily comfort should be evaluated on an individual basis for possible discontinuance. Medications such as antihypertensives, replacement hormones, vitamin supplements, iron preparations, hypoglycemics, long-term antibiotics, antiarrhythmics, and laxatives, unless they are essential to patient comfort, can and should be discontinued unless doing so would cause symptoms or discomfort. Accordingly, special consideration should be given to the use of diuretics with patients with end-stage heart disease and corticosteroids in patients with neuropathic pain or for the treatment of increased intracranial pressure. The control or prevention of distressing symptoms should be the guiding principle in the use of medications, especially in the final days of life. Resumption of the drug at any point is always an option that should be offered to the patient and family if the need becomes apparent. Customarily, the only drugs necessary in the final days of life are analgesics, anticonvulsants, antiemetics, antipyretics, antisecretories, and sedatives.[21]

Implantable cardioverter defibrillator

Implantable cardioverter defibrillators (ICDs) are used to prevent cardiac arrest due to ventricular tachycardia or ventricular fibrillation. Patients with ICDs who are dying of another terminal condition or are withdrawn from antiarrhythmic medications may choose to have the defibrillator deactivated, or turned off, so that there will be no interference from the device at the time of death. If the patient has an ICD it is critical to confirm its deactivation if that is in keeping with the goals of care. Some authors suggest routine screening for ICDs in out-of-institution care settings, like hospices, because of the high likelihood of preventable adverse events.[22,23] Deactivating the ICD is a simple, noninvasive procedure usually overseen by a cardiologist or an associated provider. The device is tested after it is turned off to ensure that it is no longer operational, and the test result is placed in the patient record. Patients and families often find this procedure important to provide assurance that death indeed will be quiet and easy, when it does occur.

Renal dialysis

Renal dialysis is a life-sustaining treatment, and as death approaches it is important to recognize and agree on its limitations. Discontinuation of dialysis should be considered in the following cases:

♦ Patients with acute, concurrent illness, who, if they survive, will be burdened with a great deal of disability as defined by the patient and family.

♦ Patients with progressive and untreatable disease or disability.

♦ Patients with dementia or severe neurological deficit.

There is general agreement that dialysis should not be used to prolong the dying process.[24] The time between discontinuing dialysis and death varies widely, from a matter of hours or days (for patients with acute illnesses, such as those described earlier) to days or a week or longer if some residual renal function remains.[24-25] Opening a discussion about the burden of treatment, however, is a delicate task. There may be competing opinions among the patient, family, and even staff about the tolerability or intolerability of continuing treatment. The nurse who sees the patient and family on a regular basis may be the most logical person to recognize the discrete changes in status. Gently validating these observations may open a much-needed discussion regarding the goals of care.

The discussions and decisions surrounding discontinuation or modification of treatment are never easy. Phrases such as, "There is nothing more that can be done" or "We have tried everything" have no place in end-of-life discussions with patients and families. Always reassure the patient and family members—and be prepared to follow through—that you will stand by them and do all you can to provide help and comfort. This is essential to ensure that palliative care is not interpreted as abandonment.

In addition to addressing concerns the patient and family may have as death nears, the nurse should explore and confirm wishes and preferences for after the patient dies. For example, have funeral arrangements been discussed? Have any decisions been made? Has a funeral provider been selected? Are there any special considerations for eye, tissue, or body donation? The nurse has a pivotal role in encouraging family members to carefully select a funeral provider as they would any other provider (for example a long-term care facility, a healthcare provider). Urge the family, if the choice is not certain, to take the time to call and visit funeral providers before taking advice from others and making a final decision. This is a critical nursing function regardless of the setting of care and the place of anticipated death.

Common signs and symptoms of imminent death and their management

There usually are predictable sets of processes that occur during the final stages of a terminal illness due to gradual hypoxia, respiratory acidosis, metabolic consequences of renal failure, and the signs and symptoms of hypoxic brain function.[1,9] These processes account for the signs and symptoms of imminent death and can assist the nurse in helping the family plan for the actual death.

The following signs and symptoms provide cues that death is only days away[1,9,26]:

◆ Profound weakness (patient is usually bedbound and requires assistance with all or most care).

◆ Gaunt and pale physical appearance (most common in persons with cancer if corticosteroids have not been used as treatment).

◆ Drowsiness and/or a reduction in awareness, insight, and perception (often with extended periods of drowsiness, extreme difficulty in concentrating, severely limited attention span, inability to cooperate with caregivers, disorientation to time and place, or semicomatose state).

◆ Increasing lack of interest in food and fluid with diminished intake (only able to take sips of fluids).

◆ Increasing difficulty in swallowing oral medications.

During the final days, these signs and symptoms become more pronounced, and, as oxygen concentrations drop, new symptoms also appear. Measurement of oxygen concentration in the dying person is not advocated, because it may add discomfort and does not alter the course of care. However, knowledge of the signs and symptoms associated with decreasing oxygen concentrations can assist the nurse in guiding the family as death nears.[26] As oxygen saturation drops below 80%, signs and symptoms related to hypoxia appear. As the dying process proceeds, special issues related to normalizing the dying process for the family, symptom control, and patient and family support present themselves. Table 31.1 summarizes the physiological process of dying and suggests interventions for both patients and families.

As the imminently dying person takes in less fluid, third-spaced fluids, clinically manifested as peripheral edema, ascites, or pleural effusions, may be reabsorbed. Breathing may become easier, and there may be less discomfort from tissue distention. Accordingly, as the person experiences dehydration, swelling is often reduced around tumor masses. Patients may experience transient improvements in comfort, including increased mental status and decreased pain. The family, in this case, needs a careful and compassionate

Table 31.1 Symptoms in the normal progression of dying and suggested interventions

Symptoms	Suggested interventions
Early-stage sensation	
Perception	◆ Interpret the signs and symptoms to the patient (when appropriate) and family as part of the normal dying process; for example, assure them the patient's "seeing" and even talking to persons who have died is normal and often expected.
◆ Impairment in the ability to grasp ideas and reason; periods of alertness along with periods of disorientation and restlessness are also noted.	◆ Urge family members to look for metaphors for death in speech and conversation (e.g., talk of a long journey, needing maps or tickets, or in preparing for a trip in other ways) and using these metaphors as a departure point for conversation with the patient.
	◆ Urge family to take advantage of the patient's periods of lucidity to talk with patient and ensure nothing is left unsaid.
	◆ Encourage family members to touch and speak slowly and gently to the patient without being patronizing.
	◆ Maximize safety; for example, use bedrails and schedule people to sit with the patient.
◆ Some loss of visual acuity	◆ Keep sensory stimulation to a minimum, including light, sounds, and visual stimulation; reading to a patient who has enjoyed reading in the past may provide comfort.
◆ Increased sensitivity to bright lights while other senses, except hearing, are dulled.	◆ Urge the family to be mindful of what they say "over" the patient, because hearing remains present; also continue to urge family to say what they wish not to be left unsaid.

(continued)

Table 31.1 Continued

Symptoms	Suggested interventions
Cardiorespiratory	
◆ Increased pulse and respiratory rate.	◆ Normalize the observed changes by interpreting the signs and symptoms as part of the normal dying process and ensuring the patient's comfort.
◆ Agonal respirations or sounds of gasping for air without apparent discomfort.	
◆ Apnea, periodic, or Cheyne-Stokes respirations.	◆ Assess and treat respiratory distress as appropriate.
◆ Inability to cough or clear secretions efficiently, resulting in gurgling or congested breathing (sometimes referred to as the "death rattle").	◆ Assess use and need for parenteral fluids, tube feedings, or hydration. (It is generally appropriate to either discontinue or greatly decrease these at this point in time.)
	◆ Reposition the patient in a side-lying position with the head of the bed elevated.
	◆ Suctioning is rarely needed, but when appropriate, suction should be gentle and only at the level of the mouth, throat, and nasal pharynx.
	◆ Administer anticholinergic drugs (transdermal scopolamine, hyoscyamine) as appropriate, recognizing and discussing with the family that they will not decrease already existing secretions.
Renal/urinary	
◆ Decreasing urinary output, sometimes urinary incontinence or retention.	◆ Insert catheter and/or use absorbent padding.
	◆ Carefully assess for urinary retention, because restlessness can be a related symptom.
Musculoskeletal	
◆ Gradual loss of the ability to move, beginning with the legs, then progressing.	◆ Reposition every few hours as appropriate.
	◆ Anticipate needs such as sips of fluids, oral care, changing of bed pads and linens, and so on.
Late-stage sensation	
Perception	
◆ Unconsciousness.	◆ Interpret the patient's unconsciousness to the family as part of the normal dying process.
◆ Eyes remain half open, blink reflex is absent; sense of hearing remains intact and may slowly decrease.	
	◆ Provide for total care, including incontinence of urine and stool.
	◆ Encourage family members to speak slowly and gently to the patient, with the assurance that hearing remains intact.
Cardiorespiratory	
◆ Heart rate may double, strength of contractions decrease; rhythm becomes irregular.	◆ Interpret these changes to family members as part of the normal dying process.
◆ Patient feels cool to the touch and becomes diaphoretic.	◆ Frequent linen changes and sponge baths may enhance comfort.
◆ Cyanosis is noted in the tip of the nose, nail beds, and knees; extremities may become mottled (progressive mottling indicates death within a few days); absence of a palpable radial pulse may indicate death within hours.	
Renal/urinary	
◆ A precipitous drop in urinary output.	◆ Interpret to the family the drop in urinary output as a normal sign that death is near, usually 24–72 hours away.
◆ Carefully assess for urinary retention; restlessness can be a related symptom.	

explanation regarding these temporary improvements and encouragement to make the most of this short but potentially meaningful time. There are multiple patient and family educational tools available to assist families in interpreting the signs and symptoms of approaching death (Figure 31.1). However, as with all aspects of palliative care, consideration of the individual perspective and associated relationships of the patient or family member, the underlying disease course trajectory, anticipated symptoms, and the setting of care is essential for optimal care at all stages of illness, but especially during the final days and hours.[27]

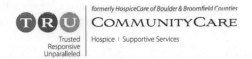

formerly HospiceCare of Boulder & Broomfield Counties

COMMUNITYCARE

Hospice | Supportive Services

TRU
Trusted
Responsive
Unparalleled

SIGNS AND SYMPTOMS OF APPROACHING DEATH

This list of symptoms and what to do about them may appear frightening, but knowing what to expect may reduce some of your anxiety about the approaching death.

Each person approaches death in their own way, bringing to this last experience their own uniqueness. Our list of "Symptoms and What To Do" is a map to the goal of a peaceful death. Like all maps, there are many different routes to the same destination.

You may see all of these symptoms or none. Death will come in its own time, and its own way to each of us. It is important to remember that **dying is a natural process**.

1. <u>Withdrawal</u> - Physical and emotional, and increased sleep.

   Natural process of withdrawing from everything outside of one's self, looking inward, reviewing one's self and one's life. Your loved one may turn inward, withdraw physically and emotionally. This occurs in an attempt to cope with the many changes that are occurring.

2. Reduced food and fluid intake.

   Decreased <u>need</u> because body will naturally begin to conserve energy. Dehydration is a <u>natural comfort measure</u>, since the body systems can't process fluids effectively. At no time should food/fluids be <u>forced.</u>

3. Confusion/Agitation can vary from mild to end stage agitation which may include trying to get out of bed, picking at covers, seeing things that are not apparent to us.

   Talk calmly and assuredly. Keep lights on, use times when patient is alert for meaningful conversation. Music can be very calming. Medication often used to control this symptom.

Figure 31.1 Continued

4.	Change in breathing patterns.	This is common. You may see irregular breathing: very rapid, very slow, and/or 10 to 30 seconds of no breathing at all (called apnea). These symptoms are very common and indicative of a decrease in circulation. It does not mean that your loved one is uncomfortable or struggling.
5.	Oral secretions collect in back of throat causing noisy respiration.	Swallowing reflex may be absent. Patient may be breathing through the secretions. • This may be more uncomfortable for us as observers than patient experiencing it. • Elevate head of bed or turn patient on side.
6.	Incontinence of urine and stool.	Reduced intake results in reduced output with darker color. Bedpads and diapers can be used to protect bed linens. Cleanse patient and change linens frequently to maintain comfort and protect skin.
7.	Changes in skin temperature and color.	Decreased circulation can cause coolness and discoloration of skin. Use light covers, turn side to side frequently to maintain comfort and prevent skin breakdown (bedsores). Heating pads and electric blankets NOT recommended.

Hearing is the last sense to be lost, so the patient can hear all that is being said. This is a good time to say good-bye, reassure them that you will be all right even though you will miss them greatly. (You may tell them it's OK to "let go".) This permission is often helpful for a peaceful death.

How would you know death has occurred?
1. No breathing
2. No heartbeat or pulse

If you believe that death has occurred, call Hospice at 449-7740. **Do not call 911 or the physician**. We will come to your home to help you. (You may want to use the time until we arrive to say your last good-byes.)

signs & symptoms death: 7/04

Figure 31.1 Sample handout for families responsible for end-of-life care. Source: Courtesy of TRU Community Care, Colorado (formerly HospiceCare of Boulder and Broomfield Counties), Colorado, March 2013.

Care at the time of death, death rituals, and facilitating early grieving

At the time of death, the nurse has a unique opportunity to provide information helpful in making decisions about organ and body donation and autopsy. In addition, the nurse can support the family's choice of death rituals, gently care for the body, assist in funeral planning, and facilitate the early process of grieving. Family members' needs change around the time of death, just as the goals of care change. During this important time, plans are reviewed and perhaps refined. Special issues affecting the time of death, such as cultural influences, decisions regarding organ or body donation, and the need for autopsy, are also reviewed.

Under U.S. federal law, if death occurs in a hospital setting, staff must approach the family decision-maker regarding the possibility of organ donation.[28] Although approaching family at this time may seem onerous, the opportunity to assist another is often comforting. Some hospital-based palliative care programs include information about organ donation in their admission or bereavement information. Readers are urged to review their own organizations' policies and procedures.

In any case, it is important to clarify specifically with family members what their desires and needs are at the time of death. Do they wish to be present? Do they know of others who wish to now say a final goodbye? Have they said everything they wish to say to the person who is dying? Do they have any regrets? Are they concerned about anything? Do they wish something could be different? Every person in a family has different and unique needs that, unless explored, can go unmet. Family members recall the time before the death and immediately afterward with great acuity and detail. As mentioned earlier, there is no chance for a dress rehearsal—we only have the one chance to "get it right" and make the experience an individualized and memorable one.

Although an expected death can be anticipated with some degree of certainty, the exact time of death is often not predictable. Death often occurs when no healthcare professionals are present. Often, dying people seem to determine the time of their own death—for example, waiting for someone to arrive, for a date or event to pass, or even for family members to leave—even if the leave-taking is brief. For this reason, it is crucial to ask family members who wish to be present at the time of death whether they have thought about the possibility they will not be there. This opens an essential discussion regarding the time of death and its unpredictability. Gently reminding family members of that possibility can assist them in preparing for any eventuality.

Determining that death has occurred

Death often occurs when health professionals are not present at the bedside or in the home. Regardless of the site of death, a plan must be in place for who will be contacted, how the death pronouncement will be handled, and how the body will be removed. This is especially important for deaths that occur outside a healthcare institution.

Death pronouncement procedures vary from state to state, and sometimes from county to county within a state. In some states, nurses can pronounce death; in others, they cannot. In inpatient settings, the organization's policy and procedures are followed. In hospice home care, generally the nurse makes a home visit, assesses the lack of vital signs, contacts the physician, who verbally agrees to sign the death certificate, and then contacts the funeral home or mortuary. Local customs, the ability of a healthcare agency to ensure the safety of a nurse during the home visit, and provision for "do-not-resuscitate" orders outside a hospital setting, among other factors, account for wide variability in the practices and procedures surrounding pronouncement of death in the home. Although practices vary widely, the police or coroner may need to be called if the circumstances of the death were unusual, were associated with trauma (regardless of the cause of the death), or occurred within 24 hours of a hospital admission.

The practice of actual death pronouncement varies widely and is not often taught in medical school or residencies. The customary procedure is to first identify the patient, then note the following:

- General appearance of the body
- Lack of reaction to verbal or tactile stimuli
- Lack of pupillary light reflex (pupils will be fixed and dilated)
- Absent breathing and lung sounds
- Absent carotid and apical pulses (in some situations, listening for an apical pulse for a full minute is advisable)

Documentation of the death is equally important and should be thorough and clear. The following guidelines are customary:

- Patient's name and time of call
- Who was present at the time of death and at the time of the pronouncement
- Detailed findings of the physical examination
- Date and time of death pronouncement (either pronouncement by the nurse, or the time at which the physician either assessed the patient or was notified)
- Who else was notified and when—for example, additional family members, attending physician, or other staff members
- Whether the coroner was notified, rationale, and outcome, if known
- Special plans for disposition and outcome (e.g., organ or body donation, autopsy, special care related to cultural or religious traditions)

Care of the body after death

The care of the patient does not end with the death, but rather continues during the immediate postmortem period as the body is prepared for transport into the care of the funeral provider. Regardless of the site of death, therefore, care of the patient's body is an important nursing function. In gently caring for the body, the nurse can continue to communicate care and concern for the patient and family members, and model behaviors that may be helpful as the family members continue their important grief work. Caring for the body after death also calls for an understanding of the physiological changes that occur. By understanding these changes, the nurse can interpret and dispel any myths and explain these changes to the family members, thereby assisting the family in making their own personal decisions about the time immediately following death and funeral plans.

A classic article regarding postmortem care emphasized that, although postmortem care may be a ritualized nursing procedure, the scientific rationale for the procedure rests on the basics of the physiological changes that occur after death.[29] These changes occur at a regular rate depending on the temperature of the body at the time of death, the size of the body, the extent of infection (if any), and the temperature of the air. The three important physiological changes—rigor mortis, algor mortis, and postmortem decomposition—are discussed along with the relevant nursing implications in Table 31.2.

Care of and respect for the body after death by nursing staff should clearly communicate to the family that the person who died was indeed important and valued. Often, caring for the body after death provides the needed link between family members and the reality of the death, recognizing that everyone present at the time of death and soon after will have a different experience and a different sense of loss. Many institutions no longer require nursing staff to care for patients after death or perform postmortem care. Further, there are few professional resources related to postmortem care and the most recent ones are not easily accessible.[31] Those

available are largely found in the British nursing literature and do not reflect a thorough knowledge of postmortem changes.[32–34] A recent analysis of postmortem policies in California hospitals found that the focus was primarily on legal procedures and the physical preparation of the body.[35] Postmortem care is clearly more than attention to the legal imperatives and physical care. A kind, gentle approach and meticulous attention to detail grounded in knowledge of the physiology of dying and death is imperative.

Rituals that family members and others present find comforting should be encouraged. Rituals are practices within a social context that facilitate and provide ways to understand and cope with the contradictory and complex nature of human existence. They provide a means to express and contain strong emotions, ease feelings of anxiety and impotence, and provide structure in times of chaos and disorder. Rituals can take many forms—a brief service at the time of death, a special preparation of the body, as in the Orthodox Jewish tradition, or an Irish wake, where, after paying respect to the person who has died, family and friends gather to share stories, food, and drink. Of utmost importance, however, is to ensure that family members see the ritual as comforting and meaningful. It is the family's needs and desires that direct this activity—not the nurse's. There are, again, no rules that govern

Table 31.2 Normal postmortem physiological changes and their implications for nursing and care of the body after death

Change	Underlying mechanisms	Nursing implications
Rigor mortis	Approximately 2 to 6 hours after death, adenosine phosphate (ATP) ceases to be synthesized due to the depletion of glycogen stores. Because ATP is necessary for muscle fiber relaxation, the lack of ATP results in an exaggerated contraction of the muscle fibers that eventually immobilizes the joints. Rigor begins in the involuntary muscles (heart, gastrointestinal tract, bladder, arteries) and progresses to the muscles of the eyelids, head and neck, trunk, and lower limbs. After approximately 96 hours, however, muscle chemical activity totally ceases, and rigor passes. Persons with large muscle mass (e.g., body builders) are prone to more pronounced rigor mortis. Conversely, frail elderly persons and persons who have been bed bound for long periods are less subject to rigor mortis.[30]	The guiding principle is to understand rigor mortis is a natural and temporary postmortem change and immediate positioning of the deceased does not impact the appearance of the body long term. After death, position the person in as relaxed and peaceful a manner as is possible. For example, close the eyes (using petroleum jelly on the eyelids can help to keep them closed), position the patient with the head on a pillow or on his/her side so the jaw does not hang open, and fold the hands. If rigor mortis does occur, it can often be "massaged out" by the funeral director.[30] Finally, by understanding this physiology, the nurse can also reassure the family about the myth that due to rigor mortis, muscles can suddenly contract and the body can appear to move.
Algor mortis	After the circulation ceases and the hypothalamus stops functioning, internal body temperature drops by approximately 1°C or 1.8°F per hour until it reaches room temperature. As the body cools, skin loses its natural elasticity. If a high fever was present at death, the changes in body temperature are more pronounced and the person may appear to "sweat" after death. Body cooling may also take several more hours.[30]	The nurse can prepare family members for the coolness of the skin to touch or the increased moisture by explaining the changes that happen after death. The nurse may also suggest kissing the person on their hair instead of their skin. The skin, due to loss of elasticity, becomes fragile and easily torn. If dressings are to be applied, it is best to apply them with either a circular bandage or paper tape. Handle the body gently as well, being sure to not place traction on the skin.
Postmortem decomposition or "liver mortis"	Discoloration and softening of the body are caused largely by the breakdown of red blood cells and the resultant release of hemoglobin that stains the vessel walls and surrounding tissue. This staining appears as a mottling, bruising, or both in the dependent parts of the body as well as parts of the body where the skin has been punctured (e.g., intravenous or chest tube sites).[34] Often this discoloration becomes extensive in a very short time. The remainder of the body has a gray hue. In cardiac-related deaths, the face often appears purple in color regardless of the positioning at or after death.[30]	As the body is handled (e.g., while bathing and dressing), the nurse informs the family member about this normal change that occurs after death. Prop the body up with pillows under the head and shoulders or raise the head of the bed approximately 30°. Remove heavy blankets and clothing and cover the deceased with a light blanket of sheet.[30]

the appropriateness of rituals; rituals are comforting and serve to begin the process of healing and acceptance.

To facilitate the grieving process, it is often helpful to create a pleasant, peaceful, and comfortable environment for family members who wish to spend time with the body, according to their desires and cultural or religious traditions. The nurse should consider engaging family members in after-death care and ritual by inviting them to either comb the hair or wash the person's hands and face, or more if they are comfortable. Parents can be encouraged to hold and cuddle their baby or child. Including siblings or other involved children in rituals, traditions, and other end-of-life care activities according to their developmental level is also essential. During this time, family members should be invited to talk about their family member who has died, and encouraged to reminisce—valuable rituals that can help them begin to work through their grief.

The family should be encouraged to touch, hold, and kiss the person's body, as they feel comfortable. Parents may wish to clip and save a lock of hair as a keepsake. The nurse may offer to dress the person's body in something other than a hospital gown or other nightclothes. Babies may be wrapped snugly in a blanket. Many families choose to dress the body in a favorite article of clothing before removal by the funeral home. It should be noted that, at times, when a body is being turned, air escapes from the lungs, producing a "sighing" sound. Informing family members of this possibility is wise. If the eyes remain open they can often be closed by applying petroleum jelly to the eyelids.[30] Again, modeling gentle and careful handling of the body can communicate care and concern on the part of the nurse and facilitate grieving and the creation of positive and long-lasting memories.

Postmortem care also includes, unless an autopsy or the coroner is involved, removal of any tubes, drains, and other devices. In home care settings, these can be placed in a plastic bag and given to the funeral home for disposal as medical waste or simply double-bagged and placed in the family's regular trash. Placing a waterproof pad, diaper, or adult incontinence brief on the patient often prevents soiling and odor as the patient's body is moved and the rectal and urinary bladder sphincters relax. Packing of the rectum and vagina is considered unnecessary, because not allowing these areas to drain increases the rate of bacterial proliferation that naturally occurs.[30]

Occasionally families, especially in the home care setting, wish to keep the person's body at home, perhaps to wait for another family member to come from a distance and to ensure that everyone has adequate time with the deceased. If the family wishes the body to be embalmed, this is generally best done within 12 hours. If embalming is not desired, the body can, in most cases, remain in the home for approximately 24 hours before further decomposition and odor production occur. However, state laws vary on the amount of time a body can remain in the home and not be refrigerated. If the family wishes to have the body remain in the home, the nurse can suggest to the family that they adjust the temperature in the immediate area to a comfortable but cooler level and remove heavy blankets or coverings.[30] Be sure, however, to inform the funeral director that the family has chosen to keep the body at home a little longer. Finally, reputable funeral directors are a reliable source of information regarding postdeath changes, local customs, and cultural issues.

Care of the body after death is a significantly meaningful experience for nurses. In addition to mindfully providing support for the family, including preparing the body for viewing, many nurses regard care of the body as a sacred act, communicating dignity for the person who died and his/her family. Support of coworkers and management in providing after death care is critical and enhances job satisfaction and coping with the demands of caring for persons and their families/close others at the end of life.[36]

The care of patients and families near the time of death and afterward is an important nursing function—arguably one of the most important. As the following case studies are reviewed, consider how the nurse interceded in a positive manner, mindful of the changing tempo of care and the changing patient and family needs, desires, and perspectives.

Case study

Tom, a 68-year-old man with end-stage liver disease

Tom, an unemployed veteran of the Vietnam War, had married twice in his life, and divorced twice. Tom had two adult sons who live in nearby towns. He and his second wife were best of friends but "just could not live together." At the time of their divorce, he returned to his parents' home to live. Although that was initially disconcerting for his parents, he fulfilled an important role in helping them during the decline and death of his father. After the death of his father, his mother welcomed Tom's presence in the home even more. They were able to establish a respectful relationship that allowed each other to continue to function in their different communities of friends. Tom was a smoker and a former heavy drinker and, by all accounts, had a pretty unhealthy life. His mother and he were able to work out the details of their coexistence, basically tolerating each other's quirks. Tom's mother was grateful for some help around the house and yard and Tom was grateful for a place to live.

Over time, Tom's mother noticed he was losing weight and had a slight yellowing of his skin. Tom would not answer when questioned about it, saying that he was fine. She persisted and urged him to go to a clinic and get it checked out. He resisted her "nagging," but promised he would see someone soon. He finally relented, made an appointment, and saw someone in within a week. His provider told him she suspected cirrhosis and ordered more testing, including an abdominal ultrasound. Tom left the clinic without stopping at the lab or scheduling the ultrasound. He couldn't help thinking of a good friend who had died of liver disease a few years ago. He was frightened and didn't know where to turn.

Goals and framework of care: Upon Tom's return home from his first appointment, his mother asked, "so what is wrong and what is the plan?" Tom responded that he might follow up with a few tests, but wanted to wait and see. . . . His mother responded that she was really scared of what was going on, and hoped he would follow up as soon as possible. There was tension between the two, as both had different goals.

The tension lasted for 2 weeks. Tom simply did not schedule appointments or plan to follow through. Then, one night, his mother found him collapsed on the bathroom floor. She called an ambulance, and he was admitted to the hospital, where he agreed to the previously ordered tests. He was diagnosed with end-stage cirrhosis.

After receiving the diagnosis, Tom refused consultation with a specialist. He just wanted to go home and get strong enough so he could hang out with his friends. He went home and was able to enjoy some time with his friends. After 2 weeks, he became confused and he collapsed again at home after vomiting frank blood.

He was again admitted to the hospital, where esophageal varices were discovered; the bleeding stopped, and he received transfusions for his severe anemia.

Goals and framework of care: The shift in goals started at this time. Tom agreed to meet with a gastroenterologist, who evaluated the source of his bleeding and was able to ligate the source of the hemorrhage. Tom was also told he could lengthen his life by strictly adhering to the recommendations of diet and medications.

Tom would not share his diagnosis with friends or his children. His mother decided she would. She told the staff simply, "I should tell them if he won't." Tom's former wife and children "stepped to the plate" quite well and talked to Tom openly about what they would like to do to help him and asked him to continue to dialogue with them.

Tom did experience a sense of control of his disease. Over the following 6 months, Tom was able to go hunting and fishing and help his mother with some of the projects that needed to be done on her house. At the end of 6 months, he again began to notice his stools were darker and again underwent ligation of his esophageal varices. He began exploring the chance of liver transplantation and, even though he was not considered an optimal candidate, met with the liver transplant center closest to home. He was hopeful this would work out—and started to work on stopping smoking. He was discouraged when he learned he was indeed not eligible for transplant but figured he would explore other options until he found a center that would be willing to put him on the transplant list.

Goals and framework of care: Suddenly there seemed to truly be a very large "elephant in the room." Death was the unspoken word. After a few days of this, his mother called his former wife and asked her if she would talk to Tom about his wishes. At her next visit, his former wife, Dixie, suggested that they speak with a lawyer, together. He agreed, and then next day, working together, Tom and Dixie, "put his affairs in order." He also was able to talk with her about his preferences for care in the event (which to him seemed unlikely) he would not be able to make decisions for himself. He designated Dixie as the person he wanted to make decisions for him and completed the necessary documentation for the state they lived in.

Tom continued to contact transplant centers but became increasingly weaker and fell several times while trying to get up out of his bed or chair. He also became delirious and began again to vomit frank blood. He returned to the hospital, where it was determined that he was in the end stages of liver failure and near death. Guided by his advance directive, the conversations he had with Dixie, and the prognostic estimation of the palliative care team, he was referred to a hospice program and transferred to an inpatient hospice facility. His delirium and pain were assessed and managed. Massive hemorrhage was anticipated and his mother and other visitors, including Dixie and his children, were prepared for the possibility. Additional medications were ordered and were readily accessible should hemorrhage occur. Five days later, he died quietly, about 10 minutes after his mother had left his bedside following an 8-hour vigil. Dixie later told his mother that dying alone was important to him.

His words, "I DID IT MY WAY." are on his gravestone, at his request.

Critical points

- Minimizing symptoms until they reach a critical point may be a conscious decision of patients who have few remaining life goals.

- Open discussion of goals is controlled by the readiness of the patient.

- Recognizing the "moment" for the open discussion is critical. Encouraging family members to listen and "seize the moment" when it comes is an important family education point.

- Patients will do it their way. Helping them find their way is an important role of the nurse.

Case study

Susan, a 30-year-old woman with breast cancer

Susan was breastfeeding her first child, a son, 8 months old, when she noted a mass in her breast. She immediately saw her physician, who was not certain of the mass's relationship to lactation but ordered an ultrasound of the breast to be "on the safe side." The ultrasound was completed and was soon followed by a mammogram, biopsy, and diagnosis of stage II breast cancer with one positive lymph node. Susan underwent a staging workup, surgery, and started chemotherapy within 3 weeks of noticing the breast lump. It was difficult for her to see past the positive lymph node; all discussions seemed to come back to it, and the meaning of one positive node. Her anxiety was apparent during her interactions with care providers. Program staff worked to provide extra time and strong emotional support for her. Family and friends were present and expressed the desire to be ready to help at any time.

Goals and framework of care: Despite Susan's positive lymph node, the cancer was still considered "early" and very treatable. Susan successfully completed chemotherapy and radiation therapy and was set up for routine surveillance. She was encouraged to use the program's psychosocial resources to help her with any questions and particularly when her fears of recurrence and a dismal future seemed to immobilize her.

Susan openly talked of what would happen if her cancer did reoccur. Who would assist her husband in raising her child? What would be important for her to leave her child? She was encouraged to think these things through, so she could have the appropriate discussions with her husband and then move forward as best she could. Slowly, she was able to do this.

Susan focused on regaining her past lifestyle. She returned to community work on a part-time basis and often talked of the value of her work in helping others. She had a great sense of "giving back." Life seemed to settle for her, until one day when she called reporting a sudden onset of back pain. Bone scan and CT showed bone and early lung metastasis. Susan and her husband received imaging results together in the clinic and then opted to return the next day to speak with the medical oncologist.

Goals and framework of care: Together with her medical oncologist, Susan and her husband mapped out a plan for initial treatment. Although she was not eligible for clinical trials, she was interested in looking for any opportunity that would give her the best chance of quality time. She clearly stated her goal "to receive treatment that would buy as many days of 'quality time' that was available, defining quality time as being present, participating, and enjoying her son's daily life." Her goal had been well thought out.

Susan started on chemotherapy. She responded well for 9 months, and had an "almost normal" life. When the second-line chemotherapy failed to control her disease, she agreed to the third-line chemotherapy. Although she tolerated the third line well, her disease progressed in spite of the treatment. Scans and lab work were not necessary to tell the staff that her liver function was rapidly declining. Ascites from her new liver metastasis complicated her comfort level and functional status. She agreed to hospitalization for symptomatic evaluation.

Goals and framework of care: During her admission to the hospital, Susan was offered a fourth-line chemotherapy regimen. After a quick discussion with her husband, she refused. She asked only that a plan for management of her discomfort be addressed, and that hospice be arranged for her.

Susan said her good-byes to the staff. She was discharged with a home hospice program, stating she simply wanted to have the freedom to have her son with her to hug and cuddle without any restrictions or expectations. She died at home, surrounded by prepared, loving and caring family and friends, 48 hours later.

Critical points

◆ Patients will often process their disease trajectory with minimal help other than the supportive, listening ears of their care providers.

◆ Patient fears are based in their reality, and we, as care providers, must not minimize or dismiss them.

◆ Patients who set clearly defined goals and are given the opportunity to share them with their care providers are generally observed to have a higher quality death experience for themselves, their family members, and the staff who care for them.

Summary

Assisting and walking alongside dying patients and their families, especially near and after death, is an honor and privilege. Nowhere else in the practice of nursing are we invited to be companions on such a remarkable journey as that of a dying patient and his or her family. Likewise, nowhere else in the practice of nursing are our words, actions, and guidance more remembered and cherished. Caring for dying patients and families is indeed the essence of nursing. Take this responsibility seriously, understanding that although it may be stressful and difficult at times, it comes with personal and professional satisfaction beyond measure. Listen to your patients and their families. They are the guides to this remarkable and momentous journey. Listen closely to them with a positive regard, empathy, and genuineness, and approach their care with an acute attention to every detail and always remember, we often only have one chance to "get it right." The patients we care for and their families—in fact, all of us—are counting on *you*.

References

1. Twycross R, Lichter I. The terminal phase. In: Hanks G, Cherny NI, Christakis NA, Fallon M, Portenoy R (eds.), Oxford Textbook of Palliative Medicine. 4th ed. Oxford: Oxford University Press; 2009:977–994.
2. Kehl KA, Kowalkowski JA. A systematic review of the prevalence of signs and symptoms of impending death and symptoms in the last 2 weeks of life. Am J Hosp Palliat Med. 2013;30(6):601–616.
3. Currow DC, Smith J, Davidson PM, Newton PJ, Agar MR, Abernathy AP. Do the trajectories of dyspnea differ in prevalence and intensity by diagnosis at end of life?: A consecutive cohort study. J Pain Symptom Manage. 2010;39:680–690.
4. Hendricks SA, Smakbrugge M, Hertogh CMPM, van der Steen JT. Dying with dementia: symptoms, treatment, and quality of life in the last week of life. J Pain Symptom Manage. 2013. Epub ahead of print. doi: 10.1016/j.jpainsymman.2013.05.015.
5. Moyer DD. Review article: terminal delirium in geriatric patients with cancer at end of life. Am J Hosp Palliat Care. 2011;28(1):44–51. doi: 10.1177/1049909110376755.
6. King S, Forbes K, Hanks GW, Ferro CJ, Chambers EJ. A systematic review of the use of opioid medication for those with moderate to severe cancer pain and renal impairment: a European Palliative Care Research Collaborative opioid guidelines project. Palliat Med. 2011; 25(5): 525–552.
7. Cambell ML, Yarandi HN. Death rattle is not associated with patient respiratory distress: is pharmacological treatment indicated? J Palliat Med. 2013;16(10):1255–1259. doi: 10.1089/jpm.2013.0122. Epub 2013 Sep 18.
8. Bailey FA, Williams BR, Goode PS, Woodby LL, Redden DT, Johnson TM 2nd, et al. Opioid pain medication orders and administration in the last days of life. J Pain Symptom Manage. 2012;44(5):681–691. doi: 10.1016/j.jpainsymman.2011.11.006. Epub 2012 Jul 4.
9. Ferris F. Last hours of living. Clin Ger Med. 2004;20:641–67.
10. Rogers C. On Becoming a Person: A Therapist's View of Psychology. Boston: Houghton Mifflin; 1961.
11. National Consensus Project for Quality Palliative Care. Clinical Practice Guidelines for Quality Palliative Care. 3rd ed. Pittsburgh, PA; 2013. http://www.nationalconsensusproject.org. Accessed November 1, 2013.
12. Du Boulay S. Cicely Saunders: Founder of the Modern Hospice Movement. London: Hodder and Stoughton; 1984.
13. Ambuel B, Weissman D. Fast Fact and Concept #016: Conducting a Family Conference (2nd ed). 2009. Available at http://www.eperc.mcw.edu/EPERC/FastFactsIndex/ff_016.htm. Accessed June 30, 2013.
14. Osenga K, Cleary JF. Fever and sweats. In: Berger AM, Shuster JL, Von Roenn JH (eds.), Principles and Practice of Palliative Care and Supportive Oncology. 3rd ed. New York: Lippincott Williams & Wilkins; 2007:105–116.
15. Kazure HS, Roman SA, Sosa JA. Epidemiology and outcomes of in-hospital cardiopulmonary resuscitation in the United States, 2000–2009. Resuscitation. 2013;84(9):1255–1260. doi: 10.1016/j.resuscitation.2013.02.021. Epub 2013 Mar 5.
16. Kjorstad OJ, Haugen DF. Cardiopulmonary resuscitation in palliative care cancer patients. Tidsskr Nor Laegeforen. 2013;133(4):417–421. doi: 10.4045/tidsskr.12.0378.
17. Dunn H. Hard Choices for Loving People: CPR, Artificial Feeding, Comfort Care and the Patient with a Life-Threatening Illness. 5th ed. Herndon, VA: A & A; 2009.
18. Zerwekh J. Do dying patients really need IV fluids? Am J Nurs. 1997;97:26–31.
19. Raijmakers NJH, van Zuylen L, Costantini M, Caraceni A, Clark J, Lundquist G, et al. Artificial nutrition and hydration in the last week of life in cancer patients: a systematic literature review of practices and effects. Ann Oncol. 2011;22(7):1478–1486. doi: 10.1093/annonc/mdq620.
20. Hospice and Palliative Nurses Association. HPNA Position Statement: Withholding and/or Withdrawing Life Sustaining Therapies. Pittsburgh: Hospice and Palliative Nurses Association; 2011.
21. Working Party on Clinical Guidelines in Palliative Care. Changing Gear—Guidelines for Managing the Last Days of Life. London: National Council for Hospice and Specialist Palliative Care Services; 2010.
22. Fromme, EK, Stewart, TL, Jepperson, M, Tolle, SW. Adverse experiences with implantable defibrillators in Oregon hospices. Am J Hosp Palliat Care. 2011;28(5):304–309.

23. National Hospice and Palliative Care Organization. Position Statement on the Care of Hospice Patients with Automatic Implantable Cardioverter-Defibrillators. Arlington, VA: National Hospice and Palliative Care Organization; 2008.

24. Davison, SN, Rosielle DA. Fast Fact and Concept #207: Withdrawal of Dialysis: Decision-Making. 2008. Available at http://www.eperc.mcw.edu/EPERC/FastFactsIndex/ff_207.htm. accessed June 30, 2013.

25. Davison, SN, Rosielle DA. Fast Facts and Concepts #208: Clinical Care Following Withdrawal of Dialysis. 2008. Available at http://www.eperc.mcw.edu/EPERC/FastFactsIndex/ff_208.htm. Accessed June 30, 2013.

26. Hwang IC, Ahn HY, Park SM, Sim JY, Kim KK. Clinical changes in terminally ill cancer patients and death within 48 h: when should we refer patients to a separate room? Support Care Cancer. 2013;21:835–840. doi 10.1007/s00520-012-1587-4.

27. Kehl KA, Kirchoff KT, Finster MP, Cleary JF. Materials to prepare hospice families for dying in the home. J Palliat Med. 2008;11(7):969–972.

28. Department of Health and Human Services, Health Care Financing Administration. Medicare and Medicaid Programs; Hospital Conditions of Participation; Identification of Potential Organ, Tissue, and Eye Donors and Transplant Hospitals' Provision of Transplant-Related Data. Final rule. 63 Federal Register 119 (1998) (codified at 42 CFR §482.45).

29. Pennington EA. Postmortem care: more than ritual. Am J Nurs. 1978;75:846–847.

30. Tjaarda, Natasha, AAS, Licensed Funeral Director and Embalmer, Young's Funeral Home, Tigard, OR, personal communication, June, 2013.

31. Caramanzana H, Wilches P. The final act of nursing care. J Contin Educ Nurs. 2012;43(7):295–296.

32. Beattie S. Hands-on-help: post-mortem care. RN. 2006;69(10): 24ac1–24ac4.

33. Higgins D. Clinical practical programs: carrying out last offices, Part 1—Preparing for the procedure. Nurs Times. 2008;104(37):20–1.

34. Higgins D. Clinical practical programs: Carrying out last offices, Part 2—Preparation of the body. Nurs Times. 2008;104(38):24–5.

35. Smith-Stoner M, Hand MW. Expanding the concept of patient care: analysis of postmortem policies in California hospitals. Med Surg Nurs. 2012;21(6) 360–366.

36. Olausson J, Ferrell BR. Care of the body after death: nurses' perspectives of the meaning of post-death patient care. Clin J Oncol Nurs. 2013;17(6) 647–651.

CHAPTER 32

Spiritual assessment

Elizabeth Johnston Taylor

Spiritual assessment questions are unbelievably intrusive to me. If a health professional asked me such questions as part of their professional activities, I would tell them to mind their business. Asking a patient about personal spirituality or religion is like asking about their sex life. We are nurses!

I say to my patients, "It takes a lot of strength to go through an illness like yours. Where do you get your strength from?" I find a simple question like this very easy to remember, and it takes the word religion out of the assessment. This is important to do because people who do not have a formal religion could get confused or feel that their spirituality doesn't count. ... Because I care for people in their own homes, this can often give many clues to their spirituality. Our patients have very low energy levels and tire very easily so a simple question is often all that is appropriate.

Hospice registered nurses' responses to a survey about spiritual assessment

My husband and I are private about these [spiritual] things. We both know that there are chaplains available if we want to talk to them. My husband is very nonreligious and would not want to be asked these questions. Nurses have got enough to do already without bothering with religion.

I believe that any way [a nurse inquired about spiritual well-being] would be appropriate. If you are open about your belief, then there is no way an inquiry will be taken in offense.

Hospice care recipients' responses to a survey about nurse spiritual assessment

Key points

◆ Spiritual assessment precedes effective spiritual caregiving. Because palliative care patients and their family members use spiritual coping strategies, and spiritual well-being can buffer the distress of dying, spiritual care is integral to palliative care.

◆ Numerous typologies identifying the dimensions of spirituality exist and provide guidance for what to address in a spiritual assessment.

◆ A two-tiered approach to spiritual assessment allows the nurse to first conduct a superficial assessment to screen for spiritual problems or needs.

◆ If needed, a more focused or comprehensive spiritual assessment should be conducted by a competent professional, typically a trained chaplain. Need for further assessment is evidenced by manifestations of spiritual distress that are relevant to health.

◆ Most experts recommending a spiritual screening question agree that it is first important to assess how important or relevant spirituality is to the patient.

◆ Salient spiritual screening questions include: "How does your spirituality help you to live with your illness?" and "What can I/we do to support your spiritual beliefs and practices?"

◆ Spiritual assessment strategies include obtaining spiritual histories, life stories, and pictorial depictions of spiritual experience, as well as asking simple questions.

◆ Although spirituality should be assessed near the time of admission to palliative care service, the process of assessment should be ongoing.

◆ Spiritual assessment data should be documented to at least some extent.

To solve any problem, one must first assess what the problem is. Consequently, the nursing process dictates that the nurse begin care with an assessment of the patient's health needs. Although palliative nurses are accustomed to assessing patients' pain experiences, hydration status, and so forth, they less frequently participate in assessing patients' and family members' spirituality.

Because spirituality is an inherent and integrating, and often extremely valued, dimension for those who receive palliative nursing care, it is essential that palliative care nurses know to some degree how to conduct a spiritual assessment. This chapter reviews models for spiritual assessment, presents general guidelines on how to conduct a spiritual assessment, and discusses what the nurse ought to do with data from a spiritual assessment. These topics are prefaced by arguments supporting the need for spiritual assessments, descriptions of what spirituality "looks like" among the terminally ill, and risk factors for those who are likely to experience spiritual distress. But first, a description of spirituality is in order.

What is spirituality?

Numerous analyses of the concept of spirituality have identified key aspects of this ethereal and intangible phenomenon. Conceptualizations of spirituality often include the following as aspects of spirituality: the need for purpose and meaning, forgiveness, love and relatedness, hope, creativity, and religious faith and its expression. A classic nursing definition for spirituality, authored by Reed,[1] proposed that spirituality involves meaning-making through intrapersonal, interpersonal, and transpersonal connection. More recent definitions of spirituality accepted by healthcare scholars emphasize not only the human search for ultimate meaning but also the human desire for harmonious connectedness with self, others, an ultimate Other, and for some, the environment.[2]

Usually, spirituality is differentiated from religion—the organized, codified, and often institutionalized beliefs and practices that express one's spirituality.[3] To use Narayansamy's metaphor: "Spirituality is more of a journey and religion may be the transport to help us in our journey."[4(p. 141)] Definitions of spirituality typically include transcendence—that is, spirituality explains persons' need to transcend the self, often manifested in recognition of an Ultimate Other, Sacred Source, Higher Power, divinity, or God. Although these definitions allow for an open interpretation of what a person considers to be sacred or transcendent, some have argued that such a definition for spirituality is inappropriate for atheists, humanists, and those who do not accept a spiritual reality.[5] Indeed, a pluralistic definition of spirituality (however "elastic" and vague it is) is necessary for ethical practice, and hence a spiritual assessment process that is sensitive to the myriad of world views is essential—if it is even appropriate for those who reject a spiritual reality.[6]

The spiritual assessment methods introduced in this chapter are all influenced inherently by some conceptualization of spirituality. Some, however, have questioned whether spiritual assessment is possible, given the broad, encompassing definition typically espoused by nurses.[7,8] Bash contended that "spirituality" is an "elastic" term that cannot be universally defined. Because a patient's definition of spirituality may differ from the nurse's assumptions about it, Bash argued that widely applicable tools for spiritual assessment are impossible to design. It is important to note, therefore, that the literature and methods for spiritual assessment presented in this chapter are primarily from the United States and United Kingdom, influenced most by Western Judeo-Christian traditions and peoples. Hence, they are most applicable to these people.

Why is it important for a palliative care nurse to conduct a spiritual assessment?

Spiritual awareness increases as one faces an imminent death.[9,10] Although some may experience spiritual distress or "soul pain," others may have a spiritual transformation or experience spiritual growth and health. There is mounting empirical evidence to suggest that persons with terminal illnesses consider spirituality to be one of the most important contributors to quality of life.[11]

For example, research findings from various studies indicate that spiritual well-being may protect terminal cancer patients against end-of-life despair; it also has moderately strong inverse relationships with the desire for a hastened death, hopelessness, and suicidal ideations. Religious beliefs and practices (e.g., prayer, beliefs that explain suffering or death) are also known to be valued and frequently used as helpful coping strategies among those who suffer and die from physical illness.[3] Family caregivers of seriously ill patients also find comfort and strength from their spirituality that assists them in coping.[12,13]

The above themes from research imply that attention to the spirituality of terminally ill patients and their caregivers is of utmost importance. That is, if patients' spiritual resources assist them in coping, and if imminent death precipitates heightened spiritual awareness and concerns, and if patients view their spiritual health as most important to their quality of life, then spiritual assessment that initiates a process promoting spiritual health is vital to effective palliative care. It is for reasons such as these that the National Consensus Project (NCP) and National Quality Forum, included guidelines and preferred practices for supporting spirituality in palliative care.[14] The NCP guidelines (5.1) state: "Spiritual and existential dimensions are assessed and responded to based upon the best available evidence, which is skillfully and systematically applied."

Providing even stronger motivation perhaps for systematically including spiritual assessment in palliative care is The Joint Commission mandate.[15] The Joint Commission stipulates that for clients entering an approved facility, a spiritual assessment should, at least, "determine the patients denomination, beliefs, and what spiritual practices are important." They also require that the institution define the scope and process of the assessment and who completes it. Often nurses are charged with completing the spiritual assessment as part of an intake assessment.

Why, as the nurse quoted at the top of this chapter argued, should palliative care nurses be conducting spiritual assessments? After all, chaplains and clergy are the spiritual care experts. Although chaplains are the trained experts in spiritual care, current mainstream thinking on this topic espouses that all members of a hospice team participate in spiritual caregiving. This position was crystalized during a multidisciplinary consensus project that offered the following guidelines for spiritual care in end-of-life care:

- All patients should be screened for spiritual distress upon admission, and a referral made if support is needed

- Structured assessment tools are recommended to aid documentation and evaluation of care

- All palliative care clinicians should be trained to recognize and report spiritual distress

- All clinicians should be trained to perform a spiritual screening; more thorough assessments are to be completed by a certified chaplain

- Screenings and assessments should be documented

- Patients should be reassessed when there is a change in their condition.[16]

Not only do professional palliative care recommendations include nurses in the process of spiritual assessment but also generic nursing ethics and professional standards support the nursing role in health-related spiritual and religious assessment.[3] Indeed, considering nurses' frontline position, coordination role, and intimacy with the concerns of patients; the holistic perspective on care; and even their lack of religious cloaking, nurses can be the ideal professionals for completing an initial spiritual assessment if they have some preparation for doing so.

However, nurses must recognize that they are not specialists in spiritual assessment and caregiving; they are generalists. Most oncology and hospice nurses perceive that they do not receive adequate training in spiritual assessment and care. In fact, it is this lack of training, accompanied by role confusion, lack of time, and other factors that nurses often cite as barriers to completing spiritual assessments.[17,18] Therefore, when a nurse's assessment indicates need for further sensitive assessment and specialized care, it is imperative that a referral to a spiritual care specialist (e.g., chaplain, clergy, patient's spiritual director) be made.

How does spirituality manifest itself?

To understand how to assess spirituality, the palliative care nurse must know for what to look. What subjective and objective observations would indicate spiritual distress or well-being? Numerous descriptive studies have identified the spiritual needs of patients and their loved ones facing the end of life.[19] Likewise, clinicians have written articles that describe the spiritual concerns of these persons. Whereas any listing of what spiritual issues might arise at the end of life would be incomplete, Puchalski and colleagues[2] provide a fairly comprehensive listing:

Lack of meaning and purpose (e.g., "Why do I have to suffer on the way to death? Why couldn't I just go to my death in my sleep?" [meaninglessness of suffering]; "I feel like I never really did anything important in life, and now it's too late")

Despair and hopelessness (e.g., "I just want to give up ... its not worth it anymore" [although some would argue that complete hopelessness is incompatible with life, hopefulness is sometimes hard to feel])

Religious struggle (e.g., "Sometimes it is hard to believe there is a loving God upstairs that has my best interests in mind" [religious struggles can arise for those who have not been religious during their adulthood, as they may struggle with the beliefs instilled in them during childhood])

Not being remembered (e.g., "Death is just so final; I know my friends will eventually move on and I'll have been like a blip on the monitor.")

Guilt and shame (e.g., "I think my cancer is a punishment for something I did when I was young")

Loss of dignity (e.g., "Look and smell this body! It's so embarrassing ... it's not me anymore")

Lack of love, loneliness (e.g., "Everyone is so busy ... too busy to take care of me")

Anger at God/others (e.g., "Why would a loving God allow this to happen to me?")

Perceiving abandonment by God/others (e.g., "I feel like my prayers aren't being answered ... where is God?")

Feeling out of control (e.g., "I'm ready to go ... but it's not happening.")

Distress secondary to misinterpretation of religious dogma or religious or spiritual community actions that impede full development of human potential

Reconciliation (e.g., desire to be reunited with estranged family members)

Grief/loss (spiritual issues often accompany the various losses persons mourn when living with a terminal illness, such as the loss of independence, social roles and vocation, body image and function)

Gratitude (e.g., "Now I have learned to appreciate the little things in life, and I'm just so happy for each new day that dawns")

Although the terminology "spiritual need" may suggest a problem, spiritual needs can also be of a positive nature, as the final bullet above illustrates. For example, patients can have a need to express their joy about sensing closeness to others, or have a need to pursue activities that allow expression of creative impulses (e.g., artwork, music making, writing). The following models for conducting a spiritual assessment will provide further understanding of how spirituality manifests.

Spiritual assessment models

Healthcare professionals from multiple disciplines offer models for spiritual assessment. The most useful models from chaplaincy, medicine, social work, and nursing will be presented here. Although some assessment models have been published during the past few years, many were developed in the 1990s, when the research about spiritual care began to proliferate. Although some were developed by clinicians caring for the terminally ill, others—easily adapted or used with those at the end of life—were developed for general use for those with an illness.

Many advocate a two-tiered approach to spiritual assessment.[2,3,20] That is, a brief assessment for screening purposes is conducted when a patient enters a healthcare institution for palliative care. If the screening assessment generates an impression that there are spiritual needs, then spiritual care can only be planned if further information is collected. The second tier of assessment allows for focused, in-depth assessment. Some chaplains further distinguish a spiritual assessment from a spiritual history, an in-depth review of one's spiritual journey through life (best done by a trained chaplain or spiritual care expert). After reviewing recommended spiritual screening questions, more comprehensive models or approaches to spiritual assessment will be presented.

Screening

Recognizing the spiritual plurality within society, and that some persons may not experience a spiritual reality, an initial screening must therefore assess for this basic orientation.[3] Others assume spirituality is universal and posit that a spiritual screening should check for the significance of the beliefs and practices to the present illness circumstances and ascertain how the patient may want spiritual support from the healthcare team. Various clinical authors proffer single questions for broaching the topic of spirituality with a patient. For example:

- How important is spirituality or religion to you?[21] Kub and colleagues,[22] in their research with 114 terminally ill persons, found a single question about the importance of religion to be more discriminating than a question about frequency of attendance at religious services—a question that has often been the sole "spiritual assessment" in some institutions.

♦ What do you rely on in times of illness?[23]

♦ Are you at peace? This question was found to correlate highly with spiritual and emotional well-being in large a study of terminally ill patients.[24]

Two other screening approaches that are very concise have been proposed by physicians Lo and colleagues,[25] who suggested the following questions for use in palliative care settings:

♦ Is faith/religion/spirituality important to you in this illness? Has faith been important to you at other times in your life?

♦ Do you have someone to talk to about religious matters? Would you like to explore religious matters with someone?

Striving to have an even more streamlined spiritual assessment, Matthews and colleagues'[26] proposed initial spiritual assessments could be limited to asking "Is your religion (or faith) helpful to you in handling your illness?" and "What can I do to support your faith or religious commitment?"

Several clinicians have devised mnemonic tools for use in spiritual assessment (see Table 32.1). Although some of these are fairly comprehensive, some of them are designed so as to collect superficial information—to screen. The most widely cited tool is likely Pulchaski's[27] FICA tool.

Hodge[33] essentially proposed the same content for his brief assessment, arguing that it well meets the Joint Commission requirement. Hodge's assessment questions include the following:

♦ I was wondering if spirituality or religion is important to you?

♦ Are there certain spiritual beliefs and practices that you find particularly helpful in dealing with problems?

♦ I was wondering if you attend a church or some other type of spiritual community?

♦ Are there any spiritual needs or concerns I can help you with?"[33(p. 319)]

The nonintrusive tone with which these questions are worded is exemplary.

A German medical researcher, using basically the same content (i.e., Would you describe yourself—in the broadest sense of the term—as a believing/spiritual/religious person? What is the place of spirituality in your life? How integrated are you in a spiritual community? What role would you like to assign to your healthcare team with regard to spirituality?), found that these questions were helpful for both patients and physicians.[34]

A prototype for a spiritual screening tool is offered in Box 32.1. This tool can be adapted to meet the unique needs of any palliative care context. It can be completed by either the patient or with the assistance of a nurse. Because it is unknown how well family can serve as proxies for measurements of spiritual health, and because responses may be easily swayed by social desirability, it is best to not have family complete such a tool. Such a tool can be inserted in the patient chart and guide ongoing spiritual assessment and care. This tool is purposefully concise to accommodate the palliative care patient who is often weak and suffering from symptom distress.

Comprehensive models

If the screening assessment, or subsequent observation, provides preliminary evidence that a spiritual need exists that might benefit from spiritual care from a member of the palliative care team, then a more comprehensive assessment is in order. Depending on the situation, a more in-depth assessment regarding the specific spiritual need or a grand tour assessment that covers multiple aspects of the patient's spirituality, will provide the evidence on which to plan appropriate spiritual care.[2] For example, if a nurse observes a terminally ill patient's spouse crying and stating, "Why does God have to take my sweetheart?," then the nurse would want to understand further what factors are contributing to or may relieve this spiritual pain. To focus the assessment on the pertinent topic, the nurse would then ask questions that explore the spouse's "why" questions, beliefs about misfortune, perceptions of God, and spiritual coping strategies.

Criteria for a tier 2 spiritual assessment

When should clinicians probe more deeply? Hodge[28] suggested four criteria for determining whether to move on to a more comprehensive assessment:

♦ First, consider patient autonomy. The patient must give informed consent. A comprehensive assessment may drill into inner depths the patient does not wish to expose to a clinician.

♦ Second, consider the competency of the clinician with regard to discussing spiritual matters. Is the clinician culturally sensitive and aware of how a personal worldview might conflict with the patient's? Might the clinician suffer from religious counter-transference and inappropriately relate to the patient from personal biases?

♦ Third, consider if the spiritual issue identified is relevant to the present healthcare situation. If not, it may not be in nurses' purview. For patients at the end of life, however, many past and diverse spiritual struggles can resurface; although these struggles may seem tangential to present caregiving, the patients may benefit from spiritual expertise that aids them to address these issues before death. (The nurse's curiosity or desire to evangelize the patient is never an ethical rationale for spiritual assessment.[3])

♦ Finally, consider the importance of spirituality to the patient. The extreme illustration of this would be if a patient states spirituality is personally irrelevant, then a comprehensive spiritual assessment would be inappropriate.

Observing these guidelines can prevent inappropriate and time-consuming assessment and care.

Although a comprehensive spiritual assessment may well be beneficial to many patients at the end of life, it is likely that few palliative care nurses are competent or able to conduct such an assessment.[2,3] Fowler posits that a person's spiritual or religious experience is arranged in layers like an onion. The outer layers of public and semipublic spiritual belief and practice are an appropriate domain for the nurse negligibly trained in spiritual assessment and care, whereas the deeper, more intimate—and often pain-filled—inner layers are best assessed and addressed by spiritual care experts.[35]

Models for comprehensive spiritual assessment

The screening models presented thus far are most relevant for palliative care nurses. By reviewing more comprehensive models,

Table 32.1 Mnemonics to guide a spiritual assessment

Author/s	Components (mnemonic)	Illustrative questions
Maugens[28]	S (spiritual belief system)	What is your formal religious affiliation?
	P (personal spirituality)	Describe the beliefs and practices of your religion or spiritual system that you personally accept. What is the importance of your spirituality/religion in daily life?
	I (integration with a spiritual community)	Do you belong to any spiritual or religious group or community? What importance does this group have to you? Does or could this group provide help in dealing with health issues?
	R (ritualized practices and restrictions)	Are there specific elements of medical care that you forbid on the basis of religious/spiritual grounds?
	I (implications for medical care)	What aspects of your religion/spirituality would you like me to keep in mind as I care for you? Are there any barriers to our relationship based on religious or spiritual issues?
	T (terminal events planning)	As we plan for your care near the end of life, how does your faith impact on your decisions?
Anandarajah and Hight[29]	H (sources of hope)	What or who is it that gives you hope?
	O (organized religion)	Are you a part of an organized faith group? What does this group do for you as a person?
	P (personal spirituality or spiritual practices)	What personal spiritual practices, like prayer or meditation, help you?
	E (effects on medical care and/or end-of-life issues)	Do you have any beliefs that may affect how the healthcare team cares for you?
Puchalski[27]	F (faith)	Do you have a faith belief? What is it that gives your life meaning?
	I (import or Influence)	What importance does your faith have in your life? How does your faith belief influence your life?
	C (community)	Are you a member of a faith community? How does this support you?
	A (address)	How would you like for me to integrate or address these issues in your care?
LaRocca-Pitts[30]	F (faith)	What spiritual beliefs are important to you now?
	A (availability/accessibility/applicability)	Are you able to find the spiritual nurture that you would like now?
	C (coping/comfort)	How comforting/helpful are your spiritual beliefs at this time?
	T (treatment)	How can I/we provide spiritual support?
Skalla and McCoy[31]	M (moral authority)	Where does your sense of what to do come from? What guides you to decide what is right or wrong for you?
	V (vocational)	What gives your life purpose? What work is important to you? What mission or role do you fell passionate about?
	A (aesthetic)	What brings beauty or pleasure to your life now? How are you able to express your creativity? How do you deal with boredom?
	S (social)	What people or faith community do you sense you belong with most? Do you belong to a community that nourishes you spiritually?
	T (transcendent)	Who or what controls what happens in life? Who/what supports you when you are ill? Is there an Ultimate Other (an entity that is sacred, for example)? If so, how do you relate to It?
McEvoy (pediatric context)[32]	B (belief system)	What religious or spiritual beliefs, if any, do members of your family have?
	E (ethics or values)	What standards/values/rules for life does your family think important?
	L (lifestyle)	What spiritual habits or activities does your family commit to because of spiritual beliefs? (e.g., Any sacred times to observe or diet you keep?)
	I (involvement in spiritual community)	How connected to a faith community are you? Would you like us to help you reconnect with this group now?
	E (education)	Are you receiving any form of religious education? How can we help you keep up with it?
	F (near future events of spiritual significance for which to prepare the child)	Are there any upcoming religious ceremonies that you are getting ready for?

Source: Taylor EJ. Spiritual assessment. In: Ferrell B, Coyle N (eds.), *Textbook of Palliative Nursing Care.* 3rd ed. New York: Oxford University Press; 2010:651, 652, 657; Tables 33.1, 33.2, 33.3.

Box 32.1 Self (or nurse-assisted) spiritual screening for palliative care patients

Dear _____,

Your palliative care team wants to make sure you receive the physical, emotional, and spiritual care and comfort you need.

Typically, persons receiving palliative care find themselves becoming more aware of their spirituality or religion. Please help us to understand what are your spiritual care and comfort needs.

Directions: Place an "X" on the lines to show the answer that comes closest to describing your experience.

1. How important is spirituality and/or religion to you now?

/ _____ /

               Not at all important very important

2. Recently, my spirits have been ...

/ _____ /

              Awful. ... low. ... okay. ... good. ... great

What can a nurse do that would help to nurture your spirit? (check all that apply)

— pray with me

— allow time and space for my private prayer or meditation

— bring art or music that will nurture me

— bring or read inspiring things to me

— listen to my thoughts about certain spiritual matters

— provide assistance so I can record my life story

— just be with me

— help me to stay connected to my spiritual community by contacting:

    ♦ my church/temple/mosque/local faith community's name and location _____

    _____

    ♦ my clergy or spiritual leader's name (any contact information will be helpful)_____

    _____

Is there anything else about your spiritual beliefs or practices that the palliative care team should know about? (e.g., diet or lifestyle encouraged by your religion? beliefs guiding your preparation for death?) Please write here (or on the back side) or tell your nurse.

Source: Taylor EJ. Spiritual assessment. In: Ferrell B, Coyle N (eds.), *Textbook of Palliative Nursing Care*. 3rd ed. New York: Oxford University Press; 2010:651, 652, 657; Tables 33.1, 33.2, 33.3.

---

however, nurses can extend their knowledge and gain appreciation for the territory that spiritual care experts may travel with patients. Nurses are in a pivotal position to refer patients to chaplains or other spiritual care specialists who can conduct a comprehensive assessment.

Fitchett,[36] a chaplain, developed the "7-by-7" model for spiritual assessment with a multidisciplinary group of health professionals. In addition to reviewing seven dimensions of a person (medical, psychological, psychosocial, family system, ethnic and cultural, societal issues, and spiritual dimensions), Fitchett advances seven spiritual dimensions to include in an assessment:

♦ Beliefs and meaning (i.e., mission, purpose, religious and non-religious meaning in life);

♦ Vocation and consequences (what persons believe they should do, what their calling is);

♦ Experience (of the divine or demonic) and emotion (the tone emerging from one's spiritual experience);

♦ Courage and growth (the ability to encounter doubt and inner change);

♦ Ritual and practice (activities that make life meaningful);

♦ Community (involvement in any formal or informal community that shares spiritual beliefs and practices); and

♦ Authority and guidance (exploring where or with whom one places trusts, seeks guidance).

This model likely offers chaplains and spiritual care experts the most comprehensive of all approaches to assessment.

Possibly the first comprehensive spiritual assessment model was that developed by Pruyser,[37] the patriarch of modern chaplaincy. Pruyser's original model identified seven aspects that each can be viewed as a continuum. These aspects of spirituality included:

♦ Awareness of the holy, or the lack thereof

♦ Sense of providence, or the lack thereof

- Faith, or the lack thereof
- A sense of grace or gratefulness, in contrast with a lack of appreciation and entitlement
- Repentance, versus unrepentant stance toward others and the world
- Communion (or feeling part of a whole), or on the continuum towards sensing no connection with others or the world
- Sense of vocation (purpose) versus meaninglessness.

Although this model is clearly influenced by a Christian worldview and may therefore be limited in its applicability, it offers a beautiful approach to thinking about spirituality comprehensively.

Standardized questionnaires

Paper-and-pencil-type questionnaires for measuring spirituality for research purposes abound; some of these have also been recommended for clinical assessment purposes. This approach to conducting a spiritual assessment allows for identification, and possibly, measurement, of how one spiritually believes, belongs, and behaves. This type of tool, however, should not "stand alone" in the process of spiritual assessment; rather, it can be the springboard for a more thorough assessment and deeper encounter with a patient, as appropriate. A quantitative tool should never replace human contact; instead it should facilitate it. Although a quantitative spiritual self-assessment form provides an opportunity for healthcare teams to glean substantial information when screening for spiritual beliefs and practices, without spending any professional's time, it also is limited by its mechanistic, rigid, and non-individualized nature.

For example, the Functional Assessment of Chronic Illness Therapy-Spiritual Well-being (FACIT-Sp) is a short 12-item instrument that assesses both religious and existential/spiritual well-being that has used considerably for health-related research purposes.[38] More recent testing suggests the tool measures not only faith (religious well-being) and meaning (existential/spiritual well-being), but also peace.[39] The FACIT-Sp has received considerable validation in numerous studies among persons with cancer. Examples of items include "I feel peaceful" and "I am able to reach down deep into myself for comfort." The 5-point response options range from "not at all" to "very much."

Another possible standardized screening tool is the Daily Spiritual Experience (DSE) scale.[40] The DSE is designed to measure "the individual's perception of the transcendent (God, the divine) in daily life and the perception of interaction with, or involvement of, the transcendent in life rather than particular beliefs or behaviors; therefore [it is] intended to transcend the boundaries of any particular religion."[40(p. 23)] The DSE is a 16-item scale with Likert-type response options measuring frequency. Like the FACIT-Sp, this instrument has been used often in research investigating patient spiritual responses and has well-established validity.

More recently developed for patients in general is the Spiritual Needs Assessment for Patients (SNAP).[41] This tool was likewise systematically developed, psychometrically tested, and found to have good support for its validity and reliability. It consists of 5 items assessing a psychosocial domain (e.g., needs related to "sharing your thoughts and feelings with people close to you?"), 13 items measuring spirituality (e.g., needs related to "resolving old disputes, hurts or resentments among family and friends"), and 5 items about religious needs (e.g., "religious rituals such as chant, prayer, lighting candles or incense, anointing, or communion"). Response options range from 1, "not at all," to 4, "very much."

The Brief RCOPE is a 14-item instrument that measures the degree of positive and negative religious coping.[42] This tool evolved from a longer version and a program of research examining the psychology of religious coping. Substantial psychometric testing affirms the validity of the tool. Positive religious coping items refer to a secure attachment to God, a sense of connectedness, and benevolence. The negative religious coping subscale items inquire about perceptions of abandonment and punishment by God, sense of isolation from faith community, questioning related to the power of God, and attributing poor coping to the devil. Pargament's program of research firmly establishes negative religious coping as maladaptive and positive religious coping as adaptive in illness contexts.

Although not so brief, the Royal Free Interview Schedule developed in the United Kingdom by King, Speck, and Thomas[43] is a 2½-page self-report questionnaire. The tool showed acceptable reliability and various forms of validity when it was tested among 297 persons, who were primarily hospital employees and church members. Questionnaire items assess both spiritual and religious "understanding in life" (1 item), religious/spiritual beliefs (8 items), religious/spiritual practices (3 items), and "intense" spiritual or "near death" experiences (6 items). Response options for items include Likert scales, categorical options, and space for answering open-ended questions.

Whereas these tools may offer the best approaches to a quantification of spiritual needs in a palliative care setting, know that other tools do exist. For further discussion of these tools (mostly developed for research purposes), consider the reviews provided by Monod and colleagues,[44] Draper,[45] and Lunder, Fulan, and Simonic.[46] Monod and colleagues observed that only 2 of the 35 scales measuring spiritual could have clinical usefulness. If spirituality is indeed a vital sign, as Lunder and colleagues posit, then careful consideration of how this vital essence of personhood can be screened and assessed by nurses is imperative.

Other spiritual assessment methods

Other approaches to spiritual assessment have been described in addition to the interview and questionnaire techniques. LeFavi and Wessels[47] described how life reviews can become, in essence, spiritual assessments. Life reviews are especially valuable for persons who are dying, as they allow patients to make sense of and reconcile their life story. By doing a life review with a terminally ill patient, the nurse can assess many dimensions of spirituality (e.g., worldviews, commitments, missions, values) in a natural, noncontrived manner. Life reviews can be prompted by questions about the significant events, people, and challenges during the life span. A life review can also occur when inquiring about personal objects, pictures, or other memorabilia the patient wants to share.

Chochinov and various colleagues around the world have developed and tested dignity therapy, which basically allows persons at the end of life an opportunity to do a life review.[48] The semistructured questions of dignity therapy include the following: "Tell me a little about your life history, particularly the parts you either remember most or think are most important? When did you feel most alive? Are there specific things that you would want your family to know about you? What are the most important roles you have played in life? What are your most important accomplishments? Are there particular things that you feel still need to be said? What are your hopes and dreams for your loved ones? What have you learned about life that you would want to pass along? Are there other things that you would like included?" The patient responses to these questions, potentially asked by a trained volunteer, are recorded and transcribed into a permanent record that the patient helps to design and that can be left as a legacy for loved ones. Although dignity therapy is reminiscence therapy, these questions overlap with what could be included in a comprehensive spiritual assessment.

Hodge[21] identified several creative approaches to collecting information about client spirituality. As a social worker, Hodge is well aware that some patients are not verbal or are not comfortable expressing their spirituality in words. Thus, he explained more visual ways for a patient to describe their spiritual experiences. These methods for assessments include:

- Spiritual lifemaps, or a pictoral depiction of where the patient has been spiritually, where the patient is presently, and where the patient expects to go. It can be a simple pencil drawing on a large piece of paper; words and illustrations can be used to convey the spiritual story—the spiritual highs and lows, blessings and burdens, and so forth.

- Spiritual genogram, like a standard genogram, depicts the issues and influences over one to three generations. Sources of spiritual influence from certain relationships (including those external to the family) can be drawn. Words that identify key spiritual beliefs and practices that were transmitted via relationships, and significant spiritual events that contribute to the patient's spiritual life can be noted around this spiritual family tree.

- Spiritual ecomaps, rather than focusing on past spiritual influences, direct the patient to consider present spiritual experiences. In particular, the patient can diagram (with self portrayed in the center) the relationship with God or transcendent other/value, rituals, faith community, and encounters with other spiritual entities.

- Spiritual ecograms allow the patient to diagram present perspectives on both family and spiritual relationships; it is a fusion of the spiritual genogram and ecomap.[45]

Other strategies include having clients draw a spiritual timeline that includes significant books, experiences, events, and so forth. Another unusual approach involves sentence completion. For example, a client may fill in the blank of sentences like "My relation to God ..." or "What I would really like to be ..." or "When I feel overwhelmed. ..." Having verbally oriented assessment strategies as well as these nonverbal methods provides clinicians with a "toolbox" for assessing spirituality, allowing the clinician to choose an approach that fits the patient personality, circumstances, and purpose for assessment.

Summary of spiritual screening and assessment models

Box 32.2 provides a case study to illustrate a few of these spiritual screening approaches. Comparing the four screening techniques

reveals that different data were generated. Other assessment approaches could be taken. Each would offer yet other emphases or angles for making sense of assessment data. It should be remembered, therefore, that each approach to spiritual assessment is one lens and may fail to address other important areas of spirituality (e.g., spiritually comforting practices and preparation for death are omitted from the above FICA and MVAST approaches).

The above summaries of various models for spiritual assessment identify spiritual dimensions that may be included in a spiritual assessment. Many of the dimensions identified in one model are observed (often using different language) in other models. Except for Hodge's[33] diagrammatic methods, these assessment approaches generally require the professional to make observations while asking questions and listening for the patient's response. The vast majority of questions recommended for use in following such a model are open ended. Several of the questions—indeed, the dimensions of spirituality—identified in this literature use "God language" or assume a patient will have belief in some transcendent divinity. All these models are developed by professionals who are influenced predominantly by Western, Judeo-Christian ways of thinking.

General observations and suggestions for conducting a spiritual assessment

When to assess

The spiritual assessment consensus project advocated that spiritual screening should be done at admission and whenever there is a change in patient status.[16] Furthermore, when the spiritual screening suggests potential for spiritual distress, a trained chaplain should be called for a more complete assessment within 24 hours. However, spiritual assessment should also be an ongoing process. The nurse does not complete a spiritual assessment simply by asking some questions about religion or spirituality during an intake interview. Instead, spiritual assessment should be ongoing throughout the nurse-patient relationship. A nurse tuned to know how spiritual health is manifested will be able to see and hear patient spirituality as it is embedded in and suffuses the everyday encounter.[49]

Gaining entrée

Spiritual needs are complex and often difficult to acknowledge and, more so, to describe with words. Furthermore, the patient may not yet feel comfortable divulging such intimate information to a nurse with whom rapport has not been established. Indeed, some patients may not want to share such inner, heart-touching experience.

Two studies provide evidence regarding what patients are looking for in a clinician if they are going to talk openly about their spirituality.[50,51] Survey responses from cancer patients and family caregivers ($n = 224$) about what requisites they would want in a nurse who provided spiritual care revealed that relationship (i.e., "show me kindness and respect" and "get to know me first") were ranked highest, with a nurse's training in spiritual care or sharing similar beliefs as the patient being less important.[52] Likewise, a small qualitative study of chronically and terminally ill patients observed that these informants

Box 32.2 Case study

Mr. T, entering hospice service with Parkinson's disease

Mr. T, is a 74-year-old Protestant man who was diagnosed about 13 years ago with Parkinson's disease. Until 8 months ago, he lived alone. When he realized he could no longer safely live alone, he moved to an assisted living facility. Now his condition has deteriorated further, requiring his admission to a skilled nursing facility. This facility has obtained hospice services for Mr. T. He is receiving antiparkinsonian and antidepressive medications.

Mr. T is divorced from his third wife and estranged from his only son and a stepson. The son lives 7 hours away (by car), and usually reenters Mr. T's life when he needs financial assistance. The only family that appears to show interest in supporting Mr. T is a niece and her husband, who live 2 hours away. Since Mr. T's divorce 10 years ago, he has been befriended by a middle-aged woman, Darlene, who has entered several business ventures with Mr. T's money.

The following are excerpts from conversations the author had with Mr. T:

"My dad was a doctor. He practiced until he was 91! He was very respected and well-known. He loved to yacht; he won the Trans-Pac race one year. I was a teen then, and could only travel with him if I was the crew's cook. So my mom taught me to peel potatoes. ...!

I wanted to be a doctor. I just couldn't get the grades, got kicked out of college ... never could have gotten into med school. So I sold cookware instead. They said I could sell snow in Alaska—I was good at selling. ...

I was born and raised in the church. Went to Christian schools all the way through college. I was an elder at my little church before I moved down here. I've got the church even in my will. ...

I know Darlene is using me, but I love her. I would marry her if I could. [She was married.] My head says one thing, but my heart says another. ...

I remember once making love to a woman and her reaction was, "Oh my God!" I guess that was a spiritual experience I helped her have!

There's not much for me to do here. Just a bunch of old people around here. Sometimes I wonder, "Why? Why keep going?'. ... I don't have anymore money to give. ... My body doesn't work anymore. ..."

[During a conversation Mr. T related he felt anxious:] I'm having a hard time ... really worried about how its all going to end. How will it? ... [When asked, "How at peace do you feel inside?":] Not at all. [When asked, "Is there anything you can think of that would bring comfort to you now?":] No, nothing.

Screening (using FICA):

F (faith)—verbalized about some indicators of adherence to a faith tradition; inward (or intrinsic) faith is fundamentally challenged as he faces his end; his faith appears to lean toward an extrinsic faith (e.g., attendance at services, donating money).

I (importance)—states it is important.

C (community)—until institutionalized, was a leader in a local Protestant congregation; desires to continue to attend.

A (address)—readily responds positively to query regarding having local pastor visit him; also accepts offer of loaned spiritual viewing materials (e.g., videos of dramatized Gospels) and musical CDs. When asked how the staff can spiritually support, he states, "No, they don't need to butt into this part of my life."

Screening (using MVAST)

Moral authority—He states the Bible is the guide for what is right or wrong. He admits struggling about how to morally relate to Darlene and yearns to reconnect with his sons.

Vocational—He excelled as a salesman during mid-adult years. More recently, his business ventures have failed. During his youth, he aspired to be a physician, yet failed to attain that goal. His life seems to have been lived in the shadow of his father, perhaps challenging his sense of worth. His financial failure also seems to challenge his sense of success and purposefulness.

Aesthetic—Loves "cars, motorcycles, and beautiful women!" His disease now prevents his ability to enjoy these interests, as he can no longer drive or attract women for a date. He does enjoy eating and listening to jazz.

Social—until institutionalized, was a leader in a local congregation; desires to continue to attend as he enjoys the opportunity to see old friends and meet people there.

Transcendent—says he prays before each meal and at bedtime, and then at times when he is very distressed, but reports that "sometimes it feels like the prayers don't go anywhere." Never describes a time in his life when there was an affective experience of God; rather, his descriptions of religious experience seem cerebral and prescribed. He does describe several times in his life when he believes his life was spared, and interprets these events as showing God intervening in his life.

Screening using FACIT-sp

Mr. T's score might indicate low peace, low existential/spiritual well-being, and perhaps slightly higher (but still low) religious well-being.

Screening using brief RCOPE

Mr. T's score likely would have indicated moderately high negative religious coping and low positive religious coping.

viewed relational characteristics (e.g., caring, honor and respect, rapport/trust) as prerequisites for discussing spirituality with a physician.[51] Ellis and Campbell's study identified other factors that patients perceive facilitate spiritual assessment by a physician: a conducive setting, sharing life priorities or values, perceived receptivity of physician to spiritual questions, and sensing that spiritual health was considered by the physician to be integral to health.[53]

Because spirituality and religiosity are sensitive and personal topics (as are most other topics nurses assess), it is polite for a nurse to preface a spiritual assessment with an acknowledgment of the sensitivity of the questions and an explanation for why such an assessment is necessary.[28,49] For example, Maugens[28] suggested this preface: "Many people have strong spiritual or religious beliefs that shape their lives, including their health and experiences with illness. If you are comfortable talking about this topic, would you please share any of your beliefs and practices that you might want me to know as your physician?"[28(p. 12)] Such a preface undoubtedly will help both the patient and the clinician to feel at ease during the assessment.

Assessing nonverbal indicators of spirituality

Although this discussion of spiritual assessment has thus far focused on how to frame a verbal question and allow a patient to verbalize a response, the nurse must remember that most communication occurs nonverbally. Hence, the nurse must assess the nonverbal communication and the environment of the patient.[2,3,49] Does the patient appear agitated or angry? What does the body language convey? What is the speed and tone of voice? Assessment of the patient's environment can provide clues about spiritual state. Are there religious objects on the bedside table? Are there religious paintings or crucifixes on the walls? Get-well cards or books with spiritual themes? Are there indicators that the patient has many friends and family providing love and a sense of community? Are the curtains closed and the bedspread pulled over the face? Many of the factors a palliative care nurse usually assesses will provide data for a spiritual assessment as well as the psychosocial assessment.

Language: religious or spiritual words?

One barrier to spiritual assessment is the nurse's fear of offending a nonreligious patient by using religious language. However, when one remembers the nonreligious nature of spirituality, this barrier disappears. Patient spirituality can be discussed without God language or reference to religion. Also, using the terms "need" or "distress" immediately after "spiritual" could be denigrating for a patient. Especially with spirituality, patients may be upset when they hear others consider them to be with need. Nurses can easily avoid such jargon.

To know what language will not be offensive during a spiritual assessment, the nurse must remember two guidelines. First, the nurse can begin the assessment with questions that are general and unrelated to religious assumptions. For example, "What is giving you the strength to cope with your illness now?" or "What spiritual beliefs and practices are important to you as you cope with your illness?" Second, the nurse must listen for the language of the patient, and use the patient's language when formulating more specific follow-up questions. If a patient responds to

a question with "My faith and prayers help me," then the nurse knows "faith" and "prayer" are words that will not offend this patient. If a patient states that the "Great Spirit guides," then the sensitive nurse will not respond with, "Tell me how Jesus is your guide." Questions using nonreligious language are presented in Box 32.3.

Asking questions

Because asking a patient questions is an integral part of most spiritual assessments, it is good to remember some of the basics of formulating good questions. Asking closed-ended questions that allow for short factual or yes/no responses is helpful when a nurse truly has no time or ability for further assessment. Otherwise, to appreciate the uniqueness and complexity of an individual's spirituality, the nurse must focus on asking open-ended questions. The best open-ended questions begin with "How," "What," "When," "Who," or phrases like "Tell me about. ..." Generally, questions beginning with "Why" are not helpful; they are often mixed with a sense of threat or challenge (e.g., "Why do you believe that?").[49]

Listening to the answers

Although it is easy to focus on and to worry about what to say during an assessment, the palliative care nurse must remember the importance of listening to the patient's responses. Discussion of active listening is beyond the scope of this chapter, yet a few comments are in order. Remember that silence is appropriate when listening to a patient's spiritual and sacred story; silence has a work.[49] Remain neutral, nonjudgmental. View the patient as a

---

Box 32.3 A collection of nonreligious questions to broach the topic of spirituality with palliative care patients

You've gone through so much lately. Where do you get your inner strength and courage to keep going?

What is helping you to cope?

What comforts are most satisfying for you now?

As you think about your future, what worries you most?

Some people seem more to live while they are dying, while others seem to die while they are living. Which way is it for you? What makes it that way?

What kind of person do you see yourself as? (Note: Chaplains suggest that how one views self parallels how one views their Creator or God.)

What do you see as the purpose for your life now, given your body isn't allowing you to do all you used to do?

What hopes and dreams do you have for your future? For your family?

What legacy would you like to leave? How can we make sure that that happens?

As I've gotten to know you, I've noticed you speak often of (spiritual theme [e.g., betrayal, yearning for love]). How do you think this theme has influenced your life, or will influence your future? How happy with your life's theme are you?

Tell me about times during your life where faced a huge challenge. What got you through? Is that resource still available to you now?

fellow sojourner on the journey of life. Recognize that you are not the authority or savior for the patient expressing spiritual pain. Rather you are a companion, or a supporter if so privileged. Listen for more than words; listen for metaphors, listen for a spiritual theme that keeps reemerging throughout life stories, listen for where the patient places energy, listen for emotion in addition to cognitions. The nurse will do well to listen to his or her own inner response. This response will mirror the feelings of the patient.[49]

Overcoming the time barrier

Healthcare professionals may believe that they do not have enough time to conduct a spiritual assessment. Indeed, Maugens[28] observed that completing his spiritual history with patients took about 10 to 15 minutes. Although this is much less time than Maugen and his colleagues expected it to take, it is still a considerable amount of time in today's healthcare context. One response to this time barrier is to remember that spiritual assessment is a process that develops as the nurse gains the trust of a patient. The nurse can accomplish the assessment during "clinical chatterings."[28] Furthermore, data for a spiritual assessment can be simultaneously collected with other assessments or during interventions (e.g., while bathing or completing bedtime care). And finally, it can be argued that nurses do not have time to not conduct a spiritual assessment, considering the fundamental and powerful nature of spirituality. Skalla and McCoy (a nurse and a chaplain) remind the users of their MVAST model that the questions are a guide, and not prescriptive; they can be threaded into the natural course of a conversation.[31]

Overcoming personal barriers

Nurses can encounter personal barriers to conducting a spiritual assessment. These barriers can include feelings of embarrassment or insecurity about the topic or can result from projection of unresolved and painful personal spiritual doubts or struggles. Every nurse has a personal philosophy or worldview that influences his or her spiritual beliefs. These beliefs can color or blind the nurse's assessment techniques and interpretation. Hence, an accurate and sensitive spiritual assessment presumably correlates with the degree of the nurse's spiritual self-awareness. Put another way, your ability to hear your own spiritual story is directly related to your ability to hear a patient's spiritual story.[49] Nurses can increase their comfort with the topic and their awareness of their spiritual self if they ask themselves variations of the questions they anticipate asking patients. For example, "What gives my life meaning and purpose?" "How do my spiritual beliefs influence the way I relate to my own death?" "How do I love myself and forgive myself?" Recognizing how one's spiritual beliefs motivate one's vocation as a nurse is also extremely helpful.

Concluding cautions

Although the presented models and evidence supporting spiritual assessment imply that it is an unproblematic and simple process, it would be naive to leave this impression. Several experts suggest potential problems associated with spiritual assessment. These include:

- The process of taking spiritual assessment data to make a spiritual diagnosis pathologizes what may be a normal process of spiritual growth.[54] Assessment tools often assume that spiritual well-being correlates with feeling good, that spiritual health and suffering cannot coexist.[6] (A more appropriate way to evaluate spirituality may be to ask how harmful one's spirituality is to self and others.[49])

- A "tick box" approach to spiritual assessment could freeze patient spirituality to the time when the assessment was completed; spiritual assessment would be considered complete and fail to continue in an ongoing manner.[54]

- A fairly prescribed assessment tool could have the unintended outcome of disempowering a patient. That is, the clinician controls (overpowers) the agenda by determining what spiritual matters are discussed.[55] A tool used for assessment could end up limiting and controlling patient expression.[56]

- A spiritual assessment to some degree will reflect the assumptions influencing the clinician (a major one being that spirituality is universal). Thus, a spiritual worldview will be imposed to some degree on a vulnerable patient. An ethical spiritual assessment would be nonalienating, nondiscriminating, and would engage and respect the patient.[57,58] Indeed, existent standardized spiritual assessment tools generally have not been tested in many cultures, so it is unknown how culturally appropriate or sensitive they are.[46]

Thus, a spiritual assessment tool—if a tool is needed—should be able to generate helpful data for guiding patient care, encourage patient participation, be flexible, easy to use, take little clinician time, be nonintrusive, allow for a patient's unique story to be understood to some degree, and be simple and clear.[58] A tall task? Perhaps. But important to strive toward.

Assessing special populations

Assessing impaired patients

Although verbal conversation is integral to a typical spiritual assessment, some terminally ill patients may not be able to speak, hear, or understand a verbal assessment. Patients who are unable to communicate verbally may feel unheard. In such situations, the nurse again must remember alternative sources of information. The nurse can consult with the family members and observe the patient's environment and nonverbal communications. For example, Telos[59] proposed that for some patients, terminal restlessness was a manifestation of spiritual distress. Ruling out other causes, and relying on previous spiritual assessment opportunities that have revealed unresolved spiritual issues, supports the palliative care team to draw this conclusion. (Hence, the importance of proactively conducting spiritual assessments for those with terminal illness.) Alternative methods for "conversing" can also be used. For patients who can write, paper-and-pencil questionnaires can be very helpful. Always be patient and be unafraid of the tears that can follow. Questions that demonstrate concern for their innermost well-being may release their floodgates for tears.

For persons with dementia or other cognitive impairments, it is helpful to recognize that communication can still occur on an emotional or physical level if not intellectually. Their disjointed stories will still offer you a window to their world. Even if you cannot sew the pieces together, trying will help you to remain curious and engaged.[49]

Assessing children

Several strategies can be employed to assess the spirituality of children. The clinician must remember, however, that building trust and rapport with children is essential to completing a helpful spiritual assessment. Children are especially capable of ascertaining an adult's degree of authenticity. Children also are less likely to be offended by a question about religion. If a nurse creates a comfortable and non-judgmental atmosphere in which a child can discuss spiritual topics, then the child will talk. Never underestimate the profoundness of a child's spiritual experience, especially a dying child's.

In addition to asking assessment questions verbally, the nurse can use play interviews, picture drawings, observations, and informal interviews.[60] The nurse may need to be more creative in formulating questions if the child's vocabulary is limited. For example, instead of asking the child about helpful religious rituals, the nurse may need to ask questions about what they do to get ready to sleep or what they do on weekends. When asking, "Does your mommy pray with you before you go to sleep?" or "What do you do on Sunday or Sabbath mornings?" the nurse can learn whether prayer or religious service attendance are a part of this child's life. An assessment question that Sexson's[60] colleague Patricia Fosarelli found to be particularly helpful with 6- to 18-year-olds was: "If you could get God to answer one question, what one question would you ask God?"

While assessing children, it is vital to consider their stage of cognitive and faith development.[60,61] Questions must be framed in age-appropriate language (a 4-year-old will likely not understand what "spiritual belief" means!). Toddlers and preschoolers talk about their spirituality in very concrete terms, with an egocentric manner. School-aged and adolescent children should be addressed straightforwardly about how they see their illness. Inquiring about the cause of their illness is especially important, as many children view their illness and impending death as punishment.

As with adults, nonverbal communication and behaviors are also significant forms of information for a spiritual screening or assessment. Mueller[61] advises that extensive crying, withdrawal, regressive and resistant behaviors are potential indicators of spiritual distress. Likewise, difficulty with eating or sleeping (nightmares), and somatic complaints can be reflective of an undergirding spiritual distress.

Assessing families

Understanding the family's spirituality is pivotal to understanding the child's. Structured interviews or unstructured conversations with parents and even older siblings will inform the healthcare team about the child's spirituality.[60,62] Similarly, knowing the spiritual or religious family context of an adult patient can also inform clinicians about a patient's faith context. Furthermore, studies document the spiritual distress of family caregivers is not unlike that of their beloved.[12,63,64] Given the provision of 24/7 physical care, the unrelenting uncertainty and anxiety, and the constellation of stressors family caregivers endure, it is not surprising they may feel angry at God,[12] isolated from their faith community, and challenged to have a meaningful outlook on life.[63] Indeed, in Delgado Guay and colleagues' study, 58% of family carers surveyed reported some spiritual pain.[64]Although it is highly unlikely that a nurse will be completing a comprehensive spiritual assessment of a family, an awareness of this process can give the nurse a richer perspective with which to conduct a screening when it is appropriate.

Barnes and colleagues[65] suggested the following questions as guides for assessing how a family's spirituality affects illness experience:

- How does the family understand life's purpose and meaning?
- How do they explain illness and suffering?
- How do they view the person in the context of the body, mind, soul, spirit, and so forth?
- How is the specific illness of the child explained?
- What treatments are necessary for the child?
- Who is the qualified person to address these various treatments for the various parts of the child's healing?
- What is the outcome measurement that the family is using to measure successful treatment (good death)?

Ferrell and Baird[66] offer a couple of family spiritual assessment questions that are specific to the caregiving role many family members often perform:

- We recognize that often family caregivers' spirituality may be similar to or very different from the patient's spirituality. Are there spiritual needs you have as a family caregiver?
- Many family caregivers tell us that while caring for a loved one … is very difficult, caregiving can also be a very meaningful experience. What has it been like for you?[66(p. 257)]

These questions will likely be welcomed by the family carer who is engaged in providing much health-related care to a loved one. Asking such questions will acknowledge to this caregiver that their role is recognized and appreciated. It will also provide the family caregiver opportunity to express and reflect on their needs, a therapeutic experience.

Buck and McMillan took the Spiritual Needs Inventory (SNI) developed by Hermann for patients, and tested its validity with 410 family caregivers of hospice patients.[63] This 17-item instrument assesses religious needs (e.g., for devotional practices and service attendance), outlook needs (e.g., "think happy thoughts," "be with friends," "see smiles"), community needs (e.g., knowing about or being with family and friends). The SNI offers a possible method for a standardized approach to family caregiver spiritual screening and assessment.

Assessing diverse spiritualties

Spiritual assessment methods must be flexible enough to obtain valid data from persons with diverse spiritual and religious backgrounds. Although the questions and assumptions presented in this chapter will be helpful for assessing most patients living in Western, Euro-American cultures, they may not be for some patients who do not share these presuppositions. For example, some may believe it is wrong to discuss their inner spiritual turmoil as they face death and will refuse to fully engage in the process of spiritual assessment. (Whereas some Buddhists and Hindus may believe they must be in a peaceful state to be reincarnated to a better state, African-American Christians may think it is sinful to express doubts or anger toward God.) Framing spiritual assessment in a positive tone may overcome this type of barrier (e.g., "Tell me about how you are at peace now.") Others may assume they are void of spirituality and therefore decline any questions regarding their "spirituality." This barrier to assessment can be overcome with questions that are void of such language (e.g., "What gives your life meaning?" or "How is your courage?").

For patients who are religious, it is important to remember that no two members of a religious community are exactly alike.[3] For example, one orthodoxly religious person may believe he should never consume any mind-altering drugs, such as morphine, while a less conservative member of the same denomination may understand that such drugs are a gracious Godly gift. Although having a cursory understanding of the world's major religious traditions provides nurses with some framework for inquiry, remaining open to the variation of religious experience and expression is essential.

The next step: what to do with a spiritual assessment

Interpreting the data

Even a spiritual screening can generate a lot of information. This information must be processed to identify what, if any, spiritual need exists and to plan spiritual care. Several points can be considered while processing the data. These include:

- What patients tell you at first reflects not how well you have asked a good question; rather it shows how safe and respected the patient feels with you.

- Consider what incongruities exist. Do the affect, behavior, and communication (ABCs) line up?

- Consider the level of concreteness or abstractness in the patient's talk about spiritual matters. Healthy spirituality straddles between these opposites.

- Consider how defensive or threatened the patient is by talk about spirituality. Did the patient change the topic? Give superficial answers? Become competitive? Analyze feelings?

- Keep in mind that crises (e.g., illness) expose the gaps in a patient's spiritual development. Did significant events earlier in life in effect stunt the patient's spiritual growth?

- Remember that religion offers a lens for interpreting life. Likewise, when patients tell meaningful stories, legends, or passages from their holy scripture, they are telling you about themselves.

- Reflect on how helpful versus harmful a patient's spiritual beliefs and practices are. Do they create inner anxiety? Do they limit the patient from using other helpful coping strategies?[49]

Although an in-depth analysis is beyond the scope of most palliative care nurses, having an awareness of these various ways to evaluate what a patient says will help the nurse to begin to make sense of the data.

Documentation

Although assessments of physiological phenomenon are readily documented in patient charts, assessments and diagnoses of spiritual problems are less frequently documented. However, for many reasons, spiritual assessments and care should be documented to at least some degree. These reasons include: (1) to facilitate the continuity of patient care among palliative care team members and (2) to document for the monitoring purposes of accrediting bodies, researchers, quality improvement teams, and so forth. Power[54] recognized that the data collected during spiritual assessments is often very private, sensitive material; to document such may breach confidentiality and thus pose an ethical dilemma. As with other sensitive charted information, nurses must treat spiritual assessment data with much respect and observe applicable privacy codes.

Formats for documenting spiritual assessments and diagnoses can vary. Some institutions encourage staff to use SOAP (Subjective, Objective, Assessment, Plan) or similar formatting in progress notes shared by the multidisciplinary team. Others have developed quick and easy checklists for documenting spiritual and religious issues. Perhaps an assessment format that allows for both rapid documentation and optional narrative data is best. However, merely documenting one's religious affiliation and whether one desires a referral to a spiritual care specialist certainly does not adequately indicate a patient's spiritual status and need.

Institutional approaches to spiritual screening and assessment

A 2-year demonstration project to improve spiritual assessment in palliative care settings was recently completed.[67,68] Funded by the Archstone Foundation and convened by the City of Hope National Medical Center, this project provided significant funding to nine southern California healthcare organizations with palliative care services. This project allowed experts to share information, resources, and change strategies with each site so they could accomplish the goal of better instituting spiritual assessment and spiritual care.

Each site, of course, developed its unique method. Typically, each site constructed a screening tool comprised of a very few open-ended screening questions. These questions were embedded into the healthcare system's standardized admission assessment, typically electronically. The electronic medical record system often was designed then to allow the clinician to not only insert patient responses to screening questions (sometimes requiring the nurse to translate a qualitative response into a yes/no tick box response) but also submit a referral or add to a care plan if a spiritual need was identified. Palliative care service clinicians were educated at each site about spiritual screening and the newly implemented process for screening and documenting patient spiritual status.[29]

Summary

Spirituality is an elemental and pervading dimension for persons, especially those for whom death is imminent. Spiritual assessment is essential to effective and sensitive spiritual care. Indeed, spiritual assessment is the beginning of spiritual care. While the nurse questions a patient about spirituality, the nurse is simultaneously assisting the patient to reflect on the innermost and most important aspects of being human. The nurse is also indicating to the patient that grappling with spiritual issues is normal and valuable. The nurse also provides spiritual care during an assessment by being present and witnessing what is sacred for the patient.

References

1. Reed PG. An emerging paradigm for the investigation of spirituality in nursing. Res Nurs Health. 1992;15:349–357.

2. Puchalski CM, Ferrell B. Making Health Care Whole: Integrating Spirituality into Patient Care. West Conshohocken, PA: Templeton Press; 2010.

3. Taylor EJ. Religion: A Clinical Guide for Nurses. New York: Springer; 2012.

4. Narayansamy A. The puzzle of spirituality for nursing: A guide to practical assessment. Br J Nurs. 2004;13(19):1140–1144.

5. Paley J. Spirituality and secularization: nursing and the sociology of religion. J Clin Nurs. 2008;17:175–186.

6. Pesut B, Fowler M, Reimer-Kirkham S, Taylor EJ, Sawatzky R. Particularizing spirituality in points of tension. Nurs Inquiry. 2009; 16:337–346.

7. Bash A. Spirituality: the emperor's new clothes? J Clin Nurs. 2004;13: 11–16.

8. McSherry W, Ross L. Dilemmas of spiritual assessment: Considerations for nursing practice. J Adv Nurs. 2002;38:479–488.

9. Williams AL. Perspectives on spirituality at the end of life: a meta-summary. Palliat Support Care. 2006;4:407–417.

10. Taylor EJ. Spiritual responses to cancer (Chapter 73). In: Yarbro CH, Wujcik D, Gobel BH (eds.), Cancer Nursing: Principles and Practice. 7th ed. Sudbury, MA: Jones and Bartlett; 2010.

11. Taylor EJ, Davenport F. Spiritual quality of life. In: King CR, Hinds PS (eds.), Quality of Life: From Nursing and Patient Perspectives. 3rd ed. Sudbury, MA: Jones and Bartlett; 2012.

12. Exline JJ, Prince-Paul M, Root BL, Peereboom KS. The spiritual struggle of anger toward God: a study with family members of hospice patients. J Palliat Med. 2013;16:369–375.

13. Newberry AG, Choi CW, Donovan HS, Schulz R, Bender C, Given B, et al. Exploring spirituality in family caregivers of patients with primary malignant brain tumors across the disease trajectory. Oncol Nurs Forum. 2013;40(3):E119–E125.

14. National Consensus Project for Quality Palliative Care (2013). Clinical Practice Guidelines for Quality Palliative Care, 3rd ed. Pittsburgh, PA. Available at http://www.nationalconsensusproject.org. Retrieved July 2, 2013.

15. The Joint Commission. Spiritual Assessment. Available at http://www.jointcommission.org/AccreditationPrograms/HomeCare/Standards/09_FAQs/PC/Spiritual_Assessment. htm. accessed December 31, 2008.

16. Puchalski C, Ferrell B, Virani R, Otis-Green S, Baird P, Bull J, et al. Improving the quality of spiritual care as a dimension of palliative care: the report of the Consensus Conference. J Palliat Med. 2009; 12:885–904.

17. Kalish N. Evidence-based spiritual care: a literature review. Curr Opin Support Palliat Care. 2012;6:242–246.

18. Taylor, EJ. New Zealand hospice nurses' self-rated comfort in conducting spiritual assessment. Inter J Palliat Care Nurs. 2013;19:178–185.

19. Cobb M, Dowrick C, Lloyd-Williams M. What can we learn about the spiritual needs of palliative care patients from the research literature? J Pain Symptom Manage. 2012;43:1105–1119.

20. Hodge DR. Administering a two-stage spiritual assessment in healthcare settings: a necessary component of ethical and effective care. J Nurs Manage. 2013. Epub ahead of print.

21. Hodge D. Developing a spiritual assessment toolbox: a discussion of the strengths and limitations of five different assessment methods. Health Social Work. 2005;10:314–323.

22. Kub JE, Nolan MT, Hughes MT, et al. Religious importance and practices of patients with a life-threatening illness: implications for screening protocols. Appl Nurs Res. 2003;16:196–200.

23. Lawrence RT, Smith DW. Principles to make a spiritual assessment work in your practice. J Fam Pract. 2004;53:625–631.

24. Steinhauser KE, Voils CI, Clipp EC, Bosworth HB, Christakis NA, Tulsky JA. "Are you at peace?": One item to probe spiritual concerns at the end of life. Arch Intern Med. 2006;166(1):101–105.

25. Lo B, Quill T, Tulsky J. Discussing palliative care with patients. Ann Intern Med. 1999;130:744–749.

26. Matthews DA, McCullough ME, Larson DB, Koenig HG, Swyers JP, Milano MG. Religious commitment and health status: a review of the research and implications for family medicine. Arch Fam Med. 1998;7:118–124.

27. Borneman T, Ferrell B, Puchalski CM. Evaluation of the FICA tool for spiritual assessment. J Pain Symptom Manage. 2010;40:163–173.

28. Maugens TA. The SPIRITual history. Arch Fam Med. 1996;5:11–16.

29. Anandarajah G, Hight E. Spirituality and medical practice: using the HOPE questions as a practical tool for spiritual assessment. Am Fam Physician. 2001;63:81–89.

30. LaRocca-Pitts M. A spiritual history tool: FACT. Available at http://www.professionalchaplains.org/uploadedFiles/pdf/FACT%20spiritual%. Accessed December 29, 2008.

31. Skalla KA, McCoy JP. Spiritual assessment of patients with cancer: the moral authority, vocational, aesthetic, social, and transcendent model. Oncol Nurs Forum. 2006;33:745–751.

32. McEvoy M. An added dimension to the pediatric health maintenance visit: the spiritual history. J Ped Health Care. 2000;14:216–220.

33. Hodge D. A template for spiritual assessment: a review of the JCAHO requirements and guidelines for implementation. Social Work. 2006;51:317–326.

34. Frick E, Riedner C, Fegg MJ, Hauf S, Borasio GD. A clinical interview assessing cancer patients' spiritual needs and preferences. Eur J Cancer Care (Engl). 2006;15:238–243.

35. Taylor, EJ. Religion and patient care (Chapter 16). In: Fowler M, Kirkham-Reimer S, Sawatzky R, Taylor EJ (eds.), Religion, Religious Ethics, and Nursing. New York: Springer; 2011:313–338.

36. Fitchett G. Assessing Spiritual Needs: A Guide for Caregivers. Lima, OH: Academic Renewel Press; 2002.

37. Pruyser, P. The minister as diagnostician: personal problems in pastoral perspective. Philadelphia, PA: Westminster Press, 1976.

38. Peterman A, Fitchett, G, Brady MJ, Hernandez L, Cella D. Measuring spiritual well-being in people with cancer: the Functional Assessment of Chronic Illness Therapy-Spiritual Well-Being Scale (FACIT-Sp). Ann Behav Med. 2002;24(1):49–58.

39. Murphy PE, Canada AL, Fitchett G, Stein K, Portier K, Crammer C, Peterman AH. An examination of the 3-factor model and structural invariance across racial/ethnic groups for the FACIT-Sp: a report from the American Cancer Society's Study of Cancer Survivors-II (SCS-II). Psycho-Oncol. 2010;19:264–272.

40. Underwood LG, Teresi JA. The Daily Spiritual Experience Scale: development, theoretical description, reliability, exploratory factor analysis, and preliminary construct validity using health-related data. Ann Behav Med. 2002; 24(1):22–33.

41. Sharma RK, Astrow AB, Texeira K, Sulmasy DP. The Spiritual Needs Assessment for Patients (SNAP): development and validation of a comprehensive instrument to assess unmet spiritual needs. J Pain Symptom Manag 2012;44:44–51.

42. Pargament K, Feuille M, Burdzy D. The Brief RCOPE: current psychometric status of a short measure of religious coping. Religions. 2011;2(1): 51–76

43. King M, Speck P, Thomas A. The royal free interview for spiritual and religious beliefs: development and validation of a self-report version. Psychol Med. 2001;31:1015–1023.

44. Monod S, Brennan M, Rochat E, Martin E, Rochat S, Bula CJ. Instruments measuring spirituality in clinical research: a systematic review. J Gen Intern Med. 2011;26:1345–1357.

45. Draper P. An integrative review of spiritual assessment: implications for nursing management. J Nurs Manage. 2012;20:970–980.

46. Lunder U, Furlan M, Simonic A. Spiritual needs assessments and measurements. Curr Opin Support Palliat Care. 2011;5:273–278.

47. LeFavi RG, Wessels MH. Life review in pastoral care counseling: background and efficacy for the terminally ill. J Pastoral Care Council. 2003;57:281–292.

48. Chochinov HM, Kristjanson LJ, Breitbart W, McClement S, Hack TF, Hassard T, et al. Effect of dignity therapy on distress and end-of-life

experience in terminally ill patients: a randomised controlled trial. Lancet Oncol. 2011; 12:753–762.

49. Taylor EJ. What do I say?: Talking with Patients About Spirituality. Philadelphia, PA: Templeton Press; 2007.

50. Taylor, EJ, Mamier I. Spiritual care nursing: what cancer patients and family caregivers want. J Adv Nurs. 2005;49(3):260–267.

51. Kvale K. Do cancer patients always want to talk about difficult emotions?: A qualitative study of cancer inpatients communication needs. Eur J Oncol Nurs. 2007;11(4):320–327.

52. Taylor EJ. Client perspectives about nurse requisites for spiritual caregiving. App Nurs Res. 2007;20(1):44–46.

53. Ellis MR, Campbell JD. Patients' views about discussing spiritual issues with primary care physicians. South Med J. 2004;97:1158–1164.

54. Dudley JR, Smith C, Millison MB. Unfinished business: assessing the spiritual needs of hospice clients. Am J Hospice Palliat Care. 1995;12:30–37.

54. Power J. Spiritual assessment: developing an assessment tool. Nurs Older People. 2006;18(2):16–18.

55. Pronk K. Role of the doctor in relieving spiritual distress at the end of life. Am J Hospice Palliat Med. 2005;22:419–425.

56. Byrne M. Spirituality in palliative care: what language do we need? Learning from pastoral care. Int J Palliat Nurs. 2007;13(3):118–121.

57. Rumbold BD. A review of spiritual assessment in health care practice. Med J Austr. 2007;186(10):S60–S62.

58. Timmins F, Kelly J. Spiritual assessment in intensive and cardiac care nursing. Nurs Crit Care. 2008;13(3):124–131.

59. Telos N. Proactive: spiritual care for terminal restlessness. Palliat Support Care. 2005;3:245–246.

60. Sexson SB. Religious and spiritual assessment of the child and adolescent. Child Adolesc Psychiatr Clin N Am. 2004;13:35–47.

61. Mueller CR. Spirituality in children: understanding and developing interventions. Pediatr Nurs. 2010;36:197–203, 208.

62. Heilferty CM. Spiritual development and the dying child: the pediatric nurse practitioner's role. J Pediatr Health Care. 2004;18:271–275.

63. Buck HG, McMillan SC. A psychometric analysis of the spiritual needs inventory in informal caregivers of patients with cancer in hospice home care. Oncol Nurs Forum. 2012;39(4):E332–E339.

64. Delgado Guay MO, Parsons HA, Hui D, De la Cruz MG, Thorney S, et al. Spirituality, religiosity, and spiritual pain among caregivers of patients with advanced cancer. Am J Hosp Palliat Care. 2012 Sep 4. Epub ahead of print.

65. Barnes LP, Plotnikoff GA, Fox K, Pendleton S. Spirituality, religion, and pediatrics: intersecting worlds of healing. Pediatrics. 2000;104:899–908.

66. Ferrell B, Baird P. Deriving meaning and faith in caregiving. Sem Oncol Nurs. 2012; 28:256–261.

67. Otis-Green S, Ferrell B, Borneman T, Puchalski C, Uman G, Garcia A. Integrating spiritual care within palliative care: an overview of nine demonstration projects. J Palliat Med. 2012;15;154–162.

68. Improving the quality of spiritual care as a dimension of palliative care. [Conference proceedings.] March 6–7, 2013; Los Angeles, CA.

CHAPTER 33

Spiritual care intervention

Rev. Pamela Baird

The most basic and powerful way to connect to another person is to listen. Just listen. Perhaps the most important thing we ever give each other is our attention.... A loving silence often has far more power to heal and to connect than the most well-intentioned words.

Rachel Naomi Remen

Key points

- Recognizing and addressing patients' spiritual needs is fundamental to palliative care.

- Spiritual care addresses issues of religion, existential suffering, and humanity.

- Nurses provide spiritual care through deep listening, presence, bearing witness, and compassion.

Spiritual care is perhaps the most mysterious and often misunderstood part of palliative care. There is much discussion about what constitutes good spiritual care, and to date there is no agreed on definition of terms. The misunderstanding is caused, in part, by this lack of agreement. It is important to establish clear definitions to demystify spiritual care. For the purposes of this chapter the terms are defined as follows:

- *Spirituality:* "Spirituality is the aspect of humanity that refers to the way individuals seek and express, meaning and purpose, and the way they experience their connectedness to the moment, to self, to others, to nature and to the significant or sacred."[1]

- *Religion:* An organization that has a set of rites, rules, practices, values, and beliefs that prescribe how individuals should live their lives and "includes a relationship with a divine being."[2]

- *Spiritual Care:* Allowing our humanity to touch another's by providing presence, deep listening, empathy, and compassion.[3]

- *Compassion:* The ability to be empathetically present to another while he or she is suffering and is trying to find meaning.[4,5]

- *Existential:* Relating to human existence and experience.[6]

Although the literature is trending toward defining them separately, some use the terms "spiritual" and "religious" interchangeably, implying they are the same. It is sometimes assumed that spiritual care is only about a person's religious traditions and beliefs. Using the definitions above, not everyone would describe him or herself as religious, but everyone is spiritual.[7] In fact, these definitions can determine the care given to patients. If a person does not identify as "religious" and the spiritual care offered is only about religious issues, then the person is denied this care, which could, in fact, provide compassion, peace, and comfort in the midst of the fear, pain, and chaos of illness. There is much spiritual care that can be given to support a person's relationship with him or herself, others, nature, and the transcendent even when religion is not a factor.

Case study

A 65-year-old woman dying at home of breast cancer

A 65-year-old woman, dying of breast cancer, was being cared for by her husband and the hospice team. The couple had been married for 43 years, had no children and at present, very few family members or friends to support them in her dying. The woman was attended by hospice for a couple of months before she died. She was lethargic and bed-bound and slept many hours of the day. She said she didn't want or need to see a chaplain but her husband did. The chaplain met the woman very briefly one time to introduce herself, but after that all visits concentrated on providing spiritual care to the husband, who despite his best efforts was being overcome by anticipatory grief.

The husband was a retired navy cook. He was high energy, engaging, talkative ... and very guarded when it came to feelings and emotions. He was eager for the chaplain's visits. He was of Italian heritage, raised in the Catholic Church but not a particularly religious person. Spiritual care for this man consisted of listening to his stories about cooking for the troops on a ship; stories about his life in the navy and with his wife; and allowing him to feed the chaplain. The first few visits the chaplain tried diligently to avoid eating, not wanting to inconvenience the husband or cause him undue concern, thinking he had to feed her. But after a couple of visits when he insisted she sit down and eat she realized that cooking for and feeding someone was just what he needed. His wife was no longer interested in food and certainly couldn't hold a conversation for very long. What he *knew* was cooking and feeding people and now that his life was unraveling he needed to engage in something pleasant and familiar that would help him cope with the grief he was trying so hard to ignore.

It was over the bowls of homemade soup that this husband, at times, felt safe enough to engage in some bits of conversation about his grief, his feelings, and his dying wife.

What is spiritual care?

Spiritual care is simply meeting the other person, human to human, providing compassionate presence, and being available for whatever comes up. In the aforementioned case study, not only was it unnecessary to talk about God, or anything religious, it would have been inappropriate and perhaps off-putting. The spiritual interchange took place just by being with the person, understanding where he was—emotionally and spiritually—and taking care of what was important to him.[8]

At other times, with other people, spiritual care might include saying prayers, reading from holy texts, or talking about God and the mysteries of the universe. It is not for us to decide what the spiritual care looks like. On some level, what we do to provide spiritual care is less important than who we bring into the room. Good spiritual care requires that the person who walks into the room put aside his/her own expectations and agenda and, instead, focus on the patient—doing whatever is needed, at the time, for the person receiving the care.

At its core, spiritual care is about being honest, being authentically human, and allowing our own humanity to touch the humanity of another[9] (Box 33.1). In the course of offering spiritual care, God and religious beliefs and ideas may emerge, but they do not have to. Religion is one way, one very important and significant way, that we express our spirituality. But religion is not a prerequisite. Spirituality can be expressed in a million ways: sitting quietly by the side of the road, taking food to a friend, watching a toddler learn to walk, working in the garden, praying, or crying with a man whose wife just died.

Rachel Naomi Remen speaks to the essence of spiritual care when she writes about the difference between "helping" and "serving." When we "help" someone, we assume they are broken and need fixing—they are weak, we are stronger, and we have the answers. But when we go to the bedside not to help or fix, but to serve, we allow our humanness, our wholeness, our brokenness, our compassion, and our vulnerability to be present and forefront. When we "help" or "fix" patients, they are in our debt. Service requires no payment. Service is mutually beneficial. When we serve, we create a space where healing can occur, both for the served and the server.[10]

"I'm only the nurse. What do I know about providing spiritual care?"

Spiritual care is in the purview of everyone: the medical staff, the palliative care team, and the patient's family and friends.[11] Given the mystery and misunderstanding surrounding spiritual care, it is understandable that many people feel unqualified and uncomfortable to provide spiritual interventions. Many feel that because they, themselves, are not religious, they could not possibly be of spiritual support to anyone. Others, although defining themselves as religious, do not feel comfortable to pray out loud or with someone else, or they think they do not know the Bible or the Quran, or any of the holy books, well enough. Here again, the religious interventions are only a part of spiritual care, and they are often best handled by the chaplain or professional spiritual caregiver. If patients are asking questions about God, expressing concerns, or ruminating over existential issues, then an appropriate intervention would be to make a referral to the chaplain (Box 33.2).[12] Chaplains are trained to address spiritual and existential concerns, both the religious and nonreligious. However, a chaplain referral is not the only spiritual intervention that can, or should, be made.

Because nurses are at the bedside 24/7 and, generally, are the medical professionals who spend the most time with patients and their families, it is important for nurses to know how to provide spiritual care and to do it well. It does not require a special degree, but it does take awareness of oneself, and the other, and it takes effort and a strong commitment. As stated earlier, at its core spiritual care is about being human and allowing our humanity to touch the humanity of another. Our humanity is expressed, in part, by providing presence, deep listening, bearing witness, and putting our compassion into action.[13] This is the foundation of spiritual care (Box 33.3).[14]

Compassionate presence and deep listening

It is not possible for the medical community to promise that a patient will never experience pain or suffering or to guarantee a

---

Box 33.1 The essential elements of spiritual care

Spiritual care encompasses

- Authenticity
- Kindness
- Compassion
- Respect
- Dignity
- Humanity
- Vulnerability
- Service
- Honesty
- Empathy

Box 33.2 Questions requiring chaplain referral

- What have I done to deserve this?
- I pray but I'm still sick.
- I used to believe in God, but now I'm not so sure.
- How will my family get along without me?
- What did my life mean?
- I'm scared.

Box 33.3 Spiritual interventions

- Compassionate presence
- Listening deeply
- Bearing witness
- Compassion at work

calm and peaceful death. But it is possible to promise to accompany the patient for the journey. This does not mean that an individual nurse should promise to always be at the patient's side, but it does mean the medical team can assure the patient it will do everything possible to alleviate pain and suffering and that the patient and family will not be abandoned.[15]

Being present is much more than just being in the room. In the words of John H. Kearsley, "it is insufficient merely to be physically present. I have had to realize that to make my presence count … I need to be *really* present, psychologically and emotionally."[16] Psychological presence entails work and effort on the part of the caregiver. Kindness, deep listening, and empathy are required for psychological or compassionate presence.[17]

Providing compassionate presence is more than just showing up or walking into a room. There is a quality to the presence that gives the message, "There is no where else I would rather be at this moment than here with you." It is not just about being physically in the room with another, but being present in that room—body, mind, and spirit. It is about "exhibiting empathy and focused attention."[18,19] Presence does not take any more time than just showing up, but it does take a lot more effort, energy, and intention, and it makes an enormous difference to the person who is the recipient. A nurse can go into a patient's room, walk directly to the IV pole, hang the medication, turn, and walk out. Or, that same nurse can go into the patient's room, walk over to the patient, make eye contact, smile, gently touch the patient's hand, walk to the IV pole, hang the medication, look directly into the patient's eyes once again, smile, turn, and walk out the door.

Human beings have a need to be seen and heard. "When dying patients are seen, and know that they are seen, as being worthy of honour and esteem by those who care for them, dignity is more likely to be maintained."[20] Spiritual care is about preserving dignity and truly seeing the other person. It is also about hearing the spirit of the message. It is not enough just to see the body or to hear the words. Spiritual care is about connecting to the heart and mind and soul because that connection says, "I see you. I hear your concerns. You matter. You are important. You are not alone. I care."

A woman and her family were going through hard times. There were children to feed, a mortgage, and all the usual expenses that go along with supporting a family of six. The woman and her husband owned a business that had been floundering for four years, and they were close to losing everything. They had $2.48 in the bank, creditors calling, and no guarantee of when the next money would arrive. The woman was in her minister's office, embarrassed, telling her story, crying, and feeling terrified by life. As she was pouring her heart out, someone walked by the minister's door, caught the attention of the cleric, and the pastor immediately stood up and waved and said, "Oh, hello!" and began talking to the passerby. The woman never again shared anything of importance or consequence with her minister.

To deeply listen means hearing what is being said and what is not being said and trying to understand the emotions and feelings behind the words. It means to "tune in" to another person so that we understand who that person really is on a deep, authentic level.[21] Listening deeply also requires the ability to hold the pain and suffering of another. When someone trusts us enough to be vulnerable in our presence and then goes even further, explaining the circumstances of the pain and suffering, he/she has offered us

a gift. It is our responsibility to embrace and protect that gift and treat it with the utmost respect, care, and deference.

The minister dismissed the woman's pain and trivialized her suffering by allowing herself to be distracted when being present was so crucial. It could have been a time of healing. Although the minister could not change the woman's circumstances, she had the opportunity to be truly present, thereby offering a human connection to the woman who was in such despair. The minister missed the moment and ensured that she would never again be given the chance to connect with her parishioner in such an intimate way.

Talking, listening, and telling our stories are all part of the human experience. In a study to investigate spiritual pain, Mako, Galek, and Poppito found that patients were more likely to request someone to sit and talk and be with them than they were to ask for religious interventions. "Patients asked that the chaplain 'stay with me as long as possible,' and 'stop by every now and then and talk to me.'"[22] Listening deeply and being "psychologically" or compassionately present are spiritual interventions that anyone can learn. But it takes time, practice, effort, willingness, and intention to be truly available to another human being. For many receiving palliative care, they have been told that there is no cure for them. A cure may not be possible, but the opportunity for healing is. Healthcare professionals can be the conduit to healing simply by being present and listening deeply.

Bearing witness

The term "bearing witness" may seem a foreign concept to some, but it is integral to spiritual care and a part of our experience as human beings. A friend is diagnosed with cancer, a coworker dies, an airplane crashes. These sad, life-changing events, and those that are happy and joyous as well, generally stimulate a response. That response is to tell the story of what happened. We feel the need to share our experiences, and we feel compelled to hear other people's stories. To bear witness is to be present to the events and the emotions of another's life and experience. We find strength and comfort in knowing that other human beings bear witness to the significant events of our lives—the good and the bad.

It may seem that bearing witness is a passive event, such as just watching and observing. But, indeed, beneficially bearing witness takes focus and intention just like compassionate presence and deep listening. Bearing witness is not "fixing," "helping," or imparting answers or platitudes. Platitudes are seldom healing, and "answers" can function to alienate the one we seek to serve. People seek medical attention looking for answers. There are some things in medicine that have definitive answers and some that do not. In the spiritual/existential realm there are very few, if any, absolutes. Two people asking the question, "Why did I get sick?" will most likely have two different answers, if they can find answers at all. Our spiritual/existential answers are our own, revealed to us through years of living life through our own lens and experience. Nurses and healthcare providers might find it a relief to know that they do not have to have the answers to patients' spiritual questions. Furthermore, offering an answer to another's spiritual questions, or providing meaning, is not in the purview of healthcare professionals and generally is not helpful or beneficial.[23] We cannot know the answers to others' questions, so to assume we do and to assert those "answers" might be harmful to the patient or, at the very least, stop them from their own process of finding meaning.

So what does it really mean to bear witness? Bearing witness means compassionate presence, deep listening, watching, observing—being with. "Your job is to offer not only compassion but also to accompany as best as you can those dying on their journey."[24] Bearing witness means to compassionately accompany another.

Like presence and listening, bearing witness does not mean taking away the person's pain or suffering. Bearing witness means being present to the pain and suffering. In fact, if our primary goal is to take away the suffering, then that itself can interfere with our ability to be present in the moment.[25] Bearing witness is the ability to sit in the midst of whatever is happening. We often betray our own discomfort while listening to the stories of patients' suffering when we jump up to get a tissue for their tears. We tell ourselves that the tissue is for the one who is crying, to make him/her more comfortable, when in fact it can say more about our own desire to step back and move away from the pain. The message we risk sending is, "Stop crying. I don't want to hear anymore. I need you to stop crying now."

When someone is sharing an intense story, if we are truly present in the moment, then we can find ourselves almost not breathing, listening to, or attending to the other. When we move, we break the moment and it can stop the process, the story, and the tears. Something as simple as reaching over and touching a person while he/she is telling the emotion-filled story can stop the flow and interrupt the process. When these interruptions occur, there is a good chance that the story, which was so important to tell, might never again find the opportunity to be told. It takes time, experience, and thoughtful awareness to learn when to speak, or move, or get tissues.

Bearing witness means being comfortable enough in our own pain and suffering that we can just sit quietly, be with another human being who is suffering, and not run. It also means being aware of our own grief and being in touch with that grief so that it does not spill over and leak out onto the patients and families we serve.

Case study

A 42-year-old female patient with stage 4 ovarian cancer with metastases to the lungs

A 42-year-old female patient, Mrs. S, with advanced ovarian cancer was readmitted to the hospital experiencing severe nausea, vomiting, pain and weight loss caused by a blockage in her intestines. She was weak, frightened and very anxious. She was married with two children, whose ages were five and seven. This was the first time the medical staff who had been caring for her for the past five years could remember this patient exhibiting behavior of fear or anxiety. Her physician had the reputation of being uncomfortable with the "human" side of cancer. She would not address questions about a patient's mortality or inquiry of, "What will happen if the chemo doesn't work and the cancer keeps growing?" This oncologist would either ignore the question and move on to something else or would minimize her patient's concern with, "Now let's not worry about that. You just keep strong and keep doing what we tell you to do and you'll be fine."

Mrs. S, who had always acquiesced to her physician's will, was now unwilling to be dismissed as her fear and anxiety escalated. The doctor was described as "cold" and some said "rude" when attempting to allay her patient's anxiety and agitation upon admission. The doctor, appearing upset and frustrated, gave an order for medication to sedate Mrs. S. The sedation was given for the next two days with the patient's agitation and anxiety returning each time the medication wore off.

The social worker and chaplain, who knew this woman well, discussed with one another the high likelihood that the reason for the anxiety was Mrs. S's desire to know what was really happening in her body so she could plan for her family's future. Her husband and children were of paramount importance to her, and Mrs. S had discussed with the chaplain and the social worker, on more than one occasion, her desire to know what was likely to happen so she could prepare her family. If she was going to die from this disease she did not want it to be a surprise to everyone, especially her husband and children.

The social worker and chaplain each met with Mrs. S to assess her psychosocial and spiritual needs and concerns. They concurred that their primary intervention would be to ask Mrs. S what she thought was causing her anxiety and to carefully listen to what the patient had to say. She reported to both of them that she felt like she was going to die and she just needed the doctor to tell her the truth. Both social worker and chaplain strongly encouraged the patient to tell her doctor that she wanted, and *needed*, to know what might happen to her.

The social worker and chaplain, together, spoke with the physician. They explained to the doctor that the patient's anxiety might be significantly decreased if she could sit and speak with Mrs. S and give her an honest prognosis. The doctor listened and somewhat reluctantly agreed before saying how hard it is for her to lose a patient. She did not like the "dying part" of being a doctor.

After the physician and Mrs. S had a conversation about the patient's poor prognosis, the anxiety dramatically decreased, eliminating the need for sedation.

It is not easy for caregivers to manage both their own grief and the grief of their patients. But to ensure that professional caregivers are providing the best care for their patients and are caring for themselves as well, it is incumbent on them to be aware of, work with, and reconcile their own grief.[26] This will be addressed more fully later in the chapter.

Compassion at work

Being present, listening deeply, and bearing witness require a commitment from the one who serves. After these interventions, the next step in providing good spiritual care is action based on compassion. Is there anything missing? Is there something more to be done? Deep listening can reveal a patient's hopes, desires, and longing. Sometimes what is needed is very simple but it can make a huge difference in the quality of the patient's life.

For many, healthcare professionals and laypersons alike, being unsure of what to say can cause discomfort at the thought of spending any quality time with one who is dying. Empathy is vital to spiritual care. The capacity to put ourselves in the place of another is paramount. We can never know what another person is really feeling, but we can, in our own mind, imagine what it might be like for us to be in the patient's situation. "How would I feel if I was the one who was dying?" "What would I want?" "What would I want someone to say ... or not say?" "What would feel supportive?"

To ask ourselves these kinds of questions is the first step in being attuned to the other person's suffering and pain. Although we can only guess what a patient might or might not want to talk about, we can ask some open-ended, leading questions that will give the patient the opportunity to express his/her feelings if he/she chooses. If we ask a question or two and the patient seems reticent or reluctant to talk, then we can assume that either this is not a good time or it is not something he/she wants to talk about with us. It does not mean we never ask another question but that we take our cues from the patient, listening carefully for a time when he/she might be open and willing to talk.

We often hear "Mrs. White just does not want to talk about it." This may or may not be true. When we are experiencing pain and suffering, it is not uncommon for us to be very particular with regard to whom we share our feelings and innermost thoughts with. We want to make sure that the person we tell will have some understanding of what we are going through and will respect our feelings and care for them. So, although Mrs. White "does not want to talk about it" with just anyone, she might be willing, even eager, to talk if the right person walked into her room—a person who would listen deeply, be present, and bear witness to her deepest fears and concerns. This would likely also be a person who would know when to honor the silence and say nothing and then would know what to say at the appropriate time.

How do we know what to say? This is something we can learn with time and experience. It is vital to be observant when we are with other people, listening to what they say, when they say it, and how the message is delivered. Watching to see what "works" and what "does not" can be a wonderful way for us to learn how to listen and communicate effectively, especially in sensitive circumstances. To learn this skill requires that we be acutely aware—aware of our own responses and the responses, verbally and nonverbally, of the ones we are observing.

It is almost always appropriate to ask a person to tell us more about the story. "How did you feel when that happened?" "What happened next?" "Tell me more about that." There are times when we are so touched or overwhelmed by a story that we honestly do not know what to say. It is an authentic response and it is not inappropriate to say, "I have no idea what to say at this moment." Because it is genuine and honest, people usually respond well to a statement that bears such candor. It is certainly preferable to making a casual remark that runs the risk of trivializing the person's feelings or the situation.

Even when a person is open and wants to talk about his/her experience and feelings, it can be difficult to know just how far to take the conversation. What questions are appropriate to ask? Questions that inquire about a person's feelings or experience are generally welcomed (Box 33.4). If a question is asked that a patient does not want to talk about, then he or she usually finds a way to "talk around" the question without actually giving an answer. Listening carefully to what is "not" said is crucial. It can tell us that the patient, at this moment, does not want to go there.

Box 33.4 Spiritual care questions

Are you scared?
What makes life worth living?
Is there anything you haven't done that you need to do?
What do you hope for?
What are you most afraid of?
Is there anything worse than death?
What are you most proud of in your life?
Do you have regrets?

Sometimes talking and listening are not enough. What a patient has to say may reveal that he or she needs more: a chaplain referral, a phone call to a family member, prayer, a walk in the garden, or a feeling of urgency to leave the hospital and go home. Just as advocating for patients is a standard component of nursing care, it is also a vital element of spiritual care and is a spiritual care intervention.

Case study

A 58-year-old woman in the hospital undergoing bone marrow transplant for leukemia

A 58-year-old single woman, with no children or close family members, was admitted to the hospital to receive a bone marrow transplant for the treatment of leukemia. The woman was fairly isolated, having only two or three friends who might visit during her hospital stay, which could last anywhere from weeks to months. When the chaplain went in to meet with the patient the first day, the woman did not identify herself as "religious" but did remark that being out in nature gave her a sense of connection to the universe, calmed her, and helped her to feel at ease. She spent most of her days outside in her garden and felt better there than anywhere else. She was wondering how she was going to survive being inside for the next few weeks. She told the chaplain she was feeling scared about the transplant and depressed at the thought of being cooped up inside unable to see her garden.

After hearing just how important nature was to her spiritual well-being, the chaplain noticed the room the woman had be given had a very large window but it overlooked a free-way with nothing in view but thousands of cars and high tension wires ... no trees or flowers or anything that could be even loosely referred to as nature. The chaplain was very aware that the transplant unit was full, however, this was a real potential for spiritual distress and might easily be averted with a simple remedy. The opposite side of the unit also had large windows ... that overlooked a beautiful mountain range with green trees and flowers and plants ... nature at its finest! The chaplain met, that afternoon, with the people who could make the room transfer possible. It was not easy convincing those who assigned the rooms that this change was not just, "Oh, I think it would be nice if she could have a pretty view while she's here" ... but rather a necessary spiritual intervention that could impact the patient's ability to cope and heal from the transplant. It took 3 days, but the change was made and the woman was delighted that she could commune with nature during her transplant, in the comfort of her hospital bed.

Presence, deep listening, and bearing witness were important and vital, but in this case more was needed. Sometimes just engaging in life review—telling the story of one's life—is what brings a sense of peace, and there is nothing more to be done. In other cases, it is not enough to just be with, be present, and listen. Sometimes, as with this patient, the situation calls for action, for doing something more.

Patients often give us specific information when we engage them in conversation, but it is not the only way we discover who patients are and what is important to them. Sometimes the clues are more subtle. They can be as simple as noticing a rosary on the bed or pictures of grandchildren on the wall. Sometimes just being aware of who visits the patient can provide insight about his/her spirituality. Noticing that a rabbi visited the patient can be a perfect entrée to asking about a person's spiritual/religious beliefs. "I noticed a rabbi came to see you this morning. It made me wonder if you're Jewish, and if you are, if there is anything we can do here in the hospital to support you in your faith?" It is important to ask and not just assume that because a rabbi was in the room that the person is Jewish. But it does give the healthcare provider a place to start in an effort to determine what kind of spiritual care, if any, the person may want or need.

One man had been hospitalized for the better part of a year, and it had been extremely difficult for him and his family. He was a bone marrow transplant patient, which meant he could not have plants or flowers in his room and could not go outside for much of that year he was in the hospital. Only after the "spiritual intervention" from his daughter did the staff discover that he was quite a gifted rose gardener. It was somewhat ironic because the hospital was known for its huge rose gardens. Unfortunately, not being allowed outside meant this patient was not able to enjoy them. However, his daughter had the idea of photographing the roses in his yard as well as some on the hospital grounds. She took beautiful, close-up pictures of individual roses in all stages of unfolding, had the prints enlarged, cut around each one of them, and taped those hundreds of roses all over the walls of his room. It was beautiful! It gave enjoyment to not only the patient and his family but to the medical staff as well. Moreover, it told something significant about the man and generated conversation with him, as a person, apart from his identity as a patient. It made him more than just another body in a bed, with no particular identity other than his diagnosis. He was the one in the hospital who loved to be outside and knew how to grow beautiful roses. It gave the staff another way to connect with him, besides just his illness.

A week before Christmas, the chaplain was paged back to the hospital shortly after leaving for the night. A 35-year-old patient was about a week away from dying and her mother and father, who were at her bedside, requested the chaplain come pray with them. The patient, who for medical reasons could no longer speak, was not particularly interested in a prayer, but she did want to sing Christmas carols. She couldn't make a sound to talk but was able to make a little noise when she tried to sing. The words were completely unintelligible, but some of the tune made itself known. The patient, her mother, and the chaplain sang for the better part of the evening, one carol after another, frequently joined by a nurse, phlebotomist, or other healthcare professional as they entered the room to give care. Before leaving for the night, the chaplain rushed out to buy Christmas CDs, which the family played all night according to the parents' report the next day.

An elderly woman, dying at home with hospice care, told the team that years before, she and her husband had raised English Setters. She spoke longingly about that time in their lives. The chaplain had a friend who had an English Setter. He and his dog, Sarah, were a part of the local hospital's pet team. Sarah was very comfortable being with people who were sick in bed. With the patient and her husband's consent, the chaplain made arrangements for Sarah to visit and lie beside the woman in her last days. The pleasure and the memories were apparent on the patient's face as she hugged and petted Sarah.

Some patients clearly verbalize what they need physically, mentally, emotionally, and spiritually and are eager to talk and share their feelings. Try as we might, others just do not express who they are, and what they need, quite so obviously. But when we do discover something that will provide comfort, or a way for a person to more fully express his or her spirituality, it is important to do

whatever we can to make it available. The clues, and the outcomes, do not have to be dramatic. One patient told everyone who would listen about her favorite nurse. The reason the nurse was so special? Whenever she went into the room to provide care, she sang the patient a song. These signs are merely ways to start a conversation about what is meaningful in a person's life.

The nurse does not have to be the only one to provide spiritual interventions. The nurse may be the one to learn what is needed, but sometimes another member of the healthcare team might be better suited to make it happen. If a patient wants someone to come and pray, perhaps, the chaplain would be the best person to provide the intervention. If the patient's goal is to complete a will or advance directive, then maybe the social worker would be best to call. Sometimes it takes more than one person to help the patient achieve his/her goal. One nurse discovered that a patient did not want further medical treatment and really just wanted to go home to die. The nurse offered spiritual intervention when she advocated for the patient by informing the physician and the medical team, who made it possible for the patient to leave the hospital and go home.

Spiritual care means finding a way to make a connection, discovering any needs or desires that might improve quality of life, and then advocating and making arrangements for the fulfillment of those needs and desires. The job of a spiritual caregiver is always to be open (absent an agenda), listen, observe, and, when in doubt, ask questions. Assuming anything, without asking, leaves open the possibility that we will get it wrong. We never can be certain what is inside someone else's mind and heart. To ask is always best.[27]

The use of rituals in spiritual care

Often when we think of rituals we speak of religious traditions that have been practiced and passed down for hundreds or thousands of years. Some of the most obvious rituals are: Holy Communion; Anointing of the Sick; prayer; and Scripture reading, chanting, singing, or saying the rosary.

But rituals do not have to be religious in nature and can be created spontaneously, in the moment, to meaningfully acknowledge a person, event, or circumstance in our lives. Angeles Arrien stated, "Ritual is recognizing a life change, and doing something to honor and support the change."[28] We engage in nonreligious, yet spiritual, rituals everyday when we bake a birthday cake for a friend and sing "Happy Birthday," read a bedtime story to our children each night, or even read the newspaper over a cup of coffee in the morning.

When patients are receiving palliative care they have often been sick for a long time and sometimes forget who they were before the illness began. Many times, the disease becomes the descriptor by which they identify themselves. For patients to avoid losing their identity to the disease, it can be especially helpful to maintain as much normalcy as possible, particularly when they have been confined to the hospital for long periods of time. Birthday cakes, bedtime stories, and reading the morning paper with a cup of coffee are simple rituals that can remind us of what we held dear before the onset of the disease.

In a cancer hospital where bone marrow transplants require patients to be hospitalized for weeks—even months—at a time, a group of patients created a ritual that served them well. Every evening after dinner they met in a lounge area and played cards. This ritual was the highlight of their hospital stay. They looked forward to an activity that under "normal" circumstances might seem ordinary and routine. But under these circumstances, this ritual afforded them the opportunity to not only get out of their rooms but allowed them to be with other people (people who had a good understanding of what they were going through) to forget they had cancer for a while, to participate in an activity that felt "normal" again, to socially engage with other people, ... and the list goes on. The nursing staff was incredibly supportive, adjusting the schedules of what needed to be done so that these patients could be free in the evenings to participate in their nightly ritual.

Nurses can be invaluable in suggesting, and supporting, "rituals" for patients. When professional caregivers are aware of their patients as unique individuals with distinct wants, needs, and desires, then caregivers can offer meaningful suggestions for rituals that might be supportive to the patient's life and experience. Listening to music during unpleasant treatments might be soothing to a musician or a teenager who loves music. Getting a patient dressed early each morning, before breakfast, might be a practice that helps the person feel more able to take on the day. Sitting at the bedside to hear a patient's stories could be important to a young mother who wants to talk about the time she spent with her children who visited earlier in the day. The list of rituals is endless.

Although religious rituals are fewer in number, they can be equally important and beneficial. Caregivers cannot be expected to know all the religious rituals people practice, so it can be beneficial for the nurse, and others, to ask patients about any traditions or rituals that may be meaningful or important to them. Although the healthcare professional may not be involved with the rituals themselves, they can play a vital role in making sure the patient has some time alone, uninterrupted, so that the ritual will have the opportunity to be fully expressed and experienced. Rituals are a part of each of our lives. By recognizing the importance of ritual and by facilitating their expression nurses can be the conduit through which palliative care patients can find support and meaning.

Spiritual care near the time of death

As death draws near, it is even more important that professional caregivers attend to patients and their families with kindness, authenticity, and deep awareness. This awareness hears what is being said, and not said, and sees the visual signs of want, need, desire, and distress. Even those families who cannot begin to entertain the possibility of death are aware, on some level that life is changing. So it is a great kindness to be especially insightful and responsive to their wants, needs, desires, feelings, and fears. Patients may not be able, or willing, to ask for what they want, but if nurses and other healthcare professionals are attentive and perceptive, clues are frequently obvious and reveal what is needed. When providing spiritual care for those who are imminently dying, the three most important things to remember are (1) don't wait, (2) intently watch and listen, and (3) trust your instincts.

A grandmother, who had been in relatively good health until 3 weeks prior, fell and broke a hip, was bedridden at home on hospice, and was declining rapidly. Some days she was alert and oriented; other days she was wildly confused. This particular morning began with her mind and memory cloudy. While sleeping, her breathing pattern changed and it caught the attention of her granddaughter. The elderly woman was being cared for around the clock by her three daughters and a granddaughter, who also worked as a hospice

chaplain. Becoming aware of the subtle changes, the granddaughter instinctively felt they should call the rest of the family to the bedside. They did just that, and within a couple of hours there were dozens of grandchildren, great-grandchildren, family members, and friends assembled in the old woman's tiny house. When the family began to arrive the grandmother perked up and became much more alive and alert than she had been in weeks. This woman, who loved her family deeply but was never one to hug or kiss or show affection of any kind—and certainly had never been described as having a sense of humor—blossomed and came to life in front of her family. She was affectionate, chatty, warm, and funny, and her family saw a side of her no one there had witnessed, ever, in the grandmother's 90 years. The day was filled with stories and great humor. She lived another ten days. They were quiet days, and she was withdrawn and frequently confused. Although the family never again experienced the joy, affection, and laughter of that Friday, the family continues to describe it as the best time they ever had with her, and they are exceedingly grateful for the gift. Had the granddaughter ignored the almost imperceptible signs of decline and neglected to call in the family, who knows if they would have ever had another opportunity to experience their loved one in such a significant way?

It is easy to doubt and question ourselves, or dismiss signs and clues that are often barely visible and unclear. Good spiritual care, especially for the dying, requires caregivers to hone their skills in assessing these subtleties. Don't wait; intently watch and listen; and trust your instincts. To not do these things risks missing the moment and the opportunity that, literally, might never come again for the one who is dying.

Healthcare professional grief and well-being

Everyday, healthcare professionals deal with their patients' grief, but that does not make the caregivers immune to their own. The death of a loved one or friend is not the only kind of grief we experience. All people who are alive and aware experience grief, whether or not they have ever known someone who has died. When someone is disrespectful and rude to us, when we do not get the job we want, or when we are transferred to another part of the country, we experience grief. Grief can be the belief that we are not enough or that we failed, or the realization that life is changing and our hopes and dreams will never be realized.[29] When a loved one dies or when we experience extreme disappointment and loss, the grief never completely goes away, but, with time and effort, it is possible to come to terms with the loss, establish a new relationship with the deceased or circumstance, and move on.[30]

Although time does have its own way of easing suffering, it is not the only thing required to heal our grief. Grief is not an event. Grief is not linear. It is a process and it takes not only time, but effort, energy, work, and intention. It is most often a sequence of "two steps forward, one step back." Individual grief therapy or grief support groups can be useful tools in teaching us how to deal with our grief.

It is also important for us to be patient and have mercy for ourselves.[31] There is no set time frame for grief. It takes as long as it takes. One man's wife died and he felt it took about 3 years to reconcile the loss. Another woman died and her husband did not feel like he had moved forward at all, even after 5 years.

Many hospices, which have served to educate our society on the importance of the grief process, give their employees only 3 days paid bereavement—and then only for very immediate family members. Very often the person has not been buried, or a service conducted, in those three days, and the shock of the death can delay active grieving for some time. Three days is not enough time to face the world after a painful loss and then be expected to act as though everything is just fine. Just being familiar with death and grief does not guarantee understanding, or ease, in dealing with the process. Healthcare professionals can have just as much difficulty as their patients—maybe more—given the frequency with which they come face to face with dying, death, and grief. It can be difficult to care for someone who is grieving when the caregiver is in the midst of his/her own grief journey. A caregiver's grief can be triggered just by being in the presence of a patient who is also grieving. It is sometimes challenging for a busy caregiver to distinguish between the patient's grief and his/her own. For the well-being of all concerned, it is essential for healthcare professionals to be aware of and deal with their own grief and loss. Nurses and others are better able to serve when they have acknowledged their own pain and have made the effort to work through their own grief process.[32]

Nurses providing spiritual care

Deep listening, presence, bearing witness, and compassion are all simple ideas. Although simple, these interventions are not easy. To provide these interventions in a way that invites healing requires, from the caregiver, a willingness to learn, the ability to be without agenda, and the commitment to be ever vigilant and self-introspective. Nurses, who are called on to provide these interventions, are at the forefront of patient care. They are asked, every day, to deal with the medical, emotional, social, and spiritual crises and burdens of others' lives. They are expected to ease suffering whenever, and wherever, possible. At best, nursing is difficult work. We seem to be asking almost superhuman acts from nurses, who want deeply to provide all that is asked of them. Fortunately, quality spiritual care does not require superhuman acts. It does require human kindness, compassion, and caring.

References

1. Puchalski C, Ferrell B, Virani R, et al. Improving the quality of spiritual care as a dimension of palliative care: the report of the consensus conference. J Palliat Med. 2009;12(10):885–904.
2. Pulchalski C, Ferrell B. Making Health Care Whole. West Conshohocken: Templeton Press; 2010.
3. McSherry W, Ross L. Nursing. In: Cobb M, Puchalski CM, Rumbold B (eds.), Oxford Textbook of Spirituality in Healthcare. New York: Oxford University Press; 2012:211–217.
4. Bryson KA. Spirituality, meaning, and transcendence. J Palliat Support Care. 2004;2:321–328.
5. Post SG. Unlimited Love: Altruism, Compassion and Service. Philadelphia, PA: Templeton Foundation Press; 2003.
6. www.macmillandictionary.com/dictionary/american/existential. Accessed June 20, 2013.
7. Puchalski C, Ferrell B, Virani R, et al. Improving the quality of spiritual care as a dimension of palliative care: the report of the consensus conference. J Palliat Med. 2009;12(10):885–904.
8. Bryson KA. Spirituality, meaning, and transcendence. J Palliat Support Care. 2004;2:321–328.
9. Remen RN. In the service of life. Noetic Sciences Review. 1996;37:24–25.
10. Remen RN. In the service of life. Noetic Sciences Review. 1996;37:24–25.
11. Puchalski C, Ferrell B, Virani R, et al. Improving the quality of spiritual care as a dimension of palliative care: the report of the consensus conference. J Palliat Med. 2009;12(10):885–904.
12. Puchalski C, Ferrell B, Virani R, et al. Improving the quality of spiritual care as a dimension of palliative care: the report of the consensus conference. J Palliat Med. 2009;12(10):885–904.
13. Halifax J. Project on Being with Dying Training for Health Care Professionals. Santa Fe, New Mexico, 2001.
14. Halifax J. Project on Being with Dying Training for Health Care Professionals. Santa Fe, New Mexico, 2001.
15. Sulmasy DP. Ethical principles for spiritual care. In: Cobb M, Puchalski CM, Rumbold B (eds.), Oxford Textbook of Spirituality in Healthcare. New York: Oxford University Press; 2012:465–470.
16. Kearsley JH. Wal's story: reflections on presence. J Clin Oncol. 2012;30(18):2283–2285.
17. Neff KD. Self-compassion: an alternative conceptualization of a healthy attitude toward oneself. Self Identity. 2003;2:85–102.
18. McDonough-Means S, Kreitzer MJ, Bell I. Fostering a healing presence and investigating its mediators. J Altern Complement Med. 2004;10(S1):S-25–S-41.
19. Guenther, MB. Healing: the power of presence a reflection. J Pain Symptom Manage 2011;41(3):650–654.
20. Chochinov HM, Cann BJ. Interventions to enhance the spiritual aspects of dying. J Palliat Med. 2005;8(S-1):S-103–S-115.
21. Slater V. What does "spiritual care" now mean to palliative care? Eur J Palliat Care. 2007;14(1):32–34.
22. Mako C, Galek K, Poppito SR. Spiritual pain among patients with advanced cancer in palliative care. J Palliat Med. 2006;9(5)1106–1113.
23. Guenther, MB. Healing: the power of presence a reflection. J Pain Symptom Manage. 2011; 41(3):650–654.
24. Halifax J. Personal communication. December 12, 2008.
25. Millspaugh D. Assessment and response to spiritual pain: Part II. J Palliat Med. 2005;8(6):1110–1117.
26. Ferrell BR, Baird P. Deriving meaning and faith in caregiving. Semin Oncol Nurs. 2012;28(4):256–261.
27. Pronk K. Role of the doctor in relieving spiritual distress at the end of life. Am J Hosp Palliat Med. 2005;22(6):419–425.
28. Arrien A. The Four-fold Way. San Francisco, CA: Harper San Francisco; 1993.
29. Klaus D, Silverman PR, Nickman SL. Continuing Bonds: New Understandings of Grief. Philadelphia, PA: Taylor and Francis; 1996.
30. Klaus D, Silverman PR, Nickman SL. Continuing Bonds: New Understandings of Grief. Philadelphia, PA: Taylor and Francis; 1996.
31. Levine S, Levine O. The grief process. Boulder, CO: Sounds True; 1999.
32. Feldstein CBD. Bridging with the sacred; reflection of an MD chaplain. J Pain Symptom Manage. 2011;42(1):155.

CHAPTER 34

Meaning in illness

Tami Borneman and Katherine Brown-Saltzman

Life is defined as "BC" or "AC"—before cancer or after cancer.

Cancer patient

Uncertainty—the next step of the journey with chemo-maintenance therapy. Not knowing how treatments are going to be and how it will affect me. There's this tunnel but there's no light yet. Did I repent my sins enough to beat the cancer? Why did you do this to me? What did I do to deserve this? Sometimes I feel like it's a punishment. God is mysterious. I get tears in my eyes when I see the kids with cancer and think, God why would you do this to kids? How long will the drugs last and work? How much time do I have? And quality of life? As long as I do the patient log and keep the positive going, I'm pretty good.

Cancer patient

In the driest whitest stretch

Of pain's infinite desert

I lost my sanity

And found this rose

Galal al-Din Rumi; Persia, 1207–1273

Key points

◆ Finding meaning in illness is an important issue when facing the end of life.

◆ The process of finding meaning in illness involves a journey through sometimes very difficult transitions.

◆ A terminal illness can greatly impact the patient-caregiver relationship.

◆ It is essential for nurses to experience their own journey regarding the dying process and bring with them a willingness to be transformed by it.

Is it possible to adequately articulate and give definition to meaning in illness? Or is meaning in illness better described and understood through using symbolism and metaphors such as the above poem? To try to define that which is enigmatic and bordering on the ineffable seems almost sacrilegious. The unique individual journey of finding meaning in illness experienced by each patient facing the end of life and their family caregiver would seem to be diminished by the very process that seeks to understand through the use of language.

Is it that we seek to find meaning in illness or is it that we seek to find meaning in the life that is now left and in those relationships and things we value? Do we seek to find meaning in illness itself as an isolated event or that which is beyond the illness, such as how

to live out this newly imposed way of life? Terminal illness often forces us to reappraise the meaning and purpose of our life. If we allow space in our lives for the process of meaning in illness to unfold, we then move from the superficial to the profound.

Terminal illness also forces us at some point to look directly at death, yet we resist getting in touch with the feelings that arise. Everything in us seeks life. Everything in us hopes for life. Everything in us denies death. There is something very cold, very unmoving, and very disturbing about it all. Does the end of one's human existence on Earth need to be the sole metaphor for death?

Although end-of-life issues have progressed nearer to the forefront of healthcare, the dying patient is still the recipient of an impersonal, detached, and cure-focused system, thereby exacerbating an already catastrophic situation. As necessary as it is for nurses to use the nursing process, it is not enough. The patient's illness odyssey beckons us to go beyond assessment, diagnosis, intervention, and evaluation to a place of vulnerability, not in an unprofessional manner but, rather, in a way that allows for a shared connectedness unique to each patient-nurse relationship. We need to be willing to use feelings appropriately as part of the therapeutic process. Separating ourselves from touching and feeling to protect ourselves only serves to make us more vulnerable, because we have then placed our emotions in isolation. Nurses can be a catalyst for helping the patient and family find meaning in the illness and, in the process, can help themselves define or redefine their own meaning in life, illness, and death.

Meaning defined

Johnston-Taylor[1] presents several definitions for meaning (Table 34.1). In the dictionary,[2] one finds meaning defined simply as "something that is conveyed or signified" or as "an interpreted goal, intent, or end." But it is the etymology of the word "mean"

Table 34.1 Definitions of meaning

Meaning	"refers to sense, or coherence.... A search for meaning implies a search for coherence. 'Purpose' refers to intention, aim, function.... however, 'purpose' of life and 'meaning' of life are used interchangeably"[4]
	"a structure which relates purposes to expectations so as to organise actions.... Meaning ... makes sense of actions by providing reasons for it"[5]
[Search for] meaning	"is an effort to understand the event: why it happened and what impact it has had ... [and] attempts to answer the question(s), What is the significance of the event? ... What caused the event to happen? ... [and] What does my life mean now?"[6]
	"is an attempt to restore the sense that one's life [is] orderly and purposeful"[7]
Personal search for meaning	"the process by which a person seeks to interpret a life circumstance. The search involves questioning the personal significance of a life circumstance, in order to give the experience purpose and to place it in the context of a person's total life pattern. The basis of the process is the interaction between meaning in and of life and involves the reworking and redefining of past meaning while looking for meaning in a current life circumstance."[8]

that helps nursing come to understand our potential for supporting patients in the process of finding meaning in their lives, even as they face death. "Mean" comes from the Old English *maenan*, "to tell of." One does not find meaning in a vacuum; it has everything to do with relationships, spirituality, and connectedness. While the process of finding meaning depends greatly on an inward journey, it also relies on the telling of that journey. The telling may use language, but it may also be conveyed by the eyes, through the hands, or just in the way the body is held. Frankl[3] reminds us that the "will to meaning" is a basic drive for all of humanity and is unique to each individual. A life-threatening illness begs the question of meaning with a new urgency and necessity.

Cassell[9] tells us that "all events are assigned meaning," which entails judging their significance and value. Meaning cannot be separated from the person's past; it requires the thought of future and ultimately influences perception of that future.[9(p. 67)] Finding meaning is not a stagnant process; it changes as each day unfolds and the occurrences are interpreted. As one patient reflected on his diagnosis, "Even though I have this I am still a whole person. My thoughts are different, my ambitions are a little different because I want to spend as much time as I can with my grandkids."[10] Coming face to face with one's mortality not only defines what is important but also focuses the poignancy of the loss of much that has been meaningful.

One's spirituality is often the key to transcending those losses and finding ways to maintain those connections, whether it is the belief that one's love, work, or creativity will remain after the physical separation or the belief that one's spirit goes on to an afterlife or through reincarnation. Meaning in life concerns the individual's realm of life on Earth. It has to do with one's humanness, the temporal, and the composites of what one has done in life to give it meaning. Meaning of life has more to do with the

existential. It is looking beyond one's earthly physical existence to an eternal, secure, and indelible God or spiritual plane. The existential realm of life provides a sense of security whereby one can integrate experiences.[11]

Spirituality has been defined as a search for meaning.[12,13] One of the Hebrew words for meaning is *biynah* (bee-naw), which is understanding, knowledge, meaning, and wisdom. It comes from the root word *biyn* (bene), which means to separate mentally or to distinguish.[14] How is it that one can come to knowledge and understanding? Patients receiving palliative care often describe a sense of isolation and loneliness. They frequently have endless hours available while at the same time experiencing a shortening of their life. It is here that the nurse has a pivotal role as the listener, for when the ruminations of the dying are given voice, there is an opportunity for meaning. Important life themes are shared, and the unanswerable questions are at least asked. As the stranger develops intimacy and trust, meaning takes hold.

Suffering creates one of the greatest challenges to uncovering meaning. For the dying patient, suffering comes in many packages: physical pain, unrelenting symptoms (nausea, pruritus, dyspnea, etc.), spiritual distress, dependency, multiple losses, and anticipatory grieving. Even the benefits of medical treatments given to provide hope or palliation can sometimes be outweighed by side effects (e.g., sedation and constipation from pain medication), inducing yet further suffering. The dictionary defines suffering in this way: "To feel pain or distress; sustain loss, injury, harm, or punishment."[2] But once again, it is the root word that moves us to a more primitive understanding—the Latin sufferer, which comprises *sub*, "below," and *ferre*, "to carry." The weight and isolation of that suffering now becomes more real at the visceral level. Cassell[9] reminds us that pain itself does not foreordain suffering; it is, in fact, the meaning that is attributed to that pain that determines the suffering. In his clinical definition, "Suffering is a state of severe distress induced by the loss of the intactness of person, or by a threat that the person believes will result in the loss of his or her intactness."[9(p. 63)] Clinicians can further unnecessary suffering, as attested in the research of Berglund et al., by making patients feel objectified or providing fragmented care.[15] Suffering is an individual and private experience and will be greatly influenced by the personality and character of the person; for example, the patient who has needed control during times of wellness will find the out-of-control experience of illness as suffering.[9] In writing about cancer pain and its meaning, Ersek and Ferrell[16] provide a summary of hypotheses and theses from the literature (Table 34.2).

Although not always recognized, it is the duty of all who care for patients to alleviate suffering and not just treat the physical dimensions of the illness. This is no small task, as professionals must first be free from denial and the need to self-protect to see the suffering of another. Then, they must be able to attend to it without trying to fix it or simplify it. The suffering needs to be witnessed; in the midst of suffering, presence and compassion become the balm and hope for its relief.

The process of finding meaning in illness

From years of working with terminally ill patients and their families, the authors have found that the process of finding meaning in illness invokes many themes. The title given to each theme is an

Table 34.2 Summary of hypotheses and theses from the literature on meaning

Hypothesis/thesis	Authors
The search for meaning is a basic human need.	Frankl 1959[3]
Meaning is necessary for human fulfillment.	Steeves and Kahn 1987[17]
Finding meaning fosters positive coping and increased hopefulness.	Ersek 1991[18]; Steeves and Kahn 1987[17]; Taylor 1983[7]
One type of meaning-making activity in response to threatening events is to develop causal attributions.	Gotay 1983[19]; Haberman 1987[20]; Steeves and Kahn 1987[17]; Taylor 1983[7]; Chrisman and Haberman 1977[21]
Meaning making can involve the search for a higher order.	Ersek 1991[18]; Ferrell et al. 1993[22]; Steeves and Kahn 1987[17]
Making meaning often involves the use of social comparisons.	Ferrell et al. 1993[22]; Taylor 1983[7]; Ersek 1991[18]; Haberman 1987[20]
Meaning can be derived through construing benefits from a negative experience.	Ersek 1991[18]; Haberman 1987[20]; Taylor 1983[7]
Meaning sometimes focuses on illness as challenge, enemy, or punishment.	Barkwell 1991[23]; Ersek 1991[18]; Lipowski 1970[24]
Pain and suffering often prompt a search for meaning.	Frankl 1959[3]; Steeves and Kahn 1987[17]; Taylor 1983[7]
Uncontrolled pain or overwhelming suffering hinder the experience of meaning.	Steeves and Kahn 1987[17]
One goal of care is to promote patients' and caregivers' search for and experiences of meaning.	Ersek 1991[18]; Ferrell et al. 1993[22]; Steeves and Kahn 1987[17]; Haberman 1988[25]

attempt to represent observed transitions that many terminally ill patients seem to experience. Not all patients experience the transitions in the same order, and not all transitions are experienced. However, we have observed that these transitions are experienced by the majority of patients. Issues faced by family caregivers and healthcare professionals are discussed in later sections. The themes shared in this section are the imposed transition, loss and confusion, dark night of the soul, randomness and absence of God, brokenness, and reappraisal. In experiencing some or all of these transitions, one can perhaps find meaning in this difficult time of life.

The imposed transition

Being told that you have a terminal illness can be like hearing the sound of prison doors slam shut. Life will never be the same. The sentence has been handed down, and there is no reversing the verdict. Terminal illness is a loss, and there is nothing we can do to change the prognosis even though we may be able to temporarily delay the final outcome. The essence of our being is shaken, and our souls are stricken with a panic unlike any other we have ever felt. For the first time, we are faced with an "existential awareness of nonbeing."[26] For a brief moment, the silence is deafening, as if suspended between two worlds, the known and the unknown. As one "regains consciousness," so to speak, the pain and pandemonium of thoughts and emotions begin to storm the floodgates of our faith, our coping abilities, and our internal fortitude, while simultaneously the word "terminal" reverberates in our heads. There is no easy or quick transition into the acceptance of a terminal diagnosis.

Facing the end of life provokes questions. The self-reflective questions include both the meaning *of* life and the meaning *in* life. Whether we embrace with greater fervor the people and things that collectively give us meaning in life or we view it all as now lost, the loss and pain are real. Nothing can be done to prevent the inevitable. There is a sense of separation or disconnectedness in that while I am the same person, I have also become permanently different from you. Unless you become like me, diagnosed with

a terminal illness, we are in this sense separated. In a rhetorical sense, the meanings we gain in life from relationships and the material world serve to affirm us as participants in these meanings.[26] When these meanings are threatened by a terminal diagnosis, we fear the loss of who we are as functioning productive human beings. The affirmations we received from our meanings in life are now at a standstill.

A 65-year-old retired military man, although accepting of his prognosis, fought to delay the inevitable for as long as possible. As a military man, he was not afraid of dying. The relationship with one of his grown children was very good, and he adored his grandchildren. They were the reason he was fighting the cancer. He felt that life was most enjoyable when he spent time with them. His concern about dying was that because the grandchildren were young, there would not be enough time with them for them to remember him after he died. "My grandkids are more important than you know so cause they got to remember their grandpa. I want them to think about me, what grandparents did you know?"[27] When we discussed ways that he might be able to leave them a legacy, he began to understand that he saw himself and his remaining time in limited ways. He feared losing what had come to define his life. Encouraging him to redefine his life in terms of meaning through leaving a legacy for his grandchildren gave him new insights and provided a practical way to spend the rest of his days.

In addition to questioning meaning *in* life, those facing the end of life also question the meaning *of* life. A life-threatening illness makes it difficult to maintain an illusion of immortality.[28] What happens when we die? Is there really a God? Is it too late for reconciliation? For those believing in life after death, the questions may focus on uncertainty of eternal life, fear of what eternal life will be like, or the possibility of this being a test of faith. No matter what the belief system, the existential questions are asked. We reach out for a connection with God or something beyond one's self to obtain some sense of security and stability. Then, in this ability to transcend the situation, ironically, we somehow feel a sense of groundedness. Frankl[3] states, "It denotes the fact that being human always points, and is directed, to something or someone, other than oneself—be it a meaning to fulfill or another human being to encounter." There is an incredibly strong spiritual need to find meaning in this new senseless and chaotic world.

Loss and confusion

One cancer patient stated, "Our lives are like big run-on sentences and when cancer occurs, it's like a period was placed at the end of the sentence. In reality, we all have a period at the end of the sentence, but we don't really pay attention to it."[29] With a terminal diagnosis, life is changed forever, for however long that life may be. Each day life seems to change as one is forced to experience a new aspect of the loss. There is a sense of immortality that pervades our lust for life, and when we are made to look at our mortality, it is staggering. With all of the many losses, coupled with the fear of dying, one can be left feeling confused from the infinite possibilities of the unknown. The panorama of suffering seems to be limitless.

The pain of loss is as great as the pleasure we derived from life.[30] The pain is pure and somewhat holy. The confusion comes not only from one's world having been turned upside down but also from those who love us and care about us. It is not intentional; nevertheless, its impact is greatly felt. In trying to bring encouragement or trying to help one find meaning, the loss and pain are sometimes minimized by comparing losses, attempting to save God's reputation by denying the one hurting the freedom to be angry at God, or by immediately focusing on the time left to live. The hurting soul needs to feel the depth of the loss by whatever means it can. The pain from loss is relentless, like waves from a dark storm at sea crashing repeatedly against rocks on the shoreline.

A 55-year-old woman with terminal lung cancer experienced further physical decline each day. She was supported by a husband who lovingly doted on her. She was one who loved life and loved her family. Many losses were experienced because of her comorbid conditions along with the cancer. The fact that her family wanted her to focus on life and not her disease or death added to these losses. Her husband informed us that they knew she was going to die but felt that her quality of life would be better if these issues were not discussed. The patient had many thoughts and feelings to sort through and wanted to talk, but no one was listening. Her loss was not just physical; it also was an imposed emotional loss caused by a loving family trying to do the right thing. Many times the patient ended up in tearful frustration. The communications with her family were different, constantly reminding her that nothing was the same and, in turn, reminded her of her losses and impending death.

Captured in Tolstoy's *The Death of Ivan Ilyich*, we hear the agony of Ivan's similar experience, "This deception tortured him—their not wishing to admit what they all knew and what he knew, but wanting to lie to him concerning his terrible condition, and wishing and forcing him to participate in that lie.... And strangely enough, many times when they were going through their antics over him he had been within a hairbreadth of calling out to them: 'Stop lying! You know and I know that I am dying. Then at least stop lying about it!' But he had never had the spirit to do it."[31]

Dark night of the soul

The descent of darkness pervades every crack and crevice of one's being. One now exists in the place of Nowhere surrounded by nothingness that is void of texture and contour. One's signature is seemingly wiped away, taking with it the identification of a living soul.[30] Job states, "And now my soul is poured out within me; days of affliction have seized me. At night it pierces my bones within me, and my gnawing pains take no rest .... My days are swifter than a weaver's shuttle, and come to an end without hope."[32] "One enters the abyss of emptiness—with the perverse twist that one is not empty of the tortured feeling of emptiness."[33] This is pain's infinite desert.

Darkness looms as one thinks about the past, full of people and things that provided meaning in life, that will soon have to be given up. Darkness looms as one thinks about the future, because death precludes holding on to all that is loved and valued. Darkness consumes one's mind and heart like fire consumes wood. It makes its way to the center with great fury, where it proceeds to take possession, leaving nothing but a smoldering heap of ashes and no hope of recovering any essence of life.[34]

A woman with fairly young children relapsed after several years free of colon cancer. She received several months of treatment with an experimental protocol. She suffered greatly, not only from the effects of the chemotherapy but also from the long periods of time not being able to "be there" for her children. When it became clear that the chemo was not working as expected, she became tortured by the thought of abandoning her children at a time when they so greatly needed a mother and the fact that she had gambled with the little time she had left and had lost. Now in her mind, her children had the double loss of months of quality time she could have had with them and her impending death. She became inconsolable because of this darkness. Time to intervene was very limited. Allowing her the room for suffering and being "present" to this suffering as a nurse was essential. In addition, moving back into her mothering role and providing for her children by helping to prepare them for her death became the pathway through the darkness and into meaning.

Although one might try, there are no answers—theological or otherwise—to the "whys" that engulf one's existence. Death moves from an "existential phenomenon to a personal reality."[35] All our presuppositions about life fall away, and we are left emotionally naked. There is neither the physical, the emotional, nor the spiritual strength to help our own fragility. The world becomes too big for us, and our inner worlds are overwhelming.[30] The enigma of facing death strips order from one's life, creating fragmentation and leaving one with the awareness that life is no longer tenable.

Randomness and the absence of God

The pronouncement of a terminal diagnosis provokes inner turmoil and ruminating thoughts from dawn to dusk. Even in one's chaotic life, there was order. But order does not always prevail. A young athlete being recruited for a professional sport is suddenly killed in a tragic car accident. A mother of three small children is diagnosed with a chronic debilitating disease that will end in death. An earthquake levels a brand new home that a husband and wife had spent years saving for. A playful young toddler drowns in a pool. There seems to be no reason. It would be different if negligence were involved. For example, if the young athlete were speeding, or driving drunk, although the loss is still quite devastating, a "logical" reason could be assigned to it. But randomness leaves us with no "logical" explanation.[33]

The word "random" comes from the Middle English word *radon*, which is derived from the Old French word *randon*, meaning violence and speed. The word connotes an impetuous and haphazard movement, lacking careful choice, aim, or purpose.[2] The feeling of vulnerability is overwhelming. In an effort to find shelter from this randomness, meaning and comfort is sought from God or from something beyond one's self, but how do we know that God or something beyond ourselves is not the cause of our loss? Our trust is shaken. Can we reconcile God's sovereignty with our loss?[33] Can we stay connected to and continue to pull or gain strength and security from something beyond ourselves that may be the originator of our pain? There is a sense of abandonment by that which has been our stronghold in life. Yet to cut ourselves off from that stronghold out of anger would leave us in a state of total disconnection. A sense of connection is a vital emotion necessary for existence, no matter how short that existence may be. But facing death forbids us to keep our existential questions and desires at a distance. Rather, it seems to propel us into a deeper search for meaning as the questions continue to echo in our minds.

Brokenness

Does one come to a place of acceptance within brokenness? Is acceptance even attainable? Sometimes. Sometimes not. Coming to a place of acceptance is an individual experience for each person. In a wonderful analogy of acceptance, Kearney states, "Acceptance is not something an individual can choose at will. It is not like some light switch that can at will be flicked on or off. Deep emotional acceptance is like the settling of a cloud of silt in a troubled pool. With time the silt rests on the bottom and the water is clear."[36(p. 98)] Brokenness does, however, open the door to relinquishing the illusion of immortality. Brokenness allows the soul to cry and to shed tears of anguish. It elicits the existential question "Why?" once again, only this time not to gain answers but to find meaning.

A woman in her mid-60s, dying of lung cancer, shared how she came to a place of acceptance. When she was first diagnosed, the cancer was already well advanced. Her health rapidly declined, and she was more or less confined to bed or sitting. Out of her frustration, anger at God, sadness, and tears came the desire to paint again. It was her way of coping, but it became more than that. It brought her to a place of peace in her heart. She had gotten away from painting because of busyness and was now learning to be blessed by quietness. She was very good at creating cards with her own designs in watercolor, leaving the insides blank to be filled in by the giver. She would give these cards away to many people as her gesture of love and gratitude.

If we go back to the poem at the beginning of this chapter, it wasn't until "sanity" was lost that the rose was found. A gradual perception occurs, whereby we realize that the way out is by no longer struggling.[36] When we come to the end of ourselves and the need to fight the inevitable that is death, we give space for meaning to unfold. It is not that we give up the desire but that we relinquish the need to emotionally turn the situation around and to have all our questions answered. Sittser, a minister who experienced a sudden loss of several immediate family members, states, "My experience taught me that loss reduces people to a state of almost total brokenness and vulnerability. I did not simply feel raw pain; I was raw pain."[33(p. 164)] Pain and loss are still profound, but in the midst of these heavy emotions there begins to be a glimmer of light. Like the flame of a candle,

the light may wax and wane. It is enough to begin to silhouette those people and things that still can provide meaning.

Reappraisal

It is here where one begins to realize that something positive can come from even a terminal diagnosis and the losses it imposes. The good that is gained does not mitigate the pain of loss but, rather, fosters hope—hope that is not contingent on healing but on reconciliation, on creating memories with loved ones, on making the most of every day, on loving and being loved.[37] It is a hope that transcends science and explanations and changes with the situation. It is not based on a particular outcome but, rather, focuses on the future, however long that may be. Despair undermines hope, but hope robs death of despair.[38]

A male patient in his late 30s, facing the end of life after battling leukemia and having gone through a bone marrow transplant, shared that he knew he was going to die. It took him a long time to be able to admit it to himself. The patient recalled recently visiting a young man who had basically given up and did not want his last dose of chemotherapy. He talked awhile with this young man and encouraged him to "go for it." He told him that there is nothing like watching the last drop of chemo go down the tube and into his body, and the sense of it finally being all over. The patient shared with the young man that when he received his own last dose of chemotherapy, he stayed up until three in the morning to watch the last drop go down the tube. Although the chemotherapy did not help him to the extent that he wanted, he wanted to encourage the young man to hope and not give up. Life was not yet over. He had tears in his eyes when he finished the story.

Facing end of life with a terminal diagnosis will never be a happy event. It will always be tragic because it causes pain and loss to everyone involved. But at a time unique to each person facing death, a choice can be made as to whether one wants to become bitter and devalue the remaining time or value the time that is left as much as possible.

An important choice to be made during this time is whether to forgive or to be unforgiving—toward oneself, others, God, or one's stronghold of security in life. Being unforgiving breeds bitterness and superficiality. As we face the end of life, we need both an existential connection and a connection with others. Being unforgiving separates us from those connections, and it is only through forgiveness that the breech is healed. Forgiveness neither condones another's actions nor does it mean that this terminal diagnosis is fair. Rather, forgiveness is letting go of expectations that one somehow will be vindicated for the pain and loss. Whether by overt anger or by emotional withdrawal, in seeking to avoid vulnerability to further pain and loss, we only succeed in making ourselves more vulnerable. Now we have chosen a deeper separation that goes beyond facing the death of the physical body—that of the soul.[33] Positive vulnerability through forgiveness provides a means of healing and, when possible, reconciliation with others. It always provides healing and reconciliation with one's God or one's stronghold of security. Forgiveness allows both physical and emotional energy to be used for creating and enjoying the time left for living.

A 30-year-old woman was admitted to the hospital with advanced metastatic breast cancer. She was unknown to the hospital staff but had a good relationship with her oncologist. During the admissions assessment, the young woman could not give the name of anyone to contact in the event of an emergency. When pressed, she stated that she was alienated from her family and chose not to be in touch. She agreed that after her death her mother could be called, but not before. A social worker was summoned in the hope that something could be done to help with some unification. However, the social worker came out of the room devastated by the woman's resolve. The chaplain also found no way to reconnect this woman's family. The nursing staff experienced moral distress as they watched this woman die, all alone in the world. One of the authors worked with the staff to help them realize that they had become trusted and in a sense were her substitute family. One may not always be able to fix the pain of life's fractures or bring people to a place of forgiveness, but it is important not to underestimate what is happening in the moment. Healing for this patient came through the relationship with her doctors and nurses, and she died not alone but cared for.

There are many emotions and issues with which those facing death must contend. It is not an easy journey, and the process is wearing; nevertheless, the rose can be found.

Impact of the terminal illness on the patient-caregiver relationship

Each of us comes to new situations with our life's experiences and the meanings we have gained from them. It is no different when being confronted with illness and the end of life. However, in this special episode of life, there are often no personal "reruns" from which to glean insight. Patient and family come together as novices, each helping the other through this unknown passage. Because different roles and relationships exist, the impending loss will create different meanings for each person involved.

Facing the loss of someone you love is extremely difficult. For the family caregiver, the process of finding meaning is influenced by the one facing death. One example experienced by one of the authors of this chapter involved a wife's discussion with her terminally ill husband over several months regarding his outlook on life. As Christians, they knew where death would take them, but she was curious as to what that meant to him and how he was handling the unknown. She felt strong in her own faith but also felt like she was giving lip service to it at times. He described life as having even more meaning in that although he loved her very much and the life they had together, he could now "cherish" every moment of that time. He was sad knowing that he would eventually die from the cancer, but until that time came, he just wanted to enjoy life with her. She shared that while what he said seemed obvious when he said it, for some reason this time it really spoke to her soul and she felt peace.

In another example, a woman helped her family create meaning for themselves from the picture she had painted of herself sitting on the beach as a little girl next to a little boy. She explained that the little boy had his arm around her as they stared out at the sea. Each time the waves covered the surface of the beach and then retreated, the sea would carry with it bits and pieces of her fears and disease. The birds circling overhead would then swoop down to pick up and carry off any pieces not taken by the sea. The little boy's arm around her signified all the loving support she had received from others. When the time would come for her to die,

she would be ready because she had been able to let go of life as she knew it. She had let the waves slowly carry that which was of life out to sea and yet had learned to hold on to the meaning that that life had represented. In doing so, she enabled her family to hold on to the meaning of their relationship with her and enabled them to remain symbolically connected after her death.

A final, poignant story offers a different perspective. A 60-year-old woman with stage IV ovarian cancer was very angry at her husband and perplexed at God. She had troubles finding any positive meaning in anything in life. She was upset that her life would be cut short, and she would not live to see her grandchildren grow. She blamed her husband for not wanting to have children after the surgeon told her that never having children increased the risk for ovarian cancer. She resented the fact that she had lived in a difficult marriage and now "this" was happening to her. She felt horrible for having these feelings because she didn't like feeling this way. She also dealt with an obsessive compulsive disorder (OCD) regarding cleanliness that made life miserable for herself and those around her. This presented problems for the family in trying to care for her because as the cancer got worse, she needed more physical care but the OCD presented a barrier not easily maneuvered around, leaving family members exhausted and frustrated. The family felt like they could give her much better care but were prevented from doing so. This was extremely difficult for her family. When the patient died, the relationships were very good, but the family had spent a lot of time talking about what all of this meant to them. They were able to talk about the positives and negatives and realized that they did the best they could given the imposed limitations by the patient.

These actual patient stories were presented to exemplify how the patient's meaning in illness affects the meaning held or created by family members. Differing or divergent meanings can be detrimental in a relationship, or they can be used to strengthen it, thereby increasing the quality of time left together. That is not to imply that the patient is responsible for the meaning created by family members; rather, they are responsible for how one affects the other. Germino, Fife, and Funk[39] suggest that the goal is not merely converging meanings within the patient-family dyad but, rather, encouraging a sharing of individual meanings so that all can learn and relationships can be deepened and strengthened.

There are many issues that family caregivers face in caring for a loved one nearing the end of life. They are discussed at length in the literature. There is one issue, however, that warrants more attention: the loss of dreams. The loss of dreams for a future with the person is in addition to the loss of the person. It is the loss of the way one used to imagine life and how it would have been with that person. It is the loss of an emotional image of oneself and the abandonment of chosen plans for the future and what might have been.[40]

For a child and the surviving parent, those losses of dreams will be played out each time Mother's or Father's Day arrives and important life-cycle events, such as graduations, weddings, or the birth of the first grandchild. As her mother lay dying, one child expressed that loss in the simple statement, "Mommy, you won't be here for my birthday!" The mother and child wept, holding and comforting each other. Nothing could change the loss, but the comforting would remain forever.

The loss of dreams is an internal process, spiritual for some, and seldom recognized by others as needing processing.[29,40–42] Nurses have a wonderful opportunity at this point to verbally recognize the family caregivers' loss of dreams and to encourage them in their search to find meaning in the loss. The ability to transcend and connect to God or something greater than one's self helps the healing process.

Transcendence: strength for the journey that lies ahead

Transcendence is defined as lying beyond the ordinary range of perception; being above and independent of the material universe. The Latin root is *trans-*, "from or beyond," plus *scandere*, "to climb."[2] The images are many: the man in a pit climbing his way out one handhold at a time; the story of Job as he endured one loss after another and yet found meaning; the climber who reaches the mountaintop, becoming closer to the heavens while still having the connection to the earth; or the dying patient who, in peace, is already seeing into another reality. The ability to transcend truly is a gift of the human spirit and often comes after a long struggle and out of suffering. It is often unclear which comes first—does meaning open the door for transcendence, or, quite the opposite, does the act of transcendence bring the meaning? More than likely, it is an intimate dance between the two, one fueling the other. In the Buddhist tradition, suffering and being are a totality, and integrating suffering in this light becomes an act of transcendence.[43]

Transcendence of suffering can also be accomplished by viewing it as reparation for sins while still living—preparing the way for eternity, as in the Islamic tradition. In other traditions, transcendence is often relationship based, involving the connection to others and sometimes to a higher power.[3] For example, the Christian seeing Christ on the cross connects one to the relationship and endurance of God and the reality that suffering is a part of life. For others, it is finding meaning in relating to others, even the act of caring for others. And for some, that relationship may be with the Earth, a sense of stewardship and leaving the environment a better place. It is rare that patients reach a state of transcendence and remain there through their dying. Instead, for most it is a process in which there are moments when they reach a sense of expansion that supports them in facing death. The existential crisis does not rule, because one can frame the relationship beyond death; for example, "I will remain in their hearts and memories forever, I will live on through my children, or my spirit will live beyond my limited physical state."

Nursing interventions

If one returns to the root word of meaning, *maenan*, or "to tell of," this concept can be the guide that directs the nurse toward interventions. Given the nature of this work, interventions may not be the true representation of what is needed. For intervention implies action—that the nurse has an answer and she can direct the course of care by intervening. "Intervention" is defined as "To come, appear, or lie between two things. To come in or between so as to hinder or alter an action."[2] But finding meaning is process oriented; while finely honed psychosocial skills and knowledge can be immensely helpful, there is no bag of tricks. One example would be of a chaplain who walks in the room and relies only on offering prayer to the patient, preventing any real discourse or relationship-building. The patient's personhood has been diminished, and potentially, more harm than good has been done.

So let us revisit "to tell of." What is required of the professional who enters into the healing dimension of a patient's suffering and search for meaning? It would seem that respect may be the starting point—respect for that individual's way of experiencing suffering and attempts of making sense of the illness. Second, allow for an environment and time for the telling. Even as this is written, the sighs of frustration are heard, "We have no time!" If nursing fails at this, if nurses turn their backs on their intrinsic promise to alleviate suffering, then nursing can no longer exist. Instead, the nurse becomes simply the technician and the scheduler—the nurse becomes a part of the problem. She has violated the American Nurses Association's Code of Ethics for Nurses that assert that nurses are obligated to address the alleviation of suffering and provide supportive care to the dying, "The measures nurses take to care for the patient enable the patient to live with as much physical, emotional, social, and spiritual well-being as possible. This is particularly vital in the care of patients and their families at the end of life to prevent and relieve the cascade of symptoms and suffering that are commonly associated with dying."[44]

If patients in the midst of suffering receive the message, nonverbally or directly, that there is no time, energy, or compassion they will, in their vulnerability, withdraw or become more needy. When patients feel distrusted, objectified, and overlooked, they suffer at the hands of those who were to provide care.[15] Their alienation becomes complete. On the other hand, if privacy and a moment of honor and focused attention are provided, this allows for the tears to spill or the anguish to be spoken. Then the alienation is broken, and the opportunity for healing one dimension is begun. The terminally ill are a vulnerable population. They die and do not complete patient satisfaction surveys; their grievances and their stories die with them. But the violation does not, for each nurse now holds that violation, as does society as a whole. The wound begets wounds, and the nurse sinks further into the protected and unavailable approach, alienated. The work holds no rewards, only endless days and demands. She or he has nothing left to give. The patient and family are ultimately abandoned. In the work of Kahn and Steeves,[45] one finds a model for the nurse's role in psychosocial processes and suffering. It represents the dynamic relationship of caring, acted out in caregiving as well as in the patient's coping, which transform each other.

For the nurse to provide this level of caregiving, he/she must understand the obstructions that may interfere. It is essential that the nurse undergo his/her own journey, visiting the intense emotions around the dying process and the act of witnessing suffering. We can serve the suffering person best if we ourselves are willing to be transformed through the process of our own grief as well as by the grief of others.[46] Presence may, in fact, be our greatest gift to these patients and their families. Still, imagine charting or accounting for presence on an acuity system! Presence "transcends role obligations and acknowledges the vulnerable humanness of us all ... to be present means to unconceal, to be aware of tone of voice, eye contact, affect, and body language, to be in tune with the patient's messages."[46] Presence provides confirmation, nurturing, and compassion and is an essential transcendent act.

Touch becomes one of the tools of presence and is valued by the dying and their families.[47,48] Used with sensitivity, it can be as simple as the holding of the hand or as powerful as the holding of the whole person. Sometimes, because of agitation or pain, direct touch becomes intrusive; even then touch can be invoked, by the touching of a pillow or the sheet or the offering of a cold cloth. Healing touch takes on another level of intention through the directing energy of prayer.

If a key aspect of meaning is to tell, then one might be led to believe that the spoken word would be imperative. However, over and over, it is silence that conveys the meaning of suffering, "a primitive form of existence that is without an effective voice and imprisoned in silence." Compassionate listeners in respect and presence become mute themselves.[46] They use the most intuitive skills to carry the message. This may also be why other approaches that use symbols, metaphors, and the arts are the most potent in helping the patient to communicate and make sense of meaning. The arts, whether writing, music, or visual arts, often help the patient not only gain new insight but convey that meaning to others. There are many levels on which this is accomplished. Whether it is done passively, through reading poetry, listening to music, or viewing paintings, or actively through creation, thoughts can be inspired, feelings moved, and the sense of connectedness and being understood can evolve. What once was ubiquitous can now be seen outside of one's soul, as feelings become tangible. It can be relational, because the act of creation can link one to the creator, or it can downplay the role of dependency, as the ill one now cares for others with a legacy of creational gifts.[49]

Meditation and yoga are other acts of transcendence that can be extremely powerful for the dying.[50–53] Even those who have never experienced a meditational state can find that this new world in many ways links them to living and dying. The relaxation response from meditation or yoga allows the anxious patient to escape into a meditative state, experiencing an element of control while relinquishing control. Many patients describe it as a floating state, a time of great peace and calm. Some who have never had such an experience can find the first time frightening, as the existential crisis, quelled so well by boundaries, is no longer confined. Most, given a trusting and safe teacher, will find that meditation will serve them well. The meditation can be in the form of prayer, guided imagery, breathing techniques, or mantras.

Prayer is well documented in the literature[54–56] as having meaning for patients and families; not only does it connect one to God, but it also again becomes a relational connection to others. Knowing that one is prayed for not only by those close at hand but by strangers, communities, and those at a great distance can be deeply nurturing. Often forgotten is the role in which the patient can be empowered, that of praying for others. One of the authors experienced her patient's prayers for her as the tables were turned, and the patient became the healer. The patient suddenly lost the sense of worthlessness and glowed with joy.

Leaving a legacy may be one of the most concrete ways for patients to find meaning in this last stage of their lives.[57] It most often requires the mastering of the existential challenges, in which patients know that death is at hand and choose to direct their course and what they leave behind. For some patients, that will mean going out as warriors, fighting until the end; for others, it will mean end-of-life planning that focuses on quality of life. Some patients will design their funerals, using rituals and readings that reveal their values and messages for others. Others will create videos, write letters, or distribute their wealth in meaningful ways. Blogging is a way to decrease a sense of isolation for patients as they record their experiences and also leaves a permanent imprint of their lives on the Internet.[58] It becomes a diary of the illness and has been shown to increase a sense of purpose and meaning as they share with others.[58,59] Parents who are leaving young children sometimes have the greatest difficulty with this aspect. On one hand, the feelings of horror at "abandoning" their children are so strong that they have great difficulty facing their death. Still, there is often a part of them that has this need to leave a legacy. The tug-of-war between these two willful emotions tends to leave only short windows of opportunity to prepare. The extreme can be observed in the young father who began to push his toddler away, using excuses for the distancing. It was only after a trusting relationship had been established with one of the authors that she could help him to see how this protective maneuver was, in fact, harming the child. The father needed not only to see what he was doing but to see how his love would help the child and how others would be there for the child and wife in their pain and grief. With relief, the father reconnected to his young son, creating living memories and a lifetime protection of love.

Another courageous parent anticipating the missed birthdays, bought cards, and wrote a note in each one, so that the child would be touched not only by the individual messages, but the knowledge that the parent found a way to be there for him with each new year. A mother wrote a note for her young daughter so that if she should ever marry, she would have a gift to be opened on her wedding day. The note described the mother's love, wisdom about marriage, and her daughter's specialness, already known through a mother's eyes. An elderly person may write or tape an autobiography or even record the family tree lest it be lost with the passing of a generation. The nurse can often be the one who inspires these acts, but it must always be done with great care so as not to instill a sense of "should" or "must," which would add yet another burden.

Helping patients to reframe hope is another important intervention.[60] Dr. William Breitbart, chief of the Psychiatry Services at Memorial Sloan-Kettering Cancer Center in New York City, designed and conducted research on a meaning-centered psychotherapeutic intervention to help terminally ill patients with cancer maintain hope and meaning as they face the end of their lives.[4] This research was inspired by the works of Dr. Victor Frankl, a psychiatrist and Holocaust survivor. Cancer patients attended an 8-week, group-focused, standardized course of experiential exercises that addressed constructs of despair at the end of life, such as hopelessness, depression, loss of meaning, suicidal ideation, and desire for a hastened death. The study revealed that the patient's spiritual well-being and loss of meaning, was more highly correlated to the components that made up despair at the end of life than either depression or hopelessness alone. As a result, if the patient could manipulate or reframe his/her sense of meaning and spiritual well-being, this would positively affect the foundational elements of despair at the end of life. When patients are able to do this, their hope is sustained because they have been able to reframe the focus of their hope.

The healthcare professional

Although the healthcare professional can be educated about death and grieving, like the patient and family, it is in living out the experience that understanding is reached. It is a developmental process, and given the demands of the work, the nurse is at great risk for turning away from her feelings. There is often little mentoring that accompanies the first deaths, let alone formal debriefing or counseling. How can it be that we leave such important learning to chance? And what about cumulative losses and the years of witnessing suffering? Healthcare needs healing rituals for all of its healthcare professionals to support and guide them in this work. Individual institutions can develop programs that address these needs.

At one institution, "Teas for the Soul" (sponsored by the Pastoral Care Department) provide respite in the workplace on a regular basis, as well as after difficult deaths or traumas. A cart with cookies and tea, as well as soft music, are provided as physical nurturance and nurture the emotions of the staff and legitimize the need to come together in support. Another support is a renewal program, the "Circle of Caring." This retreat supports healthcare professionals from a variety of institutions in a weekend of self-care that integrates spirituality, the arts, and community building. The element of suffering is a focal point for a small-group process that unburdens cumulative effects of the work and teaches skills and rituals for coping with the ongoing demands.

Perhaps one of the most challenging aspects of finding meaning for a nurse is when nonbeneficial treatment is continued and palliative care is forestalled. The nurse experiences not only the emotional burden of the normal emotions of caring for the dying, but now has the added weight and guilt of feeling that she/he is contributing to harming the patient. While efforts must be made to address the nonbeneficial treatment and a refocusing on appropriate goals of care, during that gap it is essential that nurses and the entire healthcare team attend to the moral distress. Research has demonstrated that speaking up clearly makes a lasting impact on moral distress and yet often it is not addressed. The potential for elevation of the crescendo effect is significant, as is detaching from patients or even leaving the profession.[61-63] Ultimately, even if constrained by a lack of do not resuscitate orders or continued burdensome treatments, the nurse can focus her/his intentions on what she/he is able to do for the patient and family. Whether it is treating the patient with respect and tenderness or humanizing the experience through the simplest of acts (offering music, the reading of a poem, or comfort to those at the bedside), an awareness of the moral action of caring, so essential to nursing, will not only improve the care but the resiliency of the nurse.

Clearly, there is much that can be done to support nurses individually and to support organizations. There are many opportunities for assisting nurses in their own search for meaning and for enhancing the care of patients and families. When the nurse takes the time to find meaning in this work, she/he is finding a restorative practice that will protect him/her personally and professionally. Like the patient, she/he will need to choose this journey and find pathways that foster, challenge, and renew.

As long as we can love each other,

And remember the feeling of love we had,

We can die without ever really going away.

All the love you created is still there.

All the memories are still there.

You live on—in the hearts of everyone you have

Touched and nurtured while you were here.

Morrie Schwartz[64]

References

1. Taylor EJ. Whys and wherefores: adult patient perspectives of the meaning of cancer. Semin Oncol Nurs. 1995;11(1):32–40.
2. American Heritage. American Heritage Dictionary of the English Language. Boston: Houghton Mifflin; 2013.
3. Frankl VE. Man's Search for Meaning: An Introduction to Logotherapy. Boston: Beacon; 1959.
4. Breitbart W. Reframing hope: meaning-centered care for patients near the end of life. Interview by Karen S. Heller. J Palliat Med. 2003;6(6):979–988.
5. Yalom ID. Existential Psychotherapy. New York: Basic Books; 1980.
6. Marris P. Loss and Change. 2nd ed. London: Routledge and Kegan Paul; 1986.
7. Taylor SE. Adjustment to threatening events: a theory of cognitive adaptation. Am Psychology. 1983;38:1161–1173.
8. O'Connor AP, Wicker CA, Germino BB. Understanding the cancer patient's search for meaning. Cancer Nurs. 1990;13(3):167–175.
9. Cassell EJ. The relationship between pain and suffering. Adv Pain Res Ther. 1989;11:61–70.
10. Cindy Putnam. Personal interview. 2007.
11. Koestenbaum P. Is There an Answer to Death? Englewood Cliffs, NJ: Prentice-Hall; 1976.
12. Puchalski C. Spirituality. In: Berger A, Shuster J, Roenn JV (eds.), Principles and Practice of Palliative Care and Supportive Oncology. Philadelphia: Lippincott Williams & Wilkins; 2013:702–718.
13. Vachon ML. Meaning, spirituality, and wellness in cancer survivors. Semin Oncol Nurs. 2008;24(3):218–225.
14. Concordance: Strong's Exhaustive Concordance. 2013. Accessed June 27, 2013. http://www.biblestudytools.com/concordances/strongs-exhaustive-concordance/
15. Berglund M, Westin L, Svanstrom R, Sundler A. Suffering caused by care—patients' experiences from hospital settings. Int J Qualitative Stud Health Well-being. 2012;7:1–9.
16. Ersek M, Ferrell BR. Providing relief from cancer pain by assisting in the search for meaning. J Palliat Care. 1994;10(4):15–22.
17. Steeves RH, Kahn DL. Experience of meaning in suffering. Image J Nurs Scholarship. 1987;19(3):114–116.
18. Ersek M. The process of maintaining hope in adults with leukemia undergoing bone marrow transplantation. Unpublished doctoral dissertation. Seattle: University of Washington; 1991.
19. Gotay CC. Why me? Attributions and adjustment by cancer patients and their mates at two stages in the disease process. Soc Sci Med. 1985;20(8):825–831.
20. Haberman MR. Living with leukemia: the personal meaning attributed to illness and treatment by adults undergoing bone marrow transplantation. Unpublished doctoral dissertation. Seattle: University of Washington; 1987.
21. Chrisman H. The health seeking process: an approach to the natural history of illness. Culture, Med Psychiatry. 1977;1(4):351–377.
22. Ferrell BR, Taylor EJ, Sattler GR, Fowler M, Cheyney BL. Searching for the meaning of pain: cancer patients', caregivers', and nurses' perspectives. Cancer Pract. 1993;1(3):185–194.

23. Barkwell DP. Ascribing meaning: a critical factor in coping and pain attenuation in patients with cancer-related pain. J Palliat Care. 1991;7(3):5–10.

24. Lipowski Z. Physical illness, the individual and their coping processes. Int J Psychiatr Med. 1970;1(9):101.

25. Haberman MR. Psychosocial aspects of bone marrow transplantation. Semin Oncol Nurs. 1988;4(1):55–59.

26. Tillich P. The Courage To Be. New Haven, CT: Yale University Press; 1952.

27. Personal. Personal interview. 1997.

28. Benson H. Timeless Healing. New York: Simon and Schuster; 1997.

29. Putnam C. Personal communication. 1999.

30. O'Donohue J. Eternal Echoes. New York: HarperCollins Publishers; 1999.

31. Tolstoy L. The Death of Ivan Ilyich. 1886. Translated by Louise and Aylmer Maude. Available at: http://www.ccel.org/ccel/tolstoy/ivan.txt. Accessed November 1, 2013.

32. New American Standard Bible. Grand Rapids, MI: World; 1995.

33. Sittser G. A Grace Disguised. Grand Rapids, MI: Zondervan; 1995.

34. Cross SJ. Dark Night of the Soul. Kila, MT: Kessinger; 1542.

35. Kritek P. Reflections on Healing. Boston: Jones and Bartlett; 2003.

36. Kearney M. Mortally Wounded. New York: Simon and Schuster; 1996.

37. Martins L. The silence of God: the absence of healing. In: Fundis GCaR (ed.). Spiritual, Ethical and Pastoral Aspects of Death and Bereavement. Amityville, NY: Baywood; 1992:25–31.

38. Pellegrino E, Thomasma D. The Christian Virtues in Medical Practice. Washington, DC: Georgetown University Press; 1996.

39. Germino BB, Fife BL, Funk SG. Cancer and the partner relationship: what is its meaning? Semin Oncol Nurs. 1995;11(1):43–50.

40. Bowman T. Facing loss of dreams: a special kind of grief. Int J Palliat Nurs. 1997;3(2):76–80.

41. Garbarino J. The spiritual challenge of violent trauma. Am J Orthopsychiatry. 1996;66(1):162–163.

42. Rando TA. Treatment of Complicated Mourning. Champaign, IL: Research Press; 1993.

43. Kallenberg K. Is there meaning in suffering?: An external question in a new context. Paper presented at: Cancer Nursing Changing Frontiers1992; Vienna.

44. ANA. American Nurses Association Code for Nurses with Interpretive Statements. Washington, DC: American Nurses Publishing; 2001.

45. Kahn DL, Steeves RH. The significance of suffering in cancer care. Semin Oncol Nurs. 1995;11(1):9–16.

46. Byock I. When suffering persists. J Pall Care. 1994;10(2):8–13.

47. Kuhl D. What dying people want. In: Chochinov H, Breitbart W (eds.), Handbook of Psychiatry in Palliative Medicine. New York: Oxford University Press; 2009:141–156.

48. Downey L, Engelberg RA, Curtis JR, Lafferty WE, Patrick DL. Shared priorities for the end-of-life period. J Pain Symptom Manage. 2009;37(2):175–188.

49. Bailey SS. The arts in spiritual care. Semin Oncol Nurs. 1997;13(4):242–247.

50. Baldacchino D, Draper P. Spiritual coping strategies: a review of the nursing research literature. J Adv Nurs. 2001;34(6):833–841.

51. Sellers SC. The spiritual care meanings of adults residing in the midwest. Nurs Sci Q. 2001;14(3):239–248.

52. Zhang B, Nilsson ME, Prigerson HG. Factors important to patients' quality of life at the end of life. Arch Intern Med. 2012;172(15):1133–1142.

53. van Uden-Kraan CF, Chinapaw MJ, Drossaert CH, Verdonck-de Leeuw IM, Buffart LM. Cancer patients' experiences with and perceived outcomes of yoga: results from focus groups. Support Care Cancer. 2013;21(7):1861–1870.

54. Albaugh JA. Spirituality and life-threatening illness: a phenomenologic study. Oncol Nurs Forum. 2003;30(4):593–598.

55. Taylor EJ. Nurses caring for the spirit: patients with cancer and family caregiver expectations. Oncol Nurs Forum. 2003;30(4):585–590.

56. Smith AR, DeSanto-Madeya S, Perez JE, et al. How women with advanced cancer pray: a report from two focus groups. Oncol Nurs Forum. 2012;39(3):E310–E316.

57. Kaut K. Religion, spirituality, and existentialism near the end of life. Am Behav Scientist. 2002;46(2):220–234.

58. Ressler PK, Bradshaw YS, Gualtieri L, Chui KK. Communicating the experience of chronic pain and illness through blogging. J Med Internet Res. 2012;14(5):e143.

59. Keim-Malpass J, Steeves RH. Talking with death at a diner: young women's online narratives of cancer. Oncol Nurs Forum. 2012;39(4):373–378, 406.

60. McClement S, Chochinov H. Hope in advanced cancer patients. Eur J Cancer. 2008;44(8):1169–1174.

61. Balvere P, Cassessl J, Buzaianu E. Professional nursing burnout and irrational thinking. J Nurses Staff Dev. 2012;28(1):2–8.

62. Epstein EG, Hamric AB. Moral distress, moral residue, and the crescendo effect. J Clin Ethics. 2009;20(4):330–342.

63. Hamric AB. Empirical research on moral distress: issues, challenges, and opportunities. HEC Forum. 2012;24(1):39–49.

64. Albom M. Tuesdays with Morrie. New York: Doubleday; 1997.

SECTION IV

Special patient populations

CHAPTER 35

Caring for those with chronic illness

Terri L. Maxwell

I have had COPD for 20 years but I have been living with COPD. Now I'm dying with COPD. I just don't want to suffocate. I think this is worse than cancer.

A 48-year-old

Key points

◆ Patients with advanced chronic conditions frequently have an uncertain illness trajectory and many live for years in chronically poor health marked by declining functional status and intermittent disease exacerbations.

◆ Communication about end-of-life issues is particularly challenging in the chronically ill population because of prognostic uncertainty, poor understanding among patient and family members about the terminal nature of the condition, and lack of recognition of the benefits of palliative or hospice care.

◆ Patients with chronic conditions experience myriad symptoms that diminish the quality of life and require a combination of pharmacological and nonpharmacological approaches.

◆ The provision of hospice and palliative care should be based on patient need, especially with regard to symptom management and declining functional status.

◆ Individuals with chronic progressive illness and their families benefit from an interdisciplinary palliative approach to care, and as the disease advances, hospice care should be considered.

Introduction

Although hospice programs were initially developed to care for cancer patients, cancer represents less than a quarter of all deaths in the United States.[1] Individuals suffering from life-limiting illnesses, such as end-stage cardiac or pulmonary disease, advanced dementia, and other neurological conditions, also need palliative care. For many with progressive chronic illness, the dying process has become so prolonged that it is sometimes viewed as a distinct stage of life.[2] The healthcare system and society are confronted with the challenge of providing cost-effective, high-quality, compassionate care for the rising numbers of individuals whose deaths occur after months of gradual debilitation resulting from chronic illness.

Recognizing the growing needs among those with chronic illness and their families, palliative care programs have sprung up across the county, and the hospice industry has gone beyond primarily caring for those with cancer to include all patients with life-limiting illness. The number of patients enrolling in hospice with noncancer diagnoses has been steadily climbing; in 2012, noncancer diagnoses accounted for more than half of all hospice admissions (63.1%) with debility unspecified (14.2%), dementia (12.8%), heart disease (11.2%), and lung disease/chronic obstructive lung disease (8.2%) representing the top five noncancer conditions in hospice.[3]

Despite the growing number of patients with noncancer conditions accessing hospice and palliative care, there are numerous barriers leading to their underutilization among the chronic care population. According to Medicare and Medicaid requirements for admission to hospice, patients must have a diagnosed terminal illness with a limited life expectancy and written certification by a physician of a life expectancy of 6 months or less.[4] However, determining a 6-month prognosis or determining when someone is terminal is difficult for those with life-limiting diseases such as end-stage cardiac, hepatic, pulmonary, renal, or neurological diseases. Individuals with these conditions have prognoses that are commonly much more difficult to predict than those with advanced cancer. Persons with cancer generally experience a more precipitous decline in the weeks and months before their death, whereas those with noncancer conditions often have a much less predictable course and may have a long period of survival, including survival with a reasonable quality of life. Individuals with noncancer diseases also commonly die suddenly or unexpectedly from other causes, such as multiple organ failure or persistent recurrent infection, rather than directly from their primary diagnosis. Also, some elderly persons have multiple medical problems; though none of these problems individually may amount to a terminal diagnosis, when taken together they may create a terminal condition that is difficult to prognosticate or identify as in need of hospice or palliative care.

Recognizing these challenges, the National Hospice and Palliative Care Organization (NHPCO) published medical guidelines for determining prognosis in selected noncancer diseases to aid clinicians with prognostication.[5] These guidelines are based on the premise that the prognosis of terminal illness depends on clinical judgment combined with the following: objective assessment of the natural history of the disease; treatments and response to-date; performance status; thorough physical assessment, including neurological and orthopedic; and knowledge of the psychological and sociological factors of the patient, family, and physician. Alternatively, others[2] have suggested using the question "Do you think the patient is likely to die within the next year?" as a marker for determining if palliative or hospice care might be appropriate. Subsequently, the Centers for Medicare and Medicaid Services (CMS) developed hospice Local Coverage Determination (LCD) guidelines for determining a patient's prognosis of six months or less. These guidelines, based on the original NHPCO guidelines, are used by Medicare Administrative Contractors (MACs) in reviewing claims and by hospice providers for documenting medical eligibility. This chapter reviews the palliative management of common noncancer conditions.

Heart failure

Heart failure is a clinical syndrome that results from an underlying disease that causes structural or functional damage to the heart so that the heart's pumping function grows weaker and the heart is unable to deliver a sufficient supply of oxygenated blood to meet the body's demands. It is estimated that 5.1 million Americans have heart failure,[6] and the number of new cases is rising, especially as the population ages. Among elderly patients admitted to the hospital for heart failure, 1-year mortality is over 60%, which is higher than with most cancers.[7] Heart failure has a devastating effect on patients' quality of life and functional status, yet both hospice and palliative care are underutilized in this population.

The American College of Cardiology (ACC) and the American Heart Association (AHA) published a new staging system for heart failure in 2001 that is useful in describing disease progression, exercise capacity, and symptom status[8] (Box 35.1). The first two stages (A and B) identify persons at risk to develop heart failure. Stage C designates patients with current or previous symptoms of heart failure that represent the bulk of the heart failure population. Stage D denotes persons with advanced heart failure whose symptoms progress despite maximal medical therapy with diuretics, angiotensin-converting enzyme (ACE) inhibitors, beta blockers, and possibly digoxin. Stage D patients should be evaluated for specialized therapies such as cardiac transplantation, inotropic infusions, mechanical circulatory support, and/or palliative or hospice care.[8]

Heart failure is a consequence of cardiac damage from a number of underlying diseases, such as coronary artery disease, myocardial infarction, hypertension, dilated cardiomyopathy,

valvular heart disease, and so forth. The heart attempts to compensate for the damage through a process called remodeling. Remodeling leads to enlargement of the heart and/or hypertrophy of the ventricles, resulting in decreased cardiac output and an increase in afterload. The abnormal loading induces dilatation of the ventricles that changes the shape of the ventricle, decreasing the pumping ability of the heart and contributing to symptoms despite treatment.[9]

Heart failure can be characterized based on ventricular involvement. Systolic dysfunction is the most common, whereas diastolic dysfunction is estimated to occur in 20% to 50% of cases.[10] Most patients, however, have abnormalities of both systolic and diastolic dysfunction.[8] Patients with preserved systolic function have normal ejection fractions but have abnormal ventricular filling, leading to pulmonary congestion, dyspnea, and symptoms of anorexia, fatigue, and depression; those with right-sided (systolic) dysfunction present with symptoms of weight gain, edema, dyspnea, and early satiety. Persons with diastolic heart failure are typically elderly, generally female, usually obese, and have hypertension and diabetes.[10]

Patients with heart failure have an uncertain illness trajectory, and many live for years in chronically poor health marked by declining functional status and unpredictable episodes of heart failure. Although models have been developed to predict mortality in patients with advanced heart disease, they lack specificity, making determining prognosis very difficult. This variability in prognosis was illustrated by the Study to Understand Prognoses and Preferences for Outcomes and Risks of Treatment (SUPPORT), in which over half of those with heart failure had an estimated 6-month survival prognosis within 3 days of death.[11] In addition, patients with heart failure have an array of treatments available, and they become accustomed to good treatment responses to exacerbations, making the decision to accept a palliative approach only more difficult.[12] Because of these challenges, patients with heart failure frequently lack access to specialist palliative care services and may end up being discharged alive from hospice.[13]

Persons with advanced heart failure usually have a number of disabling symptoms. Complications of heart failure include pulmonary congestion, evidenced by lung symptoms, congestive heart failure, cor pulmonale, arrhythmias, and cardiac arrest. Common symptoms of advanced heart failure are listed in Table 35.1. While shortness of breath is the hallmark symptom of heart failure, patients in outpatient heart failure clinics and those enrolled in hospice report that fatigue and lack of energy are among the most prevalent, severe, and distressing symptoms experienced.[14] Emotional issues are also paramount, including worrying, depression, and sadness.[14] The SUPPORT study

---

Box 35.1 American College of Cardiology/American Heart Association classification system

Stage A: High risk for heart failure, no structural disorder present, no symptoms

Stage B: Structural heart disorder present, no symptoms

Stage C: Current or previous heart failure symptoms associated with structural heart disease

Stage D: Advanced heart failure with symptoms occurring at rest despite maximal medical therapy

Source: Yancy et al. (2005), reference 8.

Table 35.1 Symptoms of advanced heart failure

Fatigue/weakness	Pain
Decreased appetite	Depressed mood
Shortness of breath	Anxiety
Lower extremity edema	Difficulty sleeping
Ascites	Decreased sexual interest
Cough	

described symptoms in patients hospitalized with heart failure at the end of life. Severe dyspnea was experienced by 63% of patients, and 41% had severe pain within the last 3 days of life. During the last month of life, 70% of patients with heart failure perceived their quality of life as poor.[11]

Management

There is an array of pharmacological and nonpharmacological therapy options for heart failure. The primary goals of therapy are to improve survival, slow disease progression, minimize risk factors, and reduce symptoms. Early recognition of signs and symptoms of heart failure can decrease hospitalizations and improve quality of life.

The 2013 ACC/AHA guidelines outline treatment options based on heart failure stage.[8] Patients with structural disease and previous or current symptoms (stage C) should be prescribed ACE inhibitors and beta blockers, diuretics, digoxin, sodium-restricted diet, and exercise as appropriate. The ACE inhibitors and beta blockers have demonstrated improvements in survival, morbidity, ejection fraction, remodeling, quality of life, rate of hospitalization, and incidence of sudden death. They are generally recommended for all patients, even those entering hospice.[10,12] Diuretics help to control volume overload and enhance urinary sodium excretion. Loop diuretics, such as furosemide, are generally the drugs of choice. Digoxin has been shown to reduce the risk of heart failure–associated hospitalizations. Aldosterone antagonists, such as spironolactone, have demonstrated improvements in symptoms and reductions in death and hospitalization in some patients with advanced heart failure. According to ACC/AHA guidelines, patients with advanced disease should be considered for cardiac resynchronization devices such as implantable cardioverter defibrillators (ICDs) to prevent sudden death from conduction defects, inotropic therapy to manage refractory symptoms, and ventricular assist devices (VADs) or cardiac transplantation as indicated.[8] However, implantation of ICDs is of uncertain benefit in prolonging survival in patients who are at high risk of sudden death as predicted by frequent hospitalizations, frailty, or significant prognosis impacting comorbidities such as renal dysfunction or malignancy.[8] Goals of care for patients with refractory heart failure in stage D (those with symptoms at rest and recurrent hospitalizations despite treatment) include controlling symptoms, improving quality of life, reducing hospital admissions, and establishing end-of-life goals. Options include heart transplant, advanced care measures, chronic inotropes, temporary or permanent mechanical circulatory support (MCS), experimental therapies, and palliative care and hospice.[8] The benefit and burden of each for a particular patient must be weighed carefully.

Patient education is also a central component of heart failure management. The importance of adhering to their medication regimen should be underscored with all patients. They should be placed on a moderate sodium-restricted diet, and some patients with advanced disease may benefit from restricting fluids. Patients should be encouraged to monitor their weight daily so that volume changes can be identified before symptoms occur. Patients should also be taught to avoid nonsteroidal anti-inflammatory drugs (NSAIDs), as these can worsen or exacerbate heart failure symptoms and are associated with heart failure hospitalizations.[15]

Symptom management

Symptom management in patients with advanced heart disease begins with optimal treatment with ACE inhibitors or angiotensin-receptor blockers (ARBs) and beta blockers, as described above.[12] Less-than-optimal treatment may result in premature referrals to hospice or palliative care programs.

Pain is commonly experienced by those with advanced heart disease because of immobility, edema, or ischemia. Patients may also have comorbidities such as arthritis, diabetic neuropathy, or other conditions that cause discomfort. Nitrates and opioids are indicated for anginal pain. As described earlier, NSAIDs should be avoided because of the possibility of worsening kidney function and subsequent fluid retention. Other than avoiding NSAIDs, nonopioids and opioids should be prescribed according to guidelines used for other chronic conditions.

Dyspnea is a prominent symptom among those with severe heart failure (see chapter 14). Nonpharmacological therapies such as creating a calm environment, employing techniques to manage anxiety, and using a fan to improve air circulation may reduce symptoms of dyspnea. Supplemental oxygen therapy may be helpful in those with ischemic symptoms but does not necessarily decrease the sensation of breathlessness among nonhypoxemic patients and is associated with hemodynamic deterioration in severe heart failure.[16] The primary treatment of dyspnea involves managing fluid status with cardiac medications. Oral and parenteral opioids have demonstrated substantial benefit in reducing the feeling of breathlessness in patients with advanced disease of any cause,[17] but they are often overlooked for use in those with heart failure. In fact, opioids should be considered a first-line therapy for those with advanced heart disease, as they have been proven safe and effective.[18] Although the exact mechanism by which opioids alleviate dyspnea is unknown, one popular theory is that they decrease respiratory distress by altering the perception of breathlessness and by decreasing ventilatory response to declining oxygen and rising CO_2 levels. Contrary to popular belief, opioids do not improve dyspnea through inhibition of the respiratory drive; in fact, opioids improve dyspnea without causing significant deterioration in respiratory function.[19] Although the efficacy of opioids in managing dyspnea has been demonstrated in clinical studies, the optimal dosing and route of administration is highly debated. Most clinicians agree that it is best to initiate therapy with a low dose and increase the dose slowly as needed, because respiratory drive suppression can occur if serum opioid levels rise quickly. Morphine is the opioid most studied in the treatment of dyspnea; other opioids, such as hydromorphone or codeine, are also effective. The usual dose of morphine in the opioid-naïve patient is 5 mg orally (preferred route) every 4 hours, which can be titrated upward in 25%–50% increments until symptoms are controlled.[20] Nebulized morphine has been used to relieve dyspnea with some success, but at this time, evidence to support its use is weak and it should not be used in place of oral or parenteral dosing.[17] If dyspnea causes anxiety, the addition of a short-acting benzodiazepine such as lorazepam may be beneficial.

Benzodiazepines may also help manage symptoms of anxiety or insomnia commonly experienced by patients with heart failure. Depression is also a common but frequently unrecognized comorbidity among those with advanced heart failure. Depression can be treated with selective serotonin reuptake inhibitors (SSRIs); however, they should be carefully titrated, as they can elevate blood pressure and worsen tachycardia. Tricyclic antidepressants should be avoided because they are poorly tolerated in the elderly and have negative effects on cardiac rhythms. Fatigue, often accompanied by depression, can have a profound effect on quality of life. Fatigue usually results from the heart failure itself, although the clinician should carefully assess for reversible causes or the need for more diuretic. Patients should be encouraged to be as active as possible and to reset goals of physical activity to accommodate changes in energy levels.

Patients with advanced heart failure frequently experience early satiety and nausea resulting from pressure from an enlarged, congested liver or as a result of gastric stasis. Patients with a congested liver should be treated with a loop diuretic or spironolactone and may require inotropic support. Metoclopramide may be effective in patients with gastroparesis. Patients may also benefit from antiemetics such as haloperidol or prochlorperazine.

Specialized interventions for refractory heart failure

Inotropic and vasoactive agents such as neosynephrine, dobutamine, or milrinone work by forcing the contractility of the myocardium and improving cardiac output, thereby improving patient symptoms. They are frequently initiated in patients with systolic heart failure with the expectation that brief support during a period of decompensation will enhance diuresis and accelerate hospital discharge. However, some patients cannot be weaned without clinical deterioration and progressive renal dysfunction. Unfortunately, there are no approved oral versions of inotropic agents; digoxin is the only oral positive inotropic agent available for chronic outpatient use. The routine use of intermittent inotropic infusions administered in outpatient clinics has not been supported by clinical trials,[21] and survival on home inotropic infusions is poor.[22] Symptom improvement associated with the provision of inotropic therapy is believed to result primarily from the increased clinical contact that could be accomplished in less resource intensive ways. Guidelines developed by the ACC/AHA Task Force do not support the widespread use of intravenous positive inotropic agents as outpatient treatment for heart failure due to lack of efficacy and concerns about toxicity except as "bridge therapy" in patients with stage D heart failure who are eligible and awaiting cardiac transplantation or MCS.[8] Most hospices do not support the use of inotropic therapy because of cost considerations and concerns about efficacy and patient harm.[12]

Implantable cardioverter defibrillators are inserted to prevent sudden cardiac death in those with an otherwise good prognosis and a predicted life expectancy of at least 1 year.[23] The mortality benefit of these devices has been demonstrated by a number of clinical trials. However, ICDs do not slow progression of heart failure, so increasing numbers of patients are approaching end of life with these devices in place and are at risk to have painful shocks delivered during the dying process.[24] A study from one hospice reports that 64% of ICD patients received shock therapy during the dying phase, and some received shocks even after death.[25] Therefore, physicians should discuss ICD deactivation when the device is placed; unfortunately, this rarely occurs.[26] According to guidelines, specialized staff such as the cardiologist or electrophysiologist treating the patient should deactivate ICDs, and magnets placed over the device should not be used to deactivate an ICD except as an absolute last resort.[27]

Fewer than 5% of patients with advanced heart failure are eligible for cardiac transplantation, which is partially limited by the number of organs available.[25] Some patients awaiting transplantation, or select patients who are ineligible or choose not to undergo transplant, may opt for a left VAD. A VAD is a surgically implanted mechanical pump to improve ventricular functions. Although originally used as a bridge to transplantation, now that VADs are more compact and portable, they are increasingly used as destination therapy for patients with end-stage heart disease[28] but are only indicated for carefully selected patients.[8] Despite increases in survival, the morbidity and mortality associated with the use of a VAD is high, mainly because of infection or mechanical failure of the device.[29] Before placing the device, clinicians should discuss scenarios with the patient and family to determine under what circumstances they would want the device deactivated.[30]

Advance care planning/communication challenges

There is also a notable lack of advance care planning and dialogue between heart failure patients and their providers regarding end-of-life care. In the context of prognostic uncertainty, communication is particularly challenging because of the unpredictable nature of the disease trajectory, poor understanding among patient and family members about the disease itself, and lack of recognition that heart failure is a terminal condition. To enhance end-of-life decision-making and the provision of palliative care, the 1995 ACC/AHA practice guidelines recommend (1) ongoing patient and family education regarding prognosis for functional capacity and survival; (2) patient and family education about options for formulating and implementing advance directives; (3) discussion regarding the option of inactivating ICDs; (4) continuity of medical care between inpatient and outpatient settings; (5) components of hospice care to relieve suffering, including opiates; and (6) examination of and work toward improving approaches to palliative care.[9]

Hospice eligibility criteria and referral

Hospice is underutilized by patients with advanced heart failure for a number of reasons. The inability to predict actual time to death and the patient's preference for resuscitation orders compared with cancer patients are important barriers to hospice referral. Physicians may be reluctant to engage in end-of-life discussions with their patients or may lack the skills to do so. Furthermore, there is still a misconception among many healthcare providers that hospice care is for cancer patients and they are unaware of the benefits of hospice for patients with heart failure.[31] Although helpful, LCD guidelines for determining hospice eligibility for patients with heart failure do not adequately predict short-term prognosis, so patients may be on hospice service for a long time.[32] It is important to remember that those who stabilize while on hospice care can be discharged and readmitted when their condition deteriorates. In addition to hospice, interdisciplinary palliative care should be more available to patients during hospitalization and thereafter. Reinforcement that access to palliative care is based on need rather than closeness to death may improve referral rates. Doing so may improve quality-of-life outcomes for patients and families and reduce hospitalizations and costs.

Chronic Obstructive Pulmonary Disease

Chronic Obstructive Pulmonary Disease (COPD) is a respiratory disorder characterized by chronic airway obstruction and lung hyperinflation resulting from chronic bronchitis and emphysema. During the last 30 years, the death rate for COPD has doubled.[33] It is the fourth leading cause of chronic morbidity and mortality in the United States[1] and in the world, largely as a result of the cumulative exposure to tobacco smoke.[34] The prevalence of COPD increases with age and occurs more often in men, although death rates for women have been rising since the 1970s. Chronic obstructive pulmonary disease is a progressive illness, and even with treatment, lung function generally worsens over time.

Assessment of the severity of COPD is based on the patient's level of symptoms, future risk of exacerbations, the severity of spirometric abnormality, and the presence of comorbidities than can lead to complications.[35] The Global Initiative for Chronic Obstructive Lung Disease (GOLD) guidelines describe four stages of COPD characterized by worsening airflow limitation as measured by forced ventilator volume (FEV_1) readings calculated through spirometry (Box 35.2).[35]

Symptoms

Reductions in airflow, as evidenced by declining FEV_1 readings, primarily result from inflammation, fibrosis, and exudates in small airways. As air gets trapped, the lungs hyperinflate and alveoli are destroyed. Hyperinflation results in decreased inspiratory capacity and increased functional residual capacity, causing dyspnea. Gas exchange abnormalities bring about hypoxemia and rising CO_2 levels. Some patients, especially those with chronic bronchitis, have mucous hypersecretion resulting in a chronic productive cough. Exacerbations of respiratory symptoms are common, usually triggered by bacterial or viral infections, environmental pollutants, or other unknown causes. Patients with advanced COPD are at risk to develop pulmonary hypertension that may progress to right ventricular hypertrophy and cor pulmonale (right-sided heart failure). In addition to respiratory symptoms, persons with COPD frequently have significant comorbidities such as cardiovascular disease and have systemic features such as weight loss and skeletal muscle wasting and are at risk for osteoporosis, myocardial infarction, respiratory infection, depression, sleep disorders, diabetes, and glaucoma.[35] Those with severe disease also experience fatigue, weight loss, anorexia, and severe coughing spells.

Box 35.2 Stages of Chronic Obstructive Pulmonary Disease

Stage I: Mild COPD: $FEV_1/FVC < 0.70$; $FEV_1 \geq 80\%$ predicted. Patient unaware lung function is abnormal.

Stage II: Moderate COPD: $FEV_1/FVC < 0.70$; $50\% \leq FEV_1 < 80\%$ predicted. Patient typically seeks medical attention because of pulmonary symptoms.

Stage III: Severe COPD: $FEV_1/FVC < 0.70$; $30\% \leq FEV_1 < 50\%$ predicted. Greater shortness of breath, reduced exercise tolerance, decreased quality of life.

Stage IV: Very severe COPD: $FEV_1/FVC < 0.70$; $30\% \leq FEV_1 < 50\%$ predicted. May have signs of cor pulmonale.

Source: Adapted from GOLD Guidelines, reference 36.

Management

The primary goals of COPD management are to relieve symptoms, ameliorate disease progression, improve exercise tolerance and health status, and prevent and treat complications and disease exacerbations. Treatment varies based on the impact of symptoms on the patient's quality of life and degree of disability.

The comprehensive management of COPD as outlined by the GOLD guidelines consists of a combination of pharmacotherapeutic and nonpharmacotherapeutic interventions, although it should be noted that none of the existing therapies have been shown to modify the long-term decline in lung function associated with COPD.[35] Patients should be counseled to stop smoking and to monitor their symptoms for signs of exacerbation. Nonpharmacological therapies include pulmonary rehabilitation/exercise training as tolerated and nutritional counseling. Patients with very severe (stage IV) disease with severe hypoxemia may benefit from oxygen therapy, which has been shown to increase survival and may prevent progression of pulmonary hypertension.[36] Oxygen therapy also improves alertness and may have positive effects on quality of life, including mood. The GOLD guidelines recommend oxygen treatment for at least 15 hours or more per day provided from a fixed oxygen concentrator with piping to allow the patient to move throughout their home.[35]

In patients with advanced COPD, various medications are used to prevent and control symptoms and to reduce the frequency and severity of exacerbations. These medications are generally added as the disease and symptoms worsen. By the time a patient's disease is advanced, they will likely be prescribed a long-acting and short-acting bronchodilator such as albuterol; anticholinergics such as ipratropium bromide or tiotropium; methylxanthines such as aminophylline or theophylline; and combination inhaled therapies such as formoterol/budesonide. Long-acting inhaled bronchodilators reduce exacerbations and related hospitalizations and improve symptoms and health status. Combining bronchodilators of different pharmacological classes is recommended to improve efficacy and decrease risk of side effects. Whereas regular treatment with inhaled corticosteroids reduces exacerbations and improves symptoms and lung functions, long-term treatment with oral corticosteroids is not recommended because of lack of benefit and high risk of adverse effects. In patients with severe and very severe COPD and a history of exacerbations and chronic bronchitis, the phosphodiesterase-4 inhibitor (PDE-4) roflumilast, reduces exacerbations treated with oral glucocorticosteroids.[35]

Other recommended pharmacological treatments include yearly inoculation with influenza vaccines and mucolytics for those with viscous sputum, although the benefits of the latter are very small. Antitussives for cough and prophylactic, continuous use of antibiotics have not been shown to be effective; antibiotics should be reserved to treat infectious exacerbations and other bacterial infections only. Oral and parenteral opioids are used to treat dyspnea in patients with advanced COPD, but well-designed, prospective clinical trials are limited.[37] A study by Abernethy and colleagues[15] demonstrated improved dyspnea and sleep scores for those prescribed sustained-release oral morphine. Nebulized opioids have not demonstrated a reduction in breathlessness in patients with COPD[38] and should not be used in place of oral or parenteral routes. Anxiolytics may be helpful in managing anxiety that can accompany severe dyspnea.

Decisions about the use of invasive ventilation are frequently based on the patient's prognosis, which can be difficult to determine. In patients where invasive ventilation is not deemed to be in the best interest of the patient, noninvasive ventilation (NIV) is being used as a first-line treatment for acute respiratory failure among patients with COPD. Noninvasive ventilation devices rhythmically blow air into the lungs through a mask attached over the nose and mouth. Whereas the benefits of NIV for acute exacerbations is known, its value among those with stage IV (very severe) COPD has not been demonstrated[35] although it may have a time-limited role for some patients at the end of life. The GOLD guidelines also recommend communication with advanced COPD patients about end-of-life care and advance care planning to give patients and their families the opportunity to make informed decisions, including opting for hospice care.

End-of-life issues

As in other chronic conditions, prognosis in patients with COPD is difficult to predict. When an illness trajectory is uncertain, clinicians tend to procrastinate initiating discussions about palliative and end-of-life care.[39] The provision of palliative care should be based on patient need, especially with regard to symptom management and declining functional status. Pulmonologists and palliative care teams should work together to improve communication at the end of life, especially related to goals of care and advance care planning. Hospice should be considered for stage IV patients who prefer a palliative approach to care.

End-Stage Renal Disease

End-stage renal disease (ESRD) is the most feared consequence of kidney disease. End-stage renal disease results when kidney function deteriorates to the point where it is no longer adequate to sustain life. Patients with kidney function less than 10% of normal are considered to have ESRD, usually following a long history of chronic kidney failure.[40] Diabetes and hypertension are the most common causes of ESRD, with African Americans disproportionately affected.[41] The rate of new cases of ESRD in the United States has been relatively stable since 2000 and decreased in 2010.[41] Patients with ESRD have a high percentage of comorbidities such as coronary artery disease, congestive heart failure, peripheral vascular disease, and malnutrition. Dialysis and kidney transplantation are the only treatments for ESRD. The number of those treated with peritoneal dialysis is rising due to changes in Medicare payments.[41]

Signs of ESRD include oliguria, high blood urea nitrogen (BUN) and serum creatinine levels, severe anemia, and electrolyte imbalances. Common symptoms of those undergoing dialysis include chronic pain (especially musculoskeletal pain), fatigue/lack of energy sleep disturbances, nausea and vomiting, dyspnea, and anorexia. In addition to these physical symptoms, emotional symptoms include worrying, anxiety, feeling sad, and feeling irritable.[42] The addition of other comorbidities heightens the symptom burden and makes prognosis even more uncertain. All anuric postdialysis patients die within days, but those who produce even small amounts of urine may have residual renal function that can enable them to live for weeks or, in rare cases, months. However, 6-month survival is extremely rare.

Palliative and hospice care services

Although palliative and hospice care have the potential to improve the quality of life of ESRD patients and their families, access to these services is limited. In fact, patients with kidney disease made up only 2.7% of hospice admissions in 2012.[3] The underutilization of hospice services by patients with ESRD has been attributed to the Medicare payment structure; however, it does not explain the underutilization of palliative care services among this group.[43] Patients with ESRD who elect hospice are required to forgo dialysis treatment; however, patients receiving care for a terminal condition not related to ESRD may receive covered services under both the ESRD benefit and hospice benefit.[44] Death attributed to withdrawal of dialysis has increased to 25%–34% in patients 75 years and older, and older patients have high rates of regret for choosing hemodialysis over supportive care.[45] Conservative management should be considered in some patients, as dialysis does not always confer a survival benefit for patients who are elderly or for those with multiple comorbidities.[46] All patients who are discontinuing dialysis for ESRD or those with ESRD who refuse to initiate dialysis should be considered for hospice. Recognizing the need for improved palliative care, some dialysis clinics and hospitals are developing palliative care initiatives with the goal of integrating palliative care into routine nephrology practice.[45]

Palliative management

The primary components of palliative care in ESRD are outlined in Box 35.3.

Communication and care planning

Advance care planning is an important consideration in ESRD because patients are likely to face important treatment decisions as their disease progresses, including potentially deciding to forego dialysis. Although most dialysis patients discuss their end-of-life wishes, far fewer complete advance directives. As with others with progressive conditions, discussions of advance care planning should focus on health states that the patient would deem unacceptable, rather than on treatment interventions.[48]

Withdrawal of dialysis

The goal of dialysis goes beyond life prolongation to include quality-of-life benefits. However, when the burdens associated with treatment outweigh the benefits, or if dialysis is only serving to prolong a patient's death, discontinuation of dialysis should be considered. Once considered a form of suicide, stopping dialysis is now an accepted practice with a sound ethical basis. Today, approximately 25% of patients with ESRD decide to withdraw dialysis.[49]

Patients and families who are considering stopping dialysis should be informed that the average survival time following dialysis withdrawal is 8 to 10 days but, depending on reserve

---

Box 35.3 Components of Palliative Care in End-Stage Renal Disease

Advance care planning
Symptom management
Psychosocial and spiritual support
Ethical issues in dialysis decision-making

Source: Adapted from Poppel et al. (2003), reference 47.

Box 35.4 Guidelines for discussing dialysis withdrawal

1. Identify patients who may benefit from withdrawal.
   a. Very limited prognosis
   b. Poor quality of life
   c. Pain unresponsive to treatment
   d. Progressive untreatable disease
   e. Dialysis technically difficult
2. Discuss goals of care with patient and family.
3. Discuss quality of life.
4. Discuss possible symptoms and their management.
5. Clarify that dialysis withdrawal is an option.
6. Reassure that it can result in a peaceful death.
7. Make recommendation to stop dialysis and request family support.
8. Provide reassurance that the decision is reversible.

Source: Cohen et al. (2003), reference 49.

Box 35.5 Dementia subtypes and prevalence

Alzheimer's disease 40%–75%
Cerebrovascular dementia 15%–30%
Lewy Body dementia 10%–15%
Frontotemporal dementia <1%

---

renal status, could be weeks.[50] Box 35.4 describes guidelines for discussion about dialysis withdrawal. Uremic death is typically preceded by progressive encephalopathy. Symptoms that may be experienced in the last 24 hours of life include confusion/agitation, nausea, pain, anxiety, pruritus, and edema.[51]

Symptom management

Pain and other symptoms are common and severe in ESRD and are comparable to those dying of cancer.[52] Pain should be managed as in other chronic conditions, but opioids that are metabolized by the kidneys such as morphine, propoxyphene, codeine, and meperidine should be avoided. Morphine use can lead to the accumulation of active metabolites that are neurotoxic, and chronic use can lead to myoclonus. Fentanyl and methadone are safe and effective in patients with renal insufficiency, whereas hydromorphone and oxycodone should be used with caution.[53]

Delirium resulting from uremic encephalopathy frequently manifests itself as mild confusion. Haloperidol is effective and will help to manage nausea and vomiting as well. Pruritus is treated with diphenhydramine or benzodiazepines, in addition to nonpharmacological approaches. Tube feedings and hydration should be avoided as they may contribute to peripheral edema and excessive secretions. Dyspnea should be managed with opioids, and anticholinergic medications such as atropine will help to control secretions.

Alzheimer's disease/dementia

Alzheimer's dementia is an irreversible, progressive brain disease that slowly destroys memory and thinking skills. Alzheimer's disease accounts for approximately half of all dementias. Other types of dementia are listed in Box 35.5. Typical of other progressive chronic illnesses, the course of dementia is one of continuing gradual decline. The median survival after diagnosis of Alzheimer's disease is 4 to 6 years, with younger patients living several years longer.[54,55] The incidence of Alzheimer's disease is rising, and it is now the fifth leading cause of death in the United States for those aged 65 and older.[56] Actual mortality statistics for Alzheimer's dementia are difficult to determine because acute conditions such as pneumonia are often recorded as the cause of death. In 2013, approximately 5.2 million people in the United States were estimated to have Alzheimer's disease; by the year 2050, this number may reach 16 million.[56]

There are a number of causes of dementia, including neurodegenerative changes in the brain, strokes, head injuries, drugs, and nutritional deficiencies. In Alzheimer's disease, abnormal protein deposits in the brain destroy cells that control mental functions and memory. Vascular dementia is caused by atherosclerosis in the brain, leading to multiple strokes. Lewy body dementias are caused by abnormal deposits of Lewy body protein in the brain. Patients with Lewy body dementia have symptoms similar to patients with Parkinson's disease, including tremor and muscle rigidity, and are more likely to experience delirium and hallucinations. The diagnosis of dementia is not straightforward and is largely established by a combination of clinical findings and confirmed by physiological changes in the brain seen on MRI or on autopsy.

Symptoms

Alzheimer's disease progresses slowly, and its symptoms are variable depending on the area of the brain affected. One of the first areas to be affected is the hippocampus, located in the temporal lobe. The hippocampus plays an essential role in processing new memories and in spatial navigation. Areas of the brain responsible for reasoning, emotional responses, language, and memory are also commonly involved, whereas the occipital lobe, which is responsible for visual processing, as well as primary sensory and motor neurons, are usually spared. Once the dementia has reached the severe stage, most memory is lost and patients experience incontinence, eating difficulties, and motor impairment. In the advanced/terminal stage, patients are usually bedfast, mute, and dysphagic and suffer from infections. At this stage, patients usually die from complications such as pneumonia, urinary tract infections, hip fractures, or as a consequence of malnutrition. Box 35.6 lists the clinical presentation of severe dementia.

Symptom management

Behavioral symptoms

Patients with dementia frequently exhibit behavioral symptoms such as agitation, depression, delirium, and, in some cases, hallucinations and psychosis. The management of these behaviors is important to the quality of life of the patient and his/her caregiver.[56]

Box 35.6 Clinical presentation of severe dementia

Neurocognitive
Progressive worsening of:
- Memory
- Confusion/disorientation
- Combativeness
- Inability to communicate
- Incoherent and unresponsive
- Inability to recognize self

Functional
- Loss of ability to walk or maintain posture
- Totally dependent on others for care

Nutritional
- Progressive loss of appetite
- Loss of ability to recognize food
- Loss of capacity to swallow

Miscellaneous
- Bowel and bladder incontinence
- Fevers and infections
- Decubitus ulcers
- Development of contractures

In the mid-1990s, a group of medications called cholinesterase inhibitors (e.g., glanatamine, donepezil, and rivastigmine) were approved by the FDA for the treatment of mild-to-moderate Alzheimer's disease. Donepezil was also later approved for use in patients with moderate-to-severe disease. These agents may improve neuropsychiatric symptoms such as agitation, hallucinations, depression, nighttime behaviors, and appetite disorders and may delay disease progression in some patients.[57] The clinical significance of cholinesterase inhibitors is debated and they are estimated to benefit only about half of those who take them, although a small percentage of patients may benefit dramatically.[58] A Cochrane review of donepezil, galantamine, and rivastigmine found efficacy for mild-to-moderate Alzheimer's disease with no evidence of any differences between them with respect to efficacy. Treatment effects were small, and adverse effects requiring discontinuation occurred in 29% in treatment groups compared with placebo groups (18%). Donepezil is better tolerated compared with rivastigmine.[59] Memantine, a N-methyl-D-aspartic acid (NMDA) receptor antagonist was approved by the FDA in 2003 to help slow progression of symptoms in the severe stages of illness.[60] Because of a lack of data describing the value of these medications in patients with disease advanced enough to meet hospice eligibility criteria, clinicians generally rely on clinical experience and patient/family preferences to evaluate whether to recommend continuing or discontinuing these therapies in hospice patients. A study of a large national hospice pharmacy database indicated that 21% of patients were prescribed either a cholinesterase inhibitor or an NMDA receptor antagonist at the time of hospice enrollment.[61] In addition to questionable efficacy, the high cost is likely a deterrent to their use in hospice.

Agitation and delirium

"Agitation" is an imprecise term that refers to restlessness accompanied by mental tension. Patients who are agitated are often seen pacing or may pull off their clothes or have vocal outbursts.

Common causes of agitation in dementia patients include untreated or mismanaged pain, urinary retention, or social isolation. Agitation can be confused with delirium, which is an acute symptom characterized by disturbances in attention, cognition, and perception.[62] Delirium frequently goes unrecognized and has many underlying causes. It is often difficult to differentiate between dementia and delirium as they share common clinical features, such as impaired memory or thinking. Patients experiencing delirium have a fluctuating level of consciousness, altered attention span, and disturbed sleep-wake cycle, whereas dementia is characterized by little to no clouding of consciousness; chronic, progressive symptoms; and less impaired sleep-wake cycle. Resolution of delirium depends on the resolution (when possible) of the underlying cause. Nonpharmacological approaches, such as providing sensory stimulation, reorientation, and reassurance, are important. When a pharmacological approach is needed, a benzodiazepine such as lorazepam is generally used to manage agitation. Although not approved for this indication, antipsychotic agents such as haloperidol or risperidone are frequently used to treat delirium or psychosis in dementia patients. These medications should be used judiciously, as recent meta-analyses have revealed that treatment with either typical or atypical antipsychotics increases the risk of death in patients, especially among those taking higher than conventional doses.[63] Despite these warnings, when used appropriately, antipsychotic drugs can have quality-of-life benefits in patients with advanced dementia and should be prescribed based on the goals of care and at the discretion of the prescriber after sharing the potential risk with the caregiver. It is important to recognize that patients with Lewy body dementia can be very sensitive to the effects of neuroleptic and anticholinergic medications, and they should be avoided in this patient population. Quetiapine is the first-line atypical antipsychotic agent for these patients or for those with Parkinson's disease; however, it should be used with caution and only when benefits clearly outweigh risks.

Depression

Depression is prevalent in approximately 20% to 25% of persons with dementia although, because of the difficulties associated with assessing depression, it may be underreported.[64] Depression may also be confused with apathy, which is commonly seen in Alzheimer's disease, especially in more advanced stages. In addition to nonpharmacological approaches such as providing social interaction and activity, pharmacological management might be indicated. The medications of choice for depression are SSRIs because of their low side-effect profile and reasonable tolerability in the elderly. If the patient has a poor prognosis, then a trial of a psychostimulant is recommended. Because of the risk for adverse effects in the elderly, start with the lowest dose and slowly titrate upward.

Pain

Patients with dementia tend to be older and are at risk to experience chronic pain commonly associated with aging. In addition to pain from comorbid conditions, patients with advanced disease may have pain resulting from immobility or as a consequence of complications such as urinary tract infections or decubitus ulcers. Pain perception and pain thresholds of persons with dementia are thought to be similar to those of the cognitively intact older adult.[65] Cognitively impaired persons are at increased risk for undertreatment of their pain.[66] Persons with dementia might not be able to report pain because of reduced verbal capacity and thinking, so pain assessment in this population can be especially challenging. Although some patients with dementia are able to self-report, for those who are unable, a variety of assessment strategies should be employed. These include searching for potential causes of pain or discomfort or monitoring behaviors indicative of pain.[67] Pain in advanced dementia may present as agitation or social withdrawal and may be accompanied by vocalizations, grimacing, or bracing. There are a number of validated observation scales to assess pain in persons with dementia, such as the Pain Assessment in Advanced Dementia (PAIN-AD) tool. The PAIN-AD scale consists of five items: negative vocalization, facial expression, body language, consolability, and a scale that allows the practitioner to assign a score to a particular behavior in a standardized manner. Each element of the scale can be scored from 0 to 2, for a total score of 0 to 10 (maximal pain).[68] However, the lack of specificity when observing pain behaviors remains a challenge; therefore, pain experts recommend an empirical analgesic trial if pain is suspected.[65] Furthermore, patients who require opioids should not have them withheld because of concerns about worsening confusion, as this concern is not supported by the literature.[69]

End-stage issues

In the advanced stage of dementia, the patient becomes totally dependent on others for care and is at risk for developing complications such as urinary tract infections, pneumonia, fractures, and swallowing difficulties. When possible, advance care planning should take place early in the disease course, and a surrogate decision-maker should be appointed to make treatment decisions when the patient loses decisional capacity.

Nutrition and hydration

One of the more challenging end-stage concerns for family members relates to the problem of nutrition and hydration. Persons in the advanced stages of dementia experience a progressive loss of appetite, loss of ability to swallow, and increased aspiration risk. Eventually, they resist or become indifferent to eating, have difficulty handling food in their mouths, and are at high risk for choking when swallowing.[70] The use of artificial nutrition and hydration in the final stages of dementia is not recommended due to a number of studies detailing the burdens associated with tube feeding, including increased mortality.[71] Various studies have demonstrated that feeding tubes are not associated with good outcomes; specifically, they have not been demonstrated to prevent malnutrition, pressure ulcers, or aspiration pneumonia nor do they provide comfort or prolong survival.[70] Caregivers are encouraged to hand-feed as long as possible and to use a variety of strategies to improve food intake. Caregivers need to be reassured that patients with end-stage dementia can be kept comfortable without the use of feeding tubes.

Treatment of infections

Infections are common among persons with end-stage dementia. Like other end-of-life management issues, the use of antibiotics to treat infections is not without controversy. A recent study showed that antibiotics are frequently used in patients with advanced dementia, particularly in the last 2 weeks of life.[72] However, in addition to public health concerns about the spread of antimicrobial-resistant bacteria, the provision of antibiotics can be burdensome and although they may delay death, they may also prolong the dying process.[73]

Hospice care for dementia

As the dementia approaches the end-stage, hospice should be considered, as hospice enrollment is associated with improved patient and caregiver outcomes compared with routine care.[74] Given the shifts in disease prevalence and benefits of hospice, it is not surprising that dementia now represents the third most common noncancer diagnosis for hospice services. In 2012, dementia accounted for approximately 13% of hospice admissions, compared with only 6.9% in 2001.[3]

Like those with other chronic illnesses, patients with Alzheimer's disease or other subtypes of dementia meet Medicare hospice eligibility requirements once they have a predicted life expectancy of 6 months or less and have decided not to continue cure-focused therapies. According to Medicare guidelines, hospice-eligible patients with dementia are those who are unable to walk, are unable to dress or bathe without assistance, have urinary and fecal incontinence, and cannot speak more than five intelligible words daily (FAST stage 7c).[75] In addition to these functional limitations, hospice eligibility requirements include the presence of coexisting medical complications such as aspiration pneumonia, urinary tract infections, sepsis, decubitus ulcers, or weight loss.[76] Caregivers of dementia patients endure many losses throughout the disease process and require a great deal of support.

Neurodegenerative Diseases: Amyotrophic Lateral Sclerosis and Parkinson's Disease

Amyotrophic lateral sclerosis

Amyotrophic Lateral Sclerosis (ALS) is a progressive, incurable neurodegenerative disease that affects both upper and lower motor neurons and causes progressive muscular weakness. Although rare, with an incidence of 1 to 2 cases per 100,000, it is estimated that up to 30,000 Americans have ALS at any given time. ALS is more common among males and usually develops between the ages of 40 and 70 years, although cases can develop in younger persons.[77] Development of ALS is usually sporadic with no known cause, although 5% to 10% of cases are familial.[78] The course and prognosis of ALS is variable and may depend on whether patients opt for therapies that can prolong survival, such as mechanical ventilation. Median survival is approximately 3 years, although patients may live 15 years or longer with long-term mechanical ventilation.[78] Respiratory failure resulting from progressive respiratory muscle weakness is the most common cause of death from ALS.

ALS usually presents with arm or leg weakness. Over time, the weakness increases in severity and affects more areas of the body until only sphincter control and eye movements are spared. Although cognition usually remains intact, cognitive impairment and dementia has been noted to occur in close to one-third of individuals with ALS.[79] There is no definitive diagnostic test for ALS, and it is frequently a diagnosis of exclusion, which may take months. Currently, riluzole, a glutamate antagonist is the only FDA-approved treatment for ALS. Riluzole may slow down symptoms and prolong survival by 3 to 6 months in some patients, but does not improve functional status.[79]

Table 35.2 Symptoms of Amyotrophic Lateral Sclerosis

Direct	Indirect
Progressive muscle weakness and atrophy	Depression
	Anxiety
	Sleep disturbances
Fasciculations and muscle cramps	Thick secretions and/or drooling
	Pain/muscle aches
Spasticity	Symptoms of chronic hypoventilation (morning headache, anorexia, weight loss, depression/anxiety, dyspnea, severe fatigue)
Slurred or slowed speech	
Pathological laughter or crying	
Dyspnea	
Dysphagia	

Individuals with ALS suffer numerous symptoms that are directly or indirectly related to the disease (Table 35.2). An interdisciplinary approach, preferably at a specialized ALS center, is helpful in addressing the myriad of issues that persons with ALS and their families face. Physical and occupational therapists assist patients in performing activities of daily living by improving mobility, reducing spasticity, and providing adaptive equipment. Speech therapists help to facilitate communication. Symptomatic treatments include anticholinergics such as atropine drops to reduce drooling,[80] quinine sulfate or carbamazapine for muscle cramps, baclofen for spasticity, and tricyclic antidepressants such as amitriptyline to help reduce uncontrollable laughing or crying. Depression, insomnia, and anxiety are also common and should be treated accordingly. As swallowing problems emerge, patients may benefit from placement of a percutaneous endoscopic gastrostomy tube.[81] When breathing difficulties develop, patients require some type of ventilatory support. Most patients opt for bilevel positive airway pressure support, which has been found to improve symptoms of hypoventilation, quality of life, and survival.[82] Fewer patients agree to the use of mechanical ventilation because of concerns about prolonged immobilization, limited communication, and family burden.[78] Home hospice can provide much-needed physical, psychological, and spiritual support and should be discussed before lung capacity considerably declines.

Parkinson's Disease

Parkinson's disease is a degenerative motor system disorder that results from the progressive loss of dopamine-producing brain cells. Without dopamine, the nerve cells cannot properly transmit messages, resulting in loss of muscle function. Hallmark symptoms include trembling of hands, arms, legs, jaw and face; stiffness of the arms, legs, and trunk; slowness of voluntary movement; and poor balance and coordination. As symptoms progress, individuals with Parkinson's disease may develop depression, sleep disorders, difficulty swallowing or speaking, delayed gastric emptying, constipation, bladder dysfunction/incontinence, pain, psychosis,

and dementia. There is no specific test to diagnose Parkinson's disease. Diagnosis depends on the presence of at least two of three major signs: tremor at rest, rigidity, and bradykinesia in the absence of secondary causes such as dopamine-depleting medications. Parkinson's disease prevalence increases with age and it usually has a long, chronic course. The most common causes of death are pulmonary infection/aspiration, urinary tract infection, pulmonary embolism and complications of falls, fractures, and immobility.

Currently, there are numerous treatments that improve motor function and quality of life; however, there is no known cure for Parkinson's disease, and persons affected with the disease become increasingly disabled over time. Patients sometimes need to be cared for in long-term care settings, as they become increasingly functionally disabled.[83] Parkinson's disease is treated with a variety of drugs such as carbidopa/levodopa, dopamine agonists, and MAO-B inhibitors. Unfortunately, long-term levodopa use results in dyskinesias, such as writhing, twisting, and shaking, and over time, the effects of levodopa wear off.[84] Dyskinesias are a dose-limiting effect of these agents over time. Some patients are candidates for deep-brain stimulation to block electrical signals in the brain that cause Parkinson's disease symptoms. When effective, patients treated with deep-brain stimulation experience significant improvements in motor function and quality of life without troubling side effects associated with medical therapy.[85] Once the patient becomes increasingly disabled despite optimal therapy, goals of care may shift more toward palliation. Patients usually die as a result of complications of the disease, such as from pneumonia or other infections. Like those with ALS, patients with Parkinson's disease require a multidisciplinary approach to address the debilitating and distressing aspects of the disease.

Good nursing care, including skin care, oral hygiene, positioning, incontinence and constipation management, and support for end-of-life decision-making, is an important part of care for a patient with Parkinson's disease. Pain is a common problem arising from restricted movement, rigidity, or spasms and should be treated with analgesics as in other chronic diseases. Psychosis or hallucinations are traditionally treated by reducing the dose or eliminating dopaminergic or anticholinergic drugs used to treat Parkinson's disease, even if motor symptoms worsen as a consequence.[83] If an antipsychotic is required, then quetiapine is preferred because the use of risperidone or olanzapine or haloperidol is associated with worsening of Parkinsonian symptoms,[86] although its efficacy is limited.[87]

Coping with chronic illness

Family caregivers play an important role in helping their loved one to manage their symptoms, adhere to their treatments, and cope with the psychosocial impact of illness. It's vitally important that the nurse assess how well caregivers are handling the many demands placed on them. Caregivers often feel unprepared for their caregiving responsibilities, especially as their loved one's needs increase as their physical health declines. Caregiver duties include managing with their loved one's declining mobility and changing appetite, need for assistance with toileting, bathing and showering, managing medications, and coordinating doctor's appointments, just to mention a few.

In palliative care, the patient and the family are the unit of care. Palliative care nurses play an important role in reducing the stress of caregiving by providing information about community resources and making referrals to outside support agencies, teaching family members how to assess and manage symptoms, and advocating for the patient and family's wishes and preferences. Patients with chronic illness and their caregivers often are socially isolated and lonely. By addressing the myriad of psychosocial and spiritual needs, while integrating cultural values into the plan of care, nurses can help to lessen some of these burdens.

Increasingly, palliative care nurse practitioners are assuming an important role in community-based palliative care for patients with multiple co-morbid conditions. The transitional care model (TCM), designed by Dr. Mary Naylor and colleagues at the University of Pennsylvania, is an example of a program designed to improve care coordination and prevent the negative effects associated with breakdowns in care when older adults transition from an acute care setting to home or to a nursing facility. This evidence-based approach to care has resulted in fewer hospital readmissions for primary and complicating conditions; improved the health, functioning, and quality of life of patients; and lessoned the burden among family members.[88]

Conclusion

The prevalence of chronic illness is increasing as the population ages. Despite differences in illness trajectories and difficulty estimating prognosis, patients with chronic noncancer conditions experience similar symptoms and have common needs as the illness progresses. Individuals with chronic progressive illness and their families benefit from an interdisciplinary palliative approach to care, and as the disease advances, hospice care should be considered.

References

1. Hoyert DL, Xu J. National Vital Statistics Reports. Deaths: Preliminary Data for 2011. 2012;61. Available from http://www.cdc.gov/nchs/data/nvsr/nvsr61/nvsr61_06.pdf.
2. Lynn J, Schuster JL, Kabcenell A. Improving Care for the End of Life: A Sourcebook for Healthcare Managers and Clinicians. New York: Oxford University Press; 2000.
3. National Hospice and Palliative Care Organization. NHPCO Facts and Figures: Hospice Care in America, 2013 Edition. Available from http://www.nhpco.org/sites/default/files/public/Statistics_Research/2013_Facts_Figures.pdf.
4. Centers for Medicare and Medicaid Services Conditions of Participation (COPs) Hospice. June 8, 2008. Available from http://www.cms.gov/Regulations-and-Guidance/Legislation/CFCsAndCoPs/Hospice.html.
5. National Hospice Organization. Medical Guidelines for Determining Prognosis in Selected Non-cancer Diseases. Arlington, VA: National Hospice Organization; 1995.
6. Kane GC, Karon BL, Mahoney DW, et al. Progression of left ventricular diastolic dysfunction and risk of heart failure. JAMA. 2011;306:865–863.
7. Jong P, Vowinckel E, Liu P, Gong Y, Tu JV. Prognosis and determinants of survival in patients newly hospitalized for heart failure: a population-based study. Arch Intern Med. 2002;162:1689–1694.
8. Yancy CY, Jessup M, Bozkurt B, et al. 2013 ACC/AHA guideline for the management of heart failure: executive summary: a report of the American College of Cardiology/American Heart Association Task Force on Practice Guidelines. Circ. 2013 62:e147–e238.
9. Hunt SA, Abraham WT, Chin MH, et al. Chronic heart failure in the adult: ACC/AHA 2005 guidelines for the evaluation and management of chronic heart failure in the adult: executive summary: a report of the American College of Cardiology/American Heart Association Task Force on Practice Guidelines. (Committee to revise the 1995 Guidelines for the Evaluation and Management of Heart Failure). J Am Coll Cardiol. 2005;46:1116–1143.
10. Jessup M, Bronza S. Heart failure. N Engl J Med. 2003;348:2007–2018.
11. Levenson JW, McCarthy EP, Lynn J, Davis RB, Phillips RS. The last six months of life for patients with congestive heart failure. J Am Geriatr Soc. 2000;48(5 Suppl):S101–S109.
12. Shah AG, Morrissey RP, Baraghouse, A, Bharadwaj, P, Phan A, Hamilton M, Kobashigawa J, Schwarz ER. Failing the failing heart: a review of palliative heart failure care. Rev Cardiovasc Med. 2013;14(1):41–48.
13. Bain, KT, Maxwell TL, Strassels SA, Whellan DJ. Am Heart J. 2009:158:118–125.
14. Wilson J, McMillan S. Symptoms experienced by heart failure patients in hospice care. J Hosp Palliat Med. 2013;15:13–21.
15. Amer M, Bead VR, Bathon J, Bluenthal RS, Edwards DN. Use of non-sterioidal anti-inflammatory drugs in patients with cardiovascular disease: a cautionary tale. Cardiol Rev. 2010; 18(4):204–2010.
16. Haque WA, Boehmer J, Clemson BS, Leuenberger UA, Silber DH, Sionway LI. Hemodynamic effects of supplemental oxygen in congestive heart failure. J Am Coll Cardiol. 1996:27:353–357.
17. Mahler DA. Opioids for refractory dyspnea. Expert Rev Respir Med. 2013;7(2):123–134.
18. Kamal AH, Maguire JM, Wheeler JL, Currow DC, Abernathy AP. Dyspnea review for the palliative care professional: treatment goals and therapeutic options. J Palliat Med. 2012;15(1):106–114.
19. Hallenbeck JL. Non-pain symptom management: dyspnea. In: Hallenbeck JL (ed.), Palliative Care Perspectives. New York: Oxford University Press; 2003.
20. DiSalvo WM, Joyce MM, Tyson LB, Culkin AE, Mackay K. Putting evidence into practice: evidence-based interventions for cancer-related dyspnea. Clin J Oncol Nurs. 2008;12(2):341–352.
21. Cuffe MS, Califf RM, Adams KF Jr, et al. Outcomes of a prospective trial of intravenous milrinone for exacerbations of chronic heart failure (OPTIME_CHF) investigators. JAMA. 2002;287:1541–1547.
22. Nohria A, Lewis E, Stevenson LW. Medical management of advanced heart failure. JAMA. 2002;287(5):628–640.
23. Epstein AE, DiMarco JP, Ellenbogen KA, Estes NA 3rd, Freedman RA, Gettes LS, et al. ACC/AHA/HRS 2008 guidelines for device-based therapy or cardiac rhythm abnormalities. J Am Coll Cardiol. 2008;51:e1–e62.
24. Borne RT, Varosy PD, Masoudi FA. Implantable cardioverter-defibrillator shocks: epidemiology, outcomes, and therapeutic approaches. JAMA Intern Med. 2013;(173(10):859–865.
25. Fromme EK, Lugliani Stewart T, Jeppesen M, Tolle SW. Adverse experiences with implantable defibrillators in Oregon hospices. Am Hosp Palliat Care. 2001;28:304–309.
26. Kelley AS, Mehta SS, Reid MC. Management of patients with ICDs at the end of life (EOL): a qualitative study. Am J Hosp Palliat Med. 2009;25:440–446.
27. Lambert R, Hayes DL, Annas GJ, et al. Heart Rhythm Society expert consensus statement on the management of cardiovascular electronic devices (CIEDs) in patients nearing the end of life or requesting withdrawal of therapy. Heart Rhythm. 2010;7:1008–1026.
28. Rodrigues LE, Suarez EE, Loebe M, Bruckner BA. Ventricular assist devices (VAD) therapy: new technology, new hope? Methodist DeBakey Cardiovasc J. 2013;(9(1):32–37.
29. Rose EA, Gelijns AC, Moskowitz AJ, et al. Long-term use of a left ventricular assist device for end-stage heart failure. N Engl J Med. 2001;345:1435–1443.
30. Padeletti, L, Amar DO, Boncinelli L, Brachma J, Camm JA, Daubert JC, et al. EHRA expert consensus statement on the management of cardiovascular implantable devices in patients nearing the end of life. Europace. 2010;12(10):1480–1489.

31. Berry JL. Hospice and heart disease: missed opportunities. J Pain Palliat Care Pharmacother. 2010;24:23–26.

32. LeMond L, Allen LA. Palliative care and hospice in advanced heart failure. Prog Cardiovasc Dis. 2011;54(2);168–178.

33. Jemal A, Ward E, Hao Y, Thun M. Trends in the leading causes of death in the United States, 1970–2002. JAMA. 2006;295(4):393–394.

34. Lopez AD, Shibuya K, Rao C, et al. Chronic obstructive pulmonary disease: current burden and future projections. Eur Respir J. 2006;27:397–412.

35. Global Initiative for Chronic Obstructive Lung Disease (GOLD). Global Strategy for the Diagnosis, Management, and Prevention of Chronic Obstructive Pulmonary Disease. Updated 2013. http://www.goldcopd.org/uploads/users/files/GOLD_Report_2013_Feb20.pdf. Accessed July 2013.

36. COPD Working Group. Long-term oxygen therapy for patients with chronic obstructive pulmonary disease (COPD). Ont Health Tech Assess Ser. 2012;12(7):1–84.

37. Varkey B. Opioids for palliation of refractory dyspnea in chronic obstructive pulmonary disease patients. Curr Opin Pulm Med. 2010;16(2)150–154.

38. Uronis HE, Currow DC, Abernathy AP. Palliative management of refractory dyspnea in COPD. Int J Chron Obstruct Pulm Dis. 2008;1(3):289–304.

39. Curtis JR, Engelberg RA, Nielsen EL, et al. Patient-physician communication about end-of-life care for patients with COPD. Eur Respir J. 2004;24:200–205.

40. Mitch WE. Chronic kidney disease. In: Goldman L, Ausiello D (eds.), Goldman: Cecil Medicine. 23rd ed. Philadelphia, PA: Saunders Elsevier; 2007: chap 131.

41. US Renal Data System. USRDS 2012 Annual Data Report: Atlas of Chronic Kidney Disease and End-Stage Renal Disease in the United States. National Institutes of Health; National Institute of Diabetes and Digestive and Kidney Diseases, Bethesda, MD, 1012. Available from http://www.usrds.org/adr.htm.

42. Gamondi C, Galli N, Schonholzer C, Marone C, Zwaheln H, et al. Frequency and severity of pain and symptom distress among patients with chronic kidney disease receiving dialysis. Swiss Med Wkly. 2013;143:w13750.

43. Owens DA. Palliative and end stage renal disease. J Hosp Palliat Nurs. 2006;8(6):318–319.

44. CMS. Pub 100–2. Medicare Benefit Policy Manual (2004). Chapter 9, Coverage of Hospice Services Under Hospital Insurance, §10, 10/21, 40.19, 40.24; Chapter 11, End Stage Renal Disease (ESRD), § 50.6.1.4.

45. Thorsteinsdottir B, Swetz KM, Feely MA, Mueller PS, Williams AW. Are there alternatives to hemodialysis for the elderly patient with end-stage renal failure? Mayo Clin Proc. 2012;87:514–516.

46. O'Connor NR, Kumar P. Conservative management of end-stage renal disease without dialysis: a systematic review. J Palliat Med. 2012;15: 230–235.

47. Poppel DM, Cohen LM, Germain MJ. The renal palliative care initiative. J Palliat Med 2003;321–326.

48. Kane PM, Vienen K, Murtagh FE. Palliative Care for advanced renal disease: a summary of the evidence and future direction. Palliat Med. 2013;27(9):817–821.

49. Cohen LM, Germain MJ, Poppel DM. Practical considerations in dialysis withdrawal: "To have that option is a blessing." JAMA. 2003;289(16):2113–2119.

50. Davison SN, Rosielle DA. Withdrawal of dialysis: decision-making. Fast Facts and Concepts. September 2008; 207. Available from http://www.eperc.mcw.edu/fastfact/ff_207.htm.

51. Cohen LM, Germain M. Poppel D, Woods A, Kjellstrand CM. Dialysis discontinuation and palliative care. Am J Kidney Dis. 2000;36(1):140–144.

52. Murtagh, FE, Addington-Hall J, Edmonds P, Donohoe P, Carey I, Jenkins K, et al. Symptoms in the months before death for stage 5 chronic kidney disease patients managed without dialysis. J Pain Symptom Manage. 2010;40(3):342–352.

53. King S, Forbes K, Hanks GW, Ferro CJ, Chambers EJ. A systematic review of the use of opioid medication for those with moderate

54. to severe cancer pain and renal impairment a European Palliative Care Research Collaborative opioid guidelines project. Palliat Med. 2011;25(5):525–552.

54. Wolfson C, Wolfson DB, Asgharian M, et al. Clinical Progression of Dementia Study Group. A reevaluation of the duration of survival after the onset of dementia. N Engl J Med. 2001;344(15):1160–1161.

55. Xie J, Brayne C, Matthews FE; the Medical Research Council Function and Aging Study collaborators. Survival times in people with dementia: analysis from population based cohort study with 14 year follow-up. BMJ. 2008;336:258.

56. Alzheimer's Association. 2013. Alzheimer's Disease Facts and Figures 2013;9(2). http://www.alz.org/downloads/facts_figures_2013.pdf. Accessed July 10, 2013.

57. Molino I, Colucci L, Fasanaro AM, Traini E, Amenta F. Efficacy of menantine, donepezil, or their association in moderate-severe Alzheimer's disease: a review of clinical trials. Scientific World J. 2013; 2013:925702.

58. Kaduszkiewicz H, Wiese B, Van den Bussche H. Self-reported competence, attitude and approach of physicians towards patients with dementia in ambulatory care: results of a postal survey. BMC Health Serv Res. 2008;8:54.

59. Birks J. Cholinesterase inhibitors for Alzheimer's disease. Cochrane Database Syst Rev. 2006;1. Edited (no change to conclusions); 2012;(5).

60. FDA News. FDA Approves Memantine (Namenda) for Alzheimer's Disease; 2003. Available at http://www.fda.gov/bbs/topics/news/2003/new00961.html. Accessed December 19, 2008.

61. Weschules DJ, Maxwell TL, Shega JW. Acetylcholinesterase inhibitor and N-Methyl-D-aspartic acid receptor antagonist use among hospice enrollees with a primary diagnosis of dementia. J Palliat Med. 2008;11(5):738–745.

62. Elici-Evcime Y, Breitbart W. An update on the use of antipsychotics in the treatment of delirium. Palliat Support Care. 2008;6:177–182.

63. Rochon PA, Normand S-L, Gomes T, Gill SS, Anderson GM, Melo M, et al. Antipsychotic therapy and short-term serious events in older adults with dementia. Arch Int Med. 2008;14:1090–1096.

64. Landes AM, Sperry SD, Strauss ME. Prevalence of apathy, dysphoria, and depression in relation to dementia severity in Alzheimer's disease. J Neuropsychiatry Clin Neurosci. 2005;17:343–349.

65. AGS Panel on Persistent Pain in Older Persons. The management of persistent pain in older persons. J Am Geriatr Soc. 2002;50:1–20.

66. Monroe TB, Carter MA, Feldt KS, Dietrich MS, Cowan RL. Pain and hospice care in nursing home residents with dementia and terminal cancer. Geriatr Gerontol Int. 2013;13(4):1018–1025.

67. Herr K, Coyne PJ, Key T, et al. Pain assessment in the nonverbal patient: position statement with clinical practice recommendations. Pain Manage Nurs. 2006;7(2):44–52.

68. Lane P, Kuntupis M, MacDonald S, et al. A pain assessment tool for people with advanced Alzheimer's and other progressive dementias. Home Healthc Nurse. 2003;21(1):32–37.

69. Ersek M, Cherrier MM, Overman SS, Irving GA. The cognitive effects of opioids. Pain Manage Nurs. 2004;5(2):75–93.

70. Li I. Feeding tubes in patients with severe dementia. Am Fam Physician. 2002;65:1605–1610.

71. Daniel K, Rhodes R, Vitale C, Shega J. American Geriatrics Society (AGS) Feeding tubes in advanced dementia position statement. May 2013 http://www.americangeriatrics.org/files/documents/feeding.tubes.advanced.dementia.pdf. Accessed July 10, 2013.

72. D'Agata E, Mitchell S. Patterns of antimicrobial use among nursing home residents with advanced dementia. Arch Intern Med. 2008;168(4):357–362.

72. van der Steeen JT, Lane P, Kowall NW, Knol DL, Volicer L. Antibiotics and mortality in patients with lower respiratory infection and advanced dementia. J Am Med Dir Assoc. 2012;13(2):156–161.

74. Shega JW, Hougham GW, Stocking CB, Cox-Hayley D, Sachs GA. Patients dying with dementia: experience at the end of life and impact of hospice care. J Pain Symptom Manage. 2008;35(5):499–507.

75. CMS Hospice Care Guidelines. http://www.nhpco.org/cms-medicare-hospice-regulations. (accessed December 12, 2013).

76. Jayes RL. Arnold RM, Fromme EK. Does this dementia patient meet the prognosis eligibility requirements for hospice enrollment? J Pain Symptom Manage. 2012;44(5):750–756.

77. Amyotrophic Lateral Sclerosis (ALS) Association. Who Gets ALS. 2008 Sep 1(1):[1 screen] Available from http://www.alsa. org/als/who.cfm. Accessed December 30, 2008.

78. Gordon PH. Amyotrophic lateral sclerosis: an update for 2013 clinical features, pathophysiology, management and therapeutic tools. Aging Dis. 2013(4(5):295–310.

79. Miller RG, Mitchell JD, Moore DH. Riluzole for amyotrophic lateral sclerosis (ALS)/motor neuron disease (MND). Cochrane Database Syst Rev. 2012;3:CD000147.

80. De Simone GG, Eisenchlas JH, Junin M, Pereyra F, Brizuela R. Atropine drops for drooling: a randomized controlled trial. Palliat Med. 2006;20(7):665–671.

81. Miller RG, Rosenberg JA, Gelinas DF, et al. Practice parameter: the care of the patient with amyotrophic lateral sclerosis (an evidence-based review). Neurology. 1999;52(7):1311–1323.

82. Siirala W, Aataa R, Oikkola KT, Saaresranta T, Vuori A. Is the effect of non-invasive ventilation on survival in amyotrophic lateral sclerosis age-dependent? BMC Palliat Care. 2013;12(1):23.

83. Chen JJ, Trombetta DP, Fernandez HH. Palliative management of Parkinson's disease: focus on nonmotor, distressing symptoms. J Pharm Pract. 2008;21:262–272.

84. Fernandez HH. Updates in the medical management of Parkinson's Disease. Cleve Clin J Med. 2012;79(1):28–35.

85. Weaver FM, Follett K, Stern M, et al. Bilateral deep brain stimulation vs best medical therapy for patients with advanced Parkinson disease. JAMA. 2009;301(1):63–73.

86. Friedman JH, Fernandez HH. Atypical antipsychotics in Parkinson's sensitive populations. J Geriatr Psychiatry Neurol. 2002;15:156–170.

87. Kurlan R, Cummings J, Raman R, Thal L. Quetiapine for agitation or psychosis in patients with dementia and parkinsonism. Neurology. 2007;68:1356–1363.

88. Toles MP, Abbott KM, Hirschman KB, Naylor MD. Transitions in care among older adults receiving long-term care services and supports. J Gerontol Nurs. 2012;38(11):40–47.

CHAPTER 36

Cultural considerations in palliative care

Polly Mazanec and Joan T. Panke

Culture consists of connections, not of separations.
Carlos Fuentes, 1988[1]

Key points

- Quality palliative care requires attention to patient and family cultural values, practices, and beliefs.

- A multidimensional assessment of an individual and family's culture is essential to providing palliative care.

- An individual's culture encompasses multiple components, including race, ethnicity, gender, age, differing abilities, sexual orientation, religion and spirituality, and socioeconomic status.

This chapter defines culture and the complexity of its components as they relate to palliative care. It emphasizes how recognizing one's own values, practices, and beliefs impacts care. Finally, it discusses selected palliative care concepts and issues influenced by culture. This chapter is intended to be not a "cookbook" approach to describing behaviors and practices of different cultures as they relate to palliative care but rather a guide to raising awareness of the significance of cultural considerations in palliative care.

Culture and palliative care nursing

The essence of palliative nursing is to provide holistic supportive care for the patient and the family living with a serious or life-limiting illness. Palliative nursing strives to meet the physical, emotional, social, and spiritual needs of the patient and family across the disease trajectory.[2] To meet these needs, nurses must recognize the vital role that culture has on one's experience of living and dying. The beliefs, norms, and practices of an individual's cultural heritage guide one's behavioral responses, decision-making, and actions.[3] Culture shapes how an individual makes meaning out of illness, suffering, and death.[3,4] Nurses, along with other members of the interdisciplinary team, partner with the patient and family to ensure that patient and family values, beliefs, and practices guide the plan of care.[5]

The National Consensus Project (NCP) Clinical Practice Guidelines for Quality Palliative Care[5] define the core concepts and structures for quality palliative care delivery. The guidelines comprise eight domains with corresponding criteria that reflect the depth and breadth of the specialty. Cultural aspects of care constitute one of the eight domains, emphasizing the central role that culture plays in providing strength and meaning for patients

and families facing serious illness.[5] Within this domain, two overarching guidelines define culture and outline cultural competences for interdisciplinary team members (Box 36.1).

Clinical implications of the NCP guidelines

Culture is a source of resilience for patients and families and plays an important role in the provision of palliative care. It is the responsibility of all members of the palliative care program to strive for cultural and linguistic competence to ensure that appropriate and relevant services are provided to patients and families. The following case illustrates the distress experienced by the patient, family, and healthcare team when cultural implications of care are not considered.

Case study

Mrs. S is a 79-year-old female admitted to the hospital with decompensated congestive heart failure. She and her husband moved to the United States from China in the early 1970s and raised a daughter and son in the United States. Her 85-year-old husband is in good health. On morning rounds, the medical team spoke to the patient about her diagnosis, prognosis, likely disease course, and advance care planning concerns without any other family present. The palliative care service was consulted in the afternoon to assist the primary team after the nurse found Mrs. S's husband helping her to dress and stating he was taking her to another hospital which would respect their ways.

Questions to consider in this case

1. What cultural issues are likely the basis for the conflict between the husband and medical team in this case?

2. What cultural, religious, and/or spiritual issues might impact decision-making?

3. Whom might the palliative team involve to assist in ascertaining religious or cultural aspects of care?

4. What are some techniques that the nurse and other health providers might use to both respect the patient's right to be involved in their care and ascertain what she wants to know as well as who makes decisions for this patient?

Box 36.1 Clinical practice guidelines for quality palliative care—cultural aspects of care

Guideline 6.1 The palliative care program serves each patient, family, and community in a culturally and linguistically appropriate manner.

Criteria:

- Definition of culture and cultural components
- Cultural identification of patient/family
- Assessment and documentation of cultural aspects of care
- The plan of care addresses the patient's and family's cultural concerns and needs.
- Respect for the patient's/family's cultural perceptions, preferences, and practices
- Palliative care program staff communicate in a language and manner that the patient and family understand and take into account
  - Literacy;
  - Use of professional interpreter services and acceptable alternatives;
  - Written materials that facilitate patient/family understanding.
- Respects and accommodates dietary and ritual practices of patients/families
- Palliative care staff members identify and refer patients/families to community resources as appropriate.

Guideline 6.2 The palliative care program strives to enhance its cultural and linguistic competence.

Criteria:

- Definition of cultural competence
- Valuing diversity in the work environment. Hiring practices of the palliative care program reflect the cultural and linguistic diversity of the community it serves.
- Palliative care staff cultivate cultural self-awareness and recognize how their own cultural values, beliefs, biases, and practices inform their perceptions of patients, families, and colleagues.
- Provision of education to help staff members increase their cross-cultural knowledge and skills and reduce health disparities.
- The palliative care program regularly evaluates and, if needed, modifies services, policies, and procedures to maximize its cultural and linguistic accessibility and responsiveness. Input from patients, families, and community stakeholders is integrated into this process.

Source: Adapted from National Consensus Project for Quality Palliative Care. Clinical Practice Guidelines for Quality Palliative Care 2013. www.nationalconsensusproject.org.

Increasing diversity in the United States population

As the United States becomes increasingly diverse, the range of treasured beliefs, shared teachings, norms, customs, and languages challenges the nurse to understand and respond to a wide variety of perspectives. The total US population in 2013 was estimated to be 317.3 million and was projected to cross the 400 billion mark by 2051.[6] (Population statistics from the US Census Bureau illustrate that cultural diversity is increasing among the five most common panethnic groups, which are federally defined as American Indian/Alaska Native, Asian/Pacific Islander, Black or African American, Hispanic, and White (Table 36.1).[7]

Asians and Hispanics are the nation's fastest growing race or ethnic groups. From 2012 to 2013 the fastest-growing racial group was Asian, with more than 60% of the growth stemming from international migration. By comparison, Hispanics represent the second-fastest-growing group, with the population increase mostly owing to births. Hispanics remain the second largest racial/ethnic group in the United States behind non-Hispanic Whites. Rates of growth in 2013 for other groups were as follows: Native Hawaiians and Other Pacific Islanders (climbing 2.3% to about 1.4 million), American Indians and Alaska Natives (rising 1.5% to a little over 6.4 million), and Blacks or African Americans (increasing 1.2% to 45 million) followed Asians and Hispanics in percentage growth rates.[8]

Census projections suggest that by 2060 the combined minority groups, which currently make up 37% of the US population, will constitute the majority (57%).[7] Diversity among age groups is also changing as the population ages. By 2060 the number of citizens aged 65 years and older will more than double and the number of the "oldest old," the 85-and-older age group, is expected to more than triple. It is likely that intergroup diversity will also increase, adding to the complexity of culturally competent care and the potential for cultural clashes.

With the changes in cultural diversity in the US population come increasing diversity in the nursing workforce. Nurses must be aware of how their own cultural beliefs and norms shape their professional practice and differ from the beliefs and norms of the patients and families for whom they care.

Culture defined

Culture is the "learned, shared and transmitted values, beliefs, norms and life ways of a particular group that guide their

Table 36.1 Ethnic groups, Census 2013

White	197.8 million
Hispanic	54 million
Black or African American	45 million
Asian	19.4 million
American Indian/Alaska Native	6.4 million
Hawaiian and Other Pacific Islanders	1.4 million

Source: https://www.census.gov/newsroom/releases/archives/population/cb14-118.html (accessed July 6, 2014).

thinking, decision, actions in patterned ways—a patterned behavioral response."[9] Culture is shaped over time in a dynamic system in which the beliefs, values, and lifestyle patterns pass from one generation to another.[4] This dynamic organizing system of life is adaptive, designed to ensure survival and well-being and to find a common purpose or meaning throughout life.[4]

Although culture is often mistakenly thought of as simply race and ethnicity, the definition of culture is multidimensional, encompassing such components as gender, age, differing abilities, sexual orientation, religion, and socioeconomic factors (financial status, residency, employment, and educational level).[3] Each cultural component plays a role in shaping individual responses to life and in particular to serious illness and death.[3,4]

A broad definition of culture recognizes the various subcultures within the dominant culture an individual may associate with that shape experiences and responses in any given situation. The nurse must be constantly aware that the culture of the healthcare system and the culture of the nursing profession, as well as personal beliefs, shape how he or she responds to interactions with patients, families, and colleagues.

Components of culture

Race

The commonly held misconception that "race" refers to biological and genetic differences and "ethnicity" refers to cultural variation is outmoded. Race exists not as a natural category but as a social construct.[10] Any discussion of race must include the harsh reality of racism issues and disparities that have plagued society and continue to exist even today. Recent studies have demonstrated the discrimination of persons of certain races regarding healthcare practices, treatment options, and hospice utilization.[11-14] When viewed in relation to specific races, morbidity and mortality statistics point to serious gaps in access to quality care. Racial disparities are still evident even after adjustments for socioeconomic status and other access-related factors are taken into account.[15]

There is often an underlying mistrust of the healthcare system. Memories of the Tuskegee syphilis study and segregated hospitals remain with older African Americans.[16] The combination of mistrust and numerous other complex variables influence palliative care issues such as medical decision-making and advance care planning.[4,17] Compounding the situation is the fact that healthcare providers often do not recognize existing biases within systems or themselves.[15,18] These unknown biases may add to the perceived discrimination experienced.[15,18,19]

Researchers have tried to identify causal mechanisms for healthcare disparities in psychosocial, cultural, and spiritual palliative care; however, the work is sparse and limited by methodological flaws. Evans and Ebere[13] recommend using a conceptual framework such as that used in the National Healthcare Disparities Report to explore causal mechanisms, which include access to care, receipt of care, quality of care, and examination of barriers, usage, and costs of care and effectiveness, safety, timeliness, and patient centeredness.

Ethnicity

Ethnicity refers to "a group of people that share a common and distinctive racial, national, religious, linguistic, or cultural heritage."[19] The values, practices, and beliefs shared by members of the same ethnic group may influence behavior or response. Ethnicity has been identified as a significant predictor of end-of-life preferences and decision-making.[20] Currently, there are more than 100 ethnic groups and more than 500 American Indian Nations in the United States.[19]

Ethnicity has been shown to influence utilization of hospice and palliative care service. Ethnic minority groups are less likely to use hospice services when compared with non-Hispanic Whites. Furthermore, there has been little increase in hospice utilization in Black, Hispanic, or Asian populations in recent years.[17,21] Researchers have demonstrated an understanding of disparities in quality end-of-life care among ethnicities but have not yet identified why this is happening.[13] Further study into the multiple factors influencing utilization of these services is needed.[22]

It is important to note that although an individual may belong to a particular ethnic group, he or she may not identify strongly with that group.[3,9] Members of the same family from the same ethnic group may have very different ideas about what is acceptable practice concerning important palliative care concepts such as communication with healthcare professionals, medical decision-making, and end-of-life rituals. In multigenerational families, some members may hold to traditional beliefs and practices of their ethnic community of origin. Other family members may have a bicultural orientation, moving between the family culture of origin to the host society, and others may have left their cultural roots and identify with the host society.[24]

For example, in the United States, second- and third-generation members of immigrant families may be more assimilated into Western culture than first-generation members. This can lead to cultural conflicts around sensitive palliative care concepts.

The tendency to assume that an individual will respond in a certain way because he is a member of an ethnic group contributes to stereotyping. This can lead to inappropriate interventions and unnecessary distress. The nurse should assess each individual's beliefs and practices rather than assuming that he or she holds the beliefs of a particular group. Note that many studies have demonstrated that regardless of race or ethnicity, all persons share common needs at the end of life: being comfortable, being cared for, sustaining or healing relationships, having hope, and honoring spiritual beliefs.[23-26]

Gender

Cultural norms dictate specific roles for men and women. The significance of gender is evident in areas such as decision-making, caregiving, and pain and symptom management. It is important to have an awareness of family dominance patterns and determine which family member or members hold that dominant role. In some families, decision-making may be the responsibility of the male head of the family or eldest son; in others, the eldest female may hold that responsibility. For example, those of Asian ethnicity who follow strict Confucian teaching believe that men have absolute authority and are responsible for family decision-making.[27] Discussing prognosis and treatment with a female family member is likely to increase family burden and distress and may result in significant clashes with the healthcare team.[3,23]

In addition to decision-making, cultural expectations exist regarding the responsibilities of caregiving. In many families, women have traditionally been expected to take on the role of caregiver when someone in the family is facing a serious illness.

This responsibility, in addition to responsibilities at work and for children has been overwhelming for many, affecting their physical and emotional well-being. Research has demonstrated that female caregivers tend to experience greater caregiver burden, anxiety, and depression than male caregivers.[28,29] Support for family caregivers is an essential component of palliative care.

Age

Age has its own identity and culture.[3] Age cohorts are characterized by consumer behaviors, leisure activities, religious activities, education, and labor force participation.[24] Each group has its own beliefs, attitudes, and practices, which are influenced by their developmental stage and by the society in which they live. The impact of a life-limiting illness on persons of differing age groups is often influenced by the loss of developmental tasks associated with that age group.[24,30] As the US population ages, the importance of addressing the unique needs of elders becomes more evident. Consider also the cultural impact of this aging population on caregiving issues, medical decision-making, healthcare resources, and end-of-life choices.

Myths about the impact of age on pain management continue to exist, with some professionals believing that children and older adults do not perceive pain as strongly as the middle-aged population.[31,32] These beliefs result in undertreatment of pain and unnecessary suffering of patients in these vulnerable age groups.[26]

Differing abilities

Individuals with physical disabilities or mental illness are at risk of receiving poorer quality healthcare. Those with differing abilities constitute a cultural group in themselves and often feel stigmatized. This discrimination is evident in cultures where the healthy are more valued than the physically, emotionally, or intellectually challenged.[3] If patients are unable to communicate their needs, then pain and symptom management and end-of-life wishes are not likely to be addressed. Additionally, this vulnerable population's losses may not be recognized or acknowledged, putting individuals at risk for complicated grief. Challenges to providing palliative care and hospice services to those with intellectual disabilities have been identified and include limited knowledge about palliative care among providers in residential facilities as well as a need for increasing the palliative care providers' knowledge about caring for patients with intellectual disabilities.[33] Taking time to determine an individual's goals of care—regardless of differing abilities—and identifying resources and support to improve quality of life is essential.

Sexual orientation

Sexual orientation may carry a stigma when the patient is gay, lesbian, or transgendered. In palliative care, these patients have unique needs because of the legal and ethical issues of domestic partnerships, multiple losses that may have been experienced as a result of one's sexual orientation, and unresolved family issues. Domestic partnerships, which are sanctioned by many cities and states in the United States, grant some of the rights of traditional married couples to unmarried homosexual couples who share the traditional bond of the family.[3]However, many cities and states do not legally recognize the relationship. A Durable Power of Attorney for Health Care form must be completed. Without such documentation, decision-making follows state guidelines. If legal documents have not been drafted prior to death of a partner, then survivorship issues, financial concerns, and failure to acknowledge bereavement needs may cause additional distress and complicate grief.[34,35]

Unresolved family issues can make end-of-life complicated. The patient who is gay, lesbian, or transgendered may have been estranged from his/her family of origin. Reconciliation with family, old friends, or children may be desired as the patient prepares for coming to the end of life, or it may be challenging and distressing when family dynamics prohibit this opportunity for healing.[34]

Religion and spirituality

Religion is the belief and practice of a faith tradition, a means of expressing spirituality. Spirituality, a much broader concept, is the life force that transcends our physical being and gives meaning and purpose.[30] Although religion and spirituality are complementary concepts, these terms are often mistakenly used interchangeably. It should be noted that an individual may be very spiritual but not practice a formal religion. In addition, those who identify themselves as belonging to a religion may not necessarily adhere to all the practices of that religion. As with ethnicity, it is important to determine how strongly the individual aligns with his or her identified faith and the significance of its practice rituals.

Religious beliefs can significantly influence a person's decisions regarding treatment and care. These beliefs can be at the cornerstone of decisions regarding continuation or discontinuation of life-prolonging therapies for some people.[11,27] Additionally, religious beliefs can strongly influence how patients and families understand illness and suffering.[4,11]

Chaplains, clergy from a patient's or family member's religious group—ideally their own community clergy—are key members of the interdisciplinary palliative care team. Those who turn to their faith-based communities for support may find the emotional, spiritual, and other tangible support they need when dealing with a life-limiting illness.[13,25] Keep in mind, however, that some individuals who are struggling with misconceptions of the tenets of their own faith may experience spiritual distress and need spiritual intervention from caring chaplains or spiritual care counselors. Also be aware that many community clergy are not trained in end-of-life care and may need assistance from the palliative care team in order to support the patient's spiritual journey.

Spirituality is in the essence of every human being. It is what gives each person a sense of being, meaning, purpose, and direction.[36,37] It transcends the self to connect with others and with a higher power, independent of organized religion.[13,30,36] One's sense of spirituality is often the force that helps transcend loss and suffering.[25,26,30] Spiritual distress can cause pain and suffering if not identified and addressed. Assessing spiritual well-being and attending to spiritual needs, which may be very diverse, is essential to quality of life for patients and families confronting end of life.

Socioeconomic status

One's socioeconomic status, place of residence, workplace, and level of education are important components of one's cultural identity and play a role in palliative care. For example, those who are socioeconomically disadvantaged face unique challenges when seeking healthcare and when receiving treatment. Financial costs, including pain medications, medical tests, treatments and drugs not covered by limited insurance plans, transportation, and childcare, add additional burden.

It is important to note however that regardless of financial status, an estimated 25% of families are financially devastated by a serious terminal illness.[3] Patients experiencing disease progression, or in whom treatment side effects preclude the ability to work, are forced to confront profound losses: loss of work and income, loss of identity, and loss of a network of colleagues.

Those who are educationally disadvantaged struggle to navigate the healthcare system and to find information and support. The educationally disadvantaged may lack knowledge about resources such as palliative care services and may not have the skills or access to the global Internet and social networking. Access to services is challenging for some depending on their geographic location. For those living in rural areas, access to palliative care services is inadequate when compared to urban areas.[38] Only 57% of public hospitals, which serve those without health care insurance or those in rural areas, provide palliative care services.[39] Hospice services are also lacking, with 62%-92% of rural counties in selected states reporting no access to community-based hospice services.[40] Patients and families in a supportive community have increased access to resources at end-of-life compared to other more vulnerable populations.[3] A very vulnerable population with limited community resources are the unauthorized immigrants. It is presumed that there are about 11.5 million unauthorized immigrants in the United States, (2012), most of whom are educationally and socioeconomically disadvantaged and living in the country without access to healthcare.[41] Most of unauthorized immigrant care is emergent only; little is known about access to palliative care within this population.

Conducting a cultural assessment

There are many tools available to help with cultural assessment. These tools include the components of culture discussed in this chapter. However, doing a cultural assessment involves questions that necessitate the development of a trusting relationship. When meeting the patient and family early in the disease trajectory, the palliative care nurse has the advantage of time to establish such a relationship. This luxury of time is not always available. Using the skill of presence and active listening is often more beneficial than using a standardized tool. Checklists do not necessarily build trust and can be burdensome. Simple inquiries into patient and family practices and beliefs can assist the nurse in understanding needs and goals. Asking the patient and/or the family member to tell you about him/herself or the family and then listening to those narratives is powerful. The patient and family often give clues that trigger important questions to ask to clarify patient and family needs and goals. Box 36.2 provides examples of trigger questions.

Selected palliative care issues influenced by culture

Culture impacts all aspects of palliative care. This section focuses on cultural considerations regarding selected palliative care issues and concepts.

Communication

Communication is the foundation for all encounters between clinicians, patients, and family members.[42] When the clinicians and the patient-family unit are from different ethnic or cultural

---

Box 36.2 Key cultural assessment questions

Formal cultural assessments are available for the nurse to use (see resources in Box 36.4). Remember that a checklist does not always instill trust. Below are some suggestions for ascertaining key cultural preferences from both patients and family caregivers.

- Tell me a little bit about yourself (e.g., your family, your mother, father, siblings, etc.).

- Where were you born and raised? (If an immigrant, "How long have you lived in this country?")

- What language would you prefer to speak?

- Is it easier to write things down, or do you have difficulty with reading and writing?

- To whom do you go for support (family friends, community, or religious or community leaders)?

- Is there anyone we should contact to come to be with you?

- I want to be sure I'm giving you all the information you need. What do you want to know about your condition? To whom should I speak about your care?

- Whom do you want to know about your condition?

- How are decisions about healthcare made in your family? Should I speak directly with you, or is there someone else with whom I should be discussing decisions?

- (*Address to patient or designated decision-maker*) Tell me about your understanding of what has been happening up to this point? What does the illness mean to you?

- We want to work with you to be sure you are getting the best care possible and that we are meeting all your needs. Is there anything we should know about any customs or practices that are important to include in your care?

- Many people have shared that it is very important to include spirituality or religion in their care. Is this something that is important for you? Our chaplain can help contact anyone that you would like to be involved with your care.

- We want to make sure we respect how you prefer to be addressed, including how we should act. Is there anything we should avoid? Is it appropriate for you to have male and female caregivers?

- Are there any foods you would like or that you should avoid?

- Do you have any concerns about how to pay for care, medications, or other services?

Death rituals and practices

- Is there anything we should know about care of the body, about rituals, practices, or ceremonies that should be performed?

- What is your belief about what happens after death?

- Is there a way for us to plan for anything you might need both at the time of death and afterward?

- Is there anything we should know about whether a man or a woman should be caring for the body after death?

- Should the family be involved in the care of the body?

backgrounds, relating news regarding serious illness or a poor prognosis can be challenging. Communication disparities may lead to poorer outcomes and reduced patient and family satisfaction.[4,43] Increasing diversity in the US population challenges clinicians to gain competency in cultural aspects of communication. Each individual brings his or her own cultural experiences and assumptions about the world, health, and illness to each new encounter. It is important to assess and respect differing viewpoints.[10,24] The establishment of a relationship with the clinician, where the clinician seeks to understand individual concerns of the patient and family provides a foundation for all future communication and decision-making.[23]

Communication is an interactive, multidimensional process, often dictated by cultural norms, and provides the mechanism for human interaction and connection. Given the complexities of communicating diagnosis, prognosis, and progression of a life-limiting disease, there is no "one size fits all" approach.[44] Cultural assessments, including cultural norms related to communication, should occur early in the initial assessment, and findings should be clearly documented and shared with all health providers involved in the care of the patient and family (Box 36.3).

General communication principles should be utilized at all times. These include (1) adequate preparation for communicating medical facts; (2) selecting a setting that is private and free from distractions; (3) using appropriate nonverbal communication styles, sitting down, maintaining eye contact, and conveying that the clinician is not rushed; and (4) expressing empathy and responding to patient and family emotional responses.[45]

Box 36.3 Culturally competent communication skills and best practices for palliative care clinicians

1. **Foster respect.** Baseline assessment and documentation should include primary language/dialect; determine need for professional interpreter services. Determine who is involved in giving/receiving information and decisions and how individuals prefer to be addressed.

2. **Perform person-centered interviews through active and reflective listening.** Hearing, understanding, retaining, analyzing, and evaluating information. Use information gleaned to guide future questions. Do not ask too many questions. Demonstrate active listening through an open body posture and eye contact (if culturally appropriate) and provide a private setting that is conducive to open communication. Reflect and restate essential content and determine other questions or concerns. Reaffirm intent to honor and respect individual/groups decisions and plans.

3. **Provide presence.** Know your own beliefs and values and your level of comfort in engaging in conversations regarding illness and distress. Assist individuals to meet realistic goals when facing a serious illness, challenging situation, and/or uncertain future. Listen to the stories, life goals, and values. Pay attention to interpretation time, for example, how long it takes to make decisions, time needed to complete individual goals, imminence of death. Show empathy and compassion; be quiet/reflective during times of silence.

4. **Assess clinical knowledge of disease trajectories.** Assess and address distressing symptoms, side effects of treatment, and likely disease progression. Reaffirm goals of care and attempt the relief of symptoms and other concerns. Incorporate preferred healing practices and traditions. Discuss early access to hospice care to support goals as disease progresses.

5. **Determine learning styles and provide education to patient and family.** Determine learning style and any learning deficits. Provide educational materials in preferred language and/or arrange for professional interpreter when providing education. Do not overwhelm the patient and family with too much information at one time.

6. **Address nonverbal communication.** Nonverbal communication makes up the majority of communication between individuals. Assessing appropriate forms of nonverbal communication (for example, eye contact) will assist in enhanced communication, demonstrate respect, and may avoid cultural conflict.

7. **Assess the individual's interpretation of what is important in life, what gives life meaning for them.** Understanding what is important to the individual and those closest to him/her will assist in individualizing the palliative care plan. Support patient's strengths and encourage the patient to maintain hope. Life review can help identify what gives life meaning.

8. **Assess and address religious and spiritual preferences and concerns.** It is important to understand the role a religious/faith community and spiritual beliefs and practice play in the patient's life. Consider including clergy and others that the individual/family identifies as key supports. Offer spiritual care (books, music, rituals, meditation etc.) to enhance healing and peace.

9. **Demonstrate consideration of patient's privacy, decision-making strategies, and experience of loss and grief.** Early assessment of cultural issues related to beliefs about disclosure of diagnosis and decision-making preferences will ensure that care is given in ways that respect patient and family values. Observe for signs and symptoms of anticipatory or complicated grief and refer to appropriate interdisciplinary team members.

10. **Anticipate times when communication will be difficult.** Dealing with serious illness is often stressful. Be pro-active by anticipating situations when communication may be difficult (i.e. breaking bad news, holding family meetings, and helping patients and family members communicate last wishes at end-of-life). Utilize appropriate interdisciplinary team members to provide support to the patient and family during these difficult times.

Source: Adapted from C. Long. Ten best practices to enhance culturally competent communication in palliative care.[24]

One of the most important cultural communication assessments involves determining how information is shared within the family unit. Determine who the decision-maker is, whether it is the patient or a specific family member or members, and with whom information should be shared. For example, relating a diagnosis or poor prognosis to the patient may go against some cultural norms. Ideally, preferences for communication, including full disclosure of a terminal diagnosis and poor prognosis, are best discussed early in the clinician-patient relationship when the patient is relatively healthy. When this is not possible, clinicians should take time to reflect on their own bias, listen to patient and family concerns, determine individual and group norms, and engage in an ongoing dialogue about such preferences. Such measures will strengthen the relationship and show respect for the unique ways in which a family group functions.[45,46]

Determine the dominant language and dialect spoken and the literacy level of both the patient and the family. If there is a language barrier, a professionally trained interpreter of the appropriate gender should be contacted. If such services are not available, health providers, ideally trained in palliative care, may serve as interpreters. Family members should only act as interpreters in emergency situations and only if they agree to do so, as family members placed in this role may feel uncomfortable should sensitive issues or questions arise.[3,5] Always determine what is culturally appropriate to disclose prior to discussion regardless of who is involved in the communication of medical information.[4] When using an interpreter, direct all verbal communication to the patient/family rather than the interpreter. Ongoing clarification that information is understood is critical.

Active listening is one of the most important communication techniques to master for the palliative care nurse. Elicit patient and family concerns, customs, norms, beliefs, and values, and take time to reflect back what is heard. Encourage patients and families to also reflect back what they have heard. Listening to words alone is not enough. Pay attention to nonverbal cues (e.g., gestures, posture, use or avoidance of eye contact). Nonverbal communication will give valuable information and insight into the emotional impact of what is being said, and will help inform the clinician regarding how to behave as well. The reader is referred to chapter 5 for a further discussion on communication in palliative care.

Medical decision-making

Over the past 45 years in the United States, ethical and legal considerations of decision-making have focused on patient autonomy.[11,20] This focus replaced the more paternalistic approach, decision-making as solely the physician's responsibility, with an approach that emphasizes a model of shared responsibility with the patient's active involvement.[17] The Patient Self-Determination Act of 1991 sought to further clarify and to protect an individual's healthcare preferences with advance directives.[47] The principle of respect for patient autonomy points to a patient's right to participate in decisions about the care he/she receives. Associated with this is the right to be informed of diagnosis, prognosis, and the risks and benefits of treatment to make informed decisions. Inherent in the movement for patient autonomy is the underlying assumption that all patients want control over their healthcare decisions. Yet, in fact, for some individuals, patient autonomy may violate the very principles of dignity and integrity it proposes to uphold and may result in significant distress.[4,11]

This European American model of patient autonomy has its origin in the dominant culture, a predominantly white, middle-class perspective that does not consider diverse cultural perspectives.[4] In fact, in some cultures, patient autonomy may not be viewed as empowering but rather as isolating and burdensome for patients who are too sick to have to make difficult decisions.[4,11]

Emphasis on autonomy as the guiding principle assumes that the individual, rather than the family or other social group, is the appropriate decision-maker.[4,17] However, in many non-European-American cultures, the concept of interdependence among family and community members is valued more than individual autonomy.[4,11,20] Cultures that practice family-centered decision-making, such as the Korean American and Mexican American cultures, may prefer that the family, or perhaps a particular family member rather than the patient, receive and process information.[11,13,48] For example, the traditional Chinese concept of "filial piety" requires that children, especially the eldest son, are obligated to respect, care for, and protect their parents.[49] Based on the values and beliefs of this culture, the son is obligated to protect the parent from the worry of a terminal prognosis.

Although full disclosure may not be appropriate, it is never appropriate to lie to the patient. If the patient does not wish to receive information and/or telling the patient violates the patient's and family's cultural norms, the healthcare provider may not be respecting the patient's right to autonomously decide not to receive the information. Some cultures believe that telling the patient he has a terminal illness strips away any and all hope and causes needless suffering and may indeed hasten death.[11,24] For example, imposing negative information, such as prognosis of a life-limiting illness, on the person who is ill is a dangerous violation of traditional Navajo values.[11]

The nurse must consider the harm that may occur when the health system or providers violate cultural beliefs and practices. Assessing and clarifying the patient and family's perspectives, values, and practices may prevent a cultural conflict.[3,46] The nurse is in a key position to advocate these critical patient and family issues (see Box 36.2 for examples of questions to ask). By asking how decisions are made and whether the patient wishes to be involved in both being told information or participating in the decision-making process, clinicians respect patient autonomy and honor individual beliefs and values.[46]

Discontinuation of life-prolonging therapies

Another issue with the potential for cultural conflict surrounds decision-making regarding the discontinuation or withholding of life-sustaining treatments. Inherent in the decision is that the patient will most likely die. Attitude surveys evaluating initiating and terminating life-prolonging therapies have demonstrated differences among several ethnic groups. Research suggests that groups including African Americans, Chinese Americans, Filipino Americans, Iranian Americans, Korean Americans, and Mexican Americans were more likely to start and to continue such therapies than were European Americans when such measures were felt by the healthcare team to be futile.[11,20,48,49]

When making difficult decisions, family members often feel that by agreeing to withdrawal of life-prolonging therapies, they are in fact responsible for the death of their loved one. For families who believe that it is the duty of children to honor, respect, and care for their elders, they may feel obligated to continue futile life-sustaining interventions. Allowing a parent to die may violate the principles of "filial piety" and bring shame and disgrace on the family.[49]

Religious beliefs may also play a role in the complexity of withholding or withdrawing medical interventions. For example, in the Christian Philippines, removing the ventilator is synonymous with euthanasia.[20] For those practicing Orthodox Judaism, the values that all life is precious and only God can decide our time to die, agreeing to withdrawal of life-prolonging therapies may be in violation of their beliefs.[50] In both examples, involving a priest or rabbi may help the families and the healthcare team integrate religious tenets into the culturally appropriate plan of care.

A shared decision-making conversation emphasizing goals of care rather than focusing on "medical futility" may help the family struggling with discontinuing life-prolonging therapies.[20,42] Recognize also that the words used by the healthcare team in these decisions, including "do not resuscitate" and "withdrawal of life support" all have negative connotations and involve the removing of something or the withholding of a particular intervention. Words and phrases that may seem clear to the health professional often literally get lost in translation regardless of whether the parties are speaking the same language. "Withdrawal of life support" may easily be confused with stopping all care, which is not the intention. Feelings of abandoning or "giving up on the patient" can be the result of this misinterpretation, resulting in family suffering, isolation and distress.[24] The nurse is encouraged to be acutely aware of how information and/or questions are phrased. A suggestion is to use words that convey benefit versus burden of all therapies, always beginning the conversation with what the team will do to care for the patient rather than what burdensome interventions should be stopped.

Because many ethical conflicts arise from differences in patients', families', and providers' values, beliefs, and practices, it is critical that individual members of the healthcare team be aware of their own cultural beliefs, understand their own reactions to the issue, and be knowledgeable about the patients' and families' beliefs to address the conflict.[3,46]

Meaning of food and nutrition

Across cultures, there is agreement that food is essential for life to maintain body function and to produce energy.[27] Food serves another purpose in the building and maintaining of human relationships. It is used in rituals, celebrations, and rites of passage to establish and maintain social and cultural relationships with families, friends, and others. Culturally appropriate foods may be used to improve health by groups who have strong beliefs about particular foods and their relationship to health.[27] Because of food's importance for life and life events, a loss of desire for food and subsequent weight loss and wasting can cause suffering for both the patient and family.

Families need clear guidance and explanations when a patient is no longer able to enjoy favorite foods or family mealtime rituals because of declining physical ability. Families often struggle when the patient is no longer taking in any nourishment or fluids, fearing that the patient will "starve to death" or suffer from dehydration. It is imperative that the healthcare team understand the meaning attached to food and nutrition when decisions regarding the potential burden of providing artificial nutrition and hydration for an imminently dying patient are discussed. Exploring alternative ways in which the family can care for the patient through physical, spiritual, or emotional means of support will allow families to interact with the patient in ways that are meaningful to them and reflect individual beliefs, values, and preferences. The Hospice and Palliative Nurses Association Position Statement on Artificial Nutrition and Hydration in Advanced Illness can assist the nurse in understanding the benefits and burdens associated with this medical intervention.[51]

Pain and symptom management

Pain is a highly personal and subjective experience. Pain is whatever the person says it is and exists whenever the person says it does.[52] Culture plays a role in the experience of pain, the meaning of pain, and the response to pain. The biopsychosocial model of pain suggests that pain perception and response is influenced by biological, psychological, social and cultural factors.[18] The meaning of pain varies among cultural groups. For some, pain is a positive response that demonstrates the body's ability to fight against disease or the dying process. For others, pain signifies punishment and its value lies in the patient's ability to withstand the suffering and work toward resolution and peace.[18,53]

Strong beliefs about expressing pain and expected pain behaviors exist in every culture.[53] Pain tolerance varies from person to person and is influenced by factors such as past experiences with pain, coping skills, motivation to endure pain, and energy level. Western society appears to value individuals that exhibit a high pain threshold. As a result, those with a lower threshold, who report pain often, may be labeled as "difficult patients."

Pain assessment should be culturally appropriate, using terms that describe pain intensity across most cultural groups. "Pain," "hurt," and "ache" are words commonly used across cultures. These words may reflect the severity of the pain, with "pain" being the most severe, "hurt" being moderate pain, and "ache" being the least severe.[3] The healthcare team should focus on the words the patient uses to describe pain. To help facilitate an understanding of the severity of the pain experienced by someone who does not speak English, the providers should use pain-rating scales that have been translated into numerous languages.[52] Although it is important to base the assessment on the patient's self-report of pain intensity, it may be necessary to rely on nonverbal pain indicators such as facial expression, body movement, and vocalization to assess pain in the nonverbal, cognitively impaired patient, the older adult, or the infant, who are all at risk for inaccurate assessment and undertreatment of pain.[3,52] A consistent approach to assessing pain and pain relief in a particular patient should be used by all those caring for the patient and documented in that manner.

Racial, ethnic, age, and gender biases in pain management have been identified and documented.[31,53] Studies of gender variations in pain response have identified differences in sensitivity and tolerance to pain as well as willingness to report pain.[53] Compared with men, women are more likely to report pain and have a lower pain threshold and tolerance in experimental settings.[53] Underidentification and undertreatment of pain is a well-recognized phenomenon in elder care.[54] Studies reveal that Hispanics, African Americans, and females are less likely to be prescribed opioids for pain or may be unable to fill opioid pre-scriptions depending on community access to pharmacies.[18]

Like pain, symptoms described by patients receiving pallia-tive care may have meanings associated with them that reflect cultural values, beliefs, and practices. Assessment and manage-ment of symptoms such as fatigue, dyspnea, depression, nausea and vomiting, and anorexia/cachexia should be addressed within a cultural framework. For example, some cultural groups may be hesitant to disclose depression because it is considered a sign of weakness; instead, it may be referred to as a "tired state." Using culturally appropriate language, the nurse will need to evaluate whether the symptom experienced is fatigue or depression.

Incorporating culturally appropriate nondrug therapies may improve the ability to alleviate pain and symptoms. Herbal rem-edies, acupuncture, and folk medicines should be incorporated into the plan of care if desired. Keep in mind that certain nondrug approaches, such as hypnosis and massage, may be inappropriate in some cultures.[46]

Death rituals and mourning practices

The loss of a loved one brings sadness and upheaval in the fam-ily structure across all cultures. Each culture responds to these losses through specific rituals that assist the dying and the bereaved through the final transition from life.[30,46] It is impor-tant to note that rituals may begin before death and may last for months or even years after death. Respecting these rituals and customs will have tremendous impact on the healing process for family members following the death and leave a positive last-ing memory of the loved one's end-of-life experience. The nurse should make sure that any required spiritual, religious, or cul-tural practices are known so that there is appropriate care of the body after death.

For example, dying at home is especially important for Hmong American elders who follow traditional beliefs.[55] The nurse in an acute care setting can be the advocate to ensure this tradi-tion is honored. The family may consult a shaman to perform a ceremony to negotiate with the "God of the sky" to extend life. Additional ceremonies follow. Request for an autopsy or organ donation at the time of death is inappropriate because of the belief that altering the body will delay reincarnation. After the death, there is often much wailing and caressing of the body. The family prepares for an elaborate funeral with rituals to ensure that the loved one will "cross over" and continues with ceremonies for days following the funeral to make sure the soul joins its ancestors.[55]

The tasks of grieving are universal: to accept the reality of the loss, to experience pain of grief, to begin the adjustment to new social and family roles, and to withdraw emotional energy from the dead individual and turn it over to those who are alive.[56] The expressions of grief, however, may vary significantly among cultures. What is acceptable in one culture may seem unaccept-able, or even maladaptive, in another. Recognizing normal grief behavior (vs. complicated grief) within a cultural context there-fore demands knowledge about culturally acceptable expressions of grief.[3,56]

Consider the following case study scenario and questions from a cultural perspective having read about the components of cul-ture and some of the culturally important topics in palliative care.

Case study

Mr. M. is a 62-year-old Vietnam War veteran who came to the Veteran's Affairs Medical Center for an evaluation of a cough, fatigue, weight loss and pain in his right hip. He had not sought medical care for these symptoms, which had been going on for over three months. The out patient oncology team was con-sulted for a new diagnosis of stage IV non-small-cell lung can-cer at the same time the palliative care service was called to assist with his care. Despite increasing pain in his hip and later in his chest wall, he refused any pain medication other than ibu-profen. He repeatedly stated, "I am a tough Marine, I can take it, this is nothing compared to what some of my buddies went through in Nam." He confided in the chaplain that, "I deserve this, after all the people I hurt and killed in the war—this is pay-back." His anxiety and depressive symptoms worsened as the disease progressed. His wife and adult daughters were extremely distressed witnessing his suffering.

Questions to consider in this case

1. What cultural issues may be contributing to the challenges of pain and symptom management for Mr. M.?

2. What spiritual issues need to be addressed for a peaceful death?

3. What are some techniques that the nurse and other health care providers might use to help the family as well as the staff with moral distress surrounding poor pain control?

Striving for cultural competence

Palliative care nurses value the importance of being culturally sensitive and striving for cultural competence. This sensitivity and competence is critical when working with patients with a life-limiting illness and their families.

Cultural competence refers to a dynamic, fluid, continuous process of awareness, knowledge, skill, interaction, and sensitiv-ity.[57] The term remains controversial, as some question whether one can ever become "culturally competent."[3] However, cultural competence is an ongoing process, not an endpoint or something to be mastered.[23] It is more comprehensive than cultural sensitiv-ity, implying not only the ability to recognize and respect cultural differences but also to intervene appropriately and effectively. According to Campinha-Bacote's model for enhancing cultural competence, there are five components essential in pursuing cul-tural competence: cultural awareness, cultural knowledge, cul-tural skill, cultural encounter, and cultural desire.[57]

Integrating cultural considerations into palliative care requires, first and foremost, awareness of how one's own values, practices, and beliefs influence care. Cultural awareness begins with an examination of one's own heritage, family's practices, experiences, and religious or spiritual beliefs.[57] Because culture is a dynamic concept, it is important to reassess one's own beliefs on a regular basis, reflecting on beliefs that may have changed with increasing knowledge and cultural encounters.

Each nurse brings his or her own cultural and philosophical views, education, religion, spirituality, and life experiences to the care of the patient and family. Cultural awareness challenges the nurse to look beyond his or her ethnocentric view of the world, asking the question "How are my values, beliefs, and practices dif-ferent from those of the patient and family?" rather than "How is this patient and family different from me?" Exploring one's own beliefs will raise an awareness of differences that have the potential to foster prejudice and discrimination and limit the effectiveness of care.[3,46] Exploring answers to the same cultural assessment questions used for patients and families increases self-awareness (Box 36.2). Often this exploration identifies more similarities than differences. The universal aspects of life, family, trust, love, hope, understanding, and caring unite us all.

Acquiring knowledge about different cultural groups is the second component to striving for cultural competence, but knowledge alone is insufficient in providing culturally appropriate care.[57] No one can expect to have in-depth knowledge of all cultural variations of health and illness beliefs, values, and norms. A suggested strategy is to identify the most common ethnic group/cultures living in the nurse's community and to integrate a basic understanding of norms and practices impacting issues likely to arise in palliative and end-of-life situations. To strengthen knowledge, one should seek out community members, organizations, faith communities, and leaders in a shared understanding of needs and concerns.

It is important to be aware that knowledge gained of a particular group should serve only as a guide to understanding the unique cultural needs of the patient and family, which comes through individualized assessments. Other resources, such as cultural guides, literature, and Web-based resources, are available to assist the nurse in acquiring knowledge about specific groups.[27] Box 36.4 lists several useful Web-based resources. It is important to remember that relying on culturally specific knowledge to guide practice, rather than individual assessment, is incongruent with culturally competent care.

This list offers suggestions of several useful resources. The list is not intended to be exhaustive but serves as a starting point for gaining more information.

Cultural skill is the third component of cultural competency.[57] Skills in cultural assessment, cross-cultural communication, cultural interpretation, and appropriate intervention can be learned. Multiple tools are available to assess cultural behavior and beliefs. For the new nurse, key assessment questions, applicable in the palliative care setting, may be helpful in guiding the assessment (Box 36.2). However, nothing can replace sitting with the patient and family and asking them to tell the story of their heritage/family history and their cherished practices and beliefs.

The fourth component encompasses the concept of cultural encounters.[57] Individuals with different ways of relating often misunderstand each other's cues. The more opportunities we have to engage with persons with differing values, practices, and beliefs, the more we learn about others and ourselves and the less likely we are to draw erroneous conclusions about each other. Active engagement with community leaders and use of learning tools such as case studies and role plays all help expose nurses to varied cultural experiences.[57] Increasing exposure to cultural encounters may also improve confidence in one's ability to meet the needs of diverse populations.[57]

The fifth and final component of Campinha-Bacote's model for cultural competence is cultural desire.[57] This is the interest and openness with which the nurse strives to understand patients and families and the communities from which they come. Cultural desire is motivation to "want to" engage in the process of cultural competence as opposed to being "forced to" participate in the process. The desire is genuine and authentic and encourages the

Box 36.4 Web resources for acquiring knowledge about cultural issues affecting healthcare

Cross Cultural Health Care Program (CCHCP): www.xculture.org

CCHCP addresses broad cultural issues that impact the health of individuals and families in ethnic minority communities. Its mission is to serve as a bridge between communities and healthcare institutions

Diversity Rx: http://www.diversityrx.org

This is a great networking website that models and practices policy, legal issues, and links to other resources.

EthnoMed: http://ethnomed.org/

The EthnoMed site contains information about cultural beliefs, medical issues, and other related issues pertinent to the healthcare of recent immigrants to the United States.

Fast Fact & Concept #78; Cultural Aspects of Pain Management: http://www.eperc.mcw.edu/EPERC/FastFacts Index/ff_078.htm

This website contains many "fast facts" regarding palliative care. Number 78 addresses important cultural considerations and provides assessment questions when working with patients in pain.

Fast Fact & Concept # 216: Asking About Cultural Beliefs in Palliative Care: http://www.eperc.mcw.edu/EPERC/FastFactsIndex/ff_216.htm

This resource offers a framework for assessing patient and family cultural needs by taking a "cultural history."

Office of Minority Health: https://minorityhealth.hhs.gov

This website has training tools for developing cultural competency.

Transcultural Nursing Society: http://www.tcns.org

The society (founded in 1974) serves as a forum to promote, advance, and disseminate transcultural nursing knowledge worldwide.

nurse to take advantage of cultural encounters and explore worlds beyond his/her own ethnocentric perspective. Such experiences lend opportunities for the nurse to grow both personally and professionally.[57]

Some researchers suggest that the term "cultural humility" is more acceptable than cultural sensitivity or cultural competence when trying to provide culturally appropriate.[58] They have suggested that multiple generations of blended families and intercultural marriages have made it nearly impossible to know all about healthcare practices of particular communities. These social scientists and writers recommend that nurses strive to mindfully respect each patient/family member as unique individuals rather than the components of culture (ethnicity, religion/spirituality, place of residence, etc.) that might label them.[23] We believe that integrating the proposed model of cultural competence with cultural humility into clinical practice will strengthen nurses' ability to respect and support patient and family wishes in palliative care settings.

Summary

Given the changing population of the United States, we as nurses must advocate for the integration of cultural considerations in providing comprehensive palliative care. It is imperative that each of us move beyond our own ethnocentric view of the world to appreciate and respect the similarities and differences in each other. We are challenged to embrace a better understanding of various perspectives. Striving for cultural competence first requires an awareness of how one's own cultural background impacts care. In addition, acquiring knowledge about cultures and developing skill in cultural assessment and communication are essential to improving palliative care for patients with life-limiting illnesses and their families. Most importantly, maintaining a sense of cultural humility, caring for each patient/family member as a unique human being with unique needs, and attending to those needs with dignity and respectfulness is the essence of providing culturally sensitive care.

This chapter encourages nurses to integrate cultural assessment and culturally appropriate interventions into palliative care. It is the hope of the authors that readers will enrich their practice by seeking new knowledge about different cultures through available resources and, most importantly, by respectfully interacting with the most valuable resources on cultural considerations we have— our patients and their families.

References

1. Fuentes C. Myself with Others: Selected Essays. London: Deutsch Limited; 1988.
2. Coyle N. Introduction to palliative nursing care. In Ferrell BR, Coyle N, eds. Textbook of Palliative Nursing (3rd ed). New York, NY: Oxford University Press; 2010:3–12.
3. End-of-Life Nursing Education Consortium (ELNEC), http://www. aacn.nche.edu/elnec/ (accessed June 23, 2014).
4. Kagawa-Singer M. Impact of culture on health outcomes. Pediat Hematol Oncol. 2011:33(suppl 2):S90–S95.
5. National Consensus Project for Quality Palliative Care. Clinical practice guidelines for quality palliative care. 3rd ed. Pittsburgh (PA). National Consensus Project for Quality Palliative Care; 2013.
6. United States Census Bureau. Census Bureau projects U.S. Population of 317.3 million on New Years Day 2014. Washington, DC: December. 30, 2013. http://www.commerce.gov/blog/2013/12/30/census-bureau-projects-us-population-3173-million-new-year%E2%80%99s-day (accessed July 6, 2014).
7. United States Census Bureau. U.S. Census Bureau Projections show a slower growing, older, more diverse nation a half century from now. December 12, 2012. https://www.census.gov/newsroom/releases/archives/population/cb12-243.html (accessed June 27, 2014).
8. United States Census Bureau. Census Bureau Reports June 26, 2014. Washington, DC: http://www.census.gov/newsroom/releases/archives/population/cb14-118.html (accessed July 6, 2014).
9. Leininger M. Quality of life from a transcultural nursing perspective. Nurs Sci Quart 1994;7:22–28.
10. Koffman J, Crawley L. Ethnic and cultural aspects of palliative care. In: Hanks G, Cherney NI, Christakis NA, Fallon M, Kaasa S, Portenoy RK, eds. Oxford Textbook of Palliative Medicine, 4th ed. New York: Oxford University Press; 2011:141–150.
11. Johnstone MJ, Kanitsaki, O. Ethics and advance care planning in a culturally diverse society. J Transcult Nurs. 2009;20:405–416.
12. Cohen LL. Racial/ethnic disparities in hospice care: A systematic review. J Palliat Med 2008;5:763–767.
13. Evans BC, Ebere U. Psychosocial, cultural, and spiritual health disparities in end-of-life and palliative care: where we are and where we need to go. Nursing Outlook 2012;60:370–375.
14. Hulme, PA. Cultural considerations in evidence-based practice. J Transcult Nurs. 2010;21:271–280.
15. Smedley B, Stith A, Nelson A. Unequal treatment: confronting racial and ethnic disparities in health care (Report of the Institute of Medicine). Washington, D.C.: National Academy Press; 2003.
16. Brandon DT, Isaac LA, LaVeist TA. The legacy of Tuskegee and trust in medical care: is Tuskegee responsible for race differences in mistrust of medical care? J Natl Med Assoc 2005;97:951–956.
17. Bullock K. The influence of culture on end-of-life decision making. J Social Work in End-of-Life Palliat Care. 2011;7:83–98.
18. Anderson KC, Green CR, Payne R. Racial and ethnic disparities in pain: causes and consequences of unequal care. J Pain 2009;10:1187–1204.
19. The Office of Minority Health: National Center on Minority Health and Health Disparities. http://www.ncmhd.nih.gov (accessed June 29, 2013).
20. Manalo, MF. End-of Life decisions about withholding or withdrawing therapy: medical, ethical, and religio-cultural considerations. Palliat Care: Res Treat. 2013;7:1–5.
21. Mazanec PM, Daly BJ, Townsend A. Hospice utilization and end-of-life decision making of African Americans. Amer J Hosp Palliat Med. 2010;27:560–566.
22. The Science of C: Future Directions in EOL & Palliative Care. Executive Summary: NINR 2011:1–18. www.ninr.nih.gov/sites/www.ninr.nih.gov/files/ (accessed June 28, 2012).
23. Wittenberg-Lyles E, Goldsmith J, Ferrell BR, Ragan SL. Communication in Palliative Nursing. New York, NY: Oxford Press:2012;59–92.
24. Long CO. Ten best practices to enhance culturally competent communication in palliative care. Pediatr Hematol Oncol. 2011:33(suppl 2):S136–S139.
25. Prince-Paul MJ. Relationships among communicative acts, social well-being, and spiritual well-being on the quality of life at the end of life in patients with cancer enrolled in hospice. J Palliat Med. 2008;11:20–25.
26. Ferrell B, Coyle N. The Nature of Suffering and the Goals of Nursing. New York, NY: Oxford University Press; 2008.
27. Spector R. Cultural Care: Guides to Heritage Assessment and Health Traditions (7th ed). Upper Saddle River, NJ: Pearson Education; 2009.
28. Northouse L, Williams A, Given B, McCorkle R. Psychosocial care for the caregivers of patients with cancer. J Clin Oncol. 2012;30(11):1227–1234.
29. Otis-Green S, Juarez G. Enhancing the social well-being of family caregivers. Semin Oncol Nurs. 2012;28(4):246–255.
30. Sherman D. Culture and spiritual domains of quality palliative care. In Matzo M, Sherman D, eds. Palliative Care Nursing: Quality Care to the End of Life. New York;2010:3–38.
31. Krok, JL, Baker, TA, McMillan, SC. Age differences in the presence of pain and psychological distress in younger and older cancer patients. J Hosp Palliat Nurs. 2013;15:107–113.
32. Soltow D, Given BA, Given CW. Relationship between age and symptoms of pain and fatigue in adults undergoing treatment for cancer. Cancer Nurs. 2010;33(4):296–303.
33. Stein, GL. Providing palliative care to people with intellectual disabilities: services, staff knowledge, and challenges. J Palliat Med. 2008;11:1241–1249.
34. Rawlings D. End-of-life care considerations for gay, lesbian, bisexual, and transgender individuals. Int J Palliat Nurs. 2012;18:29–34.
35. Higgins A, Glacken M. Sculpting the distress: easing or exacerbating the grief experience of same-sex couples. Int J Palliat Nurs 2009;15(4):170–176.
36. Puchalski CM, Ferrell BR, Virani R, Otis-Green S, Baird P, Bull J, et al. Improving the quality of spiritual care as a dimension of palliative care: The report of the consensus conference. J Palliat Med 2009;12(10):885–904.
37. Puchalski CM, Ferrell BR. Making Health Care Whole: Integrating Spirituality into Patient Care. 2010. Templeton Press.
38. Lynch, S. Hospice and palliative care access issues in rural areas. Amer J Hosp Palliat Med. 2012;30:172–177.
39. Morrison RA, Meier DE. Report Card: America's care of serious illness. A state by state Report card on access to palliative care in our nation's hospitals. 2011 New York, New York Center to Advance Palliative Care; National Palliative Care Research Center.

40. Madigan EA, Wiencek CA, Vander Schrier AL. Patterns of community-based end-of-life care in rural areas of the United States. Pol, Polit Nurs Pract 2009:10(1):71–81.

41. Heflt PR. To keep them from injustice: reflections on the care of unauthorized immigrants with cancer. J Oncol Pract 2012:8(4):212–214.

42. Dahlin CM. Communication in palliative care: An essential competency for nurses. In: Ferrell BR, Coyle N, eds. Oxford Textbook of Palliative Nursing. 3rd ed. New York: Oxford University Press; 2010:107–133.

43. Butow P, Bella M, Goldstein D, et al. Grappling with cultural differences; Communication between oncologists and immigrant cancer patients with and without interpreters. Patient Educ Couns. 2011:84:398–405.

44. Williams SW, Hanson LC, Boyd C, et al. Communication, decision making, and cancer: What African Americans want physicians to know. J Palliat Med 2008;11:1221–1226.

45. Barclay JS, Blackhall IJ, Tulsky JA. Communication strategies and cultural issues in the delivery of bad news. J Palliat Med 2007;10: 958–977.

46. Foley H, Mazanec P. Culture and considerations in palliative care. In Panke JT, Coyne P, eds. Conversations in Palliative Care, 3rd ed. Hospice & Palliative Nurses Association; Pittsburg PA; 2011:157–163.

47. Federal patient self-determination act 19090, 42 U.S.C. 1395 cc(a).

48. Taxis JC. Mexican Americans and hospice care: Culture, control, and communication. J Hosp Palliat Nurs 2008;10:133–161.

49. Hsiung YY, Ferrans CE. Recognizing Chinese Americans' cultural needs in making end-of-life treatment decisions. J Hosp Palliat Nurs 2007;9:132–140.

50. Schultz M, Bar-Sela G. Initiating palliative care conversations: lessons from Jewish bioethics. J Supp Onc. http://dx.doi.org/10.1016j. suponc.2012.07.003 (accessed June 20, 2013).

51. HPNA Position Statement on Artificial Nutrition and Hydration in End-of-Life Care. http://www.hpna.org/pdf/Artifical_Nutrition_and_Hydration_PDF.pdfHPNA (accessed June 24, 2014).

52. Pasero C, McCaffery M. Pain Assessment and Pharmacologic Management. St. Louis, MO: Elsevier Mosby, 2011.

53. Wadner, LD, Scipio, CD, Hirsch, AT, Torres, CA, Robinson, ME. The perception of pain in others: how gender, race and age influence pain expectations. J Pain 2012;13: 220–227.

54. Reynolds KS, Hanson, LC, Henderson M, Steinhauser, KE. End-of-life care in nursing home settings: Do race or age matter? Palliat Support Care 2008;6:21–27.

55. Gerdner LA, Yang D, Tripp-Reimer T. The circle of life: end-of-life care and death rituals for Hmong-American elders. J Gerontol Nurs 2007;33:20–29.

56. O'Mallon MO. Vulnerable populations: exploring a family perspective of grief. J Hosp Palliat Nurs 2009;11:91–98.

57. Campinha-Bacote J. A model and instrument for addressing cultural competence in health care. J Nurs Educ 1999; 38:203–207.

58. Nyatanga B. Cultural competence: a noble idea in a changing world. Intern J Palliat Nurs 2008;14:315.

CHAPTER 37

Elderly patients

Susan Derby, Roma Tickoo, and Reggie Saldivar

You are never too old to have new goals, new hopes or dreams.

An 80-year-old palliative care patient

Key points

♦ The majority of people who suffer from chronic disease are elderly.

♦ The trajectory of illness for the elderly is usually one of progressive loss of independence, with the development of multiple comorbid problems and symptoms.

♦ The last years of a frail elderly person's life are often spent at home in the care of family, with approximately 50%–60% of the elderly dying in a hospital or long-term care facility.

♦ Evidence suggests that the end of life for many elderly is characterized by poor symptom control, inadequate advance care planning (ACP), and increased burden on caregivers.

♦ Clinicians caring for the elderly often lack skills in providing palliative and end-of-life care.

♦ If we are committed to providing good end-of-life care to our population, clinicians must improve their care of elderly patients in all practice settings.

Aging is a normal process of life, not a disease, and infirmity and frailty do not always have to accompany being old. It is expected that most of us will live well into our 70s or 80s, and the aging of the population is projected to continue well into the 21st century. Projected growth for the elderly population is staggering. During the next 20 years, the fastest-growing segment of the population will be in the group aged 85 years and older. During past decades, this increase in life expectancy has mainly resulted from improvements in sanitation and infectious disease control through vaccinations and antibiotics. Death from heart disease and atherosclerosis has decreased for all age groups in the elderly. Deaths from cancer in men over 65 years decreased in the 1990s after increasing for two decades. Hypertension decreased in white men but increased markedly in African-American men.[1]

Presently, the older population is growing older because of positive trends in the treatment of chronic diseases—cardiovascular and neurological as well as cancer. This "swelling" of the older segment of the population reinforces the need for nurses, physicians, and all healthcare professionals to understand the special palliative care needs of the elderly. In our society, the majority of people who have chronic disease are elderly. One of the major differences from younger groups in treating illness in the elderly population is the need for extensive family support and care during the last weeks and months of life.

The burden of chronic illness and care for the elderly has fallen on the shoulders of families and friends—informal caregivers. The majority of these caregivers are elderly themselves who endure the burden of caring for both the individual and themselves. Care may involve providing care coordination, hands-on care with bathing and dressing, financial support or assistance with bill paying, shopping, transportation to doctor visits, supervision with home maintenance, and communication with healthcare providers.[2-4] They are involved in providing care tasks for which they have little knowledge or skill. At the end of life care responsibilities may include assisting with complex medical and nursing care such as intravenous therapies, administering medications, tube feedings, and providing for complex symptom management for pain, delirium, or dyspnea.[5] Negative health effects and psychiatric symptoms only worsen over time and with intensity of involvement, and with end-of-life caregiving. At the end of life caregivers may suffer fear and dread, anger, disillusionment, anxiety, grief, helplessness, and hopelessness.[6]

Caregiving does not stop once the patient is placed in a long-term care facility. Families continue to provide day-to-day management with physical care, feeding, decision-making, and being a presence at the bedside. Even with placement, caregiving is demanding and physically and emotionally draining.[7] This chapter is organized into two main sections. The first section provides an overview of special concerns of older patients at the end of life. The second section focuses on the assessment and management of common symptoms experienced by this population at the end of life.

Comorbidity and function

The elderly have many comorbid medical conditions that contribute an added symptom burden to this palliative care population. Sixty-six percent of older noninstitutionalized persons live in a family setting; this decreases with increasing age. Three of every five women older than 85 years live outside of a family arrangement. Rates of institutionalization are estimated to be 4% to 5% in the United States; this increases to 23% in the over-85-year-old population. The wide range of care settings for the elderly is reflected in the sites of death of the elderly.[8] Place of death varied by race in 2007. Among decedents 65 years of age and over, non-Hispanic white decedents were less likely to die while hospitalized and more likely to die in nursing homes than Hispanic or non-Hispanic black, American Indian or Alaska Native, or Asian or Pacific Islander decedents. Among decedents under age 65, non-Hispanic whites were more likely to die at home.[9]

Palliative care in nursing homes

Today 1.5 million people reside in the 16,000 nursing homes in the United States. According to the 2010 census, 3.2% of those ages 75 to 84 years, 10.4% of those ages 85 to 94, and 24.7% of those ages 95 years and older live in nursing homes nationwide. In 2006, close to 520,000 deaths occurred in nursing homes, which represented approximately one in five of all deaths in the United States.[10] The average length of nursing home residence for those who died in these institutions was 2 years, compared with the 2.28-year average length of residence for all nursing home admissions.[10,11] The need for quality palliative care at the end of life for these decedents in nursing homes is apparent given these figures.

The use of palliative care in the setting of nursing homes is often synonymous with hospice care. While the definition of palliative care encompasses symptom management throughout a patient's disease course, hospice care is palliative care specifically for patients with less than 6 months of life expectancy if the course of disease were to continue naturally. Between 1999 and 2006 there has been 137% growth in the number of Medicare-certified hospices providing care in nursing homes with 33% of residents receiving hospice.[10] The use of nursing home Medicare hospice benefit has been seen as a means of addressing the palliative care needs of residents, but gaps in symptom management remain. Although there has been substantial growth in the utilization of hospice services in nursing homes there still remain barriers to adequate palliative care for nursing home residents. Barriers to palliative care in the nursing home include institutional, patient-, and staff-related barriers (Box 37.1).

Pain management and end-of-life care in nursing homes represent management of the frailest individuals, often with minimal physician involvement. Most mild pain in nursing homes is related to degenerative arthritis, low-back disorders, and diabetic and postherpetic neuropathy. Cancer pain accounts for the majority of severe pain.

Ethical issues in providing palliative care in nursing homes

Although symptom management should be an integral part of the entire therapeutic continuum, intensive focus on palliation for elderly nursing home residents is typically an indication that the end of life is approaching. The issues that are raised and the decisions they require are some of the most difficult encountered in nursing homes. These decisions are often made by the older patient or, more often, the patient's family and the care team. Sometimes, however, the complex nature of such decisions and their profound consequences create confusion or disagreement. Issues confronting staff include questions surrounding the patient's decisional capacity, how to best promote the patient's interests, and differences in goals and plan of care. When these clinical conflicts occur, a bioethics consultation can be especially helpful in clarifying the issues and determining the goals of care.

Uncertainty of prognosis and the provision of palliative care

Providing palliative care to elderly patients is limited by the uncertain prognoses of many chronic illnesses in this population (congestive heart failure [CHF], chronic obstructive pulmonary

Box 37.1 Barriers to palliative care in nursing homes

Institution related

Limited physician involvement in care, weekly or monthly assessments
Limited pharmacy involvement, no on-site pharmacy
Limited RN involvement in care; inadequate nurse-patient staff ratios
Primary care being administered by nonprofessional nursing staff
Limited radiological and diagnostic services, which impairs determination of a pain diagnosis
Cost related issues—expensive drugs

Patient related

Physiological changes of aging, which affects distribution, metabolism, and elimination of medications
Multiple chronic diseases
Polypharmacy
Impaired cognitive status and Alzheimer's-type dementia, which impedes assessment
Underreporting of pain because of fear of addiction, lack of knowledge, fear of being transferred
Sensory losses that impede assessment
Increased incidence of depression, which may mask reporting and assessment of pain

Staff related

Lack of knowledge of symptom management at the end of life
Lack of knowledge in the assessment and management of chronic cancer pain
Lack of knowledge in use of opioid drugs, titration, and side-effect management
Fear of using opioids in elderly residents
Lack of knowledge in use of nonpharmacological techniques
Lack of experience with other routes of administration including PCA, transdermal, rectal, subcutaneous, and intravenous routes

disease [COPD], cerebrovascular disease, and dementia). Because of the difficulty of accurately prognosticating and many other factors, most patients who have fatal illnesses do not use the Medicare hospice benefit until shortly before death.[12]

The prediction of survival in end-stage dementia is particularly challenging for hospice providers, who must make difficult decisions regarding eligibility for the Medicare hospice benefit when patients "outlive" the hospice benefit. Unlike patients with terminal cancer, in whom decline is typically a straight downward course, the disease trajectory for patients with end-stage dementia is marked by slow deterioration in function over several years, with reduced levels of activities of daily living interspersed with periods of marked deterioration in parallel with urosepsis and pneumonia; this is in contrast to cancer, where death is usually heralded by a period of pronounced functional deterioration in the last 3 months of life.

The uncertain prognoses of chronic nonmalignant medical conditions can affect clinical decision-making. It may also lead to overuse of healthcare resources in acute care settings, even when death is imminent. Routine use of screening measures such as the palliative performance scale in primary care, in the emergency department, and in long-term care settings may help distinguish between patients who are chronically ill and persons in whom death is likely in the following 12 months.[13]

Advance directives and decision-making in the elderly

Advance directives are especially important in elderly patients who are at high risk of morbidity and mortality. In one study of advance care planning (ACP) among nursing home residents, two variables found to be associated with the reduced likelihood of having do-not-resuscitate (DNR) and do-not-hospitalize orders or restricting feeding, medication, or other treatment were African-American ethnicity and less time in the facility. Some studies support the notion that a patient's prior decision regarding treatment choices accurately reflects future choices.[14,15] However, others show that patient preferences are subject to change and may be influenced by a number of factors. This was demonstrated by a 2-year prospective study conducted by McParland et al.[16] to evaluate the durability over time of decisions made regarding terminal care of mentally intact nursing home patients and the influence of such factors as intervening illness, loss of significant others, and cognitive, emotional, and functional decline. Results of the study revealed that preferences regarding cardiopulmonary resuscitation and parenteral and enteral nutrition changed over both the 12- and 24-month study periods. Only degree of change in cognitive status proved to be predictive of changes in decision. Gender, presence or absence of depression, change in level of functional abilities, and intercurrent illness or stressor did not influence change regarding life-sustaining therapy.

This study suggests that periodic reevaluation of advance directives should be performed and that ongoing discussions should be initiated with patients by healthcare professionals.[16] Although this study focused on institutionalized patients, the principle of reevaluation of goals of care should be practiced by healthcare providers in all healthcare settings. As per the philosophy of palliative care, these discussions should include the caregivers and the significant others in the patient's life as a means of providing holistic support via shared decision-making. It goes without saying that this would require time allocated toward having these discussions with the healthcare teams, which could pose a challenge and constraint on addressing ACPs.

Dilemmas and challenges surrounding advance care planning in the elderly

With the evolution of advanced treatment modalities, people are living longer. However, there exists a notable discrepancy in the dynamics at the end of life. While most elderly patients prefer only comfort measures at the end of life, life-sustaining technologies are increasingly being used in the final stages of life.[17] In a randomized controlled trial conducted at two centers in Wisconsin in which patients and surrogates were recruited as pairs, eligible patients had a diagnosis of CHF or end-stage renal disease (ESRD). Patients and their surrogates were randomized to receive patient-centered ACP (PC-ACP) or usual care. The PC-ACP interview

was conducted by a trained facilitator and lasted 1 to 1.5 hours. The interview was designed to assess patient and surrogate understanding of and experiences with the illness, provide information about disease-specific treatment options and their benefits and burdens, and assist in documentation of patient treatment preferences. Assistance to surrogates in understanding patient's preferences and to prepare surrogates to make decisions that honor those preferences was provided. Of the 313 individuals and their surrogates who completed entry data, 110 died. It was found that 74% patients frequently continued to make their own decisions about care to the end. The experimental group had fewer (1/62) cases in which patients' wishes about cardiopulmonary resuscitation were not met than in the control group (6/48) but not significantly so. Notably more experimental patients withdrew from dialysis than controls. In conclusion most patients received the care they desired at the end of life or altered their preferences to be in accord with the care they would receive.[18]

In the patient's best interest

Clinicians who work in nursing homes face increasing caseloads and often rely on decisions and opinions of caregivers that may ultimately not reflect the values or goals of the patient. Advance directives are often unavailable or lack sufficient specificity and clarity to impact decisions such as transfer to the acute care setting or the institution of life-prolonging treatments. The presence, stability, and willingness to discuss ACP appears to depend on several factors, including communication issues, value differences, cultural issues, ethnicity, and mental capacity. Although much literature points toward the relationship between a patient's prior decision regarding future treatment choices, stability of nursing home residents' preferences for some life-prolonging therapies may vary over time. One study suggested that although a majority of residents consistently desired cardiopulmonary resuscitation over a 2-year period, fewer than half favored medical hydration and nutrition. However, as time progressed the proportion of residents willing to consider such interventions rose.[19,20] The majority of residents in nursing homes at the end of life are unable to make treatment decisions for themselves. This results in reliance on surrogates. The burden of decision-making about withdrawal of life-prolonging therapies may be lessened by affording the family the opportunity to explore goals of care with nursing home clinicians who have cared for their loved one over months or years, rather than being faced by unfamiliar hospital staff at critical times and in an emergent situation.

A qualitative semistructured interview study was conducted by Fritsch et al.[21] on the experience and process of decision-making in the hospitalized older adults with impaired cognition who rely on surrogates to make major medical decisions. Information on what factors surrogates actually consider when making decisions was obtained. Participants were 35 surrogates with a recent decision-making experience for an inpatient aged 65 or older. Interview transcripts were coded and analyzed using the grounded theory method of qualitative analysis. Surrogates considered patient-centered factors and surrogate-centered factors. Patient-centered factors included (1) respecting the patient's input, (2) using past knowledge of the patient to infer the patient's wishes, and (3) considering what is in the patient's best interests. Some surrogates expressed a desire for more information about the patient's prior wishes. Surrogate-centered factors included (1) surrogate's wishes as a guide, (2) surrogate's religious beliefs and/or spirituality, (3) surrogate's interests, and (4) family consensus. The study indicated that surrogate decision-making is more complex than the standard ethical models, which are limited to considerations of the patient's autonomy and beneficence. Because surrogates also imagine what they would want under the circumstances and consider their own needs and preferences, models of surrogate decision-making must account for these additional considerations.

While this study had weakness in terms of low response rate of 35% and a preponderance of female surrogates it made some pertinent points. Surrogate decision-makers for hospitalized older adults rely heavily on the standard ethical concepts of patient preferences and best interests, but also consider other factors such as their own preferences, interests, emotions, experiences and religious beliefs, factors which are not traditionally included in ethical models of surrogate decision-making. Surrogates' desire for more information about the patient's preferences points to a need for more ACP. When such information is not known, surrogates may use their wishes for themselves as a decision-making guide, but may also consider their own beliefs and interests. More work is needed to understand the implications of expansion of the ethical models of surrogate decision-making, including how to better address these important issues and to consider how they ought to be weighed in the decision-making process.

State initiatives on advance care planning: why is it relevant to the elderly?

As the population ages, it will place tremendous pressure and challenge on clinicians and members of the multidisciplinary teams to have constant and continuous conversations regarding ACP and goals of care with their patients. The growing population in the setting of advanced health care technology is likely to face complex end-of-life issues. With increasing time constraints and regulations there is need for clear and simple approaches to goals of care conversations and documentation of the same.

In 1991, Oregon State developed the "Physician Orders for Life-Sustaining Treatment" (POLST: www.polst.org), to honor end-of-life treatment preferences and to overcome some of the limitations of advance care directives.[22] Though not specific to the elderly, the POLST paradigm is designed to improve end-of-life care by converting patients' treatment preferences into medical orders that are transferable throughout the healthcare system. This paradigm is now implemented in multiple states, with many considering its use. It is designed to convert patient preferences for life-sustaining treatments into immediately actionable medical orders. The centerpiece of the program is a standardized, brightly colored form that provides specific treatment orders for cardiopulmonary resuscitation, medical interventions, artificial nutrition, and antibiotics. It is complemented based on conversations among health-care professionals with the patient and/or the appropriate proxy decision makers, in conjunction with any existing advance directive for incapacitated patients. The POLST form is recommended for persons who have advanced chronic progressive illness, who might die in the next year, or who wish to further define their preferences for treatment.

On July 7, 2008, in the state of New York, Governor David Paterson signed Chapter 197 of the Laws of 2008 allowing the use of an alternative DNR form, which is the Medical Orders for Life Sustaining Treatment (MOLST) form. The MOLST is an alternative form and process for patients to provide their end-of-life care preferences to healthcare providers across the spectrum of the healthcare delivery system. The MOLST may be honored by emergency medical services (EMS), hospitals, nursing homes, adult homes, hospices, and other healthcare facilities and their healthcare provider staff. The MOLST form is a bright pink form that was piloted by the Rochester Health Commission under previous legislation for use by the EMS community in Onondaga and Monroe Counties.[23] The MOLST has been reviewed annually since 2005 and has been adapted to meet clinical needs of the patients. The success of the MOLST Pilot Project resulted in Governor Paterson signing a bill (PHL§2977(3)) that made MOLST a statewide law, thereby changing the scope of practice for EMS across New York State.[24] The MOLST can be used in the community in lieu of the New York State Nonhospital DNR form. In signing the legislation, Governor Paterson said, "People should be allowed as much say in their end-of-life care as they would have at any other time. This bill will allow many people who are critically ill to make enduring decisions on the care they will receive."

Araw and Araw conducted a cross-sectional study of 182 long-term care residents of two skilled nursing facilities with and without MOLST in the New York Metropolitan area. The sample size was based on feasibility rather than a formal power calculation. Of the residents studied, 68.7% were females and 91% were Caucasians, and 91.8% were > 65 years of age with a mean age of 83. The median time from admission to MOLST signing was 21 days for the Caucasians and 229 days for the non-Caucasians, and the overall median time was 48 days. Almost one-third of the residents signed a MOLST on their first day of admission, indicating that there was a purposeful staff approach to ascertain patient wishes. Among the 68 subjects who signed a MOLST and died, 87% had their wishes met. A limitation of this study was the utilization of a convenience sample.[25]

Addressing ACP can be complex and challenging especially in the elderly and should be considered a dynamic process where the goals of care may need to be reset from time to time as the health status of the individuals and the resources available for their care change. Also, it would help to hold these discussions early and at the level of the community. To do so, the healthcare providers may need to incorporate these discussions in their practice as a standard of care. This may further require a motivation and commitment by educational institutions to prime the future nurses, doctors, and perhaps social workers in addressing ACP in their patients.

The last weeks and days of life: special considerations in care of the elderly

Care during the last hours of life should be a fundamental component of every nurse and physician's training. Both patients and family members are in special need of assistance with decision-making about end-of-life care. Sykes has identified the need to make a diagnosis of dying, not only so that goals of care may be established and interventions tailored but also so that patients may be made aware, if they wish, so that end-of-life decisions can be made.[26]

Decisions about a place to die—either in hospital or at home—should be made, if possible, by the patient and their family. In a recent study in British hospitals, only 45% of 2673 patients from 118 hospitals were informed by staff that they were dying.[27]

The concern about discussing death is the problem of prognostication. Physicians consistently overestimate patients' survival, and familiarity with the patients tends to decrease their ability to prognosticate. Predictors of death within days include the inability to take drinks larger than sips, semicomatose state, inability to swallow pills, being bedridden, and, in some cases, death rattle. Other signs include mottled skin color in the extremities, irregular breathing, and loss of the radial pulse. The complex symptomatology experienced by elderly patients, especially those with cancer and multiple comorbidities, demands that an aggressive approach to symptom assessment and intervention be used. Elderly patients differ from younger patients in all domains of care. At the end of life, the geriatric patient who is dying may also have a have a higher incidence of certain syndromes, including dementia, urinary incontinence, falls, hearing and visual problems, as well as limited family support. Devising a palliative plan of care for the elderly patient who is highly symptomatic or who is actively dying requires ongoing communication with the patient and family; assessment of patient and family understanding of goals of care and religious, cultural, and spiritual beliefs; access to community agencies; psychological assessment; and knowledge of patient and family preferences regarding advance directives. Box 37.2 outlines dimensions of a palliative care plan for the elderly. The management of three prevalent and distressing symptoms experienced by the elderly at the end of life—dyspnea, pain, and delirium—is reviewed below. Each of these symptoms is discussed in greater detail in other chapters.

Special considerations in managing symptoms commonly experienced by the elderly at end of life

Pharmacological considerations in providing symptom management

Pharmacological intervention is the mainstay of treatment for symptom management in the elderly palliative care patient. Knowledge of the parameters of geriatric pharmacology can prevent serious morbidity and mortality when multiple drugs are used to treat single or multiple symptoms or when, in the practice of chronic pain management, trials of sequential opioids (opioid rotation, or opioid switch) are used. With normal aging there is a steady decline in physiological reserve capacity in most organ systems and dysregulation in others.[28] These changes become apparent under stress and play an important role at the end of life, when the goal is symptom control and comfort. Important physiological changes in the elderly patient will be outlined below.

Pharmacokinetics

The four components of pharmacokinetics are absorption, distribution, metabolism, and excretion. In the absence of malabsorption problems and obstruction, oral medications are well tolerated in the elderly population. With aging, there is some decrease in gastric secretion, absorptive surface area, and splanchnic blood flow. Most studies show no difference in oral bioavailability—the extent to which a drug reaches its site of

> **Box 37.2** Dimensions of a palliative plan of care for the elderly patient
>
> 1. Assess extent of disease documented by imaging studies and laboratory data.
> 2. Assess symptoms, including prevalence, severity, and impact on function.
> 3. Identify coping strategies and psychological symptoms, including presence of anxiety, depression, and suicidal tendencies.
> 4. Evaluate religious and spiritual beliefs.
> 5. Assess overall quality of life and well-being. Does the patient feel secure that all that can be done for them is being done? Is the patient satisfied with the present level of symptom control?
> 6. Determine family burden. Is attention being paid to the caregiver so that burnout does not occur? If the spouse or caregiver is elderly, is he or she able to meet the physical demands of caring for the patient?
> 7. Determine level of care needed in the home if the patient is dying.
> 8. Assess financial burden on patient and caregiver. Is an inordinate amount of money being spent on the patient and will there be adequate provisions for the elderly caregiver when the patient dies?
> 9. Identify presence of ACP requests. Have the patient's wishes and preferences for resuscitation, artificial feeding, and hydration been discussed? Has the patient identified a surrogate decision-maker who knows their wishes? Is there documentation regarding advance directives?
> 10. Identify goals of care of the patient, family, and healthcare team.

action. There is little literature on the absorption of long-acting drugs in the elderly, including controlled or sustained-release opioids, and transdermal opioids commonly used in the treatment of chronic cancer pain in the elderly patient. Generally, it is safer to use opioids that have shorter half-lives in the elderly cancer patient.

Distribution refers to the distribution of drug to the interstitial and cellular fluids after it is absorbed or injected into the bloodstream. There are several significant physiological factors that may influence drug distribution in the elderly palliative care patient. An initial phase of distribution reflects cardiac output and regional blood flow. The heart, kidneys, liver, and brain receive most of the drug after absorption. Delivery to fat, muscle, most viscera, and skin is slower; it may take several hours before steady-state concentrations are reached. Although cardiac output does not change with age, chronic conditions, including congestive heart failure, may contribute to a decrease in cardiac output and regional blood flow. This second phase of drug distribution to the tissues highly depends on body mass. Body weight generally decreases with age, but more importantly, body composition changes with age. Total body water and lean body mass decrease, whereas body fat increases in proportion to total body weight. The volume-of-distribution changes are mostly for highly lipophilic and hydrophilic drugs, and the elderly are most susceptible to drug toxicity from drugs that should be dosed on ideal body weight or lean body weight. Theoretically, highly lipid-bound drugs (e.g., long-acting benzodiazepines and transdermal fentanyl, both commonly prescribed to elderly patients) may have an increased volume of distribution and a prolonged effect if drug clearance is constant.[29]

Water-soluble drugs (e.g., digoxin) may have a decreased volume of distribution and increased serum levels and toxicity if initial doses are not conservative. To avoid possible side effects in a frail elderly patient, it may be safe to start with one-half the dose usually prescribed for a younger patient.

Another host factor that influences drug distribution is plasma protein concentrations.[30,31] Most drugs, including analgesics, are extensively bound to plasma proteins. The proportion of albumin among total plasma proteins decreases with frailty, catabolic states, and immobility, which are commonly seen in many elderly patients with chronic conditions. A decrease in serum albumin can increase the percentage of free (unbound) drug available for pharmacological effect and elimination. In this setting, standard doses of medications lead to higher levels of free (unbound) drug and possible toxicity.

The liver is the major site of drug metabolism. Hepatic metabolism of drugs depends on drug-metabolizing enzymes in the liver. The hepatic microenzymes are responsible for this biotransformation. With advanced age, there is a decrease in liver weight by 20% to 50%, and liver volume decreases by approximately 25%.[32] Associated with these changes in liver size and weight is a decrease in hepatic blood flow, normalized by liver volume. This corresponds to a decrease in liver perfusion of 10% to 15%. Drugs absorbed from the intestine may be subject to metabolism and the first-pass effect in the liver, accounting for decreased amounts of drug in the circulation after oral administration. The process of biotransformation in the liver largely depends on the P-450 cytochrome. During biotransformation, the parent drug is converted to a more polar metabolite by oxidation, reduction, or hydrolysis. The resulting metabolite may be more active than the parent drug. The cytochrome P-450 has been shown to decline in efficiency with age. These altered mechanisms of drug metabolism should be considered when treating the elderly palliative care patient with opioids, long-acting benzodiazepines, and neuroleptics.

The effect of age on renal function is quite variable. Some studies show a linear decrease in renal function, amounting to decreased glomerular function; other studies indicate no change in creatinine clearance with advancing age.[33] Renal mass decreases 25% to 30% in advanced age, and renal blood flow decreases 1% per year after age 50.[33] There are also decreases in tubular function and reduced ability to concentrate and dilute the urine. Generally, the clearance of drugs that are secreted or filtered by the kidney is decreased in a predictable manner.

Delayed renal excretion of meperidine's metabolite, normeperidine, may result in delirium, central nervous system stimulation, myoclonus, and seizures. Meperidine is not recommended for chronic administration in any patient but is of special concern for elderly patients with borderline renal function. Other drugs that rely on renal excretion include nonsteroidal antiinflammatory agents, digoxin, aminoglycoside antibiotics, and contrast media.

Medication use in the elderly: problems with polypharmacy

Older individuals use three times more medications than younger people do. Advancing age alone does not explain the risk of adverse drug reactions, and polypharmacy is a consistent predictor. At the end of life, elderly patients with multiple comorbid medical conditions, necessitating treatment with many medications, places them at greater risk of adverse drug reactions. In addition, new medications not only place the elderly at risk of adverse drug reactions, they also increase the risk of significant drug interactions. For example, the addition of an antacid to an elderly patient already on corticosteroids for bone pain may significantly decrease the oral corticosteroid effect because of decreased absorption.

Risk factors for medication use in the elderly are outlined in Box 37.3. When multiple drugs are used to treat symptoms, the side-effect profile may increase, potentially limiting the use of one or more drugs. For example, when using an opioid and a benzodiazepine in treating chronic pain and anxiety in the elderly patient, excessive sedation may occur, limiting the amount of opioid that can be administered.

Box 37.3 Risk factors for medication problems in the elderly palliative care patient

1. Multiple healthcare prescribers (e.g., multiple physicians, nurse practitioners) who may have little or no communication between them
2. Multiple medications
3. Refills without face-to-face assessment
4. Age-related physiological changes
5. Sensory losses: visual, hearing, or neuropathy in hands and fingers
6. Cognitive defects: delirium, dementia, memory loss
7. Depression, anxiety
8. Knowledge deficits related to indication, action, dosing schedule, and side effects of prescribed medication
9. Complex or different dosing schedule of multiple drugs
10. Comorbid medical conditions: frailty, cerebrovascular disease, cardiac disease, musculoskeletal disorders, advanced cancer
13. Self-medication with over-the-counter medications, herbal remedies
14. Lack of support with medication administration or social isolation
15. Alcoholism or active substance abuse
16. Financial concerns
17. Illiteracy
18. Misconceptions about specific medications (e.g., addiction)
19. Language barrier
20. Cultural issues—misconceptions, culture-related beliefs

Symptoms commonly experienced by the elderly at end of life—dyspnea, pain, and delirium

Dyspnea

Dyspnea may be one of the most frightening and difficult symptoms an elderly patient can experience. A subjective feeling of breathlessness or the sensation of labored or difficult breathing, dyspnea contributes to severe disability and impaired quality of life. Dyspnea and fear of dyspnea produce profound suffering for dying patients and their families. Breathlessness has been described as a "total" experience affecting all domains of life, similar to the experience of chronic pain.[34,35]

The American College of Chest Physicians published a Consensus Statement on the Management of Dyspnea in Patients with Advanced Lung or Heart Disease because it was felt that patients with advanced lung or heart disease were not currently being treated consistently and effectively for relief of dyspnea.[36] Their suggestions include the measurement of patient-reported dyspnea, the use of supplemental oxygen for patients who are hypoxic during minimal activity, nonpharmacological therapies, and opioid therapies.

Physiological correlates in the elderly that increase risk of dyspnea

The effects of aging produce a clinical picture in which respiratory problems can develop. With aging, the elastic recoil of the lungs during expiration is decreased because of less collagen and elastin. Alveoli are less elastic and develop fibrous tissue. The stooped posture and loss of skeletal muscle strength often found in the elderly contribute to reduction in the vital capacity and an increase in the residual volume of the lung. Table 37.1 outlines the pulmonary risk factors for the development of dyspnea in the elderly palliative care patient.

Respiratory muscle weakness may play a major role in some types of dyspnea. Palange and colleagues[37] found that malnutrition significantly affected exercise tolerance in patients with COPD by producing diaphragmatic fatigue. In patients with cachexia, the maximal inspiratory pressure, an indicator of diaphragmatic strength, is severely impaired. Cachexia and asthenia occur in 80% to 90% of patients with advanced cancer and are also prevalent in elderly patients with multiple comorbid psychiatric and medical conditions. These mechanisms may affect the development of dyspnea and fatigue in the elderly who have advanced nonmalignant and malignant disease.

The multiple etiologies of dyspnea in the dying elderly patient with cancer include malignant (e.g., tumor infiltration, superior vena cava syndrome, pleural effusion), treatment-related (adriamycin-induced cardiomyopathy, radiation-induced pneumonitis, pulmonary fibrosis), and nonmalignant causes (e.g., metabolic, structural). Typically breathlessness may be episodic, worsened by exertion, but with rapid disease progression it often occurs at rest. Even if breathlessness can be relieved at rest, exertional dyspnea will often be present. Some clinicians have recommended that reduction is likely to be stepwise and a clinically important reduction should be the primary therapeutic aim.[39] Often dyspnea at the end of life occurs with other prominent end-of-life symptoms including cachexia, fatigue, and weakness, and decline in the cancer patient is more predictable and steadily downward.[40] Two causes of dyspnea, deep venous thrombosis

Table 37.1 Risk factors for dyspnea in the elderly palliative care patient

Risk factor	Comment
Structural factors	
Increased chest wall stiffness	Increase in the work of breathing Decrease in maximum volume expired
Increase in anteroposterior diameter	Decrease in elasticity of alveoli Decrease in vital capacity
Other factors	
Anemia	
Cachexia	
Dehydration	Drier mucous membrane, increase in mucous plugs
Ascites	
Atypical presentation of fever	Reduced febrile response
Immobility	Increased risk of aspiration, DVT, PE
Obesity	
Recent abdominal, pelvic, or chest surgery	Increased risk of DVT, PE
Lung disease (COPD, lung cancer)	
Heart failure	

Sources: Adapted from Palange et al. (1995), reference 37; Eliopoulos (1996), reference 38.
COPD-chronic obstructive pulmonary disease; DVT—deep venous thrombosis; PE—pulmonary embolism.

(DVT) and pulmonary embolism (PE), are prevalent in the elderly and are often unrecognized and undiagnosed. They may present as pleuritic chest pain with or without dyspnea and hemoptysis. The risk factors in the elderly include increased venous stasis in the legs, impaired fibrinolysis, coagulopathies, recent surgery, immobility, and CHF. Treatment depends on accurate diagnosis, and an estimate of risks versus benefits should be considered in deciding on a course of action.

Treatment of dyspnea

When possible, relief of dyspnea is aimed at treatment of the underlying disease process, whether malignant or nonmalignant in origin. When these causes are no longer reversible, symptom relief is the goal of treatment. Symptomatic interventions are used when the process is not reversible. Both pharmacological and nonpharmacological interventions should be employed. One patient may present with multiple etiologies; therefore, multiple interventions are indicated. Often dyspnea occurs in the setting of other symptoms—symptom clusters and other stressors—and these other symptoms must also be addressed. The elderly patient at the end of life who is experiencing profound dyspnea should have their anxiety, depression, and existential distress addressed, if occurring concomitantly.[41]

Therapeutic interventions are based on the etiology and include pharmacological (e.g., bronchodilators, steroids, diuretics, vasodilators, opioids, sedatives, antibiotics), procedural (e.g., thoracentesis, chest tube placement), nonpharmacological (e.g., relaxation, breathing exercises, music), radiation therapy, and oxygen. At the end of life, the pharmacological use of benzodiazepines, opioids, and corticosteroids remains the primary treatment.

Using opioids to manage dyspnea can both relieve the sensation of breathlessness and relieve other objective and subjective symptoms including anxiety, pain, and cough.[42]

Some studies have suggested the use of nebulized furosemide (not for its diuretic effect) because it appears to limit bronchospasm and may be a mild bronchodilator.[43]

Benzodiazepines and selective serotonin reuptake inhibitors (SSRIs) have been used to treat dyspnea, and their use is based on the fact that anxious patients report dyspnea, and that when it occurs, dyspnea often occurs with anxiety or depression.[41]

In one study looking at advanced cancer patients with moderate to severe dyspnea, patients had their dyspnea relieved with either oral morphine or oral midazolam.[44]

In a systematic review and meta-analysis of 18 randomized trials assessing all interventions for dyspnea in palliative care patients, Ben-Aharon et al. found a positive effect for opioid administration and a lack of benefit of oxygen to improve dyspnea; the role of benzodiazepines remains unclear.[45]

Please refer to chapter 14 for an in-depth discussion on the management of dyspnea.

Case study

Management of dyspnea in an elderly patient with metastatic breast cancer

An 80-year-old woman with recurrent breast cancer presents to her palliative care team with increasing shortness of breath, which has grown progressively worse over the past week. The patient has been home with mild shortness of breath, which was managed successfully with morphine sulfate 15 mg every 3–4 hours prn. In the past she has received chemoradiation therapy to the tumor, and treatment concluded about 2 months ago. She started experiencing radicular pain in the lower spine and pelvis, and imaging studies revealed recurrent disease. She has declined further treatment. A right pleural effusion was found 3 weeks ago, and she underwent two thoracentesis procedures (the last one 5 days ago, when 1500 mL of pleuritic fluid was drained).

Past medications for dyspnea include fentanyl patch 50 mcg, which had produced sedation and delirium. She is also receiving 30 mg of prednisone orally two times daily for bronchospasm, albuterol inhaler, senna, and a stool softener. Physical examination has revealed breath sounds decreased bilaterally, an inspiratory stridor, and mild bilateral wheezing. She is anxious and short of breath and cannot sleep. Pulse oximetry was 92% at rest, and she is using nasal oxygen (4 L/min). She has refused further aggressive intervention and has signed a home DNR order.

At-a-glance assessment

◆ Determine goals of care and clarify understanding between patient, family, and healthcare providers.

◆ Management of dyspnea in the elderly patient at the end of life should be focused on the physical, psychological, and spiritual domains of care. Relief of suffering should be a primary goal.

◆ Comprehensive management of dyspnea in the elderly patient at the end of life includes use of opioids, anxiolytics/sedatives, steroids, and nonpharmacological interventions.

Suggestions for assessment and intervention

1. Determine the etiology of the dyspnea in this patient. In this elderly cancer patient, dyspnea is multifactorial, including pleural effusion requiring thoracentesis.

2. Review goals of care with the patient. It is clear to the staff that this patient is determined to not undergo further aggressive treatment, but is willing to have X-rays or another thoracentesis if it would make her feel better. She wants to die at home, and her family is supportive of this decision.

3. Excessive fatigue is present in this patient, and a complete blood count has revealed a mild anemia, with no indication for a transfusion. A trial of a low-dose stimulant such as Ritalin administered 2.5 to 5 mg orally daily or twice a day is discussed but the patient declined, saying she "is ready to die."

4. The patient is receiving morphine for dyspnea. The dose is increased to 15–30 mg orally every 4 hours.

5. An anxiolytic—(0.5 mg of lorazepam) is prescribed orally every 4 to 6 hours with rescue doses if necessary.

6. Consider the benefit versus burden of additional interventions that are employed. The patient has refused further medical interventions, but the use of an intermittent draining pleural catheter may be an option for her.

7. Reduce the need for physical exertion. The patient has 24-hour home care, including family support, and an 8-hour daily home health aide. She has a hospital bed at home, is using a wheelchair, and has a bedside commode.

8. Address anxiety, providing support and reassurance. Reassure patient that symptoms can be controlled. The patient's son has asked what will happen if the patient becomes worse at home. The members of the palliative care team review the potential need for increasing sedating medications that would produce sedation at the end of life. The son feels greatly reassured.

9. Incorporate nonpharmacological interventions (e.g., progressive relaxation, guided imagery, and music therapy). The patient felt dyspnea relief from a fan, and used classical music to assist with her anxiety.

10. The patient is followed daily by a member of the palliative care team. After 5 days, the patient agrees to a pleural catheter, which is inserted and immediately drains 1000 mL. Over the next 2 weeks, the catheter drains approximately 300 mL daily, which allows her a great deal of symptomatic relief. The patient dies 2 1/2 weeks later at home, in her bed.

Pain

The physiological changes accompanying advanced age have been discussed earlier in this chapter; however, it is important to emphasize that the elderly are more sensitive to both the therapeutic and toxic effects of analgesics.[29,46]

The prevalence of pain in older persons consistently demonstrates a substantial burden of pain both in the community[47,48] and in nursing homes.[49]

Please refer to chapter 7 for an in depth discussion on the management of pain at the end of life. Specific areas are highlighted below that have special relevance for the elderly.

Acetaminophen

Acetaminophen is one of the safest analgesics for long-term use in the older population and should be used for mild-to-moderate pain. It is particularly useful in the management of musculoskeletal pain and is often used in combination with opioids. Guidelines developed by the American College of Rheumatology, the European League Against Rheumatism, and Osteoarthritis Research Society International concur that the initial treatment of osteoarthritis pain should be with acetaminophen.[50-52] In older patients with normal renal and liver function, it can be used safely and is highly effective for the treatment of osteoarthritis. In the setting of renal insufficiency, hepatic failure, or with patients who are drinking heavily or have a history of alcohol abuse, avoidance of acetaminophen is recommended.

Nonsteroidal antiinflammatory drugs

Elderly patients with a history of ulcer disease are most vulnerable to the side effects of nonsteroidal antiinflammatory drugs (NSAIDs), which can also cause renal insufficiency and nephrotoxicity. They should be given with caution to patients with reduced creatine clearance, gastropathy, cardiovascular disease, or congestive heart failure.[29] In the palliative setting, consideration should be given to the risks versus the benefits to the elderly patient. If, for example, the use of NSAIDs provides effective analgesia and the life expectancy of the patient is limited (days to weeks), then it is probably prudent to initiate this therapy.

Opioids

In older patients with moderate-to-severe pain who have limited prior treatment with opioids, it is best to begin with a short-half-life agonist (morphine, hydromorphone, and oxycodone). Shorter half-life opioids are generally easier to titrate than longer half-life opioids such as levorphanol or methadone and may have fewer side effects in the elderly. Recent research has demonstrated the importance of both liver biotransformation of metabolites and renal clearance of these metabolites. Most opioids are converted to substances that may have a higher potency than the parent compound or produce more adverse effects with repeated dosing and accumulation.[53]

When prescribing opioids in the older population, it is be helpful to obtain baseline renal function studies. A normal serum creatinine does not indicate normal renal function; it is prudent to determine a 24-hour creatinine clearance to accurately determine renal function.

Morphine is the most commonly prescribed opioid because of its cost and ease of administration. Morphine can be administered as an immediate-release tablet or a liquid formulation in a controlled-release tablet administered every 8 to 12 hours, or every 24 hours. Plasma clearance of morphine decreases with age; therefore, elderly patients should be carefully monitored for any signs of sedation or confusion. In the setting of impaired renal function, morphine should not be used in the elderly patient. When administering morphine for long-term use, the metabolites of morphine—morphine-3 and -6 glucuronide—may accumulate with repeated dosing, especially in the setting of impaired renal or hepatic function.[54,55] If, after a few hours of initiation with morphine, the elderly patient develops side effects that include agitation or delirium, it may mean that there is an accumulation of these metabolites, and the opioid should be changed.

Fentanyl is a highly lipophilic soluble opioid, which can be administered spinally, transdermally, trans-mucosally, and intravenously. The fentanyl patch can be used safely in the older patient, but patients should be monitored carefully. The fentanyl patch should only be used in opioid-tolerant patients who are taking at least the equivalent of 60 mg of oral morphine in a day for at least 5 to 7 days, which is equivalent to a 25 mcg/h fentanyl patch. If, after initiation with the fentanyl patch, side effects develop, it is important to remember that they may persist for long periods (hours or even days) after the patch is removed. However, the frail elderly, who have experienced multiple side effects from other opioids, may not do well with this route of administration.

Methadone can be safely used in the older adult, provided they are carefully monitored. Methadone is a mu-receptor agonist with a long half-life (ranging from 8 to 90 hours) and allows for prolonged dosing intervals.[56] The long half-life increases the potential for drug accumulation and side effects before the development of steady state blood levels, thus placing the patient at risk for sedation and possible respiratory depression. Therefore, close monitoring of these patients should be done during the first 7 to 10 days of treatment. From a cost perspective, it is one of the less costly opioids, making it appealing to some patients on limited incomes. As in younger individuals, the use of meperidine for the management of chronic cancer pain is not recommended due to the potential accumulation of metabolites, which can produce adverse effects.[57]

The parenteral route of drug administration should be considered in elderly patients who require rapid onset of analgesia or require high doses of opioids that cannot be administered orally. They may be administered in a variety of ways, including the IV and subcutaneous route, using a patient-controlled analgesia (PCA) device. A careful evaluation of the skin in the elderly patient should be done before initiation of subcutaneous administration. If the patient has excessive edema, a very low platelet count, or skin changes related to chronic steroid use, then absorption may be impaired or subcutaneous tissue may not sustain repeated dosing, even with a permanent indwelling butterfly catheter. Infusion devices with the capability of patient-administered rescue dosing can be safely used in the elderly cancer patient provided that they have clear understanding on how to use the rescue button. It is important to remember that severe cognitive impairment should not deter the use of IV administration, especially in the elderly patient at the end of life. In patients who are cognitively impaired, the PCA button should be removed. Choice of analgesics and routes of administration must be based on individual assessment of each patient.

Case study

An 80-year-old man with metastatic liver cancer

An 80-year-old man with metastatic liver cancer with known metastases to the lumbar spine is continuing to complain of pain in his lower back despite a recent rotation from tramadol to fentanyl patch. He was previously on tramadol (50 mg) every 6 hours but had worsening pain in the lower back and was rotated to a fentanyl 25 mcg patch about 1 week ago and morphine sulfate 15 mg every 4 h as needed. His family at the bedside reported that in addition to his poor pain control he appeared confused and was experiencing intermittent nausea and vomiting. Since starting on morphine, he has reported having bad dreams, confusion, and agitation, which have been corroborated by his family, who have also noted some intermittent jerking movements in his hands. He has been in bed most of the time. The family also reports constipation, with no bowel movement for 5 days. Today he was admitted to the local emergency room and was given lorazepam (1 mg IV) for agitation and morphine sulfate (2 mg IV) two times for pain. His confusion and agitation worsened and he was admitted. The patient's family mentions that he had a DNR order several months ago when he had fallen at home and fractured a rib. The family wants an aggressive evaluation for the delirium, and a brain MRI is done and is normal except for some age-related changes.

Once on the unit, he becomes more agitated and complains of severe pain. An opioid infusion of morphine sulfate (1 mg/h) is started but fails to produce analgesia, and his agitation worsens. A psychiatry consult is called, and the patient is started on lorazepam (1 mg every 6 h) around the clock. By day 2 the patient is worse, with worsening agitation and delirium.

At-a-glance assessment and management

- A comprehensive assessment of the elderly patient with delirium should include a determination of the etiology of delirium, including common predisposing factors (fever, infection, tumor, altered metabolism of drugs, alcohol, comorbid conditions, urinary/bowel retention). Often the cause is multifactorial.

- A careful history of onset and duration of symptoms as well as severity of symptoms should be determined, and dementia should be ruled out.

- When possible, the underlying cause should be identified and treated.

- In this patient, the goals of care are reviewed with the family members, who decide to aggressively try to reverse the delirium. The patient is already DNR.

- Pharmacological management should always include administration of a neuroleptic as a first-line treatment.

- Incorporate nonpharmacological interventions when appropriate.

Case analysis: what evaluation of this patient should be done and how should his delirium be managed?

1. The etiology of the confusion should be determined. A careful review of all medications should be done and all centrally acting medications discontinued. In this patient, the only recent additional medication is morphine.

2. Appropriate laboratory data (electrolytes, renal and liver function) should be obtained to determine whether there is any metabolic etiology for his confusion. Electrolytes and liver function studies are normal. BUN is 65 and serum creatinine is 3.0, which is more than doubled from 3 months ago.

3. A review of all medications is done, with careful attention to centrally acting medications. There does not seem to be any other etiology to the delirium other than the recent switch to morphine. In this patient an opioid rotation is indicated, because morphine metabolites—namely morphine-6 glucuronide—may be accumulating in the setting of worsening renal function, causing his delirium.

4. The lorazepam is stopped because it is felt to be contributing to his agitation, and the patient is started on a neuroleptic—haloperidol (1 mg every 6 h) around the clock.

5. An evaluation for the etiology of the nausea and vomiting is done. A history of onset, duration, temporal characteristics, and exacerbating/relieving factors is obtained from his family. A thorough physical examination is performed, with special attention to the abdominal and rectal examination. The physical examination reveals that bowel sounds are present, and the rectal exam reveals retained feces in the rectal vault.

6. An abdominal X-ray is done and shows extensive retained feces but no bowel obstruction.

7. It has been determined that the etiology of the nausea and vomiting is related to severe constipation.

8. The severe constipation may also be contributing to the development of confusion.

9. The decision is made to switch the patient to another opioid. In selecting another opioid, factors to consider include half-life, duration of action, and route of administration. The decision is made to start the patient on a continuous infusion of fentanyl. The equianalgesic dose table should be used as a guide. Because of the existence of incomplete cross-tolerance between drugs, advanced age, and cognitive changes, the alternative opioid should be reduced by 50%.

10. Disimpaction is attempted but cannot be tolerated. A bowel regimen of an oil-retention enema followed by a Fleets enema is tolerated, and the patient has a large bowel movement. The plan is to start the patient on an oral regimen of Senna (2 tabs orally twice a day) and Colace (300 mg orally daily) when the delirium clears.

11. Within 24 hours of discontinuation of morphine and lorazepam, the patient's mental status begins to clear and his agitation calms significantly. By day 3 he is almost back to baseline and is tolerating regular oral intake without further nausea or vomiting. With his resumption of regular oral intake and supplemental IV hydration his renal function tests return to his baseline serum creatinine of 1.1.

The use of adjuvant analgesics for pain

Several nonopioid medications have been found to be analgesic. These drugs alter, attenuate, or modulate pain perception. They may be used alone or in combination with opioids or nonopioid analgesics to treat many different pain syndromes, including neuropathic pain. Included in this category are antidepressants, anticonvulsants, N-methyl-D-aspartate (NMDA) antagonists, corticosteroids, and local anesthetics. All of these medications have side-effect profiles that can be especially harmful to the older patient, and careful monitoring is required.

Nonpharmacological approaches: complementary therapies

Physical and psychological interventions can be used as an adjunct with drugs and surgical approaches to manage pain in the older adult. These approaches carry few side effects and, when possible, should be tried along with other approaches. In selecting an approach in the dying patient, factors that should be considered include physical and psychological burden to the patient, efficacy, and practicality. If the patient has weeks to live, these strategies may allow for a reduction in systemic opioids and diminish adverse effects.

Cognitive-behavioral interventions include relaxation, guided imagery, massage, distraction, and music therapy. The major advantages of these techniques are that they are easy to learn, safe, and readily accepted by patients. Cognitive and behavioral interventions are helpful to reduce emotional distress, improve coping, and offer the patient and family a sense of control. Other physical interventions such as reflexology and massage therapy have been shown to relieve pain and produce relaxation.[58,59]

Cognitive changes: the challenges of a diagnosis of delirium or dementia

Delirium may often be superimposed on dementia in the elderly patient. In clinical practice, it is important to distinguish whether the delirious patient has an underlying dementia. When an elderly demented patient becomes delirious, it should be assumed that an organic precipitating factor—metabolic, drug-induced, acute illness—is the cause, and the patient should be evaluated for the etiology and treated. The distinction is not always apparent.

Please refer to chapter 21 for an in-depth discussion on the assessment and management of delirium. Specific areas are highlighted below that have special relevance for the elderly.

Both delirium and dementia feature global impairment in cognition. Obtaining a careful history from family members or caregivers to learn about the onset of symptoms is probably the most important factor in making the distinction. Generally, acute onset of cognitive and attention deficits and abnormalities, whose severity fluctuates during the day and tends to increase at night, is typical of a delirium. Delirium, in general, is a transient disorder that seldom lasts for more than a month, whereas dementia is a clinical state that lasts for months or years.[60] Dementia implies impairment in short- or long-term memory associated with impaired thinking and judgment, with other disturbances of higher cortical function or with personality change.[61]

Older adults with chronic illnesses are especially vulnerable to delirium as a result of inter- and intrahospital transfers, intensive care unit psychosis, and delirium associated with medication errors.

Delirium in the elderly at the end of life

In all settings, delirium is a common symptom in the elderly medically ill and cancer patient. The presence of delirium contributes significantly to increased morbidity and mortality. In elderly hospitalized patients, delirium prevalence ranges from 10% to 40% and up to 80% at the end of life. One of the major problems in the treatment of delirium in the elderly patient is lack of assessment by hospital staff, especially if the patient is quiet and noncommunicative. The etiology of delirium in the medically compromised and dying elderly patient is often multifactorial and may be nonspecific. The increased prevalence of delirium in older adults may result from a combination of physiological changes that occur as the brain ages, making it more susceptible to noxious stimuli.[62] In an elderly patient, delirium is often a presenting feature of an acute physical illness or exacerbation of a chronic one or of intoxication with even therapeutic doses of commonly used drugs.[61] Numerous factors appear to make the elderly more susceptible to the development of delirium (Table 37.2).

Various drugs can produce delirium in the medically ill or elderly patient (Table 37.3). In the palliative care setting, multiple medications are generally required to control symptoms at the end of life. Given the projected increase in the numbers of elderly patients, healthcare providers will encounter the need for management of delirium in the elderly more frequently. In cancer patients, risk factors that have been identified include advanced age, cognitive impairment, low albumin level, bone

Table 37.2 Factors predisposing the elderly to delirium

Factor	Comments
Age-related changes in the brain	Atrophy of grey and white matter; senile plaques in hippocampus, amygdala, middle cerebral cortical layers;
	Cell loss in frontal lobes, amygdala, putamen, thalamus, locus coeruleus; Alzheimer's disease, cerebrovascular disease
Brain damage	
Reduced regulation and resistance to stress	
Sensory changes	Visual, hearing loss
Infection	Foley catheters
	Pulmonary and urinary tract infections
	Intravenous lines
Impaired pharmacokinetics	Reduced ability to metabolize and eliminate drugs
Malnutrition	Vitamin deficiency as a result of prolonged illness
	Folate deficiency may directly cause delirium
Multiple comorbid diseases	Cancer and cardiovascular, pulmonary, renal, and hepatic disease
	Endocrine disorders, including hyperthyroidism and hypothyroidism
	Fluid and electrolyte abnormalities
Reduced thirst	Hypovolemia
Reduction of protein-binding of drugs	Enhanced effect of opioids, diuretics
Polypharmacy	Use of sedatives, hypnotics, major tranquilizers

Sources: Adapted from Lipowski (1989), reference 60; Inouye et al. (1996), reference 63; and Fong et al. (2009), reference 64.

metastases, and the presence of hematological malignancy. In one study that determined risk factors for delirium in oncology patients, specific etiological factors in the elderly were identified and included reduced cholinergic reserves of the brain, high prevalence of cognitive impairment and comorbid disease, visual and hearing loss, and impaired metabolism of drugs.[65,66] The diagnosis of delirium in an elderly patient carries serious risks. Delirium produces distress for patients, families, and healthcare providers. Depending on the severity of symptoms (fluctuating cognitive changes, hallucinations, agitation, or emotional lability), patients often require one-to-one observation, chemical, and—rarely—physical restraints. Falls and pressure ulcers are associated with the hyperactive and hypoactive subtypes.[67]

Delirium in terminally ill patients is a reliable predictor of approaching death within days to weeks, and hospital mortality rates among elderly patients with delirium range from 22% to 76%.[68] In one study looking at delirium in hospitalized older patients, the authors concluded that many of the poor outcomes of delirium may be related in large part to the persistence of delirium rather than the occurrence of an index episode of delirium per se and that a significant number of patients have only partial or no recovery.[69]

Table 37.3 Drugs commonly causing delirium in the elderly

Classification	Example
Antidepressants	Amitriptyline, doxepin
Antihistamines	Chlorpheniramine, diphenhydramine, hydroxyzine, promethazine
Diabetic agents	Chlorpropamide
Cardiac	Digoxin, dipyridamole
Antihypertensives	Propranolol, clonidine
Sedatives	Barbiturates, chlordiazepoxide, diazepam, flurazepam, meprobamate
Opioids	Meperidine, pentazocine
Nonsteroidal antiinflammatory agents	Indomethacin, phenylbutazone
Anticholinergics	Atropine, scopolamine
Antiemetics	Trimethobenzamide, phenothiazine
Antispasmodics	Dilomine, hyoscyamine, propantheline, belladonna alkaloids
Antineoplastics	Methotrexate, mitomycin, procarbazine, Ara-C, carmustine, fluorouracil, interferon, interleukin-2, L-asparaginase, prednisone
Corticosteroids	Prednisone, dexamethasone
H_2-receptor antagonists	Cimetidine
Lithium	
Acetaminophen	
Salicylates	Aspirin
Anticonvulsant agents	Carbamazepine, diphenylhydantoin, phenobarbital, sodium valproate
Antiparkinsonian agents	Amantadine, levodopa
Alcohol	

Source: Adapted from Lipowski (1989), reference 60.

Given the projected increase in the numbers of elderly patients, healthcare providers will encounter management of delirium in the elderly more frequently. To reduce the risk of polypharmacologically induced delirium, it is prudent to add one medication at a time, evaluating its response before adding another medication.

Delirium in the elderly patient is often undertreated for several reasons, including lack of assessment tools, inadequate knowledge of early signs of confusion, and inadequate time spent with the patient to determine cognitive function—all factors that lead to underdiagnosis.[70] In addition, behavioral manifestations of delirium may include a variety of symptoms that may be interpreted as depression or dementia. Inouye established a multifactorial model of delirium in the elderly, with baseline predisposing factors and the addition of various insults.[63] The factors that have been identified to be contributory to baseline vulnerability in the elderly include visual impairment, cognitive impairment, severe illness, and an elevated blood urea nitrogen/creatinine ratio of 18 or greater. Other factors that have been identified in the elderly include advanced age, depression, electrolyte imbalance, poor functional status, immobility, Foley catheter, malnutrition,

dehydration, alcohol, and medications, including neuroleptics, opioids, and anticholinergic drugs. Finally, delirium in an elderly patient is often a precursor to death and should be viewed as a grave prognostic sign.[71]

Alcohol withdrawal may be a cause of delirium in the elderly. Illness, malnutrition, or concurrent use of a hepatotoxic drug or one that is metabolized by the liver may result in increased sensitivity of the elderly to alcohol. Alcohol, combined with other medications, especially centrally acting medications, can produce delirium in the elderly.

The diagnosis of delirium in an elderly patient carries with it serious risks. An agitated delirious patient may climb out of bed; pull out Foley catheters, IV lines, and sutures; and injure staff in an attempt to protect themselves from a perceived threat. Mental status questionnaires are relatively easy to administer, and an examination should be performed on all patients with mental status changes. The Mini-Mental State exam, a 10-item test, is easy to administer to an elderly patient.[72] Other delirium screening and evaluation tools have been developed, including the Delirium Rating Scale-Revised,[73] Confusion Assessment Method,[74] Cognitive Test for Delirium,[75] and Memorial Delirium Assessment Scale.[76]

Treatment of delirium

Treatment of delirium includes an identification of the underlying cause, correction of the precipitating factors, and symptom management of the delirium. In the very ill or dying patient, however, the etiology may be multifactorial, and the cause is often irreversible. At the end of life the goals of care should be identified, and an intervention based on the goal of care should be employed. Maintaining comfort, allowing for a natural, peaceful death should be the end result. When the goal is to relieve suffering and allow a peaceful death diagnostic evaluations (imaging and laboratory studies) would not prove beneficial.

Ensuring safety is critical, and specialized training is needed to monitor these patients; often these patients cannot be managed at home. When caregivers are elderly, it may be necessary to advise hospitalization so that the elderly patient can be given the support and care they require.

If delirium is occurring in the dying elderly patient and the goal of care has been identified as the promotion of comfort and relief of suffering, diagnostic evaluations (imaging and laboratory studies) would not prove beneficial.

Interventions that may be helpful include restoration of fluid and electrolyte balance, environmental changes, and supportive techniques such as elimination of unnecessary stimuli, provision of a safe environment, and measures that reduce anxiety. These multicomponent interventions should also include strategies such as optimizing sensory input, orientation protocols if indicated, provision of familiar items, family presence, avoidance of restraints, and use of antipsychotic agents for hyperactive symptoms.[77] In many cases, the etiology of delirium may be pharmacological, especially in the elderly patient. All nonessential and central nervous system–depressant drugs should be stopped. The use of Foley catheters, IV lines, and physical restraints should be minimized; consider the use of gentle massage or music to facilitate sleep hygiene.

Pharmacological treatment includes the use of sedatives and neuroleptics. Breitbart and Jacobsen[78] demonstrated that the use of lorazepam alone in controlling symptoms of delirium was ineffective and contributed to worsening cognition. These authors advocate the use of a neuroleptic such as haloperidol, along with a benzodiazepine, in the control of an agitated delirium. Evidence indicates that the use of benzodiazepines should not be considered in patients with a history of psychiatric illness or alcohol withdrawal due to poor outcomes.[79] Other neuroleptics, such as risperidone and olanzapine, have also been used to treat delirium in the elderly and may have fewer side effects. The oral route is preferred, although in cases of severe agitation and delirium, the parenteral route should be used. In one study by Breitbart, 79 cancer patients were treated for delirium with olanzapine and age over 70 years was found to be the most powerful predictor of poorer response to olanzapine treatment. Other factors included history of dementia, central nervous system spread of disease, and hypoxia as delirium etiologies.[80]

Summary

Elderly patients who are dying should be able to receive skillful and expert palliative care. This means that clinicians must become knowledgeable about the aging process—the physiological changes that normally occur with aging and the impact of progressive disease on an already frail system. Management of symptoms at the end of life in the elderly patient is different from that in younger age groups because of their altered response to medications, their fear of taking medication, and the need to involve and educate informal and formal caregivers, who are often elderly themselves.

Pain, respiratory distress, and delirium are the three most common distressing symptoms in the elderly patient who is dying. Relief of these symptoms is a basic priority for care of the dying elderly patient. Continued assessment of the patient will allow for drug changes, dose adjustments, and relief of distressing symptoms. Providing relief from these symptoms will help facilitate a peaceful death, one that is remembered as such by family and friends.

References

1. Roger VL, Go AS, Lloyd-Jones DM, et al. Heart disease and stroke statisticsM2012 update: a report from the American Heart Association. Circulation. 2012;125(1):e2–e220.
2. Schulz R TC. Informal Caregivers in the United States: Prevalence, Characteristics, and Ability to Provide Care. Human Factors in Home Health Care. Washington DC: National Academies of Sciences Press; 2010.
3. Wolff JL, Roter DL. Hidden in plain sight: medical visit companions as a resource for vulnerable older adults. Arch Intern Med. 2008;168(13):1409–1415.
4. Levine C, Halper D, Peist A, Gould DA. Bridging troubled waters: family caregivers, transitions, and long-term care. Health Aff (Millwood). 2010;29(1):116–124.
5. Schulz R. Research priorities in geriatric palliative care: informal caregiving. J Palliat Med. 2013;16(9):1008–1012.
6. Funk L, Stajduhar K, Toye C, Aoun S, Grande G, Todd C. Part 2: Home-based family caregiving at the end of life: a comprehensive review of published qualitative research (1998–2008). Palliat Med. 2010;24(6):594–607.
7. Williams SW, Zimmerman S, Williams CS. Family caregiver involvement for long-term care residents at the end of life. J Gerontol B Psychol Sci Soc Sc. 2012;67(5):595–604.
8. Fried T, Pollack D, Drickamer M, Tinetti M. Who dies at home?: Determinants of site of death for community-based long-term care patients. J Am Geriatr Soc. 1999;47:25–29.
9. Health, United States, 2010: With Special Feature on Death and Dying. Hyattsville, MD: 2011.
10. Bercovitz A, Decker FH, Jones A, Remsburg RE. End-of-Life Care in Nursing Homes: 2004 National Nursing Home Survey. US Department of Health and Human Services, Centers for Disease Control and Prevention, National Center for Health Statistics; 2008.
11. National Nursing Home Survey 2004. http://www.cdc.gov/nchs/data/nnhsd/nursinghomefacilities2006.pdf. Centers for Disease Control; 2006.
12. Riley G, Lubitz J, Prihoda R, Rabey E. The use and costs of Medicare services by cause of death. Inquiry. 1987;24:233–244.
13. O'Mahony S. Cancer Pain, Prevalence and Undertreatment. In: Portenoy R, Breura E (eds.), Cancer Pain. New York, NY: Cambridge University Press; 2003:38–47.
14. McAuley W, Travis S. Advance care planning among residents in long-term care. Am J Hos Palliat Care. 2003;20:429–530.
15. Rosenfeld K, Wenger N, Phillips R, et al. Factors associated with change in resuscitation preference of seriously ill patients: The SUPPORT Investigators: Study to Understand Prognoses and Preferences for Outcomes and Risks of Treatment. Arch Intern Med. 1996;156(14):1558–1564.
16. McParland E, Likourezos E, Chichin E, Castor, Paris B. Stability of preferences regarding life-sustaining treatment: a two-year prospective study of nursing home residents. Mount Sinai J Med. 2003;70:85–92.
17. Heyland DK, Barwich D, Pichora D, et al. Failure to engage hospitalized elderly patients and their families in advance care planning JAMA Intern Med. 2013;173(9):778–787.
18. Kirchhoff KT, Hammes BJ, Kehl KA, Briggs LA, Brown RL. Effect of a disease-specific advance care planning intervention on end-of-life care. J Am Geriatr Soc. 2012;60(5):946–950.
19. Emanuel L, Madelyn I, Webster J. Ethical aspects of geriatric palliative care. In: Morrison RS, Meier DE (eds.), Geriatric Palliative Care. New York, NY: Oxford University Press; 2003.
20. Phipps E, True G, Harris D, et al. Approaching the end-of-life: attitudes, preferences and behaviors of African-American and white patients and their family caregivers. J Clin Oncol. 2003;21(3):549–554.
21. Fritsch J, Petronio S, Helft PR, Torke AM. Making decisions for hospitalized older adults: ethical factors considered by family surrogates. J Clin Ethics. 2013;24(2):125–134.
22. Hickman SE, Sabatino CP, Moss AH, Nester JW. The POLST (Physician Orders for Life-Sustaining Treatment) paradigm to improve end-of-life care: potential state legal barriers to implementation. J Law Med Ethics. 2008;36(1):119–140, 114.
23. Shoemaker LK, Estfan B, Induru R, Walsh TD. Symptom management: an important part of cancer care. Cleve Clin J Med. 2011;78(1):25–34.
24. Rezk Y, Timmins PF 3rd, Smith HS. Review article: palliative care in gynecologic oncology. Am J Hosp Palliat Care. 2011;28(5):356–374.
25. Araw AC, Araw AM, Pekmezaris R, et al. Medical orders for life-sustaining treatment: Is it time yet? Palliat Support Care. 2013;12(2):1–5.
26. Sykes N. End of life issues. Eur J Cancer. 2008;44(8):1157–1162.
27. NCDAH. Royal College of Physicians: Summary Report. December 5, 2007.
28. White HK, Cohen HJ. The older cancer patient. Med Clin N Amer. 2006;90(5):967–982.
29. American Geriatrics Society Panel on Pharmacological Management of Persistent Pain in Older Persons. Pharmacological management of persistent pain in older persons. J Am Geriatr Soc. 2009;57(8): 1331–1346.
30. Vestal RE, Montamat SC, Neilson CP. Drugs in special patient groups: The elderly. In: Melmon KL, Morrelli HF, Hoffman BB, and Nierenberg DW (eds.), Clinical Pharmacology: Basic Principles in Therapeutics. 3rd ed. New York, NY: McGraw-Hill; 1991:851–874.
31. Avorn J, Gurwitz HH. Principles of pharmacology. In: Cassel CK, Cohen HJ, Larson EB, et al. (eds.), Geriatric Medicine. 3rd ed. New York, NY: Springer; 1997:55–70.
32. Vestal RE. Aging and pharmacology. Cancer. 1997;80(7):1302–1310.
33. Aparasu RR, Sitzman SJ. Inappropriate prescribing for elderly outpatients. Am J Health Syst Pharm. 1999;56(5):433–439.
34. Abernethy AP, Wheeler JL. Total dyspnoea. Curr Opin Support Palliat Care. 2008;2(2):110–113.

35. von Leupoldt A, Sommer T, Kegat S, et al. Dyspnea and pain share emotion-related brain network. NeuroImage. 2009;48(1):200–206.

36. Mahler DA, Selecky PA, Harrod CG, et al. American College of Chest Physicians consensus statement on the management of dyspnea in patients with advanced lung or heart disease. Chest. 2010;137(3):674–691.

37. Palange P, Forte S, Felli A, Galassetti P, Serra P, Carlone S. Nutritional state and exercise tolerance in patients with COPD. Chest. 1995;107(5):1206–1212.

38. Eliopoulos C. Respiratory problems. Gerontological Nursing. Philadelphia, PA: Lippincott; 1996:277–290.

39. Johnson MJ, Bland JM, Oxberry SG, Abernethy AP, Currow DC. Clinically important differences in the intensity of chronic refractory breathlessness. J Pain Symptom Manage. 2013;46(6):957–963.

40. Booth S, Moosavi SH, Higginson IJ. The etiology and management of intractable breathlessness in patients with advanced cancer: a systematic review of pharmacological therapy. Nat Clin Pract Oncol. 2008;5(2):90–100.

41. Kamal AH, Maguire JM, Wheeler JL, Currow DC, Abernethy AP. Dyspnea review for the palliative care professional: treatment goals and therapeutic options. J Palliat Med. 2012;15(1):106–114.

42. Viola R, Kiteley C, Lloyd NS, Mackay JA, Wilson J, Wong RK. The management of dyspnea in cancer patients: a systematic review. Support Care Cancer. 2008;16(4):329–337.

43. Newton PJ, Davidson PM, Macdonald P, Ollerton R, Krum H. Nebulized furosemide for the management of dyspnea: does the evidence support its use? J Pain Symptom Manage. 2008;36(4):424–441.

44. Navigante AH, Castro MA, Cerchietti LC. Morphine versus midazolam as upfront therapy to control dyspnea perception in cancer patients while its underlying cause is sought or treated. J Pain Symptom Manage. 2010;39(5):820–830.

45. Ben-Aharon I, Gafter-Gvili A, Leibovici L, Stemmer SM. Interventions for alleviating cancer-related dyspnea: a systematic review and meta-analysis. Acta Oncol. 2012;51(8):996–1008.

46. Chou R, Fanciullo GJ, Fine PG, et al. Clinical guidelines for the use of chronic opioid therapy in chronic noncancer pain. J Pain. 2009;10(2):113–130.

47. Krueger AB, Stone AA. Assessment of pain: a community-based diary survey in the USA. Lancet. 2008;371(9623):1519–1525.

48. Maxwell CJ, Dalby DM, Slater M, et al. The prevalence and management of current daily pain among older home care clients. Pain. 2008;138(1):208–216.

49. Torvik K, Kaasa S, Kirkevold O, Rustoen T. Pain and quality of life among residents of Norwegian nursing homes. Pain Manage Nurs. 2010;11(1):35–44.

50. Recommendations for use of selective and nonselective nonsteroidal antiinflammatory drugs: an American College of Rheumatology white paper. Arthritis Rheumat. 2008;59(8):1058–1073.

51. Zhang W, Doherty M, Arden N, et al. EULAR evidence based recommendations for the management of hip osteoarthritis: report of a task force of the EULAR Standing Committee for International Clinical Studies Including Therapeutics (ESCISIT). Ann Rheum Dis. 2005;64(5):669–681.

52. Zhang W, Moskowitz RW, Nuki G, et al. OARSI recommendations for the management of hip and knee osteoarthritis. Part II: OARSI evidence-based, expert consensus guidelines. Osteoarthr. Cartil. 2008;16(2):137–162.

53. Mercadante S, Arcuri E. Opioids and renal function. J Pain. 2004;5(1):2–19.

54. Andersen G, Jensen NH, Christrup L, Hansen SH, Sjogren P. Pain, sedation and morphine metabolism in cancer patients during long-term treatment with sustained-release morphine. Palliat Med. 2002;16(2):107–114.

55. Smith MT. Neuroexcitatory effects of morphine and hydromorphone: evidence implicating the 3-glucuronide metabolites. Clin Exp Pharmacol Physiol. 2000;27(7):524–528.

56. Shaiova L, Berger A, Blinderman CD, et al. Consensus guideline on parenteral methadone use in pain and palliative care. Palliat Support Care. 2008;6(2):165–176.

57. Hanlon JT, Aspinall SL, Semla TP, et al. Consensus guidelines for oral dosing of primarily renally cleared medications in older adults. J Am Geriatr Soc. 2009;57(2):335–340.

58. Rhiner M, Ferrell BR, Ferrell BA, Grant MM. A structured nondrug intervention program for cancer pain. Cancer Pract. 1993;1(2):137–143.

59. Weinrich SP, Weinrich MC. The effect of massage on pain in cancer patients. Appl Nurs Res. 1990;3(4):140–145.

60. Lipowski ZJ. Delirium in the elderly patient. N Engl J Med. 1989;320(9):578–582.

61. Costa PT, William TD, Somerfield M, et al. Recognition and initial assessment of Alzheimer's disease and related dementias. US Department of Health and Human Services, Public Health Service, Agency for Health Care Policy and Research; 1996.

62. Rathier MO, Baker WL. A review of recent clinical trials and guidelines on the prevention and management of delirium in hospitalized older patients. Hospital Pract. 2011;39(4):96–106.

63. Inouye SK, Charpentier PA. Precipitating factors for delirium in hospitalized elderly persons: predictive model and interrelationship with baseline vulnerability. JAMA. 1996;275(11):852–857.

64. Fong TG, Tulebaev SR, Inouye SK. Delirium in elderly adults: diagnosis, prevention and treatment. Nat Rev Neurol. 2009;5(4):210–220.

65. Massie MJ, Holland J, Glass E. Delirium in terminally ill cancer patients. Am J Psychiatry. 1983;140(8):1048–1050.

66. Foreman MD. Acute confusion in the elderly. Ann Rev Nurs Res. 1993;11:3–30.

67. O'Keeffe ST, Lavan JN. Clinical significance of delirium subtypes in older people. Age Ageing. 1999;28(2):115–119.

68. Maltoni M, Caraceni A, Brunelli C, et al. Prognostic factors in advanced cancer patients: evidence-based clinical recommendations: a study by the Steering Committee of the European Association for Palliative Care. J Clin Oncol. 2005;23(25):6240–6248.

69. Cole MG. Persistent delirium in older hospital patients. Curr Opin Psychiatry. 2010;23(3):250–254.

70. Collins N, Blanchard MR, Tookman A, Sampson EL. Detection of delirium in the acute hospital. Age Ageing. 2010;39(1):131–135.

71. Lawlor PG, Fainsinger RL, Bruera ED. Delirium at the end of life: critical issues in clinical practice and research. JAMA. 2000;284(19):2427–2429.

72. Folstein MF, Folstein SE, McHugh PR. "Mini-mental state": a practical method for grading the cognitive state of patients for the clinician. J Psychiatr Res. 1975;12(3):189–198.

73. Trzepacz PT. The Delirium Rating Scale: its use in consultation-liaison research. Psychosomatics. 1999;40(3):193–204.

74. Inouye SK, van Dyck CH, Alessi CA, Balkin S, Siegal AP, Horwitz RI. Clarifying confusion: the confusion assessment method; a new method for detection of delirium. Ann Intern Med. 1990;113(12):941–948.

75. Hart RP, Levenson JL, Sessler CN, Best AM, Schwartz SM, Rutherford LE. Validation of a cognitive test for delirium in medical ICU patients. Psychosomatics. 1996;37(6):533–546.

76. Breitbart W, Rosenfeld B, Roth A, Smith MJ, Cohen K, Passik S. The Memorial Delirium Assessment Scale. J Pain Symptom Manage. 1997;13(3):128–137.

77. Holroyd-Leduc JM, Khandwala F, Sink KM. How can delirium best be prevented and managed in older patients in hospital? CMAJ: Can Med Assoc J. 2010;182(5):465–470.

78. Breitbart W, Jacobsen PB. Psychiatric symptom management in terminal care. Clin Geriatr Med. 1996;12(2):329–347.

79. Campbell N, Boustani MA, Ayub A, et al. Pharmacological management of delirium in hospitalized adults: a systematic evidence review. J Gen Intern Med. 2009;24(7):848–853.

80. Breitbart W, Tremblay A, Gibson C. An open trial of olanzapine for the treatment of delirium in hospitalized cancer patients. Psychosomatics. 2002;43(3):175–182.

CHAPTER 38

Poor, homeless, and underserved populations

Anne Hughes

I don't want to die . . . but living like this isn't good. I want to be more comfortable. Do everything you can to keep me going but I'm not going to dialysis if I don't feel like it. . . . Yeah . . . without dialysis, they tell me I'll die.

Johnny, 65-year-old African-American man with end-stage renal disease on dialysis and suspected occult malignancy

Key points

- Poor people are at risk for a poor quality of living and a poor quality of dying.

- People whose lives have been filled with physical and emotional deprivation, may be suspicious of efforts to engage them in "shared" decision-making to limit therapy, regardless of the therapy's burdens and limited benefits.

- Many persons who are poor have multimorbidities and other marginalizing social characteristics.

- Poor people's interactions with the healthcare system are frequently marked by rejection, shame, and discontinuity of care.

Poverty is inextricably linked to increased morbidity, premature mortality, and limited access to both preventive healthcare and ongoing medical care. Beyond the medical outcomes of poverty, the personal and social costs are substantial and often invisible. People who are poor constitute a *vulnerable population*, a term used in community health to describe social groups at greater risk for adverse health outcomes. The root causes of this vulnerability typically are low socioeconomic status and a lack of access to resources.[1] Vulnerable populations by definition are underserved by the healthcare system in terms of access to and quality of healthcare. Underserved communities for palliative care include not just the poor and those without adequate health insurance but also the unbefriended elderly, non-English speaking persons, the mentally ill, those with dementia, the developmentally delayed, nursing home residents, and those persons with limited health literacy.[2] When individuals or groups are denied what is regarded as standard-of-care interventions, moral questions about social justice appropriately must be asked.

The Institute of Medicine's report, which evaluated racial and ethnic disparities in healthcare, failed to address the role of poverty in disparities.[3] However, the role of poverty in contributing to inequalities, independent of race and ethnicity, is difficult to decipher because class and race are often closely intertwined.[4,5] Some believe poverty may be most responsible for disparities in healthcare.[5] In a systematic review of social determinants of death in the United States, the researchers concluded that low education, poverty (at both the individual and community level), racial segregation, limited social support, and income inequality were as likely causes of death as pathophysiological and behavioral causes.[6] In other words, being poor is as an important cause of mortality as are pathophysiological and behavioral explanations.

Although much has been written about state of end-of-life care in the United States, until recently not much has been said about those in our society who live at its margins, such as the urban poor.[7–19] Lewis (2011) conducted a systematic review of the barriers to accessing quality palliative care among the poor. Compared with those receiving palliative care who were not economically disadvantaged, the poor had less access to specialty care (often because of transportation), received fewer home visits and hospice service if they lived in high crime areas, and were at higher risk of dying in institutions. Additionally, as a result of limited health literacy, more of the economically disadvantaged received more aggressive medical interventions, had fewer discussions clarifying goals of care, and were challenged negotiating complex care delivery systems.[20]

To be poor and to have a progressive, life-threatening illness presents more challenges than either one of these conditions alone. As Taipale elegantly notes, "Poverty means the opportunities and choices most basic to human development are denied."[21(p54)] Consider the following questions: What type of death would a person hope for when that person doesn't have a home or lives in a room without a phone, a toilet, or kitchen? What are the meanings of life-threatening illness and death when premature death is an all-too-common part of life? What matters at the end of life if most of your life has been spent trying to survive day to day? All of these questions, in part, introduce us to the worlds of the poor who are confronting a life-threatening illness. Physical, psychological, and spiritual deprivation are not all that poor people contend with—deprivation also harms the moral self and the ability both to act and to live autonomously.[22]

The purpose of this chapter is to consider characteristics of the poor as an underserved population that place them at risk when seriously ill and when palliative care is indicated.[9] In particular, this chapter looks at a subset of the poor who are homeless or marginally housed and how this affects both access to and quality of care at the end of life. The economic downturn affecting the United States and the world in recent years increased the numbers of persons "doing without." However, this chapter focuses on persons whose "membership" in this group is more long term and not the result of an identifiable global economic crisis; similarly, this chapter does not address the experiences of persons living in extreme poverty in resource-limited countries around the globe.

The experience of being poor is not singular nor it is universal; poor persons are as diverse a population as the nonpoor. Case studies are used to illustrate the concepts discussed and to demonstrate the need for more research to guide practice. The cases described were modified to disguise identifying characteristics; the cases are reflective of the author's clinical practice and research in an urban area that is greatly impacted by HIV/AIDS and homelessness.[23] Therefore, these cases are not generalizable to all the poor or even to all the homeless. Poverty is only one social determinant that affects health status and access to resources. Persons with many vulnerabilities (e.g., being poor and a member of a minority community, elderly, or having other medical problems) are at the greatest risk for adverse outcomes at the end of life.[24]

Epidemiology of poverty in the United States

More than 46 million Americans (approximately one in seven) are poor.[25] The poverty line established by the federal government is based on annual household income. In 2011, a single adult under age 65 years was considered poor if his/her income was less than $11,702, and a family of four (with one adult and three children under age 18 years) was considered poor if their annual income was less than $22,891. Most experts believe the federal definition of poverty underestimates the true prevalence of poverty in the United States. For example, the poverty line (annual household income) does not capture cost-of-living differences across the country nor out-of-pocket medical costs. Table 38.1 lists states in which the poverty level exceeded the national average by almost 15% in 2011.[26]

The faces of the poor in the United States disproportionately include persons of color, children, foreign-born individuals, and single-parent families. African Americans have the highest rates of poverty in the United States (27.4%), followed by Hispanics (26.5%), Asian/Pacific Islanders (12.2%), and non-Hispanic white (9.9%), according to the US Census Bureau Report for 2011.[25] Children have greater rates of poverty than young and middle-aged adults and the elderly. Almost 48% of children under age 18 years living in a female-headed household were poor compared with 10.9% of children living with two married parents.[25]

Although poverty is not confined to urban areas, as evident in Table 38.1, which includes many states with large rural populations, nearly 85% of the poor live in or near the more populous metropolitan areas, and 52% of all the poor live in inner (or principal) cities.[25] Most of the poor have access to some type of housing or shelter, even if the basic accommodations (telephone, cooking and refrigeration, heat, water, private toilet, and bathing facilities) are inadequate. However, for a small subset, housing is marginal or unavailable. This subset is the focus of the following discussion.

Table 38.1 States whose poverty rates exceeded national average (14.9%) in 2011

State	Rate of poverty (%)
Mississippi	21.2
Louisiana	20.1
Arkansas	19.4
Kentucky	19.3
New Mexico	19.2
West Virginia	18.9
Alabama	18.5
South Carolina	17.3
Georgia	17.3
Tennessee	17.1
District of Columbia	16.5
Texas	16.4
North Carolina	16.2
Oklahoma	16
Arizona	15.8
Michigan	15.8
Ohio	15.8
New York	15.7

Source: Macartney and Mykyta (2012), reference 26.

Definition and prevalence of homelessness

Homelessness is defined in the Stewart McKinney Homeless Act as a condition under which persons "lack fixed, regular and adequate night-time residence" or reside in temporary housing such as shelters and welfare hotels.[27] Calculating the number of Americans homeless or marginally housed is extremely difficult. Most cross-sectional studies fail to capture persons transiently homeless—the hidden homeless, or those staying with family members, those living in cars or encampments, and others living in single-room occupancy hotels (SROs), sometimes known as welfare hotels.[28] Many of the poor and, in particular, the chronically homeless avoid contact with social and health services.

According to the National Coalition for the Homeless, on any given night between 440,000 to 840,000 Americans are homeless; as many as 3.5 million Americans experience homelessness in a given year.[27] Persons who are homeless are not members of a homogeneous group. Some are street people and chronically homeless, whereas others are homeless because of a financial crisis that put them out of stable housing (this number climbed with the great recession and home foreclosures). Street people may be more reluctant to accept services and may have much higher rates of concurrent substance abuse and mental illness, that is, dual diagnoses.[29] Homeless persons frequently are veterans, victims of domestic violence, the mentally ill, and substance abusers. Although the rates of mental illness and substance abuse are higher in the homeless than among persons who are stably housed, assuming that all the poor or, for that matter, all the homeless suffer from these problems only contributes to stereotypes that fail to see the person who is before us. Domestic violence, mental illness, and substance abuse are not confined to the poor; while poverty does not cause these problems, poverty may well exacerbate them.

Health problems associated with homelessness and poverty

Numerous health problems are associated with homelessness. Many of these problems are related to environmental factors such as exposure to weather conditions, poorly ventilated spaces, unsafe hotels and street conditions, and high-crime neighborhoods, where the poor are forced to live.[30] These health problems (Table 38.2) include malnutrition, lack of access to shelter and bathing facilities, problems related to drug and alcohol use, chronic medical conditions, chronic mental illness, and violence-related injuries.[28] One fourth of the homeless have a major psychiatric illness; about one in three persons who are homeless abuse drugs and alcohol.[31] Drugs and alcohol are often used to self-medicate distressing psychiatric symptoms (e.g., anxiety, depression, post-traumatic stress disorder [PTSD]).

The individual effects of poverty on health status are irrefutable.[32] Consider the case of coronary artery disease (CAD): The link between onset of CAD and low socioeconomic status has been established and is believed to be related to lifestyle factors, such as poor dietary habits, tobacco use, and limited physical activity.[33] Poor cardiac outcomes among the poor may also be related to limited access to standard medical care.[33,34] Persons who are poor, on average, have shorter life expectancies than those whose incomes are higher.[6] A survey of the "hidden homeless" in Canada to identify housing, health, and social needs reported that for many in the sample (aged 15–69 years), their first experience of homelessness occurred when they were in their teens.[28] Similar to other studies, most study participants were male, all had addiction problems, one-third had experienced violence in the prior 6 months, and about 25% reported avoiding being housed in shelters. The medical problems most often cited were: addiction problems, mental illness, dental problems, chronic pain, respiratory

conditions, and sleep disorders.[28] Health and social needs identified included access to nutritious food, transportation, money management, addiction and mental health treatment, and healthcare services/providers that were respectful and not stigmatizing or demeaning.[28] Curiously housing was not identified as a priority, perhaps in part because the researchers recruited most subjects from homeless service agencies, which would have attempted to link services with housing.

In urban areas, healthcare services for the poor are often provided by public health departments, teaching hospitals, faith communities, and nongovernmental organizations—the so-called safety net providers. These services typically are overburdened and unable to meet the needs of the poor and the growing number of Americans who are uninsured who access them. For many of the poor, the emergency department (ED) has become the primary source of medical care.[12,35]

Where and how homeless people die

Limited data are available regarding the socioeconomic factors, places of death, and immediate causes of death of the homeless.[36] Similar to those who are not poor, most poor people die in institutions. For those who are homeless, dying on the street or in jail is also a fact of life.[37]

In the past, causes of death among the homeless included drug overdose, alcohol-related deaths, and hypothermia; accidents such as fires, falls, and pedestrian-motor vehicle accidents; and violent deaths related to homicide and suicide. Researchers in Boston analyzed mortality among the homeless for shifts in patterns from previous reports.[36] Electronic databases of a program that serves the homeless were searched along with the state death registry for causes of death noted on death certificates. For the 6-year study period (2003–2008), there were 1302 deaths among the homeless. Drug overdose was the leading cause of death, with opioids implicated in 81% of the drug related deaths. Younger homeless persons (25–44 years) were most likely to die of drug overdose. Besides opioids, 43% of drug-related deaths occurred in persons who were polysubstance users; alcohol was found in almost one-third of all drug overdoses.

Heart disease and cancer (in particular trachea/bronchus/lung) were also significant causes of death in this population. Compared with matched adults in Massachusetts, the homeless aged 45 to 64 years, had a two- and threefold higher rate of death related to these chronic diseases. Most of the deaths occurred in the hospital (53%) compared with community residence (27%) or nursing home (10%). The demographic profile of the decedents was similar to past reports: male (81%), mean age 51 years (range 19–93), and white (60%). Compared with prior studies, fewer homeless persons died of HIV disease; instead drug overdose was the leading cause of mortality and tobacco contributed to other potentially preventable chronic disease-related deaths.[36]

Table 38.2 Health problems common among the homeless

Causes	Manifestations
Malnutrition	Dental problems, tuberculosis, wasting
Lack of shelter and access to bathing facilities	Skin infections, lice, podiatric problems, hypothermia, tuberculosis, respiratory infections, sleep disorders
Drug and alcohol use	Overdose, seizures, delirium, sexually transmitted infections (such as HIV, hepatitis B, hepatitis C), trauma, falls, cirrhosis, heroin nephropathy, esophageal varices
Chronic mental illness	Paranoid ideation, antisocial behaviors, psychosis, suicide
Chronic medical conditions	Hypertension, arthritis, venous stasis ulcers, cellulitis
Violence-related injuries	Assaults, homicides, rape

Case study

Al, 70-year-old white vet with lung cancer with central nervous system metastasis

Al was a 70-year-old white, Vietnam vet who was diagnosed with lung cancer after coughing up blood. His initial cancer treatment included surgical resection and chemotherapy. Al wasn't surprised by the diagnosis after smoking for almost 50 years. One year after the lung cancer diagnosis, he experienced numbness on one side of his body, got on the bus to the emergency room (transferred to a second bus to the hospital), where he was admitted and diagnosed with brain metastasis (not the stroke he feared while riding the bus, calling 911 was "expensive"). Al was estranged from his middle-class family after his mother's death while he was in his late teens. He joined the military and was sent to Vietnam. His difficult background included loss of his mother and family, alcohol abuse, loneliness, and shame about having been homeless.[11] When the elevator in his SRO was broken, Al was forced to carry his portable oxygen tank up three flights of stairs to his room. The most difficult impact of his illness, Al reported, was the weakness and 40-pound weight loss that made him feel more vulnerable when he was outside of his SRO in a high-crime neighborhood. Al was concerned that if someone bumped into him, he might fall, and he could not defend himself. He had never felt vulnerable like this before his illness, ". . . cause I've been through a war. Why would I be scared about anything?" Never married, Al approached his illness and dying matter of factly, he was grateful that he was not leaving a family behind who might be burdened, and yet at the same time regretted not having a family. Al died in a residential hospice program less than 3 days after he was transferred from a public hospital where he had received care.

Al's story reminds us that persons who are seriously ill and marginally housed are trying to manage their illness, its treatment demands, and its impact on function while simultaneously struggling with their basic needs that impact their well-being, such as negotiating stairs when an elevator is not working in an SRO hotel, using public transportation to get to the emergency department or to medical appointments, feeling more vulnerable when frail and navigating high-crime neighborhoods, and internally feeling shame for being homeless. Al, like many who are homeless, used alcohol and tobacco to cope with life's demands. His death from lung cancer occurred days after discharge from the hospital; fortunately for Al, he died in a residential hospice, where we can only hope, he finally experienced compassion and community.

Poverty, life-threatening illness, and quality of life

An enormous body of evidence has demonstrated health inequities related to race and ethnicity; indeed eliminating health disparities is a federal policy priority.[3,35] Understanding the role race and ethnicity play in the end-of-life experience of the urban poor however is complex, in no small part because as Crawley observed, race and ethnicity have been conflated with socioeconomic status (SES).[38] For the purposes of this chapter a more focused review of the literature is presented without attempting to untangle the role of race/ethnicity from SES in explaining the poorer outcomes such as quality of life.

In a systematic review of the incidence, treatment and mortality related to heart failure and SES, the researchers evaluated 28 studies that met inclusion criteria. The review concluded that disadvantaged persons had increased incidence of heart failure, higher rates of admissions and rehospitalizations, inconsistent use of beta blockers for treatment, and overall higher mortality rates than their comparison groups who were more advantaged.[39]

Solid organ transplantation is standard of care for end-stage organ diseases that would otherwise compromise quality of life

and shorten survival. The literature has documented disparities among racial and ethnic minorities related to both access to organs, and poorer graft outcomes for those who receive organs.[40,41] Risk factors for poorly functioning kidney grafts match the profile of the urban poor: African American, male, older aged, unmarried, unemployed, low income, living in poor neighborhoods, and geographic distance from transplant center.[40] Lacking a kidney transplant for example, results in a person with end-stage renal disease (ESRD) being required to get to the dialysis center (if poor this usually means on bus or on foot), and endure lengthy, uncomfortable hemodialysis treatments usually three times a week indefinitely. This kidney function replacement therapy surely compromises the quality of life.

Poor people endure a heavier burden of cancer according to several reports from the American Cancer Society and other researchers.[42] In a special report on cancer disparities and premature deaths, the American Cancer Society stated categorically that poverty was responsible for cancer disparities and premature cancer deaths regardless of race/ethnicity.[43] Edwards and colleagues used a community-based participatory research design to understand the factors that impact cancer disparities in East and Central Harlem compared with more affluent neighborhoods of New York City.[42] Forty study participants' interviews uncovered a number of themes. Many of those interviewed in Harlem believed information needs were vast and included available community resources, prevention and early detection of cancer, accessing cancer care, and symptom management. Additional themes that impacted cancer disparities in their community included unmet support needs that allowed discussion of cancer's impact and ways to cope, secrecy about the diagnosis, mistrust of healthcare systems and strongly held beliefs of stigma, fear, and fatalism. Generally, poor people encounter substantial barriers to obtaining quality cancer care, present with more advanced disease, experience more pain and suffering, and are more likely to die earlier of cancer than their economically advantaged counterparts.[43] Findings of the impact of poverty on cancer care are summarized in Box 38.1.

Barnoto and colleagues conducted a national telephone/mail survey of community-dwelling Medicare beneficiaries to explore racial and ethnic differences regarding preferences for and concerns about end-of-life treatment.[44] The sample of 2847 adults included: 2105 whites (non-Hispanic), 489 blacks (17.4%), and 113 Hispanics (4%). When most subjects were asked about their preferences if they were diagnosed with terminal illness with less than 1 year to live, the responses were quite similar: to die at home, without life-prolonging medications with adverse effects, and without mechanical ventilation if such treatment extended life by 1 week to 1 month. However, compared with white respondents, minority subjects were more likely to prefer more medical interventions, including dying in the hospital, possible life-extending medications regardless of their side effects, and mechanical ventilation for 1 month or 1 week.[44]

In the ethnographic study *Dancing with Broken Bones: Portraits of Death and Dying Among Inner City Poor*, Moller (2004) poignantly recounts and photographically documents the stories of poor patients followed by an oncology clinic in a Midwest city. His insights about the suffering of the urban poor are profound: "the dying poor are the quintessential violators of the American dream; they live in the shame of poverty and with the unpleasantness of dying."[12(p. 10)] Because much of a person's worth in

---

Box 38.1 Poverty and cancer

- Poor people lacking access to quality healthcare are more likely to die of cancer than nonpoor people.

- Poor people experience greater cancer-related pain and suffering.

- Poor people facing significant barriers to getting health insurance often do not seek necessary care if they are unable to pay for it.

- Poor people and their families make extraordinary sacrifices to obtain and pay for care.

- Poor people lack knowledge of available community resources, lifestyle factors that contribute to poorer health outcomes, warning signs of cancer, symptom management strategies, and how to access follow-up cancer care.

- Psychosocial support, both individual and group, and outreach efforts at community level are lacking.

- Mistrust of healthcare professionals, teaching hospitals, and researchers is common and a barrier to health seeking.

- Fatalism, fear, and stigma about cancer are commonly held beliefs that prevent accessing care.

- Secrecy about cancer interferes with accessing care that may even be available in nearby community.

- Cultural barriers between healthcare professionals and the community may result in services that do not take into account the community needs, including health literacy. Many in impoverished neighborhoods are certain that environmental pollution may contribute to cancer rates.

Sources: Adapted from Edwards (2013), reference 42, and Freeman (2004), reference 5.

Box 38.2 Insights about the dying poor

- Poverty inflicts substantial harm throughout life.

- Poverty exacerbates indignity and suffering throughout dying.

- Patients/families are often mistrustful and angry about the care received.

- Patients, at the same time, may be grateful for the care received.

- Spirituality plays an important role in providing strength and resilience when dying.

- Social isolation increases suffering.

- Hidden and sometimes unexpected sources of support can emerge from family and community.

- The emergency room is the front door to healthcare.

- The organization of medical care is frequently fragmented and lacks continuity.

- Funerals are important rituals, and their cost creates enormous stress for survivors.

Source: Adapted from Moller (2004), reference 12.

American society is connected with social status indicators such as occupation, income, and home ownership, the poor represent those who have not made it, have not lived up to their potential. Being poor then becomes a matter of personal failure rather than a social problem requiring public policy changes.[45] From Moller's longitudinal qualitative study of poor inner-city patients, their families, and their healthcare providers, the researcher drew a number of conclusions, which are listed in Box 38.2. His work can perhaps be summed up by saying that the indignities of being poor in America are only intensified when that person is also dying. Unlike persons who are not poor, dying is not always feared in the same way, because for some persons who are socially or economically disadvantaged, dying may represent freedom from the misery of living.[11]

Clinical presentations of advanced disease in the poor

Persons who are poor frequently present with advanced disease in part related to delays in diagnosis, mistrust of healthcare systems, and late discussions of advance directives and end-of-life care options.[46] In addition to the late-stage disease presentation, many have significant comorbidities that affect both the palliation of symptoms and the course and treatment of underlying illnesses. These clinical management issues usually occur within the context of complex psychosocial situations, as the following case illustrates.

Case study

Tiffany, 34-year-old biracial woman with AIDS-related highly aggressive non-Hodgkins lymphoma

Tiffany was a frail 34-year-old woman living with HIV disease who was intermittently homeless. When she was stably housed, she was followed by a case management program for HIV+ former sex workers who had been released from prison, typically incarcerated because of drug charges. With the support of her case manager, and in spite of some minor side effects, Tiffany was able to take antiretroviral medications (ARVs) that were delivered/prepoured and was virologically suppressed. She kept her medical and social service appointments and she was able, for the most part, to remain clean, sober, and safe. When her boyfriend, who was suspected of abusing her, showed up, Tiffany would disappear for weeks to months at a time. Eventually after being off ARVs treatment, she would present to the emergency room and would be hospitalized with an infection and in a debilitated state. After being lost to follow-up for almost a year, Tiffany presented to the emergency department with eye pain, decreased vision, and swelling that inverted her eyelid and partially exposed the globe. Tiffany underwent an MRI, and a mass, suspicious of a malignancy, was discovered. Her CD4 count was 17 and HIV viral load > 300,000. A biopsy confirmed highly aggressive non-Hodgkins lymphoma (NHL). The medical oncologist recommended systemic chemotherapy, which Tiffany accepted, and the radiation oncologist recommended external beam radiation therapy. Tiffany tolerated inpatient chemotherapy despite some side effects. She was most embarrassed by the appearance of her face when the tumor enlarged. Besides the body image disturbance, Tiffany reported moderate-severe pain, odynophagia, and anorexia. In the past, Tiffany was known to sell her opioids for crack and for heroin she shot up (injected intravenously). The case manager, who knows her, is torn seeing that Tiffany is in pain and emotionally and spiritually suffering with this new diagnosis, and yet at the same time is worried that if Tiffany is given large amounts of opioids, Tiffany's boyfriend will reappear and Tiffany will stop treatment. Tiffany only got to her first radiation therapy appointment. She has had no consistent primary care provider given her disjointed connection with a public health clinic; her medical care was being comanaged by the oncologist and HIV physician consultant. Tiffany's wishes about end-of-life care are unknown. The oncology social worker who has been assigned to work with Tiffany reports that Tiffany does not want to talk about her cancer diagnosis or prognosis. According to the case manager, other than her parole officer and her boyfriend, Tiffany has no known family or friends involved in her life.

Multimorbidities, especially those related to drug use and domestic violence, complicate therapeutic engagement, symptom management, and other medical management.[47] As Tiffany's case study illustrates, there are many pressing clinical needs: NHL management, decisions about resuming ARV therapy in a person with history of nonadherence and likely drug-resistant virus, engaging Tiffany (with the support of her care manager) in advance care planning, her safety given the possibility of domestic violence, risk of continued drug use, and symptom management and high risk of aberrant use of opioids. In Tiffany's case the latter proved most challenging for her providers. Tiffany was sent home with long-acting morphine for twice-a-day dosing, dexamethasone, and an as-needed antiemetic. Her providers considered starting Tiffany on methadone for pain, but she refused. Ultimately Tiffany presented with tumor recurrence; she was unable to see and refused further cancer treatment; she had stopped taking her ARVs. Tiffany was hospitalized, started on intravenous opioid infusion, and died in the hospital with her case manager and some volunteers at her bedside. Her boyfriend, who was unreachable, never showed up before she died.

Symptom management is critical to engaging a patient in care, to developing therapeutic connection, and then to negotiating about how to begin tackling the other issues. However in Tiffany's case there are competing factors that influenced providers' willingness to aggressively manage her pain. Persons known to be chemically dependent may be denied treatment for pain because of providers' concerns of aberrant or drug-hoarding behaviors. In recent years, increases in opioid prescriptions has resulted in a commensurate increase in drug overdoses; this trend has resulted in calls by the Centers for Disease Control and Prevention alerting prescribers and the public about the heightened risk.[48]

Will Tiffany take the medication as ordered? Is she likely to try again to sell her opioids for crack or heroin? Will she give her prescribed opioids to her boyfriend? How does one manage the severe pain of a patient with aggressive cancer who has diverted opioids in the past? Who will prescribe/monitor opioid medications? Does the local pharmacy even carry the medications? In one study pharmacies in predominantly nonwhite neighborhoods in New York City were less likely to carry opioids for pain management than were pharmacies in neighborhoods serving predominantly white communities.[49] Poor social conditions, criminal activity, and the threat of violence are significant barriers to effective pain management for persons with life-threatening illnesses.[50] While Tiffany was an inpatient receiving chemotherapy, her opioid access was controlled and her response monitored. However her nurses at times expressed concern about giving scheduled opioids, and responding to her requests for PRNs, when Tiffany seemed drowsy and yet was insisting that her pain was poorly controlled. How can the nurse know for sure that a patient is in pain, and not merely "drug seeking" or attempting to self-medicate the suffering of her everyday existence? Some questions are philosophical and often cannot be answered clinically or with psychometrically validated measurements.

Fortunately researchers and clinicians are recognizing the clinical dilemma of treating pain in persons with cancer and with HIV disease with addiction disorders and offering recommendations.[51-55] Refer to chapter 41 for a detailed discussion on caring for the dying drug-addicted patient at the end of life.

Beyond accurately diagnosing and treating the specific cause of the pain when possible, and psychologically screening for addiction and the risk for aberrant drug behaviors, Kircher and colleagues (2011) advise (1) obtaining informed consent for opioid use in those with cancer diagnosis and addiction disorder, (2) specifying prescription access in agreements, (3) selecting medications based on underlying pain mechanism and disease course, and (4) incorporating adjuvants. Other recommendations include (1) observing for aberrant behaviors such as injecting oral formulations, selling drugs, or an unexplained deterioration in function; (2) monitoring for concurrent alcohol or illicit drug abuse; (3) requiring mental health and addiction counseling; and (4) promoting the use of complementary therapies such as massage, acupressure, meditation, and support groups.[52,53] Additionally the clinician is advised to frequently evaluate the pain management plan using an acronym called the 4As: analgesia, activity (function), adverse effects, and aberrant behaviors. Given the potential risks, thorough documentation of assessment and interventions is essential for medicolegal reasons. Clinicians are further advised to remember that relapse can be expected, particularly when the person is under increased stress.[51] Such was the case with Tiffany's diagnosis of an aggressive and disfiguring lymphoma.

In addition to these quandaries, for many persons who are poor or lacking adequate health insurance, access to treatment is a significant factor that influences symptom management. For example, if an antiemetic prescribed to relieve the recurrent nausea experienced by a poor person with hepatocellular cancer is not covered on the Medicaid formulary, or the person is not eligible for any drug-assistance program, then the range of medications used to manage the nausea is limited. High-tech methods to control symptoms are not an option for the person who lives in a tent encampment. Most poor persons are institutionalized to manage uncontrolled symptoms and to provide both chronic and terminal care that cannot be managed sufficiently on the street or in the shelter.[12] Hopefully changes in healthcare insurance and healthcare delivery systems with the Affordable Care Act will result in early access to care, and improved clinical outcomes for more persons underserved by our current healthcare system.

The management of symptoms associated with progressive illness is further complicated by end-organ diseases, such as liver or renal disease, that may alter the pharmacokinetics of medications used to palliate symptoms. Clinically significant drug–drug interactions are common with the ARVs that Tiffany restarted.

The Department of Health and Human Services guidelines about initiating and modifying antiretroviral therapies are elaborated in great detail, discontinuing ARVs is barely addressed and is not recommended even for the patients who are terminally ill and very debilitated.[56] Determining whether a patient is experiencing an adverse drug reaction is not easy when the person has multimorbidities, has rapidly progressive disease, is malnourished, or may be continuing to use alcohol or other substances. When Tiffany refused to continue taking ARVs, despite being warned about the risk of viral rebound and immune decompensation, her wishes were honored. Her decision was difficult, however, for some her HIV providers.

Comorbidities also affect the healthcare providers' ability to realistically estimate prognosis and the nature of symptoms or problems that might occur down the road. Tiffany lived with HIV disease for years. Prior to the introduction of antiretroviral therapy and prophylaxis of opportunistic infections in the mid-1990s, in all probability Tiffany would not have survived as long as she did, particularly given her risky life on the street without case management. Charting the dying trajectory for the chronic progressive illness may be conceivable, but superimposing the other illnesses and injuries that the very poor live with and manage creates jagged peaks and valleys in a downward course. How quickly the life-threatening illness will progress becomes a prognostication puzzle; some persons who have been living on the street truly seem to have had nine lives.

On the other hand, despite the prevalence of substance abuse among the poor, lack of attention to self-care activities cannot be assumed in all drug users. Some homeless persons who use drugs manage complex HIV antiretroviral regimens that require scrupulous adherence and must take into account possible interactions with other medications or illicit drugs and the need for routine lab monitoring of CD4 counts and HIV viral loads.[57] Race, class, and housing status cannot be used as surrogate predictors of who abuses drugs and alcohol or who will adhere or not adhere to treatment demands.

Barriers and challenges to providing palliative care

As suggested, there are many barriers (structural or community factors) that limit access to quality palliative care for the urban poor and an equal number of challenges (individual and illness-related factors) that are common among the urban poor with advanced disease.[12]

Barriers that influence the health status of anyone living in an inner city include high rates of violent crime and drug use; marginal or substandard housing; limited public transportation; convenience stores that sell more tobacco and alcohol than fresh fruits and vegetables; environmental pollution; oversubscribed and often charity-dependent community health services, if even available; lack of pharmacies and or restricted drug formularies; and lack of insurance or a reliable income source to meet basic needs.[17,49,58]

Challenges to providing palliative care to the urban poor with advanced disease include person-specific or illness-related factors, summarized in Table 38.3. Illness-related challenges include the prevalence of serious mental illness, addiction, and PTSD; multiple comorbidities including end-organ disease and other chronic diseases, and presenting for care with advanced disease that may be

Table 38.3 Psychosocial challenges in providing palliative care to the urban poor with serious illness

Illness related	◆ Prevalence of concurrent mental illness and substance abuse
	◆ Decisional incapacity
	◆ Presentation with advanced disease
	◆ Multiple comorbidities
	◆ End-organ diseases altering pharmacodynamics
Resource challenges	◆ Health literacy
	◆ Family or friend caregiver availability
	◆ Need for designated health proxy/agent in the event of decisional incapacity
	◆ Chaotic lives that have little space for day-to-day illness demands
	◆ Limited ongoing therapeutic relationships with health or social service providers
	◆ Survival or addiction may overshadow illness management
	◆ Competing role responsibilities
	◆ Functional impairments, geographic distances, and transportation limitation compromise appointment keeping
Relationships with healthcare system or providers	◆ Cultural history of racism, discrimination, or rejection in healthcare system
	◆ As a result of disrespectful, rude, or dismissive interactions in past, may present as angry, avoidant, suspicious, or nonadherent with care recommendations
	◆ Healthcare providers often have different cultural and ethnic backgrounds/worldviews
End-of-life preferences	◆ Reluctance to relinquish aggressive medical management
	◆ Different assumptions about optimal end-of-life care, particularly in communities of color
	◆ Lack of advance care planning, as life is experienced moment to moment
	◆ Tendency to equate goals of care modification with abandonment or continued poor care
	◆ Spirituality may be a hidden resource for comfort and in guiding decision-making

Source: Hughes (2013), reference 2, reprinted with permission of Hospice and Palliative Nursing Association.

less responsive to disease modifying interventions even were such therapies available. Social resource challenges include fragile support systems, health literacy concerns, need for healthcare proxy or agent if a family member or friend is not available, and chaotic lives in which survival frequently overshadows illness management. Relationships with healthcare providers and systems may be frayed if existent; and providers may come with quite different worldviews and cultural backgrounds than the person presenting for care. In general, the barriers to providing quality palliative care to this population require community level or policy interventions while some of the challenges noted require person-centered interventions. Both levels of approaches will be discussed following a review of the evidence base for providing palliative care to the urban poor.

Evidence-based palliative care for the urban poor

The evidence base to guide palliative care for the urban poor is sparse and includes reviews, program evaluations, and research that used both descriptive and clinical trial designs. The reviews were found in textbooks and journal articles.[8,19,59] The program evaluations described shelter-based, home care[61] palliative care programs, and the impact of hospital-based palliative care consultation services on family satisfaction and do-not-resuscitate (DNR) status.[62,63] Researchers used in-depth individual and group interviews, survey, and clinical trial approaches. Researchers explored attitudes and beliefs about end-of-life care[13,14,64] and barriers to palliative care among low-income cancer patients,[17] tested methods for promoting advance directive completion among this population using low-literacy version[65] or other methods,[18] and described the experiences of the urban poor with advanced disease who were community dwelling or in a dedicated AIDS nursing home unit[10,11] and the hopes and concerns about care at the end of life for inpatients at public hospital with serious illness.[16]

Of the available "evidence" evaluated, only advance care planning using a 5th-grade reading level version, or other methods including one-to-one coaching or self-completion, was of a sufficient quality to support its translation into practice.[18,64,65]

Clinical interventions and community/policy-level approaches

Clinical interventions: importance of relationships

Developing trusting therapeutic relationships is at the very heart of all clinical interventions regardless of whether the person is impoverished and marginally housed, or has social and financial resources. Therapeutic relationships take on a particular salience with those facing serious illness and death. However developing trusting relationships with persons who have experienced rejection, abandonment, or felt unwelcomed in healthcare settings requires patience and time—scarce resources in busy clinical settings. Moreover, some groups seeking medical care may value and trust relationships more highly than data-driven guidelines,[66] increasing their importance for patient-centered, culturally sensitive palliative care.

Multiple qualitative studies of the urban poor with serious illness have demonstrated a desire for therapeutic relationships with healthcare professionals characterized by respect, by "sitting down and listening," and by honesty and consistency.[10,11,16,64,67] When patients and providers come from different life experiences, the most basic principles of therapeutic communication are crucial (see Box 38.3 for suggestions). These include addressing the person formally unless given permission to use the familiarity of first names, sitting at eye level when interacting, and appreciating that the palliative care philosophy and principles guiding care approach may be quite foreign or even suspect as a means of denying care (again) or as an "ethically charged" clinical intervention.[59,66]

Davis and colleagues interviewed homeless chronically ill adults about the case management services they received to stabilize their medical conditions and social situations.[67] Four themes emerged from the interview data: (1) participants described profound isolation prior to receiving case management services,

> **Box 38.3** Helpful suggestions when engaging a difficult-to-engage client
>
> ◆ Address anyone older than 40 years of age by the title of Mr. or Ms. Ask permission to be on a first-name basis.
> ◆ Do not hesitate to shake hands.
> ◆ Be prepared to meet people who are more intelligent, more perceptive, and more wounded than you expect.
> ◆ Be tolerant. How would you react if you were in that situation?
> ◆ Don't make promises you can't keep.
> ◆ Don't take it personally.
> ◆ Taking time out helps prevent burnout.
> ◆ Get to know the community.
> ◆ If you feel you have to save the human race, do it one person at a time.
> ◆ Providing material assistance (e.g., clean socks, food, hygiene kits) opens people up.
> ◆ Usually the most difficult clients are those most in need. Throw the word "noncompliant" out of your vocabulary.
> ◆ Make eye contact. If the person does not like eye contact or becomes agitated, avoid using it.
> ◆ Keep in mind that people who live intense lives may not particularly like unasked-for physical contact.
> ◆ Don't be afraid to ask "stupid" questions; patients' answers are better than your assumptions.
> ◆ Adjust your expectations and accept small victories with satisfaction.
>
> *Source:* Patchell (1977), reference 75.

(2) caring relationships with case managers were key to the program's benefit, (3) case managers assisted participants to navigate medical and social service systems, and (4) participants perceived improved health because of the interpersonal and practical interventions. The title of the study report perhaps says it all, "Because somebody cared about it. That's how it changed things."[67]

Assessment considerations

A comprehensive assessment by a nurse includes history of illness, treatment, comorbidities, medication, self-care abilities, symptom management, and a physical examination appropriate to the presenting complaint and history, and psychosocial information that may shape end-of-life care options. Obtaining psychosocial information over time, rather than in a single session, is more likely to promote a therapeutic connection and to uncover a richer narrative. Admittedly, appointment follow-up difficulties often justify trying to get as much information as possible during an initial encounter. While various screening or assessment tools for specific aspects of care are available, and recommended in many practice guidelines, the timing of when, or whether, to use such standardized instruments needs to be evaluated on a case by case basis in a population who may be more hesitant to engage in care and suspicious of how this information may be used.

In addition to illness, treatment, comorbidities, medication, self-care, and symptom-related assessment, psychosocial areas to assess include but are not limited to (1) housing (Where do you usually stay at night?), (2) food (Are there times when you are hungry from not having enough to eat?), (3) transportation (How do you get to appointments or to the hospital?), (4) income (Are you receiving any income or benefits?), (5) preferred communication methods (How can we get in touch with you?), (6) caregiver availability (Is there someone you can count on when you need help?), (7) use of other resources (Do you have a case manager, peer advocate, sponsor, or patient navigator?), (8) literacy (Are you much of a reader? How do you like to get information about your health?), (9) spirituality (What role does faith or religion play in your life?), (10) cultural identity (What beliefs or practices about health and healing are important for us to incorporate into your care?), (11) safety (Do you feel safe where you're staying?), (12) coping resources (How have you coped in the past when dealing with challenges?) and (13) substance use (Have you used alcohol or drugs to cope? If so, what difficulties has their use presented in your life?).[19]

In addition to the interpersonal interventions to engage the client in a therapeutic interaction, nurses are often required to become knowledgeable about the availability of services provided by community agencies. Are pharmacies available, what are their hours, are they willing to accept telephone orders, and what medications are kept on hand? What supportive services are available, such as food/meal programs, case management services, representative payee programs, supportive housing, and crisis mental health and substance abuse programs? What home health or hospice program serves the community, and are there any restrictions on services because of concerns related to staff safety? Knowing which agencies or services are involved with a client and communicating with them assures consistency of approach and continuity of care. Advocacy is often required to access services such as pain management, substance abuse treatment, mental health services, and social services for housing and money management.

In summary, developing therapeutic relationships with the poor and homeless requires: (1) expecting the person's trust to be earned over time (sometimes a long time) and not taking it for granted; (2) respecting the person's humanity, no matter how they look, what they say, and what feelings in us they evoke; (3) appreciating the person's unique story as influencing his/her response to illness and death; and, finally, (4) recognizing and addressing maladaptive behaviors. The case study below may serve to underscore the importance of relationships and knowing the person over time.

Case study

Johnny, a 65-year-old African-American man with end-stage renal disease on dialysis and suspected occult malignancy

Johnny was a 65-year-old African-American man with ESRD, managed by hemodialysis treatments three times a week for several years. Johnny was never considered a candidate for kidney transplantation. Other medical problems included hepatitis C and cirrhosis, hypertension, s/p CVA with left hemiparesis, COPD, polysubstance abuse, depression, vertebral lytic lesion, and recurrent lower gastrointestinal (GI) bleed. He has lived in an SRO until after repeated hospitalizations, he reluctantly agreed to placement in a long-term care facility. Johnny was a self-described loner; he

liked to watch people but avoided social events or groups when invited. His social worker described Johnny as not liking to be hassled and wanting to be left alone. Johnny was raised Baptist and periodically would speak to a minister who came to the facility. He described his faith as important and private. After a lower GI bleed resulted in his needing to be transfused, Johnny declined colonoscopy or other work up. An incidental finding on an X-ray after a noninjurious fall revealed vertebral lytic lesion, Johnny declined further work up. Johnny began to refuse transport to the dialysis center despite being told the implications of his refusal. When he became more symptomatic (fatigue, nausea, malaise, mental slowing) he agreed to dialysis; sometimes his condition would have deteriorated to the point when the dialysis center sent Johnny to the emergency room and he was admitted. This pattern repeated a few times. Johnny had been estranged from his family; his mother died in the past year and he'd only recently connected with his brother who lived on the other side of the country, where Johnny was born and raised. He was seen by a psychologist who determined that Johnny understood the risks of his refusal of dialysis; the psychologist confirmed that Johnny had decisional capacity and further determined his actions were not passive attempts at suicide. Johnny told the palliative care consultant," I don't want to die. . . but living like this isn't good. I want to be more comfortable. Do everything you can to keep me going but I'm not going to dialysis if I don't feel like it. . . . Yeah. . . without dialysis, they tell me I'll die." Johnny was tired of dialysis and the demands of this treatment. At the same time and seemingly contradictory, Johnny was not looking forward to death and wanted everything done to postpone his dying (except for dialysis). Johnny wanted to be kept comfortable but he finally agreed to a DNR order. Johnny understood that at some time his thinking would be affected by not having dialysis and his family would likely be consulted because he had no formal advance directive. Johnny gave permission for his brother to be contacted and to be advised of his condition. Additionally Johnny asked to see the minister to read the Bible to him and to pray with him. After refusing almost 2 weeks of dialysis, Johnny agreed to be dialyzed. Immediately after his arrival at the dialysis center, the nephrologist called the paramedics to take Johnny to the emergency room for admission. By that time, Johnny was no longer able to make his own decisions. After consultation between the medical admitting team, the facility staff, and Johnny's brother, the decision was reached to accept Johnny's action (refusal of dialysis after years of treatment) as likely more reflective of his values and wishes than his contradictory remarks about wanting everything done to keep him going, to honor his wish for comfort and his insistence on declining treatments. Johnny's goals of care were switched to comfort and he was discharged back to the long-term care facility, where he died peacefully within 48 hours.

Johnny's story reveals contradictions not uncommonly seen in many persons with progressive life-threatening illnesses: not wanting to die but no longer wanting to live in their current situation. His story illustrates several of the psychosocial issues outlined in Table 38.3. Johnny had multiple serious end-organ diseases: ESRD, COPD, cirrhosis, and a suspected metastatic malignancy that complicated understanding the trajectory and symptom management given his ambivalence regarding goals of care. His manner of coping to avoid being "hassled" was challenged by a treatment required three times a week. His relationship with family was fragile and just reestablished after years of estrangement. Assuming that a family member who had not been in Johnny's life for years is in the best position to assume the responsibility of surrogate decision maker seems both unfair and unlikely to provide the most reliable "substituted" judgment. Johnny's behaviors were inconsistent with his words: his nonadherence to dialysis would likely shorten his life, at the same time he wanted to be kept going. While Johnny had decisional capacity, before the delirium associated with uremia set in, he might have expressed his wishes for end-of-life care in an advance healthcare directive. This did not occur in spite of his social worker's encouragement to consider articulating his wishes. Johnny also reminds us of the resilience of a black man who had no doubt experienced years of discrimination who acted in a manner that was consistent with what mattered to him.[68] Johnny may have been drawing on his faith as "an important and private" source of support. Many researchers and scholars have reported on the role of spirituality as source of comfort for the African-American community.[12,16,68,69,73] Johnny died the way he wanted. What was also true that for those taking care of Johnny was that his nonadherence and reluctance to engage about his apparent ambivalence about goals of care presented a moral dilemma that required reflection and debriefing.

Program, community, or policy-level approaches

While there are no clinical practice guidelines developed specifically to define palliative care of the underserved, *Clinical Practice Guidelines for Quality Palliative Care* does serve as a useful framework for developing and evaluating services to meet the unique needs of these populations.[70] In particular, preferred practices addressing social aspects of care (Domain 4); spiritual, religious, and existential aspects of care (Domain 5); and cultural aspects of care (Domain 6) can be used to shape program development and service evaluation.

Two programs designed to meet the palliative care of the poor, one home-care based program in Hawaii[61] and a shelter-based program in Canada,[60] documented cost savings and favorable results for other quality indicators. These may serve as models for other communities with different needs and resources to consider in program development. Additionally palliative care services in safety net hospitals have demonstrated improved family satisfaction and increased the likelihood of patients/surrogate decision makers agreeing to DNR status when the patient is seriously ill and unlikely to survive this intervention.[62,63]

Obviously, at a policy and community level, stable housing is critical to providing a decent quality of life for any human being. Researchers noted the benefits of supportive housing to minority elders in East Harlem, including better psychological outcomes and increased use of informal supports,[71] and to persons who were chronically homeless with severe alcohol problems in Seattle, which demonstrated cost savings.[72] Housing First is a policy advocated by advocates for the homeless and for professionals caring for them, as the initial step in turning around the lives and hopefully preventing the premature deaths of those who are without a home (http://www.endhomelessness.org/pages/housing_first). Advocating for housing for the urban poor and those who are homeless is as critical as advocating for preventive care,

advocating for chronic disease management, advocating for symptom management, advocating for the opportunities to articulate wishes about end-of-life care, advocating for spiritual care and for mental health and addiction services. Without safe housing, the opportunities for a good enough death may not be possible.

Several scholars have argued regarding the social justice implications of palliative and end-of-life care. Crawley noted that within the African-American community premature deaths have been associated with both individual and institutional injustices.[73] Racism, discrimination and health disparities, and research abuses such as the Tuskegee syphilis study have betrayed the trust of many African-Americans and in part explained the determination among some to "go down fighting" rather than embrace some notion of a good death. A provocative essayist, Krakauer warned that advocating for palliative care in situations when disease modifying therapies was standard of care for resourced communities or countries was unjust, unacceptable, and perhaps unethical.[74] His argument was based on concerns about global efforts to offer palliative care to persons suffering with cancer or HIV disease because the costs of disease therapies were exorbitant and unattainable by resource-strapped developing economies. The same argument could be made for the poor in the United States. Palliative care should not be promoted as a substitute for society's failure to provide all Americans, rich and poor alike, with their basic needs for food, clothing, shelter, education, employment, community, or promising futures. In that way, palliative care must be part of a healthcare system and social contract that includes indicators of socioeconomic well-being alongside of safe environments, food and shelter, meaningful employment, support for families and communities, health promotion, disease prevention, chronic disease management, and palliative care.

Summary

Providing palliative care to the poor, especially the homeless, is extremely challenging. Comorbid illnesses, illnesses associated with poverty, and clarifying the etiology of presenting symptoms may seem almost impossible at times. Psychosocial risk factors and strained relationships with healthcare providers sometimes result in the client receiving futile or unwanted medical interventions at an advanced stage of illness. Clarifying with a patient what constitutes a good death for him/her can be humbling when the patient tells you he or she wants simply to have shelter and to feel safe. Meeting the palliative care needs of this underserved population will require innovative practice and education models. To truly improve end-of-life care for the poor, nurses need to advocate for public policies that assure access to safe and stable housing, health insurance, and client-centered, community-based primary care.

Acknowledgments

The author gratefully acknowledges the research and educational grant support of the American Cancer Society Doctoral Scholarship in Nursing; National Institute of Nursing Research, Ruth L. Kirschstein National Research Service Award F31NR079923; Oncology Nursing Society (ONS) Foundation Small Research Grant Award; ONS Doctoral Scholarship; UCSF Alpha Eta Research Award, Sigma Theta Tau Chapter and UCSF Graduate Student Research Award. She dedicates this chapter to the memory of Al, Tiffany, and Johnny—though they are no longer in this world, their stories and the stories of others like them continue to illuminate.

References

1. Flaskerud JH, Winslow BJ. Conceptualizing vulnerable populations health-related research. Nurs Res. 1998;47(2):69–78.
2. Hughes A. Meeting the palliative care needs of the underserved in core curriculum for the advanced practice hospice and palliative care registered nurse. In: Dahlin CM, Lynch MT (eds.), Pittsburgh, PA: Hospice and Palliative Nurses Association; 2013: 529–544.
3. Smedley BD, Stith AY, Nelson AR. Unequal treatment: confronting racial and ethnic disparities in health care. Washington, DC: National Academy Press; 2003.
4. Koenig BA, Gates-Williams J. Understanding cultural difference in caring for dying patients. West J Med. 1995;163(3):244–249.
5. Freeman HP. Poverty, culture and social injustice: determinants of cancer disparities. CA Cancer J Clin. 2004. 54(2):72–77.
6. Galea S, et al. Estimated deaths attributable to social factors in the United States. Am J Public Health. 2011;101(8):1456–1465.
7. Gibson R. Palliative care for the poor and disenfranchised: a view from the Robert Wood Johnson Foundation. J R Soc Med. 2001;94:486–489.
8. Hughes A. Poverty and palliative care in the US: issues facing the urban poor. Int J Palliative Nursing. 2005;11:6–13.
9. Hughes A. Meeting the palliative care needs of the underserved in core curriculum for the advanced practice hospice and palliative care registered nurse. In: Dahlin CM, Lynch MT (eds.), Pittsburgh, PA: Hospice and Palliative Nurses Association; 2013: 529–544.
10. Hughes A, Davies B, Gudmundsdottir M. "Can you give me respect?": Experiences of the urban poor on a dedicated AIDS nursing home unit. J Assoc Nurses AIDS Care. 2008;19:342–356.
11. Hughes A, Gundmundsdottir M, Davies B. Everyday struggling to survive: experiences of the urban poor living with advanced cancer. Oncol Nurs Forum. 2007;34:1113–1118.
12. Moller DW. Dancing with Broken Bones: Portraits of Death and Dying Among Inner-City Poor. New York: Oxford University Press; 2004.
13. Song J, et al. Dying on the streets: homeless persons' concerns and desires about end of life care. J Gen Intern Med. 2007;22(4):435–441.
14. Song J, et al. Experiences with and attitudes toward death and dying among homeless persons. J Gen Intern Med. 2007;22(4):427–434.
15. Lewis JM, et al. Dying in the margins: understanding palliative care and socioeconomic deprivation in the developed world. J Pain Symptom Manage. 2011;42(1):105–118.
16. Dzul-Church V, et al. "I'm sitting here by myself. . .": experiences of patients with serious illness at an Urban Public Hospital. J Palliat Med. 2010;13(6):695–701.
17. Lyckholm LJ, et al. Barriers to effective palliative care for low-income patients in late stages of cancer: report of a study and strategies for defining and conquering the barriers. Nurs Clin North Am. 2010;45(3):399–409.
18. Song J, et al. Engaging homeless persons in end of life preparations. J Gen Intern Med. 2008;23(12):2031–2036; quiz 2037–2045.
19. Kushel MB, Miaskowski C. End-of-life care for homeless patients: "She says she is there to help me in any situation." JAMA. 2006;296(24):2959–2966.
20. Lewis JM, et al. Dying in the margins: understanding palliative care and socioeconomic deprivation in the developed world. J PainSymptom Manage. 2011;42:105–118.
21. Taipale V. Ethics and allocation of health resources: the influence of poverty on health. Acta Oncol. 1999;38:51–55.
22. Blacksher E. On being poor and feeling poor: low socioeconomic status and the moral self. Theor Med Bioethics. 2002;23:455–470.
23. Hughes AM. "Can you give me respect?": Experiences of the urban poor with advanced disease. University of California San Francisco: School of Nursing; 2007:202.
24. Aday LA. At risk in America: the health and health care needs of vulnerable populations. 2nd ed. San Francisco: Jossey-Bass; 2001.
25. DeNavas-Walt C, Proctor BD, Smith JC. Income, Poverty, and Health Insurance Coverage in the United States: 2011. In: US Census Bureau (ed.), Current Population Reports, P60-243. Washington, DC: Government Printing Office; 2012.
26. Macartney S, Mykyta L. Poverty and Shared Households by State: 2011. In: US Dept. of Commerce, E.A.S. Administration, and US Census Bureau (eds.), American Community Survey Briefs, 2012.
27. National Coalition for the Homeless. How Many People Experience Homelessness? 2009. http://nationalhomeless.org/about-homelessness/ Accessed june 26, 2013
28. Crawley J, et al. Needs of the Hidden Homeless—No Longer Hidden: A Pilot Study. Public Health, 2013;127(7):674–680.
29. Fellin P. The culture of homelessness. In: Manoleas P (ed.), Cross-Cultural Practice of Clinical Case Management in Mental Health. New York: Haworth Press; 1996:41–77.
30. Strechlow AJ, Amos-Jones T. The homeless as a vulnerable population. Nurs Clin North Am. 1999;34(2):261–274.
31. National Coalition for the Homeless. Who Is Homeless? 2009. http://nationalhomeless.org/about-homelessness/ Accessed June 26, 2013
32. Lynch J, et al. Is income inequality a determination of population health? Pt 2: U.S. national and regional trends in income inequality and age- and cause-specific mortality. The Millbank Quarterly. 2004;82(2):355–400.
33. Horne BD, et al. Less affluent area of residence and lesser-insured status predict an increased risk of death or myocardial infarction after angiographic diagnosis of coronary disease. Ann Epidemiol. 2003;14:143–150.
34. Fang J, Alderman MH. Is geography destiny for patients in New York with myocardial infarction? Am J Med. 2003;115:448–453.
35. Hossain WA, et al. Healthcare access and disparities in chronic medical conditions in urban populations. South Med J. 2013;106(4): 246–254.
36. Baggett TP, et al. Mortality among homeless adults in Boston: shifts in causes of death over a 15-year period. JAMA. 2013;173(3):189–195.
37. Patchell T. Nowhere to run: portraits of life on the street. Turning Wheel: Journal of Socially Engaged Buddhism. 1996:4–21.
38. Crawley LM. Racial, cultural, and ethnic factors influencing end-of-life care. J Palliat Med. 2005;8(Suppl. 1):S58–S69.
39. Hawkins NM, et al. Heart failure and socioeconomic status: accumulating evidence of inequality. Eur J Heart Fail. 2012;14(2):138–146.
40. Gordon EJ, et al. Disparities in kidney transplant outcomes: a review. Semin Nephrol. 2010;30(1):81–89.
41. Smith AK, Ladner D, McCarthy EP. Racial/ethnic disparities in liver transplant surgery and hospice use: parallels, differences, and unanswered questions. Am J Hosp Palliat Care. 2008;25(4):285–291.
42. Edwards TA, et al. Cancer care in East and Central Harlem: community partnership needs assessment. J Cancer Educ. 2013;28(1):171–178.
43. American Cancer Society. Cancer Facts and Figures 2011. Atlanta: American Cancer Society; 2011.
44. Barnato AE, et al. Racial and ethnic differences in preferences for end-of-life treatment. J Gen Intern Med. 2009;24(6):695–701.
45. Kiefer CW. Health Work with the Poor: A Practical Guide. New Brunswick, NJ: Rutgers University Press; 2000.
46. Bender M, et al. Missed opportunities in providing palliative care for the urban poor: a case discussion. J Palliat Med 2013;16:587–590.
47. O'Connor PG, Selwyn PA, Schottenfeld RS. Medical care for injection drug users with human immunodeficiency syndrome. N Engl J Med. 1994;331:450–459.
48. Centers for Disease Control and Prevention. Opioids Drive Continued Increase in Drug Overdose Deaths. 2013. http://www.cdc.gov/media/releases/2013/p0220_drug_overdose_deaths.html, Accessed June 30, 2014
49. Morrison RS, et al. "We don't carry that": Failure of pharmacies in predominantly nonwhite neighborhoods to stock opioid analgesics. N Engl J Med. 2000;342:1023–1026.
50. Soares LGL. Poor social condition, criminality and urban violence: unmentioned barriers for effective cancer pain control at the end of life. J Pain Symptom Manage. 2003;26(2):693–695.
51. Kircher S, et al. Understanding and treating opioid addiction in a patient with cancer pain. J Pain. 2011;12(10):1025–1031.

52. Newshan G, Staats JA. Evidence-based pain guidelines in HIV care. J Assoc Nurses AIDS Care. 2013;24(1 Suppl):S112–S126.

53. Passik SD. Issues in long-term opioid therapy: unmet needs, risks, and solutions. Mayo Clin Proc. 2009;84(7):593–601.

54. Chou R, et al. Opioids for chronic noncancer pain: prediction and identification of aberrant drug-related behaviors: a review of the evidence for an American Pain Society and American Academy of Pain Medicine clinical practice guideline. J Pain. 2009;10(2):131–146.

55. Miaskowski C, et al. Occurrence and characteristics of chronic pain in a community-based cohort of indigent adults living with HIV infection. J Pain. 2011;12(9):1004–1016.

56. Panel on Guidelines for Adults and Adolescents, Guidelines for the Use of Antiretroviral Agents in HIV-1-Infected Adults and Adolescents. Dept. of Health and Human Services; 2013. http://aidsinfo.nih.gov/contentfiles/lvguidelines/AdultandAdolescentGL.pdf, downloaded 6/30/2014

57. Bangsberg D, Tulsky JP, Hecht FM, Moss AR. Protease inhibitors in the homeless. JAMA. 1997;278:63–65.

58. United Way, The Bottom Line: Setting the Real Standard for Bay Area Working Families. San Francisco: United Way of Bay Area; 2004:28.

59. Hughes A. Poor, homeless and underserved populations. In: Ferrell BR, Coyle N (eds.), Oxford Textbook of Palliative Nursing. New York: Oxford University Press; 2010:745–755.

60. Podymow T, Turnbull J, Coyle D. Shelter-based palliative care for the homeless terminally ill. Palliat Med. 2006;20(2):81–86.

61. Fernandes R, et al. Home-based palliative care services for underserved populations. J Palliat Med. 2010;13(4):413–419.

62. Kaufer M, et al. Family satisfaction following the death of a loved one in an inner city MICU. Am J Hosp Palliat Care. 2008;25(4):318–325.

63. Sacco J, Carr DR, Viola D. The effects of the palliative medicine consultation on the DNR status of African Americans in a safety-net hospital. Am J Hosp Palliat Care. 2013;30(4):363–369.

64. Tarzian AJ, Neal MT, O'Neil JA. Attitudes, experiences, and beliefs affecting end-of-life decision-making among homeless individuals. J Palliat Med. 2005;8(1):36–48.

65. Sudore RL, et al. An advance directive redesigned to meet the literacy level of most adults: a randomized trial. Patient Educ Couns. 2007;69(1–3):165–195.

66. Dula A, Williams S. When race matters. Clin Geriatr Med. 2005;21(1):239–253, xi.

67. Davis E, Tamayo A, Fernandez A. "Because somebody cared about me. That's how it changed things": homeless, chronically ill patients' perspectives on case management. PLoS One. 2012;7(9): e45980.

68. Teti M, et al. "I'm a keep rising. I'm a keep going forward, regardless": exploring Black men's resilience amid sociostructural challenges and stressors. Qual Health Res. 2012;22(4):524–533.

69. Born W, et al. Knowledge, attitudes, and beliefs about end-of-life care among inner-city African Americans and Latinos. J Palliat Med. 2004;7(2):247–256.

70. National Consensus Project. Clinical Practice Guidelines for Quality Palliative Care. 3rd edition. Pittsburgh, PA: National Consensus Project for Quality Palliative Care; 2013.

71. Cleak H, Howe JL. Social networks and use of social supports of minority elders inn East Harlem. Soc Work Health Care. 2003;38(1):19–38.

72. Larimer ME, et al. Health care and public service use and costs before and after provision of housing for chronically homeless persons with severe alcohol problems. JAMA. 2009;301(13):1349–1357.

73. Crawley LM. Palliative care in African American communities. J Palliat Med. 2002;5(5):775–779.

74. Krakauer EL. Just palliative care: responding responsibly to the suffering of the poor. J Pain Symptom Manage. 2008;36(5):505–512.

75. Patchell T. Suggestions for Effective Outreach. San Francisco: Department of Public Health, Homeless Death Prevention Project; 1997.

CHAPTER 39

End-of-life care for patients with mental illness and personality disorders

Betty D. Morgan

She had a history of bipolar disease and had been treated for that for a long time. She had a history of suicidal ideation with her severe depressive episodes and also attempted suicide. She felt that was no longer an issue; that the prominent issue right now was that her life was going to end. And she wasn't ready for that to happen.

Key points

- Enhanced communication skills with an emphasis on therapeutic communication are needed to work with patients with serious mental illness (SMI) and personality disorders (PDs)

- Ethical issues including capacity/competency may arise when working with people with SMI and PD, however, simply having a diagnosis of SMI or PD does not necessarily indicate lack of capacity or competency

- Redefinition of family may need to take place in order to include the patient's support system in their care

- Consultation/collaboration is essential in caring for the population of people with SMI or PD to meet the needs of the patient and their support system

Approximately 26.2% of Americans (about one in four) aged 18 years and older are diagnosed with a mental disorder in any given year. This translates to more than 57 million people in the United States. A smaller number of people, approximately 6% of Americans (1 in 17) suffer from an SMI such as schizophrenia, bipolar disease, or severe depression.[1] Comorbidity is common; almost half of the people who are diagnosed with a mental disorder meet criteria for a second mental disorder, with mood, anxiety, and addictive disorders being the most common comorbid illnesses.[1] The Global Burden of Disease study presented data revealing that mental illness accounted for 7.4 % of all disease-adjusted life years that measure disease burden.[2]

People with SMI reportedly die 20 to 25 years earlier than the general population worldwide.[3] The increase in mortality has been associated with both natural and "unnatural" causes of death, with unnatural causes defined as suicide, homicide, and accidental death.[4] Comorbid medical illnesses that are commonly observed in those with SMI include hypertension, cardiac disease, diabetes and other metabolic conditions, respiratory illnesses, obesity, renal disease, cerebrovascular disease, cancer, and HIV/AIDS.[4,5] Additionally, an estimated one-third to one-half of the homeless people in the world have schizophrenia.[6-9]

Sixty percent of premature deaths in persons with schizophrenia are due to medical conditions such as cardiovascular, pulmonary and infectious diseases.[3] Since these illnesses may be related to lifestyle factors such as tobacco use and obesity, in these instances they can be viewed as preventable.

This chapter examines what is known about palliative care and the mentally ill, including those with SMI and PDs. Special issues related to communication and treatment are presented as well as strategies for care for this population. Ethical issues including capacity and competency for decision-making as it relates to those with SMI and end-of-life care are also discussed. Collaboration and consultation between providers is essential in providing end-of-life care for those with SMI.

Research related to serious mental illness and end-of-life care

Little research has been conducted in end-of-life issues with people with SMI, and those who have SMI have been underserved in terms of palliative care. Barriers to both care and research have been cited as capacity of patients to make end-of-life decisions, provider concerns that end-of-life discussions would be upsetting, and lack of provider training and comfort in conducting discussions about end-of-life care.[9,10] However, Foti and colleagues demonstrated that a group of community-residing adults with SMI were able to designate treatment preferences for end-of life care in response to scenarios involving end-of-life situations.[11] Participants chose aggressive pain management in a scenario including pain and incurable cancer and were divided in their responses between waiting for a defined period before turning off life-support, terminating life support immediately, and keeping the person alive indefinitely for a patient with an irreversible coma. The researchers also provided follow-up with participants who were distressed by the research questions but found that none required crisis intervention or were so distressed that psychiatric decompensation was a risk.[12]

Much of the existing research has focused on identifying the increase in morbidity and mortality in this population and understanding what factors contribute to the increase. The majority of these studies were conducted in inpatient psychiatric settings, where the sickest patients and those with the most comorbid illnesses may be found. Piatt, Munetz, and Ritter broadened the discussion about the higher death rates among those with SMI by examining a population not restricted to the sickest of patients with SMI. The researchers found, by looking at case files from a community mental health center and examining years of potential life lost (YPLL), that people with SMI had a mean/standard deviation of 14.5 YPLL +/- 10.6 compared with the general population YPLL of 10.3 +/- 6.7.[10] This study also revealed that despite the fact that more people with SMI died from unnatural causes such as suicide, accidents, and assaults than the general population, most of the deaths were actually attributed to natural causes. Four specific causes contributed to the increased death for people with SMI: cancer, chronic lower respiratory diseases, dementia, and pneumonia.

Barriers to care for patients with mental illness

There are several barriers to consistent medical care for those with a mental illness; these barriers exist in primary care settings and apply to palliative care settings as well. Lack of preventive care or an ongoing relationship with a medical provider is a key issue for people with mental illness. People with SMI often seek care later in the course of the disease, resulting in costly services and complex care needs. Inadequate support systems that are common among those with SMI affect their ability to access medical care and navigate the complex health system. Adherence is a major problem in the treatment of people with SMI, and adherence to medical regimes for this population is compounded by mental health and addictive problems, homelessness, or lack of transportation to get to medical providers. Lack of financial resources may complicate the patient's ability to receive timely care or treatment.

Symptoms of SMI can have profound effects on communication, which can result in problems with development of the therapeutic relationship. In addition, symptoms of SMI can have an impact on reporting of problematic symptoms or the effect of treatment on the symptoms. One study in the Veterans Affairs (VA) system posited that people with SMI may not be able to tolerate lengthy and difficult life-sustaining treatments and might lack the supportive network that helps people endure such treatment. Therefore patients with SMI may also accept comfort care earlier on than patients who do not have SMI.[6] Finally, stigma affects communication about all aspects of care of the medical illness, including assessment, explanation of treatment options, adherence, and the development of a trusting relationship with the patient.[5,6]

Serious mental illness

Psychotic symptoms may occur as a result of certain medical conditions, substance abuse, schizophrenia, schizoaffective disorder, mania, dementia, and depression. Serious mental illness includes illnesses such as schizophrenia and other psychotic disorders, bipolar disease, and severe depression. A brief discussion of each of these illnesses will be presented; however, depression is described in detail in chapter 20. Treatment issues and special concerns in communication will be discussed as they relate to palliative care.

Schizophrenia and other psychotic disorders

Schizophrenia affects approximately 1% of the US population. However, it accounts for 40% of mental health facility beds and 9% of all hospital beds. It is a devastating illness to those who are affected—both the patient and the family of the patient. The symptoms of schizophrenia include what are referred to as positive symptoms (exaggerated or distorted function) and negative symptoms (diminution or loss of normal function). The positive symptoms include delusions, hallucinations, and disorganized and bizarre behavior and speech as well as deterioration of social behavior. The negative symptoms include flattened affect, decreased range and intensity of expression, anhedonia, restricted thought and speech, amotivation, apathy, and difficulty in mental focus and ability to sustain attention.[7,8] Other psychotic disorders, including schizoaffective disorder, delusional disorder, brief psychotic disorder, and shared psychotic disorder (folie à deux), share many of the same psychotic symptoms with schizophrenia.[6,7]

Psychotic symptoms may also be due to medications, substances, withdrawal syndromes from substances, and delirium due to other medical conditions. Such etiologies for the presenting symptoms must always be ruled out before assuming that there is a psychotic disorder present. At the end of life people with SMI may appear to have a worsening of their condition when the issue may really involve an acute mental status change due to delirium, in addition to their underlying illness.

Some of the more limiting symptoms of psychotic disorders that are of particular concern in palliative care settings are the ability to participate in decision-making, perceptual difficulties that can affect sensory integration, concrete thought processes, and difficulty in attention and concentration. The effect of perceptual difficulties has been demonstrated in research related to pain sensation in people with schizophrenia. Patients with schizophrenia may have reduced sensitivity to pain, and this could lead to delays in care or treatment.[13]

Treatment of schizophrenia and other psychotic disorders

Treatment is based on symptom management. As in palliative care, there is no curative treatment for serious mental illness and all treatment can be considered palliative in nature. Pharmacological and nonpharmacological interventions are both used to treat psychotic disorders; however, nonpharmacological interventions may not be effective unless interfering hallucinations or delusions are brought under some degree of control. The patient may then be able to participate in nonpharmacological interventions.

Pharmacological treatment

Table 39.1 lists first-generation or typical antipsychotics. These medications, developed in the 1950s and 1960s, were very effective in the treatment of the positive symptoms, and some—but not all—of these medications had an effect on negative symptoms. The negative side effect profiles of these medications, including extrapyramidal symptoms (EPS), tardive dyskinesia (TD), and anticholinergic effects, had a profound effect on quality of life and medication adherence.[8,14]

Table 39.1 Antipsychotic medications

First generation (typicals)	Second generation (atypicals)
Chlorpromazine (Thorazine)	Clozapine (Clozaril)
Thioridizine (Mellaril)	Risperidone (Risperidol)
Perphenazine (Trilafon)	Olanzapine (Zyprexa)
Trifluoperazine (Stelazine)	Quetiapine (Seroquel)
Fluphenazine (Prolixin)	Ziprasidone (Geodon)
Thiothixene (Navane)	Aripiprazole (Abilify)
Haloperidon (Haldol)	
Loxapine (Loxitane)	
Molindone (Moban)	
Pimozide (Orap)	

Sources: Adapted from Beebe (2012), reference 8; Chan (2008), reference 14.

In the 1980s the second-generation or atypical antipsychotics were developed (Table 39.1). These medications reduced both the positive and negative symptoms associated with schizophrenia, improved cognition, and were useful in treatment for patients who were considered treatment-refractory. The side-effect profile of the second-generation drugs showed lower rates of EPS and TD and fewer anticholinergic effects. However, the emergence of metabolic syndrome, including pronounced weight gain, diabetes, hyperlipidemia, and hypercholesterolemia, has resulted in the need for close monitoring of their use in treating psychotic disorders.[14] These medications result in cardiovascular problems and compound the existing higher prevalence of cardiovascular problems in people with schizophrenia.

Pharmacological treatment of psychotic symptoms in conjunction with palliative care treatment should be closely monitored by consultation with the psychiatric providers. Any change in mental status should be immediately evaluated. Screening for the presence of delirium, which can occur frequently at the end of life, should occur with any change in mental status. It should not be assumed that the psychiatric illness is the cause of a mental status change until a physical cause is ruled out. Several of the typical and atypical antipsychotic medications share common metabolic pathways with opioid analgesics. Inhibition or potentiation of the antipsychotic or the opioid medication is possible; therefore, close monitoring is essential.[14]

Nonpharmacological treatments

Nonpharmacological interventions include psychotherapeutic strategies such as supportive psychotherapy, cognitive-behavioral therapy (CBT), group therapy, skills training, and complementary therapies. Collaborative care with psychiatric providers can include additional supportive therapy to assist patients facing a terminal illness. People with SMI face the same end-of-life concerns as patients without mental illness, such as dealing with pain and suffering, fear of what lies ahead, fear of becoming a burden, spiritual concerns, financial concerns, and difficulty "saying goodbye."[15] People with schizophrenia may need additional support and extra time to process medical information. This extra support is best provided by professionals who already have a relationship with the patient, and the psychiatric providers should be included in discussions of treatment options in the palliative care setting.

Ethical issues in caring for people with serious mental illness at the end of life

There are several ethical issues related to the care of people with SMI at the end of life that require consideration over and above the consideration given to people without SMI. Care of vulnerable populations such as those with SMI carries a greater obligation for nurses to provide advocacy and protection from violation of the patient's autonomy and right to make decisions about care.

Right to refuse medication

In the 1970s psychiatric patients filed lawsuits related to their rights to refuse medication treatment. Legal decisions in Massachusetts and New York, the states where the most prominent cases were filed, resulted in different approaches to the problem. The Massachusetts decision resulted in the *Rogers* decision, which decreed that a guardian needed to be appointed for incompetent patients to deal strictly with the psychiatric medication in question and that the final decision would be left to a judge. The concept of substituted judgment—that is, what the person would consent to if they were competent—is how the judge evaluated the question of whether to give the guardian the right to overrule the patient's right to refuse medication.[16] Other states have panels, independent consultants, or psychiatrists make the decision about right to refuse medication. It is important to know the state law about the right to refuse medication so that each nurse can practice within the rules and regulations under which he/she is governed.

Advance directives

Advance directives, in terms of decisions about psychiatric care in a future emergency situation, have been a focus of concern over the last decade. Providing a patient with the opportunity to discuss their wishes, in advance, has assisted with the need to have a legal competency hearing to determine a course of treatment. Including a discussion of the patient's wishes for end-of-life care is an area that needs further exploration in psychiatric settings. Research has indicated a low rate of advance directives for either psychiatric care or medical care in patients with SMI.[6,10,17]

Capacity and competency

The ability to make decisions about treatment is a cornerstone of good palliative care. Controversy can occur when a person loses the capacity to participate in informed decision-making or a competent person refuses life-sustaining treatments. A general rule is that all competent persons have the right to make their own decisions, even when decisions conflict with what a majority would decide under similar circumstances.[17] When the patient is a person who has schizophrenia or another psychiatric disorder, the ability to make decisions may be compromised by psychotic thought processes. However, having a diagnosis of a mental illness, even one with psychotic features, does not automatically mean that a person is incompetent.[15] When treatment decisions of the patient are questioned by providers and there is no advance directive about treatment wishes, then a psychiatric evaluation must be requested.

Capacity indicates the ability to understand the problem and make decisions. A psychiatric provider makes a "clinical assessment of the patient's capacity to function in certain areas."[17]

"Competency" is a legal term and is decided by a court of law based on the capacity assessment of a psychiatric provider. Competency is usually confined to a specific area or task, such as the ability to make a will, the ability to testify in court, decision-making capacity, or the right to refuse treatment.[17] Applebaum and Grisso outlined four criteria used to determine capacity to consent to treatment[18]:

♦ Patient expression of a preference

♦ Ability to understand the illness, the prognosis with and without treatment, and the risks and benefits of the treatment (factual understanding)

♦ An appreciation of the significance of the facts (significance of the facts)

♦ Ability to use the information in a rational way to reach a decision in a logical manner (rationality of the thought processes)

Intense pain, depression, delirium, dementia, and psychosis are the most common causes of incompetence.[17] However, the existence of one of these conditions does not necessarily mean that a person is incompetent. Careful assessment of each individual is necessary to determine capacity and competency. "Competency" is a legal term, but most courts do accept the evaluation of capacity provided by the psychiatric professional. A patient is not deemed competent or incompetent until a court of law rules.

Aggression and psychotic disorders

Patients enter healthcare systems in great distress, and palliative care settings are no exception. When the patient has a SMI the distress may be even greater than in the general population, because people with SMI may have inadequate coping resources and are in a crisis state when dealing with a life-threatening illness. Most often, people become aggressive when they feel threatened in some way. The aggressive behavior may be the result of perceptual problems, such as hallucinations or delusions, and the aggressive behavior often masks a lack of confidence in self. Aggressive behavior may be a way to enhance self-esteem by overpowering others.[19,20]

There are some important predictors of aggressive behavior, including impulsivity, hostility, family history of violent or abusive behavior, substance use, and irritability.[19,20] Prevention of aggressive behavior focuses on early recognition of escalating behaviors, such as pacing, nonverbal expressions, yelling, or an angry tone of voice. Allowing the person a chance to talk may defuse the situation. It is important for the nurse to use nonthreatening body language, and to communicate with a calm but firm voice while conveying respect for the patient and his/her feelings. Allowing the patient some choice about the situation is often a way to help the patient gain some control.[19]

Communication issues and psychotic disorders

The cornerstone of both palliative care and psychiatric care is the importance of communication and the establishment of a trusting, therapeutic relationship between the nurse and the patient. Traditionally, psychiatric providers are not comfortable with medically ill patients and medical providers are not comfortable with psychiatrically ill patients. Additionally, many people with mental illness are housed in nontraditional settings. Staff of any of these settings, including medical hospital units, palliative care units, or psychiatric units as well as the homeless shelters, prisons, and nursing homes may be ill equipped to deal with psychiatric problems in the face of terminal illness. Education of all staff about mental illness and end-of-life care in these settings will result in better care for patients with SMI.[5]

There are additional communication issues and strategies involved when providing palliative care to those with psychotic illnesses. The role of stigma affects all aspects of care and communication. Patients may conceal or not report pain and other symptoms because of fear of the meaning of the symptom, self-blame, guilt, anger, or denial. As mentioned previously, mental status changes should be evaluated for a medical cause of delirium before assuming that altered perceptions or hallucinations are the result of psychotic disorder.

If the patient is delusional or hallucinating, then a safety assessment should be completed and arrangements made to keep the patient safe from self-harm. The content of the hallucinations or delusions can be very important. Any thoughts or hallucinations that the patient expresses concerning the need to die or presence of command hallucinations telling the person to die require immediate psychiatric consultation. Patient safety mechanisms, such as evaluation by emergency services (for outpatient settings) or use of sitters or frequent observation (for inpatient settings) should be instituted until the psychiatric assessment can occur.

Maintaining a calm presence and use of a quiet tone of voice, nonthreatening demeanor, and stance are important strategies when dealing with all patients who are psychotic. Decrease of environmental stimuli, such as turning off a radio or television, will decrease distractions and help the patient focus on the immediate medical care. Because the ability to concentrate or pay attention may be affected by the mental illness, detailed explanations may be needed, with additional time allowed for the patient to process the information. Conversations focused on understanding what the patient has processed about the information may need to take place over lengthened periods of time. Patients may also tend to focus on concrete parts of the information, and it can be helpful to provide alternative ways to view the situation if a patient appears to be stuck or focused on one particular aspect of the issue. Occasionally, people with psychotic disorders may become more focused and less psychotic in the face of a life-threatening illness.

Patients with SMI who are actively hallucinating or delusional, as well as those who may be delirious and experiencing altered perceptions, should receive explanations of all physical care to be delivered. Before touching the patient, it is important to let him or her know what is to be done, as the patient might misinterpret the touch and react as if he or she is being assaulted. Patients with SMI may have a different sense of private space and may also react to violations of personal space.

Family issues

For many people with SMI there are strained, distant, or nonexistent ties with their family of origin. Some of this disconnection may result from years of strain, disappointment, financial burden, and fear caused by threatening behavior. Families of patients with SMI may also have their own mental health issues and may use defensive strategies such as denial or anger in dealing with the medical problems. Additionally, family members may have been dealing with chronic sorrow related to the mental health issues of the family member, may be overprotective, and/or may be psychologically fatigued due to years of care-taking responsibilities. Careful assessment of family functioning in these situations may be beyond the scope of the hospice and palliative care nurse and may require consultation with psychiatric mental health providers.

When the patient is competent and there is discord in the family, conflict may arise if providers are restricted about the information they can give to the family due to Health Insurance Portability and Accountability Act (HIPPA) concerns and/or patient refusal for family inclusion in healthcare discussions. A family member who has been the caregiver for the patient for years and is then shut out from information about the medical illness and treatment options may respond with anger and frustration. Family meetings may be of help in these situations; if there has been an involved mental health provider, this person should definitely be included in the meetings; if there has been no mental health provider, then consultation for the patient and/or family with a mental health provider, prior to a family meeting may be useful. Finding out which supportive services, if any, have helped the family in dealing with the mental health issues is vital. Groups such as the National Alliance on Mental Illness (NAMI, www.nami.org) have been a tremendous support to families with a member with a mental illness. The National Alliance on Mental Illness also runs support groups for family members, and families may have established connections with these groups; if so, they should be encouraged to increase their participation in these groups. These NAMI groups may not be focused on end-of-life issues but are familiar with many of the ethical/legal aspects of caring for someone with a mental illness and may be more appropriate than a support group for families focused only on end-of-life issues. As with any patient and family, careful assessment will be key in developing the best treatment approach for the individual and their family.

Many people with SMI are cared for by the state government, and long-term relationships with psychiatric providers or staff of mental health housing programs may have become a substitute for family. The inclusion of these staff into the palliative care team is essential to ensuring that the treatment will be properly performed and for providing the day-to-day intensive support that may be required for the patient. Like family, staff will also have their own particular needs for support because most psychiatric providers do not have end-of-life care experience or education. Fellow patients with SMI make up the other component of family that needs to be considered in palliative care of people with SMI. Occasionally, long-term relationships with other people with SMI are the most significant relationships in the person's life. Special needs for support should be considered for this group of people as well. Although palliative care staff may not be involved in delivering this support, the collaborative partnerships with psychiatric providers should be available for support for this group of people.

Case study

A 47-year-old man with schizophrenia

JD is a 47-year-old Hispanic male with a long-term diagnosis of schizophrenia who is single and is currently living in a group home for people with SMI. Both of his parents are deceased, and he has had no contact with his siblings for over 20 years. He has had multiple hospitalizations, has lived in homeless shelters, and has been in prison twice for aggravated assaults and theft. He has been stabilized on Clozaril for the last 8 years and is adherent with his medication regime as long as he is in the group home and is given his medication by staff members. He has a long history of

polysubstance abuse including alcohol and was diagnosed with pancreatic cancer 5 months ago. He has had increasing amounts of abdominal pain since that time, and the staff at the group home are currently having trouble managing his needs for pain medication.

He is followed by a psychiatric nurse practitioner (PMHNP) at the mental health clinic where he has received care for the last decade. The NP decides to make a home visit (which she has done in the past) so that she can see the patient in his home setting as well as meet with the group home staff. On the visit she finds that his apartment/room in the house is dirty and that he has not emptied trash including old food for over a week, his personal hygiene is less than optimal, and the staff are very uncomfortable with the opioid medication that they are giving him and have concerns about the addictive potential of the medication as well as concerns that other patients may try to steal the medication.

The NP talks with both the staff and JD about a referral for home hospice care, emphasizing the help this would provide for personal care, homemaker services, and closer attention to pain management. This initial discussion is very upsetting—more so for the staff than to JD! JD is clear that he does not have that long to live and has capacity to make his own decisions and voices a clear desire to stay in the group home rather than be transferred to a nursing home for care. The staff are shocked to hear that he may die within 6 months and are initially resistant to the idea of hospice care. In talking more with the staff (many of whom are in their early 20s) the NP finds that none of them have seen someone die and are very reluctant to take on this kind of care. The NP contacts the group home director following her visit to find out what the policy of the group home is for caring for someone at the end of life (there is no policy) and discuss JD's wishes as well as the staff concerns. The group home director agrees to meet with the NP and the staff the following week to discuss JD's care.

The NP establishes contact with the area home hospice organization to find out what services would be available and discusses the care with the primary care physician who has only seen the patient once since the diagnosis of pancreatic cancer. The physician states that the prognosis for JD is 6 months or less and is agreeable to the hospice referral.

At the meeting the following week with the group home staff several staff members express their hesitation about caring for JD "till he dies" but are willing to learn more about hospice care and pain management for the time being. The psychiatric NP agrees to be involved with more home visits and coordinating care with the hospice nurses as well as providing some support to the group home staff. As time passes at least one of the group home staff becomes a strong advocate for JD and influences the other staff to continue to care for JD in the group home as his disease progresses. The staff from the hospice provided some educational sessions about pain/addiction that addressed the staff concerns and provided a lock-box for the opioid medication to ensure safety.

Five months later JD has a quiet and peaceful death in his group home surrounded by his fellow house mates and staff members.

This case illustrates several issues of importance:

- Capacity and the ability of patients to make their own decisions should be assumed despite diagnosis, unless there is a clear reason to suspect impaired capacity
- The need for regular medical care of patients with SMI

◆ The need for expansion of definition of family—often residential treatment staff are the ones with daily contact and may best know the patient's wishes regarding care

◆ The need for education of group home staff in care of the dying

◆ The need for attention to grief and bereavement of the staff and other group home residents

Bipolar disease

Bipolar disease has a fluctuating course and often results in recurrent episodes of depression, hypomania or mania. People with bipolar disease frequently discontinue their medication because of unwanted side effects and/or the feelings associated with hypomania that may result in increased productivity and pleasure. Bipolar disorder is often comorbid with other psychiatric disorders, particularly with alcohol or substance use disorders. People with bipolar disorder have more co-occurring medical conditions—especially cardiovascular disease and other problems related to metabolic syndrome—than those with other chronic mental illnesses.[21] As with psychotic disorders like schizophrenia, the use of second-generation antipsychotic medications as mood stabilizers for those with bipolar disease has increased the risk of diabetes and subsequent cardiovascular disease among people with this diagnosis.[21]

Bipolar and related disorders is a separate and new category in the DSM-5. In past issues of the DSM, bipolar disorder was included in the mood disorders category along with major depressive disorder.[7] Depression is discussed in detail in chapter 20. Bipolar I is described as having at least one episode of elevated, expansive mood for at least 1 week, causing impairment in occupational, or social functioning. "The manic episode may have been preceded by, and may be followed by, hypomanic or major depressive episodes."

Symptoms of hypomania or mania include an inflated self-esteem, grandiosity, decreased need for sleep, pressured speech, flight of ideas, increase in activities, and excessive involvement in pleasurable activities that have a high potential for consequences.[7] Severe mania can present more with symptoms of agitation than euphoria and often includes psychotic episodes as well.

Bipolar II disorder is characterized by at least one current or past hypomanic episode and a current or past major depressive episode.[7] In past years Bipolar II was considered to be a less severe form than Bipolar I. This is no longer considered true given the amount of time that people with Bipolar II disorder are depressed along with the accompanying social and occupational altered functioning that can occur with this disorder.[7]

Treatment of bipolar disorder

As with any psychiatric illness, careful assessment is the first step of any treatment. This is of particular concern in treating mood disorders. Inaccurate assessment of depression/bipolar disorder may result in initiation of antidepressant medication and precipitate a manic episode in someone with bipolar disorder. Additionally, people with bipolar disorder are at a higher risk for suicidal ideation than those with any other psychiatric disorder.[22] Treatment of bipolar disorder includes mood-stabilizing medications such as lithium and other drugs (Box 39.1). When patients are in a manic state or a severe depression, they may lack decision-making capacity but are then often capable of making decisions when they

Box 39.1	Mood stabilizers

◆ Lithium (Eskalith, Lithobid)

◆ Lithium citrate

Benzodiazepines

◆ Alprazalam (Xanax)

◆ Chlordiazepoxide (Librium)

◆ Clonazepam (Klonopin)

◆ Diazepam (Valium)

◆ Lorazepam (Ativan)

◆ Oxazepma (Serax)

◆ Prazepam (Centrax)

Anticonvulsants

◆ Valproic Acid (Depakene, Depakote)

◆ Lamotrigine (Lamictal)

◆ Carbamazepine (Tegretol)

◆ Gabapentin (Neurontin)

◆ Oxcarbazepine (Trileptal)

◆ Topiramate (Topamax)

◆ Tiagabine (Gabatril)

Calcium channel blockers

◆ Verapamil (Calan)

◆ Nifedipine (Adalat, Procardia)

◆ Nimodipine (Nimotop)

Source: Perese (2012), reference 22.

become stable. A psychiatric provider should be a part of the palliative care team and provide close follow-up for people with bipolar disorder. Any medications used in treatment of the underlying medical illness should be reviewed for their potential to induce a manic episode.[14] As with psychotic disorders, there are many psychotherapeutic interventions that are utilized in treatment of people with bipolar disorder, but patients frequently need to be stabilized with medications before these treatments are able to be used effectively.

Additional medications

Treatment of bipolar disorder in the acute phase of either a depressive episode or a manic episode may include medications in addition to the mood stabilizers indicated in Box 39.1. Use of atypical antipsychotic medication is often necessary for stabilization of a person in an acute manic episode. Benzodiazepines may also be used to supplement the use of antipsychotics and mood stabilizers. Antidepressants may also be used in treatment of the depressive symptoms along with the mood stabilizers.[22]

Nonpharmacological interventions in treatment of bipolar disease

A variety of psychotherapies have been utilized with bipolar disease; most often therapies are used in conjunction with psychopharmacological interventions. Interpersonal therapy and CBT are two of the most widely used therapies with this disorder. Provision of patient and family education is essential as well as social and coping skills training.[22]

Communication issues and bipolar disorder

Communicating with someone during a manic episode can be difficult because patients may be emotionally labile and very talkative (with pressured speech), may not be able to stop and listen or concentrate, and often reject help.[23] Patients can be quite charming and even entertaining during some stages of a manic episode. Staff members need to see these presentations as a part of the illness and not join in grandiose discussions or plans. Patients may need to be gently redirected so that they do not go off on tangents unrelated to the medical issue at hand. They may also need firm but caring limits set on behaviors that might affect others' care, such as wandering into other patients' rooms, becoming inappropriately involved in others' care, and intrusion in staff conversations with other patients. Assisting patients in calming behaviors such as sitting quietly with the patient or closing the door to the room to decrease external stimuli are strategies that maybe helpful. Inclusion of the psychiatric provider in the team will allow for communication of information about the best approach to take with an individual suffering with bipolar disorder.

Often, one of the first symptoms of a manic episode is the decreased need for sleep. Early reporting of change of sleep habits is important because it is easier to help someone regain stability early in the course of a manic episode. If the patient is beginning to exhibit signs of mania and/or psychosis, then assessment of safety issues and the potential for suicide must be considered. The importance of early intervention in escalating symptoms and good interteam communication cannot be emphasized enough when caring for someone with bipolar disorder.

Case study

A 45-year-old woman suffering from bipolar disease

Jill is a 45-year-old white female suffering from bipolar disease. She has had a very difficult course of her disease, with multiple hospitalizations following suicide attempts. Additionally, she has HIV due to a long history of heroin abuse. Her HIV has progressed over the last 12 years and her viral load has not been suppressed sufficiently by the last four medication regimens. For the last 2 years, she has been followed for supportive therapy by a psychiatric clinical nurse specialist.

Jill lives with her older brother, who is the only family member who has remained involved in her life. He has had to act as her guardian for a number of years because of Jill's psychosis during manic episodes as well as her severe depression. The physician discusses options for care with Jill and her brother and suggests a referral for hospice care. Shortly after this meeting, Jill stopped taking all of her medications and was rehospitalized with severe depression and suicidal thoughts. She has recompensated and returned to her brother's home. She now wants to live and is very meticulous in adhering to her psychiatric medication. The psychiatric clinical nurse specialist meets with Jill and her brother and brings up the issue of a hospice referral again.

Jill's brother has been unable to accept the prognosis and does not want to involve hospice services at this point. Jill becomes less able to care for herself over the next month and is eventually admitted to the hospital for severe dehydration and unresponsiveness. She is never discharged from the hospital and dies with her brother at her side a week and a half after the hospital admission. Jill's brother is despondent and blaming himself for not helping her more. The hospital social worker refers Jim to the area mental health center for counseling.

This case highlights several factors that are important in the palliative care of patients with mental illness:

- Some patients with suicidal histories may put suicidal tendencies aside in the face of a terminal illness and fight to live, in a different way than their history would indicate, as long as their quality of life is satisfactory.

- Chronic severe mental illness may have depleted family coping resources.

- Family may be in a crisis as a result of unexpected medical illness in addition to mental illness.

Personality disorders and palliative care

People with PDs can present major challenges for palliative care providers, partly because of the stigma associated with PDs. Personality traits are enduring patterns of perceiving, relating to, and thinking about the world and how one relates to the world.[7] The enduring patterns of response and behavior deviate from social norms and present in the areas of:

- Cognition (ways of perceiving self, others, events)
- Affectivity (range, intensity, lability, appropriateness)
- Interpersonal functioning
- Impulse control

There is a lack of flexibility and maladaptive behavior that can cause impairment in function and distress for the person.[7]

All humans have vulnerabilities that are accentuated when the person is under stress. Approaching personality traits as vulnerabilities that are accentuated by stress, and therefore result in the use of predictable coping mechanisms, can be a useful way to change stigmatized attitudes toward people with PDs. It is important to identify traits or vulnerabilities and move beyond labels so that treatment can be geared to preparing for the expected response, minimizing maladaptive coping mechanisms and replacing them with more functional coping mechanisms.

Personality disorders are grouped into three clusters based on some descriptive similarities. Cluster A PDs include paranoid PD, schizoid PD, and schizotypal PD. People with Cluster A disorders often appear odd, eccentric, or paranoid. People with paranoid PD have a pervasive distrust and suspiciousness of others. The person will be reluctant to trust or confide in anyone and may suspect that others are trying to cause him/her harm.[7] The person with schizoid PD has a pervasive pattern of detachment from relationships, even with family. This person prefers solitary activities, lacks close relationships, and may be emotionally detached or have a flat affect. People with schizotypal PD are uncomfortable with close relationships and have cognitive distortions, including ideas of reference, odd beliefs or magical thinking, unusual perceptions, odd thinking and speech, inappropriate affect, and social anxiety.[7]

Cluster B PDs include antisocial PD, borderline PD (BPD), histrionic PD, and narcissistic PD. People with this group of PDs often appear dramatic, emotional, or erratic, and it is this cluster that often presents the biggest challenge to healthcare providers.[7] The person with antisocial PD has a pervasive disregard for, and violates, the rights of others. They fail to conform to most social norms and can be impulsive, irritable, and aggressive at times. People with BPD have a lifelong pattern of instability of interpersonal relationships and self-image and either idealize or devalue others, or fluctuate between the two views of the same person. People with BPD are impulsive in ways that are damaging to themselves and frequently have recurrent suicidal behavior. They have a chronic feeling of emptiness and therefore constantly seek attention and contact with others to fill themselves.[7] People with histrionic PD have a pattern of excessive emotionality and attention-seeking and can be inappropriately provocative or sexually seductive. People with these traits are easily influenced by others and often consider relationships to be more intimate than they actually are. People with narcissistic PD need admiration, have a lack empathy for others, and have a sense of entitlement.[7]

Cluster C PDs include avoidant PD, dependent PD, and obsessive-compulsive PD. These disorders share anxiety and fear as their major characteristics.[7] The person with avoidant PD is hypersensitive to negative evaluation, has feelings of inadequacy, and is severely restrained in relationships. This person is reluctant to take personal risks or engage in new activities.[7] Someone with dependent PD has an excessive need to be taken care of that exhibits itself by submissive and clinging behavior and fear of separation. People with this PD have difficulty making decisions and need a lot of advice and reassurance from others. They have difficulty expressing disagreement with others because of fear of loss of support.

Finally, obsessive-compulsive PD is evidenced by a preoccupation with orderliness, perfectionism, and control. The person with obsessive-compulsive PD shows perfectionism that interferes with completion of tasks, is inflexible and overly conscientious, may be unable to throw out useless objects, and is miserly toward spending for self and others. This person may be quite rigid and stubborn in thought and behavior.[7]

Treatment of personality disorders

By description, PDs are enduring patterns and, therefore, are not likely to change rapidly. Current evidence does suggest that people with PDs can be treated, but realistic goals must be established for treatment. Symptom management and specific therapies such as CBT and dialectical behavioral therapy (DBT) have demonstrated effectiveness with specific PDs.[24] The relationship with a psychiatric provider is a primary tool in the treatment of people with PDs. There is no medication with an FDA indication for treatment for personality disorders. Comorbid psychiatric conditions are common with PD, so symptom management of anxiety, depression, and other psychiatric symptoms is important to improve quality of life.[24]

Communication issues and personality disorders

Some general principles related to communication with patients with PD can be identified. Clear information provided verbally and in writing with repeated discussions about the information can help with distortions and misinterpretation that are common in people with PDs. A calm and nonjudgmental approach is also the cornerstone of good communication in the process of developing a therapeutic relationship with patients. All discussion of suicidal ideation should be taken very seriously and a thorough psychiatric assessment should be performed, even when repeated threats of suicide occur. The therapeutic alliance may take a long time to develop, but nonetheless the development of this alliance is a goal for treatment. The techniques of CBT are helpful for people with PD to examine maladaptive ways of viewing their environment. Supportive therapy is useful in helping people with PD adjust to the issues that arise in palliative and end-of-life care.

Obstacles to therapeutic communication that occur with people suffering with PD include issues such as resistance, transference, countertransference, and boundary violations.[20] Resistance is often unconscious and is usually employed to avoid anxiety. Transference also occurs when a patient unconsciously transfers feelings or attitudes from one person in their life onto the healthcare provider.[25] Countertransference is the emotional reaction of the healthcare provider toward the patient, stimulated by their own past feelings toward someone in their personal life. Boundary violations occur when the healthcare provider goes beyond the standards of a therapeutic relationship and enters a more social relationship with a patient.

Communication issues with patients suffering from Cluster A disorders focus on the establishment of a therapeutic relationship, because distrust, suspiciousness, and withdrawal from interpersonal interactions are common. Engaging a nonthreatening approach and allowing the patient to engage with the provider at his or her own speed is very important. The intensity of a one-to-one conversation may be difficult for those with Cluster A PDs; therefore, focusing conversation on an external issue or task may be a helpful way to lessen the intensity.

Communication with people with Cluster B disorders are often the most problematic for healthcare providers. People with these disorders tend to have an increased risk of suicide, violence toward others, and self-mutilating behaviors as well as chronic low self-esteem, ineffective coping, and impaired social interactions.[24] Volatile changes in emotion as well as splitting behaviors are characteristic of BPD. Development of a consistent approach will minimize the patient's ability to split staff and minimize the heightened feelings that can arise in caring for this population.

Providers should be alert for their own countertransference reactions toward patients with PD, as this is a common issue. Patients with PD can evoke strong reactions from staff that may interfere with delivery of quality care. Staff support in working through these reactions so that care is not affected can be provided through consultative relationships with psychiatric providers. Many psychiatric clinical nurse specialists have experience with staff support groups to handle such issues.

Communication issues with people suffering from Cluster C diagnoses also focus on the development of a therapeutic relationship geared toward assisting patients in identifying their fears and anxiety as it relates to palliative care treatment and issues.[25] Helping people identify their anxiety, decrease the maladaptive response to the anxiety, and increase their supportive relationships with others are essential issues in dealing with people with in this cluster.

Case study

A 44-year-old woman with colon cancer

Lorraine is a 44-year-old woman suffering from colon cancer with metastasis to the lung. She has been hospitalized twice in the last 6 months and is now readmitted to the oncology unit. The staff is not pleased to hear about her readmission because she was a management problem on her last admission. She was frequently upset with the night shift nurses and called the patient advocate several times a week to complain about them. She also left the unit frequently and was not available at treatment times. She complained bitterly about one nurse and demanded someone else care for her when that nurse was assigned her care. This caused a great deal of dissatisfaction among the nursing staff, and most of the nurses were relieved when she was discharged.

The nurse manager greets Lorraine as she arrives for readmission to the unit and sees how frightened Lorraine appears to be. The nurse manager is able to spend a few minutes with Lorraine during which time the patient is tearful and exhibiting signs of air hunger. She is able to assist Lorraine in becoming more comfortable and discuss her plan of care. Lorraine acknowledges that "I really gave the nurses a hard time the last time I was here. . . . I don't want to do that again . . . I am really scared and I don't want to die! Please don't leave me alone."

The nurse manager is able to assure Lorraine that staff will be with her and temporarily asks one of the unit volunteers to sit with Lorraine while she discusses the care with the doctor and gets medication orders to manage Lorraine's anxiety and air hunger. She then calls the psychiatric consultation nurse and asks for help in developing a plan of care and sets up a meeting with the nursing staff to discuss the plan and their feelings about Lorraine as a patient. She updates the nurses who are able to relate to the frightened Lorraine in a compassionate way and put the negative feelings from the last hospitalization aside.

This case highlights several factors in the care of people with personality disorders:

1. The labeling and stigma associated with personality disorders and/or "difficult patients" can result in less than optimal care unless someone is able to be a "role model" in terms of providing the best care possible for the patient

2. Each encounter with patients with PD may be quite different;

3. Identification of maladaptive coping mechanisms may help staff understand patient behavior and assist them in developing a nonjudgmental approach to the patient

4. Allowing time for staff to vent and examine their reactions/feelings in dealing with patients who make them upset can help nurses improve care to patients with PD

Summary

Palliative care providers often feel poorly prepared to deal with people with SMI and/or PD. Conversely, psychiatric providers feel poorly prepared to deal with medical care and end-of-life care. Collaborative partnerships can enhance the care given to people with SMI who are in need of palliative care services. Care delivery sites need to be examined for the optimal situation to provide both palliative care and treatment in an environment that also is able to provide optimal support and treatment by psychiatric providers. If the patient has a preference for a place to receive end-of-life care, all attempts possible can be made to address this preference. If the person considers a halfway house or psychiatric unit to be their home, and they desire to die at home, providing end-of-life care in that setting should be discussed just as it would be with a person wanting to die in their more traditional home. Nurses have often been instrumental in making this kind of care possible in a situation that has not previously involved this level of care. As strong advocates for their patients, nurses have found a way to insert themselves into new arenas of care and have developed new collaborative partnerships for the ultimate benefit of their patients. Collaboration between psychiatric providers and palliative care providers is a new area in which nurses can lead the way to ultimately provide new skills for each other and meaningful end-of-life experiences for people with SMI as well as their families.

References

1. National Institute of Mental Health (AU) Mental Disorders in America. http://www.nimh.nih.gov/health/publications/the-numbers-count—mental-disorders-in-america/index.shtml#intro. Accessed June 18, 2013.

2. Murray CJL, Vos T, Lozano R, Naghavi M, Flaxman AD, Michaud C, et al. Disability-adjusted life years (DALYS) for 291 diseases and injuries in 21 regions, 1990-2010: a systematic analysis for the Global Burden of Disease Study 2010. Lancet. 2012;380:2197–2223.

3. Parks J, Svendsen D, Singer P, Foti M. 2006. Morbidity and Mortality in People with Serious Mental Illness. National Association of State Mental Health Program Directors (NASMHPD) Medical Directors Council. Alexandria, VA. 22314. http://www.nasmphd.org/generalFiles/publications/ med_directors.pub. Accessed May 20, 2013.

4. Chang C, Hayes RD, Broadbent M, Fernandes AC, Lee W, Hotopf M, et al. All-cause mortality among people with serious mental illness (SMI), substance use disorders, and depressive disorders in southeast London: a cohort study. BMC Psychiatry. 2010;10:77. www.biomed-central.com/1471-244X/10/77. Accessed August 8, 2013.

5. Baker A. Palliative and end-of-life care in the serious and persistently mentally ill population. J Am Psych Nurses Assoc. 2005;11(5): 298–303.

6. Ganzini L, Socherman R, Duckart J, Shores M. End-of-life care for veterans with schizophrenia and cancer. Psychiatr Serv. 2010;61(7):725–728.

7. American Psychiatric Association (APA). Diagnostic and Statistical Manual of Mental Disorders. 5th ed. (DSM-5). Washington DC: APA; 2013.

8. Beebe LH. Schizophrenia. In: Perese EF (ed.), Psychiatric Advanced Practice Nursing: A Biopsychosocial Foundation for Practice. Philadelphia, PA: Davis; 2012:467–509.

9. Roshanaei-Moghaddam B, Katon W. Premature mortality from general medical illness among persons with bipolar disorder: a review. Psychiatr Serv. 2009;60:147–156.

10. Piatt EE, Munetz MR, Ritter C. An examination of premature mortality among decedents with serious mental illness and those in the general population. Psychiatr Serv. 2010;61(7):663–668.

11. Foti ME. "Do it your way": A demonstration project on end-of-life care for persons with serious mental illness. J Palliat Med. 2003;6(4):661–669.

12. Foti ME, Bartels SJ, Van Citters AD, Merriman MP, Fletcher KE. End-of-life treatment preferences of persons with serious mental illness. Psychiatr Serv. 2005;56(5):585–591.

13. Kudoh A, Ishihara H, Matsuki A. Current perception thresholds and postoperative pain in schizophrenic patients. Reg Anesth Pain Med. 2000;25(5):475–479.

14. Chan P. Psychopharmacology. In: Fortinash KM, Holoday Worret PA (eds.), Psychiatric Mental Health Nursing. 4th ed. St. Louis, MO: Mosby; 2008.

15. Kuhl D. What Dying People Want. In: Chochinov HM, Breitbart W (eds.), Handbook of Psychiatry in Palliative Medicine. 2nd ed. New York: Oxford University Press; 2009.

16. Laben JK, Yorker BC. Legal issues in advanced practice psychiatric nursing. In: Burgess AW (ed.), Advanced Practice Psychiatric Nursing. Stamford, CT: Appleton and Lange; 1998.

17. Schouten R, Brendel RW. Legal aspects of consultation. In: Stern TA, Fricchione GL, Cassem HNH, Jellinek MS, Rosenbaum JF (eds.), Massachusetts General Hospital Handbook of General Hospital Psychiatry. 5th ed. Philadelphia, PA: Mosby; 2004:356.

18. Applebaum PS, Grisso T. Assessing patient's capacities to consent to treatment. N Engl J Med. 1988;319:1635–1638.

19. American Psychiatric Nursing Association (APNA). Coping with aggressive behavior in patients with schizophrenia: a roundtable discussion. Counseling Points: Enhancing Patient Communication for the Psychiatric Nurse. September 2006. Ridgewood, NJ: Delaware Media Group.

20. Perese EF. Prevention of psychiatric disorders. In: Perese EF (ed.), Psychiatric Advanced Practice Nursing: A Biopsychosocial Foundation for Practice. Philadelphia, PA: Davis; 2012.

21. Kilbourne AM, Post EP, Nossek A, Drill L, Cooley S, Bauer MS. Improving medical and psychiatric outcomes among individuals with bipolar disorder: a randomized controlled trial. Psychiatr Serv. 2008;59(7):760–768.

22. Perese EF. Bipolar disorders. In: Perese EF (ed.), Psychiatric Advanced Practice Nursing: A Biopsychosocial Foundation for Practice. Philadelphia, PA: Davis; 2012:427–464.

23. McCasland LA. Providing hospice and palliative care to the seriously and persistently mentally ill. J Hosp Palliat Nurs. 2007;9(6):305–313.

24. Perese EF. Personality disorders. In: Perese EF (ed.), Psychiatric Advanced Practice Nursing: A Biopsychosocial Foundation for Practice. Philadelphia, PA: Davis; 2012:601–638.

25. McDonald SF. Therapeutic communication. In: Fortinash KM, Holoday Worret PA (eds.), Psychiatric Mental Health Nursing. 4th ed. St. Louis, MO: Mosby; 2008.

CHAPTER 40

Patients with acquired immunodeficiency syndrome

Carl A. Kirton and Deborah Witt Sherman

I thought like so many of my friends that I would die young well before my time. There were moments that I was hanging on by just a thread. When I could not eat or drink, I became like a walking skeleton. On the AIDS unit, some other patients asked that I not walk around because I was too scary looking. Thank God, the protease inhibitors were discovered. They pulled me back from the edge of death. Over the years, I have changed my AIDS medication many times, but learned to live a healthier life to give me the best chances of staying well. I am just grateful to be alive. People are no longer as afraid of me when they know I am HIV positive. This disease changed my life, a horrible illness through which I have been transformed in many ways.

Anonymous patient

Key points

♦ With HIV/AIDS, the severity, complexity, and unpredictability of the illness trajectory have blurred the distinction between curative and palliative care.

♦ The focus of AIDS care must be on improving quality of life by providing care for the management of pain and other symptoms, while addressing the emotional, social, and spiritual needs of patients and their families throughout the illness trajectory.

♦ With up-to-date knowledge regarding HIV disease, including changes in epidemiology, diagnostic testing, treatment options, and available resources, nurses can offer effective and compassionate care to patients and families at all stages of HIV disease.

In 30+ years, AIDS has escalated from a series of outbreaks in scattered communities in the United States and Europe to a global health crisis. Although the biomedical paradigm of antiretroviral therapy has significantly reduced the mortality from HIV in the developed world and has transformed AIDS into a manageable chronic illness, the reality in developing countries is that people are not "living with AIDS" but, rather, "dying from AIDS" because of a lack of access to medications and appropriate healthcare.[1] In the late stages of HIV, there is a false dichotomy created between disease-specific, curative therapies and symptom-specific palliative therapies.[2] It is now realized that the palliation of pain, symptoms, and suffering must occur throughout the course of a life-threatening disease, not just in the final stages near the end of life. AIDS has stimulated the need to evaluate clinical practice when curative and palliative care interface. No longer should there be an abrupt demarcation between palliative care and treating disease in individuals with life-threatening, progressive illnesses.[3]

Both the public and health professionals have been troubled by the reality of over- and undertreatment of pain and symptoms in individuals with life-threatening illnesses who may suffer severe, unremitting pain in their final days.[4] Such concern extends to the care of patients with HIV and the resultant illness of AIDS because no cure has yet been found. Therefore, the focus of care must be on improving quality of life by providing palliative care for the management of pain and other physical symptoms while addressing the emotional, social, and spiritual needs of patients and their families throughout the illness trajectory. Although current therapies have increased the life expectancy of people with HIV/AIDS, the chance of experiencing symptoms related not only to the disease but to the effects of therapies also increases. Furthermore, palliative measures can be beneficial in ensuring tolerance of and adherence to difficult pharmacological regimens.[5]

Because patients are surviving longer in the latter stages of illness, an integrated model must be developed to provide comprehensive care for patients with advanced AIDS and their families.[5] This chapter provides an overview and update of the comprehensive care related to HIV/AIDS and addresses the palliative care needs of individuals and families living with and dying from this illness. With this information, nurses and other healthcare professionals will gain the knowledge to provide effective and compassionate care, recognizing the need for both curative and aggressive care as well as supportive and palliative therapies to maximize the quality of life of patients and their family caregivers.

Incidence of HIV/AIDS

HIV/AIDS is a worldwide epidemic affecting more than 34 million people. An estimated 2.5 million acquired HIV in 2011, and an estimated 1.7 million people died from AIDS.[6] In the United

States an estimated 1.1 million people are living with HIV infection (CDC, 2013). HIV incidence has remained relatively stable in the United States at about 50,000 infections per year since the mid-1990s. Certain groups, including African Americans, Latinos, and gay and bisexual men of all races/ethnicities, still continue to be disproportionately affected.[7]

Historical background of HIV/AIDS

In the early 1980s, cases were reported of previously healthy homosexual men who were diagnosed with *Pneumocystis carinii* (now known as *Pneumocystis jiroveci*) pneumonia and an extremely rare tumor known as Kaposi's sarcoma (KS). The number of cases doubled every 6 months, with further occurrence of unusual fungal, viral, and parasitic infections, and researchers realized that the immune systems of these individuals were being compromised. Over time, reports began to emerge of the appearance of similar unusual infections and immune system destruction beyond the homosexual community. This new disease was also seen among heterosexual partners, IV substance users, persons with hemophilia, individuals receiving infected blood products, and children born to women with the disease.

Origins of HIV can be traced through serum studies to 1959, when crossover mechanisms between humans and primates via animal bites or scratches in Africa led to HIV transmission. In 1981, the virus was identified and named lymphadenopathy-associated virus (LAV). By 1984, the term had been changed to human T-lymphocytic virus type III (HTLV-III), and in 1986 renamed the human immunodeficiency virus type 1 (HIV-1). HIV-1 accounts for nearly all the cases reported in the United States, whereas a second strain, HIV-2, accounts for nearly all the cases reported in West Africa. During 1988, a total of 242 HIV-2 cases were reported to the Centers for Disease Control and Prevention (CDC). Of these, 166 met the working definition. These HIV-2 cases were concentrated in the Northeast (66%, including 46% in New York City) and occurred primarily among persons born in West Africa (81%).[8]

Globally, AIDS is characterized as a dynamic epidemic that has spread to every continent in the world and has multiple and varied socioeconomic, cultural, and political dimensions. To date, the following scientific progress has been made in combating the infection: (1) the virus has been identified; (2) improved and easier methodologies for screening for HIV infection have been implemented; (3) vaccines have been tested; (4) biological and behavioral cofactors have been identified related to infection and disease progression; (5) prophylactic treatments are available to prevent opportunistic infections; (6) quantitative assays are readily available to measure viral replication and have become a standard measure to evaluate the response of the disease to treatment; (7) better and simpler treatments exists to treat HIV disease and have raised life expectancy; and (8) international collaborations have provided HIV treatments in many underdeveloped nations.

HIV pathogenesis and classification

Like all viruses, the HIV virus survives by reproducing itself in a host cell, usurping the genetic machinery of that cell, and eventually destroying the cell. The HIV is a retrovirus whose life cycle consists of (1) attachment of the virus to the cell, which is affected by cofactors that influence the virus's ability to enter the host cell;

(2) uncoating of the virus; (3) reverse transcription by an enzyme called reverse transcriptase, which converts two strands of viral RNA to DNA; (4) integration of newly synthesized proviral DNA into the cell nucleus, assisted by the viral enzyme integrase, which becomes the template for new viral components; (5) transcription of proviral DNA into messenger RNA; (6) movement of messenger RNA outside the cell nucleus, where it is translated into viral proteins and enzymes; and (7) assembly and release of mature virus particles out of the host cell.[9]

These newly formed viruses have an affinity for any cell that has the CD4 molecule on its surface, such as T lymphocytes and macrophages, which become major viral targets. Because CD4 cells are the master coordinators of the immune system response, chronic destruction of these cells severely compromises individuals' immune status, leaving the host susceptible to opportunistic infections and eventual progression to AIDS.

HIV and AIDS are not synonymous terms but, rather, refer to the natural history or progression of the infection, ranging from asymptomatic infection to life-threatening illness characterized by opportunistic infections and cancers. The end of the continuum of the illness is associated with a marked decrease in CD4 cell count and a rise in HIV-RNA viral load (VL).

The natural history of HIV infection begins with primary or acute infection. This occurs when the virus enters the body and replicates in large numbers in the blood. This leads to an initial decrease in the number of CD4 cells. Viral load climbs during the first 2 weeks of the infection. Within 5 to 30 days of infection, the individual may experience a flu-like symptom characteristic of a viremia such as fever, sore throat, skin rash, lymphadenopathy, and myalgia. Other manifestations of primary HIV infection include fatigue, splenomegaly, anorexia, nausea and vomiting, meningitis, retro-orbital pain, neuropathy, and mucocutaneous ulceration.[9] The production of HIV antibodies results in seroconversion, which generally occurs within 6 to 12 weeks of the initial infection. The amount of virus present after the initial viremia and the immune response is called the viral set-point.

Clinical latency refers to the chronic, clinically asymptomatic state in which there is a decreased VL and resolution of symptoms of the primary infection. During this period there is continuous viral replication in the lymph nodes at the rate of more than 10 billion copies of the virus made every day. It is for this reason that early medical intervention with combination antiretroviral therapy is recommended.[10] Al-Harthi et al.[11] demonstrated that when antiretroviral therapy is used as an early intervention in nonacute HIV infection, it potentially reverses immune-mediated damage.

The early symptomatic stage occurs after years of infection and is apparent by conditions indicative primarily of defects in cell-mediated immunity. Early symptomatic infection generally occurs when CD4 counts fall below 500 cells/mm³. In the absence of effective treatment, there are frequently mucosal clues, ranging from oral candidiasis and hairy leukoplakia to ulcerative lesions. Gynecological infections are the most common reasons women have a medical examination. There are also dermatological manifestations, which include bacterial, fungal, viral, neoplastic, and other conditions such exacerbation of psoriasis, severe pruritus, or the development of recurrent pruritic papules.

The late symptomatic stage begins when the CD4 count drops below 200 cells/mm³. This CD4 level is recognized by the CDC as meeting the case definition for AIDS. In the absence of effective treatments, opportunistic infections or cancers characterize this stage and result in multiple symptoms. In addition to such illnesses as KS, *Pneumocystis jiroveci* pneumonia, HIV encephalopathy, and HIV wasting, diseases such as pulmonary tuberculosis, recurrent bacterial infections, and invasive cervical cancer are sometimes seen. The advanced HIV disease stage occurs when the CD4 cell count drops below 50 cells/mm^3. In the absence of treatment common conditions seen are central nervous system (CNS) non-Hodgkin's lymphoma, KS, cytomegalovirus (CMV) retinitis, or *Mycobacterium avium* complex (MAC). In the late stages of the disease, most individuals have health problems such as pneumonia, oral candidiasis, depression, dementia, skin problems, anxiety, incontinence, fatigue, isolation, bed dependency, wasting syndrome, and significant pain.[12] Research regarding AIDS patients experiencing advanced disease confirms the multitude of patient symptoms and factors that contribute to mortality. In a study of 230 patients with advanced AIDS referred to a large urban medical center over a median of 126 days, 120 patients died; 54% of these died of late-stage HIV disease and/or bacterial pneumonia or sepsis, 19% of non-AIDS-defining cancers, 13% of liver failure and/or cirrhosis, and 12% of other progressive end-organ disease (e.g., cardiac, pulmonary, renal). On multivariate analysis, death was predicted only by age (>65 years), baseline number of ADL impairments, and Karnofsky score (P < 0.0001 for all) and not by any AIDS-specific variables.[13] Given the large number of both pre-HAART (highly active antiretroviral therapy) era and post-HAART era symptoms in AIDS, it is worth a review of the prevalent symptoms. The five most prevalent symptoms reported among AIDS patients are fatigue, weight loss, pain, anorexia, and anxiety. Other less prevalent symptoms include insomnia, cough, nausea/vomiting, dyspnea, depression, diarrhea, and constipation.[14]

Palliative care as a natural evolution in HIV/AIDS care

From the earliest stages of HIV disease, symptom control becomes an important goal of medical and nursing care to maintain the patient's quality of life. Therefore, palliative care for patients with HIV/AIDS should be viewed not as an approach to care only in the advanced stage of the illness but as an aspect of care that begins in the early stage of illness and continues as the disease progresses.[5]

With the occurrence of opportunistic infections, specific cancers, and neurological manifestations, AIDS involves multiple symptoms not only from the disease processes but also from the side effects of medications and other therapies. Patients with AIDS present with complex care issues because they experience bouts of severe illness and debilitation alternating with periods of symptom stabilization.[15] In one model of care, AIDS palliation begins when active treatment ends. Although this model limits service overlap and is economical, it creates not only the ethical issue of when to shift from a curative to a palliative focus but also promotes discontinuity of care and possible discrimination. Conversely, a second model of AIDS care recognizes that AIDS treatment is primarily palliative, directed toward minimizing symptoms and maximizing the quality of life, and necessitates the use of antiretroviral drugs, treatment of infections and neoplasms, and provision of high levels of support to promote the patient's quality of life over many years of

the illness.[16] Selwyn and Rivard[17] emphasize that although AIDS is no longer a uniformly fatal disease, it is an important cause of mortality, particularly for ethnically diverse populations with comorbidities such as hepatitis B and C, end-organ failure, and various malignancies. Further, Shen, Blank, and Selwyn[18] conducted a study based on patients (n = 230) in a large urban New York medical center who had been referred to the HIV palliative care team. They reported that close to half of all deaths for these patients were attributable to non-AIDS-specific causes, including cancer and end-organ failure. Further, age and markers of functional status were more predictive of mortality than traditional HIV prognostic variables, suggesting the need to reconsider the current value of prior prognostic variables.

Although thousands of individuals continue to suffer and die from AIDS, the division between curative-aggressive care and supportive-palliative care is less well defined and more variable than in other life-threatening illnesses such as cancer. With HIV/AIDS, the severity, complexity, and unpredictability of the illness trajectory have blurred the distinction between curative and palliative care. Other continuing challenges associated with HIV/AIDS are the societal stigmatization of the disease and, therefore, the greater emotional, social, and spiritual needs of those experiencing the illness, as well as their family and professional caregivers, who experience their own grief and bereavement processes.

Palliative care is therefore a natural evolution in AIDS care. Core issues of comfort and function, which are fundamental to palliative care, must be addressed throughout the course of the illness and may be concurrent with restorative or curative therapies for persons with AIDS. The management decisions for patients with advanced AIDS revolve around the ratio between benefits and burdens of the various diagnostic and treatment modalities and the patient's expectations and goals, as well as anticipated problems. In the face of advanced HIV disease, healthcare providers and patients must determine the balance between aggressive and supportive efforts, particularly when increasing debility, wasting, and deteriorating cognitive function are evident. At this point, the complex needs of patients with HIV/AIDS and the needs of their families require the coordinated care of an interdisciplinary palliative care team, involving physicians, advanced practice nurses, staff nurses, social workers, dietitians, physiotherapists, and clergy. Because in palliative care the unit of care is the patient and family, the palliative care team offers support not only for patients to live as fully as possible until death but also for the family to cope during the patient's illness and in their own bereavement.[19] Palliative care core precepts of respect for patient goals, preferences, and choices; comprehensive caring; and acknowledgment of caregivers' concerns support the holistic and comprehensive approach to care needed by individuals and families with HIV/AIDS. The components of high-quality HIV/AIDS palliative care, as identified by healthcare providers, include competent, skilled practitioners; confidential, nondiscriminatory, culturally sensitive care; flexible and responsive care; collaborative and coordinated care; and fair access to care.[19]

Barriers to palliative care

The neglect of the palliative care needs of patients with HIV also relates to certain barriers to care, such as reimbursement issues. Specifically, public and private third-party payers have reimbursed end-of-life care only when physicians have verified a life expectancy of less than 6 months to live. Beyond six months, patients must be classified as terminal by a licensed provider as terminal to continue to receive services and eligible for comprehensive care, with control of pain and other symptoms along with psychological and spiritual support offered by hospice/palliative care. Without a terminal diagnosis patients may be discharged from hospice care. Additionally, long-term cost of HIV medications and other therapies may outpace monthly reimbursement. HIV treatments range from $2000–$5000 monthly.

An additional barrier to palliative care use is that HIV is now seen as a chronic illness. Although palliative care is appropriate throughout the trajectory of a disease, the current emphasis is on beginning palliative care only at the end of life. A review of the evidence of barriers and inequality in HIV care by Simms et al.[20] found that there is increased complexity in the balance of providing concurrent curative and palliative therapies given the prolongation of life span as a result of antiretroviral therapy. Simms and colleagues believe that palliative care should not solely be associated with terminal care and propose four recommendations:

1. The need for multidimensional palliative care assessment for differing populations;

2. Basic palliative care skills training for all clinical staff in standard assessments;

3. Development of referral criteria and systems for patients with complex palliative care needs; and

4. The availability of specialist consultation across all settings.

Criteria for palliative care

The need for palliative care of patients with HIV care has evolved since the start of the epidemic. Traditional criteria such as decrease in functional ability, declining CD4 count and rising VL, and history of opportunistic infections were important drivers of worsening disease and perhaps end-of-life, indicating the need for palliative interventions. The complex needs of patients with HIV also indicate the need for an interdisciplinary approach to care offered by palliative and hospice care early in the course of the disease. The continual review of hospice policies in accordance with the changes in the disease is encouraged. Indeed, developing different models of care, such as enhanced home care, hospice care, day care, or partnerships with community hospitals or agencies, and conducting cost-benefit analyses will be important in meeting the healthcare needs of patients with AIDS and their families in the future.

Important advances are currently being made in the field of palliative medicine and nursing, involving an active set of behaviors that continue throughout the caregiving process to manage the pain and suffering of individuals with HIV/AIDS. Health professionals have the responsibility to be knowledgeable about the various treatment options and resources available for pain and symptom management. They must know about pharmacological agents' actions, side effects, and interactions, as well as alternative routes of medication administration. And they must be able to inform patients of their options for care—documenting their preferences, wishes, and choices; performing a complete history and physical assessment; and collaborating with other members of the interdisciplinary team to develop and implement a comprehensive plan of care.[19]

Health promotion and maintenance in promoting the quality of life of persons with HIV/AIDS

As palliative care becomes an increasingly important component of AIDS care from diagnosis to death, and given the definition of palliative care as the comprehensive management of the physical, psychological, social, spiritual, and existential needs of patients with incurable progressive illness, palliative care must involve ongoing prevention, health promotion, and health maintenance to promote the patient's quality of life throughout the illness trajectory.[19] With HIV/AIDS, health promotion and maintenance involves promoting behaviors that will prevent or decrease the occurrence of opportunistic infections and AIDS-indicator diseases, promoting prophylactic and therapeutic treatment of AIDS-indicator conditions and preventing behaviors that promote disease expression.

With no current cure, the health management of patients with HIV/AIDS is directed toward controlling HIV disease and prolonging survival while maintaining quality of life. Quality of life may be defined as the impact of sickness and healthcare on an ill person's daily activities and sense of well-being.[21,22] Furthermore, quality of life varies with disease progression from HIV to AIDS. To understand quality of life means to understand the patient's perceptions of his/her ability to control the physical, emotional, social, cognitive, and spiritual aspects of the illness. Quality of life is therefore associated with health maintenance for individuals with HIV/AIDS, particularly as it relates to functioning in activities of daily living, social functioning, and physical and emotional symptoms.[23] In a study regarding the functional quality of life of 142 men and women with AIDS, Vosvick and colleagues[24] concluded that maladaptive coping strategies were associated with lower levels of energy and social functioning and that severe pain interfered with daily living tasks and was associated with lower levels of functional quality of life (physical functioning, energy/fatigue, social functioning, and role functioning). Therefore, health promotion interventions should be aimed at developing adaptive coping strategies and improving pain management.

Health promotion in HIV/AIDS

Health promotion and maintenance for patients with HIV/AIDS must acknowledge patients' perceived healthcare needs. Based on a study of 386 HIV-infected persons, it was determined that the healthcare challenges perceived by patients with HIV/AIDS across hospital, outpatient, home, and long-term care settings included decreased endurance and physical mobility, changes in sensory perception, and financial issues—specifically lack of income and resources to cover living and healthcare expenses.[25] Furthermore, based on a sample of 162 hospitalized men and women with AIDS, Kemppainen[26] reported that the strongest predictor of decreased quality of life was depression, which accounted for 23% of the variance, with other symptoms accounting for 9.75% and female gender accounting for an additional 8%. Additionally, active involvement in the process of nursing care contributed 13.4% to the variance in quality of life. These results indicate the healthcare challenges and physical, emotional, and interactional needs of patients with AIDS. In addition to managing pain and other symptoms, a comprehensive and compassionate approach to care is necessary as the illness progresses. Furthermore, enhancing immunocompetence is critical at all stages of illness, as is treating the symptoms brought on by the disease or related to prophylactic or treatment therapies. Palliation of physical, emotional, and spiritual symptoms—particularly as experienced in the late symptomatic and advanced stages of HIV disease—is considered the final stage of a health-and-disease-prevention approach and will be discussed later in this chapter.

Through all stages of HIV, health can be promoted and maintained through diet, micronutrients, exercise, reduction of stress and negative emotions, symptom surveillance, and the use of prophylactic therapies to prevent opportunistic infections or AIDS-related complications.

Diet

A health-promoting diet is essential for optimal function of the immune system. Deficiencies in calorie and protein intake impair cell-mediated immunity, phagocytic function, and antibody response. Therefore, an alteration in nutrition is associated with impaired immune system function, secondary infections, disease progression, psychological distress, and fatigue. In patients with AIDS, common nutritional problems are weight loss, vitamin and mineral deficiencies, loss of muscle mass, and loss or redistribution of fat mass. The redistribution of fat is characterized by increased abdominal girth, loss of fat from the face, and a "buffalo hump" on the back of the neck, which may result from the administration of antiretroviral therapy.[27] Patients with HIV/AIDS often have reduced food or caloric intake, malabsorption, and altered metabolism. Reduced food or caloric intake frequently results from diseases of the mouth and oropharynx, such as oral candidiasis, angular cheilitis, gingivitis, herpes simplex, and hairy leukoplakia. Metabolic alterations may result from HIV infection or secondary infections, as well as abnormalities in carbohydrate, fat, and protein metabolism. A good diet is one of the simplest ways to delay HIV progression and will bolster immune system function and energy levels and help patients live longer and more productive lives.[28,29] Recommended protein intake is 1.25–1.5 g/kg of body weight; recommended energy intake (calories from protein, carbohydrate, and fat) is 25 kcal/kg of body weight.[30]

Micronutrients

Adequate nutritional intake is considered an important part of the clinical care of patients with HIV. Early HIV research indicated that HIV-infected individuals with lower levels of micronutrients had faster disease progression and mortality.[31] However, a recent meta-analysis based on fourteen small trials, evaluating different macronutrient supplements, found limited evidence that balanced macronutrient formulas increase protein and energy intake and no evidence that such supplementation translates into reductions in disease progression or HIV-related complications, such as opportunistic infections or death.[32] While micronutrient supplementation has not been demonstrated to affect clinical outcomes, clinicians should encourage a balanced and adequate nutritional intake throughout the course of the disease.

Exercise and massage

Exercise is considered an essential part of health maintenance, and it is hypothesized that exercise has a beneficial effect on immune function and overall health. A meta-analysis of 14 studies concluded that aerobic and resistive exercise, both alone and in combination, were associated with increased muscle mass (1.1 to 6.9 kg) and improvements in cardiovascular fitness and depression; improvements were contingent on adhering to an activity regimen for a minimum of 20 minutes/day, 3 days/week for 5 weeks. No adverse effects or immunological or virological parameters were found.[33] Resistive exercise alone for 16 weeks has been shown to increase lean body mass and muscle strength and to reduce serum triglycerides.[34] Furthermore, there is some evidence to support the use of massage therapy to improve quality of life for people living with HIV/AIDS (PLWHA), particularly in combination with other stress-management modalities, and that massage therapy may have a positive effect on immunological function.[35]

Stress and emotions

Stress and negative emotions have also been associated with immunosuppression and vulnerability to disease. In a study of 96 HIV-infected homosexual men without symptoms or antiretroviral medication use, Leserman and colleagues[36] reported that higher cumulative average stressful life events, higher anger scores, lower cumulative average social support, and depressive symptoms were all predictive of a faster progression to both the CDC AIDS classification and a clinical AIDS condition. Stress of living with HIV/AIDS is related to the uncertainty regarding illness progression and prognosis, stigmatization and discrimination, and financial concerns as disabilities increase with advancing disease.[37] Persons with AIDS frequently cite the avoidance of stress as a way of maintaining a sense of well-being.[38] The use of exercise and massage and other relaxation techniques, such as imagery, meditation, and yoga, have been reported as valuable stress-management techniques.[39] Cognitive-behavioral interventions have also been shown to improve certain aspects of quality of life, emotional status, and CD4 cell counts.[40]

Health promotion also involves health beliefs and coping strategies that support well-being despite protracted illness. Long-term survivors used numerous strategies to support their health, such as having the will to live and positive attitudes, feeling in charge, maintaining a strong sense of self and a sense of humor, and expressing their needs. Other health-promotion strategies frequently used by these patients included remaining active, seeking medical information, talking to others, socializing and pursuing pleasurable activities, finding good medical care, and seeking counseling.[41] Stress can also be associated with the financial issues experienced by patients with HIV/AIDS. Therefore, health promotion may involve financial planning, identification of financial resources available through the community, and public assistance offered through Medicaid.

It must also be recognized that additional physical and emotional stress is associated with the use of recreational drugs such as alcohol, chemical stimulants, tobacco, and marijuana because these agents have an immunosuppressant effect and may interfere with health-promoting behaviors.[42,43] The use of such substances may have a negative effect on interpersonal relationships and is associated with a relapse to unsafe sexual practices.[43] Interventions for health promotion include encouraging patients to participate in self-health groups and harm-reduction programs to deal with substance abuse problems.

Symptom surveillance

Throughout the course of their illness, individuals with HIV require primary care services to identify early signs of opportunistic infections and to minimize related symptoms and complications. This includes a complete health history, physical examination, and laboratory data, including determination of immunological and viral status.

Health history

In the care of patients with HIV/AIDS, the health history should include the following:

- History of present illness, including a review of those factors that led to HIV testing

- Medical history, particularly those conditions that may be exacerbated by HIV or its treatments, such as diabetes mellitus, hypertriglyceridemia, or chronic or active hepatitis B infection

- Childhood illnesses and vaccinations for preventing common infections, such as polio, diphtheria, pertussis, and tetanus (DPT), or measles

- Medication history, including the patient's knowledge of the types of medications, side effects, adverse reactions, drug interactions, and administration recommendations

- Sexual history, regarding sexual behaviors and preferences and history of sexually transmitted diseases, which can exacerbate HIV progression

- Lifestyle habits, such as the past and present use of recreational drugs, including alcohol, which may accelerate progression of disease, or cigarette smoking, which may suppress appetite or be associated with opportunistic infections such as oral candidiasis, hairy leukoplakia, and bacterial pneumonia

- Dietary habits, including risks related to food-borne illnesses such as hepatitis A

- Travel history to countries in Asia, Africa, and South America, where the risk of opportunistic infections increases

- Complete systems review to provide indications of clinical manifestations of new opportunistic infections or cancers, as well as AIDS-related complications both from the disease and its treatments

Physical examination

A physical exam should begin with a general assessment of vital signs and height and weight, as well as overall appearance and mood. A complete head-to-toe assessment is important and may reveal various findings common to individuals with HIV/AIDS, including those mentioned below.

- Oral cavity assessment may indicate candida, oral hairy leukoplakia, or KS.

- Funduscopic assessment may reveal visual changes associated with CMV retinitis; glaucoma screening is also recommended.

- Lymph node assessment may reveal adenopathy, detected at any stage of disease.

- Dermatological assessment may indicate various cutaneous manifestations that occur throughout the course of the illness such as HIV exanthema, KS, or infectious complications such as dermatomycosis.

- Neuromuscular assessment may indicate various disorders of the central, peripheral, or autonomic nervous systems and signs and symptoms of conditions such as meningitis, encephalitis, dementia, or peripheral neuropathies.

- Cardiovascular assessment may reveal cardiomyopathy.

- Gastrointestinal (GI) assessment may indicate organomegaly—specifically splenomegaly or hepatomegaly—particularly in patients with a history of substance abuse, as well as signs related to parasitic intestinal infections; annual stool guaiac and rectal examination, as well as sigmoidoscopy every 5 years, are also parts of health maintenance.

- Reproductive system assessment may reveal occult sexually transmitted diseases or malignancies and vaginal candidiasis, cervical dysplasia, pelvic inflammatory disease, or rectal lesions in women with HIV/AIDS. Assessments may also reveal urethral discharge and rectal lesions or malignancies in HIV-infected men. Health maintenance in individuals with HIV/AIDS also includes annual mammograms in women, as well as testicular exams in men and prostate-specific antigen screening annually.

Laboratory data

Evaluation of laboratory data are important in assisting health practitioners in making therapeutic decisions. The following laboratory tests performed during initial patient visits can be used to stage HIV disease and in the selection of antiretroviral therapy:[44]

- HIV antibody testing (if prior documentation is not available or if HIV RNA is below the assay's limit of detection);

- CD4 T-cell count (CD4 count);

- Plasma HIV RNA (VL);

- Complete blood count, chemistry profile, transaminase levels, blood urea nitrogen (BUN), and creatinine, urinalysis, and serologies for hepatitis A, B, and C viruses;

- Fasting blood glucose and serum lipids; and

- Genotypic resistance testing at entry into care, regardless of whether antiretroviral therapy will be initiated immediately. For patients who have HIV RNA levels <500 to 1,000 copies/mL, viral amplification for resistance testing may not always be successful.

The DHHS's Panel on Clinical Practices for the Treatment of HIV[44] recommends that the CD4 count and the VL be measured upon entry into care and every 3–6 months subsequently. Immediately before a patient is started on antiretroviral therapy, the patient's HIV-RNA (VL) should be measured, and again 2–8 weeks after treatment is initiated, to determine the effectiveness of the therapy. With adherence to the medication schedule, it is expected that the HIV-RNA will decrease to undetectable levels (<50 copies/mL) in 16–24 weeks after the initiation of therapy. If a patient does not significantly respond to therapy, the clinician should evaluate adherence, repeat the test, and rule out malabsorption or drug-drug interactions.

The decision regarding laboratory testing is based on the stage of HIV disease, the medical processes warranting initial assessment or follow-up, and consideration of the patient benefit-to-burden ratio. Complete blood counts are often measured with each VL determination or with a change of antiretroviral therapy, particularly with patients on drugs known to cause anemia. Chemistry profiles are done to assess liver function, lipid status, and glycemia every 3–6 months or with a change in therapy, and are determined by the patient's antiretroviral therapy, baseline determinations, and coinfections. Abnormalities in these profiles may occur as a result of antiretroviral therapy. Increasing hepatic dysfunction is evident by elevations in the serum transaminases (AST, ALT, T. bilirubin). Blood work should also include hepatitis C serology (antibody), hepatitis B serology, and Toxoplasma IgG serology.

Urine analysis should be done annually unless the person is on antiretroviral therapy, which may require more frequent follow-up to check for toxicity. Syphilis studies should be done annually; however, patients with low positive titers should have follow-up testing at 3, 6, 9, 12, and 24 months. Gonorrhea and chlamydia tests are encouraged every 6–12 months if the patient is sexually active. Annual Papanicolaou (Pap) smears are also indicated, with recommendations for Pap smears every 3–6 months in HIV-infected women who are symptomatic. In addition, HIV-infected persons should be tested for IgG antibody to Toxoplasma soon after the diagnosis of HIV infection to detect latent infection with *Toxoplasma gondii*. Toxoplasma seronegative persons who are not taking a *Pneumocystis jiroveci* prophylactic regimen known to be active against Toxoplasma encephalitis (TE) should be retested for IgG antibody to Toxoplasma when their CD4+ counts decline to <100 cells/mm³ to determine whether they have seroconverted and are therefore at risk of TE.[45]

Individuals should be tested for latent tuberculosis infection (LTBI) at the time of their HIV diagnosis, regardless of their TB risk category, and then annually if negative. An LTBI diagnosis can be achieved with the use of tuberculin skin test (TST) or by or interferon gamma release assay (IGRA) using the patient's serum. A TST is considered positive in patients with induration of greater than or equal to 5 mm. An IGRA is reported as positive or negative. Any positive test warrants chest radiograph for active disease and consideration of antituberculosis therapy based on history and laboratory, physical, and radiographic findings.

Prophylaxis

The primary strategy to prevent the development of opportunistic infections is to avoid exposure to microorganisms in the environment. Second, the immune system can be supported and maintained through the administration of prophylactic and/or suppressive therapies, which decrease the frequency or severity of opportunistic infections. Primary prophylaxis is the administration of a pharmacological agent to prevent initial infection, whereas secondary prophylaxis is the administration of a pharmacological agent to prevent future occurrences of infection. However, because of the effectiveness of antiretrovirals, there has been a significant decrease in the incidence of opportunistic infections. Therefore, prophylaxis for life for HIV-related co-infections is no longer necessary in many cases.[46] If antiretroviral therapy restores immune system function as evident by a rise in CD4 counts, then clinicians may stop administering primary prophylaxis under defined conditions.[46] The advantages to ending preventive prophylaxis for opportunistic infections in selected patients is a decrease in drug interactions and toxicities, lower cost of care, and greater adherence to antiretroviral regimens.[46] The guidelines for the prevention and treatment of opportunistic infections continue to evolve. Guidelines published by the Department of Health and Human Services provides the most up to date and authoritative resource on opportunistic infections and recommended prophylactic and alternative regimens and is available at http://aidsinfo.nih.gov/contentfiles/adult_oi.pdf.[45] In the late symptomatic and advanced stages of HIV disease, when CD4 counts are low and VL may be high, prophylaxis remains important to protect against opportunistic infections. Therefore, throughout the illness trajectory, and even in hospice settings, patients may be taking prophylactic medications, thus requiring sophisticated planning and monitoring.

Additionally, HIV-infected individuals are at risk for severe diseases that are vaccine preventable, such as hepatitis A and B, tetanus, influenza, pneumococcal and measles, rubella, and mumps. Figure 40.1 presents vaccine-preventable illnesses and interventions.

Indications for antiretroviral therapy across the illness trajectory

Without a cure for HIV, all treatments are essentially palliative in nature to slow disease progression and limit the occurrence of opportunistic infections, which adversely affect quality of life. The goal of initiating antiretroviral therapy is to achieve maximum long-term suppression of HIV-RNA and to restore or preserve immune system function and thereby reduce morbidity and mortality and promote quality of life. Historically, assessment of the CD4 cell count was used to determine the initiation of antiretroviral therapy with antiretroviral therapy primarily reserved for CD4 counts below 350 cells/mm³. Currently, antiretroviral therapy is recommended for all HIV patients regardless of CD4 cell count.[44] The benefits of early therapy include earlier suppression of viral replication, preservation of the immune system functioning, prolongation of disease-free survival, and a decrease in the risk of HIV transmission.[44] However, the risks of early therapy initiation include lower quality of life caused by the adverse effects of therapy, problems with adherence to therapy, and subsequent drug resistance, with the potential limitation of future treatment options. There is further concern regarding the risks of severe toxicities associated with certain antiretroviral medications, such as elevations in serum levels of triglycerides and cholesterol, alterations in fat distribution, or insulin resistance and diabetes mellitus.[44] The decision to start therapy involves discussion with the patient regarding his/her willingness, ability, and readiness to begin therapy and the risk for disease progression given the VL as well as CD4 count. When prescribed, HIV regimens must be maximally suppressive regimens and should be used guided by resistance assays. The use of drug resistance testing has become an integral part of HIV clinical care and is an important component of choosing the most effective antiretroviral regimens.

Antiretroviral therapy used to treat HIV infection

Antiretroviral drugs are broadly classified by the phase of the retrovirus life-cycle that the drug inhibits.

- Nucleoside reverse transcriptase inhibitors (NRTIs) interfere with the action of an HIV protein called reverse transcriptase, which the virus needs to make new copies of itself.

Immunization Schedule for Human Immunodeficiency Virus (HIV)-Infected Adults

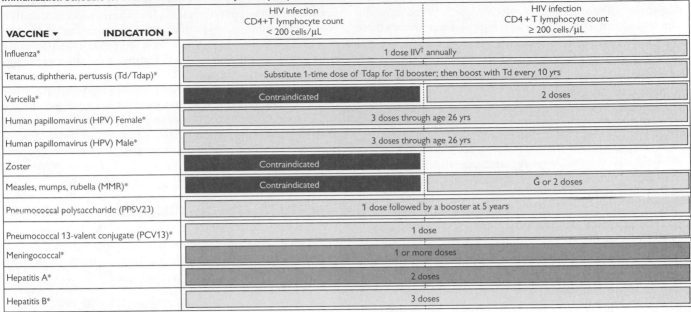

VACCINE ▼ INDICATION ▶	HIV infection CD4+T lymphocyte count < 200 cells/μL	HIV infection CD4 + T lymphocyte count ≥ 200 cells/μL
Influenza*	1 dose IIV† annually	
Tetanus, diphtheria, pertussis (Td/Tdap)*	Substitute 1-time dose of Tdap for Td booster; then boost with Td every 10 yrs	
Varicella*	Contraindicated	2 doses
Human papillomavirus (HPV) Female*	3 doses through age 26 yrs	
Human papillomavirus (HPV) Male*	3 doses through age 26 yrs	
Zoster	Contraindicated	
Measles, mumps, rubella (MMR)*	Contraindicated	G or 2 doses
Pneumococcal polysaccharide (PPSV23)	1 dose followed by a booster at 5 years	
Pneumococcal 13-valent conjugate (PCV13)*	1 dose	
Meningococcal*	1 or more doses	
Hepatitis A*	2 doses	
Hepatitis B*	3 doses	

* Covered by the Vaccine Injury Compensation Program
†IIV-Inactivated Influenza Vaccine. LAIV (live attenuated influenza) is not recommended for HIV-infected persons.

For all persons in this category who meet the age requirements and who lack documentation of vaccination or have no evidence of previous infection;

zoster vaccine recommended regardless of prior episode of zoster

Recommended if some other risk factor is present (e.g., on the basis of medical, occupational, lifestyle, or other indications)

No recommendation

Adapted from the Advisory Committee on Immunization Practices (ACIP) 2013 Adult Immunization Schedule. A summary of the adult immunization schedule vaccines and their primary indications, adverse events and contraindications can be found at: www.cdcgov/vacciness/schedules/downloads/adult/mmwr-adult-schedule.pdf. For more detailed information on immunization of persons with HIV infection against influenza, pneumococal disease, hepatitis B, human papillomavirus, varicella, and hepatitis A, see disease-specific sections in the text and in Table 1. For additional information on these and other vaccines (tetanus, diphtheria, pertussis, measles, mumps, rubella, and meningococcal disease), refer to recommendations of the ACIP at: www.cdc.gov/vaccines/pubs/acip-list.htm.

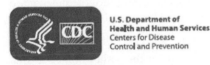

U.S. Department of Health and Human Services
Centers for Disease Control and Prevention

Figure 40.1 Vaccine preventable illnesses and immunization schedule for HIV-infected adults.[45]

♦ Non-nucleoside reverse transcriptase inhibitors (NNRTIS) inhibit reverse transcriptase directly by binding to the enzyme and interfering with its function.

♦ Protease inhibitors (PIs) target viral assembly by inhibiting the activity of protease, an enzyme used by HIV to cleave nascent proteins for final assembly of new virons.

♦ Integrase inhibitors inhibit the enzyme integrase, which is responsible for integration of viral DNA into the DNA of the infected cell.

♦ Entry inhibitors (fusion inhibitors and CCR5 antagonist) interfere with binding, fusion, and entry of HIV-1 to the host cell by blocking one of several targets. Maraviroc and enfuvirtide are the two available agents in this class.[45]

Recommended antiretroviral therapy for patients naïve to antiretroviral therapy

When patients are naïve to antiretroviral therapy, it is recommended that they begin a combination antiretroviral regimen.

As of this writing, the preferred regimens are either NNRTI, protease inhibitor, or integrase inhibitor based. The exact combinations recommended constantly change based on the emergence of high-quality evidence that supports the effectiveness in naïve patients. The reader should refer to the Department of Health and Human Services website to obtain the latest approved medications and the combination recommendations based on the latest evidence (http://aidsinfo.nih.gov/guidelines).

Reasons to change a regimen

It is appropriate to change a medication regimen when there is insufficient viral suppression, evident by an increase in VL, an inadequate increase in CD4 cell counts, evidence of disease progression, adverse clinical effects of therapy, or compromised adherence caused by the inconvenience of difficult regimens. The decision to change therapy involves consideration of whether other drug choices are available, the results of baseline resistance assays and the patient's commitment to adhere to therapy.

More specifically, the criteria for considering changing a patient's antiretroviral regimen include the following[44]:

- When there is virological or incomplete failure: When the HIV VL fails to fall to a level < 200 copies/mL or < 50 copies/mL by 48 weeks after starting therapy; virological rebound when there is HIV RNA > 200 copies after complete suppression

- When there is immunological failure: Persistent decline in CD4 cell or failure to achieve an adequate CD4 response despite virological suppression

- The occurrence or recurrence of HIV-related events after at least 3 months on an antiretroviral regimen (excluding immune reconstitution syndrome)

A change in an antiretroviral regimen can also be guided by drug-resistance tests, such as genotyping and phenotyping assays. Consultation with an HIV specialist is essential.

Concern regarding drug interactions

Considerations should also be given to possible drug interactions such as pharmacokinetic interactions, which occur when administration of one agent changes the plasma concentration of another agent, and pharmacodynamic interactions, which occur when a drug interacts with the biologically active sites and changes the pharmacological effect of the drug without altering the plasma concentration. For example, in palliative care, drug interactions have been reported for patients who are receiving methadone for pain management and who begin therapy with several different HIV drugs in several different classes, particularly the NNRTI and protease inhibitor classes of drugs. Individuals may experience symptoms of opioid withdrawal within 2–3 days of starting therapy because of its effect on the cytochrome P-450 metabolic enzyme CYP3A4 and its induction of methadone metabolism (see Figure 40.2).

Use and continuation of antiretrovirals in the hospice/palliative care setting

The current aims of antiretroviral therapy are to prevent progression to AIDS, prevent the direct effects and symptoms of HIV disease (such as dementia, neuropathy, and diarrhea), and to prevent the complications of AIDS. At the end of life, it is typical to consider only those medications that are necessary to minimize suffering and symptoms. Considering whether or not to continue antiretroviral therapy is be best made in consultation with an HIV specialist and a in focused discussion with the patient and family members. Patients can be asked, "How do you feel when you take your antiretroviral medications?" Because medications may still symbolize hope, patients who enter hospice may have a greater acceptance of their mortality and wish to stop antiretrovirals because of the side effects. Other patients may wish to continue antiretroviral therapy because of its symptom relief and the prevention of future symptoms related to opportunistic infections. Still consistent with today's perspective, Von Gunten and colleagues suggest the following plan[47]:

1. If the drug causes burdensome symptoms, then discontinue.

2. If the patient no longer wants the drug, then discontinue.

3. If the patient is asymptomatic and wants the drug, then continue with close clinical assessment.

4. Discontinue the measurement of VLs and CD4 counts and help the patient focus on relief of symptoms.

In the hospice and palliative care settings, it is important for clinicians to discuss with patients and families their goals of care to make important decisions regarding the appropriateness of curative, palliative, or both types of interventions. More specifically, examples of clinical decisions about palliative or disease-specific care include[48]:

- The use of blood transfusions, psychostimulants, or corticosteroids to treat fatigue in patients with late-stage AIDS

- Aggressive antiemetic therapy for PI-induced nausea and vomiting or discontinuation of such antiretroviral therapies, given severe side effects

- Continued suppressive therapy for opportunistic infections

- Continued use of antiretrovirals or the withdrawal of antiretrovirals after evidence of treatment failure, with assessment of medical risk-benefit and emotional value of therapy

- Decisions to initiate antiretroviral in newly diagnosed late-stage patients

Interaction of Methadone and Non-Nucleoside Reverse Transcriptase Inhibitors (NNRTIs)		
Medication	Effect on Methadone or NNRTI	Dosage Recommendation
Efavirenz	Methadone AUC ↓ 52%	Opiate withdrawal common; increased methadone dose often necessary.
Etravirine	No significant effect	No dosage adjustment necessary.
Nevirapine	Methadone AUC ↓ 37–51% Nevirapine: no significant effect	Opiate withdrawal common; increased methadone dose often necessary
Rilpivirine	R-Methadone AUC ↓ 16%	No dosage adjustment necessary, but monitor for withdrawal symptoms.

Figure 40.2 Potential drug-drug interactions with methadone and non-nucleoside reverse transcriptase inhibitors. Source: This figure is adapted from information obtained from a panel on antiretroviral guidelines for adults and adolescents. Guidelines for the use of antiretroviral agents in HIV-1-infected adults and adolescents. Department of Health and Human Services. March 27, 2012;1–239.

Selwyn and Rivard[48] suggest that decisions regarding these issues need to be based on the specific goals of care, such as quality of life or life prolongation, the use of palliative care interventions to relieve the side effects of other medications, and the use of certain disease-specific therapies to enhance quality of life, as well as the decision to not prolong life when a certain threshold is met, such as progressive dementia.

Adherence to therapy

Adherence, which is "the extent to which a person's behavior coincides with medical and health advice,"[49] is essential to health maintenance for patients with HIV/AIDS because nonadherence to antiretroviral therapy may lead to HIV drug resistance. Medication adherence is defined as the ratio of medication doses taken to those prescribed. The gold standard for medication adherence requires that more than 95% of the regimen be taken to achieve full supression.[50,51] Simplifying the patient's regimen to decrease the number of medications taken and the number of times the patient has to take medications can improve adherence.[52,53] Assessment of adherence is most often done by self-report, with studies showing that it is a valid indicator of adherence.[54] Important aspects of assessment include asking patients to bring their medications to a health visit, to describe their pill-taking regimens, to review the number of doses taken in 24 hours, and to ask about problems taking the medications and effects of the medications.[55] Factors not predictive of adherence include age, sex, race, education, occupation, and socioeconomic status,[56] whereas factors predictive of adherence include the following:[57]

◆ Patient characteristics, such as physical and emotional health, material resources, cultural beliefs, self-efficacy, social support, personal skills, and HIV knowledge

◆ Clinician factors, including interpersonal style and availability, as well as assessment, communication, and clinical skills

◆ Medication regimen factors, such as frequency, number, and size of pills, taste of pills, storage, side effects, effectiveness, and cost

◆ Illness factors, including symptoms duration, severity, and stigma

Adherence to medication regimens can be improved through educational, behavioral, and social interventions specific to the patient, clinician, and medication regimen (Table 40.1).[58] An established partnership and an open, trusting, and supportive relationship between patient and clinician remain key factors in promoting not only adherence to medication regimens but support of all health-promotion and management initiatives to delay disease progression and AIDS-related complications.

AIDS-related opportunistic infections and malignancies

Opportunistic infections are a great cause of morbidity in individuals with HIV. Given the compromised immune system of HIV-infected individuals, there is a wide spectrum of pathogens that can produce primary and sometimes life-threatening infections, particularly when the CD4 cell counts fall below 200 cells/mm^3 (see Figure 40.3). Given the weakened immune systems of

Table 40.1 Interventions to improve antiretroviral medication adherence

Type of intervention	Specific examples
Interventions addressing the patient	
Key patient education topics	Dynamics of HIV infection
	Purpose of antiretroviral therapy
	All names of medications
	Reasons for dose and administration requirements
	Potential side effects
	Techniques for managing side effects
Cues and reminders for patient	Detailed daily schedule
	Doses planned to coincide with daily habits (favorite TV program, morning news)
	Medication boxes and timers (available from some pharmaceutical companies)
	Prepoured medications
	Unit-of-use packaging
Patient involvement in therapeutic plan	Contributes to choice of antiretroviral combination
	Self-control of medications for side effects
	Anticipatory planning for weekends, vacations
Rewards and reinforcements	Positive feedback: falling HIV RNA level, rising CD4+ cell count, fewer clinic appointments
Social support for adherence	Involvement of significant others
	Support groups
	Peer counseling and buddy plans
	Treatment of concomitant conditions such as substance abuse, depression
	Case management and financial assistance
	Home visits and telephone follow-up
Interventions addressing the clinician	
Continuing education regarding	Importance of adherence
	Factors associated with adherence
	Techniques to increase adherence
	Teaching skills
	Communication skills
	Effective management of side effects
Cues and reminders for the clinician	User-friendly medication review forms
	Tables and checklists in the clinical chart
	Patient teaching tools
Social support	Involvement of colleagues
	Team approach
	Administrative approval for additional time spent with patient on adherence concerns
Interventions addressing the regimen	Once- or twice-a-day dosing regimens
	Use of fewer pills per day
	Use of smaller pills or capsules
	Improved taste
	Simpler storage requirements
	Fewer side effects
	Increased effectiveness
	Decreased cost

Source: Williams (1999), reference 55. Copyright 1999 with permission from Elsevier.

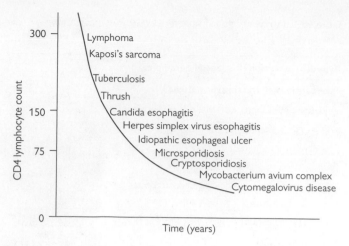

Figure 40.3 Natural history of untreated HIV infection and relationship of specific opportunistic infections to CD4 count.

HIV-infected persons, even previously acquired infections can be reactivated. Most of these opportunistic infections are preventable through treatment and can at best be palliated to control the acute stage of infection and prevent recurrence through long-term suppressive therapy. Additionally, patients with HIV/AIDS often experience concurrent or consecutive opportunistic infections that are severe and cause a great number of symptoms. The most comprehensive and authoritative review on specific opportunistic infections and their treatments can be found at http://aidsinfo. nih.gov/contentfiles/adult_oi.pdf.

Patients with HIV/AIDS require symptom management not only for chronic debilitating opportunistic infections and malignancies but also for the side effects of treatments and other therapies. There are five broad principles fundamental to successful symptom management: (1) taking the symptoms seriously, (2) assessment, (3) diagnosis, (4) treatment, and (5) ongoing evaluation.[59]

- Taking the symptoms seriously implies that symptoms often are not observable and measurable. Therefore, self-report of the patient should be taken seriously by the practitioner and acknowledged as a real experience of the patient. An important rule in symptom management is to anticipate the symptom and attempt to prevent it.[30] Assessment and diagnosis of signs and symptoms of disease and treatment of side effects require a thorough history and physical examination. Questions regarding when the symptom began and its location, duration, severity, and quality, as well as factors that exacerbate or alleviate the symptom, are important. Patients can also be asked to rate the severity of a symptom by using a numerical scale from 0 to 10, with 0 being "no symptom" and 10 being "extremely severe." Such scales can also be used to rate how much a symptom interferes with activities of daily life, with 0 meaning "no interference" and 10 meaning "extreme interference."

- Many patients seek medical care for a specific symptom, which requires a focused history, physical exam, and diagnostic testing. Throughout the continuum of HIV, CD4 counts, VLs, and blood counts and chemistries may provide useful information for the management of the disease and its symptoms. Assessment of current medications and complementary therapies, including vitamin therapy, past medical illness that may

be exacerbated by HIV disease, and the administration regimen of chemotherapy and radiation therapy, should also be ascertained to determine the effects of treatment, side effects, adverse effects, and drug interactions. However, when treatment is no longer effective, as in the case of extremely advanced disease, practitioners must reevaluate the benefits versus burden of diagnostic testing and treatments, particularly the need for daily blood draws or more invasive and uncomfortable procedures. When the decision of the practitioners, patient, and family is that all testing and aggressive treatments are futile, their discontinuation is warranted.

- Treatment of opportunistic infections and malignancies often requires support of the patient's immune system, antiretroviral therapy to decrease the VL and improve CD4 cell counts, and medications and therapies to cure the patient of opportunistic infections or merely palliate the associated symptoms. Indeed, the treatment of symptoms to improve quality of life plays an important role in the management of HIV throughout the course of the illness.[18] In the case of many infections, acute treatment is followed by the regular dosing or maintenance therapy to prevent symptom recurrence. To maximize the quality of life, each patient's treatment regimen and plan of care should be individualized, with documentation of the treatment response and ongoing evaluation.

- Ongoing evaluation is key to symptom management and to determining the effectiveness of traditional, experimental, and complementary therapies. Changes in therapies are often necessary because concurrent or sequential illness or conditions occur.[59]

Holzemer and others[60,61] emphasize a number of key tenets related to the symptoms experienced by patients: (1) the patient is the gold standard for understanding the symptom experience; (2) patients should not be labeled "asymptomatic" early in the course of the infection, because they often experience symptoms of anxiety, fear, and depression; (3) nurses are not necessarily good judges of patients' symptoms, as they frequently underestimate the frequency and intensity of HIV signs and symptoms; however, following assessment, they can answer specific questions about a symptom, such as location, intensity, duration, and so forth; (4) nonadherence to treatment regimens is associated with greater frequency and intensity of symptoms; (5) greater frequency and intensity of symptoms leads to lower quality of life; (6) symptoms may or may not correspond with physiological markers; and (7) patients use few self-care symptom management strategies other than medication.

Symptom assessment and management have been related to quality of life in patients with HIV/AIDS. Using data from a nationally representative cohort of HIV patients ($n = 2267$), Lorenz et al.[62] reported that symptoms were significantly related to health-related quality of life and that the functional status and well-being of patients with HIV was inextricably linked to their symptoms.

The experience of pain in HIV

Pain management must become more integrated in the comprehensive care offered to patients with AIDS. Management of chronic pain syndromes is the most common reason for referral to palliative care.[63] Patients with HIV infection present various painful manifestations: (1) GI pain syndromes: oropharyngeal pain, esophageal, abdominal pain, biliary tract and pancreatic pain, and anorectal pain; (2) chest pain syndromes; (3) neurological pain syndromes: headache and neuropathies; and (4) rheumatological pain syndromes: arthritis and arthropathies, myopathy, and myositis.[64] In a longitudinal study based on 95 patients with AIDS, Frich and Borgbjerg[65] reported the overall incidence of pain as 88%, with 69% suffering moderate-to-severe constant pain that interfered with daily living. The survival rate of patients without pain was significantly higher than in those who reported pain.[65]

Pain may be undertreated in certain HIV populations, particularly in HIV patients who are intravenous drug users. Providers may view reports of pain as drug-seeking behavior. A vicious cycle ensues whereby this view may actually lead to drug-seeking behaviors.[64] When caring for active drug users and those on methadone maintenance it must be assumed that they have tolerance to opioids and may require higher doses of pain medications.

The inadequate assessment and treatment of pain often occurs because of societal, practitioner, and patient barriers and limitations. For example, with regard to pain management, society fears addiction to opioids and has not distinguished between the legitimate and illegal use of drugs. Practitioners may have inadequate knowledge and misconceptions about pain management, whereas patients often fear pain because it is suggestive of advanced disease, and they are reluctant to report pain because they desire to be perceived as "good" patients.

Pain syndromes in patients with AIDS are diverse in nature and etiology. For patients with AIDS, pain can occur in more than one site, such as pain in the legs (peripheral neuropathy reported in 40% of AIDS patients), as well as pain in the abdomen, oral cavity, esophagus, skin, perirectal area, chest, joints, muscles, and head. Pain is also related to HIV/AIDS therapies such as antiretroviral therapies, antibacterials, chemotherapy (such as vincristine), radiation, surgery, and procedures.[66] Following a complete assessment, including a history and physical examination, an individualized pain management plan should be developed to treat the underlying cause of the pain.

The principles of pain management in the palliative care of patients with AIDS are the same as for patients with cancer and include regularity of dosing, individualization of dosing, and using combinations of medications. The three-step guidelines for pain management (as outlined by WHO) should be used for patients with HIV disease.[67] This approach advocates for the selection of analgesics based on the severity of pain. For mild-to-moderate pain, antiinflammatory drugs such as nonsteroidal antiinflammatory drugs (NSAIDs) or acetaminophen are recommended. However, the use of NSAIDs in patients with AIDS requires awareness of toxicity and adverse reactions because they are highly protein-bound, and the free fraction available is increased in AIDS patients who are cachectic or wasted.[67] For moderate-to-severe pain that is persistent, opioids of increasing potency are recommended, beginning with opioids such as codeine, hydrocodone, or oxycodone (each available with or without aspirin or acetaminophen), and advancing to more potent opioids such as morphine, hydromorphone (Dilaudid), methadone (Dolophine), or fentanyl either intravenously or transdermally. In conjunction with NSAIDs and opioids, the following adjuvant therapies are recommended[67]:

- Tricyclic antidepressants, heterocyclic and noncyclic antidepressants, and serotonin reuptake inhibitors for neuropathic pain
- Psychostimulants to improve opioid analgesia and decrease sedation
- Phenothiazine to relieve anxiety or agitation
- Butyrophenones to relieve anxiety and delirium
- Antihistamines have minimal effect on analgesia but increase sedation and relieve anxiety, insomnia, and nausea
- Corticosteroids to decrease pain associated with an inflammatory component or with bone pain
- Benzodiazepines for neuropathic pain, anxiety, and insomnia

Caution is noted, however, with use of protease inhibitors (PIs) because they may interact with some analgesics. For example, Ritonavir has been associated with potentially lethal interactions with meperidine, propoxyphene, and piroxicam. The PIs must also be used with caution in patients receiving codeine, tricyclic antidepressants, sulindac, and indomethacin to avoid toxicity. Furthermore, for patients with HIV who have high fevers, the increase in body temperature may lead to increased absorption of transdermally administered fentanyl.

To ensure appropriate dosing when changing the route of administration of opioids or changing from one opioid to another, the use of an equianalgesic conversion chart is suggested. As with all patients, oral medications should be used, if possible, with round-the-clock dosing at regular intervals and the use of rescue doses for breakthrough pain. Often, controlled-release morphine or oxycodone are effective drugs for patients with chronic pain from HIV/AIDS. In the case of neuropathic pain, often experienced with HIV/AIDS, tricyclic antidepressants such as amitriptyline or anticonvulsants such as Neurontin can be very effective.[67] However, the use of neuroleptics must be weighed against an increased sensitivity of AIDS patients to the extrapyramidal side effects of these drugs.[67] If the cause of pain is increasing tumor size, radiation therapy can also be very effective in pain management by reducing tumor size, as well as the perception of pain. Please refer to the chapter 7, on pain management, which presents the nonopiate analgesics for pain management in patients with pain and opioid analgesics for the management of mild-to-moderate pain and from moderate-to-severe pain in patients.

Tolerance, dependence, and addiction

Physiological tolerance refers to the shortened or diminished effect of a drug resulting from exposure to the drug and, therefore, the need for increasing doses to maintain effect. In the case of opioids, tolerance to analgesic properties of the drug appears to be uncommon in the clinical setting, whereas tolerance to adverse effects such as respiratory depression, somnolence, and nausea is common and favorable. Most patients can remain on stable doses of opioids for prolonged periods of time. If an increase in opioid dosage is needed, it is usually because of disease progression. Another expected physiological response to opioids is physical dependence, which occurs after 3 to 4 weeks of opioid administration, as evidenced by withdrawal symptoms after abrupt discontinuation. If a drug is to be discontinued, halving the daily dose every 1 to 2 days until the dose is equivalent to 15 mg of morphine will reduce withdrawal symptoms.[68]

Tolerance and physical dependence to opioids does not imply addiction, as addiction is a compulsive craving for a drug for effects other than pain relief and is thought to be uncommon in patients who are terminally ill. Furthermore, studies have demonstrated that although tolerance and physical dependence commonly occur, addiction (psychological dependence) is not common and occurs infrequently in individuals who do not have histories of substance abuse.[68] However, it should be noted that a certain percentage of patients with HIV/AIDS will have a history of substance abuse, either past or current, that needs to be recognized so that their pain can be managed appropriately, as well as other symptoms for which they are self-medicating. Healthcare providers in palliative care are often concerned with the administration of opioids to patients who have a history of substance abuse, who are in methadone maintenance programs, or who currently are abusing drugs. Therefore, these patients often receive ineffective pain management. Consistent use of a standard pain scale and regular monitoring of drug consumption by one nurse and one physician can be helpful in ongoing assessment and pain management because it limits potential abuse. Oral administration of medications also lowers abuse potential. Given that substance-abusing patients have greater tolerance to morphine derivatives and benzodiazepines because of previous exposure to these drugs, increased dosage may be necessary for effective pain management, or the interval between doses should be shortened. Furthermore, the dosages of medications should be carefully monitored to avoid overdosing, given the possibility of hepatic failure in substance-abusing patients. Simultaneous use of agonists and antagonists are avoided in all populations because they provoke withdrawal symptoms.[66]

Alleviating opioid side effects

Although opioids are extremely effective in pain management for patients with HIV, their common side effects must be anticipated and minimized. In medically fragile populations, such side effects may also result from other comorbid conditions rather than from opioid analgesia itself; therefore, a complete assessment is warranted. Medications and treatments to alleviate opioid side effects include:

- Nausea and vomiting, treated with prochlorperazine (Compazine), metoclopramide (Reglan), haloperidol (Haldol), granisetron (Kytril), and ondansetron (Zofran); (a change in the opioid may also be necessary)

- Constipation, treated by increasing fiber in the diet, stimulating cathartic drugs such as bisacodyl or senna, or hyperosmotic agents such as sorbitol or lactulose

- Sedation, treated by reducing the opioid in each dose or decreasing the frequency, as well as the ingestion of caffeine, and administering dextroamphetamine or methylphenidate (again, a change in the opioid may be warranted)

- Confusion, treated by lowering the opioid dose, changing to a different opioid or haloperidol

- Myoclonus, treated with clonazepam (Klonopin), diazepam (Valium), and baclofen (Lioresal), or a change in the opioid

- Respiratory depression, prevented by starting at a low dose in opioid-naïve patients and being aware of relative potencies when changing opioids, as well as differences by routes of administration. Naloxone (Narcan) may be administered to reverse respiratory depression but should be used with caution in patients who are opioid-tolerant because of the risk of inducing a withdrawal state. Dilute one ampule of naloxone (0.4 mg) in 10 mL of normal saline and titrate to the patient's respirations.[68]

Nonpharmacological and complementary interventions for pain

Nonpharmacological interventions for pain management can also be effective in the care of patients with HIV. Bed rest, simple exercise, heat or cold packs to affected sites, massage, transcutaneous electrical stimulation, and acupuncture can be effective physical therapies with this patient population. Psychological interventions to reduce pain perception and interpretation include hypnosis, relaxation, imagery, biofeedback, distraction, and patient education. Newshan and Staats[69] performed a comprehensive review of the literature on the effectiveness of complementary therapies for pain. Only acupuncture has been adequately studied in the HIV population, and the effectiveness of acupuncture for pain management is inconsistent. Other modalities such as acupressure, massage, yoga, and energy-based therapies have the most evidence to support their use in pain management.

Management of other symptoms experienced with HIV

Patients with HIV/AIDS require symptom management not only for chronic debilitating opportunistic infections and malignancies but also for the side effects of treatments and other therapies. The most prevalent symptoms in AIDS population are fatigue (54%–85%), pain (63%–80%), nausea (43%–49%), and constipation (34%–35%); other symptoms include depression, breathlessness, insomnia, diarrhea, anorexia and anxiety.[12,70] Personal characteristics that interact with both HIV diagnosis and its medical management can influence symptom experience. In a prospective longitudinal study, of 317 men and women living with HIV/AIDS in the San Francisco Bay Area completed the Memorial Symptom Assessment Scale, which is designed to estimate prevalence, severity, and distress of each symptom and global symptom burden. The median number of symptoms was nine, and symptoms experienced by more than half the sample population included lack of energy (65%), drowsiness (57%), difficulty sleeping (56%), and pain (55%). Global symptom burden was unrelated to age or CD4 cell count. Those with an AIDS diagnosis had significantly higher symptom burden scores, as did those currently receiving antiretroviral therapy. African Americans reported fewer symptoms than Caucasians or Mixed/ Other race, and women reported more symptom burden after controlling for AIDS diagnosis and race.[12] Symptom and comfort measures at the end of life for HIV-infected patients share many of the features seen in non-HIV-infected patients at the end of life, because a large percentage of late-stage AIDS patients are now dying of non-AIDS-defining illnesses. Therefore, translation of basic principles in pain and symptom management should be used for HIV-infected patients at the end of life.[71]

Table 40.2 lists selected symptoms in HIV, common presentations, and selected interventions.

Table 40.2 Selected symptoms associated with HIV/AIDS

Symptom	Cause	Presentation	Interventions
Fatigue (asthenia)	HIV infection Opportunistic infections AIDS medications Prolonged immobility Anemia Sleep disorders Hypothyroidism Medications	Weakness Lack of energy	Treat reversible causes. Pace activities with rest periods/naps. Ensure adequate nutrition. Use relaxation exercises and meditation. Take warm rather than hot showers or baths. Use cool room temperatures. Administer dextroamphetamine 10 mg/day PO.
Anorexia (loss of appetite) and cachexia (wasting)	Metabolic alterations caused by cytokines and Interleukin-1 Opportunistic infections Nutrient malabsorption from intestines Chronic diarrhea Depression Taste disorders	Diminished food intake Profound weight loss	Treat reversible causes. Consult with dietician about choice of food. Make food appealing by color and texture. Avoid noxious smells at mealtime. Avoid fatty, fried, and strong-smelling foods. Offer small, frequent meals and nutritious snacks. Encourage patients to eat whatever is appealing. Provide high-energy, high-protein liquid supplements. **? Antidepressants** Use appetite stimulants such as megesterol acetate 800 mg/day PO or dronabinol 2.5 mg PO qd or bid. Testosterone administered by 5 mg transdermal patch to increase weight gain and muscle mass.
Fever (elevated body temperature)	Bacterial toxins Viruses Yeast Antigen–antibody reactions Drugs Tumor products Exogenous pyrogens	Body temperature >99.5°F (oral), 100.5°F (rectal), or 98.5°F (axillary) Chills, rigor Sweating, night sweats Delirium Dizziness Dehydration	Treat reversible causes. Maintain fluid intake. Use loose clothing and sheets, with frequent changing. Avoid plastic bed coverings. Exceptionally high temperature may require ice packs or cooling blankets. Administer around-the-clock antipyretics such as acetaminophen or ASA, 325–650 mg PO q6–8 h.
Dyspnea (shortness of breath) and cough	Bronchospasm Embolism Effusions Pulmonary edema Pneumothorax Kaposi's sarcoma Obstruction Opportunistic infections Anxiety Allergy Mechanical or chemical irritants Anemia	Productive or nonproductive cough Crackles Stridor Hemoptysis Inability to clear secretions Wheezing Tachypnea Gagging Intercostal retractions Areas of pulmonary dullness Anxiety	Treat reversible causes. Elevate bed to Fowler's or high Fowler's position. Provide abdominal splints. Administer humidified oxygen therapy to treat dyspnea. Use fans or open windows to keep air moving for dyspnea. Remove irritants or allergens such as smoke. Teach pursed-lips breathing for patients with obstructive disease. Use frequent mouth care to decrease discomfort from dry mouth. Treat bronchospasm. Suppress cough with dextromethorphan hydrobromide 15–45 mg PO q4 h PRN, or opioids such as codeine 15–60 mg PO q4 h even if taking other opioids for pain, or hydrocodone 5–10 mg PO q4–6 h PRN, or morphine 5–20 mg PO q4 h PRN (may be increased) to relieve dyspnea, cough, and associated anxiety. For hyperactive gag reflex use nebulized lidocaine 5 mL of 2% solution (100 mg) q3–4 h PRN.

(continued)

Table 40.2 (Continued)

Symptom	Cause	Presentation	Interventions
Diarrhea	Idiopathic HIV enteropathy Diet Bowel infections (bacteria, parasites, protozoa) Chronic bowel inflammation Medications Obstruction with overflow incontinence Stress Malabsorption	Flatulence Multiple bowel movements/day Cramps/colic Hemorrhoids	Treat reversible causes. Maintain adequate hydration. Replace electrolytes by giving Gatorade or Pedialyte. Give rice, bananas, or apple juice to reduce diarrhea. Increase protein and calories. Avoid dairy products, alcohol, caffeine, extremely hot or cold foods, spicy or fatty foods. Maintain dignity while toileting. Provide ready access to bathroom or commode. Maintain good perianal care. Administer medications such as Lomotil 2.5–5.0 mg q4–6 h; Kapectolin 60–120 mL q4–6 h (max 20 mg/day); Imodium 2–4 mg q6 h (max 16 mg/day); or aregoric (tincture of opium) 5–10 mL q4–6 h.
Insomnia (inability to fall asleep or stay asleep)	Anxiety Depression Pain Medications Delirium Sleep disorders such as sleep apnea Excess alcohol intake Caffeine	Early-morning awakening Nighttime restlessness Fear Nightmares	Treat reversible causes. Establish a bedtime routine. Reduce daytime napping. Avoid caffeinated beverages and alcohol. Take a warm bath 2 h before bedtime. Use relaxation techniques. Provide an environment conducive to sleep (dark, quiet, comfortable temperature). Administer anxiolytics such as benzodiazepines (use for <2 wk because of dependency), antidepressants (helpful over long term), or other sedatives such as Benadryl.
Headache	Infections such as encephalitis, herpes zoster, meningitis, toxoplasmosis Sinusitis	Pain in one or more areas of the head or over sinuses	Treat reversible causes. Suggest chiropractic manipulation. Provide message therapy. Use relaxation therapy. Apply TENS. Use stepwise analgesia. Administer corticosteroids to reduce swellings around space-occupying lesions.

Source: Coyne et al. (2002), reference 72.

Psychosocial issues for patients with HIV/AIDS and their families

Uncertainty is a chronic and pervasive source of psychological distress for persons living with HIV, particularly as it relates to ambiguous symptom patterns, exacerbation and remissions of symptoms, selection of optimal treatment regimens, the complexity of treatments, and the fear of stigma and ostracism. Such uncertainty is linked to negative perceptions of quality of life and poor psychological adjustment.[73] However, many practitioners focus on patient's physical functioning and performance status as the main indicators of quality of life, rather than on the symptoms of psychological distress such as anxiety and depression.[74] Based on a sample of 203 patients with HIV/AIDS, Farber and colleagues[75] reported that positive meaning of the illness was associated with a higher level of psychological well-being and lower depressed mood and contributed more than problem-focused coping and

social support to predicting both psychological well-being and depressed mood. In a sample of 99 HIV-infected persons, perceived stress, total mood disturbance, present health, and HIV status were independently associated with both frequency of symptoms and symptom distress. The strongest correlates were observed between fatigue and symptom frequency, as well as fatigue and symptom distress. After conducting a backward stepwise regression analysis that included perceived stress, sex, age, HIV status, race, and income, researchers showed that predictor variables of symptom distress included symptom frequency, depression/dejection, anger/ hostility, and fatigue, explaining 79% of the variance in symptom distress after controlling for variables that were removed from the model.[76]

Nurses must also be cognizant of issues such as the experience of multiple losses, complicated grieving, substance abuse, stigmatization, and homophobia, which contribute to patients' sense of alienation, isolation, hopelessness, loneliness, and depression.

Such emotional distress often extends to the patient's family caregivers as they attempt to provide support and lessen the patient's suffering yet are often suffering from HIV themselves. Reciprocal suffering is experienced by family caregivers as well as patients, and there is the need to improve their quality of life through palliative care.[77]

Psychosocial assessment of patients with HIV

Psychosocial assessment of patients with HIV is important throughout the illness trajectory, particularly as the disease progresses and there is increased vulnerability to psychological distress. Psychosocial assessment includes the following:

♦ Social, behavioral, and psychiatric history, which includes the history of interpersonal relationships, education, job stability, career plans, substance use, preexisting mental illness, and individual identity

♦ Crisis points related to the course of the disease as anxiety, fear, and depression intensify, creating a risk of suicide

♦ Life-cycle phase of individuals and families, which influences goals, financial resources, skills, social roles, and the ability to confront personal mortality

♦ Influence of culture and ethnicity, including knowledge and beliefs associated with health, illness, dying, and death, as well as attitudes and values toward sexual behaviors, substance use, health promotion and maintenance, and healthcare decision-making

♦ Past and present patterns of coping, including problem-focused and/or emotion-focused coping

♦ Social support, including sources of support, types of supports perceived as needed by the patient/family, and perceived benefits and burdens of support

♦ Financial resources, including healthcare benefits, disability allowances, and the eligibility for Medicaid/Medicare.

Depression and anxiety in patients with HIV

Because AIDS is a life-threatening, chronic, debilitating illness, patients are at risk for such psychological disorders as depression and anxiety. Among persons living with HIV/AIDS, the prevalence of depression has been estimated at 20%–30% and is characterized by depressed mood, low energy, sleep disturbance, anhedonia, inability to concentrate, loss of libido, weight changes, and possible menstrual irregularities.[78] It is also important to assess whether depressed patients are using alcohol, drugs, and opioids.

Patients with HIV who are diagnosed with depression should be treated with antidepressants to control their symptoms. Selective serotonin reuptake inhibitors (SSRIs) are as effective as tricyclic antidepressants but are better tolerated because of their more benign side-effect profile.[79] Further, SSRIs may interact with such antiretroviral medications as protease inhibitors and NNRTIs; therefore, initial SSRI dosage should be lowered with careful upward titration and close monitoring for toxic reactions.[79] Serotonin and norepinephrine reuptake inhibitors such as venlafaxine and duloxetine are newer antidepressants that also are useful in treating chronic pain. Tricyclic antidepressants are indicated for treating depression only in patients who do not respond to newer medications.[79] It is noted that monoamine oxidase

inhibitors may interact with multiple medications used to treat HIV and should therefore be avoided. Medication interaction and liver function profiles should be considered before antidepressant therapy is initiated.

Because depression is a common symptom in patients with HIV/AIDS, research studies have also focused on other factors that relate to depression in this patient population. Schrimshaw examined whether the source of unsupportive social interactions had differential main and interactive relations with depressive symptoms among ethnically diverse women with HIV/AIDS ($n = 146$).[80] After controlling for demographic variables, Schrimshaw[80] found that unsupportive social interactions with family had a major effect in predicting more depressive symptoms and that there was a significant interaction between unsupportive interactions from a lover/spouse and friends, which predicted high levels of depressive symptoms. Arrindell[81] examined differential coping strategies, anxiety, depression, and symptomatology among African-American women with HIV/AIDS ($n = 30$). The results indicated that the majority of women used emotion-focused coping; however, there were no main effects for coping strategies on psychological distress and no significant difference between symptomatology and coping strategies. An inverse relationship was reported between psychological distress and social support, with less distress reported when women had financial assistance from their families and friends. There was a relationship reported between symptomatology and anxiety, with those who were asymptomatic reporting no anxiety.

Anxiety disorders are more prevalent in people with HIV than in the general population. The prevalence rate of anxiety disorders in people with HIV has been estimated to be as high as 38%.[82] Generalized anxiety disorder is manifested as worry, trouble falling asleep, impaired concentration, psychomotor agitation, hypersensitivity, hyperarousal, and fatigue.[82]

The treatment for patients with anxiety is based on the nature and severity of the symptoms and the coexistence of other mood disorders or substance abuse. Short-acting anxiolytics such as lorazepam (Ativan), and alprazolam (Xanax) are beneficial for intermittent symptoms, whereas buspirone (BuSpar) and clonazepam (Klonopin) are beneficial for chronic anxiety.[83]

For many patients experiencing psychological distress associated with HIV, participation in therapeutic interventions such as skill-building, support groups, individual counseling, and group interventions using meditation techniques can provide a sense of psychological growth and a meaningful way of living with the disease.[84–86] Such interventions are particularly helpful for patients with HIV/AIDS who may not have disclosed their sexual orientation or substance-abusing history to their families. Often, significant stress is associated with sharing such information, particularly when such disclosures occur during the stage of advanced disease. However, the need for therapeutic communication and support from all health professionals caring for the patient and their family exists throughout the illness continuum.

Often many members of a single family are infected and die because of the transmission of the disease from sexual partners and through childbirth. In the homosexual community and substance-abusing community, multiple deaths resulted in complicated mourning. The anxiety, depression, sadness, and loneliness associated with multiple deaths and unending experiences of loss must be recognized and support must be offered. Community resources and referrals to HIV/AIDS support groups and bereavement groups are important in emotional adjustment to these profound losses.

Spiritual issues in AIDS

As health professionals, assessment of the patient's spiritual needs is an important aspect of holistic care. Learning about patients' spiritual values, needs, and religious perspectives is important in understanding their perspectives regarding their illnesses and their perceptions and meaning of life and its purpose, suffering, and eventual death. Spirituality is a way of being or experiencing that comes about through an awareness of a transcendent dimension and values with regard to self, others, nature, and God.[87] An understanding of the patient's relationship with self, others, nature, and God can inform interventions that promote spiritual well-being and the possibility of a "good death" from the patient's perspective.

Some patients living with HIV have the spiritual needs of meaning, value, hope, purpose, love, acceptance, reconciliation, ritual, and affirmation of a relationship with a higher being.[87] Kremer[88] found that spirituality was a prime factor in determining whether the individual viewed HIV as a positive or negative turning point in their life. Those with increased spirituality felt chosen by a Higher Power to have HIV and perceived their infection as a positive turning point in their life. In contrast those with lower spirituality viewed HIV as a negative point in their life. Other investigators have also found a relationship between spirituality and HIV disease progression.[88] Ironson et al.[89] conducted a large, longitudinal study that documented the effects of perceptions of God on the health status of PLWH. In this study, positive perceptions of God were associated with slower while negative perceptions of God were associated with faster HIV disease progression.

Assisting patients to find meaning and value in their lives, despite adversity, often involves a recognition of past successes and their internal strengths. Respectful behavior toward patients demonstrates love and acceptance of the patient as a person. Encouraging open communication between the patient and family is important to work toward reconciliation and the completion of unfinished business.

As with many life-threatening illnesses, patients with AIDS may express anger with God. Some may view their illness as a punishment or are angry that God is not answering their prayers. Expression of feelings can be a source of spiritual healing. Clergy can also serve as valuable members of the palliative care team in offering spiritual support and alleviating spiritual distress. The use of meditation, music, imagery, poetry, and drawing may offer outlets for spiritual expression and promote a sense of harmony and peace.

In a grounded-theory study of hope in patients with HIV/AIDS, Kylma and colleagues[90] found that patients had an alternating balance between hope, despair, and hopelessness based on the possibilities of daily life. They experienced losses such as loss of joy, carefree time, safety, self-respect, potential parenthood, privacy, and trust in self, others, systems, and God. However, there was hope as they received strength by seeing their life from a new perspective as well as an acceptance of the uncertainty of life and the value of life. Hope was described as a basic resource in life and meant the belief that life is worth living at the present and in the future, with good things still to come. Despair meant losing grip,

unable to take hold of anything, whereas hopelessness implied giving up in the face of an assumably nonexistent future, which was the opposite of hope.

For all patients with chronic, life-threatening illness, hope often shifts from hope that a cure will soon be found to hope for a peaceful death with dignity, including the alleviation of pain and suffering, determining one's own choices, being in the company of family and significant others, and knowing that their end-of-life wishes will be honored. Often, the greatest spiritual comfort offered by caregivers or family for patients comes from active listening and meaningful presence by sitting and holding their hands and showing them that they are not abandoned and alone.

Spiritual healing may also come from life review, as patients are offered an opportunity to reminisce about their lives, reflect on their accomplishments, reflect on their misgivings, and forgive themselves and others for their imperfections. Indeed, such spiritual care conveys that even in the shadow of death, there can be discovery, insight, the completion of relationships, the experience of love of self and others, and the transcendence of emotional and spiritual pain. Often, patients with AIDS, by their example, teach nurses, family, and others how to transcend suffering and how to die with grace and dignity.

Advance care planning

Advance planning is another important issue related to end-of-life care for patients with HIV/AIDS. Most patients with AIDS have not discussed with their physicians the kind of care they want at the end of life, although more homosexual men have executed an advance directive than injection-drug users or women.[91] Nonwhite patients with AIDS report that they do not like to talk about the care they would want if they were very sick and are more likely to feel that if they talk about death, it will bring death closer. Conversely, white patients were more likely to believe that their doctor was an HIV/AIDS expert and good at talking about end-of-life care and to recognize they have been very sick in the past and that such discussions are important.[81,92] According to Ferris and colleagues,[93] healthcare providers can assist patients and families by (1) discussing the benefits of healthcare and social support programs, unemployment insurance, worker's compensation, pension plans, insurance, and union or association benefits; (2) emphasizing the importance of organizing information and documents so that they are easily located and accessible; (3) suggesting that financial matters be in order, such as power of attorney or bank accounts, credit cards, property, legal claims, and income tax preparation; (4) discussing advance directives or power of attorney for care and treatment, as well as decisions related to the chosen setting for dying; and (5) discussing the patient's wishes regarding their death—Whom does the patient want at the bedside? What rituals are important to the dying patient? Does the patient wish an autopsy? What arrangements does the patient want regarding the funeral services and burial? Where should donations in remembrance be sent? It is important to realize that these issues should be discussed at relevant stages in the person's illness, in a manner that is both respectful to the patient's wishes and strengths and that promotes the patient's sense of control over his/her life and death.

Healthcare providers must also understand the concept of capacity. In assessing the patient's capacity to make healthcare decisions (a clinical assessment) the health provider must question whether the decision-maker knows the nature and effect of the decision to be made and understands the consequences of his/her actions and determine whether the decision is consistent with an individual's life history, lifestyle, previous actions, and best interests.[93]

When an individual has capacity, and in anticipation of the future loss of capacity, he/she may initiate advance directives such as a living will and/or the designation of a healthcare agent who will carry out the patient's healthcare wishes or make healthcare decisions in the event that the patient loses capacity. The patient may also give an individual the power of attorney regarding financial matters and care or treatment issues. Advance directives may include the patient's decisions regarding such life-sustaining treatments as cardiopulmonary resuscitation, use of vasoactive drips to sustain blood pressure and heart rate, dialysis, artificial nutrition and hydration, and the initiation or withdrawal of ventilatory support. The signing of advance directives must be witnessed by two individuals who are not related to the patient or involved in the patient's treatment. Individuals who have capacity can revoke their advance directives at any time. If a patient is deemed mentally incompetent (by the Court), state statutes may allow the Court to designate a surrogate decision-maker for the patient.

Palliative care through the dying trajectory

Death from AIDS usually results from multiple causes, including chronic infections, malignancies, neurological disease, malnutrition, and multisystem failure. However, even for patients with HIV/AIDS for whom death appears to be imminent, spontaneous recovery with survival of several more weeks or months is possible. The terminal stage is often marked by periods of increasing weight loss and deteriorating physical and cognitive functioning. In the terminal stage of HIV, decisions related to prevention, diagnosis, and treatment pose ethical and clinical issues for both patients and their healthcare providers because they must decide on the value and frequency of laboratory monitoring, use of invasive procedures, use of antiretroviral and prophylactic measures, and patients' participation in clinical trails.

The dying process for patients with advanced AIDS is commonly marked by increasingly severe physical deterioration, leaving the patient bed-bound and experiencing wasting, dyspnea at rest, and pressure ulcers. Ultimately, patients become dependent on others for care. Febrile states and changes in mental status often occur as death becomes more imminent. Maintaining the comfort and dignity of the patients becomes a nursing priority. Symptomatic treatments, including pain management, should be continued throughout the dying process, as even obtunded patients may feel pain and other symptoms.

The end of life is an important time for individuals to accept their own shortcomings and limitations and differences with significant others so that death may be accepted without physical, psychosocial, and spiritual anguish. At the end of life, patients with AIDS may have a desire for hastened death. Based on a sample of 128 terminally ill patients with AIDS who were receiving palliative care, Pessin[94] found that there was a significant association between desire for a hastened death and cognitive impairment, with memory impairment providing an independent and unique contribution to desire for hastened death. Curtis and colleagues[95] also examined the desire of AIDS patients for less life-sustaining treatment as associated with the medical futility rationale. It

was reported that 61% ($n = 35$) of patients with advanced AIDS accepted the medical futility rationale as it applied to their medical care at the end of life, including the use of mechanical ventilation. However, because 26% ($n = 15$) thought the medical futility rationale was probably acceptable and 10% ($n = 5$) said it was definitely not acceptable, clinicians invoking the medical futility rationale should consider the diversity of these patient attitudes toward care at the end of life. Through an interdisciplinary approach to care, health professionals can assist patients with the following: reducing their internal conflicts, such as fears about the loss of control, which can be related to a desire for hastened death; making end-of-life decisions regarding medical treatments that are consistent with their values, wishes, and preferences; promoting the patient's sense of identity; supporting the patient in maintaining important interpersonal relationships; and encouraging patients to identify and attempt to reach meaningful but limited goals.

Because palliative care also addresses the needs of family, it is important to consider the vulnerability of family members to patients' health problems at the end of life. In a study of the health status of informal caregivers ($n = 76$) of persons with HIV/AIDS, Flaskerud and Lee[96] found that caregiver distress regarding a patient's symptoms, anxiety, and education was related to depressive symptoms and that depressive symptoms, anger, and functional status of patients with AIDS were related to poorer physical health of informal caregivers. Therefore, members of the palliative care team can provide much-needed assistance not only to patients but their families.

As illness progresses and death approaches, health professionals can encourage patients and family members to express their fears and end-of-life wishes. Encouraging patients and families to express such feelings as "I love you," "I forgive you," "Forgive me—I am sorry," "Thank you," and "Good-bye" is important to the completion of relationships.[97] Peaceful death can also occur when families give the patient permission to die and assure them that they will be remembered.

Loss, grief, and bereavement for persons with HIV/AIDS and their survivors

Throughout the illness trajectory, patients with HIV disease experience many losses: a sense of loss of identity as they assume the identity of a patient with AIDS; loss of control over health and function; loss of roles as the illness progresses; loss of body image because of skin lesions, changes in weight, and wasting; loss of sexual freedom because of the need to change sexual behaviors to maintain health and prevent transmission to others; loss of financial security through possible discrimination and increasing physical disability; and loss of relationships through possible abandonment, self-induced isolation, and the multiple deaths of others from the disease.[98] In a study of AIDS-related grief and coping with loss among HIV-positive men and women ($n = 268$), Sikkema and colleagues[98] reported that the severity of grief reaction to AIDS-related losses was associated with escape-avoidance and self-controlling coping strategies, the type of loss, depressive symptoms, and history of injection drug use. For healthcare professionals, each occurrence of illness may pose new losses and heighten the patient's awareness of his or her mortality. Therefore, each illness experience is an opportunity for health professionals to respond to cues of the patients in addressing their concerns and approaching the subject of loss, dying, and death. Given that grief is the emotional response to loss, patients dying from AIDS may also manifest the signs of grief, which include feelings of sadness, anger, self-reproach, anxiety, loneliness, fatigue, shock, yearning, relief, and numbness; physical sensations such as hollowness in the stomach, tightness in the chest, oversensitivity to noise, dry mouth, muscle weakness, and loss of coordination; cognitions of disbelief or confusion; and behavior disturbances in appetite, sleep, social withdrawal, loss of interest in activities, and restless overactivity.

Upon the death of the patient, the patient's family and significant others enter a state of bereavement, or a state of having suffered a loss, which is often a long-term process of adapting to life without the deceased.[97] Family and significant others may experience signs of grief, including a sense of presence of the deceased, paranormal experiences or hallucinations, dreams of the deceased, and a desire to have cherished objects of the deceased and to visit places frequented by the deceased. The work of grief is a dynamic process that is neither time-limited nor predictable.[99] It may be that those left behind never "get over" the loss but, rather, find a place for it in their life and create through memory a new relationship with their loved one.

Families and partners of patients with AIDS may experience disenfranchised grief, defined as the grief that persons experience when they incur a loss that is not openly acknowledged, publicly mourned, or socially supported.[100] Support is not only important in assisting families in the tasks of grieving but is also important for nurses who have established valued relationships with their patients. Indeed, disenfranchised grief may also be experienced by nurses who do not allow themselves to acknowledge their patient's death as a personal loss or who are not acknowledged by others, such as the patient's family or even professional colleagues, as having suffered a loss.

For all individuals who have experienced a loss, Worden[101] has identified the tasks of grieving as (1) accepting the reality of the death; (2) experiencing the pain of grief; (3) adjusting to a changed physical, emotional, and social environment in which the deceased is missing; and (4) finding an appropriate emotional place for the person who died in the emotional life of the bereaved.

To facilitate each of Worden's tasks, Mallinson[99] recommends the following nursing interventions:

- Accept the reality of death by speaking of the loss and facilitating emotional expression.

- Work through the pain of grief by exploring the meaning of the grief experience.

- Adjust to the environment without the deceased by acknowledging anniversaries and the experience of loss during holidays and birthdays; help the bereaved to problem-solve and recognize their own abilities to conduct their daily lives.

- Emotionally relocate the deceased and move on with life by encouraging socialization through formal and informal avenues.

The complications of AIDS-related grief often come from the secrecy and social stigma associated with the disease.[102] Reluctance to contact family and friends can restrict the normal support systems available for the bereaved.

In addition to a possible lack of social support, the death of patients with AIDS may result in complicated grief for the bereaved, given that death occurs after lengthy illness, and the relationships may have been ambivalent. Through truthful and culturally sensitive communication, health professionals can offer families support in their grief and promote trust that their needs are understood and validated.

Case study

Maria Jackson, a patient with MAC

Maria Jackson, a 34-year-old woman, was seen in the emergency room for fever, fatigue, anorexia, nausea and vomiting, and weight loss, having 30 episodes of liquid diarrhea each day. As a differential diagnosis, she was tested for HIV. Findings indicated a CD4 count of 45 cells/mm^3 and a VL of 142,000 mL, indicative of the advanced stage of HIV. Her laboratory work indicated anemia and an elevated alkaline phosphatase. Disseminated MAC was confirmed by culture of her blood. Physical examination revealed hepatosplenomegaly and inguinal lymphadenopathy. Maria was started on azithromycin and rifabutin to treat MAC, as well as a regimen of combination antiretroviral agents one potent PI and two NRTIs—specifically atazanavir + ritonavir (PI)—and emtricitabine and tenofovir disoproxil fumarate (Truvada) to treat her advanced stage of AIDS. Maria had lived with Juan for the last five years, but they were not married as he had a drug history and two incarcerations for drug possession. Maria did not know his criminal history when she met him. After Maria's infection improved she still had difficulty "holding down" food but ate small frequent meals. She lost two dress sizes, going from a size 8 to a size 4. Maria had all she could do to take care of herself and two young children.

The diarrhea improved with medications, but Maria was still too insecure to leave the house because she was more comfortable having immediate access to a toilet. Within the month, Maria became more depressed and isolated. Although a home health aide visited for a few hours each day, there was minimal verbal interaction between them. She began to stay in bed for long periods of time during the day, wondering if she was ever going to get better. Maria was treated with an antidepressant, and within weeks her mood improved. Her appetite also increased and her physician was encouraged by her response to therapy. Maria's physician discussed advance directives, and Maria asked her sister to be her healthcare proxy and she also wanted her sister to be her children's guardian, as Juan was not the children's father.

Over the next 2 months, Maria's quality of life improved because she was free of opportunistic infections, and although unemployed she kept busy with household activities. Maria understood the fragility of her condition and was adherent to her medication regimen. However, night sweats, fever, and diarrhea returned, and she was readmitted to the hospital within 6 months of her initial hospitalization with an exacerbation of MAC and severe dehydration. The palliative care team was asked for a consultation by the AIDS specialist. The advanced practice nurse developed a very supportive relationship with Maria and her family. She listened attentively to Maria's fears and concerns and provided a caring presence that helped her to relax. They discussed her relationship with Juan, her children, and her sister. Maria asked the nurse to call her sister and tell her about her hospitalization. Maria was coming to terms with her diagnosis and was ready to move beyond old hurts in her life. Maria had a strong religious faith, and asked for the chaplain to visit because she was trying to come to terms with her own suffering and the fears she had about leaving her children and family.

Although Maria appeared to be recovering, her condition took an unexpected turn for the worse as her fever began to rise and she became delirious. Several tests were conducted to identify other potential sources of the infection, and other possible reasons for the delirium. Her symptoms were treated with Haldol and antipyretics. However, within the next day, Maria slipped into a coma and died. At her bedside was found a letter written by Maria to thank her physicians and the members of the palliative team for their care. She said she knew that her illness was advanced and did not expect to regain her health. Maria told her children how much she loved them, to be good for their aunt, and that she would watch over them from heaven. Members of the palliative care team were surprised at her sudden death but also understood the uncertainty of living with advanced AIDS. They had a celebration of her life on the palliative care unit, remembering her special smile, the gratefulness she expressed even for the small comforts offered and how their own lives were touched as they watched her quiet strength even in the face of death.

Summary

The care of patients with HIV/AIDS requires both active treatment and palliative care throughout the disease trajectory to relieve the suffering associated with opportunistic infections and malignancies. With up-to-date knowledge regarding HIV, including changes in epidemiology, diagnostic testing, treatment options, and available resources, nurses can offer effective and compassionate care to patients, alleviating physical, emotional, social, and spiritual suffering at all stages of HIV. Patients can maintain a sense of control and dignity until death by establishing a partnership with their healthcare professionals in planning and implementing their healthcare, as well as through advanced care planning to ensure that their end-of-life preferences and wishes are honored. The control of pain and symptoms associated with HIV/AIDS enables the patient and family to expend their energies on spiritual and emotional healing and the possibility for personal growth and transcendence, even as death approaches. Palliative care offers a comprehensive approach to address the physical, emotional, social, and spiritual needs of individuals with incurable progressive illness throughout the illness trajectory until death. Therefore, palliative care preserves patients' quality of life by protecting their self-integrity, reducing a perceived helplessness, and lessening the threat of exhaustion of coping resources. Through effective and compassionate nursing care, patients with AIDS can achieve a sense of inner well-being even at death, with the potential to make the transition from life as profound, intimate, and precious an experience as their birth.

References

1. Piot P, Quinn TC. Global health: response to AIDS pandemic. N Engl J Med. 2013;368:2210–2218.
2. Selwyn P, Forstein M. Overcoming the false dichotomy of curative vs palliative care for late-stage HIV/AIDS: "Let me live the way I want to live, until I can't." JAMA. 2003;90:806–814.
3. Strand JJ, Mihir KM, Crey EC. Top 10 things palliative care clinicians wished everyone knew about palliative care. Mayo Clin Proc. 2013;88(8): 895–865.
4. King NB, Fraser V. Undertreated pain, narcotics regulations, and global health ideologies. PLOS. 2013;10(4):e1001411.
5. Selwyn PA, Rivard M. Palliative care for AIDS: challenges and opportunities in the era of highly active antiretroviral therapy. J Palliat Med. 2003;6(3):475–487.
6. UNAIDS. The global HIV/AIDS epidemic/fact sheet/december 2012. UNAIDS. http://www.unaids.org/en/media/unaids/contentassets/documents/epidemiology/2012/gr2012/2 0121120_FactSheet_Global_en.pdf. Accessed August 24, 2013.
7. Centers for Disease Control and Prevention. HIV surveillance report. 2011; vol. 23. http://www.cdc.gov/hiv/topics/surveillance/resources/reports/. Accessed March 24, 2013.
8. CDC. HIV-2 infection surveillance, United States 1987–2009. MMWR. 2011;60(29):958–988.
9. Orenstein R. Presenting syndromes of human immunodeficiency virus. Mayo Clin Proc. 2002;77:1097–1102.
10. Department of Health and Human Services (DHHS). Panel on Antiretroviral Guidelines for Adults and Adolescents. Guidelines for the Use of Antiretroviral Agents in HIV-1-Infected Adults and Adolescents. Available at http://aidsinfo.nih.gov/contentfiles/lvguidelines/AdultandAdolescentGL.pdf. Accessed August 24, 2013.
11. Al-Harthi L, Siegel J, Spritzler J, Pottage J, Agnoli M, Landay A. Maximum suppression of HIV replication leads to the restoration of HIV-specific responses in early HIV disease. AIDS. 2000;14(7): 761–770.
12. Lee K, Gay C, Portillo CJ, Coggins T, Davis H, Pullinger C, Aouizerat B. Symptom experience in HIV-infected adults: a function of demographic and clinical characteristics. J Pain Symptom Manage. 2009;38(6):882–893.
13. Shen JM, Blank A, Selwyn PA. Predictors of mortality for patients with advanced disease in an HIV palliative care program. J Acquir Immune Defic Syndr. 2005;40:445–447.
14. Selwyn P. Palliative care for patient with human immunodeficiency virus/acquired immune deficiency syndrome. J Palliat Med. 2005;8:1248–68.
15. Huang YT. Challenges and responses in providing palliative care for people living with HIV/AIDS. Int J Palliat Nurs.2013;19(5): 220–225.
16. Malcolm JA. What is the best model for AIDS palliative care? Annual Conf Aust Soc HIV Med. 1993;5:60.
17. Selwyn P, Rivard M. Palliative care for AIDS: challenges and opportunities in the era of highly active anti-retroviral therapy. J Palliat Med. 2003;6:475–487.
18. Shen JM, Blank A, Selwyn PA. Predictors of mortality for patients with advanced disease in an HIV palliative care program. J Acquir Immune Defic Syndr. 2005;40:445–447.
19. National Consensus Project for Quality Palliative Care. Clinical Practice Guidelines for Quality Palliative Care. National Consensus Project for Quality Palliative Care. http://www.nationalconsensusproject.org/guideline.pdf. Accessed September 28, 2013.
20. Simms V, Higginson IJ, Harding R. Integration of palliative care throughout HIV disease. Lancet Infect Dis. 2012;12(7):571–575.
21. Ragsdale D, Morrow J. Quality of life as a function of HIV classification. Nurs Res. 1992;39:355–359.
22. Ragsdale K, Kortarba J, Morrow J. Quality of life of hospitalized persons with AIDS. Image. 1992;24:259–265.
23. Nichel J, Salsberry P, Caswell R, Keller M, Long T, O'Connell M. Quality of life in nurse case management of persons with AIDS receiving home care. Res Nurs Health. 1996;19:91–99.
24. Vosvick M, Koopman C, Gore-Felton C, Thoresen C, Krumboltz J, Spiegal D. Relationship of functional quality of life to strategies for coping with the stress of living with HIV/AIDS. Psychosomatics. 2003;44:51–58.
25. Baigis-Smith J, Gordon D, McGuire DB, Nanda J. Healthcare needs of HIV-infected persons in hospital, outpatient, home, and long-term care settings. J Assoc Nurses AIDS Care. 1995;6:21–33.
26. Kemppainen J. Predictors of quality of life in AIDS patients. J Assoc Nurses AIDS Care. 2001;12:61–70.

27. Guaraldi G, Stentarelli C, Zona S, Santoro A. HIV-associated lipodystrophy: impact of antiretroviral therapy. Drugs. 2013;73(13):1431–1450.

28. Hussein R. Current issues and forthcoming events. J Adv Nurs. 2003;44:235–237.

29. Campa A, Yang Z, Lai S, Xue L, Phillips JC, Sales S, et al. HIV-related wasting in HIV-infected drug users in the era of highly active antiretroviral therapy. Clin Infect Dis. 2005;41:1179–1185. http://dx.doi.org/10.1086/444499?

30. Ockenga J, Grimble R, Jonkers-Schuitema C, Macallan D, Melchior JC, Sauerwein HP, et al. ESPEN guidelines on enteral nutrition: wasting in HIV and other chronic infectious diseases. Clin Nutr. 2006;25:319–329. http://dx.doi.org/10.1016/j.clnu.2006.01.016.

31. Semba R, Graham P, Caiaffa J. Maternal vitamin A deficiency and mother-to-child transmission of HIV-1. Lancet. 1994;343:1593–1597.

32. Grobler L, Siegfried N, Visser ME, Mahlungulu SSN, Volmink J. Nutritional interventions for reducing morbidity and mortality in people with HIV. Cochrane Database Syst Rev. 2013;2: CD004536. Doi: 10.1002/14651858.CD004536.pub3.?

33. O'Brien K, Nixon S, Tynan AM, Glazier, G. Aerobic exercise interventions for adults living with HIV/AIDS. Cochrane Database Syst Rev. 2010;8. http://dx.doi.org/10.1002/14651858.CD001796.pub3 Art. No.: CD001796.

34. Yaresheski K, Tebas P, Stanerson B, Claxton S, Martin D, Bae K, et al. Resistance exercise training reduces hypertriglyceridemia in HIV-infected men treated with antiviral therapy. J Appl Physiol. 2001;90(1):133–138.

35. Hillier SL, Louw Q, Morris L, Uwimana J, Statham S. Massage therapy for people with HIV/AIDS. Cochrane Database Syst Rev. 2010;20(1):CD007502. doi: 10.1002/14651858.CD007502.pub2.

36. Leserman J, Petitto J, Gaynes B, et al. Progression to AIDS, a clinical AIDS condition and mortality: psychosocial and physiological predictors. Psychol Med. 2002;32:1059–1073.

37. Corless IB, Voss J, Guarino AJ, Wantland D, Holzemer W, Jane Hamilton M, et al. The impact of stressful life events, symptom status, and adherence concerns on quality of life in people living with HIV. J Assoc Nurses AIDS Care. 2013 Mar 6. Epub ahead of print. pii: S1055-3290(12)00259-2. doi: 10.1016/j.jana.2012.11.005.

38. Sherman DW, Kirton C. Hazardous terrain and over the edge: the survival of HIV-positive heterosexual minority men. J Assoc Nurses AIDS Care. 1998;9:23–34.

39. Lorenc A, Robinson N. A Review of the use of complementary and alternative medicine and HIV: issues for patient care. AIDS Patient Care STDS. 2013;27(9):503–510. doi: 10.1089/apc.2013.0175.

40. Gonzalez-Garcia M, Ferrer MJ, Borras X, Muñoz-Moreno JA, Miranda C, Puig J, et al. Effectiveness of mindfulness-based cognitive therapy on the quality of life, emotional status, and CD4 cell count of patients aging with HIV infection. AIDS Behav. 2013 Sep 28. Epub ahead of print.

41. Slomka J, Lim JW, Gripshover B, Daly B. How have long-term survivors coped with living with HIV? J Assoc Nurses AIDS Care. 2013;24(5):449–459. doi: 10.1016/j.jana.2012.09.004. Epub 2012 Dec 17.

42. Grover KW, Gonzalez A, Zvolensky MJ. HIV symptom distress and smoking outcome expectancies among HIV+ smokers: a pilot test. AIDS Patient Care STDS. 2013;27(1):17–21. doi: 10.1089/apc.2012.0333.

43. Carrico AW, Pollack LM, Stall RD, Shade SB, Neilands TB, Rice TM, et al. Psychological processes and stimulant use among men who have sex with men. Drug Alcohol Depend. 2012;123(1-3):79–83. doi: 10.1016/j.drugalcdep.2011.10.020. Epub 2011 Nov 15.

44. Panel on Antiretroviral Guidelines for Adults and Adolescents. Guidelines for the Use of Antiretroviral Agents in HIV-1-Infected Adults and Adolescents. Department of Health and Human Services. http://aidsinfo.nih.gov/ContentFiles/Adultand AdolescentGL.pdf. Accessed October 15, 2013, B-1.

45. Panel on Opportunistic Infections in HIV-Infected Adults and Adolescents. Guidelines for the Prevention and Treatment of Opportunistic Infections in HIV-Infected Adults and Adolescents: Recommendations from the Centers for Disease Control and Prevention, the National Institutes of Health, and the HIV Medicine Association of the Infectious Diseases Society of America. http://aidsinfo.nih.gov/contentfiles/lvguidelines/adult_oi.pdf. Accessed June 30, 2014.

46. Murphy R, Flaherty J. Contemporary Diagnosis and Management of HIV/AIDS Infections. Newtown, PA: Handbooks in Health Care; 2003.

47. Von Gunten CF, Martinez J, Neely KJ, Von Roenn JH. AIDS and palliative medicine: medical treatment issues. J Palliat Care. 1995; 11:5–9.

48. Selwyn P, Rivard M. Palliative care for AIDS: challenges and opportunities in the era of highly active anti-retroviral therapy. J Palliat Med. 2003;6:475–487.

49. Haynes RB, Taylor DW, and Sackett DL. Compliance in Health Care. Baltimore, MD: Johns Hopkins University Press, 1979.

50. Bangsberg DR. Less than 95% adherence to nonnucleoside reverse-transcriptase inhibitor therapy can lead to viral suppression. Clin Infect Dis. 2006;43(7):939–941.

51. Raffa JD, Tossonian HK, Grebely J, et al. Intermediate highly active antiretroviral therapy adherence thresholds and empirical models for the development of drug resistance mutations. J Acquir Immune Defic Syndr. 2008;47(3):397–399.

52. Flexner C, Plumley B, Brown Ripin DH. Treatment optimization: an outline for future success. Curr Opin HIV AIDS. 2013;8(6):523–527.

53. Aldir I, Horta A, Serrado M. Single-tablet regimens in HIV: does it really make a difference? Curr Med Res Opin. 2013 Oct 4. Epub ahead of print.

54. Chesney M. Adherence to HIV/AIDS treatment. In: Program of Adherence to New HIV Therapies: A Research Conference. Office of AIDS Research, Washington, DC: National Institutes of Health; 1997.

55. Williams AB. Adherence to highly active antiretroviral therapy. Nurs Clin North Am. 1999;34:113–127.

56. Meichenbaum D, Turk C. Facilitating Treatment Adherence: Practitioner's Guidebook. New York, NY: Plenum; 1987.

57. Haynes RB, McKibbon KA, Kanani R. Systematic review of randomized trials of interventions to assist patients to follow prescriptions for medications. Lancet. 1996;348:383–389.

58. Williams AB. Adherence to highly active antiretroviral therapy. Nurs Clin North Am. 1999;34:113–127.

59. Newshan G, Sherman DW. Palliative care: pain and symptom management in persons with HIV/AIDS. Nurs Clin North Am. 1999;34(1):131–145.

60. Holzemer W. HIV/AIDS: the symptom experience: what cell counts and viral loads won't tell you. Am J Nurs. 2002;102:48–52.

61. Willard S, Holzemer WL, Wantland DJ, Cuca YP, Kirksey KM, Portillo CJ, et al. Does "asymptomatic" mean without symptoms for those living with HIV infection? AIDS Care 2009;21(3):322–328. doi: 10.1080/09540120802183511.

62. Lorenz KA, Cunningham WE, Spritzer LK, Hays RD. Changes in symptoms and health-related quality of life in a nationally representative sample of adults in treatment for HIV. Quality Life Res. 2006;15:951–958.

63. Perry BA, Westfall AO, Molony E, Tucker R, Ritchie C, Saag MS, et al. Characteristics of an ambulatory palliative care clinic for HIV-infected patients. J Palliat Med. 2013;16(8):934–937. doi: 10.1089/jpm.2012.0451. Epub 2013 Mar 11.

64. Fontes AS, Gonçalves JF. Pain treatment in patients infected with human immunodeficiency virus in later stages: pharmacological aspects. Am J Hosp Palliat Care. 2013; Mar 15. Epub ahead of print.

65. Frich LM, Borgbjerg FM. Pain and pain treatment in AIDS patients: a longitudinal study. J Pain Symptom Manage. 2000;19:339–347.

66. Margolis AM, Heverling H, Pham PA, Stolbach A. A Review of the toxicity of HIV medications. J Med Toxicol. 2013 Aug 21. Epub ahead of print.

67. Breitbart W. Pain. In: O'Neill J, Selwyn A, Schietinger H (eds.), A Clinical Guide to Supportive and Palliative Care for HIV/AIDS; 2003:85–122 (chap 4). http://hab.hrsa.gov/deliverhivaidscare/files/palliativecare2003.pdf. Accessed October 15, 2013.

68. Manchikanti L, Abdi S, Atluri S, Balog CC, Benyamin RM, Boswell MV, et al. American Society of Interventional Pain Physicians (ASIPP) guidelines for responsible opioid prescribing in chronic non-cancer pain. Part 2: Guidance. Pain Physician. 2012;15(3 Suppl):S67–S116.

69. Newshan G, Staats JA. (2013). Evidence-based pain guidelines in HIV care. J Assoc Nurses AIDS Care. 2013;24(1 Suppl):S112–S126. doi: 10.1016/j.jana.2012.05.006.

70. Solano JP, Gomes B, Higginson IJ. A comparison of symptom prevalence in far advanced cancer, AIDS, heart disease, chronic obstructive pulmonary disease and renal disease. J Pain Symptom Manage. 2006;31(1):58–69.

71. Fausto JA Jr, Selwyn PA. Palliative care in the management of advanced HIV/AIDS. Prim Care. 2011;38(2):311–326, ix. doi: 10.1016/j.pop.2011.03.010.

72. Coyne P, Lyne M, Watson AC. Symptom management in people with AIDS. Am J Nurs. 2002;102:48–57.

73. Brener L, Callander D, Slavin S, deWit J. Experiences of HIV stigma: the role of visible symptoms, HIV centrality and community attachment for people living with HIV. AIDS Care. 2013;25(9):1166–1173.

74. Grassi L, Sighinolfi L. Psychosocial correlates of quality of life in patients with HIV infection. AIDS Patient Care STDS. 1996;10:296–299.

75. Farber E, Mirsalimi H, Williams K, McDaniel J. Meaning of illness and psychological adjustment to HIV/AIDS. Psychosomatics. 2003;44:485–491.

76. Jaggers JR, Dudgeon WD, Burgess S, Phillips KD, Blair SN, Hand GA. Psychological correlates of HIV-related symptom distress. J Assoc Nurses AIDS Care. 2013 Oct 5. Epub ahead of print. pii: S1055-3290(13)00120-9. doi: 10.1016/j.jana.2013.06.003.

77. Sherman DW. Reciprocal suffering: the need to improve family caregiver's quality of life through palliative care. J Palliat Med. 1998;1:357–366.

78. Edwards M, Byrd Quinlivan E, Bess K, Gaynes BN, Heine A, Zinski A, et al. Implementation of PHQ-9 depression screening for HIV-infected patients in a real-world setting. J Assoc Nurses AIDS Care. 2013 Oct 5. Epub ahead of print. pii: S1055-3290(13)00092-7. doi: 10.1016/j.jana.2013.05.004.

79. Primeau MM, Avellaneda V, Musselman D, St Jean G, Illa L. Treatment of depression in individuals living with HIV/AIDS. Psychosomatics. 2013;54(4):336–344. doi: 10.1016/j.psym.2012.12.001. Epub 2013 Feb 4.

80. Schrimshaw R. Relationship-specific unsupportive social interactions and depressive symptoms among women living with HIV/AIDS: direct and moderating effects. J Behav Med. 2003;26:297–313.

81. Arrindell J. Differential coping strategies, anxiety, depression, and symptomatology among African-American women with HIV/AIDS. Dissertation Abs Int. Section B: The Sciences and Engineering. 2003;64:1481. US: Univ MicroFilms International.

82. Bing EG, Burnam MA, Longshore D, Fleishman J, Sherbourne C, Longon A, et al. Psychiatric disorders and drug use among human immunodeficiency virus-infected adults in the United States. Arch Gen Psychiatry. 2001;58, 721–728. http://dx.doi.org/10.1001/archpsyc.58.8.721

83. Gallego L, Barreiro P, López-Ibor JJ. Psychopharmacological treatments in HIV patients under antiretroviral therapy. AIDS Rev. 2012;14(2):101–111.

84. De Santis JP, Florom-Smith A, Vermeesch A, Barroso S, DeLeon DA. (2013). Motivation, management, and mastery: a theory of resilience in the context of HIV infection. J Am Psychiatr Nurses Assoc. 2013;19(1):36–46. doi: 10.1177/1078390312474096.

85. Casale M, Wild L, Kuo C. "They give us hope": HIV-positive caregivers' perspectives on the role of social support for health. AIDS Care. 2013;25(10):1203–1209. doi: 10.1080/09540121.2013.763893. Epub 2013 Jan 29.

86. Kerr ZY, Miller KR, Galos D, Love R, Poole C. Challenges, coping strategies, and recommendations related to the HIV services field in the HAART era: a systematic literature review of qualitative studies from the United States and Canada. AIDS Patient Care STDS. 2013;27(2):85–95. doi: 10.1089/apc.2012.0356. Epub 2013 Jan 22.

87. Szaflarski M. Spirituality and religion among HIV-infected individuals. Curr HIV/AIDS Rep. 2013 Sep 1. Epub ahead of print.

88. Kremer H, Ironson G, Kaplan L. The fork in the road: HIV as a potential positive turning point and the role of spirituality. AIDS Care. 2009;21:368–77.

89. Ironson G, Stuetzle R, Ironson D, et al. View of God as benevolent and forgiving or punishing and judgmental predicts HIV disease progression. J Behav Med. 2011;34:414–425.

90. Kylma J, Vehvilainen-Julkunen K, Lahdevirta J. Hope, despair and hopelessness in living with HIV/AIDS: a grounded theory study. J Adv Nurs. 2001;33:764–775.

91. Curtis R, Patrick D, Caldwell E, Collier A. Why don't patients and physicians talk about end of life care?: Barriers to communication for patients with acquired immunodeficiency syndrome and their primary care clinicians. Arch Intern Med. 2000;160:1690–1696.

92. Wenger NS, Kanouse DE, Collins RL, Liu H, Schuster MA, Gifford AL, et al. End-of-life discussions and preferences among persons with HIV. JAMA. 2001;285(22):2880–2887.

93. Ferris F, Flannery J, McNeal H, Morissette M, Cameron R, Bally G. Palliative Care: A Comprehensive Guide for the Care of Persons with HIV Disease. Toronto, ON: Mount Sinai Hospital/Casey House Hospice; 1995.

94. Pessin H. The influence of cognitive impairment on desire for hastened death among terminally ill AIDS patients. Dissertation Abs Int. 2001;62:2963.

95. Curtis R, Patrick D, Caldwell E, Collier A. The attitudes of patients with advanced AIDS toward use of the medical futility rationale in decisions to forgo mechanical ventilation. Arch Intern Med. 2000;160:1597–1601.

96. Flaskerud J, Lee P. Vulnerability to health problems in female informal caregivers of persons with HIV/AIDS and age-related dementias. J Adv Nurs. 2001;33:60–68.

97. Byock I. Dying Well: The Prospect for Growth at the End of Life. New York, NY: Riverhead Books; 1997.

98. Sikkema K, Kochman A, DiFrancesico W, Kelly J, Hoffman R. AIDS-related grief and coping with loss among HIV-positive men and women. J Behav Med. 2003;26:165–181.

99. Mallinson RK. Grief work of HIV-positive persons and their survivors. In: Sherman DW (ed.), HIV/AIDS Update. Nurs Clin North Am. Philadelphia, PA: W.B. Saunders; 1999:163–177.

100. Doka K. Disenfranchised Grief: Recognizing the Hidden Sorrow. Lexington, MA: Lexington Books; 1989.

101. Worden J. Grief Counseling and Grief Therapy: A Handbook for the Mental Health Practitioner. New York, NY: Springer; 1991.

102. Maxwell N. Responses to loss and bereavement in HIV. Prof Nurse. 1996;12:21–24.

CHAPTER 41

Caring for the patient with substance use disorder at the end of life

Kenneth L. Kirsh, Peggy Compton,
Kathy Egan-City, and Steven D. Passik

> As soon as I heard that I had stage IV cancer the first thing I thought was not, Oh my God I might die, or I might leave my family or even an existential crisis of what to do with the time I have left . . . no it was, "Great now I can have narcotics again."
>
> A 68-year-old patient with 35 years of sobriety being told of a lung cancer diagnosis; his story is related at the end of the chapter

Key points

- With the changing face of cancer and other advanced diseases progressing, patients are living for longer periods of time, which creates new challenges in treating pain and potential addiction issues on a longer term basis.

- Identifying addiction in patients with advanced disease is not an easy task, and old conceptions of addiction such as tolerance and dependence need to be reexamined.

- Patients with advanced disease and comorbid addiction are difficult to manage but can be successfully treated with careful documentation and planning.

- Remember that the patient with advanced disease and comorbid addiction has two diseases that need treatment: one of drug addiction and one of chronic pain.

Substance use disorders are a consistent phenomenon in the United States, with estimated base rates of 6% and 15%.[1-4] This prevalence of drug abuse certainly touches medically ill patients and can negatively influence how pain is treated. Because of these issues and despite the fact that national guidelines exist for the treatment of pain disorders such as cancer, pain continues to be undertreated, even at the end of life.[5-7] In cancer, approximately 40% to 50% of patients with metastatic disease and 90% of patients with terminal cancer or other advanced diseases are reported to experience unrelieved pain.[5-7] Furthermore, inadequate treatment of cancer pain is an even greater possibility if the patient is a member of an ethnic minority, female, elderly, a child, or a substance abuser.[8] Therefore, for multicultural patients, we sometimes have conflicting multiple biases in pain treatment that can lead to poor management, mutual suspicion and alienation, and suffering unless these biases are adequately addressed. Finally, although we

must consider the potential of abuse, misuse, and diversion with palliative patients, we must never let this worry generate fear on the part of the practitioner, which could ultimately lead to further undertreatment of pain as discussed above. The following case is an extreme example of when this fear, combined with a failure to understand the nuances of aberrant behaviors, can lead to poor patient care.

Case study

A 74-year-old woman with breast cancer

A 74-year-old married woman with breast cancer and posttraumatic stress disorder related to early life abuse, had undergone a lumpectomy when she later developed severe hip pain. She was seen by the psychologist on the palliative care team who referred her to the pain clinic. Initial studies ruled out a metastatic cause of the pain. Epidural steroid injections were ineffective, and the patient found both the MRI scans and the injections to be quite noxious due to her history of traumatization. She required psychological support and clonazepam to weather them. Ultimately she responded to low doses of oxycodone and clonazepam and was quite stable entering her survivorship continuing in psychotherapy. However, significant problems later developed in consistently being able to obtain her low doses of controlled substances when she fell between the cracks—her interventional pain physician did not want to prescribe on an ongoing basis; her oncologist was no longer seeing her frequently enough to comply with new state laws; when the laws changed in the neighboring state wherein her internist of 40 years had been willing to prescribe but then later stated he was afraid he could not any longer, the patient was panicked. She then learned that she had had a relapse and was going to require a mastectomy. A nurse practitioner at the original pain clinic assumed the mantel of caring for her for a time, but insisted that the patient see a psychiatrist for the (0.5 mgs BID) of clonazepam she was taking. A urine drug test around this revealed no oxycodone despite the fact that the patient reported taking it "most of the time" adding "I don't hurt every day. I don't need it 3–4 times every day." Her husband later revealed that he had found a large cache of pills, perhaps 50 or more. The nurse practitioner then refused to prescribe the medications. The patient revealed to the psychologist that she had starting skipping doses and hoarding for fear of untreated postoperative pain. She revealed that she had seriously considered not having the surgery at all. It was only with reassurances that her pain would be addressed by the team as a whole, and the identifying of an internal medicine doctor who had agreed to provide postoperative and ongoing pain medication and anxiety medication that she was able to find the strength to proceed with the surgery.

Incidence of substance use disorders in patients with advanced disease

Although few studies have been conducted to evaluate the epidemiology of substance abuse in patients with advanced illness, substance use disorders appear to be relatively rare within the tertiary-care population with cancer and other advanced diseases. Findings from a consultations review performed by the psychiatry services at Memorial Sloan-Kettering Cancer Center revealed that requests for management of issues related to substance abuse consisted of only 3% of the consultations.[9,10]

While the incidence of substance use disorders is much lower in patients with advanced disease than in society at large, in community-based medical populations, and in emergency medical departments, this may not represent the true prevalence in the advanced illness spectrum overall. Institutional biases or a tendency for patients' underreporting in tertiary care hospitals may be reflective of the relatively low prevalence of substance abuse among advanced patients. Social forces may also inhibit patients' reporting of drug use behavior. Many drug abusers are of lower socioeconomic standing and feel alienated from the healthcare system and, therefore, may not seek care in tertiary care centers. Furthermore, those who are treated in these centers may not acknowledge drug abuse for fear of stigmatization.[9–11] In addition, minority patients are treated in such settings less often than are Caucasians.

Issues in defining abuse and addiction in the medically Ill

It is difficult to define substance abuse and addiction in patients with advanced illness, as the definitions of both terms have been adopted from addicted populations without medical illness. Furthermore, the pharmacological phenomena of tolerance and physical dependence continue to be commonly confused with abuse and addiction. The use of these terms is so strongly influenced by sociocultural considerations that it may lead to confusion in the clinical setting. Therefore, the clarification of this terminology is necessary to improve the diagnosis and management of substance abuse when treating patients with advanced disease.[10]

Substance abuse concentrates on the psychosocial, physical, and vocational harm that occurs from drug-taking, which makes identifying drug-taking behaviors more difficult in patients with advanced illness who are receiving potentially abusable drugs for legitimate medical purposes. In contrast, substance dependence emphasizes chronicity and includes the dimensions of tolerance and physical dependence. Because of the possibility that patients may develop these effects as a result of therapeutic drug use, it is inapplicable to use this terminology in the medically ill. Not only does the existing nomenclature complicate the effort to distinguish the drug-taking behaviors of patients with advanced disease that are appropriately treated with potentially abusable drugs, it also impedes the communication that is fundamental for proper pain management and medical care.[9,10]

Theoretical problems in the diagnosis of substance use disorders

Because substance abuse is increasingly widespread in the population at large, patients with advanced disease who have used illicit drugs are more frequently encountered in medical settings. Illicit drug use, actual or suspected misuse of prescribed medication, or actual substance use disorders create the most serious difficulties in the clinical setting, complicating the treatment of pain management. However, the management of substance abuse is fundamental to adherence to medical therapy and safety during treatment. Also, adverse interactions between illicit drugs and medications prescribed as part of the patient's treatment can be dangerous. Continuous substance abuse may alienate or weaken an already tenuous social support network that is crucial for alleviating the chronic stressors associated with advanced disease and its treatment. Therefore, a history of substance abuse can impede treatment and pain management and increase the risk of hastening morbidity and mortality among advanced patients, which can only be alleviated by a therapeutic approach that addresses drug-taking behavior while expediting the treatment of the malignancy and distressing symptoms, as well as addiction.[11]

When assessing drug-taking behaviors in the patient with advanced disease, issues exist that increase the difficulty in arriving at a diagnosis of abuse or addiction. These issues include the problem of undertreatment of pain, sociocultural influences on the definition of aberrancy in drug-taking, and the importance of cancer-related variables.[9,10]

Pseudoaddiction

Various studies have provided compelling evidence that pain is undertreated in populations with advanced disease.[5–7] Clinical experience indicates that the inadequate management of symptoms and related pain maybe the motivation for aberrant drug-taking behaviors. Pseudoaddiction, coined by Weissman and Haddox, is the term used to depict the distress and drug-seeking that can occur in the context of unrelieved pain, such as similar behaviors in addicts.[12,13] The main factor of this syndrome is that sufficient pain relief eliminates aberrant behaviors.

The original paper on pseudoaddiction was a four-page, single case study of a 17-year-old man presenting with leukemia and complaining of chest wall pain. The case was made that undertreated pain created behavioral changes that looked much like iatrogenic addiction in the patient and resulted in a crisis regarding the clinical interactions between the healthcare team and patient. Clinically, pseudoaddiction is not uncommonly seen in outpatients, those with and those without histories of chemical dependency. Interestingly, patients with chemical dependency are often set up for pseudoaddiction. Their unique pharmacological needs, combined with the ambivalence clinicians feel about their treatment, render them a likely to be underdosed. With regard to the range of behaviors to which the term has been applied, it is important to note that the original patient's behaviors as described in the paper were relatively tame. In pain lectures and case discussions, it would not be uncommon to hear the use of illicit drugs and alcohol described as evidence of pseudoaddiction. That they might be desperate attempts to improve analgesia is not categorically impossible, but the degree of conviction that clinicians express about it as a possibility has clearly changed.

More recent scientific advances have also provided new insight into behaviors that may be considered pseudoaddiction. Pharmacogenetic variances in the enzymes that metabolize pain medications help to explain individual differences in medication response and side effects experienced. If a patient is an ultrarapid metabolizer, they may complain that the medication is effective for a shorter period of time than is common for that medication. If a patient is a poor metabolizer, they may complain that the medication is not working or possibly continue to ask for increased amount of medication. Pharmacogenetic variations should be considered and pharmacogenetic testing implemented when a patient has an unusual response to a medication, more than expected side-effect profile, and/or inefficacy at usual dosages.[14]

The potential for pseudoaddiction creates a challenge for the assessment of a known substance abuser with an advanced illness. Clinical evidence indicates that aberrant behaviors impelled by unrelieved pain can become so dramatic in this population that some patients appear to return to illicit drug use as a means of self-medication. Others use more covert patterns of behavior, which may also cause concerns regarding the possibility of true addiction. Although it may not be obvious that drug-related behaviors are aberrant, the meaning of these behaviors may be difficult to discern in the context of unrelieved symptoms.[9,10]

Distinguishing aberrant drug-taking behaviors

Whereas abuse is defined as the use of an illicit drug or a prescription drug without medical indication, addiction refers to the continued use of either type of drug in a compulsive manner regardless of harm to the user or others. However, when a drug is prescribed for a medically diagnosed purpose, less assuredness exists as to the behaviors that could be deemed aberrant, thereby increasing the potential for a diagnosis of drug abuse or addiction. Although it is difficult to disagree with the aberrancy of certain behaviors, such as intravenous injection of oral formulations, various other behaviors are less blatant, such as a patient experiencing unrelieved pain who is taking an extra dose of prescribed opioids.[9,10]

The ability to categorize these questionable behaviors as apart from social or cultural norms is also based on the assumption that certain parameters of normative behavior exist. Although it is useful to consider the degree of aberrancy of a given behavior, it is important to recognize that these behaviors exist along a continuum, with certain behaviors being less aberrant (such as aggressively requesting medication) and other behaviors more aberrant (such as injection of oral formulations). Empirical data defining these parameters do not exist regarding prescription drug use (Table 41.1). If a large portion of patients were found to engage in

Table 41.1 Sample behaviors more or less likely to indicate aberrancy

Less indicative of aberrancy	More indicative of aberrancy
Drug hoarding during periods of reduced symptoms	Prescription forgery
Acquisition of similar drugs from other medical sources	Concurrent abuse of related illicit drugs
Aggressive complaining about the need for higher doses	Recurrent prescription losses
Unapproved use of the drug to trea another symptom	Selling prescription drugs
Unsanctioned dose escalation one or two times	Multiple unsanctioned dose escalations
Reporting psychic effects not intended by the clinician	Stealing or borrowing another patient's drugs
Requesting specific drugs	Obtaining prescription drugs from nonmedical sources

a certain behavior, it may be normative, and judgments regarding aberrancy should be influenced accordingly.[9,10]

We know more scientifically about aberrant behaviors and their prevalence and meaning today than we did in the mid-1990s. We know that many patients will have at least a few aberrant behaviors in a 6-month period.[15] We also know that once a patient has demonstrated four behaviors in their lifetime, they have an 85% likelihood of meeting diagnostic criteria for substance use disorder.[16] But there is still much to be learned, confirmed, replicated, and studied.

The importance of social and cultural norms also raises the possibility of bias in the determination of aberrancy. A clinician's willingness to classify a questionable drug-related behavior as aberrant when performed by a member of a certain social or ethnic group may be influenced by bias against that group. Based on clinical observation, this type of prejudice has been found to be common in the assessment of drug-related behaviors of patients with substance abuse histories. Regardless of whether the drug-abuse history is in the past or present, questionable behaviors by these patients may immediately be labeled as abuse or addiction. The possibility of bias in the assessment of drug-related behaviors also exists for patients who are members of racial or ethnic minority groups different from that of the clinician.[9,10] The following case study illustrates the point that aberrant behaviors do not have a universal interpretation (including the illegal and obviously worrisome ones) and must be understood in the context of the patient's care.

Case study

A 33-year-old woman with a history of ovarian cancer

A 33-year-old woman with a recent history of locally advanced ovarian cancer was undergoing chemotherapy and was status post-surgery. She had ongoing abdominal pain for which she required escalating doses of opioids (hydromorphone) and adjuvants (duloxetine) despite what appeared to be stable and, indeed, responsive cancer. At a routine follow-up visit with her oncological team a urine drug test was ordered. There was neither pain medication nor duloxetine present in her urine. When the team engaged her in discussion about this finding, the patient vehemently denied misusing her medications (i.e., binging on them and then running out) or selling them. Her husband, who was in attendance, was a veteran of three tours of duty in Iraq and Afghanistan who suffered a traumatic amputation of his leg below the knee when his Humvee ran over an improvised explosive device (IED) in his final tour. He also suffered a head injury and had symptoms of PTSD. He explained that he wasn't able to consistently receive opioids from his VA doctors because he had tested positive for synthetic cannabinoids and marijuana that he had been using. His wife explained how he had had a bad few weeks and she had given him virtually all of her medications to take. She ultimately exclaimed, "I couldn't stand to see my husband suffer. He served his country and we couldn't afford both my pain medications and his so we shared them sometimes." Ultimately she was educated about the absolute necessity of not sharing her medications and the husband was provided with a referral to pain and trauma services.

Disease-related variables

Changes caused by progressive diseases, such as cancer, also challenge the principal concepts used to define addiction. Alterations in physical and psychosocial functioning caused by advanced illness and its treatment may be difficult to distinguish from the morbidity associated with drug abuse. In particular, alterations in functioning may complicate the ability to evaluate a concept that is vital to the diagnosis of addiction: "use despite harm." For example, discerning the questionable behaviors can be difficult in a patient who develops social withdrawal or cognitive changes after brain irradiation for metastases. Even if diminished cognition is clearly related to pain medication used in treatment, this effect might only reflect a narrow therapeutic window rather than the patient's use of analgesic to acquire these psychic effects.[9,10]

To accurately assess drug-related behaviors in patients with advanced disease, explicit information is usually required regarding the role of the drug in the patient's life. Therefore, the presence of mild mental clouding or the time spent out of bed may have less meaning than other outcomes, such as noncompliance with primary therapy related to drug use or behaviors that threaten relationships with physicians, other healthcare professionals, and family members.[9,10]

Appropriate definitions of abuse and addiction for advanced illness

A more appropriate definition of addiction would exemplify that it is a chronic disorder characterized by "the compulsive use of a substance resulting in physical, psychological, or social harm to the user and continued use despite the harm."[17] Although this definition is not without fault, it emphasizes that addiction is essentially a psychological and behavioral syndrome.[9,10]

A differential diagnosis should also be considered if questionable behaviors occur during pain treatment. A true addiction (substance dependence) is only one of many possible interpretations. A diagnosis of pseudoaddiction should also be taken into account if the patient is reporting distress associated with unrelieved symptoms. Impulsive drug use may also be indicative of another psychiatric disorder, the diagnosis of which may have therapeutic implications. On occasion, aberrant drug-related behaviors

appear to be causally remotely related to a mild encephalopathy, with perplexity concerning the appropriate therapeutic regimen. On rare occasions, questionable behaviors imply criminal intent. These diagnoses are not mutually exclusive.[9,10]

Varied and repeated observations over a period of time may be necessary to categorize questionable behaviors properly. Perceptive psychiatric assessment is crucial and may require evaluation by consultants who can elucidate the complex interactions among personality factors and psychiatric illness. Some patients may be self-medicating symptoms of anxiety, depression, insomnia, or problems of adjustment (such as boredom caused by decreased ability to engage in usual activities and hobbies). Yet others may have character pathology that may be the more prominent determinant of drug-taking behavior. Patients with borderline personality disorders, for example, may impulsively use prescription medications that regulate inner tension or improve chronic emptiness or boredom and express anger at physicians, friends, or family. Psychiatric assessment is vitally important for both the population without a prior history of substance abuse and the population of known substance abusers who have a high incidence of psychiatric comorbidity.[18]

Cultural issues in the treatment of substance use disorders

As noted earlier, cancer pain continues to be grossly undertreated despite the availability of guidelines for its clinical management, with patients who are members of an ethnic minority or substance abusers having a greater risk of inadequate treatment of cancer pain.[5-7] In fact, various studies have documented that minority patients receive insufficient pain treatment compared with nonminority patients when being treated for pain caused by a variety of sources.[19-21] Because minority patients with advanced illness are undertreated for pain, they may be at greater risk of being misdiagnosed if exhibiting behaviors of pseudoaddiction.

Recently, more attention has been given to the significant influence that age, gender, and ethnicity have on the issues and treatment of substance abuse. Certain issues must be considered when implementing substance abuse treatment with the minority patient who is suspected of having a substance use disorder.[22]

First and foremost, it must be recognized that immense diversity exists within the different sociocultural groups themselves. Any given minority patient may possess beliefs, values, or drug-taking behaviors that greatly differ from the majority of the sociocultural group of which the patient is a member. In addition to ethnic orientation, attention must also focus on other sociocultural factors such as age, gender, sexual orientation, income, education, geographic location, and level of acculturation.[22] Ascribing certain cultural characteristics to all patients of a particular minority group may lead to stereotyping, alienating patients, and compromising treatment effectiveness.[23] Although the perfect scenario would be to accurately understand all of the possible cultural issues that influence the patient within the context of his/her life circumstances, this is difficult and may be impractical.[1,22] Therefore, it is particularly important to respond to cultural needs in the treatment of substance abuse, because sociocultural factors greatly affect the manifestation of the disease. Consequently, clinicians must often acclimate their therapeutic approaches to accommodate the patient's sociocultural orientation.[22]

Risks in patients with current or remote histories of drug abuse

There is a lack of information regarding the risk of abuse or addiction during or subsequent to the therapeutic administration of potentially abusable drugs to medically ill patients with a current or remote history of abuse or addiction.[9] The possibility of successful long-term opioid therapy in patients with cancer or chronic nonmalignant pain has been indicated by anecdotal reports, particularly if the abuse or addiction is remote.[24–26]

Because it is commonly accepted that the likelihood of aberrant drug-related behavior occurring during treatment for medical illness will be greater for those with a remote or current history of substance abuse, it is reasonable to consider the possibility of abuse behaviors occurring when using different therapies. For example, although no clinical evidence exists to support that the use of short-acting drugs or the parenteral route is more likely to cause questionable drug-related behaviors than other therapeutic strategies, it may be prudent to avoid such therapies in patients with histories of drug abuse.[9] Box 41.1 presents a basic set of principles pertaining to prescribing controlled substances to this patient population.

Summary of issues

Clinicians should understand that essentially any drug that acts on the central nervous system or any route of administration has the potential to be abused. Therefore, a more comprehensive approach that recognizes the biological, chemical, social, and psychiatric aspects is necessary to effectively manage patients with substance abuse histories. Using this strategy extends beyond merely avoiding certain drugs or routes of administration—it also affords practical means to manage risk during cancer treatment.[9]

Clinical management of advanced-disease patients with substance use histories

The most challenging issues in caring for patients with advanced disease typically arise from patients who are actively abusing

---

Box 41.1 Basic principles for prescribing controlled substances to patients with advanced illness and issues of addiction

Choose an opioid based on around-the-clock dosing.

Choose long-acting agents when possible.

As much as possible, limit or eliminate the use of short-acting or "breakthrough" doses.

Use nonopioid adjuvants when possible, and monitor for compliance with those medications.

Use nondrug adjuvants whenever possible (e.g., relaxation techniques, distraction,

biofeedback, transcutaneous nerve stimulation (TNS), communication about thoughts and feelings of pain).

If necessary, limit the amount of medication given at any one time (i.e., write prescriptions for a few days' worth or a week's worth of medication at a time).

Use pill counts and urine toxicology screens as necessary.

If compliance is suspect or poor, refer to an addictions specialist.

---

alcohol or other drugs. This is because patients who are actively abusing drugs experience more difficulty in managing pain.[27] Patients may become caught in a cycle where pain functions as a barrier to seeking treatment for addiction with another addiction, possibly complicating treatment for chronic pain.[28] Also, because pain is undertreated, the risk of binging with prescription medications and/or other substances increases for drug-abusing patients.[27]

General guidelines

The following guidelines can be beneficial, whether the patient is actively abusing drugs or has a history of substance abuse. The principles outlined assist clinicians in establishing structure, control, and monitoring of addiction-related behaviors, which may be helpful and necessary at times in all pain treatment.[29]

Recommendations for the long-term administration of potentially abusable drugs, such as opioids, to patients with a history of substance abuse are based exclusively on clinical experience. Research is needed to ascertain the most effective strategies and to empirically identify patient subgroups who may be most responsive to different approaches. The following guidelines broadly reflect the types of interventions that might be considered in this clinical context.[10,29]

Multidisciplinary approach

Pain and symptom management is often complicated by various medical, psychosocial, and administrative issues in the population of advanced patients with a substance use disorder. The most effective team may include a physician with expertise in pain/palliative care, nurses, social workers, and, when possible, a mental healthcare provider with expertise in the area of addiction medicine.[10,29]

Assessment of substance use history

In an effort to not offend, threaten, or anger patients, many times clinicians avoid asking patients about drug abuse. There is also often the expectation that patients will not answer truthfully. However, obtaining a detailed history of duration, frequency, and desired effect of drug use is vital. Adopting a nonjudgmental position and communicating in an empathetic and truthful manner is the best strategy when taking patients' substance abuse histories.[11,29]

In anticipating defensiveness on the part of the patient, it can be helpful for clinicians to mention that patients often misrepresent their drug use for logical reasons, such as stigmatization, mistrust of the interviewer, or concerns regarding fears of undertreatment. It is also wise for clinicians to explain that in an effort to keep the patient as comfortable as possible, by preventing withdrawal states and prescribing sufficient medication for pain and symptom control, an accurate account of drug use is necessary.[11,29]

The use of a careful, graduated-style interview can be beneficial in slowly introducing the assessment of drug abuse. This approach begins with broad and general inquiries regarding the role of drugs in the patient's life, such as caffeine and nicotine and gradually proceeds to more specific questions regarding illicit drugs. This interview style can also assist in discerning any coexisting psychiatric disorders, which can significantly contribute to aberrant drug-taking behavior. Once identified, treatment of comorbid psychiatric disorders can greatly enhance management strategies and decrease the risk of relapse.[11,29]

Use of risk assessment tools

As stated above, potential opioid use must be accompanied by risk stratification and management. Given time constraints, a full psychiatric interview may not be feasible and thus time-sensitive measures are clearly needed to help in this endeavor. However, until very recently, there were nearly no validated screening tools for the prediction of aberrant behaviors in pain patients. This need has been acknowledged and there has been a substantial increase in addiction-related screening tools.[30] Many screening tools contain items on personal and family history of addiction as well as other history-related risk factors, such as preadolescent sexual abuse, age, and psychological disease. Some of the tools are particular to pain management, whereas others are simply risk factors for addiction in general. The rather sudden and large volume of tools available is both a blessing (in that we have choices) and a curse (in that it is sometimes difficult to determine which is most applicable to a particular practice). As a final note, it must be remembered that these are tools for clinical decision-making and should not be viewed as necessarily diagnostically accurate. Whatever tool the clinician chooses, it is advised that the screening process be presented to the patient with the assurance that no answers will negatively influence effective pain management.

Setting realistic goals for therapy

The rate of recurrence for drug abuse and addiction is high. The stress associated with advanced illness and the easy availability of centrally acting drugs increases this risk. Therefore, total prevention of relapse may be impossible in this type of setting. Gaining an understanding that compliance and abstinence are not realistic goals may decrease conflicts with staff members in terms of management goals. Instead, the goals might be perceived as the creation of a structure for therapy that includes ample social/emotional support and limit-setting to control the harm done by relapse.[11,29]

There may be some subgroups of patients who are unable to comply with the requirements of therapy because of severe substance use disorders and comorbid psychiatric diagnoses. In these instances, clinicians must modify limits on various occasions and endeavor to develop a greater variety and intensity of supports. This may necessitate frequent team meetings and consultations with other clinicians. However, pertinent expectations must be clarified, and therapy that is not successful should be modified.[11,29]

Evaluation and treatment of comorbid psychiatric disorders

Extremely high comorbidity of personality disorders, depression, and anxiety disorders exist in alcoholics and other patients with substance abuse histories.[18] The treatment of depression and anxiety can increase patient comfort and decrease the risk of relapse or aberrant drug-taking.[11,29]

Preventing or minimizing withdrawal symptoms

Because many patients with drug abuse histories use multiple drugs, it is necessary to conduct a complete drug-use history to prepare for the possibility of withdrawal. Delayed abstinence syndromes, such as those that may occur after abuse of some benzodiazepine drugs, may be particularly diagnostically challenging.[11,29]

Considering the therapeutic impact of tolerance

Patients who are active substance abusers may be tolerant to drugs administered for therapy, which will make pain management more difficult. The magnitude of this tolerance is never known. Therefore, it is best to begin with a conservative dose of therapeutic drug and then rapidly titrate the dose, with frequent reassessments until the patient is comfortable.[9,26] Also, it must be remembered that opioids, pharmacologically speaking, still have no ceiling.[31] Cancer patients and those with progressive disease can still be treated with gradually increasing doses, and opioids can still be titrated to effect or toxicity with no arbitrary number of milligrams constituting a limit.

Applying pharmacological principles to treating pain

Widely accepted guidelines for cancer pain management must be used to optimize long-term opioid therapy.[32,33] These guidelines stress the importance of patient self-report as the basis for dosing, individualization of therapy to identify a favorable equilibrium between efficacy and side effects, and the value of monitoring over time.[29] They also are strongly indicative of the concurrent treatment of side effects as the basis for enhancing the balance between both analgesia and adverse effects.[34]

Individualization of the dose without regard to the size, which is the most important guideline for long-term opioid therapy, can be difficult in populations with substance abuse histories.[29] Although it may be appropriate to use care in prescribing potentially abusable drugs to these populations, deciding to forego the guideline of dose individualization without regard to absolute dose may increase the risk of undertreatment.[35] Aberrant drug-related behaviors may develop in response to unrelieved pain. Although these behaviors might be best understood as pseudoaddiction, the incidence of such behaviors serves to verify clinicians' fears and encourages greater prudence in prescribing.[29]

Another common misconception concerns the use of methadone. Clinicians who manage patients with substance abuse histories must comprehend the pharmacology of methadone because of its dual role as a treatment for opioid addiction and as an analgesic.[36,37] Methadone impedes withdrawal for significantly longer periods than it relieves pain. That is, abstinence can be prevented and opioid cravings lessened with a single dose, whereas most patients appear to require a minimum of three doses daily to obtain sustained analgesia. Although patients who are receiving methadone maintenance for treatment for opioid addiction can be administered methadone as an analgesic beyond the guidelines of the addiction treatment program, this usually necessitates a substantial modification in therapy, including dose escalation and multiple daily doses.[11,29]

From a pharmacological stance, the management of such a change does not pose difficult issues. It can, however, create substantial stress for the patient and clinicians involved in the treatment of the addiction disorder. Because the drug has been classified as addiction therapy, as opposed to pain therapy, some patients express disbelief in the analgesic efficacy of methadone. Others wish to continue the morning dose for addiction even if treatment throughout the remainder of the day uses the same drug at an equivalent or higher dose. Some clinicians who work at methadone clinics are willing to continue to be involved and prescribe opioids outside the program, and others wish to relinquish care.[29]

Selecting appropriate drugs and route of administration for the symptom and setting

The use of long-acting analgesics in sufficient amounts may help to minimize the number of rescue doses needed, lessen cravings, and decrease the risk of abuse of prescribed medications, given the possible difficulty of using short-acting formulations in patients with substance abuse histories. Rather than being overly concerned regarding the choice of drug or route of administration, the prescription of opioids and other potentially abusable drugs should be carried out within limits and guidelines.[11,29]

Many clinicians now respond to particularly high doses with rotation to another opioid. This practice is based on capitalizing on incomplete cross-tolerance, or the unique pharmacology of methadone in particular, to bring doses down while maintaining or improving efficacy and changing the balance of efficacy to toxicity.[38,39] Some clinicians set arbitrary dose limits for the various opioids. Others stopped using certain opioids they perceived as of higher risk or street value. Still others became so disillusioned as to stop using opioids altogether.

Recognizing specific drug abuse behaviors

In an effort to monitor the development of aberrant drug-taking behaviors, all patients who are prescribed potentially abusable drugs must be evaluated over time. This is particularly true for those patients with a remote or current history of drug abuse, including alcohol abuse. Should a high level of concern exist regarding such behaviors, frequent visits and regular assessments of significant others who can contribute information regarding the patient's drug use may be required. To promote early recognition of aberrant drug-related behaviors, it may also be necessary to have patients who have been actively abusing drugs in the recent past submit urine specimens for regular screening of illicit, or licit but unprescribed, drugs. When informing the patient of this approach, explain that it is a method of monitoring that can reassure the clinician and provide a foundation for aggressive symptom-oriented treatment, thus enhancing the therapeutic alliance with the patient.[11,29]

Using nondrug approaches as appropriate

Many nondrug approaches can be used to assist patients in coping with chronic pain in advanced illness. Such educational interventions may include relaxation techniques, ways of thinking of and describing the experience of pain, and methods of communicating physical and emotional distress to staff members (see Box 41.1). Although nondrug interventions may be helpful adjuvants to management, they should not be perceived as substitutes for drugs targeted at treating pain or other physical or psychological symptoms.[11,29]

Inpatient management plan

In designing the inpatient management of an actively abusing patient with advanced illness, it is helpful to use structured treatment guidelines. Although the applicability of these guidelines may vary from setting to setting, they provide a set of strategies that can ensure the safety of the patient and staff, control possible manipulative behaviors, allow for supervision of illicit drug use, enhance appropriate use of medications for pain and symptom control, and communicate an understanding of pain and substance abuse management.[11,29]

Under certain circumstances, such as actively abusing patients who are scheduled for surgery, patients should be admitted several days in advance, when possible, to allow for the stabilization of the drug regimen. This time can also be used to avoid withdrawal and to provide an opportunity to assess whether modifications to the established plan are necessary.[11,29]

Once established, the structured treatment plan for the management of active abuse must proceed conscientiously. In an effort to assess and manage symptoms, frequent visits are usually necessary. It is also important to avoid drug withdrawal, and to the extent possible, prescribed drugs for symptom control should be administered on a regularly scheduled basis (see Box 41.1). This helps to eliminate repetitive encounters with staff that center on the desire to obtain drugs.[11,29]

Treatment management plans must be designed to represent the clinician's assessment of the severity of drug abuse. Open and honest communication between clinician and patient to stress that the guidelines were established in the best interest of the patient is often helpful. However, in cases where patients are unable to follow these guidelines despite repeated interventions from the staff, discharge should be considered. Clinicians should discuss this decision for patient discharge with the staff and administration, while considering the ethical and legal ramifications of this action.[11,29]

Outpatient management plan

Alternative guidelines may be used in the management of the actively abusing patient with advanced illness who is being treated on an outpatient basis. In some instances, the treatment plan can be coordinated with referral to a drug rehabilitation program. However, patients who are facing end-of-life issues may have difficulty participating in such programs. Using the following approaches may be helpful for managing the complex and more difficult-to-control aspects of care.

Using written agreements

Using written agreements that clearly state the roles of the team members and expectations for the patient is helpful when structuring outpatient treatment. Basing the level of restrictions on the patient's behaviors, graded agreements should be enforced that clearly state the consequences of aberrant drug use.[11,29] Figure 41.1 provides a sample agreement for the initiation of opioid therapy. This template can be modified and structured to fit individual practices and palliative or hospice care settings, but it is a good general indication of the responsibilities of the patient as well as the provider or palliative care/hospice team.

Guidelines for prescribing

Patients who are actively abusing must be seen weekly to build a good rapport with staff and afford evaluation of symptom control and addiction-related concerns. Frequent visits allow the opportunity to prescribe small quantities of drugs, which may decrease the temptation to divert and provide a motive for not missing appointments[11,29] (see Box 41.1).

Procedures for prescription loss or replacement should be explicitly explained to the patient, with the stipulation that no renewals will be given if appointments are missed. The patient should also be informed that any dose changes require prior communication with the clinician. Additionally, clinicians who are covering for the primary care provider must be advised of

Opioid Medication Consent Form

PATIENT NAME: _____   SSN: _____

The purpose of this Agreement is to clarify expectations and prevent misunderstandings about certain medicines I will be taking for pain management. This is to help both my doctor and I comply with the law regarding controlled prescription drugs. I understand that this Agreement is essential to the trust and confidence necessary in a doctor/patient relationship and that my doctor will treat me based on this Agreement.

I understand that if I break this Agreement, my doctor may decide to stop prescribing these pain-control medicines. In this case, my doctor may taper off the medicine (i.e., slowly decrease) over a period of several days, as necessary to avoid withdrawal symptoms. Also, a drug-dependence treatment program may be recommended.

GOALS OF OPIOID TRIAL/TREATMENT
The purpose of this medication is to increase your ability to function at work and at home. Success will be measured by your activity level, not your report of pain.

RISKS OF OPIOID TRIAL/TREATMENT
This medication has the potential to cause an addiction. Physical tolerance and dependence occurs with regular use of a narcotic, but this is different from addiction. For a person's health, safety and protection, this medication may be stopped if there is a concern about addiction.

ADDICTION BEHAVIOR
- a lot of time & energy focused on obtaining medication
- continuing to take medications despite being told to stop
- decline in family and/or work functioning
- loss of interest in other life activities (e.g., hobbies, social activities)
- consistent misuse of medications (see below)

MISUSE OR ABUSE OF MEDICATION
- taking more medication than prescribed
- use of pain medications that have not been prescribed by this program
- use of alcohol to manage pain
- high number of emergency room visits seeking medication
- failing to use other recommended pain management techniques (e.g., physical therapy, relaxation techniques, TNS unit)
- getting medication from more than one doctor
- using someone else's opioid medication
- reports of lost or stolen medication
- asking only for medications with a high street value

GUIDELINES FOR OPIOID PRESCRIPTIONS

Our Responsibility
- Medication will only be prescribed by a SINGLE PROVIDER.
- Medication will be prescribed on a "by-the-clock" schedule.
- Lost or stolen prescriptions or medications will not be replaced.
- OPIOID MEDICATIONS WILL NOT TYPICALLY BE FILLED OVER THE PHONE.
- If an opioid taper is unsuccessful, medical care will be provided. Referral to facilities specializing in medication detoxification may be necessary.

Figure 41.1 Continued

Opioid Medication Consent Form (Continued)

Your Responsibility

- A person is responsible for his or her medications, and needs to make sure that prescriptions are filled correctly. Therefore, they need to make certain that the pharmacy gives them the correct number prescribed.
- No increases in medication doses will be made without the approval of the prescribing physician.
- If a person takes more medication than is prescribed, he or she will run out of medication before being given more.
- Narcotic medication use questions should be made during normal business hours, Monday through Friday, 8:00 A.M. to 4 P.M.
- Patients are expected to be on time for all appointments including those not related to refills medications. You will be asked to come in before a medication is to be refilled at times.

Informed Consent

- I will communicate fully with my doctor about the character and intensity of my pain, the effect of the pain on my daily life, side effects, and how well the medicine is helping to relieve the pain.
- I may be asked to bring unused medications to clinic with me for a "pill count" to ensure that I am using the medication as prescribed.
- I consent to submit to a blood or urine test if requested by my doctor to determine my compliance with my program of pain control medicine.
- I will not use any illegal controlled substances, including marijuana, cocaine, etc., as these will interact poorly with my pain medications.
- I will not share, sell, or trade my medication with anyone as these are dangerous to use when not under a doctor's care.
- I will not attempt to obtain any pain medicines, including opioid pain medicines, stimulants, or anti-anxiety medicines from any other doctor.
- I authorize the doctor and my pharmacy to cooperate fully with any city, state or federal law enforcement agency, including this state's Board of Pharmacy, in the investigation of any possible misuse, sale, or other diversion of my pain medicine. I authorize my doctor to provide a copy of this Agreement to my pharmacy. I agree to waive any applicable or right of privacy or confidentiality with respect to these authorizations.

If these guidelines are not met, you may be discharged from the program.

I, the undersigned, agree that the above guidelines have been explained to me, and that my questions and concerns regarding this treatment have been adequately answered. I agree to comply with the above guidelines. I have a copy of this document.

Signed: _____ Date: _____

Physician/Clinician: _____ Date: _____

Witness: _____ Date: _____

Figure 41.1 Pain management guidelines: opioid medication consent form.

the guidelines that have been established for each patient with a substance abuse history to avoid conflict and disruption of the treatment plan.[11,29]

Using 12-step programs

Depending on the patient's stage of advanced illness and functional capabilities, the clinician may want to consider referring the patient to a 12-step program with the stipulation that attendance be documented for ongoing prescription purposes. If the patient has a sponsor, the clinician may wish to contact the patient's sponsor, depending on the stage of illness and individual capabilities, in an effort to disclose the patient's illness and that medication is required in the treatment of the illness. This contact will also help to decrease the risk of stigmatizing the patient as being noncompliant with the ideals of the 12-step program.[11,29] If the patient is unable to participate in a 12-step program, other psychosocial and/or spiritual team members can provide care that supports sobriety.

Urine medication monitoring

The physician or hospice team may want to order a test to see how medications are being metabolized, and to see whether other medications are present that may present a safety risk for the patient. This could be done with a urine specimen or oral swab specimen. This practice, as well as finding nonprescribed medications or illicit substances should be clearly explained to the patient at the beginning of therapy. A response to an unexpected result generally involves increasing the guidelines for continued treatment, such as more frequent visits and smaller quantities of prescribed drugs.[11,29] If the patient is being cared for at home, it may involve daily deliveries of controlled substances, or a safe in the home to prevent others from obtaining the patient's medications.

Family sessions and meetings

The clinician, in an effort to increase support and function, should involve family members and friends in the treatment plan. These meetings will allow the clinician and other team members to become familiar with the family and additionally assist the team to identify family members who are using illicit drugs. Offering referral of these identified family members to drug treatment can be portrayed as a method of gathering support for the patient. The patient should also be prepared to cope with family members or friends who may attempt to buy or sell the patient's medications. These meetings will also assist the team in identifying dependable individuals who can serve as a source of strength and support for the patient during treatment.[11,29] A final case study illustrates how a highly complicated patient with advanced cancer was managed when access to opioids and other controlled substances was initiated in a man with a known addiction history.

Case study

A 68-year-old man with lung cancer

A 68-year-old man with metastatic lung cancer was referred to the psychologist on the palliative care team to help structure care for his burgeoning pain, anxiety, and substance abuse issues in the setting of advancing cancer. The patient was recently diagnosed and learned from the outset that he had stage IV disease and a life expectancy of less than 1 year. He had previously had problems with alcoholism and heroin addiction but became sober through ongoing participation in 12-step programs for 35 years. Indeed,

it was there he met his wife, who was also sober for this length of time, and the couple had a college-aged daughter. When he was initially seen he was withdrawn and worried. He knew his prognosis was grave and he was concerned about leaving behind his wife and daughter, though he was forthcoming and open to discussing these issues. But when it came time to discuss the approach to his anxiety and pain treatments he became more obstinate. He had been given some oxycodone and acetaminophen IR, which he said he liked and he was unclear whether he was using it strictly for pain, anxiety, or to elevate mood. He was also taking alprazolam IR. The psychologist discussed the need for clarity around these issues of drug taking and that the team needed to plan to help the patient not lose control of his medication taking in the setting of advancing pain and worsening psychological concerns, given his history of both alcohol and heroin addiction however remote. The plan would include a switch to methadone or long-acting morphine, clonazepam, both supplied in small quantities with urine drug testing and counseling and frequent meetings while he continued to "work his program." Despite his rapport with and like for the psychologist, he refused and stated he wanted to continue taking "these drugs because they are working." A standoff was created between the patient and the team and he left the institution, going to an outside oncologist from whom he withheld details of his drug addiction history. He remained on alprazolam and oxycodone and acetaminophen IR precipitating a 6-month long spiral into drug abuse, overuse of his medications, missing of medical treatment and withdrawal from family members, who were grief stricken at the missed opportunity to spend quality time with him for the short duration of his life. Ultimately, his wife brought him back to the original institution's ER, where he was seen by the psychologist. His wife had set limits and said, "If you don't do everything this doctor says, you don't have a place to live tonight." His daughter added, "For the past 6 months, you haven't felt the pain of your cancer, we have." The patient was disheveled, disheartened, and contrite. He agreed to the abovementioned plan, spent the end of his days comfortable and interacting with his family and rekindling ties to his 12-step friends. It was in a psychotherapy session with the psychologist that he stated, "As soon as I heard that I had stage IV cancer the first thing I thought was not, Oh my God I might die, or I might leave my family or even an existential crisis of what to do with the time I have left . . . no it was, 'Great now I can have narcotics again.'" He discussed how he realized what a tenacious disease his addiction was, and was able to impart this knowledge in meetings to younger members, which he considered his legacy.

Summary

Treating patients who are experiencing chronic pain from advanced illness and a substance use disorder is both complicated and challenging, because each can significantly complicate the other. Patients are living longer with advanced disease and pain concerns. We are no longer able to justify high-dose opioid therapy in a vacuum without trying to assess and manage addiction and abuse behaviors. In addition, the management of an advanced patient who is actively abusing drugs and is a member of an ethnic minority is more perplexing because of cultural differences that may exist. Using a treatment plan that involves a team approach that recognizes and responds to these complex needs is the optimum strategy to facilitate treatment. Although pain management may continue to be challenging even when all treatment plan procedures are implemented, the healthcare team's goal should be providing the highest level of pain management for all patients with substance use disorders.

References

1. Substance Abuse and Mental Health Services Administration, Office of Applied Studies. Treatment Episode Data Set (TEDS). Highlights—2007. National Admissions to Substance Abuse Treatment Services, DASIS Series: S-45, DHHS Publication No. (SMA) 09-4360, Rockville, MD, 2009. Available at: http://wwwdasis.samhsa.gov/teds07/TEDSHigh2k7.pdf Accessed October 2013.

2. Esteban S, Schulenberg JE, O'Malley PM, Patrick ME, Kloska DD. Nonmedical use of prescription opioids during the transition to adulthood: a multi-cohort national longitudinal study. Addiction. 2013 Sep 3. Epub ahead of print. doi: 10.1111/add.12347.

3. Khan S, Okuda M, Hasin DS, Secades-Villa R, Keyes K, Lin KH, et al. Gender differences in lifetime alcohol dependence: results from the national epidemiologic survey on alcohol and related conditions. Alcohol Clin Exp Res. 2013;37(10):1696–1705.

4. Blanco C, Rafful C, Wall MM, Jin CJ, Kerridge B, Schwartz RP. The latent structure and predictors of non-medical prescription drug use and prescription drug use disorders: a national study. Drug Alcohol Depend. 2013 Aug 17. Epub ahead of print. doi:pii: S0376-8716(13)00276-7. 10.1016/j.drugalcdep.2013.07.011.

5. Mori M, Elsayem A, Reddy SK, Bruera E, Fadul NA. Unrelieved pain and suffering in patients with advanced cancer. Am J Hosp Palliat Care. 2012;29(3):236–240.

6. O'Connor M, Weir J, Butcher I, Kleiboer A, Murray G, Sharma N, et al. Pain in patients attending a specialist cancer service: prevalence and association with emotional distress. J Pain Symptom Manage. 2012;43(1):29–38.

7. Swarm RA, Abernethy AP, Anghelescu DL, Benedetti C, Buga S, Cleeland C, et al. Adult cancer pain. J Natl Compr Canc Netw. 2013;11(8):992–1022.

8. Rupp T, Delaney KA. Inadequate analgesia in emergency medicine. Ann Emerg Med. 2004;43(4):494–503.

9. Passik SD, Portenoy RK. Substance abuse issues in palliative care. In: Berger A, Portenoy R, Weissman D (eds.), Principles and Practice of Supportive Oncology. Philadelphia, PA: Lippincott Williams and Wilkins; 1998:513–524.

10. Passik SD, Portenoy RK, Ricketts PL. Substance abuse issues in cancer patients. Part 1: Prevalence and diagnosis. Oncology. 1998;12:517–521.

11. Passik SD, Portenoy RK. Substance abuse disorders. In: Holland JC (ed.), Psycho-oncology. New York, NY: Oxford University Press; 1998:576–586.

12. Weissman DE, Haddox JD. Opioid pseudoaddiction: an iatrogenic syndrome. Pain. 1989;36:363–366.

13. Passik SD, Webster L, Kirsh KL. Pseudoaddiction revisited: a commentary on clinical and historical considerations. Pain Manage. 2011;1(3): 239–248.

14. Argoff CE. Clinical implications of opioid pharmacogenetics. Clin J Pain. 2010;26(1 Suppl):S16–S20.

15. Passik SD, Kirsh KL, Whitcomb LA, Schein JR, Kaplan M, Dodd S, et al. Monitoring outcomes during long-term opioid therapy for non-cancer pain: results with the pain assessment and documentation tool. J Opioid Manage. 2005;1(5):257–266.

16. Fleming MF, Balousek SL, Klessig CL, Mundt MP, Brown DD. Substance use disorders in a primary care sample receiving daily opioid therapy. J Pain. 2007;8(7):573–582. Epub May 11, 2007.

17. Rinaldi RC, Steindler EM, Wilford BB. Clarification and standardization of substance abuse terminology. JAMA. 1988;259:555–557.

18. Gros DF, Milanak ME, Brady KT, Back SE. Frequency and severity of comorbid mood and anxiety disorders in prescription opioid dependence. Am J Addict. 2013;22(3):261–265.

19. Anderson KO, Mendoza TR, Valero V, Richman SP, Russell C, Hurley J, et al. Minority cancer patients and their providers. Cancer. 2000;88:1929–1938.

20. Reynolds KS, Hanson LC, Henderson M, Steinhauser KE. End-of-life care in nursing home settings: do race or age matter? Palliat Support Care. 2008;6(1):21–27.

21. Burgess DJ, Crowley-Matoka M, Phelan S, Dovidio JF, Kerns R, Roth C, et al. Patient race and physicians' decisions to prescribe opioids for chronic low back pain. Soc Sci Med. 2008;67(11):1852–1860. Epub October 15, 2008.

22. Seale JP, Muramoto ML. Substance abuse among minority populations. Subst Abus. 1993;20:167–180.

23. Cintron A, Morrison RS. Pain and ethnicity in the United States: a systematic review. J Palliat Med. 2006;9(6):1454–1473.

24. Dunbar SA, Katz NP. Chronic opioid therapy for nonmalignant pain in patients with a history of substance abuse: report of 20 cases. J Pain Symptom Manage. 1996;11:163–171.

25. Laroche F, Rostaing S, Aubrun F, Perrot S. Pain management in heroin and cocaine users. Joint Bone Spine. 2012;79(5):446–450.

26. Burton-MacLeod S, Fainsinger RL. Cancer pain control in the setting of substance use: establishing goals of care. J Palliat Care. 2008;24(2):122–125.

27. Kirsh KL, Whitcomb LA, Donaghy K, Passik SD. Abuse and addiction issues in medically ill patients with pain: attempts at clarification of terms and empirical study. Clin J Pain. 2002;18(4 Suppl):S52–S60.

28. Savage SR, Kirsh KL, Passik SD. Challenges in using opioids to treat pain in persons with substance use disorders. Addict Sci Clin Pract. 2008;4(2):4–25. Available at: http://www.drugabuse.gov/PDF/ascp/vol4no2/Challenges.pdf. Accessed December 10, 2009).

29. Passik SD, Portenoy RK, Ricketts PL. Substance abuse issues in cancer patients. Part 2: Evaluation and treatment. Oncology. 1998; 12:729–734.

30. Passik SD, Kirsh KL, Casper D. Addiction-related assessment tools and pain management: instruments for screening, treatment planning, and monitoring compliance. Pain Med. 2008;9(S2):S145–S166.

31. Coluzzi F, Pappagallo M; National Initiative on Pain Control. Opioid therapy for chronic noncancer pain: practice guidelines for initiation and maintenance of therapy. Minerva Anestesiol. 2005;71(7–8):425–433.

32. Christo PJ, Mazloomdoost D. Cancer pain and analgesia. Ann N Y Acad Sci. 2008;1138:278–298.

33. American Pain Society. Principles of Analgesic Use in the Treatment of Acute Pain and Cancer Pain. 6th ed. Glenview, IL: Author; 2008.

34. Dy SM, Asch SM, Naeim A, Sanati H, Walling A, Lorenz KA. Evidence-based standards for cancer pain management. J Clin Oncol. 2008;26(23):3879–3885.

35. Cohen MJ, Jasser S, Herron PD, Margolis CG. Ethical perspectives: opioid treatment of chronic pain in the context of addiction. Clin J Pain. 2002;18(4 Suppl):S99–S107.

36. Kilonzo I, Twomey F. Rotating to oral methadone in advanced cancer patients: a case series. J Palliat Med. 2013;16(9):1154–1157.

37. Smith HS, Kreek MJ, Johnson C, Kirsh KL. Methadone and methadone issues. In Smith HS, Passik SD (eds.), Pain and Chemical Dependency. New York, NY: Oxford University Press; 2008:113–122.

38. Wirz S, Wartenberg HC, Elsen C, Wittmann M, Diederichs M, Nadstawek J. Managing cancer pain and symptoms of outpatients by rotation to sustained-release hydromorphone: a prospective clinical trial. Clin J Pain. 2006;22(9):770–775.

39. Zimmermann C, Seccareccia D, Booth CM, Cottrell W. Rotation to methadone after opioid dose escalation: how should individualization of dosing occur? J Pain Palliat Care Pharmacother. 2005;19(2):25–31.

CHAPTER 42

Palliative care of cancer survivors

Mary S. McCabe and Stacie Corcoran

I am adjusting to the fact that recovery takes time. I feel stronger mentally in facing challenge, and I value my relationships with family and friends even more, which I didn't think was possible. I feel humble and honored that I have been given this new gift of life.

Cancer survivor

It isn't accomplished by knowing every curve in the road ahead. Instead, the headlights shine a light on what's immediately in front of us—that's all. And that's what's necessary—shining a light on the few feet ahead, and then the next few feet, and on and on . . . and before we know it we have traveled the whole trip in the dark.

Cancer survivor

Key points

- There are over 14 million cancer survivors in the United States.
- Being told you are cancer-free does not mean you are free of the consequences of the disease.
- Seventy-six percent of cancer survivors are over age 60 years and have coexisting medical conditions that complicate post-treatment recovery to maximum health.
- Childhood cancer survivors carry a heavy burden of medical and psychological problems resulting from their experience with cancer.
- Improvements are needed in the coordination of care for cancer survivors to assure optimal quality of life.
- Cancer diagnosis and treatment affects the family as well as the patient.

Just as palliative care has faced many challenges in reaching its full potential as a specialty within the healthcare continuum, so it is with survivorship care. Until recently, the primary focus in oncology was on the diagnostic and treatment phases of care. It wasn't until the 2006 publication of the seminal report by the Institute of Medicine (IOM), *From Cancer Patient to Cancer Survivor: Lost in Transition*, that national attention has been given to the specific health issues and resulting care needs of cancer survivors[1] (see Table 42.1). Fortunately, there is a growing body of knowledge about the lingering and late consequences of cancer and its treatment, greater understanding about the interventions needed to address these problems, a focus on developing models for optimal care delivery, and an awareness of the key role nurses play in the delivery of survivorship care.[1–8]

The intersection of palliative care and cancer survivorship

The essentials of palliative care—attention to physical pain and suffering, including existential distress; the inclusion of the family as a unit of care; and interdisciplinary care—are all relevant to and needed by the cancer survivor.[9] Although many survivors recover quickly and completely from the toxicities of cancer treatment, the words of one survivor—"being free of the cancer is not being free of its consequences"—ring true for many others. Survival after a cancer diagnosis can come at a price in terms of medical, psychosocial, and existential problems.[10,11] For example, chronic pain may be the result of surgery and radiation in a young adult treated for a rare head and neck tumor; fatigue may last for years in a survivor treated for Hodgkin's disease; severe anxiety may prevent the social reintegration of a patient treated for leukemia with a stem cell transplant; and lymphedema of the leg may impede the function of a person treated for a sarcoma. In each of these cases, the application of palliative care strategies can reduce and/or eliminate the problems.

Challenges of survivorship

In discussing the palliative care needs of cancer survivors, it is important to first understand who is considered a cancer survivor and what cancer survivorship means. As reported by the President's Cancer Panel, the time at which a person diagnosed with cancer becomes a survivor has a variety of interpretations depending on the focus of the group doing the defining.[12] A widely embraced definition states that a person is a survivor from the moment of diagnosis and that family members are included in

Table 42.1 The cancer control continuum

Prevention	Early detection	Diagnosis	Treatment	Survivorship	End-of-life care
Tobacco control	Cancer screening	Oncology consultations	Chemotherapy	Long-term follow-up/ surveillance	Palliation
Diet	Awareness of cancer signs and symptoms	Tumor staging	Surgery	Late-effects management	Spiritual issues
Physical activity		Patient counseling and decision-making	Radiation therapy Adjuvant therapy		Hospice
Sun exposure			Symptom management	Rehabilitation	
Virus exposure				Coping	
Alcohol use			Phychosocial care	Health promotion	
Chemoprevention					

Source: With permission, Hewitt and Stovall (2006), reference 1.

the survivorship experience throughout the trajectory. Both the National Coalition for Cancer Survivorship and the National Cancer Institute's Office of Cancer Survivorship have adopted this definition.[1]

> An individual is considered a cancer survivor from the time of diagnosis, through the balance of his or her life. Family members, friends and caregivers are also impacted by the survivorship experience and are therefore included in this definition.

For the purposes of highlighting a set of often neglected issues requiring palliative care interventions, this chapter focuses, as did the IOM report, on the survivorship experience following diagnosis and treatment of the initial cancer and prior to the development of a recurrence. This phase of care has been given relatively little attention until recently, often because the care ends abruptly once treatment is completed or because the follow-up care becomes episodic and focuses on disease recurrence and not on a comprehensive approach to posttreatment needs.

The acute toxicities associated with cancer treatment (chemotherapy, radiation, and surgery) are well characterized, and considerable research has appropriately focused on their amelioration. Professional medical and nursing societies have made the education about these interventions a central focus. Now, with the rapidly growing number of cancer survivors, it is time to do the same for the long-term and late effects of cancer treatment. The long-term effects are those that begin during treatment and become chronic, continuing well beyond the end of treatment. As defined by Aziz, the late effects of treatment are those that occur after treatment has ended but "manifest later with the unmasking of hitherto unseen injury to immature organs by developmental processes or as a result of failure of compensatory mechanisms because of the passage of time or organ senescence."[13]

Fortunately, these long-term and late effects are becoming better understood and, increasingly, research is being conducted that focuses on reducing and/or preventing these problems.[14,15] At the same time, professional societies and cancer organizations are developing much needed guidance for clinicians. Some groups such as the Children's Oncology Group have taken an exposure-based approach to the guidance for follow-up care of survivors of pediatric cancer, while the American Cancer Society

is taking a disease-based approach to surveillance guidelines. The National Comprehensive Cancer Network and the American Society of Clinical Oncology are both taking a symptom-based approach (e.g., fatigue, depression, sleep disturbances) to the clinical management of cancer survivors. This symptom-based approach will be extremely useful in identifying problems requiring palliative care interventions.

Because cancer is a disease of the elderly, with the overwhelming majority of survivors being over age 60 years, these long-term and late effects add significant morbidity to the lives of elderly cancer survivors, and if not identified and treated, they may not only add to the burden of illness but also significantly impact quality of life (QOL) and even survival itself.[16-18]

The negative consequences of cancer treatment are not restricted to physical domains. There is a known set of important psychosocial concerns as well.[19,20] In addition, although the diagnosis and treatment phases are widely recognized as being psychologically challenging for all patients and their families, there are a subset of survivors who experience long-term psychological distress or problems later in their survivorship. Studies have identified risk factors for developing these problems, including anxiety, depression, and poor adjustment—all of which influence posttreatment recovery, health, and overall well-being.[21-23]

Special at-risk groups

Pediatric survivors

One of the most important successes in oncology has been in pediatrics, where over 80% of children and adolescents treated for cancer become long-term survivors.[24] However, as these young people grow into adulthood, they face (often serious) health consequences of their cancer treatment that may not become evident for many years.[25,26] Both the organ system damage and psychological impact of having been treated at such a young age creates a need for ongoing care focused on prevention, surveillance, early detection, and management of late treatment effects.

Numerous seminal survivorship studies have been conducted with participants who are in the Childhood Cancer Survivor

Study (CCSS; a multi-institutional cohort of long-term cancer survivors diagnosed with a pediatric malignancy from 1970 to 1986) to determine the prevalence, incidence, and severity of chronic health conditions in adult survivors of pediatric cancers; the risk of chronic conditions compared with their siblings; and the subpopulations of survivors at highest risk for severe, debilitating, or life-threatening health conditions.[25,27] Major studies have reported that the risk of chronic health conditions is high—particularly for second cancers, cardiovascular disease, renal dysfunction, musculoskeletal problems, and endocrinopathies—and that the incidence of these conditions and others increases over time.[11,25,28,29] Survivors were eight times as likely as their siblings to have severe or life-threatening conditions, and there were particular treatment combinations, especially those including chest, abdominal, or pelvic radiation, that were associated with a 10-fold increase in risk for severe or life-threatening conditions. Overall, in patients treated 30 years ago, almost three-fourths have a chronic health condition; one-third have multiple conditions; and more than 40% experience severe, life-threatening, disabling, or fatal conditions, such as heart attacks or second cancers.[25]

The important future challenge in survivorship care is the identification and treatment of these conditions to assure the long-term health and well-being of this unique group of survivors. One well-established effort exists at academic medical centers, where long-term follow-up clinics for pediatric cancer survivors provide the specialized care required for their complex problems. Unfortunately, it has been reported that less than 20% of adult survivors of childhood cancers are followed at a cancer center or by a knowledgeable professional such as an oncologist.[30] This leaves much work to be done in educating the survivor and other healthcare providers about needed surveillance, symptom identification, and proper management. Fortunately, an important resource for assuring quality care for this group of survivors that can be made widely available for use by any provider of survivorship care are the Long-Term Follow-Up Guidelines for Survivors of Childhood, Adolescent, and Young Adult Cancers developed by the Children's Oncology Group. The guidelines are available at (http://www.survivorshipguidelines.org/) and represent an important guide to the management of survivors of pediatric cancers.[31] The dissemination of this resource to both survivors of pediatric cancers and the healthcare community involved in their care is a critical next step in which nurses can play a crucial role when caring for these individuals.

Bone marrow transplant/hematopoietic stem cell transplantation survivors

Bone marrow transplant, or the more current term *hematopoietic stem cell transplantation* (HSCT), is a curative treatment for many patients with cancer, including those with relapsed and/or high-risk acute and chronic leukemia and subsets of patients with lymphoma and multiple myeloma.[32] Advances in therapeutic approaches over the last decade, including the use of diverse sources of stem cells, reduced-intensity conditioning regimens, and improvements in supportive care, have decreased the morbidity and mortality rates for most HSCT recipients and increased the number of eligible patients, including the elderly and those without suitably matched donors.[33] As a result, there are increasing numbers of transplants performed annually and greater

expectations for long-term survival. A recent study of patients who are disease-free at 2 years after allogeneic HSCT indicated a 90% probability of surviving 5 years and an 80% probability of surviving 15 years after transplant.[34]

Despite these advances in toxicity reduction, the physical late effects of transplant continue to include the risk of secondary malignancies, pulmonary complications, cataracts, sterility, and graft-versus-host disease (GVHD).[35] A comprehensive analysis of disease- and treatment-related factors associated with late mortality in a large cohort of allogeneic HSCT recipients demonstrated mortality rates twice as high as that of the general population and that survivors face challenges affecting their overall health and well-being.[34] As the number of survivors increases, the long-term effects on the QOL of patients and families becomes more important. Although many transplant recipients report normal QOL, the majority indicate a poorer QOL relative to premorbid status and when compared with healthy peers, including low energy levels and sleep difficulties, low self-esteem, sexual difficulties, psychological distress, and impaired social relationships.[35,36] Functional well-being is reported as lower in transplant recipients in comparison with siblings, as measured by decreased likeliness to be married, greater likeliness to have difficulty holding a job because of a health problem, lower household income, and more difficulty obtaining health and life insurance.[34] A study of the presence of posttraumatic stress disorder (PTSD) in HSCT recipients revealed that patients at risk were those with a pretransplant measurement of poor social support combined with avoidance coping.[37]

Chronic graft-versus-host disease (cGVHD) remains the most significant complication affecting QOL and overall outcomes in long-term survivors after transplant.[32] It is the chief cause of nonrelapse-related death.[34] Incidence of cGVHD has increased along with the number of allogeneic HSCTs performed, affecting an estimated 50% of long-term survivors.[34] While cGVHD can involve almost any organ, it most commonly affects the skin, mouth, mucosa, liver, eyes, and lungs in addition to the hematopoietic and lymphoid organs. Clinical manifestations can vary in both severity and clinical course.[33] Traditionally, treatment requires immunosuppression with corticosteroids (prednisone) along with calcineurin inhibitors (cyclosporin or tacrolimus) as the primary therapy. Newer agents and techniques are under study for prevention, primary treatment, and treatment of steroid refractory or dependent disease.[38] Balancing the treatment of symptoms while maintaining sufficient immune function to protect against opportunistic pathogens is the greatest challenge because infections that occur as a result of lymphopenia are the major cause of death in cGVHD.[33]

A multidisciplinary approach to the supportive care of patients with cGVHD is essential. Potential side effects of treatment include infections, osteoporosis, hypertension, hyperglycemia, renal insufficiency, and hyperlipidemia as well as reduced QOL and psychosocial disturbances.[38] Care includes antimicrobial and antifungal prophylaxis as well as nutritional support and physical therapy. The National Institutes of Health Consensus Development Project for Clinical Trials in Chronic Graft Versus Host Disease published recommendations for standardized monitoring and treatment with an emphasis on supportive care.[39] Identification of patients at greatest risk for posttransplant difficulties—whether physical, psychological, or functional—and implementing appropriate interventions for prevention and management is an important step in achieving a better QOL for this ever-growing number of long-term survivors.

Elderly survivors

Of the over 14 million cancer survivors in the United States, 60% (6.5 million) are age 65 years and older.[40] By 2030 there will be 71 million Americans age 65 years and older, accounting for 20% of the population.[40] If current trends continue, then the increase in survival rates coupled with the aging population present a major challenge to our healthcare system charged with the posttreatment care of this rapidly growing number of Americans.

The posttreatment health of older cancer survivors is influenced by multiple factors, including toxicity of treatment, presence of symptoms and/or late effects, comorbid health conditions, social resources, and normative aging.[18] Physical and social functioning are the most common health domains adversely affected. A recent review of the research literature found that older cancer survivors reported higher rates of comorbid health problems compared with older adults without a cancer history.[18] Although it is unclear whether these conditions are late treatment effects, it appears that the coexistence of comorbid health conditions (whatever their cause) can exacerbate the effects of cancer treatment on the posttreatment health of older adults.[24] With respect to mental health, cancer in older adults may occur in the context of other losses, isolation, and constraint on social resources, thus putting strain on coping mechanisms.

Care for the projected numbers of older cancer survivors presents new challenges with predictions of shortages in the number of oncologists and geriatricians. The role of nurses, particularly geriatric nurse practitioners, will grow in importance as the complexities of posttreatment and comorbid conditions of aging converge. There is much to be studied in elderly cancer survivors so that appropriate guidelines for surveillance and follow-up interventions can be developed. Research on physiological and psychological effects of therapy; QOL and physical function; risk of coexistence of comorbid conditions and disability; and control and prevention of late effects have all been identified as important to the provision of care to this expanding population.[41,42]

Socioeconomically disadvantaged survivors

Cancer patients who are socioeconomically disadvantaged face greater challenges compared with patients who have adequate resources.[43–45] The stress of a cancer diagnosis adds enormous burden to the physical, psychological, and financial deprivation already experienced by the poor.[46] With limited healthcare choices already, the complexity and expense of therapies can become overwhelming for disadvantaged cancer patients. Often, essentials such as food and shelter remain the first priority. Cancer survivors who live in poverty remain vulnerable even after the acute treatment period has ended. They have limited access to ongoing medical care and may not be aware of the importance of ongoing follow-up. Therefore, they are less likely to receive treatment for comorbidities and are less likely to receive psychosocial services. Follow-up care for needed services of long-term and late effects are most often not attainable. Palliative care services needed by the survivor, in particular, may be overlooked because access to healthcare may abruptly end once cancer treatment is completed. Sadly, these barriers faced by the socioeconomically underserved survivor mirror the problems faced by the poor in general and are outlined in an American Cancer Society report: poor people experience more cancer-related pain; poor people often do not seek necessary care if they are unable to pay for it; cancer education and outreach efforts are often insensitive and irrelevant to the lives of many poor people; and fatalism about cancer is common among the poor and often prevents them from accessing care.[43]

The challenges to improving the care of the disadvantaged cancer survivor are tied to the important issue of assuring access to quality care for the poor in general. It requires community-based approaches that incorporate healthcare access into a broader plan for housing, social services, and job training.

Selected symptoms of importance in survivor care

Fatigue

Fatigue is the most common symptom associated with cancer and its treatment.[47,48] Cancer-related fatigue is defined as a "distressing, persistent, subjective sense of tiredness or exhaustion related to cancer or cancer treatment that is not proportional to recent activity and interferes with usual functioning."[49] Prevalence and severity depend on the disease stage, treatment type, and treatment phase. It occurs most frequently among patients receiving chemotherapy with or without radiation therapy.[50,51] Fatigue is multidimensional and reported by patients in terms of perceived energy, mental capacity, and psychological status. Fatigue can interfere with normal functioning and lead to negative effects on QOL.[52] Although the study of fatigue generally is focused on the active treatment period, fatigue may persist for a significant time afterward.[53] A national survey of cancer patients more than 1 year post treatment using consensus-based diagnostic criteria for cancer-related fatigue (CRF) showed a prevalence of CRF of 17%, with 64% of survivors reporting some fatigue-related problem.[54]

Fatigue has been well documented in specific survivor populations. Minton and Stone conducted a literature review to characterize and quantify the phenomenon of posttreatment fatigue (PTF) in breast cancer survivors that is distinguishable from fatigue related to aging and comorbidities seen in the general population.[55] In studies of women less than 2 years after treatment completion, prevalence of PTF has been as high as 20% to 30%, with a significant difference between treated women and controls. Longer term studies, longer than 2 years posttreatment, have shown significant disturbances compared with the general population up to 5 years after treatment, most notably in respect to physical functioning and mental fatigue. Data suggest that in affected women, any improvement is seen only after 2 years and that fatigue may continue up to 5 years. Longitudinal studies suggest the existence of ongoing PTF but with improvement in fatigue symptoms over time. A significant minority of women still experience PTF up to 5 years, with a wide variation in prevalence. The authors conclude that fatigue is not a phenomenon that occurs solely during breast cancer treatment and should not be dismissed without palliative care interventions.

Prevalence of chronic fatigue (CF), defined as elevated fatigue levels lasting longer than 6 months, is 2.5 to 3 times higher in Hodgkin's lymphoma (HL) survivors than in the general population.[56] Most studies attribute excess fatigue to cancer treatment.

However, prospective data suggest that fatigue is a significant problem at diagnosis and does not remit with effective treatment. Fatigue in HL survivors may be multifactorial and could relate to ongoing disruption of proinflammatory cytokines that are part of the underlying disease as well as endocrine, respiratory, and circulatory alterations as well as comorbid conditions.[56] Survivors of HL do report a reduced QOL related to fatigue, persistent after resolution of treatment effects.[56] Further research is needed to understand the etiology of this long-term complication of HL so that effective assessment and interventions can be employed.

Evaluation of CRF is difficult because of the subjectivity of measurement and is complicated by a wide range of symptoms consistent with psychological impairment, low physical performance, pain, and depression. Surveys of patients, caregivers, and oncologists have revealed that fatigue is rarely discussed and that few recommendations for treatment are offered, particularly with survivors.[35] Assessment of fatigue at follow-up visits is important to determine the impact on the patient's adjustment after treatment. Identification of physiological conditions (such as persistent anemia) or psychological factors (such as depression) can help in initiating appropriate management. Educating patients and caregivers about pharmacological and nonpharmacological strategies to reduce symptoms is essential. The National Comprehensive Cancer Network (NCCN) incorporated specific interventions for fatigue monitoring and management for cancer survivors into the latest version of their Cancer-Related Fatigue guidelines. The guidelines Cancer Related Fatigue: Interventions for Patients on Long Term Follow-up are available on the NCCN website http:/www.nccn.org/professionals/physician_gls/PDF/survivorship.pdf.[49] A further in depth discussion on fatigue can be found in chapter 8.

Chronic pain

Although chronic pain is common in cancer survivors, it is an underappreciated and underreported symptom and its etiology, characteristics, and impact on QOL are still not well understood.[57] Until recently, there was limited focus by the healthcare team on pain as an important consequence of treatment, and previously, patients were often reluctant to discuss this symptom for fear it was a poor prognostic sign about their survival.[58] The types of pain experienced by survivors are complex, are difficult to diagnose, and may begin during treatment (e.g., taxane neuropathy) or occur many years later (e.g., radiation-induced plexopathy).[59] In a recent study, the authors found that 20% of a diverse group of cancer survivors had cancer-related chronic pain and 43% had experienced pain since diagnosis.[17] They also found racial and sexual disparities in cancer-related chronic pain's incidence and impact on QOL. Chronic pain caused by cancer therapy may be further complicated by preexisting pain in the elderly and further intensified by untreated anxiety and depression.

Chemotherapy

As highlighted by Paice, painful peripheral neuropathies caused by the chemotherapy agents (CIPN, for chemotherapy-induced peripheral neuropathy) are increasing in frequency as more neurotoxic agents are being used to treat a wide variety of cancers. These include the platinum-based drugs; taxanes; Vinca alkaloids; and protease inhibitors thalidomide, ixabepilone, and lenalidomide.[60] Although this pain most often resolves over time without intervention, it can remain intensely painful in a small group of survivors.[61,62] Its severity may be increased by preexisting neuropathy

caused by diabetes or alcoholism. Although a definitive treatment does not yet exist, clinicians rely on antiepilepsy drugs, antidepressants, opioids, and other pharmacological therapies. Physical therapy is an important component of a plan of care focused on rehabilitation to maximize functioning and assure safety.

Corticosteroids are an integral part of treatment regimens for some cancers, such as leukemia and myeloma, and are known to cause osteonecrosis. Usually occurring within 3 years of steroid treatment, osteonecrosis primarily affects the bones of the weight-bearing joints, leading to limited range of motion and pain. In children treated for acute lymphoblastic leukemias, the reported incidence of osteonecrosis ranges between 5%–10% and 20%–30%.[63] Unfortunately, there is often limited awareness of this significant problem and no consistent diagnostic standards exist. Because adolescents may be more susceptible to the development of osteonecrosis as a result of maturing bones, particular attention should be paid to joint pain symptoms in young adults who have received steroids as part of cancer treatment.[64]

Radiation

A number of late effects of radiation therapy can result in significant chronic pain. These include plexopathies, osteoradionecrosis and fractures.[65] Radiation-induced brachial plexopathies are most common in breast cancer, followed by lung cancer and lymphoma survivors.[60] The initial presentation of this painful syndrome varies in time to initiation and types of symptoms. The incidence of painful, disabling brachial plexopathy ranges from 1% to 5% depending on the radiation dose, technique, and concurrent chemotherapies, and 9% of women have at least a mild plexopathy.[66] Lumbosacral plexopathy is seen most frequently in survivors of colorectal and gynecological cancers and can have a disabling array of symptoms, such as pain, paresthesias, hypoesthesia, and weakness.

In each of these patient groups, the presentation of new onset pain requires a careful assessment that includes a review of prior cancer treatment because the chronic pain syndrome resulting from radiotherapy has a delayed onset of many years. This is one of the key reasons for ongoing careful assessment of the cancer survivor and for healthcare providers to be knowledgeable about the survivor's prior cancer therapy.

Surgery

Chronic pain syndromes in cancer survivors are associated with persistent nociceptive pain or neuropathic pain, or a combination of both. Chronic postoperative pain has been described after procedures such as thoracotomy, breast surgery, modified-radical neck dissection, limb amputations, nephrectomy, and inguinal lymph node dissection and is most common in survivors who have undergone an amputation and who have been treated for thoracic and breast cancers.[57]

There is significant variability in the incidence of chronic postsurgical pain, ranging from 13% to 24% for phantom breast pain to 30% to 80% for phantom limb pain.[57] The predisposing factors for phantom limb pain include preamputation pain, severe postoperative pain, and a more proximal amputation.[67] The interplay between chronic pain and physical disability in amputees is a complex one, and researchers have found that ongoing functional impairment is most closely correlated with severe stump pain, the level of the amputation, and significant phantom sensation.[68] This information provides an important guide for the focus of combined pain and rehabilitation interventions.

Numerous studies have evaluated the incidence of chronic post-thoracotomy pain in patients with lung cancer. Although there is usually gradual improvement over time, 60% of patients continue to report pain significant enough for analgesic use at one year, and prolonged chronic pain may have an incidence of as high as 50%, with half of these individuals reporting moderate-to-severe pain.[69] In a study by Dajczman, the patients with severe pain required daily analgesics, nerve blocks, or referral to a pain clinic.[70] This intensity and chronicity of pain then leads to functional limitations that become an impediment to the survivor's recovery and may also affect psychological domains.

Chronic pain after breast cancer surgery is seen in as many as 50% of mastectomy patients and is characterized into specific types: phantom breast pain, intercostobrachial neuralgia, neuroma pain, and other nerve injury pain.[57] Studies have identified that the pain can be present in the arm, neck, shoulder, axilla, chest, or breast, and it is influenced by the type of surgical procedure.[57] Although it was hoped that the newer breast-conserving surgical procedures would reduce the incidence of chronic pain, this has not been demonstrated as true. In fact, in one survey, women undergoing a breast-sparing surgery with axillary node dissection had a higher incidence of chronic pain.[71] Tasmuth et al. have shown that the best predictor of chronic pain in breast cancer survivors is the severity of acute postoperative pain.[72] This acute pain may be related to anxiety and depression and postoperative complications—all issues that require palliative care interventions. In-depth discussions on pain assessment and management can be found in chapters 6 and 7.

Sleep disorders

Although sleep disorders are known to be associated with various medical conditions, only limited attention has been paid to the impact of sleep quality in cancer patients—particularly in cancer survivors. Insomnia has been reported in adult cancer patients beginning during treatment with a prevalence of 30% to 50% and remaining as high as 23% to 44% following treatment.[73] In a unique study of survivors of pediatric cancers, the prevalence was much lower (16.7%) but varied greatly by diagnosis, with 50% of survivors of pediatric leukemia reporting sleep difficulties.[74] Not only are sleep difficulties common in cancer patients, they are also of major concern as a source of emotional and physical distress in these individuals.[75–77]

There are numerous important factors that contribute to the experience of sleep disorders. In particular, fatigue, physical pain, and depression all are known to impact sleep in adults and are specifically known to increase the likelihood of insomnia.[78] Unfortunately, far less is known about these symptoms in the cancer population. Servaes et al. have shown that fatigue is a distressing and common symptom estimated to be as high as 70% to 96% in recently treated adult cancer patients across diagnoses, but it also has been found to be present years after completion of cancer therapy.[79] Chronic pain in cancer survivors is also an understudied and underreported problem and contributes significantly to sleep disorders when unrelieved. Although many surveys have identified the relationship between depressive feelings and insomnia, studies in cancer patients have been rare. In a recent study of cancer patients, Davidson et al. found that individuals who experienced "ups and downs" of mood were prone to insomnia, thus suggesting that mood variability is associated with insomnia.[78]

In addition, recent studies suggest that fatigue, sleep disturbance, and depression may stem from distinct biological processes in posttreatment survivors.

While continuing to describe the prevalence and type of sleep disorders and their relationship to other cancer-related symptoms and treatment exposures, it is critical that studies be conducted focusing on the formal assessment of sleep quality in cancer patients along with adaptive interventions that can be evaluated and made part of a palliative care plan. For example, Hoyt et al. have proposed that an avoidance-oriented coping style may negatively impact mood and sleep, thus having implications for psychological interventions in this group.[80] In addition, given the complex nature of sleep disorders in survivors, treatments focused on reducing cognitive arousal and pain would be useful palliative care strategies. Most importantly, because of the immensely negative impact of sleep disturbance on the QOL of cancer survivors, palliative care interventions targeted to the array of related and contributory symptoms are essential for recovery. An in-depth discussion on insomnia can be found in chapter 22.

Cognitive dysfunction

Increasingly, research is focused on the identification and understanding of the cognitive changes associated with cancer and its treatment.[81,82] Although it is known that cancers involving the central nervous system (CNS) and treatments involving cranial surgery and radiation cause cognitive impairment, most research to date has focused on non-CNS cancers.

Breast cancer has been the focus of the greatest number of studies in response to the anecdotal reporting of changes in memory and concentration, termed "chemo brain," in breast cancer survivors that received adjuvant chemotherapy and hormonal therapy.[83] Although most breast cancer patients report some cognitive changes during active treatment, recent prospective studies have demonstrated that some degree of cognitive dysfunction exists prior to breast cancer treatment, suggesting that the disease may contribute to the cause.[84] The cognitive changes may lessen and even resolve over time, but there is now evidence that, for a subset of breast cancer survivors, cognitive changes may be long-lasting or even have a delayed onset.[85] Increasingly research is being expanded to include other patient groups, such as the survivors of pediatric cancer and transplant survivors. In each of these groups, the resulting neurocognitive deficits result in unique impairments, such as poor employment and a need for physical rehabilitation.[86,87] Multiple factors have been found to influence, and possibly increase, risk for cognitive changes, either independently or in interaction with chemotherapy. These include older age at treatment, lesser intelligence and education, anxiety and depression, fatigue, menopause, and prior hormonal therapy. Overall, the symptoms of cognitive dysfunction are often subtle and complex. They are related to memory, concentration, and executive functioning.[81] Such impairment can impact a survivor's ability to function normally, impeding the attainment of personal, professional, and general QOL goals.

Various interventions are being evaluated to reduce or prevent chemotherapy-induced cognitive decline. Pharmacological interventions (including psychostimulants, cholinesterase inhibitors, and gingko biloba) and cognitive rehabilitation may improve memory and concentration.[88] To guide the development of future interventions of this distressing symptom, the results of longitudinal studies are needed to provide greater understanding of the extent of cognitive deficits created by cancer and chemotherapy, the number of patients affected, and the factors that contribute.[89] Studies using neuroimaging techniques and animal models have begun to examine structural and functional correlates of cognitive changes associated with therapy.[81] The use of functional MRI may add a new dimension to pre- and posttreatment assessment in understanding the patterns of regional brain activation, and greater understanding of genetic factors may identify targets for agents that could prevent or reduce cognitive effects.[19,82] Future research hopefully will provide answers to the many questions about this pervasive problem in cancer survivors.

Psychological effects

Nearly all cancer patients experience some level of psychological distress, including depression, sadness, anxiety, fear, worry, anger, or panic.[19] For most individuals, distress remits during the first 24 months after diagnosis, and individuals experience few late or long-term psychological effects.[90] For some, however, the cancer experience triggers a psychological response that has a lasting impact, leading to poor adjustment and functional limitations extending across the survivorship trajectory.[91] Fortunately, efforts are growing nationally to include screening for emotional distress as the sixth vital sign so that these important issues can be identified and treated early as part of the growing emphasis on patient-centered care.

Psychological response to cancer is a function of two classes of variables: the stress and burden posed by the cancer experience and the resources available to cope with the stress and burden. The balance of these variables determines the psychological health of the cancer survivor in the short and long term.[91] Overall, certain factors can predict poor adjustment and functional limitations over time. These include such factors as receipt of chemotherapy, social isolation or conflict, expectancies for low level of control and negative outcomes, and avoidance of thoughts and feelings about cancer.[90] Protective factors that can be incorporated into interventions to treat anxiety include counseling survivors about having emotionally supportive relationships, using active coping strategies such as problem solving, positive reappraisal, and emotional expression.[90] It is important to note that many individuals extract positive meaning and benefit from their experience with cancer such as enhanced personal relationships, deepened appreciation for life, increased personal strength, greater spirituality, valued change in life priorities and goals, and greater attention to health-promoting behaviors.[92] Survivors also report that the positive and negative sequelae of cancer coexist.[93]

Assessment of long-term psychological effects in cancer survivors at follow-up visits is essential for implementation of effective interventions. Research shows that survivors who receive an intervention designed to improve function or well-being do better than those who do not.[10] The majority of interventions studied include the use of support groups, which have been shown to reduce distress, not only in patients but also in families. Physical activity can have positive effects on psychosocial measures, including depression, anxiety, self-esteem, and QOL.[94] In the last decade, long-term cancer survivors have higher rates of mental healthcare utilization than controls, but this usage of services and support group interventions may not address the real need.[95] Lack of insurance coverage is a factor limiting access and should be addressed locally for the individual and nationally as part of the Affordable Care Act implementation.

Depression

Estimates of the prevalence of depression in cancer survivors vary from 0% to 38% for major depression and 0% to 58% for depression spectrum syndromes.[96] Variability is attributable to multiple factors, including variations in cancer site, cancer treatment, age, disease, stage at diagnosis, and time from diagnosis and completion of treatment.[97] It is likely that many people affected by subclinical depression go undetected. Depression symptoms are more common in those with cancers of the head and neck, pancreas, lung, and breast and are less common in colon and gynecological cancers and lymphoma.[10] Depressive symptoms are reported in cancer survivors with unique concerns, such as loss of fertility and sexuality issues.[98,99]

Posttraumatic stress disorder can be a debilitating effect of cancer and the majority of studies suggest a prevalence of PTSD in the range of 5% to 15%, which exceeds the prevalence in the general population.[100] Symptoms include cognitive avoidance, emotional reactivity, hypervigilance, sleep disruption, difficulty concentrating, intrusive thoughts related to cancer and treatment, fear of recurrence, and physical reactions such as heart palpitations or nausea.[93] Risk factors for the development and severity of depression and PTSD are reported as persistent physical problems; poor psychosocial or familial adjustment to cancer; avoidant coping style; lower socioeconomic status, educational, or financial resource level; younger age at diagnosis; female gender; poor premorbid physical and mental health; prior traumas or a current or prior negative stressful event; inadequate social support; cancer stage and type; and treatment severity.[10] Although many patients do not meet the full criteria for cancer-related depression and PTSD, subclinical syndromes are not uncommon.[93] A recent study of adult survivors of childhood cancers found that those with physical health problems are at risk for suicidal ideation (SI). Of survivors, 7.8% reported SI compared to 4.6% of controls. Because both depression and PTSD are treatable problems, it is critical to assess individuals with symptoms and those who are at risk as part of routine survivorship care. To address these important conditions, the NCCN has developed guidelines for the screening and treatment of depression as part of their Survivorship Guidelines.[101]

Anxiety

Like other psychological effects of cancer, anxiety is not disabling in the majority of cancer survivors. However, recent publications suggest that after a diagnosis of cancer, increased rates of anxiety tend to persist compared with healthy controls, whereas increased rates of depression are less long-lasting.[102] Thus, these findings suggest that anxiety, rather than depression, is likely to be the most common psychological problem in long-term cancer survivors. Most cancer survivors experience anxiety over the possibility of a cancer recurrence. Anxiety related to posttreatment surveillance visits and testing is commonly reported. Although fear of recurrence is normal after cancer treatment, fear that is severe and persistent can significantly impact QOL and diminish everyday functioning.[96] Anxious individuals experience and report more symptoms related to their cancer than others. They monitor their bodies for symptoms of relapse and may use maladaptive patterns of reassurance-seeking as a coping mechanism, which can perpetuate anxiety. Possible predictors of anxiety after cancer include poor social support, impaired quality of life, pain, and burden of disease.[103,104] However, until recently, screening for anxiety has been overlooked compared with screening for distress and depression, but in 2013, NCCN developed and published screening and treatment guidelines for anxiety.[101]

An in-depth discussion on anxiety and depression can be found in chapter 20.

Case study

Surviving is not survivorship: the future contribution of palliative care

Michael is a 49-year-old man who was diagnosed with stage 3 colon cancer 8 years ago. His treatment included chemotherapy and radiation therapy followed by an extensive surgical resection. Since treatment completion Michael has experienced mild-moderate peripheral neuropathy. A regimen of antineuropathic medication along with physical therapy have significantly improved his pain and enabled him to function without any significant limitations. Approximately 3 years ago Michael began noticing changes in his bowel habits including increased flatus and constipation followed by diarrhea. As a salesperson spending 2–3 weeks per month traveling, these symptoms created considerable stress and anxiety for Michael. The survivorship nurse practitioner advised Michael on diet modification including increased fiber intake. Michael followed these instructions and was relieved to note an improvement in his bowel regularity and consistency. One year ago at his follow-up visit Michael described new onset of bowel incontinence, which again triggered feelings of anxiety and embarrassment, causing him to refrain from many social activities and even curtail his work travel. He stated "I want to be able to go to meetings and go out in the community with my family and friends without worrying about accidents." The survivorship nurse practitioner referred him to physical therapy, where a program was designed to address Michael's pelvic floor dysfunction. She also referred him for counseling to address his anxiety, with the goal of improving his coping ability during symptomatic episodes as well as better long-term stress and anxiety management. The prescribed physical therapy improved his bowel control and enabled him to return to his usual professional and personal activities. Counseling has also helped Michael identify and manage stress more effectively, allowing him to feel greater control and quality of life.

As one can see from this case study, the challenges for cancer survivors as they become a greater and larger force in the American population are many. First is the education of healthcare providers—particularly nurses—about the medical, psychological, social, and spiritual problems facing cancer survivors. Second is the development of communication tools to be shared between the survivor and healthcare professionals outlining these potential problems, along with plans for follow-up care. Third is greater professional education and training about how to conduct a careful assessment to identify these long-term and late effects of treatment. Fourth, survivors should receive aggressive palliative care interventions for their symptoms. Finally, there should be greater public discussion and debate about how best to employ and provide insurance reimbursement for the comprehensive approach used by palliative care experts to individuals living with and beyond their cancer.

References

1. Hewitt M, Greenfield S, Stovall E. From Cancer Patient to Cancer Survivor: Lost in Transition. Washington, DC: Institute of Medicine and National Research Council of the National Academies; 2006.
2. McCabe MS, Bhatia S, Oeffinger KC, et al. American Society of Clinical Oncology statement: achieving high-quality cancer survivorship care. J Clin Oncol. 2013;31(5):631–640.
3. Lewis R, Neal RD, Williams NH, et al. Nurse-led vs. conventional physician-led follow-up for patients with cancer: systematic review. J Adv Nursing. 2009;65(4):706–723.
4. Campbell MK, Tessaro I, Gellin M, et al. Adult cancer survivorship care: experiences from the LIVESTRONG centers of excellence network. J Cancer Surviv. 2011;5(3):271–282.
5. Pollack CE, Platz EA, Bhavsar NA, et al. Primary care providers' perspectives on discontinuing prostate cancer screening. Cancer. 2012;118(22):5518–5524.
6. McCabe MS, Jacobs LA. Clinical update: survivorship care—models and programs. Semin Oncol Nurs. 2012;28(3):e1–e8.
7. Oeffinger KC, McCabe MS. Models for delivering survivorship care. J Clin Oncol. 2006;24(32):5117–5124.
8. Howell D, Hack TF, Oliver TK, et al. Models of care for post-treatment follow-up of adult cancer survivors: a systematic review and quality appraisal of the evidence. J Cancer Surviv. 2012;6(4):359–371.
9. Ferrell BR, Coyle N. For every nurse–a palliative care nurse. In: Ferrell BR, Coyle N (eds.), Textbook of Palliative Nursing. New York: Oxford University Press; 2013:IX.
10. Alfano CM, Rowland JH. Recovery issues in cancer survivorship: a new challenge for supportive care. Cancer J. 2006;12(5):432–443.
11. Hudson MM, Ness KK, Gurney JG, et al. Clinical ascertainment of health outcomes among adults treated for childhood cancer. JAMA. 2013;309(22):2371–2381.
12. President's Cancer Panel. Living Beyond Cancer: Finding a New Balance. Bethesda, MD: National Cancer Institute; 2004.
13. Aziz NM, Rowland JH. Trends and advances in cancer survivorship research: challenge and opportunity. Semin Radiation Oncol. 2003;13(3):248–266.
14. Siegel R, DeSantis C, Virgo K, et al. Cancer treatment and survivorship statistics, 2012. Cancer. 2012;62(4):220–241.
15. Miller KD, Triano LR. Medical issues in cancer survivors: a review. Cancer J. 2008;14(6):375–387.
16. Rowland JH. Cancer survivorship: rethinking the cancer control continuum. Semin Oncol Nurs. 2008;24(3):145–152.
17. Green CR, Hart-Johnson T, Loeffler DR. Cancer-related chronic pain: examining quality of life in diverse cancer survivors. Cancer. 2011;117(9):1994–2003.
18. Grov EK, Fossa SD, Dahl AA. Short-term and long-term elderly cancer survivors: a population-based comparative and controlled study of morbidity, psychosocial situation, and lifestyle. Eur J Nur Oncol. 2011;15(3):213–220.
19. Andrykowski MA, Lykins E, Floyd A. Psychological health in cancer survivors. Semin Oncol Nurs. 2008;24(3):193–201.
20. Armes J, Crowe M, Colbourne L, et al. Patients' supportive care needs beyond the end of cancer treatment: a prospective, longitudinal survey. J Clin Oncol. 2009;27(36):6172–6179.
21. Meyerowitz BE, Oh S. Psychosocial response to cancer diagnosis and treatment. In: Miller SM, Bowen DJ, Croyle RT (eds.), Handbook of Behavioral Science and Cancer. Washington, DC: American Psychological Association; 2008:110–128.
22. Dalton SO, Laursen TM, Ross L, Mortensen PB, Johansen C. Risk for hospitalization with depression after a cancer diagnosis: a nationwide, population-based study of cancer patients in Denmark from 1973 to 2003. J Clin Oncol. 2009;27(9):1440–1445.
23. Recklitis CJ, Diller LR, Li X, Najita J, Robison LL, Zeltzer L. Suicide ideation in adult survivors of childhood cancer: a report from the Childhood Cancer Survivor Study. J Clin Oncol. 2010;28(4):655–661.
24. Howlander N, Noone AM, Krapcho M, et al., eds. SEER Cancer Statistics Review, 1975–2010. Bethesda, MD: National Cancer

Institute. http://seer.cancer.gov/csr/1975_2010. Based on November 2012 SEER data submission, posted to the SEER website, April 2013.

25. Oeffinger KC, Mertens AC, Sklar CA, et al. Chronic health conditions in adult survivors of childhood cancer. N Engl J Med. 2006;355(15): 1572–1582.

26. Sun CL, Francisco L, Kawashima T, et al. Prevalence and predictors of chronic health conditions after hematopoietic cell transplantation: a report from the Bone Marrow Transplant Survivor Study. Blood. 2010;116(17):3129–3139; quiz 3377.

27. Mertens AC, Yasui Y, Neglia JP, et al. Late mortality experience in five-year survivors of childhood and adolescent cancer: the Childhood Cancer Survivor Study. J Clin Oncol. 2001;19(13):3163–3172.

28. Freyer DR. Transition of care for young adult survivors of childhood and adolescent cancer: rationale and approaches. J Clin Oncol. 2010;28(32):4810–4818.

29. Casillas J, Kahn KL, Doose M, et al. Transitioning childhood cancer survivors to adult centered healthcare: insights from parents, adolescent, and young adult survivors. Psychooncology. 2010;19(9):982–990.

30. Oeffinger KC, Mertens AC, Hudson MM, et al. Health care of young adult survivors of childhood cancer: a report from the Childhood Cancer Survivor Study. Ann Fam Med. 2004;2(1):61–70.

31. Children's Oncology Group Long-Term Follow-Up Guidelines for Survivors of Childhood, Adolescent, and Young Adult Cancers. Available at: http://www.survivorshipguidelines.org. Accessed February 18, 2009.

32. Appelbaum FR. Hematopoietic-cell transplantation at 50. N Engl J Med. 2007;357(15):1472–1475.

33. Joseph RW, Couriel DR, Komanduri KV. Chronic graft-versus-host disease after allogeneic stem cell transplantation: challenges in prevention, science, and supportive care. J Support Oncol. 2008;6(8):361–372.

34. Bhatia S, Francisco L, Carter A, et al. Late mortality after allogeneic hematopoietic cell transplantation and functional status of long-term survivors: report from the Bone Marrow Transplant Survivor Study. Blood. Nov 15 2007;110(10):3784–3792.

35. Pidala J, Anasetti C, Kharfan-Dabaja MA, Cutler C, Sheldon A, Djulbegovic B. Decision analysis of peripheral blood versus bone marrow hematopoietic stem cells for allogeneic hematopoietic cell transplantation. Biol Blood Marrow Transplant. 2009;15(11):1415–1421.

36. Sun C-L, Kersey JH, Francisco L, et al. Burden of morbidity in 10+ year survivors of hematopoietic cell transplantation: report from the bone marrow transplantation survivor study. Biol Blood Marrow Transplant. 2013;19(7):1073–1080.

37. Cooke L, Gemmill R, Kravits K, Grant M. Psychological issues of stem cell transplant. Semin Oncol Nurs. 2009;25(2):139–150.

38. Reddy P, Arora M, Guimond M, Mackall CL. GVHD: a continuing barrier to the safety of allogeneic transplantation. Biol Blood Marrow Transplant. 2009;15(1 Suppl):162–168.

39. Couriel D, Carpenter PA, Cutler C, et al. Ancillary therapy and supportive care of chronic graft-versus-host disease: national institutes of health consensus development project on criteria for clinical trials in chronic graft-versus-host disease: V. Ancillary Therapy and Supportive Care Working Group Report. Biol Blood Marrow Transplant. 2006;12(4):375–396.

40. Vincent GK, Velkoff VA. 2010. The Next Four Decades: The Older Population in the United States: 2010 to 2050. Population Estimates and Projections. http://www.census.gov/prod/2010pubs/p25-1138.pdf. Accessed June 21, 2013.

41. Becker H, Jung S. Health promotion among older cancer survivors with prior disabling conditions. J Gerontol Nurs. 2012;38(7):38–43.

42. Bellury LM, Ellington L, Beck SL, Stein K, Pett M, Clark J. Elderly cancer survivorship: an integrative review and conceptual framework. Eur J Nur Oncol. 2011;15(3):233–242.

43. Freeman HP. Poverty, culture, and social injustice: determinants of cancer disparities. Cancer. 2004;54(2):72–77.

44. Holm LV, Hansen DG, Larsen PV, et al. Social inequality in cancer rehabilitation: a population-based cohort study. Acta Oncol. 2013;52(2):410–422.

45. Fu MR, Rosedale M. Breast cancer survivors' experiences of lymphedema-related symptoms. J Pain Symptom Manage. 2009;38(6):849–859.

46. Ell K, Xie B, Wells A, Nedjat-Haiem F, Lee P-J, Vourlekis B. Economic stress among low-income women with cancer: effects on quality of life. Cancer. 2008;112(3):616–625.

47. Andrykowski MA, Donovan KA, Laronga C, Jacobsen PB. Prevalence, predictors, and characteristics of off-treatment fatigue in breast cancer survivors. Cancer. 2010;116(24):5740–5748.

48. Mitchell AJ, Baker-Glenn EA, Granger L, Symonds P. Can the Distress Thermometer be improved by additional mood domains? Part I. Initial validation of the Emotion Thermometers tool. Psychooncology. 2010;19(2):125–133.

49. Cancer-Related Fatigue: Interventions for Patients on Long-Term Follow-Up. V.1.2013 National Comprehensive Cancer Network, Practice Guidelines in Oncology. Available at: http://www.nccn.org/professionals/physician_gls/PDF/survivorship.pdf. Accessed June 23, 2013.

50. Hung R, Krebs P, Coups EJ, et al. Fatigue and functional impairment in early-stage non-small cell lung cancer survivors. J Pain Symptom Manage. 2011;41(2):426–435.

51. Goedendorp MM, Andrykowski MA, Donovan KA, et al. Prolonged impact of chemotherapy on fatigue in breast cancer survivors: a longitudinal comparison with radiotherapy-treated breast cancer survivors and noncancer controls. Cancer. 2012;118(15):3833–3841.

52. Banthia R, Malcarne VL, Ko CM, Varni JW, Sadler GR. Fatigued breast cancer survivors: the role of sleep quality, depressed mood, stage and age. Psychol Health. 2009;24(8):965–980.

53. Cavalli Kluthcovsky ACG, Urbanetz AA, de Carvalho DS, Pereira Maluf EMC, Schlickmann Sylvestre GC, Bonatto Hatschbach SB. Fatigue after treatment in breast cancer survivors: prevalence, determinants and impact on health-related quality of life. Supportive Care Cancer. 2012;20(8):1901–1909.

54. Cella D, Davis K, Breitbart W, Curt G, Fatigue C. Cancer-related fatigue: prevalence of proposed diagnostic criteria in a United States sample of cancer survivors. J Clin Oncol. 2001;19(14):3385–3391.

55. Minton O, Stone P. How common is fatigue in disease-free breast cancer survivors?: A systematic review of the literature. Breast Cancer Res Treat. 2008;112(1):5–13.

56. Daniels LA, Oerlemans S, Krol ADG, van de Poll-Franse LV, Creutzberg CL. Persisting fatigue in Hodgkin lymphoma survivors: a systematic review. Ann Hematol. 2013;92(8):1023–1032.

57. Levy MH, Chwistek M, Mehta RS. Management of chronic pain in cancer survivors. Cancer J. 2008;14(6):401–409.

58. Sun V, Borneman T, Piper B, Koczywas M, Ferrell B. Barriers to pain assessment and management in cancer survivorship. J Cancer Surviv. 2008;2(1):65–71.

59. Lu Q, Krull KR, Leisenring W, et al. Pain in long-term adult survivors of childhood cancers and their siblings: a report from the Childhood Cancer Survivor Study. Pain. 2011;152(11):2616–2624.

60. Paice JA. Chronic treatment-related pain in cancer survivors. Pain. 2011;152(3 Suppl):S84–S89.

61. Boland B, Sherry V, Polomano R. Chemotherapy-induced peripheral neuropathy in cancer survivors. Oncology. 2010;24(2):33.

62. Nurgalieva Z, Xia R, Liu C-C, Burau K, Hardy D, Du XL. Risk of chemotherapy-induced peripheral neuropathy in large population-based cohorts of elderly patients with breast, ovarian, and lung cancer. Am J Ther. 2010;17(2):148–158.

63. McNeer JL, Nachman JB. The optimal use of steroids in paediatric acute lymphoblastic leukaemia: no easy answers. Brit J Haematol. 2010;149(5):638–652.

64. Mattano LA, Jr., Sather HN, Trigg ME, Nachman JB. Osteonecrosis as a complication of treating acute lymphoblastic leukemia in children: a report from the Children's Cancer Group. J Clin Oncol. 2000;18(18):3262–3272.

65. Burton AW, Fanciullo GJ, Beasley RD, Fisch MJ. Chronic pain in the cancer survivor: a new frontier. Pain Med. 2007;8(2):189–198.

66. Olsen NK, Pfeiffer P, Johannsen L, Schroder H, Rose C. Radiation-induced brachial plexopathy: neurological follow-up in 161 recurrence-free breast cancer patients. Int J Radiat Oncol Biol Phys. 1993;26(1):43–49.

67. Smith J, Thompson JM. Phantom limb pain and chemotherapy in pediatric amputees. Mayo Clinic Proc. 1995;70(4):357–364.

68. Borsje S, Bosmans JC, van der Schans CP, Geertzen JH, Dijkstra PU. Phantom pain: a sensitivity analysis. Disabil Rehabil. 2004;26(14-15):905–910.

69. Perttunen K, Tasmuth T, Kalso E. Chronic pain after thoracic surgery: a follow-up study. Acta Anaesthesiol Scand. 1999;43(5):563–567.

70. Dajczman E, Gordon A, Kreisman H, Wolkove N. Long-term post-thoracotomy pain. Chest. 1991;99(2):270–274.

71. Tasmuth T, Kataja M, Blomqvist C, von Smitten K, Kalso E. Treatment-related factors predisposing to chronic pain in patients with breast cancer--a multivariate approach. Acta Oncol. 1997;36(6):625–630.

72. Wallace MS, Wallace AM, Lee J, Dobke MK. Pain after breast surgery: a survey of 282 women. Pain. 1996;66(2-3):195–205.

73. Savard J, Morin CM. Insomnia in the context of cancer: a review of a neglected problem. J Clin Oncol. 2001;19(3):895–908.

74. Mulrooney DA, Ness KK, Neglia JP, et al. Fatigue and sleep disturbance in adult survivors of childhood cancer: a report from the childhood cancer survivor study (CCSS). Sleep. 2008;31(2):271–281.

75. Fleming L, Gillespie S, Espie CA. The development and impact of insomnia on cancer survivors: a qualitative analysis. Psychooncology. 2010;19(9):991–996.

76. Sharma N, Hansen CH, O'Connor M, et al. Sleep problems in cancer patients: prevalence and association with distress and pain. Psychooncology. 2012;21(9):1003–1009.

77. Clanton NR, Klosky JL, Li C, et al. Fatigue, vitality, sleep, and neurocognitive functioning in adult survivors of childhood Cancer: a report from the childhood cancer survivor study. Cancer. 2011;117(11):2559–2568.

78. Davidson JR, MacLean AW, Brundage MD, Schulze K. Sleep disturbance in cancer patients. Soc Sci Med. 2002;54(9):1309–1321.

79. Servaes P, van der Werf S, Prins J, Verhagen S, Bleijenberg G. Fatigue in disease-free cancer patients compared with fatigue in patients with chronic fatigue syndrome. Support Care Cancer. 2001;9(1):11–17.

80. Hoyt MA, Thomas KS, Epstein DR, Dirksen SR. Coping style and sleep quality in men with cancer. Ann Behav Med. 2009;37(1):88–93.

81. Vardy J, Wefel JS, Ahles T, Tannock IF, Schagen SB. Cancer and cancer-therapy related cognitive dysfunction: an international perspective from the Venice cognitive workshop. Ann Oncol. 2008;19(4):623–629.

82. Correa DD, Ahles TA. Neurocognitive changes in cancer survivors. Cancer J. 2008;14(6):396–400.

83. Ganz PA. Cognitive dysfunction following adjuvant treatment of breast cancer: a new dose-limiting toxic effect? J Natl Cancer Inst. 1998;90(3):182–183.

84. Wefel JS, Witgert ME, Meyers CA. Neuropsychological sequelae of non-central nervous system cancer and cancer therapy. Neuropsychol Rev. 2008;18(2):121–131.

85. Koppelmans V, Breteler MM, Boogerd W, Seynaeve C, Gundy C, Schagen SB. Neuropsychological performance in survivors of breast cancer more than 20 years after adjuvant chemotherapy. J Clin Oncol. 2012;30(10):1080–1086.

86. Syrjala KL, Stover AC, Yi JC, et al. Development and implementation of an Internet-based survivorship care program for cancer survivors treated with hematopoietic stem cell transplantation. J Cancer Surviv. 2011;5(3):292–304.

87. Kirchhoff AC, Krull KR, Ness KK, et al. Physical, mental, and neurocognitive status and employment outcomes in the childhood cancer survivor study cohort. Cancer Epidemiol Biomarkers Prev. 2011;20(9):1838–1849.

88. Ferguson RJ, Ahles TA, Saykin AJ, et al. Cognitive-behavioral management of chemotherapy-related cognitive change. Psychooncology. 2007;16(8):772–777.

89. Ahles TA, Saykin AJ. Candidate mechanisms for chemotherapy-induced cognitive changes. Nat Rev Cancer. 2007;7(3):192–201.

90. Stanton AL. Psychosocial concerns and interventions for cancer survivors. J Clin Oncol. 2006;24(32):5132–5137.

91. Stein KD, Syrjala KL, Andrykowski MA. Physical and psychological long-term and late effects of cancer. Cancer. 2008;112(11 Suppl.):2577–2592.

92. Stanton AL, Bower JE, Low CA. Posttraumatic growth after cancer. In: Calhoun LG, Tedeschi RG (eds.), Handbook of Posttraumatic Growth: Research and Practice. Mahwah, NJ: Erlbaum; 2006:138–175.

93. Cordova MJ, Andrykowski MA. Responses to cancer diagnosis and treatment: posttraumatic stress and posttraumatic growth. Semin Clin Neuropsychiatry. 2003;8(4):286–296.

94. Schwartz AL. Physical activity after a cancer diagnosis: psychosocial outcomes. Cancer Invest. 2004;22(1):82–92.

95. Earle CC. Cancer survivorship research and guidelines: maybe the cart should be beside the horse. J Clin Oncol. 2007;25(25):3800–3801.

96. Massie MJ. Prevalence of depression in patients with cancer. J Natl Cancer Inst Monographs. 2004(32):57–71.

97. Pasquini M, Biondi M. Depression in cancer patients: a critical review. Clin Pract Epidemiol Ment Health. 2007;3:2.

98. Gorman JR, Malcarne VL, Roesch SC, Madlensky L, Pierce JP. Depressive symptoms among young breast cancer survivors: the importance of reproductive concerns. Breast Cancer Res Treat. 2010;123(2):477–485.

99. Mosher CE, DuHamel KN, Rini C, Corner G, Lam J, Redd WH. Quality of life concerns and depression among hematopoietic stem cell transplant survivors. Support Care Cancer. 2011;19(9): 1357–1365.

100. Kangas M, Henry JL, Bryant RA. Posttraumatic stress disorder following cancer: a conceptual and empirical review. Clin Psychol Rev. 2002;22(4):499–524.

101. Anxiety and Depression. V.1.2013 National Comprehensive Cancer Network, Practice Guidelines in Oncology. Available at: http://www.nccn.org/professionals/physician_gls/PDF/survivorship.pdf. Accessed June 23, 2013.

102. Mitchell AJ, Ferguson DW, Gill J, Paul J, Symonds P. Depression and anxiety in long-term cancer survivors compared with spouses and healthy controls: a systematic review and meta-analysis. Lancet Oncol. 2013;14(8):721–732.

103. Hill J, Holcombe C, Clark L, et al. Predictors of onset of depression and anxiety in the year after diagnosis of breast cancer. Psychol Med. 2011;41(7):1429–1436.

104. Mehnert A, Berg P, Henrich G, Herschbach P. Fear of cancer progression and cancer-related intrusive cognitions in breast cancer survivors. Psychooncology. 2009;18(12):1273–1280.

CHAPTER 43

Veterans

Deborah Grassman

Hoping and wishing you can settle this whole thing in your mind about this war resolving it within yourself before the time of atonement comes, weeping and crying at the end of your life.[1]

A population with unique hospice and palliative care needs: Veterans

In many ways, veterans face the end of life in a similar manner to civilians. In some ways, however, they experience death differently. This chapter identifies some of these differences in the hopes that readers will come to understand the unique hospice needs of veterans and their families. For example, the value of stoicism so earnestly and necessarily indoctrinated in young soldiers, may interfere with a peaceful death for veterans, depending on the degree to which stoicism had permeated their later lives.

Key points

◆ Veterans who served in dangerous duty assignments may have their deaths complicated by traumatic memories or paralyzing guilt, depending on the extent to which they were able to integrate and heal traumatic or guilt-inducing memories. This sometimes manifests as agitation at the end of life;

◆ A high incidence of alcohol abuse or other "flighting"-type behaviors are often used either to avoid confronting locked-up feelings or to numb traumatic memories.[2] These factors may contribute to "unfinished business" as veterans face the end of their lives;

◆ Veterans often acquire wisdom because they have reckoned with trauma, stoicism, and addictions. Understanding these three elements helps access their wisdom and has been referred to as "post-traumatic growth."[3]

◆ Veterans and their families have unique bereavement needs to consider when providing care.

Vantage point: Veteran Inpatient Hospice Unit

Military experiences often change veterans in fundamental ways that shape, mold, destroy, and redeem the rest of their lives, including the end of their lives. The following excerpt provides an overview of patients cared for by the author, a nurse practitioner on a hospice unit at a Veterans Affairs (VA) medical center.

It allows the reader a bird's-eye view into the unique and not-so-unique needs of veterans at the end of life:

> To help you imagine my everyday world, let me tell you the stories of the nine patients on the Hospice and Palliative Care unit at the time of this writing. Then, you can understand the context from which the lessons that you are going to read are derived. You will also understand the privilege that it is to care for veterans.
>
> Mark is dying of liver failure from alcohol abuse, his skin yellow as a low-glowing lamp. He came to the Hospice and Palliative Care unit semicomatose; we will not get to know him except through his brother's eyes. I comment on his brother's devotion. The brother responds, "I look at Mark and know why I'm in Alcoholic's Anonymous."
>
> Donnie is 50 years old and has lung cancer. He has been a quadriplegic since he was 27, when an automobile accident detoured his career as a professional football player. "I spent three years in despair. Then I found God and salvation," he tells me. He says he is thankful for his suffering: "I never would have found Jesus if the accident hadn't happened."
>
> In the next room, an embittered, lonely man sits sullenly. Alcohol has estranged Zachary from his family. At 82, he is angry at his body for failing him. He has been afraid of death since he was 10 years old, when a neighbor died falling through a skylight on his roof. Bitterly, he tells me, "My only solace is knowing that someday all the rest of you are going to be in this bed too." A gathering of team members provided a turning point as he experiences the concern of four staff who were willing to love him. "Why aren't we talking about my breathing, and the 16 pills I'm taking?" Zachary asks us. "Because you are more than just your breathing, and we are more than just pill-givers" I reply, leaning in and daring to touch him tenderly. A tear comes; features soften for the first time. "I can't argue with that," he says quietly.
>
> In the room next to Zachary is Marvin. He was a photographer to a general in World War II. He has been a physician, sailboat racer, and builder of piers, driveways, and roofs "made with my own hands." Marvin's wife and four children sit at his bedside supporting his journey into the next world and supporting each other. Near death, he says little except the Lord's Prayer. There is no need for us to intervene with anything other than supportive care.
>
> In the adjoining bed is Jim, a Vietnam War veteran who has lived a colorful life. He is intermittently confused; sometimes he is argumentative. He has no family; a few close friends are his source of comfort. His first days on the unit were filled with agitation. He was convinced the Vietcong had put a bomb in the stereo. Nurse Suzanne responded creatively. She called the security officer and said, "I want you to inspect the stereo and declare it bomb-proof. Tell the patient

you're pulling guard so you've got his back and the perimeter is safe. Let him know that another guard will be on patrol when you leave duty." The police officer responded convincingly, and Jim's agitation subsided.

Then there's Bruce, a 67-year-old man who came for pain control. He had not wanted to come to the Hospice unit "because I'm afraid I'll never get out." His early days of anxiety and impatience were manifested with frequent summons on the call light. Probably because he realizes he is in a safe, loving environment his spirit is now emerging bright and full. He simply needed a little time and a little love to know that he need not fear. He has grown closer to his family as he approaches death and tells us, "I wouldn't trade these last few weeks in my life for anything."

His roommate, Richard, suffers respiratory distress from a tumor encroaching on his trachea. He awaits his daughter's arrival from Indiana tomorrow. He says his suffering will be redeemed when he can rejoin his wife who died 2 years ago. "That will be a happy day," he says with tears. We share his anticipated joy.

Ben has a history of drug use and actively continues with alcohol abuse. He identifies himself as a loner who has witnessed much violence. "My family doesn't care about me," he told me. We've had some difficult sessions confronting his suffering. He's going to be discharged next week. I do not know what is going to happen with him. What I *can* tell you is that his brow unfurls after prayer, he plans to go to Alcoholic Anonymous meetings, and he wants to reach out to a faith community. Seeds planted and good intentions—they are not enough to withstand the ravages of alcohol. His suffering's redemption awaits a courageous decision that only he can make every day for the rest of his life.

The last patient, Edwin, has severe COPD and is ready to die but he worries about his wife of 54 years. His needs are increasing rapidly but he does not acknowledge them because he does not want to worry her. "I can't hold on much longer though," Edwin says while making plans to hold on for his wife's sake. We talk about the advantage of letting go so he can prepare himself and his wife for his death; we talk about the damage his denial is causing them both. Edwin cries; his grieving begins.[4]

Military tenets that facilitate healthcare provider understanding

There are 1800 veterans dying every day in America—that represents about 25% of all dying Americans. Only 4% of these veterans die within the VA medical system. Many of the remaining 96% receive end-of-life care in community hospice programs.[5] Hopefully, many of these community hospice providers have the requisite information about veterans to provide that care.

Stoicism: early indoctrination that continues at the end of life

Veterans are often noncomplaining, "grin-and-bear-it" types who endure their sufferings silently. The few times tears or fears break through their stoic facades, they feel embarrassed, apologize, and quickly re-retreat; these walls offer protection. Unfortunately, their "fight to the bitter end" attitudes sometimes mean just that—fighting until a death that is, indeed, bitter. Their "attack and defend" instincts make death the enemy and dying a battle. Survival-mode mentality interferes with letting go. When backed into a corner, soldiers are not conditioned to surrender; they are conditioned to fight.

Breaching facades can be important because these walls of stoicism might contribute to agitation and lack of peace as veterans die. It is important that clinicians know how to create safe emotional environments to breach stoic facades. Otherwise, dying veterans will underreport their physical and emotional pain as well as any fear they are experiencing.

Stoicism is necessary on the battlefield, as it is in many life situations, but the walls that stoicism erects can outlast its usefulness. The walls keep out necessary feelings—and other people. Although it is important to respect veterans' silence when they choose to maintain stoic fronts, it is also important to offer alternatives. Helping veterans use stoicism like a door instead of a wall can be useful. A door can be opened or closed at will and as often as they want, leaving the safety of their stoicism available to them.

Stoicism might be conceptualized as comprising three components: pride, control, and independence. Anything threatening pride, control, or independence can incite anger and defensive fight/flight responses. Dying is a humbling experience that challenges all of these. Control is lost, pride takes a blow, and independence is gradually taken away. Sooner or later, the wall has to crumble. Later means fighting to the bitter end; sooner means a weary soldier is finally able to surrender to hope for a peaceful death.

An inability to let go of pride, control, and independence so that a veteran can reach out for help increases suffering. Physical limitations and emotional displays can embarrass veterans and create fears that others will perceive them as weak. They might feel helpless and vulnerable to attack. Letting go might be viewed as admitting defeat or an act of surrender—something good soldiers do not do. Yet, mature mental health includes identifying needs and asking for help when it is needed. Both require vulnerability. Stoicism often keeps people from saying what they need or allowing others to meet their needs. This mask of invulnerability sometimes will not even allow them to admit they *have* needs. This can cause frustration for family members and professional caregivers who desperately want to do whatever they can to help.

Many dying veterans are able to let go of control, allowing themselves to become completely human, growing in humility as they learn how to ask for help and how to become a gracious receiver, discovering connection and compassion in the process. This takes courage and it is as heroic as facing any enemy in battle.

The culture of combat

Embedded within the stoic, military culture is another culture: the culture of war.[6] Although a few soldiers were motivated for self-glorification and promotion in combat zones, most were motivated for different reasons. They did not fight for themselves; they were selflessly motivated to fight for a *cause* and to fight for *comrades*. They were willing to lay down their lives for each other. Many exhibited extraordinary acts of bravery to preserve their buddies' survival or accomplish an important mission. Many effects, however, were not good. Soldiers sustained emotional, mental, social, spiritual, and moral injuries that sometimes caused a lifetime of suffering. This suffering might be kept submerged in unconsciousness, but at the time of death, wartime memories sometimes emerge unbidden.

Combat culture is not universal. Each war was different. Each had its own culture that exerted a different influence on young soldiers. World War II was enthusiastically supported by Americans. Some veterans joined the military when they were as young as 14, lying about their ages so they could fight.

Virtually everyone sought a way to support the war effort. People grew "victory gardens" and the Red Cross sent pictures of the gardens to the soldiers so they could see their country's support. Women worked in munitions factories while others stayed home and made clothing for the soldiers. No one was left untouched.

Without televisions, the public could be shielded from war's brutality. War could be glamorized, which increased its appeal and fostered national unity. The mission of World War II enhanced this unity; it was clear and largely undisputed—especially after Pearl Harbor. The soldiers knew they were in the war for its duration. This fostered cohesion and a determination to get the mission accomplished—a "we're in this together until the job gets done" attitude. When the war was over, troops came home *together*. They were greeted as heroes by a public eager to hear their victorious wartime stories.[7]

While the adulation was gratifying, the soldiers needed more from their friends, families, and the media. They had been through horrors they could not have imagined; they had done things they never thought they would do. They needed the approval they were getting, but they also needed to give voice to the traumas they had suffered. The awaiting public, however, only wanted to hear about acts of bravery and heroism, not of trauma and moral confusion. The soldiers themselves often downplayed their acts of courage: "The *real* heroes were those that didn't come home" or "I was just doing my duty." This kind of reticence was sometimes taken for modesty, but some veterans say that it was not modesty. They did not feel like heroes because they knew the ugly, despairing, or cowardly acts of war: "If you knew what I did, you wouldn't think I was so heroic." These stories often remained untold, lurking in the veterans' consciousness; they often hid guilt and shame.

The Korean War was different. Korean War veterans are often more tight-lipped. Known later as the "Forgotten War," it was never an officially declared war; rather, it was called a "Conflict" or "Police Action." There were no ticker tape parades for these returning soldiers; this time was the happy 1950s and people wanted to forget about war and focus on growing prosperity. Korean War soldiers' trauma had been minimized or neglected and their combat contributions sometimes forgotten.[8]

If Korea taught the American public how to ignore soldiers, Vietnam taught the public how to shame and dishonor them. There was extensive television coverage from Vietnam. Americans now understood the brutality of war, and many were at odds with its politics. Protests were organized across college campuses.

Many young men had mixed feelings about the Vietnam War, and some opposed it. The draft forced these and others into military service and then into combat. Also, imposed beliefs from fathers who were World War II veterans sometimes prompted unwilling sons to volunteer for Vietnam. For others, sons sought the hero status their World War II fathers had held in the family (and usually came back disappointed).

These soldiers often became more cynical by their experience in Vietnam, and their cynicism affected the soldiers who believed the war was necessary. This prevailing mood is depicted by a caption on a painting by Dale Samuelson in the National Vietnam Veterans Art Museum in Chicago. It reflects the bitterness that corrodes the souls of some veterans. It reads:

We the willing

Led by the unknowing

Do the necessary

For the ungrateful

In addition to political influences, there were pragmatic factors. Although they could volunteer for more, soldiers were required to do only 1-year tours in Vietnam. Rather than the "we're in this together until we get the job done" attitude of World War II soldiers, they tended to think in terms of "rotating through until my tour's up." Reports of antiwar protests at home shook their confidence in the war as well.[7]

War tactics also varied in different wars. Before Vietnam, there was a certain level of safety "behind the lines" (if there can be any safety in a war), which allowed a small degree of mental and emotional recuperation between battles. In Vietnam, however, it was guerrilla warfare; there was no safe place to let defenses down; there were no "front lines" to fight behind. The enemy easily infiltrated, making it difficult for soldiers to distinguish friend from foe. Soldiers were on guard even in their sleep. Explosives were sometimes hidden on dead bodies, blowing up when soldiers came to retrieve them. Commonly, soldiers would carry food so they could give it to village children; but this could be used against them. Sometimes, the children were booby-trapped to explode while in the soldiers' midst!

As important as any of the military factors was how the nonmilitary public treated Vietnam veterans. Unlike World War II veterans, these men and women were *not* welcomed as heroes. Often they were not welcomed home at all. Antiwar protests had grown, and people who had advocated bringing the soldiers home now turned their anger against the soldiers themselves. They greeted returning soldiers at the airports by spitting on them and shouting "baby killers" or "murderers." As a result, soldiers often hid their history about Vietnam.

The public did not want to hear about Vietnam. As a result, soldiers' stories had nowhere to go. They could not even talk with each other much of the time. Unlike World War II soldiers who often came home in boats or trains that gave them time to share their experiences and "debrief" each other along the way, Vietnam soldiers were flown home into a hostile civilian culture in a single day. Their suffering was never validated, their souls left burdened, their stories left untold until the end of life, when the stories sometimes surface.

World War II veterans rightfully swell up with pride when Adolf Hitler is mentioned. "We got him," they will say, feeling the satisfaction of being part of a successful campaign to protect the world from evil. Vietnam veterans rarely feel this kind of satisfaction. Uncertainty and ambiguity about the goals and outcomes of the war often erode any sense of achieved purpose. Without a convincing victory, veterans felt their sacrifices had been meaningless. The political nature of the war added to their sense of injustice: "We could have won that war if the politicians had stayed out of it" or "They never financed the war so that we could have the resources to do what needed to be done. They sent us in there knowing we couldn't win." This sense that their sufferings had been futile could linger for years, corrupting their civilian lives and even their deaths years later.

Memories of killing other people can also corrupt peaceful dying. Combat veterans sometimes come to the end of their lives with unresolved grief or guilt related to military duty. Hospice can serve as a last chance to develop peace with unpeaceful memories and to reckon with the guilt of deeds inhumanly committed during human wars. For some veterans, consciously suppressed memories can no longer be kept at bay; memories sometimes come forth unbidden because as people come to the end of their lives, their conscious mind gets weaker and their unconscious gets stronger.

Making peace with wartime memories begins by acknowledging guilt that veterans sometimes harbor. Some feel guilty about killing. This moral injury they sustain can sometimes haunt them if they have not reckoned with it previously. Others feel guilty for *not* killing: "They had to take me off the front lines. I was such a coward."

Noncombat veterans sometimes feel guilty when fellow soldiers volunteer for dangerous missions. For example, one veteran was a talented trumpeter assigned to the Navy band, playing as ships left harbor for Vietnam: "Here I was with this cushy job playing an instrument I loved to play. It wasn't fair." Another veteran said he vicariously sustained trauma with his job handling body bags. "Each of these guys could have been me, except that I was in the USA counting their corpses." Combat guilt can even sabotage people who were never soldiers at all. One man was sitting at his World War II father's bedside on a Hospice unit. The son had been a conscientious objector during the Vietnam War. Later, he became a psychologist and found himself working with Vietnam veterans: "I have a lot of guilt about the impact my actions had on them."

Military nurses and medics can also experience guilt about the life-and-death decisions they made. One nurse said she was not afraid of hell: "I've already been there. I have to live every day with the faces of those soldiers who didn't have a chance during mass casualties. The doctor left it up to me, a 21-year-old nurse, to decide which ones got surgery and which ones were left to die."[8]

Survivor's guilt is common. It can interfere with veterans' ability to enjoy their lives. One World War II veteran said, "When I landed on the beach, there were all these dead bodies. The sand underneath them was pink with their blood." Then he tearfully added, "They didn't get to have grandkids the way I did." The pleasure he felt with his grandkids was tainted with guilt. "It's not fair that I should have this enjoyment when they can't."

The forgiveness process includes those on the other side—the "enemy." Many veterans have been able to forgive the enemy they fought; others harbor hatred that continues to poison their vitality.

Some loved the rush of the killing and later have guilt for having enjoyed it. One veteran who had been an especially effective sniper during the Korean War, tearfully lamented his pride in his expertise: "I won many awards for marksmanship, but now I can't believe how much *pride* I took in being able to pick them off. *That's* what hurts the most." Although snipers can be a long way off from their victims, the killing is very graphic because the scope magnifies the target. Others have guilt for killing women and children. Killing enemy soldiers can at least be justified; civilians' deaths cannot, nor can the accidental killing of comrades in what is called "friendly fire." There can also be the intentional killing of officers who consistently made poor judgments that jeopardized lives of those they commanded.

Some Vietnam veterans struggle with forgiving the government for using and betraying them. Korean and Vietnam veterans might have to forgive the American public for ignoring or scorning them.

Forgiveness is not just between people either. Soldiers have to forgive the world for being unfair and for having cruelty and war in it; they have to forgive God for allowing the world to be like it is with war in it.

It is too soon to know how hospice care will need to be modified for veterans of more recent wars. No doubt, many factors will be the same and some factors will be different. It is also important to remember that many veterans who did not serve in a declared "combat zone" have also experienced the consequences of a combat culture. Dangerous missions are required for numerous military assignments. In fact, sometimes the trauma they sustain can be even more damaging because it often goes unacknowledged or is minimized because "I didn't see combat." All veterans set aside prime years in their lives, delayed personal goals, separated from loved ones, and went to strange and sometimes dangerous parts of the world. They were expected to do difficult jobs they may or may not have been inclined to perform, all the while "grinning and bearing it" or "biting the bullet." All were trained to defend their country and be willing to risk their lives if necessary to do so. Most of the American public declined those "opportunities."

A combat subculture: posttraumatic stress disorder

Stoicism permeates military culture, whether a veteran served in combat or not. Combat veterans, and others who have served in dangerous-duty assignments, have to additionally cope with traumatic memories.[7] For some, the memories crystallize into a constellation of symptoms known as posttraumatic stress disorder (PTSD). The *Diagnostic and Statistical Manual* (DSM)[9] identifies six criteria that must be present for the diagnosis (see Box 43.1).

Many people with PTSD have successfully suffered their traumatic experiences by learning lessons that help them live their lives, deal with trauma, and reckon with PTSD.[8] If they have received PTSD treatment, they can often say what helps them feel better. They might already have a PTSD network of friends who can provide support. Family members usually know how to respond to breakthrough episodes of PTSD because it is familiar territory.

Other people with PTSD have not had this experience. They have compartmentalized the trauma, banishing it into unconsciousness. They might have increased difficulty as death approaches—haunted by residual memories or corroding guilt. Others seem less affected.

When patients with PTSD are admitted to a hospice unit, they are sometimes anxious, suspicious, or angry. Leaving their home to enter an unknown hospital environment is threatening, increasing their feelings of danger. The hospital environment itself can act as a trigger with its militarized processes. Their own anticipated death can act as a PTSD trigger. And PTSD, especially when combined with alcohol abuse, has often taken its toll on their relationships, leaving much unfinished business to be resolved so a peaceful death can ensue. Sometimes they arrive at the end of their lives broken, bitterness poisoning their souls. However, it is never too late. Opportunities for growth abound when death approaches, and many people—even those who are bitter—avail themselves of the lessons.

Interventions: responding to the unique hospice needs of veterans

Penetrating stoic facades

Stoicism is important, even essential, especially on a battlefield. It creates protection from untrustworthy influences. It is the

---

Box 43.1 Posttraumatic stress disorder

- Exposure to actual or threatened death, serious injury, or sexual violence that is either directly experienced or witnessed as it occurred to others; learning that a violent or accidental death occurred to a loved one; or exposure to repeated aversive details of traumatic events

- The traumatic event causes at least one of the following intrusion symptoms:
  - Recurrent, involuntary, distressing recollections of the trauma
  - Recurrent, distressing dreams that relate to the trauma
  - Flashbacks or dissociative reactions
  - Distress at cues that symbolize the trauma
  - Physiological responses when confronted with cues reminiscent of the trauma

- Avoidance behaviors: evidenced by at least one of the following:
  - Avoidance of thoughts, feelings, or conversations related to the trauma

- Negative cognitive and mood alterations after the trauma, as evidenced by at least two of the following:
  - Inability to recall certain critical aspects of the trauma
  - Exaggerated negative beliefs about self, others, or the world
  - Persistent, distorted perceptions about the cause or consequences of the trauma causing blame of self or others.
  - Persistent negative emotional state (fear, horror, anger, guilt, shame)
  - Lack of interest in significant activities formerly enjoyed
  - Feelings of detachment or emotional distancing from others
  Persistent inability to experience positive emotions

- Persistent symptoms of increased arousal manifested by at least of the following:
  - Irritability and outbursts of anger
  - Reckless or self-destructive behavior
  - Hypervigilance (staying on guard and unable to calm down or relax)
  - Exaggerated startle response
  - Difficulty concentrating
  - Alterations in sleep patterns

- Symptoms persist for at least one month.
- The disturbance of symptoms causes significant distress or impairment. No physiological medical conditions or substances are causing the disturbance.

---

relationship to stoicism that might need modification. It can be used inappropriately to block energy and emotion from the self or can interfere with expressing love to others. Stoicism can also contribute to veterans' underreporting their fear, emotional pain, and physical pain. The healthcare provider can help reeducate veterans by offering alternatives for them to consider, such as: "I know a lot of veterans put on a macho front and don't want to take pain medication, but pain can consume your energy. You need your energy for other things now."

Encourage veterans not to confuse stoicism with courage: "Anyone can hide behind a stoic wall of silence. It takes courage to reach out to connect with others or to ask for help."

Helplessness and losing control are especially threatening: "Sometimes veterans tell me feeling helpless makes them angry. I imagine it's hard for a soldier to learn how to surrender, to let go," or "Some veterans tell me asking for help is humiliating. Tell me how helplessness makes *you* feel."

Creating environments of comfort for combat veterans

Veterans might talk about past experiences with death—deaths that were often violent and mutilating. They bring these experiences with them when they are enrolled in hospice programs. To allay these fears, it can be helpful to discuss the peacefulness of their expected death and the plan for how that will be achieved.

It can be important to eliminate as many "triggers" for PTSD as possible. Coming into a hospital (especially a VA hospital) can trigger past military memories of barracks, procedures, unsafe environments, past combat hospitalizations, and visiting injured comrades. A government hospital and its employees may not be trusted by Vietnam vets. On the other hand, a VA might be a source of comfort, belonging, security, and camaraderie, especially if the veteran previously received care there.

Loud or unexpected sounds will startle people with PTSD, and they should not be touched without warning—the clinician should first call the patient's name or make sure that the clinician is within their line of sight. The use of bed alarms should be limited; they exacerbate the startle response. Restraints should also be avoided; even tight bed clothes or linens can trigger memories of being confined in prison if the veteran was a prisoner of war.

Trust plays an important role in helping veterans with PTSD, because these veterans do not trust easily. They have been taught *not* to trust. Anyone who can betray someone with PTSD once can become the enemy. These veterans can sniff out a phony instantly, so authenticity is important. In a hospice program, trust may need to be gained quickly because the veteran may not have long to live;

time to build a trusting relationship is simply a luxury that is not always available. The clinician's movements, tone of voice, and open language become important opportunities to convey trustworthiness. Additionally, people with PTSD will often "test" clinicians to see if they are trustworthy.[8] Thus, dialogues about death should be done openly and directly when a veteran with PTSD is admitted to a hospice program. Covering up "death" or "hospice" with euphemisms might trigger suspicion by the veteran. Telling them that "hospice is for the living" when they know that a life-threatening illness is required in order to receive services, breeds distrust. These veterans faced death before when they were in combat. In fact, they were required to complete advanced directives and wills *whenever* they went into a combat zone, so they are used to open dialogue about dying. They do not like "sugar coating" difficult issues; they often prefer direct language.

Some veterans with PTSD use colorful language. This, too, can be an opportunity to build trust quickly. For example, a newly admitted veteran to a hospice program might say, "I've been through a lot of shit in the last few weeks." The clinician has an opportunity to connect with the veteran by responding, "What is the most difficult shit you've had to deal with?" This helps the veteran know that the clinician is not scared of him, nor is the clinician judgmental about his language. Although it seems like a small gesture, it can go a long way to help the clinician pass the veteran's "muster test." In no way, does this imply that the clinician should curse to personally express him- or herself around the veteran. It simply means using the veteran's context to respond to a clinical situation because it helps trust develop more quickly.

Facilitating forgiveness

Experiencing or witnessing violence can be disturbing for anyone; but the difference with veterans is that they *committed* much of the violence. That is a deeper level of traumatization. Guilt and shame can manifest itself in the final days of life with agitation as the anguish is acted out. Although this only occurs in a small percentage of dying veterans, when it does occur, it can greatly complicate peaceful dying because it can cause anguish and agitation. Forgiveness can bring peace with this kind of painful past. Although the past cannot be changed, the *relationship to* the past can. Forgiveness is the means to that end.

It is essential that clinicians know how to create a safe emotional environment that invites the veteran to consider forgiveness. However, this needs to be done carefully and cautiously. At no time, should the clinician overtly, covertly, or subtly convey to the veteran that he "needs to forgive." This can actually add another layer of damage by causing the veteran to feel additional guilt about not being able to achieve forgiveness. Rather, the clinician should simply offer the consideration of forgiveness and invite the veteran to stay open to its possibility. "Now is a time to look back over your life. Is there anything that might still be troubling you? Anything about the war that might still haunt you?" Then, sit quietly. These are not the kind of answers that can be hurried. This question might elicit stories that had previously been locked behind a facade. After the story is told, it is not unusual for a family member to comment, "I've never heard that story before. I had no idea."

Additionally, clinicians need to be aware of their own hostile acts they commit. If clinicians are unaware or are disconnected from personal hostility they express in everyday life, then they will have a difficult time understanding the hostilities committed by the veteran. The veteran, consciously or unconsciously, will sense this, feel judged, and not disclose. If clinicians justify their own misdeeds, they will tend to do the same with the veteran, bypassing important opportunities to precipitate healing. For example, it is important to not minimize a veteran's guilt or soothe it with rationalizations: "That was a long time ago" or "You were just obeying orders." These kinds of clinician responses essentially say to the veteran: "Don't tell me about your guilt and shame. Put it back behind that stoic wall." Veterans know when and why they killed, and whether or not it violates their deepest-held moral beliefs. What they need is to have the guilt acknowledged and accepted so that finally they can forgive themselves.

Not all staff members can be expected to be facilitators of forgiveness. Many agencies have developed teams of chaplains and social workers who specialize in responding to issues of forgiveness. Thus, all staff need to know how to initially respond to issues of guilt and shame, and then they can make a referral to specialized team members who can follow up with assessment and intervention.

If the veteran becomes agitated with wartime memories, especially if he is in the last several days of life, the hand-heart connection can support emotional safety.[10] In this technique, the clinician places their hand firmly on the veteran's chest. This is usually very calming for the veteran because anxious energy usually rises: the voice gets higher pitched and energy gets flighty. A calm, centered person's energy usually resides lower and deeper. If a calm person places his/her hand on an unsettled person's sternum, it can often help the anxious person to feel secure, more stable, less anxious, and safe to feel whatever they are experiencing. (This securing gesture is often practiced *unconsciously* when people get excited. They will place their palm over their own sternum to anchor themselves.) Family members can be taught to do the hand-heart connection with the veteran. It not only helps the agitated veteran, it helps family members with their own sense of helplessness.

Box 43.2 provides resources that can help veterans, their families, and professional caregivers. These resources provide clinicians with tools that will develop their skill and confidence in not only providing care for veterans but also learning principles about end-of-life care for *anyone* who has been traumatized.

Honoring veterans: a portal for healing

Many community hospices participate in National Hospice and Palliative Care Organization's We Honor Veterans program.[11] This program offers resources and tools that help agencies provide services to veterans.

Honoring veterans and thanking them for their service to their country is a simple act that often precipitates the story-telling process. Bearing witness to a veteran's story can begin the healing process. There are many ways to honor veterans. Ceremonially pinning veterans with an American flag pin or presenting them with a military certificate that cites their service and displays the seal of their branch of service are simple, yet effective ways. If the veteran served in Korea and Vietnam and they express sentiments about not being welcomed home or being mistreated by the American public, it is not too late to apologize: "I am so sorry for the indignities you've had to suffer because of our nation's ignorance about war. I want you to know that you *are* a hero. And *unsung* heroes are the *most* worthy kind."

Box 43.2 Resources for veterans, their families, and care providers

Opus Peace is a nonprofit organization committed to responding to the unique needs of veterans and their families at the end of life by providing resources, tools, and events surrounding veteran issues. Additionally, Opus Peace helps communities and agencies provide Soul Injury ceremonies to heal unmourned grief and unforgiven guilt that aging veterans may still be carrying. Go to www.OpusPeace.org or www.SoulInjury.org for more information.

We Honor Veterans is a program by the National Hospice and Palliative Care organization that provides information and tool kits to provide end-of-life care for veterans. Learn how to "earn your stars" as an agency who cares about veterans. Go to www.WeHonorVeterans.org for more information.

Soldiers Heart is a nonprofit organization whose purpose is to "alleviate the symptoms of PTSD by developing a new and honorable warrior identity." They also promote, train, and guide community-based efforts to heal the effects of war. Go to www.SoldiersHeart. net for more information.

Hospice Foundation of America. Living with Grief series 2013 focuses on improving care for veterans facing illness and death. Go to www.Hospice Foundation.org for more information on their educational program.

Honor Flight is an organization that flies combat veterans to Washington DC to see their memorial monuments. This program is provided free of charge to veterans. It currently emphasizes World War II veterans, but serves any war veteran nearing the end of life. In subsequent years, it will focus on post–World War II vets. Go to www.HonorFlight.org for more information.

Veterans Families United Foundation (405-535-1925) helps veterans and their families cope with the aftermath of war and provides information about accessing benefits. Go to www.VeteransFamiliesUnited.org for more information.

Military One Source (1-800-342-9647) provides counselors 24 hours/day. Go to www.militaryonesource.com for more information.

National Center for Posttraumatic Stress Disorder provides information about PTSD. Go to www.ncptsd.va.gov for more information.

National Alliance on Mental Illness (NAMI) describes various mental health issues affecting veterans. Go to www.nami.org/veterans for more information.

America Supports You is a Department of Defense website that connects veterans with organizations willing to provide services: www.americasupportsyou.mil.

Vet Centers (1-800-905-4675;1-866-496-8838) provide readjustment counseling and outreach services to all veterans who served in any combat zone, as well as services for their family members for military-related issues. Services are provided at no cost. There are 232 community-based Vet Centers located in all fifty states. Go to www.vetcenter.va.gov for locations.

www.goldstarmom.com. Support for mothers who have had a child killed in the military.

www.goldstarwives.org. Support for wives who have had husbands killed in the military.

www.va.gov/oaa/archiva/ Va_Transforms_End_of_ Life_Care.pdf. Monograph written by Larry Beresford about veteran issues surrounding the end of their lives.

Bereavement care for veterans and their families

Veterans have much unresolved grief.[6] On a battlefield, there is no time or space to grieve. A comrade dies and grief must be numbed so fighting can continue. Attention and energy are needed for survival; grief is a distraction that could be fatal. With grief on hold, their bereavement needs may stagnate. Facing their own death decades later or the death of a loved one, however, can trigger PTSD or activate grief from the many past losses during combat—deaths which were often mutilating or guilt-laden. When this occurs, there may be a disproportionate grief response. This exaggerated grief response is good if the veteran uses it as an opportunity to go back and mourn the deaths of his comrades. If he does not, he can become depressed instead.

Veterans may be aware that they have unresolved grief. This awareness can cause a fear of grieving when a member of their own family dies. "If I start crying, I may not be able to stop." This fear compounded by the stoic culture of the military sometimes interferes with veterans' willingness to receive bereavement services. They might fear being a "cry baby," losing control, or becoming vulnerable. Bereavement groups are sometimes viewed as a "pity party" that they want no part of. One-on-one approaches or providing bereavement groups strictly for veterans may be more effective. However, if the veteran has PTSD, he probably does not trust easily or is reticent to reach out to strangers trying to provide bereavement care. They might cope with grief by isolating or "bunkering down," which is often counterproductive. Initial approaches by bereavement counselors may need to be modified, focusing on gaining trust. For veterans who have a mental illness, the mental illness might become exacerbated when there is a death in their family. Bereavement programs need to be an integral part of mental health programs for veterans.

Veterans often confuse stoicism with courage. Helping them see another kind of courage—the courage to face uncomfortable emotions head on—can help them express their grief. However, the goal is not to make veterans cry; the goal is to help them grieve in whatever way they can. Sometimes actions such as planting a memorial tree, visiting the surviving family members, or going to a grave site may be more effective. However, it is still important to give veterans permission to cry so they can feel free to do so: "I see you choking down tears. I want you to know that it's okay to cry. We say here that the only bad tears are uncried tears," or "This is a very sad time. Tears are welcome here."

Soul Injury ceremonies can help address the unmourned grief and unforgiven guilt that combat veterans may still be carrying from the deaths of comrades killed in war. The hole this leaves in surviving comrades' hearts continues to exert its influence throughout their lives until the deaths are acknowledged, honored, mourned, and redeemed. Soul Injury Ceremonies can help restore wholeness to a nation broken by war. *Opus Peace*, a nonprofit organization, helps agencies and communities plan, organize, and implement ceremonies so that the unmet bereavement needs of veterans can be healed. (Go to www.SoulInjury.org or www.OpusPeace.org for more information.)

Bereavement for families of veterans

Stoicism can affect whole family systems. Grief might be hidden by a silent or angry facade. If the veteran was "career military," the family may have lived in numerous places for short periods of time. This can have different effects on bereavement. Because they have no established roots, there may not be a network of support that facilitates effective grieving. On the other hand, because of frequent moving, families of veterans may readily reach out for support because they have learned how to ask for help and form new bonds quickly.

If the veteran had PTSD, especially if it became exacerbated during their dying process, the family caregivers may be exhausted and not have the energy required for grief work. They may have become so consumed with caregiving that they lost their own life or sense of self, which makes grief recovery more difficult.

If PTSD is identified for the first time as a veteran is dying, the impact on the family needs to be factored into their bereavement needs. Some feel relieved saying, "I'm so glad to know it has a name. I knew something was wrong but I didn't know what. Now this makes sense." Others might feel guilty. "I wish I would've realized this sooner, I would have _____(listened more carefully, gotten him help, been more patient and understanding, etc.)"

Understanding the military culture as a context for delivering hospice care: application

If a patient maintains his identity as a veteran, then the military culture will probably form a significant context to provide end-of-life services. The following story written by the author, a hospice and palliative care nurse practitioner, reflects this contextual significance[8]:

Phil had been in World War II. His health was failing and the past few years had become frustrating, taking its toll on his relationship with his daughter Carol.

"He has to have everything just right," Carol told me. "He yells whenever things don't go his way. I hate to see his life end with our relationship like this," she said ruefully.

I asked Carol about her father's childhood as well as his military experience, searching for clues to what was causing his lack of peace and his escalation of distrust. Carol said she knew little about his childhood, and she knew little about his military career other than he had served in World War II. So I met with Phil to ascertain these things directly. As he told me his history, I had little trouble understanding why he tried to keep his world ordered, controlled, and rule-driven.

"I never told Carol about my childhood because I'm ashamed of it," Phil said hesitantly when I met with him. "You see, my father was the town drunk." Phil had been laughed at and humiliated. "I'll never forget my mother looking up one day and seeing a horse eating grass on the side of the road and saying, 'Look. Someone at the bar must have strapped your Dad on the horse and sent him back in

our direction.' Of course, Mom would bring him in and wait until his drunkenness wore off and life would go on." There was also a lot of violence. "Mom won the physical assaults because Dad didn't fight back. I guess he thought he deserved it," Phil said forlornly. "I'm not sure what he told the doctors when he was hospitalized with the broken ribs and bones; I'm sure it wasn't the truth because everyone covered up for each other. One thing I know. There was no love in our home growing up."

I felt sad just listening to Phil. At age 75, the pain still stabbed Phil's heart. "Later, it was cars instead of horses. I can't tell you how many times we would find Dad's car pulled over to the side of a road with him laying half in and half out." Through it all, his mother covered up for him, beat his dad up, and left Phil and his brother unprotected and without any sense of emotional security. "All the activities and awards I got at school, my Dad never knew about. Actually, he didn't even know if I was in school or not. All he knew was how to get his next drink and how to make it home after his last drink and how to endure my mother's verbal and physical assaults in between."

When he got older, his relationship with his father remained based on hurt and shame. "One of my worst memories was when my bosses took me out to a restaurant to tell me they were promoting me. It was a great time of celebration and I was on top of the world," he said lighting up with the memory. "When we came out of the restaurant, there was a large crowd gathered in the street with the police. To my shocked dismay, there Dad was, stone drunk in the middle of the street. I didn't know what to do. If I said anything, my bosses would know." But Phil told the policeman it was his father and he'd take him home. However, the policeman had already called the black Mariah to take his father to jail. "So I stood by helplessly and watched as they slung my father, unconscious, into the back of the truck like a piece of meat. The indignity of it hurt all the way through me. Of course, my mother bailed him out, and it all started over again."

Phil said his military years were difficult too. He tried not to think about them. "I really can't describe how lonely military life is. One day you're a young man in familiar surroundings, and the next, you're plucked up with hundreds of other soldiers and you don't know a one of them. You find yourself overseas where nothing is familiar in the midst of a war, a war that has given me a lifetime of memories I've tried to shut out and run from as best I could. No man should see some of the things I've seen." He paused a long time before resuming. He said the only time he wasn't scared was the week he went on pass in France. "Anybody who says they aren't scared when bullets are hitting all around you and shells are coming down upon you, is lying." He said he was also afraid of friendly fire. "Some of the new guys were trigger-happy, and they weren't afraid to shoot at anything that moved. It's hard to see your buddies shot up because a new guy was too scared to see who they were shooting."

His role in the war was to run telephone wires. One of the jobs that scared him the most was when tanks got tangled up in wire and he was sent in to take care of it. "I figured that the enemy knew the tank was there and that someone would be sent to retrieve it so I was an easy target. Each time I approached, I really did expect death. Even if I escaped that, what greeted me was almost as bad. Sometimes it was the soldiers shot. Sometimes they were stabbed. You just can't believe what humans can do to each other," he said haltingly, his voice cracking with emotion. "I was only a boy myself. It really made me sick. Still does. But I don't want to get my mind in some of these places." Then he added proudly, "Meanwhile, we kept the wires up. A lot depended on that!"

The military taught him self-control. "Growing up, I had little self-control. For years after I got out, family members commented how much I had changed because I had learned self-control." He said learning self-control was good but "war changes you in ways that can't be described. Maybe a few ways are good. Many are bad. And probably most are not even known."

I asked Phil about how his experiences had shaped his relationship with Carol. "As I grew up, I knew one thing for sure: I would never put my kids through what I had been through," he said. "I made a decision not to drink or smoke. I would not bring shame to the family name. I would hold a steady job. I would be successful. My children would be proud of their father. They would never have to know the humiliation of neighbors and strangers laughing at the town drunk. They would never have to wonder where Dad was." He was proud that he was a self-made man. "I rose against the odds and I made it. God's been good to me. He made up for the childhood I had."

We talked at length about how he had covered up his shame with success. He said he felt certain that the way to achieve success was through strict self-control. As we spoke, he realized how his fear of shame ended up controlling him. He began to see how this had imprisoned him in a rigid lifestyle that constrained his relationships. Once he realized this, he had little trouble seeing the effect this had on his daughter.

Quickly he agreed to write a letter to his daughter so he could leave a different legacy than the one he had begun. He started the letter by telling his daughter the details of his history. Then he provided Carol his new perspective: "I didn't want pain and shame to touch my own family. Unfortunately, it did anyway. It just wore a different mask of shame and hurt. I like most about myself those things I liked least about my father. As a little kid, it's so scary to not know where your Dad is, if he will show up, what he will look like when he's found or even if he will be alive, or what rampage your mother will go on that will land your Dad in the hospital or jail. My brother and I only had each other to cling to helplessly while we watched and silently cried out for it to stop. I thought if I worked hard enough and became successful enough, my children would be proud of their father. I thought that would be the best gift I could ever give. Now, I realize working long hours at work and renting the farm and being with the horses all the time left you alone and feeling forgotten. I thought I was making people happy. Neighbors were proud of us. You kids didn't have to hang your head in shame every time you walked down the street. You didn't have to be laughed at when you walked by someone. There was laughter and no loneliness. I thought that was love. You see, when I was a child, I don't ever remember laughter in my house. I don't ever remember a house without loneliness. I don't even remember a house that anyone visited. You are helping me see that this was not such a gift after all. My preoccupation with making you proud of me meant you didn't see me much. I didn't realize that was important. I liked it when my Dad wasn't home. It may have been lonely but it was quiet. I thought as long as I was out working hard, staying busy, being responsible, and bringing honor to our name, I was being a good father. It never really dawned on me until now that you suffered my neglect. It never really dawned on me how much it hurt you to be ignored because of my need to make you proud of me. It never really dawned on me until now how much I didn't pay attention to how different you are than me. I didn't see you as a little girl with your own thoughts and feelings. I assumed your needs were the same as mine had been when I was a kid. I still have trouble with that. I still want to tell you how to think and feel because I forget you are your own person. I realize now how self-centered that is. I thought I was giving you the father you always wanted. Now I realize I was giving you the father *I* always wanted and I cheated you out of the father you needed. I'm ashamed of the verbal attacks I've had with you over the past few years. I don't believe you deserved that. My pride and my thinking you should think like me made me blind to what I was doing. I ask your forgiveness for that now. Carol, I love you. I showed love in the best way I knew how: to work hard, be responsible, be punctual, be honorable, maintain my senses and control, all so you would feel proud and not suffer embarrassment and humiliation. I'm so sorry this left you ignored and abandoned. I'm so sorry it has meant that I didn't see you as your own person and assumed you would want for yourself what I wanted for you which was really what I had longed for as a child for me. I'm sorry I cheated you out of the Dad you needed me to be because I was too blind to find out what that was. I'm ready to die. Waiting. Glad for it. I say that out of joy. Joy for my Maker and his Son. In recent years, I have tried to live my life as a good Christian as best I can. I still have many potholes, but if you look for the potholes, you'll always see them. I know that God forgives me for the potholes I've created. He's filled them up with love and peace and He doesn't even see them. I'm ready to be with Him. My only hope is that you can forgive me for the ways in which I have let you down. Certainly, the last thing I ever wanted was to hurt or disappoint you or make you not feel proud to have me as your father. Please forgive me. Dad."

Carol was extremely grateful for the insights her father provided her. The letter provided explanations that filled in unknown gaps. "I knew Dad's childhood had been bad, but I didn't know how bad it was. I'd always assumed it was me, that I was unlovable. Now, I realize it had nothing to do with me. The funny thing is I realize now how much he *did* love me. He was trying to protect me from experiencing what he had experienced. That was love and I just didn't know it."

I was also grateful for Phil's insights. I told him how his courage, honesty, and humility were teaching me things I needed in my own life. He seemed pleased, adding yet another bit of wisdom. "Learning is what I take with me when I die," he said with a twinkle in his eye. "What I have taught others is what I leave behind."[8]

References

1. *Atoning*, by Ron Mann. Displayed in the National Vietnam Veterans Art Museum in Chicago.
2. Grossman D. On Killing: The Psychological Cost of Learning to Kill in War and Society. NY: Little, Brown; 1996:260.
3. www.apa.org/ptgi.
4. Grassman D. The Hero Within: Redeeming the Destiny We Were Born to Fulfill. St. Petersburg, FL: Vandamere Press; 2012.
5. VHA Directive 2003–008. Palliative Care Consult Teams. Washington DC: Department of Veterans Affairs; 2003, Feb 4
6. Tucci A, Doka K, eds., Improving Care for Veterans: Facing Illness and Death. Hospice Foundation of America; 2013.
7. Amana J, Hendricks A, eds. Military Healthcare. New York: Routledge; 2013.
8. Grassman D. Peace at Last: Stories of Hope and Healing for Veterans and Their Families. St. Petersburg, FL: Vandamere Press; 2009.
9. American Psychiatric Association. Diagnostic and Statistical Manual of Mental Disorders. 5th ed. Arlington, VA: Author; 2013:271–276.
10. Simpson M. (1999). Grief and the Healing Arts. Amityville, NY: Baywood. Also, go to www.OpusPeace.org under "tools" for a pictorial description.
11. www.WeHonorVeterans.org

SECTION V

End-of-life care across settings

CHAPTER 44

Improving the quality of care across all settings

Marilyn Bookbinder and Romina Arceo

The world as we have created it is a process of our thinking. It cannot be changed without changing our thinking.

Albert Einstein

Key points

- Quality palliative care is a result of intelligent systematic efforts to raise standards of care throughout an organization.

- Tools are available to assist in the monitoring and measurement of structure, process, and competency in the delivery of palliative care.

- Outcome measures are needed to evaluate the impact of innovative change on patient and family quality of life, healthcare systems, and professional practice.

One system for addressing health and end-of-life (EOL) care is the inclusion of quality methodologies designed to improve education, streamline healthcare bureaucracies, help measure costs, and even address how people feel about their jobs. Whether or not your organization is accredited by The Joint Commission (TJC), formerly the Joint Commission on Accreditation of Health Care Organizations (JCAHO) or mandated to use a quality improvement (QI) methodology, a planned-change approach is needed to achieve positive outcomes and to cultivate an infrastructure that maintains optimal standards of care for those at the end of life.

This chapter provides perspectives on QI-based initiatives in US healthcare organizations across settings and populations and discusses their impact on patient, professional, and system outcomes in palliative care. Principles of QI and structural, process, and outcome approaches to conducting QI studies are introduced. A case study is presented of a care-path for the end of life that the author and colleagues pilot-tested. An algorithm addressing dyspnea, a distressing symptom at end-of-life, will be offered for testing, and a new approach to evaluating care at end-of-life using TJC's tracer methodology will be introduced. These examples are used to establish the linkages between QI principles and practice to improve EOL care. The chapter closes by showcasing nurses within interdisciplinary teams who are building evidence and providing leadership in the field of quality and palliative care.

The terminology turmoil

Quality improvement is increasingly commonplace in the lexicon of industry and government healthcare systems in the United States. Typically, QI is used to describe a process for improving things. Although the terms vary, distinct vocabulary, tools, and techniques used to conduct QI studies are the same. Other labels include continuous quality improvement (CQI), total quality management (TQM), total quality systems (TQS), quality systems improvement (QSI), total quality (TQ), and performance improvement (PI).[1]

Because consensus regarding these terms is unlikely, it is recommended that each organization define a methodology and terms that apply across the board and be consistent in their use. This will encourage users of QI to read beyond labels and to examine the meaning behind concepts and the value of teamwork in achieving goals. For the purposes of this chapter, QI is defined generically as the label for the philosophy driving a systematic approach to improving clinical practice, systems, issues, education, and research.

Quality improvement in healthcare

What is quality improvement?

As a philosophy, QI is broadly defined as "a commitment and approach used to continuously improve every process in every part of an organization, with the intent to exceed customer expectations and outcomes." As a management approach, QI is a way of doing business—a way to stimulate employees to become part of the solution by improving the ways care is delivered, identifying the root causes of problems in systems, designing innovative products and services, and evaluating and continuously improving.[2]

The concepts of QI go back to the 1920s, with pioneers in the field such as Deming, Shewhart, Juran, and Ishikawa. W. Edwards Deming, an American engineer and statistician most widely known for his efforts to assist Japan in its quest for quality after World War II, was all but unknown in his own country (United

States) until the 1980s. In fact, the Deming prize, Japan's highest award for industrial productivity and quality, was first awarded to an American company, Florida Electric and Light Company, in 1989. To date, no healthcare organizations have received the Deming prize. Joseph Juran, also involved in the Japanese quality transition in the 1940s and 1950s, added the concepts of planning and control to the quality process and addressed the "costs" of poor quality, which includes wasted effort, extra expense, and defects. Readers wanting more detail about the rationale and statistical methods behind QI philosophy and methods are referred to the writings of Deming and others.[2] The first to apply statistical methods to the problem of quality control was Walter A. Shewhart of the Bell Telephone Laboratories. He issued a memorandum on May 16, 1924, that featured a sketch of a modern control chart.

Although Deming's quality method has been used extensively in industry with much success, it has only been adapted to education and healthcare since the early 1990s. The US Health Care Reform Act of 1992 fueled the need for QI methods and better control over inconsistencies in services. Effects of the reform include: (1) increased managed-care contracts in health systems and reductions in reimbursement; (2) reorganization and downsizing of hospitals and staff; (3) cross-training and the development of multipurpose personnel; (4) shorter hospital stays for patients; and (5) a shift in the provision of services from hospital care to ambulatory and home care. Some countries have expanded their quality measures to include palliative care and end-of life care. The quality of death index, for example, measures the current environment for end-of-life care on 27 indicators across 40 countries.[3]

The most recognized symbol of quality in healthcare remains the TJC, a nonprofit organization which accredits and certifies more than 20,000 healthcare organizations and programs in the United States to meeting certain performance standards.

The urgent need for healthcare reform in the United States has propelled private and professional organizations to form coalitions to assist the United States in making Healthy People 2010 become a reality (i.e., improve quality and years of *healthy* living). In the last decade, organizations such as the Institute for Healthcare Improvement spurred by the Rand Corporation and Don Berwick, leader in QI, have provided leadership for healthcare professionals striving to improve quality and costs in their organizations. With the help of Web-based learning systems, virtual teams of professionals can join national and regional collaborative efforts around specific content areas, offering mentorship and resources.

Introducing the Beth Israel Medical Center case to improve end-of-life care

Table 44.1 describes six key principles of QI, based on the doctrines of Deming. These principles were applied to a QI project to improve EOL care at Continuum's Beth Israel Medical Center (BIMC) in New York City in early 2001 and are still applicable today.[4] At BIMC, chart reviews of inpatient deaths and other sources of data provided evidence that EOL care could be improved. The purpose of the 1-year pilot study, funded by a New York State Quality

Measurement grant, was to create a benchmark for the care of the imminently dying inpatient.

The QI process begins and ends with customers, determining their needs and creating products that meet or exceed their expectations. To achieve the necessary improvement, multidisciplinary teams are to break down barriers between disciplines and departments, promote collaboration and mutual respect among healthcare workers, and encourage "buy-in" from front-line staff. In the BIMC pilot study, to determine the root causes of variation in EOL care, a 28-member team was formed to involve staff integral to the EOL process on five pilot units: oncology, geriatrics, hospice, medical intensive care, and step-down unit. Early in the study, QI techniques of brainstorming and flowcharting were used to identify health system barriers and to identify possible strategies for dealing with them.

Quality improvement teams use a systematic, scientific approach and statistical methods to study problems and make decisions. This paradigm encourages an environment of lifelong learning and promotes a team approach to identifying and developing the "best practices." The BIMC project identified a critical need for multidisciplinary education and team-building. For example, monthly QI meetings included a segment of the American Medical Association's (AMA's) Education for Physicians on End-of-Life Care[5] training program. Discussions, led by Russell K. Portenoy, MD, a coinvestigator for the AMA project and leader in palliative care, provided team members fundamental information about the components of good EOL care, as well as opportunities to voice their own ideas and concerns.

The QI team worked in four subcommittees over a 5-month period to reach the implementation schedule of the project. One subcommittee developed the Palliative Care for Advanced Disease (PCAD) pathway, which has three parts: a multidisciplinary care path, a flow sheet for daily documentation of care, and a physician's order sheet that includes suggested medications for treating 15 of the most prevalent symptoms at EOL. The other three subcommittees addressed (1) education of nurses, physicians, other staff, patients, and families; (2) a timeline and detailed plan for implementation, education, and evaluation of PCAD; and (3) tools and methods for evaluating patient, family, staff, and system outcomes of the project.

The effectiveness of quality improvement

Those wanting to improve quality by using best evidence quickly learn the value of the Cochrane Collaboration, an international not-for-profit organization, providing up-to-date high-quality research evidence about the effects of healthcare. Readers are encouraged to search the Cochrane Library for the results of an interventional protocol reviewing CQI and its effects on professional practice and healthcare outcomes. One of the principle objectives of the review was to determine the relative effectiveness of CQI approaches compared with standard healthcare practices, the sustainability of the outcomes, and the associated costs. The review concludes that CQI efforts produce positive results, including the effects of modifying information flows (e.g., paper or electronic records), material flows (e.g., a blood sample sent to a laboratory), patient flows (e.g., patient experiences through

Table 44.1 Principles of quality and application for improving end-of-life care

Principle	Discussion	Application
1. Customer-driven	The focus is on customers, both internal and external, and understanding them. Teams strive to achieve products/services to better meet needs and exceed expectations of customers.	Chart reviews of patient deaths reveal areas to improve: Documentation regarding advance directive discussions, symptom management effectiveness, spiritual and psychosocial care, treatment decisions in last 48 hours of life. Focus groups with caregivers reveal need for better communication with health professionals about patient's progress.
2. System optimization and alignment	Organizations/teams are systems of interdependent parts, with the same mission and goals for customers.	Hospital-wide multidisciplinary CQI team is formed to reduce variation in EOL care with three standardized tools that provide guidelines for care (care path), documentation, and physician orders.
	Optimizing performance of the entire system means aligning the processes, technology, people, values, and policies to support team efforts to continually improve.	Ongoing resources from Pain and Palliative Care available to pilot unit staff (one advanced practice nurse).
3. Continual improvement and innovation	Focus shifts to processes of care and using a systematic and scientific approach. Methods seek to reduce and control unnecessary process variation and improve outcomes.	Flowcharting and brainstorming techniques help identify current activities and unit norms for EOL care regarding establishing goals of care, advance directives, respecting patient and family preferences, and barriers to implementing goals of project.
4. Continual learning	Resources are available to develop a culture in which people seek to learn from each other and access new sources of evidence. Feedback mechanisms support the use of evidence to drive improvements.	Extensive literature searches and team expertise guide development of clinical tools and educational materials. Team members receive education regarding issues in EOL care, viewing of Education in Palliative and End-of-Life Care (EPEC, ELNEC). Adult learning principles guide sequencing and content of educational sessions for unit staff (e.g., physiology of dying).
5. Management through knowledge	Decision-making is based on knowledge, confirmed with facts about what is "best practice," and guided by statistical thinking.	Team uses FOCUS-PDSA methodology to structure study processes. Content experts in EOL, measurement, outcomes, and QI guide sampling, selected outcome measures, and graphic display of data.
6. Collaboration and mutual respect	Organizations/teams engage everyone in the process of improvement and in the discovery of new knowledge and innovations. Mutual respect for the dignity, knowledge, and potential, contributions of others is valued by members.	Team forms subcommittees to develop materials in four areas based on expertise and interest: Care-path development, flow sheet, physicians' orders. Implementation (timeline for phases of planning, launching, rollout, evaluation, dissemination, and decisions to adopt practice changes). Education (staff, patient, and family). Outcomes (patient, family, staff knowledge, process audit of new tools).

outpatient department), or combinations of these (e.g., reviews of specific patient groups). Strategies used for implementing the approaches included educational materials, educational meetings, educational outreach, or opinion leaders/product champions, marketing, or use of other media.[6]

A direct effort to improve quality in palliative care in US hospitals can be attributed to the Joint Commission's Advanced Certification Program for Palliative Care certifying their five hospitals in 2012.[7] These include (1) Regions Hospital in St. Paul, Minn.; (2) Strong Memorial Hospital in Rochester, N.Y.; (3) Mt. Sinai Medical Center, New York City; (4) St. Joseph Mercy Oakland, Pontiac, Mich.; and (5) The Connecticut Hospice, Inc. in Branford, Conn. The certification program is designed to recognize inpatient programs that demonstrate exceptional patient and family-centered care that aim to optimize the quality of life for patients with serious illnesses.

Given the emphasis in healthcare on using QI to achieve high quality at reduced costs, nurses and colleagues can expect to see increases in accountability in the following areas: performance monitoring, participation in multidisciplinary team meetings, education in quality improvement, implementation of process improvement approaches, use of algorithms and other technologies and techniques for decision-making and data gathering, restructuring of workflow patterns and removal of barriers to patient care, development and use of quality indicators, and focus on patient and caregiver outcomes.

The need for quality improvement in palliative care

The World Health Organization defines palliative care as the "the active total care of patients whose disease is not responsive to curative treatment.... when control of pain, of other symptoms and of psychological, social and spiritual problems is paramount."[8] Palliative care is often referred to as supportive care or comfort care that seeks to prevent, relieve, alleviate, lessen, or soothe the symptoms of disease without effecting a cure.

The Institute of Medicine's (IOM's), landmark report *Approaching Death: Improving Care at End of Life*, published by a 12-member medical nursing expert committee, summarized four areas needing improvement: the state-of-the-knowledge in EOL care, evaluation methods for measuring outcomes, factors impeding high-quality care, and steps toward agreement on what constitutes "appropriate care" at the end of life. These major findings and the World Health Organization report *Palliative Care for Older People: Best Practices*[9] suggest starting points for QI work needed in palliative care:

- *Patient care:* Too many people suffer needlessly at the end of life, both from errors of omission (when caregivers fail to provide palliative and supportive care known to be effective) and from errors of commission (when caregivers do what is known to be ineffective and even harmful).

- *Organizations:* Legal, organizational, and economical obstacles conspire to obstruct reliably excellent care at the end of life.

- *Education:* The education and training of physicians and other healthcare professionals fail to provide them with knowledge, skills, and attitudes required to care well for the dying patient.

- *Research:* Current knowledge and understanding are inadequate to guide and support consistent practice of evidence-based medicine at the end of life.

The IOM report includes results from the national SUPPORT study, which produced over 104 publications supporting the deficiencies in care and citing the frequency of aggressive medical treatment at the end of life (deaths occurring in the ICU) and the lack of adequate symptom management (conscious patients with moderate to severe pain).[10]

The need to identify quality care measures at EOL for oncology patients has also been a priority. Through its evidence-based practice centers (EPCs), the Agency for Healthcare Research and Quality'(AHRQ) sponsored the development of a technical evidence report (TEP) titled "Cancer Care Quality Measures: Symptoms and End-of-Life Care."[11] The TEP identified evidence-based quality measures to support quality assessment and improvement in the palliative care of cancer patients in the areas of pain, dyspnea, depression, and advance care planning. Of the 537 articles that met the TEP criteria for review, only 25 contained quality measures: 21 on advance care planning, 4 on depression, 2 on dyspnea, and 12 on pain, of which only a few had been specifically tested in a cancer population. These findings suggest that little progress has been made in standardizing the assessment of the quality of care delivered and quality measures are key research areas in which nurse researchers can make a difference.[11]

More recently, the cost of EOL care has become a major priority in the United States as we move away from fee for service reimbursement structures to capitation models. In a recent hospital review newsletter,[12] Diane Meier, Director for the Advance of Palliative Care and a national authority on palliative care programs in the United States, reports on why hospital executives need to pay attention to the 5% of patients who are driving 50% of their spending budgets. This 5% group are the over-85 elders expected to reach 8.5 million by 2030. It is estimated that 27% of Medicare dollars are spent on their last year of life, when most of them will spend some time in the hospital. Emphasis will be placed on managing this 5% of the population well and palliative care.

The number of hospitals with palliative care programs has tripled over the last decade. In 2000 roughly 500 hospitals had a program; by 2011, 1900 were documented. Dr Meier and others recommend to those starting programs to make the argument that palliative care increases patient satisfaction and quality of care and supports better bedside care and resource allocation. Hospital leaders also face the pressures of Medicare's value-based purchasing programs, which emphasize use of quality metrics, and patient satisfaction measures. Dr Meier asserts that palliative care outcomes are a natural offshoot to accompany these efforts.

The Joint Commission's Advanced Certification Program for Palliative Care that began September 2011 has propelled hospital-based palliative care programs to develop infrastructures and quality indicators using evidence-based guidelines.[7] Dr. Joe Contreras, Chairman of the Pain and Palliative Care Institute at Hackensack (New Jersey) University Medical Center, helped Hackensack become the first TJC certified program in New Jersey. He proposes three steps for those moving toward certification and a quality program:

- Identify a palliative care champion; someone who is a leader in how the palliative care program functions and promotes the notion of transdisciplinary teams. Roles and functions of various members are a shared responsibility in efforts to get the patient's story and develop a personal plan of care.

- Assemble a committee and team to educate stakeholders, patients, families, and the community about what palliative care is.

- Expand palliative care to the home setting to reduce patients calling 911 or asking relatives to take them to the hospital. More palliative care at home can reduce hospital-acquired infection, mortality, and other adverse events.

- Focus on quality and certification in the next decade to achieve standardization of guidelines (e.g., national consensus project) that penetrate the healthcare system.

The next segment of this chapter highlights approaches to improving quality palliative care in the IOM's four areas of identified need: patient care, organizations, education, and research. Donabedian's classic framework for defining and improving quality will be used: structure, process, and outcome components.[13]

Improving structure, process, and outcomes in palliative care

Structure

Quality improvement models can provide structure to an EOL-care program. In addition to explaining the interrelationship of program parts, a systematic approach guides the activities of people performing QI as well as assuring the validity and relevance of a study. Quality improvement experts agree that "quality is never an accident" and that it is "always the result of intelligent effort, intent, and vigilance to make a superior thing." To achieve this, QI teams need a systematic methodology to follow. Although various models have evolved, all of them support the notion of QI as an unceasing, organization-wide effort that focuses people and systems on improving the processes of work. They are not intended for policing or blaming people for errors after the fact.

The oldest and most frequently used methodology designed to support "intelligent effort" is the FOCUS-PDCA cycle, which illustrates the BIMC team's application of each step in the cycle (see

Appendix 44.1). The details and application of the FOCUS-PDCA cycle and tools and techniques for conducting QI studies have been described more fully elsewhere.[14] The PDCA (plan–do–check–act) portion of the cycle, will be called by its more commonly used name today, the PDSA (plan–do–study–act). The FOCUS-PDSA methodology is briefly described below using the BIMC example. Its first five steps are aimed at team-building, clarifying the nature and scope of the improvement needed, and gathering information about the culture and setting in which the study will be done.

Focus

- *Find a process to improve.* The focus for the BIMC study was care of imminently dying inpatients on the five hospital units known to have the highest volume of patient deaths. Chart reviews of patient deaths investigated 2 years earlier identified the need for the study.

- *Organize to improve a process.* A 28-member QI team of stakeholders spanned departments and disciplines to address EOL issues such as ethics, social work, chaplains, pharmacists, nurses, and physicians. Experts in the Department of Pain and Palliative Care and End of Life took the lead.

- *Clarify what is known.* Flowcharts were created to map the ideal process of care and increase dialogue among the team's disciplines about "why" EOL care varied. Based on the results, the team regrouped into four concurrent subcommittees: (1) care-path development; (2) implementation; (3) education; and (4) evaluation, including searches of internal and external sources of evidence and rationale in EOL care.

- *Understand variation.* Brainstorming techniques helped the team elicit reasons for variations in the care process and identify potential barriers. An Ishikawa diagram (to display cause and effect) was used to show the barriers; materials, methods, people, and equipment categories were used. Subcommittees considered the barriers when planning and implementing the program.

- Select a process improvement. The four subcommittees developed evidence-based interventions, including the three-part PCAD care path, educational materials, a timeline for implementation, and tools to measure professional, patient and family, and system outcomes. The FOCUS step prepares the team for the PDSA cycle.

The PDSA cycle: Plan–Do–Study–Act

Also known as the Shewhart Cycle and Deming Wheel,[2] the PDSA cycle constitutes the evaluation aspect of the study and its iterative problem-solving process. Once a team has set an aim, established its membership, and developed measures to determine whether a change leads to an improvement, the next step is to test a change in the real work setting. The PDSA cycle is shorthand for testing a change—by planning it, trying it, observing the results, and acting on what is learned. This is the scientific method, used for action-oriented learning. Here is the PDSA cycle used by the education subcommittee:

- *Plan.* In this step, a timeline of activities for the 1-year pilot prepared administration, team members, and others with direction, goals, and resources. The sample timeline in Appendix 44.1 illustrates the various phases involved in launching the pilot project: the planning phase, rollout or introduction phase, and the implementation, evaluation, and dissemination and reporting phases. Then the study design is crafted. This includes determination of sample size and selection, what data will be collected and by whom, what tools will be used and when they will be applied, what training will be conducted and by whom, and who will perform data analysis. Table 44.2 outlines principles for assuring the quality of data.

- *Do.* The interventions are implemented and data collection begins. In the BIMC study, several premeasures were obtained, including baseline knowledge, using Ross's Palliative Care Quiz for Nurses,[15] chart reviews, and focus groups with staff to obtain baseline data.

Table 44.2 Principles for assuring the quality of data

Principle	Key point
Validity/reliability	There is accuracy and consistency in data collection.
Completeness	Measurement system includes a policy for missing data and timeliness of collection.
Sampling method	Sample size is determined by power analysis to ensure representativeness of population.
Outlier cases	Measurement systems make efforts to validate or correct outliers.
Data specification	There are standardized definitions and terminology for transmission/use of data across departments.
Internal standards	Prespecified data-quality standards are tailored for individual performance measures.
External standards	There is a commitment to implementing data sets, codes, and methodologies developed by accrediting bodies (e.g., government, professional organizations) for data use across healthcare systems.
Auditability	Data are traceable to the individual case level.
Monitoring process	Ongoing data-measurement process in place is based on prespecified standards.
Documentation	Data standards and findings are recorded and available for review.
Feedback	Performance systems regularly provide summary reports on data quality to organization leadership.
Education	Performance systems provide support through education, on-site visits, and guidelines to ensure quality data.
Accountability	Measurement systems are responsible for data quality and dissemination to participating members.

- *Check/Study.* The results of data collection are checked and analyzed by the team and the next steps formulated. For example, the BIMC group used the findings from the knowledge pretest to identify areas for continuing education. Through consensus, members agreed that knowledge items answered incorrectly by 15% of staff would be targeted for continued education.

- *Act.* Action plans are developed. The BIMC team gave monthly feedback to the QI team, pilot units, and the hospital QI department in a quarterly report. Knowledge scores on pilot units were lowest on items about the dying process. The pretest scores and staff requested education in "the physiology of dying." To address an educational need at the BIMC team level, videos from the End of Life Care for Physicians Education Consortium were shown at monthly meetings. Discussions were led by the department's palliative care experts. Knowledge scores were monitored at 3- and 6-month intervals for additional gaps in understanding palliative care and EOL-care principles.

Measures and repeated use of the cycle

The PDSA rapid cycle process has been used successfully by many QI teams in national Improvement for Healthcare Initiative (IHI) collaboratives to improve EOL care.[16] In this model, teams are formed, including senior leadership, acknowledging buy-in and support for the effort from the start. During a designated time period, members are coached by IHI faculty with additional three 1-day educational sessions, online discussions groups, on-site visits by faculty, and telephone conference calls of frequently discussed topics, such as advance directives, pain and symptom management, and bereavement care. Figure 44.1 shows the general approach to sequential PDSA cycles. Teams are encouraged to make small changes rapidly and, once goals are met, to repeat the PDSA cycle with the next phase of the process or move to another process. This rapid cycle method has helped many achieve positive results within weeks to months. Encouraging teams to reach their targeted goals quickly reinforces team-building and motivates the teams to examine other processes. More detailed readings on the rapid cycle approach can be found in *Improving Your Office Testing Process: A Toolkit for Rapid Cycle Patient Safety and Quality Improvement.*[17]

Standards of care provide structure

Quality in clinical settings begins with well-defined standards of care that are accepted as authoritative by professionals. Such standards represent acknowledged conditions against which comparisons can be made and levels of excellence are judged. They serve to establish consistency, expectations, and patterns for practice. They articulate what healthcare professionals do and whom they serve, and they define what clinical services and resources are needed. Standards also provide a framework against which quality of care can be measured and constantly improved.

In QI, the term "benchmark" is used to refer to "the search for the best practices that consistently produce best-in-the-world results"[18]—the gold standard. Nurses leading QI teams are increasingly joining benchmarking associations, such as the Association for Benchmarking Health Care[18] (http://www.abhc.org/) and the Six Sigma Health Care Benchmarking Association (http://www.sixsigmabenchmarking.com/6shcba. html),[19] that offer mentorship, education, newsletters, and participation in benchmarking studies relevant to their healthcare needs. Clinicians seeking to make improvements in the appropriateness, effectiveness, and cost-effectiveness of care can look to several evidence-based documents by national and specialty organizations, including standards, guidelines,[20-22] position papers,[23-26] and research models for EOL care.[27-29] If explicit, guidelines can describe appropriate management of specific symptoms and provide a basis for assessment, treatment, and possible outcomes. However, if the evidence is weak, as is the case for much of EOL care, guidelines or standards need to be supported with recommendations made through consensus.

In 2004, two leading documents containing standards for palliative care clinicians were released. The first, published by the Center to Advance Palliative Care (CAPC), was the "Crosswalk

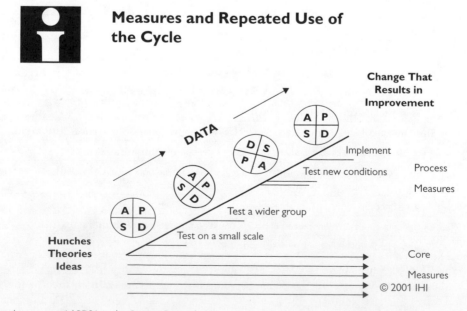

Measures and Repeated Use of the Cycle

Figure 44.1 General approach to sequential PDSA cycles. Source: Copyright IHI.

of JCAHO Standards and Palliative Care—with PC Policies, Procedures and Assessment Tools" and is updated frequently.[30] This document provides hospitals with the policy and administrative foundation for delivering palliative care services that are consistent with TJC standards. Its intent is to assist programs in implementing quality palliative care in accordance with TJC standards. The document can be accessed at www.capc.org.

One example of a standard from the crosswalk relative to palliative care is within the provision of care standards (PC.5.50). It states that care, treatment, and services are provided in an interdisciplinary, collaborative manner. To implement this standard, a palliative care team would provide documentation of assessments, planning, and treatments from physicians, nurses, social work, and perhaps a chaplain. The team has policies and procedures that address the standard, including the timing and scope of performing initial assessments and reassessments, patient care planning and guidelines for staff about patient and family meetings, and assessment and treatment and relief of pain and symptoms. The document suggests tools to implement the standards and document how they've been met, such as a consultation report, progress notes, spiritual care assessment, social work consultation note, initial assessment, plan of care, patient and family care conference record, and a palliative care intervention form.

The second document is the National Consensus Project for Quality Palliative Care.[20] This project produced guidelines for quality palliative care programs that represent a consensus opinion of the major palliative care organizations and leaders in the United States and that are based on both the available scientific evidence and expert professional opinion. These clinical practice guidelines have become the accepted means of promoting consistency, comprehensiveness, and quality across eight domains of healthcare. Processes that cross all domains include assessment, information sharing, decision-making, care planning, and care delivery at the end of life. Adoption of these guidelines in the United States will help to promote high-quality care to persons living with life-threatening and debilitating chronic illness. In 2006, a third document was endorsed by the National Quality Forum (NQF): the National Framework and Preferred Practices for Palliative and Hospice Care Quality. The framework serves as a foundation on which a quality measurement and reporting systems are currently being built. The report includes a set of preferred practices designed to improve palliative and hospice care. The NQF continued to endorse both the framework and the preferred practices in 2012.

Evidence from these earlier documents have been incorporated by two main organizations providing hospitals today with guidance on structuring quality palliative care programs, TJC's Advanced Certification Program for Palliative Care and CAPC.

Process

Answering the question "What are the key processes for delivering "best practices" to a dying patient?" can generate many ideas for QI work. Process refers to the series of linked (but not necessarily sequential) steps that by design deliver a set of results. Quality improvement operates on the principle that people do their best but are constrained by faulty healthcare processes that need to be addressed. Nurses' routine processes for assessment, diagnosis, reassessment, treatment, documentation, and evaluation of patient care are critical to producing positive patient and family outcomes. Specifically, assessment and reassessment of pain, dyspnea, agitation, delirium, nausea, diarrhea, and constipation are important symptoms leading to nursing interventions that can reduce the suffering of dying patients.

As clinicians have been challenged to deliver high-quality care at lower cost, there has been an explosion of tools designed to reduce variability in the processes of care. Algorithms and clinical pathways are two such tools that offer streamlined strategies for multidisciplinary teams to monitor and manage the processes of patient care. These tools define desired patient outcomes for specific medical conditions and delineate the optimal sequence and timing of interventions to be performed by healthcare professionals.

Algorithms and standardized orders streamline processes

Algorithms are step-by-step guides used by busy clinicians in their day-to-day work. The Providence Hospice in Yakima, Washington, is a model program of QI thinking applied in daily practice and service. Their pocket-size handbook of standing orders and algorithms, "Symptom Management Algorithms for Palliative Care,"[31] is widely used by clinicians. The symptom-management algorithms allow for a team approach involving the referring physician, medical director, nurse, pharmacist, patient, and family caregivers. Quality improvement results have been positive thus far at Yakima. In one study, use of an algorithm reduced the turnaround time of medication delivery to home hospice patients from 24 to 48 hours to less than 2 hours. Other topics in the handbook include algorithms for pain and other distressing symptoms, such as mucositis, anxiety, and terminal agitation and dyspnea. Figure 44.2 shows an example of an algorithm to improve the management of dyspnea developed at Dartmouth-Hitchcock Medical Center (Lebanon, New Hampshire).[32] The approach offers clinicians a methodology for assessing and directing treatment options and includes pharmacological and nonpharmacological interventions. Others are available at http://www.intelli-card.com/photos/Dyspnea.pdf.[33–34]

Clinical pathways reduce variation in processes of care

The term "pathway" refers to clinical trails that form a structured, multidisciplinary action plan. It defines the key events, activities, and expected outcomes of care for each discipline during each day of care. Pathways are evidence-driven, reflect best practices, and delineate the optimal sequence and timing of interventions. The goal of using a pathway is to "reduce variation" in services and practices, thus reducing costs and negative patient outcomes."[4,35,36] Box 44.1 shows a six-step process for developing pathways. Box 44.2 lists commonly used elements of care and interventions. Reducing variation in any process (clinical decision-making or care delivery) takes three steps. The first step is to study the process as it currently operates (usually done through flowcharting) to identify potential sources of variation and to learn about which activities are likely to achieve the desirable outcomes. The second step is to stabilize the process by getting everyone to use the same procedures, equipment, and materials, and also to recognize the need for individualized patient care. This is usually done by giving prompt feedback to users, educating about procedures, and involving them in tweaking the process and in individual responses. The third step is to measure again and again and repeat the process until control within agreed-on limits is reached. Standardizing care should not compromise individual's care needs.

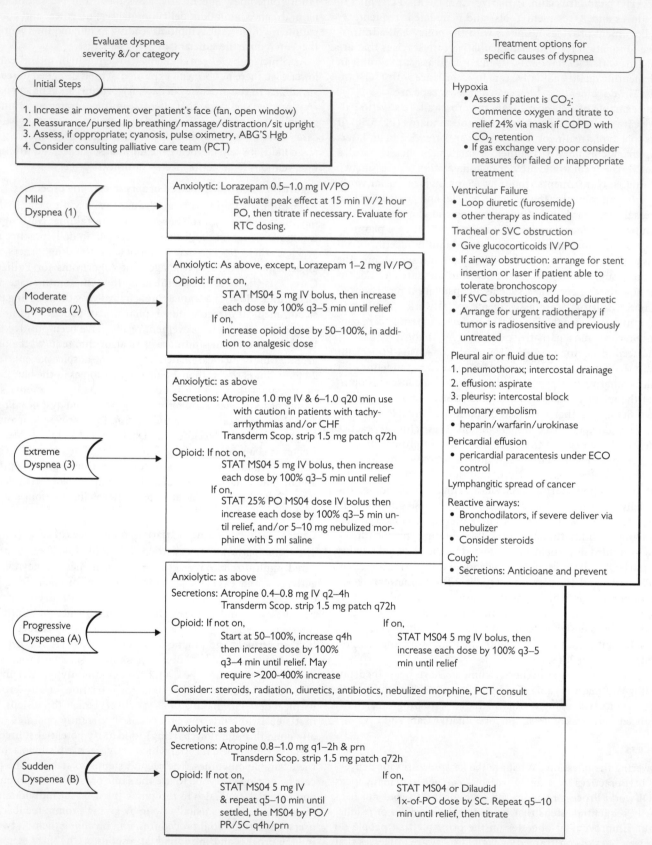

Evaluate dyspnea
severity &/or category

Initial Steps

1. Increase air movement over patient's face (fan, open window)
2. Reassurance/pursed lip breathing/massage/distraction/sit upright
3. Assess, if oppropriate; cyanosis, pulse oximetry, ABG'S Hgb
4. Consider consulting palliative care team (PCT)

Mild Dyspnea (1)

Anxiolytic: Lorazepam 0.5–1.0 mg IV/PO
　　　　　Evaluate peak effect at 15 min IV/2 hour
　　　　　PO, then titrate if necessary. Evaluate for
　　　　　RTC dosing.

Moderate Dyspenea (2)

Anxiolytic: As above, except, Lorazepam 1–2 mg IV/PO
Opioid: If not on,
　　　　　STAT MS04 5 mg IV bolus, then increase
　　　　　each dose by 100% q3–5 min until relief
　　　If on,
　　　　　increase opioid dose by 50–100%, in addi-
　　　　　tion to analgesic dose

Extreme Dyspnea (3)

Anxiolytic: as above
Secretions: Atropine 1.0 mg IV & 6–1.0 q20 min use
　　　　　with caution in patients with tachy-
　　　　　arrhythmias and/or CHF
　　　　　Transderm Scop. strip 1.5 mg patch q72h
Opioid: If not on,
　　　　　STAT MS04 5 mg IV bolus, then increase
　　　　　each dose by 100% q3–5 min until relief
　　　If on,
　　　　　STAT 25% PO MS04 dose IV bolus then
　　　　　increase each dose by 100% q3–5 min un-
　　　　　til relief, and/or 5–10 mg nebulized mor-
　　　　　phine with 5 ml saline

Progressive Dyspenea (A)

Anxiolytic: as above
Secretions: Atropine 0.4–0.8 mg IV q2–4h
　　　　　Transderm Scop. strip 1.5 mg patch q72h
Opioid: If not on,　　　　　　　　　　　If on,
　　　　　Start at 50–100%, increase q4h　　　STAT MS04 5 mg IV bolus, then
　　　　　then increase dose by 100%　　　　increase each dose by 100% q3–5
　　　　　q3–4 min until relief. May　　　　　min until relief
　　　　　require >200-400% increase
Consider: steroids, radiation, diuretics, antibiotics, nebulized morphine, PCT consult

Sudden Dyspenea (B)

Anxiolytic: as above
Secretions: Atropine 0.8–1.0 mg q1–2h & prn
　　　　　Transderm Scop. strip 1.5 mg patch q72h
Opioid: If not on,　　　　　　　　　　　If on,
　　　　　STAT MS04 5 mg IV　　　　　　STAT MS04 or Dilaudid
　　　　　& repeat q5–10 min until　　　　1x-of-PO dose by SC. Repeat q5–10
　　　　　settled, the MS04 by PO/　　　　min until relief, then titrate
　　　　　PR/5C q4h/prn

Treatment options for
specific causes of dyspnea

Hypoxia
• Assess if patient is CO_2:
Commence oxygen and titrate to
relief 24% via mask if COPD with
CO_2 retention
• If gas exchange very poor consider
measures for failed or inappropriate
treatment

Ventricular Failure
• Loop diuretic (furosemide)
• other therapy as indicated

Tracheal or SVC obstruction
• Give glucocorticoids IV/PO
• If airway obstruction: arrange for stent
insertion or laser if patient able to
tolerate bronchoscopy
• If SVC obstruction, add loop diuretic
• Arrange for urgent radiotherapy if
tumor is radiosensitive and previously
untreated

Pleural air or fluid due to:
1. pneumothorax; intercostal drainage
2. effusion: aspirate
3. pleurisy: intercostal block

Pulmonary embolism
• heparin/warfarin/urokinase

Pericardial effusion
• pericardial paracentesis under ECO
control

Lymphangitic spread of cancer

Reactive airways:
• Bronchodilators, if severe deliver via
nebulizer
• Consider steroids

Cough:
• Secretions: Anticioane and prevent

Figure 44.2 Continued

Figure 44.2 Algorithm designed to improve the management of dyspnea. Source: Developed at Dartmouth-Hitchcock Medical Center, Lebanon, NH, 198, used with permission.

MARY HITCHCOCK MEMORIAL HOSPITAL
Lebanon, NH
Last Breaths (Resource #)
DOCTOR'S ORDERs
DATE/TIME:

Draft

1. Evaluate severity of dyspnea: (see reverse side for scale description)

   0   1   2   3   4   5   6   7   8   9   10
   no dyspnea   mild dyspnea   moderate dyspnea   extreme dyspnea

2. Useful nonpharmacological methods to reduce dyspnea
   ☐ Positioning (sit, lean forward, elevate head)   ☐ Reassurance
   ☐ Direct fan toward patient   ☐ Nasal cannula (c O2 _____
   ☐ Breathing strategies (Pursed lip breathing)   ☐ Mask (c O2 _____
   ☐ Guided imagery, desensitization

3. Medication Categories   Dose   Route   Frequency
   EXPECTORANTS
     ☐ Glycerol Bualacolate   _____   _____   _____
   MUCOLYTIC AGENTS
     ☐ Acetylcysteine (Mucomyst)   _____   _____   _____
   OPIOIDS (BE SURE TO FOLLOW-UP WITH BOWEL ORDERS WHEN PRESCRIBING OPIOIDS)
     ☐ Morphine Sulfate   _____   _____   _____
   SEDATIVES/ANXIOLYTICS
     ☐ Diazepam (Valium)   _____   _____   _____
     ☐ Lorazepam (Ativan)   _____   _____   _____
     ☐ Midazolam (Versed)   _____   _____   _____
     ☐ Promethazine (Phenergan)   _____   _____   _____
     ☐ Chlorpromazine (Thorazine)   _____   _____   _____
   STEROIDS
     ☐ Prednisone   _____   _____   _____
     ☐ Dexamethasone (Decadron)   _____   _____   _____
   ANTIMUSCARINICS
     ☐ Atropine   _____   _____   _____
     ☐ Scopalamine patch   _____   _____   _____
     ☐ Levsin   _____   _____   _____
   DIURETICS
     ☐ Furosemide (Lasix)   _____   _____   _____
     ☐ Bumelanide (Bumex)   _____   _____   _____
   COUGH SUPPRESSANTS
     ☐ Benzonate (Tessalon)   _____   _____   _____
     ☐ Codeine   _____   _____   _____
   NEUROLEPTICS
     ☐ Haloperidol (Haldol)   _____   _____   _____
   INHALED MEDS (nebulizer for patients with COPD and hypercapnia should be air and not oxygen)
     ☐ Morphine   _____   _____   _____
     ☐ Lidocaine   _____   _____   _____
     ☐ Saline   _____   _____   _____
   BRONCHODILATORS
     ☐ Albuterol   _____   _____   _____

   _____ / _____   _____
   Physician Signature   RN Signature   Secretary Signature

   Print Physician Name: _____   Beeper Number: _____

DYSPNEA SCALE

MILD DYSPNEA (1–3)
Usually can sit and lie quietly
May be intermittent or persistent
Worsens with exertion
No or mild anxiety during SOB
Breathing not observed as laboured
No cyanosis

MODERATE DYSPNEA (4–7)
Usually persistent
May be new or chronic
SOB worsens if walk or exert; settles partially with rest
Pause while talking q30 sec
Breathing mildly laboured
Cyanosis usual

EXTREME DYSPNEA (8–10)
Agonizing air hunger
Talk only 2–3 words between gasps for air
Very frightened
Exhausted—tries to sit and lean forward, falls back
Total concentration on breathing
Cyanosis usual
+/– resp. congestion
+/– confusion
Maybe cold, clammy

PROGRESSIVE DYSPNEA (A)
Often acute on chronic
Worsening over few days/wks
Anxiety present
Often awoken suddenly with SOB.
+/– cyanosis
+/– onset confusion
Laboured breathing awake & asleep
Pause while talking q15 sec
Cough often present

SUDDEN DYSPNEA (B)
Sudden onset (min. to few hrs.)
High anxiety & fear
Agitation with very laboured respirations
Pause while talking
+/– resp. congestion
~+/– acute chest pain
+/– diaphoresis
+/– confusion

Use incremental titration until, when asked, "Is your breathing easy now?" the patient replies, "Yes."

MEDICATION CATEGORIES	DOSE	ROUTE	FREQUENCY
Acetylcysteine (Mucomyst)	10% 2–20 ml	nebulizer	Q6H prn
Albuterol (Proventil, ventolin)	1–2 puffs	MDI	Q8H/prm
Atropine	0.4–1.0 mg	PO/SC	Q4-12H
Benzonate (Tessalon)	100 mg	PO	Q4-6H
Butemide (Bumex)	0.5–2.0 mg	IV	prn
Chlorpromazine (Thorazine)	25–100 mg	PO	Q4-6H/prm
Codeine	30 mg	PO	Q3-4H
Dexamethasone (Decadron)	1–4mg	PO	QID
Diazepam (Valium)	2–10 mg	PO	prn
Furosemide (Lasix)	20–80 mg	IV	prn
Glycerol guaiacolate	5 ml	PO	Q4H
Haloperidol (Haldol)	.5–30 mg	IV	I6H
Levsin			
Lidocaine 2%	2.5–5 ml	nebulizer	Q6H prn
Lorazepam (Ativan)	1–2 mg	PO	Q6-8H
Metaproterenol (Alupent)	20 mg	PO	Q10min
Midazolam (Versed)	1–10 mg	IV	Q4H or 4 hourly prn
Morphine	5–10 mg	nebulizer	Q15 min
Morphine Sulfate	5–10 mg (initial bolus), or	IV	
	2.5–5 mg/hr (infusion), or		
	5–10 mg, or	SC	
	2–5 mg		
Prednisone	10–15 mg	PO	Q4H
Promethazine (Phenergan)	25–50 mg	PO	~ TID
Saline	5 ml	nebulizer	Q4-6H/prn
Scopalamine	1.5 mg	patch	Q72H
Theophylline	100 200 mg	PO	Q6H

Box 44.1 The six-step process for developing a care path

1. Identify high-volume, high-priority case types, review medical records, review and evaluate current literature to characterize the specific problems, average length of stay, critical events, and practical outcomes.

2. Write the critical path, defining the sequence and timing of functions to be performed by physicians, nurses, and other staff.

3. Have nurses, physicians, and other disciplines involved in the process review the plan of care.

4. Revise the pathway until consensus on care components is reached.

5. Pilot-test the pathway and revise as needed.

6. Incorporate pathway patient management into quality-improvement programs, which include monitoring and evaluating patient care outcomes.

Box 44.2 Routine elements of care paths

- Physical elements
- Medications
- Nutrition and dietary
- Vital signs, intake and output, weight
- Comfort assessment
- Safety and activity
- Diagnostic lab work
- Intravenous use
- Transfusions
- Diagnostic tests
- Psychosocial and spiritual needs
- Referrals and consultations
- Patient and family counseling and education

The BIMC QI team's pilot test of a clinical pathway is described in the next section. The PCAD pilot was on three units—oncology, geriatrics, and the hospice units—and two medical units served as control units.

Pilot test of a pathway to improve end-of-life care

The BIMC QI team's care path subcommittee designed an evidenced-based PCAD pathway consisting of three parts: (1) a Care Path—the interdisciplinary plan of care; (2) a Daily Patient Care Flow Sheet for documentation of assessments and interventions (including automatic referrals to social work and chaplaincy); and (3) a standardized Physician Order Sheet, with suggestions for medical management of 15 symptoms prevalent at the end of life (see Appendix 44.1 or go to http://www.StopPain.org/professional).[37] This three-part pathway was designed to guide interdisciplinary management of the imminently dying inpatient, using

a tailored approach, once the patient's primary physician had ordered PCAD (Box 44.3).

Implementation of PCAD in daily care on the three pilot units confirmed the enormous complexity of "implementation" and predicting the timing of a patient's death.[34] Although "imminently dying" was defined for the study as "hours to two weeks until death," nurses and physicians reported discomfort about making this decision. Each patient was assessed for eligibility during daily morning report or at weekly discharge planning rounds by answering the question "Whose death would not surprise you this admission?" Designated nurse leaders on each unit served as the liaisons between staff and primary physicians to request a patient's enrollment into PCAD. During the 3-month start-up period, multidisciplinary teams reported that their greatest challenge was identifying patients who were imminently dying. As patients were identified by nurses as candidates, barriers to implementing PCAD began to surface: patients and families wanted "everything done" to continue curative treatment; a physician evaluated a patient as "fragile" and unable to hear "bad news"; a patient's physical status changed dramatically in 24 hours, from dying to "rallying" and preparing for discharge; or a house staff physician felt that he was already prescribing PCAD and could not see the benefit of enrollment.

There were several positive outcomes of the PCAD pilot. Results included (1) a heightened awareness by staff of the disease trajectory (such as initial diagnosis, curative treatment, life-prolonging treatment, palliative care, symptomatic palliative care, and care of the imminently dying) and the importance of knowing patient wishes for this admission; (2) increased discussions about the goals of care and the rationale for treatment orders; (3) increased symptom assessments and interventions; and (4) increased awareness of the need to identify patients requiring referral to hospice and pain medicine and palliative care for symptom management and family support following discharge.

Debriefing was included in the implementation of the care path. Sessions held with staff after a patient died became an important aspect of the PCAD process. Staff were encouraged to discuss their satisfaction or dissatisfaction with the experience of the PCAD pathway. Such questions as "Were the patient's wishes honored?", "Were unnecessary tests/procedures performed?", "Did the patient

---

Box 44.3 Goals of the palliative care for advanced disease pathway

- Respect patient autonomy, values, and decisions.
- Continually clarify goals of care.
- Minimize symptom distress at the end of life.
- Optimize appropriate supportive interventions and consultations.
- Reduce unnecessary interventions.
- Support families by coordinating services.
- Eliminate unnecessary regulations.
- Provide bereavement services for families and staff.
- Facilitate the transition to alternate care settings, such as hospice, when appropriate.

have a peaceful death?", "Were symptoms controlled?", and "What is the family's likelihood for complicated grieving and the need for follow-up?" generated much dialogue and opportunities for teaching and grief resolution. Overall, staff expressed appreciation for the opportunity to talk about experiences of patient care and the personal involvement in caring for a patient and family whom they may have known over several admissions. Another positive outcome for unit nurses was using the PCAD Daily Flow Sheet. Hospice nurses reported that the pathway got all disciplines on the same page in terms of goals of care and patient and family wishes. They said it provided them with an easy and comprehensive system for documenting the assessment and intervention of key elements in EOL care: comfort; physical, psychosocial, and spiritual care as well as tailoring patient and family support.

Quality improvement team members also identified several areas that the hospital needed improvement during the pilot period: (1) clearer definition and measure of the concept of "comfort care"; (2) the need for a forum for educating voluntary physician staff, who have less unit/hospital involvement than staff physicians; (3) documentation of spiritual care and issues; (4) systematic identification of families at risk for complicated grieving; and (5) resources about local bereavement services and education for families.

At the organizational level, results of the pilot suggested that PCAD is a means for (1) increasing multidisciplinary team discussions of patients' goals of care during hospitalization; (2) reducing the variation in the documentation of care of imminently dying patients, placing emphasis on comfort, patient and family wishes, and closure for caregivers; (3) increasing staff awareness of patients who are imminently dying or in need of palliative care services, long-term care, hospice, and bereavement care; (4) improving symptom assessment and the use of evidence-based interventions, and (5) identifying areas in EOL care for continual improvement in BIMC's organizational, education, practice, and evaluation systems.[35–37]

The PCAD pathway, education, and evaluation tools have been disseminated widely. As of January 2009, nearly 25,000 clinicians, from all settings, have downloaded the pathway and materials from http:/www.stopPain.org. A replication study of the PCAD project was conducted by the Veterans Administration of Brooklyn, New York.[38] The VA team has translated PCAD for the electronic medical record and reported similar positive results such as increased documentation of goals of care, decreased length of stay in ICU, and fewer interventions in the last days of life.

Outcomes

Outcomes refer to results of actions or nonaction to structures, processes, patients and caregivers, professionals, and systems in the organization. Reduced symptom distress, improved family satisfaction, and improved perceived support of professional caregivers reduced costs of EOL care are all examples of outcomes relevant to quality EOL care.

Clinicians will need to become competent at measuring outcomes of their care. Federal and state governments, private purchasers, physicians, nurses, insurers, labor unions, health plans, hospitals, and accreditation organizations, among others, have placed pressure on organizations to address some of the significant quality problems in US healthcare systems (http://www.ahcpr.gov/qual).[39] The Centers of Medicare and Medicaid

Services' pay-for-performance initiative is designed to support better quality care of Medicare beneficiaries. About 100 such initiatives are in progress across the country. The general intent is to reward hospitals and doctors for providing better care. We will need to improve our ability to measure and report the quality of care being delivered. Such reporting prompts a closer look at provider and healthcare practices, both as feedback for clinicians and as publicly available score cards for consumer evaluation. With just a click of a mouse, consumers can instantly access free performance data that allow them to compare the standards of care provided by hospitals, home health agencies, nursing homes and health maintenance organizations, and emergency rooms (http://consumers.ipro.org/index/compare-hosp).[40]

Two approaches are described for measuring outcomes in palliative care at the unit level. Teams can use a single indicator of a quality of service or multiple measures.

Quality improvement indicators: measures of organizational performance

A clinical indicator is typically defined as a quantitative measure that evaluates the quality of important patient care and support-service activities. Indicators that directly affect quality services typically include such factors as timeliness, efficiency, appropriateness, accessibility, continuity, privacy and confidentiality, comfort, participation of patients and families, and safety and supportiveness of the care environment. Although they are not direct measures of quality, indicators serve as "screens" or "flags" that direct attention to specific performance areas that should be targets for ongoing investigation within an organization.

Institutions recently surveyed by TJC have experienced the shift in focus of performance from competence and skills ("Is the organization able to provide quality services?") to productivity and outcomes ("To what extent does the organization provide quality services?") and efficiency (To what extent does the organization use resources efficiently?"). For example, rather than requesting a review of the institution's policy and procedure manual for a pain or palliative care program, surveyors might evaluate whether pain standards have been implemented and to what extent they have had an effect on patients' satisfaction with care or patient understanding of side effects associated with analgesics. Surveyors are now using a tracer methodology, whereby the surveyor may interview the nurse caring for the patient, the doctor, a social worker, and if more information seems needed, the surveyor may interview the patient and/or family member about their satisfaction with care. Nurses and other clinicians will need to be knowledgeable in systems of care as the accreditation process promises to get more rigorous in areas affecting our largest and most costly group of citizens: the ill elderly.

Indicators can reflect a performance measure such as competence or safety. Competence means that individuals or the organization have the ability (e.g., education, behavioral skills) to provide quality services; safety means that those abilities are translated into actions that achieve quality outcomes. Results of indicators can reveal deviations from the norm and may warn of impending problems. Indicators may require a single-item measure, multiple items, or multiple tools. Indicators are typically expressed as an event or ratio (percentage).

Examples of structure, process, and outcome indicators that are clinical (patient care), professional (competence), and administrative (satisfaction) are described here.

1. *Structural indicators* are derived from standards of care and need to be aligned with the mission, philosophy, goals, and policies of a hospital, department, or unit. Structure standards measure whether the authorized norms are being followed. For example, a standard and its accompanying policy may read that all (100%) patients admitted to the hospital require discussion and documentation about advance directives within 48 hours of admission. The percentage obtained would indicate the extent to which adherence to the 100% goal is being met. A structural indicator on an oncology unit might read:

INDICATOR: Number of records with documentation of a discussion of advance directives/Total number of patients who were admitted to the oncology unit (determined period)

Another structural indicator relates to staff competence. This indicator may reflect a standard and policy that requires all staff working on a geriatrics unit pass a competency in EOL care. The competency might consist of written exam (cognitive) and demonstration of skill (behavioral) in the use of an EOL pathway (see Appendix 44.1 for sample knowledge quiz in palliative care). For this indicator, a threshold is determined for successful completion, such as 90% on the written exam plus three return demonstrations in the use of the pathway. Low results on this indicator might suggest the need to send key nurses to an EOL care training for nurses (End-of-Life Nursing Education Consortium [ELNEC]). Readers can visit http://www.aacn.nche.edu/ELNEC/ to read more about ELNEC's national effort and courses available.[41]

2. *Process indicators* measure a specific aspect of nursing practice that is related to flow of work: flow of information, materials, or patient care. Examples of process indicators might include pain screening, assessments, implementation of an intervention, reassessment, prompt management of complications, and documentation. These indicators describe "how care is to be delivered and recorded." Sometimes it may be difficult to separate process indicators from outcome indicators. For example, if an improvement study is directed toward reducing discomfort related to dyspnea in dying patients, then the indicator might involve the process of assessment of respirations, obtaining an order, and giving appropriate medication within a designated time period. The indicator might read that 100% of patients with severe dyspnea will be assessed and treated with appropriate medications within a 2-hour period. Another segment of the same process may produce an indicator that reads that 100% of patients treated for severe dyspnea will achieve relief (reduction to mild dyspnea) within 8 hours. The indicator would read: Time severe dyspnea treated to time of relief (mild dyspnea) (in minutes)/Each patient reaching mild relief within 8 hours is scored a yes.

INDICATOR: Number of patients with severe dyspnea reaching mild dyspnea within 8 hours/The total number of patients experiencing severe dyspnea (designated period)

Low results on this indicator might prompt a special QI team to investigate the barriers to adherence. The team may learn that the dyspnea measure is too difficult to administer, too time-consuming, or too confusing to assess mild, moderate, and severe dyspnea. Is the computer screen's field for documenting care not easy to use? Were physician's orders not appropriate for treating severe dyspnea? Were calls made to providers with delays in answering? Any of these pieces of the process could trigger a new look at the process of reaching mild relief of this symptom, including testing the use of a dyspnea algorithm.

3. *Outcome indicators* measure what does or does not happen after something is or is not done. Many organizations have shifted their focus from examining the documentation of processes of care to measuring outcomes of care and learning which treatment works best, under what conditions, by which individuals, and at what cost. Examples of outcome indicators for quality EOL care include family satisfaction with care (family), symptom control (patient), respect for patient cultural and religious preferences, family support and communication at the time of the patient's death, and referral for ethics consultation if no healthcare agent is identified. Outcome indicators such as these might be appropriate following the implementation of a multidisciplinary pathway to improve care of dying inpatients. The goal might be to achieve a family satisfaction with care rating of 90% very satisfied, using a 0 to 5 scale (0 = very dissatisfied to 5 = very satisfied). An oncology unit might decide that designated family members will be contacted at 3 to 4 months following the patient's death for an interview about satisfaction with care. The indicator would read: 90% of families will report being very satisfied with care when asked about overall satisfaction with the patient's care in the last days of life. In this example, the response rate from families should ideally be over 50% so that findings are used with confidence and not viewed as biased.

INDICATOR: Number of families scoring very satisfied with overall care/Number of persons completing satisfaction surveys following the death of a family member (Designated Period)

Although few tested methods currently exist to adequately measure the quality of care at the end of life, Twaddle et al. reported one of the first attempts at benchmarking the quality of palliative care services in 35 academic hospitals.[42] The research team used a multicenter, cross-sectional, retrospective design, and reviewed 1596 patient records against 11 key performance measures (KPMs; Box 44.4) derived from evidence-based practice standards. Results suggested wide variability in adherence among hospitals, ranging from 0% to 100% (with 0% meaning no adherence and 100% meaning complete adherence). Greater improvement in KPMs indicated greater improvement in quality outcomes, cost, and length of stay. Institutions that benchmarked above 90% did so by incorporating KPMs into care processes and using systematized triggers, forms, and default pathways. Results of this study suggest that a "palliative care bundle" (i.e., selected KPMs) leads to improvement in areas of deficiency when all components of care are given to patients. For example, patients who had pain and other symptoms and who were assessed within 48 hours of admission were more likely to report relief of the symptom within the same timeframe than those patients who were not assessed.

Building evidence in quality palliative care

A synthesis of the evidence in key elements of palliative care was recently published by palliative care experts and the British

---

Box 44.4 Areas for improving quality care at the end of life

1. Physical and emotional symptoms
2. Support of function and autonomy
3. Advance planning
4. Aggressive care near death, including preferences about site of death, CPR, and hospitalization
5. Patient and family satisfaction
6. Global quality of life
7. Family burden
8. Survival time
9. Provider continuity and skill
10. Bereavement

Source: American Geriatrics Society (1996), reference 29.

Journal Publishing Group. The review addressed the control of common symptoms such as pain, dyspnea, and fatigue; communication and goal setting; and effective efficient transition management. Readers are encouraged to consult "Putting Evidence into Practice: Palliative Care" as a resource when searching for best practices.[43] In terms of coordination of care, the review found moderate-quality evidence that specialized palliative care services improved family satisfaction, but evidence on patient satisfaction, quality of life, and symptoms control was less clear-cut. A systematic review of specialized palliative care found 22 randomized controlled trials. Problems with study implementation or analysis were common. Insufficient power, including high withdrawal rates, typically limited the potential for finding a positive effect. The best evidence of effectiveness was family satisfaction, with 7 of 10 studies indicating a positive effect. The review identified no good evidence that specialist care improved symptoms. Indications that usual care was not sufficient included indicators such as patient and/or family distress and symptoms not responding to usual management.[44]

A new area of study for researchers interested in improving quality patient care is implementation, the work of putting the evidence into practice (i.e., evidence-based practice) on a routine basis. The science of nursing implementation, according to Achterberg, Shoonhovern, and Grol[44] requires an analytical, deliberate process of identifying the determinants of implementation and choosing the appropriate strategies to achieve successful behavior change. They describe common determinants of success to include factors such as knowledge, cognitions, attitudes, routines, social influence, the organization, and its resources. The authors of this chapter showed that strategies such as reminders, decision support, and use of information and communication technology, records, and combined strategies are often effective in encouraging implementation of innovations. The authors recommend using relevant theories to go from identification of determinants to selection of strategies. For example, if a team is interested in improving knowledge deficits in advance care planning, active learning strategies derived from social cognitive theory (such as role modeling or observing an ethics committee at work) might

prove more beneficial than traditional lectures. The authors also recommend the need to pilot an innovation and conduct evaluations to assure that the intended changes are delivered as planned. Without this check, a lack of effect may be attributed to inadequate implementation of the strategy.

Joan Teno, MD, of the Center for Gerontology and Health Care Research at Brown University, together with faculty and staff at the Center to Improve Care of the Dying, has assembled a comprehensive annotated bibliography of instruments to measure the quality of care at the end of life. The Toolkit of Instruments to Measure End-of-Life Care includes a Patient Evaluation, After-Death Chart Review, and After-Death Caregiver Interview.[45] Included in the toolkit is the mortality follow-back survey of family members or other knowledgeable informants representing 1578 decedents' perceptions of the last place of care.[45] Teno's research section "Data Analysis and Reports for Toolkit Instruments" refines the toolkit and measures for users. Box 44.5 shows additional outcome measures suggested for improving EOL care.

Donabedian stated that "achieving and producing health and satisfaction,...is the ultimate validator of the quality of care." There has been limited research in examining satisfaction among terminally ill patients and families. However, for most dying patients, satisfaction may be the most important outcome variable for themselves and their families. Professor Irene J. Higginson, PhD, an international leading researcher for more than two decades, has been using the audit cycle, a feedback process similar to QI methods, to improve outcomes in palliative care. Currently at King's College School of Medicine and Dentistry and St. Christopher's Hospice in London, England, she notes the difficulties in obtaining outcome information, such as quality of life, from the weakest group of patients.[47] She supports the need to test the use of proxies to obtain this important information. The Palliative Outcome Scale is one such measure that can be used to measure physical and psychological symptoms, spiritual considerations, practical concerns and psychosocial needs.[48] Readers seeking

---

Box 44.5 Executive summary of the Toolkit of Instruments to Measure End-of-Life Care

Chart review instrument, surrogate questionnaires, patient questionnaires
  Measuring quality of life
  Examining advance care planning
  Instruments to assess pain and other symptoms
  Instruments to assess depression and other emotional symptoms
  Instruments to assess functional status
  Instruments to assess survival time and aggressiveness of care
  Instruments to assess continuity of care
  Instruments to assess spirituality
  Bibliography of instruments to assess grief
  Bibliography of instruments to assess caregiver and family experience
  Instruments to assess patient and family member satisfaction with the quality of care

Source: Teno (1998), reference 46.

measures and indicators to be used in clinical audits are referred to "Clinical and Organizational Audit in Palliative Medicine."[47]

Measures of family satisfaction in palliative care such as the FAMCARE scale[49] are also available. FAMCARE is based on qualitative research that asks family members to list indicators of quality of palliative care from the patient's perspective and their own. The Family Assessment of Treatment at the End of Life (FATE)[50] tool is a 14-item instrument with one global rating and assesses the following domains: communication; treatment preferences; dignity; spiritual support; psychosocial support; pain control, planning for death; overall care to patient. The FATE-S has been rolled out nationally in the VA system and at least 70 hospitals and 60 nursing homes are currently using it.

Figure 44.3 presents a model used by the BIMC Department of Pain Medicine and Palliative Care for outcomes research in the medically ill. The model illustrates the feedback loop between outcomes and healthcare. Outcomes research requires ongoing data collection and analysis that feeds into the modification of guidelines for clinical practice, resulting in improved patient, caregiver, professional, and systems outcomes, including costs.[51] Appendix 44.1 presents an early BIMC Palliative Care Initial Consultation Tool. The tool can be used to screen patients for key components of palliative care and resources needed from an interdisciplinary team. The symptom assessment portion of the form is a validated instrument, the Memorial Symptom Assessment Scale-Condensed.[52] This data can be used to evaluate changes in symptoms and effectiveness of treatments within individuals and among groups of patients.

Summary

Nurses are poised to have pivotal roles in improving the quality of care of the dying in the decades ahead. As nurses, we need to continue to learn what works and what does not work for patients and families and professional caregivers in our practice settings and to stay active in developing and testing QI models, tools, and interventions toward better EOL care. Nurses are providing leadership in areas of clinical practice,[53–55] education,[41,56–58] and research.[59–62]

Nurses need to continue to test interventions for improved symptom management,[63–66] developing models for assuring "best practices" using research,[67] and integrating QI methods into palliative care practices.[68] Palliative and end-of life care needs to be integrated into basic and advanced practice nursing (APN) curricula.[56] The number of graduates from APN fellowships in pain and palliative care are increasing, providing leadership in academic and clinical settings.[69] Nurses will need to strengthen their involvement in national and international efforts that educate professionals and consumers and influence healthcare policy in EOL-care issues.

To survive, healthcare systems must be able to change and improve rapidly. Healthcare, as with any other service operation, requires systematic innovation efforts to remain competitive, cost-efficient, and up-to-date. If the quality of EOL care is to improve, nurses will need to have expert knowledge about making change: how to encourage it and how to manage and to evaluate it within and across organizations and settings. This knowledge needs to be coupled with the methods and know-how to produce change. Clinical audits and feedback are a means to encourage dialogue among all ranks of staff, disciplines, and services. Nurses with expertise in QI methods and tools can provide necessary leadership in designing and testing strategies to improve EOL care.

References

1. Kelly DL. Applying Quality Management in Healthcare: A Systems Approach (3rd ed). Chicago, IL: Health Administration Press; Association of University Programs in Health Administration; 2011.
2. Deming WE. Out of the Crisis. Cambridge, MA: The MIT Press; 2000.
3. Economist: A report from the Economist Intelligence Unit. The quality of death: Ranking end-of-life care across the world. 2010. Available at http://www.eiu.com/site_info.asp?info_name=qualityofdeath_lienfoundation&page=noads. Accessed October 28, 2013.
4. Bookbinder M, Blank AE, Arney E et al. (2005). Improving end-of-life-care: Development and pilot-test of a clinical pathway. J Pain Symp Manage. 2005;29(6):529–543.
5. Education for Physician's on End-of-Life Care (EPEC) (2013). EPEC distance learning. Available at http://www.epec.net. Accessed September 25, 2013.

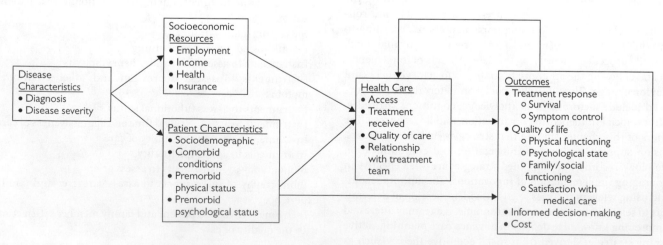

Figure 44.3 Model of outcomes research in the medically ill. Source: Kornblith (1999), reference 51, with permission.

6. Brennan S, McKenzie J, Whitty P, Buchan H, Green, S. Continuous quality improvement: effects on professional practice and healthcare outcomes (Protocol). Cochr Datab Syst Rev, 2009; Issue 4. Art. No.: CD003319. doi: 10.1002/14651858.CD003319.pub2.

7. The Joint Commission (TJC) (2013). Certification: Advanced certification for palliative care programs. Available at http://www.jointcommission.org/certification/palliative_care.aspx. Accessed June 12, 2013.

8. World Health Organization. (1990). Cancer Pain Relief and Palliative Care: Report of a WHO expert committee (Technical reports no. 804). Geneva: WHO.

9. Hall S, Petkova H, Tsouros AD, Costantini M, Higginson IJ. Palliative Care for Older People: Better Practices. Geneva: World Health Organization; 2011.

10. SUPPORT Principal Investigators. A controlled trial to improve care for seriously ill hospitalized patients: The Study to Understand Prognoses and Preferences for Outcomes and Risks of Treatments (SUPPORT). JAMA. 1995;274(23):1591–1598.

11. The Advisory Board Company (2013). Cancer quality dashboards: Metrics, definitions, and benchmarks spanning the cancer care continuum. Washington, DC: The Advisory Board Company.

12. Herman B. Palliative care: Why it has become a growing specialty within hospitals. Becker's Hospital Review. Available at http://www.beckershospitalreview.com/hospital-key-specialties/palliative-care-why-it-has-become-a-growing-specialty-within-hospitals.html. Accessed September 1, 2013.

13. Donabedian A. Evaluating the quality of medical care. Milbank Quart. 2005;83(4):691–729.

14. Hughes RG. Patient Safety and Quality: An Evidence-Based Handbook for Nurses. Chapter 44: Tools and strategies for quality improvement and patient safety. 2008. Rockville, MD: Agency for Healthcare Research and Quality. Available at http://www.ahrq.gov/professionals/clinicians-providers/resources/nursing/resources/nurseshdbk/index.html. Accessed September 25, 2013.

15. Prem V, Karvannan H, Kumar SP, et al. Study of nurses' knowledge about palliative care: A quantitative cross-sectional survey. Ind J Palliat Care. 2012;18(2):122–127.

16. Institute for Healthcare Improvement. (2009). Cambridge, MA. Available at http://www.ihi.org. Accessed January 10, 2009.

17. Improving your office testing process: A toolkit for rapid cycle patient safety and quality improvement. 2013. Rockville, MD: Agency for Healthcare Research and Quality (AHRQ) Available at: http://www.innovations.ahrq.gov/content.aspx?id=4023. Accessed November 30, 2013.

18. Association for Benchmarking Health Care. 2009. Houston, TX. Available at http://www. abhc.org. Accessed January 2, 2009.

19. Six Sigma Health Care Benchmarking Association. 2009. Houston, TX. Available at http://shcba.sixsigmabenchmarking.com. Accessed September 25, 2013.

20. Dahlin C. Clinical Practice Guidelines for Quality Palliative Care, 3rd ed. Pittsburgh, PA: National Consensus Project for Quality Palliative Care; 2013.

21. Berlinger N, Jennings B, Wolf SM. The Hastings Center Guidelines for Decisions on Life-Sustaining Treatment and Care near the End of Life: Revised and Expanded, 2nd ed. Garrison, NY: Oxford University Press; 2013.

22. Registered Nurses' Association of Ontario (RNAO). 2011. End-of-life care during the last days and hours. Toronto, ON: RNAO. Available at http://rnao.ca/sites/rnao-ca/files/End-of-Life_Care_During_the_Last_Days_and_Hours_0.pdf. Accessed September 25, 2013.

23. American Academy of Hospice and Palliative (AAHPM). 2010. Position statement: Requirements for the successful development of academic palliative medicine programs. Chicago, IL: AAHPM. Available at http://www.aahpm.org/positions/default/academicprgms. html. Accessed September 26, 2013.

24. Reynolds J, Drew D, Dunwoody C. American Society for Pain Management Nursing Position Statement: Pain management at the end of life. Pain Manage Nurs. 2013;14(3):172–175.

25. American Nurses Association (ANA). 2011. Revised position statement: Foregoing nutrition and hydration. Available at http://www.nursingworld.org/MainMenuCategories/Policy-Advocacy/Positions-and-Resolutions/ANAPositionStatements/Position-Statements-Alphabetically/prtetnutr14451.pdf. Accessed September 25, 2013.

26. Oncology Nursing Society (ONS). 2013. ONS and Association of Oncology Social Work joint position on palliative and end-of-life care. Revised 3/2010. Available at http://www.ons.org/publications/media/ons/docs/positions/endoflife.pdf. Accessed September 25, 2013.

27. Bruera E, Billings JA, Lupu D, Ritchie CS and Academic Palliative Medicine Task Force of the American Academy of Hospice and Palliative Medicine. AAHPM position paper: requirements for the successful development of academic palliative care programs. J Pain Sympt Manage. 2010;39(4):743–755.

28. National Institute for Health and Clinical Excellence (NICE). NICE quality standards: Information for adults who use NHS end of life care services and their families and carers. 2011. Available at www.nice.org.uk/nicemedia/live/13845/60322/60322.pdf. Accessed October 28, 2013.

29. Statement regarding the value of advance care planning: A position statement from the American Geriatrics Society. 2011. Available at http://www.americangeriatrics.org/files/documents/Adv_Resources/AGS.Statement.On.Advance.Care.Planning.01.2011.pdf. Accessed November 1, 2013.

30. The Joint Commission. 2013. Advanced certification for palliative care: Performance measurement requirements for palliative care. Available at http://www.jointcommission.org/certification/performance_measurement_requirements_palliative_care.aspx. Accessed October 25, 2013.

31. National Quality Forum (NQF). 2012. Palliative care and end-of-life care: A consensus report. Washington, DC: NQF. Available at http://www.qualityforum.org/Publications/2012/04/Palliative_Care_and_End-of-Life_Care%e2%80%94A_Consensus_Report.aspx. Accessed October 27, 2013.

32. Wrede-Seaman L. Symptom Management Algorithms: A Handbook for Palliative Care, 3rd ed. Yakima, WA: Intellicard; 2008.

33. Dartmouth-Hitchcock Medical Center: Hematology/Oncology Group. A Dyspnea Algorithm. Lebanon, NH: Dartmouth-Hitchcock Medical Center; 1998.

34. Wrede-Seaman L. Dyspnea treatment algorithm. In: Symptom management algorithms: A handbook for palliative care, 3rd ed. Yakima, WA: Intellicard; 2008. Available at http://www.intelli-card.com/photos/Dyspnea.pdf. Accessed January 2, 2009.

35. Costantini M, Pellegrini F, Di Leo S, et al. The Liverpool Care Pathway for cancer patients dying in hospital medical wards: A before-after cluster phase II trial of outcomes reported by family members. Palliat Med published online 7 May 2013. DOI: 10.1177/0269216313487569

36. National Hospice and Palliative Care Organization (NHPCO). 2010. A pathway for patients and families facing terminal illness. Arlington, VA: NHPCO. Available at http://www.nhpco.org/sites/default/files/public/quality/Standards/PFC.pdf. Accessed September 25, 2013.

37. Continuum Health Partners, Inc., Beth Israel Medical Center, Department of Pain Medicine and Palliative Care. Palliative Care for Advanced Disease (PCAD) Care Path. (CQI Team on End-of-Life Care), NY. Available at http://www.stoppain.org. Accessed November 30, 2013.

38. Luhrs CA, Meghani S, Homel P, et al. Pilot of a pathway to improve the care of imminently dying oncology inpatients in a Veterans Affairs Medical Center. J Pain Symp Manage. 2005;29(6):544–551.

39. Agency for Healthcare Research and Quality (AHRQ). Quality and patient safety. Rockville, MD: AHRQ. Available at http://www.ahrq.gov/professionals/quality-patient-safety. Accessed September 25, 2013.

40. Health Care Reports. Compare the standards of care provided by hospitals, home health agencies, nursing homes and HMOs in New York State and beyond. Albany, NY: IPRO. Available at http://dev2.ipro.org/index/compare-hospitals/printable. Accessed September 25, 2013.

41. American Association of Colleges of Nursing (AACN) and City of Hope, CA. The End-of-Life Nursing Education Consortium (ELNEC) project. Available at http://www.aacn.nche.edu/elnec. Accessed January 1, 2009.

42. De Roo ML, Leemans K, Claessen SJJ, Cohen J, Pasman HRW, Deliens L, Francke AL. Quality indicators for palliative care: Update of a systematic review. J Pain Symp Manage. 2013;*46* (4): 556–572.

43. Brunnhuber K, Nash S, Meier DE, Weissman DE, Woodcock J. Putting Evidence into Practice: Palliative Care. London, England: BMJ; 2008.

44. Achterberg TV, Schoonhoven L, Grol R. nursing implementation science: How evidence-based nursing requires evidence-based implementation. J Nurs Scholar. 2008;*40*(4):302–310.

45. Center for Gerontology and Health Care Research, Brown Medical School. 2004. Choosing an instrument. Providence, RI: Brown Medical School. Available at http://as800.chcr.brown.edu/pcoc/Choosing.htm#Toolkit%20as%20Resource. Accessed September 26, 2013.

46. Teno JM, Clarridge BR, Casey V, Welch LC, Wetle T, Shield R, Mor V. Family perspectives on end-of-life care at the last place of care. In: Meier DE, Isaacs SL, Hughes RG. Palliative Care: Transforming the Care of Serious Illness. San Francisco: Jossey-Bass; 2009.

47. Higginson J. Clinical and organizational audit and quality improvement in palliative medicine. In: Hanks G, Cherny NI, Christakis NA, Fallon M, Kaasa S, Portenoy RK. Oxford Textbook of Palliative Medicine (4th ed). Oxford, England: Oxford University Press; 2011.

48. Hearn J, Higginson IJ. Development and validation of a core outcome measure for palliative care: The palliative care outcome scale. Palliative Care Core Audit Project Advisory Group. Qual Health Care. 1999;*8*(4):219–227.

49. Aoun S, Bird S, Kristjanson LJ, Currow D. Reliability testing of the FAMCARE-2 scale: Measuring family carer satisfaction with palliative care. Palliat Med. 2010;*24* (7):674–681.

50. Casarett D, Pickard A, Bailey FA, et al. A nationwide VA palliative care quality measure: The family assessment of treatment at the end of life. J Palliat Med. 2008;*11*(1):68–75.

51. Kornblith A. Outcomes research in palliative care. Newsletter, Department of Pain Medicine and Palliative Care. 1999;*2*: 1–2. New York, NY: Beth Israel Medical Center.

52. Chang VT, Hwang SS, Kasimis B, Thaler HT. Shorter symptom assessment instruments: The Condensed Memorial Symptom Assessment Scale (CMSAS). Cancer Invest. 2004;*22*(4):526–536.

53. Pasero C, McCaffery M. Pain Assessment and Pharmacologic Management (1st ed). St. Louis, MO: Mosby; 2010.

54. Duggleby WD, Williams A, Holstlander L, et al. Evaluation of the living with hope program for rural women caregivers of persons with advanced cancer. BMC Palliat Care. 2013;*12*:36.

55. Graves ML, Sun V. Providing quality wound care at the end of life. J Hosp Palliat Nurs. 2013;*15*(2):66–74.

56. Matzo ML Sherman DW. Palliative Care Nursing: Quality Care to the End of Life (3rd ed). New York, NY: Springer; 2009.

57. Hospice and Palliative Nurses Association (HPNA). 2013. Core curriculum for the advanced practice hospice and palliative registered nurse (2nd ed). Pittsburgh, PA: HPNA. Available at http://hpna.org/Item_Details.aspx?ItemNo=978-1-934654-31-6. Accessed September 26, 2013.

58. Prem V, Karvannan H, Kumar SP, Karthikbabu S, Syed N, Sisodia V, Jaykumar S. Study of nurses' knowledge about palliative care: A quantitative cross-sectional survey. Ind J Palliat Care. 2012;*18*(2):122–127.

59. Ferrell BR, Coyle N. The nature of suffering and the goals of nursing. Oncol Nurs Forum. 2008;*35*(2):241–247.

60. Ferrell BR, Grant M, Sum V. Nursing research. In: Ferrell BR, Coyle N. Oxford Textbook of Palliative Nursing (3rd ed). Oxford, England: Oxford University Press; 2010.

61. Hospice and Palliative Nurses Association (HPNA). 2013. HPNA research agenda for 2012–2015. Pittsburgh, PA: HPNA. Available at http://www.hpna.org/DisplayPage.aspx?Title=Research. Accessed September 26, 2013.

62. The National Institute of Nursing Research (NINR). 2012. Research and funding: Spotlight on end-of-life research. Bethesda, MD: NINR. Available at http://www.ninr.nih.gov/researchandfunding/spotlight-on-end-of-life-research. Accessed September 26, 2013.

63. Chan R, Webster J. End-of-life care pathways for improving outcomes in caring for the dying. Cochr Datab Syst Rev, 2010; Issue 1. Art. No.: CD008006. doi: 10.1002/14651858.CD008006.pub2.

64. Gries CJ, Curtis JR, Wall RJ, Engelberg RA. Family member satisfaction with end-of-life decision making in the ICU. Chest. 2008;*133*(3):704–712.

65. Bookbinder M, McHugh M. Symptom management: A systematic review in palliative care and end-of-life care. Nurs Clin N Amer. 2010;*45* (3), 271–327.

66. Smith EM, Bakitas MA, Homel P, et al. Preliminary assessment of a neuropathic pain treatment and referral algorithm for patients with cancer. J Pain Symp Manage. 2011;*42*(6):822–838.

67. Bookbinder M, Glajchen M, McHugh M, et al. Nurse practitioner based models of specialist palliative care at home: Sustainability and evaluation of feasibility. J Pain Symp Manage 2010;*23*(8):544–551.

68. Gordon DB, Polomano RC, Pellino TA, et al. Revised American Pain Society Patient Outcome Questionnaire (APS-POQ-R) for quality improvement of pain management in hospitalized adults: Preliminary psychometric evaluation. J Pain. 2010;*11*(11):1172–1186.

69. Hospice and Palliative Nurses Association (HPNA). 2013. Nursing fellowships: Description of seven fellowship programs. Pittsburgh, PA: HPNA. Available at http://www.hpna.org/DisplayPage.aspx?Title=Nursing%20Fellowships. Accessed September 26, 2013.

*F*ind *a process to improve.*

Set the boundaries by defining the beginning and end points of the process.

Opportunity statement
An opportunity exists to improve EOL care for the imminently dying inpatient,
(Name the process.)
beginning with a physicians' order for the Palliative Care for Advanced Disease care path
ending with death or discharge to homecare, hospice, or residential facility.
(Set boundaries.)
This effort should improve patient comfort and family satisfaction with EOL care
(Name outcome measure)
for hospitalized oncology, geriatric, hospice, and intensive care unit patients.
(Name the customers.)

The process is important to work on now because good EOL care is an institutional priority, no
benchmarks are currently available in the US, and no standard approach is used at BIMC* to
assess and treat patients who are imminently dying.
(State significance.)

*O*rganize *to improve the process.*

Form a multidisciplinary CQI team; establish roles, rules, and meeting times.

Multidisciplinary Team (22 members)
Department of Pain Medicine and Palliative Care
MDs, nurses, social workers, psychologist, chaplain
Hospital departments
Ethics
Pediatrics
Nutrition
Quality improvement
Pharmacy
Outcomes measurement (research grants and contracts)
Pilot units (Oncology, Geriatrics, Intensive Care, Hospice)
Nurse managers, case managers, clinical nurse specialists

_____

* BIMC: Beth Israel Medical Center

Figure 44A.1 The FOCUS portion of the FOCUS-PDCA cycle. Source: Continuum Health Partners, Inc., Beth Israel Medical Center, Department of Pain Medicine and Palliative Care. Palliative Care for Advanced Disease (PCAD) Care Path. (CQI Team on End-of-Life Care), NY. Available at http://www.stoppain.org. Accessed November 30, 2013.

C *larify what is known.*

**FLOWCHART OF PALLIATIVE CARE FOR
ADVANCED DISEASE (PCAD) CARE PATH**

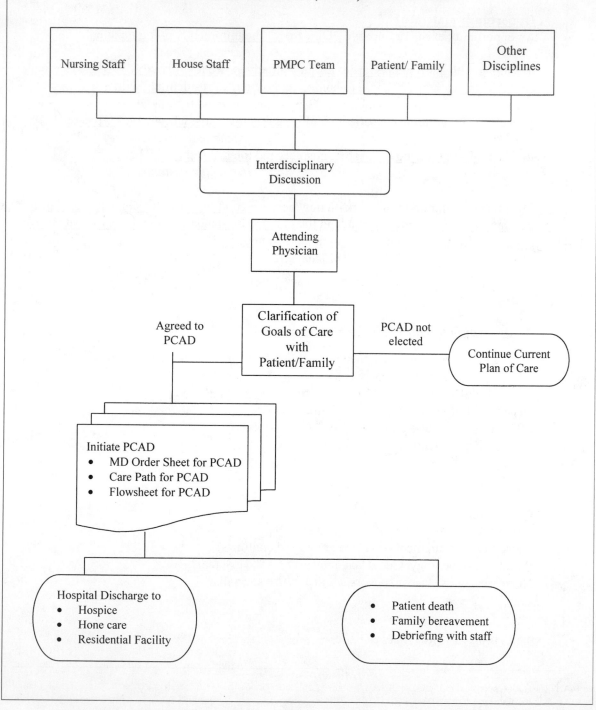

Understand the variation

Brainstorm with those at the grass roots level about why the process varies. Categorize sources of variation by people, materials, methods, and equipment. Display data using a cause-and-effect diagram.

Brainstorming Session with CQI Team on End-of-life (EOL) Care Question:
What barriers could be encountered in implementing an EOL Pathway at BIMC?

EOL awareness/ discomfort/readiness:
> What is "end-of-life care?" When is treatment palliative vs. life ending? How do we choose?
> Patient, family, readiness/awareness of dying
> Physician, family, patient willingness to acknowledge that death is imminent
> Issues of truth telling: family may not know status of patient prior to the pathway
> Physician discomfort with stopping treatment
> Medical uncertainty about when to stop treatment

Team communication:
> Physician and nurse discomfort in discussing change in treatment strategy
> Is it the physician's decision alone? The heath care team as a whole needs to be acknowledged in decision.
> Definition of terms. Need to define who the team is. May need a new model.
> Nurses' comfort—may be put in the middle of team/family attending and decisions.

Unit resistance:
> Resistance of unit teams. May see this project as "another thing to do."
> Large-scale resistance. Some may not see that there is something to "fix."
> Organizational pressure to discharge quickly.

Knowledge deficit:
> Assumptions about pastoral care (patient, family, staff) and what the experience will be.
> Knowledge deficit about medical and nursing interventions
> How to implement the care path and encourage people to speak up front rather than later
> Large cultural diversity at BIMC
> Education needed about biomedical analysis and ethical problems
> Physician/patient and physician/family communication skills

Cause and Effect (Ishikawa) Diagram (Barriers to implementing PCAD)—Themes above

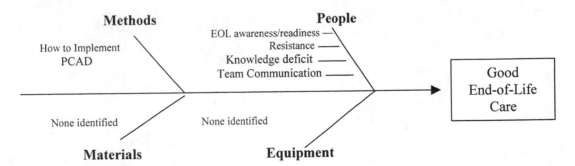

Select the process improvement.

Describe the new intervention in detail. Palliative Care for Advanced Disease (PCAD) Care Path: Care Path, Flow Sheet, and Physicians' Order Sheet **(see following pages)**

BETH ISRAEL HEALTH CARE SYSTEM

☐ PETRIE DIVISION   ☐ NORTH DIVISION   ☐ KINGS HWY DIVISION

Care Path: *PALLIATIVE CARE for ADVANCED DISEASE*

PLAN:	PRE-ADMISSION CONSIDERATION/ ADMISSION CRITERIA	DISCHARGE OUTCOMES	STAMP ADDRESSOGRAPH NAME OF SERVICE/ATTENDING/ HOUSE MD

	☐ Disease at Advanced Stage – limited life expectancy
	
	☐ HCP: Agent _____
	☐ DNR
	☐ Primary Caregiver _____
	☐ Next of Kin
		☐ Discharge to Community:
		  _ Hospice _ Home Care
		  _ Alternative Care Facility _ Home
		  or
		☐ Patient expired/Bereavement resources provided to family	

	START DATE:		ONGOING DAYS:

TREATMENTS/ INTERVENTIONS/ ASSESSMENTS	1) CLARIFY GOALS OF PALLIATIVE CARE FOR ADVANCED DISEASE (PCAD) WITH PATIENT AND/OR FAMILY
	2) FACILITATE DISCUSSION & DOCUMENTATION OF ADVANCE DIRECTIVES:
	Identify designated individuals & roles in decision-making:
	  1) Health Care Agent 3) Primary Caregiver
	  2) Durable Power of Attorney 4) Next-of-kin
	Identify patient/family preferences regarding:
	  • Health Care Proxy • Resuscitation Status/DNR
	  • Living Will
	3) INITIATE PHYSICIAN ORDER SHEET/REVIEW DAILY
	4) COMFORT ASSESSMENT to include
	  • Pain and symptom management needs
	  • Psychosocial coping, anticipatory grieving, and social/cultural needs
	  • Spiritual issues and distress
	5) VS – None unless useful in promoting pt/family comfort
	6) ASSESS FOR AND PROVIDE ENVIRONMENT CONDUCIVE TO MEET PATIENT & FAMILY NEEDS
			REPEAT CARE PATH DAILY
			
			DOCUMENT IN:
			DAILY PATIENT CARE FLOW SHEET
			PROGRESS NOTES

PAIN MANAGEMENT	1) ASSESS PAIN Q 4 HR and evaluate within 1 hr post intervention. Complete pain assessment scale. Anticipate pain needs.		
TESTS/PROCEDURES	1) USUALLY UNNECESSARY for patient/family comfort (All lab work and diagnostic work is discouraged)		
MEDICATIONS	1) Medication regimen focus is the RELIEF OF DISTRESSING SYMPTOMS.		

FLUIDS/NUTRITION	1) DIET: Selective diet with no restrictions
	  • Nutrition to be guided by patient's choice of time, place, quantities and type of food desired. Family may provide food.
	  • Educate family in nutritional needs of dying patient
	2) IVs for symptom management only
	3) TRANSFUSIONS for symptom relief only
	4) INTAKE AND OUTPUT – consider goals of care relative to patient comfort
	5) WEIGHTS – consider risks/benefits relative to patient comfort		

©Continuum Health Partners, Inc., Department of Pain Medicine & Palliative Care 1999

Figure 44A.2 A Care Path—the interdisciplinary plan of care. Source: Continuum Health Partners, Inc., Beth Israel Medical Center, Department of Pain Medicine and Palliative Care. Palliative Care for Advanced Disease (PCAD) Care Path. (CQI Team on End-of-Life Care), NY. Available at http://www.stoppain.org. Accessed November 30, 2013.

		REPEAT CARE PATH DAILY DOCUMENT IN: DAILY PATIENT CARE FLOW SHEET PROGRESS NOTES	
ACTIVITY	1) ACTIVITY DETERMINED BY PATIENT'S PREFERENCES AND ABILITY. Patient determines participation in ADLs; i.e., turning and positioning, bathing, transfers		
CONSULTS	1) INITIATE referrals to institutional specialists to optimize comfort and enhance quality of life (QOL) only.		

PSYCHOSOCIAL NEEDS	1) PSYCHOSOCIAL COMFORT ASSESSMENT of:
	  • Patient
	  • Primary caregiver
	  • Grieving process of patient & family
	
	2) PSYCHOSOCIAL SUPPORT: Referral to Social Work
	  • Offer emotional support
	  • Support verbalization and anticipatory grieving
	  • Encourage family caring activities as appropriate/individualized to family situation and culture
	  • Facilitate verbal and tactile communication
	  • Assist family with nutrition, transportation, child care, financial, funeral issues
	  • Assess bereavement needs		

SPIRITUAL NEEDS	1) SPIRITUAL COMFORT ASSESSMENT
	  • Spiritual supports
	  • Spiritual needs and/or distress
	
	2) SPIRITUAL SUPPORT: Referral to Chaplain
	  • Provide opportunity for expression of beliefs, fears, and hopes
	  • Provide access to religious resources
	  • Facilitate religious practices		

PATIENT/FAMILY EDUCATION	1) ASSESS NEEDS AND PROVIDE EDUCATION REGARDING:
	  • Goals of Palliative Care for Advanced Disease
	  • Physical and psychosocial needs during the dying process
	  • Coping techniques/Relaxation techniques
	  • Bereavement process and resources		

DISCHARGE PLANNING	1) FOR DISCHARGE TO COMMUNITY: Referral to Pain Medicine & Palliative Care/ Hospice/Home Care/Social Work as needed.
	
	2) AT TIME OF DEATH:
	  • Post Mortem care observing cultural and religious practices and preferences
	  • Provide for care of patient's possessions as per family wishes
	  • Bereavement support for family and staff		

©Continuum Health Partners, Inc., Department of Pain Medicine & Palliative Care 1999

This document is to be used as a guideline only. Each case should be evaluated and treated individually based upon clinical findings.

Beth Israel Health Care System
Carepath: Palliative Care for Advanced Disease
DAILY PATIENT CARE FLOW SHEET

ADDRESSOGRAPH

DATE:

☐ DNR	☐ NO DNR	☐ HCP	☐ NO HCP	HCP AGENT:	CAREGIVER:

COMFORT ASSESSMENT: Comfort Level Patient states or appears to be
1. Always comfortable   2. Usually comfortable   3. Sometimes comfortable   4. Seldom comfortable   5. Never comfortable

TIME (per MD order)									
PATIENT Comfort Level (Indicate number)									

VITAL SIGNS ONLY AS ORDERED	T									
	P									
	R									
	BP									

P A I N	TIME										PAIN/RELIEF SCALE KEY		SEDATION SCALE
	LOCATION										NONE ◄————► WORST		0 Alert
													1 Awake but drowsy
	PAIN RATING										0 1 2 3 4 5 6 7 8 9 10		2 Drowsy/Easily awakened
													3 Sleeping/Easily awakened
	RELIEF/SEDATION										COMPLETE RELIEF NO RELIEF		4 Sleeping/Difficult to awaken
													5 Unarousable

* See Progress Note   A = Assessment   I = Intervention   Check mark = present or done   * Needs MD Order

		Time							Time							Time			
E Y E S	A	Moist/Clear				**B R E A T H I N G**	A	**Rate:** Normal				**N U T R I T I O N**	A	Full meal			
		Inflamed						Rapid						> 50%			
		Dry/Crusted						Slow						< 50%			
								Rhythm: Reg						Refused			
								Irregular						Nausea/vomiting			
	I	Routine Care						**Depth:** Normal						NPO			
		_Artificial Tears						Shallow						Dysphagia			
		_Oint/Lubricant						Labored									
								Secretions: None									
								Mild					I	Diet as tolerated			
L I P S	A	Smooth/moist						Copious						NG/G tube			
		Dry/Cracked						**Breath sounds:**						Enteral feeding			
		Ulcerated						Clear						Feeding set changed			
								Diminished						Residual vol-cc's			
								Absent						Placement check			
	I	Routine Care						Crackles						Meds as ordered			
		Topical Lubricant						Wheeze									
								Dyspnea				**I V L I N E S**	A	IV site			
														No S&S infil/phleb			
M O U T H	A	Moist												Dry & intact			
		Dry					I	None									
		Coated						Reposition					I	IV Dsg change			
		Stomatitis						_O2 via__@__lpm						IV Tubing change			
								Suctioning q__						See progress note			
								Trach Care						Cap Change			
	I	Routine Care						Elevate HOB						Huber needle change			
		*Artificial Saliva						Fan									
		_Magic Wash						Meds as ordered									
		Meds as ordered															

Figure 44A.3 A Daily Patient Care Flow Sheet for documentation of assessments and interventions (including automatic referrals to social work and chaplaincy). Source: Continuum Health Partners, Inc., Beth Israel Medical Center, Department of Pain Medicine and Palliative Care. Palliative Care for Advanced Disease (PCAD) Care Path. (CQI Team on End-of-Life Care), NY. Available at http://www.stoppain.org. Accessed November 30, 2013.

		Time						Time							Time			
M	A	Bedbound				**S**	A	Normal				**F**	A		Engaged w pt			
O		OOB Chair				**L**		Interrupted Cycle				**A**			Coping w loss			
B		Amb w Assist				**E**		Insomnia				**M**			Distressed			
I		OOB ad lib				**E**						**I**						
L		BR Privileges				**P**	I	Modify Environment				**L**						
I	I	T&P per pt comfort						Relaxation				**Y**	I		Goals of care reviewed			
T		ROM q						Meds as order							Encourage verbal			
Y		Assistive Device													& non-verbal			
		__Ted Stocking(s)				**P**	A	Awake/alert							communication w pt			
		Side Rails Up				**S**		Responds to voice							Family Meeting			
E	A	Voiding qs				**Y**		Resp to tactile stim							Bereavement			
L		Anuria				**C**		Unresponsive							support			
I		Incontinent Urine				**H**		Oriented										
M		Bowel Movement				**O**		Confused										
I		Incontinent Feces				**S**		Hallucinating										
N		Diarrhea				**O**		Calm										
A		Constipation				**C**		Anxiety				**M**			AM Care			
T						**I**		Agitated				**I**			PM Care			
I	I	__Foley Catheter				**A**		Depression				**S**			PresUlcer Prev Plan			
O		Texas Catheter				**L**		Spiritual distress				**C**			Fall Prev Plan			
N		Inc't Pads										**E**			Precautions:			
		__Enema					I	Emotional support				**L**			Isolation:			
		Meds as ordered						Verbal/tactile				**L**			Siderails Up			
								stimulation				**A**			ID Bracelet			
								Social Worker visit				**N**			Allergy Bracelet			
S	A	Normal/Intact						**Chaplain visit**				**E**			DNR Bracelet			
K		Feverish										**O**			Post Mortem care			
I		Diaphoretic										**U**						
N		Pressure Ulcer Stg___										**S**						
		Ostomy site D/I																
		Edema				Comments/Progress Notes												
		Pruritis																
		Cool/Mottled																
W	I	Site																
O		Dressing_____																
U		Dry & Intact																
N		Drain_____																
D		Drainage																
		Odor																
C		Ostomy site care																
A		Tube site care																
R																		
E																		

PATIENT/FAMILY EDUCATION: **See IPFER**

PCAD Care Path: **Initiated**   **Reviewed/Continue With Plan Of Care**   ☐ **Revised (See Progress Note)**

OTHER NURSING DOCUMENTATION:
☐ **I & O SHEET**   ☐ **RESTRAINT FLOW SHEET**   ☐ **NEURO-ASSESSMENT**   ☐ **OTHER**_____

SIGNATURE/TITLE	DATE	SHIFT	INITIALS	SIGNATURE/TITLE	DATE	SHIFT	INITIALS
1.				6.			
2.				7.			
3.				8.			
4.				9.			
5.				10.			

©Continuum Health Partners, Inc., Department of Pain Medicine & Palliative Care 1999

Beth Israel Health Care System
DOCTOR'S ORDER SHEET
PALLIATIVE CARE FOR ADVANCED DISEASE

ADMISSION HT_____   ADMISSION WEIGHT_____

ORDERS OTHER THAN MEDICATION/INFUSION	MEDICATION/INFUSION (Specify route & directions)
1 Primary Diagnosis:	1. Assess patient for the following symptoms:
2 Activate PCAD Care Path	
3 Anticipated time on PCAD Care Path: ___ hours ___days ___weeks ___unknown	
4 Allergies:	
5 Diet: ☐ No restrictions (food may be provided by caregiver) ☐ NPO ☐ Other:	
6 Activity: ☐ OOB as tolerated ☐ OOB with assistance	
7 Vital Signs: ☐ Discontinue ☐ Daily ☐ q shift ☐ q ___hours	
8 Comfort Assessment: ☐q ___ hr ☐q 2 hr ☐q 4 hr ☐q shift	

Assess patient symptoms list:

Anxiety & Insomnia   Hiccups
Confusion/Agitation   Nausea/Vomiting
Constipation   Pain
Depressed Mood   Pruritis
Diarrhea   Stomatitis
Dyspnea   Terminal Secretions
Fever   (Noisy Respirations)

See reverse side for suggestions for pain management and symptom control

2. DISCONTINUE ALL PREVIOUS MED ORDERS

3. ORDERS:

9 Weight: ☐ None   ☐ q ____ day(s)

10 I & O: ☐ None   q _____

11 Visiting: ☐ Open visiting, nurse-restrictions apply
☐ Per routine policy
☐ Other:

12 DNR: ☐ Yes   ☐ No

13 PCAD Care Path will include (specify if otherwise):
Psychosocial Care – Social Work Referral
Spiritual Care – Chaplaincy Referral

14 Consults:
☐ Pain Medicine & Palliative Care Consult
☐ Ethics Consult
☐ Hospice Consult
☐ Other:

15 Labs: ☐ Discontinue all previous standing orders
☐ Continue previous lab orders
☐ Other labs:

16 Oxygen Therapy: _____ L/min via_____

17 Other orders:

CLERK	DATE	TIME	NURSE'S SIGNATURE	PRESCRIBER'S SIGNATURE	ID#	DATE	TIME

©Continuum Health Partners, Inc., Department of Pain Medicine & Palliative Care 1999

Figure 44A.4 A standardized Physician Order Sheet, with suggestions for medical management of 15 symptoms prevalent at the end of life. Source: Continuum Health Partners, Inc., Beth Israel Medical Center, Department of Pain Medicine and Palliative Care. Palliative Care for Advanced Disease (PCAD) Care Path. (CQI Team on End-of-Life Care), NY. Available at http://www.stoppain.org. Accessed November 30, 2013.

The following are medications for consideration in treating pain and symptoms of patients on PCAD:

PAIN MANAGEMENT
For Opioid-Naïve Patient:
Morphine Sulfate 15 mg po or 5 mg SQ/IV.
Repeat q 1 hr until pain relief is adequate. Begin Morphine Sulfate 30 mg po or 10 mg SQ/IV q 4 hr ATC or begin IV Morphine Sulfate basal infusion at 2 mg per hour and 2 mg SQ/IV q 1 hr prn.

For Opioid-Treated Patient:
If pain uncontrolled, increase fixed schedule dose by 50%.

Many non-opioid analgesics are available and should be considered after opioid therapy has been optimized. If pain remains uncontrolled, consider consult to Department of Pain Medicine and Palliative Care (Beeper #6702).

ANXIETY & INSOMNIA
Lorazepam 0.5mg po/SQ/IV BID-TID q HS for anxiety.
Temazepam 15 – 30 mg po q HS for anxiety/ insomnia.
Clonazepam 0.5 – 2 mg po BID-TID for anxiety/myoclonus.

CONFUSION/AGITATION
Haloperidol 0.5 mg po/SQ/IV. Repeat q 30 minutes until symptom intensity declines.
Haloperidol 0.5 – 5 mg po/SQ/IV q 4 hr prn.

CONSTIPATION
Lactulose 30 ml po q 2 hr prn until constipation relieved.
When symptom improves, begin Lactulose 30 ml po q 12 hr.
Warm Fleets Enema TIW prn

To prevent constipation:
Senokot 1 – 2 tabs po BID and
Colace 1 – 2 tabs po BID.

SYMPTOMS OF DEPRESSION
If anticipated survival is in weeks:
Begin SSRI, e.g., Paroxetine 20 mg po daily, and titrate to effect.

If anticipated survival is in days:
Methylphenidate 2.5 mg po q morning and at noon and escalate daily to 5 – 10 mg po q morning and at noon or Pemoline 18.75 mg po q morning and at noon and escalate daily to 37.5 mg po q morning and at noon.
Higher doses may be needed.

Consider Liaison Psychiatry consultation

DIARRHEA
Loperamide 4 mg po q 4 hr prn

DYSPNEA
For Opioid-Naïve Patient:
Morphine Sulfate 5 – 15 mg po or 2 – 5 mg SQ/IV. Repeat q 1 hr, if needed. When symptom is improved, begin Morphine Sulfate 30 mg po or 10 mg SQ/IV q 4 hr ATC; or begin Morphine Sulfate basal infusion at 2 mg per hour and 2 mg SQ/IV q 1 hr prn.

For Opioid-Treated Patient:
If dyspnea uncontrolled, increase fixed schedule dose by 50%.
If breathlessness continues, add Lorazepam 0.5mg po or SQ/IV prn. Repeat q 60 minutes if needed until symptom intensity declines, then begin 1 mg po/SQ/IV q 3 hr.

Additional therapies may include:
Dexamethasone 16 mg po/IV, followed by 4 mg po/IV q 6 hr
Albuterol 2.5 mg via nebulization q 4 hr prn if wheezing present

FEVER
Acetaminophen 650 mg po/PR q 4 hr prn, and/or
Dexamethasone 1.0 mg po/SQ/IV q 12 hr prn

HICCUPS
Chlorpromazine 10 – 25 mg po/IM TID prn
Haloperidol 0.5 – 2 mg po/SQ/IV TID – QID

INTRACTABLE SYMPTOMS, MANAGEMENT OF
Consider referral to Department of Pain Medicine & Palliative Care (Beeper # 6702).

IV HYDRATION
Consider decreasing IV rate to 0.5 – 1 liter/24 hr

NAUSEA/VOMITING
Metoclopromide 10 mg po/IV q 4 hr prn, or
Prochlorperazine 10 mg po/IV q 4 hr or 25 mg PR q 8 hr prn with or without Dexamethasone 4 mg po/IVPB q 6 hr

PRURITIS
Diphenhydramine 25 – 50 mg po/IV q 12 hr
Hydrocortisone 1 % cream to affected areas q 6 hr
Dexamethasone 1.0 mg po daily alone or in combination with above

STOMATITIS
Viscous lidocaine 2 % to painful areas prn
Clotrimazole 10 mg troche 5 times daily
Nystatin S & S q 6 hr prn
Magic Mouthwash prn

TERMINAL SECRETIONS (NOISY RESPIRATIONS)
Scopolamine patches 1.5 – 3 mg 72 hr, or
Scopolamine 0.4 mg SQ q 4 – 6 hr

PLAN—DO—CHECK—ACT (the Shewhart cycle)

lan

Create a timeline of resources, activities, training, and target dates. Develop a data collection plan, the tools for measuring outcomes, and thresholds for determining when targets have been met.

Timeline for One-Year Pilot CQI EOL Project

Phase 0 – Planning

Jan – June

Formalize CQI Team for the development of a clinical pathway.
Clarify knowledge of processes: review literature and existing data sources, conduct brainstorming, flowcharting with pilot units.
Evaluate and synthesize literature, tools, other data gathered.
Identify content for Care Path.
Develop and pilot audit tool for chart reviews.
Create database, codebook, and scoring guidelines for data entry.
Identify patient outcome assessment tools.
Identify family outcome assessment tools.
Identify staff assessment tools.
Refine study tools/procedures.
Develop staff education.
Develop caregiver educational materials.

June 21   Medical Records review

Aug 2   Tools Committee review

July 3   Committee on Scientific OSA Application and Approval

Phase I – Launching the Project

August 2   Meet with hospital leadership—Introduction to Palliative
                 Care for Advanced Disease Care Path
                 • PCAD Care Path, MD Orders, and Flow sheet
                 • Timeline for Education/Evaluation

August 11   Introduction of PCAD Care Path to medical staff

Figure 44A.5 The PDCA portion of the FOCUS-PDCA cycle. Source: Continuum Health Partners, Inc., Beth Israel Medical Center, Department of Pain Medicine and Palliative Care. Palliative Care for Advanced Disease (PCAD) Care Path. (CQI Team on End-of-Life Care), NY. Available at http://www.stoppain.org. Accessed November 30, 2013.

Phase II – Unit Implementation and Education of PCAD Care Path

	Cohort 1	Cohort 2		Cohort 3
• Meet with unit leaders of pilot units	June 21	September 15	July 21	October 11
• Pre-test	August 23–25	September 27	September 14	TBS
• Unit leadership team meeting	TBS	October 5	October 12	TBS
• Introduction of PCAD Care Path to unit staff	August 31–September 1	September 27–September 30	October 22	TBS
• In-service of unit staff	September 1 September 2 September 3	October 4–October 6	October 25–October 26	TBS TBS TBS
• Rollout of Care Path	September 6	October 11	November 1	TBS
• Brainstorming—educational needs	October 11	November 8	December 13	December 6
• Educational series	September–February	October– March	November–April	November–April
• Focus groups	October & January	November & February	December & March	December & March
• Feedback / closure / continuation	March	April	May	May
• Post-test	March	April	May	May

Phase III – Evaluation

Chart Reviews using Chart Audit Tool (CAT) (Total =330)

June–Aug	• 20 retrospective audits for 5 pilot units	(Total = 100)
Sep 1999–Mar 2002	• 20 retrospective audits for 2 control units	(Total = 40)
	• 10 during implementation audits for 5 pilot units	(Total = 50)
	• 20 post implementation audits for 5 pilot units	(Total = 100)
	• 20 post implementation audits for 2 control units	(Total = 40)
	Each patient on PCAD Care Path as admitted.	
Sep 1999–Mar 2002	Tool: Teno's After Death (interview or mailed survey)	
Dates TBD	Staff survey post-tests (4 mo post-initiation of PCAD) Tool: Palliative Care Quiz	
Sep 1999–Mar 2002	Process Audits (PAT) Ongoing throughout time patient on PCAD Care Path	
Sep 1999–Mar 2002	Brainstorming sessions and focus groups with staff to identify education 1–2 mo after each unit begins PCAD	

Phase IV – Reporting

April 15, 2002	Report to grant agency, hospital, and unit staff

D_o

Collect data and monitor the intervention until fully implemented.

Palliative Care Quiz for Nurses (PCQN)

Name: _____

Background Information:

Department/ Service

1. Nursing   2. Social work
3. Medicine   4. Pharmacy
5. Surgery   6. Chaplaincy
7. Critical care   8. Other (describe)

Unit: _____

Age: _____

Sex:
1. Male
2. Female

Years of experience in discipline:
1. 0–5
2. 6–10
3. >10

Educational preparation:
1. HS diploma
2. Associate degree
3. Baccalaureate degree
4. Masters' degree
5. Postgraduate degree

Previous education/ training in palliative care:
1. No
2. Yes (describe) _____

_____

_____

_____

_____

_____

The 20-item survey that follows is used with permission. Ross, M. M., McDonald,B., & McGuinness, J. (1996). The palliative care quiz for nurses (PCQN): the development of an instrument to measure nurses' knowledge of palliative care. Journal of Advanced Nursing, 23:125-137.

Please circle your response to the items below using the following key:

T = True   **F = False**   **DK = Don't Know**

1. Palliative care is appropriate only in situations where there is evidence of a downhill trajectory or deterioration.   T   F   DK

2. Morphine is the standard used to compare the analgesic effect of other opioids.   T   F   DK

3. The extent of the disease determines the method of pain treatment.   T   F   DK

4. Adjuvant therapies are important in managing pain.   T   F   DK

5. It is crucial for family members to remain at the bedside until death occurs.   T   F   DK

6. During the last days of life, the drowsiness associated with electrolyte imbalance may decrease the need for sedation.   T   F   DK

7. Drug addiction is a major problem when morphine is used on a long-term basis for the management of pain.   T   F   DK

8. Individuals who are taking opioids should follow a bowel regime.   T   F   DK

9. The provision of palliative care requires emotional detachment.   T   F   DK

10. During the terminal stages of an illness, drugs that can cause respiratory depression are appropriate for the treatment of severe dyspnea.   T   F   DK

11. Men generally reconcile their grief more quickly than woman.   T   F   DK

12. The philosophy of palliative care is compatible with that of aggressive treatment.   T   F   DK

13. The use of placebos is appropriate in the treatment of some types of cancer pain.   T   F   DK

14. In high doses, codeine causes more nausea and vomiting than morphine.   T   F   DK

15. Suffering and physical pain are synonymous.   T   F   DK

16. Demerol is not an effective analgesic in the control of chronic pain.   T   F   DK

17. The accumulation of losses renders burnout inevitable for those who seek work in palliative care.   T   F   DK

18. Manifestations of chronic pain are different from those of acute pain.   T   F   DK

19. The loss of a distant or problematic relationship is easier to resolve than the loss of one that is close or intimate.   T   F   DK

20. The pain threshold is lowered by anxiety or fatigue.   T   F   DK

C_{heck}

Analyze findings, graph results, and evaluate reasons for variations. If targets are reached, set a date to stop or decrease the frequency of monitoring. Summarize what was learned.

Sample: Results of Palliative Care Knowledge Quiz, Preimplementation of PCAD

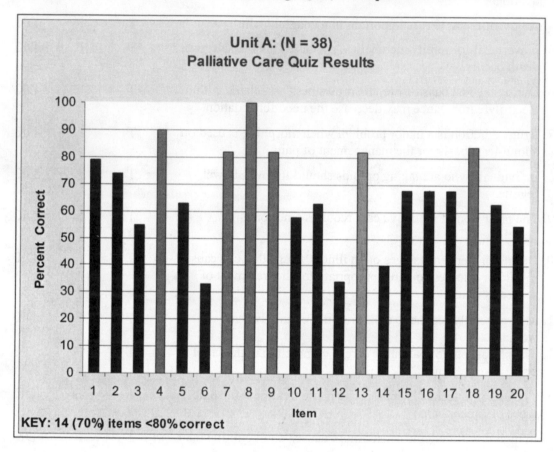

Unit A: (N = 38)
Palliative Care Quiz Results

Y-axis: Percent Correct
X-axis: Item

KEY: 14 (70%) items <80% correct

Act

Act on what is learned and determine the next steps. If successful, act to hold the gain achieved and work at making the intervention a part of standard operating procedure.. If not successful, analyze the sources of failure, design new solutions, and repeat the PDCA cycle.

Sample: Quarterly Reporting Form

BETH ISRAEL MEDICAL CENTER
PAIN MEDICINE AND PALLIATIVE CARE
QUALITY IMPROVEMENT STUDY REPORT

Title of Study: Improving End-of-Life Care

Date(s) of study:
1st Quarter ✓   2nd Quarter__   3rd Quarter__   4th Quarter __

Interdisciplinary Team: See listing of CQI Team members.

Sample: The Palliative Care Knowledge Quiz was given to all nursing staff preimplementation of the Palliative Care for Advanced Disease (PCAD) Care Path on three of five planned units thus far.

Findings: In this quarter, we report on the results of knowledge surveys. A total of 90 staff from three units has completed the survey thus far. Analyses have been completed on Unit A described below.

Analysis/interpretation: Unit A, above, is used to describe the process of providing feedback to staff. The threshold for competency was set for 80%. Fourteen of twenty items (70%) are targeted for improvement. No formal education has been given thus far. This data will be used to (a) measure change pre and post an educational series and use of the PCAD in practice, (b) determine levels of competency and targeted areas for continued education, and (c) to stimulate discussion and dialogue with the multidisciplinary team.

Conclusion: Continued education is needed to integrate palliative care principles into the mainstream of daily clinical practice.

Action Plan / Step 1: In-services are scheduled in Quarter 2, 2000. All survey answers will be shared. The Pain Medicine and Palliative Care team will lead a discussion, supported by research results, about the 14 items for which staff answered <80% correctly. Three content areas were identified: end-of-life issues, pain treatment and side effects, and philosophy of palliative care.
Step 2: Based on the dialogue and discussion, subsequent in-services using case-based teaching, will be scheduled. A post-test survey is planned following 6 months of implementation PCAD on each unit.

Follow-up plan: We will report progress at monthly CQI Team meetings. Next report will include chart audit results.

Beth Israel Medical Center-Department of Pain Medicine and Palliative Care

PALLIATIVE CARE CONSULTATION FORM

Patient's Name: _____   Date Completed: _____/_____/_____

Admission Date: _____/_____/_____   Chart # _____   Date of Follow-up: _____/_____/_____

Days from Admission: _____   Insurance: _____   Completed by: _____

I. <u>BACKGROUND</u>
1. Gender: [1] Male   [2] Female

2. Age: _____   Date of Birth: _____/_____/_____

3. Race/Ethnicity:[1] White-Non-Hispanic   [2] Black-Non-Hispanic   [3] Hispanic-White   [4] Hispanic-Black
               [5] Asian   [6] Other

4. Marital Status: [1] Single (*never married*) [2] Married (*living with partner*) [3] Separated [4] Divorced [5] Widowed

5. Household [*circle all that apply*]:   [1] Lives Alone [2] Spouse/Partner [3] Children [4] Parents [5] Other Relative

6. Religion: [1] Catholic [2] Protestant [3] Jewish [4] Muslim [5] Hindu [6] Other _____   [7] None

7. Language: [1] English as primary language [2] Other: _____, but can speak & understand English
   [3] Non-English speaking

8. Primary Medical Diagnosis: [1] _____
                               [2] _____
                               [3] _____

9. Where seen: [1] Inpatient-hospital   [2] Inpatient-nursing home   [3] Outpatient-office/clinic   [4] Home

10. Reason for consult: [1] Pain   [2] Other symptoms   [3] Management of imminent death   [4] Other _____

SECTIONS II – VII TO BE COMPLETED BY A MEDICAL HEALTH PROFESSIONAL MD/PA/RN

II. COGNITIVE STATUS

11. <u>COGNITIVE IMPAIRMENT</u>
   [1] Normal
   [2] Mild Impairment; some memory loss or cognitive disability, but does not interfere with functioning; some confusion or
       disorientation, but brief and resolves quickly
   [3] Moderate impairment; memory loss, confusion or disorientation interfering with functioning, but <u>no</u> interference with
       activities with daily living (ADL)
   [4] Severe impairment; confusion, delirium, memory loss interfering with ADL; frank mental retardation.
   [5] Comatose; vegetative state; not conscious

12. <u>DECISIONAL CAPACITY</u>
   [1] Normal – Has decisional capacity
   [2] Cognitively impaired, but has decisional capacity
   [3] Global incompetence, lacks decisional capacity

III. PATIENT SELF-DETERMINATION/ADVANCE DIRECTIVES
13. Circle all treatment preferences/advance directives, with <u>supporting documents</u>
   [1] Living will   [4] Court appointed guardian
   [2] Do not resuscitate (DNR)   [5] Patient chooses not to discuss
   [3] Health care proxy, durable power of attorney   [6] Don't know

   A. If no Health Care Proxy; Who would you like to speak for you if you were not able to speak for yourself?
      Name: _____ Phone #: _____

Figure 44A.6 Palliative Care Consultation Form. Source: Continuum Health Partners, Inc., Beth Israel Medical Center, Department of Pain Medicine and Palliative Care. Palliative Care for Advanced Disease (PCAD) Care Path. (CQI Team on End-of-Life Care), NY. Available at http://www.stoppain.org. Accessed November 30, 2013.

IV. COMMUNICATION

14. METHOD OF COMMUNICATION
    [1] Speaking [2] Language Barrier [3] Sign Language (*for hearing impaired*) [4] Writing Only [5] None

15. DEGREE OF INDEPENDENCE IN COMMUNICATING
    [1] Functional; independent with all aspects of communication (speaking, hearing, sight), with or without glasses, hearing aids, or communication devices
    [2] Moderate assist; communicates ¿ 50% of the time
    [3] Dependent; unable to communicate with others

V. PHYSICAL/ACTIVITY STATUS

16. PRESSURE ULCERS
    [1] None
    [2] Mild [Stage I/II]: Injury to skin, Partial loss of skin layers
    [3] Severe [Stage III/IV]: Deep craters in skin that extends down to but not through underlying fascia; breaks in skin exposing muscle or bone; extensive destruction, tissue necrosis, or damage to muscle, bone or supporting structures (e.g., tendons)

17. BOWEL AND BLADDER FUNCTION
    [1] Independent in bowel and bladder function, with full self-care, including ostomy/catheter, if present
    [2] *Not* incontinent, but some assistance needed in managing bathroom or bedpan or ostomy/catheter, if present
    [3] Rarely incontinent; requiring substantial assistance in managing bathroom or bedpan or ostomy/catheter, if present
    [4] Occasionally incontinent; requires full assistance in managing bathroom or bedpan or ostomy/catheter, if present
    [5] Fully incontinent or unable to assist in management of ostomy/catheter, if present
    [6] Don't know

18. PERFORMACE STATUS
    [0] Normal activity
    [1] Capable of all self-care, is ambulatory, but restricted in physicallythan 50% of waking hours strenuous activity, able to carry out work of a light or sedentary
    [2] Ambulatory, capable of all self-care activities, but unable to carry out any work activities; up and about more than 50% of waking hours
    [3] Capable of only limited self-care; confined to bed greater
    [4] Completely disabled; cannot carry on any self-care; nature (e.g., light housework, office work) totally confined to bed/chair

19. NUTRITIONAL INTAKE
    [1] Normal
    [2] Modified Independent; intake limited, need for modification unknown
    [3] Requires diet modification to swallow solid foods and liquids (puree, thickened fluids)
    [4] Combined oral and tube feeding
    [5] Tube feeding only
    [6] No oral intake (NPO) and no tube feeding

20. PRACTICAL SUPPORT WITH ESSENTIAL TASKS (e.g., cooking, cleaning, shopping)
    [1] Needs assistance in essential tasks which is not available
    [2] Needs assistance in essential tasks which is often unreliable or incomplete
    [3] Needs assistance in essential tasks which is sometimes inadequate or available only for less critical tasks such as banking
    [4] Needs assistance in essential tasks is usually available; assistance in less critical tasks is incomplete and unreliable; other responsibilities limit helper availability
    [5] Assistance is available and adequate for any need

VI. SOCIAL SUPPORT

21. The emotional support I have had from my family and friends has been:
    [1] As much as I wanted   [2] Very adequate   [3] Adequate   [4] Inadequate   [5] Very Inadequate

Beth Israel Medical Center-Department of Pain Medicine and Palliative Care

VII. SPIRITUALITY (*Skip if Patient is Globally Incompetent*)

22. How important is your religion or spiritual beliefs in your everyday life?
    [1] Not at all important   [2] A little   [3] Somewhat   [4] Important   [5] Very important

23. During your current illness, how much comfort and strength are you finding from your religion or spiritual beliefs?
    [1] None [2] A little [3] Some [4] A lot [5] Great strength/comfort [6] Not religious

NOTES:

_____

_____

_____

_____

_____

_____

SECTIONS VIII - IX TO BE COMPLETED BY PATIENT/FAMILY MEMBER OR HEALTH PROFESSIONAL

VIII. SYMPTOMS (*CMSAS-Condensed* Memorial Symptom Assessment Scale)
    If the patient has any of the following symptoms, how severe and distressing are they now?
    <u>Specify who is responding</u>: [1] Patient   [2] Family member, friend, other   [3] Health Care Professional

How much did this symptom bother or distress you in the past 7 days?

Symptom	Present	Not at all	A little Bit	Some what	Quite a bit	Very much
Lack of energy	Y N	0	1	2	3	4
Lack of appetite	Y N	0	1	2	3	4
Pain	Y N	0	1	2	3	4
Dry mouth	Y N	0	1	2	3	4
Weight Loss	Y N	0	1	2	3	4
Feeling drowsy	Y N	0	1	2	3	4
Shortness of breath	Y N	0	1	2	3	4
Constipation	Y N	0	1	2	3	4
Difficulty sleeping	Y N	0	1	2	3	4
Difficulty concentrating	Y N	0	1	2	3	4
Nausea	Y N	0	1	2	3	4

How frequently did these symptoms occur during the last week?

Symptom	Present	Rarely	Occasionally	Frequently	Almost constantly
Worrying	Y N	1	2	3	4
Feeling sad	Y N	1	2	3	4
Feeling nervous	Y N	1	2	3	4

References:
Kaasa, T, Loomis, J, Gillis, K Bruera, E, & Hanson, J. (1997) The Edmonton Functional Assessment Tool: preliminary Development and
    Evaluation for Use in Palliative Care. JPSM 13(1):10-19.
Coyle, N, Goldstein, M, Passik, S, Fishman, B & Portenoy, R. (1996). Development and validation of a patient needs assessment tool
    (PNAT) for oncology clinicians. Cancer Nursing. 19(2):81-92.
Oken, M.M, Creech, RH, Tormey, DC, Horton, J, Davis, TE, McFadden, & ET, Carbone, PP. (1982). Toxicity and Response Criteria Of the
    Eastern cooperative Oncology Group (ECOG). Am J Clin Oncol 5:649-655.
Chang, VT, Hwang, SS, Kasimis, B & Thaler, H. (2004). Shorter symptom assessment instruments: the Condensed Memorial Symptom
    Assessment Scale (CMSAS). Cancer Invest 22(4):526-36.
National Pressure Ulcer Advisory Panel Report. 1996. Pressure ulcer staging. Wound Ostomy and Continence Society. 4(3).

CHAPTER 45

Long-term care
Focus on nursing homes

Joan G. Carpenter and Mary Ersek

My mother's aunt was a widow and childless. Her health was failing and she could not take care of herself at home. Although she suffered from severe chronic back pain, her primary care provider was hesitant to treat her pain with medications, fearing that my great aunt would become dependent on the drugs and also be more likely to fall. Because of her frailty and health conditions, she reluctantly moved to a nursing home. From the first day, the nursing assistants made her feel at home, putting special photos of my late uncle on her bedside table and working with her to find her favorite foods for meals each day. The nurses talked to her about her pain and asked the facility's nurse practitioner to start stronger medicines to ease her discomfort. My great aunt was in the nursing home for about 2 years before she died. I visited her every Sunday and became close to many other residents and staff. Our family felt it was the best place for her care at the end of her life; she told us she did not want to die in a hospital. She had attentive staff, and family was encouraged to visit frequently.

Woman talking about her great aunt

Key points

◆ Over 25% of older adults and almost 70% of persons with advanced dementia live out their final days in nursing homes.

◆ While the number of hospice patients living in nursing homes has increased dramatically over the past decade, other comprehensive palliative care models have not been widely adopted or tested in nursing homes.

◆ Palliative care nurses play critical roles in collaborating with nursing home staff to enhance end-of-life care and outcomes for older persons.

Quality end-of-life (EOL) care in nursing homes is important. In 2009, over 3 million Americans lived in nursing homes.[1] More than half of these nursing home residents require extensive assistance, or are completely dependent in bathing, dressing, toileting, and transferring. Despite the efforts to keep frail elders in the community, the nursing home population is expected to increase as the numbers of older persons in the United States and other developed countries increase. As more people live in nursing homes, for short or long periods, many will also die there. Although nursing homes were not established as sites for end-of-life care, they are increasingly becoming the place where many people die.

Long-term care

Long-term care refers to a continuum of medical and other services addressing the health, personal care, and social service needs for persons who need help with activities of daily living as a result of functional impairment.[2] People of all ages receive long-term care. Services are often categorized as community-based or institutional, and may be provided in private homes, group homes, assisted living facilities, nursing homes, or day care centers. Since the late 1990s, there has been a movement to transition people receiving long-term care from nursing homes and into community settings. While this has resulted in many individuals living outside of facilities, the demand for high quality nursing home care continues and is expected to increase with the aging population.

Non-nursing-home residential long-term care settings

Assisted living facilities (ALFs) are residential settings that house people who need help coordinating day-to-day healthcare activities but do not need 24-hour skilled nursing care. Services in ALFs include meal preparation and planning, assistance with activities of daily living, medication monitoring and administration, and recreational activities. Residents in ALFs are more independent than nursing home residents; they typically need help with two activities of daily living.[3] Although individual state governments certify and regulate ALFs, there is much variation among states with regard to regulations, definitions, and Medicaid support.[4] Residents and/or their families pay most expenses, because, compared to nursing homes, there is relatively little state or federal government support for ALFs. Increasingly, ALFs are becoming a setting of end-of-life care. In 2010, the average stay in an ALF was approximately 28 months. According to the National Center for Assisted Living, 33% of those living in ALFs will die there, 59%

will move to a nursing facility for a higher level of care, and the others will move to another community setting or private home.[3] Research reveals that ALF staff feel confident caring for dying residents but may need assistance initiating EOL discussions.[5]

Continuing Care Retirement Communities (CCRCs) are for-profit or not-for-profit organizations that offer a full range of services for residents including independent living, assisted living, and nursing home care. These residences provide different levels of service in one location with a stepwise approach, as needed. For example, residents who experience physical or cognitive decline in a CCRC can receive additional ALF services such as assistance with medications and help with dressing. For postacute care or longer-term skilled nursing care, a resident can move to the CCRC's nursing home. There are many costs associated with living in a CCRC (e.g. entrance fees, buy-in fees, monthly fees, and services fees). Most costs are paid out-of-pocket. However, many facilities may require residents have Medicare coverage for skilled nursing care (if and when it is needed).

Group homes are small dwellings where residents with similar needs live and receive help with activities of daily living. Residents in group homes do not need 24-hour skilled nursing care. These facilities are not as strictly regulated as nursing homes and, like ALFs, often do not receive payments from Medicare or Medicaid programs.

Nursing homes

There are approximately 15,900 nursing homes in the United States.[1] All nursing homes provide 24-hour nursing care for residents. Many facilities provide short-term, rehabilitative care (also called skilled nursing care or postacute care) and/or long-term care. A nursing home that delivers skilled care is often referred to as a skilled nursing facility (SNF), and most are certified by Medicare. Skilled nursing facilities can be stand-alone facilities, part of an acute care hospital, or facilities within a larger campus. The purpose of an SNF is to provide a place for residents to receive intensive rehabilitation, usually after a hospitalization, for a period of days to several weeks, with a goal of returning to a more independent level of activity. Following rehabilitation, residents are discharged home or admitted to another care setting for long-term care if they are unable to return home. Some residents are transferred to another section of the same facility that is designated for long-term care.

Residents needing long-term care often receive restorative care designed to maintain their optimal level of function. Some nursing homes have specialty units for dementia care, which are often secured to prevent elopement. Staff is educated to care for people with cognitive impairment. Residents requiring long-term care often stay in this setting for the rest of their lives.

Nursing homes may be described as not-for-profit, for-profit, or government facilities. Not-for-profit and for-profit facilities may be privately owned and operated by a single owner or part of a large organization with several or hundreds of facilities (e.g., a "chain"). Government facilities include Veterans Affairs (VA) nursing homes, referred to as Community Living Centers (CLCs). These CLCs are contained on VA campuses and provide nursing home care for eligible veterans. There are 132 CLCs in the United States.[6] State veterans homes are nursing facilities for veterans that are owned and managed by individual state governments.

The VA does not operate state veterans homes; however, they do certify these facilities according to VA standards. All fifty states have a state veterans home.

In nongovernment homes, there are three sources of payment: private pay (i.e., directly paid for using the resident's financial assets or private long-term care insurance), Medicare, and Medicaid. Medicare pays for most short-term, skilled nursing care, while private pay and Medicaid covers most long-term care. As of 2009, 90% of nursing homes accepted both Medicare and Medicaid payment.[1] Long-term care residents are often obliged to exhaust their life savings (also called "spending down") and then apply for Medicaid in order to afford costs associated with nursing home care.

Up to 18% of nursing home costs are paid for by Medicare.[2] The national median daily rate for skilled nursing home care in 2013 was $207 for a semiprivate room and $230 for a private room, representing costs of almost $7000 per month. This is significantly less compared with the average monthly cost of care in an ALF ($3,450), as assisted living does not provide continuous nursing care.[7] Medicaid pays beneficiaries' costs associated with living in a nursing home and is the major payer for long-term nursing home care in the United States.

Although long-term care stakeholders are calling for increased number and type of community-based services, the majority of long-term care expenditures support nursing home short- and long-stay residents.[2] In 2007, close to 30% of adults greater than 65 years of age died in nursing homes.[8] It is estimated that by 2040, 40% to 50% of deaths will occur in long-term care settings.[8] Of those with advanced dementia, 67% die in nursing homes.[9] Much of the research about palliative care in long-term care facilities has been conducted in nursing homes.[10] For these reasons, the rest of the chapter focuses on this setting.

History and growth of nursing homes

Nursing homes have been described as the offspring of the almshouse and boarding house and the stepchild of the hospital.[11] In the mid-19th century, older people who were poor, sick, or disabled and without family support had few options other than the almshouse.[12] Private homes for the aged emerged as an alternative to public almshouses after the passage of the Social Security Act in the 1930s. Women who were caring for their ill family members at home took in other patients to help pay the bills. From these small homes, proprietary nursing homes evolved.

The growth of nursing homes from the 1930s to the 1960s was related to several key factors.[11,12] First, establishment of the Old Age Assistance (OAA) program in 1935 allowed a portion of the elderly to purchase long-term care services, although OAA payments were denied to those living in public institutions. As a result, many public facilities privatized and residents were permitted to receive OAA payments and purchase services. Second, the Hill-Burton Act was amended in 1954, granting federal support for construction of public institutions, including those that housed older adults unable to stay at home. Third, the American Association of Nursing Homes became a strong lobby for this new industry, and the federal government began to develop some standards for nursing homes. With the creation of Medicare and Medicaid in 1965, the "nursing home" became fully established.

In 1986, the Institute of Medicine published a report, titled "Improving the Quality of Care in Nursing Homes," that described many deficiencies in nursing home care and regulatory policies. In response, Congress passed the Omnibus Reconciliation Act of 1987 (OBRA-87). Contained in this bill was the Nursing Home Reform Act, which called for sweeping changes, including a focus on person-centered care and residents' quality of life.[13] Many providers, regulators, leaders, researchers, and advocates worked toward the recommendations and formed the Pioneer network in 1997, bringing together expertise, models, and other resources that embodied this "culture change."[13]

The nursing home environment

Residents

According to 2009 statistics, greater than 20% of the 5.6 million Americans 85 years and over received care in a nursing home.[1] Over 70% of nursing home residents are female. Half of residents need assistance with four activities of daily living, and the majority of older residents take nine or more medications.[14] Sixty-eight percent of residents have cognitive impairment,[1] and persons with dementia continue to use long-term care in higher numbers than other populations.[9]

Length of stay

The average length of stay in a nursing home is slightly over 2 years from admission to discharge, and over 50% of those over 65 years of age admitted to a nursing home stay for more than 1 year.[14] However, the average length of stay for nursing home decedents is 5 months.[15]

Interdisciplinary care team

Nursing home staff and providers form an interdisciplinary team (IDT), consisting of nursing administrators, directors of nursing, licensed nursing staff, certified nursing assistants, recreation therapists, and occupational and physical therapists. Other staff, such as dietary workers, environmental services personnel, and beauty shop employees, also play important roles because they are part of the resident's home.

Nursing assistants, also called direct care workers, represent over half of the staff in nursing homes; they provide personal care (e.g., bathing, grooming, toileting) and assist with activities of daily living.[14] Nursing assistants observe and report physical and psychosocial changes and problems to licensed nurses. Many nursing assistants have not completed high school, work for low pay, and receive few benefits. Because nursing assistants spend the most time with residents, they often see more death and dying than other staff and experience the accompanying grief.[16] In addition, nursing assistants have the least amount of formal training in EOL care, which may lead to job dissatisfaction and burnout.

The ratio of residents to licensed staff varies significantly from state to state, however all facilities certified by Medicare must adhere to federal guidelines for minimum licensed staffing standards. Minimum staffing standards include one registered nurse (RN) in the facility for 8 consecutive hours each day of the week (including weekends and holidays) and one RN or a licensed practical/vocational nurse (LPN/LVN) in the facility for the two remaining 8-hour shifts. Each state then sets a different standard for staffing within the federal guidelines.[17] Facilities need to adhere to set standards to avoid penalties and receive reimbursement from Medicare and Medicaid. There are no federal standards for the ratio of direct care workers (e.g., nursing assistants) to residents, and state requirements are wide ranging and vary depending on the state and the time of day. For example, in one state the day shift ratio of direct care workers to residents is 1:6, while in another state the ratio is 1:20 for all shifts.[18] Some states have no minimum direct care worker requirements, stipulating only that sufficient staff be onsite to meet the residents' needs. This results in inconsistency in quantity and quality of care delivery from one facility to another, since the leadership of each facility is at liberty to define for itself the meaning of "sufficient staffing."

Nurse practitioners (NPs), physician assistants (PAs), and physicians provide primary care for nursing home residents. The NPs and PAs are important to the quality and continuity of care, as physicians' visits are relatively infrequent, typically once a month for residents whose health and function are stable. The lack of physician involvement is a source of dissatisfaction for families who, in one study, referred to physicians as "missing in action."[19] This absence also makes licensed staff nurses responsible for communicating changes in a resident's condition to the primary care provider.

Models that enhance primary care in nursing homes, are effective at delivering more care to residents within the nursing home. Medicare managed care programs place primary care providers, usually NPs, in nursing homes to work collaboratively with staff, primary care physicians, and medical directors. The NPs spend over half of their work day on patient care, diagnosing and treating common acute illnesses, interpreting diagnostic tests and developing appropriate plans of care, and maintaining residents' chronic illness and health maintenance activities. The model emphasizes frequent communication with residents' family members.[20] These types of models have been shown to significantly increase advance directive (AD) completion rates and to reduce hospitalizations when compared with the AD completion rates and number of hospitalizations of residents not enrolled in the program.[21,22]

Licensed nursing staff include RNs and LPN/LVNs. They are responsible for providing skilled nursing care, including administering medications, delivering treatments, assessing and managing physical and psychosocial problems, and communicating with primary care providers. The RNs often manage and coordinate the overall care of residents and assume leadership positions in facilities, although the LPN/LVNs perform these duties when no RN is available. Compared with the acute care setting, nursing home staff nurses are less likely to have baccalaureate or advanced degrees, and the less educated LPNs/LVNs generally outnumber the RNs.[23] These characteristics exacerbate the lack of palliative care knowledge and skills that have been documented among long-term care nursing staff.[24]

Ethical issues unique to nursing homes

Autonomy is based on the right of an individual to make decisions freely (e.g., to accept or refuse a treatment). The media and public in general have historically criticized nursing homes for limiting autonomy. The routines, regulations, and restrictions in nursing homes result in an environment that is structured according to staff schedules; nursing focuses on medication administration and treatments; therapists focus on restorative care; and nursing assistants provide personal care. Most nursing homes use a medical model of care, which focuses on the cause and treatment of disease. There is a diminished focus on what activities and treatments are most important to the resident. This approach naturally results in a divergence from personal autonomy and person-centered care.

The physical environment of the nursing home also limits autonomy. Space is limited; residents share personal space in living areas (e.g., rooms and eating areas) and use common restrooms and shower facilities. In dementia units, residents may wander in and out of others' rooms. Private conversations are limited, as others may overhear residents talking. However, nursing homes do take steps to provide as much privacy as possible. Some couples are able to room together and share personal time alone. Allowing residents choices, especially in directing their own care, is important.[25] Nurses need to advocate for residents' ability to maintain privacy, confidentiality, and autonomy.

Nursing home residents have the right to participate in decisions about their care, including EOL care. The Patient Self Determination Act (PSDA), passed in 1990, requires Medicare reimbursed facilities to inform residents about their rights to accept or refuse medical or surgical treatment. The OBRA 87 regulations emphasized the resident's right to self-determination, including the right to participate in care planning and the right to refuse treatments. Revisiting discussions about EOL care with the resident or surrogate when there is a change in health status is crucial for maintaining the resident's right to informed decision-making.

One of the most difficult and sometimes controversial ethical issues involves decisions regarding the use of artificial nutrition (e.g., tube feeding). Food, in all societies, is part of the ongoing cycle of daily interaction, and families may continue to try to feed their relatives when they are no longer able to eat. The use of feeding tubes to provide artificial nutrition has not been shown to improve survival in individuals residing in nursing homes with end-stage dementia.[26]

Nursing home staff can assist families by explaining that it is normal to lose appetite at the end of life and that the body only takes in what it needs. Trying to force someone to eat may cause more burden than benefit to the resident and increase distress for the caregiver. Nursing staff may encourage families to offer "comfort feeding" with small amounts of favorite foods and drinks.

Challenges and opportunities for palliative care delivery in nursing homes

Despite the benefits, implementing palliative care philosophy and approaches to care in nursing homes is difficult. There are many barriers to delivering quality EOL care, although several characteristics facilitate the adoption of palliative care practices.[27]

Challenges to palliative care delivery

Regulatory structures, reimbursement policies, workforce issues, and resident characteristics hamper efforts to expand the delivery of palliative care services in nursing homes. For example, regulations favor restorative rather than palliative care. There has been a remarkable growth in postacute restorative nursing home care since 2001.[28] Efforts to administer palliative care are sometimes misinterpreted by facilities and regulators, leading to citations for poor care. For example, marked weight loss is an expected change toward the end of life and is rarely treated aggressively by palliative care and hospice teams. However, state surveyors who inspect nursing homes may interpret the loss as a sign of poor care.

Reimbursement also promotes more aggressive therapy. Generally, Medicaid and Medicare pay nursing homes a per diem for the care they provide rather than for specific care provided. Specifics of care are instead accounted for in the facility's case mix index, a composite score reflecting the complexity of care delivered to residents. In facilities providing more medical interventions, therapy services, and assistance with activities of daily living, the case mix index and the reimbursement rates are higher. Therefore, facilities are financially incentivized to accept residents requiring "skilled" treatments. Intravenous therapies and tube feedings, for example, are reimbursed at a higher rate than alternative, less invasive therapies. These policies act as disincentives to nursing homes to provide palliative care services, even though these services may improve the overall quality of care and the residents' quality of life.[27]

In addition to regulatory and financial pressures, workforce issues are challenging. Nursing home staff tends to lack training in palliative care approaches and therefore have difficulty recognizing and implementing palliative treatments as appropriate. Unlicensed nursing assistants and LPN/LVNs provide the majority of direct care to residents, and their skills related to symptom assessment and treatment, communication, and decision-making are limited. Clinical decision-making is also somewhat fragmented because LPN/LVNs and nursing assistants often are minimally involved in developing care plans, even though they may know the residents best. As a result, symptoms may be poorly assessed and managed, families are dissatisfied, and residents are frequently subject to unnecessary and distressing medical interventions and hospitalizations.[27]

Another workforce issue is staff turnover, which is staggeringly high. In 2008, the annual turnover among nursing assistants was 53%, that of LPNs and RNs was 43%, and for directors of nursing, 18%. High turnover is associated with lack of care continuity and poorer care,[29] resulting in a workforce that is constantly changing, overwhelmed, and dissatisfied. It also requires offering educational programs on a continual basis to keep knowledge and skills current.[27]

Until recently, there was little empirical research investigating the direct correlation between staff turnover and the ability of nursing home staff to deliver high-quality EOL care. Using both quantitative and qualitative data, one research team was able to link high staff turnover to residents' poorer quality of dying. This inverse relationship was magnified with higher rates of turnover resulting in even poorer EOL care. Family members believed that the lack of staff contributed to worse quality of dying for their loved one.[30]

One strategy to address nursing assistant job satisfaction and improve EOL care is through continuing education programs. Researchers found statistically significant improvement in attitudes and knowledge about EOL care after a daylong education program.[16] Additional research through surveys of hospice and palliative care nursing assistants on job satisfaction reported changes, such as better compensation and improved relationships (e.g., communication, appreciation, respect), were perceived to improve job satisfaction.[31]

Finally, many residents have complex physical and psychosocial needs that are difficult to assess and manage because of cognitive impairment. Severe impairment interferes with residents' ability to provide reliable self-report, thereby hindering pain and symptom assessment and management. When pain and other symptoms are identified, multiple comorbidities and polypharmacy further complicate effective treatment.

Facilitators to providing palliative care

Although there are hindrances, several nursing home characteristics facilitate palliative care delivery. These factors include relatively long stays and daily interaction between direct care staff and residents, the existing team approach to care, family meetings, and use of the Minimum Data Set (MDS).[27]

Daily interaction between staff and residents who are familiar with each other establishes a rich context for developing relationships congruent with palliative care philosophy. Nursing assistants who care for residents from day to day have greater knowledge of resident routines, likes and dislikes, and needs. Residents are often more comfortable and accustomed to caregivers who know them well. Nursing home staff frequently describe themselves as part of the resident's family.[32] These close relationships can improve mutual understanding of residents' goals of care, values, and preferences, and result in better symptom management.

The existing IDT—RNs, LPNs, nursing assistants, social work, rehabilitation specialists, dietitian, and wound care specialists—supports the palliative care philosophy. The best approach to care for older adults with life-limiting illness is through multiple professionals working together for a common purpose—to meet a resident's goal of care. Unmet psychosocial support and spiritual needs can be addressed in this forum by social workers and pastoral care staff.

Nursing homes are required to hold regular meetings with residents and/or their family members to discuss the comprehensive physical, emotional, mental, and social care plan for each resident. The plan focuses on objectives that maintain the resident's highest level of function. Ideally, at the point when the highest level of function is not maintained, the nursing home staff, resident and/or family should discuss revising goals of care.

The MDS is a mandated assessment tool for Medicare and Medicaid beneficiaries in nursing homes. The goal of this tool is to create a comprehensive evaluation and to identify opportunities to improve functional status. The MDS 3.0 is a revised tool that builds on previous versions using resident input or "voice" in assessments. The tool is completed by an RN at specified intervals using medical records, staff input, and observation in combination with a resident interview. The resident interview consists of discussions of preferences for routines and activities—including goals of care—and questions about pain, mood, and cognition.[33] The MDS can be used to identify residents with life-limiting illness who have unmet symptom-management and psychospiritual support needs; these residents are candidates for palliative care. The crucial next step after identifying palliative care needs is the delivery of care that matches the resident's goals of treatment.

Models to deliver palliative care in nursing homes

There is a shortage of evidence-based research in palliative care delivery models in nursing homes. In contrast, there is a great deal of evidence about the effectiveness of palliative care teams in acute care settings. Palliative care teams have been shown to reduce healthcare costs by avoiding unwanted or undesired treatments and to increase satisfaction using person-centered patient care.[34-37] Meier et al. asserted that the benefits of palliative care can be achieved in nursing homes, too.[38]

The Center to Advance Palliative Care (CAPC) compiled anecdotal evidence for successful palliative care delivery models in nursing homes and reported their findings in 2008.[39] These various programs can be categorized into three major approaches: hospice-nursing home partnerships, external palliative care consultation teams, and in-house teams and specialized palliative care units.[27]

Hospice care in nursing homes

Hospice care is the most common and well established program for delivering palliative care in US nursing homes. The Medicare Hospice Benefit (MHB) was extended to nursing homes in 1989, and by 2004, 78% of nursing homes reported a contract with a hospice agency.[40] Hospice, and the MHB, is the traditional program for delivering end-of-life care to individuals with terminal illness. Nursing home residents must meet hospice admission criteria: a life expectancy of 6 months or less should the terminal illness run its usual course and a decision not to pursue aggressive "curative" treatments.

In nursing homes, the MHB pays for the hospice agency to oversee the plan of care and provide all medical supplies and medications related to the terminal condition. Medicare pays the hospice agency for care related to the terminal illness. The facility continues to deliver 24-hour nursing care for the resident. The MHB does not provide the resident's payment for room and board—the most expensive component of nursing home care. Only rarely can residents access the Medicare SNF and MHB at the same time (e.g., unrelated diagnoses for each benefit). Some suggest that this barrier incentivizes families to choose the benefit with greater financial support.[41,42]

Hospice is often described as an "extra layer of support" for residents. The use of hospice in nursing homes is associated with improved symptom management, reduced hospitalizations, and increased satisfaction with care. Research comparing EOL care for residents with and without hospice demonstrates hospice care is associated with better psychosocial support, bereavement care, and pain management.[43,44] Facility leadership report improved ability to manage pain and symptoms, address psychosocial needs, and provide bereavement support when a formal program, such as hospice, is integrated into the facility culture.[45]

The challenge for hospice agencies, facilities, and providers is that a majority of nursing home residents have a life-limiting illness with an uncertain trajectory, making it difficult to decide when the illness is "terminal" according to existing guidelines. Persons with dementia and neurological conditions experience a long, slow disease progression with eventual complete dependence on others for daily living. Those with chronic respiratory and cardiac illness have frequent exacerbations that require acute care and result in diminished capacity during recovery. As a result, residents live with frailty and are susceptible to aggressive treatments that may not align with their values and goals of care.

There are other barriers to enrolling residents in hospice. Nursing home administrators and staff may believe that bringing hospice services into the facility indicates that their own care is inadequate.[46] Furthermore, poor communication and lack of collegial relationships can compromise care and engender ill will between nursing home and hospice staff. Additionally, there are financial disincentives for nursing homes to transfer residents who were admitted under the Medicare SNF benefit to the MHB because the reimbursement is much lower for the MHB.[27]

External consultation teams

External palliative care consultation teams provide specialized services in nursing homes and make recommendations for the resident's care. Consultation teams can be an extension of existing hospital-based teams, outpatient teams, or independent practitioners. Depending on the team and resources, consultations may focus on symptom management, advance care planning, or assisting with prognostication and/or hospice entry. Need for a consult is typically identified by staff and/or leadership, then formally requested by the primary care provider. The consultant bills under Medicare part B, and thus the costs for these services are not incurred by the nursing home.

The outcome of consultation is dependent on several factors. First the consulting clinician needs to understand the nursing home environment and have knowledge of interventions that can and cannot be carried out. For example, some palliative care medications are not on nursing home formularies. In addition, the ability to administer and titrate intravenous opioids may be limited. Second, implementing recommendations depends on the primary care provider's willingness to accept and implement palliative care recommendations.[39] Third, nursing homes are unique settings, and few are exactly the same. Depending on the underlying culture, facility staff may not be comfortable implementing EOL care.[27]

Integrated palliative care

Some nursing facilities report the presence of an internal palliative care team, services, or unit. In 2004, 27% of nursing home respondents reported having a special program and staff for hospice and/or palliative/EOL care.[40] Incorporating palliative care into daily routines requires a commitment to person-centered care and improving EOL care. Benefits of this model have been reported for residents and staff alike, including a reduction in resident medication use and staff empowerment.[47,48] Culture change and integrated palliative care share several characteristics, including person-centered care and practices that maximize choice (i.e., autonomy) and individualized care.

A major hindrance to developing internal nursing home palliative care services is the lack of resources. The need to train staff and the additional time necessary to deliver high-quality palliative care are additional barriers. In addition, there are no financial incentives to provide high-quality palliative care, since the highest reimbursement rates are for postacute, skilled care.[27]

Specific strategies for enhancing palliative care

Some nursing homes incorporate specific palliative care approaches in addition to, or instead of, comprehensive models. These targeted areas often are pain management, advance care planning, and interventions to decrease hospitalizations.

Pain and other symptoms are common in nursing home residents. Evidence from several studies show that pain occurs in 40%–86% of residents,[49] dyspnea: 11%–75%,[49,50] feeding problems: 28%–70%[49,50] delirium: 29%–47%,[49-51] incontinence: 59%,[49] and noisy breathing: 39%–59%.[49] Several studies provide evidence that these symptoms often are inadequately managed.[10,50]

Several intervention trials to improve pain management have been conducted. These studies used a variety of approaches, including quality improvement, pain management algorithms, specialized pain teams, and staff education.[10] The effectiveness of these approaches has been mixed.[10] Moreover, there are no high-quality trials of interventions aimed at nonpain symptoms.[10] Despite the lack of empirical evidence about effective ways to change pain- and symptom-management practices, many excellent resources are available to promote qualtity symptom assessment and management in nursing homes (Table 45.1.)

Advance care planning

The number of nursing home residents with advance directives (ADs) increased dramatically over the past 15 years. Jones et al.[57] reported that 65% of nursing home residents had an advance directive in 2004 (the most recent year for which there are national data). These ADs, in the form of a living will and durable power of attorney for healthcare, are completed by residents while they have decision-making capacity. When a resident lacks medical decision-making capacity, a resident's family member (acting as an appointed healthcare agent or surrogate decision maker) will ideally use the AD as guidance when making decisions regarding medical treatments and EOL care. The majority of advance directives for older nursing home residents reflect preferences for less aggressive EOL care.[57]

Although documented preferences about resuscitation are common, decisions about other interventions such as artificial nutrition and hydration, hospitalization, antibiotics, and comfort measures are not.[58] The use of the Physician's Orders for Life-Sustaining Treatment (POLST) is one effective way of encouraging discussion about, and documentation of, residents' and families' decisions about specific therapeutic approaches.[59] Moreover, the POLST paradigm increases concordance between residents'/families' preferences and care received.[60] Other effective strategies are the use of social workers, who receive specialized training in advance directves and facilitating goals-of-care discussions,[61] and implementation of the "Let Me Decide" advance directive program.[62]

End-of-life transitions

Several studies have documented that many nursing home residents are hospitalized in the final weeks of life[63,64] and receive burdensome treatments with little benefit, including tube feeding[65] and postacute, rehabilitative care.[41,42]

To address this problem, Ouslander et al.[66] used a pre-post intervention design to examine the effectiveness of several treatment algorithms and other tools designed to reduce hospitalizations. Findings from this quality improvement program indicated that these tools can decrease hospitalization rates and healthcare costs. Packaged into a program, the Interventions to Reduce Acute Care Transfers (INTERACT) tools[67] are now being examined in several ongoing nursing home demonstration projects funded by the Center for Medicare and Medicaid Innovations (CMMI) (http://innovation.cms.gov/initiatives/rahnfr/index.html).

Table 45.1 Palliative care resources for nursing home nursing staff and other providers

Resource	Description
End-of-Life Nursing Education Consortium (ELNEC) Geriatric curriculum[52]	Comprehensive training for nurses and nursing assistants, as well as social workers, chaplains, and others working in nursing homes Also useful for hospice staff who serve nursing homes Website: http://aacn.nche.edu/elnec/index.htm
Advancing Excellence in America's Nursing Homes	Initiative of the Advancing Excellence in Long Term Care Collaborative; goal of the campaign is to ensure quality of care and quality of life for nursing home residents Website contains resources on palliative care topics such as advance care planning and pain assessment and management organized within a quality improvement framework. Website: http://nursing homequalitycampaign.org/star_index.aspx?controls=welcome
Core Curriculum for the Long-Term Care Nurse	Comprehensive curriculum in detailed outline, book format Organized by the National Consensus Project Domains[53] Available from the Hospice and Palliative Nurses Association: http://hpna.org/Item_Details.aspx?ItemNo=978-1-934654-30-9
Nursing Education Computerized Education Program[54]	Comprehensive curriculum for nursing assistants working in any setting CD contains text, audio clips, video clips, a pop-up glossary, quizzes and printable pdf files. Available for the Hospice and Palliative Nurses Association: http://.hpna.org/Item_Details.aspx?ItemNo=NACDROM
Palliative Care in the Long Term Care Setting	Developed for medical directors and primary care providers in nursing homes. Contains a variety of resources to improve palliative and end-of-life care through leadership, education, best-practice guidelines, and quality assurance Available from the American Medical Directors Association: http://amda.com/resources/ltcis.cfm#LTCPC1
Geriatric Pain Website	Website containing evidence-based materials to guide nurses and other nursing home staff in assessing and managing residents' pain, including those with dementia. Website: http://geriatricpain.org/Pages/home.aspx
Palliative Care for Advanced Dementia Teaching Unit[55,56]	Developed by the Beatitudes Campus Dementia and Aging Research Department and Hospice of the Valley in Phoenix, Arizona, this interdisciplinary program specifically targets the knowledge and skills needed to provide person-centered, comfort care to persons with dementia and their families. Website: http://beatitudescampus.org/aging-research-and training/palliative-care-for-advanced-dementia-program
Consult Geri_RN	Website with articles and videos relevant to the care of older adults, including pain assessment in nonverbal persons and avoiding restraint use Website: http://consultgerirn.org/resources

Another promising approach to decreasing hospitalizations and promoting comfort was tested in a cluster randomized controlled trial conducted by Loeb and colleagues.[68] The study compared the effects of a nursing home–based clinical pathway for pneumonia treatment with usual care on hospitalizations, length of hospital stay, mortality, health-related quality of life, functional status, and cost. Results showed that the pneumonia clinical pathway was associated with significantly fewer hospitalizations, shorter lengths of hospital stay, and lower costs compared with usual care.

Resources for enhancing palliative care in nursing homes

Over the past several years, many professional and industry groups have developed curricula, websites, and other palliative care resources for nursing homes. Many of these resources are training materials that have been shown to increase nursing home staffs' knowledge and skills.[69] Table 45.1 presents information about several of these resources.

Special needs of nursing home staff

Nursing staff who care for nursing home residents at the end of life are at risk for work-related stress. Many staff members develop a bond with the residents they care for, especially during the last months and weeks of life. In addition, nursing assistants often encounter ethical dilemmas when pain is not treated optimally, when limited staffing delays care or results in poor care, and when residents' wishes for EOL care are not upheld by family members.[70]

The nursing home staff often feels the close relationship that a family feels for their loved one. It is not uncommon for staff to cope with the loss of a resident by talking to each other, reminiscing, and mourning together. Some nursing facilities offer memorials where staff can grieve together, as often a family will do, after the loss of a resident. Some family members continue to visit the nursing facility staff after the resident dies as they too develop a relationship with the staff.

Self-care for the body, mind, and spirit is important for nursing staff. In addition to attaining adequate sleep, eating healthy meals, and scheduling time for leisure activities, staff should be allotted time to discuss ethical dilemmas and distress they encounter. For successful debriefing to occur, facility leadership needs to cultivate a safe environment, where staff are not judged and feel comfortable talking openly.[70]

Conclusion

The principles of palliative care should be an integral part of nursing home care. While nursing homes represent a unique long-term care environment, modifications can help facilities in delivering high-quality EOL care. The nursing home staff should address the physical, psychological, social, and spiritual needs of all residents. Leadership should set the tone for person-centered care. Primary care clinicians need to recognize the regulations and guidelines under which facilities operate. Interdisciplinary team research by nurses is needed to improve EOL care in nursing homes. Nurses can make a difference in the quality of EOL care in nursing homes.

Case study

Ms. Jones, an 82-year-old woman

Ms. Jones is an 82-year-old woman with congestive heart failure (CHF), chronic obstructive pulmonary disease (COPD), painful arthritis in her knees and suspected mild cognitive impairment. Her lifelong partner died 1 year ago. Since that time Mrs. Jones has had three hospital admissions for complications related to CHF and COPD. During the most recent admission, she was intubated and subsequently had an extended hospitalization for 2 weeks. During discharge planning, the care coordinator, primary care nurse practitioner, and attending physician recommended nursing home placement, suspecting she would now need long-term care. Mrs. Jones has no family—her sister died several years ago—and no community support at home. She has a niece who lives close by but is busy caring for her own family. She is close to her pastor and faith network. Upon admission to the nursing home, Mrs. Jones participates in therapy, but based on MDS assessment, the staff quickly realizes she is not making gains. She fatigues easily with shortness of breath despite oxygen 24 hours/day and has constant pain in her knees. She becomes withdrawn, prefers to stay in her room, and begins to show signs and symptoms indicating progression of cognitive impairment. The staff is concerned about depression.

Ms. Jones clearly has many unmet needs. What is the first step? Can Ms. Jones make her own decisions? What should you do now to ensure that Ms. Jones' goals of care are known? How do you document these goals in writing? How do you assess her pain? How could palliative care help? What challenges do you anticipate? How can the nursing home staff support Ms. Jones? What ways can the staff ensure her pain and symptoms are controlled?

Consider her depression. How can the staff approach Ms. Jones' depression nonpharmacologically, and if unimproved, with the use of medications?

References

1. Center for Medicare and Medicaid Services. Nursing Home Data Compendium. 8th ed. 2010. https://www.cms.gov/Medicare/Provider-Enrollment-and-Certification/CertificationandCompliance/downloads/nursinghomedatacompendium_508.pdf. Accessed July 1, 2014.
2. Kaye H, Harrington C, LaPlante M. Long-term care: who gets it, who provides it, who pays, and how much? Health Affairs. 2010;29(1):11–21.
3. National Center for Assisted Living. Resident Profile. 2010. http://www.ahcancal.org/ncal/resources/Pages/ResidentProfile.aspx. Accessed June 20, 2013.
4. Stevenson DG, Grabowski DC. Sizing up the market for assisted living. Health Affairs. 2010;29(1):35–43.
5. Shaffer MA, Zwirchitz F, Keenan K, Tierschel L. End-of-life discussion in assisted living facilities. J Hosp Palliat Nursing. 2012;14(1):13–24.
6. US Department of Veterans Affairs. Geriatrics and Extended Care, Guide to Long Term Care. 2013. http://www.va.gov/GERIATRICS/Guide/LongTermCare/Nursing_Home_and_Residential_Services.asp. Accessed June 8, 2013.
7. Genworth Financial Inc. Executive Summary, Genworth 2013 Cost of Care Survey. 2013. https://www.genworth.com/dam/Americas/US/PDFs/Consumer/corporate/131168_031813_Executive%20Summary.pdf. Accessed June 15, 2013.
8. National Center for Health Statistics. Health, United States, 2010: With Special Feature on Death and Dying. Hyattsville, MD: 2010.
9. Mitchell SA, Teno JM, Miller SC, Mor V. A national study of the location of death for older persons with dementia. J Am Geriatr Soc. 2005;53(2):299–305.
10. Ersek M, Carpenter JG. Research priorities for geriatric palliative care in long-term care settings with a focus on nursing homes. J Palliat Med. 2013;16(10). Epub ahead of print.
11. Kane RL. The evolution of the American nursing home. In: Binstock RH, Cluff LE, Von Mering O (eds.), The Future of Long-Term Care: Social and Policy Issues. Baltimore, MD: Johns Hopkins University Press; 1996:145–168.
12. McTague V, Sutermaster J, D. Domain I: structure and processes of care. In: Stafford C (ed.), Core Curriculum for the Long Term Care Nurse. Hospice and Palliative Nurses Association; 2012:1–10.
13. Koren MJ. Person-centered care for nursing home residents: the culture-change movement. Health Affairs. 2010;29(2):312–317.
14. Jones A, Dwyer L, Bercovitz A, Strahan G. The National Nursing Home Survey: 2004 Overview. National Center for Health Statistics; 2009.
15. Kelly A, Conell-Price J, Covinsky K, et al. Length of stay for older adults residing in nursing homes at the end of life. J Am Geriatr Soc. 2010;58(9):1701–1706.
16. Wholihan D, Anderson R. Empowering nursing assistants to improve end-of-life care. J Hosp Palliat Nurs. 2013;15(1):24–32.
17. Collier E, Harrington C. Staffing characteristics, turnover rates, and quality of resident care in nursing facilities. Res Gerontol Nurs. 2008;1(3):157.
18. Harrington C. Nursing home staffing standards in state statutes and regulations. 2010. http://www.theconsumervoice.org/sites/default/files/advocate/action-center/Harrington-state-staffing-table-2010.pdf. Accessed October 13, 2013.
19. Shield RR, Wetle T, Teno J, Miller SC, Welch L. Physicians "missing in action": family perspectives on physician and staffing problems in end-of-life care in the nursing home. J Am Geriatr Soc. 2005;53(10):1651–1657.

20. Evercare. What is the nurse practitioner care model? 2011. http://www.myevercare.com/what_is_nurse_practitioner_model.jsp. Accessed October 13, 2013.

21. Kane RL, Keckhafer G, Flood S, Bershadsky B, Siadaty MS. Effect of Evercare on hospital use. J Am Geriatr Soc. 2003;51(10):1427–1434.

22. Lawrence JF. The advance directive prevalence in long-term care: a comparison of relationships between a nurse practitioner healthcare model and a traditional healthcare model. J Am Acad Nurse Pract. 2009;21(3):179–185.

23. Harrington C, Choiniere J, Goldmann M, et al. Nursing home staffing standards and staffing levels in six countries. J Nurs Scholarsh. 2012;44(1):88–98.

24. Whittaker E, Kernohan WG, Hasson F, Howard V, McLaughlin D. The palliative care education needs of nursing home staff. Nurse Educ Today. 2006;26(6):501–510.

25. Choi NG, Ransom S, Wyllie RJ. Depression in older nursing home residents: the influence of nursing home environmental stressors, coping, and acceptance of group and individual therapy. Aging Ment Health. 2008;12(5):536–547.

26. Teno JM, Gozalo PL, Mitchell SL, et al. Does feeding tube insertion and its timing improve survival? J Am Geriatr Soc. 2012;60(10):1918–1921.

27. Sefcik J, Rao A, Ersek M. What models exist for delivering palliative care and hospice in nursing homes? In: Goldstein N, Morrison R (eds.), Evidence-Based Practice of Palliative Medicine. Philadelphia: Elsevier; 2013:450–457.

28. Tyler DA, Feng Z, Leland NE, Gozalo P, Intrator O, Mor V. Trends in postacute care and staffing in us nursing homes, 2001–2010. J Am Med Dir Assoc. 2013 Jun 27. Epub ahead of print.

29. Harrington C, Carrillo H, Blank B. Nursing Facilities, Staffing, Residents and Facility Deficiencies, 2001 Through 2007. http://ualr.edu/seniorjustice/uploads/2008/12/Nursing%20Home%20Facilities,%20Staffing,%20Residents,%20and%20Facility%20Deficiencies%202001%20Through%202007.pdf. Accessed July 6, 2013.

30. Tilden V, Thompson S, Gajewski B, Bott M. End-of-life care in nursing homes: the high cost of staff turnover. Nurs Econ. 2012;30(3):163–166.

31. Head BA, Washington KT, Myers J. Job satisfaction, intent to stay, and recommended job improvements: the palliative nursing assistant speaks. J Palliat Med. 2013 Sep 14. Epub ahead of print.

32. Ersek M, Sefcik J, Stevenson D. Palliative care in nursing homes. In: Kelley AM, DE (ed.), Meeting the Needs of Older Adults with Serious Illness: Clinical, Public Health, and Policy Perspectives. New York: Springer;2014.

33. Saliba D, Buchanan J. Development and validation of a revised nursing home assessment tool: MDS 3.0. Santa Monica: RAND Health. 2008.

34. Smith TJ, Cassel JB. Cost and non-clinical outcomes of palliative care. J Pain Sympt Manage. 2009;38(1):32–44.

35. Morrison RS, Penrod J, Cassel B, et al. Cost savings associated with US hospital palliative care consultation programs. Arch Intern Med. 2008;168(6):1783–1790.

36. Morrison RS, Dietrich J, Ladwig S, et al. Palliative care consultation teams cut hospital costs for medicaid beneficiaries. Health Affairs. 2011;30(3):454–463.

37. Cassel JB, Webb-Wright J, Holmes J, Lyckholm L, Smith TJ. Clinical and financial impact of a palliative care program at a small rural hospital. J Palliat Med. 2010;13(11):1339–1343.

38. Meier DE, Beresford L. Palliative care in long-term care: How can hospital teams interface? J Palliat Med. 2010;13(2):111–115.

39. Center to Advance Palliative Care. Improving Palliative Care in Nursing Homes. New York, NY: Center to Advance Palliative Care; 2008.

40. Miller SC, Han B. End-of-life care in U.S. nursing homes: nursing homes with special programs and trained staff for hospice or palliative/end-of-life care. J Palliat Med. 2008;11(6):866–877.

41. Aragon K, Covinsky K, Miao Y, Boscardin J, Flint L, Smith A. Use of the Medicare posthospitalization skilled nursing benefit in the last 6 months of life. Arch Intern Med. 2012;172(20):1573–1579.

42. Miller SC, Lima JC, Mitchell SL. Influence of hospice on nursing home residents with advanced dementia who received Medicare-skilled nursing facility care near the end of life. J Am Geriatr Soc. 2012;60(11):2035–2041.

43. Miller SC, Lima JC, Looze J, Mitchell SL. Dying in U.S. nursing homes with advanced dementia: how does health care use differ for residents with, versus without, end-of-life Medicare skilled nursing facility care? J Palliat Med. 2012;15(1):43–50.

44. Huskamp H, Kaufmann C, Stevenson D. The intersection of long-term care and end-of-life care. Med Care Res Rev. 2012;69(1):45–57.

45. Rice KN, Coleman EA, Fish R, Levy C, Kutner JS. Factors influencing models of end-of-life care in nursing homes: results of a survey of nursing home administrators. J Palliat Med. 2004;7(5):668–675.

46. Stevenson DG, Bramson JS. Hospice care in the nursing home setting: a review of the literature. J Pain Symptom Manage. 2009;38(3):440–451.

47. Suhrie EM, Hanlon JT, Jaffe EJ, Sevick MA, Ruby CM, Aspinall SL. Impact of a geriatric nursing home palliative care service on unnecessary medication prescribing. Am J Geriatr Pharmacother. 2009;7(1):20–25.

48. Stone R, Harahan MF. Improving the long-term care workforce serving older adults. Health Affairs. 2010;29(1):109–115.

49. Brandt HE, Deliens L, Ooms ME, van der Steen JT, van der Wal G, Ribbe MW. Symptoms, signs, problems, and diseases of terminally ill nursing home patients: a nationwide observational study in the Netherlands. Arch Intern Med. 2005;165(3):314–320.

50. Hanson LC, Eckert JK, Dobbs D, et al. Symptom experience of dying long-term care residents. J Am Geriatr Soc. 2008;56:91–98.

51. Duncan JG, Bott MJ, Thompson SA, Gajewski BJ. Symptom occurrence and associated clinical factors in nursing home residents with cancer. Res Nurs Health. 2009;32(4):453–464.

52. Kelly K, Ersek M, Virani R, Malloy P, Ferrell B; End-of-Life Nursing Education Consortium. Geriatric training program: improving palliative care in community geriatric care settings. J Gerontol Nurs. 2008;34(5):28–35.

53. National Consensus Project for Quality Palliative Care. Clinical Practice Guidelines for Quality Palliative Care. 2013.

54. Ersek M, Wood BB. Development and evaluation of a nursing assistant computerized education programme. Int J Palliat Nurs. 2008;14(10):502–509.

55. Meade R. The sense of an ending. The New Yorker. 2013:92–103. http://www.newyorker.com/reporting/2013/05/20/130520fa_fact_mead?currentPage=all. Accessed July 1, 2014.

56. Long C, Alonzo T. Palliative care for advanced dementia: a model teaching unit. Practical approaches and results. Ariz Ger Soc J. 2008;13(2):14–17.

57. Jones A, Moss A, Harris-Kojetin L. Use of Advance Directives in Long-Term Care Populations. Hyattsville, MD: National Center for Health Statistics; 2011. NCHS Data Brief, No. 54.

58. Levy CR, Fish R, Kramer A. Do-not-resuscitate and do-not-hospitalize directives of persons admitted to skilled nursing facilities under the Medicare benefit. J Am Geriatr Soc. 2005;53(12):2060–2068.

59. Hickman SE, Nelson CA, Perrin NA, Moss AH, Hammes BJ, Tolle SW. A comparison of methods to communicate treatment preferences in nursing facilities: traditional practices versus the physician orders for life-sustaining treatment program. J Am Geriatr Soc. 2010;58(7):1241–1248.

60. Hickman SE, Nelson CA, Moss AH, Tolle SW, Perrin NA, Hammes BJ. The consistency between treatments provided to nursing facility residents and orders on the physician orders for life-sustaining treatment form. J Am Geriatr Soc. 2011;59(11):2091–2099.

61. Morrison RS, Chichin E, Carter J, Burack O, Lantz M, Meier DE. The effect of a social work intervention to enhance advance care planning documentation in the nursing home. J Am Geriatr Soc. 2005;53(2):290–294.

62. Molloy DW, Guyatt GH, Russo R, et al. Systematic implementation of an advance directive program in nursing homes: a randomized controlled trial. JAMA. 2000;283(11):1437–1444.

63. Gozalo P, Teno JM, Mitchell SL, et al. End-of-life transitions among nursing home residents with cognitive issues. N Engl J Med. 2011;365(13):1212–1221.

64. Ouslander JG, Lamb G, Perloe M, et al. Potentially avoidable hospitalizations of nursing home residents: frequency, causes, and costs: [see editorial comments by Drs. Jean F. Wyman and William R. Hazzard, pp 760–761]. J Am Geriatr Soc. 2010;58(4):627–635.

65. Teno JM, Mitchell SL, Gozalo PL, et al. Hospital characteristics associated with feeding tube placement in nursing home residents with advanced cognitive impairment. JAMA. 2010; 303(6):544–550.

66. Ouslander JG, Lamb G, Tappen R, et al. Interventions to reduce hospitalizations from nursing homes: evaluation of the INTERACT II collaborative quality improvement project. J Am Geriatr Soc. 2011;59(4):745–753.

67. Interventions to Reduce Acute Care Transfers: INTERACT. 2011. http://interact2.net/index.aspx. Accessed July 5, 2013.

68. Loeb M, Carusone SC, Goeree R, et al. Effect of a clinical pathway to reduce hospitalizations in nursing home residents with pneumonia: a randomized controlled trial. JAMA. 2006;295(21):2503–2510.

69. Ersek M, Grant MM, Kraybill BM. Enhancing end-of-life care in nursing homes: Palliative Care Educational Resource Team (PERT) program. J Palliat Med. 2005;8(3):556–566.

70. McClement S, Lobchuk M, Chochinov HM, Dean R. "Broken covenant": healthcare aides' "experience of the ethical" in caring for dying seniors in a personal care home. J Clin Ethics. 2010;21(3):201–211.

CHAPTER 46

Home care and hospice home care

Paula Milone-Nuzzo, Elizabeth Ercolano, and Ruth McCorkle

I was working full-time and caring for my ill wife when I was diagnosed with stage IV esophageal cancer. I was unprepared for the course of events that were to follow. When my symptoms became overwhelming, I was grateful for the referral to palliative care and the help of the home care nurses. Because my symptoms were controlled, I was able to remain home. I was relieved that my burdens were reduced for myself and my family.

Male with esophageal cancer

Key points

◆ Palliative home care can be used for chronically ill patients to improve their quality of life. Often, home care interventions can be provided on a short-term basis when clients experience a crisis that requires focused interventions.

◆ Nurses are the leaders and essential members of the home care team. Advanced practice nurses can have an impact on the cost, access to, and quality of care provided to chronically ill patients.

◆ Patients with complex problems need family caregivers who are taught to provide care in the home. Caregiving can be extremely stressful for family members and may adversely affect the health of the caregiver. Home care providers should assist family caregivers to maintain their health.

◆ Palliative home care should be provided by a team of providers, including physicians, mental health workers, therapists, nurses, and paraprofessionals.

Originally, palliative care in home care nursing was associated with patients who were clearly near the end of life. The contemporary philosophy of palliative care had its beginnings in England in 1967, when Dame Cicely Saunders founded St. Christopher's Hospice. Home and respite care continue to be a major component of that program. Palliative care, by definition, focuses on the multidimensional aspects of patients and families, including physical, psychological, social, spiritual, and interpersonal components of care. These components of care need to be instituted throughout all phases of the chronic illness trajectory and not only at the point when patients qualify for hospice services. Palliative care also needs to be delivered across a variety of settings and not be limited to inpatient units.

The primary purpose of palliative care is to enhance the quality and meaning of life and death for both patients and loved ones. To date, health professionals have not used the potential of palliative care to maximize the quality of life of patients in their homes. In this chapter, we discuss home care as an environment that provides unique opportunities to promote palliative care for patients and families throughout their illnesses. The chapter gives background information on what home care is, its historical roots, the types of providers available to give services, the regulatory policies controlling its use, examples of models of palliative home care programs, and recommendations to professionals for facilitating the use of home care in palliative care, concluding with a case study illustrating key elements of palliative care provision in the home.

Historical perspective on home care nursing

The period spanning the middle of the 20th century, during which patients were routinely cared for in acute care hospitals, may turn out to have been but a brief period in medical history. Before that time, patients were cared for primarily at home by their families. Today social and economic forces are interacting to avoid hospitalization, if possible, and to return patients home quickly if hospitalized. As we enter the era of value-based contracting, reducing length of stay in hospitals and preventing hospital readmissions are even more important to the fiscal health of hospitals. Although at face value these changes seem positive, they have highlighted gaps and deficiencies in the current healthcare delivery system.

Scientific advances have allowed us to keep patients with diseases such as cancer alive increasingly longer despite complex and chronic health problems. The burden of their care usually falls on families, who often are not adequately prepared to handle the physically and emotionally demanding needs for care that are inherent in chronic and progressive illnesses. In addition, family members often become primary care providers within the context of other demands, such as employment outside the home and competing family roles. The necessity among most of the nation's family members to assume employment outside the home and to alter those arrangements when faced with a sick relative has created an immeasurable strain on physical, emotional, and financial resources. The increasing responsibilities of the family in providing care in the face of limited external support and the consequences of that caregiving for patient and family raise important challenges for clinicians.[1]

The origins of home care are found in the practice of visiting nursing, which had its beginnings in the United States in the late 1800s. In 1859, William Rathbone of Liverpool, England, established the modern concept of providing nursing care in the home. Rathbone, a wealthy businessman and philanthropist, set up a system of visiting nursing after a personal experience, when nurses cared for his wife at home before her death. In 1859, with the help of Florence Nightingale, he started a school to train visiting nurses at the Liverpool Infirmary, the graduates of which focused on helping the "sick poor" in their homes.[2]

As in England, caring for the ill in their homes in the United States focused, from its inception, on the poor. Compared to the upper and middle class, who received frequent visits from the family physician, either in their homes or in the hospital pay wards, treatment of the sick poor seemed careless at best. Visiting nurse associations (VNAs) in the United States were established by groups of people who wanted to assist the poor to improve their health. In 1885 and 1886, visiting nurse services developed in Buffalo, New York, Boston, and Philadelphia that focused on caring for the sick poor.[2]

During World War II, as physicians made fewer home visits and focused instead on patients who came to their offices and were admitted to hospitals, the home care movement grew, with nurses providing most of the health and illness care in the home. Up until the mid-1960s, not-for-profit VNAs developed in major cities, small towns, and counties throughout the United States. Under their auspices, nurses focused on providing health services to women and infants and illness care to the poor in their homes, whereas most acute care was provided to patients in hospitals.[2]

The face of home care in the United States changed dramatically with the passage of an amendment to the Social Security Act that enacted Medicare in 1965. Home care changed from almost exclusively care for well mothers and children and the sick poor to a program that focused on care of the sick elderly in their homes. In 1967, there were 1753 home care agencies, a large percentage of which were not-for-profit VNAs. Almost 45 years later, in 2009, there were 10,581 home care agencies, with the largest percentage of agencies represented by the proprietary sector.[3] Not only did the types of agencies change, the acuity of patients increased and the development of technology allowed for the delivery of highly complex care in the home setting. The structural changes in the healthcare delivery system associated with the passage of the Medicare legislation in 1965 provided the foundation for the contemporary practice of home care nursing in the United States.

The 1990s brought a new challenge, managed care, to healthcare in general and home care specifically in the United States. The most significant impact of managed care on home care was a decrease in the number of visits allowed per patient per episode of illness. The result was a decline in the amount of home care patients received, causing a stabilization of the rapid growth in the home care delivery system. The American Balanced Budget Act of 1997 (PL 105–33) mandated the implementation of a prospective payment system for home care for Medicare beneficiaries. In this system, home care agencies receive a designated dollar amount per episode of illness to provide care for a Medicare patient based on the patient's admitting diagnosis and other factors related to physical and functional status. Just as the Diagnostic Related Group (DRG) system caused a significant decline in the number of hospital beds in the 1980s, the prospective payment system (PPS) for home care has resulted in significant shrinkage of the home healthcare industry as a result of patients receiving fewer visits per episode of illness. Between 1998 and 2000, Medicare Homecare spending fell from $14 billion to $9.2 billion. One of the major initiatives of PPS was the requirement that all Medicare patients be assessed on admission, every 60 days, and at discharge using a standardized assessment tool called Outcomes and Assessment Information Set (OASIS) (revised and now called OASIS-C). This tool is used to determine the patient's case mix weight, which partially defines reimbursement to the home care agency.[4] As home care agencies have become adept at working within the PPS, utilization of home care service has begun to rebound. Between 2000 and 2008, utilization of home care increased by 32%.[3]

In 2010, the Patient Protection and Affordable Care Act (also known as Obamacare) was passed into law, which we anticipate will significantly affect the utilization of all types of healthcare. The most important part of this Act required all citizens to have health insurance no later than March 31, 2014, or be subject to a tax. Previously there were 44 million citizens without health insurance. As of January 2014, that number has decreased to 35 million. As these individuals access health insurance, they might be more likely to use health services such as home care.

Definition of home care nursing

Home care, home healthcare, and home care nursing can be confusing terms to both providers and consumers, because they are often used interchangeably. Numerous definitions of home care have been provided by the many professional and trade associations that address home care issues (National Association for Home Care, Consumer's Union, American Hospital Association, American Medical Association, Center for Medicare and Medicaid Services, etc.). Common to all the definitions is the recognition that home care is care of the sick and well in the home by professionals and paraprofessionals, with the goal to improve health, enhance comfort, and improve the quality of life of clients. Home care nursing is defined here as "the provision of nursing care to acutely ill, chronically ill, terminally ill and well patients of all ages in their residences. Home care nursing focuses on health promotion and care of the sick while integrating environmental, psychosocial, economic, cultural, and personal health factors affecting an individual's and family's health status."[5]

Home care use in the United States

Home care is a diverse industry that provides a broad scope of care to patients of all ages. In 2010, it was estimated that approximately 12 million people received home care services for acute illness, long-term health conditions, permanent disability, and terminal illness.[3] The demographic picture of home healthcare recipients shows a predominately female (63.8%) and white (90.3%) population. The majority (86.1%) of home care patients are age 65 years and older, although home care is provided to patients of all ages, from birth to death. By 2050, it is estimated that 27 million people will need long-term care, the majority of which will be provided in the home. The number of elderly receiving home care is expected to increase in the coming years due to the aging of the American population and the desire of individuals to age in place.[6]

Although home care is provided to a large number of people, it still represents a very small percentage of national healthcare expenditures. Home care represented only 3% of the total national health expenditure in 2009, whereas hospital care consumed 37% and physician services 26%,[3] demonstrating the cost-efficient nature of home care practice. The majority of patients (67.5%) who received home care were discharged primarily to urban home care agencies.[6] As the reimbursement for home care visits has decreased and the cost of home visiting in rural areas has increased because of increased travel time, many rural home care agencies have been forced to close, limiting access to home care for the population in the region. The federal government has been inconsistent in its payment of additional dollars to home care agencies that provide care in rural settings.

The most common primary diagnoses for home care patients are diseases of the circulatory system, including heart disease. Other common primary diagnoses of patients receiving home care are diseases of the musculoskeletal system and connective tissue; diabetes mellitus; diseases of the respiratory system; endocrine, nutritional, and metabolic diseases; and immunity disorders.[3] Home care patients have an average of 4.2 diagnoses at the time of admission to an agency. A primary diagnosis of malignant neoplasm represents only 3.9% of home healthcare patients,[6] whereas it accounts for 47% of all patients in hospice.[7] Clearly, nonhospice home care has not been used adequately as an integral part of care for cancer patients and families as they have endured the physical and emotional demands of complex cancer treatments and move across the acute, chronic, and terminal phases of their disease. This is an ideal context in which the need for palliative care should drive an increased use of home care services.

Types of home care providers

Home care providers are traditionally characterized as either formal or informal caregivers. Informal caregivers are those family members and friends who provide care in the home and are unpaid. It is estimated that 52 million informal caregivers provide care to adults with a disability or illness[8]; 14.9 million of those care for someone who has dementia or Alzheimer's disease.[9] The majority of those providing informal home care are female, older than 49 years of age, and are providing assistance approximately 20 hours per week.[10] The type of care provided by informal caregivers ranges from routine custodial care, such as bathing, to sophisticated skilled care, including tracheostomy care and intravenous medication administration. Informal caregivers assume a considerable physiological, psychological, and economic burden in the care of their significant other in the home. When layered on top of existing responsibilities, caregiver tasks compete for time, energy, and attention resulting in serious physical and mental health consequences for the caregiver. Seventeen percent of caregivers feel that their health has gotten worse as a result of their caregiving responsibilities.[1]

The burden of caregiving for informal caregivers is complicated by the increasing expectation of highly skilled care in the home that would previously be provided by skilled home care workers. Family and friends are asked to assume responsibility for providing complex care while experiencing their own emotional response to their loved ones illness.[10] The economic cost of providing informal care in the home also places a significant burden on caregivers. With the shift toward community-based care, numerous costs have shifted to the patient and caregiver. Out-of-pocket financial expenditures include medications, transportation, home medical equipment, supplies, and respite services, all of which increase in utilization as the patient's condition worsens.[11] These costs are nonreimbursable and often invisible but are very real to families who are trying to provide care on a fixed income.

Formal caregivers are those professionals and paraprofessionals who are compensated for the in-home care they provide. In 2009, an estimated 958,000 persons were employed in home health agencies. In home care, nurses represent 32% of the formal caregivers providing care to patients in Medicare-certified home care agencies.[3] Home health aides and personal care aides also represent a large proportion of the formal caregivers in home care and are expected to increase in number in upcoming years. These two occupations represent the fastest growing occupations during the period of 2010–2020.[12] Table 46.1 describes the professionals and paraprofessionals who represent the range of home care providers in home health agencies.

Reimbursement mechanisms

Home health services are reimbursed by both commercial and government third-party payers as well as by private individuals. Government third-party payers include Medicare, Medicaid, Tricare, and the Veterans Administration system. These government programs have specific requirements that must be met for the coverage of services. Commercial third-party payers include insurance companies, health maintenance organizations (HMOs), preferred provider organizations (PPOs), accountable care organizations (ACOs) and case management programs. Commercial insurers often allow for more flexibility in their requirements than Medicare. For example, the home care nurse may negotiate with an insurance company to obtain needed services for the patient on the basis of the cost-effectiveness of the home care plan, although that service may not be routinely covered.

Medicare

Medicare is a federal insurance program for the elderly (65 years and older), the permanently disabled, and persons with end-stage renal disease in the United States and is the single largest payer for home health services. To be eligible for this program, an individual or spouse must have paid into Social Security. Medicare is a federal program and, as such, the benefits are the same from state to state. The Centers of Medicare and Medicaid Services (CMS), a department in the federal government, regulates payments for services under Medicare. The Centers of Medicare and Medicaid Services contracts with insurance companies called fiscal intermediaries to process Medicare claims that are submitted from home care agencies.

Since agencies are now reimbursed using a prospective payment methodology, home care has gained increased flexibility for the

Table 46.1 Types of providers in home care

Type of provider	Roles and responsibilities
Nurses	
Registered nurses (RNs)	Deliver skilled care to patients in the home
	Considered to be the coordinator of care
Licensed practical nurses (LPNs)	Deliver routine care to patients under the direction of a registered nurse
Advanced practice nurses (APNs)	Coordinate total patient care to complex patients, supervise other nurses in difficult cases related to their specialty, develop special programs, and negotiate for reimbursement of services
	Teach patients and caregivers special skills and knowledge
Therapists	
Physical therapists	Deliver skilled care that includes assessment for assistive devices in the home
	Perform therapy procedures with the patient, and teach the patient and family to assist in treatment. Assist patient to improve mobility. Can also serve as coordinator of care for certain patients
Occupational therapists	Focus on improving physical, mental, and social functioning
	Rehabilitation of the upper body and improvement of fine motor ability
Speech therapists	Rehabilitation of patients with speech and swallowing problems
Respiratory therapists	Provide support to patients using respiratory home medical equipment such as ventilators. Perform professional respiratory therapy treatments
Other clinical staff	
Social workers	Help patients and families identify needs and refer to community agencies
	Assist with applications for community-based services and provide financial assistance information
Dietitians	Provide diet counseling to patients with special nutritional needs
Paraprofessionals	
Home health aides Personal care aides	Perform personal care, basic nursing tasks (as opposed to skilled), and incidental homemaking
Homemakers	Perform housekeeping and chores to ensure a safe and healthy home care environment

services provided under Medicare. In the former fee-for-service model, designated and specific home care providers were paid for each visit made. Today, home care agencies are responsible for assuring that the patients achieve their health outcomes in the most efficient manner. If a home care agency suggests the most effective plan of care would be to integrate alternative and complementary therapies or mental health therapy into a patient's plan of care, it will not reduce or increase the amount of payment received from the government.

There are five criteria (summarized in Table 46.2) that a patient must meet for home care services to be reimbursed by Medicare.

Medicare is the main payer of hospice services in the United States under the Medicare Hospice Benefit, which Congress first enacted as part of Medicare Part A in 1982 under the Tax Equity and Fiscal Responsibility Act (TEFRA; P.L. 97-248). The law was in effect from 1983 until 1986, when Congress made hospice a permanent part of the Medicare program.[11] The impetus behind Medicare's hospice benefit came from the recognition that the regulations and restrictions for traditional Medicare were not well suited to meet the needs of terminally ill patients.

Medicare hospice was designed primarily as a home care benefit that included an array of services to assist care providers in the clinical management of the terminally ill in the home.[12] These services include the usual home care providers of the registered nurse, home health aide, and physician but also include medical social services, medical supplies, counseling, including dietary counseling, and any other service specified in the plan of care.[7] The regulations for hospice care also require home care providers to have in-patient hospice beds available for terminally ill patients in need of respite care, procedures necessary for pain control, or acute or chronic symptom management.[13] Recognizing that hospice is a philosophy of care rather than a place for care, it seems appropriate that hospice care is given in a variety of settings.

For a patient to elect the hospice Medicare benefit, the patient must waive the traditional Medicare benefit. By electing the hospice Medicare benefit, the patient and family are acknowledging the terminal nature of the illness and opting no longer to have curative treatment.

Medicaid

Medicaid is an assistance program for the poor, some disabled persons, and children. Unlike Medicare, Medicaid is jointly sponsored by the federal government and the individual states. Therefore, Medicaid coverage varies from state to state. These differences can often be dramatic and in some cases dependent on the state's financial solvency. Eligibility for Medicaid is based on

Table 46.2 Criteria for home care reimbursement under Medicare

Criterion	Description
Homebound	A patient is considered homebound if absences from the home are rare and short of duration and attributable to the need to receive medical treatments.
Completed plan of care	A plan of care for home care services must be completed in Centers for Medicare and Medicaid services (CMS) forms 485 and 487. The plan of care must be signed by a physician.*
Skilled service	Medicare defines skilled service as one provided by a registered nurse, physical therapist, or speech therapist. Skilled nursing services include skilled observation and assessment, teaching, direct care and management, and evaluation of the plan of care.
Intermittent and part-time	Part-time means that skilled care and home health aide services combined may not exceed 8 hours per day or 28 hours per week. Intermittent means that skilled care is provided or needed on fewer than 7 days per week or less than 8 hours of each day for periods of 21 days or less, with extensions for exceptional circumstances.
Reasonable and necessary	The services provided must be reasonable for the patient given the diagnosis and necessary to assist the patient to achieve the expected outcomes.

*In 2014 legislation was pending that will enable advanced practice nurses to order home care and sign the plan of care needed for reimbursement by Medicare.

income and assets and is not contingent on any previous payments to the federal or state governments.

Unlike the requirements of the Medicare program, Medicaid covers both skilled and unskilled care in the home and usually does not require that the recipient be homebound. To qualify for the home care benefits under Medicaid, patients must meet income eligibility requirements and have a plan of care signed by a physician, and the plan of care must be reviewed by a physician every 60 days.

Commercial insurance

Many commercial insurance companies are involved in health insurance for individuals or groups. These local or national companies often write policies that include a home care benefit. Commercial insurers often cover the same services covered by Medicare in addition to preventive, private duty, and supportive services, such as a home health aide or homemaker. Commercial insurance companies cover patients of all ages, including Medicare patients with supplemental insurance policies that cover health-care expenditures not reimbursed by Medicare.

Supplemental insurance policies are a source of confusion and anxiety among home care patients, often when families are under increased stress because of the complexity of the health situation for one of its members. Nurses should encourage families to carefully review the specifics of the supplemental insurance policy, including copays, annual review of benefits, anticipated out-of-pocket costs, and pharmacy costs. Families should recognize that when changing a supplemental insurance carrier, you may also have to change the home care provider, because some supplemental policies state which home care provider will be reimbursed for services.

The Medicare Advantage (MA) program allows Medicare beneficiaries to voluntarily elect to take their Medicare entitlement in the form of a fixed monthly payment to an authorized private insurance plan. Commercial insurance firms compete for customers by providing additional benefits that are not covered by the traditional Medicare program, such as vision and dental coverage. If their plans are less expensive than the area average for Medicare's fee-for-service program, then the insurer must pass along most of the extra savings as an incentive for beneficiary enrollment. Currently, about one in four seniors are enrolled in an MA plan.[14] In the Affordable Care Act, reimbursements to the Medicare Advantage program are significantly reduced.

Commercial insurance often includes a maximum lifetime benefit as part of the policy. The high cost of high-technology care forces a growing number of patients to reach this maximum rather quickly and face the loss of coverage. This has resulted in the development of case-management programs administered by insurance companies. The case manager projects the long-term needs and costs of care for the patient and develops a plan with the patient to meet those needs in a cost-efficient manner. Consideration is given to the life expectancy of the patient in relationship to the maximum lifetime benefit.

Unlike the Medicare program, in which negotiation for services is not an option, it may be important for home care nurses to identify the needed services for a patient with a commercial insurance plan and intervene to obtain funding for those services. When working with an insurance case manager, the home care nurse must be specific about the services the patient will need, the overall cost of those services, and the expected outcome related to the services requested. The more precisely the home care nurse can describe the impact of the care plan on the patient outcomes with objective data, the more inclined the case manager will be to authorize services. Insurance companies are very concerned with the satisfaction of their enrollees. Patients and families should be empowered to make their voices heard about the services they need to remain safe in the home. If out-of-network services or special pricing is negotiated with the insurance case manager, written documentation of the agreement should be included in the patient's record. Ideally, the patient should be given a copy of this agreement in the event that any disputes over payment occur.

Hospice care

Hospice care is a philosophy of supportive and palliative care provided to people at the end of their life. Although most of hospice care is provided in the home, because hospice care is an approach to care, it can be provided in any setting. The focus of hospice care is on the management of symptoms, providing comfort care and supporting quality of life rather than curative treatments. A team of interdisciplinary professionals (i.e. medicine, nursing, recreation, social work, arts, spiritual care) coordinates an individual plan of care that addresses the physical, emotional, and spiritual needs of the patient and the patient's family.

Hospice legislation was enacted in 1982 as an addition to the Medicare benefit for terminally ill patients with a life expectancy of 6 months or less if the disease ran its normal course. In order to be eligible for hospice care, the patient must have a prognosis of 6 months or less, certified by their own provider and the hospice medical director. The patient must waive their traditional Medicare benefit (that includes curative treatments) in order to participate in the hospice Medicare benefit. The hospice benefit consists of an initial 90-day period, a subsequent 90-day period and an unlimited number of 60-day benefit periods as long as the patient meets the eligibility requirement of a terminal diagnosis with a prognosis of 6 months or less. For a full description of hospice care, please see chapter 2 in the 2010 edition of this text.

While Medicare was the first to offer hospice services as part of its benefits, since 1982 Medicaid (in most states) and many private insurance companies have included hospice care as part of their benefits. The requirement to waive curative care applies in all programs except for one specific instance. In the Patient Protection and Affordable Care Act of 2010, terminally ill children enrolled in the Medicaid or the Children's Health Insurance Plan (CHIP) hospice benefit, will also be able to receive curative treatment while still receiving the wide array of hospice services designed to improve the quality of end-of-life care.[15] This change in regulation, specifically for children, has significant policy implications since waiving the expensive curative therapies provides the financial resources for increasing supportive care services. The impact of this change, because of its currency, has not yet been determined.

The home health–hospice connection

For a patient to receive the full array of hospice services under Medicare, the care must be provided by a certified hospice provider. To be reimbursed, home care agencies that are not certified hospice providers must refer their terminally ill patients to an agency that carries the certification. This regulation affects clinical care in several ways. Home care nurses have a long history of developing strong and intimate bonds with patients and families. As patients progress toward the terminal phase of their illnesses, it is emotionally difficult for home care nurses to refer their patients to hospice providers. At times, it is equally difficult for a family to accept the referral, knowing that they will have to give up "their nurse." The home care nurse and the family may believe that the relationship that has developed among the patient, the family, and the home care nurse is more important than any additional benefits that hospice might bring.

Although families may feel that they are getting sufficient home care in the terminal phases of the patient's life from their traditional home care agency, they are not able to take advantage of the prescription drug components of the hospice benefit, which may result in significant financial burden. They also usually do not receive supportive services such as pastoral care and bereavement follow-up, which are integral to the hospice program. Because the emotional impact of the patient's death is unknown at the time the patient makes the decision to forego a hospice referral, it is impossible to predict the significance of a service such as bereavement follow-up. In addition, hospice nurses are skilled in pain and symptom management in the terminal phases of life. This is one of the areas in which hospice care can be most effective for patients and their families. The nonhospice home health agency and the hospice provider offer important services, especially nursing care to patients at the end of life; strengthening mechanisms that facilitate transitions between these two types of services is essential.

In order to ease the transition for patients and families from traditional home care to home hospice care, home care agencies that are dually licensed as home care and hospice providers have developed bridge programs. These programs are designed for patients who have advanced disease, are homebound and in need of skilled care, yet are not ready to accept hospice care. Perhaps the patient is not ready to give up curative care or the families are not ready to think about the possibility of end of life. A bridge program allows patients and families to ease into end-of-life care and benefit from the usual hospice services without having to elect the hospice Medicare benefit. Often the home care nurse and the hospice nurse will collaborate on the care of the patient with the goal of moving the patient to hospice at the appropriate time.[16]

Cancer as a prototype for home care use in palliative care

Over the years cancer has shifted from a terminal illness to a chronic disease. Patients with advanced disease and guarded prognoses initially may be treated as if their disease is curable rather than progressive and terminal. Although the philosophical underpinnings and goals of curative and palliative treatments are quite different, an individual who has advanced disease is often treated first with a curative approach.[17] During this time, it is important that there is frequent communication among the patient, family, and health-care team as the disease, its stage, and the patient's response to treatment is understood.[18] The course of the patient's disease depends on the type of cancer and its biology. Some courses are faster than others, and some patients often experience disease-free intervals and multiple treatments before the cancer becomes terminal.[19] The experience of living with progressive disease and effects of the treatment can have physical, social, and emotional consequences that ultimately affect the patient's quality of life. Characteristics of advanced cancer that require coordinated palliative care include multiple physical needs, intense emotional distress manifested by anxiety and depression, and complex patient and caregiver needs. The goals of palliative care are best achieved if care is initiated early,[20] and one of the most efficient ways of monitoring patients' needs is to coordinate the overall plan of management with home nursing care during times of crisis to decrease fragmentation and promote continuity.

Needs of patients with cancer and their caregivers

Because of the continued trend to discharge hospitalized patients as soon as possible, the increasing use of ambulatory care services, and the increasing use of complex therapies, the need for ongoing monitoring and teaching of patients and families has never been greater. Family members, often without the assistance of any formal home care services, are assuming primary responsibility for the care of patients at home. This demand on families is not new, although the caregiver role has changed dramatically from promoting convalescence to providing high-technology care and psychological support in the home. Members of a patient's family are of vital importance in meeting the patient's physical and psychological needs and accomplishing treatment goals.[21] Cancer family caregivers represent a sizable and diverse segment of the population who are making major contributions to their families, communities, and the healthcare system, often at the expense of their own health and well-being.[22]

Research to identify patient-defined home care needs began in the 1980s and has increased steadily since the 1990s. An early study identified pain, sleep, and elimination management as major patient needs.[23] Wellisch and colleagues[24] investigated the types and frequency of problems experienced by two separate groups of seriously ill cancer patients and their families in their homes in the Los Angeles area and explored the types of interventions that helped to reduce the problems. The five most frequent problem categories identified included somatic side effects, including pain; patient mood disturbance; equipment/technology problems; family relationship impairment; and patient cognitive impairment. Interventions reported to be effective included reinforcement to the patient and family, counseling, and emotional support. They noted that patients with cognitive deficits had special needs, and their family members were at high risk for ongoing problems. Although these two studies were accomplished more than 30 years ago, the findings remain relevant today. There have been numerous review articles that have documented these needs across the disease and treatment courses.[25,26] Evidence suggests that both patients and their families benefit from home care services directed at their needs, including physical and psychological distress.[27,28] An overlooked benefit of recognizing and supporting caregivers as key members of the patient's health team is the beneficial effect caregivers can have on the patient's recovery and clinical outcomes.[22,29] Improved patient outcomes, including reduced postoperative complications, better management of side effects, increased adherence to oral medications, and early detection of adverse events, would result in reduced healthcare utilization and costs.[30]

Similarly, the needs of family members who provide care to patients with cancer have been summarized in review articles.[31,32] Generally, researchers have found that a significant number of cancer caregivers exhibit psychological distress and physical symptoms throughout all phases of the chronic illness trajectory. Predictors of caregiver distress included a number of patient-related variables, including more advanced stages of cancer, younger age, disability, and complex care needs.[33] There have been a number of individual studies to test interventions to help family members provide care and reduce their stress. For example, McMillan and colleagues designed a caregiver intervention, COPE, based on problem-solving strategies that address the specific needs of family caregivers. Patients receiving home care hospice and their caregivers were randomized to one of three groups: a control group, an attention control group, and an intervention group who received usual care plus COPE. The COPE intervention consists of four components: creativity, optimism, planning, and expert information and was administered to caregivers over nine days. Patients in the COPE intervention group reported significantly less symptom distress than the other two groups.[34]

There is no question that patients have a better quality of life when they have an informed and competent caregiver at home; however, the financial burden of caregiving may prevent many family members from assisting. In 2011, the annual cost associated with family caregiving to individuals with all types of illnesses and disabilities was conservatively estimated at $450 billion dollars.[1] The cost of family caregiving far exceeds that amount when one considers the health and social consequences incurred by the caregiver. Cancer family caregivers are a valuable and indispensable resource whose needs should be accurately identified so that interventions to support their caregiving can be efficiently tested and supplied.

Patients and caregivers consistently report the need for information.[35,36] Their search for information can be extensive, as they use many sources for obtaining information, including the Internet. Caregivers may be more active than patients in seeking information, and often initiate a search for information to supplement the information provided by health professionals. Caregivers need information about specific treatments, what to expect, the ways to manage symptoms, and available community resources. Caregivers also need information on the emotional aspects of the illness and patients' expected course of recovery, both physically and emotionally. Their information needs can vary from one phase of the trajectory to another.[37]

In general, the literature on the needs of cancer patients and caregivers of cancer patients highlights: (1) that patients are increasingly being treated in ambulatory clinics and have ongoing, unmet complex care needs with little or no use of home or palliative care referrals; (2) that caregivers are assuming more and more responsibility for monitoring patients' status and providing direct care in the home with little instruction or opportunities for respite; (3) that as patients' physical status changes, caregivers have a high proportion of unmet needs themselves; (4) that the caregiving experience encompasses both positive and negative elements; and (5) that the conceptualization of caregiver burden is linked to negative reactions to caregiving.[38]

Models of the delivery of palliative care

Although the field of palliative care is still a relatively new discipline, there have been major advances in the establishment of programs—primarily hospital-based programs with recent expansion to outpatient clinics.[39-41] Many of these programs have demonstrated significant improvements in symptom management and satisfaction with care. There has been little research specifically testing the effects of home care interventions on patient outcomes in palliative care. For palliative care to flourish in home care, there must be systems that can facilitate it and clinicians who are knowledgeable about the state of the science. A growing body of evidence suggests that input from specialists in palliative care can improve the quality of patient care and reduce costs.[42-44] Kuebler and Bruera recommend a collaborative consultative Internet relationship to support clinicians in providing comprehensive palliative interventions for patients in a timely manner. They tested the model between a rural palliative care nurse practitioner and an urban medical research physician. Preliminary results show promise, and its potential success could enhance care of the persons living within underserved or remote areas around the world.[45] Many countries, other than the United States, provide healthcare with government support and realize the potential cost savings.[46,47] These countries, which have delivered palliative care in the patient's home successfully for a number of years, include Great Britain, Canada, Sweden, Italy and Australia.

Patient and caregiver palliative care interventions

Nurse counseling or care management is the most frequently studied approach to delivering information and support to cancer patients and their caregivers. Earlier meta-analyses of randomized trials of nursing interventions suggest that many are effective in reducing symptoms of cancer or its treatment[48] as well as symptoms of anxiety, depression, and psychological distress.[49] However, because of the mixture of different intervention components, these meta-analyses are of limited help in identifying the intervention elements that contribute to their effectiveness. Randomized trials conducted by McCorkle[50] and others[51] have demonstrated that nursing interventions directed at improving patient and family self-management skills have reduced symptoms, improved function, reduced rehospitalizations, improved mood and mental health status, reduced psychological distress, and improved survival among patients during cancer treatment. Cognitive-behavioral interventions with an emphasis on problem solving delivered by trained oncology nurses have been shown to reduce symptoms.[52] To illustrate, Given and colleagues[53] tested a cognitive-behavioral intervention among solid tumor patients undergoing chemotherapy that began with collaborative problem identification by patient and nurse. The nurse would then propose interventions that would be collaboratively evaluated, and an action plan would be developed. These were supported by classes focused on self-management, problem solving, and communication with providers. Those receiving the experimental intervention reported significantly less severe symptoms at 10- and 20-week follow-ups. Efforts to give patients with cancer and their families the information, skills, and confidence needed to manage the physical, psychosocial, and communication challenges associated with cancer and its care seem warranted by the literature. Progress in this area could be accelerated by the systematic use of symptom management evidence-based guidelines by home care nurses through the Internet[54] and access to the researchers' symptom management toolkit, an evidence-based symptom management guide to support self-management which is readily on the Web for both clinicians and patients.[55]

There have also been several literature reviews of interventions conducted with caregivers of patients with cancer.[56-59] Northouse and McCorkle categorized the interventions described in these studies into four broad intervention areas: (1) supportive-educative, (2) caregiving skills/symptom management, (3) coping skills, and (4) relationship-focused interventions.[37] These are not necessarily discrete categories because some interventions address more than one area. The reviews indicate that positive results related to improvement in caregivers' coping skills and knowledge. Studies that focused on education for palliative and hospice care had a tendency to show decreases in caregiver stress.[60-62] In addition, there have been a number of programs developed to teach caregivers direct care responsibilities for patients in the home that have had positive outcomes on patients and caregivers.[63-65] Unfortunately the majority of this evidence-based research rarely is adopted into clinical practice.

Recommendations for facilitating the use of home care nursing in palliative care

Home care nursing is an ideal mechanism to deliver effective palliative care; however, for a number of reasons, it has been underutilized. Patients who need palliative care have complex and often challenging physical and psychological problems. Palliative care for specific types of diseases requires knowledgeable and competent clinicians. It is common for professional staff nurses in home care agencies to lack the knowledge and expertise to manage patients' symptoms and to teach caregivers the skills they need to manage the day-to-day problems they encounter in caregiving. And yet repeatedly, home care nurses are placed in the position of being responsible for patients who have palliative care needs. One potential solution is to teach the staff to use evidence-based research to remain current in the advances in palliative care. The rationale for promoting evidence-based palliative care is straightforward, but there are major challenges to achieving the goal of translating palliative care research into everyday clinical practice. Maybe the most difficult challenge is persuading the staff to change how they deliver care.[66] Schumacher and colleagues used standard pain management strategies to teach the staff to change their practice in the home.[67] Another successful strategy has been the use of medication kits containing prescription medications to treat pain and dyspnea to use with dying patients as they approach death.[68] In addition, for palliative care to be successful in the home, physicians and other experts must work collaboratively with nurses and be available to solve problems as they arise. It is often easier for physicians to admit patients to the hospital than to work with home care nurses to keep patients at home.

The state of the science in home care was reviewed for this chapter. Results from these studies have not been systematically incorporated into clinical practice where services are reimbursed. However, we identified critical factors in these studies that, if adopted, could become the basis of successful home care palliative nursing. These include the following:

1. *Staff nurses who are responsible for direct patient care in the home must have contact with experts who have specialized knowledge and skills related to the disease-specific needs of patients.*

Experts can include any member of a palliative care program, but usually include an advanced practice nurse (APN) or palliative care physician. The term "advanced practice nurse" used here is defined as a professional nurse, including clinical nurse specialists and nurse practitioners, who has graduated from a master's program in a specialty field such as an oncology advanced practice program. To assist the staff nurse in dealing with the complexity of palliative care, either a palliative care physician or an APN should serve as a supervisor/consultant to the team and be directly involved in clinical decisions. There may be fewer than needed opportunities for APNs working directly in home care agencies because of the perception that they are too costly to employ. As agencies move to prospective payment and greater efficiency, the role of the APN may factor more prominently in home care agencies. Advanced practice nurses may also work independently and provide care to a group of patients, for example, as case managers from an ambulatory clinic. As a result of the Balanced Budget Act of 1997 (PL 105–55), APNs—specifically clinical nurse specialists and nurse practitioners—practicing in any setting can be directly reimbursed at 85% of the physician fee schedule for services provided to Medicare beneficiaries. In home care, this change has the potential to facilitate access to care for patients who do not have access to a home care agency or other primary care provider, specifically those in rural and underserved areas.

2. *Because of the barriers to entering hospice care, home care nurses must become knowledgeable and highly skilled in providing palliative care to patients.*

This will require not only the development of skills in a new area of clinical expertise but also a paradigm shift in the way home care nurses view the episode of care for patients in the home. Home care has traditionally been viewed as a component of the long-term care delivery system. Although the number of home visits per episode of illness has decreased significantly, home visits tend to be spread out over a greater period of time, usually a 60-day certification period. For patients requiring palliation, home care may need to be very intensive over a relatively short period of time (2–4 weeks). In this model, the home care nurse can assist the patient and family in methods of managing symptoms and coping with the caregiving role. In the long term, as the patient's disease progresses, the patient and caregivers will need "booster" visits, but the majority of visits and care may be given in short periods of time, when the patient and caregivers are most in need. Telephone visits to provide care have been shown to be an effective strategy for chronic illnesses in which the needs are for support and education. Home care can also be used for short durations in crisis situations. By providing intensive home care for short durations, nurses can help patients to address current issues in the most effective way. These short but intensive interventions can improve quality of life and may also impact survival outcomes for some patients. While home health agencies are usually paid on the basis of a 60-day episode of care, the PPS has a low utilization payment for beneficiaries whose episode of care consists of four or fewer visits.[69]

3. *Patients are usually hospitalized when symptoms get out of control and their disease is unstable. When patients are hospitalized, comprehensive discharge care coordination and follow-up by nurses skilled in palliative care are needed to ensure that the plan is implemented, evaluated, and modified as needed.*

Patients with complex problems including distressing symptoms need assistance to make a smooth transition from the hospital to their homes, and caregivers need access to information, skills training, and resources to help with providing essential assistance. A referral to a home care agency may also be necessary for successful outcomes. The complexity of symptom management following hospitalization may require the advanced skills of an APN or other expert in palliative care to provide consultation to the home care nurse or to implement a plan of care with a patient and family. Access to these nurses may be based in a variety of settings, such as hospital-based clinics, private offices, and home care agencies. The multidisciplinary care provided by nurses, physicians, paraprofessionals, social workers, chaplains, and pharmacists is essential to the development of positive outcomes. As members of the multidisciplinary team, physicians must work in collaboration with other professionals across settings to provide comprehensive care to patients and families. Collaboratively, the team determines the amount of care needed, the most appropriate setting for care, and the type of interventions required to improve the patient's quality of life.

4. *Patients who have complex problems and receive home care nursing need family caregivers who are willing and able to learn the skills to provide care.*

Standardized educational programs to teach family caregivers skills to provide care are needed and should be a part of routine home nursing care. Examples of successful evidence-based programs have been cited in this chapter and can serve as an excellent beginning for nurses in home care facilities to develop a program.

In the event these caregivers are ill themselves, additional or complementary services need to be provided to help with the patients' care. Nurses providing home care for ill patients should conduct ongoing assessments of family caregivers, including willingness and skills to provide care, their health, and demands made on them.

5. *The use of innovative models must be considered as a strategy for providing care to patients and families.*

Telephone visits have been shown to be an effective strategy to help families cope with the caregiver role. Traditionally, specific criteria have been used to define the requirements for home care services. These criteria need to be reexamined in light of our increased understanding of disease patterns, treatment effects, and patient responses to illness. In the future, we need to consider alternative ways of delivering services to patients and family caregivers. Under prospective payment for home care, home care providers are no longer constrained by the per-visit method of reimbursement, and telephone visits can be integrated into the plan of care. The use of alternative and complementary therapy, nutritional counseling, or mental health therapies has been made financially reasonable as a result of the move to prospective payment. Telehealth programs have also been used effectively with patient populations at home.[70] Other technology interventions could include the use of the Internet or e-mail.[71,72] As the technology becomes less expensive, increased opportunity to implement these strategies will occur.

A growing number of cancer patients are being discharged from the hospital following surgery or other cancer treatments to be cared for at home by family caregivers who have chronic illnesses themselves, as described by the following case study. In this case study, we illustrate how patients can be admitted and discharged several times to home care throughout their illness trajectory. It is well established that patients can obtain the greatest benefit from palliative care if it is instituted early as part of their home care.

Case study

Mr. D, 61-year-old a male with stage IV esophageal cancer

Trajectory point 1 (diagnostic and hospital phase)

Mr. D is a 61-year-old executive who has worked his entire life to provide for his wife and three grown children. Overall, he had been in good health, monitoring his cholesterol and blood pressure since both his parents died of cardiac disease. Over the last decade, he gradually gained weight due to his sedentary life style, extended working hours, and increased dependency of his wife, who was diagnosed with multiple sclerosis 8 years ago About a month ago, Mr. D began having indigestion and heart burn. After ruling out cardiac problems, his primary care physician ordered antireflux medications. Subsequently, he complained of persistent pain, bloating, and difficulty getting his breath. A referral to the gastroenterologist revealed he had a large mass at the base of the esophagus. Because of the size of the tumor, it was recommended that Mr. D undergo radiation therapy to reduce the tumor prior to surgery. After completing his 6 weeks of radiation, Mr. D underwent removal of the distal end of his esophagus. Preoperatively, Mr. D experienced acute anxiety over his fear of being unable to care for his wife. His eldest daughter had come to care for her mother during his hospitalization, but she needed to leave to care for her own family and to return to work. Mr. D's postoperative recovery proceeded smoothly; he resumed a regular diet, was able to ambulate without assistance, and his pain was well controlled. During his hospital stay he and his family met with a social worker to identify postdischarge needs. Due to his improving health, he reported less anxiety about his wife, but identified a new concern related to his diagnosis of advanced cancer and requirement for additional cancer treatment. His return to near normal physical functioning and improved control of symptoms, however, resulted in his discharge after 4 days with routine postoperative instructions and no referral for home care services. He woke during his first night at home with severe pain and difficulty breathing. His wife called 911, and he was subsequently rehospitalized and diagnosed with a pulmonary embolus.

During his second hospitalization Mr. D was treated for his pulmonary embolus. He also reported increased pain related to swallowing, prompting a consult to the palliative care service. During this time, the palliative care APN recommended changes to his pain medications. He was also taught to administer his anticoagulation medication subcutaneously and was assisted by a nurse discharge coordinator to arrange home nursing services; he was considered homebound and in need of skilled nursing services. The goals of this skilled care were to ensure his safe administration of subcutaneous anticoagulation medication; help stabilize his blood coagulation; monitor signs and symptoms related to his potential for a recurrent embolus; and to provide ongoing monitoring of his postoperative recovery, particularly his pain. As part of her skilled observation and assessment, the home care nurse identified a potentially unstable situation due to Mr. D's role as primary caregiver for his wife and counseled the couple to consider arranging for homemaker services for Mrs. D. if Mr. D's condition was to worsen temporarily due to his ongoing cancer treatment with chemotherapy.

Trajectory point 2 (treatment)

Within 4 weeks after the second hospitalization, Mr. D's need for skilled nursing services lessened; he was able to return to work; his incision had healed, his stamina had improved, he was transitioned from subcutaneous anticoagulation medication to oral therapy, and his blood coagulation studies were considered within a therapeutic range. His throat pain had improved, and he was able to reduce his reliance on the analgesics. Home care services were discontinued, even though Mr. D's medical oncologist recommended he have a 6-month course of chemotherapy to reduce his chance of recurrence. Mr. D agreed and attempted to work full-time during his treatment and care full-time for his

ailing wife. Eventually, his cumulative chemotherapy treatments resulted in increasing fatigue, issues with neutropenia, and persistent and progressive neuropathic symptoms. He reported to his medical oncologist how his symptoms had resulted in a reduced work schedule as he was unable to care for both his wife and do his job. He also reported his anxiety had returned and he was having trouble sleeping. His medical oncologist contacted the palliative care team again. Mr. D met with a palliative care APN who recommended changes to his medications and self-management strategies to improve control of his physical and emotional symptoms. Also, she collaborated with the institution-based oncology nurse case manager to implement home health aide and homemaker services for his wife.

Trajectory point 3 (survivorship)

Once Mr. D's symptoms lessened, he gradually returned to work full-time and to his caregiving duties. He was discharged from the palliative care service. Mr. D remained asymptomatic and without any evidence of disease for 18 months.

Trajectory point 4 (initial recurrence)

Over time, Mr. D found he was losing weight, had a poor appetite, and became increasingly tired. His subsequent MRI demonstrated that the mass had returned and had spread to his liver. Mr. D and his family agreed to more chemotherapy to treat the symptoms associated with the return and spread of his cancer. Even with his chemotherapy, his symptoms were not adequately controlled. He continued to experience more intense weakness and loss of appetite. He developed abdominal ascites, difficulty swallowing, difficulty breathing, and generalized pain. His anxiety had also returned due to decline in physical health. In spite of his increasing physical dependency, Mr. D wanted to remain at home. The palliative care APN instituted palliative care services in the home, consisting of skilled nursing visits, home health aide support, and counseling by a palliative care social worker and pastoral staff. Mr. D's plan of care included pain management, nutritional and bowel management, support with activities of daily living, and counseling as it pertained to his job, finances, health insurance coverage issues, advanced directives, and his role as primary caregiver. Mr. D's social worker and the pastoral staff also spent time with him and his family preparing them for the inevitable outcome.

Trajectory point 5 (end of life)

Mr. D became increasingly sedentary and symptomatic, causing Mr. D's medical oncologist and his palliative care APN to initiate a discussion about stopping chemotherapy treatments. Mr. D and his family agreed—this change in treatment enabled Mr. D to be eligible for hospice-level benefits and hospice-level services at home. Fortunately, the home care agency providing services to Mr. D was certified as a hospice care agency, thereby allowing Mr. D and his family to keep the same home care providers. Within days, Mr. D's home care nurses assessed his progression toward dying and supported his decline accordingly. Two weeks after his death, Mr. D's palliative care APN met with the family to review the care that Mr. D had received. The nurse reinforced what a good job the family did with helping to keep Mr. D at home throughout his illness. Up to 6 months after his death, the palliative care APN kept in touch with the family to assist with their bereavement.

Summary

For palliative care to be a viable component of the service provided by home care agencies, changes are needed in both the structure of home care and the mechanisms for reimbursement. The regulations for the provision of home care under Medicare must be substantively modified to allow increased access to palliative care. Under the current regulations in the United States, the physician is the only provider who has the ability to order and to supervise a home plan of care through home care agencies. The literature is consistent in its description of the positive role APNs play in supporting both the patient and family caregivers in the home, yet APNs are not given the authority to direct patient care through home care agencies for patients who need palliative care. Exceptions do exist through hospital-based programs. For example, Memorial Sloan Kettering Cancer Center (New York) had a successful hospital-based supportive care program that provided palliative care in the home for high-risk cancer patients and their families. This program was directed by an APN who worked with community home care and hospice programs mainly through telephone contact and some home visits. There was no charge for the program. This program no longer exists and has been transitioned into a model where the outpatient APNs follow patients they have seen in the outpatient Pain and Palliative Care Clinic through ongoing telephone contact. Home visits are not made but contact with community nurses providing home care for the patients helps to provide continuity of care.

Regulations that support the critical role APNs play in the clinical management of patients at home who require palliative care and that legitimize the APN's ability to order and to supervise the plan of care are essential. The few successful models in hospital-based and ambulatory clinics could be implemented in home care agencies.

Additionally, the historical structure of Medicare reimbursement was a disincentive for the use of APNs in home care agencies. Because of the regulatory changes in reimbursement to prospective payment, APNs could play an increasingly important role in the delivery of effective home care. As the demographics of the home care population change and the complexity of clinical problems increases, agencies can ill afford to be without expert clinical providers or, at the very least, access to consultative services.

The earlier case study had a successful outcome, although the current home care delivery system is fragmented; however, the care in this case was effective because it was under the coordination of a palliative care team based in a cancer comprehensive center. The need for palliative care to be integrated into both home care as well as hospice care is essential for the provision of a continuum of care to patients at the end of life. For these changes to be integrated into the care delivery system, regulations need to be changed to allow home care nurses to provide end-of-life care in situations in which hospice care is unavailable, or at the request of the patient or family. Bridge programs have been developed to support the delivery of hospice-like services to traditional home care patients, but they are costly for the home care agency because Medicare will reimburse for only the traditional services. Nontraditional services such as bereavement care or counseling are not reimbursed. Creative strategies are needed to translate effective evidence-based interventions into standard clinical care, such as access to resources through the Internet.

In summary, home care is an important component of palliative care. Clinical and regulatory barriers have made palliative care in the home provided by certified hospices at the end of life the norm. Structural changes in home care are needed to fully integrate palliative care into the home care delivery system and at different times of crisis throughout the illness course. Additionally, the role of APNs must be fully acknowledged and reimbursement mechanisms established to integrate palliative care into home care for both patients and family caregivers.

References

1. American Association for Retired People. Valuing the Invaluable: The Economic Value of Family Caregiving 2011 Update. Available at: http://www.aarp.org/relationship/caregiving/info 07-2011/valueing-f.s.html (Accessed on July 22, 2013).
2. Clement-Stone S, Eigsti D, McGuire S. Comprehensive Health Nursing. 4th ed. St. Louis, MO: Mosby, 1995.
3. National Association for Home Care. Basic Statistics About Home Care. Updated 2010. Available at: http://www.nahc.org/assets/1/7/10HC_Stats.pdf (Accessed July 22, 2013).
4. Centers for Medicare and Medicaid Services, OASIS-C. Available at: http://www.cms.gov/Medicare/Quality-Initiatives-Patient-Assessment-Instruments/HomeHealthQualityInits/OASISC.html (Accessed July 22, 2013).
5. American Nurses Association. Home Health Nursing: Scope and Standards of Practice. Silver Springs, MA: American Nurses Association; 2008.
6. US Department of Health and Human Services, Home Health Care and Discharged Hospice Care Patients: United States, 2000–2007. National Health Statistics Reports Number 38. Washington, DC; 2011.
7. National Association for Home Care, Hospice Facts and Stats. Updated 2010. Available at: http://www.nahc.org/assets/1/7/HospiceStats10.pdf (Accessed July 22, 2013).
8. Coughlin, Joseph. (2010). Estimating the impact of caregiving and employment on well-being. Center for Health Research, Healthways, Incorporated. Available at http://www.healthways.com/success/library.aspx?id=615 (Accessed July 22, 2103).
9. Alzheimer's Association. Alzheimer's Disease Facts and Figures. 2011;7(2).
10. National Alliance for Caregiving. Caregiving in the United States 2009. Available at: http://www.caregiving.org/data/Caregiving_in_the_US_2009_full_report.pdf (Accessed on July 22, 2013).
11. vanRyn M, Sanders S, Kahn K, vanHoutven C, Griffin J, Martin M, et al. Objective burden, resources, and other stressors among informal cancer caregivers: a hidden quality issue. Psycho-Oncol. 2011;20:44–52.
12. US Department of Labor, Bureau of Labor Statistics. Occupational Employment Projects to 2020. Available at: http://www.bls.gov/emp/ep_table_103.htm (Accessed July 22, 2013).
13. Fleming M, Haney T. Improving patient outcomes with better care transitions: the role for home health. Cleve Clin J Med. 2013;80(1):e-S2–eS6.
14. Obamacare Watch, Medicare. Available at: http://obamacarewatch.org/primer/medicare (Accessed on July 22, 2013).
15. Lindley LC. Health care reform and concurrent curative care for terminally ill children: a policy analysis. J Hosp Palliat Nurs. 2011;13(2):81–88.
16. Lillard A. A bridge to hospice: smoothing the transition to end of life care. Advance. 2008;6(13):12–14.
17. Harrington S, Smith T. The role of chemotherapy at the end-of-life: "When is enough, enough?" JAMA. 2008;299:2667–2678.
18. Hack TF, Degner LF, Parker PA. The communication goals and needs of cancer patients: a review. Psycho-Oncol. 2005;14(10):831–845.
19. Schofield P, Carcy M, Love A, Nehill C, Wein S. Would you like to talk about your future treatment option?: Discussing the

transition from curative cancer treatment to palliative care. Palliat Med. 2006;20:397–406.

20. Murray S, Kendall M, Boyd K, Sheikh A. Illness trajectories and palliative care. BMJ. 2002;330:611–612.

21. Greer JA, Pirl WF, Jackson V, Muzikansky A, Lennes IT, Heist RS, et al. Effect of early palliative care on chemotherapy use and end-of-life care in patients with metastatic non-small cell lung cancer. J Clin Oncol. 2012;30(4):394–400.

22. Northouse L, Williams AL, Given B, McCorkle R. Psychosocial care for family caregivers of patients with cancer. J Clin Oncol. 2012,30(11):1227–1234.

23. Googe MC, Varricchio CG. A pilot investigation of home health care needs of cancer patients and their families. Oncol Nurs Forum. 1981;8:24–28.

24. Wellisch D, Fawzy F, Landsverk J, Pasnau R, Wocott D. Evaluation of psychosocial problems of the home-bound patient: the relationship of disease and sociodemographic variables of patients to family problems. J Psychosoc Oncol. 1983;1:1–15.

25. Teunissen S, Wesker W, Kruitwagen C, et al. Symptom prevalence in patients with incurable cancer: a systematic review. J Pain Symptom Manage. 2007;34:94–104.

26. Van den Beuken-van Everdinger MH, de Rijbe JM, Kessels AG, Schouten HC, van Kleef M, Atijn J. Prevalence of pain in patients with cancer: a systematic review of the past 40 years. Ann Oncol. 2007;18(9):1437–1449.

27. El-Jawahri A, Greer JA, Temel JS. Does palliative care improve outcomes for patients with incurable illness?: A review of the evidence. Support Oncol. 2011;9(3):87–94.

28. Candy B, Holman A, Leurent B, Davis S, Jones L. Hospice care delievered at home, in nursing homes and in dedicated hospice facilities: a systematic review of quantitative and qualitative evidence. Int J Nurs Stud. 2011;48:121–133.

29. McGuire DB, Grant M, Park J. Palliative care and end of life: the caregiver. Nurs Outlook. 2012;60(6):351–356.

30. McCorkle R, et al. Healthcare utilization in women after abdominal surgery for ovarian cancer. Nurs Res. 2011;60(1):47–57.

31. Finlay J, Higginson I, Goodwin D, et al. Palliative care in hospital, hospice, at home: results from a systematic review. Ann Oncol. 2002;13(Suppl):257–264.

32. Williams A, McCorkle R. Cancer family caregivers during palliative, hospice, and bereavement phases: a review of the descriptive psychosocial literature. Palliat Support Care. 2011; 9(3):315–325.

33. Goldstein NE, Concato J, Fried TR, Kasl SV, Johnson-Hurzeler R, Bradley EH. Factors associated with caregiver burden among caregivers of terminally ill patients with cancer. J Palliat Care. 2004;20:38–43.

34. McMillan SC, Small BJ, Using the COPE intervention for family caregivers to improve symptoms of hospice homecare patients: a clinical trial. Oncol Nurs Forum. 2007;34:313–321.

35. Chan Z, Kan C, Lee P, Chan I, Lam J. A systematic review of qualitative studies: patients' experiences of preoperative communication. J Clin Nurs. 2011;21:812–824.

36. Epstein RM, Street RL Jr. Patient-Centered Communication in Cancer Care: Promoting Healing and Reducing Suffering. NIH Publication No. 07-6225. Bethesda, MD: National Cancer Institute; 2007.

37. Northouse L, McCorkle R. Spouse caregivers of cancer patients in psycho oncology. In: Holland J, Jacobsen P, Loscalzo M, McCorkle R (eds.), Psycho-oncology. New York: Oxford Press; 2010:1907–1978, Chapter 72.

38. Proot I, Aby-Saad H, Crebolder H, Goldstein M, Luker K, Widdershoven G. Vulnerability of family caregivers between burden and capacity. Scand J Caring Sci. 2003;17:113–121.

39. Byock I, Twohig J, Merriman M, Collins K. Promoting excellence in end-of-life care: a report on innovative models of palliative care. J Palliat Med. 2006;9:137–151.

40. Low LF, Yap M, Brodaty H. A systematic review of different models of home and community care services for older persons. Health Serv Res. 2011;11(93):1–15.

41. Follwell M, Burman D, Le L, et al. Phase II study of an outpatient palliative care intervention in patients with metastatic cancer. J Clin Oncol. 2009;27(2):206–213.

42. Kralik D, Anderson B. Differences in home-based palliative care service utilization of people with cancer and non-cancer conditions. J Nurs Healthcare Chronic Illness. 2008;17(11):429–435.

43. Griffin J, Koch K, Nelson J, Cooley M. Palliative care consultation, quality-of-life measurements, and bereavement for end-of-life care in patients with lung cancer. Chest. 2007;132:404S–422S.

44. Given CW, Bradley C, You M, Sikorski A, Given B. Costs of novel symptom management Interventions and their impact on hospitalizations. J Pain Symptom Manage. 2010;39(4):663–672.

45. Kuebler K, Bruera E. Interactive collaborative consultation model in end-of-life care. J Pain Symptom Manage. 2000;20:202–209.

46. Corner J, Hallisday D, Haviland J, et al. Exploring nursing outcomes for patients with advanced cancer following intervention by Macmillan specialist palliative care nurses. J Adv Nurs. 2003;4:561–574.

47. Bakitas M, Lyon KD, Hegel MT, et al. Effects of a palliative care intervention on clinical outcomes in patients with advanced cancer: the Project ENABLE II randomized controlled trial. JAMA. 2009;19:741–749.

48. Meyer TJ, Mark MM. Effects of psychosocial interventions with adult cancer patients: a meta-analysis of randomized experiments. Health Psychol. 1995;14(2):101–108.

49. Sheard T, Maguire P. The effect of psychological interventions on anxiety and depression in cancer patients: results of two meta-analyses. Br J Cancer. 1999;80(11):1770–1780.

50. McCorkle R. A program of research on patient and family caregiver outcomes: three phases of evolution. Oncol Nurs Forum. 2006;33(1):25–31.

51. Given BA, Given CW, Sikorskii A, Jeon S, Sherwood P, Rahbar M. The impact of providing symptom management assistance on caregiver reaction: results of a randomized trial. J Pain Symptom Manage. 2006;32:433–443.

52. Miaskowski C, Dodd M, West C, Schumacher K, Paul SM, Tripathy D, et al. Randomized clinical trial of the effectiveness of a self-care intervention to improve cancer pain management. J Clin Oncol. 2004;22(9):1713–1720.

53. Given C, Given B, Rahbar M, et al. The effect of a cognitive behavioral intervention on reducing symptom severity during chemotherapy. J Clin Oncol. 2004;22(3):507–516.

54. Strecher VJ. Internet methods for delivering behavioral and health-related interventions (eHealth). Ann Rev Clin Psychol. 2007;3:53–76.

55. Family Care Research Program. Michigan State University. Family Education Issues: Symptom Management, 2009. Available at: http://www.cancercare.msu/edu (Accessed July 10, 2013).

56. Harding R, Higginson I. What is the best way to help caregivers in cancer and palliative care?: A systematic literature review of interventions and their effectiveness. Palliat Med. 2003;17:63–74.

57. Hudson P, Remedios C, Thomas K. A systematic review of psychosocial interventions for family carers of palliative care patients. BMC Palliative Care. 2010;9:1–6.

58. Northouse LL, Katapodi MC, Song L, Zhang L, Mood D. Interventions with caregivers of cancer patients: meta-analysis of randomized trials. CA Cancer J Clin. 2010;60:317–339.

59. Candy B, et al. Interventions for supporting informal caregivers of patients in the terminal phase of a disease (Review). Cochrane Database Syst Rev. 2011. Issue 6.

60. Budin WC, Hoskins CN, Haber J, et al. Breast cancer: education, counseling, and adjustment among patients and partners: a randomized clinical trial. Nurs Res. 2008;57:199–213.

61. Lewis FM, Cochrane BB, Fletcher KA, et al. Helping her heal: a pilot study of an educational counseling intervention for spouses of women with breast cancer. Psycho-Oncol. 2008;17:131–137.

62. Northouse LL, Mood DW, Schafenacker A, et al. Randomized clinical trial of a family intervention for prostate cancer patients and their spouses. Cancer. 2007;110:2809–2818.

63. Northouse LL, Mood DW, Schafenacker A, et al. Randomized clinical trial of a brief and extensive dyadic intervention for advanced cancer patients and their family caregivers. Psycho-Oncol. 2013;22:555–563.

64. McMillan SC, Small BJ, Weitzner M, et al. Impact of coping skills intervention with family caregivers of hospice patients with cancer. Cancer. 2006;106:214–222.

65. Ferrell B, Hudson P, Aranda S, Hayman-White K. A psycho-educational intervention for family caregivers of patients receiving palliative care: a randomized controlled trial. J Pain Symptom Manage. 2005;30:329–341.

66. Jacobsen P. Promoting evidence-based psychosocial care for cancer patients. Psycho-Oncol. 2009;18(1):6–13.

67. Schumacher KL, Koresawa S, West C, et al. Putting cancer pain management regimens into practice at home. J Pain Symptom Manage. 2002;23:369–382.

68. Bishop M, Stephens L, Goodrich M, Byock I. Medication kits for managing symptomatic emergencies in the home: a survey of common hospice practice. J Palliat Med. 2009;12:37–43.

69. Center for Medicare and Medicaid Services. Home Health PPS. Available at: http://www.cms.gov/Medicare/Medicare-Fee-for-Service-Payment/HomeHealthPPS/index.html (Accessed July 22, 2013).

70. Van den Brink JL, Moorman PW, de Boer MF, et al. Impact on quality of life of a telemedicine system supporting head and neck cancer patients: a controlled trial during the postoperative period at home. J Am Med Inform Assoc. 2007;14(2):198–205.

71. Bowles K, Baigh A. Applying research evidence to optimize tele-homecare. J Cardiovasc Nurs. 2007;22(1):5–15.

72. Kinsella A, Doughty K. Home telehospice: new tools for end-of-life care services. J Assist Technol. 2009;2:47–50.

CHAPTER 47

The intensive care unit

Jennifer McAdam and Kathleen Puntillo

> What really made it different was she [the ICU nurse] treated me with respect and dignity, and the dignity was what made it above and beyond. There were certain things that I could not do, I was not able to physically do, that were humiliating, that she had to do for me, and it was very, very, not pretty, it was very gross. But she treated me with respect and dignity and I thanked her profusely. She said it was just my job, and I know, but, thank you. You really make the difference.[1]

Key points

- All intensive care unit (ICU) patients deserve palliative care, whether the goal is cure or a peaceful end of life.

- Although an ICU is rarely the place where patients would choose to die, transition from aggressive care to end-of-life care is a frequent occurrence.

- Optimal transitional care in ICUs requires clear communication among patients, family members, and care providers from multiple disciplines.

- The appropriateness of procedures should be assessed, unnecessary procedures eliminated, and the pain associated with necessary procedures treated appropriately.

- Analgesics should be administered in the amounts necessary to decrease pain and symptoms without concern about the milligram dose required.

- Pain and symptom assessment and management, although challenging in an ICU setting, are primary roles and contributions of the ICU nurse.

- Conducting family meetings early in the ICU stay, establishing goals of care, and helping patients and family members with decision-making are important aspects of quality palliative and end-of-life care.

- Decisions to forgo life-sustaining therapies are made when the burden of aggressive treatment clearly outweighs the benefits. There are two methods of withdrawing ventilator therapy: immediate extubation and terminal weaning. Guidelines exist for each of these methods of withdrawal.

- Optimal family care occurs at any point along the patient's illness trajectory by providing access, information, support, and involvement in caregiving activities.

An ICU is, by tradition, the setting in which the most aggressive care is rendered to hospitalized patients. Patients are admitted to an ICU so that health professionals can perform minute-to-minute titration of care. The primary goals of this aggressive care are patient resuscitation, stabilization, and recovery from the acute phase of an illness or injury. However, many patients die in ICUs. It is estimated that greater than 500,000 people die after admission to ICUs in the United States each year.[2] Stated otherwise, almost one in five Americans receives ICU services before death. Researchers assessing mortality rates in seven states found that 47% of all hospital deaths involved intensive care services.[3] Investigators comparing Medicare beneficiaries' places of care and sites of death from 2000 to 2009 reported a significant increase in ICU usage during the last 30 days of life, with 29% of the decedents experiencing ICU care in the last month of life.[4] In addition, 24% of patients with poor-prognosis cancers were admitted to the ICU within 30 days of death.[5] Therefore, it is clear that management of the process of dying is common in ICUs.

In the high-technology environment of an ICU, it may be difficult for health professionals and families of dying patients to acknowledge that there are limits to the effectiveness of medical care. However, it is important to focus on providing the type of care that is appropriate for the individual patient and the patient's family, be it aggressive life-saving care, palliative care that includes symptom management, good communication, and interdisciplinary collaboration, or palliative end-of-life care. This chapter discusses the provision of palliative care in ICUs, with an emphasis on end-of-life care. Specifically, challenges and barriers to providing such care in ICUs are described, and recommendations are offered for the provision of symptom assessment and management. Current issues related to holding family meetings, establishing patient goals of care, surrogate decision-making, and withholding and withdrawing life-sustaining therapies are covered. Recommendations are offered for attending to the needs of families as well as healthcare providers who care for ICU patients at the end of life. Finally, an international agenda for improving end-of-life care in ICUs is presented.

The limitations of end-of-life care in intensive care units

Although many deaths occur in ICUs, an ICU is rarely the place that one would choose to die.[6] Health professionals in ICUs, frequently uncertain about whether a patient will live or die, are caught between the opposing goals of preserving life and preparing the patient and family for death. It is important for professionals to realize that a patient's death is not necessarily an indication of ineffective care. Yet, there remain serious limitations to the care provided to seriously ill and dying patients and their families. Communication between physicians, patients, and family members may be poor[7,8]; patients and family members may be overly optimistic about the outcomes of cardiopulmonary resuscitation (CPR)[9] and have unrealistic expectations of ICU technological treatments[10]; end-of-life decision-making can be challenging and present conflicts[11,12]; and many hospitalized patients die in moderate-to-severe pain and with other troubling symptoms.[13–15]

In a landmark study, more than 5,000 seriously ill hospitalized patients or their family members were asked questions about the patients' pain (SUPPORT).[16] Almost one-half of these patients had pain during the previous 3 days, and almost 15% had pain that was moderately or extremely severe and occurred at least half of the time. Of those with pain, 15% were dissatisfied with its control. In a more recent study measuring the symptom experiences of 171 ICU patients at high risk of dying, symptom prevalence ranged from 27% (confusion) to 75% (fatigue) and many symptoms were reported as intense (thirst) and distressful (shortness of breath, fear, confusion, and pain).[14] In a retrospective chart review of 88 ICU patients with advanced cancer referred for palliative care consultation, a significant proportion reported symptoms such as pain (84%), dyspnea (82%), fatigue (95%), constipation (60%), anxiety (65%), and depression (45%).[17] These findings stress the importance of attending to the assessment and management of pain and other symptoms in all ICU patients.

Planning palliative care for intensive care unit patients

Providing comfort to patients should accompany all ICU care, even during aggressive attempts to prolong life. However, if a patient is not expected to survive, the focus shifts to an emphasis on palliative care. It is often extremely difficult in an ICU to determine the appropriate time for a change of focus in care. A transition period occurs during which the health professionals, the patient's family, and sometimes the patient recognize the appropriateness of withdrawing and/or withholding life-sustaining treatments and begin to make preparations for death. The transition period (i.e., the time from decision to death) may be a matter of minutes or hours, as in the case of a patient who has sustained massive motor vehicle injuries, or it may be a matter of weeks, as in the case of a patient who has undergone bone marrow transplantation and has multiple negative sequelae while in the ICU. Clearly, this time difference must be recognized as a factor that can influence the experience of a patient's family members. When patients rapidly approach death, their family members may not have time to overcome the shock of the trauma and adjust to the possibility of death. On the other hand, when death is prolonged, family frustration and fatigue may be part of their experience. Health professionals who are sensitive to these different experiences can individualize their approaches and interventions for family members.

The death trajectory in the ICU usually follows one of the following patterns: a patient in good health that suffers a catastrophic event such as an intracranial bleed,[18] a patient with several comorbidities that presents with a new acute problem,[19] a patient with an exacerbation of their chronic condition,[20] or an elderly patient progressively declining with a life-threatening illness.[21] However, the transition from aggressive care to death preparation has not been well operationalized. The transition period is clearly uncomfortable for many healthcare professionals because clinically useful prediction models recognizing which patients have the highest risk of death in the ICU remain elusive.[22–25] Scenarios concerning end-of-life decision-making in the absence of patient or family input are especially challenging. Therefore, it is important for ICU professionals to hold patient and family meetings early in the ICU stay in order to address goals of care.[26] The following steps may be useful when caring for patients at risk for not surviving their ICU course:

♦ Ascertain whether the patient has developed an advance directive, whether a family member has durable power of attorney, and whether the patient has communicated a preference about CPR. In a retrospective review of 347 patients who died in the ICU, only 22% of the patients' preferences regarding life support were documented, and in 36% of the cases it was not reported whether a patient's representative existed or was involved with decision-making.[27]

♦ Hold a patient and family meeting early in the ICU stay with the goal being within the first 5 days.[26,28] Identify and communicate the goals of care for the patient and discuss and update them daily.

♦ Outline the steps that need to be taken to accomplish the goals of care and evaluate their effectiveness. Technology should not drive the goals of care. Instead, technology should be used, when necessary, to accomplish the goals, and its use should be minimized when the primary goal is achievement of a peaceful death.

♦ Use a multidisciplinary team approach to decision-making regarding transition to end-of-life care. All team members, including the patient's family, should reach a consensus—sometimes through negotiation—that the withdrawal of life support and a peaceful death are the appropriate patient outcomes.[29,30]

♦ In a situation where the patient lacks decision-making capacity and surrogate representation, it is recommended that a court appoint a guardian on behalf of the patient or that safeguards be put in place, such as mandatory ethics committee review, to protect the patient's interests. It is generally not recommended that the physician make the decision in isolation.[30–33]

♦ Develop and communicate the palliative care plan to professionals and family, and identify the best persons for implementing the various actions in the plan.

♦ Developing a plan of care may include enlisting the assistance of in-hospital palliative care staff and/or hospice services. The major goals in any palliative care plan are to provide optimal symptom management, provide psychosocial and spiritual support, provide patient- and family-centered care, coordinate care across settings, and provide staff support.[1,31,34]

Symptom assessment and management: essential components of palliative care

Pain assessment

Healthcare professionals have an ethical mandate to provide comfort to patients entrusted in their care.[35,36] However, in spite of advances in pain assessment and management techniques, hospitalized patients continue to receive inadequate pain management.[14,37] Pain research focusing specifically on dying ICU patients remains scarce, but advances that have been made in the assessment of pain in other critically ill patient populations can be applied to dying patients.[17,38–41] The patient's report of pain is still considered to be the most valid source, and seeking this information from the patient should be attempted whenever possible. Some ICU patients, even if they are being mechanically ventilated, may be able to use simple numeric or word rating scales, word quality scales, and body outline diagrams if they are provided. A 0–10 visually enlarged, horizontal numeric rating scale was found to be the most valid and feasible of five pain intensity rating scales tested in over 100 ICU patients.[42] However, many critically ill patients are unable to self-report because of their disease process, technological treatment interventions (e.g., mechanical ventilation), or the effects of medications (e.g., opioids, benzodiazepines [BZDs]). The use of BZD infusions may make patients too sedated to respond to pain, although pain may still be present. On the other hand, the use of the anesthetic agent propofol or of neuromuscular blocking agents (NMBAs) such as vecuronium may limit or entirely mask the patient's ability to express or show any behavioral signs of pain. It is essential that clinicians understand that propofol and NMBAs have no analgesic properties, although visible signs of pain disappear during their use. If these agents are used, they must be accompanied by infusions of analgesics, sedatives, or both. In these situations, the nurse may enlist the assistance of family members or friends in their evaluation of the patient's discomfort. The nurse can ask them about any chronic pain experienced by the patient or methods used by the patient at home to decrease pain or stress. This information can then be incorporated into the patient's care plan. In a recent study, the family members' ratings compared with the ICU patients' reports of pain intensity had a moderate to high level of agreement (intraclass correlation coefficient = 0.43).[43] Thus, there is early support that the family member might be a valid proxy reporter of patient pain.

When patients are too ill to communicate their pain through self-report, clinicians can conduct systematic observations of behaviors that might be indicative of pain. Li and colleagues published a systematic review of objective pain measures that can be used in critically ill patients.[44] These measures include the Behavioral Pain Scale (BPS) that was developed to quantify pain in sedated, mechanically ventilated patients.[45,46] Items on this scale include facial expressions, upper limb movements, and compliance with mechanical ventilation. A second behavior observation scale that can be considered is the Critical-Care Pain Observation Tool (CPOT).[47] It, too, prompts the assessor to view the patient's facial expressions, movements, ventilator compliance, and, additionally, muscle tension. Its psychometric properties have been evaluated in several studies.[38,48–50] The use of these scales helps clinicians assess specific pain behaviors in patients who are unable to self-report, and both the BPS and the CPOT have been recommended for patients unable to self report pain.[51,52] However, behavioral measures are only proxies for the patient's subjective reports, although they are frequently the only measures available. As another proxy measure, nurses can use their imaginations to identify possible sources of pain by asking the question, "If I were this patient and had intact sensations, what might be making me uncomfortable?" Even if patients are not exhibiting behavioral or physiological signs of pain, it does not mean that they are pain free.

Procedural pain

Before and during the transition from aggressive care to end-of-life care, critically ill patients undergo many diagnostic and treatment procedures. Many of these, such as central, arterial, and peripheral line placements, nasogastric tube placements,[53] chest tube removal,[54] and tracheal and endotracheal suctioning,[55,56] are quite painful and may be the primary cause of suffering at the end of life. Turning, one of the most ubiquitous procedures performed in acute and critical care settings, was shown to be the most painful of six commonly performed procedures.[57] Other procedures that may be unnecessary, painful, and unpleasant include central line insertions,[46] wound debridement, frequent dressing changes,[57,58] and the use of sequential compression devices.[46] Delgado-Guay and colleagues[17] demonstrated through a chart review that many ICU patients with advanced cancer had numerous procedures during end-of-life care. These procedures included chemotherapy, hemodialysis, total parenteral nutrition, and ventilators. In spite of this knowledge, routine and frequently conducted procedures continue to cause pain in ICU patients.[58,59] Nurses can act as "gatekeepers" by evaluating the appropriateness of procedures being planned for patients, especially after a decision has been made to end life support, and they can advocate for their omission. Helping patients avoid iatrogenic suffering is a fundamental part of palliative care. Practice guidelines should include recommendations that anticipating and treating pain be part of procedural instructions.[60] The most important procedures for patients to experience at the end of life are those that promote comfort. Yet, when necessary procedures must be performed, the nurse can facilitate pain management before, during, and after procedures.

Pharmacological management of pain

Numerous categories of analgesics and types of modalities exist for administration to critically ill patients.[61] As in all situations, the selection of analgesics should depend on the specific pain mechanism, and the route and modality should be matched to their predictability of effectiveness. Although no comprehensive survey of pain management techniques used for dying ICU patients has been reported, the most common analgesic intervention is use of intravenous (IV) opioids.[59] Choosing the best opioid and method of delivery will depend on factors such as the patient's body composition (e.g., amount of adipose tissue), development of tolerance, and the adverse effect profiles of the various opioids.[61] Use of a continuous infusion of an opioid allows for titration of the drug to a level of analgesic effectiveness and for maintenance of steady plasma levels within a therapeutic range. Box 47.1 presents basic principles in using opioids in critically ill patients.[61]

Box 47.1 Tenets of pain management

- Healthcare professionals should be patient advocates for effective pain control.

- Most critically ill patients will experience pain during their ICU stay.

- Healthcare professionals should assume that pain may be present especially when the patient cannot self-report or when objective measures of pain are conflicting.

- Early recognition and assessment of pain is more effective in controlling and managing pain.

- If there is any notion that the patient has pain, analgesics should be given prior to sedative agents (i.e., "analgesia first"),[63] especially with agents that possess little or no analgesic effects.

Sources: Erstad et al. (2009), reference 61; Barr et al. (2013), reference 51.

Additionally, healthcare professionals may consider the administration of intermittent opioid boluses for breakthrough pain. (See Table 47.1 for information on opioids commonly used in the ICU setting.) Please refer to chapter 7 for an in-depth discussion of pain management at end-of-life.

Clearly, concerns about patients becoming tolerant of or dependent on opioids are misplaced during terminal care. What is important is that professionals recognize the development of tolerance, which is the need for larger doses of opioid analgesics to achieve the original effect,[63] and increase the dosage as necessary. There is no ceiling effect from opioids; the dose can be increased until the desired effect is reached or intolerable side effects develop. If it is the family's wish to have the opioid infusion decreased in a sedated patient to assess that the patient is able to participate in end-of-life decision-making, this must be done slowly and carefully. Opioid-dependent patients are at high risk of developing withdrawal symptoms,[63] which would seriously increase their discomfort. In this situation, physical dependence can be addressed by gradually lowering the opioid dose while carefully assessing for signs of pain or withdrawal.

Titration of analgesics to achieve the desired effect is one of the most challenging and important contributions that ICU nurses can make to the comfort care of dying patients. The desired effect can often be described as use of the least amount of medication necessary to achieve the greatest comfort along with the optimum level of tranquil awareness. In ICU settings, there may be concerns that administration of analgesics in the amounts necessary to provide comfort could "cause" death. It is essential that ICU health professionals understand the "double-effect" principle. In brief, the double-effect principle states that administration of analgesics to dying patients in the amounts necessary to decrease pain and suffering—although possibly causing unintentional hastening of death—is a good, ethically sound way to treat a dying patient.[64] This principle, framed in ethics, provides support to such an action when the clinician's moral intent is directed primarily at alleviating suffering rather than intending to kill. In fact, critical care investigators have found no relationship between the terminal patient's duration of survival and use of opioids.[65,66] When the

Table 47.1 Pharmacology of commonly used opioids in the ICU

Agent	Equianalgesic dose (mg)	Onset		Half-life	Intermittent dose	Infusion dose range	Active metabolites	Unique concerns[a]
Fentanyl	0.1	N/A	1–2 min	2–4 h	0.35–0.5 µg/kg IV every 0.5–1 h	0.7–10 µg/kg/h	No metabolite, parent accumulates in fatty tissues	Less hypotension than morphine Accumulation in hepatic impairment Muscle rigidity
Hydromorphone	1.5	7.5	5–10 min	2–3 h	0.2–0.6 mg IV every 1–2 h	0.5–3 mg/h	hydromorphone 3 glucoronide and 6 glucoronide	May work in patients tolerant to morphine or fentanyl Accumulation in hepatic/renal impairment
Morphine	10	30	5–10 min	3–4 h	2–4 mg IV every 1–2 h	2–30 mg/h	6- and 3-glucuronide metabolite	Bradycardia/hypotension Bronchospasm Accumulation in hepatic/renal impairment
Remifentanil	N/A	N/A	1–3 min	3–10 min	N/A	1.5 µg/kg loading dose, then 0.5–15 µg/kg/h	None	Bradycardia/hypotension No accumulation in hepatic/renal failure Use ideal body weight if > 30% IBW

Abbreviations: IV, intravenous; IBW, ideal body weight; N/A, not applicable.

[a] Common adverse effects associated with all opioids, such as respiratory and central nervous system depression, are not listed.

Sources: Erstad et al. (2009), reference 61; Joffe et al. (2013), reference 62; Barr et al. (2013), reference 51.

ICU patient is approaching death, the most important aim of care should be to make the patient's dying as comfortable as possible. Effective symptom control may be one of the last interventions offered to dying patients and their families.[15]

Nonpharmacological management of pain

Nonpharmacological interventions for pain management complement, but do not substitute for, the use of pharmacological interventions. Numerous therapies may be used by critical care nurses to augment the administration of medications to promote patient comfort. They include the use of distraction (e.g., music, humor), relaxation techniques (e.g., visual imagery, rhythmic breathing), and massage.[67] Complementary therapies are low-cost, easy to provide, and safe, and many clinicians can implement them with little difficulty or resources. There is research evidence that ICU nurses do use these types of therapies in their practice.[15] A group of 22 ICU nurses caring for 24 patients were asked about their use of nonpharmacological therapies for patients' symptoms. Nurses reported the use of nonpharmacological interventions such as music, distraction, touch, and talk. However, they did not immediately recognize them as such. Family members can be encouraged to assist with the provision of comfort measures and may welcome this way of participating in care and decreasing their sense of helplessness. Family involvement is discussed in further detail in a later section of this chapter.

Anxiety, agitation, and sedation

An important part of palliative care in the ICU is assessment and treatment of anxiety and agitation. In one study of 171 ICU patients with a high risk of dying, 58% reported feeling anxious and rated this symptom at a moderate level of intensity.[14] There are many reasons for a dying patient to be anxious, agitated, or both. Assessment of anxiety and agitation provides the practitioner with information that can guide the use of specific interventions. It is imperative to assess for these symptoms because they have been associated with nosocomial infections,[68] unplanned extubations,[69,70] shortness of breath, increase in blood pressure and heart rate, and combative behavior.[71]

Assessment of anxiety and agitation

Simple numeric rating scales for anxiety can be used if the patient can self-report to identify how much the patient is psychologically bothered. Critical care clinicians and patients are familiar with the use of the 0 to 10 numeric rating scales for pain. "Anxiety" word anchors can be substituted for pain word anchors so that the numeric rating scales also can be used to quantify the degree of distress.

Common behavioral or physiological signs of anxiety include trembling, restlessness, sweating, tachycardia, tachypnea, difficulty sleeping, and irritability. Several agitation/sedation assessment scales are available (e.g., Richmond Agitation Scale, Ramsey Scale, Sedation Agitation Scale).[59,72] These scales can be printed on the patient flowsheet, on a separate form, or in the electronic medical record and used as a bedside assessment tool. Nurses can plan periodic and simultaneous assessments of pain and agitation using pain rating scales and agitation scales. The frequency with which the scales are used depends on the patient's condition and the schedule for evaluating treatment interventions.

Pharmacological management to promote sedation in anxious or agitated patients

Along with opioids, other categories of sedating drugs are frequently used in the ICU, especially for patients who are mechanically ventilated. Several guidelines,[51,73] algorithms,[74] and review articles[59,72,75,76] exist regarding the use of analgesics and sedatives. Often, the goal of combined analgesic-sedative therapy is to promote physical and psychological comfort. Practice decisions include choosing the right type and combination of medications, determining whether to use interrupted sedative infusions (which provide opportunities for patient assessment) or continuous infusions,[56,76] determining appropriate clinical endpoints for pharmacological interventions,[77] and evaluating the effectiveness of sedation protocols on practices and outcomes.[78,79]

The appropriate pharmacological agent to control agitation and anxiety is selected according to the desired effect.[77] For example, uncomplicated anxiety is best treated with BZDs, whereas paranoia, panic, and fear accompanied by delusions and hallucinations may require the addition of antipsychotic agents. The BZDs are excellent agents for anxiolysis, but they possess no analgesic or psychological properties. Concomitant use of BZDs, opioids, and certain neuroleptic agents may relieve anxiety-provoking symptoms through a synergistic action.[80] When used together, these drugs can be administered in lower doses less frequently, have fewer side effects, and can decrease or delay development of tolerance or dependence through the use of smaller doses of each drug. At lower doses, BZDs reduce anxiety without causing central nervous system sedation or a decrease in cognitive or motor function. With increasing dosages, inhibition of motor and cognitive functions as well as central nervous system depression does occur. Sufficiently high doses can induce hypnosis and coma.[80]

The most frequently used BZDs in critical care are midazolam and lorazepam.[77] When midazolam is used as a continuous infusion, the dose can be 1 to 2 mg/h for mild sedation or as high as 20 mg/h for severe agitation if the patient is mechanically ventilated (see Table 47.2). If the degree of sedation is not adequate, then the serum level of midazolam can be raised by one to three small bolus IV injections while simultaneously increasing the infusion rate.[76]

Lorazepam gives effective sedation and anxiety relief over a longer period than midazolam. Cardiovascular and respiratory effects occur less frequently with this drug than with other BZDs. It may also act synergistically with haloperidol, a neuroleptic agent discussed later in this chapter. Lorazepam can be administered intravenously, intramuscularly, or orally. Intravenous doses may be 2 to 6 milligrams every 4 to 6 hours. In the critical care setting, it can also be administered as an infusion at 1 to 10 mg/h and titrated to clinical effect.[76] As with opioids, tolerance to BZD effects can develop in critically ill patients, especially those receiving midazolam infusions. Midazolam should also be used in caution with patients with renal insufficiency.[76,80] Benzodiazepine dependence can occur, evidenced by symptoms such as dysphoria, tremor, sweating, anxiety, agitation, muscle cramps, myoclonus, and seizures on abrupt medication withdrawal.[81] Benzodiazepines should also be used with caution as they may be a risk factor in the development of ICU delirium.[51,82]

Propofol is a highly lipophilic IV sedative/hypnotic agent that has a very rapid onset of action and short duration. It is indicated for use in the ICU to control agitation and the stress response in

Table 47.2 Pharmacological symptom management

Symptom	Drug type most frequently used	Method of administration	Usual dose[*]
Pain	Opioids (e.g., morphine, fentanyl, hydrocodone, methadone)	Continuous IV infusions with use of intermittent boluses for procedure-related pain or during treatment withdrawal	Continuous infusion: 1–10 mg/h morphine equivalents[**] Bolus: 2–5 mg IV morphine equivalent slow push; titrate to effect
Anxiety/agitation	Benzodiazepines (e.g., lorazepam, midazolam)	Same as for opioids	Continuous midazolam infusion: 1–20 mg/h Bolus midazolam: 2–5 mg IV Continuous lorazepam infusion: 1–10 mg/h Bolus lorazepam: 2–6 mg IV every 4–6 hours
	Haldol	IV boluses	Bolus: 0.5–20 IV
	Propofol	Continuous IV infusion	Continuous: 50–150 mcg/kg/min
Dyspnea	Oxygen	Multiple methods (e.g., nasal cannula, mask, ventilator)	Concentration as needed See above for IV doses
	Opioids (e.g., morphine)	Continuous IV infusion and/or IV bolus; or per nebulizer	Per nebulizer: 2.5 mg in 3 mL saline (preservative free) or sterile water q4h
	Benzodiazepines	See above	See above
	Bronchodilators (e.g., metaproterenol sulfate)	Per nebulizer	Metaproterenol sulfate: 2.5 mL 0.4–0.6% solution
	Diuretics (e.g., furosemide)	IV bolus, slow push	Bolus furosemide: 20–40 mg IV
	Anticholinergics (e.g., atropine)	Per nebulizer	Atropine: 0.025 mg/kg diluted with 3–5 mL saline three or four times daily; doses not to exceed 2.5 mg

[*]Drug doses are general recommendations. Dosing should be individualized to a particular patient. Under usual circumstances, start with low doses, wait for effect, and titrate to desired effect.

[**]"Rapid titration of opioids with small incremental IV doses is the preferred initial mode of therapy for critically ill patients with acute pain" (Erstad, reference 61, p. 1079)

Sources: Erstad et al. (2009), reference 61; Kompanje et al. (2008), reference 141; Treece et al. (2004), reference 147; Hughes et al. (2012), reference 77; Campbell, M. (2012), reference 97; Campbell, M. (2011), reference 99; Mahler et al. (2010), reference 103.

patients who are mechanically ventilated and those who require deep sedation for procedures.[77] However, propofol has no analgesic properties and must always be used in conjunction with analgesics whenever the patient might experience pain. During initial use of propofol, a drop in systolic blood pressure, mean arterial blood pressure, and heart rate may occur in patients with fluid deficits and in those receiving opioids.[77] The rapid loss of clinical effect of propofol renders it a valuable sedative agent in the critical care environment. Continuous infusion doses may range from 5 to 150 mcg/kg/min (see Table 47.2).[76] The short effective half-life of propofol allows rapid clinical evaluation of the patient's level of consciousness and determination of the minimum dose required for effective sedation. This may make it a useful drug during situations in which intermittent interaction with professionals and family members is desired.[80,83]

Dexmedetomidine is a potent, centrally acting alpha 2-adrenergic agonist that can be used for ICU patients requiring light sedation.[84] Even though this medication does have analgesic properties, most patients will require additional opioids for pain management.[84,85] Sedation is often initiated with a bolus of 1 mcg/kg over 10–20 minutes followed by an infusion of 0.2–0.7 mcg/kg/h and has been FDA approved for use in sedation for less than 24 hours.[77] However,

dosages and durations of therapy exceeding those approved by the FDA may be relatively safe.[86] Continuous infusions of dexmedetomidine have been associated with bradycardia and hypotension, whereas frequent bolus doses have been associated with hypertension.[80] Due to side effects occurring from rapid bolus dosing, it may not be the preferred choice for patients with acute agitation.[84] In addition, because this medication is metabolized by the liver, it should be used with caution in those with liver disease.[87] Current pain, agitation, and delirium guidelines suggest the use of non-BZD sedatives, such as propofol and dexmedetomidine, as the preferred choice for sedation medications.[51]

It is important that patients in ICUs be routinely assessed for the presence of delirium using available and reliable tools such as the Intensive Care Delirium Screening Checklist (ICDSC) or the Confusion Assessment Method for ICU (CAM-ICU).[51,88–91] Haloperidol is a frequently used neuroleptic for critically ill patients with delirium.[92,93] In a recent study, short-term prophylactic administration of low-dose IV haloperidol given to elderly ICU patients after noncardiac surgery led to a significant decrease in the incidence of postoperative delirium.[94] However, there is no published evidence that haloperidol actually reduces the duration of delirium.[51] This drug does have the benefit of less cardiovascular effects unless given rapidly, in which case vasodilation and hypotension may occur. Haloperidol does not depress respirations; rather, it has a calming effect on agitated, disoriented patients, making them more manageable without causing excessive sedation. However, haloperidol has some significant adverse effects, such as reduction of the seizure threshold, precipitation of extrapyramidal reactions, and prolongation of the QT interval leading to torsades de pointes.[92] Clinicians may try other atypical antipsychotic medications (e.g., olanzapine, quetiapine, and ziprasidone) in treating delirium with fewer side effects than haloperidol.[93] Recent guidelines suggest evidence that atypical antipsychotics may reduce the duration of delirium however they do not prevent delirium in ICU patients.[51] More robust clinical trials are needed to justify the most appropriate pharmacological treatment of delirium.[92]

Nonpharmacological interventions for anxiety and agitation

Numerous interventions exist that may promote tranquility and sedation in a critical care environment. These include distraction, control of environmental noise and the use of clocks, calendars, and personal articles such as pictures from home.[71] Music therapy can be used to decrease anxiety and pain as well as promote sleep.[67] In a recent study, Chlan and colleagues reported that patients in a self-directed music group had a reduction in sedation frequency, intensity, and medication use when compared with patients with usual care.[95] As noted earlier, imagery and relaxation techniques also provide a means of distraction for patients and help to alleviate anxiety.[67,96]

The act of physically caring for a patient and providing gentle touch is a major source of comfort for patients in critical care. Taking the time to provide simple measures such as back rubs and massages, repositioning the patient, smoothing bed linen wrinkles, removing foreign objects from the bed, providing mouth and eye care, and taping tubes to maintain patency and inhibit pulling effectively promotes comfort and decreases anxiety. Family member participation in caregiving activities, such as bathing, massages, and back rubs, can have a powerful calming effect on patients and promote sleep and psychological integrity.

For alert patients, increasing opportunities for control is a strategy that can reduce the sense of helplessness that often accompanies patients who are critically ill. This sense of control can be promoted by allowing alert patients to make decisions about the timing of interventions. Facilitating contact and communication with clergy, psychologists, or psychiatrists, if appropriate, can help to alleviate the distress experienced by both patients and families.

Dyspnea assessment and management

Dyspnea is a subjective experience of feeling short of breath and is one of the most distressing symptoms that can be experienced by critically ill patients at high risk for dying.[97] In addition, it is often associated with other symptoms such as anxiety and pain.[98] The gold standard for assessing dyspnea is patient self-report. The simplest way is to ask the patient, "Do you feel short of breath?" A "yes" or "no" answer gives the healthcare clinician initial information. However, most critical care patients at high risk of dying cannot self-report and give a yes or no answer.[99] In

this case, the Respiratory Distress Observation Scale is the only known tool to assess dyspnea in an adult patient who cannot self-report. This tool has eight items that measure the presence and intensity of respiratory distress. Each of the items is scored from 0 to 2 with higher scores indicating higher respiratory distress. This tool has demonstrated interrater reliability, construct, convergent, and discriminant validity[100–102] and is appropriate to use on patients undergoing terminal ventilator withdrawal (discussed later in the chapter).[99] Management of dyspnea in patients at high risk of dying includes oxygen therapy, opioids, BZDs, bronchodilators, diuretics, and anticholinergics (see Table 47.2).[99,103] Please refer to chapter 14 for an in-depth discussion of dyspnea.

Other distressing symptoms

Scant research has been conducted on symptoms experienced by ICU patients who are at high risk of dying. A notable exception was the study by Puntillo and colleagues.[14] These investigators specifically focused on the self-reported symptom experiences of ICU patients who were at high risk of dying. Investigators used a 10-item symptom checklist measuring both intensity (scale 0–3) and distress (scale of 0–3) of symptoms such as pain, fatigue, shortness of breath, restlessness, anxiety, sadness, hunger, fear, thirst, and confusion. Their sample consisted of 171 patients (mean age: 58 years; 64% male); 34% were mechanically ventilated, and 19% died during their ICU stay. The most prevalent symptoms included fatigue (75%), thirst (71%), and anxiety (56%). Symptoms lower in prevalence but reported to be moderately distressful by patients included shortness of breath, pain, confusion, fear, and sadness. This study demonstrated that a significant proportion of patients at high risk of dying in ICUs experience substantial emotional and physical symptoms.

Nurses in the ICU play a major role in alleviating distressing symptoms experienced by patients at the end of life. For example, there have been several methods identified for relieving thirst and dry mouth. Nurses can use topical dry mouth products containing olive oil, betaine, and xylitol,[104] or they can use artificial saliva and salivary flow stimulants. A recent randomized trial reported that patients using a "bundle" of thirst interventions (sprays of cold water, swabs of cold sterile water, and mouth and lip moisturizer) had significantly decreased thirst intensity and distress when compared with patients in a "usual care" group.[105,106] Because nurses are the healthcare providers who are constantly at the bedside, they can assess the presence of these symptoms, advocate for effective pharmacological therapy, use additional nursing comfort measures, and provide for continuity of therapy. Symptom management is a special contribution that ICU nurses can make to their patients at the end of life.

End-of-life practice issues: withholding and withdrawing life-sustaining therapies

Limiting life-sustaining therapies in an ICU is becoming more common. It is estimated that withholding or withdrawing of life support occurs in 67%–84% of deaths in ICUs.[107,108] Generally, life-sustaining treatment is withdrawn when death is believed to be inevitable despite aggressive interventions. The American College of Physicians (ACP)[109] supports the right of a competent patient to refuse life-sustaining and life-prolonging therapy. They also note that there is no moral difference between withholding and withdrawing therapy. In addition, critical care–related professional organizations have published position papers in support of the patient's autonomy regarding withholding and withdrawal decisions.[31,110]

If patients are unable to make treatment decisions, then these decisions must be made on the patient's behalf by surrogates or by the healthcare team.[29,111] Optimally, patients' living wills or advance directives can provide the direction for decisions related to treatment withholding or withdrawal. However, completion rates of these documents remain low.[17,112,113] When surrogates are asked to participate in decision-making, it is recommended that a family-centered,[31,34] shared decision-making approach be used.[111,114] These approaches are recommended for major decisions involving limiting life-sustaining treatments when survival is unlikely but possible or when survival may come with significant impairment.[29] Holding multidisciplinary family meetings is an effective way for families to arrive at decisions about the patient's goals of care and may help reduce the burden and distress they experience during this time.[30] Because problems with decision-making and communication deficits around end-of-life care are still frequent sources of conflict in the ICU,[115] having a guideline to follow for conducting family meetings may be helpful. The following is a list of steps for conducting a family meeting when the patient is unable to participate in the decision-making process.[116–119] In addition, there are helpful mnemonic techniques that may improve the quality of the communication processes between ICU clinicians and family members during end-of-life-care family meetings (see Table 47.3).

Conducting ICU family meetings

Prepare

- Review the patient history and medical problems.
- Coordinate who on the healthcare team will attend the meeting (should be multidisciplinary and include the attending MD, bedside RN, social worker, palliative care clinician(s), and other relevant healthcare team members).[30]
- Discuss goals of the meeting with the healthcare team.
- Identify one team member as meeting leader.

Table 47.3 Helpful mnemonics for family meetings

VALUE technique	NURSE
V- Value and appreciate what the family has said	N- Name: "You seem distressed [or angry or worries, etc.]"
A- Acknowledge family emotions	U- Understand: "This must be very difficult for you."
L- Listen to the family	R- Respect: "I can see how much you are trying to honor your Dad's wishes."
U- Understand the patient as a person through the family	S- Support: "We will be there to help advise you."
E- Elicit family's concerns and questions	E- Explore: "Tell me more about what you are thinking/feeling."

Sources: Curtis et al. (2002), reference 120; Pollack et al. (2007), reference 121.

- Discuss which family members will be present.
- Arrange a private, quiet location with seating for all.

Open the meeting

- Introduce all in attendance.
- Establish the overall goal of the meeting, elicit family goals as well.
- Acknowledge that this is a difficult time and situation.
- Set rules for the discussion (e.g., time frame for the meeting).

Elicit family understanding

- Ask questions of family members and listen.
- As they respond, think about:
  - What do they understand?
  - What do they believe will happen?
  - What are their emotions?

Identify preferences for decision-making and information sharing

- Identify how family members prefer to receive information and the level of detail they would like to receive.
- Assess the family's preference for their role in decision-making (this can range from letting the physician decide to the family member assuming all responsibility for the decision).[111]

Give information

- Give brief information (e.g., two points you really want them to understand) and allow time for family to ask questions.
- Avoid medical jargon.
- Do not talk too much or focus on technical matters.
- Be transparent about uncertainty.
- If the patient is dying, be sure to use the words "death" or "dying".

Respond with explicit empathy to family emotions

- Use the N-U-R-S-E mnemonic (see Table 47.3).
- Don't fight but rather join family statements of hopefulness, using wish statements (e.g., "I wish I could promise that things would get better. I hope he gets better soon too.").
- See if the family can hope for the best but prepare for the worst.

After giving information, ask about concerns and questions

- "You just got a lot of information. What questions do you have?"

Elicit patient and family values and goals

- Ask about the patient's goals, values, and previous discussion about end-of-life care.
- Frame those wishes within the context of the current medical situation.

- Avoid asking family, "What do you think we should do?" Instead, ask what they know about their loved one's preferences and maintain focus on the patient's perspective.

- Identify pertinent cultural, ethnic, or religious beliefs that may influence communication, decision-making, family relationships, and concepts of death and dying.[122]

Deal with decisions that need to be made

- Make a recommendation based on patient and family goals.[111,123]

- Time-limited trials with clear endpoints may make sense in certain clinical situations.

- Do not offer treatments that are inappropriate, as when the burdens outweigh the benefits.

- Do not speak of "withdrawing care" or "treatment." Affirm ongoing quality of care and reassure the family that care will never be withdrawn, but the focus of care may change.

Close the meeting

- Offer a brief summary of what was discussed.

- Offer to answer questions and assure the family that the team is accessible.

- Check in to make sure the family heard what you wanted them to hear.

- Express appreciation and respect for the family.

- Facilitate referrals to support services.

- Make a clear follow-up plan, including scheduling the next family meeting.

Document and debrief

- Communicate the outcome of the meeting to the rest of the clinical team.

- Document the meeting in the medical chart.

Incorporating mnemonic communication approaches such as the ones listed in Table 47.3 or following the guidelines for conducting a family meeting have shown promise. For example, in a randomized controlled trial comparing family members who received standard care to family members who received the VALUE intervention during their end-of-life care conference, researchers found that those family members who received the intervention had significantly lower symptom prevalence of posttraumatic stress disorder (PTSD), anxiety, and depression.[124] Other investigators found that when using palliative care indicators such as physician recommendation to withdraw life support and expressions of patients' wishes, and discussion of families' spiritual needs were reported, family members satisfaction with end-of-life decision making was significantly higher.[123] Other researchers reported that the use of empathetic comments were associated with higher family satisfaction with communication.[125] In another study family members reported significant improvement in having their needs met when they participated in multidisciplinary family meetings conducted by palliative care nurses.[126]

Nurses in the ICU can be integral in family meetings and improving surrogate decision-making. One investigator discussed five ways that the ICU nurse can assist families with surrogate decision-making. They can begin by preparing the family member for the role of being a surrogate. Next, they can organize regular meetings between the family and the multidisciplinary team. Then, once the meeting is scheduled, the nurse can prepare the family before each ICU family meeting on what to expect and what questions to ask. Fourth, they can provide emotional support to the family during the ICU meetings. Finally, they can be present for the family after the meeting.[127] One mixed methods study assessing the effectiveness of using a nurse as a family support specialist found that the intervention improved communication, improved discussion of the patient's values and preferences, and improved patient-centered care.[128]

Nelson and colleagues discussed the importance of ICU nurses being involved in family meetings. The ICU nurses know the patient's condition, have knowledge of the family, and have a continuous presence at the bedside. In addition to this, they can provide continuity to the family as well as ensure that communication and decisions are consistent within the team.[129] However, this role is not always comfortable for the ICU nurse. Therefore, a group of researchers implemented an educational intervention to improve communication skills for ICU nurses to better prepare them for their role in interdisciplinary meetings. Nurses received training in key components of their role in ICU family meetings, strategies in dealing with strong emotions, and approaches to dealing with conflict. Nurses who attended this training reported more confidence in voicing concerns about patient care, better ability to initiate meetings, and less anxiety in taking part in the meetings.[130]

When a decision to forgo life-saving therapy is made in the ICU, there should be a concerted effort to evaluate all therapies, including blood products, hemodialysis, vasopressors, mechanical ventilation, total parenteral nutrition, antibiotics, IV fluids, and tube feedings, to assess whether these treatments could make a positive contribution to the patient's comfort.[31,131] Withdrawal of therapies should be preceded by chart notations of do-not-resuscitate (DNR) orders and a note documenting the rationale for comfort care and removal of life support.[132] There should be a clear plan of action and provision of information and support to the family. Adequate documentation of patient assessments, withdrawal decisions and plans, therapy withdrawal orders, and patient and family responses during and after withdrawal is essential.[29,31,132] However, there is considerable variability regarding physician recommendations and documentation of discussions with families regarding withdrawal of life support.[8,131,133–135] In addition, there is considerable variability in the standardization around the process of withdrawing life support[136,137] and decision-making.[138,139] All of these inconsistencies may infer—rightly or wrongly—the lack of quality end-of-life and palliative care in the ICU.[8]

Withdrawal of ventilator therapy with consideration of analgesic and sedative needs

It is important to understand the methods by which mechanical ventilation may be removed. Withdrawal of this treatment deserves the same clinical preparation as any other ICU procedure.[31] The primary goal during this process should be to ensure that patients and family members are as comfortable as possible, both psychologically and physically. Two primary methods of

Table 47.4 Methods of mechanical ventilation withdrawal

Immediate extubation	Terminal weaning
Description	
Abrupt removal of the patient from ventilator assistance by extubation after suctioning (if necessary). Humidified air or oxygen is administered to prevent airway drying.	Physicians or other members of the ICU team (e.g., respiratory therapists, nurses) gradually withdraw ventilator assistance. This is done by decreasing the amount of inspired oxygen, decreasing the ventilator rate and mode, removal of positive end-expiratory pressure (PEEP), or a combination of these maneuvers. Usual time from ventilator to T-piece or extubation: 15–60 min.
Positive aspects	
Patient free of technology; dying process less likely to be prolonged; intentions of the method are clear.	Allows titration of drugs to control symptoms; maintains airway for suctioning if necessary; patient does not develop upper airway obstruction; longer time between ventilator withdrawal and death; moral burden on family may be less because method appears less active.
Negative aspects	
Noisy breathing, dyspnea may be distressful to patient/family.	May prolong dying; patient unable to communicate; machine between patient and family.
Time course to death	
Unpredictable. Usually shorter than with terminal weaning.	Unpredictable.

Sources: Truog et al. (2008), reference 31; Billings (2012), reference 144; Szalados et al. (2007), reference 142; Campbell (2007), reference 143.

mechanical ventilation removal exist: immediate extubation and terminal weaning (Table 47.4). Debates continue as to which of these methods is optimal for the patient, and often the method is determined according to the physician's, patient's, or family members' comfort levels.[140-142] However, in one study, Gerstel and colleagues reported a significant increase in family satisfaction with immediate extubation before death of their loved one in the ICU.[131]

Although there is considerable variability regarding the preferred approach to withdrawal,[143] recommendations regarding specific procedures for withdrawal are available.[31,141,145,146] Box 47.2 presents a protocol for withdrawal of mechanical ventilation for the clinician's consideration that includes specific recommendations regarding use of analgesics and sedatives. Consensus guidelines on the provision of analgesia and sedation for dying ICU patients support the titration of analgesics and sedatives based on the patient's requests or observable signs indicative of pain or distress.[31] The guidelines emphasize that no maximum dose of opioids or sedatives exists, especially considering that many ICU patients receive high doses of these drugs over their ICU course. Anticipatory dosing, as opposed to reactive dosing, is recommended by some to avoid patient discomfort and distress.[31,141] Researchers surveying 143 nurses and 61 physicians on the usefulness of using a standardized order form for the withdrawal of life support, found the majority of nurses (84%) reported the form was helpful and were mostly satisfied with the sedation and mechanical ventilation sections. Almost all of the physicians (95%) reported that the form was helpful and were mostly satisfied with the sedation, mechanical ventilation, and death preparation sections.[147] Using a standardized order form is recommended,[31] however, in a more recent study, only 12% of nurses reported using standing orders to guide withdrawal of life support, and most (64%) were guided by individual physician's orders.[136]

It is important to provide comfort to dying patients who could experience pain and other distressing symptoms during withdrawal of mechanical ventilation. One group of investigators

studying patients receiving morphine or morphine equivalents and BZDs prior to mechanical ventilation withdrawal reported that these agents did not cause unintended harm and shorten survival time.[148] In another study, researchers found that increased dosages of morphine were actually associated with a longer time to death.[149] Therefore, clinicians should strive for symptom control at the end of life and assure that comfort is maintained.[141,144]

Patients should be withdrawn from NMBAs before withdrawal from life support. The use of NMBAs (such as vecuronium) makes it almost impossible to assess patient comfort; although the patient appears comfortable, he/she may be experiencing pain, respiratory distress, or severe anxiety. The use of NMBAs prevents the struggling and gasping that may be associated with dying but not the patient's suffering.[31,141,150] The horror of such a death can only be imagined. The withdrawal of these agents may take considerable time for patients who have been receiving them chronically, and patients continue to have effects from lingering active metabolites.[143,151]

As mentioned earlier, research to guide the practice of ventilator withdrawal and factors associated with withdrawal is scant. One group of researchers assessed the process of withdrawal of life support in 88 ICU patients. They reported that 10% died after removal of vasopressors, 35% died after mechanical ventilation was withdrawn, and 55% died after the withdrawal of both mechanical ventilation and vasopressors.[148] Verkade and colleagues reviewed the charts of patients who had life-support treatments withdrawn to identify factors associated with this process. They found wide variability in practice; however, overall, forgoing active life-supporting treatment decisions were associated with older patient age, being admitted with medical versus surgical reasons, higher severity of illness scores, and severe central nervous system injury.[108] Finally, other investigators reported that most ICU clinicians used a stuttering withdrawal process (removing one treatment at a time) and that on average removal of life-support treatment was prolonged (lasting longer than 1 day). In this study, they found that factors such as younger patient age,

Box 47.2 A protocol for the withdrawal of mechanical ventilation

I. Anticipate and prevent distress

    A. Review process in advance with patient (if awake), nurse, and family. Identify family goals during withdrawal (e.g., ability to communicate versus sedation). Arrange a time that allows the family to be present, if they wish.

    B. Provide for special needs (e.g., clergy, bereavement counselor). Assess respiratory pattern on current level of respiratory support.

    C. Use opioids and/or benzodiazepines* to control respiratory distress (i.e., respiratory rate >24 breaths per minute, use of accessory muscles, nasal flaring, >20% increase in heart rate or blood pressure, grimacing, clutching). In patients already receiving these agents, dosing should be guided by the current dose.

    D. In the absence of distress, reduce intermittent mandatory ventilation (IMV) rate to less than 10 and reassess sedation.

    E. Discontinue therapies not directed toward patient comfort:

        1. Stop neuromuscular blockade after opioids and/or benzodiazepines have been started or increased.[†]

        2. Discontinue laboratory tests, radiographs, vital signs.

        3. Remove unnecessary tubes and restraints.

        4. Silence alarms and disconnect monitors.

II. Optimize existing function

    A. Administer breathing treatment, if indicated.

    B. Suction out the mouth and hypopharynx. Endotracheal suctioning before withdrawal may or may not be advisable depending on patient distress and family perception. Consider atropine (1–2.5 mg by inhalation q6h), scopolamine (0.3–0.65 mg IV q4–6h), or glycopyrrolate (1–2 mg by inhalation q2–4h) for excessive secretions.**

    C. Place the patient at least 30 degrees upright, if possible.

III. Withdraw assisted ventilation[‡]

    A. In general, changes should be made in the following order[§]:

        1. Eliminate positive end-expiratory pressure (PEEP).

        2. Reduce the fractional oxygen content of inspired air (FIO_2).

        3. Reduce or eliminate mandatory breaths.

        4. Reduce pressure support level.

        5. Place to flow-by or T-piece.

        6. Extubate to humidified air or oxygen.

    B. Constant reevaluation for distress is mandatory. Treat distress with additional bolus doses of opioids and/or benzodiazepines equal to hourly drip rate and increase drip by 25%–50%.

    C. Observe for postwithdrawal distress, a medical emergency. A physician and nurse should be present during and immediately after extubation to assess the patient and to titrate medications. Morphine (5–10 mg IV q10 min) or fentanyl (100–250 µg IV q3–5 min) and/or midazolam (2–5 mg IV q7–10 min) or diazepam (5–10 mg IV q3–5 min) should be administered.

*Drug doses are difficult to specify because of the enormous variability in body weight and composition, previous exposure, and tolerance. In opioid-naïve patients, 2–20 mg morphine or 25–250 µg fentanyl, followed by an opioid infusion of one-half of the loading dose per hour, is a reasonable initial dose.

[†]Usually the effects of neuromuscular blocking agents (NMBAs) can be reversed within a short period, but it may take days to weeks if patients have been receiving NMBAs chronically for management of ventilatory failure. Neuromuscular blockade masks signs of discomfort. Therefore, clinicians should feel that the patient has regained sufficient motor activity to demonstrate discomfort.

[‡]There is no one sequence applicable to all patients because their clinical situations are so variable. The pace of changes depends on patient comfort and may proceed as quickly as 5–15 min or, in an awake patient to be extubated, over several hours.

**These measures may be started earlier or prior to extubation if the patient is having excessive secretions.

[§]Patients who require high levels of ventilatory support may die after small adjustments such as reduction or elimination of PEEP or decrease in FIO_2 to 21%. In such patients, the physician should be present during and immediately after the change in therapy to assess the patient.

Sources: Kompanje et al. (2008), reference 141; Szalados et al. (2007), reference 142; Treece et al. (2004), reference 147.

longer ICU stay, more life-sustaining interventions, and more decision makers involved led to prolonged withdrawal.[131]

Regardless of the methods, factors, or processes used to withdraw life-sustaining therapies, the critical care nurse plays a major role during the decision and implementation of withdrawal of patients from mechanical ventilation. Increased nursing involvement can help provide optimal care to these patients and their families. Specifically, the nurse can be an active member at family meetings where patient prognosis and goals of care are discussed. In addition, the nurse can ensure that a rationale for, and all elements of, the plan have been adequately discussed among the team, patient, and family. The nurse can ensure that adequate time is given to families and their support persons, such as clergy, to reach as good a resolution as possible. The family needs reassurance that they and the patient will not be left alone and that the patient will be kept comfortable with the use of medications and other measures. As discussed earlier, opioids, alone or in combination with BZDs, are used during withdrawal to ensure that patients are provided the optimal degree of comfort. Please refer to chapter 27 for a further in-depth discussion of withdrawal of life-sustaining therapies including mechanical ventilation.

Care for the family of the dying intensive care unit patient

Although the focus of care in many critical care areas is on the critically ill patient, nurses and other clinicians with family care skills realize that comprehensive patient care includes care of the patient's family. A family-centered approach to care is strongly supported by best practice recommendations,[152] and this approach acknowledges a reciprocal and all-important relationship between the family and the critically ill patient.[153] A change in one affects the other, and vice versa. Current research indicates that an ICU experience for family members can be stressful (especially when their loved one dies in the ICU) and has been associated with symptoms of PTSD, anxiety, depression, and complicated grief,[154–158] or most recently termed as post-intensive care syndrome–family.[158] Therefore, no discussion of palliative care in the ICU is complete without also discussing care of the dying patient's family. Family is defined here as any significant other who participates in the care and well-being of the patient.

The clinical course of any given critically ill, dying patient can vary tremendously, ranging from a rapid decline over several hours to a gradual decline over several days, weeks, and even months. Of course, the manner in which a family copes is also highly variable. Caring for families at any point along the dying trajectory, however, encompasses major aspects of access, information and support, and involvement in care-giving activities.

Access

A crucial aspect of family care is ensuring that the family can be with their critically ill loved one. Historically, critical care settings have severely restricted family access and discouraged lengthy family visitation. Commonly cited rationales to limiting family access include concerns regarding space limitations, patient stability, infection, rest, and privacy; the negative effect of visitation on the family; and clinicians' performance abilities.[159,160] Some of these concerns have merit, whereas others, such as adverse

patient-related issues and a negative effect on the family, have not been borne out in the research literature.[160]

Many ICUs around the world routinely limit visitors to two at any one time.[161–164] Space limitations in critical care areas can be profound, because most ICUs were designed for efficient use of life-saving machinery and staff and were not intended for end-of-life vigils by large, extended families. Ensuring that all interested family members have access to their loved one's bedside can present challenges to the often already narrow confines of the ICU. However, family members of dying loved ones should be allowed more liberal access (both in visiting time and in number of visitors allowed).[152,165,166] Patients are confronting what may be the most difficult of life passages, and therefore, they may need support from their family members. Researchers assessed 149 family members and 43 ICU workers regarding their perceptions of unrestricted visiting hours in the ICU. They reported that family members were more satisfied with this practice; however, ICU nurses and physicians reported moderate interruptions to patient care. Nurses reported a slight delay in organizing nursing care, and physicians reported greater unease when they were assessing the patient and perceived greater family stress, but they also perceived greater family trust.[161] Although healthcare professionals may feel that family visitation interferes with some aspects of patient care, the benefits far outweigh the risks.

Visitation of children should also be considered when a family member is dying. There is support for letting children visit the patient and become familiar with the care the patient is receiving and allow them to understand what is going on.[167] Visitation has the potential to help the child cope and gives the child a chance to say goodbye. If ICU clinicians account for the child's developmental status and properly prepare the child, then children can visit a critically ill family member in the ICU without ill effects.[152,168]

There is a growing body of literature that supports family access to patients during invasive procedures and resuscitation. Facilitating family access during such times has come to be known as facilitating family presence, a practice supported by the Emergency Nurses Association[169] and the Society of Critical Care Medicine.[152] Several authors have reviewed the impact of family presence during procedures and have found that family members thought their presence benefited their loved ones by being present to comfort and support them.[170–172] Studies examining family satisfaction with family presence have yielded similar results,[169] and one study demonstrated no adverse psychological effects on the part of family members after the witnessed resuscitation and as a matter of fact, found that families had lower symptoms of anxiety, depression, and PTSD.[173]

Finally, caring for the critically ill, dying patient and his/her family can call forth feelings of failure for clinicians bent on finding a cure and can force healthcare providers to reflect on their own mortality.[174] Even if family presence may be stressful for healthcare professionals and may not be fully embraced by ICU professionals,[175] current literature reveals that family presence during resuscitation may help humanize the patient, improve communication, and help families with the grief process.[176–178] Currently it has been recommended that hospitals establish formal programs that allow immediate family members to be present during resuscitation. This program should include trained staff to support the family, assess the family for distress, educate the family regarding the process, and debrief after the process.[179,180] The emotional burden for healthcare providers when providing palliative care is discussed later in this chapter.

Information and support

Information has been identified as a crucial component in family coping and satisfaction in critical care settings.[123,181] Support, in the form of clinicians' caring behaviors and interactions, is enormously influential in shaping the critical care experience for both patients and their families.[123,181] In the context of caring for a critically ill, dying patient, however, nurses and physicians alike have reported high stress related to "death-telling," or notifying family members of the patient's death or terminal prognosis.[174,182–185] In general, very few healthcare providers feel they have the skills and knowledge necessary to counsel families effectively during this emotionally charged time. The ethical principle of honesty and truth-telling collides with the limits of knowing the truth precisely when there is clinical ambiguity and also collides with the suffering imposed on a family having to face the hard truth. Compassionate truth-telling requires dialogue and relationship, timing, and attunement,[186] all of which are relational aspects that are frequently overlooked in the hectic pace of the ICU. Add patient, family, and healthcare provider culture to the equation, and one can readily understand why communication between involved parties is a less-than-perfect science. The educational implications for clinicians are addressed later in this chapter.

Overall satisfaction with end-of-life care has been shown to be significantly associated with completeness of information received by the family member, support and care shown to the patient and family, consistency in staff, and satisfaction with the amount or level of healthcare received.[181,187] Family conferences have been used extensively as a means to improve communication between healthcare providers and family members, and the few studies that have investigated best practices in relation to the timing, content, and participants necessary for optimal communication during a family conference, have shown improved satisfaction and lower emotional distress for family members.[124,146] Encouraging family members to attend rounds has been shown to improve family satisfaction with the frequency of communication with physicians and in support with decision-making.[188] In addition, diaries may help lower distress for family members. Researchers found that family members who recorded a diary during their loved one's ICU stay had lower levels of posttraumatic stress-related symptoms 12 months after the ICU experience.[189]

Some hospitals have created interdisciplinary teams to improve communication and to help work with critically ill patients and their families in an effort to meet patients' and families' physical, informational, and psychosocial needs.[30,130,190] Such teams usually include a nurse, physician, chaplain, and social worker. Working in concert with the nurses and physicians at the bedside, these interdisciplinary teams can more fully concentrate on end-of-life issues so that, theoretically, no patient or family needs go unmet during this time.

Finally, because feelings of grief in surviving family members are still commonly unresolved 1 year after a loved one's death, many critical care units across the life span have organized bereavement follow-up programs.[191–193] These programs typically involve contacting the surviving family (by telephone or mail) monthly for some period of time and at the 1-year anniversary of their loved one's death. In addition to remembering and

supporting the family, these programs have also been shown to help healthcare providers cope with the loss as well. Another suggestion that may be helpful to family members is that the ICU staff can hold memorial services twice a year for family/friends of the patient to reconnect with the critical care staff. During this service, names of those who have died in the past 6 months are read. A reception is held afterward that gives everyone, especially the staff, an opportunity to reflect on their work and to honor the people they have served.[194]

Involvement in caregiving activities

Few interventional studies have examined the effect of family involvement on critically ill patients and their families, yet families should have the opportunity to be helpful.[195] One study qualitatively assessed the roles family members assume when their loved one is at high risk of dying in the ICU.[196] Families in this study discussed their roles as patient protector, facilitator, historian, coach, voluntary caregiver, and actively present person. These roles were extremely important to family members and gave them a sense of purpose. Acknowledging the contributions of family members and involving them in caregiving activities can be beneficial. These activities can range from minor activities (such as assisting with oral care or rubbing the dying patient's feet) to major activities (assisting with postmortem care). This involvement may be helpful for family members in working through their grief by demonstrating their love in caring and comforting ways. Being involved in meaningful caregiving activities can make a family member feel useful rather than useless and helpful rather than helpless.[195,196]

Although physical death occurs in the dying patient, the social death is felt in the patient's surviving family. Because the perception of death lingers at the family level long after the physical death has occurred, involving family members who are interested in participating in their loved one's care may go far to provide closure, comfort, and connection. Nurses' facilitation of family involvement in their dying loved one's care is a practical family intervention that should be more widely employed if humane and comprehensive palliative care is desired.[196,197]

Care for the caregiver of the dying intensive care unit patient

It's only human to hurt, to cry, to grieve, when a person who's influenced you in some way has died. Please cry with your patients and their families; it's okay for you to grieve too.[198]

Numerous studies have described the tension and moral distress between the cure-oriented critical care setting and palliative care.[183,199–201] The bedside healthcare provider, typically a nurse, often feels caught between differing perceptions held by physicians and family members concerning patient progress and treatment goals.[115,202] Facilitating and coordinating dialogue and consensus between these groups as well as caring for the dying patient and family can cause conflicts and can be physically and emotionally exhausting. If the dying process is prolonged, the nurse can become frustrated and fatigued. Although healthcare providers often cope with this stress by emotionally disengaging themselves from the charged atmosphere, emotional distancing has been shown to hamper skill acquisition and the development of involvement skills and lead to burnout.[185,203,204] Involvement skills are defined here as the cluster of interpersonal skills that enable a nurse and the patient and family to establish a relational connection. This section discusses two strategies to help healthcare providers sustain their caring practices and extend their involvement skills—namely, sharing narratives and death education.

Sharing narratives

Debriefing, either formally or informally, has been used effectively in many settings to discuss and process critical incidents; analyze healthcare providers' performance in terms of skill, knowledge, and efficiency; and learn, both personally and institutionally, from mistakes and system breakdown.[205-208] Sharing stories or narratives of practice can be used to achieve the same goals, but telling stories from practice also enables clinicians to (1) increase their skill in recognizing patient and family concerns; (2) learn to communicate more effectively with patients, families, and other healthcare providers; (3) reflect on ethical comportment and engaged clinical reasoning; and (4) articulate clinical knowledge development.[206,209,210]

Creating the interpersonal and institutional space in which to both tell and actively listen to stories from practice also enables healthcare providers to share skills of involvement and sustaining strategies. These understandings can provide clinicians with guidance—and, in some cases, corrective action—to intervene in ways that are true to the patient's condition and to the patient's and family's best interests.[185,204,210,211] Through reflection and dialogue with others, nurses and other healthcare providers can pool their collective wisdom and extend their care of dying patients and their families.

Death education

Closely coupled with sharing clinical narratives are the use of seminars and other reflective exercises aimed at preparing nurses and other healthcare providers for the care of dying patients and their families. Death education often consists of didactic and experiential classes. Participants in these classes are encouraged to reflect on and share their own perceptions and anxieties about death, as well as their attitudes toward care of the dying patient and his/her family. This approach has been used with varying degrees of success with nurses, nursing students, and physicians.[182,212-215] Because many healthcare providers feel ill prepared to effectively care for terminally ill patients and have also identified barriers to delivering quality end-of-life care,[216-218] this is a promising strategy that deserves more implementation and research.

Additionally, integrating palliative care into the ICU requires preparation and education of ICU clinicians. The main components include:

- Educating critical care staff about palliative care (e.g., principles of shared decision-making, communication techniques, symptom management, and practices of withdrawal of life support).[219] This step can be accomplished through lectures, pamphlets, teaching videos, and poster boards.[146,220]

- Training local ICU champions who can serve as role models and facilitate behavior change. This can be completed through half-day or full-day training sessions.[146,210,221,222]

- Collecting feedback on quality improvement data (e.g., family members' satisfaction with care or family members' ratings of the quality of death and dying).[8,223]

- Finally, utilizing system supports and hospital resources to develop family informational pamphlets, (e.g., "get to know me" posters for patients' rooms and developing withdrawal of life support forms).[146,194]

An international agenda to improve care of dying intensive care unit patients

Considerable emphasis has been placed on improving care at the end of life for ICU patients. Several books that comprehensively and specifically address ICU end-of-life care have been published.[224,225] A Robert Wood Johnson Foundation–sponsored national ICU Peer Workgroup on end-of-life care conducted several education and research initiatives related to this topic. One of these initiatives was the development of quality indicators for end-of-life care in ICUs.[226] These quality indicators can provide a framework for interventions to improve care of the dying in ICUs. An international consensus statement and a task force guideline have been published to provide evidence on end-of-life care in ICUs and to make recommendations for research and practice improvements.[31,158] The Robert Wood Johnson Foundation funded demonstration projects in four ICUs in the United States. These demonstration projects developed palliative care models for ICUs and assessed the impact on the quality of care for patients and their families.[227] It is anticipated that findings from these demonstration projects will continue to guide national and international practice improvements. Finally, the IPAL-ICU project, with support from the National Institutes of Health (NIH) and the Center to Advance Palliative Care (CAPC), was designed to provide a central location for sharing evidence, tools, links to organizations, and informational materials. The goal is to assist ICU leaders, as well as clinicians across disciplines, to integrate palliative care and intensive care successfully.[228]

Summary

As noted by Morell, one can learn that "a death can be a good death."[229] Striving to relieve suffering from pain and other distressing symptoms, and providing a dignified death is the right of all ICU patients. Research has offered some guidance for managing the issues that surround ICU patient deaths. However, Chapple[230] presented important goals to consider during an ICU patient's dying process: (1) honor the patient's life; (2) ensure that the patient and the family are not abandoned; (3) provide a sense of moral stability; and (4) ensure the patient's safety and comfort. Intensive care unit nurses can feel privileged to strive toward the accomplishment of those goals.

Case study

Positive palliative and end-of-life care in the intensive care unit

Submitted by Kathleen Turner, RN, BSN, CHPN, CCRN CMC

Adult Medical-Surgical ICU, University of California San Francisco Medical Center

Palliative Critical Care? Using ICU Resources to Enhance Quality of Life in Serious Illness

Mrs. S had spent many years as a nurse providing primary care to underserved communities from Guatemala to Baltimore. She now lived on the coast with her husband and dog, and enjoyed swimming and hiking in the nearby national park. In 2010, she was diagnosed with multiple myeloma. She received several courses of chemotherapy, resulting in cardiomyopathy and renal failure. Mrs. S had spent 40 of the past 60 days in the hospital, receiving plasmapheresis and hemodialysis (HD) to prepare her for additional chemotherapy and possible stem cell transplant.

August 15–17: Mrs. S presented to UCSF with several days of fatigue, worsening nausea, and decreased urine output. She was admitted to the oncology floor. Over the next 3 days she received HD and plasmapheresis and was started on a new course of chemotherapy. Concern for tumor lysis syndrome necessitated aggressive intravenous (IV) hydration. Mrs. S began to develop lower extremity edema and crackles in her lung bases. Her blood pressure was becoming more tenuous, making it difficult to achieve desired fluid removal during HD.

August 18: Mrs. S had difficulty moving her legs, was unable to eat, and reported significant dyspnea. During HD, she began vomiting and became acutely hypotensive. She was transferred immediately to the medical-surgical intensive care unit (ICU). The oncology attending physician informed Mrs. S that she would not be a candidate for stem cell transplant. Nephrology ordered continuous renal replacement therapy (CRRT) to correct her electrolyte imbalances while preventing further fluid buildup.

That evening, Mrs. S had a lot on her mind, and her nurse Ron was ready to listen. Mrs. S revealed that she had made treatment decisions more for her loved ones than for herself. She had used this extra time to rebuild relationships with estranged family members and reflect on having accomplished so many of her life goals. Ron and Mrs. S rehearsed what it might be like to tell her husband that there would be no stem cell transplant and hopefully no more chemotherapy. Mrs. S spoke of walking in the hills near her home and how her current state made that seem very far away. She talked about shopping at her local farm market and memorable family dinners. She hoped to return home for her last days, able to walk and eat. Ron pulled the ICU resident aside and passed along what Mrs. S had said, suggesting that a family meeting with all the teams and the palliative care service might be helpful.

August 19: The nephrologist stopped in to check on Mrs. S during breakfast and they discussed her desire to shift to a palliative plan of care. In the last four days, Mrs. S had gained 20 pounds of water weight. In keeping with the new approach, the team began using CRRT to gently reverse her fluid excess. All services collaborated on moving IV medications and fluids to the oral route to facilitate the transition to home.

The attending physician from the palliative care service met with Mrs. S around lunchtime. She reported severe pain, primarily in her back and legs. With additional questioning, the physician determined that the pain appeared to have three main components: bone pain from a lesion in her spine, neuropathic pain emanating from her low back into all extremities, and discomfort due to edema now extending to her pelvis. He recommended starting daily methadone, with oxycodone for breakthrough pain. Dexamethasone was added as adjunctive therapy. He discussed options for additional neuropathy control, but Mrs. S was concerned that too many new medications might make her feel "woozy." She began taking senna to prevent constipation.

For Mrs. S, uncontrolled nausea permitted only small sips of water. The team started around-the-clock haloperidol, with sublingual lorazepam available for breakthrough nausea and vomiting. The new dexamethasone was expected to help as well.

When asked about her goals, Mrs. S had four that came to mind:

- Remove enough edema to allow her to walk
- Be able to swim near her home
- Spend time with her dog
- See her second grandchild, due to be born in one month

She requested palliative care service assistance in discussing expectations and plans with her husband. Mrs. S declined further chemotherapy and, at her instruction, a "Do Not Resuscitate" order was placed in her chart.

Ron returned that night to the bedside, and he and Mrs. S worked hard together to take advantage of the new medications in managing her symptoms. They talked about the interdisciplinary family meeting scheduled for the next day and reviewed the four goals she had set for her remaining time.

August 20: The morning was brightened by a visit from a familiar face, the oncology social worker. Mrs. S updated her on the whirlwind events of the past few days and said, "I've made the right decision. It's OK to die."

Nephrology increased the CRRT fluid removal rate and discontinued all nonessential lab work. When the palliative care service physician examined Mrs. S, she was still experiencing severe back pain and nausea. He increased the around-the-clock dose of haloperidol and added promethazine. Scopolamine was offered; Mrs. S declined.

At 2 PM, the family meeting was convened at the bedside. The team explained to Mr. S that there were no further curative therapies available for his wife. They offered that, under these circumstances, the current level of care could be refocused on maximizing comfort and quality of life. Mr. S was sad but said he could see why his wife was ready to go home. The palliative care chaplain arranged to visit the next day to help Mrs. S write legacy letters to her grandchildren.

Mrs. S started the oral vasopressor midodrine to enable accelerated fluid removal with CRRT. She received the Sacrament of Healing from the visiting priest. Her spirits were much improved and she expressed relief that "the end is in sight." When Ron returned for the night shift, he and Mrs. S worked with the ICU physicians to improve her pain control. Mrs. S spent several hours that night praying for the patient in crisis across the hall; she told Ron that, as a nurse herself, she wanted to help.

August 21: As morning approached, Mrs. S struggled with vomiting and was again unable to eat. When the interdisciplinary team met to formulate the day's plan of care, they decided to tackle nausea first. The oncology service ordered daily high-dose dexamethasone and another run of plasmapheresis. The palliative care service added dronabinol to the plan.

Over the course of three days in the intensive care unit, CRRT had removed 6 liters of fluid. Mrs. S had continuous cardiac and arterial blood pressure monitoring, making it possible to safely deliver this therapy. Lower extremity edema had improved to 2+, and her lungs were clear nearly to the bases. Nephrology ordered a further increase in the hourly CRRT fluid removal rate.

Mrs. S shared with the team that, for the first time, she believed she would make it home. To each person entering her room, she expressed her thanks and challenged them to keep pushing her. She and the chaplain took advantage of some down time to reflect and work together on letters to her grandchildren. During the night, her one-on-one nursing care continued—fine-tuning doses and frequencies of medications so that Mrs. S would have the best possible regimen on which to discharge home.

August 22: Mrs. S's nausea was under control and her diet was advanced to "as tolerated." She felt well enough to enjoy a long-anticipated bit of black coffee for breakfast! The day got even better when her nurse brought a walker to her room and assisted her out of bed. Together they walked to the end of the ICU, where an enormous picture window faces the Golden Gate Bridge and the sea. Standing there with her nurse, Mrs. S could almost see home.

Later that day, the teams met with Mrs. S and her family. "We're ready to get her home—this is our window of opportunity," Mr. S noted. The oncology and palliative care social workers set up home hospice referral, had durable medical equipment delivered, and located a pharmacy near the tiny town where the family lived.

August 23: When the palliative care team visited Mrs. S, she was in her bedside chair, watching the news and breathing room air. CRRT had been discontinued a few hours earlier. The attending physician completed the Physician Orders for Life Sustaining Treatment (POLST), reflecting Mrs. S's request not to be resuscitated or receive artificial nutrition and hydration. The hospice and UCSF providers coordinated next steps for symptom management and psychosocial support. Ron stopped in to say goodbye. A little while later, Mrs. S went home—to walk, swim, and relax with her dog. She died a week later, in her own bed, on her own terms.

References

1. Nelson JE, Puntillo KA, Pronovost PJ, et al. In their own words: patients and families define high-quality palliative care in the intensive care unit. Crit Care Med. 2010;38(3):808–818.
2. Angus DC, Barnato AE, Linde-Zwirble WT, et al. Use of intensive care at the end of life in the United States: an epidemiologic study. Crit Care Med. 2004;32(3):638–643.
3. Wunsch H, Linde-Zwirble WT, Harrison DA, Barnato AE, Rowan KM, Angus DC. Use of intensive care services during terminal hospitalizations in England and the United States. Am J Respir Crit Care Med. 2009;180(9):875–880.
4. Teno JM, Gozalo PL, Bynum JP, et al. Change in end-of-life care for Medicare beneficiaries: site of death, place of care, and health care transitions in 2000, 2005, and 2009. JAMA. 2013;309(5):470–477.
5. Miesfeldt S, Murray K, Lucas L, Chang CH, Goodman D, Morden NE. Association of age, gender, and race with intensity of end-of-life care for Medicare beneficiaries with cancer. J Palliat Med. 2012;15(5):548–554.
6. Lusardi P, Jodka P, Stambovsky M, et al. The going home initiative: getting critical care patients home with hospice. Crit Care Nurse. 2011;31(5):46–57.
7. Levin TT, Moreno B, Silvester W, Kissane DW. End-of-life communication in the intensive care unit. Gen Hosp Psychiatry. 2010;32(4):433–442.
8. Penrod JD, Pronovost PJ, Livote EE, et al. Meeting standards of high-quality intensive care unit palliative care: clinical performance and predictors. Crit Care Med. 2012;40(4):1105–1112.
9. Field RA, Soar J, Nolan JP, Perkins GD. Epidemiology and outcome of cardiac arrests reported in the lay-press: an observational study. J R Soc Med. 2011;104(12):525–531.
10. Millner P, Paskiewicz ST, Kautz D. A comfortable place to say goodbye. Dimens Crit Care Nurs. 2009;28(1):13–17.
11. Luce JM. A history of resolving conflicts over end-of-life care in intensive care units in the United States. Crit Care Med. 2010;38(8):1623–1629.
12. Siegel MD. End-of-life decision making in the ICU. Clin Chest Med. 2009;30(1):181–194, x.
13. Goodridge D, Duggleby W, Gjevre J, Rennie D. Exploring the quality of dying of patients with chronic obstructive pulmonary disease in the intensive care unit: a mixed methods study. Nurs Crit Care. 2009;14(2):51–60.
14. Puntillo KA, Arai S, Cohen NH, et al. Symptoms experienced by intensive care unit patients at high risk of dying. Crit Care Med. 2010;38(11):2155–2160.
15. Puntillo KA, Smith D, Arai S, Stotts N. Critical care nurses provide their perspectives of patients' symptoms in intensive care units. Heart Lung. 2008;37(6):466–475.
16. A controlled trial to improve care for seriously ill hospitalized patients. The study to understand prognoses and preferences for outcomes and risks of treatments (SUPPORT). The SUPPORT Principal Investigators. JAMA. 1995;274(20):1591–1598.
17. Delgado-Guay MO, Parsons HA, Li Z, Palmer LJ, Bruera E. Symptom distress, interventions, and outcomes of intensive care unit cancer patients referred to a palliative care consult team. Cancer. 2009;115(2):437–445.
18. Davidson GH, Hamlat CA, Rivara FP, Koepsell TD, Jurkovich GJ, Arbabi S. Long-term survival of adult trauma patients. JAMA. 2011;305(10):1001–1007.
19. Macintyre NR. Chronic critical illness: the growing challenge to health care. Respir Care. 2012;57(6):1021–1027.
20. Nelson JE, Cox CE, Hope AA, Carson SS. Chronic critical illness. Am J Respir Crit Care Med. 2010;182(4):446–454.
21. Fuchs L, Chronaki CE, Park S, et al. ICU admission characteristics and mortality rates among elderly and very elderly patients. Intensive Care Med. 2012;38(10):1654–1661.
22. Billings JA. The end-of-life family meeting in intensive care. Part II: Family-centered decision making. J Palliat Med. 2011;14(9):1051–1057.
23. Ehlenbach WJ, Cooke CR. Making ICU prognostication patient centered: is there a role for dynamic information? Crit Care Med. 2013;41(4):1136–1138.
24. Fisher M, Ridley S. Uncertainty in end-of-life care and shared decision making. Crit Care Resusc. 2012;14(1):81–87.
25. Billings JA. The end-of-life family meeting in intensive care. Part I: Indications, outcomes, and family needs. J Palliat Med. 2011;14(9):1042–1050.
26. Nelson JE, Walker AS, Luhrs CA, Cortez TB, Pronovost PJ. Family meetings made simpler: a toolkit for the intensive care unit. J Crit Care. 2009;24(4):626 e627–e614.
27. Spronk PE, Kuiper AV, Rommes JH, Korevaar JC, Schultz MJ. The practice of and documentation on withholding and withdrawing life support: a retrospective study in two Dutch intensive care units. Anesth Analg. 2009;109(3):841–846.
28. Gay EB, Pronovost PJ, Bassett RD, Nelson JE. The intensive care unit family meeting: making it happen. J Crit Care. 2009;24(4):629 e621–e612.
29. Curtis JR, White DB. Practical guidance for evidence-based ICU family conferences. Chest. 2008;134(4):835–843.
30. Machare Delgado E, Callahan A, Paganelli G, Reville B, Parks SM, Marik PE. Multidisciplinary family meetings in the ICU facilitate end-of-life decision making. Am J Hosp Palliat Care. 2009;26(4):295–302.

31. Truog RD, Campbell ML, Curtis JR, et al. Recommendations for end-of-life care in the intensive care unit: a consensus statement by the American College [corrected] of Critical Care Medicine. Crit Care Mcd. 2008;36(3):953–963.

32. White DB, Curtis JR, Lo B, Luce JM. Decisions to limit life-sustaining treatment for critically ill patients who lack both decision-making capacity and surrogate decision-makers. Crit Care Med. 2006;34(8):2053–2059.

33. White DB, Curtis JR, Wolf LE, et al. Life support for patients without a surrogate decision maker: who decides? Ann Intern Med. 2007;147(1):34–40.

34. Lanken PN, Terry PB, Delisser HM, et al. An official American Thoracic Society clinical policy statement: palliative care for patients with respiratory diseases and critical illnesses. Am J Respir Crit Care Med. 2008;177(8):912–927.

35. Brennan F, Carr DB, Cousins M. Pain management: a fundamental human right. Anesth Analg. 2007;105(1):205–221.

36. Herr K, Coyne PJ, McCaffery M, Manworren R, Merkel S. Pain assessment in the patient unable to self-report: position statement with clinical practice recommendations. Pain Manage Nurs. 2011;12(4):230–250.

37. Olden AM, Holloway R, Ladwig S, Quill TE, van Wijngaarden E. Palliative care needs and symptom patterns of hospitalized elders referred for consultation. J Pain Symptom Manage. 2011;42(3):410–418.

38. Gelinas C, Tousignant-Laflamme Y, Tanguay A, Bourgault P. Exploring the validity of the bispectral index, the Critical-Care Pain Observation Tool and vital signs for the detection of pain in sedated and mechanically ventilated critically ill adults: a pilot study. Intensive Crit Care Nurs. 2011;27(1):46–52.

39. Ahlers SJ, van Gulik L, van der Veen AM, et al. Comparison of different pain scoring systems in critically ill patients in a general ICU. Crit Care. 2008;12(1):R15.

40. Ahlers SJ, van der Veen AM, van Dijk M, Tibboel D, Knibbe CA. The use of the Behavioral Pain Scale to assess pain in conscious sedated patients. Anesth Analg. 2010;110(1):127–133.

41. Paulson-Conger M, Leske J, Maidl C, Hanson A, Dziadulewicz L. Comparison of two pain assessment tools in nonverbal critical care patients. Pain Manag Nurs. 2011;12(4):218–224.

42. Chanques G, Viel E, Constantin JM, et al. The measurement of pain in intensive care unit: comparison of 5 self-report intensity scales. Pain. 2010;151(3):711–721.

43. Puntillo KA, Neuhaus J, Arai S, et al. Challenge of assessing symptoms in seriously ill intensive care unit patients: can proxy reporters help? Crit Care Med. 2012;40(10):2760–2767.

44. Li D, Puntillo K, Miaskowski C. A review of objective pain measures for use with critical care adult patients unable to self-report. J Pain. 2008;9(1):2–10.

45. Cade CH. Clinical tools for the assessment of pain in sedated critically ill adults. Nurs Crit Care. 2008;13(6):288–297.

46. Payen JF, Bru O, Bosson JL, et al. Assessing pain in critically ill sedated patients by using a behavioral pain scale. Crit Care Med. 2001;29(12):2258–2263.

47. Gelinas C, Fillion L, Puntillo KA, Viens C, Fortier M. Validation of the critical-care pain observation tool in adult patients. Am J Crit Care. 2006;15(4):420–427.

48. Gelinas C, Fillion L, Puntillo KA. Item selection and content validity of the Critical-Care Pain Observation Tool for non-verbal adults. J Adv Nurs. 2009;65(1):203–216.

49. Gelinas C, Johnston C. Pain assessment in the critically ill ventilated adult: validation of the Critical-Care Pain Observation Tool and physiologic indicators. Clin J Pain. 2007;23(6):497–505.

50. Gelinas C, Harel F, Fillion L, Puntillo KA, Johnston CC. Sensitivity and specificity of the critical-care pain observation tool for the detection of pain in intubated adults after cardiac surgery. J Pain Symptom Manage. 2009;37(1):58–67.

51. Barr J, Fraser GL, Puntillo K, et al. Clinical practice guidelines for the management of pain, agitation, and delirium in adult patients in the intensive care unit. Crit Care Med. 2013;41(1):263–306.

52. Puntillo K, Pasero C, Li D, et al. Evaluation of pain in ICU patients. Chest. 2009;135(4):1069–1074.

53. Morrison RS, Ahronheim JC, Morrison GR, et al. Pain and discomfort associated with common hospital procedures and experiences. J Pain Symptom Manage. 1998;15(2):91–101.

54. Puntillo K, Ley SJ. Appropriately timed analgesics control pain due to chest tube removal. Am J Crit Care. 2004;13(4):292–301; discussion 302; quiz 303–294.

55. Arroyo-Novoa CM, Figueroa-Ramos MI, Puntillo KA, et al. Pain related to tracheal suctioning in awake acutely and critically ill adults: a descriptive study. Intensive Crit Care Nurs. 2008;24(1):20–27.

56. Payen JF, Chanques G, Mantz J, et al. Current practices in sedation and analgesia for mechanically ventilated critically ill patients: a prospective multicenter patient-based study. Anesthesiology. 2007;106(4):687–695.

57. Puntillo KA, White C, Morris AB, et al. Patients' perceptions and responses to procedural pain: results from Thunder Project II. Am J Crit Care. 2001;10(4):238–251.

58. Siffleet J, Young J, Nikoletti S, Shaw T. Patients' self-report of procedural pain in the intensive care unit. J Clin Nurs. 2007;16(11):2142–2148.

59. McGrane S, Pandharipande PP. Sedation in the intensive care unit. Minerva Anestesiol. 2012;78(3):369–380.

60. Czarnecki ML, Turner HN, Collins PM, Doellman D, Wrona S, Reynolds J. Procedural pain management: a position statement with clinical practice recommendations. Pain Manag Nurs. 2011;12(2):95–111.

61. Erstad BL, Puntillo K, Gilbert HC, et al. Pain management principles in the critically ill. Chest. 2009;135(4):1075–1086.

62. Joffe AM, Hallman M, Gelinas C, Herr DL, Puntillo K. Evaluation and treatment of pain in critically ill adults. Semin Respir Crit Care Med. Apr 2013;34(2):189–200.

63. American Pain Society. Principles of Analgesic Use in the Treatment of Acute Pain and Cancer Pain. 6th ed. Glenview, IL: Author; 2008.

64. Campbell ML. Treating distress at the end of life: the principle of double effect. AACN Adv Crit Care. 2008;19(3):340–344.

65. Clemens KE, Quednau I, Klaschik E. Is there a higher risk of respiratory depression in opioid-naive palliative care patients during symptomatic therapy of dyspnea with strong opioids? J Palliat Med. 2008;11(2):204–216.

66. Chan JD, Treece PD, Engelberg RA, et al. Narcotic and benzodiazepine use after withdrawal of life support: association with time to death? Chest. 2004;126(1):286–293.

67. Tracy MF, Chlan L. Nonpharmacological interventions to manage common symptoms in patients receiving mechanical ventilation. Crit Care Nurse. 2011;31(3):19–28.

68. Abad C, Fearday A, Safdar N. Adverse effects of isolation in hospitalised patients: a systematic review. J Hosp Infect. 2010;76(2):97–102.

69. Huang YT. Factors leading to self-extubation of endotracheal tubes in the intensive care unit. Nurs Crit Care. 2009;14(2):68–74.

70. Jarachovic M, Mason M, Kerber K, McNett M. The role of standardized protocols in unplanned extubations in a medical intensive care unit. Am J Crit Care. 2011;20(4):304–311; quiz 312.

71. Tate JA, Devito Dabbs A, Hoffman LA, Milbrandt E, Happ MB. Anxiety and agitation in mechanically ventilated patients. Qual Health Res. 2012;22(2):157–173.

72. Sessler CN, Grap MJ, Ramsay MA. Evaluating and monitoring analgesia and sedation in the intensive care unit. Crit Care. 2008;12 Suppl 3:S2.

73. Martin J, Heymann A, Basell K, et al. Evidence and consensus-based German guidelines for the management of analgesia, sedation and delirium in intensive care—short version. Ger Med Sci. 2010; 8:Doc02.

74. Schweickert WD, Kress JP. Strategies to optimize analgesia and sedation. Crit Care. 2008;12 Suppl 3:S6.

75. Sessler CN, Wilhelm W. Analgesia and sedation in the intensive care unit: an overview of the issues. Crit Care. 2008;12 Suppl 3:S1.

76. Sessler CN, Varney K. Patient-focused sedation and analgesia in the ICU. Chest. 2008;133(2):552–565.

77. Hughes CG, McGrane S, Pandharipande PP. Sedation in the intensive care setting. Clin Pharmacol. 2012;4:53–63.

78. Robinson BR, Mueller EW, Henson K, Branson RD, Barsoum S, Tsuei BJ. An analgesia-delirium-sedation protocol for critically ill trauma patients reduces ventilator days and hospital length of stay. J Trauma. 2008;65(3):517–526.

79. Sessler CN, Pedram S. Protocolized and target-based sedation and analgesia in the ICU. Crit Care Clin. 2009;25(3):489–513, viii.

80. Gommers D, Bakker J. Medications for analgesia and sedation in the intensive care unit: an overview. Crit Care. 2008;12 Suppl 3:S4.

81. Riker RR, Shehabi Y, Bokesch PM, et al. Dexmedetomidine vs midazolam for sedation of critically ill patients: a randomized trial. JAMA. 2009;301(5):489–499.

82. Pisani MA, Murphy TE, Araujo KL, Slattum P, Van Ness PH, Inouye SK. Benzodiazepine and opioid use and the duration of intensive care unit delirium in an older population. Crit Care Med. 2009;37(1):177–183.

83. Flower O, Hellings S. Sedation in traumatic brain injury. Emerg Med Int. 2012;2012:637171.

84. Reardon DP, Anger KE, Adams CD, Szumita PM. Role of dexmedetomidine in adults in the intensive care unit: an update. Am J Health Syst Pharm. 2013;70(9):767–777.

85. Barletta JF, Miedema SL, Wiseman D, Heiser JC, McAllen KJ. Impact of dexmedetomidine on analgesic requirements in patients after cardiac surgery in a fast-track recovery room setting. Pharmacotherapy. 2009;29(12):1427–1432.

86. Jones GM, Murphy CV, Gerlach AT, Goodman EM, Pell LJ. High-dose dexmedetomidine for sedation in the intensive care unit: an evaluation of clinical efficacy and safety. Ann Pharmacother. 2011;45(6):740–747.

87. Tan JA, Ho KM. Use of dexmedetomidine as a sedative and analgesic agent in critically ill adult patients: a meta-analysis. Intensive Care Med. 2010;36(6):926–939.

88. Luetz A, Heymann A, Radtke FM, et al. Different assessment tools for intensive care unit delirium: which score to use? Crit Care Med. 2010;38(2):409–418.

89. Jones SF, Pisani MA. ICU delirium: an update. Curr Opin Crit Care. 2012;18(2):146–151.

90. Bergeron N, Dubois MJ, Dumont M, Dial S, Skrobik Y. Intensive Care Delirium Screening Checklist: evaluation of a new screening tool. Intensive Care Med. 2001;27(5):859–864.

91. Skrobik Y. Delirium prevention and treatment. Crit Care Clin. 2009;25(3):585–591, x.

92. Cavallazzi R, Saad M, Marik PE. Delirium in the ICU: an overview. Ann Intensive Care. 2012;2(1):49.

93. Hipp DM, Ely EW. Pharmacological and nonpharmacological management of delirium in critically ill patients. Neurotherapeutics. 2012;9(1):158–175.

94. Wang W, Li HL, Wang DX, et al. Haloperidol prophylaxis decreases delirium incidence in elderly patients after noncardiac surgery: a randomized controlled trial. Crit Care Med. 2012;40(3):731–739.

95. Chlan LL, Weinert CR, Heiderscheit A, et al. Effects of patient-directed music intervention on anxiety and sedative exposure in critically ill patients receiving mechanical ventilatory support: a randomized clinical trial. JAMA. 2013;309(22):2335–2344.

96. Fitzgerald M, Langevin M. Imagery. In: Snyder M, Lindquist R (eds.), Complementary and Alternative Therapies in Nursing. 6th ed. New York, NY: Springer; 2010:63–89.

97. Campbell ML. Dyspnea prevalence, trajectories, and measurement in critical care and at life's end. Curr Opin Support Palliat Care. 2012;6(2):168–171.

98. Schmidt M, Demoule A, Polito A, et al. Dyspnea in mechanically ventilated critically ill patients. Crit Care Med. 2011;39(9):2059–2065.

99. Campbell ML. Dyspnea. AACN Adv Crit Care. 2011;22(3):257–264.

100. Campbell ML. Respiratory distress: a model of responses and behaviors to an asphyxial threat for patients who are unable to self-report. Heart Lung. 2008;37(1):54–60.

101. Campbell ML. Psychometric testing of a respiratory distress observation scale. J Palliat Med. 2008;11(1):44–50.

102. Campbell ML, Templin T, Walch J. A Respiratory Distress Observation Scale for patients unable to self-report dyspnea. J Palliat Med. 2010;13(3):285–290.

103. Mahler DA, Selecky PA, Harrod CG. Management of dyspnea in patients with advanced lung or heart disease: practical guidance from the American college of chest physicians consensus statement. Pol Arch Med Wewn. 2010;120(5):160–166.

104. Ship JA, McCutcheon JA, Spivakovsky S, Kerr AR. Safety and effectiveness of topical dry mouth products containing olive oil, betaine, and xylitol in reducing xerostomia for polypharmacy-induced dry mouth. JOR. 2007;34(10):724–732.

105. Arai S CB, Nelson J, Stotts N, Puntillo K. A thirst intervention bundle decreases the distress of ICU patients' thirst.(Abstract). Crit Care Med. 2012;40(12).

106. Puntillo KAS, Cooper B, Stotts N, Nelson J. A thirst intervention bundle decreases the intensity of ICU patients' thirst. Intensive Care Med. 2014;40(12): 235–248.

107. Jensen HI, Ammentorp J, Ording H. Withholding or withdrawing therapy in Danish regional ICUs: frequency, patient characteristics and decision process. Acta Anaesthesiol Scand. 2011;55(3):344–351.

108. Verkade MA, Epker JL, Nieuwenhoff MD, Bakker J, Kompanje EJ. Withdrawal of life-sustaining treatment in a mixed intensive care unit: most common in patients with catastropic brain injury. Neurocrit Care. 2012;16(1):130–135.

109. Snyder L. American College of Physicians Ethics Manual: sixth edition. Ann Intern Med. 2012;156(1 Pt 2):73–104.

110. American Association of Critical Care Nurses. Position Statement: Withholding and/or Withdrawing Life-Sustaining Treatment. Newport Beach, CA: AACN; 1999.

111. White DB, Malvar G, Karr J, Lo B, Curtis JR. Expanding the paradigm of the physician's role in surrogate decision-making: an empirically derived framework. Crit Care Med. 2010;38(3):743–750.

112. Halpern NA, Pastores SM, Chou JF, Chawla S, Thaler HT. Advance directives in an oncologic intensive care unit: a contemporary analysis of their frequency, type, and impact. J Palliat Med. 2011;14(4):483–489.

113. Kumar A, Aronow WS, Alexa M, et al. Prevalence of use of advance directives, health care proxy, legal guardian, and living will in 512 patients hospitalized in a cardiac care unit/intensive care unit in 2 community hospitals. Arch Med Sci. 2010;6(2):188–191.

114. White DB, Curtis JR. Establishing an evidence base for physician-family communication and shared decision making in the intensive care unit. Crit Care Med. 2006;34(9):2500–2501.

115. Azoulay E, Timsit JF, Sprung CL, et al. Prevalence and factors of intensive care unit conflicts: the conflicus study. Am J Respir Crit Care Med. 2009;180(9):853–860.

116. Strand JJ, Billings JA. Integrating palliative care in the intensive care unit. J Support Oncol. 2012;10(5):180–187.

117. Billings JA, Block SD. The end-of-life family meeting in intensive care. Part III: A guide for structured discussions. J Palliat Med. 2011;14(9):1058–1064.

118. Spinello IM. End-of-life care in ICU: a practical guide. J Intensive Care Med. 2011 Mar 24. Epub ahead of print.

119. Nelson J, Arnold RM. A Guide for Conducting an ICU Family Meeting When the Patient Is Unable to Participate. 2010. http://ipal-live.capc.stackop.com/downloads/ipal-icu-organizing-an-icu-palliative-care-initiative.pdf. Accessed May 3, 2013.

120. Curtis JR, Engelberg RA, Wenrich MD, et al. Studying communication about end-of-life care during the ICU family conference: development of a framework. J Crit Care. 2002;17(3):147–160.

121. Pollak KI, Arnold RM, Jeffreys AS, et al. Oncologist communication about emotion during visits with patients with advanced cancer. J Clin Oncol. 20 2007;25(36):5748–5752.

122. Savory EA, Marco CA. End-of-life issues in the acute and critically ill patient. Scand J Trauma Resusc Emerg Med. 2009;17:21.

123. Gries CJ, Curtis JR, Wall RJ, Engelberg RA. Family member satisfaction with end-of-life decision making in the ICU. Chest. 2008;133(3):704–712.

124. Lautrette A, Darmon M, Megarbane B, et al. A communication strategy and brochure for relatives of patients dying in the ICU. N Engl J Med. 2007;356(5):469–478.

125. Selph RB, Shiang J, Engelberg R, Curtis JR, White DB. Empathy and life support decisions in intensive care units. J Gen Intern Med. 2008;23(9):1311–1317.

126. Hudson P, Thomas T, Quinn K, Aranda S. Family meetings in palliative care: are they effective? Palliat Med. 2009;23(2):150–157.

127. White DB. Rethinking interventions to improve surrogate decision making in intensive care units. Am J Crit Care. 2011;20(3):252–257.

128. White DB, Cua SM, Walk R, et al. Nurse-led intervention to improve surrogate decision making for patients with advanced critical illness. Am J Crit Care. 2012;21(6):396–409.

129. Nelson JE, Cortez TB, Curtis JR, et al. Integrating palliative care in the ICU: the nurse in a leading role. J Hosp Palliat Nurs. 2011;13(2): 89–94.

130. Krimshtein NS, Luhrs CA, Puntillo KA, et al. Training nurses for interdisciplinary communication with families in the intensive care unit: an intervention. J Palliat Med. 2011;14(12):1325–1332.

131. Gerstel E, Engelberg RA, Koepsell T, Curtis JR. Duration of withdrawal of life support in the intensive care unit and association with family satisfaction. Am J Respir Crit Care Med. 2008;178(8):798–804.

132. Valentin A, Druml W, Steltzer H, Wiedermann CJ. Recommendations on therapy limitation and therapy discontinuation in intensive care units: Consensus Paper of the Austrian Associations of Intensive Care Medicine. Intensive Care Med. 2008;34(4):771–776.

133. Psirides AJ, Sturland S. Withdrawal of active treatment in intensive care: what is stopped—comparison between belief and practice. Crit Care Resusc. 2009;11(3):210–214.

134. Frost DW, Cook DJ, Heyland DK, Fowler RA. Patient and healthcare professional factors influencing end-of-life decision-making during critical illness: a systematic review. Crit Care Med. 2011;39(5): 1174–1189.

135. Browning AM. Empowering family members in end-of-life care decision making in the intensive care unit. Dimens Crit Care Nurs. 2009;28(1):18–23.

136. Kirchhoff KT, Kowalkowski JA. Current practices for withdrawal of life support in intensive care units. Am J Crit Care. 2010;19(6): 532–541; quiz 542.

137. Hynninen M, Klepstad P, Petersson J, Skram U, Tallgren M. Process of foregoing life-sustaining treatment: a survey among Scandinavian intensivists. Acta Anaesthesiol Scand. 2008;52(8):1081–1085.

138. Baggs JG, Schmitt MH, Prendergast TJ, et al. Who is attending? End-of-life decision making in the intensive care unit. J Palliat Med. 2012;15(1):56–62.

139. Forte DN, Vincent JL, Velasco IT, Park M. Association between education in EOL care and variability in EOL practice: a survey of ICU physicians. Intensive Care Med. 2012;38(3):404–412.

140. Curtis JR, Vincent JL. Ethics and end-of-life care for adults in the intensive care unit. Lancet. 2010;376(9749):1347–1353.

141. Kompanje EJ, van der Hoven B, Bakker J. Anticipation of distress after discontinuation of mechanical ventilation in the ICU at the end of life. Intensive Care Med. 2008;34(9):1593–1599.

142. Szalados JE. Discontinuation of mechanical ventilation at end-of-life: the ethical and legal boundaries of physician conduct in termination of life support. Crit Care Clin. 2007;23(2):317–337, xi.

143. Campbell ML. How to withdraw mechanical ventilation: a systematic review of the literature. AACN Adv Crit Care. 2007;18(4):397–403; quiz 344–395.

144. Billings JA. Humane terminal extubation reconsidered: the role for preemptive analgesia and sedation. Crit Care Med. 2012;40(2):625–630.

145. Curtis JR. Caring for patients with critical illness and their families: the value of the integrated clinical team. Respir Care. 2008;53(4): 480–487.

146. Curtis JR, Treece PD, Nielsen EL, et al. Integrating palliative and critical care: evaluation of a quality-improvement intervention. Am J Respir Crit Care Med. 2008;178(3):269–275.

147. Treece PD, Engelberg RA, Crowley L, et al. Evaluation of a standardized order form for the withdrawal of life support in the intensive care unit. Crit Care Med. 2004;32(5):1141–1148.

148. Epker JL, Bakker J, Kompanje EJ. The use of opioids and sedatives and time until death after withdrawing mechanical ventilation and vasoactive drugs in a dutch intensive care unit. Anesth Analg. 2011;112(3):628–634.

149. Mazer MA, Alligood CM, Wu Q. The infusion of opioids during terminal withdrawal of mechanical ventilation in the medical intensive care unit. J Pain Symptom Manage. 2011;42(1):44–51.

150. Truog RD, Brock DW, White DB. Should patients receive general anesthesia prior to extubation at the end of life? Crit Care Med. 2012;40(2):631–633.

151. Truog RD, Burns JP, Mitchell C, Johnson J, Robinson W. Pharmacologic paralysis and withdrawal of mechanical ventilation at the end of life. N Engl J Med. 2000;342(7):508–511.

152. Davidson JE, Powers K, Hedayat KM, et al. Clinical practice guidelines for support of the family in the patient-centered intensive care unit: American College of Critical Care Medicine Task Force 2004-2005. Crit Care Med. 2007;35(2):605–622.

153. Leon AM, Knapp S. Involving family systems in critical care nursing: challenges and opportunities. Dimens Crit Care Nurs. 2008;27(6):255–262.

154. Anderson WG, Arnold RM, Angus DC, Bryce CL. Posttraumatic stress and complicated grief in family members of patients in the intensive care unit. J Gen Intern Med. 2008;23(11):1871–1876.

155. McAdam JL, Dracup KA, White DB, Fontaine DK, Puntillo KA. Symptom experiences of family members of intensive care unit patients at high risk for dying. Crit Care Med. 2010;38(4): 1078–1085.

156. McAdam JL, Fontaine DK, White DB, Dracup KA, Puntillo KA. Psychological symptoms of family members of high-risk intensive care unit patients. Am J Crit Care. 2012;21(6):386–393; quiz 394.

157. Siegel MD, Hayes E, Vanderwerker LC, Loseth DB, Prigerson HG. Psychiatric illness in the next of kin of patients who die in the intensive care unit. Crit Care Med. 2008;36(6):1722–1728.

158. Davidson JE, Jones C, Bienvenu OJ. Family response to critical illness: postintensive care syndrome-family. Crit Care Med. 2012;40(2):618–624.

159. Adams S, Herrera A 3rd, Miller L, Soto R. Visitation in the intensive care unit: impact on infection prevention and control. Crit Care Nurs Q. 2011;34(1):3–10.

160. Whitton S, Pittiglio LI. Critical care open visiting hours. Crit Care Nurs Q. 2011;34(4):361–366.

161. Garrouste-Orgeas M, Philippart F, Timsit JF, et al. Perceptions of a 24-hour visiting policy in the intensive care unit. Crit Care Med. 2008;36(1):30–35.

162. Liu V, Read JL, Scruth E, Cheng E. Visitation policies and practices in United States intensive care units. Crit Care. 2013;17(2):R71.

163. Biancofiore G, Bindi LM, Barsotti E, Menichini S, Baldini S. Open intensive care units: a regional survey about the beliefs and attitudes of healthcare professionals. Minerva Anestesiol. 2010;76(2): 93–99.

164. Spreen AE, Schuurmans MJ. Visiting policies in the adult intensive care units: a complete survey of Dutch ICUs. Intensive Crit Care Nurs. 2011;27(1):27–30.

165. Family presence: visitation in the adult ICU. Crit Care Nurse. 2012;32(4):76–78.

166. Kirchhoff KT, Faas AI. Family support at end of life. AACN Adv Crit Care. 2007;18(4):426–435.

167. Kean S. Children and young people visiting an adult intensive care unit. J Adv Nurs. 2010;66(4):868–877.

168. Hanley JB, Piazza J. A visit to the intensive cares unit: a family-centered culture change to facilitate pediatric visitation in an adult intensive care unit. Crit Care Nurs Q. 2012;35(1):113–122.

169. Egging D, Crowley M, Arruda T, et al. Emergency nursing resource: family presence during invasive procedures and resuscitation in the emergency department. J Emerg Nurs. 2011;37(5):469–473.

170. Mortelmans LJ, Cas WM, Van Hellemond PL, De Cauwer HG. Should relatives witness resuscitation in the emergency department?: The point of view of the Belgian emergency department staff. Eur J Emerg Med. 2009;16(2):87–91.

171. Tinsley C, Hill JB, Shah J, et al. Experience of families during cardiopulmonary resuscitation in a pediatric intensive care unit. Pediatrics. 2008;122(4):e799–e804.

172. Dudley NC, Hansen KW, Furnival RA, Donaldson AE, Van Wagenen KL, Scaife ER. The effect of family presence on the efficiency of pediatric trauma resuscitations. Ann Emerg Med. 2009;53(6):777–784 e773.

173. Jabre P, Belpomme V, Azoulay E, et al. Family presence during cardiopulmonary resuscitation. N Engl J Med. 2013;368(11):1008–1018.

174. McMillen RE. End of life decisions: nurses perceptions, feelings and experiences. Intensive Crit Care Nurs. 2008;24(4):251–259.

175. Ganz FD, Yoffe F. Intensive care nurses' perspectives of family-centered care and their attitudes toward family presence during resuscitation. J Cardiovasc Nurs. 2012;27(3):220–227.

176. Demir F. Presence of patients' families during cardiopulmonary resuscitation: physicians' and nurses' opinions. J Adv Nurs. 2008;63(4):409–416.

177. McClement SE, Fallis WM, Pereira A. Family presence during resuscitation: Canadian critical care nurses' perspectives. J Nurs Scholarsh. 2009;41(3):233–240.

178. Walker W. Accident and emergency staff opinion on the effects of family presence during adult resuscitation: critical literature review. J Adv Nurs. 2008;61(4):348–362.

179. Basol R, Ohman K, Simones J, Skillings K. Using research to determine support for a policy on family presence during resuscitation. Dimens Crit Care Nurs. 2009;28(5):237–247; quiz 248–239.

180. Leung NY, Chow SK. Attitudes of healthcare staff and patients' family members towards family presence during resuscitation in adult critical care units. J Clin Nurs. 2012;21(13–14):2083–2093.

181. Stricker KH, Kimberger O, Schmidlin K, Zwahlen M, Mohr U, Rothen HU. Family satisfaction in the intensive care unit: what makes the difference? Intensive Care Med. 2009;35(12):2051–2059.

182. Khot S, Billings M, Owens D, Longstreth WT, Jr. Coping with death and dying on a neurology inpatient service: death rounds as an educational initiative for residents. Arch Neurol. 2011;68(11):1395–1397.

183. Gelinas C, Fillion L, Robitaille MA, Truchon M. Stressors experienced by nurses providing end-of-life palliative care in the intensive care unit. Can J Nurs Res. 2012;44(1):18–39.

184. Kelly E, Nisker J. Medical students' first clinical experiences of death. Med Educ. 2010;44(4):421–428.

185. Stayt LC. Death, empathy and self preservation: the emotional labour of caring for families of the critically ill in adult intensive care. J Clin Nurs. 2009;18(9):1267–1275.

186. Benner P. A dialogue between virtue ethics and care ethics. Theor Med. 1997;18(1–2):47–61.

187. Osborn TR, Curtis JR, Nielsen EL, Back AL, Shannon SE, Engelberg RA. Identifying elements of ICU care that families report as important but unsatisfactory: decision-making, control, and ICU atmosphere. Chest. 2012;142(5):1185–1192.

188. Jacobowski NL, Girard TD, Mulder JA, Ely EW. Communication in critical care: family rounds in the intensive care unit. Am J Crit Care. 2010;19(5):421–430.

189. Garrouste-Orgeas M, Coquet I, Perier A, et al. Impact of an intensive care unit diary on psychological distress in patients and relatives. Crit Care Med. 2012;40(7):2033–2040.

190. Curtis JR, Ciechanowski PS, Downey L, et al. Development and evaluation of an interprofessional communication intervention to improve family outcomes in the ICU. Contemp Clin Trials. 2012;33(6):1245–1254.

191. Milberg A, Olsson EC, Jakobsson M, Olsson M, Friedrichsen M. Family members' perceived needs for bereavement follow-up. J Pain Symptom Manage. 2008;35(1):58–69.

192. Ross MW. Implementing a bereavement program. Crit Care Nurs. 2008;28(6):88, 87.

193. Yeager S, Doust C, Epting S, et al. Embrace Hope: an end-of-life intervention to support neurological critical care patients and their families. Crit Care Nurse. 2010;30(1):47–58; quiz 59.

194. End-of-Life Nursing Education Consortium (ELNEC). http://www. aacn.nche.edu/elnec Accessed July 9, 2013.

195. Mitchell M, Chaboyer W, Burmeister E, Foster M. Positive effects of a nursing intervention on family-centered care in adult critical care. Am J Crit Care. 2009;18(6):543–552; quiz 553.

196. McAdam JL, Arai S, Puntillo KA. Unrecognized contributions of families in the intensive care unit. Intensive Care Med. 2008;34(6):1097–1101.

197. Fridh I, Forsberg A, Bergbom I. Doing one's utmost: nurses' descriptions of caring for dying patients in an intensive care environment. Intensive Crit Care Nurs. 2009;25(5):233–241.

198. Reese CD. Please cry with me: six ways to grieve. Nursing. 1996;26(8):56.

199. Browning AM. CNE article: moral distress and psychological empowerment in critical care nurses caring for adults at end of life. Am J Crit Care. 2013;22(2):143–151.

200. Espinosa L, Young A, Symes L, Haile B, Walsh T. ICU nurses' experiences in providing terminal care. Crit Care Nurs Q. 2010;33(3):273–281.

201. Robinson R. Registered nurses and moral distress. Dimens Crit Care Nurs. 2010;29(5):197–202.

202. Festic E, Wilson ME, Gajic O, Divertie GD, Rabatin JT. Perspectives of physicians and nurses regarding end-of-life care in the intensive care unit. J Intensive Care Med. 2012;27(1):45–54.

203. Jourdain G, Chenevert D. Job demands-resources, burnout and intention to leave the nursing profession: a questionnaire survey. Int J Nurs Stud. 2010;47(6):709–722.

204. Shorter M, Stayt LC. Critical care nurses' experiences of grief in an adult intensive care unit. J Adv Nurs. 2010;66(1):159–167.

205. Moola S, Ehlers VJ, Hattingh SP. Critical care nurses' perceptions of stress and stress-related situations in the workplace. Curationis. 2008;31(2):77–86.

206. Keene EA, Hutton N, Hall B, Rushton C. Bereavement debriefing sessions: an intervention to support health care professionals in managing their grief after the death of a patient. Pediatr Nurs. 2010;36(4):185–189; quiz 190.

207. Hildebrandt L. Providing grief resolution as an oncology nurse retention strategy: a literature review. Clin J Oncol Nurs. 2012;16(6):601–606.

208. Santiago C, Abdool S. Conversations about challenging end-of-life cases: ethics debriefing in the medical surgical intensive care unit. Dynamics. 2011;22(4):26–30.

209. Macpherson CF. Peer-supported storytelling for grieving pediatric oncology nurses. J Pediatr Oncol Nurs. 2008;25(3):148–163.

210. Gordon E, Ridley B, Boston J, Dahl E. The building bridges initiative: learning with, from and about to create an interprofessional end-of-life program. Dynamics. 2012;23(4):37–41.

211. Abazzia C, Adamo F, Gill B, Morrison R, Volpe K, Prata J. In the name of good intentions: nurses' perspectives on caring for a pregnant patient in a persistent vegetative state. Crit Care Nurse. 2010;30(1):40–46.

212. Schroder C, Heyland D, Jiang X, Rocker G, Dodek P. Educating medical residents in end-of-life care: insights from a multicenter survey. J Palliat Med. 2009;12(5):459–470.

213. Smith L, Hough CL. Using death rounds to improve end-of-life education for internal medicine residents. J Palliat Med. 2011;14(1):55–58.

214. Eskildsen MA, Flacker J. A multimodal aging and dying course for first-year medical students improves knowledge and attitudes. J Am Geriatr Soc. 2009;57(8):1492–1497.

215. Rose C, Bonn A, MacDonald K, Avila S. Interdisciplinary education on discussing end-of-life care. Dimens Crit Care Nurs. 2012;31(4):236–240.

216. Aslakson RA, Wyskiel R, Thornton I, et al. Nurse-perceived barriers to effective communication regarding prognosis and optimal end-of-life care for surgical ICU patients: a qualitative exploration. J Palliat Med. 2012;15(8):910–915.

217. Friedenberg AS, Levy MM, Ross S, Evans LE. Barriers to end-of-life care in the intensive care unit: perceptions vary by level of training, discipline, and institution. J Palliat Med. 2012;15(4):404–411.

218. Montagnini M, Smith H, Balistrieri T. Assessment of self-perceived end-of-life care competencies of intensive care unit providers. J Palliat Med. 2012;15(1):29–36.

219. Billings JA. Massachusetts General Hospital, Medical ICU Project: Ventilator Withdrawal Guidelines. http://www.aacn.org/WD/Palliative/Docs/mgh8.pdf. Accessed June 24, 2013.

220. Nelson JE, Cortez TB, Curtis JR, et al. Integrating palliative care in the ICU: the nurse in a leading role. J Hosp Palliat Nurs. 2011;13(2):89–94.

221. Ferrell BR, Dahlin C, Campbell ML, Paice JA, Malloy P, Virani R. End-of-life Nursing Education Consortium (ELNEC) Training Program: improving palliative care in critical care. Crit Care Nurs Q. 2007;30(3):206–212.

222. Shannon SE, Long-Sutehall T, Coombs M. Conversations in end-of-life care: communication tools for critical care practitioners. Nurs Crit Care. 2011;16(3):124–130.

223. Glavan BJ, Engelberg RA, Downey L, Curtis JR. Using the medical record to evaluate the quality of end-of-life care in the intensive care unit. Crit Care Med. 2008;36(4):1138–1146.

224. Medina J, Puntillo K, eds. AACN Protocols for Practice: Palliative Care and End-of-Life Issues in Critical Care. Sudbury, MA: Jones & Bartlett; 2006.

225. Rocker G, Puntillo K, Azoulay E, Nelson J. End-of-Life in the Intensive Care Unit. London: Oxford; 2010.

226. Mularski RA, Curtis JR, Billings JA, et al. Proposed quality measures for palliative care in the critically ill: a consensus from the Robert Wood Johnson Foundation Critical Care Workgroup. Crit Care Med. 2006;34(11 Suppl):S404–S411.

227. Robert Wood Johnson Foundation. Promoting Excellence in End-of-Life Care: An RWJF National Program. http://www.rwjf.org/content/dam/farm/reports/program_results_reports/2009/rwjf69604 2009. Accessed May 3, 2013.

228. CAPC. IPal-ICU: Improving Palliative Care in the ICU. http://www.capc.org/ipal/ipal-icu. Accessed May 3, 2013.

229. Morell EA. Learning that a death can be a good death. J Palliat Med. 2012;15(2):248–249.

230. Chapple HS. Changing the game in the intensive care unit: letting nature take its course. Crit Care Nurse. 1999;19(3):25–34.

CHAPTER 48

Palliative care nursing in the outpatient setting

Pamela Stitzlein Davies

Bob was such a fighter. I think it is why he lived so long after his diagnosis. But it also made it really hard to move through the final stages of cancer during his last 6 months. Having our palliative care nurse practitioner involved provided honest, frank and reasonable dialogue around difficult conversations. She was able to help manage expectations, recognized when it was time to hire in home help, and helped us to manage the process not only for Bob as a patient, but for our whole family. She was not only focused on the disease and its symptoms, but the emotional impacts of the final stage. I can't imagine how much harder it would have been without her. She really made our experience bearable. She helped us to grow so much. We are forever grateful.

Daughter-in-law of a 67-year-old man with metastatic renal cell carcinoma

Key points

- The ambulatory setting is an important site for provision of palliative care, as the majority of care for advanced cancer and other chronic life-limiting illnesses are provided in outpatient clinics.

- Studies show that early involvement of outpatient palliative care in the setting of advanced cancer can promote better quality of life, reduce emergency department visits, reduce inappropriate chemotherapy in the final 2 weeks of life, promote earlier hospice enrollment, and potentially prolong life.

- Algorithms to trigger a palliative care consult are helpful in selecting those who would benefit the most from specialty palliative care.

- Nurses and advanced practice nurses (APNs) play a key role in the provision of palliative care in the outpatient setting.

- "Primary palliative care" refers to the first-line management that all clinicians provide to patients in their care. Therefore, all nurses should learn the communication skills needed to talk about advanced illness and end-of-life preparation.

Introduction

The vast majority of healthcare in the United States is provided in ambulatory care clinics. Although palliative care (PC) has become incorporated into most major acute care hospitals, it is still relatively novel in the outpatient (OP) clinic, especially in noncancer settings.[1] Meier and Beresford describe the provision of PC in the outpatient setting as the "new frontier."[2] The American Society of Clinical Oncologists (ASCO) has a goal of providing PC as a routine part of comprehensive cancer care for all patients by 2020; and specifically state that PC should be available in all of the settings that care is received, including OP clinics.[3] In 2014, ASCO, in conjunction with the American Academy of Hospice and Palliative Medicine (AAHPM) launched a 3-year collaborative with 25 practice sites, designed to improve the quality of PC provided in the OP setting.[4] In addition, the Center to Advance Palliative Care (CAPC) has developed a website to promote and improve OP PC.[5] Thus, the field of OP PC is anticipated to expand significantly in this decade.

Patients are living longer and with greater disabilities than ever before.[6] In addition to advanced cancer, other terminal diseases managed in ambulatory care include end-stage heart failure, advanced cirrhosis, renal failure, and terminal neurological disorders such as advanced dementia. Primary and specialty care providers are central in the care of these advanced illnesses, but they receive minimal training on end-of-life (EOL) care, and are challenged to find the time to address these essential issues.[7-10] Nurses and APNs, with their extensive psychosocial training, and in collaboration with a multidisciplinary team, play an important role in helping ambulatory clinic patients and caregivers navigate concerns that arise as EOL approaches.[11] This chapter addresses the provision of PC in the adult OP setting, with a focus on the role of nurses and APNs.

Advantages and challenges faced in the outpatient setting

The OP setting is ideal for providing PC, as the pace is less crisis-driven than inpatient care, and typically benefits from long-term trusting relationships that form between the patient/caregiver and the medical team over months and years. These factors permit dialogues regarding advanced care planning to be held over a series of visits, allowing the patient to absorb small "doses" of information at a time, and discuss these options with loved ones in the comfort of their home environment. Other advantages of providing PC in the OP setting are listed in Box 48.1.

Challenges faced in the OP setting are described in Box 48.2. Some of these challenges are common to PC teams in any setting, such as receiving late referrals (when a patient is actively dying), and funding issues.[19] Other issues are specific to the OP setting such as coordinating OP PC visits with the primary team's appointments. A unique issue faced by some OP PC programs is referrals for management of chronic pain not related to the primary diagnosis (e.g., chronic low back pain requiring ongoing, moderately high dose opioid therapy in a patient with a curable leukemia), or for ongoing management of chronic pain in a cancer survivor years after completion of therapy.[1] Because most PC programs focus on patients with terminal illness, long-term management of complex chronic pain problems may be beyond the parameters of what the PC team can offer. However, in some institutions, the chronic pain clinic is combined with the PC clinic, and has the expertise and manpower to manage these cases on a chronic basis.

Primary, secondary, and tertiary palliative care

Primary palliative care describes the role that every nurse, APN, and other medical provider has in recognizing and addressing PC needs in ambulatory settings.[5] Also referred to as "generalist" PC,

---

Box 48.1 Advantages of providing palliative care in the outpatient setting

- Early involvement by the PC team for pain and symptom management helps build relationships with patients and caregivers; this can foster communication during times of stress or crisis.

- The OP setting is less crisis driven, thus allowing patient and caregivers to confer about advance care planning in "little doses," months or years before decisions are needed.

- Continuity of care between the inpatient PC and OP PC service allows for seamless PC involvement when the patient is admitted or discharged.

- OP PC may result in fewer emergency department visits and fewer admissions or readmissions.

- Earlier recognition and treatment of depression and anxiety in patients and caregivers.

- Improved QOL ratings in patients, despite continued physical decline.

- PC fosters less "overaggressive" chemotherapy in the final weeks of life.

- PC promotes earlier hospice referral, resulting in improved quality at EOL.

- Potential for prolonged survival benefit compared to standard care.

Sources: References 2, 6, 12, 13–18.

Box 48.2 Challenges faced when providing palliative care in the outpatient setting

- The patient may feel abandonment, or believe that a referral to PC means the clinician is "giving up" on them.

- Clinician misunderstanding of the PC role may result in late referrals to the PC service, when a hospice referral is more appropriate (e.g., the patient is actively dying).

- Providing excellent communication and seamless coordination of care with the primary team takes extra time and effort on the part of the PC team.

- Scheduling challenges occur when trying to consolidate patient appointments by coordinating PC appointments on the same day as the primary clinician's appointment.

  - PC appointments scheduled in an OP oncology infusion center may be challenging due to administration of sedating premedications, such as diphenhydramine, making the visit impossible due to sedation. In addition, lack of privacy may limit visits in this area.

- Lack of funding for clinician and support staff salaries.

- Lack of availability of clinic examination room space.

- Challenge in providing staffing for 24/7 telephone availability by the PC team.

- Determining who "owns" patient symptom management issues. For example, who manages chemotherapy-induced nausea? Who titrates the pain medicines and prescribes the opioid renewals?

  - A special issue in outpatient oncology is which team (oncologist or PC) is responsible for addressing a new pain problem. Depending on the individual setting, most PC teams in a consultant or collaborative role will defer the workup of new pain syndromes to the oncologist, as pain may be due to progression of malignancy, resulting in a change of chemotherapy or initiation of radiotherapy.

- While some OP PC programs may be able to accept all referrals, most will need to define and limit the type of consultations accepted, due to staffing limitations. If scheduled, the OP PC team might elect to limit their involvement to only a few visits. For example:

  - Referrals on patients with moderate symptom burden from chronic disease, but who are not in advanced state of illness, with anticipated life expectancy of decades

  - Management of chronic pain issues that are not related to the advanced illness, in the cancer survivor with anticipated long-term management needs, or in the patient with active substance use

Sources: References 5, 19–21.

---

this includes skill sets such as basic pain and symptom management and EOL discussions and advanced planning paperwork.[8] Because PC resources are limited, referrals should focus on patients with complex needs who require specialty consultation. In addition, the majority of community oncology care is provided in settings that lack PC resources.[9] Thus, the clinic team members act in a front-line role for the provision of the majority of PC needs.[3] For example, when a patient arrives in pulmonary clinic for a posthospitalization visit after a COPD exacerbation, his nurse may inquire whether any discussions occurred regarding advanced directives and code status during the recent inpatient stay. Oftentimes, patients receive paperwork from the inpatient social worker related to such discussions, but do not complete it. The clinic nurse can help them finalize the forms during the clinic visit or notify the social worker to assist. Another example of primary palliative care in symptom management is the oncology nurse who reminds patients to utilize a bowel management plan when taking opioids for cancer pain. Ambulatory care nurses also play a key role in providing education and support in the decision to transition to hospice care. Ongoing learning is needed to keep nurses and clinicians up to date on basic palliative care skills.[6] The essential role of the clinic nurse in addressing PC needs cannot be overemphasized: these concepts are at the very heart of nursing.[11] In other words, every nurse should be providing primary palliative care on an ongoing basis.

Secondary palliative care refers to the formal involvement of PC specialists to assist with more complex cases.[3] Problems addressed may relate to complicated pain and symptom management; maladaptive coping and distress; or assistance with particularly challenging EOL situations.

Tertiary palliative care describes major PC programs with a focus on research and teaching to advance the specialty, and may include a PC physician and APN fellowship programs.[22]

As OP PC expands into nononcology fields, such as cardiology or neurology, PC specialists must become familiar with specific PC topics that arise in various fields. Some topics are common to all fields, such as advanced care planning; other topics are unique to a specialty, such as the decision to stop dialysis. Box 48.3 lists some of these topics.

Models of care

Three basic models exist in the delivery of OP PC: collaborative, consultative, and medical home.[29] The collaborative model (also known as embedded, integrated, or concurrent model) is the most popular style found in the outpatient setting.[1] In this model, the PC team takes the lead in managing certain aspects of care, such as pain and symptoms, distress, or decision-making, thus allowing the clinician (oncologist, cardiologist) to focus on the overall management of the patient. In the collaborative model, the PC team institutes their own recommendations, including writing prescriptions, and follows patients on an ongoing basis, often in coordination with their clinic follow-up visit. Advantages of this model include combining "the best of both worlds" with specialists from both fields contributing to care and working together to improve quality of life (QOL) in distinct, yet complementary, roles.[30] Embedded clinics create the opportunity for a shared visit with the clinician, thus improving communication and coordination of care. This model is usually more convenient for the patient, especially if PC visits are held on the same day and location as their other clinic appointment. However, it creates special challenges for the scheduling of PC visits to accomplish that coordination.[20] For optimal success in this model, the PC team must consider themselves diplomats; with ongoing efforts to foster a good relationship with the referring clinician, striving for flexibility to work within the framework of that clinician's practice style.[31,32] For example, some clinicians may object to the PC team discussing questions about prognosis before they have addressed that subject themselves.

In the consultative model, the PC provider evaluates patients, and forwards management recommendations to the team for their implementation. The PC team does not write prescriptions, and does not implement the recommended plan of care. In addition, PC does not typically follow patients on an ongoing basis. Unfortunately, this model may suffer from a lack of follow through on the PC recommendations. Rabow found a low percentage of patients had the plan of care implemented when utilizing a consultative model in a primary care clinic to address pain and depression among other issues.[33] However, patients seen under this model could potentially benefit if the structure and goals of the visit are specifically defined. For example, if a nurse meets with a patient to discuss goals of care and advance planning, that single visit fulfills the PC intervention. Research is needed to further define methods to make this model work well.

The final model of care is the medical home model (defined in the literature as the "primary palliative care" model, which is different from the same term discussed above).[34] In this model, the PC team functions as the "medical home" or "primary care provider" and addresses all aspects of the patient's care; from management of the life-limiting illness, such as end-stage liver disease; to other chronic conditions, such as hypertension and osteoarthritis.[12] This model integrates PC into primary care, and is an excellent option for medically underserved populations and for patients who are not eligible for, or elect not to pursue, specialized treatments such as dialysis or chemotherapy. The clinician must have a broad knowledge base and access to specialists for formal or informal consultation. In many ways, this model is comparable to services traditionally provided by general practitioners for decades.[6,23]

Key studies in outpatient palliative care

Several important trials have shown the advantage of utilizing PC in the OP setting. The most notable is Temel et al.[13] (2010), which examined the effect of providing early PC to patients recently diagnosed with metastatic non-small-cell lung cancer (NSCLC, which typically has a prognosis of less than a year.) This was a nonblinded randomized controlled study of 151 patients, with 74 patients receiving standard care and 77 patients receiving embedded PC in addition to standard care. The PC team, consisting of six physicians and one nurse practitioner (NP), met with patients within 12 weeks of diagnosis, and saw them monthly until death. The visits focused on symptom management, psychosocial distress, goals of care, and treatment decisions. The findings, which received wide publicity, showed that patients in the PC arm lived 30% longer than the control group (11.6 vs. 8.9 months), and reported better QOL with fewer symptoms of depression, despite receiving less aggressive treatment at EOL and earlier hospice enrollment.

In a pilot study, led by an advanced practice registered nurse (APRN), Prince-Paul et al.[14] (2010) studied the impact of PC in adults with advanced cancer in an OP oncology clinic. Fifty-two patients received usual care, and 49 received usual care plus

Box 48.3 Sample topics addressed in outpatient palliative care, by specialty

- ◆ All sites
  - Pain management
  - Symptom management
  - Psychosocial-spiritual distress, coping with serious illness
    - Recognizing and addressing existential distress that contributes to the pain experience
    - Assisting the primary team in working with "challenging patients," such as those with significant psychopathology (schizophrenia, personality disorder), which create disruptions in care, or "staff splitting"
  - Treatment decisions, future planning
    - Goals of care discussions
    - Completion of advanced directives, durable power of attorney for healthcare (DPOA-HC), DNR orders
  - Caregiver issues
    - Coping, stress management, education, respite needs
  - Decision and timing of referral to hospice
  - Requests for hastened death
- ◆ Oncology
  - Decision-making related to stopping chemotherapy and other treatments. This is usually required in order to enroll in hospice.
  - Decision to move forward with a hematopoietic cell transplant when anticipated outcome is poor
  - Moral distress experienced by infusion nurses related to ongoing transfusion of blood products (a scarce resource) for transfusion-refractory anemia or thrombocytopenia (e.g., an end-stage AML patient with no active bleeding, not on treatment, who is receiving ongoing platelet transfusions 3 times a week despite a minimal rise in the posttransfusion platelet count)
- ◆ Neurology
  - Discussions regarding initiation or discontinuation of tube feedings or ventilator in end-stage dementia, amyotrophic lateral sclerosis, or multiple sclerosis
- ◆ Nephrology
  - Decision not to initiate, or to discontinue, dialysis
  - Issues around inclusion or removal from kidney transplant list
- ◆ Cardiology
  - Complex decisions regarding initiation or discontinuation of left ventricular assist devices (LVAD)
  - Turning off automatic internal cardiac defibrillator (AICD)
  - Issues around inclusion or removal from heart transplant list
- ◆ Pulmonary
  - Discussion about do-not-intubate orders
  - Issues around inclusion or removal from lung transplant list
- ◆ Hepatology
  - Issues around inclusion or removal from liver transplant list
  - Patient distress related to personal behaviors that may have contributed to the development of hepatocellular carcinoma (HCC, e.g., use of intravenous drugs decades prior, leading to development of hepatitis C, leading to higher risk of HCC)
- ◆ Primary care/geriatrics
  - Care decisions in debility, failure to thrive, dementia, including placement in skilled nursing facilities
  - Assisting the primary care provider (PCP) in explaining or confirming specialty recommendations (e.g., why treatment of breast cancer is not recommended in a frail 92-year-old woman with severe dementia)
  - Assisting the PCP with management of complex hospice cases, especially if the specialty provider (oncology, cardiology, or neurology) has signed off the case

Sources: References 5, 6, 23–28.

PC provided in a collaborative model. More than 50% of the patients received chemotherapy during the study. The PC visits focused on pain and symptom management, medicine education, psychosocial-spiritual support, and discussions about EOL preparation. Patients were followed for 5 months. Findings revealed that those in the PC arm were 84% less likely to be hospitalized and 25 times more likely to be alive at 4 months, compared with the usual care group. In addition, higher scores on social well-being scales resulted in fewer hospitalizations and lower mortality. The authors conclude that the provision of PC by an APRN in the oncology setting is beneficial; and the provision of emotional support and active presence by the PC nurse may explain some of that benefit.

Bakitas et al.[15] (2010) randomized 322 subjects with advanced cancer to either usual care, or usual care with PC, under the study name of Project ENABLE (Educate, Nurture, Advise, Before Life Ends). This APRN-led study involved four structured psychoeducational sessions, followed by monthly telephone calls. Educational topics included patient activation, self-management, self-advocacy, and communication skills to use with their oncologist. The intervention group showed improvement in QOL and mood scores, demonstrating the impact of nurse-led education to empower the cancer patient.

Murphy and colleagues[12] examined the healthcare utilization of 147 patients enrolled in a medical home PC model, compared with the 12-month period prior to enrollment. Patients received care for a variety of life-limiting illnesses, such as cancer, heart failure, COPD, dementia, and end-stage renal disease, in addition to management of other primary care issues. Most participants from this county "safety-net" academic medical center struggled with mental illness, substance use, or homelessness. The results of the chart review showed a 27% reduction in emergency department (ED) visits and a 20% reduction in hospitalizations after enrollment in the PC program. This confirmed the findings of the Owens et al.[34] (2012) pilot study in this population and again demonstrated the success of APRNs providing both primary care and PC to patients with life-limiting illness.

Muir et al.[32] (2010) examined the benefits of an embedded PC team in a private oncology practice. This study focused on provider satisfaction and time saved by the oncologist in addition to quality care outcomes. The PC involvement resulted in a 21% reduction in symptom burden, increased oncologist satisfaction and saved an estimated 170 minutes of oncologist time for each new referral seen by the PC team.

Practical details in providing outpatient palliative care

Many questions arise when developing or expanding an OP PC program. This section will address common issues in implementation, with a focus on oncology clinics, since the majority of the literature exists in the oncology setting.

Referrals to the outpatient palliative care team

Referrals to OP PC depend on multiple factors unique to the individual provider, clinic milieu, and organizational setting. In a survey of 12 OP PC centers, oncologists initiated 76% of the referrals, and 23% came from the inpatient PC team.[35] Other factors include the needs and expertise of the referring clinician (oncologist, nephrologist, neurologist), access to supportive care services in the referring clinic (such as social work), percentage of patients in the practice with complex needs, and availability of PC clinicians. Close physical proximity to the referring clinician appears to play a major role in generating consults.[36] However, each clinician has a different personal threshold regarding whom would benefit most from employing the PC team.[32] Triggers for referral may be based on diagnosis, symptoms, or psychosocial factors.[37] Box 48.4 lists common criteria for a consult to OP PC.

Establishing an ongoing referral base is important when building and maintaining a PC OP practice, because most patients die within weeks or months of an initial PC visit. The embedded PC practice model creates the most referrals, especially if PC can see a new consult soon after, or even concurrently with, the referring clinician to assist with "bad news" discussions or complex symptom management.[36] Participating in multidisciplinary clinic rounds (tumor board or heart failure clinic) can increase PC visibility and generate referrals. Palliative care rounds in which complex patient cases are discussed or educational programs on complex symptom management are other options that may act to generate referrals.

Box 48.4 Sample referral criteria to outpatient palliative care (see text)

Patient/symptom characteristics

- Limited treatment options, such as very advanced HCC

- Diagnosis of highly fatal malignancies, such as metastatic NSCLC or pancreatic or esophageal cancer

- Anticipated poor outcomes, such as elderly patients with AML, or pretransplant for a "high-risk" stem cell transplant

- Diagnosis of end-stage cardiac, pulmonary, renal, or hepatic disease

- Poorly controlled pain or other symptoms

- Declining functional level (e.g., Eastern Clinical Oncology Group [ECOG] score of 3 or 4, or Palliative Performance Scale </= 50)

- Frequent emergency department visits or hospitalizations

- Enrollment in a Phase-1 chemotherapy trial

Psychosocial circumstances

- High levels of psychological, social, or spiritual/existential distress

- Poor social support

- Inability to engage in advance care planning discussions

- Family discord in decision-making

- Requests for hastened death

Other

- Staff issues including moral distress and compassion fatigue

Sources: References 19, 29, 38–40.

In the author's setting, any clinician may send a referral to OP PC. In addition to the oncologist, clinic policy allows nurses, social workers, physical therapists, nutritionists, and chaplains to generate a consult. Infusion center nurses are a great source of referrals. These nurses form close relationships with patients over months, sometimes years, of chemotherapy, and frequently have in-depth discussions about coping with cancer. If the patient experiences worsening symptoms or distress that is not well managed at the "primary PC" level (e.g., nurse or oncologist level), the infusion or team nurse may refer to PC for expert assistance, without first obtaining the oncologist's approval. Some oncologists initially expressed concern regarding this policy, as they are in charge of the overall care and well-being of the patient, and were concerned that PC involvement might cause the patient to "lose hope." In response, the PC team made significant efforts to maintain positive relationships and close communication with the oncologists, with a focus on methods the PC team can assist and decrease their workload. In addition, research findings supporting positive outcomes of PC involvement were reviewed on a formal and informal basis. These strategies allayed oncologist concerns and significantly increased acceptance of PC involvement in their patient's care.

Finally, in the author's clinical setting, patients may self-refer to PC, with information on PC provided on the clinic website and brochures. Clinic volunteers, who assist in the waiting room, and often hear stories of suffering from the patient, are encouraged to offer a PC brochure and instruct that patients may self-refer by calling the PC phone. Referrals also come from family members or leaders of community cancer support groups. In these cases, the PC nurse or coordinator will contact the patient directly to describe the PC service and confirm their interest in scheduling an appointment. On occasion, PC will see a caregiver alone, without the patient present, to discuss EOL planning. However, verbal permission is first obtained from the patient.

Organizational recommendations for palliative care referral

In 2012, the ASCO issued a Provisional Clinical Opinion recommending that all patients with metastatic NSCLC be offered PC, along with standard oncological treatment, based on findings of Temel et al. (2010).[13,38] In addition, the National Comprehensive Cancer Network (NCCN) guidelines on PC list a broad range of referral criteria.[39] Although such widely inclusive referral criteria are ideal, they are probably not realistic for most organizations, due to limitations in PC resources. A strategy is needed to identify those most in need of a referral to secondary and tertiary level PC specialists. For that reason, algorithms are becoming more commonly used in the inpatient and OP settings.[41,42]

Glare et al.[43] developed a screening tool for PC referral in an OP gastrointestinal (GI) oncology clinic based on the NCCN PC guidelines. This one-page instrument assigned 0 to 13 possible points for 5 items: metastatic or locally advanced disease (2 points); ECOG score (0–4 points); serious complication of advanced cancer (hypercalcemia, cachexia, 1 point); serious comorbid disease (heart failure, cirrhosis, 1 point); and five specific PC problems (uncontrolled symptoms, high levels of distress, specific request for referral, complex decision-making/goals of care: 1 point each). The clinic nurse screened 119 patients over a 3 week period. Depending on the threshold used, 7% to 17% of patients would be eligible for PC consultation. The authors further determined that a score of 5 or higher had the best predictive value, and would trigger a PC consult in 13% of the GI oncology clinic population. However, the screening process took 3–5 minutes per patient, resulting in a burdensome 1–2 hours of nursing time per clinic day. The authors suggest that prepopulating the instrument with diagnosis from the electronic medical record (EMR) and having the patient self-report on symptoms and distress, could reduce the screening time. Of course, this requires the EMR to have accurate diagnostic information (e.g., "metastatic colon cancer," not just "colon cancer") and serious comorbidities (such as stage 3 congestive heart failure [CHF]) listed in the problem list. The authors suggest screening at the initial visit, post hospitalization, and every 6 months. Interestingly, the clinic nurse indicated that *all* patients met the NCCN standards for a referral to PC, further emphasizing the need to prioritize primary PC from secondary or tertiary care.

Screening new patient referrals

When receiving a PC referral, it is helpful to ascertain several key points.[20]

♦ First, *what is the purpose of the consult?* If the referral only indicates, "evaluate and treat," it is helpful to speak with the referring team to get more information. Such as: What specifically triggered the request for this patient? Are there signs of maladaptive coping with progressive disease? Is the caregiver insisting on aggressive treatment when the patient seems to want to stop chemotherapy? Is the patient experiencing ongoing severe symptoms despite standard treatment? A few minutes spent clarifying the purpose of the consult can help the PC team to better understand the situation and help to focus the visit.

♦ Second, *what is the urgency of the consult?* Should they be scheduled immediately, or can the initial PC visit be held until they return for their next chemotherapy visit in 3 weeks? An important observation is that what is deemed urgent by the referring source (oncologist, neurologist) may not appear urgent to the PC team, or even to the patient.[31] For example, the patient may call the nurse and express high levels of distress, asking for any kind of help as soon possible, but then declines to schedule a next-day appointment with the PC team, preferring to wait a few weeks.

♦ Third, *is the patient/caregiver aware of the consult?* Even if they are aware, it is surprising how many patients and caregivers perceive the PC referral as abandonment, saying to the scheduler: "I guess this is how Dr. Jones is telling me he's giving up on me." Therefore, the scheduler has an important and delicate task, when setting up the initial visit, to explain the purpose of PC involvement. If there appears to be any confusion or hesitation, the referring team should be notified and asked to assist with communication regarding the PC consult.

The wait time from referral to first PC appointment is ideally less than 1–2 weeks, with urgent consults seen even earlier.[1] This may be a challenge for many programs, due to staffing limitations. If the PC physician's schedule is filled, and an urgent same-day consult cannot be accommodated, the PC nurse may assist by assessing the patient's needs. The nurse then discusses the case with either the primary provider (oncologist), or the PC provider, and follows up with the patient by phone if needed. The PC provider is then scheduled to see the patient as soon as possible.

Maintaining a good relationship with the referring physician

Success in providing OP PC in the collaborative model requires maintenance of positive relationships with the referring specialty physician (oncologist, neurologist, cardiologist), their nurse, and other team members.[32] It may be helpful to think of that physician as the "customer" and PC as the service they are "buying." Close communication and a respectful approach are key, along with negotiation of "who does what" in patient care.[20] For example, opioids for pain management and cough are prescribed by the PC service, but the oncologist prescribes 3 days of steroids to reduce chemotherapy-induced nausea with each cycle. It is important for the PC team to respect this provider's specialized skills and acknowledge that they may have known this particular patient for years, even decades. In addition it is helpful to recognize that the physician, as the "captain of the ship," may feel a bit threatened when referrals to PC are generated by another source, especially if they believe that everything is stable.[20] To smooth this process, the author's team sends an e-mail to the oncologist informing them that a referral was received, whom it was from (infusion nurse, inpatient PC provider), what services were requested (e.g., coping with recent news of disease progression, management of symptoms), and asking for contact if there are any questions or concerns about PC involvement in the patient's care. After each visit, the oncologist and team nurse are updated on the patient status via EMR note. An e-mail with additional information is sent if there are particular points to highlight, for example, to inform the oncologist that the patient was started on an antidepressant for anxiety management. Direct personal communication with the oncologist is always attempted if there are major issues, such as when the patient requests to stop chemotherapy and enroll in hospice. Although this coordination of care takes a significant amount of time, it is immensely helpful in keeping relationships positive and assures future referrals.

Because there are many drug interactions with chemotherapy, it is incumbent on the PC team to consult with the team pharmacist, or pharmaceutical references, before writing new prescriptions. This will prevent serious drug interactions (e.g., methadone, ondansetron, and citalopram all cause QT prolongation), but may also highlight the potential inactivation of the anticancer therapy by certain drugs (such as paroxetine on tamoxifen.) To prevent creating problems, and more work, for the primary team, it is essential to check potential interactions before a prescription is written.

Team members providing outpatient palliative care

The OP PC team may range from a part-time PC nurse in the oncology clinic to a fully staffed interdisciplinary palliative care team with clinics 5 full days per week, in a range of OP clinics. In a recent survey of 20 OP PC programs in a variety of practice settings, 19 clinics used physicians, 10 sites had APRNs, 14 had a registered nurse, and 12 had a social worker.[1] The full time equivalent (FTE) staffing varied widely, ranging from a sole physician working 0.25 FTE, to an academic cancer center with 5 FTE, which included 2 physicians, 2 APRNs, and 1 RN. For physicians in particular, it is common practice to have multiple providers filling a position; for example, one academic oncology site has 6 physicians, each working 0.1 FTE, for a total physician FTE of 0.6. This may create challenges in continuity of care and team cohesiveness. Two additional surveys showed that nurses and APRNs typically represent the majority of staff appointments, with nurses the most common employees (0.9–1.7 FTE); then APRNs (0.7–0.9 FTE); social workers (0.7–0.8 FTE), and physicians (0.3–0.6 FTE).[35,44]

Other PC team members may include chaplaincy, pharmacy, nutrition, and rehabilitation medicine staff such as physical, occupational, or speech therapist.[29,36] The essential role of chaplaincy in addressing existential and spiritual distress cannot be overstated.[45,46] Reports of "pain" in the dying patient may arise from *spiritual pain*, and require the specialized input of a chaplain. Access to a board-certified chaplain is fundamental to the success of an OP PC team.[37,47] Finally, Bookbinder et al. noted that inclusion of a social worker in their study resulted in 100% completion of advance directives, in addition to providing psychosocial support.[48]

Components of the palliative care visit

Patients dealing with advanced illness have many needs impacting multiple domains of suffering. Determining what issues to address at the initial OP PC visit depends on the needs identified by the patient, the stated purpose of the consult (e.g., symptom management, assistance with goals of care), and the specialty of the PC clinician (social worker vs. pain specialist). To assess the patient's perspective on priority of issues, inpatient PC subjects were asked, "What bothers you most?" Categories of initial patient response were: physical distress, 44%; emotional, spiritual, existential, or nonspecific distress, 16%; relationships, 15%; concerns about death and dying, 15%; loss of function or normalcy, 12%; distress about being in the hospital, 11%; distress with medical providers or treatment, 9%; miscellaneous, 15% (more than one category was stated by some).[46]

To further define the components of a PC visit, Yoong et al.[30] (2013) investigated 20 randomly selected patients with lung cancer from the Temel et al.[13] study, analyzing PC and oncologist chart notes in detail. Based on panel analysis of PC notes, the following key elements of a PC visit were identified:

- Relationship and rapport building
- Symptom evaluation and management
- Coping strategies
- Illness understanding
- Discussing cancer treatments
- End-of-life planning
- Engaging family members

This study was particularly interesting. The detailed analysis found that the PC team focused initially on building relationship and illness understanding, while discussions about resuscitation preferences and hospice became more prevalent at a later time after "clinical turning points" such as disease progression occurred.[30]

In another study of OP PC, components of a supportive care team intervention were assessed in a nonrandomized study of 278 patients with advanced GI or ovarian cancer.[49] These components were identified as:

+ Assessment of patient symptoms and distress and social and spiritual concerns of the patient and caregiver

+ Documentation of the plan of care in the EMR

+ Provision of support for patient/caregiver needs

+ Advance care planning discussions as early as possible

+ Minimum of monthly contact with patient

+ Telephone availability daily

+ Regular meetings with the oncologist to review and coordinate patient care

+ Referral to home care or hospice, as appropriate

Von Roenn and Temel[50] identified five domains of care for PC visits:

+ Physical symptoms

+ Spiritual care

+ Assistance with practical needs

+ End-of-life care

+ Support for decision-making

Finally, in the author's practice, three major domains guide the framework of practice: providing pain and symptom management, addressing psychosocial-spiritual needs, and assisting with future planning for those faced with a serious illness, such as advance directives and timing of hospice enrollment. Patients are told, "Dr. Smith asked me to talk to you about your sleep problems, but I'd also like to know what you feel is most important for us to talk about today." If multiple issues are identified, the patient is asked to prioritize the top two items. In this way, the primary needs of the patient as well as the referring provider are addressed at the initial visit, with additional issues deferred to follow-up visits.

Length of palliative care visits

The literature indicates a variety of visit lengths for OP PC, but a key consensus is that providing palliative care takes time, and quality care cannot be rushed.[2,50] Initial visits are typically 60 minutes, and follow-up visits are 30–60 minutes. However, many clinicians discover that returning patients often need as much time as the initial visits.[20] Disease progression leads to an increase in the number and intensity of symptoms, news of progressive illness creates worsening distress, and EOL decision-making becomes more of a priority. In addition to the patient visits, a significant amount of PC time is spent in coordinating care with the specialty clinician (oncologist, pulmonologist), which may take as much as 5–15 minutes before and after each visit.[29] As noted above, such coordination helps to "keep everyone on the same page," assists with role delineation (e.g., who is writing the prescriptions for antiemetics), and keeps the relationship with the specialty provider strong.

In a subanalysis of the Temel et al.[13] study, Jacobsen et al.[51] (2011) described six components of the OP PC visit. These components, along with the median and range of time spent at the initial visit, include:

+ Symptom management (median 20 minutes, range 0–75 minutes)

+ Patient and caregiver coping with a life-threatening illness (median 15 minutes, range 0–78 minutes)

+ Illness understanding and education (median 10 minutes, range 0–35 minutes)

+ Decision-making (median 0 minutes, range 0–20 minutes)

+ Care planning and referrals (median 0 minutes, range 0–20 minutes)

Initial visits lasted a median of 55 minutes, with a range of 20–120 minutes. Not surprisingly, patients who rated low on QOL, as measured by the Functional Assessment of Cancer Therapy-General (FACT-G) scale, required longer visits; and higher depression scores, as measured by the Patient Health Questionnaire (PHQ-9), predicted greater time spent on symptom management.[51] A Canadian study found that initial visits utilizing a combined nurse and physician took 90–120 minutes.[52] Another paper reported combined nurse practitioner and social worker initial visits were scheduled for 90 minutes.[2] This author schedules initial visits for 60–90 minutes and return visits for 30 to 60 minutes depending on the anticipated length of time needed.

Measures used in clinic visits

A wide variety of instruments are used to gather research data in the OP PC clinic visits.[13,16,29] These fall into the major categories of functional scales, global symptom scales, pain scales, psychological and social measures, spiritual assessment, and QOL.[29] However, it is less clear which measures are typically utilized in nonresearch everyday clinical practice. Consideration should be given to utilizing a formal assessment tool, as one study found a 10-fold increase in reported symptoms with a formal tool, compared with open-ended questioning by a provider.[53] Similarly, this author has also found that use of clinical (nonresearch) tools significantly helps with symptom reporting; therefore, two scales are used regularly in practice: the Edmonton Symptom Assessment Scale (ESAS) and the Brief Pain Inventory, Short Form (BPI-SF). The ESAS[54] is a commonly used PC clinical tool that lists a variety of symptoms (pain, fatigue, appetite, anxiety), rated on a 0 to 10 scale, with 0 being no symptom and 10 being the worst symptom possible. The BPI-SF[55] includes a body diagram for indicating pain location; 0 to 10 pain intensity rating scales for worst, least, average and current pain; word descriptors of pain, and pain interference scales such as activity, mood, and sleep. Additionally, a third tool, the PHQ-9, a brief 9-item depression-screening survey is used if significant depression is suspected.[56]

Another brief clinical screening tool is the Distress Thermometer.[57] This is a simple drawing of a vertical thermometer with a 0–10 numerical rating scale labeled "no distress" at 0, "moderate distress" at 5, and "extreme distress" at 10. A score of 5 or more indicates that a consult to specialized psychosocial support is needed. This tool has been validated in multiple OP clinical settings and is recommended by NCCN as a quick measure of distress.[58]

Funding the outpatient palliative care program

A practical aspect of clinic viability is the need to secure sources of ongoing funding.[19] Billing revenue is insufficient for OP PC programs to become self-sustaining, especially for APRN-led clinics, due to lower reimbursement rates for nonphysician providers.[37,48] Most clinics require institutional support to survive.[1,2] Other sources of funding include philanthropy, private foundation support, and research grants.

Management by telephone is a major aspect of the provision of OP PC (see below). Although these calls can make the difference between a patient remaining comfortably at home, rather than making a trip to the ED, information on such cost-avoidance data is difficult to capture.[17] Thus, in some settings, the PC team may be challenged to find unique methods to demonstrate to the executive leadership that the PC nurse role makes a difference and is not simply another salary expenditure. This may be easier to demonstrate in a managed care setting.[9,29] More research is needed to support the cost benefit of OP PC, especially for nonreimbursable costs.

Telephone support

As noted above, support by telephone is a key function of the PC nurse. This role may start prior to the initial visit, when the PC nurse calls to confirm the upcoming appointment and answer any questions from the patient or caregiver.[20] It is not unusual for the patient to indicate that they do not understand why they have an appointment with PC. A simple description that works well is: "PC provides an extra layer of support for you and your family. We specialize in improving quality of life by helping with pain, symptoms, and coping with the stress of serious illness." It is important to emphasize that the patient's doctor (oncologist, neurologist, cardiologist) will remain in charge of their overall care, and the PC team will provide expert assistance (unless the patient is seen in the medical home PC model).

A phone check a few days after the initial visit is beneficial to assess whether patients are following the treatment plan, if problem is better, worse, or unchanged. The call also functions as a reminder that the PC team is now involved in their care. It is particularly important to follow up by phone after the patient received bad news (e.g., disease progression) or a referral to hospice, as such events can lead to great distress accompanied by a sense of isolation and abandonment.[59] An expression of concern for the patient and caregiver's welfare is always appropriate, and may aid in distress management.

Telephone contact may be useful in other ways. Some patients seem more amenable to addressing the scary "what if" questions via a phone conversation than in person. For example, "What is it going to be like when I die? Will I suffer?" Caregivers may have questions that concern them greatly, but they do not want to ask in front of the patient; such as: "What do I do if he starts to bleed?" "Will he choke to death?" Patients should be encouraged to call if there are questions or concerns, and be reassured that they are not "bothering" the team in any way when they call. We oftentimes tell patients, "We would much rather that you call, even if you think it is a small problem, because we can help before it becomes a bigger problem."

And finally, a condolence call or notecard sent a few days or weeks after the patient's death allows an opportunity to say a final goodbye. Family members can be encouraged to make use of hospice bereavement services to assist them in their grief. Such calls or notes are an important gesture, and may assist with closure, both for the bereaved, as well as the PC team who provided care.

Prescriptions

Renewal of opioid and other Schedule II prescriptions (oxycodone, morphine, fentanyl, methylphenidate) is a special concern for nonhospice patients, as these drugs cannot be "called in" to a local pharmacy. Because many patients come from a long distance away, they are asked to notify the PC team a week before the opioid medicine runs out to allow time to mail the prescription and fill it at a local pharmacy. Writing Schedule II opioid prescriptions, completing insurance paperwork for prescription prior approvals, and enrolling patients in the Risk Evaluation Management Strategy (REMS) program (for transmucosal fentanyl prescriptions) can be very time consuming for providers, and may be a reason for some of the consults sent to the PC service.

Patient education

An important aspect of nursing is that of patient education. This is especially true in the PC setting, when patients are often too fatigued, and caregivers are too stressed, to remember information. Simple and clearly written instructions are essential to achieve compliance with the plan of care and thus better control symptoms. A copy is given to the team nurse to communicate the PC interventions and also aids in "keeping everyone on the same page" in the collaborative care model. A follow-up call in a few days by the PC nurse can further refine patient education, check if the instructions were instituted (e.g., increased dose of pain medicine), and answer questions.[37] Preprinted instruction sheets on commonly reviewed PC topics, such as pharmacological and nonpharmacological pain management, constipation prevention and management, sleep hygiene, relaxation and coping techniques, and websites with helpful information, will streamline the provision of information for the patient.

Communication skills for the nurse

Excellent communication skills are at the heart of PC nursing.[11,60] These skills, which include both verbal and nonverbal communication, can be intentionally learned; they are not an "innate" ability possessed by a selected few.[61] However, becoming proficient takes time and practice. For the clinic nurse interested in providing "primary palliative care," learning a few basic techniques will enhance the ability to understand and address patient and caregiver needs. For nurses at the secondary and tertiary level of PC practice, expertise in complex communication practices, including conducting family meetings, is a key proficiency.

In a document titled *Peaceful Death: Recommended Competencies and Curricular Guidelines for End-of-Life Nursing Care*,[62] training is recommended for nurses to become competent in EOL communication. These skills are important in all fields of nursing, particularly in oncology, nephrology, and geriatrics, in which a significant number of deaths would be anticipated.[63] Chapter 5 is devoted to the topic of communication. In addition, Box 48.5 lists several techniques for interacting with patients and caregivers in the OP setting. Two helpful resources are Back et al. (2005)[64] and Malloy et al. (2010).[11] Nurses are encouraged to attend an End of Life Nursing Education Consortium (ELNEC) course to gain further knowledge in communication and other skills at EOL.[65]

Talking to patients and caregivers about prognosis

Ideally, physicians, APNs, nurses, and other team members are able to provide realistic prognosis estimates that are clearly communicated to patients and caregivers, with appropriate and timely

Box 48.5 Palliative care communication skills (see example in Box 48.6)

- Ask, Tell, Ask:
  - Ask a series of questions of the patient to elucidate their understanding of the situation, their hopes and concerns, and how they prefer to receive information.
  - Offer to share information ("Would it be okay if I shared some thoughts on this decision?").
  - Follow up with more questions on their response and perspective.
- NURSE: This acronym describes methods of acknowledging and responding to patient or caregiver emotion.
  - Naming: Name the emotion you are observing ("It sounds like you are upset with the news of the scan results you got today.").
  - Understanding: Seek to gain an understanding of the impact of the emotion ("This must be very disappointing.").
  - Respecting: Show empathy by use of verbal or nonverbal acknowledgment of the patient's emotion, or praise for their coping skills (with an expression of concern, "I have always been impressed with your efforts to follow the medical instructions exactly. I know you have done everything possible to fight the cancer.").
  - Supporting: Share a statement of partnership and support for the future, because patients fear abandonment. Make sure your statement is something realistic and truthful ("I will be here to support you with the road ahead.").
  - Exploring: Explore further the emotional cues ("You mentioned this was the worst thing that could ever have happened to you. I'd like to understand a bit more of what you mean by that. Can you tell me a little more?").
- Silence is golden
  - The use of silence is a key communication technique. Although it may seem like "nothing is happening," this is an important time that allows the patient/caregiver to collect their thoughts, get in touch with deep emotions, and process suffering.
  - It is appropriate to consider the use of silence when the patient/caregiver becomes tearful, when they appear to be processing information or formulating questions, or when they seem reticent to speak.
  - Use of silence should be accompanied by an active and attentive presence by the nurse (this is not a time to check the clock or catch up on charting).
  - Periods of silence may last 5–30 seconds or more. This takes practice to become comfortable! Start out by allowing short periods of silence lasting 5–7 seconds, then build the length, as appropriate.
  - Empathetic presence through silence can be a form of *witness* to the suffering that is being endured, and is thus therapeutic.
- Use communication continuers
  - Examples include: "Tell me more," "It sounds like this has been very difficult," or "Help me to understand why that upset you so much."
  - Be aware of your body language, and strive for "open" nonverbal communication by body turned toward the patient, appropriate eye contact, concerned expression, and keeping your arms and legs uncrossed.
  - When the patient is crying, after a period of silence ask, "Can you tell me about the tears?"
- Recognize conversation terminators used by the patient/caregiver
  - "I'm getting tired." "Maybe we could talk about this some other time."
  - Nonverbal cues (crossed arms, sighing, looking at watch, tapping a pencil). You can address this by simply asking, "I get the sense that you are ready to end the visit at this point." Or, "Your wife still has several questions on her list, but you look like you're getting tired. Would you prefer to rest in the waiting room while we finish talking?"
- Perceiving the unspoken message
  - Expert nurses excel in "hearing" the unspoken message. This involves paying attention to potential messages, to uncover concerns in the cultural, spiritual, or psychological domains.
  - For example, a patient question about the probability of future worsening pain may actually mean, "I'm afraid I'm going to die in terrible pain!"
  - Issues involving worsening sleep may uncover untreated anxiety or existential distress.
  - Asking the same questions repeatedly may also point to untreated depression and anxiety, as well as high levels of fear and distress about the future.

(continued)

Box 48.5 (Continued)

- ◆ Guided narrative in palliative care. These questions will help the PC team understand the patient/caregiver's perspective. (Adapted with permission from Farber and Farber.[69])

  - "What is your understanding of your current situation?"

  - "What are you hoping for?"

  - "What concerns you most?"

  - "What gives you strength to get through every day?"

  - "What do you value most in life?"

  - "Is religion or spirituality important to you?" "Are you at peace?"

  - "What are your experiences with serious illness or death?" "What do you know about hospice care?"

  - "What else would you like the team to know about you so that we can provide you with the best care?"

Sources: References 21, 61, 64, 66–69.

referrals to hospice. However, it is not uncommon for nurses to hesitate in speaking about prognosis, for a variety of reasons. In a survey of 174 experienced hospital nurses, five categories were identified that created obstacles for nurses to speak to patients and family about prognosis and hospice referral.[70] These included (1) unwillingness of patient or family to accept prognosis or hospice referral; (2) sudden death, or change in patient status, which prevented communication; (3) belief of physician hesitance, or perception that physicians did not feel it was the nurse's role to speak about prognosis; (4) nurse discomfort in speaking about death, or feeling they were too busy to address the topic; (5) nurse desire to maintain hope in the patient/family, and desire to prevent them from getting upset. Although this was an inpatient study, it is likely that these issues also impact nurses in the ambulatory care setting.

Nurses may face a dilemma when a patient or caregiver directly asks about prognosis, as some oncologists and other specialty physicians may object to a nurse (or even a PC physician) attempting to answer this question.[31] However, the literature indicates that oncologists, as well as primary care providers, are not particularly good at estimating prognosis and tend to be overly optimistic.[2,71] When there are clear signs and symptoms that the patient is moving into a terminal phase, the nurse may feel a moral obligation to speak up in order to allow appropriate preparation for death, but may also fear that this may impede the relationship with the oncologist if he or she objects to the nurse having such conversations.[31] One method of resolving this dilemma is to use a communication technique called "Ask, Tell, Ask." A technique that addresses emotion is the acronym NURSE: Naming, Understanding, Respecting, Supporting, Exploring.[61] Both of these techniques are explained in more detail in Box 48.5.

By using these methods, the nurse elucidates the patient's knowledge about prognosis without explicating stating something that the physician may find objectionable. Patients often have an "inner knowing" that their time is short and death is approaching. By using open-ended questions, the nurse can explore the patient's perception in a supportive manner. Box 48.6 has an example of this technique. In the example, the euphemistic statement, "I'm worried that your time might be shorter than we hope," allows the

nurse to address her moral dilemma by expressing her concerns about shorter prognosis without explicitly contradicting what the oncologist told the patient (or the patient's *perception* of what he was told) about prognosis. As the oncologist becomes more comfortable and trusting of the nurse's judgment and communication skills, it is hoped that moral dilemmas such as this example occur less frequently.

Maintaining hope in the face of advanced illness

As part of the human experience, we all need hope, especially when faced with a serious and life-limiting illness. The nurse may be concerned that such discussions may "destroy hope."[70] However, hope can be maintained, even at EOL, through "redefining" what is hoped for. As disease progresses, and death approaches, our hopes change.[72,73] Fanslow-Brunjes describes this process as the Four Stages of Hope: (1) hope for a cure, (2) hope for treatment that works, (3) hope for prolongation of life, and (4) hope for a peaceful death.[73] The skillful nurse can facilitate this transition of hope through the various stages, through focusing on what *can* be done to help the patient.[72] It is always essential to remember that "just being there," with empathetic nonverbal communication, provides support and comfort to the patient and family members as they face an uncertain future.[11] The impact of *presence* in the face of suffering is meaningful, and cannot be overlooked. Nurses can excel in this simple but extremely powerful intervention that can engender hope and reduce suffering.

Staff education

Providing staff education regarding the PC role is a common mission of the PC nurse, even if it is not part of the formal job description. Education on a formal or informal basis will help the clinic nurses and providers to grow in their ability to provide "primary palliative care" of symptom management, distress management, coping with advanced illness, and preparation for EOL. For example, the PC nurse gives an inservice to infusion center nurses on tips for supporting patients experiencing high levels of distress. Or, an oncology physician assistant asks for a curbside consult with the PC APRN regarding appropriateness for the

Box 48.6 Communication example: discussing prognosis

(The oncology nurse has just completed a "chemo teach" for Joe, a divorced 48-year-old male with metastatic pancreas cancer. He is being started on third-line therapy, because scans show further progression of disease and tumor markers continue to rise. He is in the clinic alone today.)

Patient: "Nancy, how much time do you think that I have left?"

Nurse: "Joe, this is a very important question. I'd like to understand a little bit more about why you are asking this. Did something come up today that prompted you to think about prognosis?"

Patient: "Well, I was reading my friend Mike's blog. He's got stage 4 pancreatic cancer like I do. I've always thought that he is doing much better than me, but his doctor just put him on hospice, and he said he is getting ready to die. Then I started thinking about dying, and. . . . it really scared me! . . ." [Patient becomes choked up and tearful.]

Nurse: "Oh dear. . . ." [Has a concerned expression, leans forward, sits attentively in silence for 10 seconds.]

Patient: "I'm sorry."

Nurse: "Oh, Joe, there's no need to apologize. Tears are a natural part of what you're going through. [Pause for a few seconds.] I'm wondering, what would you say is the hardest part of this for you?"

Patient: [Choked up] " . . . I don't want to suffer!"

Nurse: "It sounds like you are concerned about having pain?"

Patient: [Nods his head affirmatively.]

Nurse: "Joe, I want you to know that Dr. Smith and I will do everything we can to keep you as comfortable as possible as you approach the end. When the time comes, we'll bring in the hospice team. They are experts at helping you through the final weeks and months of your life, so that you do not suffer."

Patient: "OK . . . thanks. . . . I know the doc keeps saying that I still have years left to live, but I'm not so sure about that."

Nurse: "What makes you think you don't have that long to live?"

Patient: "Oh, you know, I keep losing weight, the cancer is growing on the scans, and the doc keeps changing the chemotherapy, because nothing is working."

Nurse: "Mmm. . . . [Pause several seconds] . . . Joe, would it be okay if I shared a few of my thoughts on this?"

Patient: "Sure."

Nurse: "I think you're right, these are signs that the cancer is getting worse. Doctor Smith told me that he talked to you about this at the last visit?"

Patient: "Yes."

Nurse: "These signs make me worried that your time might be shorter than we hope. [Pause] Does it surprise you to hear me say this?"

Patient: "[Sighs] No, not really. It's kind of what I was thinking."

Nurse: "It sounds like you've been thinking that things are getting worse?"

Patient: "Yeah"

Nurse: [Pause] "I wonder, if things do go more quickly, and if you die sooner rather than later, what do you think are the most important things for you to do at this point?"

Patient: "I guess I need to get around to talking to my sister about that Power of Attorney thing the social worker talked about. I don't want my parents making medical decisions for me because they're too old. . . . But I don't want to worry my sister either, that's why I keep putting it off. . . . I guess you're saying that I should get that done soon, huh?"

Nurse: "I always think it is best to get the legal paperwork completed. We all need to do it, in case we're in an accident. Then its done, and you don't have it hanging over your head."

Patient: "Yeah, you're right."

Nurse: "You said that you don't want to worry your sister. What concerns you the most about talking to her?"

Patient: "I don't know. I don't want her to be upset I guess. I hate it when women cry. I don't want to give her a shock."

Nurse: "Uh huh." [Pause] "Do you think she will be shocked with how you are doing?"

Patient: "Well, maybe not. She came to the appointment with Dr. Smith 2 weeks ago. I thought I might be getting bad news, and she insisted on coming along. She's my big sister, you know; gotta watch out for little Joey."

Nurse: [Smiles] "So, it sounds like she has an idea of where things are at for you. Maybe it won't be such a shock if you talk to her in more detail?"

Patient: "Yeah."

Nurse: "Well, I think it's a good idea to have a chat with her about the Durable Power of Attorney for Healthcare. Part of the responsibility of that role is to have an idea of what kinds of things you would want or not want for medical care, if you could not speak for yourself. This would be a good time to let her know a few of those things. Did the social worker give you the booklet called "Five Wishes"?"

Patient: "Yeah, I have it, but I haven't read it."

Nurse: "Do you think you might be able to look through it in the next few days, then give your sister a call to chat about it?"

Patient: "Yeah, sure, I can do that."

Nurse: "If you have questions about how to fill it out, either the social worker or I can help. Also, if you would like for me to talk directly to your sister, I'd be more than happy to do that. I would just need you to sign a form indicating it is okay for me to share some information with her."

Patient: "That would help. I'm not very good about talking about these things."

Nurse: "Okay Joe, let's plan on that. [Pause] Is there anything else on your mind today?"

Patient: "No, thanks, that's enough for now. I guess we need to talk about hospice too, but I've had enough for today. Thanks."

Nurse: "Okay. We can talk about hospice next time. Please feel free to call anytime. I'm here to help."

use of methylnaltrexone in a patient with severe opioid-induced constipation.

Such informal education commonly involves reassuring providers that PC involvement does not preclude use of antineoplastic therapies. For example, an oncologist may state "he's not ready for palliative care yet" in reference to a patient with stage IV NSCLC who is starting second-line therapy and was referred to PC by an infusion nurse for symptom management. This provides an excellent opportunity for the PC team to explain the benefits of PC involvement and dispel myths. It is unfortunate that many oncologists still equate palliative care with hospice.[9] This is an important distinction, because most hospice agencies require patients to stop chemotherapy in order to enroll. By explaining the broader scope of PC compared to hospice, and explaining that involvement of the PC team does not preclude the use of chemotherapy or other aggressive treatments, the conduit may be opened for additional referrals from that oncologist. Another example is a self-referral from a patient who faces a difficult but potentially curable treatment, such as a stem cell transplant for acute myelogenous leukemia (AML). The hematologist may say, "We're planning to cure this patient! We don't need PC!" Clear explanations that the goal of PC involvement is to "add an extra layer of support" to the patient and caregiver as they move through the aggressive transplant process with the goal of a cure; and reassurance that the transplant team will be kept abreast of all discussions, should reduce concerns.

Other opportunities for staff education may involve boundary-setting regarding tasks that can be handled at the "primary palliative care" level, for example, an urgent request for the PC team to immediately enroll a new patient in hospice, despite the absence of pressing physical or emotional needs. Upon further questioning, the team nurse indicated a lack of knowledge about how to enroll someone in hospice, and presumed the PC team took care of this for all patients in the ambulatory center. The PC APRN respectfully explained that this is the responsibility of the team nurse in this facility. Education was then provided regarding the necessary paperwork to collect and assistance with locating the appropriate hospice agency.

Similarly, a physician paged the OP PC APRN requesting completion of a do-not-resuscitate (DNR) order on the Physician Orders for Life Sustaining Treatment (POLST). Inquiry revealed no complex issues with this patient; however, the oncology fellow was unfamiliar and uncomfortable with this process. Discussing a DNR decision is an essential aspect of medical care, of which every provider should have a basic working knowledge. Therefore, the PC APRN provided brief coaching, then offered to join the visit while the fellow explained the form to the patient and assisted with DNR decision-making. Thus, the provider gained skill in this important task, and the PC team is available to address more complex or unusual situations that may arise in the future.

Conclusion

This is an exciting time of momentum in the field of OP PC. As the discipline grows and matures in the oncology arena, attention is turning toward expanding PC into those OP clinics with large numbers of terminally ill patients, such as cardiology, nephrology, neurology, and geriatrics. With the mandate of the Affordable Care Act, the role of OP PC in preventing ED visits, hospital admission, and readmission will become more imperative.

Because there are more patients than can be seen by the limited PC resources, use of screening methods or algorithms should be utilized to identify those who are in the greatest need of referral. For the remainder, clinicians and nurses must learn the skills for providing "primary palliative care" in the OP setting.

Nurses play an important role in the provision of OP PC, with research showing that nurses or APNs provide the bulk of staffing in these settings. Nursing skills are well adapted toward the issues commonly addressed by the PC team. With additional training in programs such as ELNEC, every nurse can indeed become a PC nurse.

Case study

Bob is a 67-year-old Caucasian man with metastatic renal cell carcinoma (RCC). He underwent left nephrectomy when initially diagnosed, and has subsequently been on a variety of chemotherapy and biological agents over the last few years. He moved to town a year ago from the Midwest, to be closer to family, but then sought experimental treatment at a major cancer center on the East Coast for a period of 4 months, which depleted much of his savings. He lives alone, but his son and his family live nearby. Bob's oncologist, Dr. J, referred him to OP PC for pain management. He presented to the initial outpatient palliative care visit accompanied by his daughter-in-law, Gina. His chief complaint was severe and uncontrolled pain, despite transdermal fentanyl 200 mcg/h every 72 hours, and oxycodone 5 mg tablets, ordered 1–2 every 4 hours as needed for pain, but he is taking 20 tablets per day (100 mg per day) with minimal relief. The most recent scan shows massive tumor invasion of the pelvis destroying a portion of the right iliac crest, involving the right iliopsoas muscle, with tumor implants invading the sciatic nerve. Bob has declined to take anticonvulsives or antidepressants for neuropathic pain, and has also deferred radiation therapy.

As the initial visit proceeded, it became apparent that Bob had a unique and "prickly" personality. He had a strong need to manage the pace and direction of the visit, frequently holding up his hands to halt discussion so that he could take meticulous notes. (He declined an offer to audiotape the visit for future reference.) Bob highly values having control of all medical decisions; he must thoroughly and carefully research each possible option for cancer treatment and pain management before he will agree to consider it, to such a degree that it appears to be interfering with his anticancer treatment and his comfort. Gina is clearly frustrated with this process, explaining that it usually takes weeks, even months for him to make any decision, and is the reason he has not yet started radiation therapy for pain control.

The APRN discussed options with Bob and recommended the addition of gabapentin for neuropathic pain, short-term dexamethasone for rapid pain control, and initiating the radiotherapy previously ordered. Since Bob did not want to change his opioid dose, she suggested switching to oxycodone 15 mg tablet to decrease the number of short-acting opioids he is taking each day. After extensive discussion and negotiation, Bob eventually agreed to start the radiation therapy, and to take dexamethasone 4 mg daily for 2 weeks. He did not agree to a trial of gabapentin, and did not want any changes in his opioid pill strength. The initial visit took over an hour, with the entire conversation involving negotiation of pain control options.

The PC team followed Bob every 2–4 weeks, coordinating visits with his oncologist appointments. The patient slowly began to trust the APRN, especially as his pain started to improve. After many visits, and with extensive negotiation, he agreed to start gabapentin for neuropathic pain, and eventually also agreed to add duloxetine for neuropathic pain and mood. Despite these strategies, his pain remained severe. The APRN started introducing the concept of existential distress as a potential significant component of Bob's pain experience. Although he did not accept that psychological or spiritual issues had any impact on him, his relationship with the APRN had developed to the point that he was willing to listen to the concept. He also appeared more comfortable and relaxed during the visits, taking notes, but no longer insisting on controlling each visit.

Bob remained strongly optimistic that he had many more years to live. However, after becoming intensely frightened during a pain crisis, which led to a 3-night hospital stay, he initiated discussions about his eventual demise. (He refused to see the inpatient PC team, indicating that he wanted to talk about these issues only with his OP PC APRN after discharge.) Bob asked detailed questions about the dying process, wanting to know what he needed to do to prepare himself. Durable power of attorney for healthcare and DNR paperwork were completed. Hospice enrollment was discussed, and Bob agreed to meet with them, but subsequently cancelled the appointment and did not return their calls.

Several weeks later, Bob called the PC team, complaining of severe pain, but refused the PC APRN's advice to come into the clinic or ED for evaluation. After multiple telephone discussions with Bob and Gina over the next 3 days, he ultimately agreed to enroll in hospice. However, this triggered significant worsening of his anxiety, and the compulsive component of his personality emerged once again. He was reluctant to follow through on the hospice team's advice for pain management, and called the OP PC APRN repeatedly, despite her ongoing reassurance that she was working closely with the hospice nurse to manage his pain. Gina also called the OP PC team several times each week, in exasperation, wondering how to best help Bob. He was still living alone, and declined to allow a hired caregiver in the home despite having total immobility of the right leg, repeated falls, and difficulty managing his medications. He refused to see the hospice social worker or chaplain despite high anxiety and distress levels.

By this time he was on high-dose methadone for cancer pain, with high doses of hydromorphone for breakthrough pain. He remained in severe pain, and appeared to be developing opioid-induced hyperalgesia. The OP PC APRN called Bob and recommended admission to the inpatient hospice center to initiate a ketamine infusion. She also reminded him of the option for an intrathecal block, which had been discussed multiple times over the months, but Bob had always declined due to the risk of leg weakness. After several days of consideration, while experiencing progressive and severe pain, Bob agreed to be transported to the inpatient hospice unit, where he stayed for 12 days. A ketamine infusion and hydromorphone PCA were started, resulting in much improvement in pain control. He was converted to oral ketamine 30 mg TID, and methadone was decreased to 30 mg TID. While he was an inpatient, the hospice social worker and chaplain were able to make explorations into existential distress as a contributor to his pain experience. Significant issues were uncovered and addressed, and Bob appeared to be more at peace. Once the pain was better controlled, he was discharged home, and he

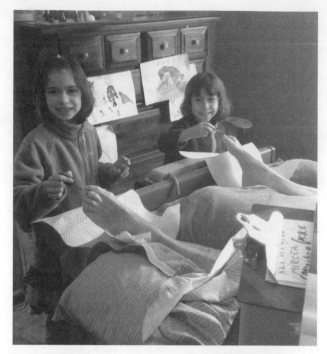

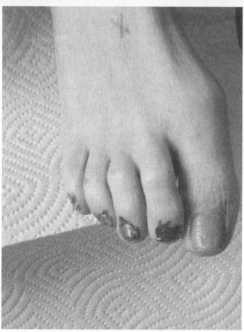

Figure 48.1A and B Bob loved playing silly games with his granddaughters. Here he is getting a pedicure while in his hospice bed at home. The infectious joy of the children kept him grounded and linked to his family. This family support ultimately helped him find peace in the end. Source: © Pamela Davies 2013.

agreed to hire a caregiver. This was a special time of bonding for Bob and his son, daughter-in-law, and two young granddaughters. He was delighted with the infectious joy of the children and would let them paint his toenails, play silly games, and snuggle with him in his hospice bed while he napped (Figure 48.1).

Bob did surprisingly well for 6 weeks, then fell and broke his pelvis, resulting in new severe pain. It took 3 days for him to agree to hospital admission. He was deeply disappointed when told by the orthopedic surgeon that the fracture could not be repaired due to extensive bone erosion. Realizing he would never walk again, he agreed to an intrathecal catheter with bupivacaine, which provided excellent pain control. Bob was discharged home after a week in the acute care hospital, and died a month later, surrounded by his family. Before his death, he was able to make amends with several estranged family members and was at peace in the end.

Although this was one of the more challenging cases ever managed by the author, it also provided a rich opportunity for professional growth during the 6 months of collaboration. Lessons learned include the power of pure acceptance of a patient, just as he is, without trying to speed up his process of adjusting to illness; the power of listening carefully and without judgment, even if the patient's rationale for delay in treatment seemed foolish; and the power of showing true kindness, warmth, and patience as a means to create a bridge to a "prickly" man's heart, which ultimately helped him to die comfortably, and at peace.

References

1. Smith AK, Thai JN, Bakitas MA, et al. The diverse landscape of palliative care clinics. J Palliat Med. 2013;16(6):661–668.
2. Meier DE, Beresford L. Outpatient clinics are a new frontier for palliative care. J Palliat Med. 2008;11(6):823–828.
3. Ferris FD, Bruera E, Cherny N, et al. Palliative cancer care a decade later: accomplishments, the need, next steps—from the American Society of Clinical Oncology. J Clin Oncol. 2009;27(18):3052–3058.
4. American Society of Clinical Oncology. ASCO Virtual Learning Collaborative. http://www.asco.org/quality-guidelines/asco virtual-learning-collaborative. Accessed November 5, 2013.
5. Center to Advance Palliative Care. Improving Palliative Care—Outpatient (IPAL-OP). 2013. http://www.capc.org/ipal/ipal-op. Accessed July 21, 2013.
6. McCormick E, Chai E, Meier DE. Integrating palliative care into primary care. Mount Sinai J Med: J Trans Pers Med. 2012;79(5):579–585.
7. Smith AK. Palliative care: an approach for all internists. comment on "Early palliative care in advanced lung cancer: a qualitative study" Palliat Care. JAMA Int Med. 2013;173(4):291–292.
8. Quill TE, Abernethy AP. Generalist plus specialist palliative care—creating a more sustainable model. N Engl J Med. 2013;368(130):01173–1175.
9. Lesperance M, Shannon R, Pumphrey PK, et al. Training mid-level providers on palliative care: bringing advanced directives and symptom assessment and management to community oncology practices. Amer J Hosp Palliat Med. 2013;31(3):237–243.
10. Janjan N. Palliative care: meaningful benefit in oncology care. Oncology (Williston Park, NY). 2011;25(13):1244–1256.
11. Malloy P, Virani R, Kelly K, Munévar C. Beyond bad news: communication skills of nurses in palliative care. J Hosp Palliat Nurs. 2010;12(3):166–174.
12. Murphy A, Siebert K, Owens D, Doorenbos A. Health care utilization by patients whose care is managed by a primary palliative care clinic. J Hosp Palliat Nurs. 2013;15(7):372–379.
13. Temel JS, Greer JA, Muzikansky A, et al. Early palliative care for patients with metastatic non–small-cell lung cancer. N Engl J Med. 2010;363(8):733–742.
14. Prince-Paul M, Burant CJ, Saltzman J, Teston L, Matthews C. The effects of integrating an advanced practice palliative care nurse in a community oncology center: a pilot study. J Supp Oncol. 2010;8(1):21–27.
15. Bakitas M, Lyons KD, Hegel MT, et al. Effects of a palliative care intervention on clinical outcomes in patients with advanced cancer: the Project ENABLE II randomized controlled trial. JAMA. 2009;302(7):741–749.
16. Groh G, Vyhnalek B, Feddersen B, Führer M, Borasio GD. Effectiveness of a specialized outpatient palliative care service as experienced by patients and caregivers. J Palliat Med. 2013 May 16. Epub ahead of print.
17. McNamara BA, Rosenwax LK, Murray K, Currow DC. Early admission to community-based palliative care reduces use of emergency departments in the ninety days before death. J Palliat Med. 2013;6(7):774–779.
18. El-Jawahri A, Greer JA, Temel JS. Does palliative care improve outcomes for patients with incurable illness?: A review of the evidence. J Support Oncol. 2011;9(3):87–94.
19. Bakitas M, Bishop MF, Caron P, Stephens L. Developing successful models of cancer palliative care services. Semin Oncol Nurs. 2010;26(4):266–284.
20. Jackson V, Kamdar M, Rinaldi S. Embedding palliative care in the oncology clinic: culture, infrastructure, and growth. CAPC Audioconference: Center to Advance Palliative Care; 2013 June 12.
21. Davies PS. Palliative care and hospice: care when there is no cure. In: Davies PS, D'Arcy Y (eds.), Compact Clinical Guide to Cancer Pain Management: An Evidence-Based Approach for Nurses. New York: Springer; 2013:301–328.
22. von Gunten CF. Secondary and tertiary palliative care in US hospitals. JAMA. 2002;287(7):875–881.
23. Johansen M-L, Holtedahl KA, Rudebeck CE. A doctor close at hand: how GPs view their role in cancer care. Scand J Prim Health Care. 2010;28(4):249–255.
24. Schell JO, Bova-Collis R, Deziel S, Moss A, H. The patient wants to stop dialysis: the latest evidence on how to respond. Nephrology News and Issues. 2012;April(4):22–28.
25. Kheirbek RE, Alemi F, Citron BA, Afaq MA, Wu H, Fletcher RD. Trajectory of illness for patients with congestive heart failure. J Palliat Med. 2013;16(5):478–484.
26. Beernaert K, Cohen J, Deliens L, et al. Referral to palliative care in COPD and other chronic diseases: a population-based study. Resp Med. 2013;107(11):1731–1739.
27. Schell JO, Patel UD, Steinhauser KE, Ammarell N, Tulsky JA. Discussions of the kidney disease trajectory by elderly patients and nephrologists: a qualitative study. Amer J Kid Dis. 2012;59(4):495–503.
28. Quill TE, Battin MP. Physician-Assisted Dying: The Case for Palliative Care and Patient Choice. Baltimore, MD: John Hopkins University Press; 2004.
29. Davies PS, Prince-Paul M. Palliative care in the outpatient cancer center: current trends. J Hosp Palliat Nurs. 2012;14(8):506–513.
30. Yoong J, Park ER, Greer JA, et al. Early palliative care in advanced lung cancer: a qualitative study. JAMA Intern Med. 2013;173(4):283–290.
31. Weissman DE, von Gunten CF. Palliative care consultations as American football: full contact, or just touch? J Palliat Med. 2012;15(4):378–380.
32. Muir JC, Daly F, Davis MS, et al. Integrating palliative care into the outpatient, private practice oncology setting. J Pain Symptom Manage. 2010;40(1):126–135.
33. Rabow MW, Dibble SL, Pantilat SZ, McPhee SJ. The comprehensive care team: a controlled trial of outpatient palliative medicine consultation. Arch Intern Med. 2004;164(1):83.
34. Owens D, Eby K, Burson S, Green M, McGoodwin W, Isaac M. Primary Palliative Care Clinic Pilot Project demonstrates benefits of a nurse practitioner directed clinic providing primary and palliative care. J Am Acad Nurse Pract. 2012;24(1):52–58.
35. Rabow MW, Smith AK, Braun JL, Weissman DE. Outpatient palliative care practices. Arch Intern Med. 2010;170(7):654–655.
36. Dennis K, Librach S, Chow E. Palliative care and oncology: integration leads to better care. Oncology (Williston Park, NY). 2011;25(13):1271–1275.
37. Alesi ER, Fletcher D, Muir C, Beveridge R, Smith TJ. Palliative care and oncology partnerships in real practice. Oncology (Williston Park, N.Y.). 2011;25(13):1287–1293.
38. Smith TJ, Temin S, Alesi ER, et al. American Society of Clinical Oncology Provisional Clinical Opinion: the integration of palliative care into standard oncology care. J Clin Oncol. 2012;30(8):880–887.
39. National Comprehensive Cancer Network. Clinical Practice Guideline in Oncology: Palliative Care. 2013. http://www.nccn.org/professionals/physician_gls/f_guidelines.asp - supportive. Accessed June 9, 2013.

40. American Cancer Society. Cancer Facts and Figures 2013. 2013. http://www.cancer.org/research/cancerfactsfigures/cancerfactsfigures/cancer-facts-figures-2013. Accessed June 2, 2013.

41. Weissman DE, Meier DE. Identifying patients in need of a palliative care assessment in the hospital setting: a consensus report from the center to advance palliative care. J Palliat Med. 2011;14(1) :17–23.

42. Imhof SL, Kaskie B, Wyatt MG. Finding the way to a better death: an evaluation of palliative care referral tools. J Gerontol Nurs. 2007;33(6):40–49.

43. Glare PA, Semple D, Stabler SM, Saltz LB. Palliative care in the outpatient oncology setting: evaluation of a practical set of referral criteria. J Oncol Pract. 2011;7(6):366–370.

44. Berger GN, O'Riordan DL, Kerr K, Pantilat SZ. Prevalence and characteristics of outpatient palliative care services in California. Arch Intern Med. 2011;171(22):2057–2059.

45. Hills J, Paice JA, Cameron JR, Shott S. Spirituality and distress in palliative care consultation. J Palliat Med. 2005;8(4):782–788.

46. Shah M, Quill T, Norton S, Sada Y, Buckley M, Fridd C. "What bothers you the most?" initial responses from patients receiving palliative care consultation. Amer J Hosp Palliat Med. 2008;25(2):88–92.

47. Puchalski C, Ferrell B, Virani R, et al. Improving the quality of spiritual care as a dimension of palliative care: the report of the consensus conference. J Palliat Med. 2009;12(10):885–904.

48. Bookbinder M, Glajchen M, McHugh M, et al. Nurse practitioner-based models of specialist palliative care at home: sustainability and evaluation of feasibility. J Pain Symptom Manage. 2010;41(1):25–34.

49. Daly BJ, Douglas SL, Gunzler D, Lipson AR. Clinical trial of a supportive care team for patients with advanced cancer. J Pain Symptom Manage. 2013 Mar 22 Epub ahead of print.

50. Von Roenn JH, Temel J. The integration of palliative care and oncology: the evidence. Oncology (Williston Park, N.Y.). 2011;25(13):1258–1266.

51. Jacobsen J, Jackson V, Dahlin C, et al. Components of early outpatient palliative care consultation in patients with metastatic nonsmall cell lung cancer. J Palliat Med. 2011;14(4):459–464.

52. Riechelmann RP, Krzyzanowska MK, O'Carroll A, Zimmermann C. Symptom and medication profiles among cancer patients attending a palliative care clinic. Support Care Cancer. 2007;15(12):1407–1412.

53. Homsi J, Walsh D, Rivera N, et al. Symptom evaluation in palliative medicine: patient report vs systematic assessment. Support Care Cancer. 2006;14(5):444–453.

54. Chang VT, Hwang SS, Feuerman M. Validation of the Edmonton symptom assessment scale. Cancer. 2000;88(9):2164–2171.

55. MD Anderson Cancer Center. Symptom Assessment Tools: Brief Pain Inventory. 2012. www3.mdanderson.org/depts/symptomresearch/. Accessed June 3, 2013.

56. Kroenke K, Spitzer RL, Williams JBW. The PHQ-9: validity of a brief depression severity measure. J Gen Intern Med. 2001;16(9):606–613.

57. Mitchell AJ. Pooled results from 38 analyses of the accuracy of distress thermometer and other ultra-short methods of detecting cancer-related mood disorders. J Clin Oncol. 2007;25(29):4670–4681.

58. Hoffman BM, Zevon MA, D'Arrigo MC, Cecchini TB. Screening for distress in cancer patients: the NCCN rapid-screening measure. Psychooncology. 2004;13(11):792–799.

59. Dyar S, Lesperance M, Shannon R, Sloan J, Colon-Otero G. A nurse practitioner directed intervention improves the quality of life of patients with metastatic cancer: results of a randomized pilot study. J Palliat Med. 2012;15(8):890–895.

60. Dahlin CM, Kelley JM, Jackson VA, Temel JS. Early palliative care for lung cancer: improving quality of life and increasing survival. Int J Palliat Nurs. 2010;16(9):420–423.

61. Schell JO, Arnold RM. NephroTalk: communication tools to enhance patient-centered care. Semin Dial. 2012;25(6):611–616.

62. American Association of Colleges of Nursing. Peaceful Death: Recommended Competencies and Curricular Guidelines for End-of-Life Nursing Care. 2011. http://www.aacn.nche.edu/elnec/publications/peaceful-death. Accessed July 21, 2013.

63. Duggleby W, Berry P. Transitions and shifting goals of care for palliative patients and their families. Clin J Oncol Nurs. 2005;9(4):425–428.

64. Back AL, Arnold RM, Baile WF, Tulsky JA, Fryer-Edwards K. Approaching difficult communication tasks in oncology. CA Cancer J Clin. 2005;55(3):164–177.

65. American Association of Colleges of Nursing. End-of-Life Nursing Education Consortium (ELNEC). 2013. http://www.aacn.nche.edu/elnec. Accessed July 21, 2013.

66. Buckman R. Communication skills in palliative care: a practical guide. Neurol Clin. 2001;19(4):989–1004.

67. Farber S, Egnew T, Farber A. A respectful death. In: Berzoff J, Silverman PR (eds.), Living with Dying: A Handbook for End-Of-Life Healthcare Practitioners. New York: Columbia University Press; 2004:102–127.

68. Farber S, Farber A. The respectful death model: difficult conversations at the end of life. In: Katz RS, Johnson TA (eds.), When Professionals Weep: Emotional and Countertransference Responses in End of Life Care. Series in Death, Dying, and Bereavement. New York, NY: Routledge; 2006:221–237.

69. Steinhauser KE, Voils CI, Clipp EC, Bosworth HB, Christakis NA, Tulsky JA. "Are you at peace?": One item to probe spiritual concerns at the end of life. Arch Intern Med. 2006;166(1):101–105.

70. Schulman-Green D, McCorkle R, Cherlin E, Johnson-Hurzeler R, Bradley EH. Nurses' communication of prognosis and implications for hospice referral: a study of nurses caring for terminally ill hospitalized patients. Am J Crit Care. 2005;14(1):64–70.

71. von Gunten CF, Lutz S, Ferris FD. Why oncologists should refer patients earlier for hospice care. Oncology (Williston Park, NY). 2011;25(13):1278–1285.

72. Evans WG, Tulsky JA, Back AL, Arnold RM. Communication at times of transitions: how to help patients cope with loss and re-define hope. Cancer J. 2006;12(5):417–424.

73. Fanslow-Brunjes C. Beyond pain: the search for hope in the patient's journey. Asian Pacific J Cancer Prev. 2010;11:63–66.

CHAPTER 49

Rehabilitation and palliative care

Donna J. Wilson and Kathleen Michael

I was diagnosed with stage 4 breast cancer 14 years ago. I have been on multiple chemotherapy drugs. Maintaining my muscular strength gives me the energy and self-confidence to maintain a quality of life and enjoy my family.

A patient

Key points

- Rehabilitation principles are applicable to palliative care to enhance quality of life.
- Interdisciplinary care is a key concept in rehabilitation.
- Rehabilitation in palliative care can prevent disability and complications.
- Mobility and self-care are the critical components of physical functioning in palliative care.

Case study

Ann, a 59-year-old woman with metastatic breast cancer

Ann was diagnosed with breast cancer at the age of 36. She had a right mastectomy with reconstruction followed by chemotherapy and radiation therapy. She tolerated the treatment and continued working in advertising. She was energetic and outgoing and enjoyed music and the arts. Ann was previously overweight (275 pounds) up to the age of 25 but then lost the weight and considered sugar toxic. After the scare of breast cancer, she started walking and going to the gym 2 times a week. She was happy and dating when, 5 years later, at a routine check-up she was diagnosed with metastatic disease to her sternum. She once again had surgery to remove the nodule on her sternum and then began an aromatase inhibitor. She was then diagnosed with osteoporosis. Ann had met the "man of her dreams," and he was not concerned about her diagnosis and asked her to marry him. Ann started exercising more and added weight-bearing and muscle-strengthening exercises to her routine. She married a year later. Ann continued to be monitored closely for recurrent disease but was enjoying life.

Ten years after her initial diagnosis, her tumor markers were on the rise and additional testing revealed nodules in her lungs and liver. For the next several years she was treated with a variety of chemotherapy agents, but managed to work full-time and to enjoy married life. Ann found that going to the gym was therapeutic, as her body felt stronger, her self-esteem improved, and the stress associated with chronic treatment was bearable. She was taking control through exercise and mind-body therapies during this time of stress and illness.

After several years of dealing with metastatic breast cancer, she had a seizure at work. She was diagnosed with metastatic disease to her brain and required a craniotomy and brain radiation leaving her with right-hand weakness. She took early retirement from work but still focused on the goal of survival. A psychiatrist was added to her team to help her with stress, anxiety, and fears of dying, and a physical therapist to help with her right-arm weakness. Over the next year she and her husband took a European trip, and continued to enjoy the theater and family visiting.

Ann now presented with shortness of breath requiring a chest Pleurx catheter for drainage. Her overall condition was deteriorating with complaints of increasing fatigue and dyspnea. She continued to do upper body flexibility exercises and breathing exercises. Ann reported that the movement decreased her generalized body pain and discomfort and the deep breathing exercises gave her some relief. She continued to fight for continued life, requesting the rehabilitation team to assist her to walk and to remain physically active. The palliative care team helped to maintain her comfort and independence and to enjoy the love of her husband. This case study demonstrates the primary principles of rehabilitation nursing care throughout a disease trajectory.

This chapter will apply the concepts of physical activity to palliative care across settings. A physical activity program for each patient should be presented at the time of diagnosis and extend to end-of-life care. Even when it is not possible to cure or reverse a disease processes, or to restore a previous level of functioning and independence, a rehabilitative approach to nursing care adds quality to the experience of living until life's completion. The language of rehabilitation nursing is a language shared with those who practice palliative care. Feelings of self-confidence, independence, hope, human dignity, and autonomy are all influenced by an individually tailored program of rehabilitation.

Rehabilitation nursing

Nursing in any context concerns itself with adaptation. As life proceeds to its end, adaptation to a new state allows people to remain whole: interact with their environment, to experience human relationships, and to achieve personally meaningful goals. Nurses find themselves at work in every phase of growth, development, and dying, as individuals strive to adapt across the continuum of life.

Rehabilitation nurses care for persons with incurable progressive disease states in a variety of settings.[1] Whether care is patient-provider or facility-centered, the merging of rehabilitation and palliative nursing approaches are evident. Rehabilitation nurses are in a key position to motivate, providing hope, physical and psychologically, to patients and their caregivers to improve the patient's quality of life.

Just as all nurses incorporate aspects of palliative care into their daily care of patients so they also incorporate aspects of rehabilitation. In the assessment, planning, implementation, and evaluation of nursing care are the concepts of independence and interdependence, self-care, coping, and quality of life.[1,2] Although the focus is on physical activity, fundamental to this practice is the acceptance of varieties of life experiences, including those at life's end. The true challenge in a rehabilitation program is to motivate and change or maintain the patient's physical performance to the best of their ability and to help them to adapt to a changing physical situation. Again the goal is to enhance self-esteem and quality of life.

Patients can lose 10% of their muscle strength during a week of bedrest. There are also many problems related to inactivity such as impaired bowel or bladder function, deep vein thrombosis and poor balance from muscular weakness. To minimize these complications nurses need to encourage patients to do some movement each day, however limited, such as walking if possible, arm movements, or chair or bed exercises. Teaching patients to coordinate their breathing with each movement will improve their performance. Breathing exercises provide increased lung capacity, calm the mind and body, and activate targeted muscles. Breathing exercises with arm or leg movements do not require any equipment and can be done anywhere (including in bed) at anytime.

Physical activity in advanced disease and the effects on symptom control

The literature demonstrates the benefits of physical activity on patients with advanced-stage cancer. Physical activity is defined as any bodily movement produced by the skeletal muscles and requires more energy than resting.

The benefits of physical activity in this population of patients is to strengthen bones and muscles, improve mental health, improve their ability to do daily activities, prevent falls, and possibly even improve survival. Physical activity is the one intervention that will address the needs of the palliative patient. The most common side effects of cancer treatment are fatigue and dyspnea. These symptoms will interfere with normal activities of daily living. Patients who complain of fatigue and dyspnea also complain of generalized weakness, anxiety, depression, poor balance, and social isolation.

Rehabilitation/integrative techniques can prevent disability and complications in advanced disease. These techniques or strategies include flexibility training, walking aerobics, weight-bearing exercises using elastic bands or hand weights, yoga, and stretching. Massage therapy is an integrative technique providing touch to the soft tissues of the body and can also be part of rehabilitation. It provides comfort, relaxation, reduced muscular tension, decreased pain, and improved circulation and increases flexibility, thus enhancing a patient's physical activity. A randomized trial with 3 interventions, massage, a nontouching intervention, and usual care for patients with metastatic cancer demonstrated patients in the massage group had beneficial effects of improved pain control and quality of sleep.[3,4]

Research in exercise programs

Research has demonstrated that exercise is an effective nonpharmacological therapy for managing fatigue, dyspnea, mobility, and self-care. A low to moderate intensity exercise program for patients and family members can be designed in an acute, subacute, long-term, or hospice care setting. Chair aerobics, chair yoga, and chair pilates include breathing exercises, stretching, arm and leg movements for flexibility, light weight training, and chair squats. These nonstressful programs help to reconnect the body and brain, deepen breathing patterns, and improve confidence with movement and use core muscles to support the spine, improve posture, and decrease muscle tension.[5] Chair exercises were documented to slow the decline of fatigue and dyspnea by improved muscular strength of the legs and chest wall muscles, thus improving quality of life in patients with severe lung disease.[6] Pulmonary rehabilitation can reduce fatigue and dyspnea by improving muscle strength of the legs and chest wall, thus improving quality of life in patients with severe lung disease.[6]

The beneficial effects of physical fitness are physiological and psychological. The physiological effects include enhanced rest, better sleep patterns, improved flexibility and range of motion, improved muscular strength, and improved delivery of oxygen-rich blood to the brain and tissues, which reduces fatigue. The psychological effects include enhanced coping ability, reduced stress, improved self-confidence, mood elevation, sharpened mental functioning, and decreased depression. The benefits may seem small, but engaging the patient and family together in an exercise program decreases feelings of helplessness by maintaining some muscle strength and physical activity.[7,8]

Another approach to maintain quadricep muscle function is neuromuscular electrical stimulation (NMES).[9] A controlled study of a home-based program was conducted with lung cancer patients. Many patients with lung cancer are deconditioned, presenting with muscle wasting. The pilot results were not significant, but more of the patients in the NMES group improved their strength as demonstrated in a walk and step test. The NMES was tolerated by the patients and may be a worthwhile treatment to preserve physical function, but further research is needed.

A pilot study by Oldervoll and colleagues provided an outpatient hospital-based structured exercise program for patients consisting of 1 hour twice a week for 6 weeks.[10] The exercise program focused on strength-promoting activities such as aerobic exercises using large muscle groups in a standing or sitting position, bicycling, upper and lower body strength exercises, chair squats, balance, and optional abdominal exercises. At the end of the 6 weeks the patients reported decreased levels of fatigue and improved ability to do self-care activities and the response to physical activity played a role in maintaining independence.

A second study by Oldervoll consisted of a randomized controlled trial of 231 patients with a life expectancy of less than 2 years. Half the group exercised two times a week for 60 minutes and the other group received usual care. The exercise group demonstrated no change in the patients' fatigue level, but their physical performance significantly improved in the 8 weeks of exercise.[11] Physical activity is an excellent approach to maintain a patient's physical performance with advanced disease.

Physical function assessment for palliative care patients has received little attention until recently. Helbostad and colleagues reviewed the literature for all existing instruments that had physical function items to assess this patient population is physical performance.[12] In response to the dearth of such tools, the first steps for the development of a new instrument to measure the physical function of cancer patients receiving palliative care was described. This instrument is planned to identify and describe specific types of exercise beneficial to this population. An individualized exercise program can then be designed for the patient.

Complementary therapies as part of exercise programs in palliative care

Selman and colleagues evaluated two complementary therapies for palliative care—yoga and dance therapy.[13] Eighteen patients participated in a once-a-week 6-week course. Ten patients participated in yoga, five in dance therapy (the Lebed Method), and three did both therapies. Fifteen of the 18 patients were receiving palliative care only. The yoga class included postures, breathing techniques, relaxation through visualization, and hand movements. The Lebed dance method consisted of a combination of movements and exercises focusing on the lymph system and flexibility for range of motion of both shoulders. Each of the programs could be performed in a standing or sitting position. In the precourse questionnaire, the patient concerns were mobility, breathing problems, arm/shoulder, neck/back problems, inability to relax, and anxiety. All of the concerns identified by patients in the preclass were self-reported as significantly improved in the postclass evaluations of both programs.

A randomized controlled clinical trial compared pranayama yogic breathing and usual care.[14] The four yogic breathing techniques were taught in weekly classes during two consecutive cycles of chemotherapy. The control group received usual care. The results of teaching the four yogic breaths approached statistical significance for improved sleep disturbances, decreasing anxiety, and improving mental quality of life.

Dru yoga has been studied with palliative care patients.[15] This is a gentle style of yoga with flowing movements that are combined with breath awareness, and relaxation. In a study of six patients, the patient attended a 40-minute weekly practice for 12 weeks. Even though their medical conditions were deteriorating, five of the patients reported physical, emotional, and mental improvement.

Although many of the research studies have small sample sizes, all of the movement-related exercise programs such as chair aerobics, yoga, chair pilates, or dance have reported positive outcomes for the palliative care patient. This suggests that noninvasive therapies that can decrease symptoms of fatigue, dyspnea, weakness, or anxiety in patients should be incorporated into the patient's care plan early on in the treatment course. Physical activity, however minimal, appears to improve a patient's quality of life throughout the disease trajectory including at the end of life. Lowe and colleagues reported patients with advanced cancer are very interested in physical activity programs.[7]

Understanding outcomes

In rehabilitation, there is a strong emphasis on the measurement of patient outcomes. Since the 1950s, many functional assessment instruments have been developed and used to help quantify the changes that occur in patients as a result of care and recovery. Some instruments to measure functional and physical outcomes are applicable to the assessment of patients within the last month of life.

There are more than a dozen functional outcome measurement tools in common use in rehabilitation settings in the United States and Canada. Measurement of self-care and mobility are central to rehabilitation, but the functions and behaviors required to lead a meaningful life are much broader. They may include cognitive, emotional, perceptual, social, and vocational function measurements as well.

For measuring function in the last 30 days of life, three scales may be particularly useful. The Rapid Disability Rating Scale (RDRS-2)[16] has a broad scope to include items related to activities of daily living, mental capacity, dietary changes, continence, medications, and confinement to bed. The Health Assessment Questionnaire (HAQ)[17] is a widely used instrument that summarizes the patients' areas of major difficulty. The Functional Independence Measure (FIM) is an ordinal scale that quantifies 18 areas of physical and cognitive function in terms of burden of care.[18,19] These scales are appropriate to palliative care because they focus on specific aspects of function that relate to patients' independence. The scales may be used to determine whether interventions at the end of life serve to foster independence and function for as long as possible.

There is also strong interest in the field of rehabilitation in measuring patients' perceptions of quality of life. When the measured domains are considered, the connection between rehabilitation and end-of-life care becomes evident. Most of the measurements of quality of life have to do with physical, cognitive, social, and spiritual function, the chief concerns of the rehabilitation practitioner.

Outcome measurements matter because they can reveal a lot about the quality of life experienced by persons near the end of life. For example, by assessing at intervals, it is possible to determine how much function patients retain as they approach death. By identifying and measuring differences in this experience, it is possible to determine the essential interventions and care activities that contribute to the highest levels of functional independence until the end of life.

Further research is needed to:

◆ Establish norms and indications for the application of rehabilitation in palliative care

◆ Determine cost-effectiveness of rehabilitation interventions

◆ Determine optimal time frames for providing rehabilitation services after the onset of disease

◆ Define variables having the greatest impact on patient outcomes

Inpatient rehabilitation, long-term care, hospice, and pediatrics

Acute comprehensive inpatient rehabilitation units are set up in such a way that complex medical-surgical issues may be managed concurrently with the functional processes of comprehensive rehabilitation.[20] For example, patients with metastatic cancer affecting their bones may have significant care needs related to mobility and activities of daily living, well addressed in an inpatient rehabilitation setting.

For many patients with terminal illness, the transition to an acute rehabilitation unit represents a crucial point in their healthcare experience. It is a time when the future comes into focus, and goals are defined based on the likely disease progression. Sometimes a short stay on an inpatient rehabilitation unit makes it possible for patients to return to a home setting, because of the gains in independent function that may be realized. Patients and family members may begin to face limited prognoses, decline in abilities, and changes in roles. Through an interdisciplinary therapeutic process, care needs are clarified, and skills and adaptation strategies are taught to patients and those who will care for them outside of the hospital.

Subacute rehabilitation facilities provide additional therapy activities, such as physical, occupational, or speech therapy, based on patient need, endurance, and tolerance. The pacing and amount of therapy are gauged according to individualized goals. As in comprehensive inpatient rehabilitation units, the aim is to facilitate improved physical function and as much independence as possible, even as the disease process moves the patient toward death. Patients with advanced disease who are too frail to participate in a full acute rehabilitation program may benefit from the slower-paced rehabilitation of a subacute setting.

Long-term care settings, such as skilled nursing facilities, are often places where lives are completed. Specialized geriatric facilities focus on the care needs of aging persons, often requiring specialized rehabilitation interventions. In both of these settings, rehabilitation nurses may plan and direct care delivery and make sure that patient and family concerns are kept in the forefront. Attention is paid to optimizing function and self-care, as well as addressing physical care issues.

Hospice settings either in the home or as an inpatient, may also provide a venue for a rehabilitative approach to end-of-life care. Careful planning of care to take into account limitations, yet promote function and autonomy, is a key factor in smoothing the transition to an inevitable death. Rehabilitative techniques and strategies make it easier for caregivers to manage increasing deficits, thereby protecting patient comfort and dignity through the dying process. Involving the family in the patient's exercise or activity program decreases feelings of helplessness.

Pediatric rehabilitation is focused on guiding the development of children to minimize disability and handicaps that may result from physical or cognitive impairment. There are situations in pediatric rehabilitation in which palliative care comes into play, and efforts are directed toward enhancing the normal function of both patient and family through the course of disease. For example, the family members of a child with progressive neuromuscular disease may learn how to use adaptive devices to position the child in a wheelchair for comfort and social interaction as well as for physiological function.[21]

Insurance issues and case management

In the insurance industry and managed care systems, rehabilitation nurses have the opportunity to advocate for the needs of persons with disease or disability and to reduce barriers to their access to care and resources. Near the end of a terminal disease course, planning and resource management are essential to ensure optimal care without undue economic and emotional burdens to families. Case management is an expanding practice area for rehabilitation nurses, usually with multidisciplinary relationships. Because palliative care needs are unique to individuals and require coordination of the care across disciplines, usual or episodic patterns of delivery and resource use may prove inadequate. The implementation of an activity program in palliative care requires careful and compassionate guidance and evaluation, tailored to meet individual strengths, abilities, needs, and preferences.[20,22] Enabling a kind of wellness to exist even at the point of death fits with the rehabilitation philosophy. Many rehabilitation nursing actions center on supporting physiological function and preventing complications, goals that are still appropriate at the end of life.

Finally, rehabilitation has long been concerned with understanding, enhancing, and measuring quality of life, whether related to physical, psychosocial, or spiritual domains.

The foundations of rehabilitation nursing practice

The real value of a rehabilitative approach to the nursing care of persons with declining health states lies in the foundations of rehabilitation nursing practice. The Association of Rehabilitation Nurses (ARN) believes cancer rehabilitation registered nurses' role is to collaborate together to provide quality patient care. "The goal of rehabilitation nursing is to assist the individual with disability and chronic illness in the restoration and maintenance of maximal health."[23] This includes:

- Attending to the full range of human experiences and responses to health and illness
- Dealing with families coping with lifelong issues
- Providing a holistic approach to care
- Facilitating team dynamics and integration
- Educating patients and their families to help them control and manage a wide range of challenges associated with chronic illness or disability
- Forming partnerships with patients and other healthcare providers to attain the best possible outcomes

The hallmark of rehabilitation is interdisciplinary collaboration. The synergy of collaboration enhances the value of rehabilitation nursing interventions and ensures that patient needs are addressed from a variety of perspectives. Typically, the rehabilitation team consists of physicians with specialized training in physical medicine and rehabilitation; rehabilitation nurses; physical, occupational, speech, respiratory, and recreation therapists; exercise physiologists; dietitians; social workers; and others as required to address particular needs. Effective teamwork requires mutual understanding and synchrony of the roles and responsibilities of each member. When the rehabilitation team works in synergy, it serves patients and families across the continuum of life.

Rehabilitation principles applied to palliative care

The rehabilitation of patients with palliative care needs should begin as early as possible. As soon as functional deficits are observed or anticipated, appropriate consultation with members of the rehabilitation team should be initiated. Certain diagnoses, such as progressive neuromuscular diseases; malignancies affecting the brain, spinal cord, or skeletal system; organ failure; and many other conditions that result in functional impairments, should trigger mobilization of the rehabilitation team.

The goals of rehabilitation are to prevent secondary disability, to enhance the function of both affected and unaffected systems, and to help patients adapt to their physical and social environments by means of physical restoration and adaptive devices.[38-42]

Rehabilitation nursing strategies focus on:

♦ Caring for whole persons in their social and physical environments

♦ Preventing secondary disability

♦ Enhancing function of both affected and unaffected systems

♦ Facilitating use of adaptive strategies

♦ Promoting quality of life

To illustrate the rehabilitation strategies as they may be applied in actual palliative nursing care situations, a variety of case studies are discussed in the following section. The stories serve to illuminate the role of rehabilitation nursing in palliative care and represent issues in common with many rehabilitation patients.

The case studies also reflect an approach to care—that of caring for whole person in their social and physical environments. Appreciating each person as a unique individual is extremely important to the rehabilitation process. Whereas it may be evident to rehabilitation professionals that certain goals and interventions would suit the patient's needs, even more important is finding congruence with the patient's own perceived and stated goals and values.

Case study

AD, a 60-year-old female with lung cancer

AD, age 60, was in her usual state of good health as a homemaker and enjoying traveling with her husband and playing cards and was a party organizer. She was slim and exercised 4 times a week even though exercise was not her favorite activity to do. She was much loved and known for giving of herself to others. AD went for her yearly routine physical. A chest X-ray showed a right upper lobe mass. A CT scan confirmed the mass and a fine needle aspiration biopsy was positive for adenocarcinoma non-small-cell lung cancer (NSCLC).

AD was completely asymptomatic. She had smoked occasionally in high school and had been exposed to second-hand smoke in her youth. At the time of surgery (a thoracotomy) she was found to have disease in four mediastinal lymph nodes. Following surgery, chemotherapy was started followed by radiotherapy. During her chemotherapy AD continued to exercise five times a week. Her exercises included breathing exercises, treadmill walking for 20 minutes, squats, upper body light-weight training, and stretching. She enjoyed doing the breathing exercises because she felt her lateral chest expand and felt the relaxation from the deep breathing. The breathing was performed slowly, rhythmically, and under control. She was taught to coordinate her breathing pattern with each exercise. When bending forward to do a stretch, she would blow out through her lips, bend forward and then breathe slowly to hold the stretch. She was reminded not to hold her breath with each exercise. AD frequently complained that her exercise workout was more painful than the chemotherapy. She refused pain medication, but continued with the exercise program saying that it maintained

her strength and allowed her to enjoy dinner with family and friends each night. Her family and friends were her great support and were always there to push, encourage, and love her. They would sometimes call when she was on the treadmill. She would put the phone on speaker and chat for 20 minutes and the time went fast.

After completing chemotherapy and radiation, her chest X-ray was clear. One year later, however, she was found to have a second lesion on her lung. A surgical resection was performed, and her postop course was uneventful. AD continued her exercise program as she felt it kept her strong.

For several years her life was normal without evidence of disease. She maintained a 15-minute exercise program and treadmill walking. One evening, however, she had a seizure and was found to have lung cancer metastasis in the right occipital lobe of the brain. The tumor was resected, and this was followed by a course of whole brain radiotherapy and chemotherapy. She continued on her exercise program. The exercises were modified, but she wanted to be strong physically to enjoy dinners with her family. Maintaining strength of the large muscle groups was important for her. She was able to do chair squats with minimal assistance and walk outside with some support. AD's family and the rehabilitation team adapted her activities of daily living to maintain as good a functional status as possible thus decreasing feelings of helplessness and hopelessness.

At this time AD demonstrated good muscle tone and strength of her arms and legs. She did, however, experience some chemotherapy-related peripheral neuropathy in her lower extremities. Reflexology provided some relief. She was alert and oriented but having difficulty with short-term memory loss. To reduce the stress from memory loss she would do things she enjoyed, such as looking at family pictures, listening to music, or talking with her closest friends. At this time she had a Karnofsky performance score of 80%.

Over the next several months AD was stable, until the cancer was found to have metastasized to her spine. She had increased back pain and muscle weakness but continued to walk with the use of a walker and continued to have dinner with family and friends. The rehabilitation team and family members adapted AD's exercise program to maintain the activities she requested, such as going to the bathroom and participating in family gatherings each evening. Many of the exercises were performed in bed and chair. Breathing exercises were performed 3–4 times a day with instruction and a family member or the home health aide providing gentle pressure to her lateral chest wall as she would breathe out to lengthen her exhalation. As she lost more control and ambulation became more difficult, her family and the rehab team were meticulous about her safety. It was during this time that the rehab team provided increased support for her family and friends discussing role changes, and coping with the loss of someone special.

AD's husband expressed the following:

"No matter the stage of her illness there was always some level of physical activity you could do to maintain her independence. The exercises rebuilt her muscular strength and endurance, reduced fatigue, regained range of motion and flexibility, and relieved anxiety, anger, and stress while restoring her energy level and hope each day we shared together. Thank you."

Case study

EW, a 60-year-old woman with a lung transplant

With a history of rapidly worsening chronic obstructive pulmonary disease, 60-year-old EW was faced with few options. As every breath became a struggle, she wondered how she could go on with her life and whether it was worth continuing the fight. She had already lost so much of what was important to her: mobility, independence, and social relationships. Now she found herself homebound, exhausted, and unable to carry on even a telephone conversation with friends and family she so cherished.

After much consultation and deliberation, she agreed that lung transplantation was the only course of treatment that would afford her the function and independence she believed made her life worthwhile. She received the transplanted lungs after a relatively short wait. But her expectations of returning to wellness were not to be fulfilled. EW began an extraordinarily complicated postoperative course and a journey that would lead her to a life's end.

Initially, EW required prolonged ventilatory support. She struggled with infection and rejection of her new lungs. She experienced shock, sepsis, and distress; her medical records thickened with stories of heroics and near misses, of technology, of miracles, of persistent argument with fate. She had established with her family that she would want everything possible done to preserve her life, and thus the critical balancing act went on for months. Just as her condition seemed to be stabilizing, she had a massive stroke, resulting in dense hemiplegia and loss of speech/language function.

She was admitted to the inpatient rehabilitation medicine service to focus on mobility, self-care, and speech functions in order to help her to return home with her family. She progressed very slowly, with numerous complications related to her pulmonary status, immunosuppression, and cardiovascular deterioration.

A second stroke left her with even more-limited language and cognitive function. She required maximum assistance for all activities of daily living, and she ceased to make progress toward her rehabilitation goals. Her pulmonary function declined. Her family recognized that they would not be able to meet her care needs at home. Further evaluation of her lungs revealed that she had developed a lymphoma, for which, in her case, no treatment could be offered. Her prognosis plummeted, with the likelihood of death in a matter of weeks.

The focus of her rehabilitation care shifted. No longer would it be reasonable to expect her to reach the level of independence she would need to return home. A rigorous exercise program was not going to change the trajectory of her disease and in fact might drain her energies and contribute to more frustration and discomfort.

By talking with family and friends, the rehabilitation team learned that EW was strong willed, stubborn, and difficult, but deeply loved. She was seen as the matriarch of the family. For most of her adult life, she had balanced her responsibilities as a single parent with her work as a postal clerk. She was characterized as determined and cantankerous, impatient, critical, and quick to frustrate. Her family was close and extremely important to her. She had a wide circle of friends. Her four sons took turns visiting her in the hospital and sincerely wanted to get her back home again.

With these facts in mind, the rehabilitation team designed communications and interventions that took into account the personal traits and values that were particular to EW. They knew that she would have difficulty tolerating frustration. They knew that she would need to feel in control as much as possible. They also knew that involvement of her family and friends would be essential. They anticipated the effects of prolonged stress on the family unit and recognized the profound loss the family would sustain as her life concluded.

Rehabilitation nursing actions focused first on communication. Because of her dense aphasia, she was unable to verbalize her thoughts or feelings. Instead, she perseverated on one word, growing increasingly agitated when people were unable to understand her. A speech therapist was involved in setting up nonverbal methods of communication, such as picture boards.

As the nursing staff worked with EW, they tuned in to behavioral cues and expressions. Family members also helped in the interpretation of her attempts to communicate. Strategies for communication included:

- Direct eye contact
- Relaxed, unhurried approach
- Slow, distinct phrases in normal tone of voice
- One thought presented at a time
- Time allowed to process information
- Gestures to convey and clarify meaning

Efforts were directed toward maintaining EW's comfort and dignity. Whenever possible, she was supported in making her own choices. Occupational and physical therapies concentrated on interventions that would promote her autonomy. Functional activities, such as dressing, grooming, and eating, allowed her opportunities to exercise her independence. Access to her physical environment was accomplished through the use of adaptive devices and wheelchair mobility skills. As her condition deteriorated, it was more difficult to ascertain her desires. Inclusion of family members became more important, both for carrying out her wishes as they knew them and for giving the family the active role in her care that they wanted.

Throughout the course of EW's final illness, spiritual and psychosocial support were priorities. With her ability to communicate so severely impaired, her needs for support might have been misunderstood or overlooked. She was suddenly unable to serve as the source of stability and strength for her family, and roles and expectations were greatly changed. The rehabilitation nurses, the psychologist, the social worker, and the chaplain worked together to counsel and care for both patient and family.

When death came, the family described a mixture of feelings of relief, sorrow, and satisfaction. Through their sadness, they recognized the efforts of the rehabilitation team to preserve EW's uniqueness and integrity as a human being. Thus they would remember her.

Preventing secondary disability

Whatever the disease process, persons in declining states of health are at risk for development of unnecessary complications. Even at the end of life, complications can be prevented, thereby enhancing a person's comfort, function, independence, and dignity. Treatment of one body system must not compromise another. For example, patients who are bed-bound are at risk for development of muscular, vascular, integumentary, and neurological compromise, which could result in secondary disability.

Case study

JB, a man with amyotrophic lateral sclerosis

JB knew his days were numbered, irrevocably ticking away with the advance of his amyotrophic lateral sclerosis. Bit by bit, his body functions eroded. Weakness began in his lower extremities, then spread to his trunk and upper extremities. He was troubled with spasticity, which soon made ambulation almost impossible. He depended on his wife to help him with all of his daily living activities but continued to get out each day in his electric wheelchair, to work with the city government on disability policies. When he went on the ventilator to support his breathing, he likened his health to driving an old truck down a mountain road: no way to stop, no way to turn around, nothing to do but drive on home.

As JB's disease progressed, he was at risk for the development of secondary disabilities. Concerns included the potential development of edema, contractures, and skin breakdown. JB lacked the normal muscular activity that would promote vascular return, and he developed significant edema in his extremities. Knowing that "edema is glue" when it comes to function, rehabilitation nursing actions included range-of-motion exercises and management of dependent edema with compression and elevation.[1]

Spasticity complicated positioning of JB's limbs. It was important to avoid shortened positions that favored the flexors, because that would allow contractures to occur. Contractures would further limit his mobility and function, so he and his wife were taught a stretching program as well as the use of positioning devices and splints to maintain joints in neutral alignment.

Because of his impaired mobility, JB was at risk for skin breakdown. He enjoyed spending a lot of time in his wheelchair. Although his sensation was basically intact, he was not able to react to the message of skin pressure and to change his position. JB learned how to shift his weight in the wheel-chair, by either side-to side shifts or tilt-backs. A small timer helped remind him of pressure releases every 15 minutes when up in his chair. In addition, a special wheelchair cushion protected bony prominences with gel pads.

Enhancing function of both affected and unaffected systems

A chief concern in rehabilitative care is enhancing function of both affected and unaffected body systems, thereby helping patients to be as healthy and independent as possible. In palliative care, many care issues involve the interconnections of body systems and the need to enlist one function to serve for another.

Case study

PO, a man with metastatic prostate cancer

PO had been a successful attorney for 30 years. A burly, loud-spoken Irishman, he prided himself in bringing life and laughter everywhere he went. Although diagnosed and treated for prostate cancer, he never slowed the hectic pace of his law practice or his busy social calendar. In fact, he had little time to pay attention to the ominous symptoms developing that indicated the advance of his disease.

When he sought medical attention at last, the cancer had metastasized to his spine, resulting in partial paralysis and bowel and bladder impairment. Orthopedic spine surgeons attempted to relieve pressure on his spinal cord with the hope of restoring motor and sensory function. However, during surgery, it was determined that the cancer had spread extensively, and they were unable to significantly improve his spinal cord function. Radiation followed, but it had little effect on the spreading cancer.

PO was stunned. He could not believe the turn his life had taken. Suddenly, nothing seemed to work. He had to depend on others for the first time in his life. He felt like "some kind of freak," unable to move his legs or even manage normal bodily functions.

His bulky frame became a heavy burden as he tried to relearn life from a wheelchair. He wrestled with the unfairness of the situation, finally promising himself that he would "go out in style." He wanted to get home as soon as possible, so as not to waste his precious remaining time.

PO spent 12 days on the inpatient rehabilitation unit, then transitioned to home with continued therapies and nursing care. He died 2 months later, at home with his family present.

In PO's case, several body systems were at risk for complications, although not all were directly affected by the disease process. Mobility was a critical concern. Bowel and bladder management also presented challenges. His neurological deficits and rapidly progressing disease, combined with his size and the need to learn new skills from a wheelchair level, placed him at risk for development of contractures, skin breakdown, and deep vein thrombosis. Problems with bowel and bladder function put him at risk for constipation, distention, and infection. He experienced severe demoralization. In keeping with his wishes, the rehabilitation nursing staff designed a plan for Mr. PO and his family to follow at home. Priority rehabilitation nursing issues included:

- Managing fatigue related to advancing disease
- Pain control
- Promoting mobility and independence
- Managing neurogenic bowel and bladder
- Alleviating social isolation related to the effects of terminal illness
- Anticipatory grieving and spiritual care

The rehabilitation team planned PO's care to protect his periods of rest throughout the day. They knew that his therapy would be more effective and his ability to carry over new learning of functional activities would be better if he were in a rested state. His sleep-wake cycle was restored as quickly as possible. Occupational therapists taught him strategies for energy conservation in his activities of daily living, including the use of adaptive devices, planning, and pacing. PO initially described his pain as always with him, dull and relentless, wearing him down. Rehabilitation nurses evaluated his responses in relation to different medications and dosage schedules, as well as nondrug pain control interventions such as positioning and relaxation. The most effective method of pain control for PO was scheduled doses of long-acting morphine, coupled with short-acting doses for breakthrough or procedural pain. This method of pain management is frequently used in rehabilitation settings, because it does not allow pain to become established, and the patient does not have to experience a certain level of pain and then wait for relief.

It also minimizes sedative effects. With his pain under better control, Mr. PO was able to actively participate in his own care and make deliberate decisions about his goals.

Positioning and supporting of the body in such a way that function is preserved and complications are prevented is an important consideration in mobility. As his disease progressed and he experienced increasing weakness and fatigue, he spent more and more time in bed. Teaching of the patient and family focused on the techniques of bed mobility and specific precautions to prevent complications.

Supine lying was minimized because of high risk for sacral skin breakdown. Even with a pressure-reducing mattress, back-lying time needed to be restricted. To reduce shearing forces, the bed was placed in reverse Trendelenburg position to raise the head, rather than cranking up just the head of the bed. Draw sheets were used to move Mr. PO, to prevent shearing. Stretching and breakage of capillaries and subcutaneous tissues contributes to the potential for deep skin breakdown.

Positioning of the lower extremities is important to prevent complications such as foot drop, skin breakdown, contractures, and deep vein thrombosis. When the patient is supine, care should be taken to support the feet in neutral position. This can be accomplished by using a footboard or box at the end of the bed or by the application of splints. Derotational splints were placed on his lower legs to keep his hips in alignment, to prevent foot-drop contractures, and to reduce the risk of heel breakdown. Range-of-motion exercises were done at least twice daily.

When Mr. PO was side-lying, pillows were employed to cushion bony prominences and maintain neutral joint position. His uppermost leg was brought forward, and the lower leg was straightened to minimize hip flexion contractures. Frequently overlooked as a positioning choice, prone lying offers advantages not only of skin pressure relief and reduction in hip flexion contractures, but also in promoting greater oxygen exchange.[17] His bed position was alternated between back, both sides, and prone at least every 2 hours.

There are many physiological benefits of upright posture. Blood pressure, digestive and bowel functions, oxygenation, and perception are geared toward being upright. Weight bearing helps to avert skeletal muscle atrophy. Sitting, standing, and walking provide for changes in scenery and enhance the ability to socialize. This was an important consideration for Mr. PO, who experienced emotional distress at the social isolation his illness imposed.

It is important to choose seating that supports the patient, avoiding surfaces that place pressure on bony prominences. A seat that is angled back slightly helps keep the patient from sliding forward. Placing the feet on footrests or a small box or stool may add comfort, as may supporting the arms on pillows or on a table in front of the patient. Sitting time should be limited, based on patient comfort, endurance, and skin tolerance. Mr. PO followed a sitting schedule that increased by 15 minutes a day until he was able to tolerate about 2 hours of upright time. That was enough time to carry out many of his personal activities, yet not so much as to overly tire him.

Planning for Mr. PO's return home involved careful assessment of his equipment needs. Physical and occupational therapists conducted a home evaluation to determine how he would manage mobility and self-care activities and what equipment would be appropriate. Family members practiced using equipment and devices under the guidance of the rehabilitation team. The objective was to simplify the care as much as possible, while still supporting his active participation in his daily activities.

Examples of home care equipment often used include commodes, wheelchairs, sliding boards, Hoyer lifts, adaptive devices such as reachers, dressing sticks, long-handled sponges, tub/shower benches, hospital beds, and pressure-relieving mattresses. Examples of home modifications include affixing handrails and grab bars, widening doors, using raised toilet seats, and installing stair lifts and ramps.

For PO, the loss of bowel and bladder function was especially distressing. It placed him in a position of dependence and impinged on his privacy. It reinforced his feelings of isolation and being different. The focus of rehabilitation nursing interventions was to mimic the normal physiological rhythms of bowel and bladder elimination. By helping him gain control of his body

functions, nursing staff hoped to promote his confidence, dignity, and feelings of self-worth.

Bowel regulation and continence were achieved by implementing a classic bowel program routine. PO was especially prone to constipation due to immobility and the effects of pain medications. The first intervention was to modify his diet to include more fiber and fluids. He also took stool softener medication twice daily. His bowel program occurred after breakfast each morning, to take advantage of the gastrocolic reflex. He was assisted to sit upright on a commode chair. A rectal suppository was inserted, with digital stimulation at 15-minute intervals to accomplish bowel evacuation. The patient and his wife were taught how to manage this program at home. Although reluctant at first, he became resigned to the necessity of this bowel program and worked it into his morning routine. His wife, eager to help in any way she could, also learned the techniques. Once a regular pattern of elimination was established, he no longer experienced incontinence.

For bladder management, nursing staff implemented a program of void trials and intermittent catheterization. The patient learned to manage his own fluid intake and to catheterize himself at 4-hour intervals, thereby preventing overdistention or incontinence. However, as his disease progressed, he opted for an indwelling urinary catheter because it was easier for him to manage. There is a continuous need to evaluate and individualize rehabilitation goals, and to alter goals as patients experience more advanced disease.

With a history of active social involvement, PO had great difficulty with the limitations his disease imposed on his energy level and his ability to remain functional. He did not want others to see him as incapacitated in any way. He did not want to be embarrassed by his failing body. The rehabilitation team concentrated on solving the physical problems that could be solved. A recreation therapist assessed his leisure and avocational interests and prescribed therapeutic activities that would build his confidence in social situations. Together, the team helped him learn to navigate around architectural barriers and helped him to practice new skills successfully from a wheelchair level.

PO concentrated on making plans and settling financial matters in preparation for his death. He continued to set goals for himself and to maintain hope, but the nature of his goals shifted. Initially, he was concerned with not becoming a burden to his family and focused on his physical functioning. As his mobility and endurance flagged and he had to rely more on others for assistance with basic care needs, he began to change his goals. Some of his stoicism fell away. He revealed his feelings more readily and described the evolution of his emotions. Now the focus became his relationships: an upcoming wedding anniversary, a son's graduation from law school. Rehabilitation nurses, home care nurses, the psychologist, and the social worker supported the patient and his family as they began to grieve the past that would never return and the future that was not to be. Pastoral care was a significant part of the process, as he struggled with spiritual questions and sought a peaceful understanding of what was happening to him. The rehabilitation team endeavored to help the patient live all the days of his life, by helping body and soul continue to function.

Facilitating use of adaptive strategies

The ability of patients to continue to participate actively in living their lives has much to do with successful adaptation to changes in function. Even at the end of life, a patient's capacity to adapt remains. Everyday activities may become very difficult to perform with advancing disease. However, rehabilitation nursing actions that promote communication, the use of appropriate tools and equipment, family participation, and modifications to the environment all enhance the process of adaptation.

Communication

Opening the doors to communication is the most important rehabilitation nursing intervention. By removing functional barriers to speech, by teaching and supporting compensatory strategies, and by allowing safe opportunities for patients and families to discuss difficult issues around death and dying, rehabilitation nurses perform a critical function in the adaptation process.

Tools and equipment

Many adaptive devices are available to patients and families that enhance functional ability and independence. Rehabilitation offers the chance to analyze tasks with new eyes and solve problems with creativity and individuality. Examples of useful tools to assist patients in being as independent as possible include reachers, dressing aids such as sock-starters, elastic shoelaces, and dressing sticks. For some patients, adapted eating utensils increase independence with the activity of eating and thereby support nutritional intake. Modifications to clothing may permit more efficient toileting and hygiene, conserving both energy and dignity.

Family participation

As illustrated in the previous case studies, the involvement of family and friends has multifaceted benefits. Because of the social nature of humankind, presence and involvement of family and friends has great importance at the end of life. Family members may seek involvement in the caring activities as an expression of feelings of closeness and love. They may try to find understanding, resolution, or closure of past issues. For the person at the end of life, the presence of family, friends, and even pets may be a powerful affirmation of the continuity of life.

Modifications to environment

Rehabilitation professionals are keenly aware of the effect of the environment of care on function, independence, and well-being. The physical arrangement of furnishings can be instrumental, not only in promoting patient access to the environment, but also in the ease with which others care for the patient. The environment can be made into a powerful tool for orientation, for spatial perception, and for preserving a territorial sense of self.

Light has a strong effect, not only on visual perception, but also on mood and feelings of well-being. Light can be a helpful tool in maintaining day-night rhythms and orienting patients to time and place. Sound is also an important environmental variable. For example, music has been implicated as a therapeutic intervention in both rehabilitation and palliative care.

Promoting quality at the end of life

The concept of quality of life is linked to function and independence. Patients often describe their satisfaction with life in terms of what they are able to do. Important determinants of quality of life include (1) the patient's own state, including physical and cognitive functioning, psychological state, and physical condition; (2) quality of palliative care; (3) physical environment; (4) relationships; and (5) outlook. Rehabilitation zeroes in on the essential components of mobility, self-care, cognition, and social interaction, which define what people can do.

Case study

LN, a 42-year-old woman with a malignant brain tumor

LN, age 42, had just started her own consulting business when she began to experience headaches and visual disturbances. At first, she attributed her symptoms to the long hours and stress related to building her business. But when she experienced weakness of her left side, she knew that something more serious was happening.

She had a glioblastoma multiforme growing deep in her brain. Surgery was performed to debulk the tumor, but in a matter of weeks it was clear that the mass was growing rapidly. A course of radiation was completed to no avail. Her function continued to decline, and it seemed that every body system was affected by the advancing malignancy. Now her left side was densely paralyzed, she had difficulty swallowing and speaking, and her thinking processes became muddled.

Her family was in turmoil. On one hand, they resented the disruption her sudden illness imposed on their previously ordered lives. On the other hand, they wanted to care for her and make sure that her remaining time was the best that it could be. As they watched her decline day by day, ambiguities in their relationships surfaced, and conflicts about what would define quality of life emerged.

Rehabilitation's part in promoting quality of life at the end of life is several-fold. Rehabilitation is a goal-directed process. Realistic, attainable goals based on the patient's own definition of quality of life drive the actions of the team. In the area of physical care, rehabilitation strategies support energy conservation, sequencing and pacing, maintaining normal routines, and accessing the environment. Beyond that, rehabilitation nurses facilitate effective communication and problem-solving with patients and families. They offer acceptance and support through difficult decision-making and help mobilize concrete resources.

When rehabilitation nurses approach care, it is with the goal of enhancing function and independence. In LN's case, the brain tumor created deficits in mobility, cognition, and perception. Also, more subtle issues greatly influenced the quality of her remaining time. It was important to understand how the patient would define the quality of her own life and to direct actions toward protecting those elements.

Promoting dignity, self-image, and participation

LN's concept of quality of life was evident in how she participated in her care and the decisions that she made about her course of treatment. The rehabilitation team learned that LN's mother had died several years earlier of a similar brain tumor. Caring for her mother had solidified her beliefs about not wishing to burden others. Part of LN's definition of quality of life was that she would not be dependent on others.

LN prided herself on being industrious and self-sufficient. To her, the ability to take care of herself was a sign of success. Rehabilitation nurses and therapists focused on helping to manage symptoms of advancing disease so that she would be able to do as much for herself as possible. This included adaptive techniques for daily living skills, pain management, eating, dressing, grooming, and bowel and bladder management. Even with her physical and cognitive decline, retaining her normal routines helped to allay some feelings of helplessness and to promote a positive self-image.

Control, hope, and reality

As her illness progressed, LN felt she was losing control. It became difficult for her to remember things, and expressing herself became more laborious and frustrating. She slept frequently and seemed disconnected from external events. Her family understood her usual desire for control and made many attempts to include her in conversations and to support her in making choices.

At first, her concept of hope was tied to the idea of cure. Radiation therapy represented the chance of cure. When that was completed without appreciable change in her tumor, some of her feelings of hopefulness slipped away. She sank into a depression. Her family was alarmed: LN's psychological well-being was a critical component in her own definition of quality of life. Treating her depression became a priority issue for the rehabilitation team. Through a combination of rehabilitation, psychological counseling, and antidepressant medications, her dark mood slowly lifted. Hope seemed to return in a different form, less connected to an event of cure and more a part of her interactions with her daughter and sister.

Family support

Another significant area that related to quality of life for LN had to do with social well-being. She struggled with the idea of becoming a burden to her family and realized that she was losing control over what was happening to her. Her relationships with others in her life were complex, and now they were challenged even further. At the same time, her family members wrestled with memories of the mother's death and feared the responsibilities for care that might be thrust on them.

The rehabilitation team tried to help the patient and her family work through their thoughts, feelings, and fears, and helped them to find ways to express them. The team arranged several family conferences to discuss not only the care issues but also the changes in roles and family structure. Whenever possible, the team found answers to the family's questions and made great effort to keep communications open. Creating safe opportunities for the family to express their ambivalence and conflict helped move them toward acceptance. The family was able to prepare in concrete ways for the outcome they both welcomed and dreaded.

Summary

Rehabilitation nursing approaches have value in palliative care. Research has demonstrated that physical activity is safe, improves stamina and quality of life, and is a feasible intervention in patients with terminal illness. Physical activity promotes and encourages enjoyment of life despite living with progressive disease to the very end, and the benefits of movement decreases and sometimes allieviates many of the common side effects of treatment and progression of disease. Regardless of the disease trajectory, nurses can do something more to preserve function and independence and positively affect perceptions of quality of life, even at its end. Rehabilitation nurses facilitate holistic care of persons in their social and physical

environments. They direct actions toward preventing secondary disability and enhancing both affected and unaffected body systems. They foster the use of adaptive strategies and techniques to optimize autonomy. The deliberate focus of rehabilitation nurses on function, independence, dignity, and the preservation of hope makes a fitting contribution to care at the end of life.

References

1. Hoeman S. Rehabilitation Nursing: Prevention, Intervention and Outcomes. 4th ed. St. Louis: Mosby; 2007.
2. American Nurses' Association. Rehabilitation Nursing—Scope of Practice: Process and Outcome Criteria for Selected Diagnoses. Kansas City, MO: American Nurses' Association; 2010.
3. Toth M, Marcantonio ER, Davis RB, Walton T, Kahn JR, Phillips RS. Massage therapy for patients with metastatic cancer: a pilot randomized controlled trial. J Alter Comp Med. 2013;19 (7):650–656.
4. Mitchinson A, Fletcher CE, Jim HM, Montagnini M, Hinshaw DB. Integrating massage therapy within the palliative care of veterans with advanced illnesses: an outcome study. Am J Hosp Palliat Care. 2013;online:1–8 (online). http://ajh.sagepub.com/content/early/2013/0 2/13/1049909113476568.
5. Headley JA, Ownby KK, John LD. The effect of seated exercise on fatigue and quality of life in women with advanced breast cancer. Oncol Nurs Forum. 2004;31:997–983.
6. Albrecht TA, Taylor AG. Physical activity in patients with advanced-stage cancer: A systematic review of the literature. Clin J Oncol Nurs. 2011;16(3):293–300.
7. Lowe SS, Watanabe SM, Baracos VE, Courneya KS. Physical activity interests and preferences in palliative cancer patients. Support Care Cancer. 2010;18:1469–1475.
8. Lowe SS, Watanabe SM, Courneya KS. Physical activity as a supportive care intervention in palliative cancer patients: a systematic review. Journal of Supportive Oncology. 2009;7:27–34
9. Maddocks M, Lewis M, Chauhan A, Manderson C, Hocknell J, Wilcock A. Randomized controlled pilot study of neuromuscular electrical stimulation of the quadriceps in patients with non-small cell lung cancer. J Pain Symptom Manage. 2009;38:950–956.
10. Oldervoll LM, Loge JH, Paltiel H, Vidvei U, Wiken AN, Hjermstad MJ, et al. The effect of a physical exercise program in palliative care: a phase II study. J Pain Symptom Manage. 2006; 31: 421–430.
11. Oldervoll LM, Loge JH, Lydersen S, Paltiel H, Asp MB, Nygaard UV, et al. Physical exercise for cancer patients with advanced disease: a randomized controlled trial. Oncologist. 2011;16(11):1649–1657.
12. Helbostad JL, Holen JC, Jordhoy MS, Ringdal GI, Oldervoll L, Kaasa MD. A first step in the development of an international self-report instrument for physical functioning in palliative cancer care: a systematic literature review and an expert opinion evaluation study. J Pain Symptom Manage. 2009;37:196–205.
13. Selman LE, Williams J, Simms V. A mixed-methods evaluation of complementary therapy services in palliative care: yoga and dance therapy. Eur J Cancer Care. 2012;21:87–97.
14. Dhruva A, Miaskowski C, Abrams D, Acree M, Cooper B, Goodman S, et al. Yoga breathing for cancer chemotherapy-associated symptoms and quality of life: results of a pilot randomized controlled trial. J Altern Complement Med. 2012;18(5):473–479.
15. McDonald A, Burjan E, Martin S. Yoga for patients and carers in a palliative day care setting. Int J Palliative Nursing. 2006; 12(11): 519–523.
16. Linn M, Linn BS. The Rapid Disability Rating Scale-2. J Am Geriatr Soc. 1982;30:378–382.
17. Steen V, Medsger TA. The value of the Health Assessment Questionnaire and special patient-generated scales to demonstrate change in systemic sclerosis patients over time. Arthritis Rheum. 1997;40:1984–1991.

18. Stineman M, Shea JA, Jette A, Tassoni CJ, Ottenbacher KJ, Fiedler R, et al. The Functional Independence Measure: tests of scaling assumptions, structure, and reliability across 20 divers impairment categories. Arch Phys Med Rehabil. 1996;77:1101–1108.

19. Quatrano LA, Cruz TH. Future of outcomes measurement: impact on research in medical rehabilitation and neurologic populations. Arch Phys Med Rehabil. 2011; 92(10 suppl):S7–S11.

20. Doloresco L. CARF: symbol of rehabilitation excellence. Sci Nurs. 2001;18:165,172.

21. Himelstein B, Hilden J, Boldt J, Weissman D. Pediatric palliative care. N Engl J Med. 2004;350:1752–762.

22. Association of Rehabilitation Nurses Position Statements. Available at: http://rehabnurse.org/advocacy/content/Position-Statement.html. Accessed October 1, 2013.

Resources

American Academy of Physical Medicine and Rehabilitation (AAPM&R) 9700 West Bryn Mawr Avenue, Rosemont, IL 60018
http://www.aapmr.org

American Congress of Rehabilitation Medicine (ACRM)
11654 Plaza America Drive, Suite 535, Reston, VA 20109
http://www.acrm.org

Association of Rehabilitation Nurses (ARN)
8735 W. Higgins Road, Suite 300, Chicago, IL 60631
http://www.rehabnurse.org

Commission for the Accreditation of Rehabilitation Facilities (CARF)
6951 East Southpoint Road, Tucson, AZ 85756
http://www.carf.org

CHAPTER 50

The emergency department

Mary Bowman

You-never-know.
Joaquin Andujar[1]

Key points

♦ Palliative care can be provided to all patients who present to the emergency department (ED).

♦ Pain is one of the most common chief complaints of patients presenting to the ED.

♦ The growing number of patients presenting to the ED at the end of life means an increase in the proportion of patients for whom the default resuscitation approach is less applicable.

♦ Rapid identification of treatment goals with the terminally ill patient or surrogate prevents unwanted resuscitation and application of burdensome life-prolonging therapies.

♦ Unrestricted access of the family to the dying patient can be successfully implemented in the ED.

The use of EDs has increased dramatically over the past decades with a large portion of this increase attributed to "inappropriate" or nonurgent visits. More individuals are using the ED as a type of primary care, and hospital EDs have become an integral part of the American healthcare system. Reasons for this "overuse" are numerous, including the progressive aging of the population and the associated increase in chronic conditions; lack of cost awareness of the use of the ED for non-emergency care; organizational problems in providing primary care; better ED convenience and accessibility for patients; and patients' subjective perception of illness severity and greater confidence in the ED compared with primary care services.[2–4] Additionally the ED has become the "safety net" of healthcare for the indigent and uninsured, a population that often lacks a primary medical provider. This difficulty in accessing primary care contributes to the 23.1% rise in ED visit rate observed from 1997 to 2007 alone. The increase is most significant among Medicaid and African-American patients.[5] Across the United States there are approximately 130 million patient visits to the ED each year. These numbers imply that 1 in 5 persons in the United States had one or more ED visits in a 12-month period.[2,3] This accounts for approximately 4% of all national healthcare spending).[4]

In addition to acting as a safety net for primary care, EDs must also be prepared to handle large volumes of patients in a short amount of time in the event of a mass casualty situation, a terrorist attack, or a natural disaster.

Providing palliative care in a fast-paced and high-stress environment

The ED is a fast-paced and high-stress environment where decisions are made quickly at times with suboptimal levels of information. Although the ED may be chaotic and relationships among providers, patients, and families hastily forged, emergency clinicians play a crucial role in influencing the trajectory of the patient's care. The ED nurse plays a primary role in this area as the one who interfaces first with the patient and family. The calm and reassuring presence of a nurse can reflect both competency and compassion. At no time is this role more important than when a patient presents to the ED with advanced illness, and curative or life-prolonging therapy is no longer possible, appropriate, or desired by the patient. Palliative care is central to good emergency nursing and medical care. This chapter is designed to assist in recognizing and addressing the palliative care needs of critically ill or injured patients and their families in the fast-paced, often chaotic conditions of an emergency department. Once emergency clinicians recognize that all patients who present to the ED are eligible to receive palliative care, nurses and physicians can tailor the plan of care from a broader range of interventions to help patients and families receive the best care possible while honoring their wishes. From this perspective, questions to be added to the basic ED assessment include the following: How ill is the patient? Is he or she terminally ill or close to death? What does the patient know about the disease and prognosis? What are the treatment options? What are their goals/preferences for care? Does the patient have an advance directive? Who is the decision maker for the patient if he or she lacks capacity? How rapidly can we establish treatment goals? What can be done to relieve distressing symptoms? What can be done to ease the family's distress and meet their needs? What other disciplines do we need to contact to help meet the needs of this patient and family (for example the palliative care team, social work, chaplain)?

End-of-life care and goals of care in the Emergency Department

As our population ages and prevalence of chronic illness increases, healthcare providers are faced with a growing number of patients in their final stages of cancer, respiratory failure, end-stage heart failure, and/or dementia.[6] These patients present in distress to

EDs, and as a result palliative care has become a critical part of ED care. The patients frequently have multiple chronic medical conditions as well as social issues they struggle with. They cycle in and out of the hospital via the ED, thus providing an opportunity for healthcare providers to discuss goals of care and treatment options during each visit, and to document the outcomes of these discussions. The ED nurse is frequently the one who initiates these conversations and or alerts the physician of the need to do so.

Although some patients complete advance directives and the completed form has become part of the chart, research on their overall use and effectiveness show mixed results. An early study found that only 27% of ED patients had completed these documents.[7] Their effectiveness in ensuring the patient's preferences for care are met has also been in question. Reasons for their ineffectiveness include that the documented advance directive is difficult to find in the patient's records, or if located may be ignored by medical personnel or overridden by a surrogate decision-maker.[7] Recent research suggests that those patients with advance directives are more likely to have their wishes fulfilled.[7]

In addition to traditional documents such as advance directives or a living will, many states have also adopted a state-specific document that helps further clarify patient's wishes during a time of critical illness. For example, the Physician Orders for Life-Sustaining Treatment (POLST) is a process that translates a patient's goals for care at the end of life into medical orders that follow the patient across care settings. It enables healthcare professionals, through a conversation with a patient or surrogate decision-maker, to assess and convey the wishes of patients with serious life-limiting illness who may have a life expectancy of less than 1 year, or of anyone of advanced age interested in defining his or her wishes for end-of-life care.[8,9] All hospitals receiving Medicare or Medicaid funding must provide inpatients with a copy of an advance directive form. There is no obligation, however, that the form be completed.

Making decisions for a patient affected by sudden devastating injury or illness traumatizes the patient's family and loved ones. Even in the absence of an emergency, individuals making end-of-life treatment decisions find it extremely difficult and can be overwhelmed by a sense of responsibility for what may seem to them like a life-and-death decision. Helping family members or loved ones with these end-of-life decisions under emergent conditions requires the healthcare team to be extremely clear when presenting information related to the patient's prognosis, as well as treatment options and recommendations.[7] It is important to break bad news with both clarity and compassion, so that family and other loved ones understand both the gravity of the situation and the benefits and burden of each treatment option. The well-being of the patient is central to the conversation, but the families need to feel heard. Box 50.1 details the core components of a discussion about end-of-life treatment options in the ED.

An ED nurse with a generalist level of palliative care and communication skills training, alongside the palliative care team can be helpful in holding these conversations, providing the assurance that attention to the patient's comfort and dignity will be paramount. This includes management of pain, dyspnea, anxiety and other symptoms that may occur[7] If and when the patient's condition stabilizes, depending on the agreed-on goals of care, arrangements can be made for in-hospital admission or referral to home hospice. The ED nurse helps facilitate these transitions. Please

---

Box 50.1 Core components of a discussion about end-of-life treatment goals in the emergency department

Prepare in advance.
- Identify the diagnosis/prognosis.
- Determine what the patient or surrogate already knows.
- Seek assistance from support personnel (e.g., chaplain, social worker, patient advocate, palliative care team).

Establish a therapeutic milieu.
- Identify a private and quiet place in the emergency department where everyone can sit and be seen and heard.
- Minimize interruptions.

Seek patient and surrogate knowledge about diagnosis and prognosis.
- Correct inaccuracies and misconceptions.
- Provide additional information.

Communicate effectively.
- Avoid jargon, slang, and acronyms.
- Demonstrate empathy.
- Be honest and direct.

Make a palliative care treatment recommendation.
- Provide rationale for recommendations.
- Answer questions.

Seek patient or surrogate agreement with recommendation.

Source: Reference 26.

---

refer to chapter 5 for an in-depth discussion on communication in palliative care.

Deaths in the Emergency Department

Deaths in the ED differ from deaths in other settings: (1) They are likely to be sudden and unexpected, as in severe trauma or the death of a child; (2) the patient may arrive in the ED unconscious, alone, and without identifying documents; (3) the patient's and family's values are often initially unknown; (4) there is commonly no previous patient-physician or patient-nurse relationship; and (5) decisions are often based on limited medical history and information.[7] A "good death" in the ED as elsewhere, requires planning and preparedness from the interdisciplinary ED and if available, palliative care teams. While the initial thought in an emergency setting is toward resuscitation and invasive procedures, it is critical that the care providers rapidly appraise the patient's situation and establish goals of care congruent with the patient's situation and wishes if known. If the patient is dying, the family and other caregivers need to be apprised of the imminence of death and assisted to face the emotions and experiences that will occur when death comes.[6] The presence and caring of a nurse is a critical part of this interaction and in making sure that the patient and family are supported and guided throughout the process.

Nursing leadership in managing the dying process often involves attempting to modify the physical environment of the ED to support the patient and family and to attempt to create a calm and peaceful place for the patient to die. For all that healthcare providers might wish that the death occurred elsewhere, the ED is the final common pathway for many difficult health issues.[6] Patients with advanced illness present to the ED in the last months, weeks, and even days of life, with the proportion of patients presenting to the ED during the final 2 weeks of life reported to be as high as 40%. All of these patients need some level of palliative care.[10] Debriefing and bereavement for the staff when a patient dies in the ED are essential components of palliative care and staff support.

Case study

KR, a 59-year-old man with metastatic lung cancer

KR, was a 59-year-old man with metastatic lung cancer who had spent a significant amount of time over the past 3 months in the hospital. During his last admission, the medical team had talked to him about hospice care, but he had stated he was "not ready." On this particular warm summer day, he had again become acutely short of breath, confused, and lethargic. His wife had called the emergency medical service (EMS) and he had arrived in the ED. He was initially placed in a room across from the nurses' station and two rooms down from the acute holding room for psychiatric patients. The room was small and did not have space for all the family members who wanted to be with KR. The ED doctors consulted with the hospital oncologist as well as the palliative care team, who agreed that KR was actively dying. The initial plan was to transfer him to the palliative care floor; however, no beds were available. One of the ED nurses, sensitive to the needs of the patient and family, suggested that the patient be moved to the 24-hour observation part of the ED. The rooms were larger and not nearly as noisy and would enable the family to stay with the patient more easily. The observation area of the ED did not typically take actively dying patients, and the nurses were initially uncomfortable with the idea. They felt unprepared to take care of a dying patient. However, after discussing the plan of care, including starting a versed drip and giving morphine as needed, and reassuring them that the interdisciplinary palliative care team would be involved in the care of the patient and family, including a chaplain and social worker, the nurses agreed. The palliative care nurses from the inpatient floor sent a handmade quilt and pillowcase down for the patient. These were gifts symbolizing caring that the family could take home with them after the patient died. The palliative care team helped put in orders for comfort care and spoke to the family and staff about the changes that would occur as KR went through the dying process. KR spent 5 hours in the observation unit before he died. He was able to experience a peaceful and dignified death, and the family was able to be by his side when he passed. The ER nurses caring for the patient admitted that while they were uncomfortable at first, by the time the patient passed they were proud that they were able to provide such good care and a dignified death to the patient.

Special issues in the management of symptoms in the Emergency Department

The management of symptoms commonly experienced by patients at the end of life is addressed in detail in Section II of this textbook. However, there are certain issues specific to the management of symptoms in the ED that warrant mentioning. The very nature of ED patient evaluation, with multitasking and frequent interruptions coupled with ED crowding, may contribute to poor symptom assessment. High ED census and the need for rapid triage may also negatively impact the quality of care delivered. For example, there may be significant delays in the assessment of pain, documentation of pain scores, and actual pain management. It is known that patient-related factors, such as age, gender, and race/ethnicity, as well as characteristics of the treating clinician are associated with disparities in pain care.[11]

The growing problem of prescription drug abuse, superimposed on a chronic national epidemic of undertreated pain, has generated unprecedented scrutiny on opioid prescribing in the United States. While there are numerous reasons why ED providers may be hesitant to provide opiate analgesia, concern about patients seeking medication for nontherapeutic purposes is among the most common. Such patients are estimated to account for as many as 20% of all ED visits, and are often labeled as "drug-seeking." Furthermore, they often present with conditions that are difficult to evaluate and easily feigned, such as headache, back pain, and dental pain.[12] Prescription monitoring programs have emerged as a means of identifying patients trying to obtain medication for nonmedical purposes. The use of prescription monitoring programs in the ED has been shown to affect prescribing behavior, and in one study such a program changed ED prescribing practice in more than 60% of cases.[13] The increase of prescription drug abuse makes it challenging for ED providers to feel confident in providing adequate pain medication while keeping patients safe. It is important for healthcare providers to remember that despite the challenges, pain management is an important part of emergency medicine, especially when seeing patients with advanced disease and terminal illness. Uncontrolled pain and other symptoms in a terminally ill and dying patient presenting to the ED should be viewed as a medical and nursing emergency and treated as such. The ED nurse, as patient advocate, must ensure that this happens.

Other acute symptoms frequently seen in the ED include dyspnea, nausea/vomiting, delirium, and agitation. The ED environment, often noisy and frenetic, can be overwhelming to any patient, especially those with a terminal illness. Patients and caregivers may experience increased anxiety, associated with the long wait times both in the ED holding area and pending admission to a hospital bed. Patients are often symptomatic while waiting and uncertain and worried as to what the exacerbation in symptoms might imply. Frequent communication by the ED nurse updating the patient and family about what is happening and what to expect can do much to allay their anxiety.

Respiratory symptoms can cause much distress and suffering in patients who present to the ED. Dyspnea is a subjective awareness of having difficulty breathing. One of the most common and most feared symptoms among cancer patients, it occurs in approximately 20% to 40% of patients at the time of diagnosis of advanced disease and increases up to 70% in the last 6 weeks of life.[14] Treatment of dyspnea or respiratory distress can be organized into three categories: prevention, treatment of the underlying cause, and palliation of symptom distress. Prevention of dyspnea in the dying ED patient warrants maximizing treatments that have proven beneficial to the patient, including enhancing ventilator synchrony if the patient is going to remain ventilated, avoiding volume overload, and continuing oxygen and nebulized bronchodilators. Measures to correct metabolic acidosis may also be useful to decrease the work of breathing and thereby decrease respiratory distress.[15,16] Treating underlying causes of dyspnea in the ED may be useful, particularly if the benefit of the treatment is not in disproportion to the burden. If death is not imminent, the patient may benefit from antibiotics, corticosteroids, paracentesis, pleurodesis, or bronchoscopy. Fear and anxiety may also be components of the respiratory distress experienced by the ED patient. Care of the patient's family and loved ones to reduce their fear, anxiety, and grief warrants as much effort as that directed to the patient's symptoms. Please refer to Section II in this textbook for in-depth discussions on the assessment and management of common symptoms in the terminally ill.

Family presence

Studies have consistently demonstrated that families want to be close to their terminally ill loved ones.[17,18] Family access promotes cohesion, affords the opportunity for closure, and may soothe the patient. Unrestricted access of the family to the dying patient is a standard of care in the majority of hospitals and nursing homes. The family of the patient who is dying in the ED should be afforded this same benefit. There is growing evidence and support for the successful implementation of families at the side of loved ones during resuscitation and invasive procedures in the ED.[19-21] Although additional "outcomes" research is needed, it is logical that if families and patients can be accommodated with open access to one another in the ED during procedures, then unrestricted visiting for the dying patient and grieving family is possible. Emergency departments may consider first implementing a family presence program in children or adults with nontraumatic cardiac arrest, and then extend successful practices to traumatic cardiac arrest. The latter involves special challenges, especially when gang violence is suspected.

Ideally, a dying patient and family should be separated from the harried milieu of the ED whether the death is expected to occur in the ED or transfer to a inpatient hospital bed is pending, yet should remain visible and accessible for close monitoring and care. Movement to a quieter area in the ED, such as the observation care unit or an isolation room, may serve this purpose, particularly if there is space for a few chairs and the attendant family. Limiting visitors to only two at a time has no rationale if the patient is dying and there is a large, loving family.

Improving palliative care in the Emergency Department

Palliative care focuses on the physical, spiritual, psychological, and social care from diagnosis of a potentially life-threatening illness to cure or death. When cure is not attainable and the end of life approaches, the intensity of palliative care is enhanced to deliver the highest quality care to both the patient and their loved ones. The ED frequently cares for patients and families during the end-of-life phase of the palliative care continuum. The intersection between palliative care and emergency care continues to be on the forefront of healthcare.

There is a mounting body of evidence to guide the most effective strategies for improving palliative care in the ED. In a workgroup session at the 2009 Agency for Healthcare Research and Quality (AHRQ)/American College of Emergency Physicians (ACEP) conference "Improving the Quality and Efficiency of Emergency Care Across the Continuum: A Systems Approach," four key research questions arose: (1) Which patients are in greatest need of palliative care services in the ED? (2) What is the optimal role of emergency clinicians in caring for patients along a chronic trajectory

of illness? (3) How does the integration and initiation of palliative care training and services in the ED setting affect healthcare utilization? and (4) What are the educational priorities for emergency clinical providers in the domain of palliative care?[22-24] Adopting the core palliative skills of symptom management, effective communication and goals of care discussions, along with a strong understanding of end-of-life issues is essential and should be melded into the skill set of all ED healthcare staff. The development of tools and protocols to identify and address the needs of terminally ill patients in the ED is also an important research priority.

Education in palliative and end-of-life care for Emergency Department Nurses and Physicians

High-quality curriculums such as the End-of-Life Nursing Education Consortium—Critical Care (ELNEC-CC) for ED nurses (described in more detail below), and the Education in Palliative and End-of-Life Care–Emergency Medicine project (EPEC-EM), funded by the National Cancer Institute of the NIH, for ED physicians, can greatly assist in teaching and improving core knowledge, skills, and attitudes in palliative care.[22-24]

The ELNEC-CC curriculum is a joint collaboration between the City of Hope National Medical Center and the American Association of Colleges of Nursing. It is designed to train emergency and critical care nurses in palliative and end-of-life care.[22] The ELNEC-CC curriculum is a comprehensive training program that covers content areas of symptom management, communication strategies, care at the end of life, ethics, cultural issues, and loss and bereavement. The goal is to assist nurses in expanding their holistic care of the patients and families. Extensive support materials such as a CD, binder of printed materials, case studies, textbooks, and other educational materials are provided to participants to educate colleagues about palliative and end-of-life care in critical care settings. Hospice and palliative care nursing is recognized at a generalist level as an integral part of all nursing care. It is also recognized as a nursing specialty requiring specific education at an advanced level and board certification. The reader is referred to chapter 66 for in-depth discussion on education opportunities in palliative care for nurses.

The EPEC-EM is another educational curriculum designed to teach emergency clinicians about palliative and end-of-life care so that clinicians can incorporate these skills and interventions into their daily practices.[24] The EPEC-EM curriculum provides core clinical competencies in palliative and end-of-life care for emergency clinicians through teaching modalities that incorporate interactive lecture, case vignettes, and role-play, among others.[24] Palliative and end-of-life topics are presented, such as trajectories of approaching death, prognoses of illnesses, rapid palliative care assessment, establishing goals of care, ethical and legal issues, withholding and withdrawing treatment, family-witnessed resuscitation, and pain and symptom management. Hospice and Palliative Medicine is now an official medical subspecialty, and the American Board of Emergency Medicine is a cosponsoring board. However, the number of board-certified emergency physicians who are also board certified in this subspecialty remains small, though the number is growing.[23] For those emergency care providers who want to learn more about this discipline, education and training is available through programs like EPEC-EM and the

Harvard Program in Palliative Care Education and Practice. The Harvard program is an interdisciplinary program in which nurses both participate and teach.[24] These training programs allow nurse and physicians to serve as palliative care champions in their own EDs. More recently, a number of pilot programs have been developed by palliative care teams to partner with EDs.[28]

Summary

Dying care in the ED can be complicated by the milieu and by the usual "resuscitative" expectations of this environment. A default view of ED success is whether the patient left the ED with return of spontaneous circulation. The fact that a growing number of patients are presenting to the ED at the end of life demands palliative care competency by ED staff. In most EDs, there are clinicians who are willing to guide terminally ill patients or their surrogates toward a palliative care approach, in which success is redefined as preventing suffering and enabling a good death.

An abundance of evidence about managing pain and dyspnea is available to guide the ED staff in reducing symptoms and distress. Similarly, optimal care for the grieving family has been informed by research and includes effective communication about prognosis or death notification and timely access to the patient before or after death. Personal and professional satisfaction with comprehensive palliative care in the ED can be achieved by ED staff. Compassionate recommendations made to decrease suffering and ensure respect for the dying patient can afford the survivors a positive experience, even in the face of loss.[25]

References

1. Baseball Almanac. 2013. *Joaquin Andujar Quotes.* Retrieved October 31, 2013, from http://www.baseball-almanac.com/quotes/quoandj.shtml.
2. Flores-Mateo G, Violan-Fors C, Carrillo-Santisteve P, Peiró S, Argimon, J. 2012. *Effectiveness of Organizational Interventions to Reduce Emergency Department Utilization: A Systematic Review.* Retrieved from http://www.plosone.org/article/info%3Adoi%2F10.1371%2Fjournal.pone.0035903.
3. Centers for Disease Control. 2013. *Emergency Department Visits.* Retrieved from FASTFACTS: http://www.cdc.gov/nchs/fastats/ervisits.htm#.
4. Centers for Disease Control. 2012. *United States Health, Emergency Department.* Retrieved from United States Health: www.cdc.gov/nchs/data/hus/hus12.pdf
5. Brown L, Burton R, Hixon B, et al. Factors influencing emergency department preference for access to healthcare. West J Emerg Med. 2012;13(5):410–415.
6. Ieraci S. Palliative care in the emergency department. Emerg Med Aus. 2013;25(2):112–113. doi:10.1111/1742-6723.12053.
7. Limehouse D, Feeser VR, Bookman K, Derse A. A model for emergency department end-of-life communications after acute devastating events—Part I: Decision-making capacity, surrogates, and advance directives. Acad Emerg Med. 2012;19(9):1068–1072. doi:10.1111/j.1553-2712.2012.01426.x.
8. Bomba P. POLST: An improvement over traditional advance directives. Clev Clin J Med. 2012;79:457–464. doi:10.3949/ccjm.79a.11098.
9. Vawter L, Ratner E. 2010. *The Need for POLST: Minnesota's Initiative.* Retrieved from Minnesota Medicine: http://www-ncbi-nlm-nih-gov.proxy.library.vcu.edu/pmc/articles/PMC2837547/
10. Wallace EM, Cooney MC, Walsh J, Conroy M, Twomey F. Why do palliative care patients present to the emergency department? Avoidable or unavoidable? Amer J Hosp Palliat Med. 2013;30(3):253–256. doi:10.1177/1049909112447285.
11. Hwang U, Richardson L, Livote E, Harris B, Spencer N, Morrison RS. Emergency department crowding and decreased quality of pain care. Acad Emerg Med. 2008;15(12):1248–1255.
12. Hawkins S, Smeeks F, Hamel J. Emergency management of chronic pain and drug-seeking behavior: an alternate perspective. J Emerg Med. 2008;34:125–129.
13. Grover C, Garmel G. How do emergency physicians interpret prescription narcotic history when assessing patients presenting to the emergency department with pain? Permenente J. 2012;16(4):32–36.
14. Hui D, Morgado M, Vidal M, et al. Dyspnea in hospitalized advanced cancer patients: Subjective and physiologic correlates. J Palliat Med. 2013;16(3):274–280. doi:10.1089/jpm.2012.0364.
15. Campbell ML. Nurse to Nurse Palliative Care. New York, NY: McGraw-Hill; 2009.
16. Navigante AH, Cerchietti LC, Castro MA, Lutteral MA, Cabalar ME Midazolam as adjunct therapy to morphine in the alleviation of severe dyspnea perception in patients with advanced cancer. J Pain Symp Manage. 2006;31(1), 38–47.
17. Hampe SO. Needs of the grieving spouse in a hospital setting. Nurs Res. 1975;24:113–120.
18. Steinhauser KE, Christakis NA, Clipp EC, McNeilly M, McIntyre L, Tulsky JA. Factors considered important at the end of life by patients, family, physicians, and other care providers. JAMA. 2000;284:2476–2482.
19. Duran CR, Oman KS, Abel JJ, Koziel VM, Szymanski D. Attitudes toward and beliefs about family presence: a survey of healthcare providers, patients' families, and patients. Amer J Crit Care, 2007;16(3):270–279.
20. Swinburn CR, Mould H, Stone TN, Corris PA, Gibson GJ. Symptomatic benefit of supplemental oxygen in hypoxemic patients with chronic lung disease. Amer Rev Resp Dis. 1991;143:913–915.
21. Booth S, Kelly MJ, Cox NP, Adams L, Guz A. Does oxygen help dyspnea in patients with cancer? Amer J Resp Crit Care Med. 1996;153:1515–1518.
22. Ferrell BR, Dahlin C, Campbell ML, Paice JA, Malloy P, Virani R. End-of-life nursing education consortium (ELNEC) training program: Improving palliative care in critical care. Crit Care Nurs Q, 2007;30:206–212.
23. Grudzen C, Byrant E. 2011. Making the Case for Palliative Care in the ED. Retrieved from ACEP News: http://www.acep.org/Content.aspx?id=79796.
24. Emanuel LL, Quest T, eds. The Education in Palliative and End-of-Life Care for Emergency Medicine (EPEC-EM) Curriculum. The EPEC Project. Chicago, IL: Author; 2007.
25. Chan GK, Campbell ML, Zalenski R. The Emergency Department. In Ferrell BR, Nessa C. The Oxford Textbook of Palliative Nursing. Oxford: University Press; 2010: 949–959.
26. Campbell ML. Communicating a poor prognosis and making decisions. In: Foregoing Life-Sustaining Therapy: How to Care for the Patient Who Is Near Death. Aliso Veijo, CA: American Association of Critical-Care Nurses; 1998: 19–41.

CHAPTER 51

The role of nursing in caring for patients undergoing palliative surgery for advanced disease

Anna Cathy Williams, Betty R. Ferrell, Gloria Juarez, and Tami Borneman

This is all too much. Even if I have this surgery, I will not be cured. Maybe I should just let the cancer take its natural course and trust that God will do His best by me and let me die sooner than later.

A patient

Key points

- Patients and their family caregivers facing surgery for advanced disease have complex physical and psychosocial needs.
- Patients and family members require support as they make decisions regarding the benefits and burdens of treatments for advanced disease.
- Palliative surgeries affect physical, psychological, social, and spiritual well-being as well as additional health system outcomes.

Palliative surgery

The probability of being diagnosed with an advanced cancer is 44% for males and 38% for females.[1] However, overall survival rates have increased in recent years, with almost 10.8 million individuals with cancer being alive in 2004, with the majority of deaths stemming from metastasis, or progression, of the disease.[1] Of these millions of patients, most are now receiving palliative care during their last months of life.

A relatively novel approach in oncology care, the field of palliative surgery is rapidly increasing with more focused educational preparation for healthcare professionals by way of algorithms, specific procedures, and surgeries. A great deal of reevaluation has been instituted in presenting new forums to underscore the need for relief of symptom burden, and to enhance quality of life (QOL), even though the process itself does not prolong a patient's life.[1]

Although newer in the traditional setting, palliative care and surgeries are emerging at a very rapid pace. As the path of the surgeon, the patient's disease trajectory, and that of palliative intervention overlap, it is possible for professional and personal conflicts to arise, with negotiations needing to take place. Surgeons and palliative care colleagues, along with other health team members and patients, will need to collaborate on a very intimate level and often.[2] With the expansion of this clinical expertise, managing such complex and end-of-life decisions in palliative care will become an increasingly crucial and integrated part of interventions in the healthcare setting.[2]

Case study
Isabella Mendez, a 28-year-old woman with stage IV renal carcinoma

Mrs. Mendez was a native Californian who was the mother of three children, the youngest being age 2. She and her spouse, Ernesto, owned a small auto repair shop, which provided a good living for the family. Approximately 4 months prior, Mrs. Mendez began to notice pink urine, back pain just below the ribs, weight loss, fatigue, and intermittent fevers. After attempting to treat the symptoms using over-the-counter medications and herbal treatments, without success, she was evaluated at a community clinic and was found to have stage IV renal cancer. The family sought care at a large university cancer center and placed great trust in the fact that Isabella's cancer would be cured, as one of her cousins had been treated successfully there the previous year. After undergoing neoadjuvant chemotherapy, to which there was little therapeutic response, she was scheduled for a surgical consult, for palliative intervention. At the oncology appointment, the surgeon explained the seriousness of her cancer, as well as results from diagnostic imaging, which showed widespread metastases to the lung. When the surgeon discussed treatment options with the family, Isabella and Ernesto, along with her extended family voiced a desire for aggressive treatment. Isabella expressed her desire to "try anything" in treating the cancer, and she repeated her confidence in the abilities of the surgeon and his team to save her life. The surgeon attempted to clarify to Isabella and her spouse that the planned surgical procedure was not curative and the procedure was primarily offered for symptom control. Both Isabella and Ernesto stated that they had faith in God, as well as the skills of the surgeon, and again articulated their confidence that her cancer would be cured. Later that evening (the day before surgery), the evening nurse approached Isabella for discussion of the surgical consent. Isabella stated that she had no questions and was eager to sign any surgical consent needed, because the sooner she had the surgery, the faster her cancer would be cured.

This case illustrates the numerous complexities of caring for patients with advanced disease for whom surgical treatment may be an option. The healthcare team, including the nurse, is faced with caring for this patient who has advanced cancer and a poor prognosis, yet both the patient and family are expecting a "miracle." There are many intricate cultural and social factors affecting her decisions for care as well. The nurse is challenged to work with the patient, her family, the physician, and other interdisciplinary colleagues to provide the best information and support. They will also be anticipating the many immediate postoperative needs as well as the longer term symptom management and disease issues. This case is only one example of the incredibly complicated and challenging needs of patients undergoing surgery for advanced disease.

Decision-making in palliative surgery

Patients confronting advanced disease are frequently in the position of making arduous choices regarding treatments. They often face a critical juncture of determining when they should continue disease-focused treatments such as chemotherapy, radiation, or surgery, and when it is time to discontinue such interventions. Even amid the recognition of advanced disease, patients frequently seek aggressive treatment with the hope of prolonging their survival, even if only for a matter of months—or of possibly enhancing their QOL through the relief of symptoms.[3-4]

Research performed on 98 individuals undergoing palliative care and surgical consultations revealed essential aspects in the comprehensive interventions of these oncology patients.[4] An indispensable part to the all-embracing care given to these individuals is the decision-making criteria chosen by the patients after their palliative consultations. This prospective observational study enrolled the cohort and dispensed open-ended questionnaires to them inquiring as to the reasons they made the decision to receive palliative surgery or not. The results of the research revealed that 44 patients elected surgical intervention and 54 did not. Reasons for the intervention were QOL and symptom relief (the two main reasons), prolonged life expectancy, and treatment of the cancer itself. Those who chose against surgery cited complication concerns, physician recommendations, religious issues, and other unclear responses.[4]

Timing is another very significant decision-making issue in palliative surgery.[5] Badgwell et al. cite a study in which researchers were interested in determining when surgical intervention was at the most favorable juncture. This prospective study enrolled 77 patients going through palliative surgical intervention consultation. Follow-up consisted of QOL assessment at 1 and 3 months. The bulk of patients were operated on due to bowel obstruction. Of the total population 44% were treated in a nonoperative fashion, whereas 44% were operated on, with 12% undergoing endoscopic intervention. Forty percent of the patients expired before the study's completion. Unfortunately, the data revealed that a larger population would be required to adequately measure for QOL differences. However, the research was interesting in the fact that it did point to anticipating the need for developing a satisfactory time frame in which to perform palliative surgery and the need for the expertise itself.[5]

Figure 51.1 is derived from research in the area of palliative surgery conducted at the City of Hope (COH) National Medical Center.[6] The model demonstrates that the process of making decisions about palliative surgery involves influences from the patient, the family, and the healthcare team. Patients and families must weigh the potential benefit versus the harm of the surgery proposed, whereas the healthcare team considers factors such as the difficulty of the procedure, the duration of hospitalization, recovery time, chance of achieving the goal, anticipated resilience of the intervention, and anticipated disease progression.[6-8] It becomes evident in reviewing these factors that much of the decision-making involves great individual variants, so that it is difficult to estimate who might profit most from more aggressive treatment. For example, the patient with a poor prognosis resulting from an extremely advanced gastrointestinal tumor, who subsequently lives twice the original duration anticipated, may well have benefited from surgery to relieve obstruction for abdominal pressure causing severe nausea, vomiting, or bowel problems.[6-8]

The process of making decisions involves a focus on goals of care, recognizing the values of the patient, acknowledging alternatives, and continuously weighing the risks versus benefits.[9] As surgeries have become more technically advanced, it is often possible to perform very extensive surgery on an outpatient basis or with very short hospitalization times. This reduced "burden" makes it more likely that patients may opt for surgical procedures. Given the many symptoms or problems resulting from advanced disease, patients consider a variety of treatment choices, including surgery, chemotherapy, radiotherapy, or a combination of treatments.

The outcomes of this process of decision-making are depicted in Figure 51.1 as affecting all dimensions of QOL. Physical well-being and symptoms, as well as function, are almost always affected by treatment choices.[10,11] Psychological well-being, including anxiety and depression as well as fear, is also influenced by treatment choices.[3,9,11,12] Patients and families have often reflected that although a particular treatment may have not prolonged survival, it gave them a tremendous sense of assurance that everything possible was being done to treat the illness. In the realm of social well-being, the choices of treatments have very significant impact on the patient's roles and relationships as well as the burden on the caregiver.[10,12-15]

Although invasive, "high-tech" treatments may be thought of as adding to the caregiver burden; in advanced disease, the failure

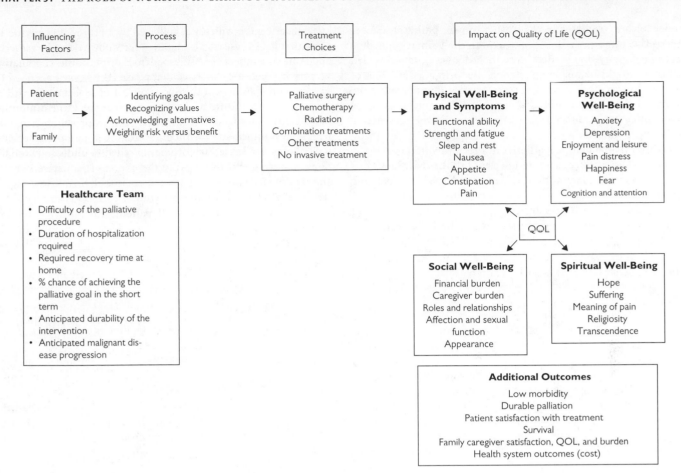

Figure 51.1 Clinical decision-making in palliative surgery. Source: Ferrell et al. (2003), reference 9.

to aggressively treat problems commonly results in heightened burden. For example, a patient who declines surgery relatively early in the course of an advanced gastrointestinal tumor may then experience much worse nausea, vomiting, diarrhea, and subsequent complications that could result in a more intense caregiver burden than would have been required after earlier surgery.

Finally, spiritual well-being is greatly influenced by decisions regarding palliative surgery, because patients rely on their faith and religion in making treatment choices.[1,3] One of the strongest themes throughout palliative care research has been the concept of hope. This concept is covered in greater detail in chapter 28, but it certainly applies closely to the topic of palliative surgery. Patients may perceive that surgery, even if presented as only palliative in nature, is still potentially curative or life prolonging, and therefore may opt for surgery with unfounded hope for a cure.[16]

The model in Figure 51.1 illustrates how important it is for nurses to provide education, counseling, and support as patients and families wrestle with treatment choices. It also is not uncommon for patients and families to have different perspectives and conflicting opinions. For example, a patient with advanced disease may opt for no further invasive treatments and instead focus on measures of comfort. At the same time, family members may press for the patient to endure continued procedures for even the smallest possibility of prolonged survival.

Research in palliative surgery

Research in the field of palliative care has been sparse with even less focus in the area of palliative surgery. Recent studies have begun to document both the lack of research in the field and the limitations of existing research.[17–19] Leaders in the field of palliative surgery have documented that few studies evaluating these procedures have included measures of patient QOL, symptom management, or psychosocial concerns.[18]

As mentioned by Geoffrey Dunn[20] regarding the aforementioned Badgwell study, the data numbers were inadequate, but they offered numerous indications for potential future QOL studies for palliative intervention, patient decision-making, and the use of multidisciplinary efforts.[20] Palliative care is becoming more expansive, and surgeons have good reason to use the expertise among palliative care health professionals. Dunn cites that surgeons alone rate as poor predictors of patient survival in palliative interventions. In the not-too-distant past, there were few options for patients with stage IV disease. It is only through research and collaboration that we will achieve any measure of promoting QOL in advanced-stage oncology patients.[20]

A research study review by Anwar et al. in 2011[21] demonstrated a survival benefit from surgery for some patients with advanced colorectal cancer. The population consisted of colorectal patients with stage IV disease. Individuals on study could choose either traditional chemotherapy or palliative resection of the tumor. Median survival was the primary outcome measure. Twenty-one studies were included, and data revealed that there might be a survival benefit for primary resection of stage IV colorectal disease. The research also mentions that the surgery should be performed according to tumor burden and the patient's performance status rather than on the presence or absence of symptoms.[21]

Research in the area of palliative surgery was initiated at the COH in 2000, and since that time a series of studies have been conducted involving collaboration between the Division of Nursing Research and the Department of Surgery. Box 51.1 summarizes phases of this research to-date. The studies included a review of surgical cases to determine the extent of palliative surgery used

at a cancer center, which was followed by a prospective review of cases that led to research evaluating decision-making by patients and family members.[22,23] To broaden understanding of palliative surgery beyond one cancer center, phase III involved a survey of 419 surgeon members of the Society of Surgical Oncology.[24,25] A very important finding of this research was the identification of ethical dilemmas faced by surgeons, such as providing patients with honest information without destroying hope and preserving patient choices. These early studies have led to clinical investigations exploring effort to capture the effects of palliative surgery and its potential impact on symptoms and QOL.[26] These inquiries have also provided an opportunity to incorporate qualitative methods for exploration of patient and family caregiver experiences.[1,3]

Box 51.1 Description of program of research

Phase I

Surgical Palliation at a Cancer Center[27]

Design: Retrospective review of surgical cases (*n* = 1915) during a 1-year period with a 1-year survival follow-up. This descriptive study began exploration of the extent of palliative surgery and identification of patient outcomes.

Key findings: Palliative surgeries (PS) made up 240 (12.5%) of 1915 surgical procedures. There were 170 major and 70 minor procedures. Neurosurgical (46.0%), orthopedic (31.3%), and thoracic (21.5%) surgical procedures were frequently PS. The most common primary diagnoses were lung, colorectal, breast, and prostate cancers. Length of hospital stay was 12.4 days (range, 0–99 days). Mortality was 21.9% for surgical procedures classified as major and 10.0% for those classified as minor. The investigators concluded that in significant numbers of PS mortality was high; however, a significant number of patients had short hospital stays and low morbidity. Thus, PS should remain an important part of end-of-life care. Patients and their families must be aware of the high risks and understand the clear objectives of these procedures.

Phase II

Advancing the Evaluation of PS for Cancer Patients[23]

Design: Prospective review of PS (*n* = 50). Pilot testing of interview guide for use with patients, family caregivers (FCG) and surgeons to explore decision-making and goals.

Key findings: Prospective design allowed expansion of outcomes to include QOL and exploration of the involvement of FCG.

Phase III

Indications and Use of Palliative Surgery—Results of Society of Surgical Oncology (SSO) Survey[24,25]

Design: Mailed survey (110 items) of members of the SSO (*n* = 419 responses). This phase was intended to provide a national perspective on the topic of PS and to expand knowledge of surgeons' decision-making.

Key findings: Surgeons estimated 21% of their cancer surgeries as PS in nature; 43% of respondents believed PS was best defined based on preoperative intent, 27% based on postoperative factors, and 30% on patient prognosis. Only 43% considered estimated patient survival time an important factor in defining PS, and 22% considered 5-year survival rate important. Patient symptom and pain relief were identified as the two most important goals in PS, with increased survival the least important. On a scale of 1 (uncommon problem) to 7 (common problem), surgeons reported that the most frequent ethical dilemmas in PS were providing patients with honest information without destroying hope and preserving patient choice. On a scale of 1 (not a barrier) to 7 (severe barrier), surgeons rated the most severe barriers to optimum use of PS as limitations of managed care and referral to surgery by other specialists. The least severe barriers were surgeon avoidance of dying patients and surgery department reluctance to perform PS.

Phase IV

A Prospective Evaluation of Palliative Outcomes for Surgery of Advanced Malignancies[26]

Design: Prospective evaluation of patients undergoing PS (*n* = 59) with longitudinal measures for 1 year. Outcomes were expanded to provide more detailed evaluation of symptom management and QOL. Qualitative evaluation included in-depth interviews of patients, FCG, and surgeons pre- and postoperatively to further describe decisions and outcomes related to surgery.

Key findings: Preoperatively, surgeons identified 22 operations (37%) as PS, 37 (63%) as curative. Thirty-three patients (56%) were symptomatic preoperatively, and symptom resolution was documented in 79% surviving >30 days. Good to excellent palliation, defined as "more than 70% symptom-free non-hospitalized days relative to postoperative days of life," was achieved in 53% of PS patients. Among patients with postoperative survival <6 months, 63% had good to excellent palliation. The majority of symptomatic patients undergoing major surgery for advanced malignancies attained good to excellent symptom relief. The researchers concluded that outcome measurements other than survival are feasible and are likely to play an important role in defining surgery as an important component of multimodality palliative care.

(continued)

Box 51.1 Continued

Phase V

A Comparison of Resource Consumption in Curative and Palliative Surgery[22]

Design: Prospective evaluations of all surgeries performed over a 3-month period ($n = 302$) with 6-month follow-up. The investigators extended the outcomes of surgery to be evaluated based on Phases I–IV.

Key findings: Over a 4-month period, the outcome and service needs of 302 consecutive patients with malignancy undergoing surgeon-defined PS or curative surgery were evaluated. Previous treatment history, comorbidities, symptoms, procedures, outcome, and use of supportive services were collected. Patients were monitored for 6 months after the surgical procedures performed for cure (breast or prostate cancer) or for palliation (breast, lung, and bone and soft tissue tumors). There were 3 (1%) curative and 4 (6%) palliative deaths during the surgical admission. Mean hospital stay was 5.1 days (range, 0–58 days) for curative surgery patients and 1.9 days (range, 0–34 days) for PS patients. After discharge, a total of 4690 encounters with the cancer center occurred, including 1676 encounters with surgery, 1595 encounters with medical oncology, 1006 encounters with radiation oncology, 226 visits to medical specialists, and 187 visits with supportive services. Mean number of encounters for curative and PS patients were 15 and 17, respectively ($P = 0.41$). Curative patients were more likely to have visits with therapeutic intent, including chemotherapy ($P = 0.01$) and radiation ($P = 0.003$). Readmission occurred in 82 (34%) of curative and 28 (48%) PS patients during the 6-month period ($P = 0.04$). PS patients were more likely to be admitted for symptom management ($P = 0.0001$), whereas curative surgery patients were more likely to be admitted for repeat procedures ($P = 0.006$).

Phase VI

Concerns of Family Caregivers of Cancer Patients Facing Surgery for Advanced Malignancies (Borneman et al., 2003)[3]

Design: FCG were assessed before planned PS and at 2 and 6 weeks after surgery. Quantitative assessment of caregiver QOL occurred at each time point. A subset of nine CG also participated in a structured interview before surgery and 2 weeks after surgery.

Key findings: The study findings indicate important FCG QOL concerns and needs for support at the time surrounding surgery for advanced disease. Psychological issues were most pronounced with common needs of uncertainty, fears regarding the future, and loss. FCG voiced concerns about surgical risks and care postoperatively and experienced recognition of the patient's declining status. The investigators concluded that surgery is an important component of palliative care and is an area requiring further research and clinical attention.

Patient perspectives

The research at COH has explored patient perspectives of surgery through in-depth individual interviews conducted pre and postoperatively, as well as assessment of symptoms and QOL. Box 51.2 includes some representative comments from patients' perspectives of QOL after surgery. As this study demonstrates, patients may believe that surgery is their only option to avoid progression and eventual death from their disease. The presence of physical symptoms has been found to be a key motivator for seeking surgical intervention. Even those patients who recognize that surgery is not curative may aggressively seek surgical approaches to relieve distressing physical symptoms such as pain, gastrointestinal symptoms, bleeding, odors, and other problems. These studies also demonstrated that tremendous psychological stress and anxiety are induced by the need to make decisions about surgical options. Also, it is not uncommon to find evidence of far more advanced disease during the surgery than was originally identified.

The COH investigators also examined differences in resource utilization of surgical patients following curative or palliative procedures. Results showed that the number of resources utilized was similar in both groups but that the nature of interactions was different.[22] This suggests that resource needs are different for the two treatment intents. In a separate analysis of advanced gastrointestinal cases, Podnos and colleagues described the effect of palliative surgical procedures on symptoms and overall QOL. The most common symptom reported was pain associated with obstruction.[27] The frequency of primary symptoms improved postoperatively, but overall QOL decreased over time.[8]

Family caregivers

The palliative surgery research at the COH has also described the concerns of family caregivers of patients undergoing palliative surgery for advanced malignancies. Family caregivers ($n = 45$) were assessed before planned palliative surgery and at 2 and 6 weeks after surgery.[10] Quantitative assessment of caregiver QOL occurred at each interval. A subset of nine caregivers also participated in structured interviews before surgery and 2 weeks after surgery. Caregiver concerns, QOL, and decision-making were evaluated. Findings of the study indicated that family caregivers have important QOL concerns and need for support before and after surgery for advanced disease. Psychological issues were most pronounced, and common concerns included uncertainty, fears regarding the future, and loss. Further analysis suggested that family caregivers also experienced disruptions in overall QOL that were similar to those experienced by patients.[28,29] Caregivers' distress levels were high prior to surgery, and overall distress continued to worsen over time after the surgery. Financial burden for caregivers included transportation, medications, and other services that were not covered by insurance. In a path analysis of variables influencing caregiver burden in palliative care, Grove and colleagues found a direct significant association between caregiver depression and caregiver burden.[30] The effects of other variables, such as patient's symptom status, social support, and caregiver overall QOL, on caregiver burden were all mediated by caregiver depression.[30]

Family caregivers had concerns about surgical risks and patient care needs after surgery and voiced recognition of the declining

---

Box 51.2 Patient perspectives on QOL and surgery

Surgery-only option:

"Because this is one of the slower—slower growing cancers, radiation and chemo wouldn't have helped at all. So there was—there was no option other than—other than the surgery—there was no option."

Gastrointestinal symptoms:

"I used to always, I had the constant urge that I was going to have a bowel movement. Well, I did not have a bowel movement, but, and this urge was so strong, I'd go in and sit on the toilet. And then, of course, I would pass some mucus and stuff. Um, there for awhile before the surgery, oh, it was just terrible. And a lot of it would be quite bloody. And, ah, you know, I had a good day yesterday. I had a good night last night and the night before that I had a good night."

Psychological well-being:

"But now I feel even the surgery's not complete. I still have my tumor in my kidney. But that is not operable based on what [the doctor] told me. Just, just a few alternatives. You know, it's a surgery, remove the whole kidney? Or do the gene therapy? Or do the freezing or burn technique, you know. So there's still a chance."

Postsurgery quality of life:

"Yeah. Every time my friend, or whoever, has cancer, I told them don't give up. Find an alternative. If you're rejected by this doctor, don't just give up. Keep on trying whatever possible, whatever you have to go through. So, that's the only way. A lot of my friends are cancer patients. When they come to the end of the tunnel, they don't know how to and they are so depressed, I say don't worry. We already have the problem. You got to face it. Your worry doesn't help. You know, you got to ask God to give you a day. Use the medical technology available . . . Somebody may save you. You know, a miracle. This could happen to you, too. It happened to me many times."

Source: Ferrell et al. (2003), reference 9.

Box 51.3 Family caregivers' perspectives

Preoperative

Concerns about surgery and risks:

"I'm scared. I worry about just him getting through it . . . for the first few days, I'll still be worried. I'll be glad to do anything, you know, just to have him come home again. I know it's good to know the truth, and I'm glad that [the doctor] was so up front with us. But it's just so hard to deal with. Surgery's very scary. The chemotherapy and radiation was not scary. I knew he would get sick, but I knew that there was no chance of him dying from it. This is a whole different animal."

Benefits of surgery:

"I think it's a good thing. Because, you know, your immune system concentrates on, like, if you have a tumor, they concentrate all over the body. By taking this out, this is a big thing that, you know, it has cancer in it. By taking that out I feel like maybe her body can concentrate on other parts a little bit better than with, you know, with this in her. And then they're going to take the one out of her hip and I, I think it's a good thing. I'm glad that she's having the surgery."

Postoperative

No change in prognosis:

"It was more of a QOL thing. They'd like to get her eating, like to get her home. Like to get her spending her time in a way that she finds, you know, enjoyable. But, um, they're not planning on curing her or anything like that, I think she is aware of the prognosis. But, you know, like she said, she wants to still be in the treatment category more than, she doesn't want hospice at this point. So, although she knows that, she's not ready to just say that's it and prepare to die. She wants to do whatever she can to keep going."

Uncertain survival:

"The last day, of course, he was sleeping. I couldn't stand to even see him because his eyes were all swollen and his face was all swollen. But he never woke up on that second day anyway. That very morning, [the doctor] told me that it would be a long, slow recovery, but he was going to do okay and he had a 50–50 chance that morning. And that was at about 9 o'clock in the morning. And at 7 o'clock that night, [the doctor] told me he wasn't going to make it through the night. Do you know how that can throw a person emotionally? Do you? You have no idea what kind of an emotional roller coaster I was on for those 13 days. One day, everything's looking better. The next day everything was just horrible. I'm surprised I didn't end up having a heart attack myself or a nervous breakdown."

Source: Borneman et al. (2003), reference 3.

---

status of patients. The needs of family caregivers are multiple and complex, requiring ongoing assessment to provide interventions that help them cope and ultimately improve their QOL. This important topic requires further research and clinical attention.

Box 51.3 includes examples of family caregivers' perspectives provided both pre and postoperatively. Families articulated their concerns about the surgery and its risks and were more concerned than patients about potential negative consequences of surgery.[10] Family members often discussed the benefits of surgery, with a strong sense from both patients and family caregivers that surgery is always a good option because "to take it out" must increase one's chance for survival. For family members, however, the postoperative period was most often one of incredible stress as they faced the reality that the patient's prognosis was not likely to have changed and that surgery may in fact have revealed more evidence of advanced disease. For many patients, the surgical experience became a "roller coaster," in which they grasped for hope for a cure from surgery, even if intended as palliative, but hope was balanced by recognition of the patient's decline in status.

Nursing care of patients undergoing palliative surgery

The care of patients undergoing palliative surgery is often focused more on the medical aspects, yet nursing care is essential throughout all phases of preoperative, intraoperative, immediate postoperative, and postoperative recovery and discharge. This is a critical time, with numerous transitions between care settings, and nurses play a vital role in ensuring continuity across settings such as the operating room, intensive care unit (ICU), postoperative surgical unit, and home care. A prime example is the role of nursing in ensuring pain management by assessing a patient's chronic pain problem at the time of admission to plan adequate analgesia as the patient is admitted for surgery. The nurse then collaborates with the physician and pharmacist to plan the analgesic orders for the transition from the oral analgesics used preoperatively to an appropriate regimen postoperatively. Additional monitoring is needed as the patient's pain may escalate after major surgery. The nurse should also ensure the appropriate changes are instituted as the patient goes from chronic oral medications taken at home, to parenteral administration required in the postoperative period and in the ICU. Maintaining adequate analgesia after discharge from the ICU to the postoperative unit and then to home care is essential for the patient's timely discharge to home and remains a requirement during recovery. This is a simple example of just one aspect of care in pain management, illustrating the vital role of nursing during this very acute phase of treatment.

Patients with advanced disease often undergo surgery with the goal of palliation to achieve a longer survival, even when cure is not a realistic goal. The following case illustrates this point.

Case study
Nathan Washington, a 57-year-old-man with rectal cancer

Nathan Washington was a 57-year-old African-American man with stage IIIb rectal cancer who underwent neoadjuvant chemoradiation followed by anterior resection of his rectum. After a prolonged postoperative course and extensive recovery phase, Mr. Washington was able to return to work as a cook at a local restaurant. About 4 months after his initial surgery, Mr. Washington was admitted to the hospital with abdominal pain, dehydration, and nausea and vomiting that was refractory to antiemetics. The final diagnosis was malignant bowel obstruction, secondary to recurrence of his rectal cancer as well as chronic adhesions, a complication from his previous surgical procedure. The surgical team met with Mr. Washington and his spouse, Etta, to explain the status of his recurrence and treatment options for the malignant bowel obstruction. Because of the extent and location of the recurrence, it was suggested that a nonsurgical approach be taken to manage the obstruction with the use of octreotide. Other options, such as surgical removal of a portion of the recurrent tumor as well as the site of adhesion, were also discussed. The surgeon also wanted to discuss the fact that the recurrence meant that any procedure would only be palliative and not curative and that his prognosis was likely to worsen. Mr. Washington and his wife expressed their strong faith and belief that God would guide the surgeon in helping him with removal of all his remaining cancer. Mr. Washington also voiced an important goal for them: to make sure, at all costs, that he would live to see their son's college graduation in 6 months. This was a particularly significant event, because Mr. Washington's son would be the first in their family ever to receive a college degree.

This case illustrates the role of palliative surgery and the benefit of extending patient survival to achieve life goals even if a cure is not possible. Nurses would play a vital role in Mr. Washington's care, including aggressive management of his existing symptoms and additional psychosocial support required at that critical time in his illness, as he and his family confronted the reality of his worsening disease. Continued attention would also be needed after surgery to monitor his progress. For example, if his disease progressed more rapidly or if he developed postoperative complications that could have lead to shorter survival, it might have been necessary to work with the family to realize what choices they could have made if he had not lived to see the graduation. Supporting Mr. Washington's faith and the spiritual crisis that might have developed if he believed that God had abandoned him, was essential. This case also demonstrates the vital role of nurses in monitoring patients after surgery to assist with transitions to home care/hospice or palliative care programs.

The goal of symptom relief

The following case study illustrates the goal of symptom relief in palliative surgery.

Case study
Beatrice Fineman, an 80-year-old woman with pancreatic cancer

Beatrice Fineman is an 80-year-old Jewish American woman who was diagnosed with advanced pancreatic cancer approximately 2 months prior. After Mrs. Fineman was evaluated and informed of her diagnosis, she opted for supportive care only and initially was not interested in the possibility of surgery or chemotherapy; however, she did express a desire for aggressive symptom management with the goal of reducing her pain and maintaining her function and independence "as long as possible." Ms. Fineman was evaluated by a pain specialist at the local hospital. She was started on a pain regimen, but the treatment alone was unsuccessful in achieving significant pain relief. At this point, Ms. Anderson was referred to a surgeon and was presented with the option of surgical debulking to lessen the tumor burden and impingement of vital organs. At first her spouse was hesitant in having her undergo such an extensive surgery at age 80 years. However, Mrs. Fineman insisted on having the surgery if it would help with achieving some pain relief. The nurse practitioner in the surgical clinic met with the patient and family, as well as the surgeon, to describe the procedure and the expected postoperative course. Mrs. Fineman underwent surgery and recovered without any major complications, with the exception of an infection acquired during her postoperative stay at the hospital. Her pain significantly improved, although she remained on pain medications on an as-needed basis. She continued to be monitored by the pain specialist at the hospital.

This case reveals the role of surgery in relieving severe symptoms that have been unresponsive to less aggressive means. It also validates the importance of evaluating the patient's goals of care and circumstances as well as the fact that quite often surgical intervention, although considered to be invasive or aggressive, may be the best option for symptom relief even in the face of advanced disease.

Psychosocial issues affecting palliative surgery

Patients facing advanced disease and critical associated decisions related to treatment options also present with compound psychosocial and spiritual needs. The following case shows complex issues in patients who are torn between the desire to survive and weariness and readiness for life's end.

Case study

Grace Nakos, a 59-year-old Native American woman with esophageal cancer

Mrs. Nakos was a 59-year-old Native American woman with advanced esophageal cancer. She and her spouse lived in a tribal community. The Nakos family consisted of five children who had all completed high school and were doing well. The family prospered as successful tribal leaders in the Arapaho Nation. Three years ago, Mr. Nakos passed away suddenly from cardiac arrest. Since then, Mrs. Nakos battled chronic depression, and the family relationships suffered greatly. Approximately 2 years after her husband's death, Mrs. Nakos was diagnosed with esophageal cancer and underwent neoadjuvant chemoradiation plus surgery to remove the primary tumor. Her postoperative course was complicated by numerous problems, including a chronic problem with digestion, swallowing, and pain. She experienced a fairly sharp decline in status 6 months later.

Mrs. Nakos made her wishes very clear: she did not want life-sustaining treatment. She felt that she had become a burden for her children. Over the past month, Mrs. Nakos developed worsening dysphasia and was found to have recurrent disease. The surgeon recommended a procedure to remove some of the tumor but stated that it might not be possible to remove the entire tumor given its location. Mrs. Nakos hesitantly agreed to the surgery. She mentioned to the nursing staff that she had hoped that it wouldn't come to this, stating, "I think I'm dying from the inside out. The spirits are not with me any longer." The surgical resident came to obtain her consent for the surgery. Mrs. Nakos became extremely angry when the resident informed her that her "do-not-resuscitate" order would have to be rescinded for her to have surgery, because it was the hospital's policy that all patients entering surgery were at full code status. Mrs. Nakos told the resident that she and her deceased husband's spirits would haunt him for the rest of his career if he should "rob her of the opportunity to die" if "The Maker" deemed it should be so during surgery. After the resident left, a nurse came to the bedside to talk with Mrs. Nakos. While in tears, Mrs. Nakos stated that she still wanted the surgery, but she couldn't imagine that the surgeons would want to resuscitate her if the need should arise during surgery. It all seemed very unnatural and at odds with her beliefs. After she became much calmer, Mrs. Nakos admitted to the nurse, "On the other hand, I wish that maybe my heart would stop during surgery so it would be easier for everyone if I would die quickly."

The case of Mrs. Nakos illustrates the difficulties of dealing with patients with advanced disease. Cultural, spiritual, and psychosocial issues are important influences. This case also demonstrates the importance of nursing leadership in creating policies and procedures that support the goals of palliative care. Many institutions have eliminated the requirement for full code status with patients undergoing surgery and now honor the request to avoid resuscitation even if its need should occur during the procedure. Mrs. Nakos's clinical signs of depression are also important to evaluate in considering her overall plan of care. A patient's wish for death should never be dismissed, and such information ought to be shared with the surgical staff. Instances such as this are also primary examples for incorporating psychiatry or psychology: evaluation of her depression is essential, and attention to her emotions would be needed before the surgery as well as in the follow-up period. Nurses play a critical role in attending to communication around this issue and in acting as the patient's advocate in all stages of care and across settings.

Summary

Nurses will often encounter end-of-life situations. During these difficult times, patients and their loved ones will desire accurate and honest information. Unassailable communication skills are an essential element in navigating these families through the cancer trajectory. Palliative nursing care extends across all treatment modalities, and patients undergoing surgery require rigorous support and care. Nurses play a critical role in patient and family communication, establishing goals of care and providing expert management of symptoms. There is a need for continued research to address this area of palliative care and for persistent advancements of clinical nursing expertise to best serve these patients and families.[17,23]

References

1. Hanna NM, Bellavance E, Keay T. Palliative surgical oncology. Surg Clin N Am. 2011;91:343–353.
2. Adolph MD. Inpatient palliative care consultation: enhancing quality of care for surgical patients by collaboration. Surg Clin N Am. 2011;91:317–324.
3. Borneman T, Chu DZJ, Wagman L, et al. Concerns of family caregivers of patients with cancer facing palliative surgery for advanced malignancies. Onc Nurs Forum. 2003;30:997–1005.
4. Collins LK, Goodwin JA, et al. Patient reasoning in palliative surgical oncology. J Surg Onc. 2013(107):372–375.
5. Badgwell BR, Krouse R, et al. Frequent and early death limits quality of life assessment in patients with advanced malignancies evaluated for palliative surgical intervention. Ann of Surg Onc. 2012;19(12):3651–3658.
6. Podnos YD, Juarez G, Pameijer C, Choi K, Ferrell BR, Wagman LD. Impact of surgical palliation on quality of life in patients with advanced malignancy: results of the decisions and outcomes in palliative surgery (DOPS) trial. Ann Surg Onc. 2007;14(2):922–928.
7. Bradley CJ, Clement JP, Lin C. Absence of cancer diagnosis and treatment in elderly Medicaid-insured nursing home residents. J Natl Cancer I. 2008;100(1):21–31.
8. Hoffman B, Haheim LL, Soreide JA. Ethics of palliative surgery in patients with cancer. Br J Surg. 2005;92(802–809).
9. Ferrell BR, Chu DZJ, Wagman L, et al. Patient and surgeon decision making regarding surgery regarding advanced cancer. Onc Nurs Forum. 2003;30:E106–E114.
10. Miner TJ, Jaques JP, Shriver CD. A prospective evaluation of patients undergoing surgery for the palliation of an advanced malignancy. Ann Surg Onc. 2002;9:696–703.
11. Burke CC. Surgical treatment. In: Miakowski C, Buchsel P (eds.), Oncology Nursing: Assessment and Clinical Care. Elsevier, St. Louis, MO; 1999.

12. Milch RA, Dunn GP. Communication: part of a surgical armamentarium. J Am Coll Surg. 2001;93:449–451.

13. Andrews SC. Caregiver burden and symptom distress in people with cancer receiving hospice care. Oncol Nurs Forum. 2001;28:1469–1474.

14. Given BA, Gicen CW, Kozachik S. Family support in advanced cancer. CA Cancer J Clin. 2001; 51:2013–2231.

15. Langenhoff BS, Krabbe PF, Wobbes T, Ruers TJ. Quality of life as an outcome measure in surgical oncology. Br J Surg. 2001;88:643–652.

16. Bruera E, Sweeney C, Calder K, Palmer L, Benisch-Tolley S. When the treatment goal is not cure: are cancer patients equipped to make informed decisions? J Clin Oncol. 2001;20:503–513.

17. Velovich V. The quality of quality of life studies in general surgical journals. J Am Coll Surg. 2001;193:288–296.

18. Dunn GP. The surgeon and palliative care. Surg Oncol Clin North Am. 2001;10:7–24.

19. Easson AM, Crosby JA, Librach SL. Discussion of death and dying in surgical textbooks. Am J Surg. 2001;182:34–39.

20. Dunn GP. Palliative surgical outcomes: are we looking through a keyhole? Ann Surg Oncol. 2012;19:3637–3638.

21. Anwar S, Peter MB, Dent J, Scott NA. Palliative excisional surgery for primary colorectal cancer in patients with incurable metastatic disease: is there a survival benefit?: A systematic review. Colorectal Dis. 2011;14:920–930.

22. Cullinane CA, Borneman T, Smith DD, Chu DZ, Ferrell BR, Wagman LD. The surgical treatment of cancer: a comparison of resource utilization following procedures performed with a curative and palliative intent. Cancer. 2003;98(10):2266–2273.

23. Krouse R, Ferrell BR, Nelson RA, Juarez G, Wagman LC, Chu D. Advancing the evaluation of palliative surgery for cancer patients. In Ferrell BR, Coyle N (eds.), Oxford Textbook of Palliative Nursing. 3rd ed. Oxford: Oxford University Press; 2010:959–967.

24. McCahill LE, Krouse R, Chu DZJ, et al. Indications and use of palliative surgery: results of Society of Surgical Oncology survey. Ann Surg Onc. 2002;9:104–112.

25. McCahill LE, Krouse RS, Chu DZJ, et al. Decision making in palliative surgery. J Am Coll Surg. 2002;195:411–423.

26. McCahill LE, Smith D, Borneman T, et al. A prospective evaluation of palliative outcomes for surgery of advanced malignancies. Ann Surg Oncol. 2003;10:654–663.

27. Krouse RS, Nelson RA, Ferrell BR, et al. Surgical palliation at a cancer center: incidence and outcomes. Arch Surg. 2001;136:773–778.

28. Podnos YD, Juarez G, Pameijer C, Uman G, Ferrell BR, Wagman LD. Surgical palliation of advanced gastrointestinal tumors. J Palliat Med. 2007;10(4):871–876.

29. Juarez G, Ferrell B, Uman G, Podnos Y, Wagman LD. Distress and quality of life concerns of family caregivers of patients undergoing palliative surgery. Cancer Nurs. 2008;31(1):2–10.

30. Grov EK, Fossa SD, Sorebo O, Dahl AA. Primary caregivers of cancer patients in the palliative phase: a path analysis of variables influencing their burden. Soc Sci Med. 2006;63(9):2429–2439.

CHAPTER 52

Palliative chemotherapy and clinical trials in advanced cancer
The nurse's role

Virginia Sun

I was given the option of going on a clinical trial for treatment, but it was also explained to me that the chance of the trial helping to shrink my cancer is small. I want to try anything possible, so that at least at the end I know that I have tried everything I can to stay alive.

A patient

Key points

♦ Patients with advanced cancer are often caught between the dichotomy of continuing aggressive treatment and the focus on quality supportive and palliative care.

♦ Faced with difficult decisions, patients and families become especially vulnerable and may experience heightened physical, psychological, social, and spiritual distress.

♦ Palliative chemotherapy uses systemic antineoplastic agents to treat symptoms of incurable malignancies and maintain quality of life.

♦ Nurses can help alleviate suffering by supporting patients and families through changes in treatment intent, the decision-making process, and supportive care needs during palliative chemotherapy.

Nurses have always been in the forefront of managing treatment-related symptoms. In an ever-changing and complex healthcare setting, optimal care requires a transdisciplinary approach. This approach is especially valued in an oncology setting, where patients frequently present with complex disease- and treatment-related symptoms. These often debilitating symptoms negatively affect the quality of life (QOL) of patients and their extended families.[1] For patients with advanced cancer, treatment options are often limited. It is usually at this stage of the cancer continuum that discussion of palliative modalities of treatment occurs. These palliative modalities often include—but are not limited to—radiation, surgery, and chemotherapy. It is also during this stage of the continuum that physicians discuss the use of investigational therapeutic agents as an attempt to control the disease. However, it is not uncommon for patients and families to be faced with difficult

decisions. Patients with advanced cancer are often caught between the dichotomy of continuing aggressive treatment and the focus on quality supportive and palliative care.[2] The debate of treatment futility often comes into play at this stage of the cancer continuum, because patients and families are faced with a shorter life expectancy and all standard therapeutic regimens have failed to control the spread and proliferation of the tumor itself. Faced with these difficult decisions, patients and families become especially vulnerable and may experience heightened physical, psychological, social, and spiritual distress.[3]

In advanced malignancies, the choice between palliative chemotherapy, clinical trial, or best supportive care may be difficult. This chapter describes the use of chemotherapy and cancer investigational agents as a palliative treatment for patients with advanced cancer. Emphasis is placed particularly on the role of palliative chemotherapy and the dichotomy between clinical trials of cancer investigational therapeutic agents and palliative care. Finally, an in-depth analysis of the role of nurses in supporting patients and families receiving palliative chemotherapy or investigational agents through clinical trials is discussed.

Definitions

Palliative chemotherapy, in its broadest sense, is the use of systemic antineoplastic agents to treat an incurable malignancy.[4] In most medical literature, the efficacy of palliative chemotherapy is reported through data regarding tumor response rate, duration of response, and survival benefit.[5] However, the purpose of these studies usually is not the investigation of these agents for palliation of symptoms, although most subjects accrued in these clinical trials are deemed incurable.[6] It is only in recent years that symptom palliation has become an important aspect in the design and evaluation of cancer clinical trials. The majority of the symptom palliation research incorporated into therapeutic clinical trials focuses on QOL as a prognostic factor for better patient outcomes.[7] Other more specific definitions used to describe palliative chemotherapy include the relief of cancer-induced symptoms.[4,8] This refers to the use of antineoplastic agents with the expectation of prolonged survival and improved QOL, which includes the relief and prevention of adverse symptoms that are indicative of advanced malignancies.[4,8]

Curative versus palliative chemotherapy

As a primary therapy, chemotherapy may be potentially beneficial in the prolongation of survival in the advanced stages of cancer. However, the majority of malignancies in adults are incurable with chemotherapy. Although the development of adjuvant chemotherapy has resulted in a decrease in recurrence rates, the data show that there is no significant difference in disease-free survival.[4] Therefore, the majority of patients living with cancer will experience recurrence of disease, and it is this population that may also receive palliative chemotherapy.

Trends in the aggressiveness of cancer care at the end of life have been explored in the literature. Earle and colleagues identified several indicators of aggressive care, including intensive use of chemotherapy, low rates of hospice use, emergency room visits, hospitalization, and intensive care unit (ICU) admissions.[9] In a subsequent study to characterize end-of-life treatment aggressiveness in older adults on Medicare, the investigators found that rates of palliative chemotherapy treatment increased from 27.9% to 29.5% between 1993 and 1996.[10] For patients who received palliative chemotherapy, 15.7% received treatments up to 2 weeks before death.[10] An increasing proportion of patients used hospice services, but the services were primarily initiated within the last 3 days of life.[10] An updated analysis published in 2004 showed that the aggressiveness of care continued to increase, with more patients being referred to hospice within 3 days of death.[11] In both sets of analyses, elderly, female, nonwhite, and unmarried patients were less likely to receive aggressive care.[10–12] Other studies reported similar trends in treatment aggressiveness at the end of life for advanced lung cancer and ovarian cancer.[12,13] Studies have also found that many palliative chemotherapy treatments are initiated within 30 days of death.[14] In a retrospective cohort analysis of Medicare beneficiaries at the end of life, Emanuel and colleagues found that palliative care chemotherapy use was similar for patients with breast, colon, and ovarian cancer compared with those with less chemosensitive cancers, such as pancreatic, hepatocellular, or melanoma.[15]

When the disease has metastasized to other organ systems, the primary goal of using chemotherapy in advanced disease is to control the patient's symptoms and maintain QOL.[8] The rationale for palliating direct or indirect symptoms of cancer is multifaceted, but it is important for practitioners to remember that not all patients are suitable for palliative chemotherapy. Standard chemotherapy should not be offered to all patients with metastatic malignancies. A predicted toxicity of treatment should preclude any consideration for the use of palliative chemotherapy.[4,8] The benefit-to-toxicity ratio of treatment should be seriously considered. Subtherapeutic doses of chemotherapy should never be given to maintain hope in a patient's prognosis.[8] Such a false sense of hope may prove to be even more distressing and may induce tremendous suffering for patients and families.

Several prognostic factors have been used in chemotherapeutic treatments of cancer to determine palliative treatment modality. One of the most important prognostic factors is performance status.[4] A severely debilitated patient with a restricted performance status is more likely to sustain excessive chemotherapy toxicity. The site of metastasis outside the primary tumor can also be prognostic of patient response to symptoms related to treatment.[8] These tumor-specific prognostic factors are crucial because they can assist nurses in defining an incurable disease.

The decision to treat or not to treat is based not only on clinical indicators but also on the patient's perspective. Chemotherapy involves a commitment on the part of the patient and family to travel to the treating institution on a scheduled basis. Repeated hospitalizations, venipunctures, cannulations, investigations, and assessments over and beyond the actual administration of chemotherapy are inevitable routines of cancer treatment. These factors need to be addressed with patients and families in an effort to facilitate the decision-making process.

Quality-of-life concerns in palliative chemotherapy

The assessment of QOL has increasingly become a key measure in cancer clinical trials, in conjunction with other measures such as tumor response, disease-free survival, and overall survival.[16,17] Some of the parameters commonly included in QOL measurement tools are factors that affect the quality of a patient's physical, psychological, social, and spiritual well-being.[4] Quality of life should be used clinically to weigh the benefit-to-toxicity ratio of palliative chemotherapy. Aside from assessing antitumor effects and the toxicity of chemotherapy, the overall positive or negative impact of the treatment on QOL must also be addressed.[18] An ideal situation in which palliative chemotherapy might be beneficial is one in which the treatment does not alter survival duration but does positively affect QOL.[8]

Very few prospective studies have investigated the QOL benefits of supportive care versus a combination of palliative chemotherapy plus supportive care for the management of advanced, incurable malignancies. The average prolongation of survival with chemotherapy compared with best supportive care has not been fully described in literature. An increasing number of studies have reported the potential palliative benefits of chemotherapy.[19–25] Shanafelt and colleagues[25] performed a systematic analysis of 25 randomized, controlled clinical trials comparing cytotoxic chemotherapy with best supportive care. Sixteen of the clinical trials involved patients with non-small-cell lung cancer. The results indicated that there is a modest relationship between response rate and both median and 1-year survival rate for patients with non-small-cell lung cancer treated with cytotoxic chemotherapy.[25]

A meta-analysis of randomized clinical trials of best supportive care versus chemotherapy for unresectable non-small-cell lung cancer was performed to allow for better determination of the actual statistical significance of the treatment effect.[26] There was a survival benefit in the range of 6 to 10 weeks for those patients treated with palliative chemotherapy. However, this benefit was seen only in patients who had an adequate performance status.

Patients with Eastern Cooperative Oncology Group (ECOG) performance status of 3 or 4 had no benefit from chemotherapy.[26] In summary, it appears that palliative chemotherapy is effective only for a select group of patients in the lung cancer population. A strong predictor of positive treatment benefit is related to the patient's performance status.[26]

In a study of patients with unresectable metastatic or locally advanced non-small-cell lung cancer, subjects were randomly assigned to receive either best supportive care or two different chemotherapy regimens ($n = 150$).[27] Survival was 8 to 15 weeks longer for the chemotherapy + supportive care arm, but improved survival was observed only in patients who had a high ECOG performance status (0 or 1) and a weight loss of less than 5 kilograms. Moreover, about 40% of subjects were judged to have sustained severe, life-threatening, or lethal toxicities.[27] Very few patients showed improvement in performance status or gained weight during chemotherapy treatment.[27] Finally, in a meta-analysis that sought to determine the benefits and harms of palliative chemotherapy in patients with locally advanced or metastatic colorectal cancer, results from the analysis of 13 randomized, controlled trials found an improvement of 16% with median survival of 3.7 months.[28] However, the investigators found that the overall quality of evidence for palliative chemotherapy in relation to treatment toxicity, symptom control, and QOL was poor.[28]

The QOL of family caregivers was addressed in a study to compare the impact of cancer caregiving in curative and palliative settings.[29] Family caregivers of patients receiving palliative care had significantly lower QOL scores and lower overall physical health scores.[29] There was no additional significant variability in caregiver QOL scores after adjustments for patient performance status and treatment status. These results suggest that patients' poor performance status is a predictor of low QOL in the palliative care setting that also affects caregivers' QOL.[29] The data reinforce the importance of supporting families as well as the impact on their QOL and on the patient's well-being when the treatment intent is palliative.

When and how long to treat?

Multiple factors need to direct the decision-making process when considering palliative chemotherapy for patients with advanced cancer. The goal at this juncture in the cancer continuum is to relieve or prevent tumor-induced symptoms, with the potential of prolonging survival.[8] Patients who are symptomatic from malignancy, and those who are expected to be symptomatic soon, are typically considered for treatment initiation within a few days or weeks.[4] This indication for palliative chemotherapy, although proven to be somewhat beneficial for effective palliation in oncological emergencies, is appropriate for only selected patients.[4] Local treatments with palliative radiation or surgery are also common treatment modalities in advanced malignancies.

A more difficult scenario of whether to delay or begin palliative chemotherapy occurs with patients who are asymptomatic from malignancy. In these circumstances, especially with tumor types that are less responsive to chemotherapy, the general consensus is that the benefit-to-toxicity ratio may be more heavily weighted toward the toxicity side.[4] In such situations, treatment may be withheld and the patient closely monitored until symptomatic progression is evident.

Case study
Mrs. K, a patient with lung cancer

Mrs. K is a 65-year-old woman who never smoked but was diagnosed with metastatic non-small-cell lung cancer. At the time of diagnosis, she had widespread disease to her bones. Because of the bone metastasis, Mrs. K has been experiencing pain that is escalating. She continues to lose weight and her energy level was decreasing to the point where she spends most of her days at home and in bed. Mrs. K has received three lines of chemotherapy for her lung cancer with disease progression. She recently started treatment with an oral targeted agent. Mrs. K has decided to continue with treatment because of her 2-year-old grandson. After approximately four months of treatment, Mrs. K's condition deteriorates, with worsening shortness of breath, increasing fatigue, and worsening of pain. Her pain is not well controlled by standard pain medications. She is finally transferred to an inpatient hospice facility, and dies 3 days following admission.

In this case, a focus on watchful waiting or aggressive supportive care was indicated. Mrs. K's performance status was gradually declining; therefore, she could be anticipated to experience more difficulties with treatment side effects if palliative chemotherapy was given. The chemotherapy did not have a long-term effect on Mrs. K's pain. Aggressive supportive care involving experts such as pain specialists would have been beneficial for symptom management and QOL for this patient immediately following diagnosis. In such cases, the healthcare team should also provide Mrs. K's family with adequate information regarding the pros and cons of palliative chemotherapy at this stage of the cancer trajectory. Another important aspect of caring for Mrs. K was to support her family. Because Mrs. K's decision to receive palliative chemotherapy was for her grandchild, supportive care experts who specialize in working with young families or children should have been included to aid Mrs. K in treatment decision-making.

Decision-making: accept, reject, or continue

After the initial shock of receiving a cancer diagnosis, patients and families must battle anxiety-provoking concerns such as dying from the disease, financial burdens, disease-related pain, and treatment-related toxicities. The general public often perceives chemotherapy as extremely toxic.[30] These concerns are very much related to patient and family decision-making processes, especially when the intent to treat is to palliate symptoms. There are also concerns about whether patients are equipped with enough information to help make informed decisions. The current evidence suggests that patients with advanced, incurable cancers are not given clear information about the survival gain of palliative chemotherapy.[31] Other evidence suggests that patients perceive themselves to be well informed, but information about prognosis and alternatives to palliative chemotherapy are still lacking.[32,33] There is also evidence that suggests that patients with advanced cancer perceive much benefit from cancer treatments in general.[34] Patients in general are willing to be treated for as little as 1 month of extra survival.[35] Slevin and associates investigated the differences between patients' attitudes to either mild or intensive cancer chemotherapy and the attitudes of healthcare providers, such as physicians and nurses.[36] Cancer patients were more likely to accept intensive treatment with debilitating toxicities in exchange for an extremely small probability of cure, prolongation of life, and symptom relief.[37–44] Medical oncologists were more likely to accept aggressive treatment than were general practitioners. Oncology nurses, not surprisingly, were more divided on the aggressiveness of treatment. The nurses' perceptions fell between aggressive treatment and wanting more information on the benefit-to-toxicity ratio.[37]

Silvestri and coworkers conducted a study to determine how patients with advanced non-small-cell lung cancer valued the trade-off between the survival benefit of chemotherapy and its toxicities.[44] Data were qualitatively collected through the use of three scripted scenarios. Patients' willingness to accept chemotherapy varied widely (n = 81). Many would choose chemotherapy for a likely survival benefit of 3 months only if the treatment positively affected QOL as well.[44] The investigators found that the conflict between patients' preferences and the actual care they received greatly affected their decision-making. It appears that some patients did not receive the treatment they would have chosen had they been fully informed in their previous choice of treatment.[44]

Koedoot and colleagues investigated patient treatment preferences and decision-making processes in regard to palliative chemotherapy or best supportive care.[45] The actual treatment decision was the main outcome of the study. At baseline, the majority of subjects preferred to undergo chemotherapy rather than watchful waiting.[45] The majority of subjects also eventually chose treatment with chemotherapy. Treatment preference and a deferring style of decision-making were predictors of actual treatment choice. Treatment preference is positively explained by striving for length of life and negatively explained by striving for QOL.[45] The results indicated that it is still questionable whether the purpose of palliative chemotherapy is made clear to patients.[46] This emphasizes the need for healthcare providers to attach further attention to the process of information-giving and shared decision-making in patients with advanced cancer.[45]

The role of nurses in palliative chemotherapy

Through randomized clinical trials and meta-analyses, the incorporation of chemotherapy into the palliative care setting has been shown to have survival benefits for patients with advanced cancer whose disease is incurable. However, these benefits are seen only in patients with higher baseline performance status and in those who are asymptomatic from their metastatic malignancies. Hence, it is evident that palliative chemotherapy, although effective in palliating certain disease-related symptoms, has limited benefits for all advanced cancer patients. Therefore, it is important for nurses, as integral team members in the transdisciplinary approach of oncology palliative care, to support patients and families through the difficult path of answering the quintessential question: to treat or not to treat? Nurses can help alleviate further anguish and suffering for patients with advanced cancer and their families in three crucial areas related to palliative chemotherapy: change in treatment intent, decision-making, and supportive care through treatment choice.

Change in treatment intent

When curative intent of treatment becomes impossible, practitioners should begin to address the intent to treat as palliation of disease-related symptoms. This initial communication is traditionally the domain of the treating physician. However, with more and more collaborative practices emerging among nurses, advanced practice nurses (APNs), and physicians, it is becoming apparent that a transdisciplinary approach offers the best support for patients and families during this difficult and vulnerable time.[1] Communication of difficult news should best be conducted in a prearranged consultation session in which the treating physician, nurse, and social worker together deliver the information to the patient, the family, and other individuals who are integral to the decision-making process. Nurses can foster this transdisciplinary approach of delivering difficult news through collaboration and communication with experts across disciplines. Nurses are often the first to recognize the need for dialogue between the health-care team and the patient/family regarding treatment intent and prognosis.[47] Therefore, nurses can advocate for patients by recommending and organizing these important communication sessions to alleviate unnecessary suffering for patients and families.

Case study

Mrs. R, a patient with locally advanced esophageal cancer

Mrs. R, a 62-year-old Hispanic female who emigrated from Mexico to the United States 20 years ago, was diagnosed with locally advanced esophageal cancer. She was treated with chemoradiation, followed by surgery. Six months later, her disease recurred. Mrs. R wants to be aggressive with treatment despite her poor prognosis. Since the recurrence, Mrs. R's functional status has gradually deteriorated, and she has lost a tremendous amount of weight due to malnutrition. An esophageal stent was placed to palliate her dysphagia. Despite all this, Mrs. R maintains a positive outlook on life for the sake of her family and wants to remain functional as long as possible. She speaks some English and is accompanied by her husband, who speaks no English, and her daughter, who speaks fluent English, to talk with the healthcare team about other treatment options.

In this case, a consultation session is warranted. The objective of the session is threefold: (1) to present the difficult news of further disease progression and failure of treatment; (2) to reevaluate treatment intent; and (3) to make recommendations for treatment. An interpreter should be on hand during the session to ensure that the patient and the family understand the situation. Before divulging the difficult news, it is important to assess for cultural needs in terms of communicating bad news. The healthcare team should understand how much information patients want to know and how much they already know. This assessment guides the consultation session. If supportive care experts such as a psychologist or chaplain are not available to be present during the session, then it is vital that they be accessible to intervene during this very difficult and sensitive time of the cancer trajectory.

Decision-making

Once the change in treatment intent has been discussed, the next step is to guide patients and families through an informed decision-making process to either continue on aggressive treatment or focus on symptom relief. Again, this information should be delivered in a setting where all practitioners involved in the care of the patient and family are present. If this scenario is not possible, it is imperative for members of the healthcare team to communicate and follow-up with each other regarding details of the information disclosed to the patient and family. In presenting this information, it is important to avoid the use of medical jargon and to use resources such as information leaflets and diagrams to assist the patient and family in informed decision-making.[8] Nurses, having expertise in educating patients and families, can facilitate the availability of these visual resources and present them to patients and families.

Some patients might find it helpful to meet other similar patients or to access supportive care services such as psychology or chaplaincy. Nurses can encourage and facilitate these desires by initiating referrals to these services. A compassionate and ethical approach to review the medical situation with the patient and family is essential to providing them with an informed assessment of possible treatment choices.[4] It is important to include in the treatment choices the use of hospice services and nonchemotherapy palliative care, depending on the patient's individual situation. Another important aspect to consider is the awareness of specific cultural needs and differences. Patient and family desires for open communication and participation in decision-making are greatly influenced by both ethnicity and religion, so it is important to assess these needs and ensure cultural sensitivity before presenting the information.[4]

When discussing the possibility of palliative chemotherapy as a treatment choice, it is essential, before presenting statistical evidence, to learn about other specific factors that may affect the decision-making process. Nurses can facilitate and perform the assessment to obtain this vital information. Questions should focus on the following factors: (1) questions and decisions that need to be addressed in the patient's or family's lives; (2) a special upcoming event or specific unfinished business that must be completed; and (3) fears about dying or spiritual issues that need interventions from other supportive care services.[4] Nurses can play a particularly important role in facilitating information-gathering on the third factor, fear of dying and spiritual needs. Fear of dying and spirituality represent a much-ignored area in the general medical literature but have been shown to have significant impact on the QOL of cancer patients, especially when disease is incurable.[48] Nurses can facilitate the patient's and family's search for spiritual understanding of their situation and alleviate existential suffering by first acknowledging patient's fears and distress. Facilitation of open communication regarding existential suffering can help alleviate fears of dying.[48] Nurses must be compassionate listeners and allow patients and families a forum to discuss their deepest fears concerning the seemingly impending and inevitable terminality of their disease.

Supportive care through treatment choice

If palliative chemotherapy is the treatment choice, support for patients and families through treatment becomes the most important objective for nurses. Education regarding the common and expected side effects of the specific chemotherapy regimens can foster a sense of control over symptom management and prevent unnecessary anxiety-provoking episodes related to poorly managed side effects. The use of written materials that list and explain common side effects can be helpful in facilitating the learning process for patients and families. Most importantly, nurses can

assist in the continuous assessment of patient and family needs, focusing not only on the physical but also on the psychological, social, and spiritual domains.[49] Communication during this difficult and vulnerable phase of the disease trajectory is key to the success of quality cancer care. Nurses can serve as a bridge of communication by fostering continued dialogue on the goals of treatment between patients/families and the healthcare team. This bridge of communication, although often difficult to sustain, is essential in a truly transdisciplinary model of care. Open and clear communication among healthcare team members can guide the assessment of patient and family needs but can also alleviate suffering by maintaining consistency in the amount and types of information provided. Inconsistencies in vital communication factors in palliative chemotherapy, such as treatment intent, often create false hopes and distress for patients and families.[4]

If palliative chemotherapy is not the chosen plan of treatment, patients and families frequently experience a profound sense of abandonment.[4] This sense of abandonment is most often directed toward healthcare providers. Patients and families, after living through the initial treatment phase of the cancer trajectory wherein follow-up with physicians and nurses is routine, suddenly lose the security of being assessed on a regular basis. Nurses can assist in alleviating this sense of abandonment through reassurance that follow-up care will remain in place. If referral to hospice is warranted, then nurses can act as a liaison to attending physicians and hospice services to foster a smooth transition between care settings and to maintain continuity of care.

Clinical trials and advanced cancer

Several reports published or commissioned by government advisory boards such as the National Cancer Policy Board and the Institute of Medicine noted that the quality of end-of-life care in the United States is seriously deficient.[6] Many oncology professional organizations assert that hospice is the best-developed model of end-of-life care in the US healthcare delivery system.[6] Hospice offers quality palliative care using a transdisciplinary approach. With the rising interest in palliative care for terminally ill patients, there has also been a dramatic increase in interest regarding palliative care specifically for advanced cancer patients.

Patients with advanced cancer are often offered the opportunity to enroll in a phase I clinical trial. Although research on new therapeutic agents is crucial to the oncology specialty, it is not uncommon that patients who enroll in phase I trials are forced to forgo the use of services such as hospice and palliative care. This dichotomy is primarily a result of US federal policy. Medicare and insurance policies deny hospice coverage to patients with terminal cancer who enroll as participants in phase I studies. However, it is precisely this population of cancer patients who would benefit from comprehensive palliative care. It is important to note that phase I studies are designed to determine the toxicity and maximum tolerated dose of potential treatments, mostly for currently incurable cancers. These studies are not designed, and do not have the intended purpose, to have a therapeutic effect. In fact, studies have shown that therapeutic effects from cancer investigational therapeutic agents occur in only 2% to 4% of subjects enrolled in a phase I clinical trial.[50,51] It is also ironic that the entry criteria for phase I trials is similar to the disease state criteria for admission into hospice—but it is precisely this dichotomy that renders a patient ineligible for the quality palliative care services that hospice provides.[6]

Patients who enter investigational cancer trials participate, in part, because of protocol eligibility such as disease and functional criteria. Many advanced-stage cancer patients who make decisions to participate in cancer clinical trials are also characterized by a highly motivated personality.[52] They feel that active treatment is best for them.[53] Other factors identified with enrollment may include altruism and the influence of the physician.[54] Patient expectations include a response to therapy, a reduction in symptoms, and improved and increased communication with their physicians.[55–57] Preliminary findings also have suggested that patients who choose to enroll in experimental trials are slightly more spiritual than other patients with advanced cancer who choose not to participate.[58] Therapeutic efforts are often equated with superior QOL and are measured against no other options. By contrast, patients and families believe palliative care is a passive choice, the equivalent of "no care."

The current evidence suggests that there is controversy about whether patients with advanced incurable cancers, when faced with decision-making regarding their plan of care, fully understand the choices that are available to them. Studies have found that patients are aware of other alternatives at the end of life, but their overwhelming need to fight their cancer at any cost prevents them from seriously considering the other alternatives.[59,60] Patients who would qualify for hospice services as regulated by Medicare have very little understanding of admission criteria and services rendered.[61] It is unlikely that patients who are potential study participants understand fully that to enroll in a clinical trial means that they must temporarily forgo the opportunity of receiving comprehensive palliative care.[6] Furthermore, there are no informed consent documents that disclose the risk of losing hospice benefits when enrolled in a clinical trial. Within the informed consent documents for cancer investigational therapeutic agents, there are no descriptions in the benefits and risks section that address the risk of temporarily losing hospice eligibility.[62] This loss of eligibility is not permanent; rather, patients and families can enroll and disenroll from hospice benefits whenever they choose.

Tensions between palliative care and clinical research

Despite significant progress in research and treatments, the diagnosis of cancer creates fear and turmoil in the lives of every cancer patient and the patient's family. Cancer disrupts all components of social integration—family, work, finances, and friendships—as well as the patient's psychological status. Over the extended course of the illness, physical changes and deterioration create multiple and complex demands on the patient and family. These demands, in conjunction with significant financial assaults, generate a negative synergy, which is often ignored in the care of patients with advanced disease.

Patients with advanced, incurable cancers are especially vulnerable and therefore have many unique needs in coping with their disease.[63] Hence, it is helpful to tailor treatment to the specific needs of each individual and family to fulfill personal goals and maintain QOL. This is precisely what a comprehensive palliative care program can provide. At the same time, many patients faced with the terminality of their disease want and seek new innovative

therapies. In the absence of further evidence-based and effective standard therapy, clinical trials offer a sense of hope for a potential cure.[63] But for patients who choose to participate in a clinical trial, there are often no guarantees of benefit, and there is the added possibility of harm and discomfort in the form of physical and psychological distress.

The impact of clinical trial participation on physical symptoms related to advanced cancer is complex, and there is a paucity of data regarding the extent of these symptoms.[63] Like standard treatment agents, experimental agents cause side effects. The difference in the side-effect profile of a well-established agent versus an experimental agent lies in the anticipation of symptoms. Well-established agents have well-documented side effect profiles that can be anticipated and predicted and therefore better controlled or even prevented in certain situations. The novelty of experimental agents, however, renders their side effects unpredictable. There is a tremendous amount of uncertainty about what effects an experimental agent might have on a particular patient.

Palliative care stands in contrast to disease-directed therapy at most cancer centers in the United States. The rift between them creates a dissonance for development of clinical research protocols and for recruitment of some groups of patients into cancer clinical trials. Only one-third of all cancer patients receive formal palliative care through hospice, and often this occurs only in the final days of life.[64] Although advanced cancer should be a time of refocusing and resolution, the hospice referral process often occurs during crisis situations. As disease advances, a positive relationship exists between increased physiological symptom severity and the patient's level of emotional distress and overall QOL. An inability to complete end-of-life tasks may lead to patient dissatisfaction as well as complicated family/caregiver stress and grief after the death.[64–66]

Quality-of-life concerns for clinical trial participants

Although the structure and requirement of a clinical trial protocol mandates the inclusion of a plan of action for unexpected physical symptoms, these plans often are focused on pharmacological interventions only. For example, if nausea and vomiting is an anticipated or expected side effect, a protocol of which antiemetic agents to use is written into the clinical trial protocol itself. However, the psychological and social distress from this side effect is not included in the plan. A clinical trial protocol generally does not include plans that specifically state the need for referrals to other allied health professionals, such as palliative care specialists and psychologists.[6]

The psychological and cognitive symptoms of patients participating in research studies vary.[63] Some patients may be distressed to be told that they are not eligible for inclusion into clinical trials. Research subjects may also have difficulty when an experimental treatment fails, which often mandates the withdrawal of subjects from the treatment protocol. One potential advantage of enrollment in clinical trials is that several members of the research team care for these patients. There are regularly scheduled visits, and that attention may affect the patient's psychological well-being. This added attention might lead to early detection of psychological symptoms that are indicative of depression, sadness, anxiety, or irritability.[63] Subtle changes in psychological effects might be readily detected by research personnel, and nurses are an integral part of this team. However, for this added attention to be beneficial to patients and families, it is important for research teams to work collaboratively with allied health professionals and palliative care specialists to address concerns in all areas of patient and family well-being.

Economic demands and caregiving needs may also be affected by clinical trial participation. Financial burdens may be increased for clinical trial participants even if the experimental agents are provided free of charge. The usual intensive monitoring and testing that can sharply increase with participation in clinical trials may not be covered by either the trial budget itself or the patient's insurance. The frequent visits for treatment, physician assessment, and various other procedures that are often mandated in clinical trial protocols may incur further economic burdens in terms of expenses for travel and room and board.[63]

The needs of caregivers and families may also change with clinical trial participation. Families experience tremendous physical, psychological, social, and spiritual concerns that are related to the patient's well-being. Physical symptoms such as fatigue can plague caregivers and families who are faced with the complex care of patients with advanced cancer.[30] The complexity of navigating through the healthcare and insurance systems can place tremendous burdens on both patients and caregivers. Social exposure may be diminished for caregivers, because much of their days are spent caring for their loved ones.[30] Finally, the agony of being a witness to a loved one's suffering and the prospect of grief and bereavement in terminal illness may present caregivers with spiritual and existential distress.

Attending to the spiritual and existential needs of patients with advanced cancer is an important factor in the overall experience of patients and families facing the inevitability of terminal illness. It is often at this point in the cancer trajectory that patients experience the needs of altruism.[63] Patients and families who recognize the diminishing hope of survival may find comfort and solace in the possibility of contributing to the advancement of science through participation in clinical trials.[63] Others may choose to focus on using precious time to concentrate on more personal goals, such as unfinished business and QOL.

Case study
Mr. G, a patient with primary liver cancer

Mr. G is a 34-year-old Asian male who was recently diagnosed with hepatocellular carcinoma. He and his wife have only been married for a year. Mr. G. underwent surgery, but experienced a recurrence in just 3 months. He was started on an oral targeted agent, but treatment effect was not long-term. Mr. G is worried about Mrs. G, and he feels guilty about getting sick so early in their marriage. A decision is made to enroll in a clinical trial. Unfortunately, Mr. G's condition continues to worsen 1 week following initiation of the clinical trial treatment. Lately, Mrs. G has become increasingly tearful when accompanying Mr. G during his clinic visits.

In this case, it is clear that the caregiver is suffering tremendously. After surviving through several bouts of treatment without much effect on the tumor, the impact of repeated discouragement weighs heavily on the patient's and caregiver's hearts. Mrs. G has probably witnessed and supported Mr. G through the agonies of treatment and continued progression of disease. One can anticipate that they

will experience tremendous difficulties with regard to grief and bereavement. It is important, therefore, to recommend or establish support for the family. In this case, referral to supportive care experts might be warranted. The family should be provided with information on other types of support, such as support groups. It might be helpful to connect them with other caregivers, and to exchange experiences on caring for a terminally ill loved one.

Perspectives toward clinical trials
Patient versus nurses

The conduct of clinical trials involving human subjects raises ethical concerns for healthcare professionals. In the process of decision-making in a clinical trial setting for patients with advanced cancer, the impact of nurses presents an additional element.[67] Nurses are involved in clinical trials both as clinical investigators and as caregivers for patients and families undergoing experimental treatments. In the clinical setting, nurses facilitate practitioner-patient communication and also serve as advocates.[67] Nurses often spend a considerable amount of time with patients and their families, and they are acutely aware of attitudes, needs, and concerns regarding participation.

Burnett and coworkers conducted a study to identify nurses' attitudes and beliefs toward cancer clinical trials and their perceptions of the factors influencing patients' participation.[67] A 59-item questionnaire was administered to nurses working in NCI-designated comprehensive cancer centers. Of the 417 nurses who responded, 96% reported that participation is important to improving standards of care, but only 56% believed that patients should be encouraged to participate in these clinical trials.[67] As a group, research nurses were more likely to have favorable views toward clinical trials and also about patient understanding regarding treatment plans and goals. On the other hand, nurses working in ICUs and bone marrow transplant settings had more concerns regarding patient understanding and patient–physician communication. Ninety-two percent of nurses reported that patients entered a clinical trial with the belief that it would cure their cancer.[67] Sixty-eight percent of nurses reported the belief that patients participate in clinical trials because they hope to receive better medical care. Nurses also indicated their perception that nurses, as professionals, are more likely to respect patients' wishes and less likely to apply pressure on patients regarding clinical trial participation.[67] These results indicate the concerns that nurses working in oncology settings have toward the informed consent process of clinical trial participation and strongly suggest the need to develop nursing interventions to better support this process.

Aaronson and associates conducted a study to test the efficacy of a telephone-based nursing intervention on improving the effectiveness of the informed consent process in cancer clinical trials.[68] This randomized study compared the effectiveness of this nursing intervention in patients who were randomly assigned to either a standard informed consent procedure based on verbal explanation and written information or the standard informed consent process plus the supplementary telephone intervention (intervention group). Results showed that the intervention group was significantly better informed about the following: (1) the risks and side effects of treatment; (2) the clinical trial context of the treatment;

(3) the objectives of the clinical trial; (4) the use of randomization in allocating treatment (if relevant); (5) the availability of alternative treatments; (6) the voluntary nature of the participation; and (7) the right to withdraw from the clinical trial. The intervention did not have any significant effect on patients' anxiety levels or on the rate of clinical trial accrual.[68]

Cox conducted a qualitative study to identify the psychosocial impact of participation in clinical trials, as experienced by the patients' themselves.[69] The study sought to interpret patients' ways of coping with their individual situations and also to identify the consequences of trial involvement. Of the 55 patients involved in the study, the offer of a trial treatment was seen as a turning point for patients. Thirty patients (54%) described the offer of participation as being "the light at the end of a tunnel" because they perceived that hope was offered.[69] On the other hand, 58% of subjects described how the trial generated uncertainty, whereas 54% felt special, privileged, pleased, lucky, and honored to have been offered participation.[69] The majority of patients interpreted the offer of trial participation as being the right plan of action because their physicians offered it. Reasons for patients to accept trial participation included the desire to be in expert hands (54%) and the desire to help others (52%).[69]

As clinical trial initiation began and patients progressed through treatment, an overwhelming sense of being burdened by trial involvement was noted in all cases. These burdens focused on side effects and additional demands, such as blood tests and scans.[69] It was evident that these trial burdens were not fully anticipated by patients at the beginning of trial involvement. Nevertheless, most of the patients desired to persevere through treatment rather than withdraw.

At the conclusion of participation, patients expressed disappointment that the trial drug was not successful. An overwhelming sense of abandonment was a feature in all patients. Subjects were also eager to receive feedback on the trial in which they had participated.[69] Trial withdrawal resulting from disease progression or toxicity was a common feature for subjects in this study. Trial withdrawal and conclusion was a deeply distressing and stressful time for all patients. In addition to having to confront the realities of having a terminal illness and the lack of response to their last hope for "cure," patients also experienced a dramatic decrease in contact from healthcare providers, which inevitably led to an overwhelming sense of abandonment.[69] These findings suggest that patients and families need support during and beyond the trial to deal with the major disruption that clinical trial participation might have on the overall dying trajectory. The investigators suggested that one way to overcome these issues is to consider early clinical trials in the context of a continuing palliative care program, in which the duty of care extends beyond trial involvement and in which death and dying concerns can be addressed.[69]

The role of nurses in caring for clinical trial patients

Clinical trials of new investigational cancer therapeutics are a necessary component to the process of translating scientific discoveries into standard practice of care.[70] Oncology nurses have many different roles in the conduct of cancer clinical trials. First and foremost, the process of obtaining true informed consent is a critical factor, not only in improving patient accrual into clinical trials but also in the overall well-being of patients and their families. The informed consent process is an opportunity to provide accurate information regarding important factors that affect the patient's and family's decision-making process in advanced cancer. These factors include trial procedures and potential risks and benefits.[71] The initial informed consent process is also a time to correct any misconceptions and allay unfounded fears and to provide sufficient time for patients and families to thoughtfully consider clinical trial participation.[70] A predecisional support process provided by oncology nurses may influence the soundness of patients' decisions to enroll in clinical trials.[70] Nursing interventions that would assist in well-considered decisions include helping patients gather additional relevant sources of information, describing patients' roles and rights in studies, encouraging patients to define their own reasons for participating in clinical trials, and supporting patients in making decisions that correspond with their personal values and wishes.[72]

Nurses can also assist in educating not only clinical trial patients but also the extended community. Interventions aimed at increasing community awareness can foster better understanding of clinical trials and their importance in the advancement of treatment options and strategies for oncology patients.[70] The formation of clinical trial support groups for patients and families considering enrollment in research is another strategy that may provide necessary education and social support.[70] Strategies such as follow-up phone calls or e-mail messages while patients are considering clinical trial participation can have a positive effect on the decision-making process.[70]

Nurses are in an ideal position to promote awareness of the importance of clinical trials and subsequent improvements in patient care. The three key roles of nurses caring for clinical trial patients and their families are educator, patient advocate, and study coordinator.[73] As patient and family educators, nurses can have a tremendous impact on a patient's experience with clinical trial participation. Nurses are clinical interpreters who provide patients and families with explanations of highly complex and intricate protocols without using medical jargon.[73] Education about the specific protocol process, expectations at each stage, management of side effects, and the importance of communicating changes in health status to practitioners is integral to the oncology research setting.

As patient advocates, nurses play an important role in the critical gateway to clinical trial participation—the informed consent process.[73] Nurses bring to this role a patient-centered, holistic method of support. The nursing perspective is important in that it provides a framework within which patients and families are treated with dignity and respect. Clarification of reasons behind decisions to participate—whether physical, psychological, social, or spiritual—should be encouraged.

Advanced practice nurses such as clinical nurse specialists and nurse practitioners can be an important factor in the conduct of clinical trials. Expertise in symptom management and clinical problem-solving is a key asset for APNs in the research setting. For example, nurse practitioners working in a clinical trial setting have an expanded scope of practice that allows them to perform routine follow-up physical examinations as well as diagnose and manage treatment complications.[26] This level of participation in patient and family care may enhance patient satisfaction, compliance, and retention.

Summary

Of all the topics to which oncology healthcare providers, palliative care specialists, and ethicists have devoted their attention, few raise as much heated debate as the dichotomy between active treatment and palliative care. The use of palliative chemotherapy and clinical trial participation as a treatment option for patients with advanced cancer has been at the heart of this debate for decades. There is a growing movement in the United States to integrate palliative care into clinical trials. However, there is still much work to be done. Frustration lies in the assumption that subjects who are actively treated for symptom palliation, whether through palliative chemotherapy or experimental agents, must forgo a coordinated plan of care that involves quality palliative care.[74] It has become increasingly evident that this dichotomy should not exist—that is, patients and families can simultaneously receive therapy for palliation of symptoms and have access to quality palliative care. It is also increasingly evident that this quality care can be provided only through a transdisciplinary model of care. Nurses can help alleviate the tension between palliative care and disease-directed therapies through education, advocacy, and coordination of care. It is only by removing this dichotomy that patients with advanced cancer and their families can be provided with the highest quality of information to facilitate their decision-making process.

References

1. Joshi TG, Ehrenberger HE. Cancer clinical trials in the new millennium: novel challenges and opportunities for oncology nursing. Clin J Oncol Nurs. 2001;5:147–152.
2. Casarett DJ, Karlawish J, Henry MI, Hirschman KB. Must patients with advanced cancer choose between a phase I trial and hospice? Cancer. 2002;95:1601–1604.
3. Chevlen EM. Palliative chemotherapy. In: Berger AM, Portenoy RK, Weissman DE (eds.), Principles and Practices of Palliative Care and Supportive Oncology. 3rd ed. Philadelphia PA: Lippincott Williams & Wilkins; 2007:549–560.
4. Peppercorn JM, Weeks JC, Cook EF, Joffe S. Comparison of outcomes in cancer patients treated within and outside clinical trials: conceptual framework and structured review. Lancet. 2004;363:263–270.
5. Byock I, Miles SH. Hospice benefits and phase I cancer trials. Ann Intern Med 2003;138:335–337.
6. Osoba D. Lessons learned from measuring health-related quality of life in oncology. J Clin Oncol. 1994;12:608–616.
7. McIllmurray M. The medical treatment of cancer in palliative care. In: Doyle D, Hanks G, Cherny N, Calman K (eds.), Oxford Textbook of Palliative Medicine. 4th ed. Oxford, England: Oxford University Press; 2010:513–525.
8. Earle CC, Park ER, Lai B, Weeks JC, Ayanian JZ, Block S. Identifying potential indicators of the quality of end-of-life cancer care from administrative data. J Clin Oncol. 2003;21(6):1133–1138.
9. Ho TH, Barbera L, Saskin R, Lu H, Neville BA, Earle CC. Trends in the aggressiveness of end-of-life cancer care in the universal health care system of Ontario, Canada. J Clin Oncol. 2011;29(12):1587–1591.
10. Earle CC, Landrum MB, Souza JM, Neville BA, Weeks JC, Ayanian JZ. Aggressiveness of cancer care near the end of life: is it a quality-of-care issue? J Clin Oncol. 2008;26(23):3860–3866.
11. Rose JH, O'Toole EE, Dawson NV, et al. Perspectives, preferences, care practices, and outcomes among older and middle-aged patients with late-stage cancer. J Clin Oncol. 2004;22(24):4907–4917.
12. Temel JS, McCannon J, Greer JA, et al. Aggressiveness of care in a prospective cohort of patients with advanced NSCLC. Cancer. 2008;113(4):826–833.
13. von Gruenigen V, Daly B, Gibbons H, Hutchins J, Green A. Indicators of survival duration in ovarian cancer and implications for aggressiveness of care. Cancer. 2008;112(10):2221–2227.
14. Braga S, Miranda A, Fonseca R, et al. The aggressiveness of cancer care in the last three months of life: a retrospective single centre analysis. Psychooncology. 2007;16(9):863–868.
15. Emanuel EJ, Young-Xu Y, Levinsky NG, Gazelle G, Saynina O, Ash AS. Chemotherapy use among Medicare beneficiaries at the end of life. Ann Intern Med. 2003;138(8):639–643.
16. Sloan JA, Cella D, Frost MH, Guyatt G, Osoba D; Clinical Significance Consensus Meeting Group. Quality of life. III: Translating the science of quality-of-life assessment into clinical practice: an example-driven approach for practicing clinicians and clinical researchers. Clin Ther. 2003;25(Suppl):D1–D5.
17. Osoba D, Slamon DJ, Burchmore M, Murphy M. Effects on quality of life of combined trastuzumab and chemotherapy in women with metastatic breast cancer. J Clin Oncol. 2002;20:3106–3113.
18. Cullen MH, Billingham LJ, Woodroffe CM, et al. Mitromycin, ifosfamide, and cisplatin in unresectable non-small-cell lung cancer: effects on survival and quality of life. J Clin Oncol. 1999;17:3188–3194.
19. Glimelius B, Ekstrom K, Hoffman K, et al. Randomized comparison between chemotherapy plus best supportive care with best supportive care in advanced gastric cancer. Ann Oncol. 1995;71:587–591.
20. Huskamp HA, Keating NL, Malin JL, Zaslavsky AM, Weeks JC, Earle CC, et al. Discussions with physicians about hospice among patients with metastatic lung cancer. Arch Intern Med. 2009;169(10):954–962.
21. Finlay E, Lu HL, Henderson H, O'Dwyer PJ, Casarett DJ. Do phase 1 patients have greater needs for palliative care compared with other cancer patients? Cancer. 2009;115(2):446–453.
22. Lang K, Marciniak MD, Faries D, Stokes M, Buesching D, Earle C, et al. Trends and predictors of first-line chemotherapy use among elderly patients with advanced non-small cell lung cancer in the United States. Lung Cancer. 2009;62 (2):264–270.
23. Lang K, Marciniak MD, Faries D, Stokes M, Buesching D, Earle C, et al. Costs of first-line doublet chemotherapy and lifetime medical care in advanced non-small-cell lung cancer in the United States. Value Health. 2009;12(4):481–488.
24. Cunningham D, Pyrhonen S, James RD, et al. Randomized trial of irinotecan plus supportive care versus supportive care alone after fluorouracil failure for patients with metastatic colorectal cancer. Lancet. 1998;352:1413–1418.
25. Saito AM, Landrum MB, Neville BA, Ayanian JZ, Earle CC. The effect on survival of continuing chemotherapy to near death. BMC Palliat Care. 2011;10:14.
26. Rapp E, Pater JL, Willan A, Cormier Y, Murray N, Evans WK. Chemotherapy can prolong survival in patients with advanced non small cell lung cancer: report of a Canadian multicenter randomized trial. J Clin Oncol. 1988;6:633–643.
27. Souquet PJ, Chauvin F, Boisel JP, et al. Polychemotherapy in advanced non-small-cell lung cancer: a metaanalysis. Lancet. 1993;342:19–30.
28. NSCLC Meta Analysis Collaborative Group. Chemotherapy in addition to supportive care improves survival in advanced nonsmall-cell lung cancer: a systematic review of meta-analysis of individual patient data from 16 randomized controlled trials. J Clin Oncol. 2008;26:4617–4625.
29. Weitzner MA, McMillan SC, Jacobsen PB. Family caregiver quality of life: differences between curative and palliative cancer treatment settings. J Pain Symptom Manage. 1999;17:418–428.
30. Comis RL, Miller JD, Aldige CR, Krebs L, Stoval E. Public attitudes toward participation in cancer clinical trials. J Clin Oncol. 2003;21:830–835.
31. Audrey S, Abel J, Blazeby JM, Falk S, Campbell R. What oncologists tell patients about survival benefits of palliative chemotherapy and implications for informed consent: qualitative study. BMJ (Clinical Research Ed). 2008;337:a752.
32. Kass NE, Sugarman J, Medley AM, Fogarty LA, Taylor HA, Daugherty CK, et al. An intervention to improve cancer patients' understanding of early-phase clinical trials. IRB. 2009;31(3):1–10.

33. Shin J, Casarett D. Facilitating hospice discussions: a six-step roadmap. J Support Oncol. 2011;9(3):97–102.

34. Stiggelbout AM, de Haes JC. Patient preference for cancer therapy: an overview of measurement approaches. J Clin Oncol. 2001;19(1): 220–230.

35. de Haes H, Koedoot N. Patient centered decision making in palliative cancer treatment: a world of paradoxes. Patient Educ Couns. 2003;50(1):43–49.

36. Slevin ML, Stubbs L, Plant HJ, Wilson P, Gregory WM, Armes PJ, et al. Attitudes towards chemotherapy: comparing view of patients with those of doctors, nurses, and general public. BMJ. 1990;300:1458–1467.

37. Balmer CE, Thomas P, Osborne RJ. Who wants second-line, palliative chemotherapy? Psychooncology. 2001;10(5):410–418.

38. Jansen LA, Appelbaum PS, Klein WM, Weinstein ND, Cook W, Fogel JS, et al. Unrealistic optimism in early-phase oncology trials. IRB. 2011;33(1):1–8.

39. Casarett DJ, Fishman JM, Lu HL, O'Dwyer PH, Barg FK, Naylor MD, et al. The terrible choice: re-evaluating hospice eligibility criteria for cancer. J Clin Oncol. 2009;27(6):953–959.

40. Harrington SE, Smith TJ. The role of chemotherapy at the end of life: "When is enough, enough?" JAMA. 2008;299(22):2667–2678.

41. Maltoni M, Amadori D. Palliative medicine and medical oncology. Ann Oncol. 2001;12(4):443–450.

42. Finlay E, Casarett D. Making difficult discussions easier: using prognosis to facilitate transitions to hospice. CA Cancer J Clin. 2009;59(4): 250–263.

43. Matsuyama R, Reddy S, Smith TJ. Why do patients choose chemotherapy near the end of life?: A review of the perspective of those facing death from cancer. J Clin Oncol. 2006;24(21):3490–3496.

44. Silvestri G, Pritchard R, Welch HG. Preferences for chemotherapy in patients with advanced non-small cell lung cancer: descriptive study based on scripted interviews. BMJ. 1998;317:771–775.

45. Koedoot CG, de Haan RJ, Stiggelbout AM, Stalmeier PF, de Graeff A, Bakker PJ, et al. Palliative chemotherapy or best supportive care?: A prospective study explaining patients' treatment preference and choice. Br J Cancer. 2003;89:19–26.

46. Keating NL, Landrum MB, Rogers SO Jr, Baum SK, Virnig BA, Huskamp HA, Earle CC, Kahn KL. Physician factors associated with discussions about end-of-life care. Cancer. 2010;116(4):998–1006.

47. Aiken JL. Quality-of-life studies. In: Klimaszewski D, Aiken JL, Bacon MA, DiStasio SA, Ehrenberger HE, Ford BA (eds.), Manual for Clinical Trial Nursing. 2nd ed. Pittsburgh, PA: Oncology Nursing Press; 2004:231–2234.

48. Karigan M. Psychosocial considerations. In: Klimaszewski D, Aiken JL, Bacon MA, DiStasio SA, Ehrenberger HE, Ford BA (eds.), Manual for Clinical Trial Nursing. 2nd ed. Pittsburgh, PA: Oncology Nursing Press; 2008:133–140.

49. Sutradhar R, Seow H, Earle C, Dudgeon D, Atzema C, Husain A, et al. Modeling the longitudinal transitions of performance status in cancer outpatients: time to discuss palliative care. J Pain Symptom Manage. 2013;45(4):726–734.

50. Seow H, Barbera L, Sutradhar R, Howell D, Dudgeon D, Atzema C, et al. Trajectory of performance status and symptom scores for patients with cancer during the last six months of life. J Clin Oncol. 2011;29(9):1151–1158.

51. Weinfurt KP, Seils DM, Lin L. Research participants' high expectations of benefit in early-phase oncology trials: are we asking the right question? J Clin Oncol. 2012;30(35):4396–4400.

52. Yates BC, Dodendorf D, Lane J, LaFramboise L, Pozehl B, Duncan K, et al. Testing an alternate informed consent process. Nurs Res. 2009;58(2):135–139.

53. Gray SW, Hlubocky FJ, Ratain MJ, Daugherty CK. Attitudes toward research participation and investigator conflicts of interest among advanced cancer patients participating in early phase clinical trials. J Clin Oncol. 2007;25(23):3488–3494.

54. Hui D, Glitza I, Chisholm G, Yennu S, Bruera E. Attrition rates, reasons, and predictive factors in supportive care and palliative oncology clinical trials. Cancer 2013;119 (5):1098–1105.

55. Miller FG, Joffe S. Benefit in phase 1 oncology trials: therapeutic misconception or reasonable treatment option? Clin Trials. 2008;5(6):617–623.

56. Wendler D, Krohmal B, Emanuel EJ, Grady C. Why patients continue to participate in clinical research. Arch Intern Med. 2008;168(12):1294–1299.

57. Daugherty CK, Fitchett G, Murphy PE, et al. Trusting God and medicine: spirituality in advanced cancer patients volunteering for clinical trials of experimental agents. Psychooncology. 2005;14(2): 135–146.

58. Daugherty CK. Ethical issues in phase I clinical trials. Clin Adv Hematol Oncol. 2004;2(6):358–360.

59. Schapira L, Moynihan TJ, von Gunten CF, Smith TJ. Phase I versus palliative care: striking the right balance. J Clin Oncol. 2009;27(2):307–308.

60. Daugherty CK, Hlubocky FJ. What are terminally ill cancer patients told about their expected deaths?: A study of cancer physicians' self-reports of prognosis disclosure. J Clin Oncol. 2008;26 (36):5988–5993.

61. Kass NE. Early phase clinical trials: communicating the uncertainties of "magnitude of benefit" and "likelihood of benefit." Clin Trials. 2008;5(6):627–629.

62. Mack JW, Cronin A, Taback N, Huskamp HA, Keating NL, Malin JL, et al. End-of-life care discussions among patients with advanced cancer: a cohort study. Ann Intern Med. 2012;156 (3):204–210.

63. Ferrell BR, Grant MM, Rhiner M, Padilla GV. Home care: maintaining quality of life for patient and family. Oncology. 1992; 6(2 Suppl):136–140.

64. BrintzenhofeSzoc KM, Smith ED, Zabora JR. Screening to predict complicated grief in spouses of cancer patients. Cancer Pract. 1999;7:233–239.

65. Schulz R, Beach SR. Caregiving as a risk factor for mortality: the Caregiver Health Effects Study. JAMA. 1999;282:2215–2219.

66. Burnett CB, Koczwara B, Pixley L, Blumenson LE, Hwang YT, Meropol NJ. Nurses' attitudes toward clinical trials at a comprehensive cancer center. Oncol Nurs Forum. 2002;28:1187–1192.

67. Aaronson NK, Visser-Pol E, Leenhouts G, et al. Telephone based nursing intervention improves the effectiveness of the informed consent process in cancer clinical trials. J Clin Oncol. 1996;14:984–996.

68. Cox K. Enhancing cancer clinical trial management: recommendations from a qualitative study of trial participants' experiences. Psychooncology. 2002;9:314–322.

69. Barrett R. A nurse's primer on recruiting participants for clinical trials. Oncol Nurs Forum. 2002;29:1091–1098.

70. Marshall PA, Magtanong RV, Leek AC, Hizlan S, Yamokoski AD, Kodish ED. Negotiating decisions during informed consent for pediatric phase I oncology trials. J Empir Res Hum Res Ethics. 2012;7(2):51–59.

71. Instone SL, Mueller MR, Gilbert TL. Therapeutic discourse among nurses and physicians in controlled clinical trials. Nurs Ethics. 2008;15 (6):803–812.

72. Ocker BM, Plank DM. The research nurse role in a clinic-based oncology research setting. Cancer Nurs. 2000;23:286–292.

73. Kapo J, Casarett D. Palliative care in phase I trials: an ethical obligation or undue inducement? J Palliat Med. 2002;5:661–665.

74. Fu S, Barber FD, Naing A, et al. Advance care planning in patients with cancer referred to a phase I clinical trials program: The MD Anderson Cancer Center experience. J Clin Oncol. 2012;30:2891–2896.

CHAPTER 53

Rural palliative care

Marie A. Bakitas, Kathleen N. Clifford,
J. Nicholas Dionne-Odom, and Elizabeth Kvale

> After Hurricane Sandy we couldn't get out of our house because the water washed away the bridge connecting us with the road to clinic. We had to get airlifted by helicopter; I went to stay with my daughter so that I could get to the clinic and get my treatments. . . . I take the Stage Coach (bus service). It takes us just over an hour each way . . . but the people on the bus are real friendly.
>
> Cancer patient in Vermont

Key points

- Providing palliative care to persons living in rural areas across the globe presents significant barriers including transportation, geographical and economic challenges, and often a lack of local clinicians with expertise and resources to provide complex palliative care services.

- Strategies are being designed and successfully implemented to meet the challenges of rural palliative care such as telehealth, phone-based care, specially trained lay community workers, and academic-community partnerships.

- Research in addressing the gaps in expanding the evidence base for palliative care should recognize the unique issues presented by a rural environment.

Case studies

John—a case of lack of local expertise

John is an unmarried 45-year-old road worker and volunteer fireman who was diagnosed with advanced lung cancer following a visit to his local physician for a cough that persisted for months after he had a cold. During the winter he would not take time to go to the doctor because he was responsible for plowing and maintaining the roads in his small town, resulting in many 12-hour work days (longer when it was snowing). Upon diagnosis his local doctor sent him to the academic center, which was over an hour away by the main highway. He underwent chemotherapy and radiation at the academic center but he did not respond. He developed spinal metastasis and severe back pain unresponsive to high dose opioids. He did not get referred to see palliative care specialists at the medical center until after he had had an intraspinal pump placed. He had relief from intraspinal opioids via the pump, but when the discharge planner contacted the only local visiting nurse hospice agency in his small town they would not accept him because they did not have policies in place to care for a patient with an intraspinal pump. Neither the local hospital nor area nursing homes would accept him also due to not having staff that were trained in caring for patients with intraspinal pumps. Offers by the palliative care staff to train nursing staff in the care of the pump were declined, as the managers at these agencies could not "afford" the time to train staff in a procedure that they were unlikely to use again in the near future. John was faced with a decision to continue getting relief from the pump without assistance at home or remove the pump and risk a painful dying.

Katie—lack of age-appropriate specialized expertise

Katie is an 8-year-old child with advanced non-Hodgkin's lymphoma. All standard and investigational treatments have been exhausted, and all agree that she is in last weeks of life. She has a chest tube for comfort to intermittently drain a large pleural effusion, a large wound in her groin with a vacuum dressing, and a central venous catheter for high-dose opioids and antiemetics. She and her parents want her to be able to spend her end-of-life at home. Fortunately her local hospice agency has been trained in caring for all of these types of interventions, but the hospice medical director is reluctant, since he does not have training in pediatrics.

Rural palliative care: what is different?

Among the many challenges that persons with serious illness face in accessing expert palliative care early in their diagnosis, a significant proportion of the population across the globe have an additional challenge of being located in a rural environment. According to the 2010 US Census data, approximately 60 million citizens (about 20% of the US population) live in rural (also called "nonurban" or "micropolitan") areas (Figure 53.1).[1] However, depending on the definition of "rural," estimates of the rural US population can be as high as 40%.[2] Twenty-five percent of Europeans, 25% of Canadians, and 11% of Australians also reside in rural areas. Asia and Africa remain the most rural continents with 58% and 60%, respectively, of the population living in rural areas.[3] Box 53.1 provides additional information about rural definitions and rural health facts.

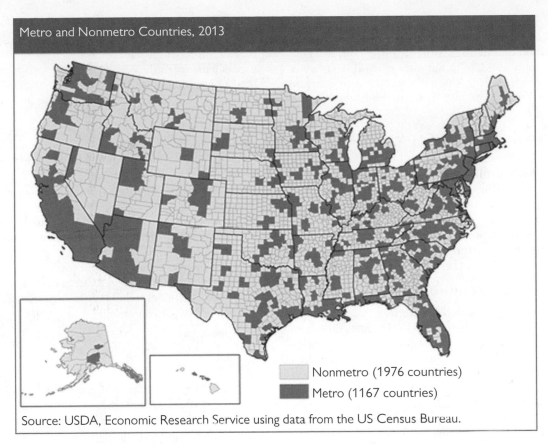

Metro and Nonmetro Countries, 2013

Nonmetro (1976 countries)

Metro (1167 countries)

Source: USDA, Economic Research Service using data from the US Census Bureau.

Figure 53.1 Nonmetropolitan counties include some combination of:
1. open countryside,
2. rural towns (places with fewer than 2,500 people), and
3. urban areas with populations ranging from 2,500 to 49,999
that are not part of larger labor market areas (metropolitan areas). The US Census Bureau uses much smaller geographic building blocks to define rural areas as open country and settlements with fewer than 2,500 residents. Most counties, whether metro or nonmetro, contain a combination of urban and rural populations.

A number of authors have provided literature reviews in the past decade to define and study the issues of palliative care access in rural areas.[4–6] In a comprehensive review, Robinson and colleagues[7] found no US studies that examined and evaluated rural palliative care programs. An updated literature review since that time identified 11 additional papers covering diverse issues, such as validating a model of rural palliative care, identifying differences in care, patient and provider perspectives, and social and ethical issues.[4]

Rural patients who are in the final stages of their illness are particularly vulnerable and at high risk to experience disparities in care and social isolation.[8] A recent report card on access to palliative care in US hospitals found that living in a region served by small rural hospitals put patients at high risk to not having access to palliative care.[9] Long distances and low population density impose logistical and financial barriers that can impede access to specialty care and diffusion of innovations. Rural hospice and palliative care programs are eclectic, and community-based hospice resources may be limited.[7] Local primary care clinicians are most often multiskilled generalists who may see few terminally ill patients, limiting their ability to develop needed palliative care expertise.[7] In small rural communities with scarce palliative care resources, clinicians may also face the challenge of being called on to care for their own family, life-long friends, and neighbors at their end-of-life.[7]

Rural location has often been related to less and later hospice use[10] and higher rates of hospitalization at end-of-life, particularly in rural nursing home residents.[11] Most rural patients in need of palliative care expertise are unlikely to have access to the "gold standard" interdisciplinary team provided by palliative and hospice services. As a result, these patients may have to choose between "going without" or being transferred to a distant site for care.[4] Patients transferred to distant tertiary care settings are at high risk of spending their last days or weeks of life far from home and loved ones. Rural patients with advanced disease, severe pain, or related symptoms who make the choice not to be transferred to a tertiary care center may suffer during their last weeks of life because many areas lack the availability of state-of-the-art techniques for treating pain or other causes of distress. The cases at the beginning of this chapter provide vivid examples of the suffering that can occur when local rural areas are not equipped and staff is not trained to handle the specialized care that can be provided at end-of-life.

Challenges to providing palliative care in rural settings

As is apparent in the case studies and Box 53.2, the challenges and barriers to accessing and providing palliative care are numerous. A survey of 23 community sites within the National Cancer

---

Box 53.1 Defining rural

Sometimes population density is the defining concern; population thresholds used to differentiate rural and urban communities range from 2,500 up to 50,000, depending on the definition. Two commonly used methods for defining rural are:

Rural urban commuting area (RUCA) classification

The rural-urban commuting area (RUCA) codes classify US census tracts using measures of population density, urbanization, and daily commuting.

They are classified as:

Metropolitan (population 50,000 or greater)

Large Rural* (10,000 through 49,999)

Small Rural* town (2,500 through 9,999)

Isolated Small Rural* town (2499 or less)

Urban, urban area, urban clusters, rural

For the 2010 Census, an urban area comprised a densely settled core of census tracts and/or census blocks that meet minimum population density requirements, along with adjacent territory containing nonresidential urban land uses as well as territory with low population density included to link outlying densely settled territory with the densely settled core. To qualify as an urban area, the territory identified according to criteria must encompass at least 2,500 people, at least 1,500 of which reside outside institutional group quarters. The Census Bureau identifies two types of urban areas:

◆ Urbanized Areas (UAs) of 50,000 or more people;

◆ Urban Clusters (UCs) of at least 2,500 and less than 50,000 people.

"Rural" encompasses all population, housing, and territory not included within an urban area.

Source: http://www.census.gov/geo/reference/ua/urban-rural-2010.html

Facts about rural health issues

◆ The rural area poverty rate was 17.0% in 2011 and has remained consistently higher than the urban poverty rate over time. This is the highest rate since 1993.

◆ Population growth was uneven across rural and small-town America: over half of the 2,053 urban counties lost population, while in over 350 others, population growth was higher than the national average rate of 0.7%.

◆ Rural America had just over 51 million residents in July 2011, a slight increase in population over the previous year compared with a slightly smaller percent in urban areas.

◆ The rate of rural population growth in America has slowed dramatically since the onset of the housing mortgage crisis in late 2006 and the recession a year later.

*Rural is also categorized/known as "micropolitan" in some US government schemas.

Source: United States Department of Agriculture (USDA), economic research service analysis using data from the Bureau of Labor Statistics. Economic Brief Number 21. December 2012.

Box 53.2 Barriers/challenges to rural palliative care

Lack of clinician acceptance

Lack of patient/family acceptance

Limited community clinician access to palliative care experts

Limited community clinician exposure to palliative care patients in their practice

Limited availability of palliative care education in the community

Poor communication/coordination of care between academic and rural community settings

Limited evidence of palliative care benefits in rural palliative care

Lack of transportation and long distances to palliative care centers (for patients and family/friend visitors)

Preference to stay in home community for care

Patient/clinician concerns that they will lose touch with community providers if they seek care at centers far from home

Lack of availability of technology/techniques used for complex patients (e.g., pain pumps)

Sources: Data from Clifford et al. (2012), reference 12; Dunham et al. (2003), reference 93; Goodridge and Duggleby (2010), reference 94.

Institute Community Cancer Center Programs (NCCCP) conducted by Clifford and colleagues identified the top barrier to integrating palliative care in 65% of their community programs as lack of physician acceptance. In that survey physicians believed that patients' needs were already being adequately addressed without the addition of palliative care services. That there was only a 17% use of palliative care resources in the communities that had such resources is no surprise.[12] "Gate-keeping" by physicians, that is lack of referral of patients for palliative care services, is not unique to rural settings; however, the reasons for this and extent have not been fully explored in rural locales. It is therefore not unexpected that patients and family members may not seek out or accept palliative care or hospice providers if a trusted physician does not advocate for these services.

Rural geography can create feelings of isolation in both patients and clinicians.[13] Community hospice providers may have to travel great distances to see patients, making visits infrequent and creating difficulty in providing a rapid response to patients' and families' feelings of distress.[14–16]

Another barrier to providing high quality palliative care in rural areas is the inaccessibility of adequate clinician education in the most current palliative care practices.[17] While distance education may soon address this issue, currently, clinicians who wish to obtain specialized palliative care training must be able to get release time and travel great distances to find high-quality programs. Access to on-line resources, current journals, and palliative care textbooks is essential. However, complex palliative care communication techniques are often most effectively learned through "in person" and role-play strategies, which may not be readily available.[17] A comprehensive review of professional development for rural palliative care nurses found very little research on the best ways to provide quality palliative care education that actually had an impact on patient outcomes; a lack of availability, use of, and satisfaction with distance technology for education; and very little use of interactive learning strategies for nurses.

These authors recommended the need for more research on the best ways to improve palliative care education through increasing information technology use and targeted education to meet the needs of rural learners.[17]

Creative strategies to meet the palliative care needs of rural patients

Telehealth

A major challenge to palliative care delivery in rural areas is the need to provide high quality care across distances with limited resources. Telehealth, or telemedicine, uses advanced information and communication technologies to improve access to care. Telehealth is not a single technology; rather, it is a large, heterogeneous collection of clinical practices, technologies, and organizational arrangements.[18] Telehealth strategies have been found to be cost-effective and have been associated with high quality clinical outcomes and high patient satisfaction in a variety of healthcare areas, including palliative care.[19,20] Barriers to telehealth, such as startup and maintenance costs and concerns over equipment costs, privacy, and security, have begun to decrease. Furthermore, adoption of electronic medical records has contributed to staff training and comfort levels with telehealth. There has also been fear that overdependence on technology will be seen as dehumanizing and impersonal, conflicting with core principles of palliative care.[21] However, increasing evidence demonstrates that it has been possible to overcome these barriers and high satisfaction has been reported as telehealth improves access to palliative care.[22] Palliative care telehealth approaches can provide access to consultations, education, and collaboration for providers, patients, families and caregivers.[23–25] Such approaches are being successfully implemented in rural areas around the world.[26–29]

Worldwide healthcare delivery systems are evolving and the telehealth industry is expanding rapidly. Health data can easily be monitored and measured over geographical, social, and cultural distances. This is facilitated by the use of the Internet and smart phones, with an increasing number of mobile applications available. In the United States an estimated 11% of Americans had a health application on their cell phone in 2012.[30] The Health Information Technology for Economic and Clinical Health (HITECH) Act, enacted by Congress in 2009, accelerated the adoption of meaningful use of information technology (IT) for clinical purposes.[31] The HITECH Act defines meaningful use objectives for participants in Medicare and Medicaid programs aimed at improving quality, safety, and efficiency; engaging patients and families; improving care coordination; improving public and population health; and ensuring privacy and security for personal health information. In 2013 the Federal Communications Commission (FCC) funded a rural healthcare support mechanism to expand access to broadband, especially in rural areas. This is intended to encourage the creation of healthcare networks and use of technology to improve care, lower costs, and improve patient experiences.[32] The use of information technology and mobile applications is still in the the early stages.[30]

Using telehealth to increase access for patients

An early application of telehealth was the use of phone and Internet videoconferencing to link regional specialists with providers in remote locations. A collaborative model using Internet conferencing between a rural palliative care nurse practitioner and an urban palliative care physician expert was able to improve access for underserved patients and families.[33] A Canadian study used regional palliative care experts to provide telehealth assessments and coordinate with local providers to improve symptom management.[25] A Canadian province developed a 24-hour telephone hotline to provide expert palliative care consultation, which was most frequently accessed by rural communities.[34]

Palliative care consultation has been used to expand access in Canada's Rural Palliative Telehealth Project.[35] Aided by provincial and national funding, the aim of the project was to examine the use of telehealth to conduct direct palliative care consultations with patients and families, conduct palliative care conferences with distant primary care teams, deliver staff education, and link rural patients with their urban specialists under circumstances where travel was no longer reasonable or possible. The project found that telehealth was particularly useful for linking with rural home care teams for palliative care case conferences. However, its utility in direct patient consultation was limited by shortage of videoconference equipment at the bedside in rural facilities, lack of technology for in-home use, and patient conditions that affected communication, such as delirium or excessive drowsiness. Telehealth was not ideal for new patient consultations but did prove helpful in follow-up discussions with rural palliative providers and urban consultants. Often difficult treatment decisions could be discussed and future plans established without the need to travel to an urban center. Telehealth was beneficial for discharge planning between the urban tertiary palliative care unit and the rural care team when patients with complex issues were being transitioned back to their home communities. Project funding was used to purchase videoconferencing equipment for the palliative care unit conference room to enable this part of the project to proceed.[35]

Rural patients' experiences with telehealth

Remote monitoring, in combination with the application of adult learning and cognitive behavioral theories applied to telehealth care delivery and practice, can promote improved patient self-efficacy with disease management.[36] The benefit of phone interventions by advanced practice nurses in providing quality palliative care to patients and caregivers in rural areas has been demonstrated.[37]

An early application of telehealth, via a primarily phone-based concurrent palliative care intervention for newly diagnosed rural advanced cancer patients, from 1999 to the present, is called Project ENABLE (Educate, Nurture, Advise, Before Life Ends).[37–39] Developed for patients with advanced cancer, ENABLE is based on the World Health Organization continuum of care[40,41] and Wagner's chronic illness care[42] models. Following a face-to-face standardized palliative care consultation, the "Charting Your Course" curriculum (see Table 53.1) is delivered by a nurse coach to patients and care partners. Approximately 1000 patients (and their family caregivers) have participated in this series of clinical trials. Published trial results have demonstrated gains in quality of life, improvement in symptoms, less depression, and improved survival.[37,43] The primary focus of the ENABLE model involves coaching patients to learn new skills of problem-solving, patient empowerment and activation, proactive symptom management,

Table 53.1 ENABLE Charting Your Course Curriculum

Patient Curriculum—Charting Your Course (CYC)	Caregiver Curriculum—COPE
Module 1 (week 1)	**Module 1 (week 1)**
Behavioral Activation/Problem Solving	Problem Solving & Self Care
Module 2 (week 2)	**Module 2 (week 2)**
Symptom Management	Focus on **symptom management**
Module 3 (week 3)	**Module 3 (week 3)**
Decision-making, Communication & Support	Focus on **decision-making**
Module 4 (week 4)	Planning for follow up
Life Accomplishments & Goals and Life Review	**Monthly & bereavement follow-up**
Module 5 (week 5)	
Accomplishments and Future Goals/ Forgiveness	
Module 6 (week 6)	
Unfinished Business/Leaving a Legacy	
Monthly follow-up	

healthcare decision-making, advance care planning, communication, and legacy/life review. Another feature is assisting the patient and family to identify local, community primary care and palliative/hospice resources to reduce dependence on distant care providers and allow them to stay in their home communities. Family caregivers participating in the program report lower depression scores, and improved symptom burdens.[44]

The Veterans Health Administration (VHA) began the VA Hospice and Palliative Care initiative in 2002, collaborating with the National Hospice and Palliative Care Organization to improve care to veterans and families. In addition to establishing hospice and palliative care teams in all its medical centers, the initiative developed a telehealth model to provide holistic end-of-life care. The Advanced Illness/Palliative Care (AIPC) program utilized text messaging and videophones to monitor patients and provide symptom management and spiritual support. Participants reported that technology helped them feel more connected to the care team.[45,46]

Videoconferencing

Videoconferencing specialists' consultation to rural cancer patients attending local health facilities was found to be feasible, required minimal equipment, resulted in cost savings and is satisfactory to participants.[47] Psychotherapy interventions can be effectively delivered with telephone or videoconferencing.[36,48] Patients who are too ill to leave their homes can benefit from Dignity Psychotherapy interventions via videophone.[49]

Web-based resources

Palliative care resources are available through the Internet to anyone with electronic access. The Center for the Advancement of Palliative Care (CAPC.org) offers Internet-based educational programs and links for patients and caregivers. The American Academy of Hospice and Palliative Medicine (AAHPM.org) and the Hospice and Palliative Nursing Association (HPNA.org) offer online resources. Healthcare networks and advocacy groups are using electronic media to make educational programs available to healthcare providers, patients, caregivers, and the general public. In Australia, oncology specialists developed an educational program on palliative oncology for health professionals that focused on the needs of rural providers. Participants reported they improved their knowledge, and 75% planned to review or change their practice as a result.[28] The Minnesota Rural Palliative Care Initiative partnered with rural communities to expand access to palliative care using Web-based educational sessions, a dedicated Web page with resources for program development, links to national guidelines, clinical tools, and shared draft documents.[23] The NCCCP (ncccp.cancer.gov) encouraged palliative care initiatives to improve access in underserved and rural areas. The group collaborated via teleconferencing and Internet file sharing to establish a program assessment tool based on established quality standards and services relevant to ambulatory community cancer care.[12,50]

Developing clinical capacity of adequately prepared clinicians in rural palliative care

As the population over age 65 doubles by 2030, a shortfall is projected over the next 20 years for many physician specialties. Distribution of palliative care resources is noted to vary by geographic region, with rural regions most frequently underserved.[14,51,52] As the need for services expands in the coming years, the interdisciplinary team will be increasingly important, including in palliative care and particularly in rural areas.[46,47,53–55] A recent survey of hospice medical directors in one rural state found that none of the responding medical directors were board certified in Hospice and Palliative Care.[56] The palliative care workforce issue among physicians is well defined with conservative models estimating the current shortfall at between 6000 and 18,000 physicians. This prediction has not taken into consideration the anticipated growth in palliative outpatient care.[57] As a result there is a need to increase expertise of all physicians in palliative care content.[58] This strategy can be combined with enhanced education in palliative care skills at the early learner level and with policy support to mandate palliative care training in all training programs. This should increase the number of physicians with adequate training to address primary palliative care needs.[59]

The Institute of Medicine[60] has called for nurses to fill new and expanded roles to increase access to care. Healthcare transformation is increasing the use of advanced practice nurses such as clinical specialists and nurse practitioners. While hospitals are establishing programs led by board-certified palliative medicine physicians, advance practice nurses have led the way in outpatient care providing symptom management and acting as a coordinator and as a resource for the interdisciplinary team.[39,61–66] Palliative care programs have been able to expand services to outpatient and home care with the use of advanced practice nurses.[54] A Pennsylvania health network utilized nurse practitioners to provide home-based nonhospice consultation that improved access to palliative care and reduced inpatient costs for end-of-life care.[47,67] The VA model for palliative care has also successfully used advanced nurse practitioners.[46] The HPNA offers educational programs, promotes networking, and provides for specialty certification for advanced practice nurses (www.HPNA.org).

As more advanced practice nurses are added to the workforce they are improving access to quality palliative care.

Lay health workers

Given that most persons with advanced illness are located in community settings,[69] and the relative scarcity of outpatient palliative care support,[70] strategies to address the palliative care needs of persons living in rural areas must include innovative health services. Lay health workers (community health advisors or community health workers) have been effective in disseminating public health and behavioral strategies and interventions to improve health outcomes.[70,71] Community health workers trained in principles of palliative care may have a role in delivering components of palliative care in regions where access to formal healthcare systems with palliative care resources is limited.[70] In developing countries, volunteer community health workers have been trained in basics of palliative care and supported in the delivery of care. Evaluations have found these programs to be beneficial to both patients and the volunteer health worker.[70] In some areas community health workers include health system "navigators," thus extending the role of the lay navigator from reduction of cancer disparities to the palliative care spectrum.

The effectiveness of this approach is being evaluated in some established cancer navigation programs. The Deep South Cancer Navigation Network, which has demonstrated important gains in cancer screening rates, is training nurse and lay navigators (community health advisors) both in communication skills related to conversations and decision-making about advanced disease and in symptom recognition and advocacy.[72] The feasibility and impact of this implementation of the cancer navigation model on palliative care outcomes is yet to be determined.

In rural regions with high levels of hospice penetration, lay health workers may also be engaged as "sitters." "Sitters" are persons without formal medical training who may assist in the care of a seriously ill person by providing companionship, assistance with activities of daily living, and assistance with other practical and logistical issues. Persons with limited healthcare training (in the United States identified as certified nursing assistants [CNAs] or in Canada they may be personal service workers) have a role in caring for persons with advanced illness. Data from Canada and Great Britain indicate that these workers find caring for palliative care patients challenging,[73] but no data were identified related to workforce capacity or rural locations in the United States. Hospice volunteers in rural regions may also have an expanded scope. This expanded role of volunteerism provides valuable assistance while interacting with both informal and formal caregivers of hospice patients.[74] The available literature indicates that in rural regions, support for palliative care patients may include a complex web of individuals including informal caregivers, community volunteers, and trained healthcare workers who form an organic and site-specific network of caring for the seriously ill and dying.[75] While literature and evidence about the role of lay health workers or community advisors in palliative care and hospice is sparse, it is likely that pressures to expand capacity for the provision of palliative care in rural regions will increase the use and evaluation of these services in coming years. Important areas for research include defining the role that community health workers or community health advisors may play in enhancing access to palliative care in rural regions. Understanding the potential impact of using lay personnel on palliative care outcomes, and defining the best way to integrate training for this potential new workforce in rural palliative care should be an active area of investigation.

The role of critical access hospitals

Rural hospitals provide essential healthcare services to nearly 54 million people, including 9 million Medicare beneficiaries, who are often in need of palliative care services. Rural hospitals care for, on average, a higher percentage of Medicare patients, since rural populations are typically older than average urban populations.[76] Medicare reimbursement issues, sustained workforce shortages, rising healthcare insurance costs, aging rural hospital facilities, and the demand for expensive new information systems all contribute to the daily challenges of providing adequate care in rural settings. To deal with some of these issues, in 1997 through the Balanced Budget Act (BBA) of 1997, a designation of Critical Access Hospitals (CAHs) was developed that would receive cost-based reimbursement. To be designated a CAH, a rural hospital must meet defined criteria (see Box 53.3).[77]

The goal of CAHs can at times be at cross purposes with the goals of palliative care. For example, there is financial incentive for brief stays to essentially stabilize and transfer the patient to a larger hospital or academic center.[78] In many cases, for these chronically ill, older adults, the more appropriate goal from a palliative care perspective, would be to establish goals of care and identify appropriate local care resources rather than transfer these patients to academic centers from which they might not ever return. In many cases it might be more appropriate for these rural hospitals

---

Box 53.3 Critical access hospital criteria

- Must be rural, located within a state participating in the Medicare Rural Hospital Flexibility program

- Must be more than a 35-mile drive from any other hospital or CAH (or, in the case of mountainous terrains or in areas where only secondary roads are available, more than 15 miles from any other hospital or CAH)

- Must have 15 or fewer acute inpatient care beds (or, in the case of swing bed facilities, up to 25 inpatient beds which can be used interchangeably for acute or SNF-level care, provided no more than 15 beds are used at any one time for acute care) as reported on the cost report

- Must restrict patient length of stay to no more than 96 hours unless a longer period is required because of inclement weather or other emergency conditions, or a physician review organization (PRO) or other equivalent entity, on request, waives the 96-hour restriction (modified the 96-hour length-of-stay limitation in 1999 to a per patient annual average)

- Must offer 24-hour emergency services

- Must be owned by a public or nonprofit entity (modified in 1999 to extend eligibility to for-profit hospitals)

Source: American Hospital Association (2013), reference 77.

to keep patients for end-of-life care or to stabilize the patient and if possible arrange for return home with hospice care. Two efforts to encourage this approach in CAHs, improve care and increase access to expert palliative care resources in rural Northern New England were the North Country Palliative Care Collaborative (NCPCC) and the Peer Observership Program (POP). The NCPCC was developed to improve rural clinician knowledge, skills, and care coordination of palliative care patients in areas served by critical access hospitals in Northern New England. The POP brought teams of rural clinicians to an academic center with an established palliative care program for 1- and 2-week experiential learning experiences. The goals of the program were to increase trust and to establish relationships and expertise in the local clinicians. In this way when future patient situations arose, more local resources and ready access to palliative care experts would increase the likelihood that patients remained in their home community for palliative care when needed.

Creating academic-community partnerships and systemwide improvements

Patients with palliative care needs located in rural or isolated areas have been able to take advantage of local community resources and to rely on local primary care and other clinicians, through partnerships with an academic or other palliative care program that is well resourced. A guide developed by the Health Research and Educational trust for small and rural hospitals, focuses strategies to improve care by using a focus on better population health management. This is achieved through well-structured relationships between rural hospitals and community care partnerships.[76] Figure 53.2 illustrates a continuum of types of population health partnerships: (1) networking, (2) coordination, (3) cooperation,

and (4) collaboration.[76] The reader is referred to the guidebook *The Role of Small and Rural Hospitals and Care Systems in Effective Population Health Partnerships* for excellent resources in developing such relationships (available at http://www.hpoe.org/small-rural-partnerships).

As can be seen in Figure 53.3, there are palliative care programs located throughout the United States that serve as tertiary centers. These centers should have, as part of their mission, strategies to bring their expertise to the community. Using community capacity development theory, a learning collaborative model, and focusing on the National Quality Forum "Consensus Report: National Framework and Preferred Practices for Palliative and Hospice Care Quality," a partnership called the Minnesota Rural Palliative Care Initiative (MRPCI) was formed between Stratis Health, an independent nonprofit organization, and Fairview Health Services' palliative care program. The goal was to improve care across 10 rural communities. The MRPCI partnered with rural communities to expand access to palliative care using Web-based educational sessions, a dedicated Web page with resources for program development, links to national guidelines, clinical tools, and shared draft documents.[23]

Another innovative partnership (mentioned previously) between an established palliative care program at the Dartmouth-Hitchcock Medical Center (DHMC) and community hospitals and clinicians across northern New Hampshire and Vermont, the NCPCC was formed to improve community awareness and expertise in end-of-life care.[78] The program brought together more than 150 individuals, representing hospitals, home health and hospice agencies, nursing homes, physicians' practices, community pharmacies, and other social service providers, to address the specific challenges of providing palliative care in rural communities. A needs assessment, the Transitions of Care Quality

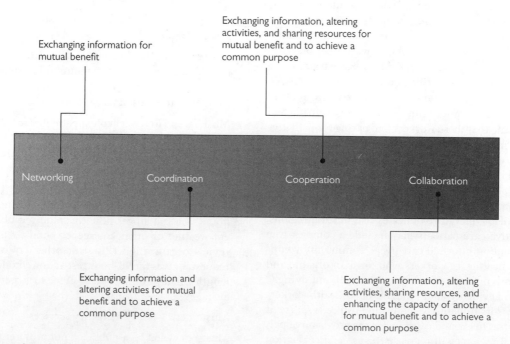

Figure 53.2 Types of population health partnerships.

Sources: Adapted from Robert Pestronk et al.'s Public health role: Collaborating for Healthy Communities, and Arthur T. Himmelman's Collaboration for a Change: Definitions, Decision-making Models, Roles and Collaboration Process Guide, 2013.

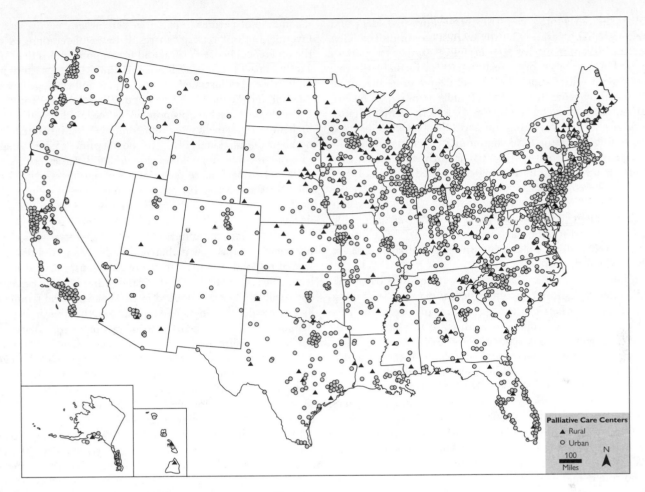

Figure 53.3 Map of rural versus urban palliative care programs.
Only 10% of the palliative care centers are in rural areas despite 20% of the population being there.
Urban = 1875
Rural = 204
Total = 2079
Map created by Heather Carlos, MS, Norris Cotton Cancer Center; Lebanon, NH, GeoSpatial Resource.
Data from: http://www.census.gov/geo/reference/ua/urban-rural-2010.html

Improvement Survey, identified areas ripe for improvement, including the following:

1. Communication between care providers in the community and DHMC, defining clearly the provider(s) ultimately responsible for each patient's local medical care;

2. Rapid transfer of all relevant medical information to and from the referral centers;

3. More consistent, timely feedback regarding a patient's care after transfer to a referral center or a patient's return to their community; and

4. Availability of common palliative care medications in community pharmacies.

The system improvement efforts of the NCPCC yielded changes in patterns of referrals, local and regional consultation with specialty services, use of assessment tools, rural pharmacy formulary guidelines to increase symptom medication availability, and a general increase in baseline knowledge of palliative care practice.[78]

Delivering palliative care in rural areas beyond the United States

Across the globe, authors note that the evidence base characterizing rural palliative care has yet to come into full maturity, and thus there is still much to discover about how current guidelines can best be applied.[79-81] However, there are both similar and dissimilar elements in delivery and receipt of palliative care in the rural United States. In industrialized nations, like the United States, the demand for palliative care services in rural areas appears to far outweigh the supply.[80] However, the gap between demand and supply is likely to become further exaggerated in developing countries as the average life expectancy and increase in populations of individuals 65 and older are expected to increase exponentially.[80] Because of the proportionally few palliative care specialists in developing countries, generalist providers and informal caregivers residing locally in rural communities often provide the bulk of palliative care services.[79] Studies from South Africa and Australia report a relative lack of formal palliative care training in international healthcare degree programs and a high demand by generalists, who feel underprepared, to receive formal palliative care education.[79,80,82] As in the United States, many rural palliative care programmatic efforts have prioritized mentoring and educating local community providers and volunteers in delivering palliative care, particularly rural home care providers, as opposed to developing centralized, hospital-based approaches whereby the larger urban centers attempt to serve the rural areas.[83–86] Unfortunately, also as in the United States, palliative care is often viewed as care provided at the very end of life after all curative treatments have been exhausted.[79,87] Hence, the patterns of underutilization and late timing of palliative care are equally prevalent.[88]

Although many challenges of rural settings outside of the United States are similar, as described above, in developing nations, they are often more pronounced and extreme. This is partly because the public and healthcare infrastructure of many developing nations is markedly less amenable to the delivery of palliative care services and medications in remote areas. Examples of this include insufficient inventory or lack of access to pain medications, especially opioids[78,80,83,84]; severely decrepit or nonexistent highways and roads combined with considerable distances between remote areas[79,82,84]; limited legal scope of practice for nurses resulting in the inability to administer pain medications[79]; and physical dangers including fear of violence and infectious disease, particularly for home care providers.[87] Thus, the role demands of the palliative care clinician or team are oftentimes vastly greater in scope and can include providing food, shelter, and transportation provisions.[82–84] Taboos can also often be more extreme than in the United States: for example Singer et al.[84] note that the Bedouin population in Israel seldom speak the word "cancer" as there is great shame associated with having this illness. The shame is such that a Bedouin girl of a family where someone has cancer may have difficulties marrying. In another study, Campbell[89] found that male palliative care health workers in South Africa were perceived by female patients as more likely to perpetrate physical abuse, thus hindering the delivery of palliative care. Finally, the types of life-threatening illnesses addressed by palliative care clinicians in foreign rural areas are often not the advanced cancer and heart failure populations seen in the United States and other developed countries but HIV/AIDS and tuberculosis, as is prevalent in sub-Saharan Africa.[87] All this said, such stark contrasts in rural palliative care are more salient when the distinction is between industrialized and developing countries as opposed to the United States and all other countries.

Clinical and research implications

There have been many outstanding efforts in the past two decades to improve and articulate standards for the emerging specialty of palliative care.[90] Yet existing guidelines and models of palliative care delivery have mostly overlooked a key multifaceted variable that is critical to achieving better outcomes at the population level: that of geography and of the unique obstacles faced by palliative care clinicians delivering care to rural populations. When it comes to disparities in palliative care, *where* one lives matters. Overlooking this reality can result in an underappreciation of the differences between rural and urban populations that significantly impact the approach one takes in delivering optimal palliative care. As illustrated in this chapter and cataloged by Hart, Larson, and Lishner,[91] rural populations in comparison with urban populations have proportionally more older adults over 65; higher unemployment rates; higher numbers of uninsured; higher numbers of individuals below the poverty line; greater sensitivity to economic downturn; lower population densities, longer travel distances to healthcare facilities; fewer numbers of healthcare specialists and generalist providers; narrower scope of available healthcare services; higher rates of chronic disease; and greater dependence on Medicare and Medicaid.

Accounting for these and other unique characteristics of rurality, the question is how palliative care clinicians and researchers should respond. For palliative care clinicians, the priority challenge will be to explicitly ask about and address any misperceptions about palliative care expressed by rural patients and families and local generalist providers. We recommend that this be a requisite item of discussion with any new interaction or consultation with patients, families, and providers. Clinicians might also consider taking a more proactive approach and initiate regular check-ins with generalist providers in outlying areas to offer expertise and consultation on difficult cases in their areas. A model from Spain suggested that development of community-based teams, with central coordination, showed promise.[92]

For palliative care researchers, a change in perspective is needed that migrates from the familiar territory of health as seen at the pathophysiological, individual, and social level to the more uncharted terrain of palliative care at the level of living conditions, communities, geography, and social and economic policies and climates. Given the growing use, prevalence, and capabilities of communications and other technologies, researchers are called on to propose and test innovative solutions that incorporate the use of such technologies in order to overcome many of the geographical obstacles of rural healthcare delivery.

If but one message comes across, we hope that it is conveyed that where one lives makes a huge difference to whether or not a patient and family receive adequate palliative care.

References

1. The Economics of Food, Farming, Natural Resources, and Rural America: Measuring Rurality: What Is Rural? 2007. (Accessed March 26, 2009, at http://www.ers.usda.gov/Briefing/Rurality/WhatisRural/.)
2. US Department of Agriculture ERS. Defining the "Rural" in Rural America; Amber Waves: The Economics of Food, Farming, Natural Resources, and Rural America. 2008 June.
3. Urban and Rural Areas. United Nations, 2009. (Accessed June 1, 2013, at http://www.un.org/en/development/desa/population/publications/pdf/urbanization/urbanization-wallchart2009.pdf.)
4. Downing J, Jack BA. End-of-life care in rural areas: what is different? Curr Opin Support Palliat Care. 2012;6:391–397.
5. Robinson CA, Pesut B, Bottorff JL. Issues in rural palliative care: views from the countryside. J Rural Health. 2010;26:78–84.
6. Wilson DM, Justice C, Sheps S, Thomas R, Reid P, Leibovici K. Planning and providing end-of-life care in rural areas. J Rural Health. 2006;22:174–181.
7. Robinson CA, Pesut B, Bottorff JL, Mowry A, Broughton S, Fyles G. Rural palliative care: a comprehensive review. J Palliat Med. 2009;12:253–258.

8. Institute of Medicine. Crossing the Quality Chasm: A New Health System for the 21st Century. Washington, DC: National Academy Press; 2001.

9. Morrison RS, Meier DE. America's Care of Serious Illness: A State-by-State Report Card on Access to Palliative Care in Our Nation's Hospitals. New York: Center to Advance Palliative Care; 2011.

10. McCarthy EP, Burns RB, Davis RB, Phillips RS. Barriers to hospice care among older patients dying with lung and colorectal cancer. J Clin Oncol. 2003;21:728–735.

11. Haller IV, Gessert CE. Utilization of medical services at the end of life in older adults with cognitive impairment: focus on outliers. J Palliat Med. 2007;10:400–407.

12. Clifford K, Tallen C, Davis MH, et al. Implementing patient-centered care: challenges in community oncology. J Clin Oncol. 2012;30:192.

13. Baltic T, Bakitas Whedon M, Ahles T, Fanciullo G. Improving pain management in a rural area. Cancer Pract. 2002;10:S39–S44.

14. Carlson MD, Bradley EH, Du Q, Morrison RS. Geographic access to hospice in the United States. J Palliat Med. 2010;13:1331–1338.

15. Campbell CL, Merwin E, Yan GF. Factors That influence the presence of a hospice in a rural community. J Nurs Sch. 2009;41:420–428.

16. Lynch S. Hospice and palliative care access issues in rural areas. Am J Hosp Palliat Care. 2013;30:172–177.

17. Phillips JL, Piza M, Ingham J. Continuing professional development programmes for rural nurses involved in palliative care delivery: an integrative review. Nurs Educ Today. 2012;32:385–392.

18. Institute of Medicine. The Role of Telehealth in an Evolving Health Care Environment: Workshop Summary. Washington, DC: Author; 2012.

19. Darkins A, Ryan P, Kobb R, et al. Care coordination/home telehealth: the systematic implementation of health informatics, home telehealth, and disease management to support the care of veteran patients with chronic conditions. Telemed JE Health. 2008;14:1118–1126.

20. Kidd L, Cayless S, Johnston B, Wengstrom Y. Telehealth in palliative care in the UK: a review of the evidence. J Telemed Telecare. 2010;16:394–402.

21. Kuziemsky C, Jewers H, Appleby B, et al. Information technology and hospice palliative care: social, cultural, ethical and technical implications in a rural setting. Inform Health Soc Care. 2012;37:37–50.

22. Whitten P, Doolittle G, Mackert M. Providers' acceptance of telehospice. J Palliat Med. 2005;8:730–735.

23. Ceronsky L, Shearer J, Weng K, Hopkins M, McKinley D. Minnesota Rural Palliative Care Initiative: building palliative care capacity in rural Minnesota. J Palliat Med. 2013;16:310–313.

24. Nesbitt TS, Dharmar M, Katz-Bell J, Hartvigsen G, Marcin JP. Telehealth at UC Davis—a 20-year experience. Telemed JE Health. 2013;19:357–362.

25. Watanabe SM, Fairchild A, Pituskin E, Borgersen P, Hanson J, Fassbender K. Improving access to specialist multidisciplinary palliative care consultation for rural cancer patients by videoconferencing: report of a pilot project. Support Care Cancer. 2013;21:1201–1207.

26. Johnston B. UK telehealth initiatives in palliative care: a review. Int J Palliat Nurs. 2011;17:301–308.

27. Johnston B, Kidd L, Wengstrom Y, Kearney N. An evaluation of the use of Telehealth within palliative care settings across Scotland. Palliat Med. 2012;26:152–161.

28. Koczwara B, Francis K, Marine F, Goldstein D, Underhill C, Olver I. Reaching further with online education?: The development of an effective online program in palliative oncology. J Cancer Educ. 2010;25:317–323.

29. Brecher DB. The use of Skype in a community hospital inpatient palliative medicine consultation service. J Palliat Med. 2013;16:110–112.

30. West DM (2012). How Mobile Devices are transforming healthcare. Issues in Technology Innovation, May(18) Center for Technology Innovation at Brookings Institute. accessed July 6, 2014. http://www.brookings.edu/~/media/research/files/papers/2012/5/22%20mobile%20health%20west/22%20mobile%20health%20west.pdf

31. DHHS. CMS. 42 CFR Parts 412,413, 422 et al. Medicare and Medicaid Programs Electronic Health Record Incentive Program Final Rule. Federal Register 2010;75:44314–44588.

32. FCC. Rural Health Care Support Mechanism, 47 CFR Part 54, Final Rule. Federal Register 2013;78.

33. Kuebler KK, Bruera E. Interactive collaborative consultation model in end-of-life care. J Pain Symptom Manage. 2000;20:202–209.

34. Ridley JZ, Gallagher R. Palliative care telephone consultation: who calls and what do they need to know? J Palliat Med. 2008;11: 1009–1014.

35. Spice R, Read Paul L, Biondo PD. Development of a rural palliative care program in the Calgary Zone of Alberta Health Services. J Pain Symptom Manage. 2012;43:911–924.

36. Hilty DM, Ferrer DC, Parish MB, Johnston B, Callahan EJ, Yellowlees PM. The effectiveness of telemental health: a 2013 review. Telemed JE Health. 2013;19:444–454.

37. Bakitas M, Lyons K, Hegel M, et al. Effects of a palliative care intervention on clinical outcomes in patients with advanced cancer: the Project ENABLE II randomized controlled trial. JAMA. 2009;302: 741–749.

38. Bakitas M, Stevens M, Ahles T, et al. Project ENABLE: a palliative care demonstration project for advanced cancer patients in three settings. J Palliat Med. 2004;7:363–372.

39. Bakitas M, Bishop MF, Caron P, Stephens L. Developing successful models of cancer palliative care services. Semin Oncol Nurs. 2010;26:266–284.

40. WHO. Definition of Palliative Care. 2010. (Accessed November, 2010, at http://www.who.int/cancer/palliative/definition/en/.)

41. World Health Organization. Cancer Pain Relief and Palliative Care. Geneva; 1990.

42. Wagner EH, Austin BT, Davis C, Hindmarsh M, Schaefer J, Bonomi A. Improving chronic illness care: translating evidence into action. Health Aff. 2001;20:64–78.

43. Bakitas M, Tosteson T, Li Z, et al. The ENABLE III randomized controlled trial of concurrent palliative oncology care. J Clin Oncol. 2014;32:9512.

44. Dionne-Odem JN, Azuero A, Lyons K, et al. Benefits of immediate versus delayed palliative care to informal family caregivers of persons with advanced cancer: outcomes from the ENABLE III randomized clinical trial. J Clin Oncol. 2014;32:LBA9513.

45. Deitrick LM, Rockwell EH, Gratz N, et al. Delivering specialized palliative care in the community: a new role for nurse practitioners. Adv Nurs Sci. 2011;34:E23–E36.

46. Maudlin J, Keene J, Kobb R. A road map for the last journey: home telehealth for holistic end-of-life care. Am J Hosp Palliat Care. 2006;23:399–403.

47. Eichmeyer JN, Zuckerman DS, Beck TM, et al. Telehealth for oncology genetic counseling: an Idaho experience. J Clin Oncol. 2012;30:288.

48. Shore JH. Telepsychiatry: videoconferencing in the delivery of psychiatric care. Am J Psychiatry. 2013;170:256–262.

49. Passik SD, Kirsh KL, Leibee S, et al. A feasibility study of dignity psychotherapy delivered via telemedicine. Palliat Support Care. 2004;2:149–155.

50. Padgett L. The oncology palliative care matrix: a community-derived evaluation tool for constructing oncology palliative care programs. J Clin Oncol. 2012;30:253.

51. Morrison RS, Augustin R, Souvanna P, Meier DE. America's care of serious illness: a state-by-state report card on access to palliative care in our nation's hospitals. J Palliat Med. 2011;14:1094–1096.

52. Goldsmith B, Dietrich J, Du Q, Morrison RS. Variability in access to hospital palliative care in the United States. J Palliat Med. 2008;11:1094–1102.

53. Bookbinder M, Glajchen M, McHugh M, et al. Nurse practitioner-based models of specialist palliative care at home: sustainability and evaluation of feasibility. J Pain Symptom Manage. 2010;41:25–34.

54. Dahlin CM, Kelley JM, Jackson VA, Temel JS. Early palliative care for lung cancer: improving quality of life and increasing survival. Int J Palliat Nurs. 2010;16:420–423.

55. Smith AK, Thai JN, Bakitas MA, et al. The diverse landscape of palliative care clinics. J Palliat Med. 2013;16:661–668.

56. Parker Oliver D, Kapp JM, Tatum P, Wallace A. Hospice medical directors: a survey of one state. J Am Med Dir Assoc. 2012;13:35–40.

57. Lupu D. Estimate of current hospice and palliative medicine physician workforce shortage. J Pain Symptom Manage. 2010;40:899–911.

58. Quill TE, Abernethy AP. Generalist plus specialist palliative care—creating a more sustainable model. N Engl J Med. 2013;368:1173–1175.

59. Bui T. Effectively training the hospice and palliative medicine physician workforce for improved end-of-life health care in the United States. Am J Hosp Palliat Care. 2012;29:417–420.

60. The Institute of Medicine (IOM). The future of nursing: leading change and advancing health. The Prairie Rose. 2010;79:6.

61. Bakitas M, Lyons KD, Hegel MT, et al. Effects of a palliative care intervention on clinical outcomes in patients with advanced cancer: the Project ENABLE II randomized controlled trial. JAMA. 2009;302:741–749.

62. Clifford K. Adding early palliative care to treatment of non–small cell lung cancer. J Adv Pract Oncol. 2011;2:195–204.

63. Griffith J, Lyman JA, Blackhall LJ. Providing palliative care in the ambulatory care setting. Clin J Oncol Nurs. 2010;14:171–175.

64. Meier DE, Beresford L. Advanced practice nurses in palliative care: a pivotal role and perspective. J Palliat Med. 2006;9:624–627.

65. Pantilat SZ, Rabow MW, Citko J, von Gunten CF, Auerbach AD, Ferris FD. Evaluating the California Hospital Initiative in Palliative Services. Arch Intern Med. 2006;166:227–230.

66. Prince-Paul M, Burant CJ, Saltzman JN, Teston LJ, Matthews CR. The effects of integrating an advanced practice palliative care nurse in a community oncology center: a pilot study. J Support Oncol. 2010;8:21–27.

67. Lukas L, Foltz C, Paxton H. Hospital outcomes for a home-based palliative medicine consulting service. J Palliat Med. 2013;16:179–184.

68. Stjernsward J, Foley KM, Ferris FD. The public health strategy for palliative care. J Pain Symptom Manage. 2007;33:486–493.

69. Rabow MW, Smith AK, Braun JL, Weissman DE. Outpatient palliative care practices. Arch Intern Med. 2010;170:654–655.

70. Jack BA, Kirton J, Birakurataki J, Merriman A. "A bridge to the hospice": the impact of a Community Volunteer Programme in Uganda. Palliat Med. 2011;25:706–715.

71. Carr SM, Lhussier M, Forster N, et al. An evidence synthesis of qualitative and quantitative research on component intervention techniques, effectiveness, cost-effectiveness, equity and acceptability of different versions of health-related lifestyle advisor role in improving health. Health Technol Assess. 2011;15:iii–iv, 1–284.

72. Lisovicz N, Johnson RE, Higginbotham J, et al. The Deep South Network for cancer control: building a community infrastructure to reduce cancer health disparities. Cancer. 2006;107:1971–1979.

73. Kaasalainen S, Brazil K, Kelley ML. Building capacity in palliative care for personal support workers in long-term care through experiential learning. IntJ Older People Nurs. 2014;9:151–158.

74. McKee M, Kelley ML, Guirguis-Younger M, MacLean M, Nadin S. It takes a whole community: the contribution of rural hospice volunteers to whole-person palliative care. J Palliat Care. 2010;26:103–111.

75. Pesut B, Robinson CA, Bottorff JL. Among neighbors: an ethnographic account of responsibilities in rural palliative care. Palliat Support Care. 2013:1–12.

76. Health Research and Education Trust. The Role of Small and Rural Hospitals and Care Systems in Effective Population Health Partnerships. Chicago, IL: Health Research and Educational Trust; 2013.

77. American Hospital Association. 2013. Critical Access Hospital Legislative History. http://www.aha.org/advocacy-issues/cah/history.shtml.

78. Byock I, Corbeil Y. Closer to Home: Challenges and Opportunities to Care for Patients with Advanced Illness and Palliative Goals in Critical Access Hospitals and Rural Communities. Lebanon, NH: Dartmouth-Hitchcock Critical Access Hospital and Palliative Care Task Force; 2011.

79. Dekker AM, Amon JJ, le Roux KW, Gaunt CB. "What is killing me most": chronic pain and the need for palliative care in the Eastern Cape, South Africa. J Pain Palliat Care Pharmacother. 2012;26:334–340.

80. Mitchell G, Nicholson C, McDonald K, Bucetti A. Enhancing palliative care in rural Australia: the residential aged care setting. Aust J Prim Health. 2011;17:95–101.

81. Smyth D, Farnell A, Dutu G, Lillis S, Lawrenson R. Palliative care provision by rural general practitioners in New Zealand. J Palliat Med. 2010;13:247–250.

82. Cumming M, Boreland F, Perkins D. Do rural primary health care nurses feel equipped for palliative care? Aust J Prim Health. 2012;18:274–283.

83. Di Sorbo PG, Chifamba DD, Mastrojohn J 3rd, Sisimayi CN, Williams SH. The Zimbabwe Rural Palliative Care Initiative: PCI-Z. J Pain Symptom Manage. 2010;40:19–22.

84. Singer Y, Rotem B, Alsana S, Shvartzman P. Providing culturally sensitive palliative care in the desert-the experience, the need, the challenges, and the solution. J Pain Symptom Manage. 2009;38:315–321.

85. Thayyil J, Cherumanalil JM. Assessment of status of patients receiving palliative home care and services provided in a rural area-kerala, India. Indian J Palliat Care. 2012;18:213–218.

86. Spice R, Paul LR, Biondo PD. Development of a rural palliative care program in the Calgary Zone of Alberta Health Services. J Pain Symptom Manage. 2012;43:911–924.

87. Campbell LM. Experiences of nurses practising home-based palliative care in a rural South African setting. Int J Palliat Nurs. 2011;17:593–598.

88. Bakitas M, Macmartin M, Trzepkowski K, et al. Palliative care consultations for heart failure patients: how many, when, and why? J Card Fail. 2013;19:193–201.

89. Campbell L. Men's experiences delivering palliative home health care in rural South Africa: an exploratory study. Int J Palliat Nurs. 2012;18:612–618.

90. National Consensus Project. Clinical Practice Guidelines for Quality Palliative Care. 3d ed. Brooklyn, NY: National Consensus Project for Quality Palliative Care; 2013.

91. Hart L, Larson E, Lishner D. Rural Definitions for Health Policy and Research. Am J Public Health. 2005;95:1149–1155.

92. Herrera E, Rocafort J, De Lima L, Bruera E, Garcia-Pena F, Fernandez-Vara G. Regional palliative care program in Extremadura: an effective public health care model in a sparsely populated region. J Pain Symptom Manage. 2007;33:591–598.

93. Dunham W, Bolden J, Kvale E. Obstacles to the delivery of acceptable standards of care in rural home hospices. Am J Hosp Palliat Care. 2003;20:259–261.

94. Goodridge D, Duggleby W. Using a quality framework to assess rural palliative care. J Palliat Care. 2010;26:141–150.

CHAPTER 54

Palliative care in mass casualty events with scarce resources

Anne Wilkinson and Marianne Matzo

Case study

I'm not really sure what to do, I know they said it was possible that the levees would break and that this Hurricane Katrina had the potential to be devastating . . . but I never expected this. As the charge nurse in a small nursing home in St. Tammany Parish, Louisiana we have no electricity or running water. Most of the people in our neighborhood have already evacuated. Some neighbors took a few of our more ambulatory elders with them, and I was able to have the rest evacuated with the nurse's aides before the floodwaters rose too high. But, I am here alone with George, a patient on the second floor who weighs over 300 pounds, cannot carry his own weight to even transfer himself, and the flood waters are now coming in the second floor windows. I can't get him down the stairs; I can't get him to the roof. We are hot and tired. He has been in the same incontinence brief for 12 hours. I have to leave and crawl to the roof if I am going to survive. Do I leave him to die alone in the rising flood? Do I give him the last dose of pain medication that I have left and try and save myself? Do I stay at his side?

Key points

- The primary goal of a coordinated response to a mass casualty event (MCE) is to maximize the number of lives saved.

- A comprehensive and humane response should also seek to minimize the suffering of those who are not expected to survive.

- Palliative care offers a humane, effective, and medically appropriate treatment choice when resources are scarce and an alternative to "doing nothing" or ineffectively utilizing scarce resources.

Catastrophic MCEs, such as pandemic flu outbreaks, earthquakes, or large-scale terrorism-related events, quickly and suddenly yield thousands of victims whose needs overwhelm local and regional healthcare systems, personnel, and resources. Such conditions require deploying scarce resources in a manner that is different from the more common "multiple" casualty event, which does not exceed the ability of local resources to provide treatment.[1] The purpose of this chapter is to offer an introduction to the topic of disaster response/emergency nursing and the role palliative care can play during an MCE for vulnerable populations not normally addressed in usual disaster planning and response. This chapter examines issues associated with providing medical care under MCE circumstances of scarce resources; the current level of preparation of nurses to respond in these emergencies; the role for palliative care in the support of individuals not expected to survive; and recommendations of specific actions for a coordinated disaster response plan. The authors recommend that, although the primary goal of a coordinated response to an MCE is to maximize the number of lives saved, a comprehensive and humane response should also seek to *minimize the suffering of those who are not expected to survive.*

In the past 50 years, there have been greater than 10,000 reported disasters, both large and small, affecting 12 billion people and resulting in 12 million deaths.[2,3] It has been estimated that there is an MCE, either naturally occurring or man-made, that requires rapid response and that exceeds the local and regional capacity to respond, somewhere in the world every day[4] and that the frequency and intensity of these large-scale disasters are increasing.[5] While the impact of MCEs are most often felt in the Asia Pacific Region, flooding across Europe and tornadoes in the United States, as well as the 2011 earthquake in New Zealand and tsunami in Japan, have demonstrated that developed nations are also subject to MCEs in which even advanced public health and emergency response systems cannot adequately respond.

Most disasters are brief, self-limited events that preserve the community infrastructure while the ability of the "system" to care for people stays intact, although stressed by the rate of casualty presentation. Mass casualty events create problems which local and regional rescue agencies rarely face in day-to-day practice and which require a distinct approach and management.[6,7] A comprehensive definition of an MCE is a challenge to synthesize from the literature, as there are multiple definitions, many based in institution-specific contexts, and they are often very broad or very narrow.[8] The US Agency for Healthcare Research and Quality (AHRQ) defines an MCE as "an act of bioterrorism or other public health or medical emergency involving thousands, or even tens of thousands, of victims that could compromise, at least in the short term, the ability of local or regional health systems to delivery services consistent with established standards of care,"[9(p. 5)] while the American Red Cross defines an MCE as:

> A threatening or occurring event of such destructive magnitude and force as to dislocate people, separate family members, damage or destroy homes, and injure or kill people. A disaster produces a range and level of immediate suffering and basic human needs that cannot be promptly or adequately addressed by the affected people, and impedes them from initiating and proceeding with their recovery efforts. Natural disasters include floods, tornadoes, hurricanes, typhoons, winter storms, tsunamis, hail storms, wildfires, windstorms, epidemics and earthquakes. Human-caused disasters—whether intentional or unintentional—include residential fires, building collapses, transportation accidents, hazardous materials releases, explosions, and domestic acts of terrorism.[8(p. 422)]

In general, MCEs fall into two major categories: (1) "big bang" single incidents with immediate or sudden impact, such as bombings or earthquakes, and (2) "rising tide" incidents, slowly developing events with a prolonged impact, such as pandemic flu or widespread ongoing exposures to chemical, biological, and nuclear agents.[10] The first type yields large numbers of casualties at the outset of the event with few added over time. The second type yields a gradual increase in the number of people affected, rising to a catastrophic number of victims and necessitating a more prolonged response.[11]

One common characteristic to all definitions of MCEs is that these are such destructive events that the need for social and health services overwhelms the local and regional public health resources and places such extraordinary burdens on fundamental societal functions, such as law and order, communication, transportation, and water and food supplies, that they require assistance from outside the community.[12] Healthcare infrastructure may be devastated, and the arrival of outside assistance delayed. Governmental agencies may be overstretched by multiple challenges, and competing demands or their ability to function may be degraded by the MCE, as in Hurricane Katrina in New Orleans in 2005. Thus, health and social service resources become "scarce."

Not so well defined is at what point in a disaster event medical and social resources are exceeded by demand.[13] For example, an MCE may result in mass fatalities but few patients in need of care, as was the case in the World Trade Center attack on September 11, 2001. A refinement of the above definitions designed to encompass both the size and the impact of the event has been suggested by Hogan and colleagues (2002) in which an MCE with scarce resources is a situation in which the number of patients presenting for care within a given time period are such that the emergency response system cannot provide care for them *in a timely manner and without external assistance.*[14] Underlying this definition is the concept of "relative" scarcity of available resources, where scarcity of resources is comparative to the local context and impact on local health and social service infrastructure.

"Crisis" standards of medical care during a mass casualty event

Irrespective of the exact definition of an MCE with scarce resources, many questions arise concerning the allocation of health and social service resources and how those decisions are justified. Should health providers treat patients with the most serious illnesses and injuries first? Will victims be treated on a first-come, first-served basis? On the basis of individual "worth" to society? Should health providers treat the most people with the available resources, recognizing that some otherwise salvageable individuals may be allowed to die?[13] What are the ethical obligations of emergency response and healthcare providers in an MCE? What optimum management and allocation of scarce resources strategy should be used under MCE conditions?[15] These and other questions were recently addressed in two publications by the US Institute of Medicine (IOM) Committee on Guidance for Establishing Standards of Care for Use in Disaster Situations: one, a conceptual framework for establishing "crisis" standards of healthcare (CRC)[16] and the second, the operationalization of the framework[17] for use by state and local public health officials and health-sector agencies and institutions to establish and implement standards of care that should apply in disaster situations—both natural and man-made—under conditions of scarce resources. As the Committee stated, "The delivery of health care under crisis standards is ultimately about maximizing the care delivered to the population as a whole under austere circumstances that may limit treatment choices for both providers and patients."[17(p. 33)]

Standards of health and medical care, broadly defined, address not only what care is given, but to whom, when, by whom, and under what circumstances or in what place.[18] The IOM Committee on Guidance for Establishing Standards of Care for Use in Disaster Situations defined "crisis" standards of care as[16(p. 2)]:

> a substantial change in usual healthcare operations and the level of care it is possible to deliver, which is made necessary by a pervasive (e.g. pandemic influenza) or catastrophic (e.g. earthquake, hurricane) disaster. This change in the level of care delivered is justified by specific circumstances and is formally declared by a state government, in recognition that crisis operations will be in effect for a sustained period. The formal declaration that crisis standards of care are in operation enables specific legal/regulatory powers and protections for healthcare providers in the necessary tasks of allocating and using scarce medical resources and implementing alternate care facility operations.

During MCE conditions, the tactical application of medical care *shifts* from providing the optimal highest level of care for each individual patient to providing the greatest good (resources) to the greatest number; that is, to maximize the number of lives saved. However, how and in what ways standards should be altered should always be based on existing conditions during the medical surge responses, which allows for flexibility and responsiveness to local conditions and does not represent a single "standard" of care.[19,20] The difference between everyday delivery of first-aid and the management of a large mass casualty situation is one of *kind*, rather than just of degree or scale.[12] For example, "crisis" standards of care could mean applying principles of field triage to determine who gets what kind of care. It could mean changing infection control standards to permit group isolation rather than single-person isolation units. It could mean limiting the use of ventilators to surgical situations. It could mean creating alternate care sites in facilities never designed to provide medical care, such as schools, churches, or hotels. It could also mean changing who provides various kinds of care or changing privacy and confidentiality protections.[18]

The IOM Committee recommended that ethical considerations and ultimate decisions made about the allocation of resources under an MCE be made explicit and transparent and be based on community consensus so that when on-the-spot decisions must be made, they are consistent with the spirit of the ethical judgments and public input that guided the planning process.[16,17] Paramount in the Committee's consideration of these issues was the recognition that plans and protocols that shift desired patient care from the individual to the population must be grounded in the ethical allocation of resources, which ensures fairness to everyone. As the Committee stated, "The emphasis in a public health emergency must be on improving and maximizing the population's health while tending to the needs of patients within the constraints of resource limitations."[17(p. 1–6)]

The IOM Committee also recommended that the basis for allocating health and medical resources under crisis standards of care with scarce resources must be fair and clinically sound. The process for making these decisions should be transparent and judged by the public to be fair. Protocols for triage also need to be flexible enough to change as the size of a mass casualty event grows or diminishes and will depend on both the nature of the event and the speed with which it occurs.[18] If health and medical care delivered under these crises standards is to be as effective as possible in saving lives, it is critically important that current preparedness planning be expanded to explicitly address this issue and to provide guidance, education, and training concerning these crisis care standards. Disaster plans need to be targeted to the epidemiology of the disaster, coordinated on a regional level and containing an organizational structure where functional job descriptions and responsibilities of all agencies and organizations involved should be clearly delineated.[21]

Challenges for healthcare providers

Under normal circumstances, the healthcare system, especially emergency care, is already strained by routine daily volumes. Furthermore, emergency departments (EDs), inpatient units, and intensive care units (ICUs) in acute care hospitals are chronically overcrowded and resource constrained. Healthcare and public health providers need to anticipate the profound challenges in adequately caring for the surge of victims following an MCE in the face of systems already stretched to the margins. Any incident in which the available resources are outstripped by the demand for care will necessarily result in a shift in the delivery of care from conventional toward "contingency" (functionally equivalent care) to "crisis" care (care may not be initiated or may be withdrawn from selected patients so it can be reallocated to others who may be considered more likely to survive).[17] Some of the issues that disaster response planners and providers will need to address during an MCE with scarce resources include (1) the challenge to some providers of making the shift from individual-based disaster care to population-based care; (2) the challenge of existing and vulnerable healthcare populations needs and those MCE emergent care needs; (3) the limits of current triage systems; and (4) the potential conflict of interest between a providers' ethical obligation to report to work versus concern for personal and familial safety faced by individual practitioners under these conditions.

Individual patient care versus population healthcare

Those with field responsibility have to make on-the-spot decisions that will require ethical judgments during an MCE. In effect, first responders, emergency response personnel, and alternative care site and hospital-based healthcare providers will be making medical decisions based on "priority for," rather than access to, services or interventions.[22,23] However, existing medical standards of care are not sufficiently flexible to encourage healthcare professionals to act appropriately and decisively in a public health emergency and, in the wake of the recent earthquake in Haiti and the tsunami in Japan, there is growing international concern regarding the lack of accountability for errors, mistakes, or outright failures that governs current global humanitarian response to mass casualty events.[16,24–27] For example, during Hurricane Katrina, practitioners struggled to treat patients against a backdrop of considerable uncertainty about the appropriate standard of care. Other research has found that during the earthquake in Haiti, Israeli physicians were "faced with the challenge of establishing an ethical and practical system of medical priorities in a setting of chaos" that hampered their ability to "treat everyone who needed care."[28] The IOM Committee was formed, in part, to address some of these concerns. The IOM Committee recommended defining crisis standards of care in advance and in a transparent, community-based process in order to empower skilled healthcare practitioners to respond and make ethically sound critical decisions on providing equitable and appropriate care to patients and populations in a public health emergency because this process will facilitate improved outcomes for the affected populations.[16,17,24]

Nevertheless, some critics argue that making the standard of care less rigorous in effect permits physicians to have even less accountability for meeting current quality expectations since they must only meet the "lower" legal standard of duty to care. Standards of care, they argue, is a well-supported metric to judge the behavior and decisions of physicians to determine whether they are acceptable and appropriate under the circumstances. Although there is a growing consensus that in an MCE the focus of care will shift from the individual to the population, it remains "unclear" how lowering the standard of care will improve patient outcomes.[26,27] Moreover, changing standards of care does not address the medical-supply logistics problems which are the core issue inherent in MCEs. Critics argue that there is no justification for crisis standards of care because the current standard of care already covers disasters by explicitly recognizing that circumstances and resources constrain what physicians can do.[29]

Existing vulnerable populations and mass casualty event victims

Clinical practitioners will have to make quick critical judgments as to who will most likely benefit from scarce life-saving treatment, as well as who will not.[30] Consider those who are not dead but, with the limited resources of an MCE, may not survive transport or, if resources to treat them may not arrive in time, may not survive? In the worst case scenario, emergency response personnel may have to ration the delivery of care in the face of extreme demand, limited resource availability, or both.[23] Some people will be so ill or injured that the clinician must conclude that they cannot survive, even if maximal resources were available (though under an MCE, they may not be available). Thus, some patients will be provided life support and definitive treatment where possible, while others will be triaged to a nonsavable category that will include at least (1) those who survived the onset of the disaster but with life-limiting critical new injury resulting in death in a relatively short period of time as well as (2) those with preexisting illness who will be severely affected by the shift in allocation of resources. These individuals are at high risk of mortality and are likely to die during an MCE with scarce resources.[31]

This second set of "casualties" that result from an MCE has received less attention in current state and regional disaster planning; that is, those existing "vulnerable populations" already residing in the community (e.g., hospice patients, children, the frail elderly, and adults with physical, intellectual, or mental disabilities) or living in institutional settings (e.g., nursing homes, group homes, and inpatient hospice) and, in either case, heavily dependent on the established healthcare delivery system for daily function. Vulnerable populations disproportionately suffer harm during and after an MCE.[32-37] These individuals may not be able to seek help, care for themselves, or pursue other survival and recovery strategies pursued by nonvulnerable populations. They also are at greater risk of suffering and death because many of the resources that usually support existing vulnerable populations will be diverted to treat newly injured persons who are likely to survive.

The term "likely to die" is defined as those people who are too sick or injured to survive hours, days or weeks; most often categorized as the "expectant/black tag," "nonsalvageable," or "nonsavable" victims. However, in practice, this category may also include those labeled "immediate" if needed medical resources are unavailable. This category could also include situations where the individual is already dependent on the usual healthcare system to survive (e.g., ventilator-dependent patients), has an existing life-threatening illness (e.g., extensive cancer), or has illness secondary to injuries sustained in the disaster situation.[31]

For example, almost 7.6 million individuals receive care in their home from 17,000 home care providers, primarily nurses, across the United States because of acute illness, long-term care conditions, permanent disability, or terminal illness.[38] Technological advances have expanded the capabilities of home care providers so that many chronic conditions that previously would have been cared for in the hospital are now being safely managed in the home. Intravenous (IV) infusion technology, parenteral nutrition, peritoneal dialysis, oxygen therapy, feeding pumps, ventilators, pulse oximeters, and hand-held blood analysis devices are just a few examples of the common devices that have allowed the expansion of home care. During an MCE, these community-dwelling patients could experience disruption of needed support services. Depending on the level of their needs, a disruption of care/services could lead to patient decompensation and increased reliance on acute care services, including emergency medical systems and hospital EDs already stretched thin by the disaster situation.[39] The general community-dwelling population also includes many individuals who do not routinely receive services from social, mental health, or aging services agencies but who have the potential to destabilize rapidly during an emergency and require medical care. Other service providers, such as adult day care programs, medical equipment suppliers, or Meals on Wheels programs, may have routine contact with such at-risk individuals and should be included in MCE disaster response and planning.

The relevance of such considerations was dramatically demonstrated after September 11, 2001. Nearly 19,000 elders lived within a three-block radius of the World Trade Center's Twin Towers on September 11. Many frail elders and persons with disabilities were trapped for days in their high-rise apartments awaiting rescue, without electricity, fresh supplies of food and medications, or any way to communicate with the outside world. While animal protection groups were on the scene within 24 hours, rescuing pets from evacuated buildings, it took up to seven days for rescuers to start rescuing the older people who were left behind in otherwise evacuated buildings. Home care workers could not get to their clients, and community service providers could not access their computers that held client information. Many frail adults were unknown to community workers because they had never sought organized services.[40-42]

Hurricane Katrina and the subsequent flooding resulted in approximately 1,836 deaths, 71% over the age of 65 and nearly half aged 75 or more.[43-46] Healthcare practitioners in marooned New Orleans hospitals worked in almost unimaginably difficult conditions while awaiting rescue. In one hospital alone, 34 elderly and critically ill patients died during and after the storm as healthcare workers struggled to care for critically ill patients in a building with no electrical power, a nonfunctional sanitation system, flooding, and an interior temperature above 100 degrees Fahrenheit.[47]

What should first responders, disaster planning personnel, and medical care providers do when many affected people cannot reasonably survive due to the scope of their injuries, the magnitude of exposure, environmental conditions, or preexisting medical conditions that will be significantly affected by the MCE itself or the resulting scarce resources? While the primary goal of an organized and coordinated response to an MCE should be to maximize the number of lives saved, *civil society demands a secondary goal of minimizing the physical and psychological suffering of those whose lives will probably be shortened by an MCE.* These issues fall under the broad rubric of nursing and palliative care, which refers to the aggressive management of symptoms and relief of suffering.

Triage

Triage is a tool by which the victims of an MCE disaster or emergency are categorized into groups; those who will do well regardless of intervention; those who will do poorly regardless of intervention; and those who might do well with intervention.[48,49] While there are approximately six mass casualty triage systems used worldwide, very little research has been conducted on their validation.[50,51] Multiple victim disaster triage operates with several dozen systems worldwide, involving more than 120 different labels and tools. The principles of these systems are similar, and all feature a label/color coded triage tool, inclusion criteria, exclusion criteria, and minimum qualifications for survival. The most widely used field triage system in the United States is the Simple Triage and Rapid Treatment (START) system, which sorts victims into four categories. "Immediate" (Red) are those patients deemed to have life-threatening or moderately severe injuries requiring immediate intervention, treatable with a minimum amount of time, personnel, and supplies, who also have a good chance of recovery. "Delayeds" (Yellow) are patients injured but not expected to die or worsen greatly within the first hour if treatment is delayed. "Expectants" or unsalvageable (Black) are patients who are presumed deceased, have injuries requiring extensive treatment that exceeds the medical resources available, or have catastrophic injuries for which survival is not expected. "Ambulatory/minimal" (Green) patients require only minor treatment and are generally walking.[52] The START system uses ability to walk to a marked place, respiratory rate, capillary refill, and mental status (state of consciousness) to classify victims.[12]

Although first responders have used the START system since the 1980s, recent research by Kahn and colleagues (2009) found that the START system overestimated injuries of 79 victims involved in a 2002 train crash and underestimated the condition of 3 patients.[53] In an examination of 148 patient records at 13 hospitals, the authors found that just 66 patients were triaged into the correct category, for an accuracy rate of 45%. The START system was found to be effective in ensuring patients who were put in the red category got to the hospital faster than those in the yellow and green categories. The authors concluded that while the system does do a good job of identifying patients with minor injuries, it does not excel at differentiating between patients who need immediate care and those who have significant but stable injuries.[53] During MCE disaster responses, this mismatch could result in a hospital system being overwhelmed by noncritical patients who use up resources needed for truly critically injured individuals.[51,54]

Established triage schemes have substantial limitations when applied to the special circumstances of an MCE and the provision of palliative care. For example, many of the schemes do not include the assessment for preexisting medical critical illness. Furthermore, little data addresses the critical question of whether correctly sorting casualties into the categories set forth by any particular triage system results in improved outcomes; and one system may not handle all MCE events in all triage settings.[52] In addition, in practice, the "expectant" category is often applied only to those patients who are not breathing after one attempt at repositioning and opening the airway; all other critically ill or injured persons are treated as "immediate" or "delayed" (Red or Yellow). Finally, the usual triage schemes do not include palliative and comfort care measures as an alternative to curative treatment.[52]

A triage system in situations of scarce resources will function best if it is transparent, fair, valid, consistent across settings and events, dynamic (is conducted at multiple places and times), and flexible enough to address changing circumstances, including responding when patients triaged as "likely to die" actually improve or when additional treatment resources become available. Research is beginning to provide a scientific underpinning for triage[42] as well as to identify basic criteria for MCE critical care triage.[4,15] Future researchers will have to address triage applicability to palliative care as well as the role of palliative care in an MCE. The arguments for including palliative care in an MCE—humane treatment, diversion of dying people away from overburdened hospitals, the more effective use of scarce resources—have moral weight on their own. However, community education will be needed in order to demonstrate that these plans are as fair and equitable as possible and to generate the necessary commitment by the public to comply with such plans. In addition, research will be needed to assess their impact.

Willingness and ability to report to duty during a mass casualty event

There is concern that in the event of a bioterrorist attack or pandemic event there would be an interruption in normal staffing resources, both due to conflicts in duty to care and due to the exacerbation of the strained staffing resources already apparent under normal circumstances. The emergency nursing workforce shortage already provides a challenge to daily hospital operations and would become a critical issue in the event of a large-scale disaster or MCE, particularly when some nurses will decide not to contribute/refuse to work.[8] Healthcare workers are a critical component of the emergency management system of prevention, mitigation, preparation, response, and recovery. Historically, most medical and emergency response personnel typically report to duty in their usual or emergency role during disasters or their immediate aftermath.[55] However, there are a number of factors that can influence the decision of a healthcare worker about whether to report to duty or not.[56] Research since the 1990s, in particular nursing research, have been exploring the willingness, ability, and intentions of healthcare workers to respond to disasters as well as identifying potential and real barriers and facilitators to this decision. Overall, the research has consistently demonstrated that healthcare workers are more likely to be willing and able to respond to natural disasters and less likely to be willing and able to respond during infectious outbreaks or incidents with potential exposure to harmful agents (e.g., biological, chemical, nuclear, or radiological).[57]

Specifically, research findings indicate that when fear of contagion with novel and/or potentially lethal agents is high, willingness to report to duty among healthcare workers is low, with predicted nonillness absenteeism rates for the United States ranging from 35% to 80%.[55] For example, a study of emergency healthcare providers in New York revealed that anywhere from 18% to 84% of workers would be willing to report to work during an MCE. The variation in willingness to report was dependent on whether or not the cause of the incident was known, a treatment or a vaccine was available, providers became ill, the agent was transmissible, and family members could receive treatment.[58] Another study looked at willingness (e.g., the personal decision of the person) and ability (e.g., the capability for the person) to report to work under different catastrophic scenarios and found a difference in willingness and ability to respond based on the type of event. The ability to report and willingness to report was highest for an MCE or environmental disaster (80+%) versus ability to report (65%) and willingness to report (48%) for a severe acute respiratory syndrome (SARS) outbreak. Obstacles to willingness included personal health problems and concern and fear for their family and themselves, child and eldercare responsibilities, pet care, and transportation.[59]

Couig (2012) conducted a literature review concerning willingness and ability to respond to disasters between 1990 and 2012 and identified more than 50 studies, 21 published by nurses.[57] Findings were consistent with other research in this area in that willingness and ability to respond varies by type of disaster, ranging from a high of 93% (willingness) and 90.6% (ability) for an MCE to a low of 10% of sampled junior and senior nursing students for an infectious disease outbreak, unless their families were provided protection.[60–62] The main barriers to response were concern for the safety of themselves or their family and caretaking commitments; availability of protective equipment, medicines, or vaccines for self and family; and their education and training in disaster preparedness.[57]

Palliative care

Palliative care is of value for all patients in that it improves quality of life, enhances patients' capacity to live optimally, and is

Table 54.1

Palliative care is:	Palliative care is *not*:
◆ Evidence-based medical treatment	◆ Abandonment
◆ Vigorous care of pain and symptoms throughout illness	◆ Euthanasia
◆ Humanitarian care when there is nothing else to offer	◆ Hastening death

cost-effective when it is an integral part of comprehensive care (Table 54.1). Palliative care uses skills from multiple disciplines to enhance quality of life and address needs of seriously ill patients and their families by providing relief from pain and other distressing symptoms; supporting dying as a normal and manageable process of living; integrating psychological and spiritual services to meet needs of patients and families; enabling patients to live as fully as possible until death; and helping the family to cope during and after the patient's illness, including bereavement counseling, when indicated.[38] Palliative care respects the humanity of those who will die soon and assures their comfort while supporting their loved ones. The incorporation of palliative care into MCE disaster response may also greatly help reassure the public that society and its healthcare professionals will not "abandon" the patient or deliberately "cause death" under dire MCE circumstances, as was alleged during Hurricane Katrina.[31]

Under normal circumstances, palliative care plays a complementary role to comprehensive medical care focused on cure or control of an underlying life-threatening disease. If the patient has a period of needing "comfort measures only," palliative care then becomes the main focus of care. Under the dire circumstances of an MCE, disaster-related palliative care would involve the aggressive management of symptoms and the relief of patient suffering, including the obvious humanitarian call to relieve the psychosocial, spiritual, and religious suffering of patients likely to die.[31] Unusually aggressive means of symptom management are, at times, appropriate at the end of life in the same way that extraordinary means of saving life are often appropriate during curative phases of medical therapy.[63] Disaster planning and response should include plans for people who will be categorized as likely to die; that is, those who may die as a result of the event as well as those in the community or institutional settings already living with limited prognoses and who will be put at increased risk by the MCE and resulting scarce resources.

Role of nurses in disasters

Nurses are an invaluable resource, both under normal conditions and during disaster emergencies. Indeed, nurses are one of the largest groups of emergency responders during a disaster, but many nurses are unprepared to respond because of a lack of knowledge or skills.[8,64–68] Recent reviews of the literature examining disaster preparedness research and nursing disaster response found much of the research focuses on health and medical surge capacity (e.g., beds, personnel, facilities, equipment and pharmaceuticals); crisis standards of medical care; population versus military triage; and the identification of "core competencies" and knowledge needed by nurses in the event of a large-scale disaster or MCE.[2,8,69] Competencies have been defined as a "combination

of knowledge, skills, and abilities demonstrated by organization members that are critical to the effective and efficient function of the organization."[70(p. 73)]

Few studies have examined the issues, concerns, and attitudes of nurses surrounding disaster response or their perceived preparedness. One study of nurses who worked during Hurricane Katrina in New Orleans found that these nurses had to cope with the great uncertainty of the situation and had to quickly adapt to the needs that arose in both patient care and self-preservation situations.[8] The study identified the primary resources needed by nurses working during a disaster included excellent basic nursing skills, intuitive problem solving, sense of staff unity/teamwork in face of challenges. In addition, the study found that a major consequence of the nurses' disaster response participation was increased problems due to stress, including changed sleep patterns, changes in mood, eating disorders, substance abuse, and avoidance behaviors while at the same time, these nurse participants were able to practice in harmony with duty to care values and demonstrated behaviors of strength, courage, and resilience.

Other research has shown that nurses are extremely concerned about their level of knowledge and skills under "difficult, disorganized and poorly resourced situations" such as large-scale disasters or MCEs and where they are required to work "outside their scope of practice . . . including carrying out unfamiliar procedures for patients with injuries rarely seen in usual practice."[65,71,72] A survey of nurses who volunteered for the Sumatra-Andaman earthquake and tsunami of 2004 found that more than 80% of the nurses had no previous experience in disaster response and no language skills other than English.[71] In addition, the lack of nursing involvement in disaster response planning and the lack of disaster response education and training left many nurses feeling "fearful of abandonment by management," unable to communicate effectively, helpless to assist some people, and working in an atmosphere of "pandemonium and uncertainty."[8,64]

There are a number of issues yet to be resolved within the nursing profession regarding disaster response and MCEs. One problem consistently identified in the literature concerns the perception by frontline nurses that they are left out of disaster response planning and decision-making. For the most part, it is administrators, community leaders, disaster response professionals and midlevel healthcare provider managers who are directly involved in a facility or organization's disaster planning and response activities, without input from those who will actually be working and taking care of patients during and after the disaster. This appears to leave the majority of nurses perceiving that their needs and concerns during disaster events have not been considered.[8] Thus, as Hughes and colleagues (2007) argue, frontline nurses should be involved at the outset of the emergency planning process.[73]

In addition, nurse responders in previous disasters have consistently identified the importance of education in emergency and disaster preparedness, arguing that it is essential that undergraduate nurse education curriculum include the content and practical experience necessary to adequately prepare nurses for this role.[74] However, healthcare professionals, including nurses, are unprepared to cope with MCEs, and concerns have been raised about their current understanding of the required knowledge skills, abilities, and competencies needed to adequately prepare for disasters.[8]

Nursing education in disaster preparedness and response

As the majority of frontline responders in disasters, nurses need to be prepared and to have the necessary knowledge and skills needed to efficiently manage large-scale disaster events.[74] Disaster medicine and emergency public healthcare are relatively new fields comprising much more than clinical medical services/issues and requiring significant contributions from many disciplines, most of them far from the usual clinical practice.[12] Even ED personnel, who are the "first receivers" of victims of a bioterrorism, chemical, or nuclear MCE, are provided no specific coursework on MCE education.[75] Prior to 2001, few schools of nursing included content related to emergency preparedness or disaster response. After the terrorist attack on the World Trade Center in New York City in 2001, this figure increased to 53% in the United States.[74] Most experts now agree that an "all hazards" approach to the education of healthcare professionals is the most effective; however, it is not known to what extent nursing faculties teach disaster preparedness in nursing programs, even though it is required.[75]

A number of international professional organizations have developed a wide range of recommendations concerning nursing education and competencies in disaster preparedness and MCEs. For example, the World Health Organization (WHO) and the International Council of Nurses (ICN) collaborated on the development of a set of competencies required for disaster nursing.[74] Educational competencies for registered nurses (RNs) related to MCEs have also been developed by the International Nursing Coalition for Mass Casualty Education (INCMCE), an international coalition of organizational representatives of schools of nursing, nursing accrediting bodies, nursing specialty organizations, and government agencies interested in promoting mass casualty education for nurses, and the National Health Professions Preparedness Consortium (NHPPC), a coalition of three universities focusing on education in MCEs for health professionals, including Vanderbilt University (nurse education), the University of Alabama-Birmingham, focusing on physician education, and Louisiana State University, focusing on emergency medical technicians (EMTs).[75]

Overall, the INCMCE and NHPPC identified 21 performance standards focusing on recognition, communication, effective decision-making, integration and management of resources, and response/recovery roles during MCE events. Specifically, the INCMCE recommends that every nurse must have sufficient knowledge to be able to recognize the potential for a MCE incident, know how to protect oneself, know how to provide immediate care for those individuals involved, be able to recognize their own role and limitations during such events, and know where to seek additional educational information and access to resources.[76] Curricula incorporating six disaster education modules specific for nurses based on the performance level competencies designed by the INCMCE and the NHPPC can be found at www.incmce.org. Another online training MCE program is at St. Louis University (http://nursing.slu.edu.cne_disaster_prep_home.html). Completion of this nurse-focused program provides a certificate in disaster preparedness.

The competencies identified by INCMCE are consistent with the American Association of Colleges of Nursing (AACN) Essentials of Baccalaureate Education for Professional Nursing Practice.[77] The AACN recommends competencies in using clinical judgment appropriately and providing timely interventions when making decisions and performing nursing care during disasters, mass casualties, and other emergency situations. In addition, the AACN recommends that nurses should understand their role and participation in emergency preparedness and disaster response with an awareness of environmental factors and the risks these factors pose to self and patients.[8]

The National League for Nurses (NLN), with support from the National Organization of Associate Degree Nursing (NOADN), have identified educational core competencies for associate degree nurses but do not specifically explicate the responsibilities of these nurses during emergency situations. Their major recommendation for educating nurses is to develop the ability to adapt patient care to changing healthcare environments.[8] Gebbe and Qureshi (2006),[78] leading international experts in disaster management nursing, with support from the US Centers for Disease Control and Prevention (CDC), developed 14 core emergency preparedness competencies for nurses. These and a number of other sets of competencies were developed for the generalist RN practicing in the hospital setting.

Polivka and colleagues (2008)[69] built on these earlier recommendations to develop a consensus set of competencies for public health nursing, resulting in 25 competencies categorized into Preparedness ($n = 9$), focusing on personal preparedness, comprehending disaster preparedness terms, concepts and roles, knowing the local health department's disaster plan, communication suitable for disaster situations, and the role of the public health nurse in a surge event; Response ($n = 8$), focusing on conducting a rapid needs assessment, outbreak investigation and surveillance, public health triage, risk communication, and technical skills such as mass dispensing; and Recovery ($n = 7$), focusing on the debriefing process, contributing to disaster plan modifications, and coordinating efforts to address the psychosocial and public health impact of the event. In addition, these competencies have not been translated into consistent nursing curricula.

Despite these and many other efforts by professional and international governing bodies to identify and establish MCE competencies and educational tools to be included in nursing curriculum, nursing schools are still lacking in the preparation of nursing students for disaster nursing.[8,75] Research from the United States and Australia have documented a serious lack of content or curricula focused on emergency and disaster response in nursing schools and have pointed to the difficulty in finding adequate teaching expertise in the area of emergency and disaster preparedness. Moreover, much of the content that is included in nursing curricula tends to be theoretical and not practice-based.[74,75] Nursing faculty continue to feel inadequately prepared to teach disaster nursing content and argue that the nursing curricula are already content packed with little room available to add emergency and disaster specific content.[64] Major gaps in the literature on clinician education in MCE planning and response include means and methods for updating and reinforcing existing clinician training; use of Web- or telephone-based central information sources for education and reporting of incidents, and how to train clinicians to communicate with other healthcare professionals during an MCE.[75]

Education needs

Depending on the scope, nature and size of an MCE, treatment for injuries or for existing conditions may be unavailable and/or delayed. Pain and other symptoms will likely be the primary issues faced by disaster response and medical personnel.[79] Therefore, effective pain and symptom management should be a basic minimum of service delivery and training for palliative care during MCEs. Clinicians must understand the use of opioid medications, free from the usual misleading myths. Education and training should be tailored to the individual's role in emergency response and should cover, at a minimum, the basic philosophy and goals of palliative care (including the principle of double effect), basic symptom management (e.g., for pain and shortness of breath); the use and titration of oral and injectable opioid medications in patients in pain and/or near death; symptom recognition in the case of pandemic flu or chemical or radiological attack; and basic psycho-social counseling and support. Basic disaster planning should include stockpiling palliative care medications at accessible sites away from acute care hospitals (e.g., in nursing homes) and should train disaster responders as to how to locate, access and use them. In addition, the broad community will need to come to understand the changes required in the standards of care under MCE circumstances.

Local disaster management initiatives could recruit and train palliative care and long-term care professionals, retired health care professionals, and lay volunteers to take on defined palliative care roles during emergencies. Local "Disaster Palliative Assistance Teams" (DPATs) could combine interdisciplinary experience from diverse practice settings (e.g. hospitals, hospice, long-term care, etc.) as part of the Medical Reserve Corps, or organized under the National Disaster Medical System (NDMS).[79] Each DPAT sponsor could recruit the team, arrange for training their members, and coordinate team deployment to supplement remaining local palliative care services rapidly.[79] Just as for other disaster response personnel, DPAT members could be paid as part-time federal employees, all states could recognize their licensure and certifications, and they could provide services under the protection of the Federal Tort Claims Act (should a malpractice claim occur).[80]

Training in palliative care must occur prior to an MCE and can be incorporated into current Community Emergency Response Team (CERT) training activities. Disaster planners should build on existing models of emergency response training to develop and implement a variety of training methodologies that incorporate generic and "just in time" palliative care services for all disaster response team members. Cross-training of personnel from other areas of expertise, other areas of the state and region, and the lay public (e.g., bus drivers, mail deliverers, etc.) could augment the work of palliative care providers by allowing these first responders to begin to offer comfort care and basic assistance to the onsite physicians and nurses until enough professional staff are available.[31] Community planners face several significant challenges in the integration of palliative care services and personnel into mass casualty event planning and response. Of special concern are the identification and location of vulnerable populations already in the community; addressing the ethical and legal issues during the development process and in the resulting MCE disaster response plan; ensuring public education regarding crisis standards of care and the appropriate use of palliative care in MCEs; and the need to generate the requisite political will to initiate and support complex, and potentially controversial, MCE community planning efforts generally and with additional palliative care issues.

Identifying and locating existing special populations

As the events following Hurricane Katrina demonstrated, the evacuation and sheltering of vulnerable and special needs populations living in the community and in institutional settings pose many challenges to disaster planners. Many vulnerable populations require separate special accommodations during evacuation, relocation, and return. One fundamental challenge is to establish criteria and implementation plans for quickly identifying special needs populations, in order to ensure their prompt evacuation and to direct them to appropriate shelter arrangements. These special needs populations include people living with frailty associated with aging, serious mental illness, intellectual or cognitive disabilities, sensory impairments (e.g., low vision, impaired hearing), mobility problems or activity limitations, dependence on special equipment such as oxygen or wheelchairs, and no available transportation.

Many special needs populations do not have regular contact with the healthcare system and essentially none are on registries appropriate for this purpose, so finding these people before and after a disaster or emergency will be very difficult without planning. For example, in the aftermath of Hurricane Katrina, people who needed stretchers or wheelchairs could not use busses or cars to get to shelters and many intellectually disabled persons could not follow instructions to move to another shelter.[31] Public health disaster planning and response agencies will need to develop registries of people who otherwise might be abandoned at home.

Ethical and legal issues related to planning and responding to a mass casualty event

Mass casualty event community planning and response should reflect the fundamental tenets of maximizing good outcomes for the greatest number of people while having agencies, organizations, and individuals act in good faith to meet their redefined duties and obligations in the face of an MCE.[11,81] The ethical frameworks and moral considerations of society are neither simple nor consistent. Utilitarian ethical principles that evaluate actions on the basis of their consequences often conflict with ethical frameworks that construct enduring rules concerning one's duties and obligations. Both have limitations when applied to an MCE with scarce resources: it will be difficult to predict consequences, and duties and obligations will be difficult to discern. For example, how should disaster planners, public health officials, and the public balance maximum gain in survival against fairness across persons when these goals conflict?

The application of ethical principles and values applies to the planning process, the actual plan, and the implementation of these plans. Planners need to understand and apply ethical principles to the planning process. The experts held that planners should at least acknowledge their ethical responsibilities of ensuring accountability, transparency, and community engagement in scarce resource decision-making and the establishment of realistic public expectations concerning fairness and equity during an MCE.[17]

Limits of conventional disaster planning

Deciding how and why to divert resources from some sector of community need to other areas should rest not only on predictions of what will produce the best outcome for the most persons but also should include considerations of how the resource distribution process will work to ensure that obligations citizens vest in their federal, state, and local governments are met. Traditional "disaster planning" has typically focused on emergency events, such as major transportation accidents likely to yield multiple casualties, rather than catastrophic events resulting in mass casualties and crippled infrastructure.[82] Until recently, efforts to integrate the wide spectrum of relevant emergency response organizations, providers, government agencies and disciplines such as health care, emergency medical services (EMS), public health, public safety, and emergency management, has not been a priority. Plans are still primarily institutional, local, or occasionally regional based and the attention paid to planning for and management of the truly catastrophic MCE, in which overwhelming numbers of casualties and cascading failures of infrastructure compound the incident are "rudimentary" at best.[17(pp. 1–31)]

Existing disaster plans assume that in any large-scale MCE emergency, healthcare delivery will continue to adhere to established standards of care and tend to concentrate on the "surge capacity" of acute care hospitals and the expansion of beds, triage space, personnel, pharmaceuticals, and supplies through the rapid mobilization and deployment of additional resources from the community, State, regional, or national levels to the affected area.[7,75] These plans seek to *stretch* the capacity of the existing system—not *restructure* the fundamental nature and interoperability of that system.[83] Inevitably, the ability to manage such a situation is highly dependent on the existing infrastructure and existing trauma and critical care systems in the affected area (region, nation).[21]

Overall, the general public does not really understand or accept the limitations that the healthcare system will have under austere circumstances. A well-prepared public should have realistic expectations of what first responders and other disaster personnel will be able to achieve and what may be asked of the community. The meeting experts recommended that disaster planners and emergency response personnel establish effective communication, education, and training strategies and systems that will enhance the community's understanding of both crisis medical standards and the provision of palliative care. Achieving these goals will require a "paradigm" shift across all sectors of society that redefines public expectations of the medical care system under MCE circumstances.[17]

Discussion

Optimal functioning of emergency response requires broad community accord about the legal, social justice, and ethical frameworks for the allocation of scarce resources and the integration of palliative care into MCE response. The rationale for resource allocation decision-making must be readily apparent to the community at large and understood to be evidence based, fair among people in need, and responsive to the circumstances of the potential patients and the capacity of the available services.[10,84,85] The provision of palliative care and a recognition of the needs of the existing "vulnerable" populations only managing with the support of the current healthcare system in the context of an MCE is a new component of disaster planning.

Little research or thoughtfully developed model plans have been available to guide planners. Only recently have official scarce resource response recommendations explicitly advocated for the provision of palliative care. Disaster response planners and palliative care professionals have yet to fully comprehend the potential utility of incorporating community-based palliative care professionals into MCE response planning efforts. Developing, planning for, and implementing any system of MCE response incorporating the delivery of palliative care services will be fraught with ethical, legal, social, and political issues. Many of these issues are discussed at length in the AHRQ reports *Altered Standards of Care in Mass Casualty*[11] and *Mass Medical Care with Scarce Resources: A Community Planning Guide*[81] and the subsequent IOM reports.[16,17]

We have identified two populations of MCE casualties for whom death can be expected within hours, days, or weeks and for whom the provision of palliative care would be an appropriate and humane response. Those who are likely to die cannot simply be consigned to holding areas or body bags while still alive; nor should they and their family advocates overwhelm hospitals and EMS transport systems that could be addressing the needs of potential survivors. If or when a disaster occurs, communities must be prepared for the possibility that the deployment of medical assistance may be delayed or downgraded and that governmental assistance may be delayed or overstretched by multiple challenges and competing demands.

Careful consideration of the special needs of those individuals who are at greatest risk of not surviving a catastrophic disaster will be challenging. The tough decisions that will have to be made in an MCE must have an ethical foundation, sanctioned by the community as a whole as well as those communities most likely to be at risk under these circumstances, and must be understood to be fair and in the best interests of the community at large. Palliative care offers a humane, effective, and medically appropriate treatment choice when resources are scarce and an alternative to "doing nothing" or ineffectively utilizing scarce resources. For these services to be readily available and successfully integrated into MCE disaster response, hospice and palliative care providers and advocates must participate in the disaster response planning process.

The ideas presented in this chapter are complex and fraught with ethical, legal, social, and political pitfalls. The investigation reported here illuminates certain important concerns and offers recommendations as a starting point for community disaster planners and public health officials. Wise policy requires sustained attention to these issues at the local, state, and federal levels, despite the potential social controversy, legal liability, and political risks surrounding the application of crisis standards of care and palliative care principles in major disaster response efforts.

References

1. Smith JS. Mass casualty events: are you prepared? Nursing. 2010 (April):41–45.
2. Chapman K, Arbn P. Are nurses ready?: Disaster preparedness in the acute setting. AENJ. 2008;11:135–144.
3. Pesik N, Keim M. Logistical considerations for emergency response resources. Pacific Health Dialog. 2002;9:97–103.
4. World Health Organization. ICN framework of disaster nursing competencies. SE Asian J Trop Med Pub Health. 2009;40(Suppl 1):57–70.
5. Pan American Health Organisation. Why Do Natural Disasters Seem to Be Increasingly Frequent And Increasingly Deadly? 2005. http://www.paho.org/English/DD/PIN/pr060109.htm. Accessed August 22, 2013.

6. Quarantelli EL. Converting disaster scholarship into effective disaster planning and managing: possibilities and limitations. Int J Mass Emergencies and Disasters. 1993;11:15–39.

7. Phillips SJ, Knebel A. Critical issues in preparing for a mass casualty event: highlights from a new community planning guide. Biosecur Bioterror. 2007;5(3):268–270.

8. Strangeland PA. Disaster nursing: a retrospective review. Crit Care Nurs Clin N Am. 2010;22:421–436.

9. Agency for Healthcare Research and Quality (AHRQ). Training of Hospital Staff to Respond to a Mass Casualty Incident. Evidence Report/Technology Assessment 2013; Number 95. http://www.ahrq.gov/downloads/pub/evidence/pdf/hospmci/hospmci.pdf. Accessed August 30, 2013.

10. Challen K, Bentley A, Bright J, Walter D. Clinical review: mass casualty triage—pandemic influenza and critical care. Crit Care. 2007;11:212–217.

11. Health Systems Research I. Altered Standards of Care in Mass Casualty Events. Washington, DC: DHHS/AHRQ; 2005.

12. Guerisse P. Basic principles of disaster medical management. Acta Anaesth Belg. 2005;56:395–401.

13. Sztajnkrycer MD, Madsen BE, Baez AA. Unstable ethical plateaus and disaster triage. Emerg Med Clin N Am. 2006;24:749–768.

14. Hogan DE, Burstein JL. Basic physics of disasters. In: Hogan DE, Burstein JL (eds.), Disaster Medicine. Philadelphia, PA: Lippincott Williams and Wilkins; 2002:3–9.

15. Timble JW, Ringel JS, Fox S, et al. Systematic review of strategies to manage and allocate scarce resources during mass casualty events. Ann Emerg Med. 2013;61(6):677–689.

16. Institute of Medicine. Guidance for Establishing Crisis Standards of Care for Use in Disaster Situations: A Letter Report-Summary. Washington, DC; 2009.

17. Institute of Medicine. Crisis Standards of Care: A Systems Framework for Catastrophic Disaster Response. Washington, DC: National Academies Press; 2012.

18. Agency for Healthcare Research and Quality (AHRQ). Altered Standards of Care in Mass Casualty Events: Bioterrorism and Other Public Health Emergencies. Rockville, MD: Agency for Healthcare Research and Quality; 2006.

19. Hodge JG, Hanfling D, Powell TP. Practical, ethical, and legal challenges underlying crisis standards of care. J Law Med Ethics. 2013;41(Suppl 1):50–55.

20. Sasser S. Field triage in disasters. Prehosp Emerg Care. 2006;10:322–323.

21. Cooper D. Mass Casualty Management in Disasters. 2006. http://www.who.int/hac/events/experts2006/D_Cooper_Mass_casualth_disasters.pdf. Accessed June 15, 2007.

22. Burkle FM. Population-based triage management in response to surge-capacity requirements during a large-scale bioevent disaster. Acad Emerg Med. 2006;13:1118–1129.

23. Hick JL, Hanfling D, Cantrill SV. Allocating scarce resources in disasters: emergency department principles. Ann Emerg Med. 2012;59(3):177–187.

24. Gostin LO, Henfling D, Hodge JG, Courtney B, Hick JL, Peterson CA. Standard of care—in sickness and in health and in emergencies: Letters to the editor. N Engl J Med. 2010;363(14):1378–1379.

25. General Accounting Office. Emergency Preparedness: States Are Planning for Medical Surge, But Could Benefit from Shared Guidance for Allocating Scarce Medical Resources. Washington, DC: GAO; 2008.

26. Schultz CH, Annas GJ. Altering the standard of care in disasters: unnecessary and dangerous. Ann Emerg Med. 2012;59(3):191–195.

27. Annas GJ. Standard of care—in sickness and in health and in emergencies. N Engl J Med. 2010;362:2126–2131.

28. Merin O, Ash N, Levy G, Schwaber MJ, Kreiss Y. The Israeli field hospital in Haiti—ethical dilemmas in early disaster response. N Engl J Med. 2010;362(11):e38.

29. Annas GJ. Standard of care—in sickness and in health and in emergencies: Author reply to letters to the editor. N Engl J Med. 2010;363(14):1379–1780.

30. Hirshberg A, Holcomb JB, Mattox KL. Hospital trauma care in multiple casualty incidents: a critical view. Ann Emerg Med. 2001;37:647–652.

31. Matzo M, Wilkinson AM, Gatto M, Lynn J. Palliative care for mass casualty events. Biosecur Bioterror. 2009;7(2):199–210.

32. Aldrich N, Benson WF. Disaster preparedness and the chronic disease needs of vulnerable adults. Prev Chron Dis. 2007;5(1).

33. Franco C, Toner E, Waldhorn R, Maldin B, O'Toole T, Inglesby T. Systemic collapse: medical care in the aftermath of Hurricane Katrina. Biosecur Bioterror. 2006;4(2):135–146.

34. Fernandez LS, Byard D, Lin CC, Benson S, Barbera JA. Frail elderly as disaster victims: emergency management strategies. Prehosp Dis Med. 2002;17(2):67–74.

35. White S, Henretig F, Dukes R. Medical management of vulnerable populations and co-morbid conditions of victims of bioterrorism. Emerg Med Clin N Am. 2002;20:365–392.

36. Buchanan J, Saliba D, Kingston RS. Disaster preparedness for vulnerable populations: the disabled, seriously ill or frail elderly. Am J Public Health. 2002;94(14):1436–1441.

37. Salerno JA, Nagy C. Terrorism and aging. J Gerontol A Biol Sci Med Sci. 2002;57A(9):552–554.511.

38. US Census Bureau. Economic Census. 2002; www.census.gov. Accessed April 26, 2010.

39. Zane R, Biddinger P. Home Health Patient Assessment Tools: Preparing for Emergency Triage. Rockville, MD: Agency for Healthcare Research and Quality; 2011.

40. O'Brien N. Emergency Preparedness for Older People. New York, NY: Mailman Center for Public Health, Columbia University; 2003.

41. Jellinek I. Perspectives from the Private Sector on Emergency Preparedness for Seniors and Persons with Disabilities in New York City: Lessons Learned from our City's Aging Services Providers from the Tragedy of September 11, 2001. New York, NY: Council of Senior Centers and Services of New York City; 2002.

42. Kleyman P. Emergency Preparedness: Lessons for All from Sept. 11 Attack. Aging Today: American Society on Aging; 2003.

43. Gibson MJ. We can do better: lessons learned for protecting older persons in disasters. Washington, DC: American Association of Retired People; 2006.

44. Parker L. What Really Happened at St. Rita's? USA Today. November 29, 2005.

45. The White House. The Federal Response to Hurricane Katrina: Lessons Learned. 2006. http://thewhitehouse.gov. Accessed July 3, 2006.

46. Byteway B. The Evacuation of Older People: The Case of Hurricane Katrina. Understanding Katrina. 2008. http://www.understandingkatrina.ssrc.org. Accessed December 28, 2008.

47. Okie S. Dr. Pou and the hurricane—implications for patient care during disasters. N Engl J Med. 2008;358(1):1–5.

48. Korner M, Krotz M, Kanz KG, Pfeifer KJ, Reiser M, Linsenmaier U. Development of an accelerated MSCT protocol (Triage MSCT) for mass casualty incidents: comparison to MSCT for single-trauma patients. Emerg Radiol. 2006;12(5): 203–209.

49. Baker MS. Creating order from chaos. Part I: Triage, initial care, and tactical considerations in mass casualty and disaster response. Military Med. 2007;172(3):232–236.

50. Goodwin Veenema T, Take J. When standards of care change in mass-casualty events. Aus J Nurs. 2007;107(9):72A–72H.

51. Turris SA, Lund A. Triage during mass gatherings. Prehosp Dis Med. 2012;27(6):531–535.

52. Cone DC, MacMillian DS. Mass-casualty triage systems: a hint of science. Acad Emerg Med. 2005;12(8):739–741.

53. Kahn CH, Shultz MD, Ken T, Miller MD, Anderson CL. Does START triage work?: An outcomes assessment after a disaster. Ann Emerg Med. 2009;54(3):424–430.

54. Agency for Healthcare Research and Quality (AHRQ). Limited Evidence on Best Strategies During a Mass Casualty Event. Rockville, MD: DHHS; 2012.

55. Gershon RRM, Magda LA, Qureshi KA, et al. Factors associated with the ability and willingness of essential workers to report to duty during a pandemic. J Emerg Med. 2010;52(10):995–1003.

56. Schroeter K. Duty to care versus duty to self. J Trauma Nurs. 2008;15(1):3–4.

57. Couig MP. Willingness, ability and intentions of health care workers to respond. Ann Rev Nurs Res. 2012;30:193–208.

58. Syrett JI, Benitez JG, Livingston WH, Davis EA. Will emergency health care providers respond to mass casualty incidents? Prehosp Emerg Care. 2007;11(1):49–54.

59. Qureshi KA, Gershon RR, Sherman ME, et al. Health care workers' ability and willingness to report to duty during catastrophic disasters. J Urban Health. 2005;82(3):413–416.

60. Adams KN, Berrym D. Who will show up?: Estimating ability and willingness of essential hospital personnel to report to work in response to a disaster. Online J Issues Nurs. 2012;17(2).

61. Chaffee M. Willingness of health care personnel to work in a disaster: an integrative review of the literature. Dis Med Pub Heal Prep. 2009;3(1):42–56.

62. Young CF, Persell DJ. Biological, chemical, and nuclear terrorism readiness: major concerns and preparedness of future nurses. Dis Manag Resp. 2004;2(4):109–114.

63. Monzon JDC. Palliative Care. 2007. http://www.carewellcommunity.org/articles-palliative.php.

64. Littleton-Kearney MT, Slepski LA. Directions for disaster nursing education in the United States. Crit Care Nurs Clin North Am. 2008;20:103–109.

65. De Jong MJ, Benner R, Benner P, et al. Mass casualty care in an expeditionary environment: developing local knowledge and expertise in context. J Trauma Nurs. 2010;17(1):45–58.

66. Medscape Medical News. Time to Plan for a Palliative Care Pandemic: An Expert Interview with Phillip E. Rodgers, MD, FAAHPM. 2010. www.medscape.com/viewarticle/718395. Accessed August 30, 2013.

67. Hearne S, Segal LM, Earls MJ. Ready or Not?: Protecting the Public's Health from Diseases, Disasters, and Bioterrorism. 2005.

68. World Health Organization. Mass Casualty Management Systems: Strategies and Guidelines for Building Health Sector Capacity. 2007; www.who.int/hac/techguidance/tools/mcm_guidelines_en.pdf. Accessed September 3, 2013.

69. Polivka BJ, Stanley SAR, Gordon D, Taulbee K, Keiffer G, McCorkle SM. Public health nursing competencies for public health surge events. Public Health Nurs. 2008;25(2):159–168.

70. Gebbie K, Merrill J. Public health worker competencies for emergency responses. J Pub Heal Manag Prac. 2002;8(2):73–81, p. 73.

71. Arbon P, Bobrowski C, Zeitz K, Hooper C, Williams J, Thitchener J. Australian nurses volunteering for the Sumatra-Andaman earthquake and tsunami of 2004: a review of experience and analysis of data collected by the Tsunami Volunteer Hotline. Aus Emerg Nurs J. 2006;9:171–178.

72. Bergin A, Khosa B. Are We Ready?: Healthcare Preparedness for Catastrophic Terrorism. 2007.

73. Hughes F, Grigg M, Fritsch K, et al. Psychosocial response in emergency situations: the nurse's role. Int Nurs Rev. 2007;54(2):19–27.

74. Usher K, Mayner L. Disaster nursing: a descriptive survey of Australian undergraduate nursing curricula. Aus Emerg Nurs J. 2011;14:75–80.

75. Weiner EE. A national curriculum for nurses in emergency preparedness and response. Nurs Clin N Am. 2005;10:469–479.

76. International Nursing Coalition for Mass Casualty Education. Educational Competencies for Registered Nurses Responding to Mass Casualty Incidents. 2003. http://www.nursing.vanderbilt.edu/incmce/competencies.html.

77. American Colleges of Nursing. The Essentials of Baccalaureate Education for Professional Nursing Practice. Washington, DC: American Colleges of Nursing 2008.

78. Gebbie K, Qureshi KA. A historical challenge: nurses and emergencies. Online J Issues Nurs. 2006;11(3):1–14.

79. Domres B, Manger A, Steigerwald I, Esser S. The challenge of crisis, disaster, and war: experience with UN and NGOs. Pain Pract. 2003;3(1):97–100.

80. Acquaviva KD. Disaster Palliative Assistance Team (DPAT), under the NDMS System. Personal communication, 2006.

81. Phillips SJ, Knebel A, eds. Mass Medical Care with Scarce Resources: A Community Planning Guide Rockville, MD: Agency for Healthcare Research and Quality (AHRQ); 2007.

82. US Department of Homeland Security (DHS). National Preparedness Guidelines. Washington, DC: Author; 2007.

83. Salinsky E. Strong as the Weakest Link: Medical Response to a Catastrophic Event. Washington, DC: NHPF; 2008.

84. Roberts M, De Renzo EG. Chapter II. Ethical Considerations in Community Disaster Planning. Mass Medical Care with Scarce Resources: A Community Planning Guide. Publication No. 07-0001. Rockville, MD: Agency for Healthcare Research and Quality; 2007:9–24.

85. Kass NE, Otto J, O'Brien D, Minson M. Ethics and severe pandemic influenza: maintaining essential functions through a fair and considered response. Biosecur Bioterror. 2008;6(3):227–236.

SECTION VI

Pediatric palliative care

CHAPTER 55

Symptom management in pediatric palliative care

Melody Brown Hellsten and Stacey Berg

What kind of God could do this to a child?

Mother of a symptomatic pediatric patient with advanced cancer

Key points

- Children are living longer with complex chronic medical conditions.
- Life prolongation is often accompanied by multiple acute and chronic health crises and challenges for the child and family.
- Symptom management presents a unique challenge to care providers.
- Skilled and compassionate management of symptoms, using a family-centered approach, is an integral part of the care of a chronically ill child.

Complex chronic conditions of childhood (Box 55.1) are medically defined as "any medical condition that can be reasonably expected to last at least 12 months, involves either multiple organs or one organ system severely enough to require specialty pediatric care, and some probability of hospitalization at a tertiary care center."[1] A needs-based definition of children with complex chronic conditions includes "children who require ongoing skilled monitoring and care from family or professional caregivers and use supportive therapies and technology to enhance health and well-being to avert death or further disability."[2] Using currently available demographic and epidemiological data,[3,4] the estimated number of children currently living with complex chronic conditions of childhood could range from 2.2 to 3.7 million.[5,6]

Ongoing advances in medical science are contributing to life-prolonging management of children with complex chronic conditions. However, this life prolongation often comes at the cost of multiple acute and chronic health crises and hospitalizations.[7] Worsening debilitation as the child's condition progresses increases the likelihood of suffering for the child and family.[7-9] It is, therefore, imperative that care providers face the challenge of recognizing and attending to suffering as a concurrent focus of care while providing curative and life-prolonging treatment. Unfortunately, fragmentation of healthcare, limited acknowledgment of terminal care needs of children, and a paucity of research on the impact of symptoms on quality of life and interventions aimed at managing distressing symptoms all create challenges in alleviating suffering for children with complex chronic conditions.[10-12]

This chapter focuses on issues related to the assessment and management of common nonpain symptoms in children and adolescents with complex medical conditions in the advanced and terminal stages. The unique issues related to children dying in pediatric and neonatal intensive care units are addressed in chapters 56 and 59, respectively.

Assessing sources of suffering in advanced childhood illness

Family-centered care

Family-centered care is based on the understanding that the family is the child's primary source of strength and support and that the perspectives and information provided by families, children, and young adults are important in clinical decision-making.[13-17] In considering symptom management within the context of family-centered care, it is necessary to assess the family system as a whole, as well as its individual members, to identify all sources of suffering that may require intervention. Interdisciplinary collaboration with chaplains, social workers, psychologists, and child-life therapists will contribute to the overall assessment of the ill child, parents, and siblings.

The focus of family-centered care is to develop a process of shared decision-making over the course of the child's and family's illness experience that is based in the interpersonal relationship between the child and family and their healthcare providers. The physician and healthcare team must come to know the child and family as individuals and provide diagnostic, prognostic, and treatment information in a manner sensitive to the particular child's and family's experiences, values, beliefs, and available social and spiritual support.[18-20] Parents and children should be respected as the experts in their illness experience and management, and value must be given to their contribution to the plan of care. The child's and family's illness experience and goals of care, as well as the impact of a particular symptom on suffering and its effect on the child's function and quality of life, will influence the types of interventions considered as symptoms occur.[21-23]

Illness experience and sources of suffering

Research exploring the experiences of families of children with complex chronic conditions provides a glimpse into their

Box 55.1 Categories of complex chronic conditions of childhood

Neurological conditions

Congenital malformations of the brain
Anencephaly
Lissencephaly
Holoprosencephaly
Cerebral palsy/Mental retardation
Neurodegenerative disorders
Muscular dystrophies
Spinal muscular atrophy
Adrenoleukodystrophy
Epilepsy

Cardiovascular conditions

Malformations of the heart/great vessels
Cardiomyopathies
Conduction disorders/dysrhythmias

Respiratory conditions

Cystic fibrosis
Chronic respiratory disease
Respiratory malformations

Renal conditions

Chronic renal failure

Gastrointestinal conditions

Congenital anomalies
Chronic liver disease/cirrhosis
Inflammatory bowel disease

Hematology/immunodeficiency

Sickle cell disease
Hereditary anemias
Hereditary immunodeficiency
HIV/AIDS

Metabolic conditions

Amino acid metabolism
Carbohydrate metabolism
Mucopolysaccharidosis
Storage disorders

Genetic conditions

Trisomy 18
Chromosome 22 deletions

Other congenital disorders

Malignancy
Leukemias/lymphomas
Brain tumors
Sarcomas
Neuroblastoma

---

technical care and negotiate the care system for needed services and information.[28-30] Over time, parents must live with ongoing uncertainty regarding the unpredictability of the illness, the ultimate outcome of their child's treatment, the challenges of parenting a seriously ill child, and the possibility of death.[19,31-34] The child may experience disability, physical pain, and other distressing symptoms as a result of the disease and treatments, severe alterations in their social world, and disruption of their developmental process.[9,35-42] Siblings may experience feelings of anger, guilt, anxiety, depression, and social isolation.[8,43-45]

Although the above picture gives an impression of tremendous struggle and individual distress in the family, there is also research that suggests there are aspects of family functioning that facilitate coping with this new family reality. Parents' adaptation and adjustment to their child's illness is facilitated by several factors, including gaining information regarding the disease, its treatment, and prognosis; good spousal communication; similar coping styles and means of emotional expression; and sufficient social support.[46-48] Factors associated with adaptation of the ill child and siblings include having open communication and emotional support from parents during times of stress, having a wide range of coping skills, seeking information about the disease, and clarifying fears.[39,44,49-50]

Assessing and understanding the child and family's unique experiences during the illness trajectory provides the care team with insight into what symptoms may contribute to the family's suffering. This assessment involves hearing the child's and family members' "story" as they have lived it during the course of the disease. It is important to elicit care that has been helpful in past experiences with the illness as well as care that was not helpful. Insight into what the family values regarding the role of spirituality or faith, the meaning they give to their experience of illness, and what activities or interactions the child and family identify as contributing to quality of life provide a context for identifying and managing symptoms that contribute to suffering for the child and family.

Expectations and goals of care

Children with complex chronic conditions are a highly diverse population, with various illness trajectories that are often characterized by prognostic uncertainty, including sudden unexpected death, death from potentially curable disease, death from lethal congenital anomaly, and death from progressive conditions with intermittent health crises. The unpredictability and uncertainty of many of these disease trajectories often result in ongoing medical treatments aimed at cure or aggressive life-prolongation, with limited attention to the suffering of the child or family.[10,11,51]

Generally, goals of care for children with serious, life-threatening or life-limiting illness as they progress through their illness trajectory include interventions aimed at cure, life prolongation with or without aggressive life-sustaining therapies, and care focused solely on treating discomfort from symptoms as the disease moves into its terminal phase. Ideally, these goals would shift as the child, family, and primary healthcare team discussed changes in quality of life, symptoms, and prognosis over the disease trajectory. It is very important that interventions aimed at maintaining maximal comfort and quality of life occur throughout the disease trajectory

---

world. Uncertainty prevails as the parents move from the initial suspicion that something is wrong with their child to the confirmation that this is indeed the case.[24-27] Parents struggle to cope with the diagnosis and learn skills necessary to provide

as well as through the terminal stages. Conversely, the presence of a do-not-resuscitate (DNR) order should not lead to care professionals' dismissing treatable illnesses or symptoms as "part of the dying process," thereby contributing to suffering for both the child and family.

The most difficult decision a parent must face is to change the focus of care from cure or aggressive life prolongation to focusing on comfort and terminal care. In 2000, Wolfe and colleague[52,53] drew attention to symptoms and suffering experienced by children with cancer as well as the disparity between parents and care providers regarding the realization that a child with progressive cancer had no realistic chance for cure. Parents who came to that realization earlier were more likely to discuss hospice care, to establish a DNR order, and to change the focus of care from cancer-directed therapies to treatments focused on controlling discomfort and an increased perception of quality care at home. As a result of the growth of palliative care for children in the past decade, studies of parents' experience of their child's treatment and end-of-life care demonstrate improvements in attention to symptoms and suffering, however concerns persist for many parents regarding understanding of prognosis and goals of care, unmanaged symptoms, and suffering for their children with complex medical conditions.[10,11,15,42,51,54–55] Parents have reported that decisions to forgo further aggressive medical treatments and instead pursue care focused on comfort and quality of life occurred only after realizing that ongoing aggressive treatment would not bring about cure or further life prolongation, and they recognized the physical deterioration and suffering of their child. Once this realization is reached, parents report that the child's wishes and quality of life are major determinants of treatment decision-making.[19,33,56,57]

The first step to managing symptoms of children with advanced and terminal illness is a thorough assessment of the child's and family's expectations and goals of care. Interventions aimed at controlling symptoms must be compatible with the family's understanding of where their child is in the disease trajectory and their expectations of care, as well as the child's overall functional status and quality of life. For example, an adolescent with advanced muscular dystrophy may be attending school and participating in a religious community despite significant physical limitations. This level of function and quality of life may lead the child and family to desire aggressive ventilatory support for life prolongation in the event of an acute respiratory infection, with the hope that the child will be cured of the infection and resume his previous level of functioning. However, if the adolescent were home-bound and seriously debilitated as a result of progressive respiratory failure, he and his family may choose to pursue home management of respiratory discomfort without the use of ventilatory support to reduce suffering associated with intensive hospital-based interventions. In determining the expectations and goals of care with the child and family, it is important to discuss the balance between relieving and contributing to the child's suffering. The prevailing decision-making framework should not be based on whether an intervention is consistent with a palliative care focus but, rather, whether the intervention under consideration would provide relief from or contribute to the child's and family's suffering.

Physical symptoms and suffering

Children dying as the result of complex chronic conditions experience numerous symptoms throughout their illness trajectory that can contribute to suffering and decreased quality of life (Box 55.2).

Managing these symptoms requires that healthcare providers remain attentive in their assessment of the child's physical and emotional symptoms. Assessment should include the child's report of symptoms and how distressing he or she finds them, information based on parent observation of their child's condition, and the healthcare provider's knowledge of the pathophysiology of the underlying disease. Diagnostic tests should be considered carefully for the potential discomfort they may cause. Tests should be ordered only if they will help determine an intervention. A test's appropriateness should be questioned if its results will not change management (e.g., MRI to document growth of known terminal tumor).

As mentioned earlier, symptoms experienced by children with advanced and terminal chronic illnesses are often interrelated. If a child reports a distressing symptom, it is necessary to obtain a thorough assessment regarding the symptom's onset, severity, and effect on function and quality of life. Standardized assessment scales for symptoms and associated quality of life in children have been reported, but they are generally used in research, with limited knowledge of their use for ongoing assessment, clinical management, and treatment decision-making.[58–61] The healthcare provider must consider the likely cause of the symptom and determine the best course of intervention. For example, pain with urination may be related to an infection and amenable to treatment with antibiotics to cure the infection. Shortness of breath in a child with cystic fibrosis may be related to infection and amenable to treatment with antibiotics, with resolution of the symptom. However, it may also be related to progressive respiratory failure or disease progression. Oxygen therapy, opioids, ventilation and/or energy-conservation techniques may assist in relieving the

---

Box 55.2 Symptoms contributing to suffering in advanced and terminal disease

General symptoms

Fatigue
Anorexia

Psychological/emotional symptoms

Anxiety/depression

Neurological symptoms

Seizures
Somnolence

Respiratory symptoms

Dyspnea

Gastrointestinal symptoms

Nausea/vomiting
Constipation
Diarrhea

severity of the symptom but will not eliminate the underlying cause. This distinction is important to discuss with the child and parent in the context of the goal of treatment and expectation of care in relation to the child's overall condition and quality of life.

Control of present symptoms and anticipation of distressing symptoms as disease progresses is imperative in attending to the suffering of children with advanced disease and their families. Following is a discussion of the most common symptoms associated with distress and suffering experienced by children with advanced illness. It is by no means an exhaustive presentation of all symptoms that children with complex chronic conditions may experience. Each symptom is discussed with regard to its general issues, causes, assessment, and pharmacological and non-pharmacological management. As discussed earlier, there is little evidence-based data on the management of nonpain symptoms in children with advanced disease. Much symptom management in pediatric palliative care is based on empirical approaches and extrapolation from adult hospice and palliative care literature.

An inherent difficulty in pharmacological management in pediatric palliative care is a lack of pharmacological dosing and side-effect information on infants, toddlers, and early school-aged children for many medications. Starting dosages of medications will vary depending on the age, weight, and clinical circumstances of the child. It is incumbent on physicians and nurses to consult with experienced pediatricians and pediatric hospice and palliative care providers for medication choices, appropriate doses, and titration for difficult cases of symptom management. For more information on pediatric pain management, see chapter 61.

Management of symptoms during disease progression and at the end of life

General systemic symptoms

Fatigue

The most comprehensive research in fatigue experienced by children with complex chronic illnesses has been in the area of childhood cancer. Fatigue has been described as a "profound sense of being physically tired, or having difficulty with body movements such as moving legs or opening their eyes" in young children with cancer; and as a "changing state of exhaustion that includes physical, mental, and emotional tiredness" in adolescents with cancer.[52–55] Fatigue, lethargy, lack of energy, and drowsiness have been reported in more than 50% of children with cancer, and has been described as moderately to severely distressing.[36,61–63] Fatigue has also been reported as a symptom of concern in children with cystic fibrosis,[64] neuromuscular diseases,[65–67] and sickle cell disease.[68]

Fatigue is a multidimensional symptom that can be related to disease, treatment, or emotional factors (Box 55.3). Assessment requires a multidimensional approach, which includes subjective and objective data to determine the degree of distress and potential causes of the child's fatigue. Subjective assessment involves asking children about their feelings of tiredness or lack of energy, how long they feel tired, when they feel most tired, and how it affected their ability to play or go to school. Objective assessment should include vital signs, presence of other symptoms such as dyspnea or vomiting, evaluation of hydration status, and muscle strength. Laboratory data may include parameters such as oxygen

Box 55.3 Factors contributing to fatigue in children with advanced disease
Disease/treatment
Pain
Unresolved symptoms
Anemia
Malnutrition
Infection
Fever
Sleep disturbance
Debilitation
Psychological factors
Depression
Anxiety
Spiritual distress

saturation, complete blood count with differential, and thyroid studies. Management of fatigue will vary depending on the underlying cause and may include both pharmacological and nonpharmacological interventions (Table 55.1). For more information on fatigue, see chapter 8.

Nausea/vomiting

The pathophysiology of nausea and vomiting is often multifactorial; can be acute, anticipatory, or delayed; and requires careful assessment to determine underlying causes. Nausea and vomiting can cause extreme exhaustion and dehydration if not well controlled. Underlying causes of nausea and vomiting may include decreased gastric motility, constipation, obstruction, metabolic disturbances, medication side effects or toxicity, and increased intracranial pressure.

A detailed assessment of the onset and duration, as well as the presence of concomitant symptoms (e.g., headache, visual disturbances) must be obtained. Medical management of nausea and vomiting is based on the suspected underlying cause (Table 55.2).

Corticosteroids may be helpful in reducing an intestinal obstruction. Antiemetic medications combined with medications to reduce secretions (e.g., glycopyrrolate) can be helpful in relieving nausea and vomiting related to intestinal obstruction. In cases of severe nausea and vomiting related to obstruction, placement of a nasogastric tube can decompress the stomach and provide comfort. Medications that promote gastric emptying (e.g., metoclopramide) or motility should not be used if obstruction is suspected. Steroids can provide relief from vomiting caused by increased intracranial pressure. Nausea and vomiting related to medications or anorexia may be managed by a number of antiemetic medications.[71–72] Relaxation techniques, deep breathing, distraction, and art therapies may assist in reducing anticipatory nausea. For more information on nausea and vomiting, see chapter 10.

Constipation

Constipation is a frequent symptom experienced by children with advanced and terminal illness and can occur even in children with limited oral intake.[73] Children and adolescents, in particular, become embarrassed if asked about bowel habits and will deny problems, leading to a severe problem. It is important to

Table 55.1 Management of fatigue in children with advanced disease

Cause	Intervention	Dose	Comments
	Pharmacological management		
Anemia	Blood transfusion	10–15 mL/kg IV over 4 h	Premedicate with diphenhydramine (1 mg/kg/IV/PO, max dose 50 mg), acetaminophen (10–15 mg/kg PO) and hydrocortisone (2 mg/kg IV, max dose 100 mg) prior to transfusion if history of reaction
	Psychostimulants		
Disease progression	◆ Methylphenidate	0.3 mg/kg/dose PO bid	Dosage information for ≥6 y. Give doses in AM and early afternoon. May titrate by 0.1 mg/kg/dose to max of 2 mg/kg/day, gauge by child's desired activity level. May decrease appetite
	◆ Dextroamphetamine	6–12 y 5 mg/day. May titrate in 5-mg increments weekly, 12 y 10 mg/day	Titrate according to child's desired level of activity Will suppress appetite
	May titrate in 10-mg increments weekly		
	Sleep agents		
Insomnia Anxiety			
	◆ Diphenhydramine	1 mg/kg IV/PO. Max dose 50 mg/dose	May cause paradoxical excitement, euphoria, or confusion
			May use in children as young as 2 y
	◆ Lorazepam	0.03–0.1 mg IV/PO. Max 2 mg/dose	Can cause retrograde amnesia. Taper dose with prolonged use
			May use in infants and young children
	◆ Zolpidem	10 mg PO qh	Use for adolescents, young adults. No dosing information for young children
	Nonpharmacological management		
Anorexia	Nutritional supplementation (e.g., Boost®, Pediasure®, etc.)		
Generalized fatigue all causes	Frequent rest, energy conservation		
Deconditioning Weakness	Physical/occupational therapies		
All causes	Play therapy		
All causes	Exploring fears/anxiety that may interfere with sleep		

Source: Ullrich et al. (2007), reference 69.

educate the child and family about the potential distress caused by constipation and determine with the child how to discuss this issue. Constipation occurs as a result of inactivity, dehydration, electrolyte imbalance, bowel compression or invasion by tumor, nerve involvement, and/or medications. Symptoms include anorexia, nausea, vomiting, colicky abdominal pain, bloating, and fecal impaction. Physical exam may reveal abdominal distention, right lower-quadrant tenderness, and fecal masses. A rectal exam should be done; however, it is important to gain the child's or adolescent's trust before such an invasive assessment. Ask the child which parent he or she would prefer to be present and have that parent sit near the child and provide reassurance and comfort. Assess the rectum for presence of hard impacted feces, an empty dilated rectum, or extrinsic compression of the rectum by a tumor, hemorrhoids, fissures, tears, or fistulas. Caution should be used in children with cancer who are neutropenic, and a digital exam should not be done unless absolutely necessary.

Management is aimed at preventing constipation from occurring, but if constipation has occurred, it should be treated immediately to avoid debilitating effects (Box 55.4).

Stool softeners should be given for any child at risk of constipation caused by opioid pain management or decreased activity. Softeners are most effective when children are well hydrated, so the healthcare provider should encourage the child to drink water as tolerated. Stimulant laxatives should be used if a child has not had a bowel movement for more than 3 days past that child's usual

Table 55.2 Management of nausea/vomiting

Agent	Dose	Comments
Ondansetron	0.15 mg/kg/dose IV or 0.2 mg/kg dose PO q4h; max: 8 mg/dose	Indicated for opioid-induced nausea/vomiting
Metoclopromide	1–2 mg/kg/dose IV q2–4h; max: 50 mg/dose	Indicated for nausea/vomiting related to anorexia, gastroesophageal reflux
		Can cause dystonia
Promethazine	0.5 mg/kg IV/PO q4–6h; max: 25 mg/dose	Indicated for nausea/vomiting related to obstruction, opioids. May increase sedation
Dexamethasone	1–2 mg/kg IV/PO initially, then 1–1.5 mg/kg/day divided q6h; max: 16 mg/day	Indicated for nausea/vomiting related to bowel obstruction, intracranial pressure, medications
		Side effects include weight gain, edema, and gastrointestinal irritation.

Sources: Santucci et al. (2007), reference 70.

Box 55.4 Management of constipation

Senna

Infants and children <12 y

Syrup: 1 month to <2 years: 1.25 to 2.5 mL (2.2–4.4 mg sennosides) at bedtime [maximum: 2.5 mL (4.4 mg sennosides) twice daily]

  2 to <6 years: 2.5 to 3.75 mL (4.4–6.6 mg sennosides) at bedtime [maximum: 3.75 mL (6.6 mg sennosides) twice daily]

  6 to <12 years: 5 to 7.5 mL (8.8–13.2 mg sennosides) at bedtime [maximum: 7.5 mL (13.2 mg sennosides) twice daily]

  Tablet: 2 to <6 years: 1/2 tablet (4.3 mg sennosides) at bedtime [maximum: 1 tablet (8.6 mg sennosides) twice daily]

  6 to <12 years: 1 tablet (8.6 mg sennosides) at bedtime [maximum: 2 tablets (17.2 mg sennosides) twice daily]

Children ≥12 years and adults:

Syrup: 10–15 mL (17.6–26.4 mg sennosides) at bedtime [maximum: 15 mL (26.4 mg sennosides) twice daily]

  Tablet: 2 tablets (17.2 mg sennosides) at bedtime [maximum: 4 tablets (34.4 mg sennosides) twice daily]

Ducosate sodium

  Children < 3 y: 10–40 mg/day PO in 1–4 divided doses
  3–6 y: 20–60 mg/day PO in 1–4 divided doses
  6–12 y: 50–150 mg/day PO in 1–4 divided doses
  Older than 12 y: 50–100 mg/day PO in 1–4 divided doses

---

pattern. If these measures are not successful, stronger cathartic laxatives (e.g., magnesium citrate) or an enema may be used. If there is stool in the rectum and the child is unable to pass it, digital disimpaction may be necessary. The child should be prepared for the procedure and premedicated with pain and antianxiety medications. For more information on constipation, see chapter 12.

Diarrhea

Although diarrhea is far less common than constipation in children with terminal illnesses, it still may occur and contribute to a diminished quality of life.[62] Diarrhea may be caused by intermittent bowel obstruction, fecal impaction, medications, malabsorption, infections, history of abdominal or pelvic radiation, chemotherapy, inflammatory bowel disease, and foods with sorbitol and fructose (found frequently in juices, gum, and candy). Diseases related to increased risk of diarrhea include HIV/AIDS resulting from infections, cystic fibrosis related to malabsorption, and malignancies related to disease progression and treatment history.

Assessment should include onset, suddenness, duration, and frequency of loose stools; incontinence; character of the stools (color, odor, consistency, presence of mucus or blood), bowel sounds, presence of palpable masses or feces, abdominal tenderness, and examination of the rectal area. Assessment of dehydration includes observation of mucous membranes for dryness, cracking, poor skin turgor, and generalized fatigue. Diet and medication history should be reviewed for potential causes of diarrhea.

Treatment is aimed at managing the underlying causes and the results of persistent diarrhea (Box 55.5). Dietary intervention should involve continued feeding of the child's regular diet as tolerated, as well as oral rehydration with electrolyte solutions as tolerated.[51] For debilitated children using incontinence garments, attention to skin condition and prevention of breakdown is imperative. For more information on diarrhea, see chapter 12.

Feeding problems/intolerance

Gastrointestinal symptoms and related feeding problems are common in children with neurological impairments.[74] Oropharyngeal dysphagia, gastroesphogeal reflux, dysmotility, retching/vomiting, aspiration, and constipation represent a common cluster of symptoms of children with both static and progressive neurological impairment.[75,76] Symptom management is focused on balancing treatment of the underlying complications as well as the nutritional needs of the child.[77,78] Children with mild forms of neurological impairment benefit from oromotor stimulation and feeding therapy to maintain optimal nutrition.[79] For children with severe or progressive neurological conditions, malnutrition and aspiration risk complicate oral feeding. Gastrostomy tubes can improve nutrition, medication delivery, and caregiver stress

---

Box 55.5 Management of diarrhea

Loperamide
Initial doses: 2–5 y: 1 mg PO tid;
6–8 y: 2 mg PO bid;
8–12 y: 2 mg PO tid; after initial dose, 0.1-mg/kg doses after each loose stool (not to exceed the initial dose);
>12 y: 4 mg PO × 1 dose; then 2 mg PO after each loose stool (maximum dose: 16 mg/day)
Diphenoxylate and atropine
2–5 y: 2 mg PO tid (not to exceed 6 mg/day)
5–8 y: 2 mg PO qid (not to exceed 8 mg/day)
8–12 y: 2 mg PO 5 times/day (not to exceed 10 mg/day)
>12 y: 2.5–5 mg PO 2–4 times/day (not to exceed 20 mg/day)

around feeding, but do not necessarily improve the overall quality of life for the patient.[76,80] Additionally, a retrospective review of fundoplication and gastrojejunal feeding tubes for prevention of aspiration pneumonia found neither option was superior for preventing aspiration pneumonia or improving overall survival.[81]

Parents experience substantial distress when deciding to use gastrostomy as a means of feeding, as well as feelings of failure as a parent, caregiving burden, and stress. Parents should be provided with accurate information regarding risks and benefits, and support through clarification of values and informed decision-making.[82–84]

Anorexia/cachexia

Loss of appetite occurs in nearly all children with terminal illness. Anorexia involves the loss of desire to eat or a loss of appetite, with associated decrease in food intake. Cachexia is a general lack of nutrition and wasting of lean muscle mass that occurs over the course of a chronic progressive disease. Anorexia and cachexia are multidimensional in nature and are influenced by disease, treatment, and emotional factors[85–87] (Box 55.6). These symptoms are particularly distressing to parents of children with illness because

they cause concern that the child is "starving to death." Food and meals have a social association with "caring" and are significant in family culture, activities, and ritual. In most instances, children will request favorite foods as a means of comfort and familiarity. It is important to assist parents in understanding their child's changing eating habits and nutritional needs as well as ways to redirect energies toward other caregiving activities. Table 55.3 provides additional suggestions for management of anorexia and cachexia.

Parents and healthcare providers often struggle with personal and ethical dilemmas regarding fluid and nutrition management for children with terminal illness. The act of withholding medically provided fluids and nutrition (enteral feeds, total parenteral nutrition) is legally and ethically permissible for children with irreversible, progressive medical conditions when it is agreed on by the healthcare providers and family that such medically provided nutrition will increase the suffering and discomfort of the child and would not alter the progression of the disease or the outcome of death.[88–91] Such decisions are highly individual to the family and influenced by culture, religious tradition, and personal values.

Providing aggressive nutritional support does not usually improve the condition and, in fact, may add additional symptom burden for the child. When medically provided nutritional interventions are chosen by a family, the challenge is balancing fluid and nutritional supplementation as appetite and metabolic needs decrease with advancing disease. Complication rates for enteral feeds are upwards of 76%, and include fluid overload, electrolyte imbalance, pain, nausea, and vomiting.[88,91]

Ideally, as the child's condition progresses, parenteral or enteral supplements can be slowly weaned to promote comfort and decrease symptoms of increased congestion or secretions. For more information on anorexia and cachexia, see chapter 9.

Psychological/emotional symptoms

Anxiety

Children with chronic illness may experience numerous anxiety-provoking events throughout their illness. Episodes of serious illness, hospitalizations, painful procedures, changes in

---

Box 55.6 Factors contributing to anorexia/cachexia in advanced disease

Physiological factors
Uncontrolled pain or other symptoms
Feeding/swallowing problems
Poor oral hygiene and infections
Mouth sores
Nausea/vomiting
Constipation
Delayed gastric emptying
Changes in taste
Psychological factors
Depression
Anger
Stress

Table 55.3 Management of anorexia/cachexia

Intervention	Dose	Comments
Pharmacological management		
Megestrol	10 mg/kg/dose PO bid	May cause headache, rash, hypertension
Dronabinol	2.5 mg/kg/dose 3–4 times/day	Provides triple effect of antiemetic, appetite stimulant, mood elevation. May be used in young children
Nonpharmacological management		
Prepare small portions of favorite foods.		
Allow child to eat "comfort" foods, don't stress "balanced diet."		
Use thickened liquids or soft foods.		
Offer shakes, smoothies, and other high-calorie foods.		
Provide nutritional drinks as tolerated.		
Assist family in limiting stress over child's eating.		

Source: Santucci et al. (2007), reference 70.

independence and physical abilities, uncontrolled pain and other symptoms, and an uncertain future all can contribute to fear and anxiety.[35,51,92] The distinction between childhood fears and anxiety is crucial—childhood fears are specific and developmentally based (e.g., fear of the dark, fear of separation, fear of death), whereas anxiety is a generalized feeling of uneasiness without a known source.[68] Anxiety and depression may be comorbid conditions.

Anxiety in terminal illness is an expected reaction and should be assessed frequently. Toddlers and young children will generally have anxiety reactions that are an extension of the stress and anxiety levels of parents and other family members around them. These reactions may include irritability, clinginess, temper tantrums, and inconsolability. School-aged children and adolescents who can cognitively comprehend their illness and impending death may experience more adult-like symptoms, such as chronic apprehension, worry, difficulty concentrating, and sleep disturbance. Chaplains, child-life workers, social workers, and psychologists are helpful in assessing children's fears, worries, and dreams. Children and adolescents under stress may regress behaviorally and emotionally; therefore, healthcare professionals should be alert to changes in the child's coping or personality.

Depression

Little is known about the incidence or prevalence of clinical depression in children and adolescents living with chronic illness. Depression can be described as a broad spectrum of responses that range from intermittent general sadness to debilitating symptoms of clinical depressive disorders."[92-95] Children are unique in their coping abilities, which are influenced by their age and developmental level. Often, during the course of terminal illness, children remain focused on future hopes and continue to plan activities, even in the final days of life. This does not represent denial or being uninformed of their circumstance, but rather a protective developmental function and should be gently supported by family and care providers.

Risk factors for depression in chronically ill children include frequent disruptions in important relationships, uncontrolled pain, and presence of multiple physical disabilities.[90-92] Existential factors related to impending death, concern for parents and other family members, and a personal or family history of preexisting psychological problems can also increase the risk for depression in chronically ill children. Suicidal thoughts or wishes are not common in terminally ill children and adolescents, but healthcare providers should be alert to comments about wishing to die and seek social workers, child-life therapists, or psychologists to assist in further assessment and management.

Assessment of depressive symptoms must account for the child's developmental level. Psychologists, clinical social workers, and child-life therapists have expertise in assisting children with life-threatening illnesses and should be consulted early in the trajectory to reduce psychological distress. Somatic complaints such as lack of appetite, insomnia, agitation, and loss of energy may be the result of disease and cannot be considered hallmark signs of depression in ill children. More appropriate signs would include a persistent sad face and demeanor, tearfulness, irritability, and withdrawal from previously enjoyed activities and relationships. Siblings may exhibit persistent and significant decrease in school performance, hypersomnolence, changes in appetite or weight, and nonspecific complaints of not feeling well.[29,43,45,49] Parents should be assessed for depressed appearance, fearfulness, withdrawal, a sense of punishment, and mood that cannot be improved with good news and should be referred for further evaluation as needed.[9,95-97]

Pharmacological management of anxiety and depression should be considered if symptoms of anxiety and depression are debilitating. Consultation with psychiatric specialists for further evaluation and choice of agents is appropriate to assist with assessment and medication recommendations. Generally, management of anxiety and depression related to terminal illness in children involves nonpharmacological interventions aimed at addressing the underlying issues that are contributing to the symptoms. Both unconditional acceptance of the child's feelings and reassurance are powerful interventions for anxiety and depression. Facilitating open communication between children and their parents may also be helpful. Creative arts therapies, play, relaxation, storytelling, music, and games may assist in helping children begin to talk about their feelings. It is important to recognize that a certain level of anxiety and sadness is normal when facing death. Healthcare providers must take caution to not be overly "cheerful" or insistent that a child discuss his/her feelings. Calm presence, active listening, and sitting quietly with a child will help to build trust. Adolescents in particular are very private about their thoughts and feelings, and if they choose to share them with a caregiver, confidentiality is an important factor in continuing a trusting relationship with the adolescent. For more information on depression, see chapter 20.

Neurological symptoms

Restlessness/agitation

Restlessness is a state of hyperarousal in which there is the sensation of not being able to rest or remain in a relaxed position. Agitation in children may present as irritability, combativeness, or refusal of attention or participation. Causes of restlessness and agitation in children with advanced disease can include a variety of physical and psychological factors (Box 55.7).

Assessment should include observing for such behaviors as frequent position changes, twitching, inability to concentrate on activities, inconsolability, disturbed sleep-wake cycles, and moaning. Spiritual distress, disturbing dreams or nightmares, fears, and comorbid anxiety or depression should also be assessed. Treatment for agitation and restlessness should use both age-appropriate pharmacological and nonpharmacological techniques (Table 55.4). Benzodiazepines may be helpful in reducing mild-to-moderate agitation and increasing effectiveness of nonpharmacological interventions.[67,68]

In rare circumstances, children may experience such distressing restlessness or agitation as the result of unrelenting pain or other symptoms that the need for palliative sedation may be considered.[98] Palliative sedation is generally indicated when distress cannot be controlled by any other means either because of limited time-frame or risk of excessive morbidity. Healthcare professionals must determine what are truly uncontrollable pain or symptoms versus undertreated pain and/or symptoms. Before considering sedation, it is important that all efforts have been made to achieve pain and symptom control. The goal of palliative sedation is to relieve obvious suffering of the child by adding medications to induce sleep, but it is not intended to hasten death.

Box 55.7 Causes of agitation/restlessness in children

Disease/treatment-related causes

Uncontrolled pain or other symptoms
Metabolic disturbances
Infections
Hypoxemia
Constipation
Sleep disturbance

Emotional causes

Depression/anxiety
Fear
Change in family routine
Reaction to stress of other family members
Withholding of information or open discussion with child

Presenting the option of sedation to a child and family requires a caring, open relationship between the treating healthcare professionals and the family. If the child and family are opposed to sedation, they should be reassured that all efforts to relieve distress will continue. If the child and family choose sedation, there

Table 55.4 Management of agitation/restlessness

Intervention	Dose	Comments
Pharmacological management		
Lorazepam	0.03–0.1 mg IV/PO q4–6h, may titrate to max 2 mg/dose	Indicated for generalized anxiety
		May increase sedation in combination with opioids
		May use in infants and young children
Midazolam	0.025–0.05 mg/kg/dose IV/SQ	Titrate to effect
	0.3–1 mg/kg (max 20 mg) PR	Indicated for myoclonus related to prolonged opioid use, mild sedation
		Short-acting, quickly reversed if overly sedated
Haloperidol	0.05–0.15 mg/kg/day PO, IV, SQ divided 2–3 times per d	Indicated for agitation not responsive to benzodiazepines
		Monitor for extrapyramidal symptoms, treat with diphenhydramine as needed
Nonpharmacological management		

Maximize pain and other symptom assessment and management.

Decrease environmental stress or stimulation.

Encourage open communication between child and family.

Provide relaxation/guided imagery.

Provide favorite books, videos, or music.

Encourage cuddling or holding by parents and other significant family members.

Source: Wusthoff et al. (2007), reference 99.

are a number of pharmacological agents available to produce the desired level of relief. Consultation with a hospice physician would be appropriate to determine the clinical appropriateness and best agents to use to achieve the desired comfort goals of the child and family.

Seizures

The risk for seizures in advanced and terminal disease is related to the nature of the underlying disease.[99,100] Children with congenital malformations of the brain such as lissencephaly and congenital hydrocephaly, as well as other neurodegenerative diseases, often have seizures throughout their disease process. Children with malignancies of the central nervous system may experience seizures as an initial presentation of their illness or during disease progression. Children with advanced illnesses may also have seizure activity as a result of metabolic abnormalities, hypoxia, and neurotoxicity from medications. Seizure activity in children can present in a number of ways (Box 55.8). No matter what the cause, uncontrolled seizure is often one of the most distressing symptoms for parents. If a child has any risk for seizure activity at the end of life, emergency medications such as diazepam suppositories should be available in the home. Management involves correcting the underlying cause when possible and adding appropriate prophylactic pharmacological agents such as phenobarbital, clonazepam, or lorazepam (Table 55.5).

Respiratory symptoms

Dyspnea

The experience of dyspnea is one of the most common nonpain symptoms reported by children and parents.[42,102–104] Dyspnea is the unpleasant sensation of breathlessness and can be particularly frightening for children. Diseases of childhood most associated with dyspnea include cystic fibrosis and other interstitial lung diseases, muscular dystrophy, spinal muscular atrophy, end-stage organ failure, and metastatic cancer. In each of these diseases, there can be a number of underlying causes (Box 55.9) that may be amenable to treatment.

The sensation of dyspnea is a subjective experience, and assessment should include the following: its effect on the child's functional status, factors that worsen or improve dyspnea, assessment

---

Box 55.8 Seizure patterns in children

Infants and neonates

Deviation of eyes
Pedaling or stepping movements of legs
Rowing movements of arms
Eye blinking or fluttering
Sucking or smacking lips
Drooling
Apnea
Tonic/clonic movements

Older children

Staring spells and deviated gaze
Unilateral or bilateral twitching, tremors
Generalized tonic/clonic movements

Table 55.5 Management of seizures at the end of life

Intervention	Dose	Comments
Phenobarbitol	*Loading dose:* Children 10–20 mg/kg IV, may titrate by 5 mg/kg increments q15–30 min until seizure controlled or to max of 40 mg/kg/dose	Generalized tonic-clonic seizures
	Maintenance dose: Infants/children 5–8 mg/kg/day in 1–2 divided doses. Therapeutic serum levels 1–50 μg/mL	Status epilepticus
Carbamazepine	*<6 y initial:* 5 mg/kg/day PO, titrate based on serum levels q5–7 d to dose of 10 mg/kg/day, then 20 mg/kg/day if necessary, give in 2–4 divided doses	Partial or complete seizures, generalized tonic-clonic, mixed seizure patterns
	6–12 y initial: 100 mg/day or 10 mg/kg/day PO in 2 divided doses, increase by 200 mg/day in weekly intervals until therapeutic serum levels reached	
	>12 y-adult initial: 200 mg PO bid, increase by 200 mg/day in weekly intervals until therapeutic serum levels reached	
Phenytoin	*Loading dose:* Infants/children 15–20 mg/kg IV	Generalized tonic-clonic seizures
	Maintenance dose: 6 mo–3 y: 8–10 mg/kg/day in divided doses; 4 y–6 y: 7.5–9 mg/kg/day in divided doses; 7 y–9 y: 7–8 mg/kg/day in divided doses; 10 y–16 y: 6–7 mg/kg/day in divided doses.	Status epilepticus
	Therapeutic levels 8–15 μg/mL for neonates, 10–20 μg/mL for children	
Diazepam	2–5 y: 0.5 mg/kg PR 6–11 y: 0.3 mg/kg PR >11 y: 0.2 mg/kg PR May repeat 0.25 mg/kg in 10 min PRN	Status epilepticus

Source: Faulkner et al. (2006) reference 101.

of lung sounds, presence of pain with breathing, and oxygenation status. Extent of disease, respiratory rate, and oxygenation status may not always correlate with the degree of breathlessness experienced; therefore, patient report is the best indicator of the degree of distress. There is no validated tool to measure dyspnea; however, using a rating similar to a pain scale has proven anecdotally to provide some measure of distress and response to interventions.

Managing dyspnea depends on the suspected underlying cause of the symptom. Early in the terminal process, interventions for respiratory discomfort are aimed at improving respiratory effort. Antibiotics, oxygen, chemotherapy, or radiation to decrease tumor burden and noninvasive ventilation for children with muscular degenerative disease may be appropriate to treat the underlying cause. As the child becomes increasingly debilitated, the focus shifts to alleviating anxiety associated with respiratory changes and shortness of breath. There are a number of pharmacological choices for managing respiratory symptoms (Table 55.6). Opioids are the treatment of choice for managing dyspnea, as well as in treating a persistent cough. Anticholinergic medications assist in minimizing secretions. Bronchodilators promote increased air exchange in the lungs and can be helpful alone or in conjunction with opioids. Anxiolytic drugs can help reduce anxiety related to the feeling of shortness of breath and improve respiratory comfort.[42,100] As in other discussions of symptom management, it is important to determine with the child and family the level of intervention that is consistent with their perceptions of the child's suffering and quality of life. For more information on dyspnea, see chapter 14.

Box 55.9 Causes of dyspnea

Physiological causes

  Tumor infiltration/compression
  Aspiration
  Pleural effusion, pulmonary edema, pneumothorax
  Pneumonia
  Thick secretions/mucous plugs
  Bronchospasm
  Impaired diaphragmatic excursion due to ascites, large abdominal tumors
  Congestive heart failure
  Respiratory muscle weakness due to progressive neurodegenerative disease
  Metabolic disturbances

Psychological causes

  Anxiety
  Panic disorder

Mechanical ventilation in pediatric palliative care

The use of long-term mechanical ventilation has increased significantly for children with chronic respiratory failure due to neuromuscular diseases and central nervous system malformations.[103–106] Approximately half of these patients had long-term ventilation initiated during a respiratory crisis,[107–109] putting families in the position to decide to let their child die or proceed with mechanical ventilation.[110] Children with complex chronic conditions are more likely to require invasive ventilation by tracheostomy, have lower levels of cognitive capacity, experience poorer quality of life and functional status, and experience death as the outcome of mechanical ventilation.[104,107,111–113]

Table 55.6 Management of respiratory symptoms

Agent	Dose	Comments
Morphine	0.1–0.2 mg/kg/dose IV/SQ	Indicated for dyspnea, cough
	0.2–0.5 mg/kg/dose PO	May need to titrate to comfort
Hydromorphone	15 µg/kg IV q4–6h	
	0.03–0.08 mg/kg/dose PO q4–6h	
Glycopyrrolate	40–100 mg/kg/dose PO 3–4 times/day	Indicated for secretions, congestion
	4–10 µg/kg/dose IV/SQ q3–4h	May give in conjunction with hyoscyamine
Hyoscyamine	Infant drops (<2 y)	
	◆ 2.3 kg: 3 gtt q4 h; max: 18 gtt/day	
	◆ 3.4 kg: 4 gtt q4h; 24 gtt/day	
	◆ 5 kg: 5 gtt q4h; max: 30 gtt/day	
	◆ 7 kg: 6 gtt q4h; max: 36 gtt/day	
	◆ 10 kg: 8 gtt q4h; 48 gtt/day	
	◆ 15 kg: 10 gtt q4h; 66 gtt/day	
	2–12 y: 0.0625–0.125 mg PO q4h; max: 0.75 mg/day	
	>12 y: 0.125–0.25 mg PO q4h; max: 1.5 mg/day	
Hydromet (solution combination of hydrocodone and homatropine)	0.6 mg/kg/day divided 3–4 doses/day	
Albuterol	*Oral:* 2–6 y: 0.1–0.2 mg/kg/dose tid; max: 4 mg tid	Indicated for wheezing, pulmonary congestion
	6–12 y: 2 mg/dose 3–4 times/day; max: 24 mg/day	Side effects include increased heart rate, anxiety
	>12 y: 2–4 mg/dose 3–4 times/day; max: 8 mg qid	
	Nebulized: 0.01–0.5 mL/kg of 0.5% solution q4–6h	

Source: Lieben et al. (2006), reference 105.

The Patient Protection and Affordable Care Act of 2010 allows for the concurrent care of children with life-limiting conditions, allowing hospice and palliative care services while the child is receiving treatment for their terminal condition.[114] Pediatric hospice and palliative care providers will be faced with the challenge of managing increasing numbers of children with medical complexity, including long-term ventilation and home ventilatory withdrawal.[115] Palliative care and hospice providers can function as the link between the hospital and community providers for children on long-term mechanical ventilation, creating a plan of care that anticipates symptoms, potential emergencies, and how to provide compassionate withdrawal of mechanical ventilation in the home.[116–118]

Terminal respirations

In the final days to hours of life, respiratory patterns often change, initially becoming more rapid and shallow, then progressing to deep, slow respirations with periods of apnea, typically know as Cheyne-Stokes breathing.[102] As the body weakens, pooling of secretions in the throat can lead to noisy respirations, sometimes referred to as "death rattle." Often at this point in disease progression, children are somnolent most of the time and do not report distress. However, these symptoms are particularly agonizing for parents and other family members to experience. Assessment should include monitoring changes in heart rate and respiratory rate, observing for distress, stridor, wheezing, and rales/rhonchi. Management should focus on managing family distress by explaining the nature of the dying process, reassuring the family that the child is not suffering, administering appropriate anticholinergic medications to decrease secretions, and decreasing or discontinuing any fluids or enteral feedings that may exacerbate the development of secretions or fluid overload.

Summary

Symptom management for children with advanced and terminal diseases presents a challenge to healthcare providers. Suffering from uncontrolled symptoms can be prevented by knowledge of the child's underlying disease process, thorough assessment of the child and family for sources of suffering, advocacy for child and family needs, and the use of an interdisciplinary approach to management that includes appropriate pharmacological and non-pharmacological interventions.

References

1. Kogan MD, Strickland BB, Newacheck PW. Building systems of care: findings from the National Survey of Children with Special Health Care Needs. Pediatrics. 2009;124(Suppl 4):S333–S336.
2. Rehm RS. Nursing's contribution to research about parenting children with complex chronic conditions: an integrative review, 2002 to 2012. Nurs Outlook. 2013;61(5):266–290.
3. Van Cleave J, Gortmaker SL, Perrin JM. Dynamics of obesity and chronic health conditions among children and youth. JAMA. 2010;303(7):623–630.
4. Demographic Background. 2013. Retrieved September 21, 2013, from ChildStats.gov: http://childstats.gov/americaschildren/demo.asp
5. Bethell CD, Read D, Blumberg SJ, Newacheck PW. What is the prevalence of children with special health care needs?: Toward an understanding of variations in findings and methods across three national surveys. Matern Child Health J. 2008;12(1):1–14.
6. Bramlett MD, Read D, Bethell C, Blumberg SJ. Differentiating subgroups of children with special health care needs by health status and complexity of health care needs. Matern Child Health J. 2009;13(2):151–163.
7. Cohen E, Berry JG, Camacho X, Anderson G, Wodchis W, Guttmann A. Patterns and costs of health care use of children with medical complexity. Pediatrics. 2012;130(6):e1463–e1470.

8. Menezes A. Moments of realization: life-limiting illness in childhood: perspectives of children, young people and families. Int J Palliat Nurs. 2010;16(1):41–47.

9. Schwab A, Rusconi-Serpa S, Schechter DS. Psychodynamic approaches to medically ill children and their traumatically stressed parents. Child Adolesc Psychiatr Clin N Am. 2013;22(1):119–139.

10. Keele L, Keenan HT, Sheetz J, Bratton SL. Differences in characteristics of dying children who receive and do not receive palliative care. Pediatrics. 2013;132(1):72–78.

11. Schmidt P, Otto M, Hechler T, Metzing S, Wolfe J, Zernikow B. Did increased availability of pediatric palliative care lead to improved palliative care outcomes in children with cancer? J Palliat Med. 2013;16(9):1034–1039.

12. Ullrich C, Morrison RS. Pediatric palliative care research comes of age: what we stand to learn from children with life-threatening illness. J Palliat Med. 2013;16(4):334–336.

13. Dokken D, Ahmann E. The many roles of family members in "family-centered care," part I. Pediatr Nurs. 2006;32(6):562–565.

14. Chen AY, Schrager SM, Mangione-Smith R. Quality measures for primary care of complex pediatric patients. Pediatrics. 2012;129(3):433–445.

15. Doorenbos A, Lindhorst T, Starks H, Aisenberg E, Curtis JR, Hays R. Palliative care in the pediatric ICU: challenges and opportunities for family-centered practice. J Soc Work End Life Palliat Care. 2012;8(4):297–315.

16. Kuhlthau KA, Bloom S, Van Cleave J, et al. Evidence for family-centered care for children with special health care needs: a systematic review. Acad Pediatr. 2011;11(2):136–143.

17. Kuo DZ, Houtrow AJ, Arango P, Kuhlthau KA, Simmons JM, Neff JM. Family-centered care: current applications and future directions in pediatric health care. Matern Child Health J. 2012;16(2):297–305.

18. Meltzer LJ, Steinmiller E, Simms S, Grossman M. The Complex Care Consultation Team, Li Y. Staff engagement during complex pediatric medical care: the role of patient, family, and treatment variables. Patient Educ Couns. 2009;74(1):77–83.

19. Renjilian CB, Womer JW, Carroll KW, Kang TI, Feudtner C. Parental explicit heuristics in decision-making for children with life-threatening illnesses. Pediatrics. 2013;131(2):e566–e572.

20. Swallow VM, Nightingale R, Williams J, et al. Multidisciplinary teams, and parents, negotiating common ground in shared-care of children with long-term conditions: a mixed methods study. BMC Health Serv Res. 2013;13(1):264.

21. Pöder U, Ljungman G, Von Essen L. Parents' perceptions of their children's cancer-related symptoms during treatment: a prospective, longitudinal study. J Pain Symptom Manage. 2010;40(5):661–670.

22. Pritchard M, Burghen E, Srivastava DK, et al. Cancer-related symptoms most concerning to parents during the last week and last day of their child's life. Pediatrics. 2008;121(5):e1301–e1309.

23. Pritchard M, Burghen EA, Gattuso JS, et al. Factors that distinguish symptoms of most concern to parents from other symptoms of dying children. J Pain Symptom Manage. 2010;39(4):627–636.

24. Jantien Vrijmoet-Wiersma CM, van Klink JM, Kolk AM, Koopman HM, Ball LM, Maarten Egeler R. Assessment of parental psychological stress in pediatric cancer: a review. J Pediatr Psychol. 2008;33(7):694–706.

25. Alvesson HM, Lindelow M, Khanthaphat B, Laflamme L. Coping with uncertainty during healthcare-seeking in Lao PDR. BMC Int Health Hum Rights. 2013;13(1):28.

26. Barrera M, Granek L, Shaheed J, et al. The tenacity and tenuousness of hope: parental experiences of hope when their child has a poor cancer prognosis. Cancer Nurs. 2013;36(5):408–416.

27. Tong A, Lowe A, Sainsbury P, Craig JC. Experiences of parents who have children with chronic kidney disease: a systematic review of qualitative studies. Pediatrics. 2008;121(2):349–360.

28. Kuo DZ, Cohen E, Agrawal R, Berry JG, Casey PH. A national profile of caregiver challenges among more medically complex children with special health care needs. Arch Pediatr Adolesc Med. 2011;165(11):1020–1026.

29. Lindahl B, Lindblad BM. Family members' experiences of everyday life when a child is dependent on a ventilator: a metasynthesis study. J Fam Nurs. 2011;17(2):241–269.

30. Murphy NA, Carbone PS. Parent-provider-community partnerships: optimizing outcomes for children with disabilities. Pediatrics. 2011;128(4):795–802.

31. Granek L, Barrera M, Shaheed J, et al. Trajectory of parental hope when a child has difficult-to-treat cancer: a prospective qualitative study. Psychooncology. 2013;22(11):2436–2444.

32. Lerret SM, Weiss ME. How ready are they?: Parents of pediatric solid organ transplant recipients and the transition from hospital to home following transplant. Pediatr Transplant. 2011;15(6):606–616.

33. Stewart JL, Pyke-grimm KA, Kelly KP. Making the right decision for my child with cancer: the parental imperative. Cancer Nurs. 2012;35(6):419–428.

34. Tong A, Lowe A, Sainsbury P, Craig JC. Parental perspectives on caring for a child with chronic kidney disease: an in-depth interview study. Child Care Health Dev. 2010;36(4):549–557.

35. Carnevale, FA, Gaudreault J. The experience of critically ill children: a phenomenological study of discomfort and comfort. Dynamics. 2013;24(1), 19–27.

36. Miller E, Jacob E, Hockenberry MJ. Nausea, pain, fatigue, and multiple symptoms in hospitalized children with cancer. Oncol Nurs Forum. 2011;38(5):E382–E393.

37. Saito Y. Reflections on the brainstem dysfunction in neurologically disabled children. Brain Dev. 2009;31(7):529–536.

38. Van Cleve L, Muñoz CE, Riggs ML, Bava L, Savedra M. Pain experience in children with advanced cancer. J Pediatr Oncol Nurs. 2012;29(1):28–36.

39. Angström-Brännström C, Norberg A, Jansson L. Narratives of children with chronic illness about being comforted. J Pediatr Nurs. 2008;23(4):310–316.

40. Taylor RM, Gibson F, Franck LS. A concept analysis of health-related quality of life in young people with chronic illness. J Clin Nurs. 2008;17(14):1823–1833.

41. McSherry M, Kehoe K, Carroll JM, Kang TI, Rourke MT. Psychosocial and spiritual needs of children living with a life-limiting illness. Pediatr Clin North Am. 2007;54(5):609–629.

42. Wolfe J, Hammel JF, Edwards KE, et al. Easing of suffering in children with cancer at the end of life: is care changing? J Clin Oncol. 2008;26(10):1717–1723.

43. Graff C, Mandleco B, Dyches TT, Coverston CR, Roper SO, Freeborn D. Perspectives of adolescent siblings of children with Down syndrome who have multiple health problems. J Fam Nurs. 2012;18(2):175–199.

44. Malcolm C, Gibson F, Adams S, Anderson G, Forbat L. A relational understanding of sibling experiences of children with rare life-limiting conditions: findings from a qualitative study. J Child Health Care. 2013 Jun 10. Epub ahead of print.

45. Wilkins KL, Woodgate RL. An interruption in family life: siblings' lived experience as they transition through the pediatric bone marrow transplant trajectory. Oncol Nurs Forum. 2007;34(2):E28–E35.

46. Kieckhefer GM, Trahms CM, Churchill SS, Kratz L, Uding N, Villareale N. A randomized clinical trial of the building on family strengths program: an education program for parents of children with chronic health conditions. Matern Child Health J. 2013 Apr 13. Epub ahead of print.

47. Stevenson M, Achille M, Lugasi T. Pediatric palliative care in Canada and the United States: a qualitative metasummary of the needs of patients and families. J Palliat Med. 2013;16(5):566–577.

48. Toly VB, Musil CM, Carl JC. A longitudinal study of families with technology-dependent children. Res Nurs Health. 2012;35(1):40–54. doi: 10.1002/nur.21454.

49. Nielsen KM, Mandleco B, Roper SO, Cox A, Dyches T, Marshall ES. Parental perceptions of sibling relationships in families rearing a child with a chronic condition. J Pediatr Nurs. 2012;27(1):34–43.

50. Redshaw S, Wilson V. Sibling involvement in childhood chronic heart disease through a bead program. J Child Health Care. 2012;16(1):53–61.

51. Ho C, Straatman L. A review of pediatric palliative care service utilization in children with a progressive neuromuscular disease who died on a palliative care program. J Child Neurol. 2013;28(1):40–44.

52. Wolfe J, Grier HE, Klar N, et al. Symptoms and suffering at the end of life in children with cancer. N Engl J Med. 2000;342(5):326–333.

53. Wolfe J, Klar N, Grier HE, et al. Understanding of prognosis among parents of children who died of cancer: impact on treatment goals and integration of palliative care. JAMA. 2000;284(19):2469–2475.

54. Feudtner C, Kang TI, Hexem KR, et al. Pediatric palliative care patients: a prospective multicenter cohort study. Pediatrics. 2011;127(6):1094–1101.

55. Gans D, Kominski GF, Roby DH, Diamant AL, Chen X, Lin W, et al. Better outcomes, lower costs: palliative care program reduces stress, costs of care for children with life-threatening conditions. Policy Brief UCLA Cent Health Policy Res (PB2012-3), 1–8.

56. Hill DL, Miller VA, Hexem KR, et al. Problems and hopes perceived by mothers, fathers and physicians of children receiving palliative care. Health Expect. 2013. doi: 10.1111/hex.12078. [Epub ahead of print].

57. Paulmichl K. Decision-making at the border of viability by means of values clarification: a case study to achieve distinct communication by ordinary language approach. J Perinat Med. 2011;39(5):595–603.

58. Dupuis LL, Ethier MC, Tomlinson D, Hesser T, Sung L. A systematic review of symptom assessment scales in children with cancer. BMC Cancer. 2012;12(1):430.

59. Vrijmoet-Wiersma CM, Van Klink JM, Kolk AM, Koopman HM, Ball LM, Maarten Egeler R. Assessment of parental psychological stress in pediatric cancer: a review. J Pediatr Psychol. 2008;33(7):694–706.

60. Wu WW, Johnson R, Schepp KG, Berry DL. Electronic self-report symptom and quality of life for adolescent patients with cancer: a feasibility study. Cancer Nurs. 2011;34(6):479–486.

61. Malcolm C, Adams S, Anderson G, Gibson F, Hain R, Morley A, et al. The symptom profile and experience of children with rare life-limiting conditions: perspectives of their families and key health professionals. 2012. C H A S—Childrens Hospice Association Scotland. Cancer Care Research Centre, University of Stirling. https://dspace.stir.ac.uk/handle/1893/12772.

62. Ullrich CK, Dussel V, Hilden JM, et al. Fatigue in children with cancer at the end of life. J Pain Symptom Manage. 2010;40(4):483–494.

63. Whitsett SF, Gudmundsdottir M, Davies B, McCarthy P, Friedman D. Chemotherapy-related fatigue in childhood cancer: correlates, consequences, and coping strategies. J Pediatr Oncol Nurs. 2008;25(2):86–96.

64. Jarad NA, Sequeiros IM, Patel P, Bristow K, Sund Z. Fatigue in cystic fibrosis: a novel prospective study investigating subjective and objective factors associated with fatigue. Chron Respir Dis. 2012;9(4):241–249.

65. Angelini C, Tasca E. Fatigue in muscular dystrophies. Neuromuscul Disord. 2012;22(Suppl 3):S214–S220.

66. Mastaglia FL. The relationship between muscle pain and fatigue. Neuromuscul Disord. 2012;22(Suppl 3):S178–S180.

67. Montes J, Blumenschine M, Dunaway S, et al. Weakness and fatigue in diverse neuromuscular diseases. J Child Neurol. 2013;28(10):1277–1283.

68. Ameringer S, Smith WR. Emerging biobehavioral factors of fatigue in sickle cell disease. J Nurs Scholarsh. 2011;43(1):22–29.

69. Ullrich CK, Dussel V, Hilden JM, Sheaffer JW, Moore CL, Berde CB, Wolfe J. Fatigue in children with cancer at the end of life. J Pain Symptom Manage, 2010;40(4):483–494. Doi:10.1177/1043454211432295

70. Santucci G, Mack JW. Common gastrointestinal symptoms in pediatric palliative care: nausea, vomiting, constipation, anorexia, cachexia. Pediatr Clin North Am. 2007;54(5):673–689.

71. Dupuis LL, Boodhan S, Holdsworth M, et al. Guideline for the prevention of acute nausea and vomiting due to antineoplastic medication in pediatric cancer patients. Pediatr Blood Cancer. 2013;60(7):1073–1082.

72. Phillips RS, Gopaul S, Gibson F, et al. Antiemetic medication for prevention and treatment of chemotherapy induced nausea and vomiting in childhood. Cochrane Database Syst Rev. 2010;(9):CD007786.

73. Hechler T, Blankenburg M, Friedrichsdorf SJ, et al. Parents' perspective on symptoms, quality of life, characteristics of death and end-of-life decisions for children dying from cancer. Klin Padiatr. 2008;220(3):166–174.

74. Stewart G, Mcneilly P. Opioid-induced constipation in children's palliative care. Nurs Child Young People. 2011;23(8):31–34.

75. Sullivan PB. Gastrointestinal disorders in children with neurodevelopmental disabilities. Dev Disabil Res Rev. 2008;14(2):128–136.

76. Chen S, Jarboe MD, Teitelbaum DH. Effectiveness of a transluminal endoscopic fundoplication for the treatment of pediatric gastroesophageal reflux disease. Pediatr Surg Int. 2012;28(3):229–234.

77. Mahant S, Friedman JN, Connolly B, Goia C, Macarthur C. Tube feeding and quality of life in children with severe neurological impairment. Arch Dis Child. 2009;94(9):668–673.

78. Marchand, V. Nutrition in neurologically impaired children. Paediatr Child Health. 2009;14(6):395–401.

79. Riley A, Vadeboncoeur C. Nutritional differences in neurologically impaired children. Paediatr Child Health. 2012;17(9):e98–e101.

80. Morgan AT, Dodrill P, Ward EC. Interventions for oropharyngeal dysphagia in children with neurological impairment. Cochrane Database Syst Rev. 2012;10:CD009456.

81. Zaidi T, Sudall C, Kauffmann L, Folaranmi S, Khalil B, Morabito A. Physical outcome and quality of life after total esophagogastric dissociation in children with severe neurodisability and gastroesophageal reflux, from the caregiver's perspective. J Pediatr Surg. 2010;45(9):1772–1776.

82. Srivastava R, Downey EC, O'Gorman M, et al. Impact of fundoplication versus gastrojejunal feeding tubes on mortality and in preventing aspiration pneumonia in young children with neurologic impairment who have gastroesophageal reflux disease. Pediatrics. 2009;123(1):338–345.

83. Brotherton A, Abbott J. Mothers' process of decision making for gastrostomy placement. Qual Health Res. 2012;22(5):587–594.

84. Mahant S, Jovcevska V, Cohen E. Decision-making around gastrostomy-feeding in children with neurologic disabilities. Pediatrics. 2011;127(6):e1471–e1481.

85. Pedrón-Giner C, Calderón C, Martínez-Costa C, Borraz Gracia S, Gómez-López L. Factors predicting distress among parents/caregivers of children with neurological disease and home enteral nutrition. Child Care Health Dev. 2013. Epub ahead of print.

86. Mak RH, Cheung WW, Zhan JY, Shen Q, Foster BJ. Cachexia and protein-energy wasting in children with chronic kidney disease. Pediatr Nephrol. 2012;27(2):173–181.

87. Rodgers CC, Hooke MC, Hockenberry MJ. Symptom clusters in children. Curr Opin Support Palliat Care. 2013;7(1):67–72.

88. Thompson A, McDonald A, Holden C. Feeding in palliative care. In: Goldman A, Hain R, Liben S, eds. Oxford Textbook of Palliative Care for Children. London and New York: Oxford University Press; 2012:284–294.

89. Diekema DS, Botkin JR. Clinical report: forgoing medically provided nutrition and hydration in children. Pediatrics. 2009;124(2):813–822.

90. Geppert CM, Andrews MR, Druyan ME. Ethical issues in artificial nutrition and hydration: a review. J Parenter Enteral Nutr. 2010;34(1):79–88.

91. Schwartz DB, Posthauer ME, O'Sullivan Maillet J. Practice paper of the Academy of Nutrition and Dietetics abstract: ethical and legal issues of feeding and hydration. J Acad Nutr Diet. 2013;113(7):981.

92. Tsai E. Withholding and withdrawing artificial nutrition and hydration. Paediatr Child Health. 2011;16(4):241–244.

93. von Lützau P, Otto M, Hechler T, Metzing S, Wolfe J, Zernikow B. Children dying from cancer: parents' perspectives on symptoms, quality of life, characteristics of death, and end-of-life decisions. J Palliat Care. 2012;28(4): 274–281.

94. Kersun LS, Shemesh E. Depression and anxiety in children at the end of life. Pediatr Clin North Am. 2007;54(5):691–708.

95. Muriel AC, McCulloch R, Hammel JF. Depression, anxiety, and delirium. In: Goldman A, Hain R, Liben S, eds. Oxford Textbook of Palliative Care for Children. London and New York: Oxford University Press; 2012:309–318.

96. Gilmer MJ, Foster TL, Vannatta K, et al. Changes in parents after the death of a child from cancer. J Pain Symptom Manage. 2012;44(4):572–582.

97. Hatzmann J, Peek N, Heymans H, Maurice-stam H, Grootenhuis M. Consequences of caring for a child with a chronic disease: employment and leisure time of parents. J Child Health Care. 2013. Epub ahead of print.

98. Jaimsell L, Kreicbergs U, Onelöv E, Steineck G, Henter JI. Anxiety is contagious: symptoms of anxiety in the terminally ill child affect long-term psychological well-being in bereaved parents. Pediatr Blood Cancer. 2010;54(5):751–757.

99. Anghelescu DL, Hamilton H, Faughnan LG, Johnson LM, Baker JN. Pediatric palliative sedation therapy with propofol: recommendations based on experience in children with terminal cancer. J Palliat Med. 2012;15(10):1082–1090.

100. Wusthoff CJ. Management of common neurologic symptoms in pediatric palliative care: seizures, agitation, and spasticity. *Pediatr Clin North Am 2007;* 54(5): 709–733. doi:10.1016/j.pcl.2007.06.004

101. Hauer JM, Faulkner KW. Neurological and neuromuscular conditions and symptoms. In: Goldman A, Hain R, Liben S, eds. Oxford Textbook of Palliative Care for Children. London and New York: Oxford University Press; 2012:295–308.

102. Faulkner KW, Thayer PB, Coulter DL. Neurological and Neuromuscular Symptoms. In: Goldman A, Hain R, Liben S, eds. Oxford Textbook of Palliative Care for Children Oxford University Press, 2006.

103. Robinson WM. Palliation of dyspnea in pediatrics. Chron Respir Dis. 2012;9(4):251–256.

104. Schindera C, Tomlinson D, Bartels U, Gillmeister B, Alli A, Sung L. Predictors of symptoms and site of death in pediatric palliative patients with cancer at end of life. Am J Hosp Palliat Care. 2013. Epub ahead of print.

105. Brook L, Twig E, Venables A, Shaw, C. Respiratory symptoms. In: Goldman A, Hain R, Liben S (eds.), Oxford Textbook of Palliative Care for Children. London and New York: Oxford University Press; 2012:319–327.

106. Lieben S, Hain R, Goldman A. Respiratory symptoms. In: Goldman A, Hain R, Liben S, eds. Oxford Textbook of Palliative Care for Children Oxford University Press, 2006.

107. Divo, MJ, Murray S, Cortopassi F, Celli BR. Prolonged mechanical ventilation in massachusetts: the 2006 prevalence survey. Respir Care. 2010;55(12);1693–1698.

108. Edwards JD, Kun SS, Keens TG. Outcomes and causes of death in children on home mechanical ventilation via tracheostomy: an institutional and literature review. J Pediatrics. 2010;157(6):955–959. e952.

109. Goodwin S, Smith H, Langton hewer S, et al. Increasing prevalence of domiciliary ventilation: changes in service demand and provision in the South West of the UK. Eur J Pediatr. 2011;170(9):1187–1192.

110. Gowans M, Keenan HT, Bratton SL. The population prevalence of children receiving invasive home ventilation in Utah. Pediatr Pulmonol. 2007;42(3):231–236.

111. Edwards JD, Kun SS, Graham RJ, Keens TG. End-of-life discussions and advance carplanning for children on long-term assisted ventilation with life-limiting conditions. J Palliat Care. 2012;(1): 21–27.

112. Ottonello G, Ferrari I, Pirroddi IM, et al. Home mechanical ventilation in children: retrospective survey of a pediatric population. Pediatr Int. 2007;49(6):801–805.

113. Wallis C, Paton JY, Beaton S, Jardine E. Children on long-term ventilatory support: 10 years of progress. Arch Dis Child. 2011;96(11): 998–1002.

114. Carnevale FA, Alexander E, Davis M, Rennick J, Troini R. Daily living with distress and enrichment: the moral experience of families with ventilator-assisted children at home. Pediatrics. 2006;117(1): e48–e60.

115. Dybwik K, Nielsen EW, Brinchmann BS. Ethical challenges in home mechanical ventilation: a secondary analysis. Nurs Ethics. 2012;19(2):233–244.

116. Kun SS, Edwards JD, Ward SL, Keens TG. Hospital readmissions for newly discharged pediatric home mechanical ventilation patients. Pediatr Pulmonol. 2012;47(4):409–414.

117. Reiter K, Pernath N, Pagel P, et al. Risk factors for morbidity and mortality in pediatric home mechanical ventilation. Clin Pediatr (Phila). 2011;50(3):237–243.

118. Lindley LC. Health care reform and concurrent curative care for terminally ill children: a policy analysis. J Hosp Palliat Nurs. 2011;13(2): 81–88.

119. Bettini L. Concurrent care for children: how this new legislation has opened hospice care to children with high technology home care needs. Home Healthc Nurse. 2013;31(2):114–115.

120. Needle JS. Home extubation by a pediatric critical care team: providing a compassionate death outside the pediatric intensive care unit. Pediatr Crit Care Med. 2010;11(3):401–403.

121. Simpson EC, Penrose CV. Compassionate extubation in children at hospice and home. Int J Palliat Nurs. 2011;17(4):164–169.

122. Zwerdling T, Hamann KC, Kon AA. Home pediatric compassionate extubation: bridging intensive and palliative care. Am J Hosp Palliat Care. 2006;23(3):224–228.

CHAPTER 56

Pediatric hospice and palliative care

Vanessa Battista and Gwenn LaRagione

Pediatric hospices are full of light and life and joy and play, and as centers or residences of care they are clearly focused on a child's LIFE and living until a child draws his or her final breath, not on a child's dying. Compassionate and loving clinical care is provided to meet physical needs and treat the symptoms associated with end-of-life processes, and death is not an unspeakable word or even an elephant in the room. Yet everyone involved in pediatric hospice care is focused on supporting a child's best life and quality thereof, despite and around and even alongside what the rest of the world might perceive as the elephant in the room. And, when the time comes, all efforts are directed toward a child's dying well, with as little suffering and as much peace as possible.

Pamela J. Mosher, M.D., M.Div., Pediatrician and Child Psychiatrist, IWK Health Centre, Halifax, Nova Scotia, Canada

Key points

- ◆ Pediatric palliative and hospice care is multifaceted care that focuses on a child's and family's well-being along a physical, psychological, emotional, spiritual, and social continuum.

- ◆ Pediatric hospice care has a unique set of parameters that should be considered a necessary part of comprehensive palliative care.

- ◆ Pediatric palliative care involves a family-centered approach to caring for infants, children, and adolescents and considers all family members as part of a dynamic web of interconnected lives and relationships.

- ◆ Initial and ongoing education and care delivered by an interdisciplinary team (IDT) of healthcare professionals is essential in addressing the complex physical, emotional, spiritual, and practical needs and concerns of children and their families.

- ◆ Relieving suffering and improving quality of life, for even a brief life, can benefit not only the young patient but all those affected by the illness or death of the child, including siblings, parents, grandparents, other relatives, teachers, school friends, faith community, and neighbors, as well as the healthcare professionals involved in their care.

- ◆ Nurses who care for dying children and their families need a significant personal and professional support system and opportunities for renewal, personal growth, and ongoing education.

- ◆ Pediatric hospice and palliative care is a rapidly developing field with many opportunities for growth and expansion.

Overview of pediatric hospice and palliative care

Most societies share a common belief that children symbolize the "future," representing dreams and the promise of accomplishments yet to be fulfilled. The experience of serious illness or death of an infant, child, or adolescent (referred to collectively as children for the purposes of this chapter) therefore generates a legitimate threat to such hopes. Bearing witness to these experiences motivates clinicians to do their best to prevent and relieve the suffering of children likely to die, both through interventions aimed at cure and, when cure is no longer possible, through the provision of interdisciplinary pediatric hospice and palliative care. Pediatric hospice and palliative care is an area of nursing that requires specialized knowledge, training, and sensitivity to the unique needs of families enduring some of the most arduous moments of their lives. Providing this type of care throughout the illness process, from the time of diagnosis until the time of death, can be simultaneously challenging, physically and emotionally draining, enriching, and meaningful. This chapter will provide an overview of pediatric hospice and palliative care, and the special considerations necessary for nurses who may be called on to provide this unique type of care to children and their families.

Definition of pediatric palliative care

The World Health Organization (WHO) developed one of the earliest and most widely accepted definitions of pediatric palliative care (PPC), describing it as the active total care of the child's body, mind, and spirit, and involving an evaluation of a child's psychological, physical, and social distress.[1] That definition has since evolved to include care aimed at improving quality of life of patients facing life-threatening illnesses, and of their families, through the prevention and relief of suffering by early identification and treatment of pain and other problems, whether physical, psychological, social, or spiritual.[2] The American Academy of Pediatrics defines PPC as care that should aim to achieve the best quality of life for patients and families, consistent with their values.[3] The Institute of Medicine states that PPC should consider the needs of patients and families in order to provide timely, accurate, and compassionate information regarding diagnosis, prognosis, and treatment options.[4] Pediatric palliative care can also be defined as both a philosophy of care and an organized, structured system of delivering care to children living with life-threatening conditions and to their families. The goal of PPC is to prevent and relieve suffering and to maximize quality of life for children of all ages and their family members/support systems.[5]

Combining all of these definitions, PPC can be described generally as a family-centered approach to care that encompasses the physical, psychological, emotional, social, and spiritual components of a child's needs and focuses on overall quality of life. To be practiced effectively and responsibly, PPC requires an IDT of professionals from medicine, nursing, psychiatry, psychology, social work, chaplaincy, child life, physical/occupational/speech therapy, art and music therapy, nutrition, pharmacy, and other areas of healthcare (e.g., acupuncture, massage therapy). Pediatric palliative care offers expert pain and symptom prevention and management and honest discussion around the child's medical condition, which serves as the foundation for collaborative decision-making regarding goals of care. This patient-focused, family centered, holistic health care should be initiated as early as possible in the illness trajectory in order to provide the child and family with the opportunity to receive supports that will enhance their capacity to cope with a life threatening condition. PPC aims to preserve the integrity of the family throughout disease progression, addresses anticipatory grief, and also includes bereavement support following death.[5]

Definition and evolution of hospice care

The word "hospice" stems from the Latin "hospes" or "hosptium," meaning guest house and referring to both guests and hosts, and is thought to have originated in the early 11th century.[6] The National Hospice and Palliative Care Organization (NHPCO) describes hospice as a model of care designed to provide quality compassionate care through a team approach (pain and symptom management, medical, spiritual, and psychosocial care/support) to people with a life-threatening/limiting illness around their individual needs and wishes. They further explain that hospice care focuses on caring for, not curing the patient, while also providing support to family, friends, loved ones, and communities.[7]

The modern hospice movement began with Dame Cicely Saunders, trained as a registered nurse, social worker, and eventually physician, who founded St. Christopher's Hospice in the United Kingdom in 1967. As her career evolved, so did her realization that a dying person needs more than symptom management; she felt they needed a holistic approach to care, that is, they needed to be treated medically, physically, emotionally, spiritually, and socially. She also pioneered the development of bereavement services, as she recognized that the patient and family were a single entity that needed support both during the dying process and after the death of the patient.[8]

As the hospice philosophy and movement grew throughout the United Kingdom and into the United States, Medicare recognized the need to cover hospice services and introduced the hospice benefit in 1983. The benefit was designed to provide nursing care, medications, medical supplies, psychosocial support, and volunteer services for end-of-life care, through a daily per diem reimbursement rate. To be eligible for the benefit, a patient had to have a life expectancy of 6 months or less, as defined by a physician, and had to relinquish aggressive, disease-related curative treatment in exchange for supportive care during the dying phase of life. As a result, society's view of death and dying changed, an economic value was placed on dying, and end-of-life care became a public policy issue.[9]

Comparing pediatric palliative and hospice care

The terms "palliative care" and "hospice care" are often used interchangeably (as in this chapter) because of their similar core values and philosophical approaches to care. However, it is important to appreciate and understand their main differences. Primarily, palliative care can be provided at any time during the course of the disease (including the time of diagnosis), whereas hospice care focuses more around true end-of-life care.[10]

When compared with adult care, there are many differences in the provision of pediatric palliative and hospice care. The NHPCO's Standards of Practice for Hospice Programs, Appendix IV: Pediatric Palliative Care (see Box 56.1), provides in-depth insight on these differences, most notably that children go through developmental stages while having more complex, lifelong chronic conditions, complicating the identification of treatment plans, trajectories, and ethical issues around legal decision-making, all while dealing with larger community involvement, less palliative and hospice care resources, and more complicated grief.[11]

Concurrent care

When first developed, state and federal regulations and standards governing hospice care and the clinical guidelines for ongoing appropriateness (Medicare and Medicaid), did not address pediatrics. Determining the required 6-months-or-less prognosis is extremely difficult for pediatric physicians because of the wide variability of prognoses in children, often varying from days to weeks or from months to years. Referral to hospice care by physicians made them feel as though they were "giving up."

In addition, there was question as to what—if any—treatments might be acceptable under hospice admission guidelines. Programs varied on whether blood products, antibiotics, infusions, lab tests, and so forth were considered "too aggressive" an approach to care, expecting parents to surrender all means of therapies before enrollment in hospice. These interventions were also a great financial burden or unfeasible for many programs without substantial foundational support. Most hospice programs did not have the financial allowance to provide these more liberal interpretations. The option of forgoing treatment in order for their child to receive palliative or hospice care was simply too difficult a decision for parents to make.

Box 56.1 Patient- and Family-Centered Care (PPC PFC) Principle

The palliative care and/or hospice interdisciplinary team provides family-centered care that includes the child and family as one unit of care, respecting individual preferences, values, and cultural beliefs, with the child and family active in decision-making regarding goals and plan of care.

Patient and Family-Centered Care (PPC PFC) Standards:

PPC PFC 1 The goals of the child and family are foremost at the center of all services provided.

PPC PFC 1.1 Services should be available to all children and families who are referred, regardless of their financial or health insurance status.

PPC PFC 1.2 Family is defined as the persons who provide physical, psychological, and spiritual comfort to the child, and who are close in knowledge, care, and affection—regardless of genetic relationships. Family members may be biological, marital, adoptive, custodial relations, friends, as well as pets. Parents, siblings, grandparents, schoolmates and others are part of the child's community who may need particular support.

PPC PFC 1.3 All aspects of care are provided in a manner that is sensitive to: the child's developmental stage; the personal, cultural, and spiritual beliefs and practices of the child and family; and their preparedness to deal with dying or its possibility.

PPC PFC 1.4 The child has the right to age-appropriate information about his or her illness, as well as potential treatments and outcomes, within the context of family decisions. The program has trained staff and a full range of clinical and educational resources that meet the needs of each child served regardless of age, cognitive and educational ability.

PPC PFC 1.5 The family and caregivers have the right to be informed about the illness, potential treatments and outcomes.

PPC PFC 1.6 Decisions are made by the family, including the child to the level of his/her capacity, in collaboration with the interdisciplinary team and additional service providers.

PPC PFC 2 Comprehensive anticipatory loss, grief and bereavement support methodologies are offered as an integral component of care to the child and all family members from diagnosis or at admission into the program.

PPC PFC 2.1 Methods to address loss, anticipatory grief and bereavement are age-appropriate and include information about the needs of dying and grieving children at all developmental stages.

PPC PFC 2.2 Educational materials describing children's grief and supportive strategies for bereaved children are made available to family members.

PPC PFC 2.3 Partnerships among palliative care providers and community agencies (e.g., schools, faith communities) are established to facilitate outreach and support for children affected by loss.

PPC PFC 2.4 The needs of siblings are an integral part of each child/family plan of care.

Ethical Behavior and Consumer Rights (PPC EBR) Principle:

The best interests of the child shall be the primary consideration in decision-making.

Ethical Behavior and Consumer Rights (PPC EBR) Standards:

PPC EBR 1 Staff communication with the child and family is open and honest, in accordance with each child's level of understanding. Without full disclosure, the child and family cannot participate in decision-making about treatment choices. When, what, and how to disclose information to children must take into account the child's and the family's cultural or religious values, the parents'/guardians' choices of what the child can be told, and the child's capacity and desire to understand.

PPC EBR 1.1 Every child has equal access to palliative care and/or hospice, irrespective of the family's financial circumstances.

PPC EBR 1.2 Children are not subjected to treatments that impose undue burden without potential benefit.

PPC EBR 1.3 Every child receives effective pain relief and symptom management, incorporating the use of pharmacological and non-pharmacological methods.

PPC EBR 1.4 Every child is treated with dignity and respect, and is afforded privacy.

PPC EBR 1.5 The needs of adolescents and young people and their role in decision-making are addressed and planned for, well in advance.

PPC EBR 1.6 The practice of physician-assisted suicide or euthanasia is not supported or endorsed.

PPC EBR 1.7 The principles of negotiation and conflict resolution are used to address disagreements among or between healthcare providers, the child and the child's family about disclosing information to the child.

PPC EBR 1.8 When resolution is not achieved, the interdisciplinary team enlists the assistance of a cultural interpreter/advisor, chaplain and/or an ethics consultant.

PPC EBR 1.9 In the event of an ethics consult, the team meets afterwards, with the family and/or child present (*as preferred by the child and his/her family*) to discuss options, and to assist in implementing changes to the plan of care.

PPC EBR 2 The interdisciplinary team provides guidance to the child/family in choosing medically and ethically appropriate treatment options that are consistent with their values and beliefs. Team members should not attempt to influence families to make decisions that are not compatible with their values. Children with chronic illness often have a level of understanding greater than would be assumed based on their age.

PPC EBR 2.1 Every child is given the opportunity to participate in decisions affecting his or her care, according to age, understanding, capacity and parental support.

(continued)

Box 56.1 Continued

Emphasizing competence or capacity to assent or dissent, rather than the age of the child, allows children to participate in decisions regarding their care whenever possible and appropriate.

PPC EBR 2.2 While most children under the age of 18 have no legal decision-making rights, they should be included in decision-making according to their capacity. For children without complete decision-making capacity, parents or guardians make decisions based on the best interests of the child, assisted by the interdisciplinary team.

PPC EBR 2.3 For older children who demonstrate some healthcare decision-making capacity, parents/guardians and the interdisciplinary team should share age-appropriate information, seek assent, and take into consideration dissent, while ensuring the child's best interests remain at the core of decisions.

PPC EBR 2.4 For adolescents under the age of 18 who demonstrate healthcare decision-making capacity, every effort must be made to obtain parental approval to include these children in the decision-making process, thus allowing them to exercise independence.

PPC EBR 2.5 Emancipated minors with demonstrated capacity have the legal right to participate in all decisions regarding their medical care.

PPC EBR 2.6 There is an established process for anticipating, identifying, and resolving conflict, including consultation with specialists and/or a bioethics committee.

Clinical Excellence and Safety (PPC CES) Principle:

Health professionals providing pediatric palliative care and/or hospice have a responsibility to pursue comfort aggressively and minimize the child's physical, psychosocial, and spiritual pain and suffering.

Clinical Excellence and Safety (PPC CES) Standards:

PPC CES 1 Clinical care will be guided by the ethical principles of beneficence, nonmaleficence and promotion of the best interests of the child.

PPC CES 1.1 In the absence of pediatric medical expertise, the palliative care and/or hospice organization will develop a collaborative consultative relationship with pediatric providers and/or a tertiary healthcare facility to support provision of care suited to the unique needs of pediatric patients.

PPC CES 1.2 A primary care coordinator for all pediatric patients is identified.

PPC CES 1.3 A plan for anticipated pain and symptom management is part of every plan of care.

PPC CES 1.4 Pain prevention and treatment should be anticipated for all procedures or interventions related to the plan of care. Procedures or interventions not related to the goals of care should be avoided.

PPC CES 1.5 Members of all disciplines providing direct services to children will complete annual competencies in pediatric pain and symptom management.

PPC CES 1.6 Utilization of age-appropriate assessment tools is confirmed in all documentation.

PPC CES 1.7 Pain and all distressing symptoms will be assessed on every visit, by each discipline.

PPC CES 1.8 Families, and the child as age-appropriate, will be educated about pain and symptom assessment and management as it relates to their child's plan of care. Education materials are made available at time of admission and/or when pain and symptoms occur.

PPC CES 1.9 A pediatric physician and/or pharmacist are available for consultation to the interdisciplinary team as needed.

PPC CES 1.10 Adequate doses of analgesics are administered "around the clock" and not only on an "as-needed" basis. Additional doses are given to treat breakthrough pain, or predicted intermittent exacerbation.

PPC CES 1.11 When indicated, a sufficient dose and an appropriate pharmacological formulation (for example, sustained-release preparation or continuous infusion) is chosen to enable children and their families to sleep through the night, without waking in pain or waking to take their medications.

PPC CES 1.12 The appropriate opioid dose is the dose that effectively relieves pain and is not based solely on doses per body weight.

PPC CES 1.13 Age-appropriate, non-pharmacological therapies are an integral part of the pain and symptom management plan of care.

Inclusion and Access (PPC IA) Standards:

No pediatric-specific additions to this standard are suggested.

Organizational Excellence (PPC OE) Principle:

Flexibility in pediatric program design and service delivery facilitates access to services for children. A pediatric palliative care and/or hospice model that offers multiple support services over time and across settings ensures enhanced access for this underserved population.

Organizational Excellence (PPC OE) Standards:

PPC OE 1 Pediatric programs may serve patients in the perinatal period, infancy, childhood, adolescence and young adulthood. The program must have policies and procedures in place to address all developmental, physical, social, psychological and spiritual needs of children served.

PPC OE 1.1 Care by providers trained in pediatric palliative care and/or hospice is available 24 hours a day, 7 days a week.

PPC OE 1.2 Families have a key contact person to assist with coordination of care, and they are instructed on how to contact the team in the event of a crisis or if they have needs after designated business hours.

PPC OE 1.3 Coordination of care among the interdisciplinary team, the family, and all sites of care occurs regularly and is discussed routinely at interdisciplinary team meetings.

(continued)

Box 56.1 Continued

PPC OE 1.4 Pediatric palliative care and/or hospice services are accessible to children and families in a setting that is appropriate to their needs and resources.

PPC OE 1.5 Respite care is recognized as a valuable need and the team makes every effort to ensure that families have access to respite care in their own home and/or in a home-away-from-home setting or facility with pediatric interdisciplinary care.

PPC OE 2 The program partners with community agencies and others that provide resources for children.

PPC OE 2.1 The program partners with local schools.

PPC OE 2.2 The program partners with social service agencies.

PPC OE 2.3 The program partners with specialty healthcare agencies.

PPC OE 2.4 The program partners with faith groups in the community.

Workforce Excellence (PPC WE) Principle:

The organization's leadership develops and monitors systems to ensure that pediatric palliative care and/or hospice interdisciplinary team members, including volunteers, are adequately trained, staffed and supported to provide the services offered by the program, and that sufficient support is in place for staff to engage in routine self-care.

Workforce Excellence (PPC WE) Standards:

PPC WE 1 All staff caring for children receive pediatric-specific orientation, training, mentoring, development opportunities and continuing education appropriate to their roles and responsibilities.

PPC WE 1.1 Pediatric-specific training is completed by all staff caring for children with life-threatening conditions.

PPC WE 1.2 Volunteers directly working with children or their families are also trained in developmental needs, family dynamics, communication challenges, and pain and symptom management.

PPC WE 1.3 When pediatric providers are not available within an organization, partnerships or consultative agreements are established with those in the community and/or at tertiary healthcare centers who are experts in working with children and adolescents.

PPC WE 1.4 Clinical policies and procedures are developed and implemented for the care of children of any age. Policies and procedures reflect evidence-based pediatric practice and guide the provision of care by all disciplines.

PPC WE 1.5 On-call or after-hours staff are competent to take pediatric calls and provide pediatric care.

PPC WE 1.6 Pediatric consultative support is made available to staff as needed 24 hours/day.

PPC WE 2 Pediatric visit frequency and length of visit is assessed and adjusted to reflect the needs of both the child and family in the plan of care.

Standards (PPC S) Principle:

Palliative care and/or hospice programs adopt the NHPCO Standards of Practice for Hospice Programs, and utilize the appendix "Standards of Practice for Pediatric Palliative Care and Hospice" as the foundation for their pediatric care.

Compliance with Laws and Regulations (PPC CLR) Standards:

No pediatric-specific additions to this standard are suggested.

Stewardship and Accountability (PPC SA) Standards:

No pediatric-specific additions to this standard are suggested.

Performance Measurement (PPC PM) Principle:

The program develops, defines and utilizes a systematic approach to improving performance. This approach is authorized and supported by the program's governing body and leaders. The approach assures that information is collected and analyzed, actively uses performance measurement data to foster quality assessment performance improvement, and is specific to pediatric patients being served.

Performance Measurement (PPC PM) Standards:

PPC PM 1 The palliative care and/or hospice organization has a quality improvement plan in place to measure and evaluate services rendered to children and their families.

PPC PM 1.1 Measures of children's clinical outcomes are developed.

PPC PM 1.2 All adverse events are documented and investigated.

PPC PM 1.3 All medication errors are documented and investigated.

PPC PM 1.4 Resource utilization is analyzed.

PPC PM 1.5 Child and family satisfaction surveys are developed and sent to families.

Source: http://www.nhpco.org/sites/default/files/public/quality/Standards/APXIV.pdf[11]

Government has since responded with the enactment of the provision "Concurrent Care for Children" in Section 2302 of the Patient Protection and Affordable Health Care Act (PPACA) on March 23, 2010.[12] This provision allows patients with state Medicaid or Children's Health Insurance Programs (CHIP) to receive hospice care while still receiving curative treatment. Its ratification demonstrated that healthcare systems and government

better understand that the needs of children with life-threatening illnesses/conditions are distinctly different from those of adults.

To better understand and interpret this new act, in 2012 a pediatric-focused continuum briefing titled "Pediatric Concurrent Care" was composed at the National Center for Care at the End-of-Life. This briefing included some barriers to the provision: (1) a physician still needs to certify that the child is expected to die in less than 6 months; (2) every state has different Medicaid covered services/resources; and (3) the provision itself does not specify what treatments/services are deemed curative.[7] The District of Columbia Pediatric Palliative Care Collaborative and the National Hospice and Palliative Care Organization also recognized these barriers as well as the effort involved for individual states to acclimate to and utilize concurrent care. In response, they developed a Concurrent Care for Children Implementation Toolkit, designed to guide providers and interested parties in understanding the effect concurrent care could have on their individual state Medicaid programs. It describes how each state has their own amendment and waiver options and encourages learning from other states' experiences to help facilitate a statewide collaborative approach in adapting and implementing effective and efficient concurrent PPC services.[7]

In "Concurrent Care for the Medically Complex Child: Lessons of Implementation," Miller, LaRagione, Kang, and Feudtner[13] discussed some general issues they identified in coordinating concurrent care for medically complex children. They found when adding hospice services to care, existing providers (some who cared for the patient for many years) needed much education and support around the concept and clinical interventions/treatment. They also discovered the high level of complexity around coordinating and integrating hospice care with the current services and providers already in place. Frequent and ongoing communication was found to be necessary to ensure a safe and effective interdisciplinary approach to care. Lastly, determining who was responsible to provide equipment, either the current durable medical equipment company or hospice agency, and what services were still covered under the primary commercial insurance (if applicable) was challenging and complex. Despite these issues and challenges, Miller et al. found the effort worthwhile in helping to improve palliative and end-of-life care.[13]

Progress and challenges

The advancement of palliative care as a model for care and professional development in the United States has reached unprecedented levels in many types of settings. Following that surge is now a robust effort to develop and integrate programs and services for those facing a life-threatening condition from a prenatal diagnosis of a lethal condition to young adults on the brink of adulthood. Growth has been evidenced on many fronts: legislative action, research, hospital-based palliative care, community-based hospice teams/programs, and specialty areas of palliative care such as prenatal palliative care and palliative care in the emergency setting. Many educational models and programs now exist for clinicians to better understand the role of PPC and how to best provide this type of care, however many challenges to delivering optimal PPC and improving the quality of life of children and families still exist. Much work remains regarding clearly defining the population served, better understanding the needs of children with life-threatening conditions and of their families, developing an approach that will be appropriate across different communities, providing care that responds adequately to suffering, advancing strategies that support caregivers and healthcare providers, and promoting needed change by cultivating educational programs.[14] Changing the pervasive stigma of how PPC and hospice are often perceived by the general public and healthcare professionals, as synonymous with "no more hope," "giving up," "there's nothing more that can be done," or "death must be near," is a long-term goal.

The ongoing painful dilemmas and struggles for families with children who are facing life-threatening illness and end-of-life remain hidden from society's view, yet the demands and challenges of caring for a dying child are being addressed continually within hospitals and homes. Individuals, institutions, universities, and community organizations, including hospices, are making a difference in addressing the needs of children with life-threatening illnesses in their communities. One of the most difficult parts of providing PPC, however, is that this type of care is often necessary at the beginning of young lives, a stage of life when almost anyone is naturally uncomfortable with the idea of serious illness or the concept of end-of-life. Nurses are instrumental in incorporating this contradiction of beginnings and endings into a realistic and compassionate framework for the care of children and families dealing with terminal illnesses. The landmark report from the Institute of Medicine, *When Children Die: Improving Palliative and End-of-Life Care of Children and Their Families*, set forward the challenge and a "call to action" to improve all aspects of end-of-life care for children and families, including improved quality and access to pediatric hospice.[4] It became the catalyst for a cascade of national initiatives, research, funding, and heightened awareness that remains potent today. In addition, The National Consensus Project Guidelines for Quality Palliative Care, originally published in 2004 and most recently updated in 2013, provide clinical practice guidelines to foster consistent and high standards in palliative care, and encourage continuity of care across settings for both children and adults living with life-threatening illness.[15]

The ultimate goal, however, is not only to promote excellent PPC for children and families from the time of diagnosis through the time of death, but also to achieve success in heightening awareness of PPC in healthcare professionals and the general public. Improving quality of life for even a brief life can benefit not only the child, but everyone affected by his or her death, which often extends beyond parents and siblings to grandparents, other relatives, teachers, friends, and neighbors, as well as the many healthcare professionals who have been involved in the child's care and treatment. Each individual involved has played a unique role in the child's life and the extensive constellation of those impacted by a child's illness and death may be exponentially greater than one might imagine (Figure 56.1). Often the individuals involved have not had any previous experience with the death of a child and thus an essential role for the PPC provider, and often the nurse directly caring for the child, is to provide guidance and support to other family members or professionals, especially at times when the goals and/or focus of care changes throughout the evolving journey of a child's illness and up to and including the time of death.

The settings where pediatric palliative care occurs

Consistent with dispelling the message that PPC is only applicable at the end-of-life, is the understanding that PPC can be implemented in a variety of both inpatient and outpatient settings, including acute, chronic, and intensive care units, the emergency department, long-term care facilities, at home, and in schools and communities (see other chapters pertinent to PPC in particular

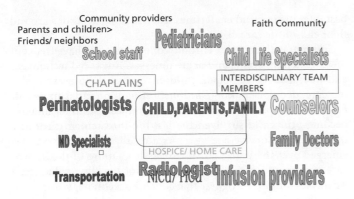

Figure 56.1 Target group for pediatric palliative care.

settings). The exact circumstances and necessary resources will vary from setting to setting, and it is important to recognize that there may be physical, organizational, philosophical, and training issues that may present challenges in some settings.[16] Because PPC is relatively new compared with other areas of medicine/nursing, and because of the misconceptions associated with PPC, part of the role of the PPC provider is to educate other providers and to work to transform the culture in other settings.[16] Many hospitals now have specialized palliative practices in particular settings (i.e., the emergency department or the special delivery unit) and some have systems in place where particular diagnoses generate an automatic referral to the PPC consult service.

Outside of the inpatient setting, PPC can take on a variety of different roles. Some hospital-based PPC teams may see patients in the outpatient/clinic setting and/or may visit with families at home. Also, "if school, service clubs, and faith and various community organizations are a part of the family's social community, and if the family wishes for them to remain an integral part of their life, these organizations should be included as part of the care giving team."[17(p433)] Studies have shown that if properly prepared and given the choice, parents would prefer to receive end-of-life care at home.[18] For this reason, it is essential that PPC teams also liaise with hospice agencies working directly in the home so that families can be better prepared and supported in caring for their children at home, if this is their ultimate goal.

PPC and hospice service availability

In evaluating the available outpatient PPC and hospice agencies that care for children, the NHPCO released facts and figures in 2009 (Table 56.1), which found of their 4000 hospice agency members, 10% served pediatric patients through either a dedicated pediatric team or individual staff members trained to care for pediatric patients. Of those 4000 members, 378 responded to a 2007 survey that provided more in-depth data: 78% reported that they served pediatric patients with 36% having a pediatric program. For the agencies without a pediatric program, 21.7% had staff members with pediatric experience providing the care/services for children.[19] Additionally they released data demonstrating the average number of pediatric patients served per year through either PPC or hospice care.

To help determine the amount of hospitals that have a PPC team, the Center to Advance Palliative Care developed a National Palliative Care Registry for Data Year 2011,[20] the only repository for national data of current hospital palliative care programs and

services. The data was analyzed with results expected to be available and published in August 2013. This data was intended to help identify the percentage of hospitals that offer PPC and through what type of venues/services.[20] Although there are fewer resources for pediatric patients than adults, there is a growing interest and number of resources to help care for children requiring PPC. The hope is to continue to build on this foundation both in quantity and quality of services.

Identifying the children that could benefit from hospice and palliative care

The most recent data available reports that there are a range of children who can benefit from PPC, and it is estimated that over 8600 children have a need for PPC on any given day, given their limited life expectancy and serious healthcare needs.[19] In the United States alone, there are about 50,000 pediatric deaths annually, and only about 5000 children receive hospice services each year.[19]

There are four generally recognized pathways of conditions that lead to death in children. In brief, they are (1) life-threatening conditions for which curative treatment may be feasible but can fail (e.g., cancer, heart disease, trauma or sudden illness, or extreme prematurity); (2) conditions with inevitable premature death, often with long periods of intensive treatment aimed to prolong life and allowing participation in normal childhood activities (e.g., cystic fibrosis, human immunodeficiency virus infection, chronic or severe respiratory failure, muscular dystrophy); (3) progressive conditions without curative treatment options, although children may live several years (e.g., severe metabolic disorders, certain chromosomal disorders, other rare diseases); and (4) irreversible but nonprogressive conditions with complex healthcare needs leading to complications and likely premature death (e.g., severe cerebral palsy, multiorgan dysfunction, severe pulmonary disability, multiple disabilities following brain or spinal cord infections, severe brain malformations). The illness trajectory of children can vary greatly depending on age and other factors, and, overall, the highest rate of death is reported as occurring in the first year, with a high proportion occurring in the first month of life.[19]

It is important to recognize that the type and length of a child's illness may impact the timing and ways in which PPC may be implemented and may also have an effect on how the family

Table 56.1 Outpatient PPC and hospice agencies serving pediatric patients

Number of pediatric patients served by agency	Hospice service	Palliative care service
None	14.9%	46.1%
1–10	56.9%	20%
11–20	8%	2.7%
21–50	3.4%	4.1%
51–100	1%	2%
>100	<1%	1.4%
Not reported	12.5%	23.7%

Source: Friebert, Sarah. (2009). NHPCO facts and figures: pediatric palliative and hospice care in America.[19]

copes with the illness and/or death and the ways in which they grieve. For example, in the first group described above, children may experience initial response to treatment, return of disease, and then poor to no response to treatments. Preoccupation with therapies, labs, or tests may overshadow any discussion about the possibility of dying, and focus remains on the tasks of managing the medical aspects of disease. Maximizing opportunities for comfort may be passed over or delayed in the intensive search for cure and life-extending alternatives. Pediatric palliative care may be necessary during periods of prognostic uncertainty, throughout the treatment course, and/or when treatment fails. In cases of death by trauma or accident, there may be little time to establish relationships, and immediate grief support might be the most helpful for the family. Conversely, children with very extended and variable pathways through illness, often referred to as complex chronically ill children, have multiple "peaks and valleys" and extensive needs over time. Life can become consumed by the constant focus on appointments, therapy, transportation, shift care, special needs, and ongoing obstacles to accessing adequate comprehensive care. Regardless of the particular condition or disease pathway, accessing PPC can be challenging for all the emotional reasons one might imagine when it is a child's life at stake. In some instances, the best introduction of PPC may be to emphasize the philosophy of comprehensive symptom management and simultaneous care for the body, mind, and spirit of both the child and family, while shifting slowly from the sole focus of preserving life to measures to relieve suffering and maintain comfort. Nurses are often present for the highest ratio of time with the child and family and, along with others members of the IDT, have an extraordinary role in adeptly guiding families through this emotionally laden course.

Barriers to accessing pediatric palliative and hospice care

Barriers to providing hospice or palliative care services for pediatric patients differ from those for adult patients. In general, society's belief that "children shouldn't die," along with denial of the process, make end-of-life care for this population a distant and mysterious concept. Within the healthcare profession, a profound silence of discomfort and denial exists regarding babies and children dying. In many cases, healthcare professionals' attitudes and denial become the greatest barrier to their patients'/families' abilities to access additional options for expert palliative care and support services. In effect, this denies families the possibility of making an informed decision regarding the range of choices available during a child's illness. Excellence in advanced illness or end-of-life care as part of the continuum of clinical expertise should be readily available for families who may transition or alternate their focus of care from a strictly curative mode to one of comfort and quality of life.

In PPC, ethical issues, law, and policy are sensitive and complex and therefore create another barrier that often intimidates providers around palliative and end-of-life care. Healthcare providers and the public need to be aware of local and state law especially around adolescents having say in their medical decision-making and goals/limitations of care. Also, the 18- to 21-year-olds who are either neurologically devastated or have the developmental age of a young child need to have advocates that understand the law (individual states may differ) and have their best interests in mind at all times when making decisions around their end-of-life care.[21]

Children with complex chronic conditions often have frequent life-threatening events and acute illnesses. Advanced technology and treatments have helped children survive these events making care, decision-making, and instituting limitations more difficult for both providers and patients/families. Common thought becomes, the child survived the last life-threatening event and therefore will survive the next. As a result another barrier has emerged over the years; death is seen as a failure of the healthcare system and not a natural process of the illness/disease.[21] Advocates for PPC recognize that advanced technology/treatment saves lives, but fear it may cloud decision-making and prolong suffering.

Pain and symptom management also have become more complex and challenging. Children with complex conditions often end up on multiple medications and/or treatment modalities making it harder to cross check interactions and determine doses and effectiveness. Primary care physicians lack expertise due to limited experience with these complex patients and therefore shy away from caring for them. Hospice agencies tend to feel their expertise in end-of-life care is insufficient in caring for the complex pediatric patient. Provider education and ongoing support from palliative care colleagues helps diffuse some of the anxiety around caring for these children and therefore should optimally remain as an integral part of caring for children and families within the context of PPC.

Lastly, the cost of caring for children with chronic life-limiting illnesses/conditions has been a barrier to pursuing pediatric hospice. Pediatric hospice or palliative care typically requires longer, more frequent home visits; longer time for family meetings and decision-making; more coordination of care with multiple physicians, other providers, and insurance companies; visits to schools by members of the team on behalf of the sick child or siblings; and hiring or access to pediatric experienced nurses, social workers, and child life specialists and aides. Ongoing therapies for palliation of distressing symptoms, including blood transfusions, antibiotics, chemotherapy, and enteral and gavage feedings typically continues longer for children than adults. The cost and responsibility for covering these therapies may be an additional factor for home-based providers in deciding whether to serve children. Now with Concurrent Care and Medicaid waiver programs, this barrier is being addressed and will hopefully become less of an issue, as implementation is more uniform and consistent across healthcare settings.

Nursing considerations

Nurses providing PPC and end-of-life care often experience emotional pain and suffering themselves around their young patients' declining conditions and poor prognoses. In programs where nurses are not clinically trained or emotionally prepared to manage pediatric patients, many issues can emerge as a result of their anguish. Previous losses of a similar nature, unresolved grief issues, conflicting beliefs regarding "supportive care-only" interventions, and insecurities and self-doubt are all common, even within the hospice setting. Personal and ethical dilemmas can emerge regarding withdrawal of aggressive care or nutritional support. Interdisciplinary ethics consultations can bring an invaluable contribution to the decision-making process and often raise the option of a PPC consult or referral to hospice care. Nurses working in predominantly adult-oriented care settings may lack pediatric physical assessment and symptom-management skills, as well as knowledge of the diverse disease processes and developmental stages and related needs essential to care for neonatal, pediatric, or adolescent patients. Those with a background in aggressive and curative care may find it difficult to support a family in transition to a palliative focus of care. It is not enough to just provide education; they need ongoing mentoring, opportunities to process and get feedback on outcomes, interventions, communication, and real-time direction from experienced palliative care nurses and others.

Hospices, palliative care teams, and hospital inpatient teams should always consider and remember that nurses have the most frequent and direct contact with patients and families. They are the frontline clinicians who provide ongoing care and education and are often the ones present during the child's death. Their support and clinical care has a high potential to greatly affect the entire experience that the family will reflect on for the rest of their lives. Nurses who are trained properly can and do report feeling honored and privileged to help patients and families during one of their most painful, private, and intimate experiences. They find it rewarding to know they were able to provide support through such a difficult experience by simply acknowledging and respecting their patient and family's pain and grief. Therefore, the better prepared, supported, and educated nurses are, the better chance for them to help influence a more positive and less traumatizing experience for all involved.[22]

Respecting what parents want and need from their healthcare providers

Nurses can support parents and families in the hospital and at home by identifying their concerns and fears regarding things such as routine care in the hospital, life outside the security of the hospital, what to expect at home, how to handle emergencies and knowing when to call for help. Nurses have an important role in creating plans for how they will communicate with the family and in helping families anticipate what may happen in different situations, as well as having appropriate medications, resources, and contacts in place when needed. In the home setting, it may be helpful to think of parents as "first responders," and as such, they need adequate access to what is needed to respond best to their child's issue when it arises. For example, having an "emergency kit" of a few basic medications in one or two doses for common crisis situations can prevent needless fear and suffering until a home care nurse arrives. Educating parents as thoroughly as possible for transitions in care and settings will reduce anxiety and unnecessary problems faced at home.

Imagine how overwhelmed parents must feel when their child is diagnosed with a serious illness. Nurses' goals are to help parents and children feel confident and competent in the hospital setting and at home; to feel cared for and connected to their care team; to be respected in how their cultural and religious or spiritual beliefs influence decision-making and provision of care; and to preserve hope. Parents also desire to remain in the role of parent to their child and may want to have control over time, routines, and ritualizing care to make their child feel safe and comfortable. They want to have their child recognized as unique and special and have some semblance of "normalcy" and intimacy allowed in the framework of their existence, whether at home or in a facility. Discussing the role and impact on siblings and/or others at home is necessary on an ongoing basis, and support for other family members may be an essential part of care. The communication between professionals and parents and children throughout the time of illness and at the end of life must be grounded in caring and compassionate relationships and mutual trust. Pediatric palliative care places special demands on healthcare providers, not the least of which is an obligation to nurture relationships that can hold both vulnerability and suffering within their embrace.[23]

Intrinsic to the adaptation of palliative care specific for children is that care is firmly anchored in developmental standards and pertinent modifications are made to care based on the individual child's cognitive, emotional, physical, and spiritual development. The NHPCO launched an effort to create pediatric-specific hospice standards to guide programs and direct how care is rendered, regardless of whether care is delivered in the home, hospital, or long-term care or respite facility.[11] Box 56.1 was created to serve as a pediatric-specific appendix to the existing NHPCO Standards of Practice for Hospice.[11]

General considerations for pediatric palliative and hospice care

As described in detail above, PPC is an approach to care for children living with life-threatening illness and for their families that aims to improve quality of life along a physical, psychological, social, emotional, and spiritual continuum and is best delivered through the collective efforts of an IDT that includes the child and the family as the center of care.

Essential components of interdisciplinary PPC include

- enhancement and promotion of quality of life;

- respect for the dignity and uniqueness of each child;

- integration of physical, psychological, spiritual, emotional, and social aspects of care;

- care provided by an IDT that includes the child's primary team;

- individualized child and family-centered approach (with child and family as center of care);

- care plans based on goals that reflect the child's and family's values and preferences;

- relationships based on trust and mutual respect between child, family, and IDT members;

- hope preserved and expressed in a variety of ways to sustain families and their beliefs;

- coordination of care between the child and family, members of the IDT, and settings of care;

- care that involves community support (i.e., schools, places of worship, community groups/teams);

- care that is introduced early and remains in place in conjunction with other therapies/treatments;

- anticipatory guidance and bereavement support;

- inpatient and outpatient hospice support and services;

- effective management of pain and other symptoms; and

- use of effective communication strategies.[24]

The essential elements of PPC (see Figure 56.2),[25] which will be reviewed in more detail below, need to be woven into every aspect of nursing care, with consideration given to how each component of care will affect each child's and family member's daily life, as well as their lives over time.

Addressing the particular needs of children and families

The philosophy of palliative care for children is similar to that for adults; however, the practical elements of palliative care differ in many ways when providing this type of care for children. Clinicians providing PPC must not only learn the nuances inherent to this type of care, but must also pay particular attention to the specific needs of children and families as they midwife them through their illness experience and death (see Figure 56.3). One must consider the reality of the burdens placed on families when caring for children with life-threatening illnesses and how their entire existence can center on details of medication schedules, treatment plans, medical appointments and trips to the hospital, and the minutiae of providing constant care, leaving little time or energy left for anyone or anything else. Taking these elements into consideration, it is the responsibility of interdisciplinary PPC providers to create individualized plans of care that are consistent with the goal of maintaining "normalcy" as much as possible while simultaneously adjusting to the "new normal" that families are often challenged to embrace. In these situations, one must consider the support and guidance that families will need when the focus of care changes as the end-of-life draws near. Nurses have a crucial role in supporting families through their fears and frustrations along with normalizing the full range of feelings that may ebb and flow throughout the course of a child's illness and death.

The team

It is widely recognized that PPC is best delivered using an interdisciplinary approach, although the make-up of inpatient PPC teams will vary, depending on available resources. Most PPC teams include physicians, nurse practitioners, nurses, social workers, chaplains, child life specialists, and therapists from different disciplines such as art and music, and some teams may

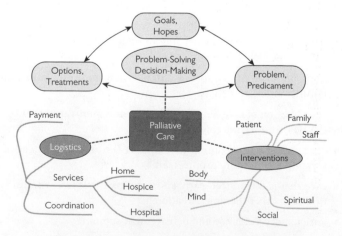

Figure 56.2 Essential elements in pediatric palliative care. Source: Feudtner (2007). Collaborative communication in pediatric palliative care: a foundation for problem-solving and decision-making. *Pediatric Clinics of North America.*[25]

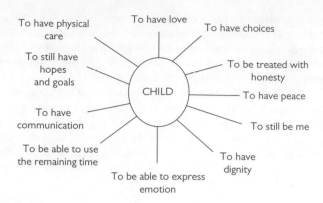

Figure 56.3 Needs of children with life-threatening illness.

also include nurse coordinators, bereavement coordinators, and/or psychologists. By definition, "effective palliative care requires a broad multidisciplinary approach that includes the family and makes use of available community resources."[14(p. 852)] Members of an interdisciplinary PPC team are professionals who have received specialized education and preparation for the care of children and families living with life-threatening illness and can serve as good resources for other allied professionals (i.e., psychiatrists, psychologists, representatives from other consulting services, primary care providers, other therapists—physical, occupational, respiratory, community representatives—teachers, coaches, religious leaders, hospice team members) who are also part of a child's care team. Together, they can provide comprehensive care for children and families, and nurses and advanced practice nurses (APNs) may serve as coordinators of such interdisciplinary care as well as the liaison between the child, family, and team. Collectively, it is the role of the IDT to accompany the child and family throughout illness, death, and bereavement and to support families in coping with the challenges of living with a life-limiting illness and the suffering that may come along with it.[26]

Building supportive relationships with families is also a crucial component of effective PPC.[27] Clinicians must be willing to listen and empathize as they build trust with families, as trust and mutual respect serve as the foundation for positive and successful interactions between members of the IDT and the child and family. Creating an open and nonjudgmental atmosphere and taking a genuine interest in the well-being of a child and family allows for the development of relationships. Once IDT members can begin to understand families' beliefs, values, hopes, wishes, expectations, fears, and worries,[28] they can support families in creating goals that are aligned with what matters to them most. Building relationships with children and families and learning about their individual and familial goals, which may not always be the same, is essential in providing quality PPC.

Family-centered care

In essence, palliative care considers the patient and family as a unique entity whose members all require care.[21] When a child is diagnosed with a life-threatening condition, the entire family, whomever that may include, is affected both on an individual and a collective level.[27] Special attention should be paid to the role of each person in the family, and how those roles may change throughout the course of a child's illness; thus, understanding existing and evolving relationships among family members is extremely important. Understanding the meaning of the illness and/or death experience must also be considered within the historical, cultural, spiritual, and environmental context of each family.[27] See Table 56.2[29,30] for guidelines for children's developmental understanding of death. Please refer to chapter 30 for more information on supporting families in palliative care.

Support for parents/guardians

Families often describe their experiences of living with a child with a life-threatening illness as "being on a roller coaster." From the first time a parent senses something is wrong, until the time of death, parents are faced with the myriad stressors associated with daily life/providing care, making difficult decisions, and often times feelings of guilt and/or failure.[27] Parents and other family members will have needs that range from needing to understand their child's diagnosis and illness course (informational), working through feelings of guilt (emotional), integrating a sense of meaning from the illness experience (meaning-making/spiritual), and requiring support for issues regarding housing, finances, childcare, work (practical).[27] Parents may feel as if they are losing control over several aspects of their lives and it is therefore helpful for nurses and other members of the IDT to find ways to continually

allow parents to remain in control, for example, by involving them in planning the child's daily routine, allowing them to participate in care, and asking if there is a certain way they would like things done. The need to feel a sense of control is also relevant to the sick child, who may be fearful from experiencing many physical and emotional changes. Nurses can assist parents with methods to help themselves and their child feel in control regarding aspects of their experience. Things such as establishing a daily routine, having children participate in conversations about care, when appropriate, and knowing what side effects to anticipate from medications, treatments, and therapies is empowering and fosters an environment of mutual trust and respect. Box 56.2 offers practical advice from the perspective of a parent.

Support for siblings

Caring for the entire family is an essential component of palliative care. Along with parents, siblings' unique needs must also be considered when caring for a child and family living with life-threatening illness. Families will have different opinions regarding sibling involvement, but it is important to always consider siblings' psychological, emotional, and social needs and to provide age- and developmentally appropriate explanations, as well as opportunities to be included in aspects of the illness experience. Siblings' individual needs will vary, depending on the age

Table 56.2 Developmental stages and perceptions of death

Age	Basic conflict	View of death	Suggestions
Birth–18 months	Trust vs. mistrust	◆ No sense of finality; death is viewed as continuous with life, child is reactive to the stress	◆ Use simple physical communication and provide comforting and nurturing care.
Early childhood: 2–3 years	Autonomy vs. shame and doubt	◆ Death is seen as reversible and not final; the child may feel that death is a punishment ◆ Children may feel that they are responsible for death.	◆ Expect regression, clinging, or aggressive behavior ◆ Encourage expression, as the child may be concerned about family function after a member dies ◆ Use honest and clear language to explain death and dying
Preschool: 3–5 years	Initiative vs. guilt	◆ Death continues to be understood as temporary ◆ The child may have a literal understanding of death, and will respond with curiosity and questioning	◆ Open communication with clear language should continue to be utilized ◆ The child should be encouraged to ask questions about death and dying
School age: 6–11 years	Industry vs. inferiority	◆ Death is understood as permanent, and the child understands that the body does not function (no breathing, heart stops beating) ◆ The child may also feel responsible and guilty for the illness ◆ The child may have spiritual ideas about afterlife ◆ The child may not want to discuss feelings	◆ Reassure the child that death is not their fault ◆ Aim to maintain as normal a structure as possible ◆ Include the child in after-life plans (funeral planning, last wishes)
Adolescence: 12–18 years	Identity vs. role confusion	◆ Adolescents understand the finality of death and may develop a mature understanding of death. They may try to take responsibility for adult concerns within the family (such as finances and caretaking) ◆ Feelings of anger may be present	◆ Allow time for the child to reflect ◆ Listen to concerns and questions ◆ Support efforts for autonomy and control

Sources: Adapted from Vern-Gross, T. (2011). Establishing communication within the field of pediatric oncology: a palliative care approach. *Current Problems in Cancer*, 35(6), 337–350. doi: 10.1016/j.currproblcancer.2011.10.008; and Foster TL, Bell CJ, & Gilmer MJ. (2012). Symptom management of spiritual suffering in pediatric palliative care. *Journal of Hospice and Palliative Nursing*, 14(2), 109–115. doi: 10.1097/NJH.0b013e3182491f4b.[29,30] Table created by Carmen Aguilar Mandac, Columbia University (2012).

Box 56.2 Family dynamics: some advice from a parent

Please know that family issues we negotiated as a well family are now under review as a family with a sick child. This is draining and difficult to handle. Therefore, please show patience with us as we struggle to manage an enormous amount of emotional turmoil on many fronts.

Please know that communicating with both parents (if possible) is always far better than each parent separately. Not only does it save you tremendous amounts of time, but even more importantly, it eliminates the he said/she said issues that can further complicate these emotionally fraught situations.

Please know that we are generally trying our best. Most of us understand the stakes and the issues and are doing our best to deal simultaneously with family issues that have often been problematic for some time.

Please remember that our family communication process may have been ineffective for years and will not improve overnight, even if we recognize that our child needs us now more than ever.

Please know that you are an instrumental part of our family dynamic now and can be of enormous assistance in helping us to heal years of emotional damage due to poor communication.

Please know that we may also be accepting new family members into our lives at this time: stepparents, stepbrothers, and stepsisters, who are also trying to cope with an extraordinarily sensitive situation.

Please know that our difficult family situation may also include issues that do not involve you professionally, but that will affect the care of our child, such as divorce, visitation, child support, and custody disputes.

and personality of the sibling, as well as the accepted behavior within a family.[31] Siblings may strive for attention and experience magical thinking (i.e., feeling they caused the illness based on something they once said or did) along with feelings of guilt, responsibility, anger, shame, and/or extreme sadness. An important component of PPC is providing resources to support and involve siblings, and some hospitals offer specific support programs for siblings.

Strategies for engaging with siblings may be as simple as including siblings during visits (e.g., greeting them by name first when entering a room), asking about their favorite toys or interests, or participating in a small activity together during a home visit. It is important to repeatedly evaluate the well child's level of understanding about the sibling's condition. Family meetings are also a good setting in which to discuss how everyone is doing (including sick and well siblings), how they each perceive the situation, how their needs are/are not being met, and how their fears and concerns can be addressed. Hospice and hospital volunteers, art therapists, and child life specialists are also extremely helpful for activities specifically with siblings such as picnics, outside play, reading stories, or memory-making activities such as handprints/molds, "memory boxes" to store keepsakes, memory beads, and/or picture collages. The goal for siblings of terminally ill children is to enhance their feelings of involvement from the time of diagnosis to the greatest degree possible to facilitate a healthy adjustment and eventual grieving process.

Interaction with schools

In addition to family members, multiple professionals are involved in the care of children living with life-threatening illnesses and are committed to maintaining their quality of life. Children living with complex chronic and/or life-threatening illnesses may also have an interdisciplinary team of caretakers at school, including teachers, healthcare providers, and a range of therapists (e.g., occupational, speech and language, physical). Because children spend significant time at school, school personnel are intimately involved in helping meet their various educational, therapeutic, medical, and basic care needs (i.e., feeding, toileting, hygiene) and play a fundamental role in advocating for them. Families often develop supportive relationships with members of their children's school-based care teams and rely on them for support and guidance as they face different care choices throughout their children's lives, as well as for responsible execution of care plans to meet children's individual needs. Thus, it is essential to keep school team members informed of any choices that families make, especially if those decisions impact the care provided to the child at school, and to include the school team in decision-making conversations. It is also important and helpful to provide education, support, and resources to members of the school team, as well as children's classmates and/or family members, whenever possible.

Components of care

This section will address some of the essential components of effective PPC. Each section is meant to give a brief overview and explain why the topic is important or relative to comprehensive palliative care. Because these topics will be reviewed in greater detail in other chapters of this text, the following sections are not meant to provide an exhaustive explanation or be all inclusive regarding all aspects of how to provide such care.

Communication

"Let us communicate with each other clearly, compassionately, and collaboratively, as we strive to improve the quality of life for children including, when necessary, that part of life that is dying."[25]

Good communication is the cornerstone of palliative care and serves as the foundation for building and maintaining relationships with families and other team members. Communication serves several purposes, among which are providing and gathering information, expressing sensitivity and/or empathy, and building partnerships.[32] Having conversations with families about goals of care as early as possible has been shown to reduce suffering.[10] Effective communication considers everyone's needs, including all family members and children, and allows for an open exchange of information and flow of emotions.[32] It involves the use of verbal and nonverbal cues, and thus it is important to pay attention to subtle cues that may be offered by both children and adult family members. In pediatrics, it is important to ask families whether and how they would like to include their child in discussions, and it is also essential to consider the child's chronological and developmental age. Effective communication is a skill that must be learned and can be developed over time by all healthcare team members so that all palliative interactions with children, families, and other healthcare team members facilitate "the development of trust, conveyance of compassion, and conduct of ethical decision making."[32(p. 170)]

Please see chapter 5 for more information on the essential components of communication.

Pain and symptom management

Pain and symptom management is another essential component of comprehensive and effective PPC, as no parent or healthcare provider wishes for children to suffer unnecessarily. Some hospitals have separate pain teams, and many primary teams will manage children's pain and symptoms independently; however, the PPC team may be consulted to recommend a plan, and it is important for nurses to be familiar with general principles of pain and symptom management in regard to PPC. It is also important to recognize that there is often reluctance to manage pain aggressively in children, based on myths and societal, cultural, and familial beliefs that may make parents leery of opioid use to treat pain.[33] Some of these beliefs include the "fear of giving up, misconceptions of opioids as 'too strong for children, fear of side effects, worry their child with become 'addicted' to pain medications, and cultural or religious beliefs."[33(p. 646)] Healthcare providers' reluctance may stem from "lack of sufficient education regarding managing pain, misconceptions about frequency and severity of side effects, such as respiratory depression, worries that opioids will shorten life expectancy, concerns that escalating opioid doses will increase the likelihood of tolerance, and thus make pain control more difficult as the disease progresses."[33(p. 646)] Being aware of these hesitancies is helpful so that fears can be addressed and healthcare team members and family members can be educated about the realities of pain management in children with life-threatening illness and at the end of life.

Aside from pain, there are three other categories of symptoms that are known to be the most distressing to children and families receiving PPC, which are dyspnea, gastrointestinal (GI) disturbances, and neurological changes.[10] Adequate symptom control is a necessary part of effective PPC, and assessment and treatment of symptoms should be done in the least invasive way possible and should not contribute to more distress and/or suffering.[10] Gastrointestinal disturbances, including nausea, vomiting, decreased appetite, and constipation, are common in children with chronic and advanced illness, and identifying and treating the underlying cause,[10] using both pharmacological and nonpharmacological techniques, is a necessary part of care.

Many of the symptoms experienced, as well as the principles and medications used for pain and symptom management, are similar in adult and pediatric palliative care. The differences stem from the age- and developmentally appropriate assessment of pain and symptoms and from dosing medications, as pediatric doses are based on children's weight. Detailed and repetitive assessment of children's pain or other symptoms is a crucial first step toward effective management. This includes a thorough evaluation and history, a detailed assessment, and a physical exam. Using a patient-specific multimodel treatment plan is also helpful, along with frequent reevaluation.[33] It is also important to recognize that a child may be playing or sleeping and not appear to be in pain, but that doesn't mean that s/he isn't experiencing pain. Many excellent resources are available to nurses for gaining competence in pain and symptom management for children, and nurses who care for children over time will become adept at recognizing when children are in pain or are uncomfortable. In addition, families require practical help, information, explanations, and support.

Attention must be paid to the practical issues of preparing for pediatric-appropriate supplies, medications, formulas, feeding tubes, medical equipment, documentation, and teaching tools for parents and children. Ongoing support and education for children and families is an essential part of delivering effective PPC.

Please see chapters 55 and 61 for more information on the essential components of symptom and pain management in PPC.

Psychological, emotional, social, religious, spiritual, and cultural care

Pediatric palliative care is best delivered by an IDT, including individuals who can provide psychological, social, emotional, and spiritual support, such as psychiatrists, psychologists, social workers and chaplains; however it is important to recognize that all members of the team are also an integral part of providing this type of support to families. Colleagues from psychiatry and/or psychology should be consulted to fully assess concerns for psychological and/or emotional distress. Although there are no validated assessment tools to gauge the precise social and emotional needs of children and families, careful assessment should be conducted regarding the following factors: the child's and family's developmental level and ability to complete developmental tasks; the experience of emotional symptoms; practical factors such as financial status, living situation, and social support; and religious or spiritual/existential background, preferences, beliefs, rituals, and practices.[34] Thus any comprehensive palliative care assessment and plan should include conversations and activities that explore all of these aspects of children's and families' lives.

Psychological symptoms and suffering

It is essential to recognize that the experience of caring for a child with a life-threatening illness may cause increased psychological and emotional distress for family members as the illness progresses and the level of care needed increases. For example, the extended time required to provide physical care for affected children may result in increased energy expenditure by parents and the feeling that time and energy necessary for other family responsibilities (e.g., other siblings) and activities (e.g., work, community activities, etc.) are being depleted. This can also be accompanied by a sense of guilt. It is important for the IDT to recognize the stresses that families endure and talk with them about this routinely. It is also important to be aware that while worry and sadness are natural in the context of having or caring for a child with a serious illness, increasing frequency of these symptoms or significant impairment in functioning are signs that the individual and/or family should be evaluated by a mental health clinician.[35]

Thus, it is appropriate for families and children to be offered early psychological and psychiatric consultations to assess the intensity of potential emotional distress, especially given that the symptoms of anxiety and depression are common, treatable, and associated with distress and morbidity, yet are often unrecognized and undertreated in this population of children.[36] Also, it is essential to offer resources for coping (via social workers, chaplains, psychologists, etc.), in an attempt to support the best functioning possible for the child and family members.[37] Consultations may facilitate open discussions, relationship-building, and survival strategies that may help to offset the emotional distress experienced by family members. Effective strategies should help equip affected children and their family members with constructive coping mechanisms (e.g., self-care activities, relaxation exercises, yoga, meditation or prayer, memory making, journal writing, expanding or enlisting community resources, reframing cognitive distortions, or limiting catastrophic thinking, etc.). Also, strategies offered by healthcare providers may enable family members to plan effectively for the future when the child's prognosis is unclear and if the child's lifespan may be limited.[38]

Anxiety and depression are forms of suffering commonly experienced by children with chronic or life-threatening illnesses and can also encumber the primary caregivers of the child as well as other family members, friends, and siblings. While there are clear differences in the treatments for anxiety and depression, both disorders/states are treatable with nonpharmacological methods such as cognitive-behavioral techniques that can be used quite easily by affected children and adults, as well as with medications in conjunction with talk therapy. Examples of nonpharmacological methods include: guided imagery, use of relaxation and breathing exercises, meditation, reframing automatic negative thoughts, and hypnotherapy (which children can learn to do themselves). Complimentary medical therapies such as physical massage, acupuncture, biofeedback, Reiki, and aromatherapy can also be extremely helpful in reducing the symptoms of anxiety and depression. Pharmacological treatment would be prescribed by a psychiatrist consulting with the primary team. As mentioned previously, it is imperative for healthcare providers to regularly monitor for the presence of psychological distress among children and family members over time, and to consult clinical colleagues who are trained to properly assess, diagnose, and provide treatment plans for patients or families struggling with anxiety and depression.[38]

Social aspects

Practical factors in a child's and family's life can have a direct impact on physical as well as psychological symptoms and treatment. Things such as family constellation, financial resources and constraints, employment status, healthcare benefits, childcare, transportation, and the ability to manage the myriad practical demands of living with and caring for a child with a life-threatening illness should be considered.[34] Social workers are usually the members of the IDT most prepared to assess these factors and to identify and connect families with the appropriate resources.

Religious/spiritual and cultural considerations

Another integral part of providing PPC is an understanding of children's and families' spiritual, religious, and cultural beliefs and how these beliefs influence the decisions that they make,[34] although addressing spiritual needs of children and families remains an area with great need for improvement.[39] Families will often have their own ways to express their beliefs—some will use the word "religious," others may say "spiritual," and others may not find it helpful to discuss their beliefs in terms of a structured or identified system of belief. Regardless, it is necessary for members of the PPC IDT to conduct spiritual assessments with families in a variety of ways, as parents of children with serious illness believe that religious or spiritual beliefs are important factors in their coping efforts and decision-making.[34] Chaplains serve to address spiritual suffering, improve family-team communication, and provide rituals that families may request such as ceremonies or sacraments.[40] Although matters of faith are often discussed with chaplains, any member of the PPC IDT should have some

level of comfort in giving families the space they need to talk about religious and spiritual beliefs, practices, and values. Having these types of discussions may be considered one of the most challenging parts of PPC, but these same discussions may also be some of the most profound, rich, and rewarding.[41] It is therefore important for PPC teams to be open to such discussions and to be aware of and utilize available hospital and community based pastoral care services.[34]

Table 56.3 provides examples of some open-ended questions to use and behaviors to observe when assessing psychosocial concerns and strengths in children and families and serves as a guideline for having conversations about such topics.

Talking to families about their cultural and ethnic beliefs, customs, and practices is also important and may or may not be tied into their religious or spiritual beliefs. Of note, using a certified interpreter (i.e., not a family member or other staff member) may be necessary and should not be overlooked when children and families do not speak English, even if they say they understand what is being said. Various cultures approach children with life-threatening illnesses differently and have different beliefs and practices, or rituals surrounding illness and/or death. It may be unacceptable to speak about illness or death or may not be acceptable to discuss medical information in front of children. Nurses and other members of the healthcare team cannot be expected to be familiar with customs from every cultural background and assuming a posture of humble curiosity is welcomed by individuals of other cultures when one does not know the culture and customs in depth. It should also not be assumed that just because someone comes from a particular cultural or ethnic background that they subscribe to the particular beliefs and practices from that group, and thus it is always important to ask children and families about their personal preferences.

Preserving hope

A common characteristic of children living with life-threatening illness and their families is a prevailing and powerful experience of hope, evidenced in their language and decision-making. It is important to preserve and nurture hope during all stages of the child's illness. No matter how grim the situation, one should always strive to deal with matters in a positive, yet realistic, manner, taking the lead from the child and family. The focus of hope may change over time, for example, from hope for cure to hope for a longer remission than previously, to hope that the child can continue to be cared for at home, or to hope that the child will die without pain. Hope may also be centered on a child-specific wish such as to return to school once more, to celebrate an important birthday, or to reach a significant milestone or rite of passage. Other expressions of hope include planning for a visit from grandparents, having friends gathered together, or even gaining the understanding for children, particularly adolescents, that their loved ones will survive and be "okay" after they die. Hope offers opportunities for growth for the child and family, yet it can also become challenging for both families and IDT members to try to balance remaining hopeful while also having realistic expectations. Thus it is important to openly discuss hopes and fears with children and family members, as well as other members of the IDT.

Please see chapter 28 for more information on the essential components of spirituality and hope in palliative care.

Table 56.3 Examples of open-ended questions and behaviors to observe when assessing psychosocial concerns and strengths in children receiving palliative care and in their families

Area being assessed	Open-ended questions	Patient behaviors to observe	Parent behaviors to observe
Developmental appropriateness and understanding	◆ Tell me about what is happening with your treatment. ◆ What questions do you have that you have been too shy/too scared to ask? ◆ Why do you think this is happening to you? (Same questions can be asked of parents)	◆ Indications of fearing sleep (will not go to sleep, resists sedative medication) ◆ Indications of fear of separation ◆ Degree to which patient can enjoy some developmentally appropriate activities (artwork, talking to peers, planning fun activities)	◆ Coddling an older child ◆ Apparent discord between treatment of child and child's developmental level ◆ Ability to let child explore some developmentally appropriate activities ◆ Ability to effectively soothe/nurture or comfort the child
Beliefs about pain	◆ What do you think is happening now that is making you hurt? ◆ How worried do you get when you feel pain? What do you worry about? ◆ What do you like (or not like) about using your pain meds? ◆ What concerns do you have about using your patient-controlled analgesia? (Same questions can be asked of parents)	◆ Use of a range of physical behaviors to demonstrate different levels of pain ◆ Behavioral manifestations of anxiety with increased pain ◆ Over- or underuse of pain medications	◆ Degree of own distress or focus on child's daily pain experience ◆ Ability to comfort and reassure the child ◆ Ability to distract the child from pain and engage in other activities
Emotional issues	◆ How are you feeling? ◆ What are the things you are sad about? ◆ What are you missing because you are sick? ◆ What are you worried about?	◆ Sadness, apathy ◆ Lethargy ◆ Unwillingness to engage in activities or conversation (must rule out physical causes for these symptoms)	◆ Hypervigilance over child's pain, labs, or physical condition ◆ Signs of anxiety or excess sadness ◆ Avoidance of discussing important issues or of seeing the child or physician ◆ Asking same questions over and over again of the medical team
Communication	◆ Sometimes it's hard to talk about some medical things. Who can you talk to about the hardest things? ◆ What things would you like to talk or hear about, but haven't been able to find someone to listen or talk to? ◆ What opportunities are people offering you to talk, and how does it work if you tell them you don't feel like talking?	◆ Patient asking questions about death, dying, prognosis, or related issues ◆ Patient becoming annoyed when people "push" him or her to talk	◆ Reluctance to talk to child or to be alone with him/her ◆ Eager insistence that child needs to talk despite child indicating need not to talk ◆ Expressing anger or exaggerated conflicts regarding the medical care
Practical issues	To parents: ◆ How have the extra medical expenses and any lost income you may have experienced affected your family? ◆ How do you get to the hospital for visits? ◆ What meals do you eat when here? ◆ Who is caring for members of the family still at home? ◆ Who lives at home? Who cares for your child when he/she is not in the hospital? ◆ What space is available in your home for hospital equipment? ◆ What would it be like for your family to have home care nursing in the house?	◆ Missed appointments ◆ Frequently bouncing back to the hospital after discharge ◆ Desire to want to stay in the hospital despite being medically cleared to go home ◆ Strong desire to have no medical intervention (including equipment or home care staff) at home	◆ Same as child observations
Spiritual needs	◆ What religious group, if any, do you belong to? ◆ What help would you like in thinking about religious or spiritual issues? ◆ What does your family believe about what happens after death? ◆ What traditions or rituals does your family practice when someone is sick or dying? ◆ What support from the hospital would be most helpful to you?	◆ Confusion or distress regarding afterlife issues ◆ Worries about what kind of service to have ◆ Unusual behaviors that may be explained or understood as cultural rituals around illness or death	◆ Same as child observations

Sources: McSherry M, Kehoe K, Carroll JM, Kang TI, & Rourke MT. (2007). Psychosocial and spiritual needs of children living with a life-limiting illness. *Pediatric Clinics of North America*, 54(5), 609–630.[34]

Ethical considerations

A large part of PPC involves helping families with decision-making. Clinical ethical dilemmas are inherent to issues surrounding palliative and end-of-life (EOL) care, and it will often be the role of the nurse and/or APN to anticipate, recognize, define, examine, and manage ethically problematic situations[42] that arise in the care of patients and families particularly during times of serious illness and/or at the end-of-life. Ethical dilemmas abound when providing such a wide array of care surrounding topics that are deeply rooted in personal, cultural, religious, and social values. Although nurses and other members of the PPC IDT are not expected to be ethicists, it is helpful to be mindful of the potential ethical dilemmas that will arise when working with families in these circumstances, and to be aware of when to consult with the hospital's ethics committee when additional support is needed. It is, therefore, also the role of the nurse/APN to recognize, contemplate, and use appropriate resources to guide such discussions and decision-making processes with patients and families.[43]

Ethical issues that are associated with end-of-life situations include decision-making under conditions of ambiguity, adequately informing patients and their families about treatment options, balancing quality of life against extending suffering, managing intractable suffering, and futile treatments. Resources are available to help guide the decision-making process, and to help children, adolescents, and adults express how they want to be treated throughout their illness and at the time of death from a medical, personal, emotional, and spiritual perspective.[44] Some helpful documents include *My Wishes* (for young children), *Voicing My Choices* (for adolescents), and *Five Wishes* (for adults) published by Aging with Dignity and available at www.agingwithdignity.org.[44]

This section does not serve to provide an all-inclusive discussion of ethics in PPC, but rather to highlight some of the dilemmas nurses may face. Please see other chapters in this text for a more thorough discussion of ethical considerations and end-of-life decision-making, such as chapter 64.

Perinatal palliative care

Although comprehensive PPC extends to children of all ages, in the United States alone, more than 15,000 children are born with conditions that are incompatible with life beyond infancy.[45] Thus, many families are faced with difficult decisions that need to be made shortly after birth and in some instances, even before a child is born, and it is necessary to recognize the unique need for palliative care in the perinatal and neonatal period. The model for perinatal palliative care has become internationally recognized and is often introduced during pregnancy. Palliative care in neonatal intensive care and other settings of infant care has evolved in many levels.[45]

Perinatal palliative and hospice care is an innovative and compassionate model of support that can be offered to parents who learn during pregnancy that their baby has a fatal condition, an unfortunate situation that occurs with increasing frequency as prenatal testing advances. This unique group of parents faces the daunting challenge of anticipating and preparing for the birth *and* the possibility of death of their baby simultaneously. For parents who receive terminal prenatal diagnoses, perinatal palliative care can be instrumental in helping them make the decision that is best for their family regarding whether or not to continue the pregnancy. For families who choose to continue their pregnancies, even if the baby may die shortly after birth, perinatal hospice helps them embrace whatever life their baby might have, before and after birth. Perinatal hospice support begins at the time of diagnosis, even before the child is born. It can be thought of as "hospice in the womb," including birth planning and preliminary medical decision-making prior to birth, as well as more traditional hospice care after birth, depending on how long the child survives. With the support of perinatal palliative care, families are given the opportunity to feel some level of control by making plans for the baby's birth, life, and death, based on their individual needs for supporting themselves, their other children, the grandparents, and friends.[46] It also provides families the opportunity to honor their baby in a way that is meaningful to them and helps families participate in memory-making experiences. Strengthening this experience during this time may help diminish long-term psychological implications for parents and siblings.

Perinatal hospice is not a place. Ideally, it is a comprehensive team approach that includes obstetricians, perinatologists, labor and delivery nurses, neonatologists, neonatal intensive care unit (NICU) staff, chaplains/pastors and social workers as well as genetic counselors, therapists, and traditional hospice professionals. Perinatal hospice is a beautiful and practical response to some of the most heartbreaking challenges of prenatal testing.[47] Some programs exist within a hospital setting, such as the labor and delivery unit, NICU, and maternal and child areas. Other times it presides within community settings. It naturally creates a seamless continuum of care across settings (office to inpatient to home) and providers, and includes advanced decision-making within the framework of a "birth plan," which includes the "who, what, when, and where" for the delivery and beyond (see Box 56.3 and Figure 56.4). Perinatal palliative care may naturally extend into neonatal palliative care, as some infants will live anywhere from days to months to years after birth.

Please see chapter 59 for more information on the essential components of neonatal palliative care.

Care at the time of death

Nothing can fully prepare families for the final moments of their loved ones' lives and the precise time of death, but there is much that can be done to help families anticipate what to expect so as to avoid unnecessary surprises when the time comes. Conversations about such sensitive topics may feel difficult to initiate, but parents are often wondering about these things and may be afraid to ask, and thus initiating the conversation after a relationship has been established and at a time that feels appropriate, is essential. Families should be reminded that PPC clinicians cannot predict exactly when and how death will occur, as it can be different for everyone, but parents and family members should be prepared for the possible range of changes that can happen, along with when they might expect such changes, and what things may look like, feel like, sound like, smell like, and so forth. Consider all the senses for both the adults and any other children who will be present. Parents also may appreciate written handouts in language that is not too clinical or frightening so that they have them to review at a time when they feel ready to do so. Having such knowledge may also prepare parents to talk with each other, other children,

---

Box 56.3 Birthing plan

Dear staff at _____:

We have received the devastating news that our baby _____ has been diagnosed with _____. However imperfect his/her little body is, he/she is still our baby whom we love and therefore we chose to continue his/her life. Your kindness, compassion, and understanding during this difficult time are greatly appreciated. We believe that precious time with _____ is the only thing that will soothe the pain of those who love him/her.

We understand that decisions may need to be made after the birth, which were not anticipated. We ask only that you keep us informed so we can make the decisions together for what is best for _____. We ask that no interventions other than those stated below be taken without approval from us and consideration be given to the precious nature of our brief time as a family.

Each of you can assist during this time by understanding and respecting our following wishes:

1. Please call our baby by his/her name _____. This is very comforting for us to hear.
2. In an effort to facilitate relaxation during labor and delivery, we would like _____ (selected music, shower, massage, etc.).
3. We prefer the same room for labor, delivery, and recovery
4. In regard to fetal monitoring, we request _____ external _____ internal _____ none.
   ◆ We may desire to hear heartbeat initially before labor progresses.
5. If there is a loss of heartbeat prior to delivery, we do/do not wish to be informed.
6. We desire the following people in attendance _____ And that the birth is videotaped.
7. Any drugs used during labor should be given to _____ in the smallest dose that will be effective, to provide maximum pain relief and comfort while still allowing _____ to remain alert. Our other preferences in regard to pain management include _____.
8. We ask that _____ be able to cut the umbilical cord.
9. We request that oral/nasal suctioning only be used for comfort and no intubation without permission of the parents.
10. After our baby is born, we ask that _____ be quickly wiped, suctioned, wrapped in a blanket and handed to _____.
11. Following delivery, we wish to hold our baby immediately and that vital signs, weighing of baby, medications, and labs are postponed if possible.
12. We understand that our baby may be born with more or fewer problems than anticipated. If this is the case, we ask that our options be discussed with us and we understand that further diagnostic testing may be needed.
13. Other than the basic care needed after delivery, my husband and I would like to be left alone without interruption to have private time with our baby. (You may prefer for staff to check on you occasionally.)
14. We request that a liaison (i.e., nurse, social worker, chaplain) periodically give updates to the waiting family.
15. Additional family and friends that are special to us may be joining us as we celebrate our child's life.
16. If our baby cannot suck and/or breastfeed, we wish to provide oral comfort with drops of expressed breast milk or formula.
17. We request that a ceremony be performed in accordance with our religious beliefs by _____ (baptism, blessing).
18. If our child is to be placed in NICU, we request that we be provided with a private space for us to care for our child in private. Help us create a *sacred space* to share his/her brief life.
19. Please discuss any medications given to our baby to relieve pain and suffering with us prior to giving them.
20. We wish to hold our baby as he/she is dying or after he/she has died.
21. We would like to bathe and touch our baby's precious little body as long as possible.
22. We would like to keep the following items as keepsakes: cord clamp, lock of hair, ID band, tape measure, crib card, baptismal certificate, weight card, hat/blanket/clothes, fetal monitor, tape, bulb syringe, footprints/handprints, thermometer, handprints of baby alone and with family, photographs-color and b/w. Anything with our baby's scent.
23. Upon discharge, please give us information on milk suppression and physical comfort measures for _____ (the mother).
24. Please allow my husband _____ or other designated person to spend the night in my room if possible.

We understand that every birthing experience is unique and offer this only as a guideline to assist you and your family to decide what feels right for you.

Source: Liz Sumner (2009). Center for Compassionate Care. The Elizabeth Hospice.[46]

---

and family members. Families may have memories from previous experiences of death of other family members and may conjure images or memories from that time, which may or may not be helpful, depending on what the particular experience was like for them.

Children and family members will likely have fears associated with death and the dying process. This may include fears about what dramatic events can unfold, fear of being alone at time of death, fear of a loved one missing the death, and fear of being unprepared for an unexpected emergency. Understanding the physical progression of events and the nearing death awareness that is common among children and adolescents may be reassuring for both members of the team and the family. It is essential to review goals for the time of death well before the time comes so that families feel as in control of the situation as possible. For example, children and families likely will have an idea of where they would like for the final hours or days of life

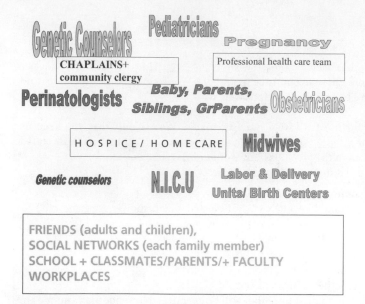

Figure 56.4 Constellation of support and providers. Perinatal palliative care.

to occur, and, when possible, nurses and other members of the IDT can try to align the proper resources to allow this to happen. If families desire to remain in the hospital, they should be given a private space or room to be together as a family. Several children's hospitals allocate a specific room or space, often called a "comfort corner" where children may be moved to spend their final hours together with their family. Typically, changing locations close to end-of-life is not desired; however, for some families it may be very important to make it home from the hospital or to get to the hospital in the event of an emergency before death and thus it is again important to talk with families about their wishes for this time. It is also crucial to consider whom a family may want to be present. In most instances, family members will be called to visit as the time of death nears and the child's bedside, whether in the hospital or at home, can become the gravitational force for loved ones to gather. Families may also have particular wishes about who should be present at the actual moment of death, as sometimes parents want to be alone with their child, with or without other children being present. Other times families may choose to get in bed with their child. The tenderness and intimacy of these final moments is beyond description and being present at this time with a family is a very precious privilege for everyone involved in the child's care, especially nurses who often spend the most time at the bedside.

Creating a sacred space

When a child is dying, regardless of their age, the very space becomes sacred ground, and it is important to maintain the holiness of that space immediately following the death for even a brief period of time. This also allows for a brief pause to honor the nurse's role in maintaining the dignity of a child and his or her family surrounding death before moving on to the next task. Some programs place a special sign on the door, or an image of a dove, butterfly, flower or leaf to subtly designate this sacred space and to minimize interruptions in and out of the room during this time. Honoring and respecting the space

also models to staff that it is not just "business as usual," for a brief time at least. At home, families may choose to have the child remain in their bed or keep the space intact for a bit of time before having the body removed. Cultural and religious practices may guide what happens at time of death and immediately following, but generally time is allowed for bathing, dressing, holding or rocking the child, offering prayers, obtaining handprints (if not obtained before), cutting a lock of hair, and gathering the clothing items that may have the child's scent on them (to be preserved in a timely manner in a zipper bag) and families may or may not choose to partake in these activities. Some families may wish to accompany their child's body to the morgue if in the hospital, and if hospital policy allows for this to happen, or out of the house if at home. Siblings and parents or others may choose to send along a note or a little something with the child's body as a symbolic way to remain connected while apart and sometimes children may have previously stated their wishes about what objects they would like to keep with them (see Box 56.4). It is also important to recognize that some families may choose to consider organ donation or autopsy, which ideally should be discussed with families before the time of death. Hospitals usually have programs that require that the option for organ donation be presented to families, and procedures are in place for representatives from the appropriate resources to be notified near or at the time of death to have these discussions with families. If families elect to donate organs or have an autopsy performed, timing will be of the essence and members of the team and the nurse should be aware of what needs to happen in what time frame to ensure that a family's wishes are met appropriately.

Self-care

It is also important to recognize that the team members caring for the child and family will need support before, during, and following the time of death. The nurses present with the family will likely have other tasks to move on to, but it is very important to have support available to allow for at least a brief respite, break, or time away from the immediate setting. In some instances, nurses may be given a lighter caseload or, when possible, have time to debrief with another colleague, chaplain, or member of the PPC IDT both immediately following and/or at a time period after the death has occurred. Great wisdom can be shared, burdens lessened, and insights and renewal gained from the time spent debriefing clinically as well as through other efforts to support colleagues. It takes a lot of energy to care for seriously ill children and members of their family physically as well as emotionally and psychologically. Preserving the meaning of and sustaining this type of work requires self-discipline and intentionality to tend to one's own centering practices and methods of self-care, whether physical, spiritual, and/or emotional. Some coping strategies may be personally beneficial, such as self-reflection and self-care, even for a few minutes throughout the day, along with building in time for ongoing renewal and reflection outside of work. Time spent focusing on other activities completely unrelated to work, and taking breaks from work on a regularly scheduled basis (i.e., vacations and time with friends and family) are necessary in order to sustain this type of intense and rewarding work.[14] Also important is professional support, as many team members find relationships with colleagues to

Box 56.4 When the time comes: how to help when a child dies in the home—by L.H. Sumner

When the call comes in that a baby or child has died in the home, it may be a challenge and even a bit overwhelming to think of what you will do to be of help and comfort to the grieving family. Below are some guidelines that may help you approach the situation a bit more prepared and thus more capable of making the process a little less painful for the parents and family.

1. Most parents may not directly ask for a home visit, but usually appreciate and often benefit from a visit at the time of the child's death. Just having someone there to help orchestrate the process when they may be feeling overwhelmed and paralyzed by their grief will be helpful. If they refuse, then there are still things to do over the phone that will be helpful for them. It is most likely that they will not need the nurse or other team members to stay for the entire time until the child is taken from the home.

2. The family should be allowed to have as much time as they need with their baby or child before the mortuary comes to take their child's body. It may seem unusual to you that they would want to keep the body for many hours, but it is a very final step to have their child taken from the home. The mortuary can be notified with the appropriate information required at time of death but informed that the family will contact them directly when they are ready.

3. Try to suggest to the parents/caregivers to take some private time alone with their child, without all the family around. This is a very intimate and personal time for them and may help to facilitate the process of "letting go" and saying goodbye. Others in the family may also wish to have some private time with the child to say a personal goodbye.

4. Encourage the parents/adults present to give any other children in the home or family the *choice* to go in and say goodbye. Children of most any age are able to decide for themselves if they want to see the child who has died. By just offering the child the choice, it has given the child a sense of control during an unfamiliar and unsettling experience. They will remember that someone thought enough of them and their relationship with the person who died to give them the chance to say goodbye. The child should be prepared in simple language for what the child will look and feel like, that they will not move, and so forth. It's a good idea to remove any tubing from infusions, oxygen tubing, catheters, and so forth to normalize the appearance at the bedside as much as possible. Someone he/she feels safe with should accompany the child. If the family plans on cremation, this may be the last opportunity for them to see their sibling, thus there may not be a second chance if not now. The child may wish to go in for just a "peek" or they may be curious and want to stay around. Whatever length of time the child chooses to stay is okay and should be up to them.

5. Allow parents to have the time they need to perform any private rituals or activities, which may include bathing the little one, redressing the child into something special, rocking, a blessing or time for prayer around the bedside. They may wish to have their priest, minister, or chaplain come to the home.

6. Offer the parents the suggestion of saving a lock of hair if they have not already done so. They may not feel comfortable doing this themselves and may wish for the staff person to do this. The nape of the neck or the back of the head is the best place to obtain a swatch of hair. It can be tied with a piece of yarn, thread, or ribbon. The hair can be placed in an envelope and sealed. Explain that they may not wish to look at it or have it now but that some day they may be glad they had this small remembrance, something tangible that connects them to their loved one, their precious child. A comfortable way to present these suggestions to the family is to say that these are some ideas and suggestions that other parents/families have found to be comforting. They may choose to do all or none of these activities, the point is to make it meaningful for themselves as a family.

7. There are instances when the family may want to take pictures of the child after death. They may wish to keep them for relatives who live away or for cultural reasons. A family may ask for your assistance to do so, or they may obtain them at the mortuary.

8. If the primary team has not already done so, it may be important to offer the suggestion of taking handprints and/or footprints of the infant or child. Someone could go out to purchase an inkpad, poster paints, or tempera paints if nothing is available in the home with which to improvise. These supplies are available to the staff in the resource area. Keep a soapy washcloth or alcohol handy to quickly remove the coloring from the extremity. It's best to try to do the prints as soon as possible before any stiffening of the body sets in. Again, if there are other children in the home it will be significant to obtain at least one print for the sibling to have for later on. Other family members can add their handprints also, creating a "family portrait" of hands.

9. When contacting the mortuary, emphasize that it was a child that died so that they will be sensitive to the situation they will face. When they arrive at the home, the family may need to say a last goodbye. Rather than have the child taken from the home by the mortuary attendants, we have found that is much less painful if one of the adults/parents carries the child out to the vehicle and surrenders over their child to the arms of the attendants. Parents have told us it felt less traumatic than if they stood back and the baby was *taken* out by "strangers." Occasionally this process becomes an informal processional to accompany the child out of the home for the last time.

10. If at all possible when the child is ready to be carried out of the home, ask the attendant to keep the child's face and head uncovered and not enclosed completely. The use of the body bag is very distressing and offensive to most parents/family. Perhaps the child can be wrapped in special blanket and/or a sheet. Sometimes the driver is willing to take the little one partially covered like this until away from the home, and then secure the child's body after leaving the area. Siblings can add a special keepsake to accompany the child's body (e.g., a note, flower, drawing, or stuffed toy).

11. Remind the family of the local bereavement support resources available to them (community or your own organization) and how/when the primary team will be following up. Request that arrangements for funeral/memorial service be communicated to the child's care team unless it is private, family-only. If visits are made after hours, notify primary team, including MDs, of how the family is coping and report on events surrounding the child's death. The primary team can follow-up with their sick child's or sibling's school with permission from the parents.

be especially supportive, even more so than relationships with friends and family outside of work in regard to PPC.[14] The burden and grief experienced from caring for children with life-threatening illness and their families can be intense and serious and requires formal and informal support to prevent burnout and to cope effectively with the challenges of this work.[14]

Ongoing professional support from other colleagues is also helpful in sustaining and gaining satisfaction from a career in PPC. Participating in professional palliative and/or pain and symptom management community-based programs, coalitions, and collaborations, joining local and national organizations, and teaching/presenting at academic centers and meetings are all excellent ways to connect with colleagues and develop vital linkages for a thriving PPC program. It is also essential to establish rapport and develop relationships with local colleagues and hospices so that one can comfortably refer families and work with community resources to ensure that families get the care they need and deserve. Children and families benefit from collaborative care provided by team members that feel well supported and are unified in their approach. Overall, appropriate and healthy self-care, along with support and collegial supervision/mentorship is essential to prevent provider burnout and to sustain providing comprehensive PPC.

Anticipatory grief and bereavement

Chapter 60 is devoted entirely to grief and bereavement in PPC, and thus it will not be discussed at length in this chapter. It would be remiss, however, to not mention the importance of anticipatory grief, grief surrounding death, and bereavement. Children and families will often begin the process of anticipatory grief at the time of diagnosis, and it is helpful for PPC team members to talk with children and families continually about the ongoing losses they are experiencing. Grief continues through and beyond the time of death, and families, community members, and team members that cared for the child and family will need ongoing bereavement support. Many hospitals have at least annual ceremonial remembrance services that families and team members find helpful for honoring and remembering the children that have died.

Overview of nursing care issues for pediatric palliative care

As evident, the responsibilities of caring for children living with life-threatening illnesses and their families are extensive and require an understanding of the interconnectedness of the myriad aspects of illness and suffering: physical, emotional/psychological, spiritual, and social. Illness unravels the pattern that belongs uniquely to each child, interrupting the ongoing stories of children's lives.[48] Nurses and members of the PPC IDT must assess for imbalances and indications of suffering in each of these areas to appropriately intervene and provide comprehensive and effective PPC. Pediatric palliative care nurses and other professionals may also experience pain and suffering,[49] and self-care, adequate support, and ongoing education and professional training are also essential components of delivering effective PPC.

Education and training

Healthcare professionals face many obstacles and challenges while providing this type of intense and unique care to seriously ill children and their families, including lack of professional education and training.[49] Nurses specifically have reported perceived lack of skill in providing PPC, including inadequate knowledge and expertise, as well as fears regarding appropriate communication with families.[49] Many educational programs exist to train nurses and other healthcare professionals in various aspects of PPC, and there are a variety of ways to implement curriculum-based training on key topics inherent to caring for children with life-threatening illness and/or at the end of life. Interdisciplinary case discussions, "lunch-and-learn" sessions, journal clubs, and/or regularly scheduled community-based educational seminars can result in a commitment from nursing and other team members to work together and support each other or form committees on specific units/other areas. Funding from small educational grants may also be available to support training programs in PPC that aim at specific topics such as pain and symptom management, communication, addressing culture and spiritual needs, bereavement, ethics, and decision-making in PPC. Children's hospitals with emerging PPC programs are now offering more palliative care seminars, conferences, "just in time" teaching sessions, and trainings for new nurses, residents, and therapists, as well as staff debriefing sessions, as a way to educate others about PPC and to allow for professional development in this emerging field. Of note, PPC has now been integrated into recent national nursing professional practice guidelines and standards, such as those of the Society of Pediatric Nursing.[50]

In recognizing that hospice and palliative nursing care has become a specialized area of nursing, the Hospice and Palliative Nurses Association (HPNA) was established in 1986. This membership organization relies on evidence-based research and data to assist members in delivering quality nursing care, symptom management, grief and bereavement support, guidance with difficult conversations, education, and encouragement in leadership and mentoring efforts. The HPNA supports credentialing for APRNs, RNs (adult and pediatric), LP/VNs, nursing assistants, and administrators through the National Board for Certification of Hospice and Palliative Nurses (NBCHPN).[51]

Additionally, recognizing that nurses need specialized training in hospice and PPC, many professional associations are supporting localized efforts by cosponsoring educational efforts with other entities. For example, End-of-Life Nursing Education Consortium (ELNEC), is a well-established and respected "train the trainer" initiative to teach nurses at all levels how to provide effective PPC, as well as how to teach this information to other nursing students and colleagues.[52] The curriculum is updated annually, and a pediatric curriculum is available that includes learning modules that highlight current practices and include cases, key references, supplemental teaching tools, and resources. A new curriculum for APNs was launched by ELNEC in 2012, which also includes pediatric-specific training modules. Although too numerous to list, there are several national professional organizations that offer specific training in both adult and pediatric palliative care for healthcare providers in all disciplines. The Center to Advance Palliative Care (CAPC) provides healthcare professionals with the tools, training, and technical assistance necessary to start and sustain palliative care programs in hospitals and other settings and includes an extensive listing of other trainings that are available on their website: http://www.capc.org. The Initiative for Pediatric Palliative Care (IPPC) sponsored by the Educational Development Center (EDC) is an interdisciplinary model of case-based experiential training, offering PPC specific training events. More information and additional training materials can be found at the IPPC website: www/ippcweb.org.[53] The NHPCO[7] also has a pediatric curriculum to address the ongoing demand for training for adult hospice programs to be prepared to care for children http://www.nhpco.org. In short, there are an increasing number of educational offerings and opportunities for nurses and other healthcare professionals to expand their knowledge of PPC.

The future unfolding for pediatric palliative care

Pediatric palliative and hospice care is a burgeoning field with a future promising to be filled with an increasing number of individual providers specializing in this type of care, growth of new and existing interdisciplinary care teams, and the expansion of available community resources.[10] Infants, children, adolescents, and their families are part of the continuum of PPC, and there is much to be done to support them and to advance the quality of pediatric palliative and end-of-life care. Each step toward increasing awareness regarding PPC is a step forward on behalf of the children who are dying without access to all of the resources that should be available to them and their loved ones. The future of PPC is aimed at improved recognition and increased utilization of PPC services and better reimbursement for palliative care providers.[10] Nurses who choose to care for seriously ill and dying children and their families need a significant support system to maintain the difficult and delicate task of balancing perspectives, as well as opportunities for ongoing personal and professional development. While challenging, this type of work is also humbling and rewarding, as those caring for children with life-threatening illnesses and their families have the privilege of being a part of families most intimate and powerful experiences both throughout children's lives and during the time of their death.

Acknowledgment

The authors gratefully acknowledge Lizabeth H. Sumner, author of this chapter in the previous edition, for her original work and ongoing contributions.

References

1. Aging with Dignity. (2012). My Wishes, Voicing My Choices, and Five Wishes. Agingwithdignity.com. Retrieved July 28, 2013 from http://www.agingwithdignity.org/index.php
2. American Academy of Pediatrics Committee on Bioethics and Committee on Hospital Care (2000). Palliative Care for Children. AAP.org. Retrieved July 28, 2013, from http://pediatrics.aappublications.org/content/106/2/351.full.   3.
3. Attig, T. (1996). Beyond pain: The existential suffering of children. *Journal of Palliative Care,12*, 20–23.
4. Battista, V., & Mosher, P.J. (2014). Palliative Care for the Infant, Child, or Adolescent with Spinal Muscular Atrophy (SMA). In V. Ferguson (Ed.), *Pediatric Life-Limiting Conditions*. Pittsburgh, PA: Hospice and Palliative Nurses Association.
5. Battista, V., Santucci, G., DeSanto-Madeya, S., & Grace, P. (2014). Nursing Ethics and Advanced Practice: Palliative and End-of-Life Care Across the Lifespan. In P. Grace (Ed.), *Nursing Ethics and Professional Responsibility in Advance Practice, Second Edition*. Burlington, MA: Jones and Bartlett Learning.
6. Browning, D. (2003). To show our humanness-relational and communicative competence in pediatric palliative care. *Bioethics Forum, 18*(3/4), 23–28.
7. Catlin, A., & Carter B. (2002). Creation of a neonatal end-of-life palliative care protocol. *Journal of Perinatology*, 22, 184–195.
8. Children's Hospice and Palliative Care Coalition (2007). Professional Advisory Committee. Retrieved June 15, 2013, from http://www.chpcc.org.
9. Crozier, F., & Hancock, L.E. (2012). Pediatric palliative care beyond the end-of-life. *Pediatric Nursing, 38*(4):198–203.
10. Davies, B., Brenner, P., Orloff, S., Sumner, L., & Worden, W. (2002). Addressing spirituality in pediatric hospice and palliative care. *Journal of Palliative Care, 18*, 59–67.
11. Dussel, V., Kreicbergs, U., Hilden, J.M., et al. (2009). The measurement of symptoms in children with cancer. *Journal of Pain and Symptom Management, 19*, 363–377.
12. End-of-Life Nursing Education Consortium (2013). ELNEC. Retrieved July 22, 2013, from http://www.aacn.nche.edu/elnec.
13. Feudtner, C. (2007). Collaborative communication in pediatric palliative care: A foundation for problem-solving and decision-making. *Pediatric Clinics of North America, 54*(5), 583–608.
14. Field, M.J., & Behrman, R.E. (2003). When Children Die: Improving Palliative and End-of-Life Care for Children and Their Families (Report of the Institute of Medicine Task Force). Washington, DC: National Academy Press.
15. Fitchett, G., Lyndes, K.A., Cadge, W., Berlinger, N., Flanagan, E., et al. (2011). The role of professional chaplains on pediatric palliative care teams: Perspectives from physicians and chaplains. *Journal of Palliative Medicine, 14*(6), 704–707.
16. Foster, T.L., Bell, C.J., & Gilmer, M.J. (2012). Symptom management of spiritual suffering in pediatric palliative care. *Journal of Hospice and Palliative Nursing, 14*(2), 109–115. doi: 10.1097/NJH.0b013e3182491f4b.
17. Friebert, S. (2009). NHPCO Facts and Figures: Pediatric Palliative and Hospice Care in America. Alexandria, VA: National Hospice and Palliative Care Organization.
18. Friedrichsdorf, S., & Kang, T.I. (2007). The management of pain in children with life limiting illnesses. *Pediatric Clinics of North America, 54*(5),645–672.
19. Himelstein, B.P., Hilden, J.M., Boldt, A.M., & Weissman, D. (2004). Pediatric palliative care. *New England Journal of Medicine, 350*, 1752–1762.
20. Hospice and Palliative Nursing Association. (2013). About Us and Certification Info. Retrieved July 29, 2013, from http://www.hpna.org/Default2.aspx.
21. Huff, S.M., Orloff, S.F., Wheeler, J., & Grimes, L. (2011). Palliative Care in the Home, School, and Community. In B.S. Carter, M. Levetown, & S.E. Friebert (Eds.), *Palliative Care for Infants, Children, and Adolescents: A Practical Handbook* (pp. 414–440). Baltimore: The Johns Hopkins University Press.
22. Initiative for Pediatric Palliative Care (2009). Pediatric Palliative Care. Ippcweb.org. Retrieved July 23, 2013, from www/ippcweb.org.
23. Jennings, P.D. (2005). Providing pediatric palliative care through a pediatric supportive care team. *Pediatric Nursing, 31*(3), 195–200.
24. Jones, B.L., Gilmer, M., Parker-Raley, J., Dokken, D.L., Freyer, D.R., et al. (2011). In J. Wolfe, P.S. Hinds, & B.M. Sourkes (Eds.), *Textbook of Interdisciplinary Pediatric Palliative Care* (pp. 135–147). Philadelphia: Elsevier Saunders.
25. Kane, J.R., Joselow, M., & Duncan, J. (2011). In J. Wolfe, P.S. Hinds, & B.M. Sourkes (Eds.), *Textbook of Interdisciplinary Pediatric Palliative Care* (pp. 30–40). Philadelphia: Elsevier Saunders.
26. Kersun, L.S., & Shemesh, E.(2007). Depression and Anxiety in Children at the End-of-Life. *Pediatric Clinics of North America, 54*(5), 691–708.
27. Kirschen, M.P., & Feudtner, C. (2013). Ethical Issues. In N.S. Abend & M.A. Helfaer (Eds.), *Pediatric Neurocritical Care* (pp. 485–493). New York, NY: DemosMedical.

28. Lanctot, D., Morrison, W., Kock, K.D., & Feudtner, C. (2011). Spiritual Dimensions. In B.S. Carter, M. Levetown, & S.E. Friebert (Eds.), *Palliative Care for Infants, Children, and Adolescents: A Practical Handbook* (pp. 227–243). Baltimore: The Johns Hopkins University Press.

29. Levetown, M., Meyer, E.C., & Gray, D. (2011). Communication Skills and Relational Abilities. In B.S. Carter, M. Levetown, & S.E. Friebert (Eds.), *Palliative Care for Infants, Children, and Adolescents: A Practical Handbook.* (pp. 169–201). Baltimore: The Johns Hopkins University Press.

30. Liben, S., Papadatou, D., & Wolfe, J. (2008). Paediatric palliative care: challenges and emerging ideas. *Lancet, 371,* 852–864.

31. National Hospice and Palliative Care Registry-Center to Advance Palliative Care. (2011). National Palliative Care Registry™ for Data year 2011. registry.capc.org. Retrieved June 22, 2013 from https://registry.capc.org

32. Mah, J.K., Thannhauser, J.E., Kolski, H., & Dewey, D. (2008). Parental stress and quality of life in children with neuromuscular disease. *Pediatric Neurology, 39*(2), 102–107.

33. McSherry, M., Kehoe, K. Carroll, J.M., Kang, T.I., & Rourke, M.T. (2007). Psychosocial and spiritual needs of children living with a life-limiting illness. *Pediatric Clinics of North America, 54*(5), 609–630.

34. MedicineNet. (2013). Definition of Hospice care. MedicineNet.com. Retrieved June 30, 2013, from http://www.medterms.com/script/main/art.asp?articlekey=24267.

35. Miller, E.G., LaRagione, G., Kang, T.I., & Feudtner, C. (2012). Concurrent care for the medically complex child: Lessons of implementation. *Journal of Palliative Medicine, 15*(11), 1281–1283.

36. Morgan, D. (2009). Caring for dying children: Assessing the needs of the pediatric palliative care nurse. *Pediatric Nursing, 35*(2), 86–90.

37. National Consensus Project. (2013). Guidelines for Quality Palliative Care. nationalconsensusproject.org. Retrieved July 22, 2013, from http://www.nationalconsensusproject.org.

38. National Hospice and Palliative Care Organization. (2010). Standards of Practice for Hospice Programs. Appendix IV PPC PFC 1: Pediatric Palliative Care (PPC PFC). NHPCO.com. Retrieved July 28, 2013, from http://www.nhpco.org/sites/default/files/public/quality/Standards/APXIV.pdf.

39. National Hospice and Palliative Care Organization. (2013). Hospice and Palliative Care, What Is Hospice? nhpco.org. Retrieved June 28, 2013, from http://www.nhpco.org/about/hospice-and-palliative-care.

40. Office of the Legislative Counsel, US House of Representatives. (2010). Compilation of Patient Protection and Affordable Care Act, As Amended Through May 1, 2010, Including Patient Protection and Affordable Care Act Health-Related Portions of the Health Care and Education Reconciliation Act of 2010, *Legislative Counsel, 111th Congress 2d Session, Print 111-1,* 202–203.

41. Orloff, S.F., Jones, B., & Ford, K. (2011). Psychosocial Needs of the Child and Family. In B.S. Carter, M. Levetown, & S.E. Friebert (Eds.), *Palliative Care for Infants, Children, and Adolescents: A Practical Handbook* (pp. 202–226). Baltimore: The Johns Hopkins University Press.

42. Wiener, L., et al. (2008). Psychological Symptoms. *Journal of Palliative Medicine, 22,* 229–238.

43. Papadatou, D., Bluebond-Langner, M., & Goldman, A. (2011). The Team. In J. Wolfe, P.S. Hinds, & B.M. Sourkes (Eds.), *Textbook of Interdisciplinary Pediatric Palliative Care* (pp. 55–63). Philadelphia: Elsevier Saunders.

44. Pediatric Palliative Care. (2012). Alexandria, VA: National Hospice and Palliative Care Organization. Perinatal Hospice: A gift of time. www.perinatallhospice.org. (accessed October 2009).

45. Society of Pediatric Nursing. Scope and Standards of Practice. July 2008..

46. Hospice and Palliative Nursing Association. (2013). About Us and Certification Info. hpna.org. Retrieved July 29, 2013 from http://www.hpna.org/Default2.aspx

47. Sumner, L., Kavanaugh, K., & Moro, T. (2006). Extending palliative care into pregnancy and the immediate newborn period: The state of the practice of perinatal palliative care. *Journal of Perinatal Neonatal Nursing, 20*(1), 113–116.

48. St Christopher's Hospice. (2013). Dame Cicely Saunders. stchristophers.org. Retrieved June 30, 2013, from http://www.stchristophers.org.uk/about/damecicelysaunder.

49. Vern-Gross, T. (2011). Establishing communication within the field of pediatric oncology: A palliative care approach. *Current Problems in Cancer, 35*(6), 337–350. doi: 10.1016/j.currproblcancer.2011.10.008.

50. Viola, D., Leven, D.C., & LePere, J.C. (2009). End-of-life care: An interdisciplinary perspective. *American Journal of Hospice and Palliliative Medicine, 26*(2), 75–77.

51. Weise, K., Levetown, M., Tuttle, C., & Liben, S. (2011). Palliative care in the pediatric intensive care setting. In B.S. Carter, M. Levetown, & S.E. Friebert (Eds.), *Palliative Care for Infants, Children, and Adolescents: A Practical Handbook* (pp. 387–413). Baltimore: The Johns Hopkins University Press.

52. Wolfe, J., Hinds, P.S., & Sourkes, B.M. (2011). The Language of Pediatric Palliative Care. In J. Wolfe, P.S. Hinds, & B.M. Sourkes (Eds.), *Textbook of Interdisciplinary Pediatric Palliative Care* (pp. 3–6). Philadelphia: Elsevier Saunders.

53. World Health Organization. (2002). Resources to Develop and Enhance Pediatric Palliative Palliative Care Services. WHO.int. Retrieved July 28, 2013, from whocancerpain.wisc.edu/old_site/eng/16_3-4/resources.html.

54. World Health Organization (1998). WHO definition of pediatric palliative care. WHO.int. Retrieved July 28, 2013, from http://www.who.int/cancer/palliative/definition/en/.

CHAPTER 57

Pediatric care

Transitioning goals of care in the emergency department, intensive care unit, and in between

Barbara Jones, Marcia Levetown, and Melody Brown Hellsten

> Be compassionate and ask how parents are. Don't fall into that detached type of working. Parents need to feel that people really care, not that it's just a job. The people at the hospital who allowed themselves to have genuine feelings helped me the most.
>
> Parent of deceased child, interviewed in Meyer et al.[1]

Key points

♦ Most children who die experience acute, unexpected death.

♦ Attention to the grieving family and organized bereavement programs can improve the outcome of emergency department (ED) deaths.

♦ Chronically ill children also often die in the intensive care unit (ICU); effective advance care planning (ACP), often beginning in the ICU and involving the child when possible, can prevent this.

♦ Compassionate, respectful, effective, consistent, bidirectional communication is a high priority for families of children who die in the ICU.

♦ Parents need to maintain a parenting role when their child is ill, even during invasive procedures and cardiopulmonary resuscitation (CPR).

♦ Parents need acknowledgment of their love and efforts and assistance with their spiritual needs.

♦ Clarity of facts and ethical principles among family and staff enables good medical decision-making and prevents regrets.

♦ The vast majority of children die after forgoing ICU interventions; this event can be transformed into a celebration of life.

♦ Grief and bereavement of family and staff must be addressed; clear evidence about effective interventions is lacking.

♦ Autopsies and postdeath conferences can be very reassuring to parents.

Palliative care is comprehensive, transdisciplinary care focused on promoting the maximal quality of life for patients living with a life-threatening illness and for their families.[2] It can and should occur from the earliest recognition of a life-threatening condition and can be concurrent with efforts to prolong life.[3,4] Palliative care is as applicable in the ED[5] and in the ICU setting[6-8] as it is in the home.[9,10] This is a critically important issue for children who die, since the vast majority of childhood deaths still occur in an ICU setting.[11,12]

Scrupulous attention to communication, symptom control, social support for the family and patient, and grief management have not been a traditional focus of healthcare delivery or training for emergency and critical care personnel.[13,14] Working together in effective interdisciplinary teams, learning new ways of communicating, using protocols where appropriate, and new tools for patient and family assessment, can assist professionals with meeting these patients' and their families' needs for a peaceful, family-centered death.[15] Efforts are being made to improve pediatric palliative care in the PICU and ED, including enhanced coordination, communication, collaboration, family-centered care, and bereavement outreach.[11,16-18] Specific suggestions for family-centered and palliative care in the ED and ICU have been published.[5-7,19] All members of the transdisciplinary healthcare team can and should play a key role in effecting this philosophy of care. Although individuals and families differ in the details and nuances of their conception of a good death, common themes emerge[20-23] (see Box 57.1).

Given that few children ill enough to be in the ICU can participate in the discussion, research has centered primarily on the needs of their families.

Epidemiology of pediatric death

Approximately 48,000 children die annually in the United States.[24] Infants (children under age 1 year), who account for close to 50% of childhood deaths, die primarily of congenital defects and

- Clear, honest, and easily accessible information provided throughout the illness
- Anticipatory guidance to limit suffering
- Compassion
- Symptom control
- Social support
- Support for parents to maintain a significant parenting role
- Unfettered access to the ill child
- Spiritual support
- Adequate space and means for self-care
- Sibling needs assessment and assistance
- Bereavement care and contact by healthcare providers

prematurity; however, sudden infant death syndrome (SIDS) and trauma (including unintentional injury and homicide) account for 13% of infant deaths.[25] For children age 1 year to 24 years, 65% of deaths are the result of trauma, while the remaining 35% are the result of cancer, congenital anomalies, infection, and metabolic defects.[25] Traumatic injury and unexpected overwhelming illness occurring in previously healthy children usually call for initial resuscitative measures provided in ED and ICU settings; many of these children may unavoidably die there, too. In fact, 20% of childhood deaths are declared in the ED each year,[5] whereas 4.6% of pediatric ICU and 10% to 20% of trauma ICU admissions end in death, together accounting for 40%–90% of childhood deaths.[8,26] Consideration of palliative care issues must therefore be a part of the care plan for critically ill or injured children at admission to the ED and the PICU, as well as at discharge if the child survives.[5–7,27] Bereavement care for families, including siblings, is a critical but often neglected need when pediatric death occurs in acute care settings.[5–7,28]

Regardless of the etiology, anticipated or unanticipated illness or injury, the care of a critically ill or injured child should be family focused, while conveying fundamental respect and a culturally appropriate commitment to shared decision-making with the parent(s).[19] All dying children and their families require appropriate facilities, information, support, and involvement in care and decision-making.[5–7,28]

Palliative care considerations in the emergency department: acute, unexpected illness or injury

Children experiencing a life-threatening event can present to the ED either having been transported by their parents or by emergency medical system (EMS) providers after a potentially dramatic "on site" resuscitation effort. The initial scene in the ED is often one of controlled chaos, with all personnel attending to the assessment and stabilization of the child. Some of these children are trauma victims, benefiting from a thorough assessment, rapid intervention, and pain control before a prognosis can be determined. For the child arriving in full arrest, the overwhelmingly likely outcome is death, whether in the ED or in the ICU a few days later.[29,30] In the absence of severe trauma, intoxication, or congenital heart disease, primary cardiac causes of arrest among children are exceedingly rare. Thus, if cardiac arrest has occurred, either the child is irreversibly dying of multiorgan failure or has sustained prolonged hypoxemia; neither of these underlying causes of arrest is amenable to resuscitation with intact survival. Misperceptions of a high likelihood of good outcomes following resuscitation from cardiac arrest have been documented and must be addressed in the care of these children and their families.[31]

Needs of parents of suddenly ill/injured children in the emergency department

Assigning a professional to guide the parents from the moment of their arrival can facilitate communication, even given the severe time pressures of the ED.[32–34] This professional should greet the parents by name, introduce himself/herself and provide a card with his or her name and contact information. The family should be apprised of the child's situation, and the child should be referred to by name.[32] This guide should also address parents' practical needs, such as offering a blanket or water and assist to gather the family's supporters. An interpreter should be summoned immediately, if needed.[5]

Especially in the ED, parents of acutely injured children prefer to be given timely, accurate, and consistent information that is easy to understand.[5,32] Information provided should be frequent, clear, and responsive to family members' questions and concerns. Extended family members or friends can often help the parents sort through the information and help them know what to ask. Although "information" emphasizes content, the nuances of "communication," or the process by which information is exchanged, demands attention as well. All family members of critically ill or dying children need to feel respected and valued. Grief and worry under these extraordinarily stressful circumstances can be incapacitating. This is the context in which parents are often asked to make decisions that, when worded poorly, imply choices between life and death; it may also be the context of their experience of the last hours with their child. Communication should ideally empower and strengthen parents' roles rather than marginalize them or imply they are outsiders in the circle of care for their child. In addition to frequent updates, nonverbal communication including eye contact and body language are the means by which the values of family-centered care are often expressed.[32,33]

Parents need to be given the opportunity to be with their child even when he or she is undergoing cardiopulmonary resuscitation or other invasive procedures.[5] Recent studies validate that parents can be present without disrupting the care process (see Box 57.2[35] for guidelines) and that their bereavement outcomes are enhanced when given this opportunity.[36] However, physicians and nurses express a wide range of opinions and comfort levels with family presence during resuscitation.[37] Written policies and staff education are needed to translate the capacity for family presence during procedures into a reality.[37,38]

Gradual disclosure of the child's condition enables the parents to better absorb the information that the child is likely to die or has died. Although it is generally recommended that the attending physician should be responsible for the disclosure of death, a study of parent preference found that parents preferred someone who is

Box 57.2 Consensus recommendations for family presence during invasive procedures and cardiopulmonary resuscitation

1. Consider family presence (FP) as an option for all families during pediatric procedures and CPR.

2. Offer FP as an option when the child's care will not be interrupted and after an assessment of the parents for:

   Combative and threatening behavior

   Extreme emotional volatility

   Behaviors consistent with intoxication or altered mental status

   Disagreement among family members

   Threat to the safety of the healthcare team

3. If family is not provided with the option for FP, document the reasons why FP was not offered.

4. Consider the safety of the healthcare team at all times.

5. In-hospital transport and transfer settings should have written policies and procedures for FP; these should include but not be limited to:

   Definition of a facilitator

   Definition of family member, legal guardian, etc.

   Definition of procedure

   Preparation of the family, including explanations, descriptions, and role of the family

   Process of escorting the family in and out of the treatment room

   Handling disagreements

   Providing support for the staff

6. Healthcare policies regarding FP should undergo legal review.

7. Educate all healthcare providers:

   Include education in FP in all core curricula for healthcare providers at all levels.

   Include this education also in healthcare settings as part of hospital orientation.

Source: Henderson and Knapp (2006), reference 35, used with permission.

knowledgeable and compassionate; they were unconcerned about the individual's title.[11] The child's usual care providers should be notified of the death as well, particularly the primary care pediatrician, who should be alerted to closely monitor the well-being of siblings in the aftermath of death.[5,11,39]

Emergency physicians typically have little to no training in the disclosure of death to a child's parents, and, not surprisingly, they find this activity to be one of the most stressful aspects of their jobs.[40] The stakes are high; every word said that day will linger in the parents' memories for the remainder of their lives, profoundly impacting their adaptation to the death. It is for this reason that the American Trauma Society has developed a program called "Second Trauma," providing interdisciplinary training on

compassionate death disclosure (www.amtrauma.org). In addition, many first responder courses now incorporate teaching about managing death and grief.[5]

When a child dies in the ED, his/her parents may prefer to be invited to be with their child's body in a private setting for as long as they need to stay; they often wish to bathe and rock or hold the child's body. This may be difficult to accommodate in the ED, but can have a tremendously beneficial effect on the family's recovery.[5,32] Ideally, the body will be cleaned up and fresh linens will be placed around it, with any disfiguring or gaping wounds covered, prior to inviting the parents to hold the child. Having the opportunity to speak with a chaplain and social worker at this time is often greatly appreciated. Even more importantly, parents need to understand the sequence of events, have their questions answered, and have supportive witnesses to their own and their child's experience.[41] Parents often want a physical memento of their child, such as a lock of hair, a mold of the child's hand, or their child's hospital bracelet and clothing.[5] Some families appreciate being assured that the child's body will not be left alone until the funeral director or coroner comes to retrieve it.

Sudden, unexpected deaths are generally coroner's cases. In some instances, there may be a criminal investigation. This circumstance may prevent the removal of medical equipment from the child's body. It is important to explain these facts to the parents and to explain the necessity and potential benefits of autopsy.[5] Autopsy is further discussed later in this chapter.

If there is the potential that the child died from neglect or abuse, this must be investigated. Sometimes death is the result of intentional abuse by the parents or caregivers. Sometimes parents do not intend to harm their child, but are ignorant of how easy it is to severely injure a child, or they may have poor impulse control. Most of the time, even if they caused the child's death, the parents did not intend to do so. They are hurting too, and their grief is all the more complex because of these factors. It may be difficult for nurses and other healthcare professionals to reach out to parents who are suspected of having contributed to the child's death. Nonjudgmental support from the healthcare team may help them begin to heal.

Sudden, unexpected death produces a high risk of complicated bereavement, regardless of the cause of death.[42,43] Parental grief commonly results in difficulty returning to work, severe anxiety, and depression.[5,11,19] It is therefore important to provide a structured bereavement program for such families, including the opportunity to review the events of that day and to understand the autopsy results, which are generally available several weeks after the death.[5] Short- and long-term interventions are called for and should address the needs of siblings as a priority.[42] At a minimum, a condolence card and a list of local grief resources should be provided.[44] Bereaved parents appreciate a phone call from direct care providers as well.[45]

Children with chronic life-threatening conditions and the Intensive Care Unit

Unfortunately, even children with chronic illnesses and anticipated deaths most often die in the ICU.[11,12] This is less often a result of the circumstances of the death than to the lack of effective anticipatory guidance and ACP,[21,46] largely related to perceptions of an uncertain prognosis (Figure 57.1).[13,14]

Ideally, the patient and family facing a chronic, progressive, and ultimately fatal illness would be provided information gradually

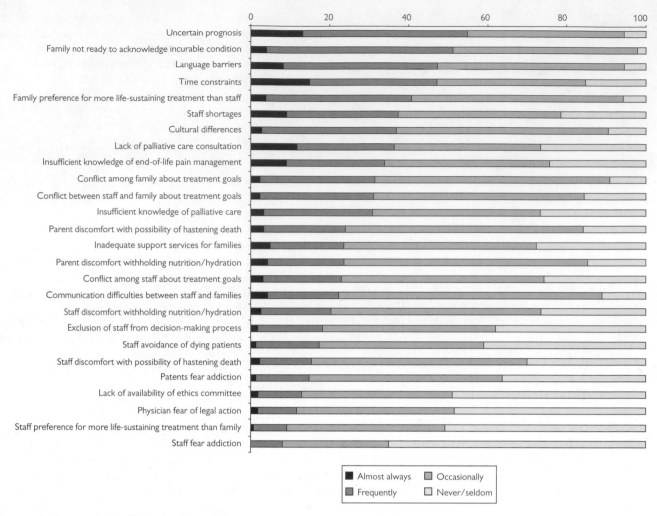

Figure 57.1 Barriers to pediatric palliative care. Source: Reference 14.

and recurrently, in an outpatient setting, tailored to the child's particular condition and the family's value system, orchestrated by a long-standing primary care or specialty physician.[2,47] Families need to understand the anticipated trajectory of the child's chronic condition and its associated symptoms; the interventions available for life-extension, their likely outcomes, benefits and burdens; the likely causes of death; the fact that symptoms can and will be controlled, regardless of the goals of care; and, most importantly, that that they will not be abandoned.[2,20,48] Preemptive discussions when the child is stable can enable the child to contribute to the discussion and aid in developing the family's preferences for care at the end of life and an associated coordinated plan of care, facilitating improved outcomes for these children and their families.[47] Parents have stated that the opportunity for ACP provides them with comfort and assurance that their child received proper care.[20,48a] Unfortunately, these conversations occur infrequently, leaving the burden to ICU personnel who have just met this chronically and now critically ill child. Crises are not the ideal time to ensure thoughtful decisions based on long-held values; nevertheless, patience and compassion can frequently lead to good outcomes.[8,11,40] Nurses often play a leading role in initiating such discussions. Ideally, the patient's medical home should be contacted to facilitate the most appropriate care plan.[17] Such shared decision-making leads to lower cost of care, fewer hospitalizations, and fewer ICU deaths.[49]

In approaching parents and children about considering limitations of medical intervention now or at a future date, it is important to understand that parents need to feel that they have done everything that is "appropriate," that they have been good, brave, and loving parents, and that the child has "been a fighter." Parents express the overt desire to be seen as a "good parent" to their critically ill or dying child.[50,51] This desire to be seen as a "good parent" can influence parental decision-making and actions. Their efforts and their concern must be acknowledged overtly.[22]

> It was terribly important for us to do exactly what was right and necessary to help our daughter. Our nurse and social worker made us feel that we WERE, in fact, doing everything in our power to take care of our daughter.
>
> *Kathleen and James Bula, parents*[52]

Table 57.1 provides suggestions regarding how to begin this discussion in the setting of a stable period of a life-threatening condition. Additional advice is found in Mack and Wolfe, 2006.[53]

Continuity and coordination of care needs

Parents need to know what care venues are available to them in the community and how to access them to avoid recurrent, no-longer-beneficial ICU admissions in the setting of a chronic,

Table 57.1 Communicating with children and families about integrating palliative care

Beginning the conversation	"What is your understanding of what is ahead for your child?"
	"Would it be helpful to talk about how his or her disease may affect him or her in the months and years ahead?"
	"As you think about what is ahead for your child, what would you like to talk about with me? What information can I give you that would be helpful to you?"
Introducing the possibility of death	"I am hoping that we will be able to control the disease, but I am worried that this time we may not be successful."
	"Although we do not know for certain what will happen for your child, I do not expect that your child will live a long and healthy life. Most children with this disease eventually die because of the disease."
	"I have been noticing that your child seems to be sick more and more often. I have been hoping that we would be able to make him or her better, but I am worried that his or her illness has become more difficult to control and that soon we will not be able to help him or her to get over these illnesses. If that is the case, he or she could die of his or her disease."
Eliciting goals of care	"As you think about your child's illness, what are your hopes?"
	"As you think about your child's illness, what are your worries?"
	"As you think about your child's illness, what is most important to you right now?"
	"You mentioned that what is most important to you is that your child be cured of his or her disease. I am hoping for that too. But I would also like to know more about your hopes and goals for your child's care if the time comes when a cure is not possible."
Introducing palliation	"Although I hope that we can control your child's disease for as long as possible, at the same time I am hoping that he/she feels as good as possible each day."
	"Although it is unlikely that this treatment will cure your child's disease, it may help him or her to feel better and possibly to live longer."
Talking about what to expect	"Would it be helpful to talk about what to expect as your child's illness gets worse?"
	"Although we cannot predict exactly what will happen to your child, most children with this disease eventually have [difficulty breathing]. If that happens to your child, our goal will be to help him or her feel as comfortable as possible. We can use medications to help control his or her discomfort."
Talking to children	"What are you looking forward to most of all?"
	"Is there anything that is worrying you or making you feel afraid?"
	"Is there anything about how you are feeling that is making you feel worried or afraid?"

Source: Mack and Wolfe (2006), reference 53.

life-limiting condition.[2,18] Children with terminal conditions and their families often want spiritual consultation and guidance, since it is very hard to understand why so tragic a thing as a child's death has to occur.[54,55] Above all, children and their families want to feel valued as individuals, with the awesomeness of the impending death duly noted and the opportunity for healing and growth at the end of life to be realized to the greatest extent possible. If end-of-life care is properly provided, fewer children with chronic, life-threatening conditions will die in the ICU, but instead will die in a setting that they or their family prefer.[21] Accurate information increases the likelihood of a decision to forgo CPR.[40] Avoidable ICU deaths are taxing to the patient and family as well as the ICU personnel, who often begin to ask, "Are we doing this *to* the child or *for* the child?."[17,54]

Therapies that are not consistent with the child's and family's goals or that will not work given the child's condition should not be offered to children who have experienced chronic, progressive illness. In addition, misperceptions about the effectiveness of CPR in life-threatening conditions must be proactively addressed.[56] Proposals to forgo medical interventions should be presented with justifications and as a recommendation, not a choice for the family to make alone. Importantly, when suggesting what should no longer be done, describe what will be added or maintained to enhance the child's and family's quality of life. Most important are the promises to care, to aggressively control symptoms, to be available, to assist (as a transdisciplinary team) in the arrangement of visits of family and friends, to facilitate the observation of important rituals, to provide spiritual guidance or affirmation (when desired), and to transfer to alternate care settings (according to the patient's condition and the child's and family's wishes).[2,18,28] One suggested phrase that captures the essence of intensified caring with new goals is: "We will help your child live to his fullest to the very last moment, regardless of when that is. His comfort and yours are our top priority."

Child participation in decision-making

Most state advance directive laws do not specifically mention children. Although there is no legal mandate to address the issues of prognosis or potential future medical interventions and their expected benefits and burdens with chronically ill children, the intent of advance directives applies equally to children with decision-making capacity as it does to adults. Developing advance directives for children ensures that the wrenching decision-making process is well considered and that the resulting care plan is enacted when the child's inevitable deterioration occurs, preventing an unwelcome ICU admission.[40] Families state that ACP for their children provides them peace and hope,[21] enabling them to decide based on the children's best interests and to include the child's perspective where possible.[57,58] It is recommended that the discussion be a longitudinal process, initiated early after the onset or discovery of life-threatening illness, maintained throughout the course of a child's illness as the family's priorities, experience and expectations change and then documented in writing.[47]

Advance care planning can prevent ED and ICU deaths for children who prefer to die at home, but ACP frequently is deferred until late in the disease or illness trajectory. Durall et al.[59] found that while 92% of providers believed that ACP should happen early or during moments of stability, 60% indicated that those conversations were more likely to occur when death was imminent or a crisis was occurring. Whenever possible, the knowing child (who may be as young as 3 years if he or she has been chronically ill) should have a voice in the discussion of the goals of medical intervention.[58] A father illustrates the importance of the child's voice well: "I think it makes it a little bit easier if they understand. In [my child's] case, he fully understands what's taking place, what's going on in his life, what's happening with his heart, and he knows that it's failing. My son says 'if I can't be me, then let me go.'"[60(p. 515)] His wife advised that all chronically ill children be involved in their own life-and-death decisions, suggesting that small amounts of information along the way facilitated good decision-making. When the child cannot be involved, the impact of parental guilt ("I can't let my child go—it would mean I failed as a parent.") and family suffering on the decision-making process should be frankly discussed.[60] Reminding parents of their obligation to decide in their child's best interests and reassuring them that letting go is a loving decision can be helpful.

In states with out-of-hospital do-not-resuscitate (DNR) laws, assuring that these forms are appropriately executed (if the family chooses this option), that the medical home physician and local EMS are involved or at least notified, and that hospice care is arranged can be very helpful to families. These activities increase the likelihood that the child will die at home, where most children and adults would prefer to die.[21]

Children and adolescents can and should be involved in end-of-life planning, and there are resources such as *My Wishes* and *Voicing My Choices* available to assist healthcare providers and family members in having these conversations with patients.[57,61,62]

In the ICU or ED, when the chronically ill child is not responding to stabilization or resuscitative efforts, the parents are often asked, "Do you want us to do 'everything'?" This question does not fully encompass the possible benefits and burdens or probable outcomes of potential interventions. From the parent's perspective, there is no reasonable answer to this question but "Yes!" However, for informed consent to occur, the goals and the understanding of likely outcomes must be discussed and aligned before proceeding. To the physician, "everything" too often means everything to prolong survival, regardless of the quality of life.[39] For parents, other goals generally take precedence.[21,54] If the child's condition is stabilized and symptoms are aggressively controlled, more rational decision-making can take place. The terms used to discuss end-of-life planning and decisions are often ambiguous and do not enable informed consent.[2] The family could, for example, choose mechanical ventilation for respiratory distress or may prefer comfort management outside the ICU if extended survival is unlikely or is unduly burdensome for the child. Common medical colloquialisms are often misinterpreted by families. Table 57.2 provides suggested phraseology to ensure clear communication and to prevent perceptions of abandonment.

Death related to chronic, progressive illness: issues relevant to Emergency Department and Intensive Care Unit personnel

Although communicating news regarding the terminal phase of chronic disease is difficult and stressful for everyone, being uninformed of the severity of the situation is even more stressful for patients and families. One of the most common complaints of patients and families is the lack of accurate and clearly communicated information.[2,6,17,54] Done well, disclosure of the prognosis associated with a chronic condition often provides confirmation for families of what was already suspected, frequently resulting in relief and reduction of anxiety.[2,54,63]

Suggestions for discussing a poor prognosis in a way that is sensitive to the needs of the child and family, as well as the medical caregivers, are found in Box 57.3. Unfortunately, even when advance directives have been thoughtfully crafted and executed, there are rarely mechanisms in place to ensure these decisions are honored. In addition, without reinforcement, parents may feel emotionally unprepared to follow through with their decisions to limit medical intervention. All too often, when the child begins to have the predicted deterioration, symptoms are inadequately controlled because no palliative care plan is in place and the patient appears in the emergency room *in extremis*.

Patient and family needs in the Intensive Care Unit

Entering an ICU or ED is a frightening experience for both the child and family, regardless of the presenting problem, prognosis, or treatment plan. The environment of care significantly impacts the ability of families to cope, particularly if the child dies.[6,11,28,54] Emergency department and critical care providers must strive to remember that the experience is new and often terrifying for children and families. Interventions to alleviate this type of suffering can improve the immediate experience of the child and the long-term outcomes for the parent.[5,17] Meert et al.[28] described several environmental needs of parents (see Box 57.4).

High levels of posttraumatic stress disorder (PTSD) have been demonstrated among family members of ICU patients.[64,65] Providing even minimal information regarding how an ICU works, identifying the personnel involved and their functions, and teaching families how to access information has a dramatically beneficial effect. A simple explanatory brochure can lower ICU family PTSD rates by 50%.[66] In addition, support and honest communication are important interventions. Compared with physicians, nurses are significantly less likely to agree that families are well-informed and that ethical issues are well discussed when assessing actual practice in their ICU.[17] More collaborative education and regular case review on bioethical issues are needed as part of standard practice in the ICU.[16]

Table 57.2 Methods of communicating sensitive healthcare information and perceptions of communication

Usual method of communicating message	How the usual communication may be perceived	Alternative method of communicating message
"Do you want us to do CPR?"	"CPR would work if you would allow us to do it"	"Tell me what you know about CPR. CPR is most helpful for patients who are relatively healthy, and even then, only 1 of 3 patients survives. Many of Lisa's organs are not working. As you know, she is getting dialysis to clean her blood like her kidneys, would have a breathing machine for her lungs, and medicine to keep her blood pressure up. If her heart were to stop, it would not be because there is a problem with her heart (it is fine), but it would be because she is dying. All of our hearts stop when we die. So pumping on her heart, or 'doing CPR' will not make her better. On the other hand, while I would recommend not doing CPR, I am not recommending stopping any other treatment she is receiving at this time. There is still a chance that she may get better. Let's hope for the best, but also plan for the worst. We will need to keep a close watch on her and keep you up to date on how she is doing. Do you have any questions? Let's talk again later today so I can update you. Is there anyone else I need to talk to?"
"Let's stop heroic treatment."	"We will provide less than optimal care." (What is heroic about performing invasive, painful, costly, nonbeneficial care?)	"At this time, I think the most heroic thing we can do is to understand how sick Jamal is and stop treatments that are not working for him. I think we should do all we can to ensure his comfort and yours, make sure there are no missed opportunities, and ensure we properly celebrate his life. I will follow your lead on this. Some ideas that have helped other families include getting him home with help for you if you wish, or you may choose to have his friends and your family come here instead and have a party; you can bring his clothes so that he will look like himself, bring in his music or a photo album and relive some of your best memories of him, make a mold of his hand so that you will always have his hand to hold, or anything else that would be a proper celebration of his life."
"Let's stop aggressive treatment."	"We will not be attentive to his needs, including symptom distress and need for comfort."	"We will do all we can to ensure he is as comfortable as possible."
"Aiesha has failed the treatment."	"The patient is the cause of the problem."	"We have tried all the proven treatments and even some experimental ones for Aiesha. Unfortunately, we did not get the results we had hoped for. I wish it were different!"
"We are recommending withdrawal of care for Marisa."	"We are going to abandon her and you."	"Marisa is too ill to get better. We need to refocus our efforts on making the most of the time she has left."
"There is nothing more we can do for Adam."	"We will allow him to suffer, we do not care about him, we only care about fighting the disease."	"We need to change the goals of our care for Adam. At this point we clearly cannot cure him, but that does not mean we can't help him and your family."
"Johnny is not strong enough to keep going."	"Johnny is weak."	"Johnny is a strong boy and he has fought hard with us to beat his disease. Unfortunately, as much as we wish we could, we cannot cure Johnny. At this point, we are hurting him rather than helping, giving him side effects, and keeping him from being at home or taking a trip, or whatever he really wants to do with the time he has left."
"We will make it so Thuy does not suffer."	"We are going to kill Thuy."	"We will do everything we can to make Thuy comfortable."
"We need to stop active treatment for Dwayne."	"We will not take care of him at all."	"The goal of curing Dwayne's disease, despite the best efforts of a lot of smart and hard-working people, is no longer possible. We are so sorry and wish that that were different! I have cared for many children who are as sick as your son. It is very hard on all of us, especially you, his parents and family when the treatments do not work as we had hoped. Many parents like you have agreed to stop efforts to cure when they are not working, as difficult as that is. Would you like me to put you in touch with some of the other parents who have been through this too?"
"Do you want us to stop Bobby's treatment?"	"You are the final arbiter of your child's death."	"Bobby is lucky to have such excellent, loving and selfless parents. I know this is hard; we will get through it together. I am glad you agree with our recommendations to change the goals of care to better meet Bobby's needs. I will let my team know what we have decided."
"I am glad you agree. Will you sign Juan's do-not-resuscitate order?"	"You are signing his death warrant."	"There is no surgery, no medicine, and all the love you clearly feel for Juan will not make him better, he is just too sick. I wish it were different." (Silence) "I will change his orders to make sure he only gets tests and treatments that can help him now."

CPR indicates cardiopulmonary resuscitation.

Source: Levetown (2008), reference 40. Used with permission.

Box 57.3 Having difficult discussions

1. Provide a "warning shot" or an introductory sentence before presenting the distressing information: "I am sorry that I have some bad news to tell you."

2. Provide an opportunity for supportive friends or family to be present when the information is shared: "Would you like to call someone to be with you when we talk?"

3. Tell the news in a private setting, with the physician, nurse, and social worker present. Bring the family (generally parents without the child first, depending on relationships and preferences) to a private conference room rather than speaking to them in the waiting room or the hall. Bring tissues. If appropriate and desired by the family, assist them in telling their children (patient and siblings) afterward.

4. Sit down near the family, not across a table. Do not stand. Children and families want to be on an even plane with their caregivers. Look the family members in the eye to engender trust unless this is culturally undesirable. Ask them to tell you about their child and about any consistent values of the child and about the things that give him or her pleasure. Ask how much they want to know about his or her medical condition and prognosis. Ask them what they understand is happening. Clarify misconceptions, particularly about the cause of the problem, and attempt to assuage any guilt that may derive from having an inherited or developmental problem ("You did not wish for your child to have this") or from trauma or other causes. Then, let them know this news is difficult for you as well. Nurses can help guide the physician to present the truth in a jargon-free manner that is consistent with the family's educational level, sophistication, and stated desire for knowledge. Ask the family to explain what they understood was said. Clarify misconceptions. Then, solicit additional questions.

5. Be unhurried. If there is only a limited time available for the physician, let the family know: "I'm sorry the doctor only has 15 minutes now, but I will stay with you and answer any questions I can, and the doctor will be back later this afternoon to answer anything I can't and to update you." Don't look at your watch. Have the charge nurse or another nurse care for your patients while you sit with the family. Remind the other team members to give their beepers to someone else during the family meeting, when possible; otherwise, switch the beepers to vibrate mode.

6. Ideally, members of the multidisciplinary team participate as full members during the family conference.[33,48] The bedside nurse, chaplain, and social worker benefit from hearing the physician-family interaction. They can solicit questions, clarify misconceptions during the meeting and after the physician leaves, and address other facets of the patient's situation that the conversation with the physician evokes. Team members can also give the physician feedback regarding his or her communication with the patient and family, such as words they did not understand, and can help the physician address any unresolved issues at the next meeting. This technique requires interdisciplinary respect and cooperation, which are essential to successful, comprehensive end-of-life care; it prevents divisive misunderstandings between disciplines regarding suspected coercion or other undesirable communication.

7. Bring trainees to the family meeting. This allows the assigned nursing or medical student and resident to learn from directly observing the interdisciplinary critical care team, as well as the patient and family responses. It keeps trainees informed so that unnecessary and often damaging miscommunications do not occur. Trainees often get lost in the minutiae of the patient's laboratory values and vital signs and may unwittingly provide contradictory information to the family. However, do not overwhelm the family with white coats—have trainees take turns attending family meetings.

8. Be specific. The physician should present the options, include a description of life-sustaining treatments, the child's current status, the chance of survival, the probability of full recovery (and the probability of significant disability), and the possible effects of the child's long-term survival on the family.

Box 57.4 Environmental needs of parents whose child is critically ill

1. Privacy and sufficient space

2. Easy access to the child, including during invasive procedures and CPR

3. Amenities enabling continuous access to the child: nearby sleeping and bathing accommodations, vending machines or other food services; a room to gather supporters in large numbers; comfortable seating in the child's room

4. Access to a phone when cell phones are not allowed

5. A clean, secure environment of care for their child and themselves

6. Secure storage

7. Need for assurance that everything that can be done to help is being done

8. Information resources, such as information on how to tell others your child has died

---

Weidner and colleagues[67] found that parents prioritize the following seven dimensions of pediatric end-of-life care:

- Respect for the family's role
- Comfort
- Spiritual care
- Access to care and resources
- Communication
- Support for parental decision-making
- Caring/humanism in providers

Needs of the child in the Intensive Care Unit

In addition to being included in ACP and having meticulous symptom control, ill children also benefit from having a member of the care team attend specifically to his or her emotional needs. Ideally, the critical care unit has a social worker or child-life specialist who is immediately accessible and able to provide critical assessment, support, distraction, and intervention for children who are alert and can participate. The benefits of this type of intervention can be seen in the following case example.

Case study

A 10-year-old girl with leukemia

Josephine, a 10-year-old African-American girl with recurrent acute myelogenous leukemia, was transferred to the pediatric ICU for a bone marrow biopsy. Because Josephine was familiar with the procedure, she was frightened. The physicians and nurses determined that it would be better to allow her time to voice her concerns before beginning the procedure. The social worker encouraged her to draw a picture of her body and indicate what she was feeling. Josephine interpreted "feelings" to represent both physical and emotional reactions, describing pain in her legs and stomach, feeling sad in her mind and confused in her intestines. She also noted that her eyes could not see. On probing, she said she could not see what her future would hold. As a result of this discussion, the medical staff understood the need to describe in more detail why the biopsy was necessary, how the results would enable a treatment plan that would likely alleviate some of her pain and discussed her overall prognosis with her. Josephine began to feel calmer, feeling some control over what was happening to her. Respect for her concerns helped her trust her caregivers, enabling Josephine to receive the care she needed with less anxiety.

Although it is not always possible to delay a medical procedure in critical care, allowing time for the child to express feelings and have questions answered will reduce the natural anxiety associated with frightening or painful procedures, resulting in better outcomes.

Compassionate, effective, consistent, bidirectional communication with the family and the patient is critical to providing care and to preventing suffering

Research on the needs and priorities of families whose child died in the ICU has found that effective and compassionate communication is of primary importance.[17,54] Parents need to retain the role of caregiver and protector of their child and to function within the context of the family unit, regardless of circumstance. Recent studies have demonstrated that the time of first discussions between medical staff and parents and definitive decision-making in the pediatric ICU (PICU) can vary from immediate to 19 days, with large variations between decision-making and actual withdrawal of ICU interventions.[68,69]

Truog et al.[70] reviewed the literature to determine evidence-based practice that will improve end-of-life care in the PICU. The six critical domains revealed were:

1. Support of the family unit;

2. Communication with the child and family about treatment goals and plans;

Table 57.3 Parents' priorities for pediatric palliative care

Honest and complete information	"What we cannot handle is not knowing what is going on."
Ready access to staff	"Set a regular time for office hours at the bedside."
Communication and care coordination	"There were too many doctors explaining things."
Emotional expression and support by staff	"People need to feel that people really care, not that it's just a job."
Preservation of the integrity of the parent-child relationship	"Show more sincere compassion for the parents' and child's needs."
Faith	"Prayer and the services of my rabbi."

Source: Meyer et al. (2006), reference 1, Table 2, used with permission.

3. Ethics and shared decision-making;

4. Relief of pain and other symptoms;

5. Continuity of care; and

6. Grief and bereavement support.

Meyer et al.[1] provided concrete examples of some of these domains of parents' preferences and priorities (see Table 57.3). Families want bidirectional communication that is timely, complete, compassionate, and consistent. Honest and accurate information is reassuring, even if it is bad news.[2,6,54]

> Things are just so unsettling that I think if you have an answer it's easier to deal with than not knowing.[39]

Information should be clearly and empathetically communicated to the family from the earliest meeting and followed by regular updates as the prognosis changes, even if the pace of change is very fast.[8] Parents want physicians to be accessible and to display a caring affect, to use lay language, and to speak at a pace in accordance with their ability to comprehend. Withholding prognostic information from parents can lead to false hopes and feelings of anger, betrayal, and distrust.[71]

Strategies for improving team communication

Nurses are often key professionals when it comes to communication with families in the ICU.[14] Being at the bedside, nurses often get to know the families and their concerns, values, and priorities well and can inform the best approach to meet the needs of each family. Participation of the bedside nurse in daily rounds and in family meetings improves continuity of care and consistency of information and communication. The information that nurses gather from patients and parents at the bedside is critically important to the entire team in understanding what the patient and family already know, what questions they have, and what further explanations or discussions are needed.[72] In addition, there is a need for excellent communication between nurses at shift change about what the family has been told and what they seem to understand. Parents often call at night to check on their children and are easily confused by conflicting messages. Strategies, such as primary nursing assignments and tools such as communication logs or a "goals of care" worksheet can improve overall communication and quality of care.[73]

Communication needs differ among families based on their education, personality, culture, experience, and expectations. The recommended way to ensure communication meets the needs of these families is to ask about their communication preferences—do you prefer one main communication director; do you prefer to hear everyone's opinion, even if there is disagreement; do you want to know any time there is a change; do you want to participate in rounds; do you prefer to have a translator present; do you want detailed information or the bigger conceptual picture?

Creative means to accommodate family communication needs may include appointments for communication, a bedside journal allowing asynchronous communication, Web-based technology including Skype, face time, e-mail, interdisciplinary family meetings, and short discussions in person or by phone when a change occurs.[55,63]

Effective communication with families

In complex environments like the ED and ICU, it is critical that members of the healthcare team also communicate effectively with each other, in order to avoid confusion and resulting distress.[15,74] Communicating in highly technical and emotional circumstances can be difficult. Factors such as the family's willingness to acknowledge or accept a potential prognosis, physician bias regarding the goals of care, the management of and tolerance for uncertainty, and the emotions of the healthcare professional and/or family all can create obstacles to open, honest communication regarding the child's condition and prognosis.[14,75] Positive communication styles are associated with being receptive to cues from patients and families, demonstrating genuine concern, moral responsibility, a caring presence, and dedication.[76,77] Many clinicians try to "shield" parents from bad news, as they are reluctant to "take away hope." However, Mack's[78,79] research has demonstrated that what parents define as hope differs from caregivers' perceptions. Parents hope for honest information that allows them to make the best decisions for and with their child and to have the capacity to ready themselves for the inevitable with the support of their loved ones[80] (for more information on communication techniques, see chapter 5).

End-of-life family conferences

Opportunities to improve end-of-life care have been identified in epidemiological and interventional studies.[74] End-of-life family conferences constitute the keystone around which excellent end-of-life care can be built. Ideally, all members of the interdisciplinary pediatric team will participate in the family conference.[14,15] Family conferences are important communication tools in the pediatric ICU that have the potential to improve care.[73]

Family conferences are formal, structured meetings between physicians, staff and family members. Guidelines for organizing these conferences take into account the specific needs of families, including reassurance that the patient's symptoms will be adequately managed. The purposes of family conferences is bidirectional communication, including honest, clear information about the patient's condition and associated treatment options and probable outcomes as well as a willingness of the care team to listen and respond to family members' concerns and emotions. Active listening promotes attention to patient and family preferences and facilitates effective shared decision-making based on the patient's actual prognosis, well-considered goals, and the construction of an associated plan of care. Such a plan allows the healthcare team and family to engage in continuous, compassionate, and technically proficient attention to the child's needs until death occurs.

Medical decision-making: shared facts and ethical principles enable good medical decision-making

Despite the benefits of formal family meetings, communication of difficult information is a process, not an event. Mutual respect of the healthcare team and family is essential for effective decision-making. This can be accomplished by encouraging patients and families share their story, concerns and preferences for care, listening without interruption, and clarifying areas of misunderstanding. Nonverbal cues such as eye contact, nodding and leaning in or touching as well as an attitude of humility and respect facilitate the development of trust. The team should then allow families to arrive at decisions in a time frame that is comfortable for them.

It is important to acknowledge family and patient concerns or potential conflicts with other healthcare professionals without indicting the colleague's competency or care. If errors in care or communication have occurred, acknowledge the errors and provide follow-up regarding the resolution for the patient and resultant approach to future patients.

Effective communication enables solicitation of families' concerns, emotional reactions, and values. Acknowledgment and validation of strong emotion is greatly appreciated by families, but is rarely offered. These ingredients allow rational decisions to be made based on the facts as well as the values of the child and his or her family, preventing regret and significant parental morbidity. Unfortunately, opportunities to communicate in this manner are often missed, particularly when strong emotions are present.[2,80]

Meert and colleagues[39] found the following elements of communication are valued by parents whose children are nearing death:

♦ Comprehensive and complete information

♦ Use of clear language and explanations

♦ Ease of access to caregivers and their explanations throughout the course of care

♦ Pacing of information. Soliciting parents' emotional responses and addressing their questions

♦ Consistency of information

♦ Honesty, lack of false hope

♦ Empathy as demonstrated by verbal, nonverbal, and affective communication

♦ Summary statements and next steps

Families of ICU patients have an increased risk of posttraumatic stress symptoms; some develop full-blown PTSD.[64,66] The risk was increased among families who felt that insufficient time was available for receiving information, who felt that information was incomplete or difficult to understand, who participated in end-of-life decision-making, and whose loved one died during the hospitalization.[64,66]

Time-limited trials

The patient's progress over the course of ICU care should be continuously reviewed with the patient (as able) and family. Monitoring the "big picture" of whether the patient is progressing along the hoped-for trajectory of improvement or whether he or she is deteriorating despite the best medical management provides real-time information to facilitate care planning and decision-making. Frequent updates, about the child's condition and reasonable medical interventions, help families avoid burdensome and unhelpful medical interventions and allow families to prepare for death as a likely outcome.[6-8] In time-limited trials, the team informs parents about the reasonable time frame to expect a response to treatment, discussing potential outcomes and associated choices in advance. There is an agreement to meet again after the interval has passed to discuss progress. This process provides the family time to adapt to the possible outcomes and to gather their supporters to hear the news with them, good or bad, and to have substantial support when making a determination of how to proceed.

Recommendations for the next clinical step should be presented based on the team's experience with similar patients, the goals and values of the patient and family, and the observations of patient and family members during the current conversation and over the course of hospitalization. The benefits and burdens (including prolongation of suffering) of each potential care option, the potential reversibility or irreversibility of the conditions being treated, the time frame for re-evaluation, the projected future quality of life, and the comfort measures available if the ICU interventions are curtailed or discontinued must be explained to the family in a manner they can understand.

When discussing the choice to forgo no-longer-beneficial medical interventions, the topic of current burdens of therapy as well as the probability of the hoped-for benefits must be clearly explained. Reassure the family that if ICU interventions are discontinued, the child will continue to receive attentive care for the relief of symptoms; describe the procedures to be undertaken, including the opportunities to observe important customs and rituals and the opportunities for visitation. Techniques to elicit family understanding, such as "teach back" enable truly informed consent.[81]

The benefits of stopping ED or ICU treatments can be presented as limiting the harm to and suffering of the child and enabling the loving presence of the family. When the option is inaccurately presented as "stopping care," it is, not surprisingly, usually rejected.[82] This shorthand phraseology is sometimes perceived as cruel and callous; patients and families fear abandonment above all else.[71,76,77] Word choice is critical. Some hospitals have begun to use AND or "Allow Natural Death" as a replacement or adjunct to DNR discussions. While there is no consensus on the use of "AND," it does provide another way to have compassionate discussions with families.[83] Stating a child died "from" the discontinuation of "life support" creates confusion for families and professionals alike. Ongoing misunderstanding (or a lack of understanding) of the bioethical tenets supporting the discontinuation of ICU interventions among even senior pediatric clinicians was recently documented.[11,39] The goals of care and the principles underlying them must be clear in everyone's mind before proceeding, in order to avoid inaccurate perceptions of wrongdoing which can create moral distress for critical care providers and family survivors.[16]

End-of-life decision-making

In most clinical situations, the justification to forgo disease-directed medical intervention in ICUs involves physician assessment of poor prognosis for survival rather than patient quality-of-life considerations.[5,14,39] Parents, however, make their decisions based on the child's quality of life, degree of pain and suffering, likelihood of improvement, and physician's recommendations, as well as the child's "will to live," knowledge of others' dying processes, and perceptions of the child's best interests.[22,71,84] Reassessing the goals of treatment only when the child is dying may deprive the patient and family of earlier choices to limit suffering rather than extend the duration of life at all costs. Children and their families often have preferences regarding the value of medical interventions. Their opinions are not knowable by the medical team a priori; they must be actively solicited.[71]

Consideration of suffering and future quality of life

Surrogates' (or parents') duties are to act on the child's wishes and in his or her best interests.[85,86] Healthcare practitioners should work closely with families to make the best decisions regarding continuation or termination of ICU interventions.[16] Thus, overriding any requests to terminate ICU interventions must be done with significant forethought and analysis. In addition, the motivation for requests to continue ICU interventions in the face of an extremely small likelihood of survival or a significantly poor quality of life must be explored fully. Guilt, fear and loss issues, in particular, should be examined:

♦ "What do you think caused his problems? You were away at work when the accident happened?"

♦ "Tell me about what has happened to your family as a result of your child's condition?"

♦ "It sounds like you've been through a lot. I wish I could make your child healthy and make it all okay again but, unfortunately, there are limits to what medicine can do. The best we can reasonably hope for, medically, is . . . . Does that change your perspective on treatment options? Our recommendation, based on all you've told us and our assessment of your child's condition is . . . ."

Eliciting and demonstrating respect for the family's and child's (where applicable) values can be helpful in resolving decisional dilemmas.

A child's[85] or surrogates' requests to stop ICU interventions must be taken seriously in order to determine current sources of suffering, eliminating them where possible, reducing them, or changing the goals of care as needed; the request may indeed signal it is time to focus on maximizing comfort, regardless of impact on life expectancy.[6] Suffering experienced by the child must play a much more prominent role in the decision-making process if maximal comfort and support are to be attained for a higher proportion of children who die.[13,14,21] The ICU physicians and nurses must be educated on ethical principles in medical practice, particularly on autonomy, beneficence, nonmaleficence, and the construct of benefits versus burdens in making and guiding decisions; there remains substantial ignorance on these issues, among even senior clinicians.[16] Personal biases regarding quality versus quantity of life, fears of litigation, and economic motivations should not play any role in decisions regarding the withdrawal of ICU interventions.[86]

Within practical limitations, the patient's comfort should be the primary determinant of the process of end-of-life care. In several studies, vasopressors were withheld first, oxygen next, and mechanical ventilation next. However, oxygen supplementation and extubation may be preferred and more comfortable, potentially providing the opportunity for a last goodbye. In addition, withholding antibiotics and allowing the peaceful death associated with sepsis, without a trip to the ICU, may be the most humane option available for some children. In other cases, forgoing nutrition may ease nausea, and forgoing hydration may decrease the discomfort of renal failure or congestive heart failure.[87] Obviously, much depends on the child's symptoms, the clinical situation, and the child's and family's values and preferences. Effecting a philosophical change among medical decision-makers to proactively solicit children's and families' perspectives may be attempted by educational intervention, although cultural changes within institutions and protocol-driven practice may have more promise.[16]

Forgoing no-longer-beneficial intensive care unit interventions: review of the patient care plan

After it has been determined that the child and family's primary goal is no longer simply the attempt to prolong life, because either the child's suffering is too great or the child will die no matter what more is done, the care plan must be reviewed in detail. The most probable mechanisms of death must be determined, possible symptoms can then be anticipated and a care plan created to address the child's comfort proactively. For example, if the child is likely to have seizures but cannot swallow, rectal or parenteral rapid-onset anticonvulsants should be written as a PRN order. It is not uncommon for the child to have several potential mechanisms for death; often, one route can be anticipated to be the most comfortable, such as dying from hyperkalemia or sepsis as opposed to hypoxemia. In attempting to enable the most comfortable dying process, kayexalate or dialysis as well as antibiotics might be discontinued, whereas oxygen supplementation might be continued. Developmentally appropriate explanations about the possible course of events should be given to the child and family unless they refuse this information. It is unwise to predict an exact time of death, but approximations (with significant margin for error—e.g., minutes to hours, hours to days, days to weeks) are helpful for the family to arrange for the child's other loved ones and friends to visit before or be present at death.[6,7,28]

All interventions that interfere with comfort or should be discontinued in favor of those aimed at promoting maximal comfort, function, and quality of life.[6,7] For example, laboratory tests are not designed to enhance comfort. In clinical practice, laboratory parameters, such as platelet counts, are sometimes monitored to "prevent" symptoms (such as bleeding) from arising. However, it is less intrusive to monitor the patient for clinical bleeding and treat if and when it arises, as desired. Medications that do not enhance comfort, including antibiotics, should be considered for discontinuation. Even feeding and IV fluids may interfere with comfort if the child has pulmonary edema, heart failure, or renal failure; a decrease in or cessation of these therapies may enhance the child's comfort.[6] Removal of no-longer-needed devices, including monitoring equipment, should also be considered.

Forgoing no-longer-beneficial critical care interventions

Forgoing mechanical ventilation precedes most ICU deaths, allowing patients to die more peacefully from their underlying conditions.[6,7] Though a common phenomenon, it remains uncomfortable for many critical care practitioners. Initiating a meeting of those involved in the care of the patient to review the choice and hear concerns, as well as to guide the care, is very helpful in minimizing distrust and maintaining cohesion among the staff.[15] The use of protocols that outline the ethical principles underlying such choices have been found to be helpful in guiding decision-making and management of the extubation by critical care physicians and nurses.[88]

Monitors, such as pulse oximeters, cardiorespiratory monitors, and the like should be removed in most cases.[6] They create physical barriers to being close, distract the family from attending to the child with their color displays and flashing lights, and emit distressing alarms that all have agreed not to respond to. They also create an excuse for caregivers to not enter the room. However, some families become so attached that removing these devices seems to them to be a form of abandonment and, in these few cases, removal should not be carried out. When a family elects to forgo treatments in anticipation of death, visitation restrictions and many of the usual rules should be reconsidered.[28] Maximization of opportunities to hold the child and even invitations to family members to climb in bed with the child should be facilitated. Letting the family bathe the child and dress him or her in clothing of the child's or family's choice is often helpful. Other requests should be honored if at all possible.

Engaging in family-centered rituals prior to forgoing critical care interventions can be helpful, allowing unhurried family time while the child is still alive. As the family is approaching readiness for extubation, they should be reminded about what changes they are likely to see in the child after extubation, making this difficult time easier. ("He may turn blue; we will treat this with morphine and oxygen if he looks uncomfortable. He may not breathe at all or may breathe comfortably for some time. His breathing may be noisy because his brain is not controlling the soft tissues in his throat. I do not know how long he will live, but I expect it will be on the order of (minutes, hours, days). I will stay with you until he is comfortable.") Positive thoughts about extubation are important to share as well. ("This will be the first time you see your daughter's beautiful face without tape and a tube interfering"; "I am giving you back your son as a child, not as a patient"; "You may be able to hear his voice for the first time in a while," depending on the age and circumstances of the child.)

Extubation technique

There is no single correct way to discontinue mechanical ventilation.[6,7] Although adult care practitioners most often wean the patient's ventilator settings and leave a "T tube" in place, it is not clear that this is what families prefer. Pediatric practitioners more often remove the tracheal tube. Although some practitioners premedicate prior to changing ventilator settings, others wait to see how the patient responds.[89,90] In a study of the concerns of parents whose child had cancer, regarding the last week of life, Pritchard[86] found that changes in consciousness were particularly disturbing. In another study, decision-making by parents of children in critical care settings was partially based on the parents' perceptions of the child's degree of suffering and "will to live".[60] It is best to understand the parents' hopes for the final minutes to hours of their child's life, to educate them about the potential likelihood of achieving them, and then make every attempt to honor their wishes. The goal of preventing any discomfort at all calls for preemptive sedation,[89,91] conflicting with a goal of a final goodbye. These considerations should be discussed in advance.

Transfer to alternative care settings

When children are acknowledged to be dying, it is common for extended family and loved ones to gather to support each other. Sometimes they may desire to perform rituals that are difficult to accommodate in the ICU setting. Thus, consideration of transferring to an alternate care setting may be helpful, even if it is only for a few hours.

If the child is anticipated to live for a few days once critical care interventions are discontinued, referral to hospice care in the home may be an option, particularly in the UK.[92] Usually a 1- to 2-day stay in the hospital to ensure "stability" and to provide family and hospice caregiver teaching is needed. Alternatively, if the child will have significant distress in his or her final days, or the child and/or family prefer to stay in the hospital, admission to the floor, or preferably a palliative care unit, may be the best plan.[17] However, an agreement to transfer out of the ICU must usually be predicated by an agreement to terminate the ventilator within hours of transfer. With the increase of pediatric palliative care programs in the United States and elsewhere, it is becoming more possible for providers to refer or collaborate with the palliative care service. As large a room as is needed to accommodate the child and his or her loved ones should be provided, if possible.[39]

Aggressive symptom management in the Emergency Department and Intensive Care Unit

For more in-depth explanations of the management of these symptoms, see Section II, "Symptom Assessment and Management." However, a few overarching principles deserve further mention.

Aggressive symptom control is a high priority for parents of children who die.[6] When critical care technologies are forgone, the most common symptom-distress risks are dyspnea, pain, and seizures.[6,7] Thus, meticulous care at the time of ventilator withdrawal, including the continuous presence of the physician and/ or nurse, and protocols for symptom management are key to the effective prevention or immediate management of symptom distress.[6,7] When attended to by a skilled interdisciplinary team that focuses on these issues as primary concerns, symptoms are usually successfully prevented or rapidly mitigated. It is helpful to most families to affirm their decision and to explain the possible events in advance of their occurrence. For example:

> You are a brave and loving family. You have recognized that Brandon will not survive, regardless of further treatments and have opted not to prolong his dying process, but, rather, enable a loving goodbye, surrounded by friends and family. This is probably the hardest thing you have ever done. Brandon is lucky you love him enough to do this for him. Do you have any concerns or questions I can address? (PAUSE) If not, let me go over the procedure for tomorrow. In order to keep Brandon comfortable, we will discontinue his IV fluids tonight so that he will breathe more comfortably. We will move him to the larger room in the morning. After your family and friends celebrate Brandon's life, when you and your family are ready, we will suction Brandon's breathing tube and then remove it from his windpipe. We will also stop the blood pressure medication. Brandon may breathe in a funny pattern—sometimes shallow and quick, sometimes like a yawn or hiccup, and sometimes not at all. He may also change color—he may become pale, red or even blue. We will stay with you; if he looks uncomfortable, we will give him medications every 5 minutes until he looks more comfortable according to you

and to me. I will not leave your side until he is looking as comfortable as possible.

Pain

> We told them she didn't do well on morphine. We saw the pain she was in. For 48 hours we kept telling them it wasn't helping. No matter how much morphine they'd give her, she was flopping around on the bed. So we stood there the whole time . . . she was moaning in pain. [Crying] Those are the images that are the most painful, that she had to suffer. We were helpless. I'm sure they thought what they were doing would work; I'm sure for most kids it works. But for her, it didn't. At that time, we felt we weren't being taken seriously. It's still the image we wake up thinking about.

> *Parent of deceased child, excerpted from Contro*[93]

Pain in the ED may be acute, related to trauma, procedures, or infections or may be related to exacerbations of chronic, painful conditions among children with complex medical illnesses. Age-appropriate assessment tools and evidence-based pain management approaches, including distraction, local anesthetics, oral analgesics, and sedation as appropriate should be employed to minimize the pain experience of children.[94]

Assessment and management of pain in the ICU setting is confounded by the likely use of sedative and paralytic agents if the child is intubated. A number of pain assessment scales are validated for the pediatric ICU patient, including the Premature Infant Pain Profile (PIPP), children's pain checklist, FLACC (Face, Legs, Activities, Cry, and Consolability) and COMFORT scales.[95] The Individualized Numeric Rating Scale can be used with children with severe cognitive impairment.[2] Primary nursing assignments facilitate symptom assessment, and parents or usual caregivers are crucial resources for pain assessment. According to the World Health Organization (WHO) pain management guidelines for children, severe pain, regardless of etiology, demands prompt treatment with a "strong opioid" such as morphine, hydromorphone (Dilaudid), fentanyl, or methadone.[96] In the vast majority of cases, pain can be rapidly controlled.[97,98] In the ICU and ED settings, parenteral administration of medications is most often indicated for moderate to severe pain.

The occurrence of pain is not well documented in the terminally ill PICU patient, but suspicion of pain must remain high, and presumptive treatment should occur if indications of pain are present. Where possible, pain needs to be categorized not only by severity, but also by character (burning, gnawing, throbbing, sharp, crampy), location and radiation, duration, continuous or intermittent nature, and precipitating and relieving factors. The quality and timing of the pain suggest the etiology of the pain and dictate the most efficacious treatment. This ideal is very difficult to achieve in young or developmentally disabled children and in sedated or intubated patients. An empirical judgment of the etiology and physiology of the pain often dictates the choice of intervention in the ICU setting.

Burning pain in a patient who received neurotoxic chemotherapy or antiretroviral agents is a sign of pain related to nerve injury (neuropathic pain). Another common source of neuropathic pain is chronic gastrointestinal pathology. Children with severe brain dysfunction also seem to have significant neuropathic visceral pain.[99,100] This pain is best treated with "adjuvant pain relievers" (medications most often used for other purposes, but which are effective in the relief of certain types of pain), such as tricyclic antidepressants and anticonvulsants, along with traditional pain-relieving agents. Some adjuvants require several days to achieve effectiveness, or may only be available as oral preparations. Thus, depending on the patient's circumstance, optimal pain management should also include nonpharmacological, surgical, and anesthetic techniques where indicated[101] and as well as traditional pain relievers, including opioids and transdermal agents such as lidocaine or clonidine patches, as appropriate.[97]

Concerns about addiction, a biopsychosocial phenomenon of craving a drug despite self-harm, are inappropriate in the ICU.[102] Around-the-clock (ATC) analgesics should be provided, particularly in the setting of surgery, multiple trauma, and recurrent procedures.[98]

Medications should be titrated to an acceptable level of pain control using acetaminophen or nonsteroidal antiinflammatory ATC dosing (unless contraindicated) in addition to opioids for more severe pain, opioids and local anesthetics for procedure-related pain, and adjuvant analgesics for neuropathic pain. "As needed" or PRN opioid doses should be ordered for the alleviation of breakthrough pain. Medications should also be available for the expected side effects of opioids, such as nausea, pruritus, urinary retention, and somnolence (when it is undesirable). Changing the specific opioid used[97,102] may also be considered for the management of refractory opioid-induced side effects when the child's expected survival is longer. Alternative routes of pain relief, such as epidurals for children who are excessively somnolent or who become delirious with systemically administered opioids may be of benefit in some cases.[2]

Respiratory depression in the face of pain is an uncommon occurrence even in children, despite aggressive use of opioids for pain relief.[102] Irregular or too rapid and shallow breathing caused by pain can often be smoothed and regulated, promoting improved gas exchange when pain is relieved.

Constipation

Constipation is very common in the ICU. Risk factors for constipation in the ICU include immobility, dehydration, and use of opioid, sedative, and paralytic medications. Nurses should consistently document bowel movement (BM) patterns, volume and consistency and report lack of BMs greater than 2 days. Stool softeners and laxatives should be initiated for any nonambulatory, sedated, or intubated patient. This is less of an issue for a child who is expected to die within 24 hours, as do most ICU patients undergoing the withdrawal or withholding of ICU interventions.[103] For more information on management of constipation see chapter 55 in this text ("Symptom Management in Pediatric Palliative Care").

Dyspnea

His breathing. It was a very shocking symptom. It was a scary symptom for us to see, and it hurt us as parents to watch because we knew how hard it was . . . he could hardly breathe. And every breath, we thought, that might be it. We kept holding our breath and thinking, "That's it. He's not coming back," and it was hard to see that, because it was so painful. It looked so painful to us. We're not sure if he was conscious enough for it to be painful for him. But as parents, it was very hard for us to watch that.[86]

When the choice is to discontinue or to not initiate mechanical ventilation, scrupulous attention to the assessment and management of dyspnea must be explained and promised to the child (if capable of participating) and the family, and the promise must be realized. The idea that there may be a trade-off between relief of dyspnea and sedation, or even a slightly earlier death, must also be broached, concerns addressed and preferences elicited. In the few studies reviewing duration of survival related to the administration of morphine during withdrawal of mechanical ventilation, however, patients of all ages actually survive longer when liberal doses of morphine are used to ease the dyspnea.[6,7] Most families opt for enhanced comfort even in the face of a potentially foreshortened survival. However, patients occasionally are much less distressed than anticipated and are able to enjoy a few hours or even days with carefully titrated opioids, as needed.[102,104]

Dyspnea is a symptom that is even more distressing than pain to experience or witness. Behavioral correlates of the sensation of dyspnea observed in ICU patients are (in decreasing order): tachypnea and tachycardia, a fearful facial expression, use of accessory breathing muscles, paradoxical (diaphragmatic) breathing, and nasal alar flaring. Dyspnea can be difficult to control and requires intensive hands-on management and reassessment. Several nonpharmacological approaches can be helpful,[105] such as limiting fluid intake, sitting the child upright, having a parent or other close family member or friend present, saying soothing words, and touching the child. In addition, having a small fan blow air across the child's face has been helpful in the hospice setting.

There are no published data on the treatment of dyspnea in children; clinical experience and the few small controlled studies done in adult patients support the use of opioids as the pharmacological agents of choice in the non-specific management of dyspnea.[106] If a specific underlying cause can be reversed, such as pulmonary edema or reactive airways disease, targeted interventions should be tried first. Various recommendations for the use of opioids in the management of intractable dyspnea exist.[6,7,15] Regardless of the protocol used, it is imperative that the child be continuously observed; the dose should be rapidly and aggressively escalated until relief is achieved. The "correct" dose is established by titration to clinical effect; there is no maximal dose of a pure opioid. Documentation should reflect dosing in response to distress and, optimally, will also note its resolution in response to treatment.[98,102,107]

The expected response to opioids is gradual slowing of rapid respirations to a more normal level; respirations do not suddenly cease unexpectedly. Reversal with naloxone or other opioid antagonists should rarely, if ever, be undertaken in palliative care. Other pharmacological aids in the management of dyspnea in the ICU include benzodiazepines to alleviate anxiety associated with, but not the sensation of, dyspnea; diuretics for children with pulmonary edema; and bronchodilators if there is an element of reactive airways disease. Withholding IV fluids or enteral feedings and adding anticholinergic agents will decrease excess secretions. Thorough suctioning of endotracheal tubes before extubation of mechanically ventilated children is helpful in preventing dyspnea and "death rattle." For more information on dyspnea, the reader is referred to chapter 14.

Palliative sedation

Occasionally, a technique known as palliative (or sometimes "total") sedation is necessary to control refractory symptoms, most often pain, dyspnea, and intractable seizures. Within the palliative care community, palliative sedation has become a generally accepted option, though infrequently used for refractory symptom management in adults. There are published articles for its use in children as well.[108,109] Palliative sedation is the extension of the tenet that, above all, the healthcare provider's duty is to relieve suffering. The intention is not to bring about the demise of the child (as in the case of physician assisted suicide and euthanasia),[110] but rather to control the symptom, even at risk of death (principle of double effect).[102,111]

Regardless of the philosophical underpinnings that lead to the practice, palliative sedation is widely regarded in palliative care circles as the only humane solution to an otherwise uncontrollable and severely distressing problem. It is only undertaken after all other attempts at symptom control by an expert have failed to bring comfort. Full agreement of the child (when possible, most often accomplished in ACP discussions) and the family is required. Explanations of the inability to reverse the underlying disease process must precede this decision.[112]

Rituals and activities that celebrate the child's life

Most communication about forgoing medical interventions concentrates on what will be stopped rather than what will be enhanced or added.[48,55] Although we cannot help the child live longer, we can help parents properly celebrate the wonder of this child, his/her relationships, value, and the impact s/he has had on the world.[6,23,54] Suggestions for accomplishing this include:

- Inviting friends and extended family to visit with the family and child

- Bringing the child's own clothing and dressing him or her in it after a bath (the parent may choose to do this or ask to have the nurse do this)

- Removing no-longer-needed medical devices ("to make him your child again, and not a patient")

- Making a three-dimensional plaster hand mold ("so you will always have your child's hand to hold")

- Reviewing photo albums to remember the good times that were shared

- Using a camera or video to commemorate the celebration

- Offering families the opportunity to invite members of their congregation or others to provide spiritual support and guidance

- Offering the child his/her favorite music, toys, videos, or other means of demonstrating the child's uniqueness

- Performing cultural, religious, or family rituals, as appropriate

Families have unique, individualized ways of acknowledging their child. One family may bring balloons and a sheet cake; another may choose to apply a teen's make-up and favorite cologne; a third might play videos of the teen's victorious football game. Easy access to a rocking chair or couch for the parent to hold the child (no matter how large) is helpful. Offer unlimited coffee, water, juice, and soft drinks.

Notification of death in the emergency department or intensive care unit when parents are not present

Unless there are extremely extenuating circumstances, even if the death is expected, most experts strongly encourage that the notification of death be done in person. ("Mrs. Smith, I am afraid I have some bad news. Could you come in to discuss it?") Empathy can be more easily expressed in person by sitting close to the parents and siblings at the time of the discussion, perhaps even giving the bereaved a hug, or shedding a genuine tear.[5-7] These small tokens of warmth and understanding help the family to know that the medical team cared about the child as a person. Additionally, insistence that the family come in allows them to see the dead child's body, facilitating the acceptance of the death and allowing the family to participate in important rituals, such as bathing the child's body, sometimes assisting in the removal of equipment, or sitting vigil, as some cultures require. These activities result in improved bereavement outcomes for the parents as well as the siblings.[11,16,39]

Autopsy and organ donation

One of the most common complaints of bereaved families is that they still, even years later, do not understand the cause of their child's death.[5] Most of the time this is because of shock preventing integration of the information or based on poor communication. However, the cause of death may not be known to the healthcare providers; in other cases, the physician is incorrect in his or her assessment. In fact, major unexpected findings related to death occurred in 28% of autopsies in a recent pediatric study. Among 100 consecutive autopsies, investigators found new information that had the potential to further clarify the cause(s) of a child's death (53% of cases); inform the future reproductive choices of either the parents (10%) or siblings (8%); affect siblings' future healthcare (6%); or contribute to patient care quality (36%) or publishable knowledge (7%).[113] For these reasons, autopsy should be encouraged. Once the body is buried or cremated, the opportunity for this helpful information is gone forever.

Autopsies can be tailored to the needs of the family. Even coroner's cases are not total body autopsies—they are limited to determining the cause of death. Most often, there is minimal disfigurement and an open-casket ceremony can still be performed, if desired. Moreover, in elective autopsies, parents can choose to limit the autopsy to the organ of interest. It is possible to take needle biopsies rather than to remove whole organs, if preferred, and a request can also be made to replace all organs back in their natural locations after the autopsy is performed. Many locales do not charge the family for the autopsy. There is generally no more than a 24-hour delay in removing the body to the funeral home if an autopsy is performed.

Many healthcare providers believe that organ donation assists families of brain-dead children to feel something good came of the death. Although this is true for some families, it has been found that the bereavement outcomes for families were more dependent on the families' perceptions of the meaning of the death, the way they were treated by hospital personnel, the way the organ donation request was broached, and their own intrinsic worldview than by the fact of organ donation.[114] In addition, donation consent was more common if the family was approached by hospital personnel who were perceived as caring, after time to absorb the fact of the death, and after time to gather supporters. Many parents of organ donors want follow-up information on the organ recipients' well-being.[115,116]

Postdeath conference

One of the most frequently recommended ways to provide needed bereavement support for families of patients who died in the ICU or ED is the postdeath conference.[5,6] Especially in sudden, unanticipated deaths, families cannot absorb new information about how and why the child died. It takes several weeks to begin to think more clearly; at that point, feelings of despair arise as the questions pour in. Parents often erroneously feel they were told nothing and can become angry about not understanding what happened. In addition, if an autopsy was performed, families may benefit from explanations provided in a face-to-face appointment with the treating physician to who explains the findings in understandable terms. This explanation can provide the bereaved family with a profound sense of peace by affirming the cause of death, affirming the irreversibility of the problems, or determining a cause of death that was unknown ante mortem.

Meert et al. studied ICU families' desires for a postdeath meeting.[11,39] The majority preferred to meet with the ICU attending physician. The reasons noted for desiring such a meeting were:

- To review the sequence of events leading to the child's death and the autopsy results in plain English
- To understand the risk to their existing or future children and any ways to prevent the same fate
- To get complete and honest information
- To be able to explain what happened to their families and friends
- To get help, reassurance, and bereavement support
- To be able to help others
- To be able to express complaints and gratitude regarding their ICU experience

The postdeath conference has even been found to improve adaptation to loss. It enables monitoring of the family's grieving process and provides the opportunity for referral to counseling, if needed, for pathological grief reactions. In the absence of a face-to-face session, families consenting to an autopsy often complain that they had no follow-up and express anger and suspicion about the motivations for the autopsy. This postdeath conference is also helpful for families who did not consent to autopsy, to answer their inevitable questions.

Bereavement care

Family-centered care is an essential approach to providing care to children and families during their stay in the PICU or ED; such care should not not end at the child's death.[5–7,17,117] Particularly after a sudden and traumatic event, the death of a child can lead to prolonged and often complicated grief for the parents, siblings, and other family members.[118] Meert and colleagues[119] found that even those parents with strong coping skills suffered prolonged and intense grief reactions after the death of a child in the PICU. Acute death predicted longer and more complicated grief as compared with death from a chronic condition.[119] In this study, the

strongest predictor of coping was the parents' level of physical health and wellness at the time of the death. Other factors that can increase the risk of complicated grief include; primary female caregiver, lack of social support, trauma, attachment style, grief avoidance, and caregiving style.[119] Compassionate care from the PICU staff also seemed to predict better outcomes for the parents.[39,120] Complicated grief does tend to decrease from 6 to 18 months after the death for some parents.[118] Research is beginning to evaluate the specific needs of parents in the PICU that can lead to less complicated bereavement.[121]

Parental grief can be further complicated by unanswered questions and confusion about the medical decisions that impacted their child.[54,118] Parents sometimes express delayed regret for not having had the opportunity to participate in organ donation.[115] For parents whose child died a violent death, attendance at a support group and maintenance of religious connection can enable better adaptation in the long term.[122,123] Bereavement programs can be particularly beneficial for parents after a traumatic death.[118]

The following factors in the PICU were reported by parents as being beneficial to their adaptation to grief: parental presence at the time of death, adequate and timely information, and kindness and empathy from staff.[28,39] When asked, bereaved parents remark that a simple card or call would have helped tremendously.[124] Healthcare professionals can positively impact the bereavement outcomes of parents by engaging in a thorough discussion of choices, provision of honest and timely information, and offering compassionate care.[11,118,121]

Recent studies have shown that after a child has died in the PICU, parents desire follow-up contact with the physicians but that this contact is not consistently available.[118,125] Meert et al. (2011) conducted a study of critical care physicians and found that one-third never had a follow-up meeting with bereaved parents, one-third participated in one to five meetings and one-third participated in more than five meetings.[118] Almost all of these meetings took place at the hospital and within the first 3 months of the death. Physicians in this study reported that the meetings were beneficial to families and also to themselves. However, they did identify a number of barriers to meetings that were both structural and interpersonal. Clearly, follow-up meetings can be a part of standard clinical practice and can benefit both the bereaved parent and members of the healthcare team.[118,125]

Studies have repeatedly shown complicated and long-lasting effects of childhood death on parents. The divorce rate among parents the first year after a child's death is higher than the national average (over the long term, however, the proportion returns to the national average of 50%). Bereaved parents often report lower quality of life, including decreased well-being, increased health problems, marital/partner struggles, and more depressive symptoms.[126,127] However, strong support and having a sense of meaning have been shown to increase positive outcomes for bereaved parents.[126] Parents have intense spiritual needs at the time of child's death in the PICU and during bereavement.[45,55] In the PICU, parents report drawing on spiritual guidance to assist them in end-of-life decision-making, to support them emotionally, and to eventually make meaning out of their loss.[55]

Memorial services

A memorial service may also be offered. This may take several forms; two are particularly suggested for the ICU. Families whose children have either come to the ICU recurrently, or those who have particularly bonded with the staff because of a child's prolonged stay or for other reasons, may be invited back to the unit with the families of a few other children who have died within the last month or 6 weeks for a ceremony of sharing. The family may bring a picture of the child, and the family and staff can exchange memories of the child. Songs may be sung, poems may be read, and prayers may be shared. Gratitude and admiration may be exchanged. In addition, all families bereaved of children could be invited to a group memorial service conducted on an annual or more frequent basis.

Grief of healthcare providers

Not only do children suffer and families and loved ones grieve but we as healthcare providers also grieve for our patients, their families, and ourselves.[13,17] We are exposed to pain and grief both vicariously and in empathy and are forced to confront the certainty of our own and our fellow humans' mortality on a daily basis. In caring for dying children, we are threatened by the reality that our own children, too, could die. The ability to share these feelings in a supportive environment, without sanction, and the ability to take leave to attend funerals can assist in increased job satisfaction and retention of highly skilled emergency and critical care personnel. It can also help to reinforce the humanity that makes us the best healthcare providers we can be.

Healthcare professionals suffer from grief and moral distress as well as from the stress of inadequate communication within the healthcare team itself.[128,129] Healthcare providers do not always feel sufficiently supported to provide the type of compassionate and open communication that they want to offer to families. Healthcare professionals from PICU, NICU, and pediatric oncology units identify the following key factors that result in increased professional comfort and knowledge when caring for children who die[130]:

- Having a palliative care network
- Attending palliative care rounds
- Having access to patient care conferences and
- Bereavement debriefing sessions

These interventions increase the staff's ability to deal with their own grief, facilitate effective communication with staff and families, and increase knowledge of coping strategies.[130] In a study of the comfort and confidence levels of pediatric intensive care staff, Jones and colleagues[131] discovered that having 8 or more years of experience increased the confidence of staff, but not their comfort level. In this same study, physicians and nurses reported higher levels of confidence and comfort in providing medical and practical aspects of care than in the psychosocial aspects of care, for which they continue to have little formal training. Parker-Raley et al.[41] found that physicians report facing a number of dialectical tensions in compassionately communicating the death of a child in the emergency room. The internal tensions included clarity and compassion, trust and blame, empathy and professionalism, intimacy and nonintimacy, and certainty and uncertainty. All of these studies point to the increased need for training and support for healthcare professionals in the PICU and ED in providing compassionate care while simultaneously addressing their own tensions, grief,

and moral distress. Interventions to improve providers' comfort and confidence in providing this care have included simulation exercises, facilitated debriefings, formal support, and institutional resources.[128-130] Clearly, standard preparatory medical and nursing education and years of experience are insufficient to mitigate the emotional challenges faced by providers in pediatric critical care. There are ongoing needs for support, debriefing, and self-compassion. In fact, the American Academy of Critical Care Medicine's (AACCM) consensus statement on end-of-life care in the ICU concluded that the unresolved grief of healthcare professionals can impact the patient care provided and called for steps to be taken to alleviate caregivers' grief and moral distress.[6]

A variety of coping strategies have been described to help professionals manage the stress of caring for seriously ill children who eventually die.[13] Some coping strategies are personal and beneficial in the short term (e.g., engaging in self-care activities such as exercise, meditation, or journal writing) or in the long term (e.g., developing a personal philosophy of care, engaging in self-reflection and self-awareness, committing to taking care of oneself). Other coping strategies are work related, the most important being the development of supportive professional relationships that promote debriefing and enhance mutual support.[128-130] Health professionals seem to rely more on their colleagues than family and friends for support. The nature of this support differs, and includes the exchange of information (informational support); the clinical collaboration to meet patient needs (clinical or instrumental support); the sharing of personal feelings and experiences (emotional support); and the reflection and attribution of meaning to one's work experiences (meaning-making support). Opportunities for formal support (e.g., participation in support groups, stress-debriefing sessions, or supervision meetings) and informal support (e.g., time out for discussions) are encouraged in different work settings, depending on the philosophy and goals of care, as well as on rules and regulations with regard to the team's functioning in the face of their patients' death.[132]

Case study

Intensive care unit management of a complex chronically ill child at the end of life

Isaiah was a 3-year-old boy with anoxic brain injury resulting from placental separation and congenital scoliosis. After a prolonged NICU admission, he was discharged home with his parents to a rural location 2 hours from an academic children's hospital. Due to the lack of available home nursing support in their home community, his mother provided necessary medically prescribed care. He developed a seizure disorder, required gastrostomy feedings due to dysphagia, and experienced chronic aspiration of secretions despite attentive suctioning and chest physiotherapy by his mother. In his first year and a half of life he experienced multiple episodes of respiratory distress related to his scoliosis and pulmonary hypoplasia, requiring local EMS interventions, intubation, and transport by life-flight to the children's hospital for ICU admission. Over the course of multiple ICU admissions and in consultation with his primary care and pulmonary teams, the option of tracheostomy was presented to the family. His mother understood her child's long-term prognosis and after discussion with her husband indicated that she did not want to pursue tracheostomy. He was sent home on aggressive pulmonary management with cough assist and chest physiotherapy. A local nurse was located, and skilled nursing services were initiated. Isaiah experienced only two brief, nonemergent hospitalizations for respiratory illness over the next year. On his final admission, he presented to the ER in respiratory distress and was admitted to the ICU. Goals of care were immediately clarified due to worsening respiratory status and need for support. His mother chose noninvasive mask ventilation, hoping that it would provide support to allow a viral infection time to improve. Isaiah's condition continued to worsen, requiring increasing pressure support on the bi-pap. Goals of care were again discussed regarding invasive ventilatory support with an ET tube or nonescalation of the current supportive measures. The parents chose nonescalation with a plan to withdraw noninvasive support and allow a natural death. Bi-pap support and medications for comfort were continued while the parents gathered family for the planned withdrawal. Isaiah's mother was seated holding him with her husband, sister, family, and friends present, and he died within 10 minutes of removing artificial ventilation.

Recommendations to enhance end-of-life care in the Intensive Care Unit and Emergency Department setting

- Admission procedures should include a values history; solicitation of any advance directives for older, chronically ill children; and discussion of expressed preferences in light of the child's current situation. This should not be reserved only for imminently dying children. Waiting until that time only increases the chances that the child's preferences will never be known and the family's guilt will be unnecessarily increased in the event they are later called on to consent to the withdrawal of no-longer-beneficial medical interventions. Good coordination with primary care providers and specialists who have cared for the chronically ill child can be enormously helpful.

- Attention to pain and the relief of other symptoms, both during procedures and more generally, must become a priority for all children. This can be accomplished only with training and appropriate policies and documentation procedures, as well as emphasis by supervisors and attending physicians.

- Improved communication techniques must be employed that allow children or their surrogates to understand their options in a supportive and unbiased way. Guilt, missed opportunities, love, and existential and spiritual issues should be included in these discussions. Again, training must be developed and carried out. The importance of truly informed consent must be emphasized, demonstrated, and reflected in the practices of the opinion leaders within the unit.

- Cooperation, respect, and regular interdisciplinary rounds among the disciplines of nursing, medicine, social work, pastoral care, and, possibly, palliative care (and others as indicated, such as pharmacy, occupational therapy, physical therapy, child life) will enhance the larger understanding of the child and his or her needs and facilitate the team's ability to assist the child with the accomplishment of his or her goals.

- Development of a celebration of life or similar protocol can transform the death of the child from a vigil to recognition of the value of the individual while supporting the family.

- Establishment of a bereavement follow-up program, including the mailing of bereavement cards, autopsy debriefing or post-death sessions, "sharing sessions," and memorial services will improve the bereavement outcome for surviving loved ones and ED or ICU staff.

- Excused, paid absences for funeral attendance, formalized staff mentoring programs and facilitation of self-care will prevent burnout and turnover and allow the retention of the ideals and values that brought each staff member to the healing professions.

Summary and recommendations for implementation

Improved end-of-life care begins with more highly focused attention on the individual child and his or her preferences and values. Pediatric and neonatal ICU and ED practitioners are the caregivers for the vast majority of children who die; thus, they must have expertise in palliative care. Infants die primarily of congenital defects, prematurity, and SIDS. Children older than 1 year of age die primarily from trauma, thus predisposing them to die in the ED or ICU settings. The principles of palliative care must be applied to all children, even those whose fate is to die in the ED or ICU. Our challenge, as practitioners of pediatric emergency and critical care medicine, is to provide each of these children a "good death" and their families a more peaceful bereavement. This can be achieved by intensive attention to the child's and family's perspectives and goals, communication within the team and with the child and his or her loved ones, dedication to the meticulous prevention and management of symptoms, particularly during procedures—the most common source of discomfort in ill children—and effective bereavement follow-up.

References

1. Meyer EC, Ritholz MD, Burns JP, Truog RD. Improving the quality of end-of-life care in the pediatric intensive care unit: parents' priorities and recommendations. Pediatrics. 2006;117(3):649–657.
2. Klick JC, Hauer J. Pediatric palliative care. Curr Probl Pediatr Adolesc Health Care.2010;40(6):120–151.
3. Baker JN, Hinds PS, Spunt SL, et al. Integration of palliative care practices into the ongoing care of children with cancer: individualized care planning and coordination. Pediatr Clin North Am. 2008;55(1):223+.
4. National Hospice and Palliative Care Organization. Pediatric concurrent care. 2012; http://www.nhpco.org/resources/concurrent-care-children, accessed July, 2014.
5. O'Malley PJ, Brown K, Krug SE. Patient-and family-centered care of children in the emergency department. Pediatrics. 2008;122(2):e511–e521.
6. Truog RD, Campbell ML, Curtis JR, et al. Recommendations for end-of-life care in the intensive care unit: a consensus statement by the American College of Critical Care Medicine. Crit Care Med. 2008;36(3):953–963.
7. Lanken PN, Terry PB, DeLisser HM, et al. An official American Thoracic Society clinical policy statement: palliative care for patients with respiratory diseases and critical illnesses. Am J Respir Crit Care Med. 2008;177(8):912–927.
8. Mosenthal AC, Murphy PA, Barker LK, Lavery R, Retano A, Livingston DH. Changing the culture around end-of-life care in the trauma intensive care unit. J Trauma Acute Care Surg. 2008;64(6):1587–1593.
9. Vollenbroich R, Duroux A, Grasser M, Brandstätter M, Borasio GD, Führer M. Effectiveness of a pediatric palliative home care team as

experienced by parents and health care professionals. J Palliat Med. 2012;15(3):294–300.

10. Bradford N, Armfield N, Young J, Smith A. The case for home based telehealth in pediatric palliative care: a systematic review. BMC Palliat Care. 2013;12(1):4.

11. Meert KL, Eggly S, Berger J, et al. A framework for conducting follow-up meetings with parents after a child's death in the pediatric intensive care unit. Pediatr Crit Care Med. 2011;12(2):147.

12. Fontana MS, Farrell C, Gauvin F, Lacroix J, Janvier A. Modes of death in pediatrics: differences in the ethical approach in neonatal and pediatric patients. J Pediatr. 2013;162(6):1107–1111.

13. Liben S, Papadatou D, Wolfe J. Paediatric palliative care: challenges and emerging ideas. Lancet. 2008;371(9615):852–864.

14. Davies B, Sehring SA, Partridge JC, et al. Barriers to palliative care for children: perceptions of pediatric health care providers. Pediatrics. 2008;121(2):282–288.

15. Curtis JR. Caring for patients with critical illness and their families: the value of the integrated clinical team. Respir Care. 2008;53(4):480–487.

16. Doorenbos A, Lindhorst T, Starks H, Aisenberg E, Curtis JR, Hays R. Palliative care in the pediatric ICU: challenges and opportunities for family-centered practice. J Soc Work End Life Palliat Care. 2012;8(4):297–315.

17. Polikoff LA, McCabe ME. End-of-life care in the pediatric ICU. Curr Opin Pediatrics. 2013;25(3):285–289.

18. Rogers SK, Gomez CF, Carpenter P, et al. Quality of life for children with life-limiting and life-threatening illnesses: description and evaluation of a regional, collaborative model for pediatric palliative care. Am J Hosp Palliat Care. 2011;28(3):161–170.

19. Meert KL, Clark J, Eggly S. Family-centered care in the pediatric intensive care unit. Pediatr Clin North Am. 2013;60(3):761–772.

20. Robert R, Zhukovsky DS, Mauricio R, Gilmore K, Morrison S, Palos GR. Bereaved Parents' Perspectives on Pediatric Palliative Care. J Soc Work End Life Palliat Care. 2012/12/01 2012;8(4):316–338.

21. Dussel V, Kreicbergs U, Hilden JM, et al. Looking beyond where children die: determinants and effects of planning a child's location of death. J Pain Symptom Manage. 2009;37(1):33–43.

22. McGraw SA, Truog RD, Solomon MZ, Cohen-Bearak A, Sellers DE, Meyer EC. "I was able to still be her mom": parenting at end of life in the pediatric intensive care unit. Pediatr Crit Care Med. 2012;13(6):e350–e356.

23. Yang SC. Assessment and quantification of Taiwanese children's views of a good death. Omega. 2012;66(1):17–37.

24. Kochanek KD, Kirmeyer SE, Martin JA, Strobino DM, Guyer B. Annual summary of vital statistics: 2009. Pediatrics. 2012;129(2):338–348.

25. Murphy SL, Xu JQ, Kochanek KD. National Vital Statistics Reports: Final Data 2010. DHHS publication; no. 2013–1120 Vol 61, No 14. Hyattsville, MD: NCHS; 2012. http://stacks.cdc.gov/view/cdc/21508/1.96%28.25

26. Sands R, Manning JC, Vyas H, Rashid A. Characteristics of deaths in paediatric intensive care: a 10-year study. Nurs Crit Care. 2009;14(5):235–240.

27. Fraser LK, Miller M, Draper ES, McKinney PA, Parslow RC. Place of death and palliative care following discharge from paediatric intensive care units. Arch Dis Child. 2011;96(12):1195–1198.

28. Meert KL, Briller SH, Schim SM, Thurston CS. Exploring parents' environmental needs at the time of a child's death in the pediatric intensive care unit. Pediatr Crit Care Med. 2008;9(6):623–628.

29. Berg MD, Schexnayder SM, Chameides L, et al. Pediatric basic life support: 2010 American Heart Association guidelines for Cardiopulmonary resuscitation and emergency cardiovascular care. Pediatrics. 2010;126(5):e1345–e1360.

30. Topjian AA, Berg RA, Nadkarni VM. Pediatric cardiopulmonary resuscitation: advances in science, techniques, and outcomes. Pediatrics. 2008;122(5):1086–1098.

31. Ford D, Zapka JG, Gebregziabher M, Hennessy W, Yang C. Investigating critically ill patients' and families' perceptions of likelihood of survival. J Palliat Med. 2009;12(1):45–52.

32. DeVader TE, Albrecht R, Reiter M. Initiating palliative care in the emergency department. J Emerg Med. 2012;43(5):803–810.

33. Hain R, Heckford E, McCulloch R. Paediatric palliative medicine in the UK: past, present, future. Arch Dis Child. 2012;97(4):381–384.

34. Mason KE, Urbansky H, Crocker L, Connor M, Anderson MR, Kissoon N. Pediatric emergency mass critical care: focus on family-centered care. Pediatr Crit Care Med. 2011;12(6):S157–S162.

35. Henderson DP, Knapp JF. Report of the national consensus conference on family presence during pediatric cardiopulmonary resuscitation and procedures. J Emerg Nurs. 2006;32(1):23–29.

36. Tinsley C, Hill JB, Shah J, et al. Experience of families during cardiopulmonary resuscitation in a pediatric intensive care unit. Pediatrics. 2008;122(4):e799–e804.

37. Jones B, Parker-Raley J, Maxson T, Brown C. Understanding health care professionals views of family presence during pediatric resuscitation: implications for family-centered care. Am J Crit Care. 2011;20(3):199–207; quiz 208.

38. Emergency Nurses Association Position Statement: Family Presence at the Bedside During Invasive Procedures and Cardiopulmonary Resuscitation. Emergency Nurses Association, Des Plaines, IL; 2005.

39. Meert KL, Eggly S, Pollack M, et al. Parents' perspectives on physician-parent communication near the time of a child's death in the pediatric intensive care unit. Pediatr Crit Care Med. 2008;9(1):2.

40. Levetown M. Communicating with children and families: from everyday interactions to skill in conveying distressing information. Pediatrics. 2008;121(5):e1441–e1460.

41. Parker-Raley J, Jones BL, Maxson RT. Communicating the death of a child in the emergency department: managing dialectical tensions. J Healthc Qual. 2008;30(5):20–31.

42. Dyregrov A, Dyregrov K. Complicated grief in children—the perspectives of experienced professionals. Omega. 2013;67(3):291–303.

43. Greer S. Bereavement care: some clinical observations. Psycho-Oncol. 2010,19(11):1156–1160.

44. Thrane S, Jones BL. Communication with families after the death of a child: a pilot study. J Hosp Palliat Nurs. 2012;14(1):6–10.

45. Wender E, Siegel BS, Dobbins MI, et al. Supporting the family after the death of a child. Pediatrics. 2012;130(6):1164–1169.

46. Craig F, Mancini A. Can We Truly offer a choice of place of death in neonatal palliative care? Semin Fetal Neonatal Med. 2013;18(2):93–98.

47. Baker JN, Hinds PS, Spunt SL, et al. Integration of palliative care practices into the ongoing care of children with cancer: individualized care planning and coordination. Pediatr Clin North Am. 2008;55(1):223–250.

48. Edlynn ES, Derrington S, Morgan H, Murray J, Ornelas B, Cucchiaro G. Developing a pediatric palliative care service in a large urban hospital: challenges, lessons, and successes. J Palliat Med. 2013;16(4):342–348.

48a. Lotz JD, Jox RJ, Borasio GD, Führer M. Pediatric advance care planning: a systematic review. Pediatrics. 2013 Mar;131(3):e873–e880.

49. Fiks AG, Mayne S, Localio AR, Alessandrini EA, Guevara JP. Shared decision-making and health care expenditures among children with special health care needs. Pediatrics. 2012;129(1):99–107.

50. Maurer SH, Hinds PS, Spunt SL, Furman WL, Kane JR, Baker JN. Decision making by parents of children with incurable cancer who opt for enrollment on a phase I trial compared with choosing a do not resuscitate/terminal care option. J Clin Oncol. 2010;28(20):3292–3298.

51. Hinds PS, Oakes LL, Hicks J, et al. "Trying to be a good parent" as defined by interviews with parents who made phase I, terminal care, and resuscitation decisions for their children. J Clin Oncol. 2009;27(35):5979–5985.

52. Field M, Behrman RE. When children die: improving palliative and end-of-life care for children and their families. Washington, DC: National Academies Press, 2003.

53. Mack JW, Wolfe J. Early integration of pediatric palliative care: for some children, palliative care starts at diagnosis. Curr Opin Pediatrics. 2006;18(1):10–14.

54. Longden JV. Parental perceptions of end-of-life care on paediatric intensive care units: a literature review. Nurs Crit Care. 2011;16(3):131–139.

55. Hexem KR, Mollen CJ, Carroll K, Lanctot DA, Feudtner C. How parents of children receiving pediatric palliative care use religion, spirituality, or life philosophy in tough times. J Palliat Med. 2011;14(1):39–44.

56. McCannon JB, O'Donnell WJ, Thompson BT, et al. Augmenting communication and decision making in the intensive care unit with a cardiopulmonary resuscitation video decision support tool: a temporal intervention study. J Palliat Med. 2012;15(12):1382–1387.

57. Wiener L, Zadeh S, Battles H, Baird K, Ballard E, Osherow J. Allowing adolescents and young adults to plan their end-of-life care. Pediatrics. 2012;130(5):897–905.

58. Fraser J, Harris N, Berringer A, Prescott H, Finlay F. Advanced care planning in children with life-limiting conditions–the Wishes Document. Arch Dis Child. 2010;95(2):79–82.

59. Durall A, Zurakowski D, Wolfe J. Barriers to conducting advance care discussions for children with life-threatening conditions. Pediatrics. 2012;129(4):e975–e982.

60. Sharman M, Meert KL, Sarnaik AP. What influences parents' decisions to limit or withdraw life support? Pediatr Crit Care Med. 2005;6(5):513–518.

61. Voicing My Choices. A Planning Guide for Adolescents and Young Adults. http://www.agingwithdignity.org/voicing-my-choices.php. Accessed July 3, 2013.

62. Lotz JD, Jox RJ, Borasio GD, Fuehrer M. Advance care planning in pediatrics: a systematic review. Pediatrics. 2013;131(3):e873–e880.

63. Gans D, Kominski GF, Roby DH, et al. Better outcomes, lower costs: palliative care program reduces stress, costs of care for children with life-threatening conditions. Policy Brief UCLA Cent Health Policy Res. 2012;(PB2012-3):1–8.

64. Kross EK, Engelberg RA, Gries CJ, Nielsen EL, Zatzick D, Curtis JR. ICU care associated with symptoms of depression and posttraumatic stress disorder among family members of patients who die in the ICU. Chest. 2011;139(4):795–801.

65. Colville G, Pierce C. Patterns of post-traumatic stress symptoms in families after paediatric intensive care. Intensive Care Med. 2012;38(9):1523–1531.

66. McAdam JL, Puntillo K. Symptoms experienced by family members of patients in intensive care units. Am J Crit Care. 2009;18(3):200–209.

67. Weidner NJ, Cameron M, Lee RC, McBride J, Mathias EJ, Byczkowski TL. End-of-life care for the dying child: what matters most to parents. J Palliat Care. 2011;27(4):279.

68. Oberender F, Tibballs J. Withdrawal of life-support in paediatric intensive care: a study of time intervals between discussion, decision and death. BMC Pediatrics. 2011;11(1):39.

69. Shore PM, Huang R, Roy L, et al. Development of a bedside tool to predict time to death after withdrawal of life-sustaining therapies in infants and children. Pediatr Crit Care Med. 2012;13(4):415–422.

70. Truog RD, Meyer EC, Burns JP. Toward interventions to improve end-of-life care in the pediatric intensive care unit. Crit Care Med. 2006;34(11):S373–S379.

71. Hinds PS. Parent-clinician communication intervention during end-of-life decision making for children with incurable cancer. J Palliat Med. 2012;15(8):916–922.

72. Foster TL, Lafond DA, Reggio C, Hinds PS. Pediatric palliative care in childhood cancer nursing: from diagnosis to cure or end of life. Semin Oncol Nurs. 2010 Nov;26(4):205–21.

73. Michelson KN, Emanuel L, Carter A, Brinkman P, Clayman ML, Frader J. Pediatric intensive care unit family conferences: one mode of communication for discussing end-of-life care decisions. Pediatr Crit Care Med. 2011;12(6):e336.

74. Uitterhoeve R, De Leeuw J, Bensing J, et al. Cue-responding behaviours of oncology nurses in video-simulated interviews. J Adv Nurs. 2008;61(1):71–80.

75. Uitterhoeve R, Bensing J, Dilven E, Donders R, Demulder P, van Achterberg T. Nurse–patient communication in cancer care: does responding to patient's cues predict patient satisfaction with communication. Psycho-Oncol. 2009;18(10):1060–1068.

76. Fineberg IC. Social work perspectives on family communication and family conferences in palliative care. Prog Palliat Care. 2010;18:213–220.

77. Fineberg IC, Kawashima M, Asch SM. Communication with families facing life-threatening illness: a research-based model for family conferences. J Palliat Med. 2011;14(4):421–427.

78. Mack JW, Smith TJ. Reasons why physicians do not have discussions about poor prognosis, why it matters, and what can be improved. J Clin Oncol. 2012;30(22):2715–2717.

79. Mack JW, Wolfe J, Cook EF, Grier HE, Cleary PD, Weeks JC. Hope and prognostic disclosure. J Clin Oncol. 2007;25(35):5636–5642.

80. Coad J, Patel R, Murray S. Disclosing terminal diagnosis to children and their families: palliative professionals' communication barriers. Death Stud. 2014 Jan–Jun;38(1–5):302–307.

81. Miller MJ, Abrams MA, Earles B, Phillips K, McCleary EM. Improving patient-provider communication for patients having surgery: patient perceptions of a revised health literacy-based consent process. J Patient Safety. 2011;7(1):30–38.

82. Bibler TM. Why I no longer say "withdrawal of care" or "life sustaining technology." J Palliat Med. 2013;16(9):1146–1147.

83. Jones BL, Parker-Raley J, Higgerson R, Christie LM, Legett S, Greathouse J. Finding the right words: using the terms Allow Natural Death (AND) and Do Not Resuscitate (DNR) in pediatric palliative care. J Healthc Qual. 2008;30(5):55–63.

84. Hinds PS, Kelly KP. Helping parents make and survive end of life decisions for their seriously ill child. Nurs Clin North Am. 2010;45(3):465–474.

85. Gerstel E, Engelberg RA, Koepsell T, Curtis JR. Duration of withdrawal of life support in the intensive care unit and association with family satisfaction. Am J Respir Crit Care Med. 2008;178(8):798.

86. Pritchard M, Burghen E, Srivastava DK, et al. Cancer-related symptoms most concerning to parents during the last week and last day of their child's life. Pediatrics.2008;121(5):e1301–e1309.

87. Diekema DS, Botkin JR, Bioethics Co. Forgoing medically provided nutrition and hydration in children. Pediatrics. 2009;124(2):813–822.

88. Levin TT, Moreno B, Silvester W, Kissane DW. End-of-life communication in the intensive care unit. Gen Hosp Psychiatry. 2010;32(4):433–442.

89. Billings JA. Humane terminal extubation reconsidered: the role for preemptive analgesia and sedation. Crit Care Med. 2012;40(2):625–630.

90. Morrison W. Titration of medication and the management of suffering at the end of life. Virtual Mentor. 2012;14(10):780–783.

91. Truog RD. Should patients receive general anesthesia prior to extubation at the end of life? Crit Care Med. 2012;40(2):631–633.

92. Gupta N, Harrop E, Lapwood S, Shefler A. Journey from pediatric intensive care to palliative care. J Palliat Med. 2013;16(4):397–401.

93. Contro N, Larson J, Scofield S, Sourkes B, Cohen H. Family perspectives on the quality of pediatric palliative care. Arch Pediatr Adolesc Med. 2002;156(1):14.

94. Fein JA, Zempsky WT, Cravero JP, et al. Relief of pain and anxiety in pediatric patients in emergency medical systems. Pediatrics. 2012;130(5):e1391–e1405.

95. Zempsky WT. Optimizing the management of peripheral venous access pain in children: evidence, impact, and implementation. Pediatrics. 2008;122(Suppl 3):S121–S124.

96. WHO. Persisting Pain in Children Package: WHO Guidelines on the Pharmacological Treatment of Persisting Pain in Children with Medical Illnesses. Geneva: World Health Organization; 2012. Accessed July 2014, http://whqlibdoc.who.int/publications/2012/9789241548120_Guidelines.pdf?ua=1

97. Johnson PN. Sedation and analgesia in critically ill children. AACN Adv Crit Care. 2012;23(4):415–434; quiz 435–416.

98. Chiaretti A, Pierri F, Valentini P, Russo I, Gargiullo L, Riccardi R. Current practice and recent advances in pediatric pain management. Eur Rev Med Pharmacol Sci. 2013 Feb;17 Suppl 1:112–126.

99. Massaro M, Pastore S, Ventura A, Barbi E. Pain in cognitively impaired children: a focus for general pediatricians. Eur J Pediatr. 2013;172(1):9–14.

100. Hauer JM. Respiratory symptom management in a child with severe neurologic impairment. J Palliat Med. 2007;10(5):1201–1207.

101. Gandhi M, Playfor SD. Managing pain in critically ill children. Minerva Pediatr. 2010;62(2):189–202.

102. Shaw TM. Pediatric palliative pain and symptom management. Pediatr Ann. 2012;41(8):329.

103. Oberender F, Tibballs J. Withdrawal of life-support in paediatric intensive care: a study of time intervals between discussion, decision and death. BMC Pediatr. 2011;11(1):39.

104. Houlahan KE, Branowicki PA, Mack JW, Dinning C, McCabe M. Can end of life care for the pediatric patient suffering with escalating and intractable symptoms be improved? J Pediatr Oncol Nurs. 2006;23(1):45–51.

105. Quill TE, Lo B, Brock DW, Meisel A. Last-resort options for palliative sedation. Ann Intern Med. 2009;151(6):421–424.

106. INCTR. International Network for Cancer Treatment and Research Palliative Care Handbook 2009. http://inctr-palliative-care-handbook.wikidot.com/dyspnea. Accessed July 2014.

107. Chidambaran V, Sadhasivam S. Pediatric acute and surgical pain management: recent advances and future perspectives. Int Anesthesiol Clin. 2012;50(4):66–82.

108. Anghelescu DL, Hamilton H, Faughnan LG, Johnson LM, Baker JN. Pediatric palliative sedation therapy with propofol: recommendations based on experience in children with terminal cancer. J Palliat Med. 2012;15(10):1082–1090.

109. Morgan C, FitzGerald M, Hoehn K, Weidner N. 872: Pediatric palliative sedation and end of life care. Crit Care Med. 2012;40(12):1–328.

110. Lloyd-Williams M, Morton J, Peters S. The end-of-life care experiences of relatives of brain dead intensive care patients. J Pain Symptom Manage. 2009;37(4):659–664.

111. Wolfe J, Hinds PS, Sourkes BM. Textbook of Interdisciplinary Pediatric Palliative Care. Elsevier/Saunders; Philadelphia, PA, 2011.

112. Anghelescu DL. Pediatric palliative sedation therapy with propofol: recommendations based on experience in children with terminal cancer. J Palliat Med. 2012;15(10):1082–1090.

113. Heller KS, Solomon MZ. Continuity of care and caring: what matters to parents of children with life-threatening conditions. J Pediatr Nurs. 2005;20(5):335–346.

114. Hogan NS, Coolican M, Schmidt LA. Making meaning in the legacy of tissue donation for donor families. Prog Transplant. 2013;23(2):180–187.

115. Corr CA, Coolican MB. Understanding bereavement, grief, and mourning: implications for donation and transplant professionals. Prog Transplant. 2010;20(2):169–177.

116. Siminoff LA, Traino HM, Gordon N. Determinants of family consent to tissue donation. J Trauma. 2010;69(4):956.

117. Liben S. Pediatric palliative care in the ICU. In: Astuto M (ed.), Basics. Anesthesia, Intensive Care and Pain in Neonates and Children. London: Springer; 2009.

118. Meert KL, Shear K, Newth CJ, et al. Follow-up study of complicated grief among parents eighteen months after a child's death in the pediatric intensive care unit. J Palliat Med. 2011;14(2):207–214.

119. Meert KL, Donaldson AE, Newth CJ, et al. Complicated grief and associated risk factors among parents following a child's death in the pediatric intensive care unit. Arch Pediatr Adolesc Med. 2010;164(11):1045.

120. Longden JV. Parental perceptions of end-of-life care on paediatric intensive care units: a literature review. Nurs Crit Care. 2011;16(3):131–139.

121. Meert KL, Templin TN, Michelson KN, et al. The Bereaved Parent Needs Assessment: a new instrument to assess the needs of parents whose children died in the pediatric intensive care unit. Crit Care Med. 2012;40(11):3050–3057.

122. Umphrey LR, Cacciatore J. Coping with the ultimate deprivation: narrative themes in a parental bereavement support group. Omega. 2011;63(2):141–160.

123. Caldwell K, Senter K. Strengthening Family Resilience Through Spiritual and Religious Resources. In: Becvar DS (ed.), Handbook of Family Resilience. New York: Springer; 2013:441–455.

124. Coleman WL, Richmond JB. After the death of a child: helping bereaved parents and brothers and sisters. In: Developmental-Behavioral Pediatrics. 4th ed. Philadelphia, PA: Saunders Elsevier; 2009:366–372.

125. Borasino S, Morrison W, Silberman J, Nelson RM, Feudtner C. Physicians' contact with families after the death of pediatric patients: a survey of pediatric critical care practitioners' beliefs and self-reported practices. Pediatrics. 2008;122(6):e1174–e1178.

126. Rogers CH, Floyd FJ, Seltzer MM, Greenberg J, Hong J. Long-term effects of the death of a child on parents' adjustment in midlife. J Fam Psychol. 2008;22(2):203.

127. Song J, Floyd FJ, Seltzer MM, Greenberg JS, Hong J. Long-term effects of child death on parents' health-related quality of life: a dyadic analysis. Fam Relat. 2010;59(3):269–282.

128. Bateman ST, Dixon R, Trozzi M. The wrap-up: a unique forum to support pediatric residents when faced with the death of a child. J Palliat Med. 2012;15(12):1329–1334.

129. Cook KA, Mott S, Lawrence P, et al. Coping while caring for the dying child: nurses' experiences in an acute care setting. J Pediatr Nurs. 2012;27(4):e11–e21.

130. Brown CM, Lloyd EC, Swearingen CJ, Boateng BA. Improving resident self-efficacy in pediatric palliative care through clinical simulation. J Palliat Care. 2011;28(3):157–163.

131. Jones BL, Sampson M, Greathouse J, Legett S, Higgerson RA, Christie L. Comfort and confidence levels of health care professionals providing pediatric palliative care in the intensive care unit. J Soc Work End Life Palliat Care. 2007;3(3):39–58.

132. Keene EA, Hsssutton N, Hall B, Rushton CH. Bereavement debriefing sessions: an intervention to support health care professionals in managing their grief after death of a patient. Pediatr Nurs. 2010;36(4):185–189.

CHAPTER 58

End-of-life decision-making in pediatric oncology

Pamela S. Hinds, Linda L. Oakes, and Wayne L. Furman

The diagnosis that the cancer came back and that there was nothing that could be done was understandable given the condition her body was in. It is more likely now that she will pass on from the infection than the cancer because the infection is in her bloodstream. It is a hard decision because you want your child to be with you. You have to think about your child and what is better for her. She already has two uncles and two baby sisters there (in heaven). She told us not to worry, that if she does die, she would go there and take care of them and she'd be OK. I just don't want her to suffer anymore. Twelve and a half years is long enough. It makes it a littler easier to put her in the hands of the Jesus and one day I'll see her again.

Mother who had made a "do not resuscitate" decision 48 hours previously on behalf of her 12-year-old daughter, who was dying of cancer

Key points

- Decision-making for parents facing the terminal illness of a child is, in most cases, extraordinarily difficult.

- Healthcare providers can influence the extent to which patients and parents participate in end-of-life decision-making by communication style and timing of the discussion.

- Children and adolescents may need assistance making decisions based on their cognitive development, and each patient should be assessed as an individual to determine his or her competence and preference for decision involvement.

- Preferences for treatment should be balanced between the child or adolescent patient and the caregiver or surrogate.

- Nurses have a professional responsibility to facilitate informed patient decisions at the end of life.

Deciding to end a child's life, and involving a child in the decision to end his/her life, are startling concepts, but we in pediatric oncology participate in those considerations with parents, patients, and other members of the healthcare team as a part of providing the highest quality care for the child or adolescent with incurable cancer. Participating in end-of-life decisions is life altering for the child or adolescent and for the family, but it can also be life altering for the healthcare provider. Clinical reports indicate that the way in which patients, family members, and healthcare providers participate in end-of-life discussions and decision-making and convey respect for the decision made can color all of their preceding treatment-related interactions, and may influence how well

parents emotionally survive the dying and death of their child.[1-3] The manner in which end-of-life decision-making processes are completed may also contribute to the well-being of parents and the survival of healthcare providers as compassionate and fully competent professionals.[4] Relationships involving the ill child, adolescent, family members, and the healthcare providers are a primary consideration in end-of-life decision-making.

Because of the significant immediate and longer-term impact of participating in end-of-life decision-making for a child or adolescent with incurable cancer, guidelines for making or for facilitating such decisions have been developed,[5] but their usefulness in clinical practice has not been fully evaluated. Additionally, these guidelines tend to be in the form of broad guidance for a certain discipline—American Nurses' Association Position Statements, "Registered Nurses" Roles and Responsibilities in Providing Expert Care and Counseling at the End of Life"[6]; American Nurses' Association Position Statements, "Nursing Care and Do Not Resuscitate (DNR) and Allow Natural Death (AND) Decisions"[7]—and are not consistently developed for use in pediatric end-of-life care. Preparation for participating in end-of-life decision-making is increasingly included in formal academic curricula[8,9] and other forms of clinician education such as workshops[10] and online materials (e.g., www.nhpco.org/;http://epec.net/epec_friendship.php; http://www.aacn.nche.edu/elnec/about/pediatric-palliative-care). There is clearly a great need for more information that can be used to develop, test, refine, and apply such guidelines into care of families whose child will not survive. The purposes of this chapter are (1) to offer a review of the current literature (both clinical and research-based) on

---

Box 58.1 Key terms used in this chapter

Decision—The final choice between two or more treatment-related options.

Phase I study—The initial stage of human testing of a drug, in which the maximum tolerated dose is established; in oncology, the subjects are usually patients who have refractory disease.

Do not resuscitate—An order written in the medical record directing that no cardiopulmonary resuscitation is to be performed in the case of an acute event such as cardiac, respiratory, or neurological decompensation.

Withdrawal of life support—Stopping a life-sustaining medical treatment such as mechanical ventilator therapy, pharmacological support of blood pressure, or dialysis, and vasoactive infusions.

Life-sustaining medical treatment—Interventions that may not control the patient's disease but may prolong the patient's life; these may include not only ventilator support, dialysis, and vasoactive infusions, but also antibiotics, insulin, chemotherapy, and nutrition and hydration provided by tubes and IV lines.

Supportive care—Comfort measures that exclude curative efforts but could include symptom management (such as pain relief and hydration) or symptom prevention (such as limited blood product support).

---

end-of-life decision-making in pediatrics, with a special emphasis on pediatric oncology, and (2) to offer guidelines for the use of healthcare professionals in assisting children, adolescents, their parents, and other healthcare professionals in making such decisions. Box 58.1 defines key terms used in this chapter.

Background

Advances in pediatric oncology have significantly increased the survival rates of patients during the past decade. The disease once thought to be universally fatal for children and adolescents is now viewed as a life-threatening, complex chronic illness that is potentially curable for many.[11] However, cancer remains the leading disease-related cause of death in children and adolescents, as ultimately 25% to 33% will die of their disease depending on the disease type.[11-14] Indeed, approximately 2,200 children and adolescents die of cancer in the United States on an annual basis.[11,14] With treatment advances come more treatment options and more treatment-related decisions for patients, their parents, and their healthcare providers.

Only a limited number of experiences with treatment decision-making occur for parents whose child is being treated for cancer, as the majority of these children will be on a therapeutic protocol according to which the child's treatment is directed. Commonly, with the exception of supportive care choices such as the type of venous access device placed, the parents' and the ill child's first experience with treatment decision-making will most likely be at the time when the disease becomes incurable. Parents and healthcare providers report that the most challenging decision-making in pediatric oncology occurs when efforts to cure the cancer have failed.[15] A few parents report that end-of-life decision-making was not complicated for them because they had already decided what they would do if their child's cancer did not respond to treatment.

However, the majority of parents and healthcare providers involved in the decision process describe this time as extraordinarily difficult. They attribute the difficulty to multiple and complex factors that must be considered, including the differing preferences of those involved in the actual decision-making or affected by it, and to intense emotions at a time when the parents' energy is depleted.

Neonatal and other pediatric specialties

End-of-life decision-making in pediatric oncology has been influenced by clinical and research reports from neonatal and other pediatric specialties and organizations. The growing commitment by professional associations to include pediatric patients and parents in end-of-life decisions marks a notable shift in care philosophy. Expectations that patients and their parents should be involved in these decisions have been formalized in policy statements of organizations such as the American Academy of Pediatrics[16]; the American Nurses Association[17]; the United Hospital Fund in its report on end-of-life care in New York offering palliative care guidance (http://www.uhfnyc.org/news/880732, 2011 release) and corresponding guidance for family caregivers (http://nextstepincare.org/left_top_menu/caregiver_Home/Hospice); the collaborative precepts statements ("Precepts of Palliative Care for Children and Adolescents and Their Families") issued by the National Association of Neonatal Nurses, the Association of Pediatric Oncology Nurses, and the Last Acts Palliative Care Task Force (www.lastacts.org/palliativecare); the recommendations from the Institute of Medicine[14]; the care guidelines issued jointly by the nurse members of the Children's Oncology Group and the members of the Association of Pediatric Oncology and Hematology Nursing[18]; and the guidelines most recently issued by the Hastings Center.[19] In these published statements, the recommended patient and parental involvement is described as participative and mutual with healthcare providers. Legislative rulings and legal decisions in some states and Canadian provinces support the participation of adolescents or mature minors in medical decision-making and in creating advance directives.[20-22] Regulatory bodies such as the Joint Commission Accreditation of Health Care Organizations (JCAHO) and health policy influencing groups such as the National Quality Forum are now becoming involved in directing or evaluating end-of-life care,[23,24] including patient and parental involvement in end-of-life decision-making. It is also likely that such involvement will be considered an indicator of the quality of end-of-life care and be linked to reimbursement for such care, as is now being proposed for adult cancer patients.[25] It is relevant to note that the sources of the above policy statements are based in the Western hemisphere in what are referred to as highly developed, industrialized nations.

The actual extent to which patients and parents participate in end-of-life decision-making varies and can be influenced by the personal and professional preferences of the healthcare provider. For example, the way the healthcare provider frames or words information about treatment options may influence the way a patient and family perceive the available alternatives.[26,27] Some advocate that the physician should assume the final responsibility for the decision, whereas others believe that the parents or even the adolescent patient should be the primary decision-maker.[19-22] Even fewer sources advocate that children should be the primary decision-makers, but several advocate that children as young as 6[28,29] should be involved in the decision-making.

The available reports on end-of-life decision-making that involve parents and healthcare providers are predominantly from neonatal settings. End-of-life decisions in these settings often reflect the presenting condition of the infant. The number of immature and critically ill neonates being admitted to neonatal intensive care units (NICUs) over the past 20 years has increased significantly, as have the corresponding recommendations from healthcare teams for end-of-life care.[30] The end-of-life decisions primarily considered include (1) limiting care, (2) withdrawing life support, or (3) withholding life support for infants who are extremely premature or have severe congenital abnormalities. Most reports describe the decision-making as having been initiated when the intensivist determined that the infant had no chance for survival or no chance for quality of life. In most cases (94% in one study),[31] parents agreed with the recommendations of the intensivist or the infant's attending physician. When bereaved parents were contacted after the death of their infant, those parents who perceived having shared in the end-of-life decision making with the physician had lower grief scores than did parents who reported being involved in other styles of end-of-life decision-making.[32]

Research findings related to end-of-life decision-making in the NICU had been primarily based on medical record reviews with notable exceptions.[32–34] In one study, Able-Boone and colleagues[33] interviewed parents and healthcare providers of seriously ill infants regarding medical decision-making and the provision of healthcare information. The parents emphasized their need and desire to be honestly informed of their child's health status. They expressed special appreciation of healthcare professionals who drew pictures to convey technical information rather than relying only on words. Parents also expressed a strong need for information that is coordinated by the healthcare team so that it is not confusing or contradictory.

In a second study that recorded the values of parents in end-of-life decisions is the grounded-theory study in which Rushton[34] interviewed 31 parents of 20 hospitalized neonates with life-threatening congenital disorders about their decisions for or against implementing or continuing life-sustaining measures for their infants. Rushton concluded that the parents made these decisions based on their understanding of what it means to be a "good parent" for a neonate with a life-threatening congenital disorder. According to these parents, the characteristics of good parents for such neonates include putting the needs of the neonate first, not giving up, not taking the "easy" way out despite the self-sacrifice involved, and courage to pursue a "good" outcome for the child.

The concept of "being a good parent to my seriously ill child" has also been studied in pediatric oncology. Hinds and colleagues interviewed more than 100 parents of children and adolescents with incurable cancers across several studies at the time of end-of-life decision making. Consistently, the majority of parents (approximately 80% within each study) identified their definition of being a good parent as influencing their end-of-life decision making on behalf of their very ill child.[5,15] Key characteristics of their definition of being a good parent to a seriously ill child have some overlap with those identified by Rushton and include "doing right by my child," "being there for my child," "conveying love to my child," "advocating for my child with staff," "having adequate knowledge of my child's medical situation to make informed and unselfish decisions," "providing the basics of food, shelter, clothing and positive health to the extent possible," "teaching my child to make good choices," "teaching my child to respect and have sympathy for others," and "to know God."[35] These characteristics did not differ by type of end-of-life decision made or by diagnosis.[36] Parents also identified the behaviors from clinicians that helped them to achieve their definition of being a good parent before their child died; primary behaviors included "respecting me and my decision," "knowing that all that can be done is being done," and "staff continue to comfort me and my child."[35] These same clinical investigators implemented a parent/clinician end-of-life communication intervention that centered on parents' definition of being a good parent to their child with incurable cancer and documented the feasibility and acceptability of this intervention to parents and clinicians and the positive outcomes including satisfaction with study participation, incorporation of the definition in clinical care, and a changed and more positive awareness in parents of having achieved their definition of being a good parent.[37] This work indicates the importance of this concept in supporting parents in their role of participating in end-of-life decision-making on behalf of their ill child.

Reviews of the medical records of patients who have died in pediatric intensive care units (PICUs) show that withdrawal of life support was chosen in 0% to 54% of cases[38–40] and that limitation of supportive care (described as not escalating care efforts but providing hydration and pain comfort measures) was chosen in 26% to 46% of cases. The wide range of these percentages may reflect cultural, ethnic, or religious differences: the lowest rate of withdrawal of life support reported was from India and the highest rates were from PICUs in Europe, the United States, and the United Kingdom. Even within a single PICU setting, decision-making can reflect cultural differences. For example, the report from a Malaysian setting noted that Muslim parents declined end-of-life options at significantly higher rates than did non-Muslim parents.[39] Reports may also reflect the research method used. For example, Meyer and colleagues[41] relied on surveys completed by parents to assess parental perceptions of pain control, decision-making, and social supports during their child's dying in a PICU. Parents reported that in most cases ($n = 56$; 90%) the physician initiated the end-of-life discussion, but in approximately half of those cases, parents had been privately considering an end-of-life decision. Factors identified by parents as influencing their decision-making included concerns about their child's quality of life, their child's chance of getting better, their child's pain or discomfort, advice of hospital staff, attitudes of hospital staff, and advice of friends or family members. Similar findings have been reported in Germany[42] and most recently in the United States.[43] Several medical record reviews of end-of-life characteristics of children dying of cancer have recently been completed. In general, the majority of these children and adolescents die of progressive disease with a medical order not to resuscitate (DNR). These characteristics indicate the child's likely death had been discussed with parents or family members. However, despite parental involvement in decision-making, the factors that influenced the decision-making and how the end-of-life discussions were initiated or facilitated were not included in the published reports. Recently published figures indicate that the majority (65% to 87%) of pediatric deaths are preceded by an end-of-life decision[44,45] and that fewer children (<10% in some reports) are dying in the pediatric intensive care setting.[42] These figures suggest that pediatric healthcare providers can correctly anticipate the likelihood of being involved in end-of-life decision-making during their careers and the need to be competent in assisting families with such decision-making.

Participation of children and adolescents

Children and adolescents are not routinely involved in making end-of-life decisions on their own behalf, largely because of doubt on the part of parents and healthcare providers that the child or adolescent has sufficient understanding of the clinical situation. This doubt is based in part on adults' belief that children and adolescents are unable to appraise their well-being and are unaware of their life goals and values and appears to have a detectable basis in culturally derived perspectives on the cognitive and reasoning capabilities of adolescents. Buchanan and Brock[46] described children who are 9 years or older as competent to make certain decisions, but they did not study children's competence in end-of-life decision-making. The same authors also indicated that children of that age may be competent to make some decisions but not others, and that competence thus depends on the specific decision. According to Ariff and Groh,[47] a child's competence to make medical decisions is an ongoing developmental process that parallels other cognitive, moral, and emotional processes and is influenced by environment and by physical and mental illness. The capacity to make an end-of-life decision cannot be determined, then, on the basis of the child's or adolescent's competence in a different situation or decision. Instead, competence must be determined for each specific decision at a defined time point and under specific circumstances. Although healthy adolescents are able to make decisions, they may be unaware of all possible options or may be unable to identify all possible consequences of those options[48] and thus may need assistance in identifying, considering, and selecting care options. A more recent study of adolescents with incurable cancer involved in an end-of-life decision on their own behalf indicated they were very able to identify end-of-life care options and the consequences of each option.[49] These differences in study findings involving healthy adolescents and adolescents experiencing a chronic or life threatening illness may indicate that serious illness experiences may facilitate adolescent awareness and understanding of the seriousness of the treatment decision-making and the related outcomes for self and others.

Experiencing a life-threatening illness such as cancer and seeing others suffer and die from it may also help a child to understand death and his or her own end-of-life circumstances.[49,50] Although they acknowledged that the competence to participate in decision-making differs with age and cognitive abilities, nearly two decades ago Burns and Truog[51] recommended that children and adolescents be involved early in the process of medical decision-making, including end-of-life decisions. In fact, Burns and Truog warned that if a child or adolescent is not involved early in the decision-making process, his or her ability to express an opinion may be lost before it can be exercised. Leikin[52] theorized that adolescents who have been treated for cancer have a clearer idea of the burdens and benefits of treatment options that are most acceptable to them. The ethical perspective is that adolescents have a conception of what is good for themselves. The treatment experience itself contributes to the adolescents' abilities to participate in end-of-life decision-making. A similar conclusion was reported by Hinds et al.[49] after analyzing data from interviews with 10- to 21-year-olds about their own end-of-life decision-making. These pediatric oncology patients were able to describe the decision they had made, the factors that influenced their decision-making, and their awareness of both likely short-term and long-term outcomes of their decision, including the effects the decision could have on others. These abilities comprise competence in participating in end-of-life decision-making on their own behalf. Impressively, the primary factor considered in their end-of-life decision-making was relationships with others and concern for them. Similarly and very recently, Miller and colleagues documented the perspectives of 20 adolescents ranging in age from 14 to 21 years who described in interview format their reasons for agreeing to participate in a Phase I clinical trial when their disease became incurable. Primary reasons included the desire for a longer life, seeking a positive clinical benefit, and hoping for an improved quality of life.[53] Preliminary findings from two other research teams led by Wiener[54] and Lyons[55] have also reported on the preferences and competence of seriously ill (in treatment for metastatic cancer or HIV) adolescents and young adults (14 to 28 years of age) for being involved in advanced care planning. Both research teams have documented that these adolescents and young adults did not find it stressful (by report of the study participants) to discuss their end-of-life planning and the majority reported such discussions to be help or very helpful to them.

Our combined clinical and research experiences have convinced us that, as a general rule, seriously ill patients age 10 years and older are able to understand that they are participating in decisions about their cancer-related treatment and their lives and are able to understand the options and the likely outcomes. Of course, some younger patients may also understand these issues and be competent to participate in end-of-life decisions, whereas some older patients may be less competent. Because of these very possible differences in understanding, each child needs to be individually assessed for his or her competence to participate. An assumption that a child is or is not competent to participate made without the assessment is not in the child's best interest.

Others have provided compelling support for the involvement of younger children in end-of-life decision-making. Nitschke and colleagues[28,29] reported that patients as young as age 6 years participated in end-of-life discussions in their pediatric oncology treatment setting. They described care conferences held with 43 families over a 6-year period in which children and adolescents with end-stage cancer, and their families, participated in discussions of therapeutic options, disease progression, lack of effective therapies, improbability of cure, and imminent death. The patients (who were ages 6–20 years) and their parents were offered the choice of Phase II investigational drugs or supportive care. According to this report, it was the patients who most frequently made the final decision. Fourteen chose further chemotherapy, 28 chose supportive care only, and 1 made no decision. Nitschke and colleagues also noted that patients younger than age 9 years understood that they were going to die soon of their disease. The authors concluded that children with cancer do have an advanced understanding of death and recommended that children as young as age 5 years have the capacity to make decisions about whether to continue therapy. This team did not investigate the specific factors considered by the patients, parents, and healthcare providers and did not describe ways in which providers may have attempted to facilitate patient and parent decision-making.

A healthcare team member who has established a relationship of trust with the child or adolescent and who has observed the child or adolescent in various challenging clinical situations is likely to be the best judge of competence in end-of-life decision-making.

However, before initiating this assessment, the healthcare team should discuss the purpose and process of the assessment, first as a group and then with the patient's parent or parents, and identify any areas of actual or potential disagreement between the team and the parents. Disagreements should be openly discussed, and participants should be allowed sufficient time to weigh the issues—another reason for initiating the end-of-life discussions in a timely manner. After the team and the parents agree on the intent and timing of the competence assessment, the team member, parent(s), and child or adolescent choose the location for the discussion. Most children younger than age 11 years prefer to have their parents present for this discussion.

Determining the child's or adolescent's competence requires establishing whether he/she understands the seriousness of the medical condition and understands that a decision point is at hand. If asked to explain the seriousness of the situation, the child or adolescent will use words or describe events that have personal, symbolic, or literal meaning. The healthcare team can then use these same words to communicate with the patient about decision-making. Throughout the assessment, the child or adolescent will need reassurance from the healthcare team member that the serious situation is not the fault of the child or adolescent.[56] The child or adolescent must also be able to indicate an understanding of the choices, including the potential consequences of each. In addition, the child or adolescent must show an understanding of how each choice made now could change future options. The healthcare team member conducting the assessment must ensure that the child or adolescent does not feel coerced to make a certain choice. The team member should also ensure that the child or adolescent has access to the information needed to make a competent decision. The team member needs to allow repeated opportunities for the child or adolescent to review the options and discuss concerns and to do so in a manner that is not rushed, and to provide different mechanisms (verbal, written, drawing) to facilitate expression of concerns or preferences.[57] It is especially important that the team member assess to what extent the child or adolescent wants to be included in the decision-making. That preference should be honored regardless of the personal preferences of team members.

Our experience is that children (some as young as age 7 years) have definite preferences regarding whether to participate in a Phase I clinical trial. Preferences most commonly reflect a desire to be home, to live a little bit longer, to play with a sibling or a friend, or to not feel sickly. Preferences regarding DNR status, although quite firmly expressed by some adolescents, tend to require more patient contemplation time. By the time this type of end-of-life decision-making needs to be considered, the members of the healthcare team are very familiar with the child and the family and already have established a style of interacting. However, it is generally useful to preface the assessment of patient preference with a statement that conveys the important nature of what is about to be said, such as, "May I ask you to be quite serious with me for a few moments? I want to tell you something important about your [insert here the term used by the child when referring to the illness]. And I want you to tell me something, too." If the child conveys an inability to be serious at that moment, the team member needs to clarify whether that means the child only wants the "serious and important" topics to be discussed with the child's family, or if it means the child wants to try to be serious at a later time. Clinicians are encouraged to allow repeated opportunities for the child or adolescent to review the care options or concerns, to provide a variety of mechanisms to facilitate the child's expressions (such as using words, drawing, or writing), and to do so in a manner that is not rushed.

Competence of surrogates

Concern about patients' competence to participate in end-of-life decisions, although valid, may sometimes be exaggerated. It is relatively easy to usurp the autonomy of children and adolescents in end-of-life decision-making. This threat lends special importance to the use of guidelines for making end-of-life decisions. Guidelines could serve as formal reminders to healthcare professionals to consider the preferences of children and adolescents to the extent that is possible or advisable. Of equal or greater concern is the competence of parents and healthcare providers to make such decisions on behalf of the child or adolescent. Making these decisions competently requires an understanding of their own values, the patient's values and goals, the treatment options, the likely outcome of each option, and the nature of the life-threatening illness. To achieve competence, surrogates such as parents need to have adequate information and awareness about their child's situation. Parents who recognize that their child will not be cured have been described as more able to say goodbye to their child in the way that they wish[3] or "letting go"[58] and are more likely to have their child treated with noncurative intent at the time of the child's death.[59] This imposes a short-term and a longer-term burden of unknown proportions on the parents and the healthcare providers. A recent report indicates that parents and pediatric oncology patients have overlapping factors in their individual end-of-life decision-making on behalf of the ill patient.[49]

There are a limited number of empirically based or theoretically based guidelines for involving children, adolescents, or their parents in end-of-life decisions, but in clinical care situations, the general assumption is that children younger than age 10 years are of doubtful competence to participate in such decision-making and that their parents are both competent and attentive to the best interests of their child. These assumptions could work to ensure that end-of-life decisions are made for seriously ill children and adolescents by their parents and healthcare professionals without involvement of the ill child. Although legal rulings and common healthcare practices support the role of parents as surrogates in treatment decision-making, there are an emerging number of position papers from professional associations that advocate for each end-of-life situation in pediatrics to be individually considered. To feel competent, to be competent, and to be satisfied with their performance as surrogate decision-makers, parents and healthcare providers need opportunities to exchange information about the child's preferences, the family's preferences, the child's chances of survival, the progression of the disease, and the intensity and intrusiveness of life-extending interventions and the likelihood of their effectiveness (including length of time gained). They also need to reflect on previous efforts to achieve cure and to question previous decisions. Competence of surrogates may also be affected by their realization of the likelihood of their child not surviving cancer. In one retrospective, descriptive study that included parent interviews and review of medical records, it was identified that physicians knew up to a year before the parents that the child would not survive.[60] Participating in end-of-life care planning is unlikely if the reality of the child's death is not yet in the parents' or surrogates' awareness. Competence of surrogate participation is also influenced by the challenges faced by healthcare providers when trying to accurately predict timing of the dying.[61] However, only in a limited number of cases is the child's dying unexpected. Because of that, some degree of planning for preferred model of end-of-life care (home, home with hospice, hospital, hospital with hospice) is possible.[62,63] Matching the surrogates' preferences for end-of-life care might contribute to decreasing the morbidity of bereaved survivors. As Mack and colleagues have documented, bereaved parents report that their communication with their child's physician was the primary basis for believing that their child did or did not receive the best possible end-of-life care and the basis of being satisfied or not with the actual care received.[64] Insuring competence of the surrogate decision maker, in most instances the parent, does mean that the parent or surrogate and the clinicians providing care to the seriously ill child need to find common ground and shared understanding of the overall clinical situation. Doing so will diminish the risk of untoward patient care outcomes and as well negative outcomes for the surrogate and healthcare provider decision makers.[65]

Participation of patients and parents

Previous studies indicate that the more informed parents become about their seriously ill child's condition, the more they are able to participate in making decisions and advocating for their child and the more certain they are of their decision/s. Parents report that information is most helpful when it is provided gradually and repeatedly,[66] and respectfully in words that are easy to understand.[30] Including information about the prognosis, likely outcomes, a commitment not to allow suffering, and to respect religious beliefs have also been identified by parents as quite helpful at the time of end-of-life decision-making.[30,67,68] In addition, seeing the healthcare team members treat the very ill neonate or child with respect and offer estimates of the appropriateness of the possible care as compared to its burdensome nature were both viewed as helpful with end-of-life decision-making.[69] Stevens[70] recommends that parents be allowed to make tape recordings or bring friends or family members to the treatment-related discussions to help them later recall the details of the discussion. Other investigators suggest that parents differ in how much detailed information they desire[71] and in how much they want to participate in the actual decision-making[72,73] during periods of crisis in their child's illness. However, parental preferences about participation in end-of-life decision-making have not been well studied and it does appear from the limited research available that parental preference for participation can vary and that occasionally may be motivated by reasons outside of the child's condition.[74,75] This does call for a case-by-case consideration[76] facilitated by decision-making guidelines.

In an international feasibility study, parents from pediatric oncology settings in Australia, Hong Kong, and the United States were interviewed about their decision-making on behalf of their ill child.[77] There were clear differences among the countries in parental preference for involvement in decision-making. Mothers in Hong Kong were reluctant to participate in end-of-life decisions because of either their gender ("Women cannot make

these decisions.") or their lack of expert knowledge ("I am only the mother. The doctor is the expert and he should decide.").[77] It remains unknown whether these parental preferences change between diagnosis and end-of-life. Regardless of their preference, all parents need reassurance from the healthcare team that their child's condition is not their fault.[70]

The factors that parents consider at decision points in the treatment of their seriously ill child have only recently been studied. Using a phenomenological approach, Kirschbaum[78] interviewed 20 parents of children who had died in the previous 6 to 12 months. The parents had all made life-support decisions on behalf of their ill child. Various diagnoses were represented, including trauma, cancer, septic shock, liver failure, and congestive heart disease. Nine factors were identified as having influenced the parental decisions: (1) wanting life as the principal good for their child, (2) avoiding suffering and pain, (3) considering current and future quality of life, (4) respecting the individuality of the child, (5) defining and redefining the family, (6) having spiritual beliefs and explanations, (7) believing in natural or biological explanations, (8) considering the child's unique personality, and (9) having a favorable view of technology in healthcare.

In a retrospective study that conducted telephone interviews with 39 parents of 37 pediatric oncology patients who had died in the previous 6 to 24 months, Hinds and colleagues[15] were able to identify the factors most frequently considered by parents in end-of-life decision-making. The end-of-life decisions that were reported most frequently by these parents were choosing between a Phase I drug study and no further treatment ($n = 14$), maintaining or withdrawing life support ($n = 11$), and giving more chemotherapy or ending treatment ($n = 8$). The factor most considered in the parents' decision-making was "information received from healthcare professionals." This information included facts, explanations, and opinions about their child's disease status, likelihood of survival, and complexities of continued care. Other factors parents frequently reported were "feeling supported by and trusting of the staff," which reflected the parents' sense that the healthcare team listened and responded to their or their child's concerns and respected the parents' decisions, and "making decisions together with my child." This factor reflected the parents' comfort in having known and respected their child's wishes.

The parents also completed a 15-item questionnaire about the importance of each factor considered in their decision-making. The parents rated eight items as "very important" at least 50% of the time. The highest-rated factors included "recommendations received from healthcare professionals," "things my child had said about continuing or not continuing treatment," "information received from healthcare professionals," "my child's breathing problems," and "sensing that my child was no longer himself [herself]." These findings clearly indicate that information and recommendations received from healthcare professionals are very important to parents who are making end-of-life decisions on behalf of their child, as is feeling certain of their child's desires about treatment.

The same research team has prospectively studied end-of-life decision-making by conducting interviews of parents, physicians, and, when possible, the children or adolescents with incurable disease who had participated in making an end-of-life decision within the past week. The same factors noted in the retrospective study—related to trust, support, information, and advice—were also identified in the prospective study. In addition, parents cited these factors: wishing for the child's survival, reassuring themselves of the correctness of their decisions, questioning certain statements or behaviors of healthcare professionals, and making decisions that would allow them to maintain communication with their dying child for as long as possible (Box 58.2).

Box 58.2 Guidelines for the healthcare team to use in assisting parents with end-of-life decision-making

1. At the time of diagnosis and throughout treatment, actively seek opportunities to provide information to the parent about treatment and the patient's response to treatment.

2. At the time of diagnosis and throughout treatment, involve the parent in treatment-related discussions and decision-making. Be available to discuss and rediscuss decisions and related concerns.

3. Ask parents if they would like to talk with parents of other pediatric oncology patients.

4. Verbally and nonverbally reassure the parents that they are "good" parents who are committed to the well-being of their child.

5. Give assurances that everything that can be done to help the patient is being done and being done well.

6. As the child's disease progresses, provide clear verbal (and written, if desired by the parent) explanations of the child's status. Provide visual sources of evidence such as actual scans.

7. Inform parents of treatment options as they become available in the treating institution or elsewhere.

8. At each treatment juncture, ask the parents what they are hoping for and anticipate that they will have more than one hope.

9. Include more than one healthcare team member in end-of-life discussions with the parents.

10. When discussing end-of-life options with parents,

    a. Strongly emphasize the team's commitment to the patient's comfort and to providing expert care at all times.

    b. Offer professional recommendations.

    c. Describe how their child is likely to respond to each option (the child's physical appearance, ability to communicate, etc.).

    d. Give information about other support resources (ethics committees, social services, other healthcare professionals, etc.).

11. When discussing end-of-life options with parents, anticipate

    a. Parents' vacillation between certainty and uncertainty about the decision.

    b. Parents' need for clarification and additional information to resolve their uncertainties.

    c. Parent's need for practical information about ways to explain the end-of-life decision to other family members.

    d. Being asked to give personal advice, i.e., what you would do if this was your child.

12. Allow parents private time to consider the options.

13. Maintain sensitivity to any specific ethnic, cultural, or religious preferences during end-of-life care.

14. Convey respect for the parents' right to change decisions, when clinically feasible.

15. Consider seeking an ethics consultation for the family and/or the healthcare team as a whole.

16. Consider seeking consultation from palliative care experts.

17. Demonstrate commitment to maintaining the child's comfort and dignity, and to affirming the parents' role.

18. Do not question the parents' decision after it has been made.

19. Carefully document the end-of-life treatment or care decision once it is made so that all clinicians can be fully informed of this decision.

Case study

A decision agreement between parents and the healthcare team

A 12-month-old infant girl has been treated for an aggressive form of leukemia. It was clear that the disease was not responding to chemotherapy. The patient was transferred to the PICU when she began to experience respiratory distress. Initially, oxygen was administered by simple mask, but her breathing difficulties persisted and became more evident within a few hours. The possibility of endotracheal intubation was first discussed among the healthcare team members and then with the parents. During the meeting with the parents, the current symptoms of the little girl were discussed, the current disease status and its unresponsiveness to treatment were reviewed, and options of intubating or not intubating were considered. The parents then discussed the options privately with each other and in less than 30 minutes reached the decision that ventilatory support not be a part of their daughter's medical care. The parents said that knowing that their daughter was not going to be cured of the leukemia and understanding that the ventilator would help reduce their daughter's respiratory distress but not the leukemia were both factors that assisted them in making the decision. They credited their discussions with the doctors as key: "From the discussion we had with the doctors, we felt if it came to that point, the only reason for using a ventilator would be just to keep her breathing." An additional factor identified by the parents as influencing their decision-making was support from the healthcare team. "Chaplain X and Dr. Y were real patient with us and understood the situation that we were in and did not seem to put pressure one way or another, or seem to think that we were making the wrong decision one way or another . . . they told us the decision was actually ours. They let us know that, but they were supportive and also gave us their opinions."

Case study
Disagreements among healthcare team providers

Rachel is a 3-year-old with multiply recurrent neuroblastoma who remains quite interactive and playful much of the time, despite being hampered with a pathological fracture of her leg, diffuse painful lower extremity edema due to lymphatic obstruction from bulky tumor-laden lymph nodes, and around-the clock prescribed opioids. Her mom is a very involved single mother who is quite large and imposing and becomes openly hostile when any member of the healthcare team tries to discuss stopping further cancer-directed therapy or the term "hospice care." Rachel's recent therapy has included several experimental, Phase I studies, one of which resulted in a nearly complete response of her tumor, although it was very short-lived. Rachel is currently receiving a course of palliative radiation to some of her bulky lymph nodes and has had several recent hospitalizations for control of pain and fever. Although Mom has had very frank discussions with Rachel's primary oncologist about what to do should Rachel acutely deteriorate, even in fact agreeing to a "DNR," she prefers that this agreement not be posted in the medical record because she fears that Rachel will then receive "different care." She is insisting on enrollment in another Phase I trial. Nurses on the clinical care team are opposed to enrolling this child on additional experimental Phase I clinical trials for fear of burdening her with the hospitalizations that are a part of the available trial. The primary oncologist believes that the mother has the right to know about the open Phase I trial. The tension among the team members is subsequently addressed by a total team meeting with Rachel's mom to review her awareness of her daughter's disease being incurable and her understanding of the purpose of the Phase I trial. Further, her understanding of the DNR status is reviewed. Members of the healthcare team in attendance repeat to the Mom their understanding of her care preferences including the actions they are to take regarding resuscitation. Although study team members remain concerned about the clinical situation, they are more settled following the total team meeting in the plan of care and their role in that plan.

Case study
Initial disagreement between parents

Tom is a 10-year-old, near genius, with progressive metastatic neuroblastoma, who has undergone multiple relapses during more than 4 years of dealing with his cancer. He has an intact loving family. His parents are well educated and very involved with Tom's care, often taking turns in bringing Tom to the hospital, although Mom is the primary caregiver a majority of the time. Recently the disease has begun to progress and is showing more and more signs of becoming unresponsive to further therapy. Tom is experiencing multiple and an increasing number of symptoms that are very troubling to him and it is apparent to all members of the healthcare team caring for Tom how well he understands his disease and his ultimate prognosis. Dad also has a very accurate and pragmatic view of Tom's prognosis, asking very appropriate questions about possible home hospice care. Mom, although admitting the bleak prognosis, continues to press for other cancer-directed therapy. It is apparent to members of the healthcare team that there is significant conflict between the parents regarding end-of-life care

decisions for Tom but they do a good job of hiding this from Tom most of the time. It is also apparent that Tom, if given the choice by *both* his parents is tired of multiple trips to the hospital and is ready to go home for good. However, he seems unwilling to voice his wishes out of respect and concern for his mother. After several experimental Phase I protocols, some palliative radiation and several hospital admissions, Tom and his parents come to the same treatment preference, which is to return home with the support of home hospice care, and Tom subsequently dies at home. Although agreement was achieved, the parents choose to separate several months later.

Case study
A decision agreement between parents and care team

A 4-year-old boy with recurrent neuroblastoma was admitted for confirmed sepsis following a course of chemotherapy as per a Phase 1 protocol. The patient was transferred to the PICU for antibiotics, fluid boluses, central venous pressure monitoring, and vasopressor support. However, over the next 48 hours he experienced renal failure followed by increased respiratory effort as his abdomen became distended. A morphine infusion was initiated to provide adequate pain control. Oxygen delivery via a mask was not sufficient to maintain normal blood gases, and his perfusion became worse despite maximum infusion rates of dopamine and dobutamine. The possibility of endotracheal intubation and hemofiltration was first discussed among the healthcare team members and then with the parents. Both the healthcare team and parents openly discussed the realization that the current chemotherapy was not controlling the neuroblastoma. The parents then discussed the options privately with each other and in less than an hour reached the decision that they did not want an endotracheal tube inserted or hemofiltration initiated. The parents said that knowing that their son was not going to be cured of neuroblastoma and understanding that the ventilator would only help reduce their son's respiratory distress but not reduce the disease were factors that assisted them in making the decision. Both parents acknowledged that having their primary oncologist being part of the discussions with the PICU team provided the needed consistency in remaining focused on how to know when adding treatments would only prolong suffering without impacting the underlying problem, that of his tumor becoming resistant to chemotherapy. Having the assurance that symptom control including infusions of opioids and anxiolytics would be continued further convinced them that their decision was best for their child as indicated by their statement: "the doctors and nurses helped us to realize our child was comfortable on the morphine infusion since we would see his heart rate as normal and he was relaxed in his bed. If we had chosen the ventilator, the need for more sedation and maybe paralytics would have made it harder for us to know he was still comfortable. Explanations of what it means to choose each option such as the ventilator was important for us to know we were really doing what was best for our child." Later that day the child asked his parents if he could see his puppy at the hospital. Arrangements were made to allow his dog into the hospital and these were interpreted by the parents as further validation that they had made a decision that would contribute to a peaceful death for their child.

Case study

Disagreement between parents

A 16-year-old girl with refractory acute lymphocytic leukemia was referred to an oncology center for a bone marrow transplant. She was accompanied by both of her parents, who were divorced with her father as the legal guardian. Upon arrival her diagnostic scans indicated disseminated disease including spinal bone involvement with multiple pathological fractures. Pain control could not be achieved with intravenous opioid infusions; therefore, an epidural infusion with fentanyl and bupivacaine was provided, resulting in improved comfort especially during movement. However, her respiratory effort became more laborious with evidence of increased pleural effusions on chest X-ray; oxygen by nasal cannula was provided. The bone marrow transplant team met daily with both parents to explain why an immediate bone marrow transplant could not be provided due to the instability of their child's medical status. Her mother understood and asked that she be provided comfort measures with the possibility of taking her home on hospice support. Her father did not want to discuss this plan and adamantly wanted to continue all medical care including the possible need for ventilatory support. When one of the transplant physicians reviewed the plan to place an endotracheal tube if necessary with the girl, she agreed to that plan as long as she would not be aware of the need for the ventilator to breathe for her. The next day while the oxygen delivery was changed to a mask due to deceased oxygen saturation, the girl told the nurse, privately, that she did not want to be "knocked out and put in the ICU." Instead, she preferred only doing what needed to be done so that "I can go home and see my friends before I die." The nurse asked her to consider explaining her preferences to her father. The 16-year-old stated she did not want to disappoint her father, as he was the one who took care of her since she was a young girl when her mother abandoned her. The nurse then made the social worker aware of what the girl had told the nurse, and a plan was made to have a patient care conference with the parents and a few members of the team. However, her father refused to attend this meeting, stating that he was aware that his daughter wanted to go home now. He added that he would not "give up on my daughter as she is all I have in my life. I had to resign from my job to come to this hospital which is 10 hours away and I had to commit to being with her for 10 months post-BMT." The mother did attend the conference and said that it would be helpful to her ex-husband if he could have more time and information to realize that a cure "was not going to happen." She further expressed that waiting for him to see that "everything was done" would help him after their daughter died. Meanwhile, chest X-rays indicated that the pleural effusions were worsening and endotracheal intubation was imminent. Gradually, the father indicated he recognized that his daughter was suffering from not being able to go home to more familiar surroundings and he then accepted more support from the healthcare team. The physician and the nurse practitioner (NP) sensed the father's coming to terms with his daughter's declining medical status. The father was then able to participate in the decision to drain her pleural effusions under sedation so that her respiratory status could possibly improve, giving him more time with her. Later that day, both parents were able to shift the goal of care from cure to comfort and return to their home community to honor their daughter's wishes. Because of her need for continuing the epidural infusion and oxygen support, the physician and NP arranged ground ambulance transport back to the community hospital where she was surrounded by more family members and friends at the time of her death 3 days later.

Case study

Adolescent and parent tension over end-of-life treatment decision-making

A 15-year-old male with progressive large B-cell lymphoma recently began a new chemotherapy and was admitted for fever and symptom control (pain, nausea, fatigue, and pruritus). He and his parents were from a non-Western country and are in the United States for treatment without any other family support. He understood and spoke English, but his parents had a very limited understanding of English. Family members who remained in the home country of this patient were opposed to having the patient treated for his cancer by Western doctors. Before coming to the United States for treatment, the patient had lived away from his parents to attend a boarding school and while there made the majority of his own life decisions. His healthcare team had arranged for his acupuncture treatments, which this adolescent regarded as beneficial for promoting his sleep. With his symptoms well controlled, he was able to concentrate and play games on his laptop computer, an activity he enjoyed. The initial treatment goal for this patient had been a cure for his lymphoma with chemotherapy and an autologous bone marrow transplant. Both the patient and his parents realized that the likelihood of cure was low and that the greater likelihood was that the adolescent would not survive his disease. As treatment progressed, his parents were making treatment decisions including interventions for pain control. This led to conflict with his parents. Increasing metastatic disease in the mediastinal space led to episodes of painful coughing. His father urged his son "to fight the pain" and not ask for as many analgesics which the father thought led to itching and sedation; the patient cried and said, "Easy for you to say," resulting in his father feeling guilty for asking his son to avoid pain medicine because he feared that the opioids were causing his son serious problems. The team learned that the parents' perceptions of pain interventions meant their son was worsening and dying. Over the last few days his life his respiratory effort increased and discussions were held with the adolescent and his parents regarding the option of discharging him with hospice support; however, the patient continued to say "I feel safer in the hospital." He had been reluctant to complete his My Wishes document, which would communicate his wishes if his disease continued to progress since he did not like to think about his dying. He wanted instead to proceed with more treatment for the lymphoma, stating "I would rather die from the chemotherapy than the cancer." He also stated "I do not like to be reminded I am sick and please talk to my parents about what is happening to me outside of my room. I just want to relax and do what I can do for fun such as play with my computer games rather than focus on my illness." Although suffering was reduced, evidenced by the patient's minimal ratings of pain, cough, pruritus, and nausea, tension between the patient and the staff with his parents existed due to their concern that their son was becoming addicted to medications. Interdisciplinary meetings were held to assure that the healthcare team was honoring the patient's preferences, controlling his pain, maintaining trust, preventing suffering, and providing emotional support for this adolescent and his family.

Twenty patients participated in individual interviews about the end-of-life decision they had made. The factors most frequently considered in their decisions included "Being influenced by relationships with others," "Information from my doctor or my parents," "Wanting to be done with treatment," and "Worrying about my family."[49] These factors convey the interconnectedness between children or adolescents with incurable diseases and their families and healthcare providers. All are affected by the decision-making process and the outcomes of the decision. This interconnectedness among the seriously ill child or adolescent, the family, and the healthcare providers contributes to more agreements on end-of-life decisions than disagreements. Although rare, disagreements between the patient and parent, or between parents and healthcare providers, do occur and are especially difficult for all involved. Disagreeing with a healthcare professional who is deemed essential for their child's well-being and with whom a care alliance is desired is at best troubling for parents but at worst disruptive to relationships and problem solving. When circumstances exist that allow a delay in the contested decision-making, a consultation with an ethicist or ethics board can facilitate decision-making. Involving the family, the patient who is deemed competent to participate in end-of-life decision-making, and the healthcare team in the same meeting with the ethicist or ethics board is particularly helpful, as all perspectives can be considered. When a family and a healthcare team do not have agreement, special measures must be initiated by the team leaders to support team members in their efforts to continue to deliver excellent care to the patient and family. Measures can include brief meetings with an esteemed institutional leader who openly acknowledges the sizable difficulty that the team is facing, having information-sharing or cathartic sessions with the ethicist, and developing strategies for handling similar future difficulties. Likewise, similar support measures need to be implemented for the family. In addition, regular opportunities to interact with the healthcare team (such as care conferences) need to be established so that trust between the family and team can be fostered.

Factors considered by healthcare providers

The factors considered by healthcare professionals in end-of-life decision-making on behalf of children and adolescents reveal important similarities and differences between nurses and physicians. Current reports indicate that nurses are more likely to reflect on the moral balance of the decision, that is, the goodness or lack thereof of extending a child's life if doing so also extends or increases the child's suffering,[79] whereas physicians first consider whether the child's life can be saved.[15,64] This difference can create tension within the healthcare team and merits discussion by the team members. Nurses and physicians also identified a factor they both consider frequently in end-of-life decision-making for pediatric oncology patients: "respecting the patient's and family's preferences." This factor reflected the healthcare professionals' efforts to inform the patient and family of all options and then to respect the choice they made. In a survey completed[77] by 21 healthcare professionals in pediatric oncology (16 physicians, 3 nurses, and 2 chaplains) regarding end-of-life decisions for patients with incurable cancer, the factors rated as most important included "discussions with the family of the patient," "thinking the patient would never get any better," "the belief that nothing else could help the patient," and "things the patient had said about continuing or not continuing treatment." Most of the participating healthcare professionals also indicated that they did not make end-of-life decisions alone but sought the input of other team members.

Strategies for facilitating child, adolescent, and parent involvement

End-of-life decision-making is a process that very likely begins at the time of diagnosis, when the patient and the parents are exposed to the seriousness of the illness, the possible risks of treatment, and the uncertainty of short-term and long-term treatment outcomes. When faced with the actual decision-making, a few parents and patients express a preference seemingly without hesitation or anguish. They are likely to have gained an earlier understanding of the situation; often, patients and parents who observe others undergoing end-of-life experiences begin to reflect on their own life values. More often, however, patients and parents require time to think after becoming aware of the impending decision point and treatment options. In both the briefer and longer contemplation periods, the decision-making capability evolves as treatment continues and understanding of the

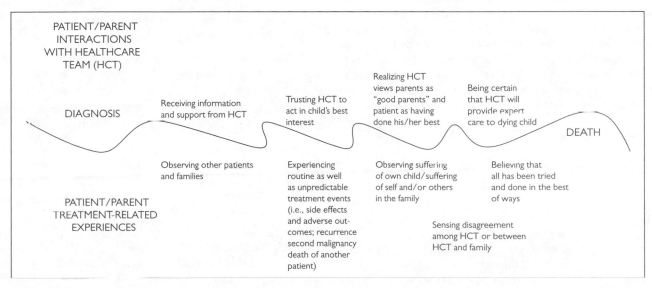

Figure 58.1 The interaction and experiences of pediatric oncology patients, their parents, and the members of their healthcare team (HCT) from the point of diagnosis forward that influences end-of-life decision-making.

patient's situation increases. End-of-life decision-making is not a single event or one well-defined point in time.

It is essential that healthcare providers realize that the end-of-life decision-making process begins early in treatment and evolves with each interaction between the provider, the patient, and the parent, and with each observation of or encounter with other seriously ill patients and their parents (Figure 58.1). Each interaction provides an opportunity for the healthcare provider to build the patient's and family's trust in him or her as a source of information and support and as a care expert who can be relied on to do what is best for the patient.[15] Each interaction is also an opportunity for the provider to facilitate parents' efforts to function fully as parents—a role that becomes increasingly uncertain as parents deal with unfamiliar decisions. Feeling competent in their parenthood is especially crucial to parents who face end-of-life decisions on behalf of their child. Believing that they have acted as "good parents" in such a situation is likely to be very important to their emotional recovery from the dying and death of their child.

Decision-making by patients and parents is influenced not only by their interactions with the healthcare team but also by the impressions they form through observations of and encounters with other patients and families in the care setting. As patients and parents learn about the treatment experiences and the positive or negative outcomes of other patients, they contemplate what it would be like to experience those situations themselves. A second type of personal experience that prompts this kind of reflection is an unexpected negative response to treatment, such as an adverse reaction or even disease progression, after positive responses. When patients and parents feel well informed by healthcare team members about disease response to treatment and are routinely involved in treatment discussions and other decisions, they are being prepared for end-of-life decision-making, should it become necessary.[80]

A third experience that prepares the patient and parents for end-of-life decision-making is the patient's experience of suffering and the parent's experience of witnessing that suffering and being unable to adequately relieve it. In our research with parents of children and adolescents who are experiencing a first or second recurrence of cancer, parents and guardians are more likely to contemplate ending curative efforts when they see their child in pain, unable to enjoy favorite activities, places, and people, or unable to find comfort.[71,73] Parents may react to the same experiences in different—even opposite—ways. The mother of a child treated for acute lymphocytic leukemia wrote in her guide for parents, friends, and healthcare providers that an end-of-life decision is an "intensely personal decision."[81] Some parents seek to exhaust all possible treatments, whereas others hope only for sufficient time to prepare themselves and their child for the dying and death.

The nurse's role

The American Nurses Association's Position Statement on Nursing and the Patient Self-Determination Act[17] asserts that nurses have a professional responsibility to facilitate informed decision-making by patients about end-of-life options. The statement does not specify patient age, but other wording, such as that describing the nurse's responsibility for knowing state laws about advance directives, suggests that the statement is oriented toward adult patients. The document also asserts that the nurse is responsible for ensuring that advance directives are current and reflect the patient's choices. The ANA makes equally explicit assertions about the nurse's role in its position statement "Nursing Care and Do-Not-Resuscitate

---

Box 58.3 Guidelines for the healthcare team to use in assisting each other with end-of-life decision-making

1. Know the guidelines offered by specific disciplines regarding roles in end-of-life decision-making (i.e., the American Nurses Association's official statements on what the nurse is expected to do to help parents and patients make decisions), because it is possible that the guidelines differ from expectations held by others outside the discipline.

2. Before initiating end-of-life discussions with patients* and parents, all members of the healthcare team should discuss and agree on

   a. The need for such a discussion.

   b. Which options are appropriate and available.

   c. Whether outside consultants, such as an ethics committee or external oncology expert, are needed to identify which options are in the best interest of the patient.

   d. Which other team members will participate in the discussion with the parents and patient.

   e. The time of the discussion and specific staff members who will participate.

   f. Which staff member will document the discussions in the medical record.

   g. Availability of the appropriate staff time and resources to address any questions parents and patients may have. Communicate to the team members who were not present at the patient-and-parent discussion what specific language was used to provide support to the parents and patient in making this decision.

3. Be available to team members and to the patient and parents to discuss and rediscuss decisions and related concerns.

4. Explore with the team all appropriate options to ensure that all that can be done is being done and being done well.

5. Consider consulting a ethics and/or palliative care expert on behalf of the entire team.

6. Inform other team members if feedback from or assessment of the patient, parents, or both indicates that any decision needs clarification or reconsideration.

7. Directly approach other team members regarding aspects of decision-making rather than seek such information from the parents.

8. Make certain that decision-making is fully documented in the healthcare record and accessible for all members of the team.

* When considering whether the patient should be present during such discussions, evaluate the developmental stage of the patient and the severity of illness and symptoms at the time of the discussion.

Decisions."[7] That position statement urges nurses to assume principal responsibility for ensuring that competent patients' preferences regarding resuscitation are honored, even if those preferences conflict with those of other healthcare professionals and family members. Nurses are further urged to facilitate explicit discussions of the resuscitation order with the patient, family members, and healthcare team, and to document the decisions clearly.

Several general studies about how nurses, physicians, and other healthcare team members perceive end-of-life decision-making have revealed differences in role responsibilities and interpretations of care priorities.[81–84] These differences contribute to tension among team members. It is important that team members be aware of official statements issued by each discipline's professional association about role expectations. For example, guidance offered by the American Academy of Pediatrics indicates that physicians are expected to provide adequate information to patients, parents, and "other appropriate decision-makers" about therapeutic options and their risks, discomforts, adverse effects, projected financial costs, potential benefits, and likelihood of success. In addition, physicians are expected to offer advice about which option to choose and to elicit questions from the patients and parents. Nurses should openly discuss expectations and team functions with other team members (Box 58.3) to prevent misunderstanding or disappointment about their perceived roles.

Guidelines for end-of-life decision-making in pediatrics

End-of-life decision-making for children and adolescents who have been seriously and chronically ill necessitates consistent and careful attention to their most meaningful relationships.[85]

Box 58.4 Guidelines for the healthcare team to use in assisting pediatric patients with end-of-life decision-making

1. Seek input of parents as to the timing and extent of information that should be offered to the patient about diagnosis, treatment options, and the likely response to treatment.

2. At the time of diagnosis and throughout treatment, actively seek opportunities to provide information to the child or adolescent that is appropriate to his or her developmental stage.

   a. For a child, ensure parental presence during such discussions.

   b. For an adolescent, ensure a discussion that includes the parents but offer to discuss with the patient alone as well.

3. Be available to discuss and rediscuss decisions and related concerns in a manner appropriate to the developmental stage of the patient.

4. With parental agreement, encourage the patient to interact with other pediatric oncology patients.

5. Convey verbally and nonverbally the recognition that the patient is trying his or her best and that the healthcare team is committed to the patient's well-being before, during, and after decision-making regardless of decision made.

6. Give assurances that everything that can be done to help the patient is being done and being done well.

7. As a patient's disease progresses, provide clear verbal (and written, if desired by the patient) explanations of the patient's status.

8. With parental agreement, inform the patient of treatment options as they become available in the treating institution or elsewhere.

9. Assess patient suffering and the need to change interventions to relieve such suffering.

10. When end-of-life options should be discussed with the patient, consult parents about the appropriate depth and timing of such discussions.

11. After receiving input from the parents and exploring the patient's readiness for information, discuss the end-of-life options, with

    a. A strong emphasis on the team's commitment to the patient's comfort and to providing expert care at all times.

    b. Professional recommendations.

    c. Descriptions about how the patient is likely to respond to each option (physical appearance, ability to communicate, etc.).

    d. Information about other support resources such as chaplains and ethicists.

12. Include more than one healthcare team member in end-of-life discussions with the patient.

13. Ask the patient what he/she is hoping for now.

14. Allow the patient private time to consider the options with his or her parents.

15. Reassess the appropriateness of the chosen end-of-life options on an ongoing basis, remaining aware that patients will

    a. Vacillate between certainty and uncertainty about the decision.

    b. Need clarification and additional information to resolve uncertainties.

16. Convey respect for the patient's right to change decisions, when such changes are clinically feasible.

17. When appropriate to the patient's comprehension level, explain to the patient the availability and value of an ethics and/or palliative care consult for the patient.

18. Maintain sensitivity to any specific ethnic, cultural, or religious preferences during the terminal stage.

19. Demonstrate continued commitment to providing symptom management, support of quality of life, and assurance of the parents' well-being.

The relationships of obvious importance are the relationship of child or adolescent with self and with family. Less obvious but also meaningful relationships are those between the patient and the healthcare professionals, and between the family and healthcare professionals (those who provide care for the child or adolescent or for the family). Because of the importance of these relationships in end-of-life decision-making, separate (although overlapping) guidelines are provided addressing how members of the healthcare team can assist parents, patients (Box 58.4), and each other in making end-of-life decisions. The overlap in the guidelines reflects the parallel, and at times interacting, decision-making processes experienced by children, adolescents, and their parents. Healthcare professionals will be most effective in implementing these guidelines if they first reflect on their feelings and concerns about the dying and death of children and adolescents and about participating in end-of-life decision-making. Research findings to date consistently indicate that when the child or adolescent participates as fully as possible in end-of-life decision-making, parents and healthcare providers are more certain and more comfortable about the decision that is made.[79] Their belief that the decision reflects the child's or adolescent's preferences helps parents and healthcare providers to make the decision and to recover emotionally from this painful experience.

References

1. Surkan P, Kreicbergs U, Valdimarsdottir U, et al. Perceptions of inadequate health care and feelings of guilt in parents after the death of a child to a malignancy: a population-based long-term follow-up. J Palliat Med. 2006;9:317–331.
2. Kreichbergs U, Valdimarsdottir U, Onelov E, et al. Care-related distress: a nationwide survey of parents having lost their child to cancer. J Clin Oncol. 2005;23:9162–9171.
3. Lannen P, Wolfe J, Mack J, Onelov E, Nyberg U, Kreicbergs U. Absorbing information about a child's incurable cancer. Oncology. 2010;78:259–266.
4. St. Ledger U, Begley A, Reid J, Prior L, McAuley D, Blackwood B. Moral distress in end-of-life care in the intensive care unit. J Adv Nurs. 2012;69:1869–1880.
5. Hinds P, Oakes L, Furman W, et al. End-of-life decision making by adolescents, parents, and healthcare providers in pediatric oncology. Cancer Nurs. 2001;24:122–136.
6. American Nurses Association Congress on Nursing Practice and Economics and Center for Ethics and Human Rights Advisory Board. Registered Nurses' Roles and Responsibilities in Providing Expert Care and Counseling at the End of Life. American Nurses Association; June 2010.
7. American Nurses Association Center for Ethics and Human Rights. Nursing Care and Do Not Resuscitate (DNR) and Allow Natural Death (AND) Decisions. American Nurses Association; March 2012.
8. Rothman M, Gugliucci M. End-of-life care curricula in undergraduate medical education: a comparison of allopathic and osteopathic medical schools. J Hosp Palliat Med. 2008;25:354–360.
9. Wallace M, Grossman S, Campbell S, et al. Integration of end-of-life care content in undergraduate nursing curricula: student knowledge and perceptions. J Prof Nurs. 2009;25:50–56.
10. Baughcum A, Gerhradt C, Young-Saleme T, et al. Evaluation of a pediatric palliative care educational workshop for oncology fellows. Pediatr Blood Cancer. 2007;49:154–159.
11. Smith M, Seibel NL, Altekruse SF, Ries L, Melbert DL, O'Leary M, et al. Outcomes for children and adolescents with cancer: challenges for the twenty-first century. J Clin Oncol. 2010; 28 (15): 2625–2634.
12. Wolfe J, Grier ME. Care of the dying child. In: Pizzo P, Poplack D (eds.), Principles and Practice of Pediatric Oncology. 4th ed. Philadelphia, PA: Lippincott Williams & Wilkins; 2002:1477–1493.
13. Wolfe J, Grier H, Klar N, et al. Symptoms and suffering at the end of life in children with cancer. N Engl J Med. 2000;342:326–333.
14. Institute of Medicine. When Children Die: Improving Palliative and End-of-Life Care for Children and Their Families. Washington DC: National Academy Press; 2003.
15. Hinds P, Oakes L, Furman W, et al. Decision making by parents and health care professionals for pediatric patients with cancer. Oncol Nurs Forum. 1997;24:1523–1528.
16. American Academy of Pediatrics, Committee on Bioethics. Guidelines on foregoing life-sustaining medical treatment for abused children. Pediatrics. 2000;106(5):1151–1153.
17. American Nurses Association, Task Force on the Nurse's Role in End-of-Life Decisions. Compendium of Position Statements on the Nurse's Role in End-of-Life Decisions. Washington, DC: American Nurses Association; 1991:1–14.
18. Ethier A, Rollins J, Stewart J, eds. Pediatric Oncology Palliative and End-of-life Care Resource. Glenview, IL: Association of Hematology and Oncology Nursing and Children's Oncology Group; 2010.
19. Berlinger N, Jennings B, Wolf SM. The Hastings Center Guidelines for Decisions on Life-Sustaining Treatment and Care near the End of Life. 2nd ed. Oxford: Oxford University Press; 2013.
20. Gilmour JM. Children, adolescents, and health care. In: Downie J, Caulfield T, Flood C, eds. Canadian Health Law & Policy, 2nd edition. Toronto: Butterworthy, 2002; 204–249.
21. Rosato JL. Foreword. Hous J Health L & Pol'Y. 2008;195–205.
22. Landsdown G. Every Child's Right to Be Heard: A Resource Guide on the UN Committee on the Rights of the Child, General Comment #12. UNICEF; 2011.
23. Joint Commission on the Accreditation of Healthcare Organizations. Standards. at http://www.jointcommission.org/standards_information/pc_requirements.aspx. Accessed September 27, 2013.
24. National Quality Forum (NQF). A National Framework and Preferred Practices for Palliative and Hospice Care Quality: A Consensus Report. Washington, DC: National Quality Forum; 2006.
25. Earle C, Park E, Lai B, et al. Identifying potential indicators or the quality of end-of-life cancer care from administrative data. J Clin Oncol. 2003;21:1133–1138.
26. Miller VA, Luce MF, Nelson RM. Relationship of external influence to a parental distress in decision making regarding children with a life-threatening illness. J Pediatr Psychol. 2011; 36: 1102–1112.
27. Miller VA, Nelson RM. Factors related to voluntary parental decision-making in pediatric oncology. Pediatrics. 2012; 129: 903–909.
28. Nitschke R, Humphrey G, Sexauer C, Catron B, Wunder S, Jay S. Therapeutic choices made by patients with end-stage cancer. J Pediatr. 1982;10:471–476.
29. Nitschke R, Meyer W, Sexauer C, Parkhurst JB, Foster P, Huszh H. Care of terminally ill children with cancer. Med Pediatr Oncol. 2000;34:268–270.
30. Williams C, Cairnie J, Fines V, et al. Construction of a parent-derived questionnaire to measure end-of-life care after withdrawal of life-sustaining treatment in the neonatal intensive care unit. Pediatrics. 2009;123:e87–e95.
31. Verhagen AAE, de Vos M, Dorscheidt JH, Engels B, Hubben JH, Sauer PJ. Conflicts about end-of-life decision making in NICUs in the Netherlands. Pediatrics. 2009;124: e112–e119.
32. Caeymaex L, Jousselme C, Vasilescu C, Danan C, Falissard B, Bourrat MM, et al. Perceived role in end-of-life decision making in the NICU affects long-term parental grief response. Arch Dis Child Fetal Neonatal Ed. 2013; 98: F26–F31.
33. Able-Boone H, Dokecki PR, Smith MS. Parent and health care provider communication and decision making in the intensive care nursery. Child Health Care. 1989;18:133–141.

34. Rushton C. Moral Decision Making by Parents of Infants Who Have Life-Threatening Congenital Disorders. Washington, DC: School of Nursing, Catholic University of America, 1994. PhD dissertation.

35. Hinds P, Oakes L, Hicks J, Powell B, Srivastava D, Spunt S, et al. "Trying to be a good parent" as defined by interviews with parents who made phase I, terminal care, and resuscitation decisions for their children. J Clin Oncol. 2009;27:5979–5985.

36. Mauer S, Hinds P, Spunt S, Furman W, Kane J, Baker J. Decision making by parents of children with incurable cancer who opt for enrollment on a phase I trial compared with choosing a do not resuscitate/terminal care option. J Clin Oncol. 2010;28:3292–3298.

37. Hinds PS, Oakes LL, Hicks J, Powell B, Srivastava DK, Baker JN, et al. Parent-clinician communication intervention during end-of-life decision making for children with incurable cancer. J Palliat Med. 2012;15(8):916–922.

38. Guglani L, Lodha R. Attitudes towards end-of-life issues amongst pediatricians in a tertiary hospital in a developing country. J Tropical Pediatr. 2008;54:261–264.

39. Goh AY, Lum LC, Chan PW, Bakar F, Chong BO. Withdrawal and limitation of life support in pediatric intensive care. Arch Disabled Child. 1999;80:424–428.

40. Burns J, Mitchell C, Outwater K, et al. End-of-life care in the pediatric intensive care unit after the forgoing of life sustaining treatment. Crit Care Med. 2000;28:3060–3066.

41. Meyer E, Burns J, Griffith J, et al. Parental perspectives on end-of-life care in the pediatric intensive care unit. Crit Care Med. 2002;30:226–231.

42. von Lutzau P, Otto M, Hechler T, Metzing S, Wolfe J, Zernikow B. Children dying from cancer: parents' perspectives on symptoms, quality of life, characteristics of death, and end-of-life decisions. J Palliat Care. 2012;28:274–281.

43. Gilmer MJ, Foster TL, Bell CJ, Mulder J, Carter BS. Parental perceptions of care of children at end of life. Am J Hosp Palliat Care. 2013; 30:53–58.

44. Zawistowski C, DeVita M. A descriptive study of children dying in the pediatric intensive care unit after withdrawal of life-sustaining treatment. Pediatr Crit Care Med. 2004;5:216–223.

45. Moore P, Kerridge I, Gillis J. Withdrawal and limitation of life-sustaining treatments in a paediatric intensive care unit and review of the literature. J Paediatr Child Health. 2008; 44:404–408.

46. Buchanan A, Brock D. Deciding for Others: The Ethics of Surrogate Decision-Making. Cambridge, MA: Cambridge University Press; 1989.

47. Ariff JL, Groh DH. In the best interests of the child: ethical issues. In: Curley M, Smith J, Moloney-Harmon P (eds.), Critical Care Nursing of Infants and Children. Philadelphia, PA: Saunders; 1996: 126–141.

48. Beyth-Marom R, Fischhoff B. Adolescents' decisions about risks: a cognitive perspective. In: Schulenberg J, Maggs J, Hurrelmann K (eds.), Health Risks and Developmental Transitions During Adolescence. Cambridge, MA: Cambridge University Press; 1997:110–135.

49. Hinds P, Oakes L, Drew D, et al. Adolescents' end-of-life care preferences. J Clin Oncol. 2005;23(36):9146–9154.

50. Hinds P, Martin J. Hopefulness and the self-sustaining process in adolescents with cancer. Nurs Res. 1988;37:336–340.

51. Burns J, Truog R. Ethical controversies in pediatric critical care. New Horizons. 1997;5:72–84.

52. Leikin S. The role of adolescents in decisions concerning their cancer therapy. Cancer. 1993;71(Suppl):3342–3346.

53. Miller VA, Baker JN, Leek AC, Hizlan S, Rheingold SR, Yamokoski AD, et al. Adolescent perspectives on phase I cancer research. Pediatr Blood Cancer 2013;60:873–878.

54. Weiner L, Ballard E, Brennan T, Battles H, Martinez P, Pao M. How I wish to be remembered: the use of an advance care planning document in adolescent and young adult populations. J Palliat Care. 2008; 11:1309–1313.

55. Lyon ME, Jacobs S, Briggs L, Cheng YI, Wang J. Family-centered advance care planning for teens with cancer. JAMA. 2013; 167:460–467.

56. Goldman A. Life threatening illnesses and symptom control in children. In: Doyle D, Hanks G, MacDonald N (eds.), Oxford Textbook of Palliative Medicine. 2nd ed. New York, NY: Oxford University Press; 1998:1033–1043.

57. Gowan D. End-of-life issues of children. Pediatr Transplant. 2003;7(Suppl 3):40–43.

58. Kars M, Grypdonck M, Korte-Verhoef M, Kamps W, Meijer-van den Bergh E, Verkerk M, et al. Parental experience at the end-of-life in children with cancer: "preservation" and "letting go" in relation to loss. Support Care Cancer. 2011;19:27–35.

59. Jalmsell L, Forslund M, Hansson MG, Henter J, Kreicbergs U, Frost BM. Transition to noncurative end-of-life care in paediatric oncology: a nationwide follow-up in Sweden. Acta Paediat. 2013;102:744–748.

60. Wolfe J, Klar N, Grier H, et al. Understanding of prognosis among parents of children who died of cancer: impact on treatment goals and integration of palliative care. JAMA. 2000;284:2469–2475.

61. Schmidt L. Pediatric end-of-life care: coming of age? Caring. 2003;22:20–22.

62. Rowa-Dewar N. Do interventions make a difference to bereaved parents?: A systematic review of controlled studies. Int J Palliat Nurs. 2002;8:456–457.

63. Contro N, Larson J, Scofield S, et al. Family perspectives on the quality of pediatric palliative care. Arch Pediatr Adolesc Med. 2002;156:14–19.

64. Mack J, Hilden J, Watterson J, Moore C, Turner B, Grier H, et al. Parent and physician perspectives on quality of care at the end of life in children with cancer. J Clin Oncol. 2005;23:9155–9161.

65. Tan A, Manca D. Finding common ground to achieve a "good death": family physicians working with substitute decision-makers of dying patients; a qualitative grounded theory study. BMC Fam Pract. 2013;14. http://www.biomedcentral.com/147-2296/14/14.

66. Kars M, Grypdonck M, Beishuizen A, Meijer-van den Bergh E, van Delden J. Factors influencing parental readiness to let their child with cancer die. Pediat Blood Cancer. 2010;54:1000–1008.

67. Robinson M, Thiel M, Backus M, et al. Matters of spirituality at the end of life in the pediatric intensive care unit. Pediatrics. 2006;118:e719–e729.

68. Meyer E, Ritholz M, Burns J, et al. Improving the quality of end-of life care in the pediatric intensive care unit: parents' priorities and recommendations. Pediatrics. 2006;117:649–657.

69. Giannini A, Messeri A, Aprile A, et al. End-of-life decisions in pediatric intensive care: recommendations of the Italian Society of Neonatal and Pediatric Anesthesia and Intensive Care (SARNePI). Pediatr Anesth. 2008;18:1089–1095.

70. Stevens MM. Care of the dying child and adolescent: family adjustment and support. In: Doyle D, Hanks G, MacDonald N (eds.), Oxford Textbook of Palliative Medicine. 2nd ed. New York, NY: Oxford University Press; 1998:1057–1075.

71. Hinds PS, Birenbaum L, Clarke-Steffen L, et al. Coming to terms: parents response to a first cancer recurrence. Nurs Res. 1996;45:148–153.

72. Pyke-Grimm KA, Degner L, Small A, Mueller B. Preferences for participation in treatment decision making and information needs of parents of children with cancer: a pilot study. J Pediatr Oncol Nurs. 1999;16:13–24.

73. Hinds P, Birenbaum L, Pedrosa A, Pedrosa F. Guidelines for the recurrence of pediatric cancer. Semin Oncol Nurs. 2002;18:50–59.

74. Cornfield DN, Kahn JP. Decisions about life-sustaining measures in children: in whose best interests? Acta Paediat. 2012;32:246–258.

75. Kilicarslan-Toruner E, Akgun-Citak E. Information-seeking behaviours and decision-making for process of parents of children with cancer. Eur J Oncol Nurs. 2013;17:176–183.

76. Gillam L, Sullivan J. Ethics at the end of life: who should make decisions about treatment limitation for young children with life-threatening or life limiting conditions? J Paediatr Child Health. 2011; 47: 594–598.

77. Hinds PS, Oakes L, Quargnenti A, et al. An international feasibility study on parental decision making in pediatric oncology. Oncol Nurs Forum. 2000;27:1233–1243.
78. Kirschbaum MS. Life support decisions for children: what do parents value? Adv Nurs Sci. 1996;19:51–71.
79. Davies B, Deveau E, deVeber B, et al. Experiences of mothers in five countries whose child died of cancer. Cancer Nurs. 1998;21:301–311.
80. Keene N. Childhood Leukemia: A Guide for Families, Friends and Caregivers. Sebastopol, CA: O'Reilly & Associates; 1997.
81. Phillips RS, Rempusheski VF, Puopolo AL, Naccarato M, Mallatratt L. Decision making in SUPPORT: the role of the nurse. J Clin Epidemiol. 1990;43(Suppl):55S–58S.
82. Randolph AG, Zollo MB, Wigton RS, Yeh TS. Factors explaining variability among caregivers in the intent to restrict life-support interventions in a pediatric intensive care unit. Crit Care Med. 1997;25:435–439.
83. Randolph AG, Zollo MB, Egger MJ, Guyatt GH, Nelson RM, et al. Variability in physician opinion on limiting pediatric life support. Pediatrics. 1999;103:S43.
84. Walter SD, Cook DJ, Guyatt GH, et al. Confidence in life-support decisions in the intensive care unit: a survey of healthcare workers. Crit Care Med. 1998;26:44–49.
85. Hume M. Improving care at the end of life. Qual Lett Healthc Lead. 1998;10:2–10.

CHAPTER 59

Palliative care in the Neonatal Intensive Care Unit

Cheryl Thaxton, Brigit Carter, and Chi Dang Hornik

There are no words to describe the feelings … when we finally got to hold our child. My husband told me later that it was the first time that he saw me relax since receiving our son's diagnosis. It was wonderful for our little family to be so close together … it was the first time the three of us were alone and it was comforting that our child could die in our arms.

Beth Seyda, mother

Key points

◆ Palliative care in the neonatal intensive care unit (NICU) is an integral component of family-centered care and patient-focused care. Palliative care gives nurses the opportunity to provide support and nurture the infant and family unit at a time of tremendous stress. It is the most intimate time that one can share with a family.

◆ Palliative care incorporates pain and symptom management for the infant, as well as emotional, psychosocial, and spiritual support for the infant and family members. Family is defined by the parents or caregivers; this may include other children, grandparents, and extended family members. Palliative care measures should be provided while maintaining cultural sensitivity and while supporting the developmental aspects of neonatal care. Palliative care is provided when a condition is life-threatening; this condition may or may not result in death.

◆ Palliative care involves a dynamic exchange of information and promotes the implementation of care that is aimed toward treatment of pain and distressing symptoms that interfere with the infant's quality of life. The nurse has a compelling role in neonatal palliative and end-of-life care.

◆ The infant mortality rate in the United States in 2009 was 6.39 infant deaths per 1000 live births, 3% lower than the rate of 6.61 in 2008. The number of infant deaths was 28,075 in 2008 and 26,408 in 2009, a decline of 1,667 infant deaths.[a] Preterm and low birth weight infants had the highest infant mortality rates and contributed greatly to overall US infant mortality; of note

the three leading causes of infant death—congenital malformations, low birth weight, and sudden infant death syndrome—accounted for 46% of all infant deaths.[1] Thus it is obvious that the death of a newborn can be a part of the nurse's sphere of practice and requires that the nurse develop competencies in providing supportive and compassionate palliative care, which can lead to a peaceful death experience for the patient and family.

Introduction

For several years there has been a substantial effort put forward to adequately address the needs of neonatal palliative care patients and families. Parents face months of anguish as they prepare for the birth of a child with a suspected lethal congenital anomaly. The sudden delivery of a prematurely born infant can also pose existential reflections within the family unit. The answer to what was a predictable and planned future suddenly can become uncertain and overwhelming. Grandparents and extended family members often standby in search of the "right things to say" to support the situation. Siblings are in the midst of the deep sense of confusion during what was once a time of anticipation; as the time draws near for the birth of the baby each family member will transition through thoughts that pose more questions than answers. Families may find it hard to acknowledge that the infant has an incurable condition, thus creating a barrier to accessing palliative care measures.[b]

American society does not have a word for a parent who has lost a child—another challenge for the nurse. For example, the term "widow" is used for the surviving female spouse, but what do we call the surviving parent? To address the fact that there is no existing

[a] Mathews TJ, MacDorman MF. Infant Mortality Statistics from the 2009 Period Linked Birth/Infant Death Data Set: National Vital Statistics Reports (vol. 61). Hyattsville, MD: National Center for Health Statistics; 2013.

[b] Catlin A. Transition from curative efforts to purely palliative care for neonates: does physiology matter? Adv Neonatal Care. 2011;11(3):216–222.

term for a parent who has lost a child in Western culture some have explored the development of this term. Other cultures may have words or strategies to support parents who have lost an infant, but American culture labels the person a bereaved parent and refers to another child in the parents' future or another living child. Tan et al. (2011) utilized a longitudinal, prospective study that incorporated parent interviews to explore the bereavement process of parents with critically ill infants.[3] The findings supported measures such as early intervention in preparation for the possible death of an infant and establishment of resources to prospectively support parent bereavement, including memory making.[3] Nurses should recognize the delicate nature of this subject and use language to promote a patient- and family-centered approach to the care of the infant during this difficult time for the family.

This chapter presents the core values of neonatal palliative care within the context of providing culturally appropriate, compassionate, individualized, family-centered developmental care (IFCDC) and patient-focused care for infants receiving care in the NICU environment. To illustrate use of palliative care with the neonatal population, the following case study was supplied by a parent.

Case study

Dylan was diagnosed in utero with congenital diaphragmatic hernia (CDH) at 16 weeks via ultrasound (this section is written entirely by his family)

Knowing about his CDH during pregnancy gave us time to adjust to the news and learn all this medical stuff, so when Dylan was born we could totally focus on him and be very present/in the moment. One objective during our pregnancy was to bond with Dylan. We wanted him to know and feel that we loved him, we wanted him and we would do everything we could to help him live. So we constantly talked to him. We thought this bonding was what we could do, our part to help when he was born. We grew to love the monthly ultrasounds. It was another way to further bond with Dylan. We were amazed at the amount of detail we could see—hair, eyelashes, nose, mouth, chin. We realize we saw him more active in the ultrasounds (e.g., swallow, suck thumb, hand pulled on ear and foot) than after he was born.

I *knew* Dylan could die, but I had to totally believe he would live. Sometimes I would think about him dying. I cried and tried to get it out of my system. I did not want to *feel* he could die, because if I could feel that, then Dylan could. And I did not want Dylan to feel he could die. Not having control or knowing the outcome was frustrating. As my due date drew nearer, I was scared because soon we'd know the outcome. But as frustrating as the unknown was, Dylan was safe during that time while he was in me—he was "healthy," alive, and kicking. It was only going to be when he was born that he'd be critically sick. I wanted to keep him in me to keep him safe.

We talked to the specialists who might be involved in Dylan's care about possible outcomes. We always got to one path where there was no progress and the machines would be what were keeping him alive. I hoped it would not get to that point. I did not think I could make the decision to let Dylan die. We got the same story from everybody (OBs/surgeon/NICU/PICU) regarding a CDH. It was good to get the same message, nothing was conflicting. But it was very depressing, we always got hit with reality. No rosy picture was painted.

Dylan was born and placed on extracorporeal membrane oxygenation (ECMO)

After we went to our room, the PICU physician visited a few times with updates, unfortunately, none of it was good news. We went through all the ventilation options and ECMO was the next and only remaining step. Did we want to proceed? Yes, we expected to give Dylan every opportunity to live. We realized later we may not have been good at communicating this up-front.

It was great to have access to the room across from the NICU to sleep. Even though we only live 10 minutes from the hospital, it was 10 minutes too far. It felt like 1,000 miles away. It was good to stay over, particularly after Dylan's surgery. When we went home at night, we were always afraid we would get a call in the middle of the night from the PICU saying Dylan had died. I couldn't bear the thought of him dying alone, all by himself.

It took me a few days to realize I had not heard a sound out of Dylan, not a peep, not a cry. And I wouldn't until the ventilator tube was removed. Up until then, my usual reaction when I heard a baby screaming was to cringe and hope the parents could quickly quiet their child. Now, Dylan's cries would be music to my ears.

Dylan turned 2 weeks old. Those 2 weeks allowed us to get to know Dylan and be his parents. We enjoyed every little thing and most of them were simple, subtle things. Dylan's face was swollen and he struggled for days to open his eyes. He finally opened his right one. It felt so good he got to see us and his eye was so expressive. Sometimes it was very curious, looking all around. Another time it pierced my heart when he was unhappy with something they were doing to him. His look was like 'Mom, how can you let them do this to me?' We could tell how strong he was when he gripped our fingers in his hands. I loved that Dylan was such a fighter. I was so proud of him. We were constantly talking to and touching Dylan. When we were told Dylan had too much stimulation, we had to just sit and watch him. That was difficult. We told Dylan that we were there with him, even if he couldn't hear or feel us. That gave me time to just adore him and look at all of his features.

It felt great that both NICU and PICU staff told us Dylan recognized our voices. They said it did not happen with our other family members present, only with his father and me. We were so happy that Dylan knew us and we seemed to have a positive effect on him. Comments were made that it must be hard for us because each day we were bonding and getting more attached to Dylan. We never thought of it that way. What we were doing, just being with him and loving him, was easy. You just can't turn off this love that is gushing out of you. What else would we do? How could any parent not be with their baby every minute they could? Again, the idea was to bond with Dylan. If he could feel all of our love for him, maybe that could carry him through. We never considered pulling away from Dylan because we thought he might die. I would never be able to forgive myself if I wasn't with him or stopped loving him. Was our attachment to Dylan noticeable because it contrasted the detachment of medicine? I kissed Dylan on his head and told him I loved him every time I left his room; I could never kiss him and tell him I loved him too much. In case something happened when I was away, I would know those were my last words to him.

We would see the medical students gather for rounds. One would come in Dylan's room and pull numbers from his chart. They never talked to us and never once stopped to even look at

Dylan. We wondered how did they learn about the human side of medicine. How did they learn to interact with patients and families? How did they learn compassionate care? We continued to learn about the human body and medicine. Such a delicate balance is required. Dylan needed to do seemingly opposite things to get better. **When I took a breath I would think, this was "all" we were trying to get him to do**.

Dylan had his surgery to repair his CDH while on ECMO. Dylan was being weaned off ECMO. We heard optimism from the docs. I think for the first time even the docs thought Dylan might pull through, but over the next few weeks, the physicians noted not much improvement and Dylan was in multiorgan system failure. It was made very clear there was no more optimism and in fact just the opposite was now true, Dylan would continue to deteriorate. We decided to give ourselves some time for that to sink in before we made any decisions.

That afternoon we were told that it was affecting his heart (it had been strong up until then). Now we had to let him go. The machines could have kept him alive for a while longer, but that was not best for Dylan. As much as we wanted more time with him, letting him die in peace and with dignity was more important. I am surprised at how "easy" it was, my husband and I barely had a conversation about it, we knew what we had to do. All I could think was—I finally was going to get to hold Dylan.

That last night we stayed up all night with Dylan. In the middle of the night I asked the respiratory therapist to suction him. She asked if I wanted to and I said yes. It felt really good to do that. Then she asked if we wanted to give him a sponge bath and we said yes. So my husband and I cleaned him up and then put lotion all over him. Doing all of these things for Dylan made me so happy but I had no idea why. What was the big deal? I was just giving him a bath. Later I figured it out. I got to be a Mom and take care of Dylan. I got to do some of the things I had planned to do with him at home.

When Dylan was getting prepped for us to hold, the nurse asked whether we had Dylan's foot/hand prints. I said I didn't think so, I had not seen them if they were done. So she did that and we cut some locks of his hair. I had not thought of these things at all. I am so glad she did.

There are no words to describe the feelings when we finally got to hold Dylan. My husband told me later it was the first time he saw me truly relax since we had gotten Dylan's diagnosis. It was wonderful for our little family to be so close together. It was the first time the three of us were alone. It was very comforting Dylan could die in our arms.

Case summary

"As much as we wanted more time with him, letting him die in peace and with dignity was more important ... it was very comforting Dylan could die in our arms." These words as stated by Dylan's parents echo the true essence of neonatal palliative care. The experiences of parents are seen through such pure insight; meaningful moments for parents can easily be missed or trampled on unknowingly by staff.

Parents are faced with challenging decisions and even some uncertainties regarding the impact of shifting their focus from curative therapies to palliative care measures.[4] Providing a seamless transition into palliative care measures requires an interdisciplinary effort and support of the entire healthcare team. The focus of the team should be to provide optimal conditions for the infant's life and death including interventions to prevent and relieve suffering.[4] Implementing a palliative care protocol involves tremendous flexibility that supports a variety of choices, moving in and out of active life-sustaining measures, up until the end of the infant's life. The nurse has a vital role in ensuring that communication with the family is not fragmented and that parents are reassured that the best effort will be made to support their wishes throughout the uncertainty of the journey. Dignity should be maintained at all costs. Patient- and family-centered care measures seek to ensure that the final hours of a dying infant are spent in a peaceful environment and in the presence of the family.

Standard of care for neonatal patients

The care of the neonatal palliative care patient is not setting specific. Care can be provided within the neonatal intensive care unit, a newborn special care unit, or through a perinatal home hospice program. The nurse is instrumental in providing goal-directed support through care that integrates curative therapies with palliative measures. Nurses work with the interdisciplinary team to ensure that the patient and family have all needs addressed. Extremely premature infants with multiple comorbidities are potential candidates for neonatal palliative care. Due to the high morbidity and mortality rate for extremely premature infants, many expectant parents are confronted during the prenatal period with the possibility that their infant may be too small for resuscitation to take place in the delivery room.[5] In order to deliver care that is interdisciplinary as well as patient- and family-centered, nurses work alongside neonatologists, nurse practitioners, social workers, geneticists, respiratory therapists, pharmacists, and many subspecialists.

Nurses can take part in neonatal palliative care discussions when there is a consultative palliative care team or specialist involved. The nurse often leads communication with the family, as they spend the most time with the infant. Wigert, Dellenmark, and Bry (2013) reported a quantitative and a qualitative analysis of strengths and weaknesses perceived by parents in their communication with doctors and nurses at the NICU.[6] The study noted that communication with nurses was described as a source of emotional support more often than communication with doctors and that nurses, because of the nature of their job, are more often physically present at the bedside and thus more available for emotional contact with families.[6] Parents and caregivers often voice concerns to the bedside nurse as they process difficult information about the infant's medical status. The neonatal nurse should be prepared to provide palliative care support within the context of the infant's trajectory while addressing issues of uncertainty and with the support of the interdisciplinary care team.

Developmental care is vital to the well-being and holistic approach to neonatal care. Core measures for developmentally supportive care in the neonatal intensive care unit have been identified. Five core measure sets for evidence-based developmental care were evaluated by Couglin et al. (2009): (1) protected sleep, (2) pain and stress assessment and management, (3) developmental activities of daily living, (4) family-centered care, and (5) the healing environment palliative care patient.[7] The terms "healing" and "suffering" have various meanings within the cultural belief

Table 59.1 Ethical principles and application to perinatal palliative care (PPC)

Ethical Principle	Definition	Application to PPC
Autonomy	The principle of self-determination in which patients participate in decisions about their lives	Provide and clarify the parents' understanding of case-specific information. Ensure informed consent.
Beneficence and nonmaleficence	The principle placing the patient's best interest first and the principle duty to first "do no harm" dictates obligation to protect patient safety and not cause injury	Identify values that each family brings to the situation; respect wishes, clarify treatment options (or lack thereof), and use bioethical principles to guide conversations.
Justice	The principle meaning to give each person or group what is "due"	Ensure equitable access to care and resources including access to staff members; palliative care protocols and support should be implemented by clinicians and supported by administrators.
Dignity	The principle that every human has intrinsic worth	The mother, fetus, and family have the right to be treated with respect and honor.
Truthfulness and honesty	The principle of veracity in which the clinician provides information regarding diagnosis and care alternatives	Recognize that some clinical scenarios involve irresolvable tragedies. Conduct an assessment of patient knowledge and offer truthful information in a compassionate, gentle, sensitive manner.

Adapted from Wool (2013), reference 8, with permission from John Wiley & Sons, Inc.

system of each individual family. The nurse should work in collaboration with the interdisciplinary team to support the needs of the family and utilize knowledge of standard ethical principles to provide a patient-focused and family-centered care (Table 59.1).

Family as the unit of care

The case study demonstrates the importance of providing comfort care measures to support the end-of-life care experiences of the patient and family (see Box 59.1). The nurse has to be present at the most difficult time for the family, to be fully attentive to the child and family, to separate personal values regarding birth, life, and death from those of the family, and to clearly ask what it is that they need from their perspective. Nurses must adapt and individualize the care so that there is as much support for the positive development as possible for the infant and family. An IFCDC approach provides the context in which to render palliative and end-of-life care. This approach reminds the nurse that within the family unit parents are first, and that they want to support their infant's development and preserve their role as parents. It is only after the parental role is solidified that parents can become the caregiver to a child that may or will die. For culturally competent care to reflect the complexity of care that is much broader than ethnicity, the nurse must be sensitive to cultural, ethnic, and religious values. A nurse must be appropriately prepared for this aspect of care. The main obstacles to good palliative care are the inability to appropriately communicate with grieving parents and a lack of knowledge about evidence-based pain management.

Cultural influences on care

Cultural values and beliefs, both religious and ethnic, influence the family's view of pain, suffering, and end of life (Table 59.2). The neonatal nurse must incorporate these values and beliefs into the plan of care if it is to be effective and benefit the patient and family. Wong and colleagues[9] and the Texas Children's Cancer Center-Texas Children's Hospital[10] address cultural influence on

---

Box 59.1 Core concepts of patient- and family-centered care

♦ **Dignity and respect.** Healthcare practitioners listen to and honor patient and family perspectives and choices. Patient and family knowledge, values, beliefs, and cultural backgrounds are incorporated into the planning and delivery of care.

♦ **Information sharing.** Healthcare practitioners communicate and share complete and unbiased information with patients and families in ways that are affirming and useful. Patients and families receive timely, complete, and accurate information in order to effectively participate in care and decision-making.

♦ **Participation.** Patients and families are encouraged and supported in participating in care and decision-making at the level they choose.

♦ **Collaboration.** Patients, families, healthcare practitioners, and leaders collaborate in policy and program development, implementation, and evaluation; in healthcare facility design; and in professional education, as well as in the delivery of care.

Source: Reprinted with permission from the Institute for Patient- and Family-Centered Care, http://www.ipfcc.org/. 2013.

---

care by outlining key aspects of health beliefs and practices that must be considered when providing any type of care.[9,10] (For further information, see refs. 9 and 10.)

For example, when working with a Native American family, the nurse must consider how to combine healing ceremonies from their tribal rituals with Western medicine to alleviate suffering. In this instance, ethnic and religious beliefs are intertwined. But in other instances, religious and ethnic values must be differentiated and incorporated into care. It must be remembered that not every family that identifies themselves with an organized religion strictly adheres to all principles of that faith. One example

Table 59.2 Religious influences

Religious sect	Birth	Death	Organ donation/ transplantation	Beliefs regarding medical care
Baptist	Infant baptism is not practiced. However, many churches present the baby and the parents to the congregation when they attend services for the first time after the birth.	It isn't mandatory that clergy be present at death, but families often desire visits from clergy. Scripture reading and prayer are important.	There is no formal statement regarding this issue. It is considered a matter of personal conscience. It is commonly regarded as positive (an act of love).	Some may regard their illness as punishment resulting from past sins. Those who believe in predestination may not seek aggressive treatment. Fundamentalist and conservative groups see the Bible as the infallible word of God to be taken literally.
Buddhist	Do not practice infant baptism.	A Buddhist priest is often involved before and after death. Rituals are observed during and after death. If the family doesn't have a priest, they may request that one be contacted.	There is no formal statement regarding organ donation/ transplantation. This is seen as a matter of individual conscience.	Illness can be used as a tool to aid in the development of the soul. Some may see illness as a result of karmic causes. Some may avoid treatments or procedures on holy days. Cleanliness is important.
Church of Jesus Christ of Latter-day Saints (Mormon)	Infant baptism is not performed. Children are given a name and a priesthood blessing sometime after the birth, from a week or two to several months. In the event of a critically ill newborn, this might be done in the hospital at the discretion of the parents. Baptism is performed after the child is 8 years old. The Church of Jesus Christ of Latter-day Saints feels that a child is not accountable for sins before 8 years of age.	There are no religious rituals performed related to death.	There is no official statement regarding this issue. Organ donation/transplantation is left up to the individual or parents.	Administration to the sick involves anointing with consecrated oil and performing a blessing by members of the priesthood. While the individual or a member of the family usually requests this if the individual is unconscious and there is no one to represent him or her, it would be appropriate for anyone to contact the church so that the ordinance may be performed. Refusal of medical treatments would be left up to the individual. There are no restrictions relative to "holy" days.
Episcopal	Infant baptism is practiced. In emergency situations, request for infant baptism should be given high priority and could be performed by any baptized person, clergy or lay. Often in situations of stillbirths or aborted fetuses, special prayers of commendation may be offered.	Pastoral care of the sick may include prayers, laying on of hands, anointing, and/ or Holy Communion. At the time of death, various litanies and special prayers may be offered.	Both are permitted.	Respect for the dignity of the whole person is important. These needs include physical, emotional, and spiritual.
Society of Friends (Quakers)	Do not practice infant baptism.	Each person has a divine nature but an encounter and relationship with Jesus Christ is essential.	No formal statement, but generally both are permitted.	No special rites or restrictions. Leaders and elders from the church may visit and offer support and encouragement. Quakers believe in plain speech.

(continued)

Table 59.2 Continued

Religious sect	Birth	Death	Organ donation/transplantation	Beliefs regarding medical care
Islam (Muslim/Moslem)	At birth, the first words said to the infant in his/her right ear are "Allah-o-Akbar" (Allah is great), and the remainder of the Call for Prayer is recited. An Aqeeqa (party) to celebrate the birth of the child is arranged by the parents. Circumcision of the male child is practiced.	In Islam, life is meant to be a test for the preparation for everlasting life in the hereafter. Therefore, according to Islam, death is simply a transition. Islam teaches that God has prescribed the time of death for everyone and only He knows when, where, or how a person is going to die. Islam encourages making the best use of all of God's gifts, including the precious gift of life in this world. At the time of death, there are specific rituals (bathing, wrapping the body in cloth, etc.) that must be done. Before moving and handling the body, it is preferable to contact someone from the person's mosque or Islamic Society to perform these rituals.	Permitted. However, there are some stipulations depending on the type of transplant/donation and its effect on the donor and recipient. It is advisable to contact the individual's mosque or the local Islamic Society for further consultation.	Humans are encouraged in the Qur'an (Koran) to seek treatment. It is taught that only Allah cures. However, Muslims are taught not to refuse treatment in the belief that Allah will take care of them because even though He cures, He also chooses at times to work through the efforts of humans.
International Society for Krishna Consciousness (A Hindu movement in North America based on devotion to Lord Krishna)	Infant baptism is not performed.	The body should not be touched. The family may desire that a local temple be contacted so that representatives may visit and chant over the patient. It is believed that in chanting the names of God, one may gain insight and God consciousness.	There is no formal statement prohibiting this act. It is an individual decision.	Illness or injury is believed to represent sins committed in this or a previous life. They accept modern medical treatment. The body is seen as a temporary vehicle used to transport them through this life. The body belongs to God, and members are charged to care for it in the best way possible.
Jehovah's Witnesses	Infant baptism is not practiced.	There are no official rites that are performed before or after death, however, the faith community is often involved and supportive of the patient and family.	There is no official statement related to this issue. Organ donation isn't encouraged, but it is believed to be an individual decision. According to the legal corporation for the denomination, Watchtower, all donated organs and tissue must be drained of blood before transplantation.	Adherents are absolutely opposed to transfusions of whole blood, packed red blood cells, platelets, and fresh or frozen plasma. This includes banking of ones' own blood. Many accept use of albumin, globulin, factor replacement (hemophilia), vaccines, hemodilution, and cell salvage. There is no opposition to nonblood plasma expanders.
Judaism (Orthodox and Conservative)	Circumcision of male infants is performed on the 8th day if the infant is healthy. The mohel (ritual circumciser familiar with Jewish law and aseptic technique) performs the ritual.	It is important that the healthcare professional facilitate the family's need to comfort and be with the patient at the time of death.	Permitted and is considered a mitzvah (good deed).	Only emergency surgical procedures should be performed on the Sabbath, which extends from sundown Friday to sundown Saturday. Elective surgery should be scheduled for days other than the Sabbath. Pregnant women and the seriously ill are exempt from fasting. Serious illness may be grounds for violating dietary laws but only if it is medically necessary.

Table 59.2 Continued

Religious sect	Birth	Death	Organ donation/ transplantation	Beliefs regarding medical care
Lutheran	Infant baptism is practiced. If the infant's prognosis is poor, the family may request immediate baptism.	Family may desire visitation from clergy. Prayers for the dying, commendation of the dying, and prayers for the bereaved may be offered.	There is no formal statement regarding this issue. It is considered a matter of personal conscience.	Illness isn't seen as an act of God, rather, it is seen as a condition of humankind's fallen state. Prayers for the sick may be desired.
Methodist	Infant baptism is practiced but is usually done within the community of the church after counseling and guidance from clergy. However, in emergency situations, a request for baptism would not be seen as inappropriate.	In the case of perinatal death, there are prayers within the United Methodist Book of Worship that could be said by anyone. Prayer, scripture, and singing are often seen as appropriate and desirable.	Organ donation/ transplantation is supported and encouraged. It is considered a part of good stewardship.	In the Methodist tradition, it is believed that every person has the right to death with dignity and has the right to be involved in all medical decisions. Refusal of aggressive treatment is seen as an appropriate option.
Pentecostal Assembly of God, Church of God, Four Square, and many other faith groups are included under this general heading. Pentecostal is not a denomination, but a theological distinctive (pneumatology)	No rituals such as baptism are necessary. Many Pentecostals have a ceremony of "dedication," but it is done in the context of the community of faith/believers (church). Children belong to heaven and only become sinners after the age of accountability, which is not clearly defined.	The only way to transcend this life is the door to heaven (or hell). Questions about "salvation of the soul" are very common and important. Resurrection is the hope of those who "were saved." Prayer is appropriate, so is singing and scripture reading.	Many Pentecostal denominations have no statement concerning this subject, but it is generally seen as positive and well received. Education concerning wholeness of the person and nonliteral aspects like "heart," "mind," etc., have to be explained. For example, a Pentecostal may have a problem with donating a heart to a "nonbeliever."	Pentecostals are sometimes labeled as "in denial" due to their theology of healing. Their faith in God for literal healing is generally expressed as intentional unbelief in the prognostic statements. Many Pentecostals do not see sickness as the will of God, thus one must "stand firm" in faith and accept the unseen reality, which many times may mean healing. As difficult as this position may seem, it must be noted that, when death occurs, Pentecostals may leap from miracle expectations to joyful hope and theology of heaven and resurrection without facing issues of anger or frustration due to unfulfilled expectations. Prayer, scriptures, singing, and anointing of the sick (not a sacrament) are appropriate/ expected pastoral interventions.
Presbyterian	Baptism is a sacrament of the Church but is not considered necessary for salvation. However, it is seen as an event to take place, when possible, in the context of a worshipping community.	Family may desire visitation from clergy. Prayers for the dying, commendation of the dying, and prayers for the bereaved may be offered.	There is no formal statement regarding this issue.	Communion is a sacrament of the Church. It is generally celebrated with a patient in the presence of an ordained minister and elder. Presbyterians are free to make their own choices regarding the use of mechanical life-support measures.

(continued)

Table 59.2 Continued

Religious sect	Birth	Death	Organ donation/ transplantation	Beliefs regarding medical care
Roman Catholic	Infant baptism is practiced. In medical facilities, baptism is usually performed by a priest or deacon, as ordinary members of the sacrament. However, under extraordinary circumstances, baptism may be administered by a layperson, provided that the intention is to do as the Church does, using the formula, "I baptize you in the name of the Father, the Son, and the Holy Spirit."	Sacrament of the sick is the sacrament of healing and forgiveness. It is to be administered by a priest as early in the illness as possible. It is not a last rite to be administered at the point of death. The Roman Catholic Church makes provisions for prayers of commendation of the dying, which may be said by any priest, deacon sacramental minister, or layperson.	Catholics may donate or receive organ transplants.	The Sacrament of Holy Communion sustains Catholics in sickness as in health. When the patient's condition deteriorates, the sacrament is given as viaticum ("food for the journey"). Like Holy Communion, viaticum may be administered by a priest, deacon, or a sacramental minister. The Church makes provisions for prayers for commendation of the dying that may be said by any of those listed above or by a layperson.

Source: Adapted from Texas Children's Cancer Center–Texas Children's Hospital (2000), reference 10.

of religious belief affecting neonatal palliative care is that of an American Caucasian family strongly tied to the Catholic Church. As their infant girl took a turn for the worst, the family was called. They immediately asked that she be baptized. The priest on call was unavailable and the family's priest was 2 hours away. Rather than take the chance that no priest would come before the infant's death, the nurse, a non-Catholic, baptized the baby. When the family arrived, they were reassured that Angela had been baptized. The infant died peacefully in her parents' arms long before either priest arrived. The family expressed comfort in knowing she was held within the religious arms of the church's beliefs.

One challenge to supporting the needs of the family is the lack of agreement among health professionals as to what constitutes palliative care.[11] Although some health professionals support children dying in their homes, the reality is that few pediatric hospice groups exist and even fewer for the neonate and family.[11,12] Catlin[13] studied 684 infants with life-threatening or chronic illnesses. She found that many infants stay 6 months or longer in the hospital, with 20% of the NICU infants transferred to the new and strange environment of the pediatric intensive care unit (PICU) to die even when care will most likely be futile. So despite having a palliative care protocol[14] supported at a national level, dissemination to individual institutions or units had not occurred. For the nurses, moral distress was noted as they were required to render futile and sometimes painful care.[13] As Anand suggests, healthcare professionals must also understand current pharmacological treatment of pain and use the most effective methods tailored to the individual infant to alleviate distress.[15]

Recognize differences in palliative care

Most neonatal health professionals recognize the unique needs of this population—their rights and their care needs. An infant has no history—as one family said, the infant does not know what the future possibilities are; there is no frame of reference. For the family, there are no memories of a past except prenatally, so palliative care is building a lifetime of memories. There are other aspects that are different as well. Box 59.2 summarizes these differences. The nurse should become familiar with the disease specific needs of patients and address the needs of the family during the implementation of neonatal palliative care measures while realizing the individual needs and uniqueness of each situation.

Palliative care plan

Catlin and Carter[14] developed a palliative care protocol that has been disseminated widely since 2002. Based on their research in neonatal palliative care, it is one of the only evidence-based plans available. It incorporates all of the elements previously discussed in this chapter. Since the 2002 creation of this protocol other dimensions of neonatal palliative care have developed. For example, the National Association of Neonatal Nurses (NANN) in 2007 published a position statement titled "NICU Nurse Involvement in Ethical Decisions Treatment of Critically Ill Newborns,"[18] and Rogers and colleagues[19] developed an educational program to address issues of moral distress in NICU nurses. The emphasis in this latter publication was to help nurses address the family needs during the dying process. It acknowledges the toll palliative care takes on the health professional.

Advocacy for support services

Nurses can serve as advocates to ensure that extensive support is being offered to the family. The benefit of providing these services is crucial for the family unit to maintain a sense of "wholeness" as they journey through this challenging period of time. The following is taken from the National Association of Neonatal Nurses position statement on Palliative Care for Newborns and Infants

Box 59.2 Differences between hospice care for newborns/infants and adults

Patient issues

- Patient is not legally competent.
- Patient is in developmental process that affects understanding of life and death, sickness and health, God, etc.
- Patient has not achieved a "full and complete life."
- Patient lacks verbal skills to describe needs, feelings, etc.
- Patient is often in a highly technical medical environment.

Family issues

- Family needs to protect the child from information about his/her health.
- Family needs to do everything possible to save the child.
- Family may have difficulty dealing with siblings.
- Family feels stress on finances.
- Family fears that care at home is not as good as care at the hospital.
- Grandparents feel helpless in dealing with their children and grandchildren.
- Family needs relief from burden of care.

Caregiver issues

- Caregivers need to protect children, parents, and siblings.
- Caregivers feel a sense of failure in not saving the child.
- Caregivers feel a sense of "ownership" of children, even at the expense of parents.
- Caregivers have out of date ideas about pain in children, especially infants.
- Caregivers lack knowledge about children's disease processes.
- Influence of "unfinished business" on style of care.

Institutional/agency issues

- There is less reimbursement or none for children's hospice/home care.
- High staff-intensity caring is required for children at home.
- Ongoing staff support is necessary.
- Children's services have immediate appeal to the public.
- Special competencies are needed in pediatric care.
- Assess how admission criteria may screen out children.
- Address unusual bereavement needs of family members.

Sources: Adapted from Kuebler and Berry (2002), reference 16 (used with permission); and Children's Hospice International, reference 17 (prepared by Paul R. Brenner).

(2010). Supporting the need for adequate services during the neonatal end-of-life care period[20]:

Appropriate family support services should be provided, including those of:

- Perinatal social workers, hospital chaplains, and clergy to provide emotional and spiritual support
- A child life specialist or family support specialist to support the infant's siblings
- A family advocate (a parent who has had a child in the NICU) to assist with navigating the NICU experience
- A lactation consultant to assist mothers who want to breastfeed their infant or donate breast milk at the end of life and to help mothers manage cessation of lactation at the end of life (Moore and Catlin, 2003)[21]

The nurse should not underestimate the impact that palliative and end-of-life care discussions can have on each member of the healthcare team during the transition through difficult clinical scenarios. The nurse can feel torn between spending quality time with a dying child and family and caring for the other neonatal patients. The emotional strain associated with end-of-life and bereavement care not only affects a nurse's health but can also affect relationships at home and with coworkers.[22] In the past decade, more attention has been paid to the role of the nurse and the sense of moral distress that can exist when a nurse is providing care for infants as they continue to decline clinically. Catlin et al. (2008) noted the most commonly reported cause of distress for nurses as having to follow orders to support patients at the end of their lives with advanced technology when palliative or comfort care would be more humane.[23] Parents may sense the moral distress when the nurse is not receiving adequate peer support during the delivery of intensive care measures. Initial distress involves feelings of frustration, anger, and anxiety when a person is faced with institutional obstacles and conflict with others about their own personal values.[24] It is vital that nurses have a forum to process their concerns within a confidential and professionally supported environment.

The implementation of debriefing sessions or clinical case reviews for difficult neonatal cases can be helpful. Team support can also come in the form of relief or "emotional rest" periods for the neonatal nurse; for example a nurse who has experienced a recent neonatal end-of-life care case may benefit from having patients with more stable clinical trajectories for the next few patient care assignments. Jonas-Simpson et al. (2013) suggest that education and support in nursing practice could be enhanced by supporting nurses to attend workshops and seminars on the topic of perinatal loss and bereavement care; incorporating discussions on supporting families, patients, colleagues, and oneself in bereavement care during orientation to the unit and ongoing education; debriefing after perinatal loss; and providing staff with a bereavement mentor.[25]

New trends

In 2003 the End-of-Life Nursing Education Consortium (ELNEC) developed a neonatal/pediatric version. To date, 650 pediatric/neonatal nurses have received this education in the United States and abroad http://www.aacn.nche.edu/elnec.

Table 59.3 Palliative care medications for neonatal patients

Medications	Usual dose	Special considerations
For pain		
Morphine	0.02–01 mg/kg IV Q2–4H PRN 0.2–0.4 mg/kg PO Q2–4H PRN 0.02–0.1 mg/kg/h	Opioid. Medication of choice for pain management in palliative and end-of-life care May use in combination with benzodiazepine More frequent doses may be needed to assure patient's comfort.
Fentanyl	1–3 mcg/kg IV or Intranasal Q1–2H PRN 1–3 mcg/kg/h	Fast onset and short-acting opioid Use injection form to administer intranasally. Bioavailability is almost 90%. Preferred in patients with renal failure
Methadone	0.05–0.2 mg/kg IV or PO Q4–24H	Long-acting opioid Usual starting frequency is every 8–12 hours scheduled. Peak onset is delayed and may require breakthrough pain medication for 48 hours after initiation or dose escalation.
Acetaminophen	10–15 mg/kg PO Q4–6H PRN 20 mg/kg PR Q6H PRN 7.5–10 mg/kg IV Q6H PRN	Analgesic. Antipyretic May give IV form undiluted over 15 minutes
Oral sucrose 24%	<1 kg: 0.1mL PO PRN 1–2 kg: 0.5mL PO PRN >2 kg: 1–2mL PO PRN	Analgesic. May administer directly into mouth or apply on pacifier
For pain/sedation		
Clonidine	1–3 mcg/kg PO Q6–8H	Alpha agonist. Has mild analgesic and sedating properties. May cause hypotension and bradycardia. Avoid use of patch in neonates.
For sedation		
Midazolam	0.05–0.1 mg/kg IV Q1H PRN 0.2 mg/kg Sublingual or Intranasal Q1H PRN 1–2 mcg/kg/min	Very short-acting benzodiazepine Anticonvulsant, sedating, produces amnesia. Rapidly penetrates the CNS. During end-of-life care, more frequent doses may be needed to ensure patient's comfort.
Lorazepam	0.05–0.1 mg/kg IV or PO Q2–4H PRN	Benzodiazepine Reduces anxiety and agitation. Anticonvulsant Consider adding to opioids for sedation
Diazepam	0.05–0.25 mg/kg PO or PR Q4–12H	Long-acting benzodiazepine. Peak onset is delayed and may require breakthrough with shorter-acting benzodiazepine for 24–48h after initiation or dose escalation. Reduces anxiety and agitation. Anticonvulsant Consider adding to opioids for sedation.
For secretions		
Glycopyrrolate	2–10 mcg/kg IV Q6H 20–100 mcg/kg PO Q6H	Decreases oral secretions through anticholinergic activity. Increase slowly to effective dose. Consider reducing dose if signs of tachycardia noted.
For constipation		
Glycerin suppository	1/8–1/4 Suppository PR Q12–24H PRN	Osmotic laxative. Consider using with opioids to reduce constipation.

Sources: References 27 to 35.

More institutions are interested in neonatal-specific content to start their own palliative care teams. Despite support from the American Academy of Pediatrics (AAP) and the World Health Organization (WHO) for the provision of palliative care, there are still many barriers. Kain[26] identified barriers to neonatal palliative care as formal educational needs on the part of staff, a feeling of failure (especially by the physicians), difficulty in communicating bad news to the parents, and ethical conflicts among the team members. The ability of the nurse to deliver care to the dying newborn is impacted by many barriers and inconsistencies to delivery of palliative care. There is demonstrated evidence through the interest in ELNEC that nurses around the world wish to provide good palliative care as a standard part of neonatal care.

Summary

Neonates who would benefit from excellent palliative care could die minutes, months, or years after birth with a life-threatening anomaly or illness. The nurse is called on to focus on providing care when the prognosis is uncertain, and this may challenge existing healthcare system structures. The trajectory can be unpredictable, and the focus needs to be on excellent pain and symptom management, while promoting developmental care of the infant as well as maintaining adequate emotional, psychosocial, and spiritual support for the family. Families and professionals have the difficult task of helping the infant live as fully as possible with complete dignity and comfort while preparing for and accepting that the infant may not live a long time. This requires a committed interdisciplinary team with community linkages as appropriate. Nurses new to palliative care should have the support of more senior nurses and staff, because the first experience of infant death can cause a considerable amount of anxiety and emotional distress for the nurse.

Regardless of the length of life or the place where that life is lived, excellent palliative care includes optimum symptom relief for the neonate, honoring the parents' wishes, providing ongoing support to parents and family, planning for the death, and honoring the life by creating memories of the life. The nurse should avoid phrases such as "withdraw care" or "nothing more can be done." There are always interventions that can be done to promote comfort during end-of-life care for infants with complex chronic conditions. For example, supporting pain, managing secretions, minimizing sleep disturbances, treatment for agitation, and optimizing time that can be spent peacefully with the family. Table 59.3 lists common medications used during the end-of-life care period for infants. The use of a neonatal scale should continue during end-of-life care.[20] Supportive care should continue throughout the bedside postmortem care and incorporate options for obtaining mementos. In some regions there are bereavement photography specialists who can assist with providing compassionately developed photographs of the deceased infant, for example "Now I lay me down to sleep" https://www.nowilaymedowntosleep.org/find-a-photog/.

Appendix 59.1

Neonatal end-of-life palliative care protocol*

*This protocol was published in Kenner C, Lott JW. *Neonatal Nursing Handbook*. St. Louis: Mosby, 2003:506–525. Adapted from Reference 10.

The purpose of this protocol of care is to educate professionals and enhance their preparation and support for a peaceful, pain-free, and family-centered death for dying newborns.

Planning for a palliative care environment

To begin a palliative care program, one must realize that some institutions find it difficult to confront the issue of a dying child. So to begin to create a palliative care environment, there must be staff education and buy-in. This education must address cultural issues that affect caregiving. Ethical issues must be addressed either by the group creating the environment or by consultants who specialize in ethics.

For the family, staff must treat the family as care partners and not visitors. They must recognize that someone needs to be available 24/7 to address issues such as advance directives and symptom and pain management both in the hospital and at home if

discharge is possible. There must be a mechanism to prepare the community for the child's entrance home or to hospice. This preparation includes what is appropriate to say to friends, relatives, and visitors.

Prenatal discussion of palliative care

It is essential that fetal development and viability be discussed with all families as a part of prenatal care packages and classes and to all families receiving assisted reproductive therapies. As the course of prenatal care progresses, pregnant women should be made aware that newborns in the very early gestational periods of 22 to 24 weeks and birth weights of less than 500 grams may not be responsive to resuscitation or applied neonatal intensive care.

Physician considerations

The families need honest, straightforward language. They need to know their options, and it is essential that they understand what to expect. Usually the physician delivers this information, but the nurse is generally the one that can help the parents sort through feelings and grasp what they were just told. If this incident is sudden, such as an unexpected premature or complicated birth, then the family's ability to comprehend and retain what is being said is limited. Reinforcement at a later time is advisable.

Family considerations

Peer support from families that have experienced a similar infant illness or death may help the family cope. If the family finds out that the pregnancy is not viable, then it is up to the healthcare team to help support their needs and to garner resources such as other family members, spiritual counselors, and friends. Helping the family to experience the normal parenting tasks such as naming the baby is very appropriate and helpful. This act helps the family gain some control and to be a parent first and to build memories of that experience.

Transport issues

It is best that mothers not be separated from their newborn infants. Transport is considered both traumatic and expensive, and if the newborn's condition is incompatible with prolonged life, then arrangements to stay in the local hospital may generally be preferred. It is best to avoid transferring dying newborns to Level III NICUs if nothing more can be done there than at the local hospital. The local area is recognized as that location at which parents have their support system, rapport with their established healthcare providers, a spiritual/religious community, and funeral availability.

The key to whatever decision is made, referral or not, requires good, clear communication with the family and between the two institutions. The family should not feel they are being sent away or given the wrong message by the nature of the transfer, or even return from a tertiary center once a referral is made if there is nothing to be done. The family needs a consistent message if trust is to be developed.

Which newborns should receive palliative care?

Although many aspects of palliative care should be integrated into the care of all newborns, there are infants born for whom parents and the healthcare professionals believe that palliative care is the most appropriate form of care. The following list includes categories of newborns that have experienced the transition from life-extending technological support to palliative care. The individual context of applying palliative care will require that each case, in each family, within each healthcare center, be explored individually. These categories of newborns are provided for educational purposes and may engender discussion at the local institutional level.

- Newborns at the threshold of viability
- Newborns with complex or multiple congenital anomalies incompatible with prolonged life, where neonatal intensive care will not affect long-term outcome
- Newborns not responding to intensive care intervention, who are deteriorating despite all appropriate efforts, or in combination with a life-threatening acute event

Introducing the palliative care model to parents

Speaking to parents about palliative care is difficult. There is heartache from the staff and heartfelt sympathy for the parents. The following points are offered to help physicians and nurse practitioners facilitate the process:

- Let the family know they will not be abandoned.
- Assist the family in obtaining all of the medical information that they want. Tell them that the entire medical team wishes the situation were different. Let them know you will support them every step of the way and that their infant is a valued and loved member of their family.
- Hold conversations in a quiet, private, and physically comfortable space.
- Give them your beeper number or telephone number to call you after they have digested the information and have more questions. Offer the ability to have a second opinion and/or an ethics consultation.
- Provide parents time to consult the local regional center that works with children with special needs or their area pediatrician, who can provide information on projected abilities and disabilities.
- Offer to introduce them to parents who have been in a similar situation.
- When possible, use lay-person language to clarify medical terms, and allow a great deal of time for parents to process the information.
- The terms "withdrawal of treatment," such as referring to the stopping of life support, or "withdrawal of care," referring to the stopping of feedings or other supportive interventions, should be avoided. The exact treatment or care that is to be terminated should be specifically explained so that the intention is clear.
- Use terms such as "change in care" or "change in treatment."
- Communicate and collaborate with parents at all times. Efforts should be made to clarify mutually derived goals of care for the infant. Give as many choices as possible about how palliative care should be implemented for their infant. Inform the parents of improved access to the infant for holding, cuddling, kangaroo care, and breastfeeding. Use of developmental care approaches such as these promotes the building of a relationship between the infant and parents.

- If the transition in care involves the removal of ventilatory support, explain that the use of ventilators is for the improvement of heart/lung conditions until cure, when cure is a likely outcome.
- Tell the parents that you cannot change the situation but you can support the infant's short life with comfort and dignity. Explain that discontinuing interventions that cause suffering is a brave and loving action to take for their infant.
- Validate the loss of the dreamed-for healthy infant, but point out the good/memorable features he/she has. Help parents look past any deformities and work to alleviate any blame they may express.
- Encourage parents to be a family as much as possible. Refer to the newborn by name. Assist them to plan what they would like to do while the infant is still alive.
- Encourage them to ask support persons to join them on the unit. Facilitate sibling visitation. Support siblings with child life specialists on staff.
- In daily conversation, avoid terms that express improvement such as "good," "stable," "better" in reference to the dying patient so as not to confuse parents.
- Prepare the family for what may happen as the infant dies.
- Introduce families to the chaplain and social worker early in the process.

Optimal environment for neonatal death

When the decision is made that a newborn infant may be close to death, there are several components to optimizing the care. These include:

- Compassionate, nonjudgmental, consistent staff for each infant, including physicians knowledgeable in palliative care. If consistent staff is not an option in a particular unit, then agreement on the plan of care is essential, with proposed revisions to care discussed with the whole team.
- Nurses and other healthcare staff educated in providing a meaningful experience for the family while caring for the family's psychosocial needs, including a period of time after the death.
- Parents who are educated in what to expect and who are encouraged to participate in, or even orchestrate, the dying process and environment of their infant in a manner they find meaningful.
- Flexibility of the facility and staff in responding to parental wishes, such as participation of siblings and other family members, and including wishes of parents and families who do not wish to be present.
- Institutional policies that allow staff flexibility to respond to parental wishes.
- Providing time to create memories, such as allowing parents to dress, diaper, and bathe their infant, feed him/her (if it is possible), take photos, and hold the infant in their arms. If they wish to take the infant outdoors to a peaceful and natural setting, that should be encouraged.
- Siblings should be made comfortable; they may wish to write letters or draw for the infant. Snacks should be available.

- Allowing the family to stay with the infant as long as they need to, including after death occurs.
- The process for treating the dying infant[14,36,37] is well described in the literature and by the various bereavement programs. Such processes include such things as having one nurse assigned to be with the family, staying with the infant while parents take breaks, and collecting mementos that families may wish to take home (e.g., pictures or videos, hand- and footprints, and locks of hair).
- Parents should be assisted in making plans for a memorial service, burial, and so forth. Some parents might wish to carry or accompany the infant's body to the morgue or to the funeral home themselves. Issues such as autopsy, cremation, burial, and who may transport the body should be discussed, especially if the parents are far from home and wish to take the body back to their home area for burial. In some states, hospitals may release a body to parents after notifying the county department of vital statistics. The family must sign a form for removal of the body. The quality assurance department should be notified. Further discussion of autopsy and organ/tissue donation issues is included.

Specific skills are needed by the staff to provide palliative care. These include

- A physician leader of the team who is familiar with family-centered care and the tenets of palliative/hospice care
- A trained nursing staff, clinical social workers, and clergy supportive of this manner of care
- Agreement to cease all invasive care, including taking frequent vital signs, monitoring, medical machinery, and artificial feeding
- Removal of all medications other than those to provide comfort or to prevent or treat a troubling symptom, with continued IV access for pain medication and anxiolytics
- Maintenance of skin care, participation in discussion on the appropriateness of feeding, and prevention of air hunger
- Use of simple blow-by oxygen or suctioning if needed for comfort
- Continuous observation and gentle assessment by nursing staff as individualized by parent wishes
- Physicians' notes describing the need for ongoing physician observation and nursing staff interventions to provide the needed level of care
- Appropriate palliative care orders on the chart

Location for provision of palliative care

Location is not as important as the "mindset" of persons involved in end-of-life care. The attitude of staff, their desire to care for dying newborns and their families, their training in observation, support, and symptom management, and their knowledge of how to apply a bereavement protocol are more important than the physical location of the patient. Many agree that an active NICU may not be the optimal place for a dying newborn. Whether the infant is moved to a room off of the unit (e.g., a family room), onto a general pediatrics ward, or kept on the postpartum floor, the best available physical space with privacy and comfort should be chosen.

The families need help to make the decision of how and where the infant is to be given care. If families take the infant home, coordination with the EMS personnel may be necessary to prevent undesired intervention. Parents need to be instructed not to call 911 because in some places emergency medical technicians (EMTs) are obligated to provide cardiopulmonary resuscitation (CPR). A letter describing the diagnosis, existence of in-hospital do-not-resuscitate (DNR) order, and hospice care plan for home with the full expectation that the patient will die should be provided to the parents, their primary physician, home-health agency/hospice, and perhaps the county EMS coordinator. Generally, hospice nurses are allowed to confirm a patient's death.

Ventilator removal, pain, and symptom management

At times, cessation of certain technological supports accompanies the provision of palliative care. The following information addresses (1) how to prepare the family, staff, and facility for discontinuation of ventilator support, and (2) the process of removing the ventilator in a manner that minimizes discomfort for the infant and the family. The latter includes who will be present at the time of extubation. A plan must be worked out with the family about what medications and support will be given to alleviate pain and suffering and what they can expect the dying process to be like for their baby. Consideration of developmentally supportive care that is attuned to ambient light and noise as well as comfort measures are important. These should incorporate cultural considerations.

Mementos can be obtained by nurses, such as a lock of hair, hand or footprints in plaster, and photos and/or videotapes of the family together if this is culturally appropriate. If the infant has serious anomalies, photos of hands, ears, lips, feet can be provided. Ear prints and lip prints are possible. Some parents have indicated that mementos of a newborn who died are not acceptable in their culture.

When death does not occur after cessation of aggressive support

A private room somewhere in the hospital is recommended where nurses trained in palliative care are available. If the expected time for expiration passes and death does not take place, the infant could be discharged to home for ongoing palliative care services. The parents, NICU staff, and the hospice staff should meet to make plans for home care, including the investigation of what services are offered and what insurance will cover. Continued palliative care/hospice services with home nursing care is essential, including the possibility of ventilator removal at home.

If the infant is to go home, a procedure for dispensing outpatient medications should be in place. All needed drugs and directions for use should be sent along with the infant so that the parents do not have to go to a pharmacy to fill prescriptions. Identifying and communicating with a community healthcare provider who will continue with the infant's home-care needs is essential.

Some families and healthcare providers feel dying newborns should be fed, and if unable to suck, should be tube fed. Others feel that artificial feeding is inappropriate. However, withholding of feedings is an ethical dilemma for many health professionals and families and needs careful consideration.[28] Recent research indicates that feeding can be burdensome and that an overload of fluids can impede respirations.[39] In all cases, infants should receive care to keep their mouth and lips moist. Drops of sucrose water have been found to be a comfort agent if the infant can swallow, and they may be absorbed through the buccal membrane. Parents who feel they cannot take the infant home should be assisted to find hospice care placement.

Discussion of organ and tissue procurement and autopsy

At some point in the course of care, organ and tissue donation and autopsy will need to be discussed. Prior to discussion with families, the regional organ donation center should be contacted to see if a particular infant qualifies as a potential donor. In some areas, only corneas or heart valves are valuable in an infant under 10 pounds, but in different locations, other organs (e.g., heart) or tissues may be appropriate. It is important to know if a newborn has no potential donor use and to communicate this respectfully. Parents often desire the ability to give this gift and may be doubly hurt if they are hoping for the opportunity to help others and are turned down.

The person who discusses organ/tissue procurement must be specially trained. While the physician usually initiates this, a nurse, chaplain, or representative from donor services may conduct the conversation with tact and compassion. The provider should be aware of cultural, traditional, or religious values that would preclude organ donation for a specific family, as many cultures and religions would consider this desecration of the dead infant.

Suggestions concerning autopsy

Requests for autopsies are not required in all states but may be considered appropriate in many instances of infant death. If the medical examiner or coroner is involved in the case, laws may require autopsy. Some providers feel that asking for an autopsy is important to potentially provide parents with some answers regarding their infant's illness and death. The placenta may also be used for testing to provide information. In the discussion, parents may wish to know all or some of the following:

- Autopsy does not cause any pain or suffering to the infant; it is done only after death.
- The body is handled with the ultimate respect.
- Some insurance companies pay for a physician-ordered autopsy.
- Final results are returned in approximately 6 to 8 weeks, at which time the primary physician can meet with the parents, conduct a telephone conference, or communicate by letter to discuss the results.

Family care: cultural, spiritual, and practical family needs

The hospital social worker is an essential component of supportive palliative care. Families may immediately need financial assistance, access to transportation, and a place to stay. Practical considerationsParents of multiples of whom some lived and one died will need special attention to validate their bereavement as well as to support their love for their living child(ren).

Time should be permitted for the parents to contact the needed authority in their culture and to plan any necessary ceremony, some of which may require special permission; for example use of incense.

Cultural sensitivityThese support needs should be anticipated and provided as much as possible:

- When using a translator, simple words and phrases should be used so that the translator can convey the message exactly as it is given. It is most appropriate to use hospital-trained and certified translators to ensure accuracy.
- Whenever possible, written materials should be given in the family's primary language, in an easy-to-read format, culturally and linguistically appropriate for the family.
- Culturally sensitive grief counseling and contact with a support group of other parents who have been through this is helpful.

Family follow-up care

Families who have experienced a neonatal death will likely leave the facility in a shocked state. Families can be best be served in these ways:

- Establishing contact with a social worker, chaplain, or grief counselor prior to discharge.
- Receiving an information packet as described and a date for a follow-up discussion with the attending physician (which maybe in conjunction with autopsy results).
- Notifying the family's obstetrician of the death no matter how long after delivery it occurred.
- A home visit by one of the staff or a public health nurse within a few days.
- Phone calls weekly, then monthly, then at 6-month intervals if parents agree. Also providing contact on significant days such Mother's Day, the infant's due date, or anniversary of death.
- Invite family to a group memorial service held by the hospital for those who have lost pregnancies or infants in the past year.
- Keep in mind that subsequent pregnancy may be difficult and offer support at that time; include genetic counseling if indicated.
- Keep snapshots and mementos on the unit if parents do not wish to take them at the time, as some parents may reconsider later.

Ongoing staff support

The work of providing end-of-life care for newborns and their families is very intense. Staff needing support must not be limited to the nursing staff, and must include physicians and all healthcare and ancillary personnel who have interacted with the infant or family. Suggested support includes the following:

- Facilitated meetings of the multidisciplinary team during the process are needed, especially if some of the team members are reluctant to change to this mode of care.
- Debriefings after every infant's death and after any critical incident will be helpful for the staff.
- Meetings or counseling sessions should be part of regular work hours and not held on voluntary or unpaid time.
- Moral support for the nurses and physicians directly caring for the dying newborn is required from peers as well as the unit director, other neonatologists, chaplain, and nursing house supervisor.

◆ Nursing staff scheduling should be flexible and allow for overtime to continue with the family or to orient another nurse to take over.

◆ If they wish, the primary nurse and physician should be called if not present at the actual time of the infant's dying. With permission by the parents, they should be allowed to attend the funeral if desired and to take time off afterward if needed.

Acknowledgments

We would like to acknowledge Beth Seyda and her family for sharing their journey and experiences with the death of their beloved son Dylan. We would also like to acknowledge Dr. Margarita Bidegain, Associate Professor of Pediatrics, Duke Children's Neonatology Division, for her support and encouragement throughout the editing of this chapter.

References

1. Mathews TJ, MacDorman MF. Infant Mortality Statistics from the 2009 Period Linked Birth/Infant Death Data Set: National Vital Statistics Reports (vol. 61). Hyattsville, MD: National Center for Health Statistics; 2013.

2. Catlin A. Transition from curative efforts to purely palliative care for neonates: does physiology matter? Adv Neonatal Care. 2011;11(3):216–222.

3. Tan JS, Docherty SL, Barfield R, Brandon DH. Addressing parental bereavement support needs at the end of life for infants with complex chronic conditions. J Palliat Med. 2012;15(5):579–584.

4. Ahern K. What neonatal intensive care nurses need to know about neonatal palliative care. Adv Neonatal Care. 2013;13(2):108–114.

5. Moro TT, Kavanaugh K, Savage TA, Reyes MR, Kimura RE, Bhat R. Parent decision making for life support decisions for extremely premature infants: from the prenatal through end-of-life period. J Perinat Neonatal Nurs. 2011; 25(1): 52–60.

6. Wigert H, Dellenmark MB, Bry K. Strengths and weaknesses of parent–staff communication in the NICU: a survey assessment. BMC Pediatr. 2013; 13: 71.

7. Couglin M, Gibbins S, Hoath S. Core measures for developmentally supportive care in neonatal intensive care units: theory, precedence and practice J Adv Nurs. 2009; 65(10): 2239–2248.

8. Wool C. Clinician confidence and comfort in providing perinatal palliative care. J Obstet Gynecol Neonat Nurs. 2013; 42(1):48–58.

9. Hockenberry MJ, Wilson D. Wong's Nursing Care of Infants and Children (8th ed). St. Louis, MO: Mosby; 2006.

10. Texas Children's Cancer Center–Texas Children's Hospital. End-of-Life Care for Children. Houston, TX: Texas Cancer Council; 2000.

11. Shipman C, Gysels M, White P, et al. Improving generalist end of life care: national consultation with practitioners, commissioners, academics, and service user groups. BMJ. 2008;337:a1720. Available at: http://www.bmj.com (accessed November 28, 2008).

12. Feudtner C, Feinstein JA, Stachell M, Zhao H, Kang TL. Shifting place of death among children with complex chronic conditions in the United States, 1989–2003. JAMA. 2007;297(24):2725–2732.

13. Catlin A. Extremely long hospitalizations of newborns in the United States: data, descriptions, dilemmas. J Perinatol. 2006;26:742–748.

14. Catlin A, Carter B. Creation of a neonatal end-of-life palliative care protocol. J Perinatol. 2002;22:184–195.

15. Anand KJS. Pharmacological approaches to the management of pain in the neonatal intensive care unit. J Perinatol. 2007;27:S4–S11.

16. Kuebler KK, Berry PH. End-of-life care. In: Kuebler KK, Berry PH, Heidrich DE (eds.), End-of-Life Care: Clinical Practice Guidelines. Philadelphia: W.B. Saunders; 2002: 25.

17. Children's Hospice International. Available at: http://www. chionline. org (accessed February 23, 2005).

18. National Association of Neonatal Nurses (NANN). NANN Position Statement 3015: NICU Nurse Involvement in Ethical Decisions (Treatment of Critically Ill Newborns). Adv Neonatal Care. 2007;7(5):267–268.

19. Rogers S, Babgi A, Gomez C. Educational interventions in end-of-life care: Part I: An educational intervention responding to the moral distress of NICU nurses provided by an ethics consultation team. Adv Neonatal Care. 2008;8(1):56–65.

20. National Association of Neonatal Nurses Palliative Care for Newborns and Infants Position Statement #3051 September 2010.

21. Moore DB, Catlin A. Lactation suppression: forgotten aspect of care for the mother of a dying child. Pediatr Nurs. (2003);29(5):383–384.

22. Zhang W, Lane BS. Promoting neonatal staff nurses' comfort and involvement in end of life and bereavement care. Nurs Res Pract. 2013. Article ID 365329, 5 pages.

23. Catlin A, Volat D, Hadley MA, Bassir R, Armigo C, Valle E, et al. Conscientious objection: a potential neonatal nursing response to care orders that cause suffering at the end of life? Study of a concept. Neonatal Netw. 2008;27(2):101–108.

24. Kain VJ. Moral distress and providing care to dying babies in neonatal nursing. Int J Palliat Nurs. 2007;13(5):243–248.

25. Jonas-Simpson C, Pilkington FB, MacDonald C, McMahon E. Nurses' experiences of grieving when there is a perinatal death. SAGE Open. 2013;3(2). 2158244013486116.

26. Kain VJ. Palliative care delivery in the NICU: what barriers do neonatal nurses face? Neonatal Netw. 2006;25(6):387–392.

27. Stevens B, Yamada J, Ohlsson S. (2004). Sucrose for analgesia in newborn infants undergoing painful procedures. Cochrane Database Syst Rev. 2004;(3):CD001969.

28. Walter-Nicolet E, Annequin D, Biran V, Mitanchez D, Tourniaire B. Pain management in newborns: from prevention to treatment. Pediatr Drugs. 2010;12:353–365.

29. Krishnan L (2012). Pain relief in neonates. J Neonat Surg. 2013; 2(2):19.

30. Harlos MS, Stenekes S, Lambert D, Hohl C, Chochinov HM. Intranasal fentanyl in the palliative care of newborns and infants. J Pain Sympt Manage. Epub 26 September 2012.

31. Allegaert K, Palmer GM, and Anderson BJ. The pharmacokinetics of intravenous paracetamol in neonates: size matters most. Arch Dis Child. 2011; 96(6):575–580.

32. van den Anker JN and Tibboel D. Pain relief in neonates: when to use intravenous paracetamol. Arch Dis Child. 2011; 96(6): 573–574.

33. Doyle D. Woodruff R. International Association for Hospice Care (IAHPC), 2nd edition; 2008.

34. Shaw TM. Pediatric palliative pain and symptom management. Pediatric Annals. 2012; 41(8): 329–334.

35. Constipation Guideline Committee of the North American Society for Pediatric Gastroenterology, Hepatology and Nutrition. Evaluation and treatment of constipation in infants and children: recommendations of the North American Society for Pediatric Gastroenterology, Hepatology and Nutrition. J Pediatr Gastroenterol Nutr. 2006; 43(3):e1–e13.

36. Oosterwal G. Caring for People from Different Cultures: Communicating Across Cultural Boundaries. Portland, OR: Providence Health System; 2003.

37. American Hospital Association (AHA). A Patient's Bill of Rights. Available at: http://www.injuredworker.org/Library/Patient_Bill_of_Rights.htm (accessed March 28, 2005).

38. McHaffie HE, Fowlie PW. Withdrawing and withholding treatment: comments on new guidelines. Arch Dis Child. 1998;79:1–2.

39. Craig F, Goldman A. Home management of the dying NICU patient. Semin Neonatol. 2003;8:177–183.

Additional resources

1. Centers for Disease Control and Prevention (CDC). Fast Stats A-Z. Available at: http://www.cdc.gov/nchs/fastats/infmort.htm (accessed February 19, 2005).

2. Centers for Disease Control and Prevention (CDC). US Infant Mortality Rate Now Worse Than 28 Other Countries. Available at: http://www.wsws.org/articles/2008/oct2008/mort-018.shtml (accessed November 28, 2008).

3. Rip MR, Dosh SA. The Neighborhood and Neonatal Intensive Care: A Population-Based Analysis of the Demand for Neonatal Intensive Care in Detroit, Michigan (1984–1988). Available at: http://www.uic.edu/sph/cade/mchepi/meetings/may2001/nicu.ppt (accessed November 8, 2003).

4. Cassel CK, Foley KM. Principles of Care of Patients at the End of Life: An Emerging Consensus Among the Specialties of Medicine. New York: Milbank Memorial Fund, 1999. Available at: http://www.milbank.org/reports/endoflife (accessed February 23, 2005).

5. Americans for Better Care of the Dying. Making Promises. Washington, DC: Americans for Better Care of the Dying, 2001. Available at: http://www.abcd-caring.org/tools/actionguides.pdf (accessed March 24, 2005).

6. Last Acts Partnership. Precepts of Palliative Care for Children, Adolescents and Their Families. National Association of Pediatric Nurse Practitioners, NAPNAP, October 2003. Available at: http://www.napnap.org/index.cfm?page=54&sec=465 (accessed November 28, 2008).

7. Institute of Medicine (IOM). To Err Is Human: Building a Safer Health System. 1999. Available at: http://www.iom.edu/CMS/8089/5575.aspx (accessed November 28, 2008).

8. Institute of Medicine (IOM). Crossing the Quality Chasm: The IOM Health Care Quality Initiative, 2001. Available at: www.iom.edu/CMS/8089.aspx (accessed November 28, 2008).

9. Lundqvist A, Nilstun T, Dykes AK. Neonatal end-of-life care in Sweden. Nurs Crit Care. 2003;8:197–202.

10. Rebagliato M, Cuttini M, Broggin L, et al. Neonatal end-of-life decision making: Physicians' attitudes and relationship with self-reported practices in 10 European countries. JAMA. 2000;284(19):2451–2459.

Grief and bereavement in pediatric palliative care

Rana Limbo and Betty Davies

In the NICU on Eliot's first day we were discussing to ourselves how the clock was creeping toward 4:59 PM and how he had been with us for 24 hours.... Minutes later, one of the nurses quietly came alongside us with what she called a "birthday hat," a small circle of tinsel she had heisted from a nearby bulletin board.... She proceeded to hand the sleep-deprived new parents, as well as each nurse, a piece of "birthday cake," otherwise known as breath mints, for Eliot's party. We laughed at her ingenuity as all who were present gathered around to sing happy birthday in hushed tones; such a familiar song rang out in such an unfamiliar setting.... And when there is no map, the smallest anchor to that present moment and now to a former reality—indeed, to a person that we love beyond measure—this tether becomes a means to bind you to what you will never forget. Ritual has served as a way to remind us and others that what we see is not all there is or was or, I believe, will be.

Matt Mooney, father of Eliot, who lived for 99 days with a diagnosis of Trisomy 13.

Key points

◆ Bereavement care for all family members is an integral component of pediatric palliative care.

◆ Grieving after a death is a normal process; however, some grief reactions become complicated, and nurses must assess for factors that put family members at risk for such reactions.

◆ Grief assessment begins at the time of diagnosis of a child's life-limiting condition, applies to all family members, and continues into the bereavement period following the child's death.

◆ Nurses have a responsibility to create supportive environments in which family members feel free to express their grief.

◆ Caring for dying children requires nurses to attend to their own personal and professional responses to death, dying, and bereavement as a basis for providing optimal care to families.

"Effective and compassionate care for children with life-threatening conditions and their families is an integral and important part of care from diagnosis through death and bereavement."[1] This guiding principle, one of seven put forth by the Institute of Medicine report on the status of palliative and end-of-life care for children and their families, emphasizes that care continues for the family following the child's death. Although medical science has contributed significantly to the treatment of children with life-limiting illnesses or conditions, children still die from cancer, cardiac disease, respiratory conditions, genetic conditions, and more. Moreover, thousands of neonates die each year and thousands more children of all ages, particularly toddlers and adolescents, die as a result of trauma. Approximately 45,000 children die annually in the United States.[2] Regardless of the cause, the death of a child is a tragedy, an incomparable life event that has an impact on all family members, friends of the family, and the community in which the family lives. A child's death also affects the physicians, nurses, social workers, and other healthcare personnel who provide care for the dying child. The purpose of this chapter is to define common words associated with grief; to describe factors that affect the grief of family members, the effects of grief on them, and the nurse's role in helping grieving individuals and their families; and to discuss the needs of nurses who work in pediatric palliative care.

Grief as a process

Death is a part of each individual life, something we all must face though we resist even the thought of our own mortality. The hoped-for pattern is that we experience deaths of others that are easier in earlier life, for us to build the skills to aid us with the more difficult deaths in later life. The death of one's child, though, sits outside of that hoped-for pattern. The grief associated with a child's death begins even before the actual death event, as the child's parents and other family members anticipate the death and experience the child's dying, and their grief continues long past the child's death. Many parents feel they never "recover" from the death of their child. They may resume daily activities, adjust to life without their child's presence, and find new pleasures in life, but many parents remain vulnerable and feel that they are not the same people they were before the child's death.[3-5] The death of a child, or any beloved person, is not something one "gets over"; rather, over time, one learns to integrate the loss into one's life. Indeed, grief is a process that is not always orderly and predictable, and given that grief is the individual experience of each human being, it manifests in many diverse ways.

Grief, bereavement, and mourning

The term *grief* is often used to refer to the emotional response to a loss.[6] But grief is much more than emotion—it is an overwhelming and acute sense of loss and despair; it is the personalized feeling and response that an individual makes to real, perceived, or anticipated death; it encompasses feelings, physical sensations, cognitions, and behaviors. Grief encompasses every domain of human life—physical, emotional, psychological, social, and spiritual. Sadness, anger, numbness, sleep and eating disturbances, inability to concentrate, fatigue, existential angst, and tension in interpersonal interactions are among the responses to a loved one's death.

Grief occurs when a loss is deemed as personally significant to the individual. For example, hearing the news about a child's death in a bicycle accident may produce sadness, but not necessarily a grief reaction. However, grief will ensue when it is learned that the child is your nephew. To a certain degree, who or what we consider to be personally significant is culturally defined. For example, in the contemporary United States, the death of one's child is expected to result in profound grief. In fact, a classic research study suggests that grief in response to a child's death is more intense than grief following the death of a spouse or parent.

The term "bereavement" refers to the state of being bereaved or deprived of something. The word derives from the Old English word *bereafian*, which means to deprive of, take away, seize, or rob.[7] This meaning implies that the lost object is a valued one, together with a suggestion of violence in the way in which the loss occurred. This definition is especially apt for bereaved parents, who often report feeling as if a part of them has been torn away. As the bereaved mother of a 22-month-old who died following a brain aneurysm sighed: "When my son died, it was as if my heart had been stolen from my breast, and my arms that held him ripped from their sockets."

Mourning refers to the outward, social expression of grief, often through ritual, and sometimes to the psychological process of adapting to loss.[8] How one expresses a loss may be dictated by cultural norms, customs, and practices, including rituals and traditions. Some cultures may be very emotional and verbal in their expression of loss, while others may appear stoic and business-like. Religious and cultural beliefs may also dictate how long one mourns and how one behaves during the bereavement period. In addition, outward expression of loss may be influenced by the individual's personality and life experiences.[9,10]

Types of grief

It is important for nurses' understanding of grief and bereavement and for the implementation of appropriate interventions to be aware of several types, or variations, of grief that have been described in the thanatology literature, including anticipatory grief, disenfranchised grief, and pathological grief reactions or complicated grief. How these concepts apply to pediatric palliative care is particularly important.

Anticipatory grief

Anticipatory grief often occurs in advance of an expected loss. Rando[11] indicates that anticipatory grief entails grieving not just for future losses, but also for losses that have already occurred and for current losses. It may be associated with the losses of expectations for a "normal" life that are associated with a particular diagnosis, with acute and chronic illness, or with death. For example, parents may fear the potential loss of health in their child when a child is being tested for unusual symptoms. All family members may grieve the expected loss of a part of the child's body, mental function, or self-image; they may grieve the loss of the child's and their own independence, choice, and dreams. Anticipatory grief occurs while the ill child is still alive, and this allows for hope. This is a subtle difference that makes anticipatory grief unique, and helps account for what parents often describe as an "emotional roller coaster," particularly for parents of children with long-term chronic illness. Their experience of witnessing the child's physical deterioration and worsening of symptoms, interspersed with remissions, "good" days, and seeming progress toward health lays fertile ground for emotional ups and downs and hope for the child's recovery. Over time, however, the focus of hope changes, and nurses can play a critical role in facilitating the expression of that hope. Initially, parents of children with cancer, for example, focus their hope on the possibility of cure. Each exacerbation chips away at the hope for the child's full recovery, and family members hope for longer remissions. Eventually, they hope their child will be able to live until he reaches a particular milestone, such as graduation, a special birthday, or the next holiday. As the child's condition worsens, parents may hope that their wish to care for their child at home will be possible, and that their child will not suffer at the end. Hope is life sustaining; healthcare providers should support family members in their hope, refraining from crushing hope with overdoses of facts. In response to a mother's proclamation that her child will overcome a serious illness, the nurse can empathize, "I certainly do hope so." The death is anticipated, but it has not occurred, and in the parents' eyes, there is a chance, no matter how small, that it might not occur:

> My son has been to the PICU three times. At his first transfer to the PICU, my sorrow was beyond description. At that time, I thought I would never see him again. But my son has fought against his cancer every time. Whenever he came back to the ward from the PICU…I remember recently that day was 3 days before his 13th birthday…it was so amazing and I prayed thanks to God for allowing me to hope for his life again.

For more information on hope, see chapter 28.

Although painful, anticipatory grieving does present an opportunity for families to begin to think about their future without the child. It can help family members begin to face the existential questions that arise when a child is dying. It can help families begin the process of reorganizing their fractured lives. Anticipatory grieving can also take its toll, especially when the child's illness endures. Rando[12] interviewed parents whose child had died from cancer, and suggests there is an optimal length of anticipatory grief of 6 to 18 months. A shorter time did not give parents enough time to prepare for the loss, and a longer period had a debilitating effect on them.

Unacknowledged grief before the death may inhibit communication and preparation for death which, in turn, may contribute to strong feelings of subsequent guilt and regret.[1] However, anticipatory grief does not mean the grieving that occurs after the child's death is somehow easier or less painful for parents and other family members. Healthcare providers cannot assume that family members whose child died following a long-term illness grieve "less" than those whose child dies suddenly and unexpectedly. In fact, every child's death is unexpected. Even when parents know their child will die, the actual moment of death is often unexpected, as reflected in parents' words: "I knew the end was near, but I really thought he would make it until his brother got home from college." Or, as the 7-year-old sister wept following her brother's death a few days before her birthday: "But, he was coming to my party."

Disenfranchised grief

Disenfranchised grief acknowledges the social context of grief. It refers to the grief that persons experience when they incur a loss that is not or cannot be openly acknowledged, publicly mourned, or socially supported.[13,14] Those at risk include, for example, classmates, teammates, teachers, coaches, school bus drivers, crossing guards, or past boyfriends/girlfriends of the child or adolescent who died—those whose relationship with the now-deceased child/adolescent is not regarded as significant. Also feeling disenfranchised are those grieving a terminated pregnancy or a neonatal death where the significance of these losses may not even be acknowledged, or if it is, comments such as "You can try again" reflect insensitive misunderstanding of the parents' grief. Families of children with serious cognitive or physical limitations, from progressive neurodegenerative illnesses, for example, may experience disenfranchised grief when others perceive the child's death as a "blessing" rather than a loss for the family. Disenfranchised grief also occurs when bereaved persons are not recognized by society as capable of grief or needing to mourn. Young children, mentally challenged children or adults, and abusing parents whose actions have caused the child's death are often disenfranchised in this way.

Complicated or troubled grief

The processes of grief and mourning are normal and healthy aspects of human living. However, all human processes can go awry, especially in particularly difficult situations, and such grief is sometimes referred to as "complicated" grieving. However, as everyone who has experienced the loss of a loved one knows, all grief is complicated. It is just that sometimes grief is more complicated than at other times. But common terminology differentiates complicated from uncomplicated grief, with the latter referring to the typical feelings, behaviors, and reactions to loss; complicated grief refers to a response to loss that is more intense and longer in duration than usual. Symptoms of complicated grief commonly include separation and/or traumatic distress, distinct from depression and anxiety.[15] Worden[16] has outlined four basic types of complicated grief: (1) chronic grief is characterized by grief reactions that do not subside and continue over long periods

of time; (2) delayed grief is characterized by grief reactions that are suppressed or postponed, and the family member consciously or unconsciously avoids the pain of the loss; (3) exaggerated grief occurs when the family member resorts to self-destructive behaviors such as suicide; and (4) masked grief occurs when the family member is not aware that behaviors that interfere with normal functioning are a result of the loss.

Those who are mourning the loss of a child are at risk for complicated grief. Other risk factors include: preexisting difficulties in the relationship with the deceased (such as between a parent and a delinquent daughter); the circumstances of the death (such as traumatic death through suicide or homicide); chronic illness; the survivor's own history of depressive illness; multiple losses or history of troubled grief reactions to previous deaths; difficulty with the dying process; when the death is socially negated; or a lack of social support system or faith system.

Factors affecting the grief process

Family responses to grief vary widely and depend on a multitude of factors. Some of these factors may be obvious, some less apparent, but all influence how individual family members cope with the pain of a child's death. Influencing factors fall into three broad categories. Individual variables have to do with attributes of the bereaved, including the relationship between the child who died and other family members; environmental factors have to do with the social, familial, and cultural environments; and situational factors pertain to the characteristics of the death. All factors interact with one another to provide the context of grief.

Individual factors

Individual, or personal, characteristics that affect the grief process may include history and relationship with the child; previous exposure to death, dying, grief, and loss; developmental level; and temperament and coping styles.

History and relationship with the child

Each parent, sibling, or grandparent has a unique history and relationship with the deceased child. Histories among siblings are closely intertwined because siblings often develop special bonds that are unlike any other. The closer two siblings are to one another before death, the more behavior problems the surviving sibling may have following the death.[17] Similarly, grandparents may be integrally involved in children's lives, whether they live geographically far apart or down the street; in other families, grandparents and children barely know one another. Some histories among the children and other family members will have been predominantly troubled (filled with tension and conflict) and others filled with laughter and harmony.

Previous experience with death

Past experiences with death and the learned response to loss also affect how each family member will grieve a child's death. Other deaths of a similar nature may have occurred in the family, such as when more than one child suffers from the same life-limiting genetic disorder. How previous losses were handled in the family will influence the current situation.

In the R family, for example, when Grandfather R was 10 years old, his older brother was killed in a car accident. No one explained to the grieving child what had happened, he was not allowed to attend the funeral, and following the death, he regretted that he had not been the one to die because he believed his brother was so much smarter than he. As a young boy, he decided unconsciously that he would hide his pain behind a wall of silence; he seldom displayed or talked about emotions. When Mr. R's grandson died from cancer at age 11 years, Mr. R was flooded with memories and sadness. His previously learned coping through silence and withdrawal resulted in his being unprepared to help his distraught son and himself with the current loss.

Developmental level

When we think of "developmental level," we often think only of children and adolescents. Variants of four subconcepts of death are commonly included in writings about children and death: irreversibility, nonfunctionality, universality, and inevitability.[18,19] But development is a lifelong process; therefore, the developmental level of each grieving individual must be considered. For example, magical thinking (i.e., the person will become alive again) is typically associated with children. Yet Joan Didion[20] entitled her book about her husband's sudden death *The Year of Magical Thinking*. She recounts numerous examples of her magical belief that he would return, such as deciding not to give away all of his shoes, since he would need them when he came home.

Young parents who are facing the death of their child have not typically experienced many life crises; elderly grandparents may be struggling under the burden of having faced too many. A teenage mother, struggling to be independent from her parents, faces new challenges when she must rely on them for assistance because her baby becomes ill and dies. A midlife father, anxious about his family's financial future following his son's long-term illness, agonizes deeply over the expenses of his son's funeral and feels guilty about his feelings. A grandmother who overcame breast cancer at age 65 years laments over why her 20-year-old granddaughter was the one to die from cancer.

Personality and coping style

Individuals of all ages vary in temperament and personality, and styles of interacting with the world are evident in even the youngest children. Some youngsters are naturally more extroverted; they talk easily with others and eagerly seek out resources and sources of support and comfort. Others are more introverted; they keep their thoughts and feelings to themselves and may prefer the solitude of reading or quiet play. Doka[13] describes styles of grieving among adults that occur along a continuum, with "instrumental" grieving at one end and "intuitive" grieving at the other. Most people fall in the middle, but describing the extremes of the continuum clarifies the differences and may be helpful in understanding how parents and other family members manifest their grief. Intuitive grievers fit the pattern of how we think individuals "should" grieve. They express strong affective reactions, their expression mirrors their inner feelings, and their adaptation involves expression and exploration of feelings. In contrast, the grief experience for instrumental grievers is primarily cognitive or physical, expressed cognitively or behaviorally, and adaptation generally involves thinking and doing. Gender, culture, temperament, and a variety of other factors influence grieving styles. Caution is advised against assuming that mothers are more intuitive in style and fathers more instrumental. Both parents must be

assessed individually to determine where on the continuum their style rests. It is important, as well, to remember that these terms represent differences, not deficiencies, in grieving styles. Most parents in pediatric palliative care are young and likely inexperienced with illness, hospitals, technologies, dying, and death. Consequently, they typically have few skills for dealing with significant loss.

Environmental factors

Environmental factors include the role of the deceased child in the family and various aspects of the family itself.

Role in the family of the child who died

Ordinal position often defines children's roles in the family. When a child dies, shifts occur among the other children. For example, Jose was the eldest of three sons. When he died, his father told Marco, the middle son, that he was now the "oldest." The three boys had shared very close relationships, and now the surviving two felt that their father was "forgetting" Jose by no longer regarding him as the eldest son. Children also play particular social, spiritual, and physical roles in the family; the child's absence leaves their role unfilled, and resultant adjustments can be difficult for remaining family members. Jose had been the "leader"; Marco did not want to assume his brother's leadership role. Also, how the child defined the other members of the family affects their grieving. Again, Jose particularly liked to joke about his "little" brother, who was growing to be taller than Jose. Marco had enjoyed the teasing and did not want to displace his admired older brother. Tension grew between father and sons.

Family characteristics

Even before their child dies, families have characteristic ways of being in the world, of solving problems, of managing crises, of interacting with one another, and of relating to those outside the family. When a child is seriously ill and dies, families respond in the ways that are typical for how they manage other life events. These ways of coping are more or less functional. Earlier research with families of adult patients[21] and with pediatric patients[17,22] documented eight dimensions of family functioning: communicating openly, dealing with feelings, defining roles, solving problems, using resources, incorporating changes, considering others, and confronting beliefs. These dimensions occur along a continuum of functionality so that family interactions tend to vary along the continuum rather than being positive or negative, or good or bad.[17] In families where thoughts and opinions are expressed freely without fear of recrimination, where a wide range of feelings is expressed and differences tolerated, where roles are flexible, where problem solving instead of blaming is the pattern for dealing with challenges, where families are able to ask for and receive assistance from others, and where beliefs and values are confronted and examined, the children and all family members are better able to manage their grief and support one another. The nurse's role is to assess each family's way of functioning, and to realize that some families are more difficult to assess and work with than others. For example, some families may not wish to share information in the presence of their children, others do not wish to discuss matters with any relatives in the room, while other families include everyone in most discussions. Thus, it is important for the nurse to gather information over time, and to talk with more than one family member to appreciate the varied perspectives. When families are less functional, practitioners may want to offer potential resources one at a time, with considerable attention paid to the possible disruption that would result from each suggestion. In more functional families, a list of possible options can be presented and considered all at once. The vast majority of families value the opportunity to tell their story, and thus listening becomes a central aspect of caring for all grieving families.

Social/cultural characteristics

No one grieves in isolation from others. Individual responses are shaped by distinct social and cultural circumstances, and, in turn, each grieving person plays many roles in shaping family and community responses. Friends, extended family, and community support also influence how the family unit and individual family members function and come to terms with a child's death. A friend with a sensitive presence and listening ear can be of significant support to a grieving parent or sibling. Or, when grieving parents are challenged by the responsibilities of parenthood, a kind and supportive aunt or uncle can help to maintain a normal routine and a safe and understanding environment for the surviving siblings.

Individuals and families grieve within broader cultural contexts. Some turn to culture and tradition to find support and comfort in the answers, rituals, ceremonies, behavioral prescriptions, and spiritual practices they provide. Others do not strongly identify with the beliefs and mores of their cultures of origin, even when other members of their own family may do so. Too often culture is thought of in prescriptive ways, as if to say that we expect a member of a given community to express and process grief in the manner typical of that group. It is broadly recognized that cultural values, beliefs, and practices play a central role in shaping how families raise and care for their children not only when they are healthy, but especially when they are seriously ill. Researchers and clinicians are paying increasingly more attention to this essential dimension of palliative care.[23-25] It is important to find out what each individual family member believes about the nature of death, the rituals that should surround it, and the expectations about afterlife. As well, we must remember that our modern healthcare systems—hospitals in particular—have their own cultural mores, which may be in conflict with the cultural beliefs and practices of families in pediatric palliative care.

Watching a child fall sick and die is a crisis of meaning for families, and it is through their cultural understandings and practices that families struggle to explain and make sense of this experience.[26-28] In fact, although research is sparse on the topic, there are some universal themes across cultures. One is the use of ritual and ceremony, and the other is the struggle for meaning and the questions that come to all bereaved families, whether they are whispered or cried out loud: "Why did my child (my sister, my brother, my grandchild) have to die?" "Where is the child now?" and "Will I ever see her again?"[10,27,29] Spiritual or religious rituals may help families find meaning when their child dies. However, such rituals may interfere with the expression of grief if they prescribe, rather than foster creation of, meaning of the child's death for individual family members.

Situational factors

Situational factors refer to characteristics of the situation or the circumstances surrounding the child's death. These variables include, for example, characteristics of the child's illness, such as its duration, and of the death, such as the cause and place of death, and the extent of involvement in death-related events.

Characteristics of the child's illness and death

Where or when a child died, decision-making about the death, memories of sights and sounds, degree of medical intervention, and the cause of death are all subject matters that families discuss during bereavement while exploring their grief. Ideally, the location (home or hospital) of a child's death is based on the family's specific needs and requests, but circumstances (insurance issues, nursing shortages, transportation issues) may preclude achieving this goal. Long-term outcomes for bereaved parents and siblings of home-care deaths suggest an early pattern of differential adjustment in favor of home-care deaths.[30-33]

Decisions at the end of life, such as withdrawal of life support, may have been made with parents feeling they had insufficient understanding of the situation. Lasting images or smells may be comforting or concerning to families depending on their associations. In fact, pain or other distressing symptoms the child might have experienced provide powerful material for families to struggle with during their grief. A full code that ends with the child's death is very different than if a child slips into death from an unconscious state. Years of treatment followed by death is experienced very differently than a situation in which a child dies quickly.

Involvement in the illness and death-related events

Growing consensus supports informing children about their medical condition and involving them in discussions and decisions about their care, appropriate for their levels of cognitive and emotional maturity.[34,35] The same is true for involving siblings in the care of the ill child and in the events surrounding the death, such as the funeral, memorial service, and burial rituals. In one study, children who were more involved in such activities had fewer behavioral problems following the death.[17] At the same time, practitioners must consider not only the individual child's capacity for involvement, but also the family's values about discussions of death, medical care, and children's roles.

Models and theories of grief

From Freud to the current day, several theories and models have been developed that offer conceptual frameworks for how grief manifests in human beings. It is not the purpose of this chapter to provide an in-depth description of these various theories and models, since that content is covered elsewhere within this text. But, since nursing practice is guided by such theories and models, it is important to outline the development of thinking about bereavement as a basis for implementing best practices. Theories and models of grief can be categorized into stage and phase models, medical models, and task models.

Stage and phase models of grief

Models of grief based on stages and phases work on the premise that there is a beginning and an end to the grief process, with some amount of sequential progression through grief. Among stage or phase theorists are Lindemann,[36] Bowlby,[37] Engel,[38] Kubler-Ross,[39] Parkes,[40] and Rando.[41] Common patterns among these theories are the sequential, although overlapping, nature they suggest and the emphasis of the physical, emotional, behavioral, social, and intellectual impact of grief.

Medical models of grief

Some models of grief liken the process to that of healing secondary to disease, injury, or psychiatric illness. Lindemann,[36] Engel,[38] Parkes,[40] and Rando[41] are among those who discuss issues of symptoms, management, or need for clinical attention with complicated forms of grief. Beverly Raphael[42] urges that although pathological complications in grieving may be more readily equated with illness, the medical analogy is more difficult to sustain with uncomplicated grief. The overall process is articulated as a form of healing that might include issues such as helplessness, resistance to the reality of the death, preoccupation with the deceased, or identification with the deceased.

Stage, phase, and medical models have been subject to numerous criticisms in recent years. In particular, critics assert that the models do not capture the diversity of how we experience grief, either from an ethnocultural approach or from the perspective of the individual. Yet the phases may be clinically useful if used descriptively, rather than prescriptively, to help those who grieve—and their healthcare providers—anticipate, predict, and understand some of the nuances of their experience of loss. Recent support for the descriptive use of the stage or phase model is provided by Maciejewski and colleagues,[43] who used a revised stage model of grief to study widowed persons whose partner had died of natural causes. Their findings suggest that disbelief, yearning, anger, and depression overlap, yet peak at distinct time periods, all within the first 6 months after loss.

Critics of the stage, phase, and medical models assert that the three types of models erroneously suggest that we come to an end in our grieving as we complete uniform or predictable stages or at last recover or reach "acceptance."[44] Yet Bowlby describes his and Parkes's final phase of "reorganization"[45(p. 93)] as the bereaved person's redefinition of self and situation, an idea compatible with reconstructed meanings.[45] Bowlby also notes that widowed persons, as part of reorganizing and redefining, "retain a strong sense of the continuing presence of their partner,"[45(p. 96)] evidence that connections and bonds continue after death as part of uncomplicated adjustment to significant loss. In truth, the questions of what happens after death or what is the meaning of life and relationship are never-ending existential mysteries for all of us. Clinicians are cautioned to avoid using these models to support the idea that grief is a passive response to loss, when, in fact, grief is hard, dynamic work that leads to maintaining, rather than ending, connections with the one who died.

Bowlby[44] specifically addresses grief in children, noting that they mourn much like adults, yearning, becoming angry, and keeping memories of the person who died close at hand. Bowlby asserts that—far from forgetting or detaching—when children establish new relationships after someone close to them dies (e.g., a parent), they do better when their attachments to the person who died are talked about and honored.

Task models of grief

Lindemann[36] was the first to coin the phrase *grief work*, and he identified three tasks: relinquish attachment to the deceased, adjust to life without the deceased, and develop new relationships. Parkes and Weiss[46] and Worden[16] have also developed task models, with a central theme being the need to loosen ties to the deceased. Attig[47,48] describes the work of grieving as an active process of relearning the world, including physical surroundings, social surroundings, aspects of self, and the relationship with the deceased.

Attig's model of relearning the world may come the closest to describing how adults, as well as children and adolescents, relearn the world by summing the many smaller tasks that together make up the complex nature of living with grief. A bereaved parent may return to normal life functioning but is never finished loving or remembering his or her child. Even if the characteristics of that grief modulate over time, there may well be some form of heartache when that child is present in parental thoughts decades after the death. In the words of a bereaved mother, "I buried my child in my heart. I will always be with him anytime and everywhere." Attig asserts that we relearn the world as whole beings, not all at once, but rather piecemeal in distinct and growth-filled encounters. Such a description aptly applies to bereaved children—they cannot take in the whole event at once, and only over time, with their whole beings, do they relearn their worlds.

A central question is how parents and other family members manage the relationship with the child who died. Given that the child is no longer physically present, what do parents, grandparents, aunts, uncles, siblings, or friends do with the bonds, feelings, thoughts, and past experiences with that child? Research studies document that grievers do, indeed, maintain lasting connections with the deceased.[17,47,49,50] In fact, nurses can do much to facilitate these ongoing connections by offering to assist the family to obtain a memento of their child, such as a lock of hair, a foot or handprint, a photograph taken in the hospital, a piece of artwork, or a poem written by the child.

Impact of grief and bereavement on family members

Dying children

Children react to their own dying as they do to most of life's experiences—within their cognitive and emotional capabilities. They live and die as children, but often with much apparent wisdom, sometimes seeming to surpass that of their adult caregivers. One of the earliest studies of seriously ill children indicated that very ill children are, indeed, aware of death and are more anxious than children hospitalized for nonserious illnesses or nonhospitalized children.[51] Bluebond-Langner,[52] based on her ethnographic study of dying children, subsequently described a process of how they become aware of their own impending death (Box 60.1). The children may experience a wide range of feelings, including but not limited to anger, anxiety, sadness, loneliness and isolation, and fear. Behaviors may include avoiding deceased fellow friends' names or staying away from their belongings; reducing attention to non-disease-related chatter and play; being preoccupied with death and disease imagery, particularly in play; engaging in open

1. I am ill. For some children there is a clear beginning to their illness although there may be a gray period before their diagnosis. For others, with a progressive disease, the realization is likely to be more gradual but it is eventually reached.

2. I have an illness that can kill people. Some children reach this stage simply because they hear a word like "leukemia" and know perhaps rather vaguely that it is associated with death. Others are told by their parents, if for no other reason than to help explain why the treatment given is so awful. The understanding that comes at this stage is virtually academic and it is possible some children do not believe what they are told.

3. I have an illness that can kill children. When there are three boys with cystic fibrosis in a school one summer term and only two in the autumn, the remaining two have had the clearest possible lesson. We should always be on guard for the ripples that come to a hospital ward or the school class when a death occurs.

4. I am never going to get better. This may follow on quite quickly after stage 3, or it may take some time. It is almost always associated with depression. This does not imply children know their death is imminent.

5. I am going to die. Some authors suggest that all children from 3 years and up are capable of reaching this stage. One must be open to the possibility that even very young children may have a full understanding not only of death but also of their own death.

Source: Goldman A. *Care of the Dying Child.* Oxford, England/New York, NY: Oxford University Press; 1994. Reprinted with permission of Oxford University Press (UK).

talk about the death only with selected persons; feeling anxious about weakened body functions and doubts about going home; evading talk of the future; being concerned with things being done right away; regressing, such as refusing to cooperate with relatively easy, painless procedures; or having estranged relationships with others, demonstrated by anger or silence.

Of course, we need to recognize individual variations within the above patterns, but this work provides some background for understanding terminally ill children, such as this 14-year-old boy whose death is imminent:

> My mother used to go to church to pray for me early every morning. I also prayed in my bed for my mother to stop her soundless sorrow. We were all sad and we pray separately in different places. Now, I am getting more worried about how sad she will be after my death, and she will feel lonely without me. How can I express my sorrow for her and thank her? She has lost so many things…money, time, and smiles, all because of me.

Parents

Parent-child relationships are not contractual, but sacred. They are unique and complex. The connectedness between parent and child has its roots in the biological and emotional bonds and attachments that precede birth. It grows as the parent begins to know and care for the child. The child is a parent's link to the future.[29,53] Parental grief is all-consuming, affecting every aspect of parents' existence. Parental bereavement after a child's death involves a level of suffering for both parents. Cacciatore, Erlandsson, and Rådestad[54] note that fathers' emotions are often overlooked in deference to the mother's grief. Yet fathers experience suffering and express gratitude when nurses and others acknowledge their level of distress.

Parents often struggle with guilt following their child's death because of deep-rooted feelings of responsibility for their child's welfare. Because parents are responsible for protecting and sustaining their children, shielding them from all danger, many parents feel they should have protected their child from illness and death. When children die from an inherited disease such as cystic fibrosis or sickle cell anemia, parents know their child's condition results from their unknowingly passing on the genetic material. When the child dies, parents may still carry the burden of knowing they "gave" their child a terminal illness. Parents whose child died from an accident may also feel guilty for abdicating their protective role. Bereaved parents may cling to irrational guilt since it is often easier to accept blame, with its fantasy of control, than the total loss of control with which they must grapple. Or, they may blame someone else for their child's death. Sometimes this guilt is targeted toward a partner or spouse, another child, or family member. Nurses need to be aware of these dynamics and help a family find an appropriate place for their anger and blame.[55] A parent may also adopt a stance of protecting the other parent from their own grief, paradoxically resulting in increased grief for both.[56]

Parents, as individuals, may have different styles of grieving, as described earlier. Nurses can help by acknowledging the "normality" of a variety of grieving styles and encouraging parents to understand each other's ways of grieving. Differences in bereavement response also may lead to a strain on the couple's sexual intimacy. Sexual abstinence is frequently reported by bereaved couples due to a lack of sexual interest; others seek out comfort through sexual intimacy. Again, pointing out that such reactions can be expected may help couples realize the "normalcy" of their reactions. Research with couples who have experienced perinatal death conflict with the previous belief that a child's death did not increase the risk of couples separating. Odds of divorce are higher in couples after miscarriage or stillbirth,[57] and relationship dissolution increases in the same circumstances for married or cohabiting couples.[58] In a recent study, researchers highlighted unique interpersonal dynamics between partners. Stroebe et al.[56] found that bereaved parents who attempted to hold in their own grief in order to spare their partner increased their own and their partner's grief over time (at 6, 13, and 20 months post death). The researchers refer to this phenomenon as "partner-oriented self-regulation (POSR)."[56(p. 395)] Nurses who work with bereaved parents often hear one parent or the other make a comment such as, "I feel like I need to be strong for her" or "If he sees how I'm hurting, I don't think he can deal with it." The paradoxical nature of the findings from this study provide nurses with insight into couple dynamics, follow-up interventions, and potential support group topics.

Professional caregivers who support bereaved parents are attuned to parents' own descriptions of being different after their child died. Through educational programs, bedside care, follow-up, support group facilitation, and numerous books written by parents, nurses learn the profound impact a child's death has on a parent forever. Gilmer et al.[5] found that changes in bereaved parents occurred primarily in two realms: their personal lives (e.g., emotions, beliefs, work habits) and in relationships. Parents themselves reported changes in priorities; their children noted the intensity of their parents' sadness. Davies and Limbo[59] share the story of a mother who asked her college-age son, who was in grade school when his brother—and a year later, his sister—were stillborn, "Did I change?" Her son was flabbergasted that she was not aware of how different she was then and subsequently. He responded, "You were never happy, you stopped being a room mother or participating with any of our sports teams. You cried all the time."[59(p. 78)]

Nurses must also be cognizant of the special needs of bereaved parents who cope with additional stressors in their everyday lives. Single parents or same-sex parents may not have as many options for support as married parents in a heterosexual relationship.

Moreover, nurses must pay attention to the indirect grief of parents who witness or coexperience the death of other terminally ill children in the same clinical setting as their child.[60]

Grandparents

The grief of grandparents is twofold: they have to bear their own grief, as well as bear the agony of the grief of their own child, the parent of the deceased child, a phenomenon termed "double pain."[61] In addition, grandparents experience "cumulative pain."[61(p. 170)] Gilrane-McGarry and O'Grady identified three sources in addition to the double pain: pain from their own past losses, pain common to all grief, and witnessing negative changes in their child. Grandparents identified two factors highly relevant to nursing care that helped them with their grief: having their loss acknowledged and being considered a part of the bereaved family.[62] Grandparents can be a source of considerable strength for parents and siblings, or they can be an additional source of stress. Their advice may be sought but then ignored; often their practical help is accepted, but their own grief is barely acknowledged. Extended family is a part of the child's team. Healthcare providers may be both challenged and gratified as they work to integrate their presence and ideas into palliative care practice and family support.[63-65] Grandparents may experience considerable helplessness and frustration; they question the meaning of life as they struggle with the "lack of order" of having the young one precede them in death.

Siblings

Siblings have been called the "forgotten grievers." They have been typically ignored when a brother or sister dies, not for lack of parental concern, but because their parents are so overcome with grief, they have little energy to devote to the needs of their surviving children. The impact of a child's death on surviving siblings is manifested in four general responses, best characterized in the words of the children themselves[66]: "I hurt inside," "I don't understand," "I don't belong," and "I'm not enough." Not all children who have a brother or sister die experience all four responses, but most children through to adolescence demonstrate all responses to varying degrees.

"I hurt inside"

The first response includes all the emotions typically associated with grief—sadness, anger, frustration, loneliness, fear, guilt, restlessness, and a host of other emotions that characterize bereavement. Unlike adults who are able to talk about their responses, children manifest their responses in various behaviors, such as withdrawing, seeking attention, acting out, arguing, fear of going to bed at night, overeating, or undereating. In response to children who are hurting inside, nurses need to allow, and even encourage, the expression of the hurt the children are feeling. They may endeavor to share their own thoughts and feelings with the children to let them know that they are not alone in this situation. If adults do not allow children to express their feelings, siblings learn there is something wrong with such feelings. When adults are impatient with children, or belittle their expression, siblings learn to stifle their feelings.

"I don't understand"

Children's difficulty in understanding death is greatly influenced by their level of cognitive development. However, once children know about death, their cognitive worlds are forever altered. If they are not helped to understand what has happened in clear, simple, and age-appropriate ways, children make up their own explanations that usually involve taking responsibility for the death and their parents' distress. Without explanations, they become more frightened and insecure. Nurses must have a solid grasp of children's cognitive development, provide appropriate explanations for events that happen, and be open to questions from children.

"I don't belong"

A death in the family tears apart the usual day-to-day activities and patterns of living. Parents are overwhelmed with their grief, with making arrangements, and with caring for their other children. Surviving children are overwhelmed with the flurry of activity and the depth of emotion surrounding them. They often feel as if they don't know what to do; they may want to help, but they don't know how, or, if they try, their efforts are not acknowledged. They begin to feel as if they are in the way, or as if they are not a part of what is happening. They feel different from their peers as well, and begin to feel as if they don't belong anymore. Nurses can play a critical role in including siblings in illness and death-related events, such as encouraging or teaching the child to participate in certain treatments (for example, by holding their sibling's hand or blowing bubbles together during painful procedures). After death, the nurse can help the parents by modeling what to say to the children.

"I'm not enough"

Assuming that they are somehow responsible for their parents' distress, siblings may feel as if they are not enough to make their parents happy ever again. They may feel that their deceased brother or sister was the favorite child, and they should have been the ones to die instead. Some siblings respond by striving to be as good as they can be, trying to prove that they are worthy. They must be made to feel special just for being themselves, and by not comparing them to their deceased brother or sister. Moreover, siblings may not want to burden their parents with their grief, knowing their parents are already overladen. Nurses can assist siblings to feel special by asking them questions about their lives and reassuring them of their value and unique characteristics or abilities.

Adolescents

Teenagers who are dying, or who are the siblings or friends of another child, are often overlooked.[67] They face a particularly complicated situation when they encounter death and bereavement because adolescents are typically engrossed in achieving independence and in proving their invulnerability. Serious illness and grief catches them by surprise, as they seldom have developed the coping skills necessary to deal with their reactions. As well, many adults believe it is difficult to help adolescents cope with death because adolescents are reputed to turn away from adults and to talk only with other adolescents. This is not entirely true, as these young people often seek out and value the input and support of adults they respect, such as a teacher, a nurse, or a friend's parent. Moreover, when adolescents turn to their peers, if they do, they may often find that their peers have no significant resources to offer because they too are inexperienced with death.

Dying adolescents with a terminal disease struggle against physical pain, are sensitive to their parents' reactions, and have a strong desire to have relationships with their friends regardless of their illness status: "I couldn't say anything with my Mom. She pretends to smile to me, but I know how she feels so sad whenever looking at me. I want to come out and share my emotions with my friend at least. But, now there is nobody around me." In such cases, nurses are in a position to help an adolescent's family members to understand adolescent cognitive and psychosocial functioning. Self-help support groups for teens, either in person or via the Internet, often prove valuable to grieving adolescents. Adolescents are often open to writing, art, or music. Adults may come along on such journeys, or share the results, but they should take care to follow the adolescents' lead, respecting confidentiality and permitting them to interpret the significance of their work in their own way.

Assessing grief

Bereavement care is interdisciplinary in nature, focusing on assessment of the comprehensive pattern and character of the whole family, as well as of individuals within the family. Grief assessment focuses on the ill child, other family members, and their significant others. Grief assessment begins when the child is admitted to the hospital or at the time of diagnosis of acute, chronic, or terminal illness. It is ongoing throughout the course of the child's illness and comes to the forefront during the bereavement period after the death. As illustrated in Figure 60.1, an integrative model of bereavement care, as opposed to a series or parallel model, highlights the central role of bereavement support for a family from the moment they suspect their child is ill. Milstein[68] emphasizes the compatibility of goals for curing and palliation that include caregiver mindsets of relationship (being with) and intervention (doing to). Nurses, in particular, play a central role in a family's initial bereavement experience, holding in mind the family's sense of loss, while pursuing with other team members care that best addresses the child's well-being. Most children's deaths still occur in the hospital; nurses are most often present at the time of death. If not with the child at the moment of death, the nurse is usually the first one called to the child's bedside. The nurse's words and actions at that time leave indelible imprints on parents. Even years after their child's death, parents

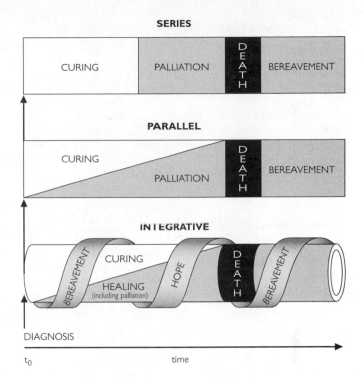

Figure 60.1 Integrative model of curing and healing (with bereavement and hope). Copyright 2010, Jay Milstein. Modified by Rana Limbo and Kathie Kobler. Used with permission.

recall vivid memories of the nurse's gentle approach in offering privacy, giving a hug, sharing the sadness, allowing families the amount of time they want with their child before leaving the hospital. Unfortunately, other parents remember the nurse who spoke abruptly to them, or rushed them away because their child's room had to be made ready for the next patient. In even these brief interactions, nurses can do so much to prevent this devastating experience from being any worse than it already is for the family.

In assessing grief, clinicians should keep in mind the range of factors that impact on the grief of family members, while noting those factors that put individuals and families at risk for disenfranchised or complicated grief. The passage of time is not a useful consideration in assessing grief responses; instead, we must assess the degree of intrusiveness into each individual's life and the extent to which family members can carry out their usual activities.

Helping bereaved families

Grief assessment leads to a plan of care with the goal of facilitating and supporting the grieving process. Understanding grief as a normal, human process that is individually expressed enables practitioners to present an accepting, nonjudgmental attitude that helps create a respectful and trusting milieu. The approach to children or other family members experiencing anticipatory grief is the same as for family members whose child has died, but the focus of some interventions may differ. For example, prior to death, families should be offered information about the signs and symptoms of disease progression and the dying process; following death, the focus may be on listening to family members review the course of the child's dying.

Grief interventions

For families

Bereaved individuals need an opportunity to express their grief in a supportive environment. Nurses have a responsibility to create such an environment for parents and other family members following a child's death so that they feel it is okay for them to express whatever they are feeling. Such comments as "It must be very difficult for you right now" give permission for expression. The form of expression may vary among family members; some will verbalize, others will cry, some may leave the room. Still others may express anger, and others appreciation.

Nurses may fear "saying the wrong thing" to a family member, or may fear not knowing what to say, or feel they must have the "right thing to say." Attitudes are conveyed through words and more importantly, through actions. Thus, it is usually best to say very little, avoiding clichés and euphemisms that can be so distressing to grieving individuals. It is not appropriate to encourage anyone to "Keep a stiff upper lip" or to "Look on the bright side." It is disrespectful, and even cruel, to say "He is no longer suffering" or "You are young; you will have more children." These messages, whether given directly or indirectly, may compound the pain by making family members think the clinicians do not understand their loss. Instead, sit or stand quietly close to the family, let them know they can stay with their child for as long as they would like, comment on the child's special qualities and acknowledge your own sadness about the child's death. Offering to help in practical and concrete ways is also helpful. However, rather than asking if "there is anything I can help you with," offer to do specific things, such as making phone calls or getting them a glass of water. Most family members have a need to share their story, telling and retelling anecdotes about the child and the events of his living and dying. Listening to their stories is probably the most helpful action. For some families, reviewing what happened with their child with the care providers is critical. Follow-up phone calls or visits with the providers who cared for the child are much appreciated by families.

Many family members who are unaware of the normal manifestations of grief can find some comfort in knowing that their pain is normal. Providing information about the common facts of grief can be helpful; having written materials to send home with families is even better. Understanding that each person's grief experience is unique helps family members understand that there is "no right way to grieve." It also helps them to realize they are not "bad" or "crazy" if they express their grief differently from other family members; it also may prevent family member from telling other family members how they "should" grieve. Clinicians should identify any need for additional assistance and make referrals as needed. For example, a family member may have spiritual concerns that would be best addressed by the pastoral care person; a social worker may assist with funeral arrangements or financial concerns. In addition, the nurse should make referrals to bereavement specialists, psychologists, or physicians as needed.

For children

Since grief is a human response, children and adults alike feel denial, anger, sadness, guilt, and longing in response to the death of a loved one, and experience lack of sleep, lack of appetite, and difficulty concentrating and maintaining usual patterns of interaction with others. However, most children have limited ability to verbalize and describe their feelings; they also have very limited capacity to tolerate the emotional pain generated by open recognition of their loss.[69] Moreover, children's cognitive developmental level interferes with their ability to understand the irreversibility, universality, and inevitability of death, and to understand the reactions of their parents. They also deeply fear being different in any way from their peers, and so are often unable to find comfort, as adults do, in sharing their discomfort with their friends. As play is the work and the language of childhood, children are able to express their feelings through their play, as well as music and art. A summary of grief reactions in children, according to age level, and corresponding suggested interventions, is presented in Table 60.1.

For parents

Before the child's death, an important emphasis for clinicians is to facilitate connections between the parents and the ill child and their other children, as well as by helping them develop memories and keepsakes that they can hold and cherish long after the death. The earlier these can be collected, the better, so they reflect a longer period of time with the child and not simply the final days of life. Facilitating communication between family members and the caregiving staff, as well as among family members themselves, also creates positive memories and optimal coping. Informing parents about the dying process, and helping them with the concept of appropriate death consistent with patient, family, cultural, and spiritual goals is necessary. Assisting with planning funeral or memorial services also can be helpful, particularly for families who have limited support systems.

After the child's death, follow-up by the clinicians who cared for the child is much appreciated by families. Such follow-up also allows ongoing assessment (see Box 60.2 for questions to ask during an initial follow-up telephone call). Parents, overcome with their own grief, may need assistance in dealing with the needs of their other children; encourage parents to enlist the support of aunts, uncles, or good friends in this regard. For parents who are willing and interested in finding additional support, provide a listing of parental support groups and other parent bereavement resources in the community, such as Compassionate Friends, a self-help organization to help parents and siblings after the death of a child (www.compassionatefriends.org).

Bereavement programs

The development of pediatric palliative care programs, including bereavement programs, in healthcare institutions has increased notably in the past decade despite budget and other resource concerns. Still, the dearth of consistency and excellence in both the training of professionals and the offering of services to families results in many gaps in the experiences of families. Such gaps must be addressed, especially for families of children who had a chronic illness that meant frequent trips to the hospital, sometimes over many years, and resulted in the development of close relationships with staff members. Such families worry that the staff will forget their deceased child; some families want to maintain an ongoing relationship with those who cared for their child. Thus, during the transition after the child's death, families and staff have to navigate the changing relationship.[3,70] A bereavement program within

Table 60.1 Grief and bereavement in children

Characteristics of age	View of death and response	What helps
Birth to 6 months		
Basic needs must be met, cries if needs aren't met	Has no concept of death	Progressively disengage child from primary caregiver if possible.
	Experiences death like any other separation—no sense of "finality"	
Needs emotional and physical closeness of a consistent caregiver		Introduce a new primary caregiver.
	Nonspecific expressions of distress (crying)	Nurture, comfort.
		Anticipate physical and emotional needs and provide them.
Derives identity from caregiver	Reacts to loss of caregiver	
View of caregiver as source of comfort and all needs fulfillment.	Reacts to caregiver's distress	Maintain routines.
Developing trust		
6 months to 2 years		
Begins to individuate	May see death as reversible	Child needs continual support, comfort.
Remembers face of caregiver when absent Demonstrates full range of emotions	Experiences bona fide grief	Avoid separation from significant others.
	Grief response only to death of significant person in child's life.	Close physical and emotional connections by significant others
Identifies caregiver as source of good feelings and interactions	Screams, panics, withdraws, becomes disinterested in food, toys, activities	Maintain daily structure and schedule of routine activities.
	Reacts in concert with distress experienced by caregiver	Support caregiver to reduce distress and maintain a stable environment.
	No control over feelings and responses; anticipate regressive behavior	Acknowledge sadness that loved one will not return—offer comfort.
2 years to 5 years		
Egocentric	Sees death like sleep: reversible	Remind child that loved one will not return.
Cause-effect not understood	Believes in magical causes	Reassure child that he/she is not to blame.
Developing conscience	Has sense of loss	Give realistic information, answer questions.
Attributes life to objects	Curiosity, questioning	Involve child in "farewell" ceremonies.
Feelings expressed mostly by behaviors	Anticipate regression, clinging	Encourage questions and expression of feelings.
	Aggressive behavior common	Keep home environment stable, structured.
Can recall events from past	Worries about who will care for them	Help put words to feelings; reassure/comfort.
		Reassure children about who will take care of them; provide ways to remember their loved one.
5 years to 9 years		
Attributes life to things that move; may fear the dark	Personifies death as ghosts, "boogeyman"	Give clear and realistic information. Include children in funeral ceremonies if they choose.
Begins to develop intellect	Interest in biological aspects of life and death	Give permission to express feelings and provide opportunities; reduce guilt by providing factual information. Maintain structured schedule, individual and family activities; child needs a strong parent.
Begins to relate cause and effect; understands consequences		
	Begins to see death as irreversible	
Literal, concrete	May see death as punishment; may feel responsible	

(continued)

Table 60.1 Continued

Characteristics of age	View of death and response	What helps
Decreasing fantasy life, increasing control of feelings		
	Problems concentrating on tasks; may deny or hide feelings, vulnerability	Notify school of what is occurring, provide gentle confirmation, reassurance.
Preadolescent through teens		
Individuation outside home	Views death as permanent	Provide unambiguous information.
Identifies with peer group; needs family attachment	Sense of own mortality; sense of future	Provide opportunities to express self, feelings; encourage outside relationships with mentors.
	Strong emotional reaction; may regress, revert to fantasy	
Understands life processes; can verbalize feelings		
	May somaticize, intellectualize, morbid preoccupation	Provide tangible means to remember loved one; encourage self-expression, verbal and nonverbal.
Physical maturation		
		Dispel fears about physical concerns; educate about maturation; provide outlets for energy and strong feelings (recreation, sports, etc.); needs mentoring and direction.

Source: Fine P, ed. *Processes to Optimize Care During the Last Phase of Life.* Scottsdale, AZ: Vista Care Hospice; 1998. Reprinted with permission.

pediatric palliative care, or as part of an agency-wide program, can be of considerable service to both families and staff. These services typically include staff with specific training in bereavement care and a follow-up component.[71] A bereavement program facilitates referral of families to grief therapists as needed; ensures that all families are made aware of the available services, such as support groups, memorial services, or grief workshops; and may facilitate bereaved families connecting with one another as a source of support. The existence of a bereavement program gives a clear message that an institution and its staff are committed to the care of families. Perinatal palliative care guidelines are provided by Limbo, Toce, and Peck.[72]

The nurse: suffering, cumulative loss, and grief

Professionals who help children and families with the serious illness and death of a child are witness to numerous heart-wrenching scenes, and are constantly reminded of the frailty and preciousness of life. Working with dying children can trigger nurses' awareness of their own personal losses and fears about their own death, the death of their own children, and mortality in general. Historically, nurses and other healthcare professionals were taught to desensitize themselves to these experiences and to maintain an "emotional detachment." This approach, which still exists today in many situations, results in the nurses' use of defenses to allay their fears, including focusing only on physical-care needs, evading emotionally sensitive conversations with children and families, and talking only superficially about topics that are comfortable for the nurse. These behaviors result in emotional distancing, avoidance, and withdrawal from dying children and their families at a time when children most need intensive interpersonal care and active

involvement by the nurse. Death anxiety occurs when clinicians are confronted with fears about death and have few resources or support systems to explore and to express thoughts and emotions about dying and death.[70,73] Thus, rather than a "desensitization" of oneself, professionals are encouraged to sensitize to this powerful human material. Caring for dying children requires nurses to explore, experience, and express their personal feelings regarding death. Personal death-awareness activities and exercises, discussion of belief systems about death/afterlife with friends and colleagues, self-exploration, and reflection may promote an understanding and acceptance of death as part of life. The process is complicated by cumulative loss, a succession of losses experienced by nurses who work with patients with life-threatening illness and their families, often on a daily basis.[70,74] When nurses are exposed to death frequently, they seldom have time to grieve one child before another child dies.

Papadatou[70] described a framework for how professionals manage grief that entails fluctuating between experiencing and avoiding intense emotions. An expert in the care of dying children, she notes that professional caregivers are profoundly affected by what is required of them in working with bereaved parents, other family members, and children. To manage the experience, a caregiver may cry at a child's bedside and be fully present to a father who has just watched the removal of his child's ventilator. Later that day, the same caregiver may avoid the intensity of the emotions garnered from the child's death to engage in a dinner out with her family. Understanding the normalcy of the grief responses provides caregivers with an awareness of how they can simultaneously support families and themselves. Papadatou proposes that meanings are attributed to death and dying through grieving, that grief complications occur when there is no fluctuation, and grief provides opportunities for personal growth.

Box 60.2 Questions for an initial follow-up telephone call to parents who have experienced the loss of a perinatal child

- "You might recall that you were told that someone from the hospital would call you in (number) weeks."

- "Is this a good time to talk?"

- "Are there any issues that you have been thinking about that perhaps I could follow-up on for you?"

- "Have you been back yet for a postpartum check-up?"

- "Some parents have noticed a change in their sleeping or eating habits. Has this been a problem for you?"

- "How has (name of other parent) responded to your loss? Sometimes it is hard for both parents to talk about it. How has it been for you?"

- "Do you have other family members or friends that you have been able to talk to? What types of things have they been able to do for you?"

- "Do you have plans to work outside of your home? The first few days at work can be especially difficult. Have you thought about how it might be for you?"

- "Did you receive any information on support groups for parents?"

- "Are there any other materials you received in the hospital that you have questions about?"

- "Are there any other questions I can answer for you?"

- "During the call you stated that . . . ."

- "I will call you again on (date)."

Source: Friedrichs J, Daly MI, Kavanaugh K. Follow-up of parents who experience a perinatal loss: facilitating grief and assessing for grief complicated by depression. *Illness Crisis Loss.* 2000;8(3):302. Reprinted with permission.

Box 60.3 The challenges of education for healthcare professionals

Challenge 1: Develop a philosophy of teaching that promotes relational learning and reflective practice.

Challenge 2: Develop curricula that include goals, learning objectives, and methods of teaching that focus on relationships with the dying, the bereaved, and coworkers.

Challenge 3: Integrate current knowledge into educational programs and supervised clinical applications.

Challenge 4: Evaluate training outcomes as well as the context and process by which learning occurs.

Challenge 5: Integrate formal and informal learning activities into the work context.

Source: Papadatou D. *In the Face of Death.* New York: Springer; 2009. Used with permission.

painful treatments they perceived as unnecessary. Grief distress occurred in response to the child's death. Both types of distress resulted from lack of open communication within the care team and lack of consideration of the nurses' viewpoints. Thus, systems of support are critical to nurses' coping with the stress of working with seriously ill children and their families.

In addition to helping bereaved families, as mentioned earlier, institutional bereavement programs also serve the needs of staff. Programs can be structured to offer help in debriefing after a death, validating staff feelings, offering support groups, and encouraging informal support through the one-one-one sharing of experiences with coworkers, peers, or pastoral care workers.[82,83] In addition, nurses can serve vital roles in cocreating ritual for both families and professional caregivers. According to Limbo and Kobler,[29] ritual creates a bridge from suffering to hope and provides all involved an awareness of the importance of "moments" in the care of bereaved families and staff. The presence of a supervisor, mentor, or instructor during the care of the dying, when a family member visits, or during the time of the child's death can greatly decrease anxiety and provide immense support to the nurse, particularly to novice nurses in pediatric palliative care.

Education that enhances knowledge and skills in end-of-life care can promote competence and self-confidence and is associated with hopeful thinking.[84] Education helps make the experience both meaningful and bearable for families.[85] Education that describes families' experiences can be invaluable because it empowers clinicians to offer care that is more sensitive to the needs of families, more humanistic, and more family centered and, thus, more rewarding to staff. Nurses have responsibilities for acknowledging their own personal and professional limitations, seeking assistance, and engaging in self-care activities. Reflection is a key process for pediatric palliative care nurses in being with the child and family before, during, and after death.[29,70,76] Education specific to grief and bereavement in palliative care can be personally and professionally transformational when designed as relationship based; inclusive of the caregiver's beliefs, values, and feelings and parents' stories; and focused on the caregiver as guide.[70,86–89] Davies et al.[90] identify the need for more education to foster

Self-awareness about one's own personal history of loss is necessary to know one's own set of beliefs about death, dying, and the afterlife. Without this awareness, our own beliefs and cultural/spiritual biases can interfere with the experience of the family. For caregivers, strong coping techniques, good self-care and ongoing education and support are necessary components not only to do the work but also to avoid burnout.

Several factors influence nurses' adaptation to the inherent grief in pediatric palliative care. They include the nurses' professional training and other training in dealing with dying, death, and grief; nurses' personal and professional history of loss and possible unresolved issues of dealing with grief; personal and professional life changes; and the presence or absence of support systems.

"Caregiver suffering" is a contemporary term that includes moral distress and grief[75,76] and encompasses bearing witness to others' suffering.[75,77,78] Suffering is part of the human condition and provides opportunities for growth and transformation for both nurses and families.[79,80] In one study[81] of nurses' experiences following the death of a child, participants described two types of distress. Moral distress resulted when the nurses knew the child's death was imminent and were required to carry out

communication skills and increase overall comfort level of nurses and physicians who work in pediatric palliative care. Papadatou[70] identifies challenges of educating healthcare professionals, a list that can be used for evaluating the content and process of effective grief and bereavement educational programs (Box 60.3).

Pediatric palliative care is a challenging field, one that demands finding the balance between providing compassionate quality care and personal satisfaction as a professional nurse. In addition, working with dying children and their families provides meaning to life. Working with these children helps to develop a clear perspective of what is really valuable; it helps us grow as persons and professionals. From the children and their families, we learn that death is part of life, that human beings are remarkably resilient, and that hope is everlasting.

References

1. Field MJ, Behrman RE, Institute of Medicine (US). Committee on Palliative and End-of-Life Care for Children and Their Families. When Children Die: Improving Palliative and End-of-Life Care for Children and their Families. Washington, DC: National Academies Press; 2003.
2. Murphy SL, Xu J, Kochanek KD. Deaths: final data for 2010. Nat Vit Stat Rep. 2013;61(4):73.
3. Meert KL, Briller SH, Schim SM, Thurston C, Kabel A. Examining the needs of bereaved parents in the pediatric intensive care unit: a qualitative study. Death Stud. 2009;33(8):712–740.
4. Hexem KR, Miller VA, Carroll KW, Faerber JA, Feudtner C. Putting on a happy face: emotional expression in parents of children with serious illness. J Pain Symptom Manage. 2013;45(3):542–551.
5. Gilmer MJ, Foster TL, Vannatta K, et al. Changes in parents after the death of a child from cancer. J Pain Symptom Manage. 2012;44(4):572–582.
6. Zisook S, Shear K. Grief and bereavement: what psychiatrists need to know. World Psychiatry. 2009;8(2):67–74.
7. Online Etymology Dictionary. Dictionary.com. http://dictionary.reference.com/browse/bereave. Accessed September 17, 2013.
8. Davies B, Limbo R, Jin J. Grief and bereavement in pediatric palliative care. In: Ferrell B, Coyle N (eds.), Oxford Textbook of Palliative Nursing. 3rd ed. New York: Oxford University Press; 2010:1082.
9. Corless IB. Bereavement. In: Ferrell B, Coyle N (eds.), Oxford Textbook of Palliative Nursing. New York: Oxford University Press; 2010:597–612.
10. Brown E, Dominica F. Around the time of death: culture, religion, and ritual. In: Goldman A, Hain R, Liben S (eds.), Oxford Textbook of Palliative Care for Children. Oxford: Oxford University Press; 2012:142–154.
11. Rando TA. Clinical Dimensions of Anticipatory Mourning: Theory and Practice in Working with the Dying, Their Loved Ones, and Their Caregivers. Champaign, IL: Research Press; 2000.
12. Rando TA. Grief, Dying, and Death: Clinical Interventions for Caregivers. Champaign, IL: Research Press; 1984.
13. Doka KJ. Disenfranchised Grief: Recognizing Hidden Sorrow. Lexington, MA: Lexington Books; 1989.
14. Doka KJ. Disenfranchised Grief: New Directions, Challenges, and Strategies for Practice. Champaign, IL: Research Press; 2002.
15. Lobb EA, Kristjanson LJ, Aoun SM, Monterosso L, Halkett GKB, Davies A. Predictors of complicated grief: a systematic review of empirical studies. Death Stud. 2010;34(8):673–698.
16. Worden JW. Grief Counseling and Grief Therapy: A Handbook for the Mental Health Practitioner. New York, London: Springer; 2008.
17. Davies B. Shadows in the Sun: The Experiences of Sibling Bereavement in Childhood. Philadelphia, PA: Brunner/Mazel; 1999.
18. Corr CA. Children's emerging awareness of death. In: Doka KJ, Tucci AS, Hospice Foundation of America (eds.), Living with Grief: Children and Adolescents. Washington, DC: Hospice Foundation of America; 2008:5–17.
19. Hunter SB, Smith DE. Predictors of children's understandings of death: age, cognitive ability, death experience and maternal communicative competence. Omega (Westport). 2008;57(2):143–162.
20. Didion J. The Year of Magical Thinking. New York: Knopf; 2005.
21. Davies B. Fading Away: The Experience of Transition in Families with Terminal Illness. Amityville, NY: Baywood; 1995.
22. Davies B, Spinetta J, Martinson I, McClowry S, Kulenkamp E. Manifestations of levels of functioning and grieving families. J Fam Issues. 1987;7(3):297–313.
23. Davies B, Larson J, Contro N, et al. Conducting a qualitative culture study of pediatric palliative care. Qual Healthc Res. 2009;19(1):5–16.
24. Davies B, Larson J, Contro N, Cabrera AP. Perceptions of discrimination among Mexican American families of seriously ill children. J Palliat Med. 2011;14(1):71–76.
25. Contro N, Davies B, Larson J, Sourkes B. Away from home: experiences of Mexican American families in pediatric palliative care. J Soc Work End Life Palliat Care. 2010;6(3–4):185–204.
26. Kenner C, Boykova M. Palliative care in the neonatal intensive care unit. In: Ferrell B, Coyle N (eds.), Oxford Textbook of Palliative Nursing. 3rd ed. New York: Oxford University Press; 2010:1065–1080.
27. Currier JM, Holland JM, Neimeyer RA. Sense-making, grief, and the experience of violent loss: toward a mediational model. Death Stud. 2006;30(5):403–428.
28. Boss R, Kavanaugh K, Kobler K. Prenatal and neonatal palliative care. In: Wolfe J, Hinds PS, Sourkes BM (eds.), Textbook of Interdisciplinary Pediatric Palliative Care. Philadelphia, PA: Elsevier/Saunders; 2011:387–401.
29. Limbo R, Kobler K. Meaningful Moments: Ritual and Reflection When a Child Dies. La Crosse, WI: Gundersen Medical Foundation; 2013.
30. Lauer ME, Mulhern RK, Bohne JB, Camitta BM. Children's perceptions of their sibling's death at home or hospital: the precursors of differential adjustment. Cancer Nurs. 1985;8(1):21–27.
31. Mulhern RK, Lauer ME, Hoffmann RG. Death of a child at home or in the hospital: subsequent psychological adjustment of the family. Pediatrics. 1983;71(5):743–747.
32. Vickers J, Chrastek J. Place of care. In: Goldman A, Hain R, Liben S (eds.), Oxford Textbook of Palliative Care for Children. Oxford: Oxford University Press; 2012:391–401.
33. Dussel V, Kreicbergs U, Hilden JM, et al. Looking beyond where children die: determinants and effects of planning a child's location of death. J Pain Symptom Manage. 2009;37(1):33–43.
34. Hinds PS, Oakes LL, Furman WL. End-of-life decision-making in pediatric oncology. In: Ferrell B, Coyle N (eds.), Oxford Textbook of Palliative Nursing. New York: Oxford University Press; 2010:1049–1064.
35. Royal Australasian College of Physicians. Decision-making at the end of life in infants, children and adolescents: a policy of the Paediatrics and Child Health Division of The Royal Australasian College of Physicians. Sydney, New South Wales, Australia: Royal Australasian College of Physicians; 2008.
36. Graham RJ, Levetown M, Comeau M. Decision making. In: Carter BS, Levetown M, Friebert SE (eds.), Palliative Care for Infants, Children, and Adolescents: A Practical Handbook. 2nd ed. Baltimore: The Johns Hopkins University Press; 2011:139–168.
37. Lindemann E. Symptomatology and management of acute grief. 1944. Am J Psychiatry. 1994;151(6 Suppl):155–160.
38. Bowlby J. Attachment and Loss. New York: Basic Books; 1969.
39. Engel GL. Grief and grieving. Am J Nurs. 1964;64:93–98.
40. Kubler-Ross E. On Death and Dying. New York: Macmillan; 1969.
41. Parkes CM. Bereavement: Studies of Grief in Adult Life. Philadelphia, PA: Routledge; 2001.
42. Rando TA. Parental Loss of a Child. Champaign, IL: Research Press; 1986.
43. Raphael B. The Anatomy of Bereavement. New York: Basic Books; 1983.
44. Maciejewski PK, Zhang B, Block SD, Prigerson HG. An empirical examination of the stage theory of grief. JAMA. 2007;297(7):716–723.

45. Bowlby J. Loss: Sadness and Depression. New York: Basic Books; 1980.
46. Neimeyer R, Burke L, Mackay M, van Dyke Stringer JG. Grief therapy and the reconstruction of meaning: from principles to practice. J Contemp Psychother. 2010;40(2):73–83.
47. Parkes CM, Weiss RS. Recovery from Bereavement. New York: Basic Books; 1983.
48. Attig T. How We Grieve: Relearning the World. New York: Oxford University Press; 1996.
49. Attig T. The Heart of Grief: Death and the Search for Lasting Love. New York: Oxford University Press; 2000.
50. Packman W, Horsley H, Davies B, Kramer R. Sibling bereavement and continuing bonds. Death Stud. 2006;30(9):817–841.
51. Klass D, Silverman PR, Nickman SL. Continuing Bonds: New Understandings of Grief. Washington, DC: Taylor & Francis; 1996.
52. Waechter EH. Children's awareness of fatal illness. Am J Nurs. 1971;7(6):1168–1172.
53. Bluebond-Langner M. How terminally ill children come to know themselves and their world. In: Princeton, NJ: Princeton University Press; 1978:166–197.
54. Arnold JH, Gemma PB. A Child Dies: A Portrait of Family Grief. 2nd ed. Philadelphia, PA: Charles Press; 1994.
55. Cacciatore J, Erlandsson K, Rådestad I. Fatherhood and suffering: a qualitative exploration of Swedish men's experiences of care after the death of a baby. Int J Nurs Stud. 2013;50(5):664–670.
56. Worden JW, Monahan JR. Caring for bereaved parents. In: Armstrong-Daily A, Zarbock S (eds.), Hospice Care for Children. 3rd ed. New York: Oxford University Press; 2009:181–200.
57. Stroebe M, Finkenauer C, Wijngaards-de Meij L, Schut H, van den Bout J, Stroebe W. Partner-oriented self-regulation among bereaved parents: the costs of holding in grief for the partner's sake. Psychol Sci. 2013;24(4):395–402.
58. Shreffler K, Hill T, Cacciatore J. The impact of infertility, miscarriage, stillbirth, and child death on marital dissolution. J Divorce Remarriage. 2012;53(2):91–107.
59. Gold KJ, Sen A, Hayward RA. Marriage and cohabitation outcomes after pregnancy loss. Pediatrics. 2010;125:1202–1207.
60. Davies B, Limbo R. The grief of siblings. In: Webb NB (ed.), Helping Bereaved Children: A Handbook for Practitioners. 3rd ed. New York: Guilford Press; 2010:69–91.
61. James L, Johnson B. The needs of parents of pediatric oncology patients during the palliative care phase. J Pediatr Oncol Nurs. 1997;14(2):83–95.
62. Gilrane-McGarry U, O Grady T. Forgotten grievers: an exploration of the grief experiences of bereaved grandparents. Int J Palliat Nurs. 2011;17(4):170–176.
63. Gilrane-McGarry U, O Grady T. Forgotten grievers: an exploration of the grief experiences of bereaved grandparents (part 2). Int J Palliat Nurs. 2012;18(4):179–187.
64. Davies B, Orloff S. Bereavement issues and staff support. In: Hanks G, Cherny NI, Christakis NA, Fallon M, Kaasa S, Portenoy RK (eds.), Oxford Textbook of Palliative Medicine. 4th ed. Oxford; New York: Oxford University Press; 2009:1361–1372.
65. Roose RE, Blanford CR. Perinatal grief and support spans the generations: parents' and grandparents' evaluations of an intergenerational perinatal bereavement program. J Perinat Neonatal Nurs. 2011;25(1):77–85.
66. Friebert S, Chrastek J, Brown MR. Team relationships. In: Wolfe J, Hinds PS, Sourkes BM (eds.), Textbook of Interdisciplinary Pediatric Palliative Care. Philadelphia, PA: Elsevier/Saunders; 2011:148–158.
67. Marshall B, Davies B. Bereavement in children and adults following the death of a sibling. In: Neimeyer RA (ed.), Grief and Bereavement in Contemporary Society: Bridging Research and Practice. New York: Routledge; 2011:107–116.
68. Balk DE. Sibling bereavement during adolescence. In: Balk DE, Corr CA (eds.), Adolescent Encounters with Death, Bereavement, and Coping. New York: Springer; 2009:199–216.
69. Milstein J. A paradigm of integrative care: healing with curing throughout life, "being with" and "doing to." J Perinatol. 2005;25(9):563–568.
70. Webb NB. Helping Bereaved Children: A Handbook for Practitioners. 3rd ed. New York: Guilford Press; 2010:408.
71. Papadatou D. In the Face of Death: Professionals Who Care for the Dying and the Bereaved. New York: Springer; 2009:330.
72. Kobler K, Limbo R. Making a case: creating a perinatal palliative care service using a perinatal bereavement program model. J Perinat Neonatal Nurs. 2011;25(1):32–41.
73. Limbo R, Toce S, Peck T. Resolve Through Sharing (RTS) Position Paper on Perinatal Palliative Care. http://www.gundluth.org/upload/docs/Bereavement/247_42805_ RTS%20Perinatal%20Palliative%20 Care.pdf. Accessed October 28, 2013.
74. Davies B, Clarke D, Connaughty S, et al. Caring for dying children: nurses' experiences. Pediatr Nurs. 1996;22(6):500–507.
75. Vachon MLS, Huggard J. The experience of the nurse in end-of-life care in the 21st century: mentoring the next generation. In: Ferrell B, Coyle N (eds.), Oxford Textbook of Palliative Nursing. New York: Oxford University Press; 2010:1131–1156.
76. Ferrell BR, Coyle N. The nature of suffering and the goals of nursing. Oncol Nurs Forum. 2008;35(2):241–247.
77. Rushton CH, Kaszniak AW, Halifax JS. A framework for understanding moral distress among palliative care clinicians. J Palliat Med. 2013;16(9):1074–1079.
78. Bateman ST, Dixon R, Trozzi M. The wrap-up: a unique forum to support pediatric residents when faced with the death of a child. J Palliat Med. 2012;15(12):1329–1334.
79. Lee KJ, Dupree CY. Staff experiences with end-of-life care in the pediatric intensive care unit. J Palliat Med. 2008;11(7):986–990.
80. Taubman-Ben-Ari O, Weintroub A. Meaning in life and personal growth among pediatric physicians and nurses. Death Stud. 2008;32(7):621–645.
81. Hogan NS. Sibling loss: issues for children and adolescents. In: Doka KJ, Tucci AS, Hospice Foundation of America (eds.), Living with Grief: Children and Adolescents. Washington, DC: Hospice Foundation of America; 2008:159–174.
82. Davies B, Clarke D, Connaughty S, et al. Caring for dying children: nurses' experiences. Pediatr Nurs. 1996;22(6):500–507.
83. Keene EA, Hutton N, Hall B, Rushton C. Bereavement debriefing sessions: an intervention to support health care professionals in managing their grief after the death of a patient. Pediatr Nurs. 2010;36(4):185–189.
84. Rushton CH, Reder E, Hall B, Comello K, Sellers DE, Hutton N. Interdisciplinary interventions to improve pediatric palliative care and reduce health care professional suffering. J Palliat Med. 2006;9(4):922–933.
85. Feudtner C, Santucci G, Feinstein JA, Snyder CR, Rourke MT, Kang TI. Hopeful thinking and level of comfort regarding providing pediatric palliative care: a survey of hospital nurses. Pediatrics. 2007;119(1):e186–e192.
86. Davies B, Contro N, Larson J, Widger K. Culturally-sensitive information-sharing in pediatric palliative care. Pediatrics. 2010;125(4):e859–e865.
87. Browning DM, Solomon MZ. Relational learning in pediatric palliative care: transformative education and the culture of medicine. Child Adolesc Psychiatr Clin N Am. 2006;15(3):795–815.
88. Browning D. To show our humanness: relational and communicative competence in pediatric palliative care. Bioethics Forum. 2002;18(3–4):23–28.
89. Ballantine A, Feudtner C. The 10 R's of clinician education: a checklist. Arch Pediatr Adolesc Med. 2010;164(4):389–390.
90. Peters L, Cant R, Payne S, et al. How death anxiety impacts nurses' caring for patients at the end of life: a review of literature. Open Nurs J. 2013;7:14–21.
91. Davies B, Sehring SA, Partridge JC, et al. Barriers to palliative care for children: perceptions of pediatric health care providers. Pediatrics. 2008;121(2):282–288.

CHAPTER 61

Pediatric pain
Knowing the child before you

Mary Layman-Goldstein and Dana Kramer

It feels like blisters you can't see burning my skin and something pressing on different parts of my leg, down to my big toe. I can't really explain it.

Casey, Age 12 with neuroblastoma, describing neuropathic pain

Key points

- Pain assessment depends on the child's age and cognitive developmental stage.

- Analgesic doses are initiated according to the child's age and body weight (milligrams or micrograms per kilogram).

- Pain management plans are based on the child's past experiences, developmental level, present response, and physical, emotional, and cultural factors.

- The child and parent are the unit of care. Parental involvement is key to successful interventions. Parents/caregivers must be included in assessment and pain management plans.

Expert pain management is a crucial part of pediatric palliative care.[1] It is possible for children of all ages to feel and express pain. A child's ability to communicate about pain is influenced by age and cognitive level,[2] but even a preverbal child can communicate about pain. To effectively manage the pain of an individual child, the nurse first must be aware of the possibility of pain, sensitively observe the child, and use developmentally appropriate, objective assessments. Developmental factors (physical, emotional, and cognitive) play an important role in both pediatric pain assessment and pain management. Through knowledge of these factors and an awareness of how they affect the child, it is possible for the nurse to better manage his or her pain (Table 61.1). Despite growing interest and research in pediatric pain management over the last 50 years, there remains a gap between what is technically possible and what is clinically practiced.[3]

Definitions of pain and other relevant terms

Pain has been described as "an unpleasant emotional experience associated with actual or potential tissue damage or described in terms of such damage."[7] Another definition, originally penned by Margo McCaffery, RN, in 1968, highlights the subjective nature of pain. According to McCaffery, pain is "whatever the experiencing person says it is, experienced whenever they say they are experiencing it."[8]

Nociception is "the perception by the nerves of injurious influences or painful stimuli."[7] This term is frequently used in discussions of pain in the neonate because of the challenges in evaluating the newborn's (preterm up to age 1 month) perception of pain.

The concept of patient-controlled analgesia (PCA) is well established. What is less understood is the term "PCA by proxy." The American Society for Pain Management Nursing (ASPMN) defines that term as the activation of the analgesic dosing button by someone other than the patient "without having been authorized and educated."[9(p. 177)] They further define the term "authorized agent controlled analgesia (AACA)" as "a method of analgesic administration (with or without a background/basal infusion) by a consistently available and competent individual who has been authorized by a prescriber and properly educated to activate the dosing button in response to pain when a patient is unable to operate an analgesic infusion pump."[9(p. 178)] The authorized agent may be the nurse who is responsible for a particular patient. In that case, AACA could be nurse-controlled analgesia (NCA). Or, the authorized agent could be a nonprofessional person such as a parent or significant other, and the method could be referred to as caregiver-controlled analgesia (CCA).[9] The term "PCA by proxy" is not encouraged, as it implies that a potentially unsafe, uneducated, unauthorized individual is activating a child's PCA pump.

One term that is frequently encountered in the subject of pediatric pain is "procedural pain." Procedural pain is pain that is caused by procedures (e.g., needlesticks, heel punctures, lumbar punctures). All children who interact with the healthcare system potentially experience procedural pain.

"Conscious sedation" has been defined by the American Academy of Pediatrics[10] as "a medically controlled state of depressed consciousness that (1) allows protective reflexes to be maintained; (2) retains the patient's ability to maintain a patent airway independently and continuously; and (3) permits appropriate response by the patient to physical stimulation or verbal command."[10(p. 1110)]

Prevalence of pain in children

Clinicians working with children in the general pediatric area will encounter pain in children who are undergoing immunizations

Table 61.1 Useful questions in evaluating a child with pain

Question	Clinical implications of answers
What is the chronological age of the child?	Age-related physiological development affects pharmacokinetic and pharmacodynamic effects of medications.
	In the neonate, normal neuroanatomical and neurobiological developmental processes occur and allow for transmission of painful stimuli.
What is the developmental stage of the child? ◆ Neonate ◆ Infant ◆ Toddler ◆ Preschooler/young child ◆ School-age child ◆ Adolescent	Developmental age helps determine: ◆ How a child might express his or her pain. ◆ Which assessment tools may be useful. ◆ What cognitive-behavioral techniques might be considered.
What type of pain does the child have? ◆ Acute pain ◆ Chronic pain ◆ Procedural pain	The particular situation can guide the clinician to a developmentally appropriate assessment tool and a situation-specific pain management plan that includes both pharmacological and nonpharmacological interventions.
Does the child have a chronic illness?	Certain painful conditions have disease-specific, validated pain assessment tools. For example, the Douleur Enfant Gustave Roussy (DEGR) scale is available to assess prolonged pain in 2- to 6-year-olds with cancer.*
Is the child neurologically impaired?	Cognitively impaired children may process information and communicate distress differently from normally developed children.†
	Besides knowing the science, and the individual child, it may help to know other children with similar conditions.†
	New pain assessment tools for children with intellectual disabilities are being validated to look at generic, procedural, and surgical pain.†
Do the child and parents speak the same language as healthcare providers?	Find ways of obtaining translators.
	Some pain assessment tools are available in translated versions.##
	It may be worth having pain assessment tools translated into languages common to certain practice settings.
What is the underlying cause of the pain?	If the underlying cause is treatable, the pain may be reduced or eliminated.
What is the child's weight in kilograms?	Dosage of analgesics is expressed in milligrams or micrograms per kilogram.
	For some medications, the starting dose depends on the child's being larger or smaller than a set weight.
Is the oral route of drug administration used whenever possible?	Besides being a cheaper and less invasive route (with less potential for pain and infection), the oral route in children provides more reliable absorption.
Are there any obvious, outstanding barriers that may be playing a role in the child's pain assessment and management?	Some barriers can be directly and quickly addressed with minimal effect and maximal positive impact.
Have nonpharmacological pain interventions been considered?	Nonpharmacological pain interventions based on the etiology of a child's pain can improve the comprehensiveness and effectiveness of a pain management plan.

Sources: *Gauvain-Piquard et al. (1999), reference 4; †Knegt et al. (2013), reference 5; ##Silva and Thuler (2008) reference 6.

and procedures and those who have pharyngitis, oral viral infections, otitis media, urinary tract infections, headache, or traumatic injuries. Pain continues to be present in children with cancer at the end of life.[11] Conditions such as meningitis and necrotizing colitis can cause pain in children. Children who experience chronic diseases such as cancer, human immunodeficiency virus (HIV) infection, sickle cell disease (SCD), hemophilia, juvenile chronic arthritis (JCA), and cystic fibrosis (CF) also will have pain.[2] Definitive studies focusing on the prevalence of pain in the pediatric population are lacking. At best, we have studies that look at the incidence of pain in various disease subpopulations. Children with certain conditions are prone to particular pain syndromes. Nurses working with children need knowledge of the pain syndromes they may commonly encounter in the populations they work with and need to feel comfortable assessing and managing those particular pain syndromes.

Etiology of pain in children

Neuropathic pain

Neuropathic pain is less common in children than in adults. Many of the neuropathic pain syndromes seen in adults are not diagnosed as frequently in children. Children may experience neuropathic pain from migraine headaches, scar neuromas after surgery, phantom limb pain after amputations for trauma, tumors, meningococcemia, autoimmune and degenerative neuropathies, and complex regional pain syndromes (reported in preteen and teenage girls).[2,12] Although diabetes is increasing in incidence in the pediatric population, it is rare to see a child who has diabetic neuropathy, a syndrome that takes years to develop. Brachial plexus avulsion, an injury that sometimes occurs to babies during childbirth, is thought by some to be less disabling and painful in babies than when it occurs (for other reasons) in adults. It is not clear whether this is due to inadequate assessment of infants or to the physical developmental functions of babies.[13] Neuropathic pain is also common in pediatric cancer patients for a number of reasons, which will be discussed in more detail below.

Burns

Burns, which can sometimes be life threatening, are thermal injuries caused by hot liquids, flames, and electricity, are among the most common causes of injury to children and are associated with pain. This injury, which destroys the skin, can have significant morbidity and mortality depending on the extent of the burn. Intact skin is necessary for protection against bacterial infection, fluid and electrolyte balance, and thermoregulation. Treatment of severe burns is associated with significant pain. Undertreatment of this pain can make it difficult for the child to cooperate with burn treatment. It is postulated that use in children of an individualized pain management plan with high-quality pain control components, such as intravenous opioids, local block, or even general anesthesia, can avoid the development of a postburn hyperalgesia syndrome caused by continuous or repeated stimulation of nociceptive afferent fibers.[13,14] Researchers are also looking to see whether aggressive pain management decreases the development of posttraumatic stress disorder, a long-term morbidity issue for some children who have been burned.[14]

Cancer

The World Health Organization (WHO) stated that 70% of children with cancer will experience severe pain during their illness.[15] The types of pain in children with cancer, whether caused by procedures, by the disease or tumor, or by anticancer treatment, have been well described for many years.[16–18] This pain can be acute or chronic. Children with chronic cancer-related pain frequently experience breakthrough pain.[2] A study by Ljungman and colleagues[19] of children receiving treatment for cancer revealed that procedure-and treatment related pain were significant problems initially and that procedure-related pain gradually decreased, but treatment-related pain remained constant. In addition, children with cancer may have pain for unrelated reasons, such as acute appendicitis.[16]

All children with cancer are at risk for procedural pain. Most procedure-related pain involves needle puncture. This procedure may be necessary for obtaining blood supplies, accessing implanted venous devices, administering intravenous chemotherapeutics, or giving intramuscular or subcutaneous medications. Lumbar punctures (using a spinal needle) or bone marrow aspiration (involving insertion of a large needle into the posterior superior iliac spine) are variations of needle puncture. Some children develop prolonged post-lumbar puncture headaches.[20] Despite significant efforts to avoid needlesticks in the pediatric population, sometimes a needle puncture is necessary and cannot be avoided. Removal of tunneled central venous catheters or implanted ports also causes procedural pain and must be addressed by clinicians caring for the children undergoing this procedure.[16]

For some children, it is the experience of tumor-related pain that leads their parents to seek medical attention and eventual diagnosis. This pain can be nociceptive or neuropathic. Nociceptive pain can be somatic, caused by tumor involvement with bone or soft tissue, or visceral, caused by tumor infiltration, compression, or distention of abdominal or thoracic viscera. Neuropathic pain can be caused by tumor involvement (i.e., compression or infiltration) with the peripheral or central nervous system.

Most children who receive a diagnosis of cancer, no matter what the stage, will receive some sort of anticancer treatment. Frequently this treatment causes some sort of pain, either acute or chronic. Surgery leads to acute, postoperative pain. Removal of limbs may lead to the development of phantom limb sensations and pain. This experience is thought to decrease over time in children. Radiation therapy may lead to an acute dermatitis or pain. Children undergoing chemotherapy are at risk acutely for mucositis pain and gastritis from repeated vomiting (if nausea and vomiting are not successfully controlled)[16] and chronically for neuropathic pain from certain chemotherapies. Children who have been treated with high doses of steroids are at risk for development of avascular necrosis, a disabling condition that eventually causes the affected bone to collapse. Some chemotherapy agents, such as vincristine, asparaginase, and cyclophosphamide, can cause pain or painful conditions such as peripheral neuropathy, constipation, hemorrhagic cystitis, or pancreatitis. Complications of intravenous chemotherapy administration may lead to pain from irritation, infiltration, extravasation, tissue necrosis (if vesicants are used), or the development of thrombophlebitis. Children receiving intrathecal chemotherapy may develop arachnoiditis or meningeal irritation, also painful conditions. The child who is immunocompromised, whether from chemotherapy or from disease, is at risk for infection and infection-related pain. Skin, perioral, and perirectal infections are common. Children seem to be at less risk for acute herpes zoster and its related pain.[2] Bone marrow transplantation may lead acutely to severe mucositis and potentially to chronic graft-versus-host disease, which may manifest as severe abdominal pain if it affects the gastrointestinal system.[16]

Medications used to prevent or modify side effects of primary disease treatment can have painful effects. Use of corticosteroids in disease treatment may lead to bone changes that cause pain.[21] Colony-stimulating factors may lead to medullary bone pain shortly after administration and before the onset of neutrophil recovery.

Nurses caring for patients receiving new treatment protocols need to be alert to the development of pain syndromes associated with particular agents. For example, in recent years, the use of 3F8, an antiganglioside monoclonal antibody, in the treatment of advanced neuroblastoma has significantly improved survival but causes an acute episode of neuropathic pain affecting random body parts during infusion.[16] As more is known about the effects of new treatment agents, more effective preventive measures can be taken to improve the quality of life of children undergoing potentially life-sustaining or life-extending therapy.

As children live longer with cancer, they may live longer with pain. Pediatric tertiary care centers, such as Children's Hospital of Boston, have reported a variety of chronic pain problems, including causalgia of a lower extremity, chronic lower extremity pain caused by a mechanical problem with an internal prosthesis, and avascular necrosis of multiple joints in long-term survivors of childhood cancers.[22]

Human immunodeficiency virus infection

Children with HIV infection may experience pain for a variety of reasons, including disease, treatment, and procedures. Some factors are quite similar to those associated with cancer-related pain, and some are unique to HIV disease. For example, children with the acquired immunodeficiency syndrome (AIDS) may have abdominal cramping pain due to AIDS-associated diarrhea.[2]

Sickle cell disease

One of the most common genetic diseases in the United States, commonly affecting individuals of African, Middle Eastern, Mediterranean, and Indian descent, is highly associated with a variety of painful conditions. Sickle cell disease is characterized by a predominance of hemoglobin S (HbS), which becomes sickle-shaped (as opposed to donut-shaped) after deoxygenation. It is this stiff, sickle-shaped red blood cell that becomes trapped in small blood vessels, leading to vaso-occlusion, tissue ischemia, and even infarction.[2]

Some of the many painful states that are commonly associated with SCD include acute painful events, acute hand-foot syndrome, acute inflammation of joints, acute chest syndrome, splenic sequestration, intrahepatic sickling or hepatic sequestration, avascular necrosis of femur or humerus, and priapism. The reader is directed to the American Pain Society's *Guidelines for the Management of Acute and Chronic Pain in Sickle Cell Disease*[23(pp. 3–7)] for a review of the clinical signs and symptoms of these and other common SCD pain states, their underlying causes, and special features or considerations. These episodes can vary in frequency and severity among and within individuals with SCD. Although most would be considered to be frequently recurring acute pain episodes, some, such as those caused by vertebral collapse or avascular necrosis of the femoral or humeral heads, can lead to chronic, debilitating painful conditions. A child with SCD may require hospitalization for pain control. Painful vaso-occlusive crisis (VOC) is the most common reason for hospitalization. Researchers in various settings are now looking to benchmark pain outcomes for children with VOC to identify areas in most need of improvement.[24–26] Inconsistent pain management for individuals with SCD clearly leads to increased morbidity and mortality for affected children and adults[27]

Other conditions associated with pain in children

Other conditions children experience that may be associated with pain include cystic fibrosis, muscular dystrophy, and other degenerative neurological diseases and severe dermatological conditions. A recent study of children with hemiplegic cerebral palsy identified from a population register revealed that 33% had mild pain and 18% had moderate-to-severe pain.[28] We continue to learn more about the prevalence, distribution, and description of pain syndromes in many life-threatening illnesses in children, but for many illnesses these facts have yet to be determined. This shortcoming may be a result of assessment difficulties in infants, preverbal children, and children with communication impairments. Or, it may be a consequence of the often single-minded focus on cure. As clinical interest broadens to also include increased attention to the comfort of these children, it is hoped that the pain and its treatment will be better defined and practiced.[29]

Physiology and pathophysiology of pain in children

Important factors relevant to the physiology and pathophysiology of pain are well covered in chapter 7. Those working with children need to be aware of the normal neuroanatomical and neurobiological developmental processes that occur in neonates and allow for the development of transmission of painful stimuli (Table 61.2). In fact, there is strong evidence to suggest that neonates have increased sensitivity to pain, because the inhibitory pain tracts are the last to develop.[30] It is possible to assess the severity of pain and the effects of analgesics in neonates. Neonates who do not cry, move, or show other behavioral response in response to painful stimuli may still be experiencing pain. It has been shown that increased neonatal morbidity and mortality may result from prolonged or severe pain. It has been shown that neonates who experience pain may respond differently to pain later on (e.g., pain from inoculation or circumcision) than do those who have not experienced previous painful events.[31]

Assessment of pain in children

Assessment of pain in pediatrics involves a conversation between the clinician, the child, and the parents. The nurse must first learn who the child is to effectively treat the child's pain. To do this, nurses evaluating pain in children of all ages must be aware of potential barriers and influencing factors that may play a role in accurate, developmentally appropriate assessment.

Barriers to pain control in children are similar to those in adults. They primarily relate to (1) lack of assessment; (2) inadequate analgesics; (3) misconceptions on the part of patients, families, or healthcare providers about pain and pain management; and (4) issues related to systems.[2,22,29] Table 61.3 reviews these barriers in detail.

Consider the child as an individual. Before pain can be properly assessed, one must take into account the child's chronological age and his or her developmental stage. Is this child a neonate, infant, toddler, preschooler, school-age child, or adolescent? When approaching pain assessment, it is important to review developmental stages and factors (see Table 61.2). The following case study may also be helpful.

Case study

Sasha, a 3-year-old girl with localized Ewing sarcoma, hospitalized with neutropenia

Sasha, had repeated episodes of distress and crying that could not be identified by her primary team. These episodes were increasing in both intensity and frequency. Immediately after these episodes, her heart rate might range from 125 to 135 bpm. At times she would talk about "itching in my bottom." The palliative care team was called to see her during one of these episodes of acute distress.

Table 61.2 Pain-related developmental milestones

Age	Development	Assessment and management implications
7 wk gestation	Pain receptors present*	
20 wk gestation	Full compliment of neurons in cerebral cortex*	
	Pain receptors spread to all cutaneous and mucosal surfaces*	
26 wk gestation	Can respond to tissue injury as demonstrated by "specific behavioral, autonomic, hormonal, and metabolic signs of stress and distress" (p. 1094) due to sufficient development of peripheral, spinal, and supraspinal afferent pain transmission pathways*	
30 wk gestation	Myelination usually complete*	
	Slower transmission of pain thought to be offset by decreased distance the impulse must travel*	
40 wk gestation	Descending, inhibitory pathways, which alter and modulate pain perception, present*	
Neonate (preterm through 1 mo)	**Acute pain responses:**	
	◆ Physiological measures, such as increase in vital signs, are similar to those of older children and adults.	◆ Challenging to differentiate symptoms of pain (a stressful situation) from other life-threatening situations such as hypoxemia[†]
	Behavioral indicators include vocalizations (crying, whimpering, groaning), facial expression changes (grimaces, furrowed brow, quivering chin, tightly closed eyes, square open mouth), body movement and posture (thrashing, limb withdrawn, fist clenched, flaccidity), and other behavior changes (sleep/wake cycle, feeding, activity, irritability or listlessness).*	◆ Validated composite measures include the Neonatal Infant Pain Scale, or NIPS[§]; the CRIES postoperative pain tool[$] (C = crying; R = requires increased oxygen administration; I = increased vital signs; E = expression; S = sleeplessness), and the Premature Infant Pain Profile, or PIPPS.♪
	◆ Chronic responses can include changes or disruptions in usual feeding, activity, and sleep/wake patterns.	◆ One-dimensional pain assessment measure: Neonatal Facial Coding System[#]
		◆ Measures do not address neonates with chronic pain, those pharmacologically paralyzed for mechanical ventilation, or those with significant facial deformity.[†]
	Physiological developmental issues*:	
	◆ Increased water and volume of distribution for water-soluble medications	◆ Need for increased dosing interval or decreased rates of infusion for many medications*
	◆ Decreased fat and muscle	◆ Vulnerable to effects of decreased ventilatory reflexes*
	◆ Immature hepatic enzyme systems, leading to decreased metabolic clearances	
	◆ Decreased glomerular filtration rates, producing accumulation of renally excreted medications and active metabolites	
	◆ Many factors in respiratory function lead to increased risk of hypoventilation, atelectasis, or respiratory failure.	
Infants (older than 1 mo)	**Acute pain responses:**	
	◆ Behavioral changes, physiological responses, and facial responses of neonates exhibited*	◆ Examine infants older than 1 mo in parent's lap.**
	◆ May cry loudly, thrash, arch, or exhibit body rigidity*	◆ Children's Hospital of Eastern Ontario Pain Scale (CHEOPS)[††]
	◆ Local reflex withdrawal of stimulated area in young infants*	
	◆ Deliberate withdrawal of affected area in older infants*	
	◆ Development of stranger anxiety after 7 mo**	

(continued)

Table 61.2 Continued

Age	Development	Assessment and management implications
	Physiological developmental issues*:	
	◆ Immature hepatic enzyme systems, leading to decreased metabolic clearances	◆ Need for increased dosing interval or decreased rates of infusion for many medications*
	◆ From birth to 7 mo, decreased glomerular filtration rates produce accumulation of renally excreted medications and active metabolites.	◆ Vulnerable to effects of decreased ventilatory reflexes in response to opioids or sedatives*
	◆ By 8 to 12 mo, renal blood flow, glomerular filtration, and tubular secretion increase to near adult values.	
	◆ Many factors in respiratory function lead to increased risk of hypoventilation, atelectasis, or respiratory failure.	
Toddlers	Behavioral changes (such as changes in eating, play/activity, and sleep/wake patterns) and physiological responses as described in neonates*	Give toddler time to get used to you and build trust.**
	May also cry intensely, be verbally aggressive, or withdraw from play or social interaction*,***	Use play and minimized physical contact during physical assessment.**
	May have words for pain by 18 mo††	Language development varies, and it is best to use words for pain that are most familiar to a particular child.**
	Stranger anxiety persists**	Often it is beneficial to have parents present during assessment and procedures.††, %
	From age 2 to 6 y, children have a larger liver mass per kilogram of body weight and this is thought to increase metabolic clearance of many medications.	By age 2 y, dosing intervals may be decreased or infusion rates increased because of increased metabolic clearance.*
Preschooler (young child, age 3–6 y)	Behavioral changes (such as changes in eating, play/activity, and sleep/wake patterns) and physiological responses are as described in neonates.*	Physical and emotional support by adults present, especially parents, may be comforting. %
	"Magical thinking" (mixes facts and fiction)‡‡	Consider building on "magical thinking" abilities when initiating nonpharmacological interventions.††
	Developmentally able to give meaningful, concrete information about location and severity of pain†,‡‡	
	Able to anticipate painful events/procedures*	Offer realistic choices if possible, and provide positive reinforcement**
	Behaviors may include clinging, lack of cooperation, and attempts to push painful stimuli away before their application.*	By age 2 y, dosing intervals may be decreased or infusion rates increased because of increased metabolic clearance.*
	Pain may be viewed as a punishment or as a source of secondary gain*	
	From age 2 to 6 y, children have a larger liver mass per kilogram of body weight and this is thought to increase metabolic clearance of many medications.	
School-age child	Behavioral changes (such as changes in eating, play/activity, and sleep/wake patterns) and physiological responses are as described in neonates.*	Child able to use more objective measures of pain, give more specific and detailed reports
		Able to use more cognitive coping methods, including educational interventions
	May exhibit rigid muscularity (gritted teeth, contracted limbs, stiff body, closed eyes, or wrinkled forehead)	Cultural beliefs may influence child's pain experience*,§§
	May demonstrate more stalling behaviors to delay potentially painful experiences	

(continued)

Table 61.2 Continued

Age	Development	Assessment and management implications
	Continued normal cognitive development influences ability to both report and learn information	
	May demonstrate influences of cultural group[§§]	
Adolescent	Behavioral changes (such as changes in eating, play/activity, and sleep/wake patterns) and physiological responses as described in neonates[*]	May deny pain in presence of peers
	May show more decreased motor activity in presence of pain	May be influenced by cultural factors regarding interpretations and expressions of pain[*§§]
	Continued normal cognitive development	Parents remain advocate for child, but teenagers, if they so desire, need to be involved in decision-making[**]
	Increased influence of peers and cultural group[**§§]	Validated multidimensional pain measurement tool is available in English and Spanish for use in adolescents and children with different medical conditions: Adolescent Pediatric Pain Tool (APPT).[+]
	Increased needs for privacy and independence[**]	
	Adolescent not legally independent (except in special cases) but needs to have a larger emerging role in his or her care[**]	

Sources: [*]Berde and Sethna (2003), reference 32; [†]American Academy of Pediatrics (2000), reference 10; [§]Lawrence et al. (1993), reference 33; [$]Krechel and Bildner (1995), reference 34; [♪]Stevens et al. (1996), reference 35; [#]Grunau and Craig (1990), reference 36; [**]Levetown (2000), reference 37; [††]McGrath et al. (1985), reference 38; [‡‡]Cramton and Gruchala (2012), reference 20; [%]Power et al. (2007), reference 39; [§§]Davies et al. (2010), reference 40; [+]Jacob et al. (2013), reference 41.

Her mother was holding her, but Sasha was inconsolable. Sasha was grimacing and guarding throughout this episode. Through careful parent history, it was learned that sometimes Sasha would hold her bottom during some of these episodes and say "Make the itching stop!" After the episode passed, Sasha was examined and found to have mucositis in her rectal area. Through careful parental interview and assessment, it was determined that Sasha was using the word "itching" to express her pain. By partnering with her mother, who was most sensitive to distress in her child, and through introduction of the Faces Pain Scale to Sasha and her mother, the team was able to better access her rectal pain and in turn, control it.

Poor communication between the pediatric patient, family, and healthcare team increases the likelihood of suboptimal pain assessment and management. Factors that may interfere with assessment include language or cultural differences between, child, family, and clinicians; the presence of chronic health conditions, developmental disabilities, cognitive, sensory, or motor impairments; and severe emotional disturbance.[13,44]

In learning who an individual child is, the nurse must interview the child as well as the parents. There is probably no more sensitive index of a change in a child's behavior than parental report. Naturally, parents are often attuned to the condition and changing needs of the child, and highly focused on his or her well-being.[45]

Choosing the appropriate pain assessment tool for a pediatric patient can be challenging. First, consider the developmental level or age of the child. Next, consider the type of pain, the context or specific illness, before selecting a tool. Attempts at measurement of pain include physiological measures, behavioral observations, composite measures, and self-report. Physiological measures may reflect the response to the stress of pain and not the pain itself.

Although they are far from ideal, physiological measures are often used in situations in which the child is unable to report pain for him or herself. Acute pain is often associated with increases of 10% to 20% in noninvasively measured blood pressure, heart rate, or respiratory rate. These changes may not be present in the child with chronic pain.

Observational pain assessment tools, also used when a child cannot self-report pain, are criticized for measuring "distress" behavior instead of pain behavior.[46] Observational or behavioral scales are most often used in preverbal or cognitively impaired children. The pain behaviors specific to certain conditions may be useful, such as the observation of guarding, bracing, and active rubbing in children with JCA.[13] The Pediatric Initiative on Methods, Measurement, and Pain Assessment in Clinical Trials (www.immpact.org) commissioned a review of observational scales of pain for children age 3 to 18 years with to identify which scales might be used as an outcome measure in clinical trials. Although this review identified tools that were useful in specific acute pain situations, such as postoperative pain in hospitalized children, it concluded that no single observational measure can be recommended for pain assessment across contexts.[46]

Self-report, the gold standard in pain assessment, can be obtained from some children as young as age 3 years and generally by 6 years. Most pediatric self-report tools are not multidimensional and measure only pain intensity.[2] To adequately report detailed ratings of pain intensity, a child, usually of school age or older, must understand the concepts of sequence and numbering. To test this knowledge, a child can be given (for example) six different-sized pieces of paper and asked to place them in order from smallest to largest.[47] If a 0-to-10 scale is used, 0 being no pain and 10 being the worst imaginable pain, older children and adolescents may be asked to rate their

Table 61.3 Pediatric-specific barriers to pain control

Issue	Barrier/misconception
Inadequate assessment	*Misconception*: Infants and children do not feel pain in the same way as adults do.*
	Misconception: Children are unable to provide useful, accurate information about the location and severity of their pain.*
	Lack of knowledge about how to assess pediatric pain[†]
	Challenge of pain assessment in preverbal or noncommunicating children
	Choosing the correct population specific tool
Inadequate analgesics ordered or administered	Need for comprehensive assessment with pain etiology and contributing or modifying factors identified
	Need to select most appropriate medications, doses, dosing intervals, and route of administration for situation[@]
	Nurses or parents may not administer the complete dose ordered or as frequently as ordered.
	Prescriber's reluctance to send children home with the effective opioids that the child received while hospitalized[†]
Incorrect attitudes or misconceptions by patients, families, or healthcare providers about pain and its management	Pain control in children too difficult or time consuming*
	Lack of knowledge or incorrect knowledge of pharmacokinetics and pharmacodynamics of analgesics, especially opioids[†]
	Lack of knowledge of the consequences of unrelieved pain[†]
	Misconception: Children can tolerate pain better than adults can (this can lead to heightened pain and anxiety about pain control).[†]
	Fear of opioid-related side effects and lack of knowledge about how to manage them can also prevent appropriate use of opioids in children.[†]
Systems-related issues	Need for systematic reevaluation and reassessment of pain management plan's effectiveness[†]
	No systematic, evidenced-based approach to pain management despite rigorous approach to other aspects of a child's care, including disease diagnosis and treatment
	Lack of appropriate use of nondrug therapies to complement or supplement the pharmacological interventions[†]
	Lack of knowledge by healthcare professionals of simple and practical physical, cognitive, or behavioral strategies that can give children and their families more control and less anxiety about pain management
	Lack of clear delineation of who is responsible for a particular child's pain control, leading to gaps in management[†]

Sources: *Levine et al. (2013), reference 42; [†]McGrath and Brown (2004), reference 43; [@]WHO (2012), reference 2, [†]Field and Behrman (2003), reference 29.

pain with an number and then asked, "Do you consider your pain to be none, slight, moderate, severe, or excruciating?" The comparison between the child's numeric pain rating and the categorical pain rating will ideally show some general agreement. Readers attempting to narrow their choices of pain assessment tools may refer to detailed reviews of tools found in several references.[13,48–50]

The case study below describes a child who is able to self-report.

Case study

Galen, a 7-year-old boy with relapsed stage IV refractory neuroblastoma admitted for abdominal pain and loose stools

On workup, Galen was found to be positive for *Clostridium difficile* and started on Flagyl. Although his abdominal pain lessened as his treatment proceeded, he continued to have severe pain as

assessed using the Faces Pain Rating scale. After these bowel movements, he consistently selected the Face 5 ("Hurts worst"). This pain would persist for about 3 hours. His mother was very fearful of giving her son strong pain medications as he had vomited in the past every time he was given IV morphine. Yet, it bothered her very much to see him in such pain. After discussion with his primary team, she agreed to let him have IV Fentanyl bolus doses. The WHO recommends a starting dose of Fentanyl 1–2 mcg/kg every 2–4 hours for opioid naïve children (age 1 to 12 years). Given his weight, 30.7 kg, a dose of 30 mcg administered slowly over 3–5 minutes every 60 minutes was ordered. An hour after the first dose, he rated his pain as Face 3 ("Hurts even more"), only a reduction of two faces. His nurse reported to the team that he tolerated the fentanyl bolus dose with no opioid-related problems (such as confusion, sleepiness, nausea, or vomiting). Galen's mother wanted her son to have better relief. His team decided that he would tolerate and benefit from a larger dose, using 2 mcg/kg as a basis for the 60 mcg IV Fentanyl over 3 to 5 minutes q 60 minutes prn ordered. When he had another bowel movement 2 hours later, again rating his pain as Face 4 ("Hurts a whole lot") he was given the higher dose of Fentanyl 60 mcg. Thirty minutes after this medication, Galen rated his pain at Face 1 ("Hurts a little bit") and at 60 minutes rated it as Face 0 ("No hurt"). As his condition improved, he had fewer bowel movements and his pain from them was managed to both Galen and his mother's satisfaction.

In any practice setting, it may be necessary to use multiple tools for patients with a broad range of developmental and cognitive abilities. Researchers are now looking at psychological responses of fear and anxiety that may influence a child's pain experience.[51] Under the stress of pain and illness, a child may show signs of cognitive and emotional regression, and may benefit from assessment with a simpler tool. A simpler tool may also be appropriate when a child is cognitively impaired secondary to medications or medical illness. At present, there is a great need for research in this area, to create more generalizable pain assessment tools with improved specificity and sensitivity.[46]

Assessment of pain begins with screening. Screening for pain can occur routinely from the time a child enters a healthcare system through simple documentation tools. Hospitalized children may be screened more than once a day for any changes in pain or for unsatisfactory pain control.[44] See below, the QUESTT approach to pediatric pain assessment. This is a simple guideline for proactive main management and reevaluation.[52]

Question the child and parent.

Use pain rating scales appropriate to developmental stage of the child and to the situation at hand.

Evaluate behavioral and physiological changes.

Secure parents' involvement.

Take the cause of pain into account.

Take action and evaluate results.

In every practice setting, a child with pain needs regular reassessment to improve or maintain safe and effective management of pain.

Management

No matter what the practice setting, clinicians involved in pediatric pain management must anticipate and prevent pain whenever possible. If not possible, it is the clinician's responsibility to minimize pain by treating the underlying cause where possible, using pharmacological and nonpharmacological modalities as appropriate, minimizing painful procedures where possible, and addressing the pain involved in necessary procedures.

Pharmacological management

Nurses caring for children with pain must be aware of physiological variations among different age groups which may affect analgesic action. Many pediatric analgesic studies in children are limited because they include a wide age range. This makes it challenging to distinguish between the effects of

developmentally dependent physiological processes that play a role in analgesia.[53] Consider the potential for pathophysiological differences in pediatric patients, including those in the body compartments, hepatic enzyme systems, plasma protein binding, renal filtration and excretion of medications and their metabolites, metabolic rate, oxygen consumption, and respiratory function.[32] Table 61.2 presents some of these developmental physiological changes and their clinical implications. Tables 61.4, 61.5, 61.6, 61.7, and 61.8 suggest starting doses for opioids and nonopioids that reflect these developmental aspects of pediatric pharmacology.

Although studies indicate that with proper age-based adjustments and dosing, children can safely receive pain medication, it is important to bear in mind that approximately 50% to 75% of medications used in pediatric medicine, including analgesics, have not been adequately studied to provide appropriate labeling information.[54] Clinicians who treat pain in children have tried to extrapolate data from the adult pain management literature.[22] This may be attributable to lack of resources. Pediatrics account for a fraction the pharmaceutical market, and there is limited financial incentive to study medications in children.[55] Fortunately, the limited pharmacokinetic data for this population is growing and will assist clinicians in making appropriate medication choices for children.[55]

There are three main groups of medications used to treat pain in children: (1) nonopioids (e.g., acetaminophen, nonsteroidal antiinflammatory drugs [NSAIDs]), (2) opioids, and (3) adjuvant analgesics. Use of these medications depends on the severity and cause of pain in an individual child. The nonopioids and opioids are most helpful in the treatment of nociceptive pain, and adjuvant analgesics work best for specific neuropathic pain. A general review of these medications and their use is presented in chapter 7. What follows in this section are factors that are most relevant to the use of these drugs in children.

In 1998, the WHO first published guidelines for cancer pain relief and palliative care in children.[15] This laid out key concepts for use of analgesics in children "by the ladder, by the clock, by the appropriate route, by the child, and with attention to detail."[15(p. 24)] In 2012, the WHO further refined the approach to the relief of pain in children with persisting pain due to medical illness when they released new pharmacological guidelines.[2] In the original guidelines, "by the ladder" refers to approaching a child's pain based on the severity of pain, with three steps clearly delineated for mild, moderate, and severe pain. In the new pediatric guidelines, the three-step ladder has been abandoned for a two-step approach, with step one being mild pain and step two being moderate to severe pain. For mild pain, nonopioids, paracetamol (acetaminophen) and ibuprofen, are indicated. The second step utilizes low starting doses of "strong" opioids such a morphine for a child with moderate to severe pain. These medications are to be administered on a regular schedule for persistent pain with addition of prn doses for intermittent or breakthrough pain. Based on reassessment of an individual child, the opioid dose will be titrated upward until satisfactory analgesia without dose-limiting side effects is achieved.[2]

The 2012 guidelines identify opioids to avoid: codeine, and tramadol.[2] Historically, in the original pediatric WHO guidelines, codeine (a "weak" opioid) was given to children with moderate pain.[15] However, codeine, an opioid with a narrow therapeutic

Table 61.4 WHO nonopioid analgesics for the relief of pain in neonates, infants, and children

Dose (oral route)				
Medicine	Neonates from 0 to 29 days	Infants from 30 days to 3 months	Infants from 3 to 12 months or children 1 to 12 years[a,b]	Maximum daily dose
Paracetamol (also known as acetaminophen)	5–10 mg/kg every 6–8 hours[a]	10 mg/kg every 4–6 hours[a]	10–15 mg/kg every 4–6 hours	Neonates, infants, and children: 4 doses/day
Ibuprofen			5–10 mg/kg every 6–8 hours	Children: 40 mg/kg/day

[a]Children who are malnourished or in a poor nutritional state are more likely to be susceptible to toxicity at standard dose regimens due to a reduced natural detoxifying glutathione enzyme.
[b]Maximum of 1 gram at a time.
Source: WHO (2012); reference 2, p. 41.

Table 61.5 Oral dosage guidelines for commonly used nonopioid analgesics

	Dose			Maximum daily dose	
Drug	Child <60 kg	Child ≥60 kg	Interval	Child <60 kg	Child ≥60 kg
Acetaminophen	10–15 mg/kg	650–1000 mg	4 h	100 mg/kg[*]	3000 mg
Ibuprofen	6–10 mg/kg	400–600 mg[†]	6 h	40 mg/kg[†,‡]	2400 mg[†]
Naproxen	5–6 mg/kg[†]	250–375 mg[†]	12 h	24 mg/kg[†,‡]	1000 mg[†]

[*]The maximum daily doses of acetaminophen for infants and neonates are a subject of current controversy. Provisional recommendations are that daily dosing should not exceed 75 mg/kg for infants, 60 mg/kg for full-term neonates and preterm neonates of >32 wk postconceptional age. Fever, dehydration, hepatic disease, and lack of oral intake may all increase the risk of hepatotoxicity.
[†]Higher doses may be used in selected cases for treatment of rheumatological conditions in children.
[‡]Dosage guidelines for neonates have not been established for ibuprofen.
Source: Berde and Sethna (2003), reference 32, with permission.

Table 61.6 WHO starting dosages for opioid analgesics for opioid-naïve neonates

Medicine	Route of administration	Starting dose
Morphine	IV injection[a] SC injection	25–50 mcg/kg every 6 hours
	IV infusion	Initial IV dose[a] 25–50 mcg/kg, then 5–10 mcg/kg/h 100 mcg/kg every 6 or 4 h
Fentanyl	IV injection[b]	1–2 mcg/kg every 2–4 h[c]
	IV infusion[b]	Initial IV dose 1–2 mcg/kg, then 0.5–1 mcg/kg/h

[a] Administer IV morphine slowly over at least 5 minutes.
[b] The intravenous doses for neonates are based on acute pain management and sedation dosing information. Lower doses are required for nonventilated neonates.
[c] Administer IV fentanyl slowly over 3–5 minutes.
Source: WHO (2012), reference 2, p. 48.

window and a higher side-effect profile than other opioids, is no longer recommended in this population, since its metabolism has been shown to be variable, which can cause safety and efficacy problems. In a study of pediatric patients, 35% of children had limited ability to metabolize codeine into morphine, the process that allows for pain relief from codeine. Conversely, children who are able to metabolize codeine quickly and effectively are at risk for toxicity.[56] The new guidelines also identify the need for more research in the use of tramadol, an analgesic with opioid effects. Until evidence emerges on the safety and efficacy of tramadol in the pediatric population, its use cannot be incorporated into the WHO guidelines.[2]

"By the clock" reflects the concept that for pain that is almost continuous, a child will benefit most from nearly continuous analgesics administered on a regular schedule, at regular intervals. This method promotes better pain control and decreases a child's anxiety regarding uncontrolled pain. "By the appropriate route" promotes the administration of analgesics by the simplest, most effective, least painful route. For most children this is the oral route, but for some situations other routes may be more

Table 61.7 Starting dosages for opioid analgesics in opioid-naïve infants (1 month–1 year)

Medicine	Route of administration	Starting dose
Morphine	Oral (immediate release)	80–200 mcg/kg every 4 hours
	IV injection[a]	1–6 months: 100 mcg/kg every 6 hours
	SC injection	6–12 months: 100 mcg/kg every 4 hours
		(max 2.5 mg/dose)
	IV infusion[a]	1–6 months: Initial IV dose: 50 mcg/kg, then: 10–30 mcg/kg/h
		6–12 months: Initial IV dose: 100–200 mcg/kg, then 20–30 mcg/kg/h
	SC infusion	1–3 months: 10 mcg/kg/h
		3–12 months: 20 mcg/kg/h
Fentanyl[b]	IV injection	1–2 mcg/kg every 2–4 h[c]
	IV infusion	Initial IV dose 1–2 mcg/kg,[c] then 0.5–1 mcg/kg/h
Oxycodone	Oral (immediate release)	50–125 mcg/kg every 4 hours

[a] Administer IV morphine slowly over at least 5 minutes.
[b] The intravenous doses for infants are based on acute pain management and sedation dosing information. Lower doses are required for nonventilated neonates.
[c] Administer IV fentanyl slowly over 3–5 minutes.
Source: WHO (2012), reference 2, p. 48.

Table 61.8 WHO starting doses for opioid analgesics in opioid-naïve children (1–12 years)

Medicine	Route of administration	Starting dose
Morphine	Oral (immediate release)	1–2 years: 200–400 mcg/kg every 4 h
		2–12 years: 200–500 mcg/kg every 4 h (max 5 mg)
	Oral (prolonged release)	200–800 mcg/kg every 12 h
	IV injection[a]	1–2 years: 100 mcg/kg every 4 h
	SC injection	2–12 years: 100–200 mcg/kg every 4 h (max 2.5 mg)
	IV infusion	Initial IV dose: 100–200 mcg/kg,[a] then 20–30 mcg/kg/h
	SC infusion	20 mcg/kg/h
Fentanyl	IV injection	1–2 mcg/kg,[b] repeated every 30–60 minutes
	IV infusion	Initial IV dose: 1–2 mcg/kg,[b] then 1 mcg/h
Hydromorphone[c]	Oral (immediate release)	30–80 mcg/kg every 3–4 h (max 2 mg/dose)
	IV injection[d] or SC injection	15 mcg/kg every 3–6 h
Methadone[e]	Oral (immediate release)	100–200 mcg/kg every 4 h for the first 2–3 doses, then every
	IV injection[g] and SC injection	6–12 h (max 5 mg/dose initially)[f]
Oxymorphone	Oral (immediate release)	125–200 mcg/kg every 4 h (max 5 mg/dose)
	Oral (prolonged release)	5 mg every 12 h

[a] Administer IV morphine slowly over at least 5 minutes.
[b] Administer IV fentanyl slowly over 3–5 minutes.
[c] Hydromorphone is a potent opioid and significant differences exist between oral and intravenous dosing. Use extreme caution when converting from one route to another. In converting from parenteral hydromorphone to oral hydromorphone, doses may need to be titrated up to 5 times the IV dose.
[d] Administer IV hydromorphone slowly over 2–3 minutes.
[e] Due to the complex nature and wide interindividual variation in the pharmacokinetics of methadone, methadone should only be commenced by practitioners experienced in its use.
[f] Methadone should initially be titrated like other strong opioids. The dosage may need to be reduced by 50% 2–3 days after the effective dose has been found to prevent adverse effects due to methadone accumulation. From then on, dosage increases should be performed at intervals of 1 week or over with a maximum dose increase of 50%.
[g] Administer IV methadone slowly over 3–5 minutes.
Source: WHO (2012), reference 2, p. 49.

effective. "By the child" indicates the need for individualization of each child's analgesic regimen, "tailoring pain treatment to the individual child."[2(p. 40)] Starting doses listed on tables are just that—starting doses. Each child's dose must be titrated up or down based on his or her response. If uncontrolled pain is present, opioids should be titrated upward until analgesic relief is obtained or unmanageable side effects occur. Although the WHO guidelines were developed for cancer pain, the same concepts can be used to guide pain management in children with chronic noncancer pain such as HIV/AIDS.

Use of nonopioids in children

Nonopioids (acetaminophen, NSAIDs, and aspirin) have a ceiling effect and cannot be safely titrated beyond the dose per weight given at drug-specific intervals. Pediatric dosage guidelines for commonly used nonopioid analgesics can be found in Tables 61.4 and 61.5.

Aspirin is not routinely used as an analgesic in infants and children because of the risk of Reye's syndrome associated with its use in this population, and it is not a preferred analgesic in pediatrics. The most widely used mild analgesic for children is acetaminophen.[57] The recommended weight-based dosing of acetaminophen in children is based on the dose response for antipyretic effects. Currently there is no safety data on long-term acetaminophen use in children.[22] The NSAIDs have been shown to be safe and effective analgesics for children. Children using NSAIDs have been shown to have greater weight-normalized clearance and volumes of distribution than adults but with similar drug half-lives. In order to decrease the change of dosage

error and toxicities, parents need to be educated regarding the proper use and administration of acetaminophen and NSAIDs.[57] Selective cyclooxygenase-2 inhibitors are now approved for limited indications in pediatrics. If traditional NSAIDs are contraindicated, drugs within this class may be used, though their safety and efficacy has only been established in children older than 2 years and for a maximum of 6 months for treatment of juvenile rheumatoid arthritis.[58]

Use of opioids in children

There is now significant data supporting the use of specific opioids in children and adolescents.[2,59–61] It takes until age 2 to 6 months for the weight-normalized clearance of many opioids to reach mature levels. Pharmacokinetic studies of morphine show an average serum half-life of 9 hours in preterm neonates, decreasing to 6.5 hours in full-term neonates and finally reaching 2 hours in the older infant. If not carefully monitored, neonates may be more likely to develop side effects from morphine due to decreased renal clearance of metabolites. The respiratory reflex response to hypoxemia, hypercapnia, and airway obstruction does not reach full maturity until 2 to 3 months after birth in both full-term and preterm infants. This can lead the nonintubated neonate receiving opioids to be at higher risk for respiratory depression.[32] Neonates receiving opioids or other agents that can compromise cardiorespiratory function must be continuously monitored in a setting equipped to provide airway management. Those receiving prolonged opioid therapy may benefit from the use of continuous infusions to avoid the variation in plasma concentrations that occurs with bolus dosing. In neonates receiving synthetic opioids, the administration of infusions over several minutes or of small, frequent aliquots is recommended to avoid the adverse effects of glottic and chest wall rigidity that are associated with rapid bolus injection of medications such as fentanyl and sufentanil.[10]

When using opioids with infants, children, and adolescents, the goal is to control pain as safely and quickly as possible. Avoid repeated administration of small, ineffective doses, which may prolong pain and worsen pain-related anxiety. For moderate to severe pain, it is appropriate to use opioids such as morphine, fentanyl, hydromorphone, and methadone in optimal doses titrated to an individual child's response.[2] Initial pediatric opioid dosing guidelines can be found in Table 61.6, Table 61.7, and Table 61.8. Meperidine, an opioid with a neurotoxic metabolite should be avoided in pediatric patients.[2]

The following case illustrates how opioids can be given and adjusted for the benefit of an individual child.

Case study

Mateo, a 12-year-old boy with a history of acute myelogenous leukemia, status post bone marrow transplant 2 years ago

At one point, Mateo had been on a prednisone maximal dose of 100 mg/day. Due to a recent graft versus host reaction, his prednisone was increased but is now being tapered. He is reporting bilateral hip pain, left greater than right. Because of this pain, he can only walk about 10 blocks, or ½ mile without severe pain, 9/10. His pain can wake him up from a sound sleep. His oncologist has started him on acetaminophen, 1000 mg po every 8 hours as needed. Mateo reports that this only helps a little bit, bring his pain down to 7/10 at best. An X-ray to his pelvis reveals severe bilateral sclerosis and collapse of his femoral heads, most severe on right. He was diagnosed with severe avascular necrosis of his hip secondary to steroid use. Mateo and his family wanted to avoid having hip replacements at this point in time. So, a plan was devised that included physical therapy and referral to the pediatric palliative care team.

The team determined a starting dose of morphine based on his weight (39.8 kg) and age (12 years). For a child from 2 to 12 years, the starting dose should be 200 to 500 mcg/kg every 4 hours. So they multiplied his weight 39.8 times 350 mcg and get a dose of 13.93 mg. But because the guidelines limit the maximum to 5 mg, the team prescribes 5 mg po q hour prn pain. Because of the dose size, it was necessary to provide this medication as a liquid solution (1 mg/mL

concentration, 5 mg dose = 5 mL) because a tablet form of this dose is not available. Mateo and his parents were instructed about how to take the morphine on an as-needed basis, how to manage opioid related constipation, and the usefulness of keeping a pain diary.

After about a week on this regimen, his pain diary was reviewed with the team. He was found to take six doses every day. His pain control had improved and ranged from 3 to 5/10. He was still waking up during the night from pain, but it was less severe. The team then started him on a prolonged-release morphine formulation. He was started on controlled-release morphine 15 mg po every 12 hours and continued on morphine sulfate 5 mg po every 4 hours as needed. On this regimen, Mateo found he only needed the prn dosing about twice a day, before his physical therapy or home exercise sessions. He tolerated the medications without problems and avoided constipation issues by staying on a bowel regimen.

PCA by proxy

Any discussion of opioid use in pediatrics would not be complete without a review of "PCA by proxy" and "authorized agent-controlled analgesia" or AACA. Patient-controlled analgesia is well established as a safe, effective method of pain control for children with moderate-to-severe pain in a variety of situations, including children in the last week of life. The risk of respiratory depression is lower because a sedated patient less likely to press the demand button.[62] Patient-controlled analgesia by proxy allows a person other than the patient to push the demand button. In 2004, JCAHO issued an alert regarding this practice, and in 2005 the ISMP also issued a sentinel alert advising against this practice. The challenge is that some children who are unable to push the dose button by themselves would benefit from use of a PCA device. Anghelescu[63] and colleagues identified four groups of patients who would benefit from AACA. They include those unable to control a PCA pump because of: (1) age (usually <5 years) or cognitive ability; (2) neuromuscular impairment; (3) the need to undergo a painful procedure; and (4) end-of-life.[63(p. 1625)] These children are often opioid tolerant. The literature and the ASPMN advocate for AACA as a means of safe, effective pain control when a designated proxy is carefully chosen and educated about appropriate use of a PCA for the child.[5,63,64] Any organization or institution setting up an AACA policy can refer to the recommendations of the ASPMN[7] along with Kenagy and Turner,[65] for guidelines in establishing proxy selection criteria, patient monitoring, and education of proxy and healthcare team members.

Use of adjuvant analgesics in children

Adjuvant analgesics are a heterogeneous group of medications that include psychostimulants, corticosteroids, anticonvulsants, antidepressants, radionuclides, and neuroleptics. Much of the evidence supporting their use in specific targeted pain syndromes comes from the adult literature. Although gabapentin has been studied as an anticonvulsant in children, it has yet to be investigated as an adjuvant analgesic in children despite widespread use as such.[2] It is recommended that a child have baseline hematological and biochemical laboratory studies and an electrocardiogram performed to rule out Wolff-Parkinson-White syndrome and other cardiac conduction defects before initiation of tricyclic antidepressants and at periodic intervals if the child receives long-term therapy or exceeds standard dose/weight guidelines.[22] Ketamine, a phencyclidine derivative, has been established a useful medication to consider for procedural sedation and analgesia when used by individuals who are trained in pediatric analgesia in pediatric settings.[66,67] Future research in the use of adjuvant analgesics in the pediatric population is needed.

The following case is an example of the usefulness of adjuvant analgesics as part of a comprehensive pain management plan.

Case study

Emily, a 17-year-old girl with recurrent, progressive germ cell tumor stage III, with severe polysensory neuropathy in lower extremities caused by carboplatin and etoposide

She has chronic, severe pain from her ankles to knees in both lower extremities which she describes as aching, sharp, and shooting. When she was first referred to the palliative care service, she was on fentanyl patches (350 mcg changed every 72 hours) but was then rotated to methadone (25 mg po q 8 hours around-the-clock) in the hopes that its NMDA receptor activity would help decrease her neuropathic pain. The methadone was gradually titrated upward to 60 mg po q 8 hours around-the-clock. She also had hydromorphone 20 mg po every 3 hours prn pain available to her. Emily typically needed to use 5 doses of prn hydromorphone a day.

Although this helped to a certain degree, Emily was not satisfied. Because of this, gabapentin was added to her regimen and gradually titrated up to a dose of 900 mg po q 8 hours. Initially, Emily found she had some problems with increased sleepiness; this problem resolved over time. With the use this adjuvant analgesia, Emily reported improved pain relief and only needed 1 to 3 prn doses of hydromorphone a day. Both Emily and her mother reported that she was more functional because of this. She and her family were open to a referral to an acupuncturist. She has started a series of acupuncture treatments as a nonpharmacological intervention. She has noticed some improvements after four sessions.

Use of local anesthetics and other anesthetic techniques

In the past, local anesthetics were not widely used in children because of concerns regarding cardiac depression and seizures. Today, they are administered by a variety of routes and have an acceptable safety profile. For bupivacaine, with or without epinephrine, the maximum recommended dose is 2 mg/kg for neonates and 2.5 mg/kg for other children. The maximum recommended dose for lidocaine in neonates is 4 mg/kg without epinephrine or 5 mg/kg with epinephrine. For children, the maximum recommended dose of lidocaine with epinephrine is 5 to 7 mg/kg.[32]

Over the past 25 years, local anesthetics have been increasingly used to help prevent pain associated with needle puncture of skin.[68] Intradermal administration of lidocaine can be effectively used for skin anesthesia if painful punctures will occur. The lidocaine can be buffered with 1 part sodium bicarbonate to 10 parts 1% or 2% lidocaine to avoid the stinging effects of lidocaine administration.[13] Several preparations of local anesthetics can be obtained for topical or transdermal administration to control procedural pain. Of these, eutectic mixture of local anesthetics (EMLA) is available as a cream or anesthetic disc and is approved for children age 37 weeks and older. One hour before puncture, the EMLA cream is placed over the site with an occlusive dressing applied to prevent or minimize puncture pain. Analgesic effectiveness is proportional to the amount of EMLA applied and the amount of time it is on prior to the needle stick. A 4% lidocaine cream (LMX4) has a quicker onset of action, 30 minutes, at a lower cost, and is approved for ages 2 years and up.[68] More expensive lidocaine/tetracaine topical patches have an onset of action of between 20 to 30 minutes

and can be used with children 3 years and older.[68] Lidocaine/adrenaline/tetracaine (LAT) or tetracaine/phenylephrine may be applied to open wounds for suturing, providing skin anesthesia for approximately 15 minutes. Because it contains adrenaline, which causes vasoconstriction, LAT must not be placed on distal arteries (located on tip of nose, earlobes, penis, fingers, and toes).[13] An iontophoretic device is commercially available that uses 10% lidocaine with epinephrine. This novel delivery sysytem only takes approximately 10 minutes of use before dermal anesthesia is achieved. This device may be somewhat frightening to young children, who may not like feeling its mild current, and it is only approved for children age 5 and older.[68] Recent advances in the technology of the noninvasive transdermal delivery systems has improved the speed of analgesic onset to the benefit of children. Widespread clinical implementation will depend on several factors including cost, adverse effects, and ease of use.[68]

The use of regional nerve blocks in anesthetized children to provide improved postoperative analgesia has expanded over the last 20 years and been shown to be both effective and safe. This technique, which involves the injection of long-acting bupivacaine or ropivacaine into nerves that innervate a designated area, can also be used to provide local anesthesia for surgical procedures such as circumcision or reduction of fractures.[69]

Long-acting anesthetics (e.g., bupivacaine, ropivacaine) can be given intraspinally (epidurally or intrathecally) in children. Administration of epidural medications (opioids, local anesthetics, clonidine) can effectively control pain in children, including preterm neonates.[70] They are often given for postoperative pain control after specific procedures or in children with chronic pain who have not tolerated or responded well to systemic therapy.[69] Readers desiring more detailed information regarding use of these interventional anesthetic techniques in the pediatric population are directed to a recent review article by Suresh, Birmingham, and Koxlowski.[69] Collaborations between pediatric anesthesia services, palliative care providers, and hospice agencies to provide safe, continuous neuraxial analgesia to children at the end of life, are now demonstrating better pain control with no limitations to where the child is discharged.[71]

A 2005 case study published in the *Journal of Clinical Oncology* by Saroyan et al. describes the role intraspinal analgesia played in the care of a 15-year-old girl with end-stage sarcoma. In this case, it was a valuable intervention for a number of reasons. It allowed the team to control her intractable pain approaching end-of-life, minimized the side effects of systemic therapy, and simplified a complex pain management plan. This ultimately allowed her to return home with her family, which was her wish.[72] The use of epidural analgesia in children requires special education and training on the part of the physicians and nurses. Careful dosing and administration of epidural medications and close postadministration observation are necessary to prevent serious complications. Nurses play a key role in setting the organizational and institutional standards for use of intraspinal analgesics in children.[31,32,69,71,73]

Nonpharmacological management

Nonpharmacological pain management interventions include psychological, physiatric, neurostimulatory, invasive, and integrative techniques. Components are frequently combined as part of a pediatric pain management plan; they are dependent on the comprehensive pain assessment of an individual child and are based on the presumed etiology of pain. In considering which nonpharmacological interventions might be beneficial, the nurse needs to look at several factors, including the child's and family's past experience with nondrug interventions. What has worked well and what has not? Are there religious or cultural issues or concerns that would make certain interventions inappropriate? Is the proposed intervention consistent with the developmental level of the child? What is the present cognitive status of the child? Has the stress and fatigue from a prolonged illness made it difficult for the child or family members to concentrate, follow directions, or learn new information? Also, the nurse should consider teaching potentially useful techniques before the skills are needed.[74]

Psychological interventions can include patient and family education, cognitive interventions, and behavioral techniques such as writing in a pain diary. Pain diaries may be especially useful in working with children who have recurrent or chronic pain, and their use has some value in pediatric pain research.[13] Children who enjoy writing may benefit from a private place to express themselves. Young children who have not mastered the written word may find drawing about their pain and pain experiences helpful. Developments in technology lend themselves to this process. For example, smart phones are being explored as a way for children and adolescents with sickle cell disease to access a Web-based e-diary to report pain and other symptoms in a timely way.[75]

The value of cognitive techniques such as distraction and relaxation is well established in children. A recent Cochrane review supports the emerging use of psychological therapies, primarily cognitive and behavioral therapies, to treat children with chronic or recurrent pain from headache and nonheadache pain.[76] Another Cochrane review of the use of psychological nonpharmacological techniques found sufficient evidence to recommend using techniques such as coaching, distraction, and hypnosis to help children cope with procedural pain.[77] Across studies, distraction has been shown to reduce children's behavioral distress during procedural pain, although it has a variable effect on pain intensity. Various distracters have been used for children's pain management, including bubble-blowing, party blowers, puppetry, video games, and listening to music. The distractor is more likely to be effective if it is age appropriate and complementary to the interests and preferences of the individual child.[4] Nurses working with infants and toddlers, to age 2 years, may distract them with mobiles, rocking, stroking, or patting. Children from 2 to 4 years of age may find blowing bubbles, breathing, puppet play, or storytelling useful distractions. Four- to 6-year-olds like these activities and may also like television shows and talking about favorite places. School-age children can be distracted with these activities and may also be receptive to humor, counting, or thumb squeezing. Progressive muscle relaxation exercise is used most effectively in older children and adolescents but can also be taught to children as young as age 5 years. Guided imagery, which ideally incorporates all of a child's senses, can help children "escape" to a safe favorite place unique to that child. Sometimes children like to imagine doing a favorite activity, such as swimming or skating.[78] It is estimated that 30% to 84% of children use complementary medicine such as acupuncture. Despite reports that acupuncture is offered in at least 30% of pediatric pain centers, there is little data regarding its use in children. It is postulated that this may be related to the possibility of fear of needles that children may have.[79] More research is needed regarding the safety, efficacy, and acceptability of the use of some complementary or integrative approaches (e.g., acupuncture) in children with pain in large,

well-designed studies before these modalities can be routinely recommended. Such data can potentially establish other credible choices for assisting children with pain as well.[80]

Nurses caring for children with pain have both collaborative and independent functions when implementing nonpharmacological interventions. Psychological interventions that a nurse should feel comfortable initiating include patient-family education and cognitive techniques such as distraction, relaxation, positive self-statements, and pain diaries. An individual nurse might initiate the use of music as a relaxation or distraction technique. Independent physiatric interventions can include movement and positioning and swaddling of neonates. Collaborative efforts may involve massage, vibration, or use of superficial heat or cold. (Protecting the child's skin by placing the heat or cold source in commercially available animal wraps or using towels decorated with favorite characters may make the experience more enjoyable for young children.) The nurse needs to know which members of a child's primary team are knowledgeable in the use of nonpharmacological techniques and which special consultants are available to help if needed.[74] The American Massage Therapy Association (AMTA) is a resource in finding an accredited massage therapist.[81] Child-life specialists can be a resource for employing distraction and other psychological pain management techniques such as providing information/preparation, medical play, and positive reinforcement in children.[82] Promising cognitive techniques such as biofeedback and hypnosis, although potentially useful for children with chronic pain, require the use of trained instructors for initiation.[79] Also, more robust clinical studies of hypnosis and its effectiveness and acceptability are needed prior to recommending it as part of a "best practice" guideline.[13,83]

The resources available to the nurse (including time available to initiate a particular intervention, education in a particular technique, availability of patient/family educational materials, and availability and affordability of particular devices) play a role in what techniques are initiated with an individual child.[74] For some children, the Internet may be a useful way to deliver family cognitive-behavioral interventions as demonstrated in a recent study by Palermo and colleagues.[84] The Institute of Medicine noted that the teaching of cognitive behavioral techniques, despite their demonstrated effectiveness, is not done in as rigorous or consistent a way as is observed for other clinical modalities.[29] A start has recently been made in teaching developmentally appropriate, cognitive-behavioral strategies to nursing students. Results of a study that looked at the effects of this type of program revealed that program participants had an improved knowledge of these strategies and were better able to implement them.[85]

Procedural pain management

Procedural pain is a widespread experience for most children interacting with the healthcare system. Hospitalized children, who may or may not be dealing with a life-threatening illness, commonly undergo painful procedures. In a recent Canadian study of hospitalized children, 78% experienced a painful procedure within a 24-hour period prior to data collection.[86] Nurses who know how to successfully address procedural pain, using both pharmacological and nonpharmacological techniques, can help a very large number of children. Procedural pain is the one area in the pain literature that is much better developed for children than for adults, who may also experience this problem. The goals of successful procedural pain management include minimizing pain, maximizing patient cooperation, and minimizing risk to the patient.[20]

Anticipation is the key word. Having procedures performed by technically competent individuals can reduce both risk of pain and risk of harm. The medical personnel involved must be knowledgeable in both pharmacological and nonpharmacological pain management appropriate to the child and the situation. Nonpharmacological interventions can focus on the immediate environment and also on behavioral techniques.[20] Both children and parents need appropriate information regarding what will happen and how they can decrease stress.[39]

How pain is avoided or managed the first time a child undergoes a particular procedure influences how the child anticipates and copes with subsequent procedures. It is recommended that pain and anxiety be maximally treated the very first time a child undergoes a procedure.[20] Depending on the procedure and the individual child, this can be as simple as providing information and topical analgesics or vapocoolant immediately before needle punctures or as complex as administering conscious sedation with the combination of an opioid analgesic and a benzodiazepine. Conscious sedation can help to manage anxiety, pain, and procedural complications in young children, and its use should be considered and advocated if a child is experiencing a heightened stress reaction.[87] It is important to bear in mind that the use of anxiolytics or sedatives alone does not provide analgesia but does render a child unable to communicate distress.

Conscious sedation/moderate sedation and analgesia are a part of the sedation continuum that is referred to as procedural sedation and analgesia (PSA). Procedural sedation and analgesia is a method of managing a child's pain and anxiety using pharmacological agents by qualified practitioners and should be tailored to each child's goal for a specific situation. Depending on the child and situation, the goal could be for analgesia, anxiety relief, or both.[87] Many institutions are considering the addition of a pediatric sedation team to promote safe and effective use of PSA.[88] A detailed review of PSA is beyond the scope of this chapter. Readers desiring practical information regarding safe and effective use of PSA for children in their practice setting are referred to articles listed in the reference section.[13,20]

It is useful to discuss coping strategies with the child and parents, if possible, long before the medical procedure. This enables them to mentally rehearse ways in which they can cope with the situation when it occurs.[39] Review of the literature by Christensen and Fatchett[89] revealed that distraction, relaxation, and imagery are effective for children in decreasing anxiety and pain associated with painful procedures. Therapeutic play and orientation to the room and equipment may help to promote patient cooperation. Risk can be minimized by having all equipment, supplies, and staff ready and available for both routine and emergency care.

Other things the nurse can do to facilitate comfort for children during stressful procedures include inviting the caregiver to be present and attending to environmental factors. This includes using a treatment room whenever possible; creating a pleasant environment; minimizing noxious noises, sounds, and sights; and maintaining a calm, positive manner. Attending to these details can not only increase the comfort of the parents and the child but also that of the healthcare personnel involved.[20] Finally, during and after the procedure, the nurse needs to

provide ongoing assessment of pain and anxiety and work to collaborate and modify the treatment plan if suboptimal control of either occurs.

Where improvement is needed

All children are vulnerable to inadequate pain assessment and management. Those most vulnerable include the preverbal child, the cognitively or neurologically impaired child, immigrant children, and children without homes or consistent caregivers. Future work may need to look at the best ways to elicit symptoms such as pain, beyond the standard aspects of validity and reliability. Researchers need to clarify the effects of culture on the experience of pain in children.[17,40] System issues that interact with the barriers discussed earlier also need to be addressed (see Table 61.3).[2] For example, children cared for in pediatric tertiary care centers may find that healthcare professionals in their home environment lack up-to-date information about pain assessment and comprehensive pain control in children.[29]

Long-term follow-up and outcome expectations and monitoring are important in preventing, anticipating, and alleviating pain in the pediatric population. Implementing a successful pediatric pain management program is more complicated than just selecting a pain assessment tool and requires a commitment of resources.[3] To follow up in a systematic way and promote the timely and adequate use of appropriate medications and behavioral interventions for children, initiatives have been started that work to develop and implement evidence-based pediatric pain assessment and management protocols.[29,90–92] A recent study looking at opioid use in dying children during the last week of life in pediatric oncology units in 33 different children's hospitals in the United States revealed much variation in continuous prescription of opioids, even after controlling for the clinical characteristics of the patients. A study such as this is the beginning of the process to determine or establish quality indicators that could be used to assess quality of pediatric end-of-life care across practice settings.[93] Disease-specific guidelines have been developed for children with SCD[23] and JCA,[53] and a position paper has been published by the Association of Pediatric Oncology Nurses for pain management of the child with cancer at the end of life.[94] Groups are focusing on the analgesic needs of the neonatal population.[95] It is hoped that pain will receive this kind of attention in other pediatric populations and that these valuable, classic guidelines and position papers will be updated to reflect the current state of the art.

Pediatric groups are striving to achieve organizational changes in pediatric pain management.[96,97] This can happen in many ways. In some settings it involves creating a formal pediatric pain or palliative care service. In other settings it may involve basic quality improvement programs.[98] To start to improve the process of pain management, it is necessary to collect information about the present process, to develop an awareness of all the various factors that may either promote or deter achievement of the desired outcome. The literature reveals several efforts to collect baseline information about pain management and areas for improvement.[95,98] One area to consider is that of pain medication errors. Sources of errors in pediatric medication administration include dilution errors, milligram-microgram errors, decimal point errors, and confusion between a total daily dose and a fractional dose.[32,99,100] Through application of the quality improvement process, nurses can play an important role in improving pain control for both the individual children they care for and other children that they may not be directly involved with.

Summary

Despite the significant increase in knowledge about assessment and management of pain in infants and children, too many suffering children do not receive proper treatment. In today's age of "powerful, invasive medicine, we can save more lives, but any wrong choice turns medicine into torture, inflicting avoidable sufferings on patients."[101(p. 2)] Pediatric palliative care exists to mitigate suffering in children with life-threatening illnesses.[1,42] To prevent suffering for children and their families, nurses and other healthcare professionals must apply the most up-to-date techniques of pain assessment and management to all children they care for, especially from the time a child receives a diagnosis of a potentially life-threatening illness through his or her survival or death. By application of an integrated treatment plan that is based on the developmental level of the individual child, involves his or her family, and uses both pharmacological and nonpharmacological interventions, optimal pain control is possible.[1]

References

1. Klick JC, Hauer J. Pediatric palliative care. Curr Probl Pediatr Adolesc Health Care. 2010;40:120–151.
2. WHO guidelines on the pharmacological treatment of persisting pain in children with medical illnesses. Geneva, Switzerland: WHO Press; 2012.
3. McGrath PJ. Science is not enough: the modern history of pediatric pain. Pain. 2011;152:2457–2459.
4. Gauvain-Piquard A, Rodary C, Rezvani A, Serbouti S. The development of the DEGR®: a scale to assess pain in young children with cancer. Eur J Pain. 1999;2:165–176.
5. Knegt NC, Pieper MJC, Lobbezoo F, Schuengel C, Evenhuis HM, Passchier J, et al. Behavioral pain indicators in people with intellectual disabilities: a systematic review. J Pain. 2013;14(9):885–896.
6. Silva FC, Thuler LC. Cross-cultural adaption and translation of two pain assessment tools in children and adolescents. J Pediatr (Rio J). 2008;84(4):344–349.
7. Pain terms: A list with definitions and notes on usage. Recommended by the International Association for the Study of Pain Subcommittee on Taxonomy. Pain. 1979;6:249–252.
8. McCaffery M, Pasero C. Pain: Clinical Manual. 2nd ed. St. Louis, MO: Mosby; 1999.
9. Cooney MF, Czarnecki M, Dunwoody C, Eksterpwicz N, Merkel S, Oakes L, et al. American Society for Pain Management nursing position statement with clinical practice guidelines: authorized agent controlled analgesia. Pain Manage Nurs. 2013;14(3):176–181.
10. American Academy of Pediatrics, Canadian Pediatric Society. Prevention and management of pain and stress in the neonate. Pediatrics. 2000;105:454–461.
11. Wolfe J, Hammel J, Edwards K, et al. Easing of suffering in children with cancer at the end of life: is care changing? J Clin Oncol. 2008;26(10):1717–1723.
12. Walco GA, Dworkin RH, Krane EJ, LeBel AA, Treede R-D. Neuropathic pain in children: special considerations. Mayo Clin Proc. 2010;85(3):S33–S41.
13. Jacob E. Pain assessment and management in children. In: Hockenberry MJ, Wilson D (eds.), Wong's Nursing Care of Infants and Children (9th ed). St Louis, MO: Elsevier Mosby; 2011:179–226.
14. Corry NH, Klick B, Fauerbach JA. Posttraumatic stress disorder and pain impact functioning and disability after major burn injury. J Burn Care Res. 2010;31(1):13–25.
15. World Health Organization. Cancer Pain Relief and Palliative Care in Children. Geneva, Switzerland: WHO; 1998.
16. Collins JJ. Management of symptoms associated with cancer: pain management. In: Carroll WL, Finlay JL (eds.), Cancer in children and adolescents. Sudbury, MA: Jones and Bartlett; 2009.
17. Ruland CM, Hamilton GA, Schjodt-Osmo B. The complexity of symptoms and problems experienced in children with cancer: a review of the literature. J Pain Symptom Manage. 2009;37(3):403–418.
18. Friedrichsdorf SJ. Pain management in children with advanced cancer and during end-of-life care. Pediatr Hematol Oncol. 2010;27:257–261.
19. Ljungman G, Gordh T, Sorensen S, Kreuger A. Pain variations during cancer treatment in children: a descriptive survey. Pediatr Hemacol Oncol. 2000;17:211–221.
20. Cramton REM, Gruchala NE. Managing procedural pain in pediatric patients. Curr Opin Pediatrics. 2012;24(4):530–538.
21. Padhyre B, Dalla-Pozza L, Little DG, Munns CF. Use of zoledronic acid for chemotherapy related osteonecrosis in children and adolescents: a retrospective analysis. Pediatr Blood Cancer. 2013;60:1539–1545.
22. Collins JJ, Berde CB, Frost JA. Pain assessment and management. In: Wolfe J, Hinds PS, Sourkes BM (eds.), Textbook of Interdisciplinary Pediatric Palliative Care. Philadelphia, PA: Elsevier Saunders; 2011:284–299.
23. American Pain Society. Guidelines for the Management of Acute and Chronic Pain in Sickle Cell Disease. Glenview, IL: APS; 1999.
24. Vijrnyhits S, Stinson J, Friedman J, Palozzi L, Taddioa A, Scolnik D, et al. Benchmarking pain outcomes for children with sickle cell disease hospitalized in a tertiary referral pediatric hospital. Pain Res Manage. 2012;17(4):291–296.
25. Po C, Colombatti R, Cirgliano A, Da Dalt L, Agosto C, Benini F, et al. The management of sickle pain in the emergency department. Clin J Pain. 2013;29(1):60–63.
26. Shah N, Rollins M, Landi D, Shah R, Bae J, De Castro LM. Differences in pain management between hematologists and hospitalists caring for patients with sickle cell disease hospitalized for vasoocclusive crisis. Clin J Pain. 2014;30(3):266–268.
27. Gillis VL, Dzingina M, Chamberlain K, Banks E, Baker MR, Longson D. Guidelines: management of an acute painful sickle cell episode in hospital: summary of NICE guidance. BMJ. 2012;344:e4063 doi;10.1136/bmj.34064.
28. Russo R, Miller M, Haan E, Cameron I, Crotty M. Pain characteristics and their association with quality of life and self-concept in children with hemiplegic cerebral palsy identified from a population register. Clin J Pain. 2008;24(4):335–342.
29. Field MJ, Behrman R, eds. When Children Die: Improving Palliative and End-of-Life Care for Children and Their Families. Report of the Institute of Medicine Task Force. Washington, DC: National Academy Press; 2003.
30. Hartley C, Slater R. Neurophysiological measures of nociceptive brain activity in the newborn infant—the next steps. Acta Paediat. 2013;doi:10.1111/apa.12490
31. American Academy of Pediatrics, Canadian Pediatric Society. Prevention and management of pain and stress in the neonate. Pediatrics. 2000;105:454–461.
32. Berde CB, Sethna NF. Analgesics for the treatment of pain in children. N Engl J Med. 2003;347:1094–1103.
33. Lawrence J, Alcock D, McGrath P, Kay J, MacMurray SB, Dulberg C. The development of a tool to assess neonatal pain expression. Neonatal Netw. 1993;12:59–66.
34. Krechel SW, Bildner J. CRIES: a new neonatal postoperative pain measurement tool: initial testing of validity and reliability. Paediatr Anaesth. 1995;5:53–61.
35. Stevens BJ, Johnson C, Petryshen P, Taddio A. Premature infant pain profile: development and initial validation. Clin J Pain. 1996;12:13–22.
36. Grunau RVE, Craig KD. Facial activity as a measure of neonatal pain expression. In: Tyler EC, Krane EJ (eds.), Advances in Pain Research Therapy: Pediatric Pain. Vol. 15. New York, NY: Raven Press; 1990:147–155.

37. Levetown M, ed. Compendium of Pediatric Palliative Care. Alexandria, VA: National Hospice and Palliative Care Organization; 2000.

38. McGrath PJ, Johnson G, Goodman JT, Dunn J, Chapman J. CHEOPS: a behavioral scale for rating postoperative pain in children. In: Fields HL, Dubner R, Cervero F (eds.), Advances in Pain Research and Therapy. Vol. 9. New York, NY: Raven Press; 1985:395–402.

39. Power N, Liossi C, Franck L. Helping parents to help their child with procedural and everyday pain: practical, evidence-based advice. J Spec Pediatr Nurs. 2007;12(3):203–209.

40. Davies B, Contro N, Larson J, Widger K. Culturally-sensitive information-sharing in pediatric palliative care. Pediatrics. 2010;125(4):e559–e865.

41. Jacob E, Mack AK, Savedra M, Van Cleve L, Wilkie DJ. Adolescent pediatric pain tool for multidimensional measurement of pain in children and adolescents. Pain Manage Nurs. 2013;S1524-9042(13)00032-5. doi: 10.1016/j.pmn.2013.03.002. [Epub ahead of print.]

42. Levine D, Lam CG, Cunningham MJ, Remke S, Chrastek J, Klick J, et al. Best practices for pediatric palliative care: a primer for clinical providers. J Support Oncol. 2013;11(3):114–125.

43. McGrath PA, Brown SC. Pain control. In: Doyle D, Hanks G, Cherny N, et al. (eds.), Oxford Textbook of Palliative Medicine. 3rd ed. New York, NY: Oxford University Press; 2004.

44. Jacob E, McCarthy K, Sambuco G, Hockenberry M. Intensity, location, and quality of pain in Spanish-speaking children with cancer. Pediatr Nurs. 2008;34(1):45–52.

45. Hockenberry MJ, Wilson D, eds. Wong's Nursing Care of Infants and Children. 9th ed. St Louis, MO: Elsevier Mosby; 2011.

46. von Baeyer C, Spagrud L. Systematic review of observational (behavioral) measures of pain for children and adolescents aged 3 to 18 years. Pain. 2007;127(1–2):140–150.

47. Anand KJ. Physiology of pain in infants and children. In: Pain in infancy and childhood. Annales Nestle. 1999;57:1–12.

48. Ghai B, Kaur Makkar J, Wig J. Postoperative pain assessment in preverbal children and children with cognitive impairment. Paediatr Anaesth. 2008;18:462–477.

49. Srouji R, Ratnapalan S, Schneeweiss. Pain in children: assessment and nonpharmacological management. Int J Pediatr. 2010;pii:474838. doi:10.1155/2010/47438. Epub 2010 Jul 25.

50. HUNT A. Pain assessment. In: Goldman A, Hain R, Liben S. (eds.), Oxford Textbook of Palliative Care for Children. 2nd ed. New York, NY: Oxford University Press; 2012:204–217.

51. Huguet A, McGrath PJ, Pardos J. Development and preliminary testing of a scale to assess pain-related fear in children and adolescents. J Pain. 2011;12:840–848.

52. Baker C, Wong D. Q.U.E.S.T.: a process of pain assessment in children. Orthop Nurs. 1987;6:11–21.

53. American Pain Society. Guideline for the Management of Pain in Osteoarthritis, Rheumatoid Arthritis, and Juvenile Chronic Arthritis. 2nd ed. Glenview, IL: APS; 2002.

54. Roberts R, Rodriquez W, Murphy D, Crescenzi T. Pediatric drug labeling: improving the safety and efficacy of pediatric therapies. JAMA. 2003;290:905–911.

55. Clarke PE. FDA encourages pediatric information on drug labeling. 2011. Last updated on May 11, 2011. Available on http://www.fda.gov/Drugs/ResourcesForYou/SpecialFeatures/ucm254072.htm.

56. Koren K. Codeine, ultrarapid-metabolism genotype, and postoperative death. N Engl J Med. 2009;8:827–828.

57. Bárzaga Arencibia Z, Choonara I. Balancing the risks and benefits of the use of over-the-counter pain medications in children. Drug Saf. 2012;35(12):1119–1125.

58. Nallani S, et al. Clinical Pharmacology BPCA Summary Review. 2006; Available at http://www.fda.gov/downloads/Drugs/DevelopmentApprovalProcess/DevelopmentResources/UCM162534.pdf.

59. Krekels EH, Tibboel D, Kanhof M, Knibbe CA. Prediction of morphine clearance in the paediatric population: how accurate are the available pharmacokinetic models? Clin Pharmacokinet. 2012;51(11):695–709.

60. Zernikow B, Michel E, Anderson B. Transdermal fentanyl in childhood and adolescence: a comprehensive literature review. J Pain. 2007;8(3):187–207.

61. Davies D, DeVlaming D, Haines C. Methadone analgesia for children with advanced cancer. Pediatr Blood Cancer. 2008;51(3):393–397.

62. Schiessl C, Gravou C, Zernikow B, Sittl R, Griessinger N. Use of patient-controlled analgesia for pain control in dying children. Support Care Cancer. 2008;16:531–536.

63. Anghelescu D, Burgoyne L, Oakes L, Wallace D. The safety of patient-controlled analgesia by proxy in pediatric oncology patients. Anesth Analg. 2005;101:1623–1627.

64. Czarnecki M, Ferrise A, Mano K, et al. Parent/nurse-controlled analgesia for children with developmental delay. Clin J Pain. 2008;24(9):817–824.

65. Kenagy A, Turner H. Pediatric patient-controlled analgesia by proxy. AACN Adv Crit Care. 2007;18(4):361–365.

66. Morton N. Ketamine for procedural sedation and analgesia in pediatric emergency medicine: a UK perspective. Paediatr Anaesth. 2008;18:25–29.

67. Dallimore D, Herd D, Short T, Anderson, B. Dosing ketamine for pediatric procedural sedation in the emergency room department. Pediatr Emerg Care. 2008;24(8):529–533.

68. Mosiman W, Pile D. Emerging therapies in pediatric pain management. J Infus Nurs. 2013;36(2):98–106.

69. Suresh S, Birmingham PK, Kozlowski RJ. Pediatric pain management. Anesthesiol Clin. 2012;30:101–117.

70. Bosenberg A, Flick RP. Regional anesthesia in neonates and infants. Clin Perinatol. 2013;40(3):525–538.

71. Anghelescu DL, Faughnan LG, Baker JN, Yang J, Kane JR. Use of epidural and peripheral nerve blocks at the end of life in children and young adults with cancer: the collaboration between a pain service and a palliative care service. Pediatr Anesth. 2010;20:1070–1077.

72. Saroyan J, Schechter W, Tresgallo M, Granowetter L. Role of intraspinal analgesia in terminal pediatric malignancy. J Clin Oncol. 2005;23(6):1318–1321.

73. Anghelescu D, Ross C, Oakes L, Burgoyne L. The safety of concurrent administration of opioids via epidural and intravenous routes for postoperative pain in pediatric oncology patients. J Pain Symptom Manage. 2008;35(4):412–419.

74. Coyle N, Layman-Goldstein M. Pain assessment and pharmacological/nonpharmacological interventions. In: Matzo ML, Sherman DW (eds.), Palliative Care Nursing: Quality Care to the End of Life. 3rd ed. New York, NY: Springer; 2010:357–410.

75. Jacob E, Stinson J, Duran J, Gupta A Gerla M, Ann Lewis M, et al. Usability testing of a smartphone for accessing a web-based e-diary for self-monitoring of pain and symptoms in sickle cell disease. Pediatr Hematol Oncol. 2012;34(5): 326–335.

76. Eccleston C, Palerma TM, Williams ACDC, Lewandowski A, Morley S, Fisher E, et al. Psychological therapies for the management of chronic and recurrent pain in children and adolescents (Review). Cochrane Library. 2013;8:1–81.

77. Uman L, Chambers C, McGrath P, Kisely S. Psychological interventions for needle-related procedural pain and distress in children and adolescents. Cochrane Database System Rev. 2006;(4):1–77.

78. Kuttner L. Pain: an integrative approach. In: Goldman A, Hain R, Liben S (eds.), Oxford Textbook of Palliative Care for Children. 2nd ed. New York, NY: Oxford University Press; 2012:260–270.

79. Johnson AM, Steinhorn DM. Integrative medicine in paediatric palliative care. In: Goldman A, Hain R, Liben S (eds.), Oxford Textbook of Palliative Care for Children. 2nd ed. New York, NY: Oxford University Press; 2012:377–390.

80. Adams D, Cheng F, Jou H, Aung S, Yasui Y, Vohra S. The safety of pediatric acupuncture: a systematic review. Pediatrics. 2011;128(6):e1575–e1587.

81. Hughes D, Ladas E, Rooney D, Kelly K. Massage therapy as a supportive care intervention for children with cancer. Oncol Nurs Forum. 2008;35(3):431–442.

82. Bandstra N, Skinner L, LeBlanc C, et al. The role of child life in pediatric pain management: a survey of child life specialists. J Pain. 2008;9(4):320–329.

83. Uman LS, Birnie KA, Noel M, Parker JA, Chambers CT, McGrath PJ, et al. Psychological interventions for needle-related procedural pain and distress in children and adolescents. Cochrane Database Syst Rev. 2013 Oct 10;10:CD005179. doi: 10.1002/14651858.CD005179.pub3. PMID: 24108531 [PubMed—in process]

84. Palermo TM, Wilson AC, Peters M, Lewandowski A, Somhegyi H. Randomized controlled trial of an internet-delivered family cognitive-behavioral therapy interventions for children and adolescents with chronic pain. Pain. 2009;146:205–213.

85. MacLaren J, Cohen L, Larkin K, Shelton E. Training nursing students in evidence-based techniques for cognitive-behavioral pediatric pain management. J Nurs Educ. 2008;47(8):351–358.

86. Stevens BJ, Abbott LK, Yamada J, Harrison D, Stinson J, Taddio A, et al. Epidemiology and management of painful procedures in children in Canadian hospitals. CMAJ: Canadian Med Assoc J. 2011;183:E403–E410.

87. Meredith JR, O'Keefe KP, Galwankar S. Pediatric procedural sedation and analgesia. J Emerg Trauma Shock. 2008;1(2):88–96.

88. Davis C. Does your facility have a pediatric sedation team? If not, why not? Pediatr Nurs. 2008;34(4):308–318.

89. Christensen J, Fatchett D. Promoting parental use of distraction and relaxation in pediatric oncology patients during invasive procedures. J Pediatr Oncol Nurs. 2002;19:127–132.

90. Zhu LM, Stinson J, Palozzi L, Weingarten K, Hogan ME, Duong A, et al. Improvements in pain outcomes in a Canadian pediatric teaching hospital following implementation of a multifaceted knowledge translation initiative. Pain Res Manage. 2012;17(3):173–179.

91. Noll RB, Patel SK, Embry L, Hardy KK, Pelletier W, Annett RD, et al; COG Behavioral Sciences Committee. Children's Oncology Group's 2013 blueprint for research: behavioral science. Pediatr Blood Cancer. 2013;60(6):1048–1054.

92. Latimer MA, Ritchie JA, Johnson CC. Individual nurse and organizational context considerations for better knowledge use in pain care. J Pediatr Nurs. 2010;25(4):274–281.

93. Orsey A, Belasco J, Ellenberg J, Schmitz K, Feudtner C. Variation in receipt of opioids by pediatric oncology patients who died in children's hospitals. Pediatr Blood Cancer. 2008. doi: 10.1002/pbc:1–6.

94. Hooke C, Hellstren MB, Stutzer C, Forte K. Pain management for the child with cancer in end-of-life care: APON position paper. J Pediatr Oncol Nurs. 2002;19:43–47.

95. Bigham MT, Schwartz HP. Ohio Neonatal/Pediatric Transport Quality Collaborative. Quality metrics in neonatal and pediatric critical care transport: A consensus statement. Pediatric Critical Care Medicine. 2013;14(5):518–524.

96. Dowden S, McCathy M, Chalkiadis G. Achieving organizational change in pediatric pain management. Pain Res Manage. 2008;13(4):321–326.

97. Oakes L, Anghelescu D, Windsor K, Barnhill P. An institutional quality improvement initiative for pain management for pediatric cancer patients. J Pain Symptom Manage. 2008;35(6):656–669.

98. Johnson D, Nagel K, Friedman D, Meza J, Hurwitz C, Friebert S. Availability and use of palliative care and end-of-life services for pediatric oncology patients. J Clin Oncol. 2008;26(28):4646–4650.

99. Broussard L. Small size, big risk: preventing neonatal and pediatric medication errors. Nurs Womens Health. 2010;14(5):405–408.

100. Tzimenatos L, Bond GR; Pediatric Therapeutic Error Study Group. Severe injury or death in young children from therapeutic errors: a summary of 238 cases from the American Association of Poison Control Centers. Clin Toxicol (Phila). 2009;47(4):348–354.

101. Facco E, Giron G. The nature of pain and the approach to the suffering child. Suffering Child. 2003;2(February):1–3. Available at: http://www.thesufferingchild.net. Accessed February 28, 2005.

SECTION VII

Special issues for the nurse in end-of-life care

CHAPTER 62

The advanced practice registered nurse

Clareen Wiencek

The advanced practice registered nurse brings a unique and essential perspective to the discipline of palliative care—to focus holistically on the patient and family as the unit of care, and to combine advanced skills in assessment, diagnosis, and management. These nurses drive team-based care for optimal patient-level and program-level outcomes.

Key points

◆ Palliative care relieves suffering and improves quality of life for patients with serious or life-threatening illness and their families by offering symptom management, care coordination, and psychosocial and spiritual support from the time of diagnosis through the period of bereavement.

◆ Advanced practice nursing builds on the strong foundation of nursing practice by incorporating advanced knowledge and expertise in assessment, diagnosis, and management of persons with serious or life-limiting illness. In addition, the palliative care advanced practice registered nurse (APRN) demonstrates skilled communication and the ability to drive treatment plans based on the goals and preferences of the patient and family.

◆ Advanced practice nursing in palliative care is recognized as a specialty with its own scope and standards of practice, education, and certification. The APRN Consensus Model, issued in 2008 and projected for full implementation in 2015, brings great potential to standardize licensure, accreditation, certification, and education of all APRNs enabling practice at the full scope and therefore ensuring greater impact on patient care and quality outcomes.

◆ Palliative care APRNs contribute to the financial viability of palliative care programs by providing cost-effective care and completing billing and reimbursement processes.

Numerous initiatives and studies over the last 2 decades have identified the critical need for better care of persons with serious or life-threatening illness and for their families.[1-3] Palliative care has grown as a discipline in response to that critical need. Palliative care means patient-family centered care that optimizes quality of life by anticipating and treating suffering. Palliative care addresses the physical, emotional, social, and spiritual needs of patients and facilitates patient autonomy and choice whether or not the patient chooses to be treated simultaneously with life-prolonging therapies.[4]

Within a changing healthcare environment, APRNs have demonstrated their ability to adapt to the challenges posed by an aging population and by the increasing prevalence of chronic and life-limiting diseases concomitant with aging. Additionally, APRNs can help patients and families to navigate an increasingly complex and fragmented healthcare system. A systematic review of APRN outcomes from 1990 to 2008 found that outcomes for APRNs are similar and in some cases better than those produced by physicians alone and that APRNs provide effective and high-quality patient care.[5]

Historical perspective and implementation of the advanced practice registered nurses consensus model

In the early 20th century, nurses who had completed postgraduate coursework, or who had extensive expertise in a particular clinical area, were called specialists.[6] They were the predecessors of today's APRNs. In 1954, the first clinical nurse specialist (CNS) program was created at Rutgers University and in 1965 the first nurse practitioner (NP) program was established at the University of Colorado.[6,7] Initially, these roles were described as extending beyond the scope of nursing due to the inclusion of some practices and procedures from medicine. It was not until the 1980s that the term "advanced practice" was adopted after growth within graduate nursing education allowed nurses to obtain advanced expertise within the field of nursing.[6] As defined by Hamric and colleagues in their textbook on the advanced practice role, APRNs have advanced knowledge and expertise in performing histories and physical examinations, ordering and interpreting diagnostic tests, and prescribing medications and other therapies appropriate for the management of particular symptoms or diseases.[8] But the rapid growth in APRN programs and practitioners during the 1980s led to concerns among the members of the National Council of State Boards of Nursing (NCSBN) about the lack of clear practice standards, inconsistency among state regulations that impacted APRN portability, and variation in educational programs.[9] These concerns led the NCSBN to develop and release the Consensus Model for APRN Regulation: Licensure, Accreditation, Certification, and Education (LACE) in 2008.[9,10] Since 2008, over 44 nursing organizations have endorsed this Model with full implementation planned for 2015.[9] The LACE regulation is the vehicle responsible for this full implementation of the APRN Consensus Model, and representatives from each of the LACE constituencies continue to work toward this goal.

The APRN Consensus Model endorses a uniform model of regulation for the legal status of advanced practice nursing designed to align licensure, accreditation, certification, and education and to support full scope of practice by all APRNs. It provides a definitive foundation for nurses who choose or plan to pursue advanced practice and has impact on licensing boards, certification corporations, schools of nursing, and accreditation entities.[9] The definition of each element of advanced practice is central to the Model. Licensure is the granting of authority to practice. Accreditation is the formal review and approval by a recognized agency of degree or certification in nursing. Certification is the formal recognition of the knowledge, skills, and experience identified by a professional association and with the intent to protect the consumer. Finally, education is the formal preparation in graduate level or postgraduate certificate programs.

The APRN Consensus Model has two main components: APRN roles and population foci with additional APRN specialties, such as palliative care.[11] "Advanced Practice Registered Nurse" or APRN is the new legal title and recognized credential to be used by any nurse licensed in any of these four roles: certified nurse practitioner (CNP), certified registered nurse anesthetist (CRNA), certified nurse-midwife (CNM), and clinical nurse specialist (CNS). The Model has helped to bring consistency to all four roles, which should include graduate level education in an accredited program; national certification; educational preparation in the core courses of advanced physiology, pharmacology, and assessment; and the provision of direct care to a patient population.[10]

The other main component of the APRN Consensus Model is the population of focus. The Model asserts that the APRN is educated in at least one of six population foci: family/individual across the life span, adult-gerontology, neonatal, pediatrics, women's health/gender related, or psychiatric-mental health. An important element of the Model is that there must be congruency between the educational program and degree and the certification exam. This is a major change for some programs and practicing APRNs.[9] Finally, the top tier of the Model refers to APRN specialties such as palliative care, oncology, and cardiology. While these specialties provide depth and reflect expertise in a specific area, these specialties have no prescribed educational criteria, no requirement for accredited certification or education and do not require Board of Nursing regulation. Thus, APRNs may specialize in the care of these populations but cannot be licensed solely within these areas of specialty. The implication for hospice and palliative APRNs is that hospice and palliative care is no longer a primary practice but rather specialty only, necessitating preparation and certification in one of the six population foci.

It is important that the palliative care APRN understand the basis for the APRN Consensus Model and the legislative and regulatory changes occurring at the state level. The overarching goal is to support the full scope of APRN practice and to improve access to APRN care by healthcare consumers, driving better outcomes for the entire population. Peer-reviewed research conducted over the past 4 decades has demonstrated the quality and safety of APRN practice, and professional associations are working to ensure consumer protection through the adoption of the Model's regulatory language.[12] Yet, at this point in the history of the full implementation of the new regulatory model, there is stiff resistance in many states that is partially explained by outdated, non-evidence-based arguments and turf issues.[12] An individual state would demonstrate full implementation of the Model by passing these statutes: the APRN title, role delineation of the four roles, educational requirement at the master's or doctoral level, required certification, licensure in the APRN role, practice autonomy for the APRN, and full prescriptive authority. As of early 2013, only six states have full implementation.[13] As work continues across the country toward full implementation of the Consensus Model, each APRN should stay abreast of the progress and refer to their state board of nursing for the most current regulations related to licensing and scope. It is the APRN's responsibility to be familiar with relevant state law and to maintain a practice that is guided by legal, ethical, and professional practice standards. The 25th Annual Legislative Update on the licensing and regulation of APRN practice in all 50 states is an excellent resource.[12]

In addition to the APRN Consensus Model, the 2010 Institute of Medicine report *Future of Nursing: Leading Change, Advancing Health* is also of important historical note in the development and growth of the APRN role.[14] This critical document strengthened the argument for the APRN role and the new regulatory structure in meeting some of the current healthcare needs and challenges and included four key messages relevant to advanced practice in all specialties and population foci:

1. Nurses should practice to the full extent of their education and training.

2. Nurses should achieve higher levels of education and training.

3. Nurses should be full partners, with physicians and other health professionals, in redesigning healthcare in the United States.

4. Effective workforce planning and policymaking require better data collection and improved information infrastructure.

There has been progress, some of which is very pertinent to the specialty of palliative care and hospice, since the publication of the Institute of Medicine's report in 2010 and the NCSBN's APRN Consensus Model regulations in 2008. Several states have amended their practice acts to bring regulatory consistency across states. New Jersey now requires APRNs to pursue education in end-of-life care and includes APRNs in the definition of "physician" when completing Physician Orders for Life-Sustaining Treatment (POLST) and includes APRNs in Hospice Licensing Standards. In addition, some states are reporting improved legal statutes related to APRN roles in pain management clinics. Seven states reported broader prescriptive authority for APRNs.[15]

In summary, the APRN Consensus Model defines a future for regulation of the APRN role and supports practice to the full extent of scope. When fully implemented, the Model will allow

APRNs to meet provider shortages across the United States.[9,15] The overarching goals are to achieve uniformity in education and licensure, remove barriers to interstate endorsement, and promote common understanding of the APRN role for optimal impact on healthcare outcomes.[9] The intent of the Model is to not disenfranchise practicing APRNs, but as graduate nursing programs, state boards of nursing and certification corporations adjust to the Model's recommendations, some impact on existing programs and individual APRNs is expected to occur.[10] Though grandfathering is a provision in the new regulatory model and should exempt those already practicing within the state of their current license, it is recognized that the requirement for current, national certification in the role and population focus may impact some APRNs.[10] It should be noted that, at this time, the APRN Consensus Model does not require or preclude the Doctorate of Nursing Practice (DNP) as an entry level degree for APRNs, a point that has caused confusion and concern in the APRN community.[9]

Developments in palliative care: the National Consensus Project, the National Quality Forum, and the Joint Commission's Advanced Certification for Palliative Care

Three significant developments, within the past decade, reflect a period of growth and standardization in the discipline of palliative care and have implications for the hospice and palliative care APRN. First, the National Consensus Project for Quality Palliative Care published the first edition of the *Clinical Practice Guidelines for Palliative Care* (NCP Guidelines) in 2004. The third edition was released in 2013.[4] The NCP is a partnership of five national palliative care organizations: The American Academy of Hospice and Palliative Medicine (AAHPM), the Center to Advance Palliative Care (CAPC), the Hospice and Palliative Nurses Association (HPNA), the Last Acts Partnership, and the National Hospice and Palliative Care Organization (NHPCO). The NCP Guidelines were intended to aid the development of palliative care programs, establish definitions of palliative care, set goals for access to quality palliative care, reduce variation, foster performance measurement and quality improvement, and promote continuity of palliative care across settings. The guidelines cover eight domains of palliative care: structure and process; physical aspects; psychological and psychiatric aspects; social aspects; spiritual, religious, and existential aspects; cultural aspects; care of the patient at the end of life; and ethical and legal aspects.[4] The third edition of the NCP Guidelines reflects current practice and is consistent with the two previous editions except that the title of Domain 7, "care of the patient at the end of life," was changed from "care of the imminently dying patient." The publication of the third edition reflects the maturation of the discipline, the changes in practice, the continued growth in the palliative care evidence base, and the impact of national seminal events such as the healthcare reform mandated in the Patient Protection and Affordable Care Act.[4] The essential underlying tenets found throughout the NCP Guidelines include patient- and family-centered care, comprehensive palliative care across care settings, early introduction of palliative care at time of diagnosis of serious illness, interdisciplinary teams, expertise in clinical and communication skills, relief of suffering,

and focus on quality.[4] The reader is referred to chapter 2 for a detailed review of the Guidelines.

While publication of the NCP Guidelines helped establish the definition and scope of palliative care, the National Quality Forum's National Framework and Preferred Practices for Palliative and Hospice Care Quality (NQF Preferred Practices) was also an essential step in the acceptance and implementation of those guidelines by the larger healthcare community.[16] The NQF is a nonprofit public-private partnership focused on improving the quality of healthcare through the establishment of voluntary consensus standards. The NQF Preferred Practices are based on the NCP Guidelines and identify 38 preferred practices that will improve the quality of palliative and hospice care. Also, the NQF framework creates a quality measurement and reporting system that may be used to support improved reimbursement for palliative care services.[16] Taken together, the NCP Guidelines and the NQF Preferred Practices set the performance standards for new and existing palliative care programs.

The third development occurred in the fall of 2012, when the Joint Commission (TJC) launched advanced certification for palliative care.[17] This certification recognizes hospital inpatient palliative care programs that demonstrate exceptional patient- and family-centered care. Over 40 standards in program management, provision of care, information management, and performance improvement are included. The Joint Commission used the NCP Guidelines to develop this certification program, which can help APRNs and their teams to build the infrastructure needed for high-quality outcomes. This 2-year certification is also a recognition of the importance of palliative care to quality healthcare outcomes and is recognized as a major landmark for the specialty.

There are several reasons why these national guidelines and TJC certification are indispensible to the professional practice of palliative care APRNs. First, the guidelines establish standards for program development and for clinical outcomes and serve as a nationally accepted benchmark of quality. Both Guidelines set the standard that palliative care teams must be interdisciplinary and that patients and families must have access to palliative care expertise 24 hours per day, 7 days per week. At the level of patient outcomes, the NQF Preferred Practices advocate for screening and assessment of symptoms with standardized scales,[16] and the NCP Guidelines call for prompt response to psychological symptoms and regular documentation of response to treatment.[4]

Second, the NQF Preferred Practices and NCP Guidelines set standards for educational preparation for APRNs and members of the palliative care team.[4,16] Advanced practice registered nurses are ideally suited to take a leadership role in providing experiences for all team members in the range of settings where patients receive care. The consensus guidelines also help graduate faculty to identify basic skills and knowledge that should be integrated into curricula and ensure that palliative care programs help advanced practice students develop specialist-level competency in all domains.[4]

An additional benefit to the use of the NCP Guidelines and NQF Preferred Practices and attainment of TJC advanced certification for palliative care is to conduct meaningful performance improvement activities using these national benchmarks. Advanced practice registered nurses as leaders on their teams can use individual standards to form the core of performance improvement measures and plans, thereby elevating the quality of the structure, processes, and outcomes at the program and patient-family level.

Finally, the NCP Guidelines and the NQF Preferred Practices serve as useful frames for palliative care research. Any APRN considering participation in research should review the recommendations made in these publications. For example, the NCP Guidelines call for new research methods to overcome the shortcomings of randomized controlled trials in palliative care, demonstration projects and multicenter research to test some of palliative care's central tenets, and more detailed studies analyzing reasons for late referrals to hospice.[4] The NQF Preferred Practices identifies gaps in palliative care's knowledge base and has extensive notes on directions for research in each of the domains and in cross-domain issues.[16]

Competency, education, and certification

Competency

The APRN's expertise is built on the strong foundation of skills possessed by the generalist registered nurse. Compared with the generalist, the APRN has broader and deeper education and expertise in the areas of assessment, diagnosis, and treatment of disease as well as prevention, health maintenance, and provision of comfort. Additionally, the APRN must hold a graduate degree in nursing, is nationally certified at the advanced practice level, and has a practice focused on care of patients and families.[8] The APRN is also expected to engage in more complex problem solving and has broader responsibility for patient care than the generalist nurse.

To address the developing role of hospice and palliative care nurses, including the growing importance of APRNs in this field, the Hospice and Palliative Nurses Association (HPNA) in collaboration with the American Nurses Association developed the *Scope and Standards of Hospice and Palliative Nursing Practice* in 2002, which included standards for advanced practice nursing.[18] These were updated in 2007. A companion document, *Competencies for Advanced Practice Hospice and Palliative Care Nurses*[19] was also produced. In the section on scope of practice, eight competencies are outlined for the generalist hospice and palliative nurse and include: clinical judgment, advocacy and ethics, professionalism, collaboration, systems thinking, cultural competence, facilitation of learning, and communication.[17] In the HPNA's companion publication on competencies for APRNs, the same eight competencies, plus a research competency, are defined and include details of additional criteria for the APRN's expanded scope of practice.[19] For example, both the generalist and APRN use the nursing process to address the multidimensional needs of patients and families but the APRN assumes greater responsibility for the evaluation, communication, and documentation of care across healthcare settings. The HPNA has supplemented the scope of practice and competency statements by providing measurement criteria for each of 15 standards.[18] There are six standards of practice (assessment, diagnosis, outcomes identification, planning, implementation, and evaluation) and nine standards of professional performance (quality of practice, education, professional practice evaluation, collegiality, collaboration, ethics, research, resource utilization, and leadership).[18] In each case, generalist standards are described first, followed by additional practices for which the APRN is responsible. The HPNA recently updated the APRN competencies.

Education

The NCP Guidelines call for improved education for all clinicians as a priority in palliative care. More than a decade ago, surveys confirmed that undergraduate and graduate nursing programs paid little attention to palliative care topics.[2,20,21] More recent data show that there is still a lack of adequate content.[22] A seminal work by Ferrell and colleagues that reviewed 50 nursing textbooks used frequently in nursing curricula found that only 2% of all pages had any end-of-life content.[23] Increased palliative care content has been endorsed by HPNA[24] and the NCSBN.[25] At the generalist level, palliative care content has already been successfully integrated into the National Council Licensure Exam for RNs (NCLEX-RN).[25] The 2013 NCLEX-RN test blueprint includes content on end-of-life care, pharmacological and nonpharmacological approaches to pain management, advance directives, ethical practice, aging, and grief and loss.[25]

At the master's level, there has also been progress in palliative care programs. The first graduate nursing programs specifically designed for training palliative care APRNs were created in the 1990s. The first palliative care nursing master's program for clinical nurse specialists was established at The Breen School of Nursing of Ursuline College in Pepper Pike, Ohio, and for nurse practitioners at New York University College of Nursing.[26] Currently, there are eight master's level programs that have specified hospice and palliative care content assimilated into population care, consistent with the APRN Consensus Model, listed on the HPNA website.[27] In 2004, the American Association of Colleges of Nursing (AACN) endorsed the Position Statement on the Practice Doctorate in Nursing[28] recommending that all advanced practice graduate nursing programs transition to DNP programs by 2015.[29] Many new DNP programs have been opened and others are in development. It remains to be seen what effect this initiative will have on advanced practice nursing in palliative care.

In addition to didactic coursework, palliative care APRNs need clinical experiences. In 2006, the HPNA published *Standards for Clinical Practicum in Palliative Nursing for Practicing Professional Nurses* (CPPN). This document sets standards for faculty, resources, curriculum, evaluation of outcomes and the teaching-learning process, and participants. It also defines the structure and content of three types of clinical practicums in palliative nursing: the observership, the preceptorship, and the fellowship.[30] Although fellowships are a standard part of physician training, they are a relatively new educational opportunity for APRNs. Currently, palliative care fellowship training is available for APRNs at six hospitals including the Beth Israel Medical Center in New York City, the Dana-Farber Cancer Institute in Boston, Massachusetts General Hospital in Boston, Memorial Sloan-Kettering Cancer Center in New York City, the University of Vermont, and the University of California-Irvine. Also, there are novel programs underway to develop palliative care specialty skills in APRNs such as the grant-funded, week-long APRN Externship being offered at Virginia Commonwealth University Health System in Richmond, Virginia, in 2013–2014. Interested APRNs can refer to the HPNA website for the most current programs that support clinical and didactic growth in the role.[31]

Continuing education is essential for the APRN to keep current in evidence based practice. All APRNs need continuing education in palliative care, which can be accomplished through self-study, clinical in-services, and professional conferences. It is important for APRNs to become active members of national, regional, and local professional organizations so they will have access to continuing education opportunities, and so that those APRNs with palliative care expertise can do the important work of providing education for the nonspecialists. In 1999, the AACN and the City of Hope National Medical Center formed the End-of-Life Nursing Education Consortium (ELNEC) to design a curriculum for teaching palliative care to nurses.[32] The ELNEC has been a successful model for improving palliative and end-of-life education for nurses across all practice specialties including pediatrics, critical care, and geriatrics.[33,34] From 2001 to 2006, ELNEC presented the ELNEC-Graduate train-the-trainer curriculum with the goal to increase the amount of education about palliative care in graduate nursing curricula.[32] This National Cancer Institute (NCI)-funded program reached a total of 300 graduate nursing program faculty members representing 63% of all graduate nursing programs in the United States and nearly tripled the average number of hours of palliative care content in their graduate curricula.[32] Such train-the-trainer programs can be particularly impactful because they have the potential to reach a much larger audience through the participants' efforts to replicate the training in other settings. Please refer to chapter 66 for a detailed review of ELNEC.

Certification: the advanced certified hospice and palliative nurse (ACHPN)

With the growth of APRN roles in hospice and palliative care, the National Board for Certification of Hospice and Palliative Nursing (NBCHPN), in partnership with the American Nurses Credentialing Center, initiated specialty certification for the advanced practice nurse in 2001. The first examination was offered in 2002, and the NBCHPN became the full proprietor of the exam in 2005. There are several benefits to obtaining national certification as an advanced certified hospice and palliative nurse (ACHPN). Certification is a marker of professional competence and assures that care meets the established standards for quality and safety. In addition, certification validates the specialty, protects the consumer, and is necessary for APRN billing and reimbursement.[8,35]

The ACHPN exam tests knowledge in five domains of practice: clinical judgment; advocacy, ethics, and systems thinking; professionalism and research; collaboration, facilitation of learning, and communication; and cultural and spiritual competence. Advanced practice nurses who wish to sit for the exam must meet eligibility criteria including graduate-level education and a minimum of 500 hours of clinical practice in palliative care.[36] The Core Curriculum for the Advanced Practice Hospice and Palliative Nurse published in 2007 and revised in 2013, provides the foundation for knowledge for APRNs who practice palliative care and is an excellent resource for exam preparation.[36] As of 2013, 803 APRNs were certified as ACHPNs.[37]

Advanced practice registered nurses outcomes across practice settings

Advanced practice registered nurses provide palliative care in a wide range of care settings including home care programs, hospices, long-term care facilities, outpatient clinics, emergency rooms, acute care hospitals, and subacute rehabilitation units. Numerous settings were highlighted in the publication "Advanced Practice Nursing: Pioneering Practices in Palliative Care."[38] Produced by Promoting Excellence in End-of-Life Care, a national program office of the Robert Wood Johnson Foundation, this publication described APRN practice in diverse palliative care programs. Because APRNs practice in such a variety of locations, they have the opportunity to reduce the fragmentation of care that can occur during transitions from one care setting to another and for specific patient populations. For example, evidence is growing that provision of expert symptom management by palliative care APRNs early in the course of cancer may improve quality of life and, in some cases, patient survival.[39,40]

Billing and reimbursement

Advanced practice registered nurse billing and reimbursement is an essential part of a palliative care program's business model, and it is easier to demonstrate and to understand the value that APRNs bring to a program through documentation of revenue generated by reimbursement from government and third-party payers. In difficult economic times this may translate into the ability to keep a palliative care program afloat or to keep an APRN on the team.[41] The following guidelines apply to reimbursement for APRN services provided in inpatient hospital settings, outpatient clinics, skilled nursing facilities, and at home. Hospice will be covered separately at the end of the section. Medicare, the federally administered health insurance available to those aged 65 years and older or who have end-stage renal disease or meet disability criteria, will be covered in some detail because it represents a large proportion of total reimbursement for hospital and office-based care, and because other third-party payers often follow Medicare's lead.[7]

Under the Omnibus Budget Reconciliation Acts of 1989 and 1990, APRNs were first granted limited ability to bill Medicare in rural areas and in skilled nursing facilities.[7,41] Prior to this legislation, APRNs could bill "incident to" physician services, but this applied only to patient encounters in which the physician provided direct personal supervision by being in the office suite at the time of the encounter, and APRNs could not bill for new patients or new problems.[7,41] In the 1997 Balanced Budget Act, APRN billing was expanded significantly. Advanced practice nurses in all geographic areas and practice sites were allowed to be reimbursed at 85% of the physician fee schedule under Medicare Part B.[7,41] "Incident to" billing continues to be an option, but applies to only a small number of encounters and is subject to numerous restrictions.[42] To qualify for Medicare reimbursement, APRNs must satisfy a variety of requirements. They must have a master's degree in nursing, advanced certification from a nationally recognized certification body, and a National Provider Identifier. The APRN must satisfy all of the state's practice requirements, including state RN and APRN licensure, and must document a collaborative arrangement with a physician even if the state does not have a collaborative practice law. The service being submitted for reimbursement must be a service for which a physician would be reimbursed, and the state must recognize the APRN's legal authority to perform that service. In addition, the practice cannot be owned by the hospital and the APRN's salary cannot be on the hospital nursing department's cost report because the hospital is reimbursed under Medicare Part A for those services.[7] The APRN who satisfies the above requirements can bill Medicare Part B. These rules apply to both nurse practitioners and clinical nurse specialists, but clinical nurse specialists may have a more difficult time meeting the requirements either because of limits or silence at the state level on their scope of practice.[7,41,42,43]

To be eligible for Medicare reimbursement, a service must be defined as a "physician service" and assigned a current procedural terminology (CPT) code to document the procedure done or the service provided.[7,41,42] The evaluation and management (E&M) CPT codes are the most frequently used in palliative care because rather than describe procedures (which make up a small part of palliative care practice), they describe cognitive services such as history taking, conducting the physical exam, decision-making, and counseling.[41] There are different sets of CPT codes for different practice settings, and each set comprises a range of numbers reflecting distinct levels of service. The level of service may be determined on the basis of either complexity or time. If greater than 50% of a clinician's time is spent in coordination and counseling, then the clinician may bill based on time. This can be an effective way to document the intensity of work in palliative care, especially if the physical exam is limited.[41] For inpatients, the total time spent on the unit is what counts toward the E&M code, and for outpatients, only face-to-face time counts.[44] For billing on the basis of complexity, the level of service is supported by documentation of the extent of the history, physical exam, decision-making, and counseling.[43,44]

A second set of codes for diagnoses is necessary to qualify a service for reimbursement. International Classification of Diseases, Ninth Revision, Clinical Modification (ICD-9-CM) codes are used to describe the disease or symptom that is treated. Examples include acute respiratory failure, pain, and nausea. It is important to note that a payer will not reimburse more than one clinician per day for the same indication. For example, a palliative care APRN who consults on a patient on a ventilator in an ICU, and who helps manage the patient's dyspnea should avoid submitting the ICD-9-M for acute respiratory failure because the critical care clinician or pulmonologist is likely to use that code. A better choice for the APRN in such a case would be to use the ICD-9-CM code for dyspnea. If two clinicians submit bills listing the same ICD-9-CM code on the same day, only the clinician whose bill is processed first will be reimbursed. It is possible to bill for concurrent care, even if the clinicians are from the same specialty, as long as each clinician is providing a different service and can bill for a different diagnosis.[44]

In addition to Medicare reimbursement, APRNs may be eligible for reimbursement from other third-party payers including Medicaid, commercial insurers, and managed care organizations (MCOs).[43] Although many of the billing and reimbursement guidelines for Medicare are applicable to these other payers, the Medicaid plans have considerable state-to-state variation, and each commercial insurer and managed care plan has its own policies.[43] The percent that Medicaid programs reimburse APRNs of the physician rate varies from as low as 70% in Alabama to 100% in California, Delaware, Maryland, and many other states.[12] All APRNs should refer to their respective Board of Nursing for the current status of reimbursement for services and for the status of implementation of the APRN Consensus Model recommendations.

The 2003 Medicare Modernization Act specifies that a nurse practitioner can directly bill Medicare Part B for services provided to hospice-enrolled patients, but only if she/he is the patient's attending, and only if she/he is not a paid or volunteer employee of the hospice. A nurse practitioner must be the patient's attending of record in order to bill and while nurse practitioners may complete hospital face-to-face encounters, they may not certify or recertify terminal illness or serve as physician replacements on hospice teams.[42,44] Nurse practitioners may order physical therapy, speech therapy, and occupational therapy but cannot order the initial referral to hospice.[45] Obviously, this statute remains a barrier to full scope of practice for the palliative APRN and contributes to fragmented transitions for patients and families.

Summary

The last decade has brought many changes for the APRN in palliative care. The growth in palliative care programs across the United States has provided more opportunities to provide care to an aging population with serious or life-limiting illnesses. Palliative care APRNs have the skills and knowledge to address healthcare challenges by contributing to interdisciplinary patient care; providing education to patients, families, and colleagues; serving as consultants; conducting research; and taking on leadership roles. In addition, reducing psychosocial and spiritual distress is a basic nursing role that palliative care APRNs fulfill by addressing symptoms and responding to suffering through compassionate presence.[46] The full implementation of the APRN Consensus Model and responses to the Institute of Medicine Future of Nursing Report is expected to promote and increase APRNs practicing to their full scope of practice, though it is recognized that these changes may be slower than desired.[13] Each APRN must keep abreast of the regulatory changes and national and state progress during this time of transition as the APRN Consensus Model is fully implemented and federal healthcare reform continues. Fortunately, the NCP Guidelines, NQF Preferred Practices, and TJC Advanced Certification for Palliative Care are excellent resources for APRNs as they lead their palliative care programs toward optimal outcomes at both the patient and program level.

Case study

JB was a 53-year-old male admitted to a Midwestern academic medical center due to intracranial hemorrhage and mass noted on a CT scan. He was transferred from an outside hospital, where he had presented with frequent falls, incontinence, right eye ptosis, hoarseness, and lower extremity weakness. A diagnosis of metastatic malignant melanoma had been made 2 months prior to this admission. An MRI was consistent with extensive intracranial and extracranial metastatic disease, and a spinal MRI showed vertebral body compression from T8 to T12. His past medical history included hypertension, osteoarthritis, and dyslipidemia. JB was married with six children and worked as an auto mechanic.

The APRN on the palliative care consult service was consulted on day 3 of JB's admission to the hematology-oncology service to address pain and constipation. The patient's current medications were morphine CR 90 q12h, hydromorphone PCA at 0.2 demand dose with 10 minute lockout and no basal rate, oxycodone 10 mg q4h prn, bisacodyl 5 mg qday, and dexamethasone 10 mg q6h. The physical examination revealed an acutely ill male reporting 10/10 sharp and numbing pain in his back and burning pain in both lower extremities. He was unable to move his legs due to pain. He had fluctuating mental status, ptosis of the right eye, hoarse voice with low volume, and hypoactive bowel sounds. His wife remarked that usually morphine was effective for pain control.

The APRN met with the patient and his wife to address goals of care. The patient preferred all aggressive measures and was being evaluated for radiation therapy, thus, his resuscitation status was full code. His strong preference was to return home and to prolong life as he was the sole breadwinner for their large family. The APRN recommended to increase the demand dose of hydromorphone PCA from 0.2 to 0.6 with 6 minute lockout, increase the morphine CR to 150 mg q12h, start roxanol 30 mg po q2h prn, and start gabapentin 100 mg TID.

Despite the changes in this regimen, JB continued to report very high levels of stabbing pain in his back. Methadone 20 mg TID was started several days later. He was using 25–45 mg of hydromorphone per day. One week after the initial consult, JB was transferred to the ICU due to change in mental status. At that time, the ICU team discontinued all opioids. Four different clinicians addressed goals of care and code status with JB's wife because he had lost decisional capacity. His wife honored his preferences for full treatment and requested that he remain a full code. It was reported that his wife was upset and angry about the repeated attempts by multiple clinicians to place a DNR order.

The palliative care APRN, having already established trust with JB's wife, held a family meeting. The APRN asked the wife how they could be most helpful and agreed to not discuss a DNR order and keep the full code order in place. JB's wife confirmed that her husband wanted every measure used to extend his life but that he very much wanted to get home and be with his children and to have the full treatment of radiation therapy. They agreed to transfer JB to a skilled nursing facility close to home with transportation arranged for radiation therapy treatments. Methadone 10 mg q12h and 10 mg q3h prn was ordered. The patient was discharged later that day.

Unfortunately, the discharge plan failed, and JB was readmitted 12 hours later for pain crisis due to the lack of availability of methadone at the outside facility. The patient was clinically unstable, minimally responsive, with tachycardia and tachypnea. The APRN knew that JB was declining quickly and that the risk of resuscitation clearly outweighed any benefit especially in light of JB's goal to be home with his children. She met with JB's wife and asked her how much time she felt her husband had remaining. When his wife responded "very little," they came to agreement that life support in the ICU was not consistent with JB's preferences. The plan moved quickly after this acknowledgment of his grave prognosis. JB's wife did agree to a DNR status and referral to hospice. JB was discharged with home hospice later that day and expired 24 hours later.

This case study illustrates the significant impact that a palliative APRN can have when using expert communication skills and pain and symptom management approaches. Though JB was clearly terminal, the APRN was able to maintain trust with his wife and honor his preferences.

References

1. Field MJ, Cassel CK. Approaching Death: Improving Care at the End of Life. Washington, DC: National Academy Press; 1997.
2. Peaceful Death: Recommended Competencies and Curricular Guidelines for End-of-Life Nursing Care. Washington, DC: American Association of Colleges of Nursing; 1998. Available at: http://www.aacn.nche.edu/publications/peaceful-death. Accessed October 24, 2013.
3. The SUPPORT Principle Investigators. A controlled trial to improve care for seriously ill hospitalized patients: the study to understand prognoses and preferences for outcomes and risks of treatments (SUPPORT). JAMA. 1995;274:1591–1598.
4. Clinical Practice Guidelines for Quality Palliative Care. 3rd ed. Pittsburgh, PA: National Consensus Project for Quality Palliative Care, 2013. Available at: http://www.national consensusproject.org. Accessed June 14, 2013.
5. Newhouse RP, Stanik-Hutt J, White KM, et al. Advanced practice nurse outcomes 1990–2008: a systematic review. Nurs Econ. 2011;29:230–250.
6. Keeling AW. A brief history of advanced practice nursing in the United States. In: Hamric AB, Spross JA, Hanson CM (eds.), Advanced Practice Nursing: An Integrative Approach. 4th ed. St. Louis, MO: Saunders; 2009:3–32.
7. Buppert C. Nurse Practitioner's Business Practice and Legal Guide. 3rd ed. Sudbury, MA: Jones and Bartlett; 2008.
8. Hamric AB. A definition of advanced practice nursing. In: Hamric AB, Spross JA, Hanson CM (eds.), Advanced Practice Nursing: An Integrative Approach. 4th ed. St. Louis, MO: Saunders; 2009:75–94.
9. Hartigan C. APRN regulation: the licensure-certification interface. AACN Adv Crit Care. 2011;22:50–65.
10. Stanley J. Impact of new regulatory standards on advanced practice registered nursing: the APRN consensus model and LACE. Nurs Clin N Am. 2012;47:241–250.
11. APRN Consensus Work Group, and National Council of State Boards of Nursing APRN Advisory Committee (2008). Consensus Model for APRN Regulation: Licensure, Accreditation, Certification and Education. Available at: http://www.aacn.nche.edu/education-resources/APRNReport.pdf. Accessed June 15, 2013.
12. Phillips SJ. 25th Annual legislative update: evidence-based practice reforms improve access to APRN care. Nur Pract. 2013;38:18–42.
13. Dahlin C. A National Perspective of Advanced Practice Registered Nursing. APRNVERVE. May 2013. http://www.hpna.org/DisplaryPage.aspx?Title=APRNVERVE.May2013. Accessed June 15, 2013.
14. Institute of Medicine. The Future of Nursing: Leading Change, Advancing Health. Washington, DC: National Academies Press; 2010.
15. Phillips SJ. 24th Annual legislative update: APRN consensus model implementation and planning. Nurs Pract. 2012;37:23–45.
16. National Quality Forum. A National Framework and Preferred Practices for Palliative and Hospice Care Quality. Washington, DC: NQF; 2006.
17. The Joint Commission Advanced Certification for Palliative Care. http://www.jointcommission.org/certification/palliative_care.aspx. Accessed June 15, 2013.
18. Hospice and Palliative Nurses Association (HPNA); American Nurses Association. Hospice and Palliative Nursing: Scope and Standards of Practice. 4th ed. Silver Spring, MD: American Nurses Association; 2007.
19. Hospice and Palliative Nurses Association (HPNA). Competencies for Advanced Practice Hospice and Palliative Care Nurses. Dubuque, IA: Kendall/Hunt; 2002.
20. Ferrell BR, Grant M, Virani R. Strengthening nursing education to improve end-of-life care. Nurs Outlook. 1999;47:252–256.
21. Hewitt M, Simone JV, eds. Ensuring Quality Cancer Care. Washington, DC: National Academy Press; 1999.
22. Paice JA, Ferrell BR, Virani R, et al. Graduate nursing education regarding end-of-life care. Nurs Outlook. 2006; 54:46–52.
23. Ferrell BR, Virani R, Grant M. Analysis of end-of-life content in nursing textbooks. Oncol Nurs Forum. 1999; 26:869–876.
24. Hospice and Palliative Nurses Association (HPNA). HPNA position statement: Value of Advanced Practice Nurse in Palliative Care.

Pittsburgh, PA: HPNA; 2006. Available at: http://www.hpna.org/PicView.aspx?ID=384. Accessed June 15, 2013.

25. NCLEX-RN Test Blueprint. https://www.ncsbn.org/nclex.htm. Accessed June 15, 2013.

26. Beach P. The evolution of hospice and palliative nursing. In: Perley MJ, Dahlin C (eds.), Core Curriculum for the Advanced Practice Hospice and Palliative Nurse. Pittsburgh, PA: Hospice and Palliative Nurses Association; 2007:3–11.

27. Hospice and Palliative Nurses Association (HPNA). Hospice and Palliative Master's Education Programs. Pittsburgh, PA: HPNA; 2009. Available at: http://wwwpna.org/DisplayPage.aspx?Title=Degree%20Program%20Listing. Last accessed June 15, 2013.

28. AACN Position Statement on the Practice Doctorate in Nursing. Washington, DC: AACN; 2004. Available at: http://www.aacn. nche.edu/DNP/DNPPositionstatement.htm. Accessed June 15, 2013.

29. DNP Roadmap Task Force Report. Washington, DC: American Association of Colleges of Nursing; 2006. Available at: http://www. aacn.nche.edu/DNP/pdf/DNProadmapreport.pdf. Last accessed June 15, 2013.

30. Hospice and Palliative Nurses Association (HPNA). Standards for Clinical Practicum in Palliative Nursing for Practicing Professional Nurses (CPPN). Pittsburgh, PA: HPNA; 2006. Available at: http://www.hpna.org/DisplayPage. aspx?Title=Standards%20for%20Clinical%20Practicum. Last accessed June 15, 2013.

31. Hospice and Palliative Nurses Association Nursing Fellowships. http://www.hpna.org/DisplayPage,aspx?Title=Nursing20%Fellowsh ips Accessed June 30, 2014.

32. Malloy P, Paice J, Virani R, et al. End-of-life nursing education consortium: 5 years of educating graduate nursing faculty in excellent palliative care. J Prof Nurs. 2008;24:352–357.

33. Ferrell BR, Virani R, Malloy P. Evaluation of the End-of-Life Nursing Education Consortium project in the USA. Int J Palliat Nurs. 2006;12(6):269–276.

34. Grant M, Wiencek C, Virani R, et al. End-of-life education in acute and critical care: the California ELNEC Project. AACN Advanced Crit Care. 2013;24(2):121–129.

35. Hanson CM. Understanding regulatory, legal, and credentialing requirements. In: Hamric AB, Spross JA, Hanson CM (eds.), Advanced Practice Nursing: An Integrative Approach. 4th ed. St. Louis, MO: Saunders; 2009:605–626.

36. Dahlin CR, Lynch MT, eds. Core Curriculum for the Advanced Practice Hospice and Palliative Nurse. 2nd ed. Pittsburgh, PA: HPNA; 2013.

37. Advanced Practice Registered Nurse (APRN) Map. Pittsburg, PA: HPNA; 2013. Available at: http://www.nbchpn.org/Certificants_Map.aspx?Cert=APRN. Accessed June 15, 2013.

38. Advanced Practice Nursing: Pioneering Practices in Palliative Care. Missoula, MT: Promoting Excellence in End-of-Life Care; 2002. Available at: http://www.dyingwell.org/downloads/apnrep.pdf. Accessed June 15, 2013.

39. Prince-Paul M, Burant C, Saltzman JN et al. The effects of integrating an advanced practice palliative care nurse in a community oncology center: a pilot study. J Support Oncol. 2010;8(1):21–27.

40. Temel JS, Greer JA, Muzikansky A, et al. Early palliative care for patients with metastatic non-small cell lung cancer. N Engl J Med. 2010;363:733–742.

41. Meier DE, Beresford L. Billing for palliative care: an essential cost of doing business. J Palliat Med. 2006;9:250–257.

42. Medicare Reimbursement Fact Sheet. Washington, DC: American Academy of Nurse Practitioners; 2009. Available at: http://www.aanp.org/NR/rdonlyres/D498CAF2-7BE6-4D89-A588-9DBC9CBD901A/0/FactSheetMedicareReimbursement108.pdf. Accessed June 15, 2013.

43. Campbell M, Dahlin C. Advanced Practice Palliative Nursing: A Guide to Practice and Business Issues. Pittsburgh, PA: HPNA; 2008.

44. National Hospice and Palliative Care Organizations. http://www.nhpco.org/physician-and-nurse-practitioner-billing/nurse-practitioner-services. Accessed June 15, 2013.

45. AANP. Fact Sheet: Ordering Medicare hospice. 2012. http://www.aanp.org/legislation-regulation/federal-legislations/medicare/68-articles/333-ordering-medicare-hospice.(accessed June 15, 2013).

46. Ferrell BR, Coyle N. The Nature of Suffering and the Goals of Nursing. New York, NY: Oxford University Press; 2008.

CHAPTER 63

Reflections on occupational stress in palliative care nursing

Is it changing?

Mary L.S. Vachon, Peter K. Huggard, and Jayne Huggard

Key points

- Hospice palliative care nursing can be both stressful and very rewarding.

- Many constructs are used to describe and measure the experience of caregiving. Each contributes to the overall understanding and articulation of the positive and negative aspects of caring.

- True compassion cannot fatigue. Compassion may be a source of resilience and hardiness and may be essential to our well-being.

- To engage in compassion for others we must first practice self-compassion.

- We can grow through the experience of trauma

- Spirituality, the amalgam of the positive emotions, including compassion, that bind us to other human beings, is associated with increased compassion satisfaction and decreased compassion fatigue and burnout.[1]

- Organizations have a responsibility to provide care for the caregivers.

Introduction and setting the stage

In this chapter the authors will combine their interests and decades of experience as well as drawing on the substantial research in the field of the stressors and rewards of work in palliative care. Recent research related to the concepts of stress, burnout, and compassion fatigue and related concepts will be reviewed, and there will be a discussion clarifying some of the concerns and overlaps with the measurement of these concepts. The literature on stress, compassion fatigue and burnout in hospice/palliative care from 2008 to 2013 will be reviewed, placing it within the context of newer work in the areas of stress, burnout, and compassion fatigue. Although the focus of this chapter is to be on work since 2008, some earlier references will be used because the more recent research draws on these sources. At some points the comments "references in

original" will be used to note the fact that the author being quoted cited other sources that are not included in this chapter because of space limitations.

The concepts of empathy and compassion will be discussed in more detail, looking at the question of whether true compassion can fatigue and discussing the concept of posttraumatic growth and resilience. There will then be a discussion of spirituality in professional caregivers in palliative care. The chapter will conclude with current research on what is being done to decrease stress and improve coping mechanisms in palliative care.

Stress, burnout, posttraumatic embitterment disorder, and compassion fatigue

Stress

This section is adapted from Vachon and Fillion (in press).[2] The European Agency for Safety and Health at Work[3] has stated, "There is increasing consensus around defining work-related stress in terms of the 'interactions' between employee and (exposure to hazards in) their work environment. Within this model stress can be said to be experienced when the demands from the work environment exceed the employee's ability to cope with them."[3](p. 1)

The French Ministry and a group of international experts[4] suggested defining occupational stress factors around six axes: intensity of work, lack of autonomy, social climate, emotional demand, conflict of values, and safety issues. Integrating these findings, Vachon and Fillion[2] suggest defining occupational stress as a mismatch between the person and the following six areas of occupational risk factors: (1) workload or intensity of work, (2) autonomy (control and reward), (3) social climate (support, communication, and community), (4) emotional demand, (5) values and meaning, and (6) safety.

Burnout and job engagement

This section is adapted from Vachon and Huggard (2010).[5] Maslach and associates[6] reviewed the research on burnout from the three decades, the 1970s through the 1990s. Burnout is a form of mental distress manifested in "normal" persons who did not suffer from prior psychopathology, who experience decreased work performance resulting from negative attitudes and behaviors.[7] The key dimensions of burnout include:

◆ Emotional exhaustion (EE), the basic *individual stress dimension* of burnout, refers to feelings of being overextended and depleted of one's emotional and physical resources. Exhaustion prompts action to distance oneself emotionally and cognitively from work, as a way to cope with work overload.[7]

◆ Feelings of cynicism and detachment from the job (depersonalization [DP]), the *interpersonal context* dimension of burnout, refers to a negative, callous, or excessively detached response to various aspects of the job. It is an attempt to put distance between oneself and various aspects of the job. Research shows a consistent strong relationship between exhaustion and cynicism from the presence of work overload and social conflict.[7]

◆ Sense of ineffectiveness and lack of personal accomplishment (PA), the *self-evaluation dimension* of burnout, refers to feelings of incompetence and a lack of achievement and productivity at work. Lack of personal accomplishment arises more clearly from a lack of resources to get the work done (e.g., lack of critical information, lack of necessary tools, or insufficient time). It may be directly related to EE and DP or be more independent.[8]

See Box 63.1 for the symptoms of burnout.

Box 63.1 Symptoms and signs of burnout

Individual

Overwhelming physical and emotional exhaustion
Feelings of cynicism and detachment from the job
A sense of ineffectiveness and lack of accomplishment
Overidentification or overinvolvement
Irritability and hypervigilance
Sleep problems, including nightmares
Social withdrawal
Professional and personal boundary violations
Poor judgment
Perfectionism and rigidity
Questioning the meaning of life
Questioning prior religious beliefs
Interpersonal conflicts
Avoidance of emotionally difficult clinical situations
Addictive behaviors
Numbness and detachment
Difficulty in concentrating
Frequent illness—headaches, gastrointestinal disturbances, immune system impairment

Team

Low morale
High job turnover
Impaired job performance (decreased empathy, increased absenteeism)
Staff conflicts

Source: References 6, 9, 10.

Six areas of work life encompass the major organizational antecedents of burnout. These include: workload, control, reward, community, fairness, and values.[6] Research in a university setting showed that fairness in the work environment might be the tipping point determining whether people develop job engagement or burnout.[7] Alternatively, people may vary in the extent to which each of the six areas is important to them. Some people may place a higher weight on autonomy than on values, or people may be prepared to tolerate a mismatch regarding workload if they receive praise and good pay, have good relationships with colleagues, and find their work meaningful.

Emotion-work variables (e.g., requirement to display or suppress emotions on the job, requirements to be emotionally empathic) account for additional variance in burnout scores over and above job stressors.[6] These stressors may be the same ones that in some situations could lead to compassion fatigue.[11,12]

Job engagement is conceptualized as being the opposite of burnout.[8] It involves energy, involvement, and efficacy. Engagement involves the individual's relationship with work. This includes a sustainable workload, feelings of choice and control, appropriate recognition and reward, a supportive work community, fairness and justice, and meaningful and valued work. Engagement is also characterized by high levels of activation and pleasure.[8] Engagement is defined as a persistent, positive-affective-motivational state of fulfillment in employees that is characterized by vigor, dedication, and absorption.[8]

More recently, Maslach quoted earlier work by colleagues that distinguished the origins of the two concepts, burnout and job engagement.[13] "The burnout concept was developed from a grass-roots, bottom-up, qualitative approach in which people were asked to describe their work experiences. The term 'burnout,' and its core components, emerged from these interviews, rather than from related theories or research. In contrast, work engagement was originally defined from a theoretical perspective, either as the opposite of burnout or as an independently positive state."[13(p. 48)]

Posttraumatic embitterment

A development in the area of burnout and the work environment is that of Michael Linden and his work on posttraumatic embitterment.[14,15] Posttraumatic embitterment disorder (PTED), described by Linden as a type of adjustment disorder, can occur following a major and exceptional single life event with the consequent development of a negative mental state. This presents with embitterment and feelings of injustice with repeated intrusive memories of the event. In this state, those experiencing PTED may not have impaired emotional modulation, therefore they have no or minimal outward appearance of their internal distress. Linden lists other symptoms and behaviors as those of helplessness, self-blame, rejection of help, suicidal ideation, aggression, sleep disturbances, and impaired performance of daily activities. He describes this embitterment as "an emotion encompassing persistent feelings of being let down, insulted or being a loser, and of being revengeful but helpless."[14(p. 197)] Linden et al.[15] have compared PTED to other mental disorders and found that PTED differed from other mental disorders with respect to both the quality and intensity of psychopathology and posttraumatic stress disorder (PTSD) symptoms. In a study by Sensky,[16] similarities between the development and presentation of PTED and PTSD were drawn, as well as differences between PTED, called "chronic embitterment" by Sensky, and burnout. Sensky "positions" chronic embitterment within a context of organizational justice within the workplace and the contribution that chronic embitterment might make toward absenteeism from the workplace. As noted above, fairness can be the tipping point as well for burnout.[7] The similarity of PTED to PTSD may suggest a link, even in the sharing of symptomatology, with those described below in the discussion on compassion fatigue.

Compassion fatigue and compassion satisfaction

Compassion fatigue is described as "'cost of caring' for others in emotional pain that has led helping professionals to abandon their work with traumatized persons."[11(p. 7)] Some researchers consider compassion fatigue to be similar to PTSD, except that it applies to those emotionally affected by the trauma of another (e.g., client or family member) rather than by one's own trauma. Compassion fatigue is also known as secondary or vicarious traumatization.[11,12] Measures of compassion fatigue involve measuring burnout as well, so the constructs can get somewhat confusing. Current thinking regarding the construct of compassion fatigue is that there is a domain of compassion fatigue that occurs when there is a combination of burnout and experiences that lead to the development of secondary traumatic stress.[17]

Comparison of constructs

Alkema, Linton, and Davies[18] quote Stamm[19] describing the differences between burnout and compassion fatigue:

> Burnout relates to feelings of hopelessness, work-related problems, high workload, lack of professional support in the workplace, and feeling as if work efforts do not make a difference in the lives of those being served.[19] Stamm stated that burnout usually has a slow onset and is the result of long-term work-related issues. Stamm[19] described compassion fatigue, however, as the result of specific secondary exposure to traumatic events (also known as vicarious trauma). Symptoms of compassion fatigue may have a rapid onset and can be related to one particular event or long-term exposure to many traumatic stories. While workers in any professional field may experience burnout, compassion fatigue is specific to those professionals in the helping professions who listen to clients' stories of traumatic events. Furthermore, burnout is a general construct describing a reaction to work-related stress; compassion fatigue is the direct result of specific experiences in the helping professions. Put simply, compassion fatigue is a professional hazard for those who choose to help others.[18(p. 104)]

Yoder[20] draws on the work of Valent[21] and Stamm[22] and notes that burnout and compassion fatigue are related but separate concepts.

> Valent believed that the two concepts arise from separate failed survival strategies; compassion fatigue arises from a rescue–caretaking response and burnout from an assertiveness–goal achievement response. He theorized that compassion fatigue occurs when one cannot rescue or save the individual from harm and results in guilt and distress. Burnout on the other hand results when one cannot achieve his or her goals and results in "frustration, a sense of loss of control, increased willful efforts, and diminishing morale."[21(p. 27)]

Compassion fatigue appears suddenly and subsides more quickly than does burnout, which arises and declines more slowly.[11,20(p. 191)]

Terms such as "burnout," "compassion fatigue," "secondary traumatic stress," and "vicarious traumatization" may all be used to describe an emotional response to stress. The latter three specifically refer to a form of secondary traumatic stress response and may differ on a phenomenological level.[23] While there are reported differences, the constructs are not mutually exclusive—each contributes to the overall understanding and articulation of the positive and negative aspects of caring.

Compassion fatigue has previously been thought of in association with an empathic process. The two concepts of compassion and empathy are different. Although various authors have previously described a relationship between empathy and compassion fatigue,[11,24,25] what is possibly operating between compassion fatigue and empathy is a process that may be regarded as a "disruption" in empathy. This has previously been reported by Wilson and Lindy.[24] They describe this as an "empathic strain" characterized by an "intrusive" empathic strain between the clinician and client that can result in overidentification and pathological bonding; and an "avoidance" empathic strain characterized by being distant and avoiding contact with the patient. These two states are not empathic in the therapeutic relationship; rather, they are dysfunctional processes. This may be what others have been describing in the discussion of the relationship between empathy and compassion fatigue.

Compassion satisfaction (CS) has been defined as "the pleasure you derive from being able to do your work well."[2,26(p. 12)] It stands in sharp contrast to compassion fatigue, which pertains to the negative effects arising from one's work. Subscales for measuring compassion fatigue, burnout, and compassion satisfaction can be found in the ProQOL: Professional Quality of Life scale.[19,26] "Compassion satisfaction (CS) may be the portrayal of efficacy: Indeed, CS may be happiness with what one can do to make the world in which one lives a reflection of what one thinks it should be."[22(p. 113)]

Stamm does not claim to actually be measuring satisfaction with compassion but rather, as noted, the ability to do one's work well, efficacy, and happiness with making the world a better place—all very important variables and goals, but perhaps misnamed as "compassion satisfaction."

The construct of CS as defined above is similar to the top coping mechanism Vachon[27] found in the 587 caregivers to the critically ill, dying, and bereaved whom she interviewed internationally. When caregivers were asked what "kept them going" in their work, the most common response was "a sense of competence, control and pleasure in one's work." Caregivers frequently commented, "I like my work. I'm good at it and I have been doing it long enough to have some control over my work environment."[27(p. 182)] These straightforward words perhaps more accurately describe what is going on than does the term compassion satisfaction. The words would also be reflective of job engagement.

Recent research in stress, burnout, and compassion fatigue in hospice/palliative care

Stress and burnout in palliative care versus other specialties

A review of the literature of stress in palliative care over the first quarter century of the movement[10] found many studies reported that staff working in palliative care had either less burnout and stress than other professionals or that they experienced no more stress than other healthcare professionals working with seriously ill and/or dying persons. This was confirmed more recently.[28] Pereira, Fonsecal, and Carvalho[29] reviewed the palliative care literature from 1999 to 2009 involving empirical studies about burnout syndrome in palliative care nurses and physicians; and articles published in Portuguese or foreign/international scientific journals. They concluded that "burnout levels in palliative care, or in health care settings related to this field, do not seem to be higher than in other contexts." [29(p. 317, from reference 2)] Huggard had similar findings in her study of New Zealand caregivers.[30]

Fillion Desbiens, Truchon, et al.[31] also confirmed these findings in Quebec nurses working in end-of-life care. Nurses working in hospital settings showed higher stress indicators (higher job demands and efforts) than did nurses working in home care settings. Further comparisons indicated that work stress indicators were higher in nurses working in critical care and oncology units compared with specialized PC units.[31(from reference 2)]

Has palliative care changed?

For his doctoral thesis,[32] Dr. Victor Cellarius, a palliative care physician has recently compared the early days of palliative care in Canada with the current situation, proposing a new palliative care ethics. His thesis asked whether Canadian palliative care ethics has changed, and if so in what regard.[32(p. 2)] Analysis of the textual data led to the descriptive themes of *person, profession*, and *well-being*. These themes, when compared across the early and late periods, generated three themes of process. Analysis of the interview data generated three similar themes of process. The themes of process from the textual and interview data were similar enough to generate three overall themes of process—*routinization, medicalization*, and *professionalization*.

Cellarius concluded that Canadian palliative care and palliative care ethics were found to have undergone rationalization, understood as the processes of *routinization, medicalization*, and *professionalization*. For palliative care, this has meant that care has become more routine, more of a career, and less of a calling; has meant that medical interventions and medical understandings are increasingly used in palliative care; and has meant that practitioners identify more with traditional professions than previously and self-identify as palliative care specialists. For palliative care ethics, this rationalization has meant a shift in emphasis in the goals of palliative care. Early palliative care emphasized the goals of *palliation, presence*, and *meaning* as a response to the sufferings and abandonment of dying persons. During rationalization, palliative care shifted to focus primarily to palliation. Cellarius proposed a revision of palliative care ethics that retrieved the earlier goals of *presence* and *meaning* as a response to abandonment.[32(pp. 2–3)]

Rates of stress, burnout, and compassion fatigue in palliative/hospice nurses

Compassion satisfaction, compassion fatigue, and burnout were studied in a national Canadian study of hospice/palliative care staff.[33] The authors note that the ProQOL[22] had not previously been used in a large study of hospice palliative care (HPC) professionals but had been used in a smaller study by Alkema et al.[18] In the Canadian study 630 clinical, administrative, allied health workers, and volunteers from hospital, community-based, and care homes responded. The ProQOL measure[34] was chosen, as the three constructs measured with this scale—compassion satisfaction, compassion fatigue, and burnout—are all processes relevant to staff working in hospice and palliative care.

In the ProQOL,

higher scores on the compassion satisfaction scale represent a greater satisfaction related to your ability to be an effective caregiver in your job. Burnout is one of the elements of compassion fatigue and is associated with feelings of hopelessness and difficulties in dealing with work or in doing your job effectively. These negative feelings usually have a gradual onset with higher scores on this scale meaning that you are at higher risk for burnout. Secondary traumatic stress, the second component of compassion fatigue, is about work-related, secondary exposure to extremely or traumatically stressful events.[19(p. 17)]

When compared with other literature, results indicate that participants in this study had higher scores for compassion satisfaction, slightly higher scores for compassion fatigue, and comparable levels of burnout. When compared with full-time staff, part-time staff were found to have lower levels of compassion fatigue and burnout with higher levels of compassion satisfaction. Professional affiliation was also found to be significant, with integrative medicine staff scoring the highest for compassion satisfaction, nursing staff the highest for compassion fatigue, and integrative medicine staff scoring the lowest for burnout.

These findings provide a valuable understanding for health professionals of the possible consequences of working in hospice and palliative care and suggest a greater attention to the provision of education and training sessions, as well as staff support initiatives, are needed.

Factors associated with burnout in palliative care

Workload

Excessive workload exhausts the individual to the extent that recovery becomes impossible. Emotional work is especially draining when the job requires people to display emotions inconsistent with their feelings. Workload relates to the exhaustion component of burnout.[7] A review of the literature[28] showed that from the early 1970s there were perceived difficulties with workload, and insufficient staff to do the job at hand in both oncology and palliative care. From the 1970s through the ensuing decades to the 21st century, oncology staff in particular report being overwhelmed with the workload imposed by the increase in cancer and the chronic nature of the illness. More recently there have been issues related to increased workload in palliative care.[31]

In a Toronto study exploring the predictive factors associated with occupational stress in oncology and palliative care staff working in an academic cancer center[35] the top two variables predicting work stress were greater perceived workload and insufficient time to grieve patients' deaths. More than half (52%) felt that their workload negatively affected patient care, and more than 80% felt that it affected their ability to provide emotional support for patients and compassionate end-of-life care. In all, 55% stated that they did not have sufficient time to grieve the death of a patient, and more than 30% felt they did not have enough resources to cope with work-related stress. The actual workplace (palliative care unit vs. oncology unit) did not predict the degree of perceived distress. Of interest is previous research conducted at the same oncology center more than 30 years earlier. In that study, nurses reported lack of resource personnel, and physicians reported "a tremendous workload imposed by the prevalence of cancer, the increased life expectancy and chronic nature of the disease."[35] (in reference 2)

Glass and Rose[37] studied 15 generalist community nurses providing palliative care to clients in their homes in Australia in order to study participant's emotional well-being and self-care. They used a qualitative design that was "emancipatory in approach. Applying a critical feminist lens, it was anticipated that the nurses' experiences of providing palliative care could be explored, increased understanding gained and opportunities for positive change(s) created. It has been argued that 'critical engagement is a means to knowledge development and emancipation of nursing.'"[38](p. 245 in reference 37) Their methods included semistructured interviews/storytelling and reflective journaling.[37] The authors reported that their results validated the finding of Vachon[39] that stress in palliative care was frequently

> derived from nurses' personal situation about their work environment, as opposed to stress resulting from working with dying patients and their families. This study reflected similar results. The nurses often spoke about their role in palliative care as being a "privilege." . . .
>
> This notwithstanding, the nurses in this study reported numerous workplace issues that impacted considerably on their emotional well-being. The nurses' relayed stories that reflected the challenges they had with regard to lack of resources and heavy workloads. One nurse highlighted the relationship between staff shortages and increased workloads and caring for herself. She asserted, "We have worked understaffed all the time and it is very, very hard to look after yourself and do all those things" [Haley].[37](p. 343)

Weissman[40] provides interesting reflections on the palliative care martyr who believes she is indispensable for managing all patient suffering and responsible to all patients in need. Recognizing that she is overworked or under personal stress, the martyr feels helpless to change the situation and feels unappreciated by those in authority, typically hospital administration. This martyrdom syndrome seems similar to the PTED referred to above, which can be the result of chronic stressors.[14–16]

Martyrs[40] are at one extreme end of the bell-shaped curve of how clinicians view their role as a responsible clinician. They devote their entire waking hours to selfless devotion to patient care, typically at the expense of their personal health and relationships with others. Part of the reason for this syndrome is the "rapid uptake of palliative care services; we generally provide exceptional care fostered by a high degree of internally driven sense of responsibility."[40](p. 1278)

Problems arise "when that sense of responsibility becomes overwhelming, obscuring our sense of self and harming our relationships with those around us. We lose the boundaries necessary for healthy professional and personal relationships. Although it is easy to blame the 'system' for failing to provide sufficient resources to lessen the burden on the martyr, I would suggest that the internal drivers that maintain the state of martyrdom are far more important to understand and ultimately address."[40](p. 1278) Similar phenomena were noted in the early days of palliative care.[2]

Autonomy, control, reward

Autonomy at work involves the worker as an active actor in work, in participation in the production of wealth, and in the driving of one's professional life. This includes[41] not only room for flexibility in the work situation but also participation in decision-making and the use and development of skills and competencies.

The mismatch occurs when there is no recognition, low control or insufficient resources to properly do the work, and lack of personal reward at work. Research suggests that restructuring high-demand, low-control jobs may enhance productivity and reduce disability costs.[42] The issue of control is related to lack of efficacy or reduced personal accomplishment. Mismatches often indicate that individuals have insufficient control over the resources necessary to do their work, or insufficient authority to pursue the work in what they believe is the most effective manner.[43](in reference 2)

A Canadian study demonstrated the importance of autonomy and acknowledgment in an occupational stress study with a sample of 209 palliative-care nurses.[44] The authors tested an integrative occupational stress model, using two hierarchical regression models, including the job demand-control-support model, the effort-reward imbalance model, and specific palliative care stressors and resources. In this model "reward" refers to the effort-reward imbalance. Rewards include job-related benefits and are divided into the following categories: money, regard, and job security/career opportunity. Efforts refer to demands placed on the employee and can include work pressure, interruptions, inconsistent demands, and task complexity."[44]

Job satisfaction, a stress-related outcome, was evaluated using the General Satisfaction subscale of the Job Diagnostic Survey.[45] The items were adapted and translated in French, using the back-translation method. Emotional distress, the second stress-related outcome, was measured using the French adaptation[46] of the Profile of Mood States, short version (POMS)[47] which calculates six emotional components: tension/anxiety, depression/dejection, anger/hostility, vigor/activity, fatigue/inertia, and confusion/bewilderment. These components provide an overall score, called "total mood disturbance," which was used to estimate emotional distress. "Professional and emotional demands" were measured with the French adaptation[48] of the Nursing Stress Scale (NSS).[49] The NSS (34 items) was initially developed to evaluate diverse situations associated with psychological stress in palliative care nursing. The initial scale included seven situations: workload, death and dying, inadequate preparation, lack of staff support, uncertainty about treatment, conflicts with physicians, and conflicts with other nurses. In the adaptation of the NSS for this study, which was originally developed to measure nursing stress in a hospice- or hospital-based setting, some statements were slightly modified to match the reality of palliative care, both in the community and at the hospital. Furthermore, in order to better represent palliative care offered at home, six items were added to obtain an accurate representation of the category of emotional stressors described in recent studies. The revised NSS (26 items) yielded five domains, which were extracted from an exploratory factor analysis: (1) exposure to death; (2) uncertainty about treatments; (3) conflicts with physicians; (4) patients' and families' emotional distress; and (5) the lack of opportunity to vent emotions. Using the mean of the items of the first four domains, an overall score was obtained, which was called "professional and emotional demands."[44] Perceived self-efficacy was measured with an instrument developed for the present study.[50] Examples of perceived self-efficacy items are "I am confident in my skills to manage physical symptoms" and "I am confident in my capacity to deal with bereavement."[44]

The best predictors of job satisfaction were reward, people-oriented culture, and appropriate workload, whereas the best predictors of emotional distress were reward, professional and emotional demands, and self-efficacy to provide good palliative care (PC).[44] If nurses felt there was a balance between their rewards and efforts they had high job satisfaction. If there was an imbalance between rewards and efforts they had distress. With a larger and more representative sample ($n = 751$),[51] the same team replicated these findings and explained even more satisfaction and distress in adding meaning at work as a mediator between autonomy and satisfaction. A new model was developed that integrates

> several key concepts: the recognition of the autonomy of the nurse, the quality of teamwork, access to skilled human resources and the relief of overall distress of the patient and the family. It helps to explain more than 80% of the job satisfaction and 40% of the distress. The lack of human resources tops the list when it comes to account for job satisfaction and distress in nurses. Finally, the meaning of work acts as a mediator between autonomy and job satisfaction of nurses. The model confirms the usefulness of taking into account the consistency between the values of caring and those of the organization.[51(p. ii)]

For the nurses in the Glass and Rose study[37] power/control and politics in the work environment were clearly of concern. "Sarah raised the issue of power and control with her nurse manager, with her story reflecting sadness between 'what is' and 'what could be.' She reflected, 'I never go and talk to my boss . . . its kind of a double-edged sword. She's offering her support but in practice, she often doesn't support you. . . . It's a big control thing.'"[37(p. 343)] Nurses may also feel out of control if they begin to get emotionally involved with patients and families without sufficient supervision and support.

The Australian palliative care nurses in Glass and Rose's[37] study had challenges with the autonomous role of the community nurse. The nurses valued autonomy but also found that working alone in situations that were emotionally challenging impacted their well-being. "Lee affirmed it: 'Can be hard when you are confronted with a particularly distressing situation when you are by yourself.'"[37(p. 342)]

Social relationship, community belonging, and fairness

Support from a supervisor, a work climate of respect and trust, and economic security are crucial. "Social relationships at work are the relationships between workers and the relationships between the worker and the employing organization. These social relations must be considered in connection with the concept of integration (in the sociological sense), justice and recognition. They were the subject of partial models, which are social support,[52] the 'effort-reward balance' (Siegrist mode[53]) and organizational justice.[4] Mismatch occurs when people lose a sense of personal connection and respect with others in the workplace or with the employing organization. Social support from people with whom one shares praise, comfort, happiness, and humor affirms membership in a group with a shared sense of values."[28,30] From early in the field of palliative care the team was seen simultaneously as being a major stressor, the place where stress was manifest, and the group to whom one turned for support.[10,27] Team communication problems have long been identified as an issue in palliative care, as in other specialties. These have occurred across time and cultures and have been documented elsewhere.[5,10,29,30]

In Australia, interpersonal communications between the community nurses and other multidisciplinary team members such as general practitioners (GPs) and specialist palliative care teams were a source of frustration. Nurses spoke of interactions with doctors that were either respectful or condescending and dismissive. One nurse recalled the emotional impact of an incident where her professional opinion was dismissed by the GP. The client subsequently needed to be admitted to the hospital to receive appropriate medication, a situation that could have been avoided.[37(p. 343)] The nurses spoke of using debriefing as a self-care strategy to help make meaning of the disempowering circumstances.

Glass and Rose[37] found that workplace politics had a "negative impact on nurses' emotional well-being. Workplace politics involved behaviors or actions by organizations and/or individuals that were perceived by participants as being destructive, blocking, or incongruent to equitable healthcare. Nurses reported that 'the politics, there is just too much of it.'"[37(p. 343)] Nurses in that study spoke of bullying within the team and noted that it particularly affected the weakest link. Similar findings with respect to scapegoating were found earlier in the field.[27]

Jayne Huggard[30] found that of the support strategies she studied, "organizational support strategies appeared to be the most important for hospice staff. The majority of participants stated that they were well supported, especially by their line managers and peers, and that they felt both supported and valued by their organization."[30(p. 143)] Table 63.1 shows the top five organizational initiatives most valued by registered nurses. Participants were asked to rank the items on a scale from 1 to 5, with 1 being "not effective" and 5 being "effective." These include manageable rosters (shifts), informal support from peers, orientation, management of staff conflict, and feedback that acknowledges that you are doing a good job.[30]

Although teamwork has been seen as being the best, and perhaps only, way of doing palliative care, some of the assumptions of palliative care teamwork have come into question.[54] A review of the literature suggests that the effectiveness of multiprofessional teams in delivering palliative care has never really been addressed[54] and more research is needed to document team functioning, staff well-being and patients' quality of care. Please refer to chapter 68 for a further discussion on team work.

Emotional demand

The emotional demands are related to the need to control and shape one's emotions, particularly in order to master and shape those felt by people with whom you interact at work. Having to hide emotions is also demanding.[4]

Palliative care has been recognized as being associated with emotional demands including multiple bereavements and grief, exposure to patients' and families' distress, and personal discomfort about suffering and death.[5,10,27–30] The mismatch may particularly appear when requirements to display or suppress emotions on the job are challenging and therapeutic relationship, human connections, or empathy could be compromised.

While the literature has been somewhat divided as to whether or not the care of the dying is a major stressor in hospice palliative care,[10,30] research in the burnout area has focused explicitly on emotion-work variables and has found these emotional factors do account for additional variance in burnout scores over and above job stressors.[6]

Table 63.1 Highest "importance" scores for organizational initiatives professional group: registered nurse

Q. No.	Organizational initiative	Importance mean	Available "yes" (%)	Effective mean
14	Manageable rosters	4.66	90.0	4.03
7	Informal support from peers	4.65	98.3	4.38
11	Orientation	4.64	98.3	3.86
17	Management of staff conflict	4.49	87.3	3.26
21	Feedback that acknowledges you are doing a good job	4.48	87.8	3.61

A survey of 479 palliative care staff from a variety of disciplines in New Zealand[30] did not identify "death and dying" issues as a major contributor to creating a stressful work environment. Participants reported that these issues were manageable as long as there were sufficient and appropriate organizational support practices, such as acknowledgment of the deaths, the use of rituals, and the availability of debriefing, if required.

In an in-depth qualitative study of palliative care nurses ($N = 11$) Melanie Vachon (no relation to the author Vachon), Fillion, and Achille[55] found that the connections nurses make with their patients in confronting death can involve both suffering and meaning. They described three patterns of nurses' experience of death confrontation: integrating death, fighting death, and suffering death. While some nurses reported feeling nourished from their contacts with dying patients (empathic resonance), others sometimes experienced feeling frustrated (discordance) or powerless (consonance).[2]

Kearney, Weininger, Vachon, et al.[9,56] reviewed the literature on the emotion-work variables associated with stress in oncology and palliative care and found the following: constant exposure to death; inadequate time with dying patients; growing workload; increasing numbers of deaths, inadequate coping with one's own emotional response; need to carry on "as usual"; communication difficulties with dying patients and relatives; identification/friendships with patients; inability to live up to one's own standards; and feelings of depression, grief, and guilt.

In the large Canadian study by Slocum-Gori et al.[33] respondents were asked which hospice/palliative care services they usually provided. The top three were:

◆ Assistance with provision of relief from physical, emotional, and/or spiritual pain or distress

◆ Providing psychosocial support to patients and/or families

◆ Providing emotional support to other team members

The respondents who provided each of these services reported higher levels of compassion fatigue and burnout and no significant difference in levels of compassion satisfaction compared with those who did not provide the service. One hypothesis was that even staff who did not provide direct clinical care derived compassion satisfaction from their work.

Sabo[57] studied palliative and hematopoietic stem cell transplant nurses and described their caring work as being included in the relationships between nurses, patients, and their families encompassing the "mental, emotional and physical effects involved in looking after, responding to and supporting others."[57(p. 24)] "This relationship requires the nurse to be fully "present" along with and for the patient and family. Within the relationship, a space is created for the patient and family to give voice to their experience(s). The sharing of the illness narrative or story involves mutual understanding and reciprocation facilitating the cocreation of reality and the meaning of life experiences for the patient and family.(refs in original) "However, what might happen when the ability to co-create meaning does not occur due to lack of resources, workload increase, or tensions between the philosophical beliefs of the nursing discipline, the nurse's beliefs and values and the overarching philosophy and beliefs of the healthcare system within which the nurses practice? What may happen when repeated listening to stories of pain and suffering becomes overwhelming for the nurse?"[57(p. 24)]

Sabo[57] suggests that helping relationships are emotionally charged and can carry a heavy emotional burden:

> Increased workloads, client acuity and complexity and ongoing contact with patients who are suffering can increase the interpersonal demands made on nurses. Emotional overload may occur when the abovementioned conditions are combined with a lack of support (professional and social), experience and skill. As a coping strategy, the nurse may become detached, a coping strategy reinforced by the medico-centric philosophy of the healthcare system and socio-cultural norms. This gives rise to a paradoxical situation wherein the palliative or H/BMT nurse struggles to maintain a balance between providing care to and caring for the patient, between balancing the potential benefits and harms of treatment provided, between quantity as opposed to the quality of life. If left unresolved, the conflict may lead to the nurse perceiving his/her patients as objects, dehumanized rather than as unique embodied beings".[57(p. 26), refs in original]

Sabo is describing the disruption in empathy or empathic strain[24,25] referred to above in the section on compassion fatigue. Over time, the nurse's sense of adequacy, effectiveness, competency and sense of accomplishment may deteriorate, resulting in burnout or compassion fatigue.[57(refs in original)]

Sabo's work can also be compared with that of Cellarius,[32] who compared the previous care *for* the patient to the present care *of* the patient.

Glass and Rose[37] found that the nurses they studied had a strong awareness of the impact that their palliative care practice had on their lives. They reported sleepless nights and feeling emotionally drained and depleted of energy. They were aware that they needed to care for themselves, but not all nurses were confident in their ability to do so. However, nurses' stories reflected an implicit leaning toward caring for themselves. At times, this involved maintaining a cognitive balance. Shae's insight was that "it's also important to keep it all in perspective. Death is not disastrous. At times there can still be funny bits, light bits and happy bits. I think that you have to keep it all on an even keel."[37(p. 344)]

Dr. Balfour Mount, a pioneer in the palliative care field, who himself has lived with metastatic esophageal cancer for many years, studied "healing connections." He and his colleagues[58] conducted a phenomenological study to explore the relevance of the existential and spiritual domains to suffering, healing, and quality of life. The themes common to patients experiencing suffering and anguish "include a sense of isolation and of being disconnected." In addition, these participants experienced an existential vacuum, a crisis of meaning, and an inability to find solace or inner peace. They often expressed feelings of victimization and a need for control. Ruminations about unsettling issues of the past and anxieties about the uncertain future consistently removed them from the potential of the present moment. These coping patterns frequently had their roots in early childhood."[58(pp. 381–382)] Analysis across cases when the participants experienced integrity and wholeness yielded strikingly different themes from those with suffering and anguish. "These individuals tended to find a sense of meaning and connectedness in the context of their illness. They also tended to experience a greater acceptance of their illness. This might even be expressed as a degree of sympathetic connection to their disease."[58(p. 382)] Mount and his colleagues note, "Although healing connections may first be experienced at any one of the four levels (with self, others, the phenomenal world, or ultimate meaning), it appears that openness to healing connections at one level fosters opening at others."[58(p. 383)]

This openness to healing connections may take place not only in the patient, but in caregivers as well. It is perhaps reflected in the fact that caregivers in oncology and palliative care with a greater sense of spirituality had greater compassion satisfaction and less burnout[59] and medical residents who practiced greater self-care had more empathy towards patients.[60] Katz[61] speaks of the alchemical reaction that occurs when two individuals engage together at the most vulnerable time in human existence—the end of life. Alchemy is "that space" that takes its own place in the poignant relationship between helper and patient. Both can be transformed through the experience. This chapter contends that, even in the midst of suffering, caregivers can have the option of healing connections that benefit both the caregiver and the patient/family member. However, in order to do this, caregivers need to engage in self-awareness practices and wellness strategies and be open to change.[9,56(from reference 62)]

Occupational health: the benefits of caring for oncology and palliative patients

Satisfaction with one's work appears to be a secondary outcome with the primary objective of studies focused on adverse consequences such as compassion fatigue (secondary trauma), burnout, moral distress and vicarious traumatization. Few occupational health studies have, as their primary objective, to determine whether or not healthcare professionals achieve personal satisfaction from their work. This backdoor approach to understanding satisfaction may result in misleading findings. For example, if a researcher assumes that a specific area of oncology practice such as hematopoietic stem cell transplant must be stress-inducing and administers an instrument to measure adverse consequences, i.e., burnout without a clear understanding of the nature of the work it may very well appear that the nature of the work is inherently distressing, emotionally overwhelming or traumatizing. The very opposite may, in fact be true. The benefits attributed to working with advanced cancer patients or individuals at end of life include compassion satisfaction, job engagement and satisfaction, vitality/hardiness/coherence, exquisite empathy, resilience and hope.[25(p. 579)]

Empathy and compassion: can compassion fatigue if we are all connected?

Reflections on empathy and compassion

First, a distinction must be made between empathy and compassion. Empathy has recently been described as "the bridge that allows us to cross into the territory of someone else's feelings. It establishes a connection between two people, and it's the reason we enjoy reading novels and watching movies."[63(p. 1337)] Landmark research by Dr. Tania Singer et al.[64(p. 1157)] showed that when the partner of a woman observed her in pain, from an electric shock to her hand, the partner's sensorimotor cortex and the insula lit up, showing the "end note" of pain "ouch, that hurt," not the part of the brain that felt the searing pain in the hand. Singer feels this overlap is the route of empathy.[64] Singer was born as a twin and says, she "was born a we." She says "we constantly resonate with each another."[63(p. 1337)] Singer is studying the difference between empathy and compassion. In doing an MRI of the brain of a French Buddhist monk, Matthieu Ricard, a meditator, with a background in molecular biology, she asked him to focus on compassion. The parts of this brain that lit up were not the ones involved with empathy, when subjects turned to the suffering of another, but the areas of the brain associated with romantic love or reward, such as the nucleus accumbens and ventral striatum. When she asked Ricard, what he had done, he said he "put himself into a state of compassion, a warm feeling of well-wishing towards the world. When Ricard went back into the scanner and concentrated on the plight of children in a Romanian orphanage . . . his brain showed the typical signature of empathy. But Ricard later said that the pain quickly became unbearable. 'I felt emotionally exhausted, very similar to being burned out.'"[63(p. 1337)]

An anecdote describing this feeling of the challenges of empathy comes from one of the nurses studied by Brenda Sabo.

> We conversed a lot in that session, about her fears and reality, her family and their way of coping. She opened up to me and I felt heroic, except that this sense of connection was overwhelmed by the breach of task-oriented nursing that so often becomes reality; I had allowed myself to imagine WG as my own mother. The thought of her suffering silently as this woman does, was becoming too much for me. I acknowledge to myself why it is so painless for us as nurses to focus on low blood pressure, increased liver function levels, fluid status and lung sounds; this is because imagining ourselves or our loved ones as a patient is too scary to fathom.

—H/BMT nurse[57(p. 26)]

Humans are more likely to empathize with those who are similar to us. Singer "acknowledges the limitations of empathy. After her experience with Ricard she changed tack and concentrated on compassion, Ricard's state of general warmth, which she also calls 'empathic concern,' as opposed to 'empathic distress. . . . Ricard taught me that compassion is something completely different from empathy.' Now she is convinced that it is this 'caring system' that needs to be used more. The general warm feelings from compassion would not be limited to friends or relatives and they are less stressful for caregivers than empathy."[63(p. 1338)]

In the Buddhist tradition, compassion is not just an isolated skill or trait, independent of others. Compassion is considered to be one of four *Brahmaviharas*, or Four Immeasurables: together with compassion, the other three are loving-kindness, joy and equanimity.

They are called immeasurables because they are virtuous qualities of the mind that can be developed limitlessly.

The four *Brahmaviharas*, . . . are defined as follows:

- **Loving-kindness** . . . is the deep-felt thought, "May all beings have happiness and the causes of happiness."
- **Compassion** . . . is the felt thought, "May all beings be free of suffering and the causes of suffering."
- **Joy** . . . is the wish, "May all beings have joy and flourish, and continuously increase their well-being."
- **Equanimity**, or impartiality, . . . is the understanding that each and every single being wants happiness, and is therefore the wish, "May all beings everywhere experience wellbeing and flourish.

. . .

The definitions of loving-kindness, compassion and joy each have two parts. The first part of the definition addresses the motivational aspect, the aspiration that you wish for something to be a certain way. It is important to realize that in this understanding and definition of compassion you are not excluding yourself. Compassion is not about excluding, or sacrificing, yourself at the cost of others' well-being. This is why it speaks of all beings, including yourself: "May I also be free of suffering and its causes." However, by the same token, one should not understand it as: "May I be free of suffering at the expense of others". It cannot be stressed enough how important it is to think that others too want to be free of suffering, be that the person in front of you or any being with whom we share a moment in life. The second part of the definition speaks about the causes. Adding the causes becomes the concrete action: it is the step that manifests the aspiration, when you engage in realizing the wish. It's not just the wish that will make a difference, but primarily changing the causes will contribute to the well-being of oneself and others. When somebody is sick, a doctor is not just wishing for that person to be well and free of suffering, but acts as best as he or she can to correct the condition. From a Buddhist perspective, the ultimate cause of suffering is ignorance—a misapprehension of reality's interdependence, and bringing insight and clarity into that delusion will lead to the eradication of suffering and its causes.[65(pp. 159,162)]

The development of compassion does not follow a single path. Compassion is not an independent skill, nor is it a tool that creates happiness; it is more a way of being. Hence one should not think of having compassion, while useful, but rather of being compassionate. Accordingly, compassion is closely related to ethical behavior and conduct. Since they are highly correlated and co-dependent, the four Brahmaviharas are always taught, trained and remembered together, as they benefit and strengthen each other.[65(p. 162)]

Roshi Joan Halifax says compassion should be the basis of medical care[66] and kindness and equanimity are essential qualities in those who care for the dying.[67] She describes kindness as being "characterized by a dispositional tenderness toward others combined with genuine concern. Equanimity is a process of stability or mental balance that is characterized by mental composure and an acceptance of the present moment."[67(p. 216)] She notes that empathy is affective attunement with another, but empathy "might or might not elicit kindness, depending on the psychological makeup of the experiencer or the capacity of the experiencer to regulate her or his arousal level and maintain equanimity."[67(p. 216, refs in original)]

Roshi Joan draws on other sources and comments, "Compassion is often associated with religion. It is also believed to be at times the cause of distress in those who experience it. And yet, recent research suggests that, on the contrary, compassion might be a source of hardiness, resilience, and well-being. It is as well an important feature of socialization essential to our individual and collective wellbeing."[67(p. 209, refs in original)]

She notes that neuroscience research on compassion is in its infancy, but "because compassion seems to be an important mental, psychophysical, and social feature in our human experience, and there appears to be a deficit of it in our society, including in our medical system, the research on compassion has become more concerted in the past several years."[67,68]

Neuroscience research on empathy is more advanced. Recent neuroscience research shows that the ability to tune into one's own body sensations activates the same brain circuits (within the insula cortex) as those of empathy.[69] Halifax suggests this may be one base for the development of empathy and compassion.[69] So, self-awareness and self-compassion may prime our brains toward empathy and compassion for others.[62,69]

As already noted, medical residents who were sufficiently attentional to their own needs to engage in self-care activities were able to care for their patients in a sustainable way with greater compassion, sensitivity, effectiveness, and empathy.[60] These self-care strategies involved relationships, work attitudes, religious/spiritual practice, personal philosophies, and strategies related to job-life balance.[60] Self-care involves self-compassion. If we are not caring for ourselves we have no energy to care for others. The heart first pumps blood to the self.[70(in reference 9),56] Dr. Brenda Sabo[71] studied 12 nurses from three Canadian stem cell transplant units. She distinguishes between compassion and empathy. Thematic analysis of her data resulted in the emergence of four core themes: bearing witness to suffering, navigating uncertainty, the need to feel supported and comfortable in one's own skin, and one overarching novel theme, *compassionate presence*. Compassionate presence challenges the notion that working with individuals who are suffering or at end-of-life inevitably leads to adverse psychosocial effects for the nurse. Sabo found that "compassionate presence emerged to suggest a potential buffering effect against adverse consequences of HSCT nursing work. This finding underscored the value of the relationship as an integral component of nursing work."[71(p. 103)] To understand what was meant by compassionate presence, one must first understand the terms compassion and empathy.

Although compassion may contain or require emotion it is not limited to emotion. Compassion includes a rational dimension—an altruistic participation in another's suffering, principally intentionality. This was reflected in the HSCT nurses' willingness to not only enter into and share the suffering of their patients and families, as reflected in the theme bearing witness to suffering, but to act to lessen or alleviate suffering.

"On the one hand you understand why they [doctors] are doing it but sometimes you just can't accept it. You see the suffering. I remember when I first started nursing; I asked one of the staff men responsible, because it was understood that this young boy was dying and there was nothing that could be done except give him supportive treatment. I remember saying to him, 'if we know this is the eventual outcome, why are we not just keeping him comfortable. Why are we not just helping him to enjoy what is left of his life with his family?'"

In this example, the HSCT nurse interpreted further active treatment as futile and increasing the suffering of the young patient. While one might suggest that advocating for a change in treatment approach is fundamental to nursing practice, her desire to ease suffering may also be considered a reflection of compassionate presence. Implicit within the notion of action is a moral dimension, relating to the needs of another and reaching beyond self-interest.[71(p. 107)]

Thus, "compassion strives for and supports a balance between standing with and working toward the elimination of suffering without taking that suffering on as our own."[71(p. 107)] Integral to compassion, however, is the recognition that all human beings are suffering, including the fact that I suffer, and a desire to alleviate the suffering of all human beings.

"In contrast, empathy, derived from the Greek *empatheia, em* (to put into or to bring about) and *patheia* (suffering), suggests a bringing about or understanding of a certain condition or state. A relatively recent term, empathy has its roots in psychology and aspects of the therapeutic process,[72] specifically the 'affective cognitive experience of understanding another person."[73(p. 65)] Rogers defined empathy as "the ability to sense the client's private world as if it were your own, but without ever losing the 'as if' quality."[74(p. 99)] Empathy is seen as an important aspect of therapeutic interactions. While empathy is an experience, it requires the nurse to "'objectify' that experience; that is, 'empathy is a means of cognitively understanding another's experiences.' "[75(p. 167)] Empathy may be thought of as a mechanism of observation to facilitate understanding but its presence does not imply good care or compassion; only that its presence is necessary for appropriate care to take place."[71(p. 108)] The research by Singer cited above shows that empathy may well be more than just a cognitive understanding of another's experience; empathy can also lead to brain changes similar to those experienced by the other.[63,64,68]

Compassionate presence

meant nurses shared in the patient and family's experience of pain and sorrow and its associated effects. In so doing, the nurse experienced a greater sense of fulfillment and enlightenment, even in the presence of pain and suffering. It became an opportunity for personal growth and enhancement of nursing practice. For the nurses, empathy and connection (which extends beyond engagement) were positive attributes of compassionate presence and enhanced caring work. HSCT nurses' experiences in this study contrasted sharply with the findings of trauma researchers who have suggested that repeated engagement with suffering individuals inevitably leads to emotional distress in the form of compassion fatigue or vicarious traumatization.[71(p. 108)]

Exquisite empathy

Harrison and Westwood[76] studied protective practices that mitigated vicarious trauma among mental health therapists, including professionals working in palliative care. There were "nine major themes salient across clinicians' narratives of protective practices: countering isolation (in professional, personal and spiritual realms); developing mindful self-awareness; consciously expanding perspective to embrace complexity; active optimism; holistic self-care; maintaining clear boundaries; exquisite empathy; professional satisfaction; and creating meaning."[76(p. 203)] One theme stood out—*exquisite empathy*. Unlike previous studies, the authors found that empathic engagement with traumatized clients appeared to be a protective practice for clinicians working with traumatized clients. Exquisite empathy "required a sophisticated balance on the part of the clinician as s/he simultaneously maintains clear and consistent boundaries, expanded perspective, and highly present, intimate, and heartfelt interpersonal connection in the therapeutic relationship with clients, without fusing, or losing sight of the clinician's own perspective."[76(p. 214)] Trauma therapists who engaged in exquisite empathy, were "invigorated rather than depleted by their intimate professional connections with traumatized clients"[76(p. 213)] and protected against compassion fatigue and burnout. Exquisite empathy seems to be similar to Singer's concept of "empathic concern."[63,68] The idea that

trauma therapists can be both invigorated and protected in their work has also been referred to as bidirectionality,[9,56,76] it refutes the commonly held notion that being empathic to dying patients inevitably leads to emotional depletion. The practice of exquisite empathy is facilitated by clinician self-awareness.[9,56,76]

Self-care and self-compassion

Alkema et al.[18] found that the caregivers they studied who used only physical approaches to self-care were more at risk of compassion fatigue. Koo et al., studying oncology and palliative care staff[59] and Peter Huggard, studying physicians[17,23,77] found greater compassion satisfaction in those who reported greater spirituality and those with little or no spirituality were at increased risk of burnout[59] as were young males.[59]

Residents studied by Shanafelt et al.[60] who had a broader repertoire of coping styles, including meditation and spirituality were more empathic. The caregivers studied by Vachon[27] reported not only the sense of competence, control and pleasure in one's work, but also a personal philosophy of illness, death and one's role in caring for dying persons and their families as well as lifestyle management techniques including: engaging in physical activities and diversions, organizing non-job-related social interactions, taking time off, attending to one's need for good nutrition and adequate sleep, and meditation and relaxation exercises.[10,27] In practicing self-compassion, we as caregivers need to practice holistic self-care and wellness strategies in order to bring compassion to others.[9,56]

The Halifax model of compassion

Roshi Joan Halifax[67] has been involved for many decades in an exploration of compassion. In distinguishing between compassion and empathy, Roshi Joan says:

The intention to transform suffering is one of the features that distinguishes compassion from empathy. From the point of view of compassion, intention is a key process in the cultivation of this mental faculty. It is based in the prosocial experience of the motivation to transform the suffering of others as well as oneself. Intention priming compassion is based in part on an ethical orientation, which is the foundation of one's motivation to not harm, do good, and to help others. This moral ground is fundamental to the practice of medicine. Even if one's motivation is altruistic, it can happen that aversive reactions and actions arise out of one's conditioning. In working with dying people, aversion is not uncommon. In this case, it is essential to override habitual responses, engage in positive and realistic appraisal, and learn how to down-regulate arousal or shift away from thoughts and behaviors that are destructive, from abandoning patients, engaging in moral outrage, or simply becoming numb to the suffering of patients, families, and colleagues. This is usually done through the experience of insight based in self-awareness and supported by the intention to decrease the suffering of the patient and all those associated with the patient.[67(p. 217, refs in original)]

Insight supports a

metacognitive perspective and mental pliancy, hardiness, and autonomy. In this cognitive dimension, self-awareness, including access to memory, can lead to insights about the nature of reality, and can foster reappraisal and down-regulation, should that be necessary, when serving those who are dying. It also primes perspective taking or cognitive attunement, which allows one to understand the mental experience of another, whether colleague, dying person or family member. A final feature in the cognitive domain that is important is that there be no attachment to an outcome. Of course, compassion entails the aspiration to transform or end suffering. At the same time, the attachment to a particular outcome can be a cause of suffering. These two valences of 1) not having an unrealistic expectation for an outcome and 2) the dedication to supporting a beneficial outcome in relation to the experience of suffering can be viewed as the "two sides of the same coin" of intention. A clinician strives diligently to alleviate disease, pain, and suffering, for example, but, at the same time, she or he has, in the best circumstances, "therapeutic humility", which leads the clinician to realize that he or she must accept the eventual course of events that may be swayed by influences beyond one's control.[67(p. 220)]

So can compassion fatigue?

From the above it can be seen that compassion is different from empathy. True compassion does not fatigue. However, for most clinicians it will be necessary to have training and supervision to truly practice compassion, compassionate care, and compassionate presence.

Posttraumatic growth

Continued efforts to help others who are suffering can lead to changes in a person's day-to-day relationship with their work, their ability to conduct their work, and overall psychological, physical, and spiritual well-being reaching far beyond the work setting. Some negative aspects are related to providing care in general and some are related to providing care to trauma survivors.[17] However, more recent research has focused on the positive changes that can occur as a consequence of being exposed to the suffering of others.

Several researchers have reported on the positive, and transformative, aspects of caring. When Vachon[27] asked caregivers to the critically ill, dying, and bereaved what kept them going in their work, the number one coping mechanism was a sense of competence, control, and pleasure in their work. Stamm[22] focused on compassion satisfaction, the positive aspects relating to providing care, and Pearlman and Caringi on the vicarious transformation that can occur.[78] Other authors have conceptualized certain positive changes resulting from trauma work as vicarious posttraumatic growth (PTG)[79,80] or vicarious resilience.[81]

Posttraumatic growth focuses on the change processes that rebuild after periods of suffering and exposure to trauma, and particularly on mechanisms that enable effective coping and managing the effects of the distressing experiences. Researchers are now exploring the notion of PTG and recovery in nurses,[82,83] physicians,[9,56] and psychotherapists.[84]

Other researchers have explored PTG from the perspective of understanding the change process and findings ways to quantify such changes. Tedeschi and Calhoun,[85] in developing their Posttraumatic Growth Inventory (PTGI) identified five dimensions within the PTG construct: personal strength, renewed appreciation of life, changes in life's priorities, in relationships with others, and religious and spiritual domains.

More recently, studies have reported on ways to enhance PTG through such practices as self-reflection,[9,56] acknowledging one's personal grief responses,[86] and engaging in one's own therapy.[87] Later in this chapter we will discuss approaches to caring for oneself in the face of exposure to those who are traumatized and suffering.

Religion and spirituality

In the early 1990s, academic medical centers, medical and nursing schools, residency programs, and hospitals began to recognize the role of spiritual care as a dimension of palliative care.[88] Puchalski, Ferrell, Virni, and their colleagues[88] reported on a consensus conference on improving the quality of spiritual care as a dimension of palliative care. The group developed the following definition: "Spirituality is the aspect of humanity that refers to the way individuals seek and express meaning and purpose and the way they experience their connectedness to the moment, to self, to others, to nature, and to the significant or sacred."[88(p. 887)] With relationship as the core of spirituality, one might infer that healthcare, by virtue of its relational quality, is inherently spiritual. As such, Puchalski and colleagues[88] proposed a model of spiritual care reflected in the transformation occurring between professional-patient relationships. For this to occur, healthcare professionals "must have an awareness of the spiritual dimensions of their own lives and then be supported in the practice of compassionate presence with patients through a reflective process."[88(p. 900)] In developing self-awareness of one's personal values, beliefs, and attitudes, a deeper, more meaningful connection may take place between the professional and the patient-family, as may enhanced coping[9,56,88,89(in reference 25)] (Box 63.2).

Religion and spirituality have been found to be helpful to caregivers in coping with work stress as well as perhaps being in a "better place" from which to meet the challenges of the work situation. Jayne Huggard's[30] respondents reported *religious support* (including faith and prayer) was received from ministers, by attendance at church services, and from the church community itself. *Spiritual support* was gained from spiritual directors, through prayer, belonging to a choir, or singing; time spent communing with nature; and time away from home (e.g., weekends

---

Box 63.2 Selected recommendations for staff providing palliative care

1. All members of the palliative care team should be trained in spiritual care. This training should be required as part of continuing education for all clinicians.

2. Team members should have training in self-care, self-reflection, contemplative practice, and spiritual self-care.

3. Healthcare systems should offer time for professional development of staff with regard to spiritual care and should develop accountability measures in spiritual care for the interprofessional team.

4. Board-certified chaplains can provide spiritual care education and support for interprofessional team members.

5. Clinical sites should offer education for community clergy members and spiritual care providers about end-of-life care procedures in healthcare facilities.

6. Chaplain certification and training in palliative care are needed.

Source: Reference 88, p. 900.

away or attending personal retreats); or reflective writing and journaling.

Vaillant[1] concludes his book by stating that "the human capacity for positive emotions is what makes us spiritual, and that to focus on the positive emotions is the best and safest route to spirituality that we are likely to find."[1(pp. 185-186)] He contrasts spirituality with religion and says, "spirituality refers to the psychological experiences of religiosity/spirituality that relates to an individual's sense of connection with something transcendent (be it a defined deity, truth, beauty, or anything else considered to be greater than self) and are manifested by the emotions of awe, gratitude, love, compassion, and forgiveness."[1(p. 187)] Where as religion arises from cultures, spirituality arises from biology.

Sinclair et al.[90] studied spirituality in an interdisciplinary palliative care team and found that caregivers struggled to define spirituality. Respondents included concepts relating to integrity, wholeness, meaning, and personal journeying. For many, their spirituality was inherently relational, might involve transcendence, was wrapped up in caring, and often manifested in small daily acts of kindness and of love. For some participants, palliative care was a spiritual calling. A collective spirituality, stemming from common goals, values, and belonging, surfaced.

In Peter Huggard's study[77] of 253 New Zealand physicians, a positive and significant correlation was found between compassion satisfaction and spirituality. This study examined the relationship between compassion fatigue, compassion satisfaction, and burnout and resilience, spirituality, empathy, emotional competence, and social-support-seeking behaviors. Huggard found a positive correlation between religion and vicarious traumatization. High scores on the "relationship with a higher power" subscale were related to high scores on the compassion fatigue subscale. He also demonstrated a negative and significant correlation between spirituality and burnout.

Coping and resilience in nurses

Time pressures, workload, multiple roles, and emotional issues are just some of the stressors that may impact on healthcare professionals.[91] These potentially negative stress outcomes can impact not only the well-being of health professionals but also their ability to care effectively for others.[92]

A literature review on resiliency in healthcare professionals revealed that in the studies reviewed researchers reported that nurses use a number of positive coping strategies. These include problem-focused coping, taking time out, and giving and receiving support from coworkers.[91,93] Results suggested that while positive coping may not be enough to reduce the negative effects of stress, maladaptive coping behaviors such as suppression and denial may significantly increase the negative effects of stress. These findings in relation to coping strategies are supported in the study by Garrosa, Rainho, Moreno-Jimenez, and Monteiro,[94] who, in a sample of 98 nurses, assessed the relationships between job stressors, hardiness, and coping resources on burnout dimensions at two time points. At the cross-sectional level, personal resources, control, and social support were negatively related to emotional exhaustion and challenge. Zander, Hutton, and King[95] investigated coping and its relationship with resilience in assisting pediatric oncology nurses. The three themes identified were (1) coping factors (social, team and organizational support; personal views, attitudes, and

circumstances; experience; and types of stressors), (2) coping processes (the contribution to effective adaptation), and (3) overcoming negative circumstances (how effective adaptation and coping are combined when dealing with workplace stressors). Supporting this research is the study by Timmermann, Naziri, and Etienne,[96] in which they quantitatively and qualitatively explored the nature of coping (emotion-focused coping) and defensive (denial, distortion, projection) strategies of nurses working in palliative care units. Their study demonstrated that in order to better understand the psychological functioning of caregivers, both of these strategies must be considered. Their results showed a relationship between different defense mechanisms and coping strategies, palliative attitudes, and the nurses' well-being, and that both defensive and coping strategies are important and functional in palliative care. The researchers believe that these defense mechanisms assist nurses to seek social support, develop a positive orientation, and engage with problem-focused and emotion-focused coping strategies.

In terms of resilience, there are a number of individual and contextual factors that contribute to levels of resilience in nurses. In a sample of Queensland nurses working in aged care, Cameron and Brownie[97] identified eight themes that impact their resilience: (1) experience; (2) amount of satisfaction attained; (3) positive attitude or a sense of faith; (4) making a difference, close intimate relationships, and sharing experiences with residents; (5) using strategies such as debriefing, validating, and self-reflection; (6) support from colleagues, mentors, and teams; (7) insight into their ability to recognize stressors and put strategies in place; and (8) maintaining work-life balance. Supervision and mentorship has been reported as enhancing resilience in nurses. These results share some similarities with those found by Ablett and Jones[98] in their study of hospice nurses. Their research resulted in 10 themes that related to interpersonal aspects and to the participant's beliefs as to their own ability to do the work required of them. The themes were (1) an active choice to work in palliative care, (2) that past personal experiences influence caregiving, (3) personal attitudes to caregiving, (4) personal attitudes to life and death, (5) awareness of one's own spirituality, (6) personal attitudes toward work, (7) aspects of job satisfaction, (8) aspects of job stress, (9) ways of coping, and (10) personal and professional issues and boundaries. Central to these 10 themes was the nurses' beliefs about their commitment to their work in palliative care and their belief that they could make a difference.

A recommendation from a literature review of personal resilience in the nursing literature by Jackson, Firtko, and Edenborough[99] was that resilience can be strengthened in nurses through strategies and mentorship programs. Their recommendation was that such programs should aim to develop positive and nurturing professional relationships, and encourage positivity, emotional insight, life balance, spirituality, and personal reflection. What is clear from these studies is that nurses working in hospice and palliative care employ a variety of strategies that enable them to positively and effectively manage the demands of this work and enhance resilience.

Interventions to decrease occupational risk factors in healthcare settings

It is clear from research previously cited that caregivers who engage in self-care and have some form of spiritual practice are more empathic[60] and are less prone to burnout[9,56] and compassion fatigue.[59,77] It is also clear that an approach to dealing with decreasing stress in caregivers will need to have a multipronged approach because the experience of stress is multifaceted.

This section describes interventions to decrease occupational risks factors and increase resilience in oncology and palliative care practitioners. This area of research is still limited and mostly aimed at reducing risks factors. Mindfulness interventions designed for health providers are briefly introduced and discussed in terms of their relevance for oncology and palliative care settings.

Emotional support is important for nurses and other health professionals working in palliative care. In order to address this as an organizational approach to best employment practice, Mercy Hospice Auckland has in place an emotional safety policy that aims to protect and promote staff members' emotional safety and reduce the impact of work-related stress.[100]

Additional organizational support practices include supervision, debriefing, pastoral support, acknowledgement of patient deaths, the use of rituals, regular performance appraisals and timely feedback.[101] The role and importance of debriefing and the variety of debriefing processes for palliative care staff have been reported by Jayne Huggard.[102] Like debriefing, supervision, either group or individual, has been shown to be an important staff support intervention.[103,104] Wallbank[105] has demonstrated the impact of supervision on reducing the level of compassion fatigue. This study has been the only one identified that measured a reduction in compassion fatigue over time as a result of supervision. Additionally at the individual level, and although often using a group format several efforts were devoted to facilitating emotional and grieving processes and active coping. Kravit et al.[106] developed and evaluated a psychoeducational program for 248 nurses in oncology that assists nurses who work in high-stress areas to develop personalized stress management plans that rely on the use of adaptive coping strategies to reduce stress and cultivate a meaning-based resilience focusing on setting creative and achievable goals and maintain positive mood. They report preliminary data on feasibility and acceptability.

Whitehead[107] evaluated the impact of the End-of-life Nursing Education Consortium at the institutional level on death anxiety, concerns about dying, and knowledge of the dying process. Participants in the experimental group significantly improved their knowledge of the dying process at posttest and 12 months later. However, no differences between experimental versus control groups were noted on death anxiety and concerns about dying, suggesting that education is not enough to enhance spiritual care competencies.

Spirituality and mindfulness-based interventions

Following the development of a meaning-centered interventions (MCI) to address emotional demands and existential issues encountered in palliative care, Fillion et al.[108] designed an experimental study (randomized waiting list design) to test its effectiveness. The intervention applied didactic and process-oriented strategies, including guided reflections, experiential exercises, and teachings based on themes of Viktor Frankl's logotherapy.[109] Spirituality, well-being, and satisfaction at work (general index and perception of benefits of working in palliative care) were measured at pre- and post-test and at 3-month follow-up. Palliative care nurses in the experimental group reported more perceived benefits of working in palliative care after the intervention and at follow-up. Spirituality and well-being remained, however, unaffected. Selection bias was suggested to explain the null findings (participants recruited were healthy workers and had higher spirituality at pretest than in some other studies. Improving access to the intervention and recruitment strategy was recommended to reach all nurses. Documenting the perceived benefits in more depth was also proposed. Two qualitative studies were designed to better understand the beneficial effect on the MCI. From the first study conducted with 11 palliative care nurses by Melanie Vachon et al.,[110] two essential themes emerged. Meaning-centered interventions (MCI) expanded nurses' spiritual and existential awareness by increasing their awareness of life's finiteness, opening them up to new meanings and purposes of suffering, having them become more aware of sources of meaning and purpose in life, and having them access a state of mindfulness. The second essential theme was the group's containing function for nurses. The group process allowed nurses to develop a shared language to talk about their spiritual and existential experience and experience validation through sharing their experience with peers.[2] Currently Melanie Vachon and her colleagues at the Montreal General Hospital are exploring MCI and being with the dying[66] approaches with staff involved in palliative care.[111]

In the second study, Leung, Fillion, et al.[112] also used an interpretative phenomenology approach with 14 nurses working in a bone marrow transplant unit. The MCI seemed to inspire participants to engage more with patients and their suffering. Three subthemes reflected this influence: (1) greater awareness of boundaries between their personal and professional involvement, (2) enhanced empathy from an awareness of a shared mortality, and (3) elevated hope when nurses linked patients' suffering with meaning. The qualitative studies also suggested the integration of a self-care component to the MCI, such as mindfulness stress reduction techniques to further self-awareness, self-care, and self-regulation of emotion.(from reference 2)

The recommendation of complementing MCI with mindfulness is in line with the Being with Dying intervention (BWD).[66,113] This is an earlier phase of the Halifax G.R.A.C.E. Model, to be discussed below. The premise of BWD, which is based on the development of mindfulness and receptive attention through contemplative practice, is that cultivating stability of mind and emotions enables clinicians to respond to others and themselves with compassion. In a survey, Rushton et al.[114] described the impact of BWD on the participants: nurses, physicians, social workers, and chaplains. Ninety-five BWD participants completed an anonymous online survey; 40 completed a confidential open-ended telephone interview. From the qualitative analyses of the interviews, four main themes emerged: the power of presence, cultivating balanced compassion, recognizing grief, and the importance of self-care. The interviewees considered BWD's contemplative and reflective practices meaningful, useful, and valuable and reported that BWD provided skills, attitudes, behaviors, and tools to change how they worked with the dying and bereaved.

Halifax initially developed the G.R.A.C.E. process designed to prime compassion for clinicians for compassion-based clinician-patient interactions and presented it in 2010. She then refined it with her colleagues Dr. Tony Black, a medical oncologist, and Dr. Cynthia Rushton, professor of nursing and clinical ethicist at Johns Hopkins University, who teach in the Upaya's end-of-life care clinician training program.[67] Based on the Halifax Model of Compassion[69] the G.R.A.C.E. intervention has been applied by clinicians, therapists, chaplains, and social workers as a means to engender compassion as they engage in clinician/patient interactions. "G.R.A.C.E. is a mnemonic device that can aid a clinician in remembering the steps to cultivate compassion, as he or she is in an interaction with a patient. The acronym G.R.A.C.E. refers to gathering attention; recalling intention; attunement to self and other; considering, in order to be open to insights and to discern what will truly serve the patient; and finally ethically engaging, enacting, and ending the interaction."[115(pp. 475–476)]

Halifax notes that "there seem to be two large categories of compassion: referential or biased compassion, i.e., compassion with an object; and non-referential or unbiased compassion, i.e., compassion that is objectless and pervasive.[116] Both of these types of compassion are important for clinicians to actualize in clinician/patient interactions."[67(p. 212)] Clinicians can understand the concept of compassion with an object from our daily work with clients and the illustrations of compassionate nurses given in this chapter. Compassion without an object was illustrated in the insights gained by Singer in her study of the Buddhist monk Matthieu Ricard.[63] Further insights into the neuroscience of empathy and compassion can be found in a collaborative article about the first- and third-person perspective on empathy and compassion by Klimecki, Ricard, and Singer.[117]

Based on insights gained while a fellow at the Smithsonian Institute, Halifax developed a model of compassion, which provides for a way of teaching compassion.[67,69] The mnemonic of the A.B.I.D.E. compassion model can assist clinicians in recalling the elements of the model, though it is important to recall that the model itself is nonlinear and compassion is an emergent process arising from the combination of all these faculties:

A.B.I.D.E. = Compassion:

A = Attention and Affect

B = Balance

I = Intention and Insight

D = Discernment

E = Embodiment and Ethical Enactment

Engagement > Equanimity/Eudaemonia[67(p. 221)]

Recently Roshi Joan wrote[113] of further insights developed when exploring with professional caregivers what they feel is important in a compassion-based interaction with their patients, fostering CMC (contemplative mindful compassion-based) care. These are:

Listening with Full Attention:

♦ Correctly discerning patient's behavioral cues

♦ Accurately perceiving patient's verbal communication

♦ Reduced use and influence of cognitive constructions and expectations...

Nonjudgmental Acceptance of Self and Patient:

♦ Healthy balance between patient-oriented, clinician-oriented, and relationship-oriented goals

♦ Sense of care-giving efficacy

♦ Appreciation of patient's traits

♦ Reduction in self-directed concerns

♦ Fewer unrealistic expectations of patient[113(p. 111)]

Emotional Awareness of Self and Patient:

♦ Responsiveness to patient's needs and emotions

♦ Greater accuracy in responsibility attributions

♦ Less dismissing of patient's or other caregivers' emotions

♦ Less withdrawal/abandonment resulting from negative emotions (e.g., anger, disappointment, shame, grief)[113(p. 114)]

Self-Regulation in the Caregiving Relationship:

♦ Emotion regulation in the caregiving context

♦ Caregiving in accordance with goals and values

♦ Less over reactive/"automatic" reactions or withdrawal

♦ Less dependence on other's emotions[113(pp. 114–115)]

Compassion for Self and Patient:

♦ Affection in caregiver/patient and colleague relationships

♦ More forgiving view of own caregiving efforts

♦ Less compromised affect displayed in the caregiving relationship

♦ Less self-blame when caregiving goals are not met[113(p. 111)]

This is an exciting time for research in mindfulness and meditation. As the deadline for the revisions for our chapter neared, we were introduced to the e-book *Compassion: Bridging Practice and Science*,[68] by Singer and Bolz.[1] We were already aware of and, with her permission, were quoting Roshi Joan Halifax's prepublication draft of one of her articles now published in the e-book.[67] Singer and Bolz's e-book is free of charge and is a rich treasure trove of recent research, photographs, soundscapes, interviews, and meditations relating to empathy and compassion. One of the chapters, by Saron,[118] describes changes from a 3-month meditation retreat, presumably not something most nurses would be able to sign up for. Compared to the control group, the participants had an increase in adaptive functioning, meaning "an increase in well-being, mindfulness, empathy, ego resiliency, and a decrease in depression, anxiety, neuroticism and difficulties in emotion regulation. Notably, this change was sustained five months later."[118(p. 351)] Importantly, at the biological level, telomerase was investigated.

Telomerase, is an enzyme responsible for restoring the length of telomeres. Telomeres are repeated DNA sequences that form a protective "cap" at the ends of chromosomes. However, the telomeres are not fully copied each time cells divide and hence grow shorter with each subsequent cell division. When telomeres grow too short, cells cannot divide. Telomerase, then, plays a crucial role in helping regulate telomere length. Furthermore, the length of telomeres in leukocytes (white blood cells) has been shown to predict longevity.... First off,

---

[1] Mary is indebted to her husband Bruce for pointing out the article in *Science* that introduced us to this e-book.

we found changes in telomerase levels between our experimental groups: the retreat group had significantly greater telomerase levels than the matched control group, about 30% more. And what did we find in attempting to link our subjective and objective measures? We found that a change in the psychological sense of purpose in life relates to the amount of telomerase you have after three months of intensive meditation practice . . . It does look like activities that foster meaningful positive psychological change, such as meditation, positively impact cellular aging.[118(p.352), refs in original]

Summary and conclusions

This chapter asked whether palliative care nursing is changing. There is some evidence that as palliative care became more of a professional academic specialty with extensive knowledge bases for the professions there may be more reliance on medical intervention and symptom relief and less on the earlier goals of *palliation, presence*, and *meaning* as a response to the sufferings and abandonment of dying persons. Cellarius proposed a revision of palliative care ethics that retrieved the earlier goals of *presence* and *meaning* as a response to abandonment[32(p. 2)] Dr. Brenda Sabo, a nurse, mentioned similar issues with the challenge of providing care to the patient versus caring for the patient.[57]

Earlier work by Kearney,[119] Doyle[120] and Georges et al.[121] also signaled changes that were potential areas of concern. Previously palliative care staff generally experienced less stress than their colleagues in other specialties.[10,28,29,30] This may be changing. Canadian hospice/palliative care staff[33] who provided direct service to palliative patients and families were more apt to be burned out and to experience compassion fatigue than were their colleagues in integrative medicine and those who did not provide direct clinical care, and they did not experience any more compassion satisfaction than their colleagues who did not provide such services. These trends will need to be watched to see whether they indicate changes internationally. The earlier concerns from Kearney[119] and Doyle[120] reflected both the European and international perspective. The important work of Georges et al.,[121] discussed in length in our previous chapter in the third edition of this textbook,[5] reflected changes in nurses in an academic European palliative care unit where many of the changes Cellarius[32] spoke of were observed.

The chapter described the numerous constructs being used to try to elucidate the positive and negative aspects of caregiving. These include stress,[3,4] burnout,[6–8,18,33] job engagement,[7] compassion fatigue,[11,12,17–23,35,77] compassion satisfaction,[18,20,22,33,34] empathic strain,[24] vicarious traumatization,[11,12,71,77] secondary traumatic stress disorder,[11,12,24] PTE,[14–16] empathy,[11,24,25,60,63,64,67–69,71–74,77] and exquisite empathy.[9,56,76] The concepts of compassion fatigue and compassion satisfaction were questioned and it was shown that the constructs are likely measuring empathy rather than compassion.

The literature on stress and burnout in palliative care was reviewed using the lenses of workload; autonomy, control, and reward; social relationships, community belonging and fairness; and emotional demand. It was seen that the workload has long been perceived as a challenge[28,36] and may be seen to be an increasing problem both in oncology and palliative care.[35,37,39] When caregivers have more autonomy and acknowledgment they are more satisfied with their jobs and able to find more meaning in their work[33,44,51,55] and when they have less control they are less satisfied[37]; and a sense of community and a good team has always been important in palliative care,[8,10,29,30] but at least some of our stress evolves from our relationships with colleagues.[5,10,28,30,37] There continue to be challenges in some relationships,[37,39] but our colleagues continue to provide a rich source of support for others.[29,101] The need to meet emotional demands is associated with burnout, however, generally care of the dying has not been a major stressor in palliative care,[33] in part because that was what we chose to do. This is not to deny that there can be stress associated with the care of the dying.[9,56,57] Our work can serve as a source of meaning in our lives, especially when work situations are good.[33,44,51,54] A sense of connectedness with others, part of compassion, is a source of the meaning in our work and sustains us.[9,56,57,59] The chapter discusses the benefits of work in palliative care including the possibility of PTG.[9,56,79,80,82–85] Nurses able to practice compassionate presence, sharing in the patient and family's experience of pain and sorrow, experienced a greater sense of fulfillment and enlightenment, which served as an opportunity for personal growth and enhancement of nursing practice.[71]

The differences between empathy and compassion are discussed in part in order to clarify that compassion fatigue, which can sound like a "noble thing to have," may actually be a reflection of empathy strain.[24] Spirituality was found to be associated with less risk of burnout and compassion fatigue and to be associated with compassion satisfaction and more satisfaction with work.[17,25,31,59,77,98,99] Resilience was associated with coping skills, self-care and self-awareness, making a conscious choice to work in palliative care, spirituality, meaning making in the work situation, social support, and pleasure in one's work.[97–99] These are similar to the top coping mechanism, a sense of competence, control, and pleasure in one's work identified by the participants in Vachon's earlier study.[27]

Staying with and coping in the field of palliative care requires good self-care, self-awareness and self-compassion. Those who practice self-care, beyond the simply physical, have more compassion and receive more rewards from their work.[18,59] Suggestions for coping are given both at the individual and organizational levels. The authors focus on mindfulness-centered interventions because these are showing evidence of making a difference in the lives of caregivers. These interventions allow caregivers to be able to practice compassionate presence, thus giving meaning to our work and returning us to our roots. Let us change the things that need to be changed-seeking to improve symptom relief and to alleviate total suffering, and have the self-awareness, wisdom, courage, equanimity, and compassion to nurture the roots of the calling of our specialty—palliative care nursing.

References

1. Vaillant GE. Spiritual Evolution. New York: Broadway Books; 2008.
2. Vachon MLS, Fillion L. Staff stress and burnout in palliative care. In: Bruera E, Higginson IJ, von Gunten CF, Morita T (eds.), Textbook of Palliative Medicine. 2nd ed. London: Hodder Arnold; in press.
3. European Agency for Safety and Health at Work. Safety at Work. 2000. http://agency.osha.eu.int/publications/factsheets/8/en/facts8_en.pdf.
4. Collège d'expertise sur le suivi des risques psychosociaux au travail. 2011. Rapport faisant suite à la demande du Ministre du travail, de l'emploi et de la santé. Mesurer les facteurs psychosociaux de risque au travail pour les maîtriser. www. college-risquespsychosociaux-travail.fr.
5. Vachon MLS, Huggard J. The experience of the nurse in end-of-life care in the 21st century: mentoring the next generation. In: Ferrell BR,

Coyle N (eds.), Textbook of Palliative Nursing. 3rd ed. Oxford: Oxford University Press; 2010:1131–1156.

6. Maslach C, Schaufeli WB, Leiter MP. Job burnout. Ann Rev Psychol. 2001;52:397–422.

7. Maslach C, Leiter M. Early predictors of job burnout and engagement. J Appl Psychol. 2008; 93:498–512.

8. Maslach C. Job burnout: new directions in research and interventions. Curr Dir Psychol Sci. 2003;13:189–192.

9. Kearney MK, Weininger RB, Vachon MLS, Mount BM, Harrison RL. Self-care of physicians caring for patients at the end of life: "Being connected . . . a key to my survival." JAMA. 2009;301:1155–1164.

10. Vachon MLS. Staff stress in hospice/palliative care: a review. Palliat Med. 1995;9:91–122.

11. Figley C. Compassion Fatigue: Coping with Secondary Traumatic Stress Disorder in Those Who Treat the Traumatized. New York, NY: Brunner-Routledge; 1995.

12. Figley CR, ed. Treating Compassion Fatigue. New York, NY: Brunner-Routledge; 2002.

13. Maslach C. Engagement research: some thoughts from a burnout perspective. Eur J Work Org Psychol. 2011;20:47–52.

14. Linden M. Posttraumatic embitterment disorder. Psychother Psychosom. 2003;72(4):195–202.

15. Linden M, Baumann K, Rotter M, Schippan B. Possttraumatic embitterment disorder in comparison to other mental disorders. Psychother Psychosom. 2008;77(1):50–56.

16. Sensky T. Chronic embitterment and organisational justice. Psychother Psychosom. 2010;79(2):65–72.

17. Huggard PK, Stamm BH, Pearlman LA. Physician stress: compassion satisfaction, compassion fatigue and vicarious traumatization. In: Figley CR, Huggard PK, Rees C (eds.), First Do No Self-Harm. New York: Oxford University Press; 2013:127–145.

18. Alkema K, Linton JM, Davies R. A study of the relationship between self-care, compassion satisfaction, compassion fatigue, and burnout among hospice professionals. J Soc Work End Life Palliat Care. 2008;4:2:101–119.

19. Stamm BH. The Concise ProQOL Manual. 2nd ed. Pocatello, ID: ProQOL.org; 2010.

20. Yoder EA. Compassion fatigue in nurses. Appl Nurs Res. 2010;23:191–197.

21. Valent P. Diagnosis and treatment of helper stresses, traumas and illnesses. In: Figley CR (ed.), Treating Compassion Fatigue. Hove, Great Britain: Brunner-Routledge; 2002:17–37.

22. Stamm BH. Measuring compassion satisfaction as well as fatigue: developmental history of the compassion satisfaction and fatigue test. In: Figley CF (ed.), Treating Compassion Fatigue. New York: Brunner-Routledge; 2002:107–19.

23. Huggard P. Compassion fatigue and dying and death: what strategies will prevent the development of compassion fatigue and what is the evidence for their effectiveness? In: Hinerman N, Fisher (eds.), Making Sense of Death and Dying. Oxfordshire: Inter-Disciplinary Net, in press.

24. Wilson JP, Lindy JL. Countertransference in the Treatment of PTSD. New York: Guilford Press; 1994.

25. Sabo BA, Vachon MLS. Care of professional caregivers. In: Davis MP, Feyer PC, Ortner P, Zimmerman C (eds.), Supportive Oncology. Philadelphia, PA: Elsevier; 2011:575–589.

26. Stamm B. The Concise Manual for the Professional Quality of Life Scale: the ProQOL. Pocatello, ID: ProQOL.org; 2009.

27. Vachon MLS. Occupational Stress in the Care of the Critically Ill, Dying and Bereaved. Washington, DC: Hemisphere; 1987.

28. Vachon MLS. Four decades of selected research in hospice/palliative care: have the stressors changed? In: Renzenbrink I (ed.), Caregiver Stress and Staff Support in Illness, Dying, and Bereavement. Oxford: Oxford University Press; 2011:1–24.

29. Pereira SM, Fonsecal AM, Carvalho AN. Burnout in palliative care: a systematic review. Nurs Ethics. 2011;18:317–326.

30. Huggard J. A National Survey of the Support Needs of Interprofessional Hospice Staff in Aotearoa/New Zealand. Unpublished Master's Thesis, University of Auckland, Auckland, New Zealand; 2008.

31. Fillion L, Desbiens JF, Truchon M, Dallaire C, Roch G. Le stress au travail chez les infirmières en soins palliatifs selon le milieu de pratique. Psycho-Oncologie. 2011;5:127–136—article in French with abstract in English.

32. Cellarius V. A Conceptual Analysis of Canadian Palliative Care Ethics. Unpublished Doctoral Thesis, University of Toronto; 2013.

33. Slocum-Gori S, Hemsworth D, Chan WWY, Carson A, Kazanjian A. Understanding compassion satisfaction, compassion fatigue and burnout: a survey of the hospice, palliative care workforce. Palliat Med. 2013;27:2:172–178. Published online 16 December 2011.

34. Stamm BH. The ProQOL Manual: The Professional Quality of Life Scale. Townsend, MD: 2005. Retrieved 9/19/2006. http://www.isu.edu/~bhstamm/documents/proqol/ProQOL_Manual_Oct05.pdf

35. Dougherty E, Pierce B, Ma C, et al. Factors associated with work stress and professional satisfaction in oncology staff. Am J Hosp Palliat Med. 2009;26:105–111.

36. Vachon, MLS, Lyall WAL, Freeman, SJJ. Measurement and management of stress in health professionals working with advanced cancer patients. Death Educ. 1978;l:365–375.

37. Glass N, Rose J. Enhancing emotional well-being through self-care the experiences of community health nurses in Australia. Holist Nurs Pract. 2008;22:6:336–347.

38. Mooney M, Nolan L. A critique of Freire's perspective on critical social theory in nursing education. Nurs Ed Today. 2006;26(3):240–245.

39. Vachon M. Occupational stress in palliative care. In: O'Connor M, Aranda S (eds.), Palliative Care Nursing: A Guide to Practice. Melbourne, Victoria, Australia: Ausmed Publication; 2003:41–51.

40. Weissman, D. Martyrs in palliative care. J Palliat Med. 2011;14:1278–1279.

41. Karasek RA. Job demands, job decision latitude and mental strain: implications for job redesign. Admin Sci Quart. 1979; 24:285–308.

42. Yandrick RM. High demand low control. Behavl Healthc Tomorrow. 1997;6:40–44.

43. Maslach C, Leiter M. The Truth About Burnout: How Organizations Cause Personal Stress and What to Do About It. San Francisco, CA: Jossey-Boss; 1997.

44. Fillion L, Tremblay I, Truchon M, et al. Job satisfaction and emotional distress among nurses providing palliative care: empirical evidence for an integrative occupational stress-model. Int J Stress Manag. 2007;14:1–25.

45. Hackman JR, Oldham GR. Development of the job diagnostic survey. J Appl Psychol. 1975;60:159–170.

46. Fillion L, Gagnon P. French adaptation of the shortened version of the Profile of Mood States (POMS). Psychol Rep. 1999;84:188–190.

47. Shacham S. A shortened version of the Profile of Mood States. J Person Assess. 1983;47:305–306.

48. Guay-Genest S. Stress et double rôle: une étude chez les infirmières [Stress and double role: a nurse's study]. Ste-Foy, Quebec, Canada: Université Laval; 1987.

49. Gray-Toft PA, Anderson JG. Stress among hospital nursing staff: its causes and effects. Soc Sci Med. 1981;5A:639–647.

50. Fillion L, Fortier M, Goupil R L. Educational needs of palliative care nurses in Québec. J Palliat Care. 2005; 21:12–18.

51. Fillion L, Truchon M, L'Heureux, et al. Rapport R-794, Montréal, IRSST, 2013, 84 pages. 2013. http://www.irsst.qc.ca/-projet-vers-l-amelioration-des-services-et-des-soins-de-fin-de-vie-mieux-comprendre-l-impact-du-milieu-de-travail-sur-la-satisfaction-et-le-bien-etre-des-0099-6050.html.

52. Johnson JV, Hall EM. Job strain, work place social support, and cardiovascular disease: a cross-sectional study of a random sample of the Swedish working population. Am J Public Health. 1988;78:1336–1342.

53. Siegrist J, Peter R, Junge A, Cremer P, Seidel D. Low status control, high effort at work and ischemic heart disease: prospective evidence from blue-collar men. Soc Sci Med. 1990;31:1127–1134.

54. Munroe B, Speck P. Team effectiveness. In: Speck P (ed.), Teamwork in Palliative Care: Fulfilling or Frustrating? Oxford: Oxford University Press; 2006:201–209.

55. Vachon M, Fillion L, Achille M. Death confrontation, spiritual-existential experience and caring attitudes in palliative care nurses: an interpretative phenomenological analysis. Qual Res Psychol. 2012;9:151–172.

56. Kearney MK, Weininger RB, Vachon MLS, Mount BM, Harrison RL. Self-Care of physicians caring for patients at the end of life: "Being connected . . . a key to my survival." In: McPhee SJ, Winker MA, Rabow MW, Pantilat SZ, Markowitz AJ (eds.), Care at the Close of Life: Evidence and Experience. New York: McGraw Hill; 2010:551–563.

57. Sabo B. Adverse psychosocial consequences: compassion fatigue, burnout and vicarious traumatization: are nurses who provide palliative and hematological cancer care vulnerable? Indian J Palliat Care. 2008;14(1):23–29.

58. Mount BM, Boston PH, Cohen R. Healing Connections: on moving from suffering to a sense of well-being. J Pain Symptom Manage. 2007;33:372–88.

59. Koo K, Zeng L, Zhang L, DasGupta T, Vachon MLS, Holden L, et al. Comparison and literature review of occupational stress in a palliative radiotherapy clinic's interprofessional team, the radiation therapists, and the nurses at an academic cancer centre. J Med Imag Rad Sci. 2013;44:14–22.

60. Shanafelt TD, West C, Zhao X, Novotny P, Kolars J, Habermann T, Sloan J. Relationship between increased personal well-being and enhanced empathy among internal medicine residents. J Gen Intern Med. 2005;20:559–564.

61. Katz R. When our personal selves influence our professional work: an introduction to emotions and countertransference in end-of-life care. In: Katz R, Johnson T (eds.), When Professionals Weep: Emotional and Countertransference Responses in End-of-Life Care. New York: Routledge;2006:3–12.

62. Vachon MLS. Reflections on Compassion, Suffering and Occupational Stress. In: Malpas J Lickiss N (eds.), Perspectives on Human Suffering. Dordrecht, The Netherlands: Springer; 2012:317–331.

63. Kupferschmidt K. Concentrating on kindness. Science. 2013;341:1336–1339.

64. Singer T, Seymour B, O'Doherty, Kaube H, Dolan RJ, Frith CD. Empathy for pain involves the affective but not sensory components of pain. Science. 2004;303:1157–1162. doi:10.1126/science.1093535.

65. Hangartner D. Human suffering and the four immeasurables: a Buddhist perspective on compassion. In: Singer T, Bolz M (eds.), Compassion: Bridging Practice and Science. eBook: Munich, Germany: Max Planck Society; 2013:153–164.

66. Halifax J. Being with Dying: Cultivating Compassion and Fearlessness in the Presence of Death. Boston: Shambala; 2008.

67. Halifax J. Understanding and cultivating compassion in clinical settings: The A.B.I.D.E. compassion model. In: Singer T, Bolz M (eds.), Compassion: Bridging Practice and Science. eBook: Munich, Germany: Max Planck Society; 2013::209–228.

68. Singer T, Bolz M, eds. Compassion: Bridging Practice and Science. eBook: Munich, Germany: Max Planck Society; 2013:download available for free.

69. Halifax J. A heuristic model of enactive compassion. Cur Opin Supp Pall Care. 2012:2:6:228–235.

70. Shapiro SL. The Art and Science of Meditation. Paper presented at: Cassidy Seminars; Skirball Cultural Center, Los Angeles, CA. June 27, 2008.

71. Sabo BM. Compassionate presence: the meaning of hematopoietic stem cell transplant nursing. Eur J Oncol Nurs. 2011;15:103–111.

72. Rogers C. Characteristics of the helping relationship. Personal Guidance Journal. 1958;37:6–16.

73. Olsen D. Empathy as an ethical philosophical basis for nursing. Adv Nurs Sci. 1991;14:62–75.

74. Rogers C. The necessary and sufficient conditions of therapeutic personality change. Journal of Counseling Psychology. 1957:21:95–103.

75. von Dietze E, Orb A. Compassionate care: a moral dimension of nursing. Nurs Inq. 2000;7:166–174.

76. Harrison R, Westwood M. Preventing vicarious traumatization of mental health therapists: identifying protective practices. Psychother Theory Res Pract Train. 2009;46(2):203–219.

77. Huggard, PK. Managing Compassion Fatigue: Implications for Medical Education. Unpublished doctoral thesis, University of Auckland, Auckland, New Zealand; 2008.

78. Pearlman LA, Caringi J. Living and working self-reflectively to address vicarious trauma. In: Courtois CA, Ford JD (eds.), Treating Complex Traumatic Stress Disorders: An Evidence-Based Guide. New York: Guilford Press; 2009:202–224.

79. Shakespeare-Finch J. Promoting resilience and posttraumatic growth in medical professionals. In: Figley CR, Huggard PK, Rees C (eds.), First Do No Self-Harm. New York: Oxford University Press; 2013:265–280.

80. Werdel MB, Wicks RJ. Primer on Posttraumatic Growth: An Introduction and Guide. New Jersey: Wiley & Sons; 2012.

81. Hernández P, Gangsei D, Engstrom, D. Vicarious resilience: a new concept in work with those who survive trauma. Fam Process. 2007;462:229–241.

82. McAllister M, Lowe P. The Resilient Nurse: Empowering Your Practice. Dordrecht, The Netherlands: Springer ; 2011.

83 Taubman–Ben-Ari O, Weintroub A. Meaning of life and personal growth among pediatric physicians and nurses. Death Stud. 2008;32(7):621–645.

84. Shiri S, Wexler I, Alkalay Y, Meiner Z, Kreitler S. Positive psychological impact of treating victims of politically motivated violence among hospital-based health care providers. Psychother Psychosom. 2008;77:315–318. doi: 10.1159/000142524.

85. Tedeschi RG, Calhoun LG. The Posttraumatic Growth Inventory: measuring the positive legacy of trauma. J Traum Stress. 1996;9:455–472.

86. Moon P. Untaming grief?: Palliative care physicians. Am J Hosp Palliat Care. 2011. doi: 10.1177/1049909111406705.

87. Bannink F. Posttraumatic success: solution-focused brief therapy. Brief Treatment Crisis Interven. 2008 8:215–225. doi: 10.1093/ brief-treatment/mhn013.

88. Puchalski C, Ferrell B, Virani R, et al. Improving the quality of spiritual care as a dimension of palliative care: the report of the Consensus Conference. J Palliat Med. 2009;12:885–904.

89. Sabo B. Nursing from the Heart: An Exploration of Caring Work Among Hematology/Blood and Marrow Transplant Nurses in Three Canadian Tertiary Care Centres. Unpublished doctoral thesis, Halifax: Dalhousie University; 2009.

90. Sinclair S, Raffin S, Pereira J, et al. Collective soul: the spirituality of an interdisciplinary palliative care team. Palliat Support Care. 2006;4:13–24.

91. Lim J, Hepworth, Bogossian F. A qualitative analysis of stress, uplifts and coping in the personal and professional lives of Singaporean nurses. J Adv Nurs. 2011;67(5):1022–1033.

92. Barnett JE, Baker EK, Elman NS, Schoener GR. In pursuit of wellness: the self-care imperative. Prof Psych: Res Pract. 2007;38(6):603–612.

93. Chang EM, Bidewell JW, Huntington AD, Daly J, Johnson A, Wilson H., et al. A survey of role stress, coping and health in Australian and New Zealand hospital nurses. Int J Nurs Stud. 2007;44(8):1354–1362.

94. Garrosa E, Rainho C, Moreno-Jimenez B, Monteiro MJ. The relationship between job stressors, hardy personality, coping resources and burnout in a sample of nurses: a correlational study at two time points. Int J Nurs Stud. 2010;47(2):205–215.

95. Zander M, Hutton A, King L. Coping and resilience factors in pediatric oncology nurses. J Pediatr Oncol Nurs. 2010;27(2):94–108.

96. Timmermann M, Naziri D, Etienne A-M. Defence mechanisms and coping strategies among caregivers in palliative care units. J Palliat Care. 2009;23(3):181–190.

97. Cameron F, Brownie S. Enhancing resilience in registered aged care nurses. Australas J Ageing. 2010;29(2):66–71.

98. Ablett JR, Jones RSP. Resilience and well-being in palliative care staff: a qualitative study of hospice nurses' experience of work. Psycho-Oncology. 2007;16:733–740.

99. Jackson D, Firtko A, Edenborough, M. Personal resilience as a strategy for surviving and thriving in the face of workplace adversity: a literature review. J Adv Nurs. 2007;60(1):1–9.

100. Huggard J, Nichols J. Emotional safety in the workplace: one hospice's response for effective staff support. Intl J Palliat Nurs. 2011;17(12):611–617.

101. Huggard J. Support for hospice nurses. Kaitaiki Nursing New Zealand. 2012;18(1):25–27.

102. Huggard J. Debriefing: a valuable component of staff support. Int J Palliat Nurs. 2013;19:5:212–214.

103. Rose J, Glass N. Nurses and palliation in the community: the current discourse. Int J Palliat Nurs. 2006;12(12):588–594.

104. White K, Wilkes I, Cooper K, Barbato M. The impact of unrelieved patient suffering. Int J Palliat Nurs. 2004;10(9):438–444.

105. Wallbank S. Effectiveness of individual clinical supervision for midwives and doctors in stress reduction: findings from a pilot study. Evidence Based Midwifery. 2010;8(2):65–70.

106. Kravit K, McAllister-Black R, Grant M, Kirk C. Self-care strategies for nurses: a psycho-educational intervention for stress reduction and the prevention of burnout. App Nurs Res. 2010;23:130–138

107. Whitehead PB, Anderson ES, Redican KJ, Stratton R. Studying the effects of the end-of-life nursing education consortium at the institutional level. J Hosp Palliat Care Nurs. 2010;12:184–193.

108. Fillion L, Dupuis R, Tremblay I, de Grace G-R, Breitbart W. Enhancing meaning in palliative care practice: a meaning-centered intervention to promote job satisfaction. Palliat Support Care. 2006;4:333–344.

109. Frankl VE. Logotherapy and the challenge of suffering. Rev Existen Psychol Psychiat. 1987;20:1–3.

110. Vachon M, Fillion L, Achille M, Duval SD. An awakening experience: an interpretive phenomenological analysis of the effects of a meaning-centered intervention shared amongst palliative care nurses. Qual Res Psychol. 2011;8:66–80.

111. Personal communication from Lise Fillion to MLS Vachon, 17 October 2013.

112. Leung D, Fillion L, Howell D, Duval S, Brown J, Rodin G. Meaning in bone marrow transplant nurses' work: experiences before and after a "meaning-centered" intervention. Canc Nurs. 2012;35(5):374–381.

113. Halifax J. Being with dying: experiences in end-of-life-care. In: Singer T, Bolz M (eds.), Compassion: Bridging Practice and Science. eBook: Munich, Germany: Max Planck Society; 2013:109–120.

114. Rushton CH, Sellers DE, Heller KS, Spring B, Dossey BM, Halifax J. Impact of a contemplative end-of-life training program: being with dying. Palliat Support Care. 2009;7:405–414.

115. Halifax J. Being with dying—curriculum for the professional training program in compassionate end-of-life care. In: Singer T, Bolz M (eds.), Compassion: Bridging Practice and Science. eBook: Munich, Germany: Max Planck Society; 2013:466–478.

116. Halifax J. The precious necessity of compassion. J Pain Symptom Manage. 2011 41(1):146–153.

117. Klimecki O, Ricard M, Singer T. Empathy versus compassion: Lessons from the 1st and 3rd person methods. In: Singer T, Bolz M (eds.), Compassion: Bridging Practice and Science. eBook: Munich, Germany: Max Planck Society; 2013:272–287.

118. Saron C. The Shamantha Project adventure: a personal account of an ambitious meditation study and its first results. In: Singer T, Bolz M (eds.), Compassion: Bridging Practice and Science. eBook: Munich, Germany: Max Planck Society; 2013:345–359.

119. Kearney M. Palliative medicine-just another specialty? Palliat Med. 1992;6:41.

120. Doyle D. The world of palliative care: one man's view. J Palliat Care. 2003;19(3):149.

121. Georges JJ, Grypdonck M, De Casterle BD. Being a palliative care nurse in an academic hospital: a qualitative study about nurses' perceptions of palliative care nursing. J Clin Nurs. 2002;11:785–793.

CHAPTER 64

Ethical considerations in palliative care

Maryjo Prince-Paul and Barbara J. Daly

> Compassion, in which all ethics must take root, can only attain its full breadth and depth if it embraces all living creatures and does not limit itself to mankind.
>
> Albert Schweitzer

Key points

- What constitutes "extraordinary care" will be almost entirely contingent on the values and clinical situation of the patient.

- Enteral and parenteral nutrition and hydration are medical treatments that can be withheld or withdrawn under appropriate medical and ethical circumstances.

- Effective palliative care that rests on a sound ethical foundation requires ongoing discussions about patient and family values and preferences.

- Decisions regarding ethical dilemmas and the choices that are necessary require thoughtful discussion and critical communication skills.

- The ethical duties of all healthcare providers include the obligation to respect diversity in the views of colleagues, as well as patients.

- Interprofessional practice, essential in quality palliative care, requires the support of formal organizational mechanisms such as ethics committees and interdisciplinary rounds.

Ethics and moral reasoning

Ethics, broadly defined, is the branch of philosophy that is concerned with the study of human conduct, with the rational analysis of how human beings ought to behave and the methods by which we can identify good and evil, right and wrong.[1]

In contrast, the term "morality" is conventionally used to refer to accepted and rational codes of conduct governing behavior, aimed to promote good and minimize evil.[2]

As can be seen, these terms are closely related and are often used interchangeably.

Much of this text is concerned with the practical sense of nursing—that is, the application of natural and behavioral sciences in designing and implementing effective processes of care. This chapter will address what Bishop and Scudder refer to as the "primary sense of nursing practice," the moral sense.[3]

The focus will be on the most common issues faced by nurses in palliative care. Our objective is to prepare the nurse for identifying, addressing, and resolving the complex questions that arise in caring for individuals and families facing life-limiting illnesses.

In confronting ethical questions, nurses may experience varying levels of moral quandaries. Given the complexity of the healthcare system and individual patient situations, nurses often are uncertain about the right or most ethically sound action. Moral uncertainty can produce discomfort, but it is the hallmark of a morally sensitive agent. It signals doubt or confusion about values or rules, but can usually be resolved with careful analysis, as we will illustrate with case studies. In contrast to uncertainty, moral dilemmas are more troublesome and occur when the nurse finds her/himself in a situation with conflicting demands or one in which every possible action seems to involve violating an ethical duty. Dilemmas may be associated with significant stress and anxiety; resolution may require assistance of others to sort through the conflicts involved. Moral distress is the most damaging state and occurs when the nurse perceives a moral duty but is unable, often because of external constraints, to fulfill that duty. Persistent moral distress can lead to disillusionment, moral apathy, and eventual resignation.

Dealing with ethical questions before moral distress occurs requires knowledge and skill in ethical reasoning. While thorough exploration of ethical theories is beyond the scope of this chapter, a brief review of the major theories that are the basis for the commonly accepted principles of autonomy, beneficence, nonmaleficence, and justice will be helpful. Following this review, specific issues that the palliative care nurse is likely to face will be explored, with particular attention to analysis of the problems.

Moral reasoning

As mentioned, ethics as a discipline has its roots in philosophy. There are many ethical theories that have been developed over the years, each with its own justification. The best known of these are deontological theories and consequentialist theories. Consequentialist theories determine the justification for actions by examining consequences. The action that produces the best consequences for the greatest number is the preferred, or "right" action. Deontological theories, in contrast, argue that actions are right or wrong according to their adherence to duties and obligations, not by virtue of the consequences of the actions. Both types of theories generate principles, such as autonomy (the right of self-determination), beneficence (the duty to promote good), and nonmaleficence (the duty to do no harm). From principles, in turn, more specific moral rules can be derived. For example, the general duty to respect autonomy and the right of self-determination is the basis of the specific rule that we obtain informed consent before interventions.

Both deontological and consequentialist theories are forms of a principlist approach to ethics. Principlist approaches, although they may rest on differing theoretical premises, all use general and relatively universal principles as the central tool for ethical analysis. Universal principles play a key role in developing mature ethical agency, provide reliable rules of thumb for responding quickly in real-life dilemmas, and reflect the considered wisdom of decades of philosophical analysis. Nevertheless, abstract and somewhat rigid principles can be insensitive to the nuances of specific clinical situations and conflict with deep intuitions of experienced clinicians. More recently, appreciation for the importance of context has grown.

Feminist ethics, an ethic of care, and narrative ethics are relatively new approaches to ethical analysis. The development of feminist ethics, an outgrowth of the feminist movement, was encouraged by the work of Carol Gilligan, who studied moral reasoning in children and found that boys relied on a rule-oriented, justice-based approach, while girls tended to analyze situations in terms of relationships and context, seeking resolution in the details of the story or narrative.[4]

Consistent with Gilligan's work, caring as a basis for ethics rests on the assumption that morality is rooted in human relationships and feelings. Nel Nodding, recognized as the originator of this theory, argues that morality must stem from the caring instinct and that the ethical ideal is located in the reciprocal caring relationship between and among persons.[5]

Narrative ethics uses the stories of patients and health professionals as the unit of analysis. In seeking understanding of ethical dilemmas from a narrative perspective, the elements of the situation are viewed as components of the story, and aspects such as the relation among participants, predominant voices, intentions of the actors, and consideration of whose voices are heard and not heard are central to developing understanding of the ethical dimensions.[6]

As with the ethic of care and feminist ethics, understanding the relationships among all participants, the meaning of what is stated and unstated, and the motives of all involved is key to the evaluation of how best to respond in ethical dilemmas.

Sara Fry has argued that the traditional approach to medical ethics, which centers on application of objective principles and simply evaluating which principle takes priority, is no longer adequate as a foundation for nursing ethics.[7]

She points out that caring, as an ideal, is a more comprehensive basis for the traditional values of autonomy and doing good for patients. Rather than relying on moral theory, Fry suggests that nursing ethics rests on a moral view of persons. Thus, in the discussion that follows, we will attempt to evaluate issues and illustrative cases with reference to the usual moral principles, but will also consider the moral obligations that may stem from the caring relationship that nurses have with their patients.

Regardless of the theoretical underpinnings of ethical analysis, the nurse who identifies ethical issues or questions will need to use a systematic process to examine the situation and reach a decision about what action to take. There are many suggested models for analyzing ethical dilemmas, and any thoughtful, deliberative process can be helpful. One approach that is similar to the problem-solving steps most nurses have learned is illustrated in Box 64.1. The process begins with identifying the issue or question; this step helps to focus the ethical issue, clarify what aspect of a complex patient care situation is raising concerns, and differentiate the ethical dilemma from clinical problems. The second step, review facts and assumptions, directs the nurse to be clear about relevant data and to be sensitive to assumptions that may not be based on adequate data. The third step, list all options, is intended to prompt the nurse to think carefully about all possible actions, rather than fall into the temptation to dichotomize the possible answers (e.g., withdraw all treatment or continue all treatment, accept the patient's decision or do not accept it, etc.). The fourth step is the point at which the nurse must bring to bear considerations related to ethical principles, relevant professional norms, laws, policies, and personal values. In this step, each option is evaluated against these touchstones or criteria. Finally, having evaluated each option, the final decision is made as the fifth step. Most ethical dilemmas are multifaceted with conflicting demands. The case studies that follow in this chapter will demonstrate the complexity of these challenges, the need to address them in a methodical and logical process, and the essential caring role of the nurse in responding to such dilemmas.

Box 64.1 Steps of ethical problem-solving

1. Define the problem.
   - Differentiate clinical problems, such as uncertainty or disagreement about prognosis, from ethical problems, such as determining how to balance duties to provide benefit and duties to respect autonomy; ensure that everyone identifies the same issue.

2. Clarify facts and assumptions.
   - Differentiate known facts from assumptions about the situation, such as presumed motives of family members; ensure that all parties have access to the same facts.

3. Develop list of all options.
   - Avoid collapsing options into "yes/no" absolutes, such as "continue all treatment" and "discontinue all treatment"; assure that all possible actions are evaluated, including intermediate steps such as continue all treatments and escalate as needed; continue all treatments but do not add anything further; discontinue ineffective interventions but continue noninvasive treatments; discontinue all interventions that do not promote comfort.

4. Evaluate all options.
   - Consider relevant laws, policies, and ethical principles; address rights, duties, and interests of all involved.

5. Choose the optimal option and implement.

Common ethical dilemmas

Case study 1

An 82-year-old man with a 15-year history of coronary artery disease, myocardial infarction, and heart failure enters the hospital with a left-sided cerebrovascular accident (CVA) that has left him partially aphasic, hemiparetic, and caused him to aspirate food of any consistency. Seven days after the stroke, his mental status is unclear, and there is disagreement as to whether or not he has decisional capacity. He is able to answer "yes" and "no," although the responses are inconsistent. The attending physician is convinced that the patient lacks decision-making capacity, while two family members (his wife and older brother) are equally convinced that he has decisional capacity. The patient does not have an advance directive. The patient's wife states that they have never held specific or detailed conversations about preferences for life-sustaining treatment. Until his stroke, he was active in his retirement and enjoyed gardening and playing bridge with friends. She believes he would not want to live in a condition that would not allow him to function as fully as he was prior to the CVA, but is ambivalent about the placement of a feeding tube. The patient's two daughters insist that a feeding tube should be placed because not doing so would be "killing him." The attending physician and the rest of the interdisciplinary healthcare team are opposed to placing the feeding tube. In fact, several nurses who have cared for this patient during previous hospitalizations for heart failure claim that the patient told them that he would not want to be sustained by artificial means. The attending physician, as well as the neurological consultant, has verified that, at this point, further significant recovery is likely to be minimal due to dense damage to the cerebral cortex. They believe placing a feeding tube would be "futile." The advanced practice nurse is not comfortable with claiming the feeding tube would be "futile" but is concerned about whether the patient would have wanted it and whether it will serve his best interests in the long term. She wonders how to get help in resolving the conflict.

Goal-setting and advance care planning

Patients with advanced disease or near the end of life, their families, and healthcare providers may encounter a variety of ethical dilemmas and subsequent choices. Although moral questions can arise about any aspect of nursing practice, including informed consent and duties to colleagues, the issues most frequently encountered in palliative care center around end-of-life decisions. These include withholding or withdrawing treatment (e.g., mechanical ventilation, hemodialysis, cardiopulmonary resuscitation, and cardiac assist devices), concerns about use of artificial nutrition and hydration (ANH), requests for hastened death (assisted suicide and euthanasia), and palliative sedation. For the most part, ethical analyses of these issues are grounded in patient choices, goals of care, preferences, prognosis, and communication. However, there are many important social, professional, and legal influences that have made these choices complex. The continual expansion of technological options and biomedical interventions, particularly over the past few decades, has enabled the medical profession to prolong life through sophisticated interventions before adequate bioethical norms have been established. As a consequence, it is usually more helpful to focus on patient preferences for *outcomes* of treatments rather than preferences or choices for *specific treatments*.[8] Clearly this requires careful and repeated discussions with patients and their families. As can be seen in Case Study 1, it would have been much more helpful to know the patient's feelings and attitudes about what states or conditions would be acceptable to him rather than general statements about use of "artificial means." The pace and demands of healthcare today add to the challenges of addressing ethical issues in the clinical setting and may lead to hasty and arbitrary decision-making. According to Levine-Ariff, "it is only with a thrust toward preventive ethics that decisions can be thoughtful and beneficial to patients and families."[9(p. 169)]

"Preventive ethics" can be thought of as standards and norms that, when adhered to, can minimize the frequency with which difficult conflicts and dilemmas occur. The use of advance care planning is an example of a "preventive ethics" intervention that nurses can implement on an individual level. The Veterans Administration, as part of their integrated ethics program, has adopted a quality improvement approach to systematizing efforts to address quality gaps, such as lack of attention to and support of advanced care planning, and nurses can be key agents in such hospital-wide efforts.[9]

Because of the many difficult decisions that will be faced by most people as they age and as they experience serious illnesses, assuring that thoughtful discussions take place before serious illness occurs can be quite helpful in preventing later uncertainties and dilemmas (see Case Study 1). Advance care planning is a process of communication and documentation to identify patients' preferences about goals of care and identify an authorized proxy who can provide competent, confident, and informed representation for choices when the patient is unable to express wishes. Advance directives are written instructions to healthcare providers that are established before the need for medical intervention. Advance directives have three major purposes: provide a mechanism to enable providers to respect patient autonomy in situations in which the patient cannot express his wishes, provide guidance to healthcare professionals and family members regarding how to proceed with decision-making about life-sustaining interventions, and provide immunity for professionals from civil and criminal liabilities when certain stated conditions are met.

A living will (LW) is one type of advance directive that is often accompanied by a durable power of attorney for healthcare (DPAHC) or health-care proxy. Living wills are used to declare wishes to refuse, limit, or withhold life-sustaining treatment under such circumstances that the individual is incapacitated or unable to communicate, while the DPAHC authorizes the agent or proxy to make all healthcare decisions, presumably acting as the patient would have. A living will, as the patient's own treatment preference, takes precedence over the DPAHC if there are conflicts. However, in many states, the LW statute specifies that this document is only in effect when the patient is terminally ill, as determined by the physician, and thus it may not be helpful in situations such as major cerebrovascular accident, persistent vegetative state, coma, or other serious illnesses that are not considered inevitably terminal.

Despite their shortcomings, advance directives are the best instruments we have to ensure that an individual's goals and preferences for care are met.[10]

Unfortunately, because predicting and outlining all possible choices regarding healthcare scenarios is difficult, advance directives are rarely defined as precisely as needed,[11] especially when a disease progresses and the context of the situation changes. Although it has been over two decades since the Patient Self-Determination Act (PSDA) was made law in 1990, empirical studies reporting effectiveness of advance directives have yielded disappointing results. Only 25% to 35% of patients have completed these, even among seriously ill populations such as persons with cancer,[12] and when present, they often do not direct care.[13,14]

Nonetheless, advance care planning is an essential process that should begin to take place at the point of diagnosis and be revisited throughout the course of the disease trajectory to ensure that patients' preferences for care are preserved.

Other forms of advance directives include out-of-hospital do-not-attempt-resuscitation (DNAR) orders (discussed below), and the Five Wishes,[15] a detailed guide for discussions of preferences for end-of-life care. The Five Wishes document, now recognized in forty-two states, helps individuals who are seriously ill and unable to speak for themselves express how they want to be treated from a medical, personal, emotional, and spiritual perspective. In addition, this unique document helps patients discuss their wishes with family and the healthcare team.

Healthcare advance directives differ widely in format and content, making the already complex issues that palliative care nurses face even more difficult. Additional barriers exist when patients transfer from one care facility to another and the requirements change or the previously existing document is not incorporated or honored.[16]

In addition, some advance directives are not sufficient to direct care in some healthcare institutions until a physician's order is written in the medical record. These barriers have led to an attempt to remedy these problems through the creation of other methods such as Physician Orders for Life-Sustaining Treatment (POLST)[17] and Medical Orders for Life-Sustaining Treatment (MOLST).[18]

The overall aim of these newer forms of advance directives is to improve the communication of personal wishes about life-sustaining treatments, resulting in higher quality medical care that is consistent with patient choice.

The POLST paradigm, as the concept is called, was originally developed in Oregon to improve end-of-life care by overcoming many of the shortcomings and pitfalls of advance directives.[16,19]

Because the POLST document is designed to be long lasting and portable across treatment settings, it can be posted on the patient's refrigerator or on the front of the patient's medical record, where it can be easily located by emergency medical personnel and other healthcare providers. The cornerstone of the program is a brightly colored standardized form that provides specific treatment orders for mechanical ventilation, antibiotics, cardiopulmonary resuscitation, and ANH. The POLST form is recommended for persons who have a life-limiting disease, who might die in the next year, or who want to further define their preferences for care and treatment. Other states have adopted similar programs with different names although all share the same core elements and with similar forms (POST in West Virginia; MOLST in New York).[20]

The National Consensus Project for Quality Palliative Care, in the third edition of the Clinical Practice Guidelines for Quality Palliative Care,[21] recommends that the POLST model be adopted nationwide because it more accurately reflects treatment goals and ensures that the information is transferable and applicable across all healthcare settings. Unfortunately, many state statutes require modification before this goal can be reached. Although the goals of these newer forms are intended to honor patients' wishes, end-of-life decisions are more nuanced and context dependent than standard "contractual" forms can adequately handle.

Nursing responsibilities related to advance care planning include initiating conversations about patient overall goals and specific wishes related to hospitalization, use of cardiopulmonary resuscitation, and other forms of advanced life support. These discussions will be most helpful if they focus on values rather than specific treatments. Patients and families should be asked about the existence of advance directives, and education about both the formal documents and the process of advance care planning is a critical responsibility in palliative care. Patients and families also frequently need assistance in the actual completion of the documents, and nurses can be effective facilitators in providing access to the documents and showing patients how to complete them, as well as helping them think through their wishes.

Do not attempt resuscitation orders

As noted, decisions about the level and type of interventions to be used must stem from consensus about the goals of care. For patients in acute care settings and those who have not yet elected to focus on comfort rather than cure, the specific issue of resuscitation status is a frequent source of distress for clinicians as well as patients and families. In addition to discomfort and inexperience with the topic, there continues to be widespread misunderstanding about the efficacy of cardiopulmonary resuscitation (CPR) efforts and the meaning of decisions to withhold CPR in the event of an arrest.

In acute care settings, cardiopulmonary resuscitation is successful in supporting survival to hospital discharge in only about 18% of instances of arrest.[22]

This success rate has changed little in the 50 years since the technique of CPR was first developed. The relative ineffectiveness of CPR reflects the inappropriate widespread use of resuscitation efforts in situations in which multiple preexisting chronic illnesses have led to an irreversible state and death is inevitable. Unfortunately, the public has little understanding of what actually occurs in CPR, the limited benefit except in situations of single-organ disease and immediate intervention, and the potential for cognitive impairment if circulation is restored.[23]

Clinicians, too, may inadvertently contribute to misunderstandings about this issue in several ways. In addition to the tendency to avoid discussions of goals of care, too often the topic of resuscitation status is raised in the form of a question to patients, or more commonly to families, as "What do you want us to do if his heart stops?" This approach reflects a well-intentioned but misguided attempt to identify patient/family preferences. It is misguided in that it places full responsibility for decision-making on the shoulders of family members and implies that it is possible to restore circulation through CPR.

As part of improving the standard of care in any institution, nurses can encourage providers to adopt the newer initialism "DNAR." The American Heart Association, the recognized experts in emergency cardiac care, converted to the initialism "DNAR" (Do Not Attempt Resuscitation) rather then the former "DNR" in their 2005 standards,[24] signaling recognition that CPR, with its current wide application, more accurately is an *attempt* to restore cardiac function. This attempt is most often unsuccessful and this change in language will hopefully facilitate recognition that a DNAR order does not entail a decision to allow a preventable death to occur. Rather, a DNAR order indicates a decision to withhold a very invasive and aggressive intervention that has little chance in promoting survival to hospital discharge.

Clarification of resuscitation status is best done as part of overall care planning. All nurses can play a key role in raising this topic, encouraging sensitive but straightforward communication, and facilitating discussion. Because the intention to use CPR in the event of an arrest is the default in virtually all healthcare settings today, resuscitation status must be addressed in every situation of life-limiting or serious illness. This is particularly important when patients change care settings or begin care with new providers, such as admission to a long-term care facility, home healthcare, or home hospice. In addition to discussion of overall goals and quality of life, the nurse can provide factual information about CPR and clarify the difference between a plan to withhold this ineffective intervention and the plan to use maximal efforts to prevent cardiac arrest.

Although use of DNAR orders is the standard method to indicate to healthcare personnel that CPR is not to be used, these orders are only effective within the facility in which they are issued. The need to have portable orders and valid indicators of DNAR status for patients moving between facilities or patients being cared for at home has led to the creation of out-of-hospital forms and identifiers. As of 2002, 42 states had passed legislation authorizing statewide "out of hospital" DNAR protocols.[25] All nurses have a responsibility to be familiar with their state's forms and protocols in order to assure that decisions to forego CPR remain in place as patients transition among care settings.

In some cases this has been specific clauses in the LW and in others, a specific out-of-hospital standard order form has been developed. Unlike most advance directives, the out-of-hospital DNAR document is a valid physician order that takes effect as soon as it is signed; it is not limited by the patient's diagnosis or terminal status. When available, these forms should be initiated when the decision to forego CPR is first made so that patients can take them with them as they are discharged or transferred among facilities.

A frequent challenge nurses face is how to manage situations in which they perceive the patient's condition is deteriorating and no one has addressed the issue of resuscitation status with the patient or family. Common concerns are that initiating such a discussion is outside the boundaries of the nursing role, that physicians will be angry if the nurse raises the topic, that patients or families will be upset. Kirchhoff and colleagues[26] reported on the perceptions of obstacles and helpful behaviors that 199 critical care nurses discussed in providing end-of-life care to dying patients. The highest ranked "helpful" was "having all physicians agree about the direction of care." This ranking may reflect the degree of distress nurses feel when "stuck in the middle." It is important for nurses to recognize that it is within the professional role of nursing to identify the need to develop consensus around goals of care and treatment plans, and to facilitate discussions surrounding difficult decision-making.

Proxy decision-making

Because patients with serious illness frequently lack cognitive capacity at some point during the illness, professionals must rely on family or friends to represent their wishes and participate in decision-making. This creates a number of possible areas of conflict and uncertainty, including the need to make careful assessments of capacity, questions about the moral authority of family and friends to make decisions for patients, and, in some cases, the need to manage conflicts among and between families and the care team, as occurred in Case Study 1.

"Incompetency" refers to a status that is conferred by a court, establishing the inability of an individual to act as an autonomous and legally responsible person. Only the court can make a determination of *competence*; clinicians provide evidence to the court regarding the *capacity* of the individual, including data about diagnosis, cognitive and functional ability, and likelihood of recovery. An individual who has been deemed "incompetent" loses the right to make all decisions, including healthcare decisions, and must have a guardian appointed by the court to manage all affairs.[27]

Clinicians, therefore, cannot establish competency, but instead do have an ongoing responsibility to assess capacity of the patient to participate in decision-making.

When patients are not able to express their wishes or make decisions and do not have a designated healthcare agent, family members are asked to act as proxies. Although this is common practice, states vary in the extent to which this is authorized by law and the precise specification of which family members have priority in decision-making. The moral basis for allowing one adult to make decisions for another is the assumption that family members are committed to furthering the best interests of the patient and family members, who share background, experiences, religion, and culture with the patient, are well equipped to represent the preferences and values of the patient. These assumptions are usually quite valid, but there are situations in which nurses question the ability of the family member to act as a valid proxy for the patient. In these cases, establishing that the assumptions that are necessary to justify relying on the proxy are, in fact, not confirmed is important in making a plan to seek another representative for that patient. These situations are difficult, and nurses must be prepared to seek guidance from the hospital ethics committee or hospital legal counsel, as well as collaborating with physicians and social workers on the care team. Proxy decision-making, even under the best of circumstances, can be very burdensome to families already stressed by the realization of the seriousness of their loved one's illness. Several studies have demonstrated that family members are not able to consistently identify the preferences of their ill relative[28,29] even when an advance directive is in place. As mentioned earlier, this is related to reluctance to discuss end-of-life issues before a crisis and, when discussion does occur, the likelihood that the discussion was of a general nature and does not necessarily apply to the very specific decisions that have to be made in situations of prognostic uncertainty. An additional common occurrence is lack of consensus among family members about specific decisions, such as limiting treatment, DNAR status, or referrals to hospice.

In the absence of formal advance directives, intrafamily conflict, as exemplified in Case Study 1, is not uncommon. In that case, the patient's wife seemed to be leaning against use of ANH, but the patient's daughters felt compelled to provide ANH. Even if the patient had completed a DPAHC that established the wife's authority as a decision maker, the nurse can provide significant assistance to the family, as a unit, in providing education, as discussed in the next section, and helping the family come to consensus.

There are several steps the nurse can take in an effort to prevent or minimize concerns related to proxy decision-making, particularly when initiating palliative care services. First, all patients who have a serious illness and do not have a DPAHC should be asked to identify a proxy to make decisions if they should become unable. This can be done on admission to the hospital or any other healthcare delivery system in a nonthreatening manner, simply pointing out that sometimes patients become too ill or too sleepy due to medication. This will enable the team to know, if there are disagreements later, who has the strongest claim to the decision-maker role. Second, the time to obtain information about the patient's lifestyle, values, and preferences is before specific decisions about pursuing invasive diagnostic tests or procedures are needed. Talking with family members about what the patient was like, what he/she enjoyed, what was important, can be helpful in later discussions. Third, when it is necessary to ask a family proxy to provide input into the plan of care, it is essential to address the task as one of helping the clinicians to know what the patient would have wanted. This can be done by referring back to earlier discussions about what was most important to the patient. The goals here are twofold: to minimize the burden of responsibility the family member might feel and to remain focused on the ethical mandate to act according to the patient's wishes, not the family members' wishes. In addition to Table 64.1, which provides some examples of ways to phrase questions that are not helpful and some ways that can be more useful in supporting family decision-making, a number of more detailed communication suggestions have been published.[8]

Table 64.1 Phrases to avoid and phrases that can be more helpful

Do not say	Do say
"What do you want us to do if your loved one's heart stops?"	"We need to talk about where we go from here if your loved one's condition continues to worsen."
"Would you want us to do CPR if your loved one's heart stops?"	"There are many things we can do, but it's very important that we talk together about what your loved one would want done in this situation. Have you and he/she ever known anyone who was this ill … did he/she say anything about what he/she would want in a situation like this?"
"We need your permission to do a (tracheostomy, PEG, angiogram, etc.)"	"Given what we've discussed about your loved one's situation and the most likely benefits and burdens of the procedure, we need your help to know if he/she would want us to proceed with the (tracheostomy, PEG, angiogram, etc.)"
"We'll do whatever you want us to … it's your decision … we'll support whatever you decide"	"We have to make some decisions about where to go from here. It's our job to give you information about the medical facts and our recommendations, and we need you to help us know what would be important to your loved one now. Then, we need to talk and come up with a plan together."

Artificial hydration and nutrition

A fundamental care-giving task is to provide food and fluids. The provision of nutrition and hydration symbolizes the essence of care and compassion, and eating serves as a symbol of health. In most societies, celebrations involve eating, and through these traditional social events we communicate sharing and well-being. Clearly, human life is represented as social and communal through the provision of food.[30]

When a loved one has an advanced illness, these opportunities wane, and when one is dying, they are often lost. However, providing ANH is not synonymous with eating or feeding another person. In health, people eat in a socially acceptable form, with others, in a social setting. Medically provided nutrition and hydration do not share these social characteristics.

The technology of feeding tubes was developed to address specific temporary medical problems (e.g., postsurgical gastric motility issues, swallowing impairment following a stroke in a patient expected to recover). However, the use of feeding tubes and medically provided nutrition and hydration have become widely used in patients with very poor prognoses and for those with little likelihood of regaining functional abilities. Few decisions are more value-laden than those to withhold or withdraw a medical intervention that is thought to be able to prolong life. As with all decisions about the use of any medical device or treatment, this decision should be based on the patient's goals of care, the medical need, and the burdens and benefits of the treatment.

In general, patients (or their surrogates) have the right to withhold or withdraw ANH if they believe that the burden or risks outweigh the benefits. There is widespread agreement in ethics and law[31–33] that patients or their surrogates have a right to choose or refuse artificial nutrition and hydration. All decisions about nutrition and hydration should be made in light of patient's goals and outcomes of care. These goals of care may change during the course of the disease or as the disease progresses and the patient's cognitive and physical functioning decline. Consequently, nurses should create opportunities for discussion and negotiation of goals and priorities of care with the patient and family/surrogate on an ongoing basis.

Artificial nutrition and hydration require the placement of a temporary or permanent feeding tube or the initiation of intravenous access. These interventions are associated with risks, including bleeding, tube displacement, and infection, as well as the potential need for repositioning and replacement.[34,35] In patients with impaired renal function, intravenous fluids may promote peripheral or pulmonary edema and increase the need for suctioning.[36] Tube feedings do not appear to prevent aspiration pneumonia and may increase the risk as compared with those patients who do not take anything by mouth.[34]

Other potential side effects of tube feeding include diarrhea, nausea, vomiting, and aspiration of the feeding into the lung.[36] Most recently, important, empirical data by Teno and colleagues concluded that feeding tubes are not associated with prevention or improved healing of a pressure ulcer.[37] In fact, hospitalized nursing home (NH) residents who received a percutaneous endoscopic gastrostomy tube (PEG) were 2.7 times more likely to develop a new pressure ulcer, and those with a pressure ulcer were less likely to show healing of the ulcer when they had a PEG inserted. Similarly, there is particularly strong evidence confirming the failure of PEGs and tube-feeding to prolong survival in states of advanced dementia.[34,35,38,39]

Many patients and family members have deep concerns about the issue of "hunger" and "starvation." Contrary to what many believe, a patient with a terminal disease, who is often anorexic from the effects of the disease may not be bothered by hunger.[40] In fact, many patients in whom the disease is progressing tend to report a complete lack of hunger. Evidence suggests that natural physiological processes that accompany the cessation of food and fluid intake naturally suppress both hunger and thirst. In addition, there is strong consensus among palliative care clinicians and oncology professionals that use of parenteral hydration in terminally ill patients is most often associated with unpleasant symptoms of fluid retention and overload.[41]

Nursing interventions that can assist with the palliation of symptoms associated with dry mouth or thirst include small sips of oral intake, ice chips, meticulous mouth care, and lubrication of the lips. Involving caregivers, family members, and loved ones in this activity may replace the family's desire and need to feed with another care-giving activity that can provide the family with the opportunity to provide physical comfort.

Financial implications of these decisions and implications for discharge planning and home care also need to be considered. Some hospice programs cover the cost of ANH, based on the individual plan of care and the goals of care, but others do not. Some extended-care facilities (i.e., nursing homes) mandate medically provided nutrition and hydration when a person stops eating and/or drinking, often related to misunderstanding and concern about state regulations or related to philosophy and religious missions. Consequently, discussions with families about decisions to use ANH, as in Case Study 1, should include consideration of these factors. In Case 1, the nurse would have several responsibilities, including clarifying the facts about the patient's previously stated wishes, educating all family members regarding the likely benefits and burdens of tube feedings, and focusing discussions with both physicians and family members on what was known about the patient's values and preferences.

Despite the lack of proven benefit in states of irreversible and advanced illness, ANH will remain an emotionally laden topic and one of the most difficult decisions. Nurses have a particularly important role in educating patients, families, and other members of the healthcare team about the benefits and burdens of tube feedings. There is a persistent widespread belief, particularly among unlicensed assistive personnel and even among physicians,[42] that we have a duty to feed all patients and that the benefits of ANH always outweigh the burdens. This misunderstanding, in combination with concerns about causing suffering, is a significant barrier to careful ethical evaluation of the decision to use or withhold ANH. Assuring informed decision-making about this aspect of the care plan often must begin with addressing the concerns of the care team before developing a plan to make clear recommendations to families and providing family members with the necessary education about this issue.

Case study 2

Withdrawal of life support in the intensive care unit

Ms. H was a 32-year-old Caucasian woman. She was divorced from her husband and had custody of her son, age 6 years, and her daughter, age 3 years. Her parents and her fiancé were her significant others. Ms. H was diagnosed with a uterine leiomyosarcoma two years ago. She had undergone two regimens of chemotherapy following a hysterectomy, but the cancer had metastasized to her hip and her mediastinum. The thoracic lesion had grown to the point where it was compressing her bronchus and she was taken to the OR for stent placement as a palliative measure. This was not able to be done, and she was then admitted to the ICU, intubated and on mechanical ventilation. Over the course of a week, several attempts were made to extubate her, but she was unable to maintain a patent airway without the positive pressure of the ventilator and the endotracheal tube. Each time the ventilator support was reduced, Ms. H became very anxious and short of breath, even with the use of increasing doses of lorazepam and morphine. She was awake and alert and able to write notes.

On rounds, the ICU attending physician mentioned to the team that it was time to think about doing a tracheostomy since it looked as if Ms. H was not able to be extubated. Ms. P, her nurse, was concerned that this would just subject Ms. H to another procedure and would not change the eventual outcome. She also was uncertain whether anyone had told Ms. H the details of her condition and the real possibility that she would never be able to leave the ICU. On the other hand, the fact that Ms. H was wide awake made it seem as if withdrawing life support (e.g., extubating her) might be cruel—how could this be done without causing suffering?

Hastening death

A central issue in decision-making in states of serious illness is the moral acceptability of actions that can be seen as hastening death. As has been noted throughout this chapter, it is well established in Western bioethics that competent patients have an almost unlimited right to accept or refuse medical interventions, regardless of the established efficacy of the intervention or its necessity for survival. Supporting and advocating for this right is a critical function of the nurse and one which has been identified as a frequent source of ethical distress.

The recognized right of the individual to elect to stop life-sustaining technology, such as mechanical ventilation or hemodialysis, has been used by some as the basis for arguing that there is no difference between this act and acts that intentionally hasten death, including both euthanasia and assisted suicide. Arguments that there is a difference usually rely on the distinction between allowing a death caused by disease, as occurs when removing unwanted or ineffective life-prolonging therapies such as mechanical ventilators and dialysis, and killing, which entails being the direct cause of death (see Case Studies 1 and 2). There is ongoing debate in the bioethics community about whether this is a morally relevant distinction and each nurse who cares for patients with life-limiting disease will have to carefully identify his/her own beliefs.

Euthanasia is defined as an intentional act performed for the purpose of causing the death of another for reasons of mercy, whereas assisted suicide is the provision of assistance in some form (e.g., supplying lethal medications or instructions) to an individual who then acts to take his/her own life. Euthanasia in all forms is illegal in the United States and is condoned by none of the professional associations (see Box 64.2). However, assisted suicide (also termed physician-aid-in-dying and physician-assisted suicide [PAS]) has been legalized in Oregon since 1997 and most recently approved by voters in Washington state.[43] At this time, professional nursing organizations do not condone nurses actively participating in assisted suicide (Box 64.2).

Nurses, as the healthcare professionals who spend the greatest amount of time with patients and their families and who often have the most intimate relationships with them, are inevitably involved in situations involving the issue of hastening death. This may take the form of explicit requests from patients for some action that would precipitate death or shorten survival, patients and families may explicitly request information or counseling from the nurse regarding hastening death, or nurses may identify more subtle clues that the patient or family are considering hastening death. The desire for hastened death at some point in terminal illness has been found to occur with relative frequency. Emanuel, Fairclough, and Emanuel[44] reported an incidence of serious consideration for either euthanasia or PAS in 10.6% of 988 terminally ill patients. O'Mahoney, Goutlet, et al.[45] found that 34% of 131 patients admitted to a palliative care service had some level of desire for hastening death. In a large Dutch survey of nurses' involvement in end-of-life decisions in hospitals,

nursing homes, and home care, the nurse was the first person with whom the patient discussed a request for euthanasia or PAS in 45.1% of cases.[46] These situations require very careful attention from the nurse, awareness of legal and ethical considerations, and a well-developed and collaborative plan for responding.

The first, and perhaps most important, responsibility of the nurse is clarification and assessment. The expression of thoughts of hastening death may be an accurate report of a serious intention, it may be a relatively off-hand comment, it may be an expression of distress prompted by unrelieved symptoms, or it maybe intended as a test of the nurse's views about hastening death. In addition to clarifying the meaning of the patient's statements, the desire for hastened death should always prompt a thorough evaluation of the adequacy of symptom management, particularly pain and depression. Ganzini et al. found that, among 58 patients in Oregon who had sought PAS, 26% were assessed as depressed on psychiatric interview.[47]

There are a number of guidelines developed by professional associations and groups to assist the clinician in responding to requests for hastened death.[48,49] All of these emphasize both the right of professionals to withdraw from situations in which they are being

---

Box 64.2 Position statements from recognized professional organizations

Artificial hydration and nutrition

◆ Hospice and Palliative Nurses Association (HPNA). Position Statement—Artificial Nutrition and Hydration in Advanced Illness. Pittsburgh, PA: Hospice and Palliative Nurses Association; 2011.

◆ National Hospice and Palliative Care Organization (NHPCO). Position Statement—Artificial Nutrition and Hydration Narrative and Statement. Alexandria, VA: National Hospice and Palliative Care Organization; 2010.

◆ American Nurses Association Position Statement (ANA). Position Statement—Foregoing Nutrition and Hydration. Washington, DC: The American Nurses Association; 2011.

◆ American Academy of Hospice and Palliative Medicine (AAHPM). Position Statement—Artificial Nutrition and Hydration Near the End of Life. Glenview, IL: American Academy of Hospice and Palliative Medicine; 2006.

Physician assisted suicide

◆ Hospice and Palliative Nurses Association (HPNA). Position Statement—Legalization of Assisted Suicide. Pittsburgh, PA: Hospice and Palliative Nurses Association, 2011.

◆ National Hospice and Palliative Care Organization (NHPCO). Commentary and Resolution—Physician Assisted Suicide. Alexandria, VA: National Hospice and Palliative Care Organization; 2010.

◆ American Academy of Hospice and Palliative Medicine (AAHPM). Position Statement—Physician Assisted Death. Glenview, IL: American Academy of Hospice and Palliative Medicine; 2007.

◆ Oncology Nursing Society Nurse's Responsibility to the Patient Requesting Assistance in Hastening Death. Pittsburgh, PA: Oncology Nursing Society; 2010.

◆ American Society for Pain Management Nursing. Position Statement—Assisted Suicide. Lenexa, KS: American Society for Pain Management Nursing; 2011.

Palliative sedation

◆ Hospice and Palliative Nurses Association (HPNA). Position Statement—Palliative Sedation. Pittsburgh, PA: Hospice and Palliative Nurses Association; 2011.

◆ American Academy of Hospice and Palliative Medicine (AAHPM). Position Statement—Palliative Sedation. Glenview, IL: American Academy of Hospice and Palliative Medicine; 2006.

◆ National Hospice and Palliative Care Organization. Position Statement—Use of Palliative Sedation in Imminently Dying Terminally Ill Patients. Alexandria, VA: National Hospice and Palliative Care Organization; 2010.

◆ National Hospice and Palliative Care Organization. Position Statement—Palliative Sedation in Hospice and Palliative Care. Alexandria, VA: National Hospice and Palliative Care Organization; 2012.

requested to act in a way, such as participating in assisted suicide, that violates their moral principles. However, the duty to assure patients that they will not be abandoned, to work diligently to investigate and address correctable factors that may be leading to the request for hastened death, and the duty to refrain from withdrawing until an alternate source of care is in place are absolute.

Special questions: cardiac assist devices, palliative sedation, futility

There are three specific issues that present particularly challenging questions in palliative care. These are the acceptability and methods of withdrawing life-sustaining interventions that consist of cardiac assistive devices (pacemakers, automatic internal cardio-defibrillators [AICD], left ventricular assistive devices [LVAD]), concerns about requests for futile therapy, and terminal sedation.

Cardiac assistive devices

One of the most concrete examples of the complexities created by advancing technologies is the situation of patients who have elected to forego continued use of cardioassistive devices in order to allow a peaceful death. There are a number of implantable mechanical assistive devices intended to either support or replace normal cardiac electrical and mechanical function, including LVADs, right ventricular assistive devices (RVADs), total implantable hearts (TIHs), AICDs, and pacemakers. Each of these raises unique issues.

Internal automatic cardiodefibrillators are very commonly used in the United States as treatment of recurrent ventricular fibrillation. Pacemakers have been a long-standing therapy for bradyarrhythmias and combined AICD-pacemakers are recommended for some forms of heart failure. In an international survey in 2005, 223,425 pacemakers and 119,121 AICDs were implanted in the United States.[50] It is therefore very likely that palliative care nurses will find themselves caring for patients with either or both of these devices. In most cases, both AICDs and pacemakers are on-demand therapy; that is, they are programmed to deliver therapy only on demand (when heart rate decreases or a lethal arrhythmia develops). Therefore, their function should be disabled when the plan of care is based on a goal of allowing a peaceful death with no further intervention. For example, AICDs should be turned off so that they will not deliver a shock as the heart rate falls or ventricular arrhythmias occur. Demand pacemakers can have the rate and sensitivity decreased so they do not prolong the dying process. Cardiologists or cardiac technicians usually must be called and requested to make these changes using the device programming magnets.

When cardiac function is dependent on active device operation, as is the case with some pacemakers and most cardiac assistive devices, there are more difficult challenges and unresolved questions. Some argue that discontinuing a cardiac assist device, with the expectation that death will follow, is no different, morally, than discontinuing mechanical ventilation for a patient who has elected (or whose family has elected) to have life-sustaining therapy discontinued. However, others believe that the fact that the device is implanted and has become, in a sense, part of the patient, makes discontinuation equivalent to an act of euthanasia and thus is impermissible.[51–53]

Since 2002, LVADs have been considered "destination therapy" for patients who are ineligible for transplant or for those patients whose estimated 1-year mortality is greater than 50% with medical therapy.[54] Moreover, LVADs will alter end-of-life trajectories.

Although intended to prolong survival related to heart failure, LVADs have the potential to decrease the overall quality of life of these patients because of serious infections, neurological complications, and device malfunction.[55–57] Numerous nurse-led research studies[58,59] have shed light on the importance of the ethical obligations nurses hold to provide significant emotional support to these patients and their families. When caring for the patient with an implanted cardiac device, the nurse has several responsibilities. First, the exact status of the device's operation has to be determined. As with all components of the palliative care plan, the plan for adjusting the device should stem from a clear understanding of the patient's goals of care. If, for example, the goal is to make the most of whatever time is left and there is hope for more time, all cardiac devices should remain active and in place. On the other hand, if the patient is actively dying or has expressed an informed desire to remove any therapy that could interfere with the dying process (whenever that might occur), the devices should be inactivated (or turned to an inactive setting). Each of these decisions, of course, must be made in collaboration with the care team. If there is consensus about discontinuing a device on which cardiac function is entirely dependent, extra care must be taken to assure that the patient, family members, and the entire care team is in agreement. Although, as with ANH, there is still some lack of consensus among healthcare professionals about the morality of discontinuing cardiac assist devices, there is formal agreement from the relevant medical professional organization (Heart Rhythm Society) that discontinuing this form of therapy is no different from the withdrawal of any other form of unwanted or ineffective therapy.[60] The timing of the discontinuation must be carefully considered and a plan to address likely symptoms put in place.

Palliative sedation

There are a very small number of situations at the end of life in which patient symptoms cannot be adequately relieved despite multiple pharmacological regimens. Despite the provision of evidence-based, state-of-the-art palliative care, some patients will continue to experience protracted, intense suffering toward the end of life. In these cases, the option of palliative sedation) is sometimes raised. Palliative sedation refers to the use of medications to induce sedation, either intermittently or continuously, for the purpose of providing relief of intractable symptoms. The intention is not to cause death. In an effort to clarify the different types of palliative sedation and how each may be used, Quill and colleagues[61] outlined three kinds of sedation: ordinary, proportionate, and palliative sedation to unconsciousness. If the goal of care is to relieve the symptom(s) without reduction of level of consciousness, ordinary sedation could serve as a treatment intervention. With proportionate palliative sedation (PPS), pharmaceutical agents such as benzodiazepines are progressively escalated to induce increasing levels of sedation during both waking and sleeping hours. This type of sedation is usually employed for intractable physical suffering in imminently dying patients. Lastly, if unconsciousness is the intended goal of care rather than a side effect, palliative sedation to unconsciousness (PSU) can be used. Although these definitions have helped to clarify the types of sedation, there remains great fear that access to these practices may become too easy. However, in a recent systematic review of the literature regarding palliative sedation and survival, Maltoni and colleagues[62] found no evidence to suggest that palliative sedation has any detrimental effect on survival of patients with terminal cancer. In fact, they suggested that it is a medical intervention that should be included in the repertoire of interventions to relieve suffering.

Despite these views and data, the wide variation in the reported use of palliative sedation and limited research evidence about best practice is likely a reflection of ambivalence and uncertainty about the ethical acceptability of the practice.[63] Perhaps the most common objection to palliative sedation is the belief that PPS and PSU will directly hasten death. However, the review of published data by Claessens et al.[64] indicates that this is not the case. Nevertheless, use of PPS and PSU does require also addressing other interventions, such as the continuation of oral medications and the administration of food and fluids. In general, these other decisions should be made separately and before palliative sedation is begun. If there are adequate reasons to stop food, fluids, and other medications (i.e., if the patient is in the final stages of dying, has been refusing food and fluids, and other medications are not needed for promotion of comfort), there is no reason to insist they be used when palliative sedation begins. On the other hand, if nutrition and hydration were indicated before sedation, there may be good reason to continue their use or sedation should be stopped or lightened intermittently to offer food and fluid.

Case Study 2 is an example of a situation in which palliative sedation might be necessary. If Ms. H, who retained decisional capacity, chose to have ventilatory support withdrawn, it might be necessary to sedate her to the point of unconsciousness in order to prevent suffering. This act certainly would shorten her survival, compared to continuing mechanical ventilation. However, this act would be morally permissible and supported by the principle of double effect. This principle, well-established in bioethics, asserts that acts that are intended to achieve a "good" effect (in this case, respecting autonomy and preventing suffering) are permissible even if the act also carries with it an unintended "bad" effect (hastened death). In addition to intending only the good effect, this principle requires that the good not be achieved by means of the bad (i.e., the relief of suffering is achieved by the sedation, not by causing death) and the weight of the good achieved must be greater than the bad effect.[30] Although the American Academy of Hospice and Palliative Medicine, the National Hospice and Palliative Care Organization, and the Hospice and Palliative Nurses Association (see Table 62.3) support the use of palliative sedation in carefully selected situations, all organizations emphasize the importance of clarity in the intended objective (relief of suffering) and the need for thorough discussion and informed consent from the patient. In addition, all organizations providing palliative and end-of-life care should have a written policy about palliative sedation and the types of sedation that will be offered to patients if requested. This policy should be provided to patients or their proxies who ask about the possibility of having PSU in the future or request it when other interventions have failed to relieve intractable suffering. Moreover, if the organization offers PSU but an individual physician objects to its provision, the organization or clinician must make alternative arrangements for the care to be transferred to another provider or institution. Given the importance of communication in the final stages of life, use of palliative sedation should be reserved for those few situations in which all other interventions have been ineffective and the patient finds continued consciousness to be intolerable.

Futility

"Futility" is a term that refers to the inability of a specific intervention to lead to its intended outcome (e.g., prolonged survival, discharge from the hospital, shrinkage of tumor). This term has gained popularity in acute care over the past decade as clinicians have increasingly encountered situations in which patients and families request or demand therapies that the clinician believes have no meaningful chance of prolonging life or improving well-being.[65-67] Over the years, there has been a growing consensus that the right of patients and families to accept or refuse therapies does not entail the right to demand therapies which the physician does not believe are medically justified.[68] The well-established right to accept or refuse therapy stems from the principle of autonomy. This principle establishes the duty to refrain from interfering in the life choices of competent persons; it is thus a "liberty right," not a right to demand access to any particular intervention.

The gradual move away from the paternalism of the past and a commitment to supporting patient autonomy has unfortunately led to a tendency to shift the responsibility for decision-making entirely to patients and families. This is sometimes seen in the reluctance of clinicians to advise or guide patients and families in decisions and, instead, to present options in a completely impartial fashion. Clinicians then may find themselves facing situations in which patients or families demand therapies that are thought to offer little benefit and significant probability of harm. Most often, this occurs with the question of resuscitation status or continued use of chemotherapy in advanced refractory cancer.[69,70] The frequency of futility dilemmas and the difficulty in resolving them has led professional organizations and many other healthcare organizations to develop policies for managing the conflict. Although these policies are important in providing general guidelines for physicians and nurses, it is far more important to attempt to prevent futility conflicts from developing. As with most ethical dilemmas, effective communication and trusting relationships are key.

Specific steps that nurses can take in working to avoid the development of irreconcilable differences begin with talking early about goals of care, learning about the values and beliefs of the patient and his/her family, and establishing a collaborative model of decision-making. Not infrequently, families will express the wish to have "everything" done for their loved one. When this is said, the nurse or physician should respond by assuring the patient and family that they are heard and that their wish to receive all therapies that have any meaningful chance of maintaining or improving the patient's condition will be used. The use of shared decision-making should be emphasized from the start. As the condition of the patient deteriorates and it becomes apparent that continued interventions will not be helpful, it is best to set the stage for later decisions by affirming that the clinicians will provide honest and direct information and will identify when there are no further curative options, with assurances that the plan of care will always be discussed before changes are made. When the situation is such that CPR or other interventions are no longer indicated, this should be stated; patients or families should not be asked to give permission to withhold an ineffective intervention. If consensus appears to be unreachable, other resources, such as clergy or ethics consultants should be utilized. Although seeking guidance from the court may be required in intractable disputes, in general this should be viewed as a last resort and thoughtful, interdisciplinary procedural approaches are preferable.[71,72]

In Case Study 2, the nurse, Ms. P, may have believed that performing a tracheostomy on Ms. H would indeed be futile. Although the procedure could be safely performed, it would not save the patient's life or even allow her to recover enough to leave the ICU—she would always require mechanical ventilation. To address this issue, Ms. P would need to first validate her assumption about the location of Ms. H's tumor and the ineffectiveness of a tracheostomy to relieve the obstruction. Next, a care conference with the entire multidisciplinary team would have to be arranged to develop consensus about the best approach. If the team reaches agreement about the lack of any effective treatment options for the cancer, a plan would have to be developed, including who would talk with Ms. H, what recommendation would be offered, what options would be acceptable, and how to manage her symptoms when she was ready to discontinue mechanical ventilation.

Although it is becoming increasingly recognized that clinicians have not only the right but also the professional duty to refrain from interventions that are harmful, it is essential to be cautious in judging interventions as "futile." There are many treatments or therapies that offer neither cure nor improvement in patient condition, but which are effective in supporting survival, such as mechanical ventilation following anoxic brain injuries. The claim of futility should not be used to justify withholding therapies in situations in which the clinician believes that the proposed therapy would accomplish its intended purpose, but the resulting quality of life would be undesirable. Judgments such as this reflect the subjective opinions and values of clinicians and are not a valid basis for withholding therapy against the wishes of patients and families.

Nursing issues, moral distress, and compassion fatigue

Decisions regarding ethical dilemmas and the choices that are necessary require thoughtful discussion and critical communication skills. Stemming from the priority of the principle of autonomy or self-determination, decisions about care should be made in accordance with patients' preferences for care, beliefs, and values. With increased medical technology, the advances in science, and conflicting interests of patients and families, nurses stand in a pivotal position to lead the way in assuring patient access to quality palliative care. This charge does not come without the risk of the nurse feeling like he/she is "in the middle," trying to provide the best possible care to the patient, and supporting the family members, while bracketing personal values.[73]

Nurses and other members of the interdisciplinary healthcare team face ethical and legal issues in decision-making related to end-of-life care daily in clinical practice. These dilemmas have a strong potential to provoke conflict among those involved in patient care, sometimes between professionals and sometimes between patients, families, and professionals. The ANA Code of Ethics states that nurses have the right to withdraw from providing care to patients when their own values conflict with that of patient, as long as the patient's care can safely be transferred to another care provider. Caring for patients with advanced illness brings with it complex clinical situations and ethical challenges;

nurses must find ways to support one another through talking and sharing experiences about moral uncertainty. The Code of Ethics for Nurses urges nurses to collaborate with colleagues to advocate for healthcare environments conducive to ethical practice and to the health and well-being of all in the setting, and to do so in ways consistent with professional behavior. The ANA goes on to discuss the importance of "preservation of integrity." Specifically, Provision 5 and 6 of the ANA Code of Ethics discusses moral self-respect and the influence of the environment on ethical obligations, moral virtues, and values. According to these provisions, nurses have a duty to remain consistent with both their personal and professional values, and possess character strengths such as compassion and patience. Although simply stated, these behaviors may become challenged when faced with ethical and moral dilemmas.

Nurses, like other licensed professionals, profess to society that they are prepared to take on certain responsibilities in safe, competent, and ethical ways. In fact, many nurses entered the profession by taking a pledge, such as the Florence Nightingale Pledge, swearing to devote themselves to others who require their care, knowledge, and expertise. Every day, hospice and palliative care nurses provide care to patients who rely on them for not only physical care needs, but also psychological, social, and spiritual care. Close, personal relationships are often formed with patients and their family as palliative care nurses care for them over a prolonged period of time. In a large survey of nurses from a variety of healthcare settings, including hospice, ICU, nursing facilities, and inpatient care, Ferrell[74] identified that nurses' greatest sources of moral distress originated from "aggressive care" and "aggressive care denying palliative care." Moral and ethical dilemmas, often associated with patient/family situations, and healthcare environments may leave the hospice and palliative care nurse feeling physically, emotionally, and spiritually drained. As nurses continue to be exposed to patients with greater healthcare needs, staff shortages, heavy and intense workloads, an aging workforce, and a lack of resources to work effectively, the opportunity to develop moral distress, moral fatigue, burnout, and compassion fatigue is glaring.

"Compassion fatigue" is a relatively new term, yet is pervasive within the nursing profession.[75] Compassion fatigue is a state in which the compassionate energy that is expended by nurses outweighs the restorative processes and the ability to recover has been lost; it is the negative aspect of helping that can be related to the actual provision of care, the environment, colleagues and/or beliefs about self.[76,77] Burnout, on the other hand, relates to work-related hopelessness; it is the inability to cope with job stress that produces feelings of inefficacy.[78] Moral distress arises when one must act in a way that contradicts personal values and beliefs; moral fatigue is the consequence of continued moral distress.[79,80] For example, nurses might act in a way that is contrary to personal and professional values or be able to translate moral choices into action. This creates anguish; the consequences can be profound and have lasting effects.[79] Nurses who appear to be at a higher risk for compassion fatigue include those who are younger nurses, who have a history of personal trauma and who have not worked through issues related to trauma, nurses working with large caseloads and/or long hours; those already experiencing professional burnout; nurses with inadequate training in effective communication or those less competent in communication, and nurses without adequate collegiate and personal support systems.[75]

Coping strategies, including self-care, are key to prevention of compassion fatigue. Integrating self-care activities, including self-compassion and mindfulness-based strategies, into professional workloads is not typically part of professional training, nor is it explicitly part of one's job description. However, if nurses do not care for themselves, they will be unable to sustain care for others.[81,82] Ethics experts recognize that moral distress is often created in situations in which nurses participate in activities that are perceived as medically futile. In fact, providing futile care undermines the core of the professional practice of nursing. One of the most crucial elements in dealing with moral distress is knowing WHAT support is available and HOW to navigate the system in place. Ethics committees are one source of support and serve to assist in resolving complicated ethical problems that affect the care and treatment of patients within healthcare organizations. The Joint Commission on Accreditation of Healthcare Organizations requires hospitals and other healthcare organizations to have a mechanism in place to address ethical issues in the provision of patient care. Healthcare organizations have different mechanisms by which to address ethical issues, and it is therefore the responsibility of all nurses to know what resources are available in their organization and how to access them. Just as preventive ethics should be used before an ethical dilemma arises, so should they be used to guide nursing practice before a crisis occurs.

Summary

There will always be new ethical dilemmas that require decision-making, and the answers to those dilemmas will not always be obvious or easily identified. It is often in states of uncertainty that serious wrongs occur. As partners in the care of patients and families with advanced illness who must make difficult decisions, nurses must be empowered to facilitate discussion and to be heard by all parties involved. The challenge for today is to ensure that all nurses acquire attributes of leadership, excellent communication skills, and self-reflection that enable them to fulfill the crucial role of nursing.

References

1. Honderich T. The Oxford Guide to Philosophy. 2nd ed. UK: Oxford University Press; 2005.
2. Gert B. Morality: Its Nature and Justification. UK: Oxford University Press; 2005.
3. Bishop AH, Scudder JR. The Practical, Moral, and Personal Sense of Nursing: A Phenomenological Philosophy of Practice. Albany: State University of New York Press; 1990.
4. Koehn D. Rethinking Feminist Ethics. New York: Routledge; 2001.
5. Nodding N. Caring. Berkeley: University of California Press; 1984.
6. Mullan F, Ficklen E, Rubin K, eds. Narrative matters. Baltimore: Johns Hopkins University Press; 2006.
7. Fry S. The role of caring in a theory of nursing ethics. In: Holmes HB, Purdy LM (eds.), Feminist Perspectives in Medical Ethics. Indianapolis, IN: Indiana University Press; 1992:93–106.
8. Sudore RL, Fried TR. Redefining the "planning" in advance care planning: preparing for end-of-life decision making. Ann Intern Med. 2010;153(4):256–261. doi: 10.7326/0003-4819-153-4-201008170-00008; 10.1059/0003-4819-153-4-201008170-00008.
9. Foglia MB, Fox E, Chanko B, Bottrell MM. Preventive ethics: addressing ethics quality gaps on a systems level. Joint Comm J Qual Patient Safety. 2012;38(3):103–111. Epub 2012 Mar 23.
10. Mack JW, Weeks JC, Wright AA, Block SD, Prigerson HG. End-of-life discussions, goal attainment, and distress at the end of life: predictors and outcomes of receipt of care consistent with preferences.

J Clin Oncol. 2010;28(7):1203–1208. doi: 10.1200/JCO.2009.25.4672; 10.1200/JCO.2009.25.4672.
11. Mack JW, Cronin A, Keating NL, et al. Associations between end-of-life discussion characteristics and care received near death: a prospective cohort study. J Clin Oncol. 2012;30(35):4387–4395. doi: 10.1200/JCO.2012.43.6055; 10.1200/JCO.2012.43.6055.
12. Detering KM, Hancock AD, Reade MC, Silvester W. The impact of advance care planning on end of life care in elderly patients: randomised controlled trial. BMJ. 2010;340:c1345. doi: 10.1136/bmj.c1345.
13. Billings JA. The need for safeguards in advance care planning. J Gen Intern Med. 2012;27(5):595–600. doi: 10.1007/s11606-011-1976-2; 10.1007/s11606-011-1976-2.
14. Yung VY, Walling AM, Min L, Wenger NS, Ganz DA. Documentation of advance care planning for community-dwelling elders. J Palliat Med. 2010;13(7):861–867. doi: 10.1089/jpm.2009.0341; 10.1089/jpm.2009.0341.
15. Five Wishes. http://www.agingwithdignity.org/five-wishes-states.php. Accessed July 2, 2013.
16. Hickman SE, Nelson CA, Perrin NA, Moss AH, Hammes BJ, Tolle SW. A comparison of methods to communicate treatment preferences in nursing facilities: traditional practices versus the physician orders for life-sustaining treatment program. J Am Geriatr Soc. 2010;58(7):1241–1248.
17. Citko J, Moss AH, Carley M, Tolle S. The national POLST paradigm initiative, 2nd edition. J Palliat Med. 2011;14(2):241–242. doi: 10.1089/jpm.2010.9730; 10.1089/jpm.2010.9730.
18. Araw AC, Araw AM, Pekmezaris R, et al. Medical orders for life-sustaining treatment: is it time yet? Palliat Support Care. 2014;12(2):101–105. doi: 10.1017/S1478951512001010.
19. Bomba PA, Kemp M, Black JS. POLST: an improvement over traditional advance directives. Cleve Clin J Med. 2012;79(7):457–464. doi: 10.3949/ccjm.79a.11098; 10.3949/ccjm.79a.11098.
20. Fast Facts. http://www.eperc.mcw.edu/EPERC/FastFactsIndex/ff_178.htm. Accessed July 2, 2013.
21. National Consensus Project. National Consensus Project Website. http://www.nationalconsensusproject.org/Guidelines_Download2.aspx. Accessed July 2, 2013.
22. Ehlenbach WJ, Barnato AE, Curtis JR, et al. Epidemiologic study of in-hospital cardiopulmonary resuscitation in the elderly. N Engl J Med. 2009;361(1):22–31. doi: 10.1056/NEJMoa0810245; 10.1056/NEJMoa0810245.
23. Jones GK, Brewer KL, Garrison HG. Public expectations of survival following cardiopulmonary resuscitation. Acad Emerg Med. 2000;7(1):48–53.
24. ECC Committee. Subcommittees and Task Forces of the American Heart Association. American Heart Association guidelines for cardiopulmonary resuscitation and emergency cardiovascular care. Circulation. 2005;112(24 Suppl):1–203.
25. American College of Emergency Physicians. "Do Not Attempt Resuscitation" Orders in the Out of Hospital Setting. http://www.acep.org/Clinical---Practice-Management/-Do-Not-Attempt-Resuscitation--Orders-in-the-Out-of-Hospital-Setting/.
26. Kirchhoff K, Spuhler V, Walker L, Hutton A, Cole BV, Clemmer T. Intensive care nurses' experiences with end-of-life care. Am J Crit Care. 2000;9(1):36–42.
27. Post LF, Blustein J, Dubler NN. Handbook for Health Care Ethics Committees. Baltimore: Johns Hopkins University Press; 2007.
28. Zettel-Watson L, Ditto PH, Danks JH, Smucker WD. Actual and perceived gender differences in the accuracy of surrogate decisions about life-sustaining medical treatment among older spouses. Death Stud. 2008;32(3):273–290. doi: 10.1080/07481180701881230; 10.1080/07481180701881230.
29. Shalowitz DI, Garrett-Mayer E, Wendler D. The accuracy of surrogate decision makers: a systematic review. Arch Intern Med. 2006;166(5):493.

30. Beauchamp TL, Childress JF. Principles of biomedical ethics. 6th ed. New York, NY: Oxford University Press; 2008.
31. New Jersey. Superior Court (Morris County), New Jersey. Supreme Court. In the Matter of Karen Quinlan: The Complete Legal Briefs, Court Proceedings, and Decision in the Superior Court of New Jersey. Vol 1. Bethesda, Maryland: University Publications of America; 1975.
32. Michael Schiavo, as Guardian of the person of Theresa Marie Schiavo, Petitioner, v. Robert Schindler and Mary Schindler, No. 90-2908GD-003 (U.S. Dist., March 2004).
33. Greer GW, Judge C. In re: The guardianship of Theresa Marie Schiavo, incapacitated. Michael Schiavo, petitioner, vs. Robert Schindler and Mary Schindler, respondents. File No. 90-2908-GD-003, Fla.6th Judicial Circuit, February 25, 2005.
34. Sampson EL, Candy B, Jones L. Enteral tube feeding for older people with advanced dementia. Cochrane Database Syst Rev. 2009;(2):CD007209. doi. 10.1002/14651858.
35. Geppert CM, Andrews MR, Druyan ME. Ethical issues in artificial nutrition and hydration: a review. J Parenter Enteral Nutr. 2010;34(1):79–88. doi: 10.1177/0148607109347209.
36. Zerwekh JV. The dehydration question. Nursing. 2012. 1983;13(1):47–56.
37. Teno JM, Gozalo P, Mitchell SL, Kuo S, Fulton AT, Mor V. Feeding tubes and the prevention or healing of pressure ulcers. Arch Intern Med. 2012;172(9):697–701. doi: 10.1001/archinternmed.2012.1200.
38. Palecek EJ, Teno JM, Casarett DJ, Hanson LC, Rhodes RL, Mitchell SL. Comfort feeding only: a proposal to bring clarity to decision-making regarding difficulty with eating for persons with advanced dementia. J Am Geriatr Soc. 2010;58(3):580–584. doi: 10.1111/j.1532-5415.2010.02740.x.
39. Teno JM, Mitchell SL, Gozalo PL, et al. Hospital characteristics associated with feeding tube placement in nursing home residents with advanced cognitive impairment. JAMA. 2010;303(6):544–550. doi: 10.1001/jama.2010.79; 10.
40. Moynihan T, Kelly DG, Fisch MJ. To feed or not to feed: is that the right question? J Clin Oncol. 2005;23(25):6256–6259.
41. Morita T, Shima Y, Miyashita M, Kimura R, Adachi I. Physician- and nurse-reported effects of intravenous hydration therapy on symptoms of terminally ill patients with cancer. J Palliat Med. 2004;7(5):683–693. doi:10.1089/jpm.2004.7.683.
42. Hanson LC, Garrett JM, Lewis C, Phifer N, Jackman A, Carey TS. Physicians' expectations of benefit from tube feeding. J Palliat Med. 2008;11(8):1130–1134. doi. 10.1089/jpm.2008.0033.
43. Washington State Death with Dignity Act. http://apps.leg.wa.gov/RCW/default.aspx?cite=70.245. Updated 2008. Accessed July 2, 2013.
44. Emanuel EJ, Fairclough DL, Emanuel LL. Attitudes and desires related to euthanasia and physician-assisted suicide among terminally ill patients and their caregivers. JAMA. 2000;284(19):2460–2468.
45. O'Mahony S, Goulet J, Kornblith A, et al. Desire for hastened death, cancer pain and depression: report of a longitudinal observational study. J Pain Symptom Manage. 2005;29(5):446–457.
46. van Bruchem-van de Scheur GG, van der Arend AJ, Huijer Abu-Saad H, van Wijmen FC, Spreeuwenberg C, Ter Meulen RH. Euthanasia and assisted suicide in Dutch hospitals: the role of nurses. J Clin Nurs. 2008;17(12):1618–1626. doi: 10.1111/j.1365-2702.2007.02145.
47. Ganzini L, Goy ER, Dobscha SK. Prevalence of depression and anxiety in patients requesting physicians' aid in dying: cross sectional survey. BMJ. 2008;337:a1682. doi: 10.1136/bmj.a1682.
48. Quill T, Arnold RM. Evaluating requests for hastened death. J Palliat Med. 2008;11(8):1151–1152.
49. Hudson PL, Schofield P, Kelly B, et al. Responding to desire to die statements from patients with advanced disease: recommendations for health professionals. Palliat Med. 2006;20(7):703–710.
50. Mond HG, Irwin M, Ector H, Proclemer A. The world survey of cardiac pacing and cardioverter-defibrillators: calendar year 2005 an international cardiac pacing and electrophysiology society (ICPES) project. Pacing Clin Electrophysiol. 2008;31(9):1202–1212. doi: 10.1111/j.1540-8159.2008.01164.
51. Mueller PS, Jenkins SM, Bramstedt KA, Hayes DL. Deactivating implanted cardiac devices in terminally ill patients: practices and attitudes. Pacing Clin Electrophysiol. 2008;31(5):560–568.
52. Hansson SO. Implant ethics. J Med Ethics. 2005;31(9):519–525.
53. Kramer DB, Kesselheim AS, Brock DW, Maisel WH. Ethical and legal views of physicians regarding deactivation of cardiac implantable electrical devices: a quantitative assessment. Heart Rhythm. 2010;7(11):1537–1542.
54. Grady KL, Shinn JA. Care of patients with circulatory assist devices. In: Moser DK, Riegel B (ed.), Cardiac Nursing. Philadelphia: Mosby; 2008:977–987.
55. Rizzieri AG, Verheijde JL, Rady MY, McGregor JL. Ethical challenges with the left ventricular assist device as a destination therapy. Philos Ethics Humanit Med. 2008;3:20-5341-3-20. doi: 10.1186/1747-5341-3-20.
56. Swetz KM, Ottenberg AL, Freeman MR, Mueller PS. Palliative care and end-of-life issues in patients treated with left ventricular assist devices as destination therapy. Curr Heart Fail Rep. 2011;8(3):212–218. doi: 10.1007/s11897-011-0060.
57. Swetz KM, Freeman MR, AbouEzzeddine OF, et al. Palliative medicine consultation for preparedness planning in patients receiving left ventricular assist devices as destination therapy. Mayo Clin Proc. 2011;86(6):493–500. doi: 10.4065/mcp.2010.0747.
58. Chapman E, Parameshwar J, Jenkins D, Large S, Tsui S. Psychosocial issues for patients with ventricular assist devices: A qualitative pilot study. Am J Crit Care. 2007;16(1):72–81.
59. Zambroski CH, Combs P, Cronin SN, Pfeffer C. Edgar Allan Poe, "The Pit and the Pendulum," and ventricular assist devices. Crit Care Nurse. 2009;29(6):29–39.
60. Lampert R, Hayes DL, Annas GJ, et al. HRS expert consensus statement on the management of cardiovascular implantable electronic devices (CIEDs) in patients nearing end of life or requesting removal. Heart Rhythm. 2010;7(7):1008–1026.
61. Quill TE, Lo B, Brock DW, Meisel A. Last-resort options for palliative sedation. Ann Intern Med. 2009;151(6):421–424.
62. Maltoni M, Scarpi E, Rosati M, et al. Palliative sedation in end-of-life care and survival: a systematic review. J Clin Oncol. 2012;30(12):1378–1383. doi: 10.1200/JCO.2011.37.3795.
63. Cassell EJ, Rich BA. Intractable end-of-life suffering and the ethics of palliative sedation. Pain Med. 2010;11(3):435–438. doi: 10.1111/j.1526-4637.2009.00786.
64. Claessens P, Menten J, Schotsmans P, Broeckaert B. Palliative sedation: a review of the research literature. J Pain Symptom Manage. 2008;36(3):310–333. doi: 10.1016/j.jpainsymman.2007.10.004;
65. Bernat JL. Medical futility. Neurocrit Care. 2005;2(2):198–205.
66. Caplan AL. Little hope for medical futility. Mayo Clin Proc. 2012;87(11):1040–1041. doi: 10.1016/j.mayocp.2012.09.003.
67. Moseley KL, Silveira MJ, Goold SD. Futility in evolution. Clin Geriatr Med. 2005;21(1):211–222.
68. Wicclair MR. Medical futility: a conceptual and ethical analysis. In: DeGrazia D, Mappes, TA, Brand-Ballard J (eds.), Biomedical Ethics. 7th ed. New York: McGraw-Hill; 2006:6:345–349.
69. von Gruenigen VE, Daly BJ. Futility: clinical decisions at the end-of-life in women with ovarian cancer. Gynecol Oncol. 2005;97(2):638–644.
70. Daly BJ. An indecent proposal: withholding cardiopulmonary resuscitation. Am J Crit Care. 2008;17(4):377–380.
71. Wilkinson DJ, Savulescu J. Knowing when to stop: futility in the intensive care unit. Curr Opin Anaesthesiol. 2011;24(2):160.
72. White DB, Pope TM. The courts, futility, and the ends of medicine. JAMA. 2012;307(2):151–152.
73. Ferrell, BR, Coyle, N. The Nature of Suffering and the Goals of Nursing. Oxford: Oxford University Press; 2008.
74. Ferrell BR. Understanding the moral distress of nurses witnessing medically futile care. Oncol Nurs Forum. 2006;33(5):922–930.

75. Aycock N, Boyle D. Interventions to manage compassion fatigue in oncology nursing. Clin J Oncol Nurs. 2009;13(2):183–191. doi: 10.1188/09.CJON.183-191.

76. Coetzee SK, Klopper HC. Compassion fatigue within nursing practice: a concept analysis. Nurs Health Sci. 2010;12(2):235–243. doi: 10.1111/j.1442-2018.2010.00526.

77. Figley CR. Treating compassion fatigue. New York: Routledge, Psychology Press; 2002.

78. Alkema K, Linton JM, Davies R. A study of the relationship between self-care, compassion satisfaction, compassion fatigue, and burn-out among hospice professionals. J Soc Work End Life Palliat Care. 2008;4(2):101–119. doi: 10.1080/15524250802353934.

79. Wiegand DL, Funk M. Consequences of clinical situations that cause critical care nurses to experience moral distress. Nurs Ethics. 2012;19(4):479–487. doi: 10.1177/0969733011429342.

80. Varcoe C, Pauly B, Storch J, Newton L, Makaroff K. Nurses' perceptions of and responses to morally distressing situations. Nurs Ethics. 2012;19(4):488–500. doi: 10.1177/0969733011436025.

81. Clark E. Self-care as best practice in palliative care. In: Altilio T, Otis-Green S (eds.), Oxford Textbook of Palliative Social Work. New York, NY: Oxford University Press; 2011:771–777.

82. Cacciatore J, Flint M. Attend: toward a mindfulness-based bereavement care model. Death Studies. 2012;36:61–82.

CHAPTER 65

Palliative care and requests for assistance in dying

Deborah L. Volker

> I was truly taken aback when the patient's mother asked me point blank about when we would give her son something to kill him.
>
> Hospital nurse caring for a dying young man

Key points

- Palliative care nurses do encounter patient and family questions, concerns, and requests for assisted dying.

- Withholding and withdrawing life-sustaining measures and provision of pain relief are not acts of assisted dying.

- Individuals with life-limiting disease who may consider assisted dying include those experiencing unrelieved pain, depression, hopelessness, psychological distress, spiritual distress, poor social support, poor quality of life, or a perception of being a burden on others.

- Nurses should respond to requests for assisted dying in a manner that reflects professional guidelines and a sense of advocacy for patient rights for quality end-of-life care.

The concept of palliative care, as described by the World Health Organization, is in direct conflict with the idea of deliberately hastening a person's death via the practice of assisted dying. Indeed, palliative care "intends neither to hasten nor postpone death."[1] Yet patients may be fearful of the extreme discomfort they anticipate as death approaches, or they may simply want some certainty as to the timing or circumstances of death. Nurses who care for patients with life-limiting disease encounter patient and family questions, concerns, and requests for assisted dying. Receiving such a request can represent a morally troubling dilemma in which there is uncertainty about how best to respond. The purpose of this chapter is to review the ethical and legal status of assisted dying, summarize empirical findings regarding both professional and lay opinions and experiences with assisted dying, and offer guidelines for responding to requests for assisted dying.

What is assisted dying?

The term "assisted dying" is typically used to describe an action in which an individual's death is intentionally hastened by the administration of a drug or other lethal substance. This may take the form of either assisted suicide or euthanasia. "Assisted suicide" indicates "the means to end a patient's life is provided to the patient (i.e. a lethal dose of medication) with knowledge of the patient's

intention. Unlike euthanasia, in assisted suicide, someone makes the means of death available, but does not act as the direct agent of death."[2] Of note, in states where assisted suicide is legal, prescriptions for lethal doses of medication, not weapons, are provided to qualified patients. *Euthanasia*, "often called 'mercy killing', is the act of putting to death someone suffering from a painful and prolonged illness or injury. Euthanasia means that someone other than the patient commits an action with the intent to end the patient's life, for example injecting a patient with a lethal dose of medication."[2] Such an action can be voluntary (e.g., requested by a competent individual) or involuntary (administered without the individual's knowledge or consent).

It is important to distinguish between the concept of assisted dying and other actions designed to allow patients to die as comfortably as possible. Withholding and withdrawing life-sustaining measures are actions designed to not interfere with the natural trajectory of an illness. That is, life-sustaining measures such as artificial ventilation, renal dialysis, cardiopulmonary resuscitation, or artificial nutrition and hydration are withheld or stopped; the patient subsequently dies because of the effects of disease. In this instance, the intent of the action is to allow a natural death, and the cause of death is the underlying illness. In assisted dying, the intent of the action is to hasten death, and the cause of death is the lethal drug or other means administered to end life. Intent and causation are the key concepts that differentiate the two actions. Some practitioners worry that administration of sufficient doses of pain medication and other drugs designed to relieve suffering may hasten death and therefore may constitute assisted dying. However, this is *not* an action of assisted dying. It does not qualify as assisted dying because the intent is to relieve suffering, even though there may be a foreseen possibility that the medications could result in a hastened death. This is an example of the ethical principle of double effect, in which a good effect (relief of pain or other symptoms) is the goal despite the possibility of an unintended, harmful effect (a hastened death). The reader is referred to chapter 7 for more information on the principles and ethics of proper pain management.

Unfortunately, the lay public and some healthcare providers continue to be confused about the definition and intent of palliative care versus actions designed to deliberately hasten death. For example, in a lay magazine article, palliative care was characterized as the "new stealth euthanasia" that is changing medical care in the United States "from lifesaving medicine to liferationing [sic] medicine."[3](p. 3) Palliative care physicians, nurses, and other practitioners may experience this sentiment in the clinical setting.[4] As such, Goldstein and colleagues conducted a survey of the frequency of formal accusations of murder and euthanasia against 663 hospice and palliative care physicians.[4] Findings revealed that over half of the sample had patient family members and/or other healthcare providers misinterpret the study participants' palliative care practices as murder or euthanasia. Most commonly reported misperceived actions included the use of opiates for symptom control and the use of palliative and sedating medications during discontinuation of mechanical ventilation to prevent suffering. Clearly, efforts to educate the public and healthcare providers about the moral and legal status of palliative care practices must be intensified.

What are the ethical and legal issues?

The ethical issues associated with assisted dying have been well described.[5–7] In essence, those who support the practice cite the patient's right to determine his/her own fate (autonomy), relieve untenable suffering, and maintain control over the end of life. Also relevant is the issue of equity, in that patients who are not dependent on life support, for example, do not have the same access to ending life as patients who can deliberately end life by discontinuing a ventilator. Those who believe assisted dying is unethical worry that the practice will erode trust in healthcare professionals, deny the sanctity of human life, discourage efforts to make palliative care available to all, and initiate a "slippery slope" in which vulnerable, underserved, disabled, or disenfranchised patients will feel pressured to take a quick way out with death. Historically, the healthcare professions' ethical codes and position statements uniformly opposed legal assisted dying. However, more recent trends reveal that a few organizations are neutral on the topic,[8] take no stand formal stand but advise members as to their ethical responsibilities as patient advocates,[9] or support patients who choose legal assisted dying.[10] Nursing organizations continue to oppose assisted dying; Table 65.1 summarizes their relevant position statements.

Euthanasia is illegal throughout the United States although physician assisted death is legal in four states, whereas the Netherlands, Belgium, and Luxembourg allow both euthanasia and assisted suicide under certain circumstances.[18] Switzerland is unique in that it (1) allows assisted suicide to be facilitated by nonphysicians (although a physician must prescribe the lethal medication, nonphysician volunteers may provide assistance such as connecting patients with physicians who are willing to prescribe a lethal drug, providing an apartment for the suicide, and so forth), (2) allows foreign citizens to engage in the practice within its borders, and (3) does not require that a person have a particular illness or prognosis.[19]

Worldwide, the Netherlands has had more experience with the practice of euthanasia than any other country. Euthanasia was legally sanctioned via a series of court decisions in the Netherlands beginning in the 1970s; euthanasia and physician-assisted suicide were legalized in 2002 by the Dutch parliament.[20] Controversy exists as to whether increasing tolerance of these practices by physicians and the public has led to an increase in their use and a lesser emphasis on palliative and hospice care. Onwuteaka-Philipsen and colleagues studied trends in end-of-life practices in the Netherlands from 1990 to 2010 via a repeated cross-sectional survey.[21] Although the overall incidence of deaths due to physician-assisted suicide did not change between 1990 and 2010, the incidence of euthanasia did increase between 2005 and 2010. Over the study period, far fewer deaths were due to physician-assisted death than euthanasia (for example, 21 versus 475 in 2010). Other trends included an increase in the use of deep sedation prior to death, an increase in the use of intensified strategies to address pain and other symptoms at the end of life, and a decrease in the frequency of ending life without a patient's request. The researchers speculated that these trends may reflect an increased interest in palliative care, and that regulations enacted in 2002 may have facilitated more open discussions between patients and physicians about end-of-life care. However, the study did not evaluate quality of end-of-life care and hospice use, nor did it obtain views of patients or family members. Ongoing study of assisted dying in the Netherlands is anticipated.

Assisted suicide was legalized in Oregon in 1997 with the passage of the Death with Dignity Act via two citizen referenda separated by 3 years. This Act allows a terminally ill person to obtain a prescription for a lethal dose of medication with the prescribing physician's understanding that the intent of the medication is to end life. Eligible patients must meet several criteria, including being at least 18 years of age, an Oregon resident, capable of making healthcare decisions, and diagnosed with a terminal illness that will cause death within 6 months. The patient who requests a prescription must make two oral requests (separated by at least 15 days) to his/her physician and provide a written request that is signed in the presence of two witnesses. The prescribing physician and a consulting physician must confirm the diagnosis and prognosis and determine whether the patient is competent to make the decision. If either physician believes the patient's judgment is in question, the patient must be referred for a psychological examination. The prescribing physician must discuss alternatives to assisted suicide (comfort care, hospice care, and pain control) with the patient and must request (but not require) that the patient notify next-of-kin of his or her plans.[22] The Act was challenged in 2001 by the US attorney general, who asserted that physicians who prescribe lethal doses of drugs are violating federal laws regarding controlled substances. The US Supreme Court ruled in 2006 that the attorney general does not have the authority to determine what constitutes a legitimate medical practice and that individual states retain this responsibility.[23] Hence, the Oregon Act remains in place and physicians may continue to prescribe controlled substances for the purpose of hastening death. Notably, only about 1 in every 1000 Oregonians who die use assisted suicide as an end-of-life option.[24]

Since Oregon legalized assisted suicide, three additional states have since approved the practice. In 2008, voters in Washington state approved a Death with Dignity Act that is modeled after the Oregon law. Although Montana does not have a similar statute, the Montana Supreme Court ruled that physician-assisted suicide was not illegal in 2009,[5] which paved the way for legal patient access to the practice. Most recently, Vermont's state legislature and governor approved a law that allows physician-assisted suicide.

Table 65.1 Position statements of nursing organizations relevant to patient requests for assisted dying

Organization	Title	Key points
American Nurses Association[7]	Euthanasia, Assisted Suicide, and Aid in Dying	The ANA "prohibits nurses' participation in assisted suicide and euthanasia because these acts are in direct violation of Code of Ethics for Nurses with Interpretive Statements" (p. 1) Nurses are obliged to provide compassionate, competent care that respects patients rights while also upholding nursing practice standards focused on "chronic, debilitating illness and the end of life" (p. 1). Although the ANA recognizes that some nurses practice in locales where assisted suicide is legal, the ANA Center for Ethics and Human Rights offers support and consultation serves to them regarding their professional responsibilities.
American Nurses Association[11]	Registered Nurses' Roles and Responsibilities in Providing Expert Care and Counseling at the End of Life	"Nurses, individually and collectively, have an obligation to provide comprehensive and compassionate end-of-life care, including the promotion of comfort, relief of pain, and support for patients, families, and their surrogates when a decision has been made to forgo life-sustaining treatments" (p. 2). "While nurses should make every effort to provide aggressive pain control and symptom relief for patients at the end of life, it is never ethically permissible for a nurse to act by omission or commission, including, but not limited to medication administration, with the intention of ending a patient's life" (p. 2).
American Society for Pain Management Nurses[12]	ASPMN Position Statement on Assisted Suicide	Supports the ANA position against nurses' participation in assisted suicide or euthanasia, and "supports improved access for pain management services and other modalities that will benefit terminally ill patients and their families" (p. 1)
Hospice and Palliative Nurses Association[13]	Legalization of Assisted Suicide	"Opposes the legalization of assisted suicide" and "affirms the value of aggressive and comprehensive end-of-life care" (p. 2). "Advises nurses practicing in states where assisted suicide is legal that they have the moral and legal right to refuse to be involved in the care of patients requesting assisted suicide" but must remain nonjudgmental and transfer the patient's care to other nurses (p. 2)
Hospice and Palliative Nurses Association[14]	Role of the Nurse When Hastened Death Is Requested	"Both patient's rights and nurses' values should be respected" (p. 2). Nurses should assess patient requests for hastened death, provide aggressive palliative care, and "share information about health choices that are legal and support the patient and family regardless of the decision that is made" (p. 2)
Oncology Nursing Society[15]	Nurses' Responsibility to Patients Requesting Assistance in Hastening Death	Does not support actions intended to hasten death but "supports continued efforts to improve compassionate, evidence-based care for the dying and encourages continued dialogue on any and all ethical dilemmas." Responses to requests for hastened death should "prompt a frank discussion of the rationale for the request, a thorough and nonjudgmental multidisciplinary assessment of the patient's unmet needs, and prompt and intensive intervention for previously unrecognized or unmet needs" (p. 1).
Oregon Nurses Association[16]	ONA Provides Guidance on Nurses' Dilemma	Does not support or oppose legalized assisted suicide. "If the patient inquires about the option of assisted suicide, one of the roles of the nurses, as healthcare provider, is to share relevant information about health choices that are legal and to support the patient and family regardless of the decision the patient makes." Provides guidelines for acceptable practices for nurses who choose to be, or not be involved with a patient who requests legal assistance to hasten death.
Vermont State Nurses' Association[17]	VSNA Position Statement on Physician-Assisted Suicide	"Opposes the legalization of physician assisted suicide and believes that the nurse should not participate in assisted suicide" (p. 12). Identifies key components of "dignified and humane end-of life care" and believes that "the focus on physician assisted suicide distracts attention and resources from the real work of helping our patients live meaningful lives in their final days" (p. 12).

Although the law has safeguards similar to those in Oregon and Washington, after a 3-year period of governmental restrictions expires in 2016, prescribing practices of physicians who write legal prescriptions for assisted suicide will become more private and guided by professional practice standards that guide physician conduct.[25]

Who wants access to assisted dying and why?

It is not unusual for terminally ill people to desire a hastened death. People who have life-limiting diseases such as cancer, degenerative neurological disorders, or end-stage cardiovascular or renal disease have been identified as individuals who may be interested in access to assisted dying. Various studies have revealed characteristics of those who have expressed a desire for hastened death. Ferrand and colleagues conducted a national survey of palliative care departments in France to describe the evolution of requests for hastened death among their patients.[26] Of the 342 teams who responded, 783 descriptions of requests were provided. Patients typically had a cancer diagnosis (72%), were terminally ill (68%), and had controlled pain (52%), a feeding impairment (65%), incontinence (49%), and/or a motor impairment (54%). Notably, less than 4% had uncontrolled pain, which may have been a reflection of care management by palliative specialists. The most commonly reported patient perceptions of their concerns included "a fear of presenting an unbearable image of oneself" (50%) and fear of becoming a burden on family (46%).

Cancer is a major risk factor for an affected person's interest in suicide. In a case–control study of suicide risk in older Americans with medical illnesses, cancer was the only illness that was associated with a higher risk of suicide.[27] The study authors conjectured that contributing factors might have included advanced disease and its treatment or social responses to progressive disease such as intractable pain, poor prognosis, use of higher doses of analgesics, or social isolation. The study focused on analysis of actual suicides and did not capture desire for suicide that was not enacted. Historically, risk for suicide in cancer patients has been associated with end-stage disease, depression, and hopelessness.[28] Further, in a study of the clinical features of suicidality in patients with advanced cancer, patients who were more likely to have suicidal thoughts (9% of the sample) than those who did not, were non-Hispanic whites, reported no religious affiliation, and were diagnosed with a current panic disorder and/or posttraumatic stress disorder.[29] However, Walker and colleagues surveyed approximately 3,000 outpatients with cancer to determine prevalence of suicidal thoughts.[30] About 8% reported suicidal thoughts. Emotional distress, substantial pain, and older age were associated with suicidal ideation in this group of patients. This finding suggests that assessment for suicidal risk in cancer patients must go beyond those with terminal illness.

Patients with amyotrophic lateral sclerosis (ALS) are at higher risk than the general population for interest in hastening death via physician-assisted suicide or euthanasia. Typically, contributing variables include severe, advanced-stage disease, treatment ineffectiveness, and increasing dependence on caregivers.[31] However, in a 40-year, case-controlled study of suicide in Sweden, people with ALS had a six-fold increased risk for over than the general population, but that the risk was higher in earlier stages of the disease.[31] The study investigators hypothesized that severe emotional burden associated with a new diagnosis of ALS and physical inability to perform suicide at later stages of disease could have accounted for their findings. In the Netherlands, death due to euthanasia is more common among people with ALS than with a cancer diagnosis.[32]

Experience with legal assisted dying in Oregon reveals another picture. During the first 15 years of the Death with Dignity Act, 673 patients took lethal medications to end their lives, whereas 1,050 Oregonians received prescriptions for assisted dying under the Act.[33] The characteristics of Oregonians who died from assisted dying have remained stable over time, including older age (median: 71 years), white race and college-level education. Most had a diagnosis of either cancer or ALS, were enrolled in hospice care, and had private or governmental health insurance. The most common end-of-life concerns voiced included loss of autonomy, decreased ability to participate in enjoyable activities, and loss of dignity.[33]

Various studies of Oregon patients, families, and healthcare providers' attitudes and experiences with assisted suicide have unfolded since the enactment of the Death with Dignity Act. In a study of the quality of death and dying in patients who requested a physician-assisted death, Smith and colleagues examined the perspective of family members of patients who had received prescriptions for assisted dying, patients who sought but did not receive such prescriptions, and patients who did not request assisted dying.[34] When comparing symptom control, connectedness with others, existential issues, preparedness for death, and global indicators of quality of life and death, the researchers concluded that "the quality of death experienced by those who received lethal prescriptions is no worse than those not pursuing physician assisted death, and in some areas is rated by family members as better."[34(p. 445)] These areas included symptom control and preparedness for death. Given that data reported to the Oregon

Public Health Division regarding patients' experiences with the Death With Dignity Act are provided by physicians, Ganzini and colleagues took a different approach and investigated Oregonians' reasons for requesting physician aid in dying.[35] In a survey of 56 individuals who had expressed interest in physician-assisted dying, the most important reasons for their interest included concerns about loss of control over independence, circumstances of death, and ability to care for self, as well as concern about physical discomfort in the future. The authors concluded that study results should prompt healthcare providers to address patient requests for assisted dying by addressing autonomy issues and worries about symptom control as the end of life unfolds.

Despite access to legal assisted dying, or perhaps because of it, Oregon is a national leader in improving planning for, and delivery of, quality of end-of-life care. Oregon is among only eight states to receive an "A" grade for access to palliative care[36] and among 13 states to receive an "A" grade for the quality of its policies that affect pain treatment.[37] The Oregon Physicians Orders for Life-Sustaining Treatment (POLST) program was created 20 years ago to implement a system that captures a patient's treatment preferences and electronically records them as medical records accessible across care settings.[38] The population of focus is those with advanced and/or chronic progressive illness or frailty. Now codified by Oregon state law, POLST has served as a model program nationally and has been adopted by 15 states, with 28 others under development.[38]

What do studies reveal about nurses and assisted dying?

Given their pivotal role in providing palliative care, nurses may encounter patient requests for assisted dying. Both survey and interview studies have captured nurses' experiences with receiving requests for assisted dying. For example, in a classic study conducted by Matzo and Emanuel,[39] the investigators surveyed 441 New England oncology nurses and discovered that 30% had received requests for assisted suicide, 1% had engaged in assisted suicide, and 4.5% had injected a drug to intentionally end a patient's life. In a national survey of more than 2,333 nurses,[40] 23% had received patient requests for assistance with obtaining a lethal prescription, and 22% had patients who requested that they be injected with a lethal dose of medication.

The experience of Oregon nurses and social workers with hospice patients who requested physician-assisted suicide or voluntary refusal of food and fluids (VSED) has also been examined. Harvath and colleagues interviewed 20 nurses and social workers regarding their experiences with patients who wished to hasten death.[41] The participants indicated that such requests presented opportunities to discuss patient concerns and fears about the dying process and to improve symptom-management strategies. But they also indicated that requests for aid in hastening death presented a dilemma between respect for patient autonomy versus honoring their commitment to uphold the goals of hospice care. In a subsequent study of policies developed by 56 Oregon hospices to manage patient requests for legal assisted dying under the Death with Dignity Act, researchers found that these policies reflect ambivalence between a commitment to care for all patients regardless of interest in assisted dying versus the traditional goals of hospice care to neither hasten death nor prolong life.[42] The question of what constitutes participation (or not) in assisted dying manifested in a variety of ways, ranging from providing information about the law to patients, to exploring patient requests for hastened death, to encouraging patient contact with their physicians. Many of the policies reflected an emphasis on the importance of maintaining neutrality during patient discussions. Almost all of the policies contained a prohibition against assistance with a lethal medication: "Hospice X will not provide, pay for, deliver, administer or assist with medications intended for physician-assisted dying,"[42(p. 233)] nor do they allow their staff to assist the patient to self-administer the medication. Nonetheless, during the investigators' site visits at participating hospices, some nurses revealed that they would "attend" a patient during an assisted death but not while "on duty."

Washington nurses are now investigating issues associated with implementation of legal assisted dying. Two years after implementation of the Washington state Death with Dignity Act, Jablonski,[43] Clymin,[44] and colleagues surveyed 582 members of the Washington State Nurses Association to determine their knowledge about the new law. Most of the respondents accurately understood some components of the law, including eligibility for assisted dying, physicians' and institutions' rights to refuse to participate, and restrictions limiting prescribing practices for lethal doses of medications to physicians only. Conversely, less than half of the respondents could accurately answer 9 of 25 knowledge items, ranging from inaccurately specifying a requirement for an interdisciplinary team evaluation of assisted dying request to misunderstanding employing institution or facility rights regarding the restriction of assisted dying practices. Only 7% of the respondents had received education about the new law when it was first enacted; many expressed concern about their lack of knowledge regarding the Act.

Given that euthanasia and assisted suicide are legal in the Netherlands, study of nurses' roles within this context is important. In a survey of 532 Dutch inpatient nurses, investigators examined the role of nurses in managing patient requests for euthanasia or assisted suicide, the decision-making process, and the administration of lethal drugs.[45] Findings revealed that patients often speak with their nurses first about their wishes for hastened death and that nurses respond by explaining legal requirements, hospital policies, and opportunities for palliative care. Most nurses reported discussing patient requests with physician colleagues. Notably, nurses administered a lethal drug with or without a physician present to 22 patients. Dutch law limits the administration of euthanatics to physicians only.

How should nurses respond to requests for assisted dying?

Of the myriad communication skills expected of nurses, responding to requests for assisted dying can be the most difficult. Not surprisingly, many nurses feel ill equipped to address a patient's interest in suicide. According to Valente,[46] barriers to appropriate nursing management of suicide risk include communication issues such as not knowing how to respond, personal judgments about the act of suicide, unresolved grief in one's personal life, uncomfortable emotions, and lack of knowledge. Regardless of his or her personal feelings about the moral acceptability of assisted dying, the professional nurse has a responsibility to skillfully respond to

a patient's request for assisted dying in a compassionate, sensitive way. The patient advocacy role of nursing is central to that response, as is the adage to never abandon the patient. Table 65.1 summarizes the guidelines that professional organizations offer to assist nurses in formulating responses to requests for assisted dying. In particular, the Oncology Nursing Society[15] has emphasized that requests for hastening death prompt a frank discussion of the rationale for the request, a thorough and nonjudgmental multidisciplinary assessment of the patient's unmet needs, and prompt and intensive intervention for previously unrecognized or unmet needs."[15(p. 1)] Box 65.1 outlines the American Academy of Hospice and Palliative Medicine's guidelines for exploring a request for assisted dying.[8] For nurses who practice in Oregon, the Oregon Nurses Association[16] has published detailed guidelines for nurses who choose to be involved in an assisted suicide, as well as guidelines for those who choose not to be involved but transfer the patient's care to another colleague. In either case, nurses may not inject or administer medication intended to end life; subject the patient, family, or other healthcare team members to judgmental comments or actions; or refuse to provide comfort and safety measures to the patient.

Are there alternatives to assisted dying?

The wish for a peaceful, comfortable death is not unreasonable. Given that assisted dying is not a viable moral or legal option for many individuals, what are the alternatives that could fulfill a desire to control the circumstances of the dying process? The obvious answer is universal access to expert palliative care. Indeed, there is strong moral consensus among healthcare providers that untreated suffering must never be a justification for assisted dying. However, there are legally and ethically sanctioned options other than assisted dying that may be palatable for some individuals. Refusal of medical treatment is a widely respected means for allowing the dying process to unfold unimpeded by treatments that will not fulfill the patient's personal goals for the end-of-life experience. Refusal may be in the form of withholding or withdrawing a life-sustaining treatment.

The individual who is not dependent on medical interventions to sustain life and wishes to control the timing of his or her death is faced with a more perplexing challenge. Voluntary refusal of food and fluids has been identified as a possible option. Although such action requires no direct participation by the healthcare team, nurses can support patients who choose this option by ensuring optimal comfort measures and family support. Depending on the patient's underlying condition, death usually occurs within 1 to 3 weeks.[47] Concern has been voiced regarding discomforts that could accompany this action. To evaluate this possibility, Ganzini and associates[48] surveyed hospice nurses who had cared for terminally ill patients who deliberately hastened death by cessation of eating and drinking. Thirty-three percent of their 307 respondents reported that they had cared for such patients. The most common reasons given by patients for this choice were readiness for death, poor quality of life or fear of poor quality of life, belief that continued existence was pointless, and desire to die at home. Most of the patients had either cancer or a neurological disease; 85% of the patients died within 15 days after ceasing intake of food and fluids. The nurses were asked to rate the quality of these patients' deaths on a scale from 0 (a very bad death) to 9 (a very

Box 65.1 Approaches to exploring a request for physician-assisted death: guidelines from the American Academy of Hospice and Palliative Medicine

◆ **Determine the nature of the request**

Is the patient seeking assistance right now? Is he seriously exploring the clinician's openness to the possibility of a hastened death in the future? Is he simply airing vague thoughts about ending life?

◆ **Clarify the cause(s) of intractable suffering**

Is there severe pain or another unrelieved physical symptom? Is the distress mainly emotional or spiritual? Does the patient feel he is a burden? Has he grown tired of a prolonged dying?

◆ **Evaluate the patient's decision-making capacity**

Does the patient have cognitive impairment that would affect his judgment? Does the patient's request seem rational and proportionate to the clinical situation? Is his request consistent with his past values?

◆ **Explore emotional factors**

Do feelings of depression, worthlessness, excessive guilt, or fear substantially interfere with the patient's judgment?

Initial responses to requests for hastened death:

◆ Respond empathically to the patient's emotions.

◆ Intensify treatment of pain and other physical symptoms.

◆ Identify and treat depression, anxiety, and/or spiritual suffering when present.

◆ Consult with specialists in palliative care and/or hospice.

◆ Consult with experts in spiritual or psychological suffering, or other specialty areas depending on the patient's circumstances.

◆ Utilize a caring and understanding approach to encourage dialogue and trust and to assure the best chance of relieving distress.

◆ Commit to the patient to work toward a mutually acceptable solution for his suffering.

When unacceptable suffering persists, despite thorough evaluation, exploration, and provision of standard palliative care interventions as outlined above, a search for common ground is essential. In these situations, the benefits and burdens of the following alternatives should be considered:

◆ Discontinuation of potentially life-prolonging treatments, including corticosteroids, insulin, dialysis, oxygen, or artificial hydration or nutrition.

◆ Voluntary cessation of eating and drinking as an acceptable strategy for the patient, family, and treating practitioners.

◆ Palliative sedation, even potentially to unconsciousness, if suffering is intractable and of sufficient severity (AAHPM Statement on Palliative Sedation: www.aahpm.org/positions/sedation.html).

Source: American Academy of Hospice and Palliative Medicine (2007), reference 8, permission granted.

good death); the median score for this sample was 8. The authors concluded that, from the perspective of the nurse participants, most of the patients died a good or peaceful death. Notably, no family or patient perspectives were obtained in this study. Future research should focus on evaluating these perspectives.

The practice of palliative sedation represents another alternative to assisted dying. Palliative sedation refers to the use of sedative medications to reduce a patient's awareness of symptoms that have not been sufficiently controlled by other therapies.[49] According to the American Academy of Hospice and Palliative Medicine, sedation to the point of unconsciousness should only be used for "the most severe, intractable suffering at the very end of life."[49(p. 1)] The goal of palliative sedation is to relieve suffering, not to cause death. A detailed discussion of this practice is provided in chapter 25. Palliative sedation may be ethically troubling for both family and professional caregivers because some do not differentiate between this practice and euthanasia. Palliative care experts can provide guidance to assist patients, families, and professionals with appropriate use of sedation and to distinguish palliative sedation from hastened death. In addition, some patients may not find this choice acceptable because they view induction of unconsciousness until the time of death as undignified and as prohibiting communication with loved ones in those final days or hours.

Case study

When a hospice patient expresses interested in suicide

In the following scenario, a hospice nurse described a patient's plan to commit suicide in the event he developed intolerable pain and dependency on others.[50]

"David, a retired stoic businessman was admitted to hospice with terminal pancreatic cancer. He told me at my first visit that he was going to commit suicide. He did not ask for my opinion or help, but I understood that he was interested in my reaction. For a time, I said nothing and then asked him what would dissuade him. He reiterated his intent after exploring his concerns about pain and dependency. We made a verbal agreement that he would take no action before my next scheduled visit. Together with the physician, we quickly increased and adjusted medications to manage David's symptoms. At each visit, for at least 3 subsequent visits, the initial contract between David and me was renewed. Gradually, David no longer talked of suicide and died with good pain control at home in the presence of his wife.

"I believe that the intense focus on David's plan and alternatives to his proposed action gave David the opportunity to explore other avenues. I believe I was able to gain David's trust, which strengthened as we worked together to assure that his final weeks were relatively pain free and that his ability to make decisions was encouraged and respected to the end. I recall my own anxiety in my first few visits to David and my resolve to remain calm, caring, and determined to help him live out his days in as much comfort and dignity as possible."

This case illustrates the disturbing consequences of a fear of untreated suffering that can occur at the end of life. The patient's discussion of his plans was the prompt for assessment and interventions to address his needs and fears. The nurse upheld professional standards by exploring the patient's concerns in a nonjudgmental manner, immediately initiating actions in consultation with the physician, and building a trusting relationship over time.

Conclusion

Although many requests for assisted dying can be resolved by the application of expert palliative care, a small subset of individuals may seek assisted dying despite such care. Nurses are responsible for responding to patient requests in a manner that reflects professional guidelines and a sense of advocacy for patient rights for quality end-of-life care. Regardless of personal values or discomfort with a request for assisted dying, nurses must apply open communication techniques that allow exploration of patients' needs and fears about the final phase of life.

References

1. World Health Organization. WHO definition of palliative care. Available at: http://www.who.int/cancer/palliative/definition/en/ (accessed June 28, 2013).
2. American Nurses Association. Euthanasia, Assisted Suicide, and Aid in Dying. 2013 Available at: http://nursingworld.org/euthanasiaand-dying (accessed June 28, 2013).
3. Mallon J. Palliative Care: The New Stealth Euthanasia. Celebrate Life November-December 2009. Available at: http://www.clmagazine.org/article/index/id/OTAwOQ/ (accessed June 28, 2013).
4. Goldstein NE, Cohen LM, Arnold RM, Goy E, Arons S, Ganzini L. Prevalence of formal accusations of murder and euthanasia against physicians. J Palliat Med. 2012;15:334–339.
5. Friend ML. Physician-assisted suicide: Death with dignity? J Nurs Law. 2011;14:110–116.
6. Jannette J, Bosek MSD, Rambur B. Advanced practice registered nurse intended actions toward patient-directed dying. JONA's Healthc Law Ethics Regul. 2013;15:80–88
7. Boudreau JD, Somerville MA. Physician-assisted suicide should not be permitted. N Engl J Med. 2013;368:1450–1452.
8. American Academy of Hospice and Palliative Medicine. Physician-Assisted Death. 2007. http://www.aahpm.org/positions/default/suicide.html (accessed June 28, 2013).
9. American Society of Health-System Pharmacists. ASHP statement on pharmacist's decision-making on assisted suicide. Am J Health-Syst Pharm. 1999;56:1661–1664.
10. American Public Health Association. Patients' Rights to Self-Determination at the End of Life. 2008. Available at http://www.apha.org/advocacy/policy/policysearch/default.htm?id=1372 (accessed June 28, 2013).
11. American Nurses Association. Registered Nurses' Roles and Responsibilities in Providing Expert Care and Counseling at the End of Life. 2010. Available at http://nursingworld.org/MainMenuCategories/EthicsStandards/Ethics-Position-Statements (accessed June 28, 2013).
12. American Society for Pain Management Nursing. Position Statement on Assisted Suicide. Nd. Available at http://www.aspmn.org/organization/position_papers.htm (accessed June 28, 2013).
13. Hospice and Palliative Nurses Association. Legalization of Assisted Suicide. 2011. Available at http://www.hpna.org/DisplayPage.aspx?Title=Position%20Statements (accessed June 28, 2013).
14. Hospice and Palliative Nurses Association. Role of the Nurse When Hastened Death Is Requested. 2011. Available at http://www.hpna.org/DisplayPage.aspx?Title=Position%20Statements (accessed June 28, 2013).
15. Oncology Nursing Society. Position Statement on Nurses' Responsibility to Patients Requesting Assistance in Hastening Death. 2013. Available at http://www.ons.org/Publications/Positions/AssistedSuicide (accessed June 28, 2013).
16. Oregon Nurses Association. Role of the Registered Nurse in Assisted Suicide. Available at http://www.oregonrn.org/displaycommon.cfm?an=1&subarticlenbr=450 (accessed June 28, 2013).
17. Vermont State Nurses Association. VSNA Position Statement on Physician-Assisted Suicide. Vermont Nurse Connection. 2004;7(1):12.
18. Shariff MJ. Assisted death and the slippery slope—finding clarity amid advocacy, convergence, and complexity. 2012. Curr Oncol. 19:143–154.
19. Andorno R. Nonphysician-assisted suicide in Switzerland. Camb Q Healthc Ethics. 2013;22:246–253.
20. Kimsa GK. Death by request in the Netherlands: Facts, the legal context and effects on physicians, patients, and families. Med Health Care Philos. 2010;13:355–361.
21. Onwuteaka-Philipsen BD, Brinkman-Stoppelenburg A, Penning C, de Jong-Krul GJF, van Delden JM, van der Heide A. Trends in end-of-life practices before and after enactment of the euthanasia law in the Netherlands from 1990 to 2010: a repeated cross-sectional survey. Lancet. 2012;380:908–915.
22. Oregon Public Health Division. Death with Dignity Act Requirements. 2006. Available at: http://public.health.oregon.gov/ProviderPartnerResources/EvaluationResearch/DeathwithDignityAct/Pages/index.aspx (accessed June 28, 2013).
23. Tucker, KL. In the laboratory of the states: The progress of Glucksberg's invitation to states to address end-of-life choices. Mich Law Rev 2008;106:1593–1611.
24. Hedberg K, Tolle S. Putting Oregon's Death With Dignity Act in perspective: Characteristics of decendents who did not participate. J Clin Ethics 2009;20:133–135.
25. McClure J. Vermont passes law allowing doctor-assisted suicide. Thomson Reuters. May 20, 2013. Available at http://www.reuters.com/assets/print?aid=USBRE94J0QC20130520 (accessed June 28, 2013).
26. Ferrand E, Drefus J, Chastrusse M, Ellien F, Lemaire F, Fischler M. Evolution of requests to hasten death among patients managed by palliative care teams in France: a multicentre cross-sectional survey (DemandE). Eur J Cancer. 2012;48:368–376.
27. Miller M, Mogun H, Azael D, Hempstead K, Solomon D. Cancer and the risk of suicide in older Americans. J Clin Oncol. 2008;26:4720–4724.
28. Quill T. Suicidal thoughts and actions in cancer patients: the time for exploration is NOW. J Clin Oncol. 2008;26:4705–4707.
29. Spencer RJ, Ray A, Pirl WF, Prigerson HG. Clinical correlates of suicidal thoughts in patients with advanced cancer. 2012. Am J Geriatr Psychiatry. 20:327–336.
30. Walker J, Waters R, Murray G, et al. Better off dead: suicidal thoughts in cancer patients. J Clin Oncol. 2008;26:4725–4730.
31. Fang F, Valdimarsdóttir U, Fürst CJ, Hultman C, Fall K, Sparén P, et al. Suicide among patients with amyotrophic lateral sclerosis. Brain. 2008;131:2729–2733.
32. Maessen M, Veldink JH, van den Berg LH, Schouten HJ, van der Wal G, Onwuteaka-Philipsen BD. Requests for euthanasia: origin of suffering in ALS, heart failure, and cancer patients. 2010. J Neurol. 257:1192–1198.
33. Oregon Public Health Division. Oregon's Death With Dignity Act—2012. Available at http://public.health.oregon.gov/ProviderPartnerResources/EvaluationResearch/DeathwithDignityAct/Pages/index.aspx (accessed June 28, 2013).
34. Smith KA, Goy ER, Harvath TA, Ganzini L. Quality of death and dying in patients who request physician-assisted death. 2011. J Palliat Med. 14:445–450.
35. Ganzini L, Goy ER, Dobscha SK. Oregonians reasons for requesting physician aid in dying. Arch Intern Med 2009;169:489–493.
36. Morrison RS, Meier DE. America's Care of Serious Illness: A State-by-State Report Card on Access to Palliative Care in Our Nation's Hospitals. New York, NY: Center to Advance Palliative Care and National Palliative Care Research Center, 2011. Available at http://reportcard.capc.org/pdf/state-by-state-report-card.pdf (accessed June 28, 2013).
37. Pain and Policies Studies Group. Achieving Balance in State Pain Policy: A Progress Report Card (CY2012). 2013. Available at http://www.painpolicy.wisc.edu/sites/www.painpolicy.wisc.edu/files/prc2012.pdf (accessed June 28, 2013).
38. Zive DM, Schmidt TA. Pathways to POLST Registry Development: Lessons Learned. Portland, OR: National POLST Paradigm Task Force, Oregon Health and Science University, 2012. Available at http://www.oregonpolst.org/wp-content/

uploads/2012/09/POLST_2012_with_cover_spreads_FINAL.pdf (accessed June 28, 2013).

39. Matzo M, Emanuel E. Oncology nurses' practices of assisted suicide and patient-requested euthanasia. Oncol Nurs Forum. 1997;24:1725–1732.

40. Ferrell B, Virani R, Grant M, Coyne P, Uman G. Beyond the Supreme Court decision: nursing perspectives on end-of-life care. Oncol Nurs Forum. 2000;27:446–455.

41. Harvath TA, Miller LL, Smith KA, Clark LD, Jackson A, Ganzini L. Dilemmas encountered by hospice workers when patients wish to hasten death. J Hosp Palliat Nurs. 2006;8:200–209.

42. Campbell CS, Cox JC. Hospice-assisted Death?: A study of Oregon hospices on Death with Dignity. J Hospice Palliat Med. 2012;29:227–235.

43. Jablonski A, Clymin J, Jacobson D, Feldt K. The Washington State Death with Dignity Act: a survey of nurses' knowledge and implications for practice, part 1. J Hospice Palliat Nurs. 2012;14:45–52.

44. Clymin J, Jacobson D, Jablonski A, Feldt KS. Washington State Death with Dignity Act: a survey of nurses' knowledge and implications for practice, part 2. J Hospice Palliat Nurs. 2012;14:141–148.

45. Van Bruchem-van de Scheur GG, van der Arend A, Abu-Saad H, van Wijmen F, Spreeuwenberg C, ter Meulen R. Euthanasia and assisted suicide in Dutch hospitals: the role of nurses. J Clin Nurs. 2008;17:1618–1626.

46. Valente S. Nurses' psychosocial barriers to suicide management. 2011. Nurs Res Pract. 2011;650765.

47. Schwarz JK. Stopping eating and drinking. 2009. Am J Nurs. 2009;109(9):52–61.

48. Ganzini L, Goy E, Miller L, Harvath T, Jackson A, Delorit M. Nurses' experiences with hospice patients who refuse food and fluids to hasten death. N Engl J Med. 2003;349:359–365.

49. American Academy of Hospice and Palliative Medicine. Statement on palliative sedation. 2006. Available at: http://www.aahpm.org/positions/default/sedation.html (accessed June 28, 2013).

50. Volker DL. Oncology nurses' experiences with requests for assisted dying from terminally ill cancer patients. Doctoral dissertation. University of Texas at Austin, 1999. Dissertation Abstracts International, 61(01), 199B.

CHAPTER 66

Nursing education

Pamela Malloy

I attribute my success to this—I never gave or took any excuse.

Florence Nightingale

Key points

- There is a need for palliative care nursing education.

- New guidelines for palliative care provide direction for nursing faculty, students, and practicing nurses.

- Updates and changes in advanced practice registered nursing will promote improved palliative care.

There has never been a more exciting time to be a nursing educator promoting palliative care education, practice, policy, and research. Opportunities are unprecedented to provide this education to the next generation of nurses and to practicing nurses. The increase in the number of palliative care teams continues to grow annually across the United States, necessitating continuing education. There are currently 1635 (66%) hospitals with more than 50 beds providing palliative care, representing a 148.5% increase since 2000.[1] The Joint Commission is now recognizing the important role palliative care plays in the healthcare system and is providing opportunities for hospitals to obtain Advanced Certification in Palliative Care.[2] Numerous documents from national and international organizations such as the National Quality Forum, National Consensus Project (NCP), Institute of Medicine (IOM), and the World Health Organization provide standards and guidelines for promoting excellent palliative care education.[3-7] Nursing faculty have a responsibility to teach palliative care to their students, as future employers will demand that nurses have this expertise. In addition, those who work in continuing education and professional development will need to promote competencies in palliative care, as their healthcare system moves forward in providing this care throughout the community.

One of the earliest responsibilities of the professional nurse was care of the dying. Florence Nightingale and other nurses provided care to soldiers dying on battlefields as well as to civilians dying as a result of epidemics. A major shift in patterns of disease and treatment began in the 20th century as more effective treatment modalities became available. Today, student nurses are exposed primarily to curative-oriented, sometimes futile care and are less likely to encounter comfort-oriented care. Although many healthcare providers work with people at the end of their lives, nurses spend the most time with the dying and their families. Most nurses will provide palliative care to patients and their families no matter where they practice. Therefore, education in palliative care should begin in the nursing schools and extend through clinical inservices, continuing education courses, and professional conferences.

History of palliative care nursing education

Nurses have a long history of leading the efforts of developing policies and guidelines regarding palliative care. For example, Dame Cicely Saunders, who began her career as a nurse, founded the very first freestanding hospice, St. Christopher's Hospice, in 1967 in London, England. Florence Wald, former dean at Yale School of Nursing, founded the first hospice in the United States in 1974. Jeanne Quint Benoliel looked at the role of nursing in caring for the terminally ill from a psychosocial standpoint, and her research has led to the way healthcare providers include families in decision-making and caregiving. Today, there are many other outstanding examples of nurses who continue the work that these pioneers began. For example, Betty Ferrell, PhD, RN, MA, FPCN, FAAN, chaired the NCP, which developed the *Clinical Practice Guidelines for Quality Palliative Care.*[4]

Nurses cannot practice what they do not know, and historically there has been a lack of palliative care content in nursing textbooks, as well as few faculty in schools of nursing with palliative care education. How can faculty teach this care if they have not been properly educated? Because of the many years of deficiencies in teaching end-of-life content in schools of nursing, nurses were working throughout all clinical settings with limited, if any knowledge of how to attend to the suffering of patients and their families facing end-of-life issues.[8] Several studies have analyzed end-of-life content in nursing textbooks.[9,10] Kirchhoff and colleagues[9] analyzed 14 critical care nursing textbooks using the American Association of Colleges of Nursing's (AACN) end-of-life competencies for undergraduate nursing education, *Peaceful Death: Recommended Competencies and Curricular Guidelines for End-of-Life Nursing Care*[11] as their framework (Box 66.1). None of the textbooks contained all of the content areas from the competencies. Although there was extensive information on ethical and legal issues, organ donation, and brain death in six or seven of the textbooks, the remaining textbooks contained no information on these topics. Pharmacological information was either mentioned briefly or absent. Approximately half of the textbooks had some information on patient/family communication.

Ferrell and colleagues completed an analysis of nine areas of end-of-life content in nursing textbooks in the late 1990s.[10] Their

Box 66.1 Competencies necessary for nurses to provide high-quality care to patients and families during the transition at the end of life

1. Recognize dynamic changes in population demographics, healthcare economics, and service delivery that necessitate improved professional preparation for end-of-life care.

2. Promote the provision of comfort care to the dying as an active, desirable, and important skill and an integral component of nursing care.

3. Communicate effectively and compassionately with the patient, family, and healthcare team members about end-of-life issues.

4. Recognize one's own attitudes, feelings, values, and expectations about death and the individual, cultural, and spiritual diversity existing in these beliefs and customs.

5. Demonstrate respect for the patient's views and wishes during end-of-life care.

6. Collaborate with interdisciplinary team members while implementing the nursing role in end-of-life care.

7. Use scientifically based standardized tools to assess symptoms (e.g., pain, dyspnea [breathlessness], constipation, anxiety, fatigue, nausea/vomiting, and altered cognition) experienced by patients at the end of life.

8. Use data from symptom assessment to plan and intervene in symptom management using state-of-the-art traditional and complementary approaches.

9. Evaluate the impact of traditional, complementary, and technological therapies on patient-centered outcomes.

10. Assess and treat multiple dimensions, including physical, psychological, social, and spiritual needs, to improve quality at the end of life.

11. Assist the patient, family, colleagues, and one's self to cope with suffering, grief, loss, and bereavement in end-of-life care.

12. Apply legal and ethical principles in the analysis of complex issues in end-of-life care, recognizing the influence of personal values, professional codes, and patient preferences.

13. Identify barriers and facilitators to patients' and caregivers' effective use of resources.

14. Demonstrate skill at implementing a plan for improved end-of-life care within a dynamic and complex healthcare delivery system.

15. Apply knowledge gained from palliative care research to end-of-life education and care.

Source: American Association of Colleges of Nursing. (1997), reference 11.

was little information on quality of life, which was surprising in view of the recent explosion of research in this area. Pain was often included in the textbooks, but usually in the context of acute rather than chronic pain. Pain and symptom management during the end of life were virtually absent. Information about communicating with patients and families at the end of life was also lacking. There was little information about the roles and needs of family caregivers or about issues of policy, ethics, and law. A paucity of information was found about death awareness, anxiety, imminent death, and preparing families for the death. The stages and process of grief were described, but there was little information about nursing interventions or the nurse's personal grief.

Shortly after reviewing the 50 nursing textbooks, Ferrell and colleagues began collaborating with the National Council of State Boards of Nursing (NCSBN).[12] The goal of this project was to improve end-of-life content in the national nursing licensure examination for registered nurses (NCLEX-RN). End-of-life content was increased in the NCLEX beginning with the April 2001 examination by incorporating the 15 competencies set forth by the *Peaceful Death* document.[11] This was a significant force in increasing end-of-life content in the nursing curriculum.

Curriculum developed to assist nursing faculty, continuing education providers, and staff development educators in providing palliative care education

Because of the development of the competencies prescribed in the *Peaceful Death* document by AACN and the work City of Hope nursing researchers had done in looking at lack of content in nursing textbooks, both organizations came together in 1999 to begin collaboration in developing a national education program on end-of-life care for registered nurses.[8,13] Nursing faculty, continuing education providers, and staff development educators had to be educated so they could teach the next generation and practicing nurses about this vital care. This national project, the End-of-Life Nursing Education Consortium (ELNEC) was originally funded by the Robert Wood Johnson Foundation (RWJF) in 2000.[8,14] A team of palliative care nurses assembled to develop the original curriculum, ELNEC-Core, which consists of nine modules: nursing care at the end of life, pain management, symptom management, ethical/legal issues, cultural considerations, communication, grief/loss/bereavement, achieving quality care, and care at the time of death (Table 66.1). The "train-the-trainer" model continues to be used today, as attendees learn about up-to-date palliative care, constructed on evidence-based practice. Education is provided through lectures, review of case studies, role plays, and use of videos. Individuals attending the ELNEC course are expected to gain knowledge of the content as well as skills in teaching the content. The RWJF funding provided eight initial courses targeted for 100 participants per course—five focused on faculty teaching in undergraduate nursing programs and three on continuing education (CE) providers and staff development educators (SDE). All totaled, over 1600 nurses attended one of these first eight RWJF-funded courses and reported 1 year post course that they had provided ELNEC training to over 19,000 student nurses, and 49% of the CE providers and SDE stated they were able to disseminate ELNEC-Core to nursing schools, various clinical

review of 50 nursing textbooks revealed that only 2% of overall content was related to end-of-life care, and much of the information was inaccurate. Deficiencies were found in all areas. Care at the end of life was usually discussed in terms of the hospice model of care rather than the broader concept of palliative care. There

Table 66.1 End-of-Life Nursing Education (elnec) Consortium modules

Module	Description of content
1. Nursing care at the end of life	Goals of care; cost issues in palliative care; use of aggressive interventions, personal death awareness, board review of end-of-life care, to encompass all age groups and across various disease trajectories or acute illness
2. Pain management	Assessment; pharmacological, nonpharmacological, and complementary therapies
3. Symptom management	Assessment; pharmacological, nonpharmacological, and complementary therapies
4. Cultural considerations in end-of-life care	Cultural assessment; beliefs regarding death and dying, after life, and bereavement
5. Ethical/legal issues	Assisted suicide, euthanasia, advance directives, decision-making, advance care planning
6. Communication	Breaking bad news; communicating with patients, families, and with other disciplines; interdisciplinary collaboration
7. Grief, loss, bereavement	Assessment; interventions; nurses' experiences with cumulative loss, grief, and moral distress
8. Preparation and care for the time of death	Nursing care at the time of death, including physical care, support of family members, saying good-bye
9. Achieving quality of life at the end of life	Physical, psychological, social, and spiritual well-being; needs of special populations

settings, and CE programs throughout their community.[15,16] This data was significant, given that nursing faculty find it difficult to add new content into a curriculum that is already robust and that CE providers and SDE also have tremendous responsibilities of maintaining and addressing quality improvement issues, orienting new staff, overseeing nursing internships/residency programs, providing CE and attending to annual competencies, and so forth.

The ELNEC project continues to provide annual national and international train-the-trainer courses. In the first 14 years of the project, over 20,000 nurses and other healthcare professionals, representing all 50 states, plus 79 international countries on six of the seven continents have received ELNEC training. The ELNEC curriculum is currently translated into seven languages: Russian, Spanish, Japanese, Korean, Armenian, German, and Romanian. By January, 2015, ELNEC will also be translated into Chinese. Both national and international ELNEC trainers have returned to their institutions and have educated over 480,000 nurses, and other healthcare providers, using the ELNEC curriculum.[17] Since its inception, the ELNEC Project has developed 11 various curricula to meet the needs of specialty nurses (Table 66.2). Opportunities to implement and disseminate ELNEC are numerous in schools of nursing and in clinical settings (Table 66.3).

In an effort to disseminate ELNEC online, the ELNEC project developed a relationship in 2006 with the Hospice Education Network (HEN), a comprehensive, innovative service that offers staff orientation programs, annual in-services, volunteer training, and specialized learning modules addressing the educational needs of nurses in all areas of clinical practice. The HEN and ELNEC offer the hospice industry, acute care facilities, schools of nursing, and other interested individuals or groups, online subscription access to eight ELNEC modules presented by national ELNEC faculty via ELNEC-Core, ELNEC-Pediatric Palliative Care, ELNEC-Critical Care, ELNEC-Geriatric, ELNEC-For Veterans, and ELNEC-For Public Hospitals. In 2014, Relias Learning acquired HEN, yet all ELNEC modules remain with this new endeavor. For more information on ELNEC curricula available on Relias Learning, go to http://academy.reliaslearning.com/.

A call to action to improve education for all nurses

There are over 3 million nurses in the United States, representing the largest segment of the healthcare workforce.[18] No healthcare provider spends more time with patients than the nurse, as they assess and manage care. The Centers for Disease Control (CDC) reported 2,468,435 deaths in the United States in 2010, with the majority of those deaths (67%) occurring from chronic illnesses such as heart failure, cancer, chronic respiratory disease, stroke, Alzheimer's, and diabetes.[19] The complexity of care for those with chronic illness, including palliative and end-of-life care, require nurses to acquire many key skills, including critical thinking, decision-making, leadership, team-building, and communication. Chronic illness is becoming an epidemic, as 75% ($1.5 trillion) of the $2 trillion in annual US healthcare is spent to meet the many challenges associated with these various diseases.[20] However, maintaining or enhancing quality of life for these individuals continues to have very little attention given to it.

While palliative care may be considered mainstream in some areas, there are still many challenges for nursing educators as they prepare the next generation to provide this care. For example, the federal government and private insurance companies are unwilling to pay for certain medical treatments and social services needed by many older Americans with multiple comorbidities. Because of this, in part, less than 2% of those graduating from US medical schools are choosing to practice in primary care.[21] Nursing faculty are providing advanced education to nurses who will be prepared to assess and manage patients needing primary care. Today, there are over 267,000 advanced practice registered nurses (APRNs) throughout the United States who are providing excellent and high-quality care to those with serious, life-threatening illness in a variety of clinical settings.[22]

Nurses are intricately involved in the evolving healthcare system and how it will be affected by the full implementation of the 2010 Patient Protection and Affordable Care Act. Because there will be many challenges associated with this Act, nurses need to be educated and well positioned to participate and lead in the changes and to promote policies that outline excellent palliative care. Nurses must be well educated and well mentored.

In 2010, *The Future of Nursing: Leading Change, Advancing Health* report was published by the IOM. This report resulted from a 2-year initiative by the RWJF and the IOM "to respond to the need to assess and transform the nursing profession."[18] The

Table 66.2 Various ELNEC curricula developed

ELNEC curricula/date of presentations	Overview of participants	# Trained	Funder
Current curricula			
ELNEC-Core (2001–Present)	Staff nurses, APRNs, undergraduate nursing students and faculty, staff development educators, unit-specific educators, community educators, administrators, researches who work in acute care settings (i.e., medical-surgical and oncology units, clinics, home care, hospice and palliative care settings	12,000	RWJF, 2000–2004
ELNEC-Pediatric Palliative Care (2003–Present)	Nurses described in ELNEC-Core are also targeted for this course. Those working in pediatric units, pediatric (PICU) and neonatal intensive care units (NICU), hospice, home care, clinics, and schools	1950	Aetna Foundation, 2005–2006
ELNEC-Critical Care (2006–Present)	Those working in intensive care (ICU), coronary care (CCU), burn, dialysis, transplant units, emergency departments and other clinical areas encompassing critical care	1110	Archstone Foundation, 2007–2010
ELNEC-Geriatric (2006–Present)	Geriatric nurses working in long-term care and skilled nursing facilities, nursing homes, undergraduate and graduate nursing faculty, hospice, community, and acute care nurses	850	California HealthCare Foundation, 2008–2010
ELNEC-APRN (2013–Present)	APRN nurses, which includes certified nurse anesthetists, certified nurse midwives, clinical nurse specialists, and nurse practitioners. There are two tracks to this course: adult and pediatric tracks	250	Cambia Health Foundation (2012—Present)
ELNEC-International (2006–Present)	Presented in 79 countries worldwide not only to nurses but also to other interdisciplinary team members. Opportunities to meet with ministers of health, nursing faculty, and other leaders generally exist, as well as to speak at international meetings.	2300	Open Society, Oncology Nursing Foundation
Integrating Palliative Oncology Care into Doctor of Nursing Practice (DNP) Education and Clinical Practice (2014–Present)	Provides DNP nursing faculty and DNP clinical practitioners with the tools and resources to prepare the next generation of DNP graduates to provide excellent, compassionate, and evidence-based palliative care to those with cancer	95	National Cancer Institute (NCI) (2013–2017)
Past curricula			
ELNEC-for Veterans (2009–2012)	Nurses who work in inpatient and outpatient veteran-specific facilities, representing over 200 institutions	745	The US Department of Veterans Affairs (2009–2012)
ELNEC-for Veterans/Critical Care (2012)	Presented to undergraduate and graduate nursing faculty	60	
ELNEC-for Veterans (2012)			Milbank Foundation for Rehabilitation (2012)
ELNEC-for Public Hospitals (2011–2013)	This 2-day course was presented to nurses in 16 public hospitals throughout California in November, 2008. Two additional face-to-face meetings took place with these trainers, as well as monthly mentoring phone calls.	58	The California HealthCare Foundation (2011–2013)
ELNEC-Oncology (2003–2007)	Nurses belonging to an Oncology Nursing Society (ONS) chapter, working in inpatient, outpatient, bone marrow transplant settings	264	National Cancer Institute (NCI) (2003–2007)
ELNEC-Graduate	Graduate nursing faculty, teaching in 285/438 (65%) schools of nursing throughout the United States	400	National Cancer Institute (NCI) (2003–2007)
TOTALS = 11 curricula		20,000+ participants	10 various funding sources

report outlined four key messages that significantly affect the future of nursing:

- Nurses should practice to the full extent of their education and training.

- Nurses should achieve higher levels of education and training through an improved education system that promotes seamless academic progression.

- Nurses should be full partners, with physicians and other healthcare professionals, in redesigning healthcare in the United States.

- Effective workforce planning and policymaking require better data collection and information infrastructure.

Two of these four key messages specifically address education. Nursing education is vital in meeting the complex needs of

Table 66.3 Examples of implementing/disseminating ELNEC in schools of nursing and clinical settings

Schools of nursing	Clinical settings
◆ Use ELNEC to develop scenarios in the simulation lab. ◆ Review details of the Terri Schiavo case and have students write a 350–500 word editorial that could be printed in a local newspaper regarding a specific component of that case. ◆ Students interview a person who has a cultural or religious background different from their own and on those rituals that provide comfort and healing and reflect his/her heritage and values. ◆ Develop an interdisciplinary oncology palliative care curriculum for nursing, medical, social work, and chaplaincy students, supported by an R-25 grant from NCI. ◆ Spearhead the collaborative development of an online interdisciplinary palliative care course at an academic medical center. ◆ Provide case studies for pharmacology class to practice using equianalgesic charts. ◆ Include ELNEC information in nursing skills lab, including signs and symptoms of impending death, preparing for autopsy and organ donation, administering culturally sensitive postmortem care, preparing the body for cremation and funeral ceremonies. ◆ Provide role-plays to practice "breaking bad news" or "picking-up the pieces after being told bad news." ◆ Chair doctoral dissertation committees with students interested in palliative care. ◆ Collaborate with other disciplines in various professional schools within the university (i.e., medicine, dentistry, pharmacy, religious studies, social work, psychology, etc.) to develop an interdisciplinary graduate course. ◆ Receive government and private grants to develop a palliative care track in a graduate nursing education. ◆ Provide content mapping of palliative care in current nursing curriculum. ◆ Forge clinical contracts with local hospices (both inpatient and homecare).	◆ Use Introduction to Palliative Nursing (ELNEC module #1) in new employee orientation. ◆ Use pain and symptom management ELNEC modules to frame annual competencies for nursing staff. ◆ When a patient is actively dying, a white wreath is placed on the outside of their door, so all staff are aware of the sacred work occurring in that room. When the patient dies, the nurse who cared for that patient at the time of death is given 1 hour of time away from the unit to eat, reminisce, and contemplate on the patient, their family, and his/her opportunity to do this work. ◆ Use the pain and symptom management, culture, and loss/grief/bereavement ELNEC modules to develop and to update a palliative care protocol for patients with heart failure. ◆ Use a brochure to introduce palliative care for all patients admitted to the nursing home, long-term care/skilled nursing facility. ◆ Provide a memorial service for family who have lost loved ones in the past 6 months and for staff. Names of those who died in the facility over the past 6 months are read, and family and staff are given opportunities to speak. ◆ Palliative care consult team makes rounds in the ICU on a daily basis. ◆ The mission of the hospital clearly states their commitment to provide excellent care at the end of life. ◆ At the time of a death in the facility, "TAPs" is played over the public address system. ◆ Families are provided an opportunity to ceremoniously bathe the body of their loved one after he or she has died, along with the nurse who cared for them.

patients and transforming healthcare systems. In order to provide safe, "seamless, affordable, and quality care," nurses must obtain higher levels of education.[18] Additional resources will be needed in planning and orchestrating care for older Americans, 65 years and older, as they will make up almost 20% (72 million) of the US population by 2030.[23] The current US healthcare system and nursing curricula focus on assessing/managing acute illnesses. However, a drastic change in curricula must take place in order to meet the needs of older adults, many who have complex, chronic comorbidities, including obesity, heart disease, hypertension, and mental illness. Schools of nursing must develop and promote "leadership, health policy, system improvement, research and evidence-based practice, and teamwork and collaboration" competencies in order to provide quality care in not only acute care settings, but also in the community, public health, and geriatric settings.[18]

According to this IOM report, schools of nursing must provide more opportunities for students to expand their clinical experiences in primary care, long-term care, and public health. Additional courses in informatics should be expanded so future nurses can improve collaboration and coordination of care with the entire healthcare team and system. An emphasis on coordination and transition of care, regulation on access, as well as negotiation with other healthcare providers in determining patients' eligibility for various health and social service programs must be included in nursing education. Instead of having students memorize various tasks, fundamental concepts need to be taught and

higher-level competencies introduced, which revolve around knowledge and decision-making that can be applied across all clinical settings and various diseases.[18]

A call for higher education

Nurses who work in palliative care must be well educated in order to orchestrate and coordinate the care of complex, seriously ill patients, to critically think, and to oversee patients as they transfer to various clinical settings. Their critical thinking skills must be astute as they assess and manage care. Their interactions with family members and other healthcare providers are critical. Educating the patient and family on the disease progression, options, and benefits and burdens of treatments is essential, so their goals of care can be articulated and understood. Managing pain, dyspnea, nausea/vomiting, constipation, anxiety, fatigue, anorexia, and caregiver needs demands the highest level of education possible for the nurse. Listening and being present are important skills to maintain. Collaborating with and referring to other interdisciplinary team members are vital in managing physical, psychological, social, and spiritual needs of the patient and family. Nurses must be encouraged to continue their education so they can meet specific needs in primary care, research, policymaking, and education related to palliative care. With all the changes that the *2010 Affordable Care Act* will bring, nurses will be called on, as never before, to practice in new and unique ways. While nurses may take advantage of advancing their education in order to respond to the transformation of care that is taking place, there are numerous cultural, regulatory, and policy barriers that prevent them from contributing to the improvement of healthcare in the United States.

Perhaps one of the leading barriers that nurses face today is legal obstacles that prohibit and prevent APRNs from practicing to the full extent of their education (i.e., Certified registered nurse anesthetist [CRNA], certified nurse-midwife [CNM], clinical nurse specialist [CNS], and certified nurse practitioner [CNP]). The *Consensus Model for APRN Regulation: Licensure, Accreditation, Certification and Education* (LACE), developed collaboratively by the Advanced Practice Nursing Consensus Work Group and the NCSBN APRN Committee, defines APRN practice, describes the APRN regulatory model, notes titles to be used, defines the specific specialty, outlines new roles and population foci, and provides strategies regarding implementation.[24] In short, an APRN is a nurse

* Who has completed graduate-level education from an accredited program, with an emphasis on preparation for one of the four APRN roles.

* Who passed a national certification examination.

* Who has advanced clinical knowledge and skills so they can provide direct and indirect care to patients. All APRNs must have a significant component of their education and practice focused on direct patient care.

* Whose practice is built on the competencies of registered nurses (RNs). They must demonstrate greater depth and breadth of knowledge and synthesis, increased complexity of skills/interventions, and greater role autonomy.

* Who has prepared themselves educationally to assume both responsibility and accountability for assessment, diagnosis, and management of patients, including the use and prescription of pharmacologic and nonpharmacologic interventions.

* Who has in-depth clinical experience

* Who has obtained the appropriate license to practice as an APRN (i.e., CRNA, CNM, CNS, CNP).[24]

Nursing educators must be on the forefront of working to lift these barriers so that these well-educated APRNs can contribute their talents to meeting the healthcare needs of the nation. Nursing faculty, CE providers, and SDE should take opportunities to speak to their interprofessional colleagues, regulatory and government agencies, and community brokers to outline the definition of the APRN, as well as the unique contributions they can make in this role. In addition, schools of nursing must be committed to provide more education regarding primary care, versus specialty care, and a greater emphasis must be made on delivering care in the community rather than in acute care settings.[18] Several schools of nursing across the United States are currently providing palliative care education tracks in their master's programs (Table 66.4).

The demand for doctoral nursing education is growing rapidly in the United States. Much of this is due to the increase of evidence-based practice; complexity of patient care due to technology and multiple comorbidities; concerns about quality of care and safety issues; shortage of nursing faculty with a doctoral degree; and an increase in the educational expectations of other

healthcare team members. Nurses have many options for increasing their education on the graduate level (i.e., clinical nurse leader [CNL], master's of science in nursing [MSN], doctor of nursing practice [DNP], doctor of philosophy [PhD]). According to the AACN's latest statistics, which reflect 754/842 (87%) nursing programs in the United States and its territories, enrollment at the master's, research doctorate (PhD, DNSc, DNS), and doctor of nursing practice (DNP) levels were 101,616; 5,110; and 11,575, respectively.[25] Growth in baccalaureate, master's, and doctoral enrollments and graduations continues (Figures 66.1 and 66.2).

In 2005, the National Academy of Sciences (NAS) developed a report, *Advancing the Nation's Health Needs: NIH Research Training Programs*, recommending that nursing develop a non-research clinical doctorate—the DNP.[26] This practice doctorate would coincide with other healthcare disciplines that have similar doctorates: medicine (MD), pharmacy (PharmD), physical therapy (PTD), and occupational therapy (OTD). The DNP degree prepares nurses not only to increase their expertise in practice but also to serve as clinical faculty in schools of nursing. In 2013, the AACN reported that there were 217 DNP programs with an additional 97 programs in the planning stages, available in 40 states, plus the District of Columbia, with the number of students enrolled in a DNP program increasing every year.[27] There are currently 131 schools of nursing with PhD programs, which stress the importance of research in practice and education with 620 graduations between August 1, 2011 and July 31, 2012.[25] Whether nurses are working as APRNs, educators, researchers, administrators, or informatics specialists, the need to remain updated on the constant changes of healthcare will be critical. This is a responsibility of all nurses, so they can provide and promote the seamless and compassionate care to the sickest-of-the-sick in our society, as well as to their families.

While the United States is in the process of transforming its healthcare system, nurses must be well educated to play a distinct role in the years ahead, as many changes will affect the way patients and their families are cared for. Nurses currently play major roles in regulatory, business, and organizational operations. Those in government, healthcare organizations, professional associations, and insurance agencies must work together to promote better care for all Americans. Nursing leaders are encouraged to continue to work with each of these organizations "to ensure that the health care system provides seamless, affordable, quality care that is accessible to all and leads to improved health outcomes."[18]

National Consensus Project's *Clinical Practice Guidelines for Quality Palliative Care*: providing a template for nursing education, practice, and research

In 2004, the NCP for Quality Palliative Care created clinical practice guidelines that have been used by numerous nursing educators, clinicians, and researchers to develop palliative care curricula, research studies, protocols, and annual competencies. Graduate nursing students have written theses, defended dissertations, and developed capstone projects using these guidelines. Administrators have accessed them to develop budgets and to plan palliative care programs or enhance present ones. Now, in its third edition, the guidelines continue to "promote quality

Table 66.4 Hospice and palliative master's educational programs in the United States

School of nursing	Comments
Boston College, Boston, MA	Goals of program to educate APN students (Peds, Adult and Family, NP, and CNS) in palliative care
Case Western Reserve University Cleveland, OH	Post-master's certificate available Symptom management classes taught in interdisciplinary format
Daemen Amherst, NY	Educates CNSs in palliative care
George Washington University, Washington, DC	An online program designed to be completed in three semesters
Loyola University, Chicago, IL	One online palliative care course, available each spring semester to all MSN students but required of Loyola Oncology CNS students
Madonna University, Livonia, MI	
Marquette University, Milwaukee, WI	
New York University, New York City, NY	500 clinical hours in diverse palliative care settings; graduates immediately eligible for palliative care certification exam
University of Alabama, Birmingham, AL	HPNA APN and NONPF competencies provide framework
University of California, San Francisco, CA	Pediatric only
University of Illinois, Chicago, IL	
University of Maryland, College Park, MD	
University of Massachusetts, Lowell, MA	Students who complete this certificate are encouraged to apply for advanced practice role preparation as an adult psychiatric mental health nurse practitioner/clinical nurse specialist, family nurse practitioner, or adult-gerontological nurse practitioner through the University of Massachusetts Lowell. Courses with grade of B or higher may be transferable to the Master's Degree in Nursing Program.
University of Pennsylvania, Philadelphia, PA	Although the minor is housed in the School of Nursing, learning experiences incorporate perspective of interdisciplinary faculty from various clinical settings.
Ursuline Pepper Pike, OH	NONPF competencies provide framework
Vanderbilt University, Nashville, TN	
Walden University, Baltimore, MD	

Source: Hospice and Palliative Nurses Association (HPNA). Graduate Program Listing. Downloaded at http://www.hpna.org/DisplayPage.aspx?Title=Graduate Program Listing.

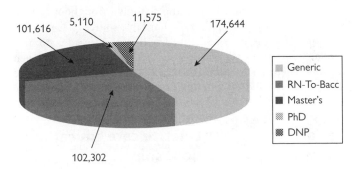

Figure 66.1 Enrollment by type of degree and student status (*N* = 742 respondent schools).

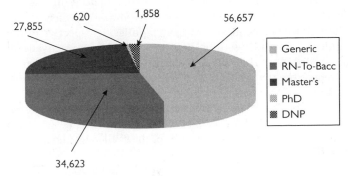

Figure 66.2 Graduations by type of degree and student status (*N* = 742 respondent schools).

palliative care, foster consistent and high standards in palliative care, and encourage continuity of care across settings."[4] These guidelines are reviewed in detail in chapter 2.

An outline and overview of how to use these guidelines has been developed (Table 66.5). This table gives specific examples regarding recommendations for implementation and dissemination, which baccalaureate/graduate nursing faculty, CE providers, and SDEs can use to strengthen palliative care content in the classroom and clinical settings and in building/maintaining palliative care teams. There is also a section dedicated to suggested content for APRN education.[28]

A call to promote oncology nursing education: tremendous needs lie ahead, cancer rates rise, and the number of oncologists decreases

While heart disease is still the number one cause of death in the United States, cancer remains the second leading cause of death, with over 597,680/574,740 deaths reported in 2011, respectively.[19] A 2009 report by the IOM/National Cancer Policy Forum outlined the future needs of the oncology workforce.[29,30] Embedded in that report were predictions from the American Society of Clinical Oncology (ASCO) that by 2020, a 48% increase in cancer incidence will occur and there will be an 81% increase of people living with/surviving cancer.[31,32] Yet, by 2020, there will only be a 14% increase in the number of practicing oncologists.[30–32] How will the tremendous needs of these oncology patients be met with not only the decline of oncologists, but also the shortage of primary care physicians and nurses entering the workforce? By instituting palliative care services, at the time of diagnosis, many cancer patients can receive better management of symptoms, and in turn this could reduce demands on the oncology workforce.[32] The American Colleges of Physicians (ACP) released an article that stated "doctors and nurse practitioners must collaborate to improve primary care."[33] The unique needs of the cancer patient and his/her family must be fundamentally in the forefront of any healthcare reform and/or redesign. Nurses, who spend more time at the bedside assessing and managing cancer patients, must continue their commitment to improve care for all Americans with cancer. By providing a highly educated nursing workforce, nurses will have opportunities to lead, to participate in decision-making, and to promote a proactive response to healthcare challenges that affect those with cancer and their families, irrespective of the clinical/community setting they may be in. Many creative ways of meeting these challenges have begun. For example, in an effort to reduce the time with the oncologist, there are academic cancer centers that provide survivorship clinics, staffed by nurse practitioners, specially trained to support the complex needs of these patients.[32] It is vital that faculty teaching in nursing programs be educated to prepare these students for the challenges and increase in responsibility that will lie ahead.

In an effort to assist nursing faculty and practicing APRNs to receive further oncology nursing education, the National Cancer Institute (NCI) provided a grant to the City of Hope Medical Center in 2013 to prepare DNP faculty to integrate palliative care content into current DNP curricula.[34] This new project, titled Integrating Palliative Oncology Care into Doctor of Nursing Practice (DNP) Education and Clinical Practice, was designed to give nursing faculty the tools and resources needed to educate DNP graduates on how to provide compassionate and evidence-based palliative care to those with cancer. Palliative care is assuming an increasing role in oncology, and DNPs will play a significant role in educating staff and planning for integration/sustainability of palliative care programs throughout the healthcare system. By preparing DNP graduates to provide evidence-based palliative care in oncology, this initiative was designed to support the commitment of nursing schools nationwide in preparing clinical experts with the skills needed to orchestrate and deliver optimal patient care to those with serious, life-threatening illnesses. These DNP graduates will play a pivotal role in leading change and transforming care for the 1.6 million Americans who will be diagnosed with cancer this year, plus the 13.7 million Americans who are living with a history of cancer.[35] As the Affordable Care Act nears full implementation, DNPs will have unprecedented opportunities to promote excellent palliative care to those with cancer. For further information on this project, which was scheduled to run from 2013 to 2017, go to www.aacn.nche.edu/ELNEC.

International efforts to educate nurses in palliative care

Educational programs for nurses in palliative care vary widely throughout the world, as the prevalence and specialty of this care are promoted differently in every country. In 2011, 58% (136/234) of the world's countries had at least one palliative care service, which is an increase of 9% (21 countries) from 2006, with the largest gain being seen in the continent of Africa.[36] The ratio of palliative care services to population ranges significantly from country to country. For example, in Austria, the ratios are 1:34,000, compared with China's 1:8.5 million.[36]

While there are tremendous variations in the establishment of palliative care services around the world, there are established courses and programs in this care at universities as well as seminars, workshops, and conferences in the Americas, Africa, Asia, Australia, the United Kingdom, northern/eastern Europe, as well as the Middle East. In other parts of the world, education in palliative care is woven into other established courses. Palliative care concepts are taught within oncology courses in Japan, South Korea, and Thailand. Since 1990, the Nairobi Hospice has provided palliative care courses for healthcare professionals and has extended this program to nursing schools throughout Kenya. An increase in the availability of charitable sources has resulted in support for the development of palliative care education in Russia, Romania, Poland, Armenia, Albania, and the Czech Republic.[37] For more information about international palliative care, see chapter 70 in this textbook, "International Palliative Care Initiatives."

Opportunities for palliative care education, certification, and scholarships

The Hospice and Palliative Nurses Association (HPNA) provides resources, educational opportunities, conferences, and support to APRNs, RNs, licensed practical/vocational nurses, nursing assistants, and administrators. There are approximately 11,000 members in the United States and in several

Table 66.5 Examples of including the 2013 National Consensus Project's *Clinical Practice Guidelines for Quality Palliative Care* in baccalaureate/graduate, advanced practice registered nurses (aprn) education, continuing education, and professional development

NCP guideline domain	Recommendations for implementation and dissemination to baccalaureate/graduate nursing education	Recommended content to be included in APRN education via didactic and clinical experiences[28]	Recommendations for implementation and dissemination to continuing education and professional development for nurses
#1: Structure and processes of care includes: ◆ Interdisciplinary team (IDT) assessment ◆ Plan of care is based on patient and family goals and values ◆ Interdisciplinary plan is orchestrated and services provided across the life span ◆ Use trained/supervised volunteers ◆ Provide and support education, training, and professional development to the team ◆ Develop, implement, and maintain data with a focus on palliative care outcomes ◆ Recognition of emotional impact of providing palliative care for the team ◆ Use of community resources for continuity of care ◆ Honoring the preference of the patient and family in regard to the physical environment **Clinical implications:** *"Palliative care occurs across the health spectrum. It necessitates the involvement of an interdisciplinary team that is trained and supported to do the work. Care focuses on promoting the physical, psychological, social and spiritual domains of quality of life. It is delivered in a safe environment with respect for the patient's and family's values, preferences, and wishes. The palliative care program strives for best practices of quality assessment and performance improvement."* (NCP, 2013)	Emphasize interprofessional education, including schools of medicine, social work, pharmacy, theology, physical and occupational therapy, etc through "ace-to-face, online, or simulation labs. Role-play scenarios that emphasize the importance of communication. Examples may include: ◆ Breaking "bad news" and/or being with patients after receiving this news ◆ Eliciting a patient's goals of care ◆ Speaking with a physician who does not believe the patient needs palliative care at this time ◆ Participating in a family meeting ◆ Answering such questions as "Am I going to die?" "Do we have to tell my wife that I am dying?" Provide education for excellent assessment and management of diseases from neonates to older adults, with an emphasis on quality of life and a review of benefits vs. burdens. This addresses not only physical needs but also psychological, social, and spiritual aspects of care. Other areas to cover include: ◆ Cultural aspects of care ◆ Compassionate and respectful care of the patient in his/her final hours and at the time of death ◆ Care of the family ◆ Ethical and legal aspects of care, with emphasis on advance care planning Recognize that neonates, children, and adolescents have unique needs, whether they are a patient, family member, or friend. Promote self-care for all students and faculty. Recognize the role of complementary and alternative therapies.	Include advanced assessment skills: ◆ Review of disease—prognosis, comorbidities ◆ Symptoms ◆ Functional status ◆ Social, cultural, and spiritual assessment ◆ Advance care planning ◆ Goals of care ◆ Collaboration with the IDT regarding assessment findings Further advanced palliative care education in the following: ◆ Communication skills ◆ Legal and ethical issues ◆ Loss, grief, and bereavement assessment and management ◆ Budgets and financial implications of end-of-life care (i.e., billing for hospice via the Medicare Hospice Benefit, billing for palliative care consult services, etc.) ◆ Development of quality improvement policies and procedures and evaluation of outcomes as it relates to palliative care	Include role of palliative care in new employee orientation for all professional staff and volunteers. Provide inservices on new policies regarding prioritizing and responding to palliative care referrals. Adapt research data in clinical practice. Include concepts of palliative care in annual competency reviews. For example: ◆ Pain and symptom assessment/management ◆ Equianalgesia ◆ Communication ◆ Ethical issues and how to respond ◆ Loss/grief/bereavement Support healthcare students in internships or fellowships as they learn concepts of palliative care and provide them with mentors to promote and sustain this care. Encourage nurses to obtain certification in hospice/palliative nursing. Review quality assessment and performance improvement (QAPI) data with staff and develop appropriate policies and procedures. Use these data to determine where further education is needed. Recognize and support the importance of self-care for the IDT.

(continued)

Table 66.5 Continued

NCP guideline domain	Recommendations for implementation and dissemination to baccalaureate/graduate nursing education	Recommended content to be included in APRN education via didactic and clinical experiences[28]	Recommendations for implementation and dissemination to continuing education and professional development for nurses
#2: Physical aspects of care Include: ◆ Use of data to assess and manage pain and other physical symptoms and their effects on quality of life for both the patient and family ◆ Assessment and management of symptoms and their side effects are circumstantial to the illness **Clinical implications:** *"Physical comfort represents a core feature of compassionate care. Expert pain and symptom management sets the foundation of palliative care and promotes psychological, social, and spiritual quality of life."* (NCP, 2013)	Provide training in pain and symptom assessment and management, using reliable and validated tools. Review documentation of pain and symptoms, recognizing that this is a vital communication tool between professions and shifts, as well as a legal document. Care of the patient who is unable to report pain and/or symptoms (e.g., unconscious, on a ventilator, confused, neonate, infant, small child). Discuss the most common symptoms seen in palliative care: ◆ Pain ◆ Dyspnea ◆ Nausea/vomiting ◆ Fatigue ◆ Anorexia ◆ Insomnia ◆ Restlessness ◆ Confusion Review treatment plan, including use of pharmacological agents, behavior and complementary therapies. Give attention to educating families in safe and appropriate care of their loved one and providing them with the necessary resources and support.	Assessment of common symptoms in palliative care: ◆ Pain ◆ Dyspnea ◆ Nausea/vomiting ◆ Fatigue ◆ Anxiety ◆ Anorexia/Cachexia ◆ Others Review of common treatments used in palliative care: ◆ Pharmacology ◆ Interventional treatments ◆ Behavioral interventions ◆ Complementary therapies Support practice with current research and encourage APRN students to contribute to ongoing palliative care research. Documentation so interdisciplinary care can be communicated across various healthcare settings In accordance with state and federal regulations and policies, develop opioid risk assessment and management for APRNs who prescribe opioids. Use assessment tools to measure and document symptoms and management in a safe and timely fashion. Research ways to provide treatments more efficaciously.	Annual competencies should include a review of pain assessment and the tools used to measure and manage it. In addition, use case studies and/or simulation to promote excellent pain and symptom assessment and management. Review and update current policies and procedures, as needed, regarding caring for patients with serious, life-threatening illness (i.e., protocols related to pain and symptom management, visitation hours, etc.).

#3: Psychological and psychiatric aspects of care include:

◆ IDT assesses and manages psychological and psychiatric issues, using evidence to provide attention to the patient and family.

◆ A grief and bereavement program must be available to patients and families receiving palliative care, based on their unique needs.

Clinical implications:

"Psychological and psychiatric assessment and services occur systematically using evidence-informed screening, assessment tools, and interventions. Education for the patient, family, and staff is an essential element of management. Grief and bereavement services are fundamental aspects of palliative care for support staff, patients, and family. Services are appropriate to patients' and families' needs, goals, ages, culture, and level of development to reflect a multidimensional intervention strategy."
(NCP, 2013)

Provide both didactic and clinical experiences, addressing depression, anxiety, delirium, and cognitive impairments that may be assessed in patients with serious/life-threatening illness and their families. When possible, provide these opportunities and experiences with other health-care professional students.

Review psychological assessment tools for patients and families. Assess for stress, anticipatory grieving, suicidal ideation, and coping mechanisms. Are there psychiatric comorbidities?

Review treatment options for psychiatric diagnoses and the role nurses play in patient and family education, promotion of informed consent, and decision-making.

Treatments may include pharmacological, nonpharmacological, and complementary therapies.

Promote interdisciplinary care in response to the developmental age of the patient—use of social workers, psychiatrists, psychologists, child life specialists.

Describe the importance of a grief and bereavement programs for both patients and families, based on their need.

Role-play scenarios that emphasize the importance of assessing/managing psychological needs and adjusting to the illness. These would be ideal in simulation. Examples may include:

◆ Explaining to a patient that throughout the illness, there will be opportunities for growth, psychological healing, and cognitive reframing

◆ Reflecting with patient and family about any unfinished business

◆ Assessing a caregiver's needs and their coping strategies

◆ Reassessing treatment efficacy

◆ Listening to a 5-year-old child who is afraid his mother is going to die and leave him alone

◆ Using verbal, nonverbal, and/or symbolic means of communicating with cognitively impaired patients (i.e., neonates, children, adolescents, older adults with dementia, etc.)

◆ Providing a family meeting where a 45-year-old wife whose husband is critically ill needs assistance with anticipatory grief

Promote the importance of self-care for all nursing students, so they can thrive amid witnessing death and dying.

Use standardized scales to assess and manage symptoms, when available:

◆ Depression

◆ Anxiety

◆ Delirium

◆ Cognitive impairments

Treatment of these symptoms should be in a timely and safe manner in collaboration with the IDT.

Development of a grief/bereavement care plan. The plan should begin prior to the patient's death and continue at least 13 months post death.

APRNs must mentor staff and lead by example in promoting self-care.

Provide interdisciplinary annual competencies related to psychological and psychiatric care at the end of life. Review various treatments, including pharmacological, nonpharmacological, and complementary therapies.

Review a recent death on a unit. What parts of the psychological domain were addressed well for the patient and family? What areas could have been addressed better? What are ways to improve this care?

Follow-up on bereavement care for family at least 12 months post death of loved one. This can be coordinated with social work and/or chaplaincy service.

Be aware of the importance and promote self-care for nurses and other interdisciplinary team members.

(continued)

Table 66.5 Continued

NCP guideline domain	Recommendations for implementation and dissemination to baccalaureate/graduate nursing education	Recommended content to be included in APRN education via didactic and clinical experiences[28]	Recommendations for implementation and dissemination to continuing education and professional development for nurses
#4: Social aspects of care includes: ◆ The IDT assessing and addressing the social aspects of care to meet patient-family needs, promoting patient-family goals, and maximizing patient-family strengths and well-being ◆ A comprehensive, person-centered interdisciplinary assessment that identifies the social strengths, needs, and goals of each patient and family **Clinical implications:** *"Each patient and family has a unique social structure. Understanding the social fabric of the patient and family promotes coping. Interventions support the social structure including culture, values, strengths, goals, and preferences. The assessment of social aspects of care is the responsibility of the IDT, which includes specialists in social aspects of care and pediatric populations."*	Collaborate with faculty from other healthcare professional schools to provide didactic instruction, skills, and/or simulation lab, stressing the importance of interdisciplinary care when assessing and managing social aspects of care for patients with serious, life-threatening illness and their families (i.e., social work, chaplaincy, child life specialists, nutrition/dietary, etc.). Arrange for students to participate in interdisciplinary rounds in clinical settings to identify social aspects of care. Emphasize special developmental needs of children—whether they are the patient or a child, sibling, or grandchild of a seriously ill loved one. Role-play scenarios that emphasize the importance of: ◆ Developing a comprehensive and interdisciplinary social assessment that includes: · family structure/function · strengths/vulnerabilities · schooling, job, financial resources · geography/location · patient and family perceptions of care · availability and opportunities/capacity to provide care · need for additional resources, financial support, and respite care ◆ Addressing unique needs of children who are facing a serious illness ◆ Communicating with children about anticipatory grief regarding potential loss of a loved one ◆ Assessing a patient/family member's financial needs due to illness ◆ Collaborating with a social worker about providing resources to assist with financial needs of the patient/family	Conduct patient/family conferences, keeping the IDT updated on goals of care and disease progression. Develop a comprehensive social care plan, including needs of the patient and the family/caregiver. Communication between family members, decision-making capabilities, financial needs, caregiver burdens, status of work. Description of community resources that can support families and patients.	Promote interdisciplinary rounds on all units, during each case review, discussing social needs of patients and families. The discussions should include: ◆ Assessing coping strategies related to grief and the impact of illness on patient and family ◆ Supporting the patient and family for decisions they have made regarding goals of care ◆ Providing emotional and social support Include in new employee orientation and annual competency reviews the importance of assessing and documenting ◆ Family structure/function ◆ Strengths/vulnerabilities of patient and family ◆ Schooling, job, financial resources and concerns ◆ Patient and family perceptions of care ◆ What is their availability and ability to provide care once the patient goes home? ◆ What are the children's needs? Who is communicating with them? ◆ How to refer the patient and family to other resources/facilities, as needed

#5: Spiritual, religious, and existential aspects of care

- The IDT assesses and addresses spiritual, religious, and existential dimensions of care.
- A spiritual assessment process, including a spiritual screening, history questions, and a full spiritual assessment as indicated, is performed. This assessment identifies religious or spiritual/existential background, preferences, and related beliefs, rituals and practices of the patient and family; as well as symptoms, such as spiritual distress and/or pain, guilt, resentment, despair, and hopelessness.
- The palliative care service facilitates religious, spiritual, and cultural rituals or practices as desired by patient and family, especially at and after the time of death.

Clinical implications:

"Spiritual, religious, and existential issues are a fundamental aspect of quality of life for patients with serious or life-threatening illness and their families. All team members are accountable for attending to spiritual care in a respectful fashion. In order to provide an optimal and inclusive healing environment, each palliative care team member needs to be aware of his or her own spirituality and how it may differ from fellow team members and those of the patients and families they serve."

- Identify and describe the difference between "spirituality" and "religion."
- Provide education to nursing students about the importance of spiritual, religious, and existential care and how it is vital they use the IDT to promote this care.
- Collaborate with other healthcare professional schools in your college/university to provide interdisciplinary education to students about honoring and respecting patient/family spiritual, religious, and existential needs and concerns. When possible, include someone from the school of religious studies.
- Demonstrate respectful and sensitive communication via role-play, case studies, simulation lab.
- Invite a chaplain/spiritual care professional to present his/her work to your students.
- Review various spiritual assessment tools. Examples include:
  - **F**aith, **I**mportance, **C**ommunity, **A**ddress **(FICA)**: www.gwish.org
  - **H**ope, **O**rganized religion, **P**ersonal spirituality and practices, **E**ffects on medical care and end of life issues **(HOPE)**: http://www.patient-centeredcare.org/chapters/chapter7g_Tool_A.pdf
  - For a listing of other resources, go to http://www.gwumc.edu/gwish/resources/spirituality-and-health-websites/index.cfm
- Demonstrate documentation of religious/spiritual/existential information, preferences, beliefs, rituals, and practices.
- Encourage students to acknowledge their own spirituality as it relates to their role as a nurse.
- Promote self-care and self-reflection to maintain and sustain their religious/spiritual/existential growth.

- Assessment of religious, spiritual, and existential concerns regarding illness.
- Document in care plan.
- Collaboration with chaplains and other spiritual advisors, respecting the wishes of patients and their families.
- Collaboration and coordination with community spiritual care professionals in providing end-of-life education and counseling, as needed.

- Promote IDT assessment of spiritual, religious, and existential care for all patients.
- Provide easily accessible list of chaplains, clergy from faith-based organizations, so nurses know how to access this information when needed.
- Encourage patient and family to display their own spiritual/religious symbols.
- In orientation and/or in annual competencies, nurses should practice:
  - Obtaining a spiritual assessment via role play, case study, simulation lab
  - Reviewing how to document a spiritual assessment
- Develop protocols for postdeath follow-up
  - Calling family to offer condolences on behalf of the staff
  - Attending funeral/wake/memorial service
  - Sending a card to the family from the staff at 1-month and at least through 12-month post death of loved one
- Encourage nurses to acknowledge their own spirituality as it relates to their role.
- Promote self-care and self-reflection to maintain and sustain their religious/spiritual/existential growth.

(continued)

Table 66.5 Continued

NCP guideline domain	Recommendations for implementation and dissemination to baccalaureate/graduate nursing education	Recommended content to be included in APRN education via didactic and clinical experiences[28]	Recommendations for implementation and dissemination to continuing education and professional development for nurses
#6: Cultural aspects of care ♦ The palliative care program serves each patient, family, and community in a culturally and linguistically appropriate manner. ♦ The palliative care program strives to enhance its cultural and linguistic competence. **Clinical implications:** "Culture is a source of resilience for patients and families and plays an important role in the provision of palliative care. It is the responsibility of all members of the palliative care program to strive for cultural and linguistic competence to ensure that appropriate and relevant services are provided to patients and families."	Define the multidimensional aspects of culture including customs, beliefs, values, race, ethnicity, age, religious/spiritual/political beliefs, sexual orientation, gender identity/expression, family status, social group, etc., and how all of these relate to palliative care. Review cultural assessment tools: ♦ American Association of Colleges of Nursing (AACN): Competencies and toolkit for undergraduate and graduate nursing students: http://www.aacn.nche.edu/education-resources/cultural-competency. ♦ Cross Cultural Health Program (CCHCP): Broad cultural issues that impact the health of individuals and families in ethnic minority communities: http://xculture.org/ ♦ Diversity Rx: Models and practices, policy, legal issues, networking and links to other resources: http://diversityrx.org ♦ Ethnomed: Information about cultural beliefs, medical issues, and other related issues pertinent to the healthcare field. Patient education materials have been translated into several languages. http://ethnomed.org/ ♦ Transcultural Nursing Society: The society serves as a forum to promote, advance, and disseminate transcultural nursing knowledge worldwide: http://tcns.org	Incorporate cultural assessment in hospice and palliative care. Examples of areas to be assessed include: ♦ Whom should information be disclosed to? ♦ Who is the decision-maker? ♦ Dietary preferences? ♦ Language? Prefer information in writing or verbally? ♦ Preference for alternative and/or complementary therapies? ♦ Role of religion and/or spirituality? ♦ Perspectives about death? ♦ What meaning does suffering have? ♦ Are there funeral and burial specifications to honor culture? Use of professional medical interpreter services as needed Develop/access education materials that are culturally sensitive, in languages of the patient/family served.	Provide tools to promote cultural assessment in all patients/families. Examples include: ♦ The Provider's Guide to Quality and Culture: Designed to help healthcare organizations and providers provide high-quality, culturally competent services to multiethnic populations: http://erc.msh.org/mainpage.cfm?file=1.0.htm&module=provider&language=english ♦ Transcultural Nursing Society: The society, serves as a forum to promote, advance, and disseminate transcultural nursing knowledge worldwide: http://tcns.org Provide interpreter services and written materials in each patient's and family's preferred language. Promote cultural humility as nurses respectfully and effectively provide care to patients from diverse cultures. Staff should be recruited, reflecting the cultural and linguistic diversity of the citizens it serves. Staff should be encouraged to reflect on their own self-awareness regarding their cultural, in an effort to prevent conflicts with the people they serve and collaborate with.

Domain 7: Care of the patient at the end of life

- The IDT identifies, communicates, and manages the signs and symptoms of patients at the end of life to meet the physical, psychosocial, spiritual, social, and cultural needs of patients and families.
- The IDT assesses and, in collaboration with the patient and family, develops, documents, and implements a care plan to address preventative and immediate treatment of actual or potential symptoms, patient and family preferences for site of care, attendance of family and/or community members at the bedside, and desire for other treatments and procedures
- Respectful postdeath care is delivered in a respectful manner that honors the patient and family culture and religious practices.

Clinical implications:

"It is essential that the IDT attends to the patient's and family's values, preferences, beliefs, culture, and religion to promote a peaceful, dignified and respectful death."

Describe and demonstrate the importance of planning for a death—assessing not only physical, but also psychological, social, and spiritual needs during the three phases of care:

- Predeath
- Perideath
- Postdeath

Identify the importance of the nurse working closely with the IDT in providing this sacred care.

Provide role-plays, case studies, and simulation labs that promote excellent care at the end of life. Examples include:

- Speaking honestly with family about their loved one's impending death, respecting their values, preferences, beliefs, culture, and religion
- Communicating with an 8-year-old child whose father is dying in the ICU. How would you talk and listen to this child who states he is afraid that his daddy will "never wake up?"
- Speaking with a family member who asks you if their brother is appropriate for hospice care. He was diagnosed 8 months ago with stage 4 pancreatic cancer, has heart disease and dementia. How would you respond?
- Communicating with family members about autopsy, organ/tissue donation, anatomical gifts before their loved one dies

Demonstrate respectful postdeath care that honors the patient/family's culture and religion.

Describe the importance of follow-up bereavement care with families after the death of their loved one.

Assessment of physical, psychological, social, and spiritual needs during the three phases of care:

- Predeath
- Perideath
- Postdeath

Communication of findings frequently with family, staff, and other IDT members

Educate the family on signs and symptoms of imminent death—keeping in mind the developmental age and culture.

Oversee/provide adequate analgesics and sedatives for comfort. Address any concerns the family may have about using these to hasten death. Reassesses frequently.

Respectful care of the body, honoring cultural and religious rites, after the death

Bereavement care plan, including community resources

Nurses must work with the IDT in identifying, communicating, and managing the patient's symptoms at the end of life and keeping family members updated on the status of their loved one.

- Address concerns, fears, and expectations that family members may have.
- Explain potential symptoms before death.
- Honor values, preferences, beliefs, culture, and religion.
- Is hospice referral appropriate for this patient and congruent with goals of care and preferences?
- Educate about signs of impending death.
- Communicate about autopsy, organ/tissue donation, and anatomical gifts.
- Document.
- Provide respectful postdeath care, honoring the patient/family culture and religion.
- Provide follow-up bereavement plan
- Update any policies/procedures that promotes care at the end of life.

Promote and participate in quality improvement (QI) issues to support education in end-of-life care.

(continued)

Table 66.5 Continued

NCP guideline domain	Recommendations for implementation and dissemination to baccalaureate/graduate nursing education	Recommended content to be included in APRN education via didactic and clinical experiences[28]	Recommendations for implementation and dissemination to continuing education and professional development for nurses
Domain 8: Ethical and legal aspects of care ◆ The patient or surrogate's goals, preferences, and choices are respected within the limits of applicable state and federal law, current accepted standards of medical care, and professional standards of practice. Person-centered goals, preferences, and choices form the basis for the plan of care. ◆ The palliative care program identifies, acknowledges, and addresses the complex ethical issues arising in the care of people with serious or life-threatening illness. ◆ The provision of palliative care occurs in accordance with professional, state, and federal laws, regulations, and current accepted standards of care. **Clinical implications:** *"Ethical and legal principles are inherent to the provision of palliative care to patients with serious or life-threatening illness. IDT members must have an understanding of the central ethical principles underlying healthcare delivery in the context of their own professional practice setting and discipline. Palliative care teams must have access to legal and ethics expertise to support palliative care practice"*	Describe the importance of eliciting patient/family goals of care in a manner that is respectful of their values, care preferences, religious beliefs, and cultural considerations. Keep in mind the ethical principles of beneficence, respect/self-determination, justice, and nonmaleficence. Document! Invite legal counsel to speak in class about specific palliative care issues—i.e., determination of decision-making capacity, use of high-dose opioids, withdrawal of ventilators and/or dialysis, palliative sedation, futile care, cessation of hydration and/or nutrition. Suggestions for role-plays, case studies, simulation labs related to ethical and legal issues: ◆ Determining decision-making capacity ◆ You have been called to see a 10-year-old patient who wishes to discontinue chemotherapy (was diagnosed 4 years ago with an osteosarcoma—had leg amputated 3 years ago and has continued with chemotherapy and multiple hospitalizations for the past 3 years. States, "I'm tired of all of this.") The parents want "everything done." How should you proceed? ◆ A homeless patient is brought into the emergency room, unresponsive. He was resuscitated in the ambulance twice on the way to the hospital. The patient has no identification. Without knowing his expressed wishes, who will make the decision about "DNR," "AND," etc.? ◆ Role-play an ethics committee and discuss a recent case that a student may have witnessed in the clinical setting. ◆ You have just admitted a patient to your unit and you suspect that she has been abused and neglected. What are your immediate legal and ethical responsibilities?	Identification and documentation of surrogate/decision maker for every patient and in every clinical/community healthcare setting. Further documentation should include: ◆ Goals of care ◆ Treatment options ◆ Setting of care Documentation of goals of care should be seamless and transferable to all care settings, adhering to Health Insurance Portability and Accountability Act (HIPAA) regulations. For minors with decision-making capacity, documentation of choices for care is made and APRN advocates that the minor's preferences be considered. When the minor's wishes are different from those of the adult decision-maker, the APRN advocates for professional staff to consult and intervene as needed. Promotion of ethics committee and development/maintenance of policies dealing with decision-making, legal issues, organ/tissue transplantation, etc. Provision of community collaboration, promoting advance care planning. Examples of how to develop advance directives include: ◆ Respecting Choices: Assists in implementing advance care planning http://respectingchoices.org/ ◆ Community Conversations on Compassionate Care: Promotes conversations that ensure patients healthcare wishes are honored http://www.compassionandsupport.org/index.php/for_patients_families/advance_care_planning/community_conversations	Remind nurses in orientation and annual competency review that state and federal law, codes of ethics, and standards of nursing practice standards provide a compass as they navigate through common issues of end-of-life care. These include: ◆ Patient and family decision-making ◆ Eliciting patient/family goals of care ◆ Honoring advanced directives ◆ Determining decision-making capacity (for all ages) ◆ Working with surrogate decision-makers ◆ Withdrawal of technology (i.e, dialysis, ventilators, etc.) ◆ Using high-dose opioids ◆ Providing palliative sedation ◆ Discontinuing hydration and/or nutrition ◆ Providing futile care ◆ Pronouncing death ◆ Requesting autopsy, organ/tissue and anatomical donation

Table 66.6 Quick palliative care links/resources for educators

Organization	Overview
Center to Advance Palliative Care (CAPC): www.capc.org	CAPC is the leading resource for palliative care program development and growth. Access essential palliative care tools, education, resources and training for healthcare professionals.
Communication curriculum live: www.CECentral.com/COMFORT	Participants earn online CE for palliative care communication curriculum live on CECentral. Four modules, each lasting 1 hour, are available through CE Central at no cost. Participants may choose to complete as many modules as they like. The purpose of this study is to assess communication curriculum for an online CE format. A certificate of completion will be provided and the activity will be added to participants' records of CE activity.
City of Hope Pain and Palliative Care Resource Center (COHPPRC): http://prc.coh.org/	The purpose of the COHPPRC is to serve as a clearinghouse to disseminate information and resources to assist others in improving the quality of pain management and end-of-life care. The COHPPRC is a central source for collecting pain assessment tools, patient education materials, quality assurance materials, end-of-life resources, research instruments, and other resources.
End-of-Life Nursing Education Consortium (ELNEC): www.aacn.nche.edu/ELNEC	The End-of-Life Nursing Education Consortium (ELNEC) project is a national education initiative to improve palliative care. The project provides undergraduate and graduate nursing faculty, CE providers, staff development educators, specialty nurses in pediatrics, oncology, critical care, and geriatrics, and other nurses with training in palliative care so they can teach this essential information to nursing students and practicing nurses.
End of Life/Palliative Education Resource Center (EPERC): http://www.eperc.mcw.edu/EPERC/FastFactsandConcepts	*Fast Facts and Concepts* provide concise, practical, peer-reviewed, and evidence-based summaries on key topics important to clinicians and trainees caring for patients facing life-limiting illnesses. *Fast Facts* are designed to be easily accessible and clinically relevant monographs on palliative care topics. They are intended to be quick teaching tools for bedside rounds, as well as self-study material for healthcare professional trainees and clinicians who work with patients with life-limiting illnesses.
Relias learning: http://academy.reliaslearning.com/	The Relias Learning offers a comprehensive and innovative solution to the challenge of providing high-quality education for hospice and other end-of-life care professionals. The Relias Learning offers courses for new staff orientation, annual inservices, volunteer training, and continuing education for nurses, social workers, and counselors. The Relias Learning is the next generation of Web-based education and it is developed specifically and exclusively for hospice and palliative care programs and professionals. Most of the ELNEC curricula are now available on Relias Learning.
Hospice and Palliative Nurses Association (HPNA): www.hpna.org. Under the arm of HPNA are two other organizations: **The National Board for Certification of Hospice and Palliative Nurses (NBCHPN):** www.nbchpn.org **Hospice and Palliative Nurses Foundation (HPNF)** www.hpnf.org	Established in 1986, HPNA is the nation's largest and oldest professional nursing organization dedicated to promoting excellence in hospice and palliative nursing care. NBCHPN offers specialty certification for all levels of the hospice and palliative nursing care team and administrators. Currently, NBCHPN certifies over 17,000 health professionals. HPNF depends on the generous spirit of individuals, businesses and foundations to support quality of life by enhancing nursing excellence. Their gift embraces hospice and palliative nursing by generating opportunities for nursing education, research, and leadership.
Joint Commission Advanced Palliative Care Certification: http://www.jointcommission.org/certification/palliative_care.aspx	Launched in September 2011, The Joint Commission's Advanced Certification Program for Palliative Care recognizes hospital inpatient programs that demonstrate exceptional patient- and family-centered care and optimize the quality of life for adult and pediatric patients with serious illness.

foreign countries. The HPNA provides educational opportunities through continuing education products such as webinars, online chats, books, seminars such as the Clinical Practice Forum, and the Annual Assembly, which is cosponsored with the American Academy of Hospice and Palliative Medicine (AAHPM). Hospice and palliative nurses can stay updated on the latest evidence-based practice through articles found in the *Journal of Hospice and Palliative Nursing* (JHPN) and through an online subscription of the *Journal of Palliative Medicine* (JPM). For more information regarding HPNA, go to www.hpna.org.

One of two affiliated organizations is the National Board for Certification of Hospice and Palliative Nurses (NBCHPN). This is the only organization that provides specialty certification for all levels of the hospice and palliative nursing care team and administrators. There are currently seven certification exams offered by NBCHPN: Advanced Certified Hospice and Palliative Nurse (ACHPN), Certified Hospice and Palliative Nurse (CHPN), Certified Hospice and Palliative Pediatric Nurse (CHPPN), Certified Hospice and Palliative Licensed Nurse (CHPLN), Certified Hospice and Palliative Nursing Assistant (CHPNA), Certified Hospice and Palliative Care Administrator (CHPCA), and Certified in Perinatal

Loss Care (CPLC). There are currently over 17,000 health professionals who are certified through NBCHPN.[38] For more information about hospice and palliative certification, go to www.nbchpn.org

The second organization affiliated with HPNA is the Hospice and Palliative Nurses Foundation (HPNF), which was incorporated in 1998. The Foundation provides scholarships for education, research, conferences, certification, and offers leadership awards. In 2014, 45 grants, scholarships, and awards were given to HPNA members. The HPNF continually seeks financial support from individuals, businesses, and foundations in an effort to provide and support a variety of professional development opportunities. For further information on the HPNF, go to www.hpnf.org.

Conclusion

There has been much progress in the past 10 years in providing palliative care education to nursing students, as well as to practicing nurses, yet still many challenges remain. Educators struggle with how best to integrate more content into an already robust curriculum. There is a tremendous need to increase the knowledge of faculty in palliative care so they can embed its content throughout the curriculum. Educators also require current teaching guides such as audiovisual materials, case studies, and other resources to present this challenging content (Table 66.6).

Teaching palliative care is not only a matter of developing didactic content, but also of providing students and practicing nurses with a vision of what excellent palliative care can look like. It provides opportunities to empower them with the knowledge to demonstrate pristine care to the most vulnerable in our society—those with serious, life-threatening illness. This necessitates attention to and respect for students and practicing nurses' values, beliefs, personal experiences, and culture. It is essential that palliative care education not only incorporate knowledge and skills but also strive to identify methods to best enhance compassion to those who suffer, empathy to those without a voice, and the "art" of palliative nursing to patients and families who desperately need this care.[39] What a privilege to provide this education!

References

1. Center to Advance Palliative Care (CAPC). Growth of palliative care in U.S. hospitals: 2012 Snapshot. http://reportcard.capc.org/pdf/capc-growth-analysis-snapshot-2011.pdf. Accessed June 5, 2013.
2. The Joint Commission (TJC). Eligibility for Advanced Certification for Palliative Care. http://www.jointcommission.org/certification/eligiblty_palliative_care.aspx. Accessed June 5, 2013.
3. National Quality Forum. A National Framework and Preferred Practices for Palliative and Hospice Care Quality. http://www.qualityforum.org/publications/reports/palliative.asp Accessed December 23, 2008.
4. National Consensus Project. Clinical Practice Guidelines for Quality Palliative Care. http://www.nationalconsensusproject.org/. Accessed June 18, 2013.
5. Field MJ, Cassel CK, eds. Approaching Death: Improving Care at the End of Life. Report of the Institute of Medicine Task Force on End of Life Care. Washington, DC: National Academy of Sciences; 1997.
6. Institute of Medicine (IOM). Priority Areas for National Action: Transforming Healthcare Quality. Washington DC: National Academy Press; 2003.
7. World Health Organization (WHO). Cancer Pain Relief and Palliative Care. WHO Technical Report Series 804. Geneva: WHO; 1990.
8. Ferrell BR, Coyle N. An overview of palliative nursing care. Am J Nurs. 2002;102(5);26–31.
9. Kirshhoff KT, Beckstand RL, Anumandla P. Analysis of end of life content in critical care nursing textbooks. J Prof Nurs. 2003;19:372–381.
10. Ferrell BR, Virani R, Grant M. Analysis of end of life content in nursing textbooks. Oncol Nurs Forum. 1999;26:869–876.
11. American Association of Colleges of Nursing (AACN). A Peaceful Death. Report from the Robert Wood Johnson End-of-Life Care Roundtable. Washington, DC: November 1997.
12. Wendt A. End-of-life competencies and the NCLEX-RN examination. Nurs Outlook. 2001;3:138–141.
13. Ferrell BR, Virani R, Grant M, Rhome A. End of life issues and nursing education. Imprint. 2000;47;43–46.
14. Malloy P, Paice J, Virani R, Ferrell BR, Bednash G. End-of-Life Nursing Education Consortium: 5 years of educating graduate nursing faculty in excellent palliative care. Prof Nurs. 2008;24:352–357.
15. Ferrell BR, Virani R, Grant M, et al. Evaluation of the End-of-Life Nursing Education Consortium (ELNEC) undergraduate faculty training program. J Palliat Med. 2005;8(1):107–114.
16. Malloy P, Ferrell B, Virani R, Wilson K, Uman G. Palliative care education for pediatric nurses. Pediatr Nurs. 2006; 32:555–561.
17. End-of-Life Nursing Education Consortium (ELNEC). Fact Sheet www.aacn.nche.edu/ELNEC. Accessed June 18, 2013.
18. Institute of Medicine (IOM). The Future of Nursing: Leading Change, Advancing Health. http://www.iom.edu/Reports/2010/The-Future-of-Nursing-Leading-Change-Advancing-Health.aspx. Accessed June 17, 2013.
19. Centers for Disease Control and Prevention (CDC). Leading Causes of Death. http://www.cdc.gov/nchs/fastats/lcod.htm. Accessed June 12, 2013.
20. Institute of Medicine (IOM). Living Well with Chronic Illness: A Call for Public Health Action. http://www.iom.edu/Reports/2012/Living-well-with-chronic-illness.aspx Accessed June 17, 2013.
21. Meier DE, Isaacs SL, Hughes RG. Palliative Care: Transforming the Care of Serious Illness. San Francisco, CA: Jossey-Bass, 2010.
22. National Council of State Boards of Nursing (NCSBN). APRNs in the U.S.: The Consensus Model for APRN Regulation, Licensure, Accreditation, Certification, and Education. https://www.ncsbn.org/4213.htm. Accessed June 5, 2013.
23. National Institute of Health (NIH). Federal Report Details Health, Economic Status of Older Americans. http://www.nih.gov/news/health/aug2012/nia-16.htm. Accessed June 17, 2013.
24. American Association of Colleges of Nursing (AACN). APRN Consensus Process. http://www.aacn.nche.edu/education-resources/aprn-consensus-process. Accessed June 17, 2013.
25. Fang D, Li Y, Bednash GD. 2012–2013 Enrollment and Graduations in Baccalaureate and Graduate Programs in Nursing. Washington, DC: American Association of Colleges of Nursing; 2013.
26. National Academy of Science (NAS). Advancing the Nation's Health Needs: NIH Training Programs. http://grants.nih.gov/training/nas_report_2005.pdf. Accessed June 7, 2013.
27. American Association of Colleges of Nursing (AACN). DNP Fact Sheet. http://www.aacn.nche.edu/media-relations/fact-sheets/dnp. Accessed June 17, 2013.
28. Dahlin C, Lentz J. National guidelines and the APRN. In: Dahlin C, Lynch M (eds.), Core Curriculum for the Advanced Practice Hospice and Palliative Registered Nurse. 2nd ed. Pittsburgh, PA: Hospice and Palliative Nurses Association; 2012:639–660.
29. Institute of Medicine (IOM). Ensuring Quality Cancer Care Through the Oncology Workforce: Sustaining Care in the 21st Century. http://books.nap.edu/openbook.php?record_id=12613. Accessed June 11, 2013.
30. Ferrell B, Virani R, Malloy P, Kelly K. The preparation of oncology nurses in palliative care. Sem Oncol Nurs. 2010;26(4):259–265.

31. Erikson C, Salsberg E, Forte G, Bruinooge S, Goldstein M. Future supply and demand for oncologists: challenges to assuring access to oncology services. J Oncol Pract. 2007;3(2):79–86.

32. Levit L, Smith AP, Benz EJ, Ferrell B. Ensuring quality cancer care through the oncology workforce. J Oncol Pract. 2011; 7(4). http://jop.ascopubs.org/content/6/1/7.full.

33. Boland BA, Treston J, O'Sullivan AL. Climb to new educational heights. Nurs Pract. 2010; 35(4):36–41.

34. American Association of Colleges of Nursing (AACN). Press Release: City of Hope and AACN Partner to Enhance Patient Care. www.aacn.nche.edu/ELNEC/news/articles/2013/city-of-hope-elnec. Accessed June 17, 2013.

35. American Cancer Society (ACS). Cancer Facts and Statistics. http://www.cancer.org/research/cancerfactsstatistics/. Accessed June 18, 2013.

36. Lynch T, Connor S, Clark D. Mapping levels of palliative care development: a global update. J Pain Symptom Manage. 2013;45(6):1094–1106.

37. End-of-Life Nursing Education Consortium (ELNEC)-International. http://www.aacn.nche.edu/elnec/about/elnec-international. Accessed June 18, 2013.

38. National Board of Certification for Hospice and Palliative Nurses (NBCHPN). Welcome. http://www.nbchpn.org/. Accessed July 1, 2014.

39. Ferrell B, Coyle, N. The nature of suffering and the goals of nursing. New York, NY: Oxford University Press, 2008:2–6.

CHAPTER 67

Nursing research

Betty R. Ferrell, Marcia Grant, and Virginia Sun

> Nurses continue to strive to integrate evidence into practice. Hospice and palliative nursing care occurs in most practice settings, at all stages of chronic illness, and for persons of all ages. Nurses are in a key position to lead research and validate effective interdisciplinary models in palliative care. This should be a key priority for our specialty.
> Remington R, Buck HG, Buck KJ, et al. (2012).[1]

Key points

- The goal of nursing research is to improve care for patients and caregivers.

- Nurses have been instrumental in the field of palliative care research.

- Palliative nursing research includes many sensitive topics such as suffering, quality of life (QOL), and life meaning.

- Nurse researchers face many obstacles in conducting research, such as obtaining informed consent, dealing with high subject attrition, and openly discussing end-of-life issues with patients and families.

- Palliative nursing research should utilize an interdisciplinary model that includes all supportive care disciplines.

- Palliative nursing research also addresses the experiences of nurses and the need for self-care.

A major component of palliative care research is nursing research.[2] The patient experience of dying is an ideal healthcare concern appropriate for nursing inquiry.[3] Because nurses are concerned with patient responses to illness, the physical, psychological, social, and spiritual responses of the terminally ill and their families are prime areas for nursing research.

The ultimate goal of nursing research, and indeed of nursing knowledge, is to improve patient care. Palliative care offers a rich opportunity for research to directly influence patient care in areas such as symptom management, psychological responses to a terminal illness, and the family caregiver experience of terminal illness.[4–7]

Some of the earliest contributions to palliative care research were made by nurses.[8] Pioneering work by Jeanne Quint Benoliel and others raised awareness of deficiencies in care of the dying.[9,10] Early descriptive studies documented the influence of nursing attitudes and beliefs about death on the care provided to patients.

From the earliest studies in the 1960s to the "awakening" of attention to palliative care in the late 1990s, research in palliative care has been limited. Nurse investigators have addressed aspects of end-of-life care such as pain management, bereavement, settings of care, and care of special populations. However, there has been a lack of support for palliative care nursing research.

In 1997, the National Institute of Nursing Research (NINR) led an initiative regarding end-of-life care research across several institutes of the National Institutes of Health (NIH). Specific recommendations of an NINR-sponsored conference on end-of-life care are described later in this chapter.[11] The NINR has been designated as the lead institute at the NIH in the area of end-of-life care. It is appropriate and commendable that the NINR is providing leadership at the NIH in this research agenda. However funding for research remains limited.[12]

As has been true in other areas of healthcare, the research agenda has lagged behind the demands of clinical practice and education. Hospice programs and palliative care settings face increased demands for improved end-of-life care with little scientific knowledge to guide clinical decisions.[13] Nursing schools have begun to develop undergraduate and graduate courses in palliative care, and some have launched degree or certificate programs in palliative care, again with limited research as a scientific foundation of their programs. Obviously, development of a solid research agenda and support of nursing science in palliative care are overdue.[14]

Goals of palliative care research

The goals of palliative care nursing research are similar to goals of other areas of nursing inquiry. Nursing research serves multiple functions, including quantification of information, discovery, description of phenomena, quality improvement, and problem solving.[1] Quantification is accomplished through descriptive studies or through epidemiological approaches. For example, there is a need to quantify the symptoms present in terminal illness, as well as their severity and impact. The field of palliative nursing care is relatively unexplored, and therefore, there is great opportunity for discovery. What are the greatest needs of terminally ill patients and their family caregivers? What is the unique role of nursing within the interdisciplinary team?

The subjective nature of terminal illness and the existential experience of dying require research methods that describe phenomena. Death, as a subject that has been avoided in society, is still a relatively unknown aspect of life. On a more specific level, palliative care is also a field that would benefit tremendously from research linked to quality improvement. Numerous reports have identified serious deficits in end-of-life care, and efforts to improve the quality of end-of-life care will undoubtedly benefit from research.[15,16] Finally, a major goal of palliative care research should be basic problem solving. What drugs are most beneficial for dyspnea or agitation? What is the best treatment for pressure ulcers in a dying patient? What education best prepares family caregivers for signs and symptoms of approaching death?

Ethical and methodological considerations in palliative care research

There are many unique aspects of research in palliative care. The multidimensional nature of care at the end of life and the vulnerability of the population are but two examples of factors that pose special challenges to this area of research.

The challenges of nursing research in palliative care should be prefaced by a discussion of the benefits. Although even the mention of conducting research with dying patients and their burdened families immediately creates concerns, there are in fact many benefits to participants. Participating in research, even at this most vulnerable and sensitive time of life, provides the opportunity for research subjects to contribute to others. Research participation often provides an opportunity to derive meaning from illness and to feel that one's suffering will provide benefit to others.[3,14,17]

In the authors' research at the City of Hope, involving numerous studies in sensitive areas such as pain, QOL, and fatigue, positive feedback has consistently been received from research subjects. Patients and family caregivers often have thanked the researchers for studying these topics, which they perceive to be of great importance. Subjects have also frequently related that completing written instruments or participating in interviews provided a mechanism for communicating needs that had not previously been voiced.

However, research in palliative care is very challenging and includes many obstacles. Nurses are often conflicted in balancing the role of clinician with that of researcher. For example, in conducting research related to pain in terminally ill cancer patients, the authors have often had to carefully balance these roles. Identifying a patient with severe pain has often meant that the patient's participation in a study must be ended in order to seek treatment for the pain. Researchers must always respect the more important ethical consideration of protecting the patient's well-being.[17]

Seeking informed consent in rapidly declining, weak patients is a challenge, as is the need to constantly protect patient and family autonomy. Subjects in palliative care research may feel obligated to participate, particularly if they have been the recipients of good care. Although all patients in palliative care are considered vulnerable, certain subgroups, such as the cognitively impaired, the poor, and the elderly, are of special concern.[18–20]

The sensitive nature of palliative care research provides inherent challenges. The areas of concern at the end of life are highly emotional and may invoke heightened distress. Exploring areas such as grief, fears, spiritual concerns, family conflict, and other common dimensions of terminal illness is highly challenging. Participation in research can bring to the forefront previously undisclosed problems. The authors have found, in their research experience, that palliative care research necessitates a highly

Box 67.1 Barriers to nursing research in palliative care

- Overall limitations in funding for nursing research and in the limited number of nurse researchers
- Research establishment and associated funding that has been focused on rehabilitation or cure
- Lack of political or consumer advocates to promote a research agenda in end-of-life care
- Limited focus on palliative care in graduate nursing education to promote end-of-life research within master's or doctoral nursing education
- Few established relationships between nurse researchers and clinical settings of palliative care
- Ethical considerations of conducting research with vulnerable populations, including issues related to ability to provide consent
- Rapidly declining status, which limits subject accrual and opportunity for longitudinal measures
- Lack of conceptual frameworks appropriate for palliative care research
- Interference with demands of patient care caused by participation in research
- Late referrals to hospice or palliative care programs, which severely restricts opportunities for accrual to studies
- Lack of research instruments and methods appropriate for this population
- Challenge of conducting research in a sensitive area
- Need to balance demands of rigorous research, such as the need for randomization, with awareness of patient needs

Sources: Adapted from Field and Cassel (1997), reference 30; and Doyle et al. (2004), reference 31.

skilled research staff. Collecting data from palliative care subjects is very different from research in healthy or chronically ill subjects. Research nurses in palliative care studies must be clinically competent, highly skilled nurses equipped to balance the rigor of research with extreme sensitivity.[13]

Palliative care research, perhaps more than any other field of inquiry, must carefully weigh subject burden. The time required of research subjects in palliative care, a precious commodity for those with terminal disease, must be carefully protected. Special consideration must be given to the selection of research instruments and procedures to minimize subject burden.[21–27]

Subject attrition is another common problem area in palliative care research.[28] Higher attrition has serious implications when determining sample sizes and also has budget implications. This problem area becomes an even greater concern in longitudinal studies, which are a definite need in palliative care. New approaches to handling data are needed to improve data analysis.

Palliative care research also necessitates diversity in research methods. The authors' experience has been that a combination of qualitative and quantitative approaches is needed.[23] Appendix 67.1 includes examples of two palliative care nursing studies (one quantitative, one qualitative) that serve as models for application of these methods for palliative care research. Quantitative approaches are essential when studying symptoms and QOL, their frequency and nature, and response to treatment. Qualitative approaches are especially important in descriptive studies, and are a useful approach in describing "the lived experience" of terminally ill patients using their own narratives.

The authors also have found that nursing research in palliative care is greatly enhanced by interdisciplinary collaboration. The problems studied are multidimensional and are best defined from the viewpoints of various members of the healthcare team. Participation from colleagues in psychology, theology, social work, and other disciplines has enhanced our work considerably.

A final special consideration in palliative care research is the importance of including family caregivers.[29] Terminal illness is a shared experience, and including family caregivers as subjects enriches the benefits to be derived from the research.[29]

Box 67.1 summarizes some of the key challenges of conducting palliative care research. Advancement of the nursing profession in palliative care will require attention to overcome these obstacles.

A research agenda in palliative nursing

The Institute of Medicine (IOM), the health arm of the National Academy of Sciences of the United States, identified priority areas for end-of-life care research, including pain, cachexia-anorexia-asthenia, dyspnea, and cognitive and emotional symptoms. Also addressed was the need for social, behavioral, and health services research. Nursing as a profession has much to contribute to each of these identified priorities.[3] The Hospice and Palliative Nurses Association has identified key priorities for research to include the following: (1) structure and processes of care, (2) physical aspects of care, and (3) psychological and psychiatric aspects of care.[1]

There is a tremendous need to bring together nurse researchers and nurse clinicians in palliative care. Historically, few nurse researchers have focused on palliative care; likewise, few expert clinicians in palliative care have had opportunities or expertise in research.

Although an exhaustive review of research methods or grant writing is not possible in this chapter, a few comments are worthy of attention. Palliative care clinicians are encouraged to seek collaboration with nurse researchers to initiate clinically relevant and scientifically sound studies.[32] Another key issue of advice is to

begin small. Conducting small pilot studies is an essential foundation to launching larger-scale studies. Potential sources for funding are found in Box 67.2.

Box 67.3 includes an example of criteria used in evaluating small-scale research projects. These criteria, adapted from the

---

Box 67.2 Funding sources for pilot studies

Hospital Continuous Quality Improvement programs

Oncology Nursing Foundation

Sigma Theta Tau

American Nursing Foundation

American Society of Pain Management Nurses

Local community foundations

Pharmaceutical companies

Hospice and Palliative Nursing Association

Box 67.3 Research proposal evaluation criteria

Abstract

- Abstract accurately reflects the proposal.
- Abstract includes problem statement and purpose.
- Abstract summarizes key variables, sample, and methods.

Study aims, hypotheses, or study questions

- Clearly stated
- Hypotheses or study questions are consistent with the study aim.
- All proposed study procedures and data to be collected are encompassed.

Significance of the study

- The research contributes to the science of palliative nursing care.
- The research has the potential to lead to further investigation.
- The research offers a unique contribution to the literature.
- The research is clinically relevant to end-of-life care.

Literature review

- Relevant and current literature is reviewed.
- Literature primarily includes research rather than opinion.
- Literature is critiqued, synthesized, and analyzed.

Conceptual/theoretical framework

- The framework identified is appropriate to the study and consistent with study questions and methods.
- The framework is consistent with the philosophy of palliative care.

Procedures

- The procedures are feasible.
- Procedures include methods for training and supervision of personnel.
- Procedures provide sufficient description of precisely what will be required of subjects.

Data analysis

- Specific statistical procedures are identified.
- Analysis is appropriate for the type of data and study design and answers the study questions.
- Computer facilities and consultation are described.
- The investigator has sought consultation if necessary in preparing the proposal.

(continued)

Box 67.3 Continued

Human subjects considerations

- Institutional Review Board approval is given or documentation of pending review is given.

- The investigator is clearly aware of the impact of participation in the study on the subject.

- The investigator addresses concerns regarding length, intrusiveness, and energy expenditure required.

- The investigator has acknowledged special considerations of terminal illness.

Investigators and research team

- Consultation is available for the less experienced researcher.

- The role of coinvestigators or consultants is established.

Overall

- The proposal strictly adheres to format restrictions and page limitations.

Source: Adapted from reference 33.

Box 67.4 General tips for preparing research proposals

- Grant writing is not a solo activity—seek consultation and collaboration from others. Seek opportunities to involve clinical palliative care settings, such as hospices, in nursing research.

- Have your proposal reviewed by peers before submitting it for funding. A proposal submitted for funding is generally the product of numerous revisions.

- Follow the directions in detail, including margins, page limits, and the use of references and appendices. Communicate directly with the funding source to clarify any directions you are unsure of.

- State ideas clearly and succinctly. Word economy is essential to a fine-tuned proposal.

- Use high-quality printing and use a good-quality copier. Give attention to spelling and grammar.

- Plan ahead and develop a time frame for completing your grant. Avoid the last-minute rush that will compromise the quality of your proposal. It is better to target a future deadline for submission than to compromise your score due to a lack of time for preparation.

- Use appendices to include study instruments, procedures, or other supporting materials. Adhere to funding agency criteria, but maximize the opportunity for a complete proposal.

- Include support letters from individuals who are important to the success of your study. This includes medical staff, nursing administration, consultants, and coinvestigators.

- Do not hesitate to contact experts in your subject area to seek their input. They are often able to review your work and direct you toward related instruments or literature.

- Start small. Successful completion of a pilot project is the best foundation for a larger study. Efficient use of small grant funding is influential when seeking larger-scale funding for major proposals.

- Be realistic. Design research projects that can be realistically accomplished within the scope of your other responsibilities and the limitations of your work setting.

- Keep focused on the patient. Design and implement research that is relevant to patient care and improves quality of life at the end of life for patients and families.

Source: Ferrell et al. (1989), reference 36.

Oncology Nursing Foundation, depict the essential elements of a research proposal.

Many professional organizations provide small grant support to novice investigators. Box 67.4 includes some general tips for preparing a research proposal. Steele and colleagues published a two-part series on their pilot study on transitioning families into pediatric hospice care. The first part of the series described the planning phase of their pilot study. The investigators described their rationale in conducting the study and provided a detailed description of the study site, recruitment of subjects, study procedures, data collection plan, and data analysis plan, as well as the challenges of conducting the study.[34] In the second part of the series, the investigators reported their findings.[35]

The authors concluded that study findings will help with the development of a nursing intervention to aid families with transitioning to pediatric hospices. Palliative care research that also publishes the study development process is helpful in assisting novice palliative care researchers to understand the challenges and limitations as well as rewards in designing quality palliative care studies.

Another useful guide for nurses initiating research proposals is included in Box 67.5. This includes the review considerations used by grant reviewers at the NIH. The five criteria of significance, approach, innovation, investigation, and environment can serve as a useful guide in designing research proposals.[11]

Several initiatives have begun to establish an agenda for palliative care research. Topics frequently identified as priority topics for palliative care research include pain, symptom management, epidemiological studies of terminal illness, family caregiver needs, bereavement, cultural considerations, spiritual needs, and health systems considerations such as costs of care.[37-39] Examples of palliative care research topics by nurse researchers include understanding the meaning of QOL domains such as social and spiritual well being,[40,41] the experience of palliative care in the urban poor,[42] providing palliative and end-of-life care for nursing-home residents,[43] and evaluating innovative end-of-life programs in nursing homes.[44]

At the City of Hope, we have developed a framework of nine areas of palliative nursing care that is used in our nursing education efforts. Table 67.1 includes a summary of these nine topic areas, with examples of potential research that is needed.[45]

Significance

Does this study address an important problem? If the aims of the application are achieved, how will scientific knowledge be advanced? What will be the effect of these studies on the concepts or methods that drive this field?

Approach

Are the conceptual framework, design, methods, and analyses adequately developed, well integrated, and appropriate to the aims of the project? Does the applicant acknowledge potential problem areas and consider alternative tactics?

Innovation

Does the project employ novel concepts, approaches, or methods? Are the aims original and innovative? Does the project challenge existing paradigms or develop new methodologies or technologies?

Investigator

Is the investigator appropriately trained and well suited to carry out this work? Is the work proposed appropriate to the experience level of the principal investigator and other researchers (if any)?

Environment

Does the scientific environment in which the work will be done contribute to the probability of success? Do the proposed experiments take advantage of unique features of the scientific environment or employ useful collaborative arrangements? Is there evidence of institutional support?

Additional considerations

In addition, the adequacy of plans to include both genders and minorities and their subgroups as appropriate for the scientific goals of the research are reviewed. Plans for the recruitment and retention of subjects is also evaluated.

Source: Adapted from reference 33.

Another excellent resource for identifying future areas of palliative care research comes from the conference convened by the NINR, described previously.[11] An excerpt of the executive summary from this NIH research workshop, which focused on symptom management in terminal illness, is included as Appendix 66.2, together with the specific recommendations from that conference, which identified research needs regarding the symptoms of pain, dyspnea, cognitive disturbances, and cachexia.[11]

Summary

Advances in the care of patients and families facing terminal illness are contingent on advances in palliative nursing research. Control of symptoms, comfort for families, and attention to psychosocial and spiritual needs will improve when nurse clinicians have a stronger scientific foundation for practice. Research will require collaboration with other disciplines and unity of nurse clinicians and researchers.

Appendix 67.1

Two examples of palliative nursing studies

Illness Perception, Symptom Distress, and Quality of Life in Advanced gastrointestinal cancers

Virginia Sun, RN, PhD
City of Hope National Medical Center

The purpose of this study was to describe the relationship between illness perception, symptom distress, and QOL in patients diagnosed with advanced GI cancers.

The burden of multiple, debilitating symptoms such as pain in advanced, incurable cancer often translates into higher levels of distress. This burden is common in GI cancers because 80% of new cases are diagnosed in advanced stages of disease. There is an emerging emphasis on exploring cancer-related symptoms from a behavioral perspective, such as an individual's perception of illness. However, the concept of illness perception has not been described in patients with advanced GI cancers. Study framework incorporates essential concepts of the common sense model and the five domains of illness perception (identity, timeline, consequences, control, cause). A cross-sectional, correlational design was used to describe the relationship between illness perception, symptom distress, and QOL in patients with three common advanced GI cancers. Study participants were recruited from the Medical Oncology Adult Ambulatory Care Clinic of two NCI-designated comprehensive cancer centers and one community cancer center, with equal stratification based on cancer diagnoses. Eligibility criteria included the following: (1) diagnosis of colorectal (CRC), pancreatic, or hepatocellular carcinoma (HCC); (2) histologically confirmed diagnosis of locally advanced or metastatic disease; and (3) able to understand English. Patients completed a one-time survey containing the following outcome measures: Illness Perception Questionnaire-Revised (IPQ-R), Memorial Symptom Assessment Scale (MSAS), and the Short-Form-12 (SF-12). Mean scores for all measures were tabulated using standard summary statistics, followed by Pearson's correlations to determine relationships between primary outcomes. Predictors of QOL were determined through regression analyses. A total of 101 patients were consented and had complete data that was evaluable. The sample included 41 patients with CRC, 30 with pancreatic cancer, and 30 with HCC. Higher overall symptom distress was correlated with beliefs about the negative consequences of cancer as well as emotional reactions to cancer. Quality of life was negatively correlated with symptoms attributed to cancer, beliefs about the cyclical nature of cancer, negative consequences of cancer, emotional reactions to cancer, and overall symptom distress. Predictors of QOL included illness identity, symptom distress, consequences of cancer, timeline, and emotional representations. Illness cognition, along with symptom distress, influences overall QOL in patients with advanced GI cancers.

Table 67.1 Potential areas for research in end-of-life (EOL) care

Critical areas of end-of-life care	Examples of area content	Examples of potential areas of inquiry
1. The concept of palliative care	A. Importance of palliative care for nurses	◆ Refinement of definitions/criteria for palliative care
	B. Definitions of palliative care	
	C. Important goals/characteristics of palliative care:	◆ Descriptive studies of interdisciplinary involvement and related outcomes
	1. Dignity/respect	◆ Evaluation of methods to provide staff support in palliative care
	2. Relief of symptoms	
	3. Peaceful death	
	4. Ethical issues	
	5. Patient control/choices	
	D. Importance of interdisciplinary collaboration	
	E. Recognition of nurses' own discomfort/anxiety	
2. Quality of life (QOL) at the end of life (EOL)	A. Recognition of multiple dimensions of QOL at the EOL	◆ Development/testing of QOL instruments for use in palliative care
	1. Physical well-being	◆ Refinement of research methods to decrease patient burden in QOL assessment
	2. Psychological well-being	
	3. Social well-being	Development/testing of QOL instruments for family caregivers
	4. Spiritual well-being	
3. Pain management at EOL	A. Definition of pain	◆ Methods of assessing pain in the nonverbal or confused patient
	B. Assessment of pain	
	C. Assessment of meaning of pain	◆ Refine methods for pain assessment to decrease patient burden
	D. Pharmacological management of pain at EOL	◆ Development of pain measures that incorporate all dimensions of pain at EOL (e.g., spiritual pain)
	E. Use of invasive techniques	
	F. Principles of addiction, tolerance, and dependence	◆ Intervention studies to treat common pain syndromes at EOL
	G. Nonpharmacological management of pain	◆ Testing of protocols to treat pain at EOL, including changing routes of analgesia
	H. Physical pain vs. suffering	
	I. Side effects of opioids	◆ Development/evaluation of teaching programs for patients/families to decrease fears regarding pain management
	J. Barriers to pain management	
	K. Fear of opioids hastening death	
	L. Equianalgesic dosing	◆ Development/evaluation of programs to educate/support nurses in managing pain
	M. Recognition of nurses' own burden in pain management at EOL	
4. Other symptom management at EOL	A. Assessment and management of common EOL symptoms	◆ Descriptive studies to better understand symptom experiences
		◆ Symptom prevalence and patterns at EOL
		◆ Evaluation of pharmacological treatments for each symptom
		◆ Development of patient/family caregiver education for symptom management, including pharmacological and nonpharmacological treatments
		◆ Evaluation of protocols/algorithms to
		◆ Enhance nurses' effectiveness in symptom
		◆ Assessment and management

(continued)

Table 67.1 Continued

Critical areas of end-of-life care	Examples of area content	Examples of potential areas of inquiry
	1. Dyspnea/cough	
	2. Nausea/vomiting	
	3. Dehydration/nutrition	
	4. Altered mental status/delirium/terminal restlessness	
	5. Anxiety/depression	
	6. Weakness/fatigue	
	7. Dysphagia	
	8. Incontinence	
	9. Skin integrity	
	10. Constipation/bowel obstruction	
	11. Agitation/myoclonus	
5. Communication with dying patients and families	A. Definition/goals of communication	◆ Descriptive studies to better determine common areas of concern regarding communication at EOL
	B. Importance of listening	◆ Studies that describe the role of nursing in communication
	C. Barriers to communication	
	D. Delivering bad news/truth-telling	◆ Evaluation of protocols for delivering/ reinforcing bad news
	E. Recognizing family dynamics in communication	
	F. Sensitivity to culture, ethnicity, values, and religion	◆ Studies that explore cultural issues influencing communication ◆ Exploration of decision-making by patients and family caregivers
	G. Discussion of options/decisions with patients/family	
	H. Communication among interdisciplinary team members/collaboration	◆ Exploration of decision-making by patients and family caregivers
	I. Responding to requests for assisted suicide	◆ Exploration of causes of requests for assisted suicide and preparation of nurses to respond to requests
6. Role/needs of family caregivers in EOL care	A. The importance of recognizing family and caregivers needs at EOL	◆ Descriptive studies to enhance understanding of the family caregiver perspective of terminal illness
	B. Assessment of family needs	◆ Studies that explore family dynamics and the family as a unit rather than focus only on single caregivers
	C. Family dynamics	
	D. Recognizing ethical/cultural influences	◆ Evaluation of educational/support approaches to enhance personal death awareness ◆ Exploratory studies to enhance understanding of cultural influences
	E. Coping strategies and support systems	◆ Evaluation of teaching approaches to prepare families for impending death
7. Care at the time of death	A. The nurse's personal death awareness	◆ Development and evaluation of protocols for care at the time of death i.e., physical and spiritual care
	B. Death as natural process	
	C. Recognizing signs/symptoms of impending death	
	D. Patient/family's fears associated with death	
	E. Preparing for the death event	

(continued)

Table 67.1 Continued

Critical areas of end-of-life care	Examples of area content	Examples of potential areas of inquiry
	1. Healthcare providers	
	2. Patient	
	3. Family caregivers	
	F. Physical care at the time of death	
	G. Spiritual care at the time of death	
8. Issues of policy, ethics, and law	A. Patient preferences/advance directives	◆ Evaluation of approaches to enhance use of advance directives
	B. Assisted suicide	◆ Testing of educational methods to enhance nurses' ability to respond to requests for assisted suicide/euthanasia
	C. Euthanasia	◆ Development and evaluation of protocols that promote patient comfort while discontinuing food/fluids and life support
	D. Withdrawing food/fluids	◆ Identification of legal and regulatory barriers to optimal EOL care
	E. Discontinuing life support	
	F. Legal issues at the EOL	
	G. Need for changes in health policy	
	H. Confidentiality	
9. Bereavement	A. Stages/process of grief	◆ Exploratory studies to enhance understanding of cultural influences ◆ Refinement of efficient methods of grief assessment ◆ Testing of approaches to facilitate staff grieving
	B. Assessment of grief	
	C. Interventions/resources	
	D. Recognition of staff grief	

The meaning of the work of nursing: Care of the Body After Death

Jill Olausson, RN, MSN, CDE
City of Hope National Medical Center

Care of the body after death is an important nursing function that occurs in a wide variety of contexts. After a patient dies, nursing care continues as physical care of the body as well as care of the family members. In this descriptive qualitative study we explored nurses' perceptions of the meaning of care of the body post death. In this descriptive study, surveys were distributed to participants attending one of several nursing education conferences. Nurses were asked to describe an example of excellent care of the body after death that they witnessed or were involved in; 196 surveys were returned for analysis. Additional information included number of years in practice and the setting in which they worked. The returned surveys were transcribed verbatim and imported to qualitative analysis software. Process coding was employed and is useful when looking for "ongoing action/inter-action/emotion taken in response to situations, or problems with the purpose of reaching a goal or handling a problem." Focused coding was then applied to develop the most salient categories. First- and second-cycle coding were constantly compared to refine codes and categories. The data was independently coded by both authors and codes were adjusted to reflect the intercoder convergence. The descriptions were coded and two overarching themes

emerged—nursing care of the body after death meant providing respectful and dignified care, sensitive to the needs of the family, and provided nurses with a mechanism for coping with care of dying patients. The findings of this study provide insight regarding nursing interpretations of what constitutes excellence in after death care (ADC) and what this care means to the nurses. Overall, excellence in ADC supported findings in the literature—care was respectful and dignified and care supported family needs. Additionally, nurses found ADC to be a mechanism for coping with death experiences. The transcendental meaning making of ADC allowed nurses to experience positive and highly rewarding death experiences. There is, however, an inherent risk that the nurse's "own agenda" may supersede the needs of the family. To ensure the prioritization of family needs, ADC planning should become standard practice. These care plans require ongoing reassessment of patient and family wishes by culturally competent nurses to enhance patient-centric rituals.

Appendix 67.2

NIH research workshop on symptoms in terminal illness—executive summary

Patients at the end of life experience many of the same symptoms and syndromes, regardless of their underlying medical condition.

Pain is the most obvious example, but others are difficult breathing (dyspnea), transient episodes of confusion and loss of concentration (cognitive disturbances and delirium), and loss of appetite and muscle wasting (cachexia), as well as nausea, fatigue, and depression. Taken together, these and other symptoms add significantly to the suffering of patients and their families, and to the costs and burden of their medical care. Yet in many cases the symptoms could be treated or prevented.

Pain, for example, is a multibillion-dollar public health problem in the United States. More than half of all cancer patients experience pain related to their disease or its treatment. Similarly, half of all cancer patients and 70% of all hospice patients experience shortness of breath in the last weeks of life. Yet dyspnea remains underdiagnosed and undertreated. Forty percent of all patients experience cognitive disturbances during the final days of life, and high numbers of terminally ill patients experience cachexia regardless of their primary disease. Significantly, these symptoms occur not in isolation but in clusters, with most patients experiencing combinations of symptoms that vary greatly in their prevalence and severity, as well as in the suffering they cause.

Basic research has improved understanding of the underlying mechanisms of symptoms that are commonly experienced at the end of life, particularly with respect to pain. Clinical research has in some cases translated this knowledge into new drugs and other interventions that can effectively relieve or prevent these symptoms, even if the underlying disease cannot be cured. However, there remain a number of important gaps in knowledge.

Clinical care would benefit from an integrative, multidisciplinary research initiative that brings basic and clinical researchers together to address the constellation of symptoms at the end of life. The following areas should receive priority:

- Epidemiology—There is a need for better data on the incidence and combinations of symptoms that are experienced at the end of life in specific populations. Epidemiological data will demonstrate the magnitude and costs of the problem and suggest specific topics for basic and clinical research.

- Basic research—Additional research is needed on the mechanisms and interactions of these symptoms, including biochemical, neuronal, endocrine, and immune approaches. The possibility of common factors, mechanisms, and pathways across different symptoms should be examined. There is also a need for research on the mechanism of action of successful therapies, with particular attention to the role of opioid receptors. This research could lead to therapies that are better targeted and more selective in their action, and thus produce fewer side effects.

- Clinical research—Because these symptoms have multiple determinants, and occur in clusters, successful interventions will also be multifactorial, including behavioral as well as pharmacological approaches. Combination therapies and off-label drugs should be explored. Researchers should be alert to differences in outcome based on age, gender, and underlying disease. Interventions to mobilize psychosocial and spiritual resources may be of help in mediating the perception and interpretation of symptoms. The goal of research should be to test a wide range of interventions that could be successfully implemented in the home or hospice, as well as in the hospital.

- Methodology—Researchers need better tests for diagnosing and assessing the level of severity of these symptoms, as well as

for monitoring the effectiveness of interventions. Standardized terminology and definitions of symptoms should be established. Particular attention should be paid to validating subjective and nonverbal measures. Better data and tools are also needed for evaluating outcomes, in order to determine costs and strengthen accountability for the quality of care at the end of life. It is important to develop and use measures that reflect the subjective experience of the effects of symptoms on quality of life.

Research is also needed on the ethical issues that may be barriers to research at the end of life, including the needs and protection of vulnerable populations, especially the role of privacy during this important phase of life. Attention must be paid to community and individual preferences about the relative value of symptom management at different points in the dying trajectory, and to the development of comprehensive strategies for early detection and treatment of the full range of symptoms at the end of life—an approach that will reduce costs as well as burdens, while preserving the patient's dignity and quality of life.

Recommendations for research on specific symptoms

The following preamble for the recommendations reflected the consensus of the entire workshop:

> To adequately address symptom control in the terminally ill, an important first step is to invest resources in the development of new methodologies for assessing symptoms and evaluating treatments. These tools will allow us to elucidate the extent of the problem and to set national priorities to improve quality of life for those facing life-limiting illness.

Pain

1. Epidemiology—There is still a great need for epidemiological data on the incidence and types of pain at the end of life. Research in this area will provide direction for researchers regarding what specific topics should be tackled next.
2. Treatment—There is a clear need to discover new drugs for the treatment of pain, including analgesic combinations. Neuropathic pain, because of its incidence and burden, should be a particular priority. There should also be studies of the relationship between disease, pain, and suffering at the end of life, which would also include psychosocial mediators. Clinical trials groups should be developed to study promising interventions.
3. Measurement—Methods should be developed for collecting valid data on pain in the home, in nursing homes, and so on, possibly using telephones or computer technology. Measurement of other outcomes of subjective experience, such as the suffering caused by pain, should also be developed and utilized.

Dyspnea

1. Epidemiology—What are the incidence and impact of dyspnea in different populations? There is some information about dyspnea in patients with cancer or chronic obstructive pulmonary disease (COPD), but almost none about patients with cardiac disease or other terminal conditions.
2. Mechanisms—Relatively little is known about the various determinants of dyspnea, including respiratory muscle strength, exercise capacity, respiratory controller, gas exchange, and psychosocial factors. Neurobiological models, like those developed for pain, will be useful, but the overall approach must be

integrative. The determinants are almost certainly multifactorial, necessitating multidisciplinary strategies.

3. Measurement—Research is needed to refine available instruments and develop new ones for measuring both the causes of symptoms and the effects of treatments. There is at present no standardized approach for assessing the degree of dyspnea in a given disease (e.g., chronic vs. acute, COPD vs. cancer). The goal would be to formulate guidelines for optimal assessment, which would point to optimal treatment.

4. Treatment—Numerous potential treatments are available, but there is little information on their relative effectiveness. Particular attention should be given to the choice and timing of anxiolytics, phenothiazines, oxygen, opiates, and exercise. Attention should also be given to the timing and management of terminal weaning (removal of ventilation), including the role of families.

The collaborative and integrative nature of this research is well suited to sponsorship and funding by NIH. It would be useful, for example, for the various NIH Institutes to sponsor a series of joint workshops that would characterize the clinical experience and impact of therapies on dyspnea in diseases other than lung cancer.

Cognitive disturbances

There is a considerable amount of epidemiological data on delirium already, and although it might be useful to gather additional information on specific patient populations, this symptom is known to be underrecognized and undertreated. Consequently, the research priorities in this symptom area are as follows:

1. Measurement—Research is needed to enhance the recognition of delirium in different treatment settings (homes, hospices, hospitals), including common diagnostic criteria and terminology. Also needed are better instruments to describe and rate the severity and course of episodes of delirium. This research will lead to a better understanding of the phenomenology of delirium—its signs, patterns, and subtypes—which in turn should produce benefits in terms of newer, more sensitive, and more effective treatments.

2. Treatment—Two aspects of treatment research deserve simultaneous attention. First, there should be randomized, placebo-controlled trials to systematically assess the efficacy of currently available therapies as well as emerging approaches, including both pharmacological and nonpharmacological strategies. Second, there should be research on the relation between the mechanism of action of these therapies and the underlying pathophysiology of delirium. In both cases, studies should include both random populations and populations with delirium of homogeneous etiology.

3. Epidemiology—Finally, there is a need for additional research on the interactions between delirium and other symptoms at the end of life.

4. A concurrent policy issue that must also receive priority attention is the need for guidelines for research in patients who are incapable of giving informed consent because of serious medical illness.

Cachexia

1. Epidemiology—High priority should go to epidemiological studies of anorexia-cachexia, to establish the magnitude of the problem, its impact on the patient and family, and its costs to society. However, it is important that cachexia not be studied in isolation from other symptoms. If the ultimate goal of cachexia research is prevention and early intervention, then it would be useful to conduct studies that examine the epidemiology of several related symptoms (e.g., pain, dyspnea, delirium) at an earlier stage in their development.

2. Mechanisms—Basic and clinical research on cachexia should be done in parallel. Basic research should emphasize the interactions among multiple underlying pathophysiological mechanisms, both central and peripheral, including biochemical, neuronal, metabolic, endocrine, and immunological. Research is also needed on the varying clinical manifestations of these mechanisms, both neuropsychiatric and gastrointestinal. This calls for a multidisciplinary approach.

3. Treatment—Similarly, because it is unlikely that any single therapeutic intervention will be successful, clinical research should emphasize multiple combination therapies that include nutritional, pharmacological, and nonpharmacological components. Combination therapies should be evaluated for their effects on other symptoms such as pain, dyspnea, and delirium. Particular attention should also be paid to differences in outcome based on age, gender, and underlying disease. In considering drug trials, NIH should concentrate on studies that would not otherwise be funded by drug companies.

Given the wide range of mechanisms and therapeutic strategies in cachexia, it would be useful to convene a preliminary, integrative workshop that would include both basic and clinical researchers.

Cross-cutting recommendations

Methods issues that need to be addressed in all four symptom areas include the following:

1. Statistical handling of missing data.
2. Proxy reporting for subjective symptoms.
3. Outcome measures that indicate quality care.
4. Ethics issues are also important. What are the barriers to research at the end of life, including the needs and expectations of vulnerable populations? What are community and individual preferences with respect to symptom management of dying persons?
5. Economics questions include the direct and indirect costs and burdens of symptoms.

References

1. Remington R, Buck HG, Buck KJ, et al. Hospice and Palliative Nurses Association 2012–2015 research agenda. J Hosp Palliat Nurs. 2012;14(2):158–163.
2. Payne SA, JM Turner. Research methodologies in palliative care: a bibliometric analysis. Palliat Med. 2008;22(4):336–342.
3. Kristjanson LJ, Coyle N. Qualitative research. In: Doyle D, Hanks G, Cherny N, Calman K (eds.), Oxford Textbook of Palliative Medicine. 4th ed. Oxford: Oxford University Press; 2010:395–402.
4. Grant M, Sun V, Fujinami R, Sidhu R, Otis-Green S, Juarez G, et al. Family caregiver burden, skills preparedness, and quality of life in non-small-cell lung cancer. Oncol Nurs Forum. 2013;40(4):337–346.
5. Cox-North P, Doorenbos A, Shannon S, Scott J, Curtis J. The transition to end-of-life care in end stage liver disease. J Hosp Palliat Nurs. 2013;15(4):209–215. doi: 10.1097/NJH.obo13e318289f4bo.
6. Freeman, B. CARES: an acronym organized tool for the care of the dying. J Hosp Palliat Nurs. 2013;15(3):147–153.
7. Krok J, Baker T, McMillan S. Age difference in the presence of pain and psychological distress in younger and older cancer patients. J Hosp Palliat Nurs. 2013;15(2):107–113. doi: 10.1097/NJH.obo13e31826bfb63.

8. Bailey C, Froggatt K, Field D, Krishnasamy M. The nursing contribution to qualitative research in palliative care 1990–1999: a critical evaluation. J Adv Nurs. 2002;40(1):48–60.

9. Benoliel JQ. Death influence in clinical practice: a course for graduate students. In: Benoliel JC (ed.), Death Education for the Health Professional. Washington, DC: Hemisphere; 1982:31–50.

10. Benoliel JQ. Health care providers and dying patients: critical issues in terminal care. Omega. 1987;18:341–363.

11. National Institutes of Health. Symptoms in Terminal Illness: A Research Workshop. September 22–23, 1997. Available at: http://www.nih.gov/ninr/end-of-life.htm (accessed December 8, 2008).

12. Prince-Paul M, Daly BJ. Moving beyond the anecdotal: identifying the need for evidence-based research in hospice and palliative care. Home Healthc Nurs. 2008;26(4):214–219; quiz 20-1.

13. Morrison RS, Maroney-Galin C, Kralovec PD, Meier DE. The growth of palliative care programs in United States hospitals. J Palliat Med. 2005;8(6):1127–1134.

14. Flemming K, Adamson J, Atkin K. Improving the effectiveness of interventions in palliative care: the potential role of qualitative research in enhancing evidence from randomized controlled trials. Palliat Med. 2008;22(2):123–131.

15. Koczywas M, Williams AC, Cristea M, Reckamp K, Grannis F, Tiep B, et al. Longitudinal changes in function, symptom burden, and quality of life in patients with early-stage lung cancer. Ann Surg Oncol. 2012. Published online November 10, 2012. doi 10.1245/s10434-012-2741-4.

16. Kelly K, Thrane S, Virani R, Malloy P, Ferrell B. Expanding palliative care nursing education in California: the ELNEC geriatric project. Int J Palliat Nurs. 2011;17(4):188–194.

17. Ritchie CS, Zulman DM. Research priorities in geriatric palliative care: multimorbidity. J Palliat Med. 2013;16:843–847.

18. American Geriatric Society Panel on Chronic Pain in Older Persons. AGS Clinical Guidelines: Management of Persistent Pain in Older Persons. 2009. Available at: http://www.americangeriatrics.org/health_care_professionals/clinical_practice/clinical_guidelines_recommendations/persistent_pain_executive_summary (accessed June 19, 2013).

19. Calman K. Ethical issues. In: Doyle D, Hanks G, Cherny N, Calman K, eds. Oxford Textbook of Palliative Medicine. Oxford: Oxford University Press; 2010:277–280.

20. Kapo J, Morrison LJ, Liao S. Palliative care for the older adult. J Palliat Med. 2007;10:185–209.

21. Ritchie CS, Currow DC, Abernethy AP, Kutner JS. Multisite studies offer a solution to recruitment challenges in palliative care studies. J Palliat Med. 2013;16:225.

22. Jimenez R, Zhang B, Joffe S, Nilsson M, Rivera L, Mutchler J, et al. Clinical trial participation among ethnic/racial minority and majority patients with advanced cancer: what factors most influence enrollment? J Palliat Med. 2013;16:256–262.

23. Gelfman LP, Du Q, Morrison RS. An update: NIH research funding for palliative medicine 2006 to 2010. J Palliat Med. 2013;16:125–129.

24. Hanson LC, Rowe C, Wessell K, Caprio A, Winzelberg G, Beyea A, Bernard SA. Measuring palliative care quality for seriously ill hospitalized patients. J Palliat Med. 2012;15:798–804.

25. Cheung YB, Goh C, Thumboo J, Khoo KS, Wee J. Variability and sample size requirements of quality-of-life measures: a randomized study of three major questionnaires. J Clin Oncol. 2005; 23(22): 4936–4944.

26. Ferrans CE. Differences in what quality-of-life instruments measure. J Natl Cancer Inst. 2007;(37):22–26.

27. Grant M, Wiencek C, Virani R, Uman G, Munevar C, Malloy P, et al. End-of-life care education in acute and critical care the California ELNEC project. AACN Adv Crit Care. 2013;24(2):121–129.

28. Steinhauser KE, Clipp EC, Hays JC, et al. Identifying, recruiting, and retaining seriously-ill patients and their caregivers in longitudinal research. Palliat Med. 2006;20(8):745–754.

29. Granda-Cameron C, Viola SR, Lynch MP, Polomano RC. Measuring patient-oriented outcomes in palliative care: functionality and quality of life. Clin J Oncol Nurs. 2008;12(1):65–77.

30. Field M, Cassel C. Approaching Death: Improving Care at the End of Life. Committee on Care at the End of Life. Washington, DC: Institutes of Medicine, National Academy Press; 1997.

31. Doyle D, Hanks G, Cherny N, Calman K, eds. Oxford Textbook of Palliative Medicine. 4th ed. Oxford: Oxford University Press; 2010.

32. Kaasa S, Loge JH. Quality of life in palliative care: principles and practice. Palliat Med. 2003;17(1):11–20.

33. NIH Announces Updated Criteria for Evaluating Research Grant Applications. Notice Number: NOT-OD-05-002. October 12, 2004. Available at: http://grants.nih.gov/grants/guide/notice-files/NOT-OD-05-002.html (accessed May 3, 2013).

34. Steele R, Derman S, Cadell S, Davies B, Siden H, Straatman L. Families' transition to a Canadian paediatric hospice. Part one: Planning a pilot study. Int J Palliat Nurs. 2008;14(5):248–256.

35. Steele R, Derman S, Cadell S, Davies B, Siden H, Straatman L. Families' transition to a Canadian paediatric hospice. Part two: Results of a pilot study. Int J Palliat Nurs. 2008;14(6):287–295.

36. Ferrell BR, Nail IM, Mooney K, et al. Applying for Oncology Nursing Society and Oncology Nursing Foundation grants. Oncol Nurs Forum. 1989;16:728–730.

37. Ferrell B, Baird P. Deriving meaning and faith in caregiving. Semin Oncol Nurs. 2012;28(4):256–261. doi:10.1016/j.soncn.2012.09.008.

38. The National Institutes of Health, the National Institute of Nursing Research. Building Momentum: The Science of End-of-Life and Palliative Care. A Review of Research Trends and Funding, 1997–2010. 2013. http://www.ninr.nih.gov/sites/www.ninr.nih.gov/files/NINR-Building-Momentum-508.pdf

39. Gelfman LP, Morrison RS. Research funding for palliative medicine. J Palliat Med. 2008;11(1):36–43.

40. Otis-Green S, Ferrell B, Borneman T, Puchalski C, Uman G, Garcia A. Integrating spiritual care within palliative care: an overview of nine demonstration projects. J Palliat Med. 2012;15(2):154–163.

41. National Consensus Project for Quality Palliative Care. Clinical Practice Guidelines for Quality Palliative Care. 3rd ed. 2013. Available at: http://www.nationalconsensusproject.org (accessed on July 1, 2013).

42. Hughes A, Gudmundsdottir M, Davies B. Everyday struggling to survive: experience of the urban poor living with advanced cancer. Oncol Nurs Forum. 2007;34(6):1113–1118.

43. Penz K, Duggleby W. It's different in the home: the contextual challenges and rewards of providing palliative nursing care in community settings. J Hosp Palliat Nurs. 2012;14(5):363–373. doi: 10.1097/NJH.obo13e3182553acb.

44. Carpenter J, Berry P. Refractory cancer pain in a nursing home resident. J Hosp Palliat Nurs. 2012;14(8):516–521.

45. American Association of Colleges Nursing. End-Of Life Nursing Education Consortium. 2002. Available from http://www.aacn.nche.edu/elnec (accessed July 9, 2013).

CHAPTER 68

Enhancing team effectiveness

Shirley Otis-Green and Iris Cohen Fineberg

With our family spread across the country, keeping the flow of information straight was really difficult. I was the only one living nearby, and was trying to juggle all of my family and work responsibilities while also visiting my mother in the hospital every day. The palliative care team helped us find a way to stay connected about what was going on for my mother. The team worked really well together, so we all got the same information, without the confusing mixed messages we had had in the past.

A 48-year-old son of patient in a cardiac care unit

Key points

- Palliative care is by definition team care. A team approach is necessary to best address the complex multidimensional biopsychosocial-spiritual concerns of patients and their families.

- The National Consensus Guidelines for Quality Palliative Care, the National Quality Forum, and the Institute of Medicine all recommend a team approach as the optimal delivery system for patient-centered and family-focused care.

- Healthcare professionals are socialized in their own unique disciplines yet are expected to work in a team environment. This makes it imperative that healthcare professionals seek opportunities to enhance the team skills necessary for effective communication, shared leadership, conflict resolution, role clarification, and addressing boundary issues and improved clinical care.

- Further research is needed to evaluate what components increase the effectiveness of team composition, leadership style, and interventions for different patient populations and settings, as well as a determination of core team competencies needed by differing staff members and how best to prepare participants for effective family meetings.

Overview

The National Consensus Project (NCP)[1] Guidelines for Quality Palliative Care, the National Quality Forum (NQF),[2] and multiple Institute of Medicine (IOM) reports[3–5] all recommend a team approach as the optimal way to provide patient-centered and family-focused care, yet our current socialization of professionals remains discipline-specific. This chapter will provide readers an opportunity to consider various strategies useful to increase team effectiveness. The use of family meetings is highlighted as an important palliative care team intervention.

Professional socialization and models of teamwork

An effective palliative care team has a collective identity and shared goals of care, recognizing that the patient and family are the "ultimate authority" whose perspective must be integrated in all assessment, implementation, and evaluation plans.[6] The complex multidimensional concerns associated with serious illness call for an integrated and collaborative team approach to care delivery to maximize opportunities to address the wide range of potential patient and family needs.[1] Palliative care teams ideally include physicians, nurses, social workers, spiritual care professionals and others with the shared goal of providing quality, comprehensive, person-centered and family-focused care. A team perspective means that individuals have consciously come together with a shared identity to address a common goal. This shared identity differentiates them from a mob (a loose grouping of people with no shared purpose); an ad hoc group (that comes together for a specified need and has typically a reactionary focus); or a single-discipline work group.

Teams exist along a continuum from a multidisciplinary team (typically a consultation-based model, with information shared passively through the medical record); an interdisciplinary team (a more collaborative model but most frequently physician or nurse led) or a transdisciplinary/interprofessional team (with intense collaboration and interaction, shared decision-making, and the recognition that there will be significant role overlap).[7]

This transdisciplinary (the term used more commonly in the United States) or interprofessional (the term more frequently used in Europe and Canada) model invites professionals to share responsibility for team outcomes, teach and learn from each other, and collaborate closely together to meet patient-identified goals and replaces hierarchical decision-making with consensus-based decisions that are reflective of the needs of the individual patient and family.[8,9] Transdisciplinary teams seek to exploit discipline diversity as a strategy to best address the complex biopsychosocial-spiritual needs of patients and their families.[10,11] This transdisciplinary approach to care evolved from the hospice philosophy with anthropological and educational roots and was adopted first in healthcare by pediatric[12] and geriatric[13] care providers. Bruder[12] describes this approach in more detail:

> A transdisciplinary approach requires the team members to share roles and systematically cross discipline boundaries. The primary purpose of this approach is to pool and integrate the expertise of team members so that more efficient and comprehensive assessment and intervention services may be provided. The communication style in this type of team involves continuous give-and-take between all members . . . on a regular, planned basis. Professionals from different disciplines teach, learn, and work together to accomplish a common set of intervention goals . . . The role differentiation between disciplines is defined by the needs of the situation rather than by discipline-specific characteristics. Assessment, intervention, and evaluation are carried out jointly by designated members of the team.[12(p. 61)]

As chronic illnesses increase and the biopsychosocial-spiritual model evolves, healthcare systems are challenged to adapt to changing contexts and diversity of expectations. Flexible boundaries and blended roles are expected and accepted based on a recognition of clinical self-awareness regarding limitations of one's skills and scope of practice. Palliative care teams are evolving now in settings where systems were designed and clinicians were trained to work in the traditional medical model that focused on acute situations.[14] This creates opportunities for new models of care delivery to be evaluated for effectiveness in different environments.

Depending on the setting, team membership might include physicians, nurses, social workers, spiritual care professionals, a variety of integrative therapists (including a range of professionals skilled in the expressive arts), dieticians, occupational therapists, pharmacists, physiotherapists, psychologists, bereavement professionals, child-life specialists, volunteers, and the patients and families themselves. Each of these professionals was socialized within their discipline and area of specialization, which results in boundary and turf issues that need to be addressed if the team is to be maximally effective. Professionals working together in teams come to that experience with training from their own disciplines, with their own theoretical perspective and culture.[15–17] Each discipline conveys to its students and members the norms, expectations, and skills of that profession.[20] Healthcare professionals typically have little formal education in team function and collaboration and may be unaware of normal team processes.[18,19]

This process of professional socialization, often subtle and unnoticed, teaches people about how to behave as a member of his or her specific discipline. Although some of this teaching is formal and explicit, much of it is conveyed by less obvious mediums such as our observations in our personal experiences and in the media, modeling of behaviors by senior colleagues, and informal discussions.[21] As a result of our professional education being separate and specific to each discipline within healthcare, most of us know relatively little about how other colleagues on the team were trained and socialized, both generally and specifically in relation to teamwork and collaboration.[22] And we know even less about the unofficial yet powerful socialization that our colleagues have received in clinical settings outside of the formal classroom. Yet, understanding that each profession socializes its

members differently is critical to realizing that the behaviors we see in other team members and behaviors that they see in us may be a reflection of deeply embedded professional norms in addition to individual views. At the same time, we must be careful to avoid stereotyping a colleague based on their professional group. It is natural to make assumptions about why people behave as they do, but making such assumptions leads us then to react in particular (and potentially prejudicial) ways (for example, we may assume that a team member's dominating approach to the team results from a lack a respect for colleagues' contributions when it may be a result of professional socialization that equates leadership and quick decision-making with a demonstration of responsibility).

If we refrain from making assumptions about why someone behaves as they do, we can use the opportunity to learn more from them about what is behind their behavior or viewpoint. Occasions where differences among team members come to light can then serve as opportunities to engage the entire team in a discussion about the norms and teachings of their professions.[23] Thus, differences may transform to strengthening opportunities for the team, especially as the team builds shared views centered on the needs of patients. Learning about the professional socialization of our team members can provide important insights into why people behave as they do, what unspoken assumptions might influence team behavior, and what areas of teamwork might be helpful to explore for the team to optimize its functioning.[22]

It is useful to remember that working in a team environment brings together a group of disciplines, each from a different professional culture.[24] If, for example, we were bringing together a group of people from different countries to work together, we would likely recognize the importance of setting aside time for intentional learning about each other's backgrounds, norms, expectations, and cultural perspectives. The awareness of cultural differences among our patients encourages us to be more open-minded when faced with a conflict, and perhaps less likely to make premature assumptions about people or their motivations with the goal of enhancing person-centered communication and tailored decision-making.[3] Taking a similar approach to our colleagues and recognizing that team members also bring a variety of professional perspectives and cultural views to the team experience will enhance the process and outcomes of teamwork.[25]

System's perspective/team evolution

Viewing the team as a system can help us to both better understand it and also more effectively influence it. A system's perspective reminds us that in a system, when any part of the system is changed or affected, there is an impact on the rest of the system. This is true for both positive and negative influences. Using the systems perspective helps us to keep in mind that in a team, no one works in isolation (even if there are people who work *as if* they are in isolation). What we do influences those around us, and because of this, we have an opportunity to influence our team toward positive change and greater effectiveness.

Teams are noted to evolve over time in typical patterns. Tuckman[26] developed a framework that postulates that teams begin with a period he characterized as "forming," in which the focus of activity is in team development. During the "storming" period that follows, the various members of the team are coming to terms with the idiosyncrasies of their talents. The "norming" phase is noted as the period during which the team develops standard operating procedures. The "performing" period is the most productive time in the life of the team as members are free to concentrate on the tasks that brought the group together. Work tends to be at its most harmonious during this period. Unfortunately, for many healthcare teams in teaching hospitals, this period is transitory, as new team members are periodically rotated through the team, resulting in frequent disequilibrium as the team adjusts to each person's coming and going.

Support for a team approach in palliative care

A consensus of leading organizations and experts recommend a coordinated interdisciplinary team approach as the best way of delivering person-centered and family-focused palliative care. The NCP[1] developed evidence-based guidelines that validate the team focus as an ideal strategy to best meet the eight domains identified as necessary for quality palliative care. The eight domains are:

- ◆ Structure and processes of care
- ◆ Physical aspects of care
- ◆ Psychological and psychiatric aspects of care
- ◆ Social aspects of care
- ◆ Spiritual, religious, and existential aspects of care
- ◆ Cultural aspects of care
- ◆ Care of the patient at the end of life
- ◆ Ethical and legal aspects of care

These domains were adopted in their entirety by the NQF[2] and have been integrated into their 38 preferred practices for the provision of palliative care. The NQF outlines ongoing training and credentialing recommendations for the various members of the team and identifies the benefits of a team approach in developing comprehensive patient-driven care plans. And in 2008, the Institute of Medicine report *Cancer Care for the Whole Patient: Meeting Psychosocial Health Needs*[5] recommended an integrated team approach as the most effective way to meet patient and families' complex, multidimensional concerns.

Common challenges to optimal team functioning

Despite this growing support for a team approach to the delivery of care, there are many challenges to effective team functioning in clinical practice. Prior to instituting actions to foster team effectiveness, it is important to recognize the unique history of each individual healthcare team and the institutional context within which it exists. Each setting brings unique demands, whether critical care, an emergency department, an ambulatory care clinic, a specialized inpatient setting, a long-term care community, a home health agency, or a hospice program.[27]

Attention to improving the functioning of the team calls on members of the team to think about the team as a whole and to dedicate time and group energy to the process of team functioning and team dynamics. Rather than focusing solely on individual professional roles, members of the team collectively determine

the shared vision and mission of the team: vision for the role of the team, vision for the organization of the team, and vision for how the team will function and act. Questions to consider when forging a shared vision may include: How do you want non-team colleagues to view the team? What kind of care do you want this team to provide and to be known for? What does this team see as standards for high-quality functioning for itself? What do team members expect from each other? Although the process of exploring and agreeing on a shared vision and mission may take some time and require reevaluation over time, it is recommended as a worthwhile investment of team effort.

When evaluating an existing team, consider its history of decision-making and its leadership style, its internal communication patterns, and how well it collaborates with others outside the team. Are members of the team considered experts within the institution? It is not uncommon for palliative care consult teams to be perceived by others as adopting an attitude of superiority that may impede collaboration. This unintended view may not be easily recognized by the existing team, but determining how others view the team provides important insights into its overall effectiveness. For those consultation teams that require formal referrals to its services, establishing a baseline measurement of where referrals come from and what types of referrals are missing also provides data for later evaluation of areas of needed growth.

The leadership type of a team has tremendous impact on how the team functions.[28,29] Although different leadership models may work better for different teams, a model that has been noted to foster team effectiveness is one of shared vision and shared accountability.[27] This differs dramatically from the model of hierarchical leadership in which one person "at the top" dictates the actions of the group; this "quarterback" model has been historically common in medicine but is no longer viewed as productive in the arena of palliative care. Team-meeting facilitators encourage positive support and pay attention to those who feel they have less power or status, building in time to regularly debrief and celebrate personal events and the professional accomplishments of one another.

The tendency for most healthcare systems is to default into personal "fiefdoms"[30] with competing and parallel tracks of care versus an integrated delivery of services. Teams constantly struggle with how to share expertise within settings filled with blurred boundaries. Most practitioners have had the experience of working with a professional who behaves like he/she "owns" a patient and may determine all aspects of care that the patient receives; with a tendency to attempt to "protect" the patient from "intrusions" by unwanted others. This can be a challenging dynamic as the remaining team members may feel they are not recognized for their expertise and professional contribution.

Although numerous professionals are caring for a patient, this does not automatically mean that people are functioning as a team.[31] How these care providers relate to each other can differ dramatically. We often see people working in their professional "silo,"[32] a situation where they practice their profession in isolation, not accounting for the holistic view of the patient or what other providers are doing for the patient. Such "silo" work leads to professionals providing parallel but disconnected and uncoordinated care and results in unnecessary gaps and services that may be redundant or competitive, minimizing potential benefit to the patient. The focus of the professionals' actions is on their particular tasks and roles regarding a patient, and although the patient might be getting reasonably "good care" from each individual professional, the focus remains on the clinicians rather than on the patient. The difficulties that arise when professionals' roles overlap and competition develops may be addressed by emphasizing care of the patient as the point of focus.

Teamwork grows from recognizing that differing members of the team will each have strengths and weaknesses, and unique areas of expertise, but that these characteristics do not exclude the place for other team members to offer patients assistance in an area of need to which they can contribute. Thus, while spiritual care might be the special expertise of the chaplain on the team, it may be beneficial for a particular patient to receive care from other team members that allows room for discussion of spiritual issues and concerns. The key to the success of the collaboration is to maintain the focus of the team on the shared goal of the well-being of the patient and family being served.[27]

It is wise to remember that systems are exquisitely designed to achieve the results they routinely get and that change will be resisted by those who are entrenched in and rewarded by the status quo. Implicit challenges to hierarchical decision-making require mutual adaptation, create confusion and ambivalence, and challenge the comfort of conformity. Sharing leadership responsibilities increases professional visibility. Less "powerful" team members may paradoxically resist efforts to increase the transparent accountability that is inherent in more transdisciplinary decision-making team models. This tendency of normal resistance makes change efforts suspect, and motives for change can be frequently misinterpreted.[33]

Healthcare is only recently integrating business and psychology models of change into its institutional change efforts. Gladwell's "Tipping Point"[34] and Hackman's "Leading Teams"[35] use successful business models to illustrate change strategies that have applicability within healthcare. Perhaps most notably, "lean" business principles derived from Toyota manufacturing have been incorporated into healthcare across the globe.[36] Identifying areas of expected resistance will assist one in leveraging change-efforts to achieve maximum team effectiveness.

Poorly functioning teams may suffer from a culture of rivalry, subsystems, scapegoating, and mutual mistrust. In this setting, role confusion and ambiguity can lead to demoralization.[37] If divergent views are not tolerated, then members may remain silent and at risk of becoming a "moral accomplice" to unethical behavior when loyalty to the team replaces loyalty to patient and family. Another danger in teamwork is that one's work becomes exposed, creating the potential for personal vulnerability by critical teammates. Fears may develop on a number of levels: concern that others will demonstrate that they can do "your" job as well as or better than you can, the sense that working closely with people will show them the areas where you feel less confident and able as a professional, the overall sense of vulnerability that accompanies inviting others into your world of practice, and the difficulty of asking others to trust you and having to trust them in return.

Recognizing one's sense of vulnerability is essential for differentiating between the treatment by others and fears of one's own. Equally essential for assuring that a sense of vulnerability does not translate to defensive or self-defeating behavior in the team is a strong understanding of one's role as a professional and the ability to convey that role to others. Confidence in one's role and value should be strengthened by the knowledge that each profession on the team needs the information and expertise of others on the team to practice successfully.

Strategies to enhance team effectiveness

Communication in teams is a critical factor impacting the functioning of the team.[38,39] As in any relationship, team communication has a tremendous impact on how team members perceive and understand each other, how coordinated the actions of the team are, how responsive the team can be, and how the team is perceived by people outside the team. Most critically, team communication has an impact on the quality and experience of patient care. Poor communication is a tremendous barrier to team behavior, making the goal of excellent communication a crucial one for any team. Communication may be enhanced using numerous approaches:

- Scheduling regular team meetings
- Finding an uninterrupted space for the team to meet
- Creating a structured approach to the team meeting
- Building in dedicated time during team meetings for discussion of team issues
- Creating ground rules for communication within the team, such as agreeing to disagree respectfully and ensuring that all members of the team have an opportunity to speak
- Giving specific attention to improving team listening skills
- Planned mini-"retreats" to periodically process team issues

Negotiation is another ongoing and central activity in teamwork. The term "negotiation" should be understood as an iterative process where multiple parties each try to have their needs met. It is not inherently adversarial though some people perceive it as such. The most effective negotiation keeps in focus an agreed-on goal, such as the best interests of the patient. With such a focus, although team members may have different approaches to the ultimate goal, discussion has the opportunity to lead to a productive outcome. Together with the ability to effectively communicate and negotiate, several additional qualities are associated with productive teams.[40,41] These attributes include:

- Clear goals and mission
- Sufficient resources including people, time, and money
- Individual expertise and a commitment to reflective practice
- Open communication and a commitment to mutual cooperation and collaboration[42]
- Commitment to both process and outcome
- Continuous evaluation of roles, norms, values, and performance
- Trust and support
- Strong leadership through empowerment of all
- Organizational support
- Systems thinking and synergy

By contrast, vicarious traumatization from chronic caregiving puts palliative care teams at special risk for members to suffer from compassion fatigue. Attrition occurs when team members feel that their talents and contributions are underappreciated and poorly rewarded. Teams with a tendency to "default" to the side of mistrust, with members' jumping to assumptions and assuming the worst about their colleagues suffer from higher rates of burnout and become decreasingly effective. Being a part of a poorly functioning team invites a downward spiral of less investment in team outcomes and poorer performance and less risk taking. Conversely, more effective teams have a willingness to "roll up one's sleeves and do what needs to be done" to achieve identified shared patient goals.

This high degree of functional nimbleness is associated with role flexibility and a conscious playing to team members' strengths while supporting other members' weaknesses (without focus on fault finding or blaming). Developing a shared network of support with like-minded individuals whom you trust and respect provides an antidote to compassion fatigue by increasing members' self-esteem and sense of self-efficacy, but requires each team member's personal and professional commitment to accountable and reflective practice.

Trust and mutual respect need to be thoughtfully built and nurtured. Just as we recognize that building a trusting relationship with patients and their families is critical to effective care, so we can understand that building trust with the team will have a major influence on the team's capacity to function well. It involves taking the time to become familiar with team colleagues as people, taking an interest in their work and their perspectives. It involves building shared experiences that enable team members to support each other and share the challenges of providing high-quality palliative care. Trust also involves being able to appreciate differences and knowing that those differences among colleagues will be handled with respect.[28]Authenticity is important if teams are to be robust and long-lived. Members do best when they feel good about their skills and feel that there is a good "fit" with what they have to give and what the team values. This authentic use of team member's individual gifts and talents comes when there is a match between team goals and a member's personal vision.

Conflicts among team members will naturally occur and require a commitment to constructive conflict resolution if they are not to impede team functioning:

- Identify symptoms, degree, and sources of conflict: competing organizational priorities, interpersonal differences, differing agendas and time constraints, differing conceptual approaches to problem solving, differing commitments, fear of change, etc.

- Explore root causes rather than having an overfocus on symptoms (identify process barriers and systems challenges)

- Explore a range of possible outcomes then identify a preferred outcome and clarify who should become involved in process

- Consider who is the "community of practice;" (both intrinsic and extrinsic members)

Teams operate best when members have a shared vision of "success." If the purpose of a palliative care team is to improve patient and family quality of life and enhance functioning, then team success should be measured accordingly. Analysis of how effectively members communicate with others (both within the team and outside of it) becomes an important indicator for team success. Establishing shared accountability for such successes requires consensual goals. Developing a perspective of "we're all in this together" (with shared credit and shared responsibility) creates an atmosphere of trust. A quick measurement of the degree to which members have a team perspective occurs when compliments or complaints are given by others regarding a team interaction. If members respond with "thanks, our team did a great job" to what could have been a personal compliment, then a team culture is in place. Similarly, if members accept accusations of blame to an individual instead of reframing the situation as an opportunity for the team to learn from its mistakes and do better next time, then the culture of the team is in need of improvement.

One of the most effective strategies for team building occurs through shared learning that supports professional development of individuals and the team. Professionals are adult learners who benefit from practical and interactive learning opportunities for skills building and reflection.[4,43] Professional education for teams can occur through numerous ways, such as:

- Regularly scheduled team trainings, such as rotating monthly "lunch and learn" sessions or annually scheduled team "retreats," offer ongoing opportunities to share responsibility to develop the training schedule, and identify topics and provide curriculum and content. These regularly occurring trainings or round-robin facilitated lectures can be focused on the internal educational needs of the team or can be an outreach effort (in the form of inservices or grand rounds) by the team toward the larger institution. In either case, increasing an understanding by constituents of what services the team offers and how the team can best be used enhances team effectiveness expands the team's common core of knowledge and increases individual expertise. The goal becomes to expand common core of knowledge while increasing individual expertise.

- Mutual mentorship encourages the transmission of expertise across disciplines and provides concrete opportunities for more junior staff to benefit from the wisdom of senior staff. Adopting a universal mentorship model demonstrates the team's commitment to support lifelong learning and institutionalizes the value of peer-to-peer training. In recognition that every team member has an area of expertise valuable to the team at large, all members are expected to develop mentorships, whether with students or colleagues. Mentorship can enhance member skills in regard to clinical care, research, patient and professional education, and advocacy skills. Team members can be encouraged to both have and be a mentor (identifying opportunities for mentorship of students, etc.).

- Journal clubs are a frequently used method to enhance team learning. These lend themselves to transdisciplinary education sessions where representatives from the differing disciplines share the responsibility to identify topics of interest and select evidence-based articles to share with the wider team. Rotating these responsibilities increases the relevancy of the materials to the greater whole.

- Inviting guests from differing disciplines to team inservices allows team members opportunities to learn from established leaders in fields outside their own. For those teams without honoraria funds, creativity may be called for in identifying speakers. Teams have successfully established networks of shared educational efforts with other community organizations to exchange presenters. Others have coordinated presentations with established organizationally funded continuing educational offerings to fold in an extra engagement at lessened or no additional expense. This strategy can allow a team the opportunity to have small-group interaction with big-name speakers for little additional institutional expense.

♦ A schedule of rotating leadership of patient-rounds or team meetings ensures that all members of a team have an opportunity to hone their leadership skills. Although initially awkward for some, developing a policy of shared leadership responsibilities demonstrates a team's commitment to honor the expertise of each team member in a concrete and tangible way. Importantly, this provides supervisors with an opportunity to identify leadership skills-training needs of supervisees that otherwise might be difficult to directly ascertain.

♦ Rotation of responsibilities for continuous quality improvement activities demonstrates the team's commitment to developing an evidence base to improve the delivery of care by each team member. Too often, the collection of data becomes optional for certain team members. Developing a broad definition of what constitutes "research" and integrating its responsibilities to the team as a whole ensures that concepts such as "continuous quality improvement" are not just the personal responsibility of a few, but a genuine priority of the palliative care team as a whole.

♦ Encouraging professional development through the attendance of courses and conferences outside of the institution or agency with an expectation that members return to the team and present "lessons learned" from the experience. This expectation that each member will contribute to the education of others through regular presentations within and beyond the team codifies the team's commitment to lifelong learning and recognizes that the best learning tool is the expectation that one will teach the skill being learned.

♦ Creating structured and intentional opportunities for periodic team debriefing and reflection (such as through Schwartz Center Rounds).[44]

Teams, like other organic systems, benefit from periodic reassessments. Setting aside time to reexamine the balance of power within the team assures that more timely adjustments can be made. Consideration of how vertical or lateral leadership and group decision-making has become allows the team to periodically recalibrate and maintain team integrity. Developing a consensus regarding what aspects of care are the shared responsibility of all team members will require frequent revisiting. Patient advocacy, cultural sensitivity, education, anticipatory guidance, and screening for pain and symptom distress are examples of concepts that may be recognized as shared responsibilities of all members of the team. Decisions about what the patient's role is in the team's collaborative dynamic will require frequent reassessment due to the myriad of factors that influence this (including culture, age, access to needed resources, etc.). This is important because, for many patients, the team is invisible and must be consciously brought into the patient and family's awareness.

Family meetings as a team intervention

Family meetings, (also called family conferences), serve as one of the most powerful communication tools available to palliative care teams.[45–48] Such meetings often involve the patient (if he or she is able to participate), multiple family members, and the care team. Family meetings are recommended as an optimal palliative care team intervention, especially useful with decision-making and in identifying goals of care. Altilio, Otis-Green, and Dahlin[49] provide concrete examples of how family meetings can be used to create a plan of care that meets the social aspects of care domain as recommended by the 2013 NCP Guidelines. Family meetings are typically held at times of transition, such as when there are changes in treatment or changes in prognosis.[50] Those patients with complicated care needs, such as those with multiple comorbidities, those for whom English is not their primary language, or those who are facing end of life are especially good candidates to benefit from a family meeting to identify shared goals of care.[51]

Family meetings offer a tremendous opportunity for coordination both within the team and between the team with other care providers and the patient and family.[52,53] Meetings usually have a particular purpose or goal, although the vision of the agenda may differ among team members and between team members, the patient, and the family.

The most effective communication from the professionals in a family meeting occurs when the team members have come together prior to the meeting to discuss their shared goals for the meeting, potential concerns, and anticipated roles of different team members at the meeting.[54] A coordinated approach from the team is important to the family meeting in a number of ways. It creates a sense of cohesion and confidence in the team that may be reassuring to patients and families. It demonstrates a holistic approach to the care of the patient and family, recognizing the complexity of people and their experiences. Further, it helps to build the basis for a shared understanding in the family meeting. Perhaps most significant about a coordinated team approach to the family meeting is what it prevents. It minimizes the likelihood that team members will argue with each other or present conflicting information in such a way that burdens stressed patients and families with team "issues." In the family meeting, the results of positive collaborative teamwork can be profound and invigorating to all who participate.

Because family meetings so often focus on difficult decision-making and education regarding complex medical options, it can be useful to structure the meeting to allow differing team members an opportunity to address each of the various issues that need to be covered. Attention to the medical indications and treatment options, identification of patient preferences, clarification regarding the social situation and family context, and attention to the quality-of-life issues important for this particular patient and family at this particular moment in time can be helpful formatting devices to ensure that the family meeting ends with an action plan that is meaningful and timely.

Potential directions for research

Although there is a growing evidence base for the effectiveness of team interventions in healthcare, more research is needed[55,56]:

♦ How do we measure the "quality" of teamwork provided? How do we evaluative the effectiveness of team interventions?[57]

♦ What is the role of team research?

♦ Is patient satisfaction with the team an adequate proxy for evaluating quality of care?[58]

- What team composition is most effective (including considerations of cost)?[59]

- What is the best way to prepare participants (including professionals, patients and families) for their roles in family meetings?

- What core competencies are necessary for each discipline to maximize team effectiveness? How should these be taught and evaluated?[60–61]

- What patient populations or settings are most helped by an integrated team approach to care?[62]

Summary

Effective transdisciplinary palliative care teams require fluid boundaries and a blending of areas of diverse expertise.[3,63] Clinicians must assess and intervene from their own individual expertise with a cross-pollination of ideas, perspectives, and knowledge. The goal is for the patient-family system to experience an enhanced relationship with the team rather than increased numbers of relationships with various team members. Ideally, leadership decisions within the team vary based on knowledge and experience rather than role functions or titles and focus on the needs of the individual patient's care plan. Successful team meetings alternate with a focus on patient care and with meetings focused on team development, team dynamics, processes, and goals.

Patient narrative 1

The complexity of interdisciplinary team work

Ms. G's persistent agitation was again the topic of conversation at the nursing station. Her nurse noted that she was tearful throughout her chemotherapy infusion and reluctant to "open up" regarding the cause of her distress. There was discussion about the possible benefit of referral, but a lack of consensus regarding the appropriate discipline to consult. The hospital had only recently established a palliative care service, and the unit was not confident of how they might assist, since her distress did not seem to be pain based and she was not near death. A new nurse suggested a referral to social work, but a temporary staff nurse thought that they were only called for complex discharge planning purposes. The charge nurse suggested chaplaincy, but there was disagreement regarding whether this was appropriate, as chaplaincy was typically called only when there was a particular religious ritual being requested. Psychology was also considered, but viewed as "too busy" to be readily available before Ms. G's discharge over the weekend. All agreed that contacting Ms. G's physician would just upset the patient, who wanted only to be "left alone." Walking to her car that evening, Ms. G's primary nurse recalled reading an article on "moral distress" and felt frustrated that she had not been able to identify an appropriate referral to address Ms. G's apparent suffering.

- How might Ms. G's primary nurse have handled this situation differently? What is the impact of unresolved moral distress?

- One of the challenges in this scenario is that people often "don't know what they don't know." This can lead to inaccurate assumptions about what services are available. The floor nurses made several assumptions about the limitations of services available to assist them with this patient. Whose "job" is it to ensure that staff have accurate information about what roles and services are available? How do nurses typically learn what services are available to assist them? How realistic is it to expect nurses to seek out additional information regarding other professionals' roles? How do "new" or "temporary" staff learn what is expected of them and whom to call under what circumstances? What roles (if any) do established staff have to assist colleagues in addressing these types of concerns in the future?

- How might the palliative care team address these inaccurate assumptions? How might the palliative care team, social worker, chaplain, or psychologist learn what assumptions others hold about them and clarify their role and services? What happens if they remain unaware of the misconceptions that others hold of their services?

Patient narrative 2

An example of the nurse's role in interdisciplinary team work

Mr. O was a 52-year-old Irish American man being cared for at a university teaching hospital for a recent diagnosis of pancreatic cancer. He had never been hospitalized before and was meeting many healthcare providers, including the palliative care team. Mr. O's wife was with him daily while she continued her full-time job, their four adult children visited on weekends, and many friends filled the visiting hours. Toward the end of one of the palliative care nurse's visits, Mrs. O expressed concern about Mr. O's mental clarity during some of his friends' visits. This was particularly distressing for her given Mr. O's long-time, deep connections with his friends. After further discussion with Mrs. O, the nurse was concerned that Mr. O may be experiencing mental status changes due to his deteriorating condition or his debilitating treatment.

At the meeting of the palliative care team the next morning, the palliative care nurse brought this issue to the attention of the team. The nurse detailed her conversation with Mr. O's wife and provided specific examples of behaviors that the wife had described. She also noted that Mrs. O had not seen these behaviors prior to the patient's current hospitalization. The team then proceeded to discuss an assessment plan to address the situation. Several suggestions arose from the team members, and a multifaceted plan was collaboratively agreed on. The team determined that the nurse and the physician on the team would meet with Mr. O and his wife for an initial mental status assessment. Having established the relationship with Mrs. O and been the person to learn about the mental status changes, the staff nurse was seen as an important team member for the assessment meeting. Further, her thoughtful preliminary gathering of information from Mrs. O enabled the team to make a collaborative and cohesive plan of care.

- Review the phases of teamwork functioning identified by Tuckman (see previous section "Team Evolution"). What phase do you think this team represents? How might the nurse's role have evolved as the team's function changed over time?

- Reflect on the teams that you have been involved in. What differences did you observe as the team evolved? How did the team adjust to these changes? What were some of the challenges that you faced as the team changed?

References

1. National Consensus Project for Quality Palliative Care. Clinical Practice Guidelines for Quality Palliative Care. 3rd ed. http://www.nationalconsensusproject.org Published 2013. Accessed on June 26, 2013.
2. National Quality Forum. National Framework and Preferred Practices for Hospice and Palliative Care: A Consensus Report. http://www.qualityforum.org/Publications/2006/12/A_National_Framework_and_Preferred_Practices_for_Palliative_and_Hospice_Care_Quality.aspx Published 2006. Accessed June 26, 2013.
3. Institute of Medicine. Delivering High Quality Cancer Care: Charting a New Course for a System in Crisis. Washington, DC: The National Academies Press; 2013.
4. Institute of Medicine. Redesigning Continuing Education in the Health Professions. Washington, DC: The National Academies Press; 2010.
5. Institute of Medicine. Cancer Care for the Whole Patient: Meeting Psychosocial Health Needs. Washington, DC: The National Academies Press; 2008.
6. Loscalzo MJ, Von Gunten C. Interdisciplinary team work in palliative care: compassionate expertise for complex illness. In: Chochinov H, Breitbart W (eds.), Handbook of Psychiatry in Palliative Medicine. 2nd ed. New York, NY: Oxford University Press; 2009:172–185.
7. Otis-Green S, Ferrell B, Spolum M, et al. An overview of the ACE project—advocating for clinical excellence: transdisciplinary palliative care education. J Cancer Educ. 2009;24(2):120–126.
8. D'Amour DE, Ferrada-Videla M, Rodriquez LSM, Beaulieu MD. The conceptual basis for the interprofessional collaboration: core concepts and theoretical frameworks. J Interprof Care. 2005; 19(Suppl 1):116–131.
9. McDaniel A, Champion V, Kroenke K. A transdisciplinary training program for behavioral oncology and cancer control scientists. Nurs Outlook.s 2008;56:123–131.
10. Grey M, Connolly C. Coming together, keeping together, working together: interdisciplinary to transdisciplinary research and nursing. Nurs Outlook. 2008;56:102–107.
11. Otis-Green S, Yang E, Lynne L. ACE project—Advocating for Clinical Excellence: creating change in the delivery of palliative care. Omega. 2013;6(1–2):5–19.
12. Bruder MB. Working with members of other disciplines: collaboration for success. In: Wolery M, Wilbers JS (eds.), Including Children with Special Needs in Early Childhood Programs. Washington, DC: National Association for the Education of Young Children; 1994:45–70.
13. Takamura J. Introduction: health teams. In: Campbell LJ, Vivell S (eds.), Interdisciplinary Team Training for Primary Care in Geriatrics: An Educational Model for Program Development and Evaluation. Washington, DC: Government Printing Office; 1985:II:64–II:67.
14. Friedman TC, Bloom AM. When death precedes birth: experience of a palliative care team on a labor and delivery unit. J Palliat Med. 2012;15:274–276.
15. Miller, SE. Professional socialization: a bridge between the explicit and implicit curricula. J Soc Work Educ. 2013;49(3):368–386.
16. Stevenson, K, Seenan, C, Morlan, G, Smith, W. Preparing students to work effectively in interprofessional health and social care teams. Qual Health Care. 2012;20(3):227–230.
17. Weaver SJ, Rosen MA, Salas E, Baum KD, King HB. Integrating the science of team training: guidelines for continuing education. J Contin Educ Health Prof. 2010;30(4):208–220.
18. Supiano KP. Weaving interdisciplinary and discipline-specific content into palliative care education: one successful model for teaching end-of-life care. Omega. 2013;67(1–2):201–206.
19. Lawrie I, Lloyd-Williams M. Training in the interdisciplinary environment. In: Speck P (ed.), Teamwork in Palliative Care: Fulfilling or Frustrating? New York, NY: Oxford University Press; 2006:153–165.
20. Bonifas, RP, Gray, AK. Preparing social work students for interprofessional practice in geriatric health care: insights from two approaches. Educ Gerontol. 2013;39(7):476–490.
21. Horsburgh M, Perkins R, Coyle B, Degeling P. The professional sub-cultures of students entering medicine, nursing and pharmacy programmes. J Interprof Care. 2006;20(4):425–431.
22. Stark D. Teamwork in palliative care: an integrative approach. In: Altilio T, Otis-Green S (eds.), Oxford Textbook of Palliative Social Work. New York, NY: Oxford University Press;2011:415–424.
23. Ekedahl M, Wengstrom Y. Coping processes in a multidisciplinary healthcare team—a comparison of nurses in cancer care and hospital chaplains. Eur J Cancer Care. 2008;17:42–48.
24. Swetenham K, Hegarty M, Grbich C. Refractory suffering: the impact of team dynamics on the interdisciplinary palliative care team. Palliat Support Care. 2011;9:55–62.
25. Terashita-Tan S. Striving for wholeness and transdisciplinary teamwork at a Pacific basin's pain and palliative care department. Omega. 2013;67(1–2):207–212.
26. Tuckman BW. Developmental sequence in small groups. Psychologic Bull. 1965;63(6):384–399.
27. Haugen DF, Nauck F, Caraceni A. The core team and the extended team. In: Hanks G, Cherny N, Christakis N, Fallon M, Kaasa S, Portenoy R (eds.), Oxford Textbook of Palliative Medicine. 4th ed. Oxford, UK: Oxford University Press; 2010:167–176.
28. Xyrichis A, Lowton K. What fosters or prevents interprofessional teamworking in primary and community care?: A literature review. Int J Nurs Stud. 2008;45(1):140–153.
29. Costa L, Poe SS. Nurse-led interdisciplinary teams: challenges and rewards. J Nurs Care Qual. 2008;23:292–295.
30. Herbold RJ. The Fiefdom Syndrome: The Turf Battles That Undermine Careers and Companies—And How to Overcome Them. New York, NY: Doubleday Business; 2004.
31. Blacker S. Deveau C. Social work and interprofessional collaboration in palliative care. Progress in Palliative Care. 2010;18(4):237–243.
32. Curtis JR. Caring for patients with critical illness and their families: the value of the integrated clinical team. Respir Care. 2008;53(4):480–487.
33. Otis-Green S. The Transitions program: existential care in action. J Cancer Educ. 2006;21:23–25.
34. Gladwell M. The Tipping Point: How Little Things Can Make a Big Difference. New York, NY: Little Brown; 2000.
35. Hackman JR. Leading Teams: Setting the Stage for Great Performances. Boston, MA: Harvard Business Press; 2002.
36. Brandao de Souza L. Trends and Approaches in Lean Healthcare: Leadership in Health Services. Bingley, UK: Emerald; 2009.
37. Speck P. Teamwork in Palliative Care Fulfilling or Frustrating. New York, NY: Oxford University Press; 2006.
38. Wittenberg-Lyles E, Goldsmith J, Ferrell B, Ragan S. Communication in Palliative Nursing. New York, NY: Oxford University Press; 2013.
39. Back A, Arnold R, Tulsky J. Mastering Communication with Seriously Ill Patients: Balancing Honesty with Empathy and Hope. New York, NY: Cambridge University Press; 2009.
40. Weaver TE. Enhancing multiple disciplinary teamwork. Nurs Outlook. 2008;56:108–114.
41. Nancarrow SA, Booth A, Ariss S, Smith T, Enderby P, Roots A. Ten principles of good interdisciplinary team work. Hum Resour Health. 2013;11(1):1–11.
42. Karnstrom S. Difficulties in collaboration: a critical incident study of interprofessional healthcare teamwork. J Interprof Care. 2008;22:191–203.
43. Caffarella R, Ratcliff Daffron, S. Planning Programs for Adult Learners: A Practical Guide. 3rd ed. San Francisco: Wiley; 2013.
44. Schwartz Center Rounds. http://www.theschwartzcenter.org/ourprograms/rounds.aspx Accessed June 26, 2013.
45. Hudson P, Quinn K, O'Hanlon B, Aranda S. Family meetings in palliative care: multidisciplinary clinical practice guidelines. BMC Palliat Care. 2008;7:12.
46. Powazki RD, Walsh D, Davis MP, Bauer A. The family conference: how we do it. J Palliat Care. 2006;22(3):240.
47. Azoulay E. The end-of-life family conference: communication empowers. Am J Respir Crit Care Med. 2005;171:803–804.

48. Fineberg IC, Bauer A. Families and family conferencing. In: Altilio T, Otis-Green S (eds.), Oxford Textbook of Palliative Social Work. New York: Oxford University Press; 2011:235–250.

49. Altilio T, Otis-Green S, Dahlin C. Applying the national quality forum preferred practices for palliative and hospice care: a social work perspective. J Soc Work End Life Palliat Care. 2008;4:3–16.

50. Deja K. Social workers breaking bad news: the essential role of an interdisciplinary team when communicating prognosis. J Palliat Med. 2006;9:807–809.

51. Fineberg IC. Social work perspectives on family communication and family conferences in palliative care. Prog Palliat Care. 2010;18:213–220.

52. Kristjanson LJ, Aoun S. Palliative care for families: remembering the hidden patients. Can J Psychiatry. 2004;49(6):359–365.

53. Fineberg IC, Kawashima M, Asch SM. Communication with families facing life-threatening illness: a research-based model for family conferences. J Palliat Med. 2011;14:421–427.

54. Lautrette A, Ciroldi M, Ksibi H, Azoulay E. End-of-life family conferences: rooted in the evidence. Crit Care Med. 2006;34(Suppl 11):364–372.

55. Fernandez R, Vozenilek JA, Hegarty CB, et al. Developing expert medical teams: toward an evidence-based approach. Acad Emerg Med. 2008;15:1025–1036.

56. Salas E, Cooke NJ, Rosen MA. On teams, teamwork, and team performance: discoveries and developments. Hum Factors. 2008;50:540–547.

57. Delva D, Jamieson M, Lemieux M. Team effectiveness in academic primary health-care teams. J Interprof Care. 2008;22:598–611.

58. Sargeant J, Loney E, Murphy G. Effective interprofessional teams: "Contact is not enough" to build a team. J Contin Educ Health Prof. 2008;28:228–234.

59. Batorowicz B, Shepherd TA. Measuring the quality of transdisciplinary teams. J Interprof Care. 2008;22:610–620.

60. Hallin K, Kiessling A, Waldner A, Henriksson P. Active interprofessional education in a patient based setting increases perceived collaborative and professional competence. Med Teach. 2009;31:151–157.

61. Salas E, DiazGranados D, Weaver SJ, King H. Does team training work?: Principles for healthcare. Acad Emerg Med. 2008;15:1002–1009.

62. Daly D, Matzel SC. Building a transdisciplinary approach to palliative care in an acute care setting. Omega. 2013;67(1–2):43–51.

63. Cuff PA, Rapporteur, Global Forum on Innovation in Health Professional Education. Establishing Transdisciplinary Professionalism for Improving Health Outcomes: Workshop Summary. Washington, DC: The National Academies Press; 2013.

CHAPTER 69

Clinical interventions, economic impact, and palliative care

Patrick J. Coyne, Thomas J. Smith, and Laurel J. Lyckholm

Healthcare is growing now at about 10% per annum in the U.S. top line, versus 3% for the economy. As someone with a sharp pencil and an eye for this kind of thing, this can't last.

James Chanos, American hedge fund manager, New York City

Key points

♦ The scope of nursing and nursing education has expanded to include multiple domains, many of which overlap other disciplines such as wellness, disease prevention, and health services administration.

♦ Economic outcome is an area in which nursing plays an essential role in providing efficient, cost-effective, and appropriate palliative care.

♦ Health services research regarding economic outcomes, while limited, may help create a framework for addressing how to make palliative care available to everyone in an ethical, economic, and effective manner.

♦ Most nurses have a major influence in clinical interventions, yet often do not consider the economic impact and in some settings may not have a voice. The impact of the Affordable Health Care Act on palliative care remains uncharted waters.

Why are economic outcomes important?

Healthcare spending and healthcare quality are major challenges in the United States, with healthcare spending reaching nearly $8000 per person per year, twice that of most other countries with similar health outcomes. In the United States, health expenditures neared $2.6 trillion in 2010, over ten times the $256 billion spent in 1980.[1] The growth rate in recent years has slowed compared with the late 1990s and early 2000s, but in the coming years is still expected to grow faster than national income.[2] Drug costs and rising hospital expenses fuel much of this spending.[1–7]

Since 2008, employer-sponsored health coverage premiums have increased by up to 97%, placing increasing cost burdens on both employers and workers.[3] Medicare covers the elderly and people with disabilities, and Medicaid provides coverage to economically challenged individuals and families. Enrollment has increased with the aging of the baby boomers, presenting ongoing economic challenges.[1,4] Twenty percent of Medicare beneficiaries have five or more chronic illnesses and consume 60% of the Medicare spending.[5] This has had a considerable impact on our government's spending, straining federal and state budgets. Health spending accounted for 17.9% of the nation's gross domestic product (GDP) in 2010.[5] Although the United States spends more on healthcare than other industrialized nations, those countries provide health insurance to all their citizens. A 2013 study found that about 25% of all senior citizens who declare bankruptcy do so because of medical expenses.[6] About 84 million Americans were uninsured or underinsured, 3 million more than when the 2010 health law was signed and 20 million more than in 2003.[9] As of January 2011 there were more than 8 million uninsured children in the United States.[7,8] Rising healthcare costs correlate to reductions in health insurance coverage.[3,9]

We spend too much money on healthcare near the end of life, the quality is often poor, and it is not what most people want. About one-fourth of all Medicare dollars are spent in the last year of life, and 40% of that is spent in the last *month* of life—at least 8% of all Medicare dollars.[10] Teno and colleagues have shown actual *increases* in intensive care unit (ICU) use in the last 30 days of life for Medicare-age people who die.[11] Of patients with a terminal illness, 29% use the ICU in the last month of life and only 42% use hospice at any time during their illness. As patients transition out of intensive care, 14% have a change of healthcare setting in the last 3 days of life. This may involve transfer from hospital to home or hospital to inpatient hospice. The last few days of life are probably the worst time to disrupt families and to expect them to form new and trusting relationships. In addition, Kelley et al. reported that even with Medicare coverage, elderly households face considerable financial risk from out-of-pocket healthcare expenses at end of life.[12]

There are substantial concerns about the quality of palliative care in our current healthcare system. The Study to Understand Prognoses and Preferences for Outcomes and Risks of Treatment (SUPPORT) showed that half of all dying patients had unnecessary pain and suffering in their final days of life while in the hospital.[13] Pooled data from 52 articles reveals that pain was prevalent in cancer patients: 64% in patients with metastatic or advanced-stage disease, 59% in patients on anticancer treatment, and 33% in patients after curative treatment. More than one-third of the patients with pain in the reviewed articles graded their pain as moderate or severe. Nearly one of two patients with cancer pain is undertreated.[14] The percentage is high, but consists of a large variability of undertreatment across studies and settings.[15] Despite 20 years of interventions, 33% of current cancer patients have inadequate analgesics prescribed, with rates even higher in minority patients.[14]

Although it is not a zero-sum situation, there is good evidence that the more that is spent on high technology care for the elderly, the less funds are available for preventive services or treatment of chronic disease conditions for the same population.[16] The drain on healthcare-directed funds is likely to increase. This is due to heightened demands from an educated elderly population, more elderly long-term survivors, new and expensive technologies, new diseases, and demands for cost cutting. Even conservative physician and ex-Senator Dr. William Frist has called on us to confront our mortality and plan for a "good death" as part of personal responsibility.[17]

The Patient Protection and Affordable Care Act (Public Law 111-148) was signed into law in the United States by President Barack Obama on March 23, 2010. Along with the Health Care and Education Reconciliation Act of 2010 (passed March 25, 2010), the Act was a product of the healthcare reform agenda of the Democratic 111th Congress and the Obama administration. The goal of the Act was to ensure that all Americans have access to affordable healthcare and to create the transformation within the healthcare system to control cost. When fully paid for, the Congressional Budget Office (CBO) has determined, the Act would provide coverage for more than 94% of Americans. The law included a large number of health-related provisions that were to take effect over the next 4 years, including expanding the role of Medicaid.

Where does palliative care fit into the economic equation?

The present average life expectancy is 78 years. Many individuals will develop chronic illnesses such as heart failure, emphysema, stroke, dementia, and cancer. They will live with these conditions for many years before they die.[6] In the adult population, degenerative diseases replaced communicable diseases as leading causes of death in the United States and most economically advanced countries. The 10 leading causes of death (in order of prevalence) accounted for 80% of all deaths in the United States in 2008.[18] The majority of individuals with degenerative disease will benefit from palliative care at some point in their disease trajectory. As we will show below, palliative care is one of the rare aspects of medicine that improves the patient experience, maintains or improves

survival, improves the quality of care especially around end-of-life care hospitalizations, and saves money.[19]

The ethics of adding economic outcomes for the provision of palliative care

While quality care is the primary goal of hospice and palliative medicine, cost control is an important consideration. Nursing and medicine aspire to promote health and provide comfort and relief of suffering in a just manner. Cost control through evidence-based disease management, or "critical paths," may actually promote these goals by making more and/or better care available.

Cost control must be differentiated from profit motivation and entrepreneurship, which have not traditionally been considered the goals of medicine. These activities in the context of healthcare are unethical in that they may make medical care more expensive and difficult to access, especially for those who are socially disadvantaged. They may also create further conflicts of interest in already precarious fiduciary relationships between clinicians and their patients. A code of ethics that covers all professionals, rather than medicine alone, might be useful.[20-24] Nursing has its own code of ethics as do other disciplines.

If palliative care can be improved and/or made less costly without sacrificing quality, it should be done in the service of promoting the values of beneficence, compassion, and respect for autonomy. Palliative care has emerged as a national movement, with the advent of several important initiatives (e.g., Oncology Nursing Society; Hospice and Palliative Nurses Association; Education for Physicians on End-of-Life Care (EPEC); and the End-of-Life Nursing Education Consortium (ELNEC)). Other well-established national resource educational programs include the National Palliative Care Resource Center; City of Hope, CA; the Center to Improve Care of the Dying at George Washington University; and the Center to Advance Palliative Care at Mount Sinai Hospital in New York. In addition, palliative care programs continue to develop all over the world. In the United States, over 80% of large hospitals have palliative care programs.[25]

Some have argued that budgets should not be balanced with penalty to one group, such as the elderly or those on Medicare.[20] Many healthcare goods are rationed justly (benefit versus risk) according to age, such as transplants, coronary bypass, and hemodialysis. This rationing is based on the theory of equality of opportunity according to ability to benefit from such procedures.[21] Palliative care is different however, in that age does not determine whether a person stands to benefit. In this circumstance, the ethic of distributive justice supports the concept that medical and social needs dictate who stands to benefit most from palliative care. Daniels reported that "it does not seem reasonable to postulate that the medical needs of the elderly terminally ill are any less than those of younger patients, and indeed they may be greater because of multiple additional pathologies associated with aging."[23] Sidgwick's argument that each moment of life is equally valuable, no matter when it occurs is most poignant in the instance of palliative care.[24] This would also apply to extending palliative care to neonates expected to live only a short time after birth. For adults, the most explicitly described guidance is from the United Kingdom's National Institute for Clinical Excellence (NICE) that gives guidance about which treatments the National

Health Service should fund, given a fixed budget. Even NICE allows for special consideration if the patient survival is short, and may waive the usual 3-month survival benefit if the treatment gives substantial palliative benefit at a reasonable cost.[26]

Patients may view benefit and toxicity in ways very different from their healthcare providers and from those who are well. Studies show that many dying cancer patients would undergo almost any treatment toxicity for a 1% chance of short-term survival, while their doctors and nurses would not; and these decisions did not change after patients experienced the toxicity of treatment.[27,28] If the patient wants to try a therapy with minimal chance of benefit, we should not assume that the oncologist or cardiologist has not adequately explained the options, risks and benefits—the patient may just have a different perspective.

What is the right amount to spend on healthcare?

How much to spend on healthcare cannot be determined without knowing the economic and cultural particulars of a country or even a health system. Blanket statements about a percentage of the gross national product (GNP) may be misleading if a comparison country spends a higher percentage on social safety net programs but less on direct medical care costs. Comments about healthcare spending as a percent of the GNP may also reflect opinions about alternative uses; for example, "We should stop spending money on defense and spend it on healthcare." In the United States, the amount spent on education has declined from 6% to 5% of the GNP, while the amount spent on healthcare (especially for the elderly) has risen from 6% to about 18%, compared with the average of 33 other developed countries of 9.5%.[29] Clearly, in all countries, the entire system of healthcare needs to be explored with policies designed to ensure that palliative care is a component of the overall healthcare system. A common threshold is the World Health Organization (WHO)'s recommended three times per-capita GNP per quality-adjusted life year, or how much we should spend to save a year of life; in the United States that would be about $140,100 in 2008 US dollars.[30]

Should there be special economic or policy considerations for palliative care?

We believe that, in general, there should be no special considerations for palliative care. Most healthcare policy analysts and economists would argue that all care should be evaluated equally. For example, a therapy that gains 1 week for 52 patients should be valued as much as a therapy of equivalent cost that gains 52 weeks for 1 patient.[31] Some health economists have argued that time given to those who are most at risk should be valued more (e.g., time added in the last 6 months of life should be given triple value).[32] The analogy was made to food and hunger: a sandwich given to a starving person would be of more intrinsic value than one given to a person who already had many sandwiches. Such discussions, while interesting, are outside the scope of this chapter and will remain unresolved.

The WHO advocates a more equal distribution of resources in developed countries, and an even greater support of palliative care in developing countries, where most of the population will experience advanced disease rather than cure or long-term survival.

One approach to funding treatments has been based on cost-effectiveness ratios. For example, Laupacis and colleagues[33] in Canada proposed explicit funding criteria: (1) treatments that are more effective and less expensive should be adopted; (2) treatments with cost-effectiveness ratios of less than C$20,000 per additional life year (LY) gained should be accepted, with the recognition that they cost additional resources; (3) treatments with cost-effectiveness ratios of $20,000 to C$100,000/LY should be examined on a case-by-case basis with caution; (4) and treatments with cost-effectiveness ratios of greater than C$100,000/LY should be rejected. These criteria are valid in a system where all resources are shared equally, such as the Veterans Administration with a fixed budget, but it is not clear how they apply to other healthcare systems, where resources may not be shared. Alternatively, patients might be allowed to purchase additional insurance for expensive treatments or pay for them out of pocket. In the United States, there has been no accepted answer, but most authorities have agreed on an implicitly defined benchmark of $35,000 to $50,000/LY saved, updated to $180,000 to $240,000 in current dollars.[34,35]

Palliative care rarely costs more and usually saves money for better care.[36] As an example, in England, home-based palliative care allowed patients to avoid emergency room (ER) visits, while promoting appropriate care with apparent cost savings of 40%.[37] A specially designed palliative care program for multiple sclerosis patients not only improved symptoms but saved the National Health Service over $2700 from reduced hospitalizations in a 12-week trial period.[38]

What are important economic outcomes?

Economic and clinical outcomes are closely related. Cost should always be considered along with clinical benefit. However, making decisions is not easy. The economic data necessary to make decisions about treatment may be collected in much the same way as clinical information, and within standard formats for collection and analysis.[39–41] Some standard definitions are listed in Table 69.1.

It is important to organize data in a way that balances clinical and cost information side by side, as shown in Table 69.2. Cost-effectiveness is the amount of money someone must pay to gain additional months or years of life. The usual benchmark is "life years gained" or LYs. If the amount of time is adjusted for quality, for instance a year with advanced metastatic disease is only valued at 50%, or 6 months, then quality-adjusted life years (QALYs) are used.

Some countries such as Canada, the United Kingdom, Australia, Germany, and France, use these metrics to inform decisions on what can be afforded. Oregon used cost-effectiveness to inform their list of covered services under Medicaid, ultimately incorporating other values into the equation.[43] The decision-making process is never easy, as it frequently means withholding some desired care. However, all health systems make such decisions now, such as a Pharmacy and Therapeutics Committee; the LY method just makes the decision-making transparent. We predict a growing emphasis on explicit sharing of effectiveness and cost information with patients as the cost of treatments goes up, in order to help them decide if something is "worth it."[44]

Table 69.1 Standard definitions for economic outcome analysis

Term	Definition	Comment
Resource utilization	Number of units used (e.g., 9 hospital days)	Best collected prospectively, using a combination of clinical research forms, hospital bills, and patient diaries for outpatient or off-site events.
Charge	What is billed to the patient	May be fair representation of the cost of service.
Cost	What it costs society to provide the service	This is different from the charge because many services cost more or less than what is billed.
Direct medical cost	Costs of standard medical interventions	Usual "cost-drivers" include hospital days, professional fees, diagnostic tests, pharmacy fees, other (e.g., blood products, operating room, emergency services).
Direct nonmedical cost	Costs of medical interventions not usually captured but directly caused	Includes transportation, time lost from work, caregiver costs, etc. Most are not covered by insurance and may be "out-of-pocket" costs.
Perspective	The viewpoint of the analysis	Should be explicitly stated. Most analyses are done from the perspective of society (valuing this intervention vs. other uses of the same money) or a healthcare system (valuing this intervention against other local healthcare needs). The perspective of the individual patient or provider may give less attention to the needs of others.[42]
Discounting	Adjusts value of intervention for future benefit to present-time amount	Health effects and costs should normally be discounted at 3% per year. Health benefits in the present are worth more than those in the future.

Source: Smith (1993)[31] Copyright © 1993, American Medical Association. All rights reserved.

Table 69.2 Ways to balance clinical evaluation and cost studies

Type of study	Advantages and disadvantages[46]
Clinical outcomes only	Ignore costs. Easy to choose among clearly superior therapies such as cisplatin for testicular cancer that do not cost much; harder among all others that give lesser benefits at high costs.
Cost only (e.g., cost of treating febrile neutropenia)	Ignores clinical outcomes. Does not help choose among clinical strategies.
Costs and clinical outcomes together	
Cost minimization	Assumes that two strategies are equal; lowest cost strategy is preferred. If generic paclitaxel is as good as expensive ixabepilone in breast cancer, choose the $60 one, not the $6000 one.
Cost effectiveness	Compares two strategies; assigns dollar amount per additional year of life (life year [LY] saved by strategy. Example: at present, cerebrospinal fluids have not improved survival, so cost must be lower for therapy to be cost-effective.
Cost utility	Compares two strategies; assigns dollar amount per additional LY saved by strategy, then estimates the quality of that benefit in cost per quality adjusted LY. No data show significant improvement in quality of life or utilities in patients who have received CSFs, so they are unlikely to have major impact.
Cost benefit	Compares two strategies but converts the clinical benefits to money (e.g., a year of life is worth $100,000). This is possible but is rarely done due to difficulty in assigning monetary value to benefit; it requires assigning a monetary value to human life. For instance, should a bus driver be valued less than a physicist, or vice versa?

Models of care and cost that maintain quality and lower cost

Coordinated care may be one of the most economically successful disease-management strategies. For instance, a large US practice created evidence-based clinical pathways with an emphasis on (1) use of generic drugs, (2) restricting treatments to those based on solid evidence, (3) incorporating more use of advance directives, and (4) earlier hospice referral. Patient survival is the same or even better with less fourth- and fifth-line chemotherapy, hospice use is increased, and cost is reduced by one-third.[45,46]

Recent randomized studies show that a modified palliative care presence (with lower costs than full hospice care per diem charges), and control over the clinical care of the patient, is associated with fewer hospitalizations, fewer ICU hospital days, and lower costs. Brumley et al.[47] studied patients in the Kaiser Permanente health maintenance organization, 161 in the Palliative Care Program and 139 in the comparison group. Palliative care patients had significantly fewer emergency department visits, hospital days, skilled nursing facility days, and physician visits. There was a 45% decrease in costs as compared with usual care patients. A randomized study showed increased satisfaction when palliative care was added to usual care. There were fewer emergency room visits, and lower costs (mean cost for patients enrolled in the palliative care group was $12,670, compared with $20,222 for usual care). The palliative care approach has been adopted by many other Kaiser Permanente groups as part of routine care for patients with advanced illness. Nationally, palliative care has demonstrated the ability to save hospitals significant amounts of money while delivering excellent, appropriate care.[48–50] Based on this experience, if New York Medicaid had palliative care services at all the New York hospitals, they would save over $84 million a year.[51]

Teaching staff about choices for ICU use can improve economic outcomes. In one setting, an ethicist in the surgical ICU addressed the issues of patient choice about dying and the ethics of futile care. The project involved giving the residents increased knowledge and skills in addressing and integrating practical ethical issues into their surgical resident practice.[52] This was associated with a decrease in length of stay from 28 to 16 days, and a decrease in surgical intensive care days from 2028 to 1003, far greater than observed in other parts of the hospital. Cost savings were estimated at $1.8 million. In a similar project, Dowdy and colleagues performed proactive ethics consultations for all mechanically ventilated patients beyond 4 days, and showed improved length of stay (less use of the ICU, either by discontinuing futile care or transferring the patient to lesser-intensity units) and a decrease in costs. In general, consultations with an expert team work better than training the existing staff in palliative care.[47,53]

Clinical practice guidelines for cancer patients now recommend concurrent palliative care as part of comprehensive cancer care. In 2012, the American Society of Clinical Oncology (ASCO) issued a provisional clinical opinion that recommended all patients with metastatic non-small-cell lung cancer (NSCLC) be offered palliative care, at the time of diagnosis, along with standard cancer therapy. The opinion further stated that palliative care should be considered early in the course of cancer for any patient with other metastatic cancers, as well as for those with a high burden of cancer-related symptoms.[54]

Several studies have demonstrated that utilizing palliative care improves quality while reducing cost.[48,49] Other data suggest that hospice care can be cost saving.[47] Hospice enrollment during the longer period of 53–105 days prior to death and the most common period of within 30 days prior to death lowers Medicare expenditures, rates of hospital and ICU use, 30-day hospital readmissions, and in-hospital death.[55] In a retrospective study of 12,000 patients at 40 centers, Aiken et al. found that hospice patients were more likely to receive home nursing care and to spend less time in the hospital than conventional care patients. Of the three models of care evaluated, conventional care was the least expensive when overall disease-management costs were calculated, but hospital-based hospice ($2270) and home care hospice ($2657) were less expensive than conventional care ($6100) in the last month of life.[56]

Advance directives

Current studies show only zero to 10% healthcare cost savings when individuals have advance directives.[57] Treatment-limiting advance directives were associated with lower probabilities of in-hospital death in high- and medium-spending regions of our country but not in low-spending regions. Cost is believed to be driven by physician practice style rather than by differences in patients' preferences for aggressiveness of treatment at the end of life.[57] Of note only one in five Americans have completed living wills and, in many cases, by the time the family decides that the living will applies, the end is indeed close (a few days), and most funds have been spent. We have missed the opportunity to put hospice in place at home, so the person dies in the hospital— not what they wanted and at great expense. Advanced directives, such as "do-not-resuscitate" (DNR) orders, have been advocated to allow patients to make autonomous choices about their care at the end of life, and possibly to reduce costs by preventing futile care. Often healthcare providers do not discuss goals of care with those patients having a life-limiting disease.[58] Determining what "futile medical care" is and when to withhold it raises an important point: Even if the patients and families at the end of life refuse life-sustaining intervention, the patient may not require less care but care of a different kind, which may be just as expensive. In fact, one retrospective from Germany purports that patients who had a palliative care consultation, compared with those who did not, are more likely to get opiates but die in the hospital and cost more.[59] Despite a belief that the use of advance directives and hospice care, along with reducing "futile care," can save our health system money, only 3.3% ($69 billion) of all health spending could actually be saved by using such practices.[60] But importantly, improvements in end of life care would not cost extra.

Nursing issues

As healthcare reform evolves, nurses have the ability to impact clinical intervention while promoting appropriate utilization of resources. Nurses play a large role in the decisions patients, families, and other healthcare providers make, and those decisions drive the cost of care. Role utilization and its potential influence will vary within each setting. For example, a complete interdisciplinary palliative care team may be necessary to meet the needs of the population in a large university-based hospital, yet a specially trained nurse with interdisciplinary support, may be adequate in a small community hospital. Such coupling of services should be examined from the standpoint of quality of care and cost-effectiveness.[61] The advanced practice nurse may play a significant role in identifying and coordinating the needs of patients/families requiring palliation. Advanced practice nurses are perfectly positioned to fill such a critical need for this population in the hospital, hospice, and nursing home.[62]

A factor not fully examined is the out-of-pocket cost that the patient's significant others bear in caring for them. These include lost work hours, expended resources, and simple care hours not reimbursed through insurance or government assistance. Also to be determined is the increased healthcare costs of those caregivers, who frequently neglect their own health while caring for others.[63]

Nursing as a profession needs to continue to advocate for this population while supporting effective quality care, and fair utilization of resources. The use of advanced technology, especially expensive diagnostic tests, may be accepted as routine in an acute care hospital, regardless of cost and goals of care. Nurses must be knowledgeable about healthcare outcomes, in particular those issues related to palliative care: the patient/family unit of care, quality of life, and decision-making around end-of-life care. Unfortunately, many nurses are largely unaware and/or uninformed about these issues. Those that are aware may not have a voice within their institutions. Greater knowledge may empower nurses to take a more prominent, collaborative place at the table when such issues are being discussed and decisions are being made. Refer to chapter 62 for an in-depth discussion of the role of the advanced practice nurse in palliative care.

Cases for consideration

Consider the following situations and how our clinical decisions impact economics and quality of life. As always, consideration of benefit/burdens and risks to patients and families needs to be paramount.

1. A 62-year-old woman is admitted for severe bone pain from advanced multiple myeloma; she has extensive bone involvement and has exhausted all standard therapy, including stem cell transplant, as well as undergone three clinical trials. She continues to have pancytopenia, but as she is minimally able to be up and around (she cannot even get into a chair as she is too weak), she does not exert herself and does not have symptoms related to anemia. She has no evidence of bleeding. She and her family request daily complete blood count (CBC) and prophylactic transfusion of blood and platelets.

2. A 58-year-old man has had multiple coronary events, has an ejection fraction of 15%, and is receiving dobutamine via infusion. When the dobutamine is decreased, he experiences severe chest pain, which resolves when the dobutamine is increased. The local home hospice agency will not support dobutamine infusion.

3. A 39-year-old woman is admitted for severe dyspnea related to very late-stage pulmonary fibrosis and pulmonary hypertension. She requires high-flow oxygen to be comfortable, which would require two concentrators at home. She is also on epoprostenol, a highly expensive IV medication for pulmonary hypertension, and the only medication that has helped her to become more comfortable, with improvement in her shortness of breath. She wants very much to go home, as she understands that her time to live is very limited.

4. A 41-year-old man is found to have stage IV colon cancer. He has an inoperable bowel obstruction and had intractable nausea until he had a nasogastric (NG) tube placed to suction and was started on subcutaneous octreotide three times a day. This led to a significant improvement in his symptoms and quality of life. He has a limited life span and would like to return home. No home health or hospice can be located that will accept him and that has access to home suction machines. The palliative care team offers to buy a home suction machine, but the hospice refuses to care for a patient with an NG tube because of fear that it will become dislodged and gastric contents will be aspirated. Furthermore, the cost of octreotide is prohibitive.

5. A 29-year-old woman has been through four chemotherapy regimens for metastatic breast cancer that has progressed relentlessly. She has been started on a new chemotherapy that requires her to be in the hospital overnight twice weekly. She lives 2 hours away from the medical center and, despite help from social services, has lost her house and car and is now living with her sister, who also has no car. She is only able to make it to the clinic about a third of her expected appointments. The clinic nurse asks her why she is being "noncompliant" with her treatments.

6. A 46-year-old man has squamous cell carcinoma of the base of tongue, which originally responded to radiation and chemotherapy. He now has recurrence of the cancer in his cervical lymph nodes as well as nodules in the lungs. The oncology team wants to perform a bronchoscopy and possibly an open biopsy of the lung nodules. This despite knowing this patient has metastatic, recurrent cancer in the neck.

7. A 46-year-old man has squamous cell carcinoma of the lung with widespread metastases to the brain, bones, pericardium, liver, and adrenal glands. He has had radiation and two cycles of chemotherapy, which made him weak and nauseated. CT scans reveal progressive disease. He is bed-bound and sleeps most of the time. He is found by a home health nurse to have an elevated calcium of 14.5 mg/dL. His oncologist calls the patient's wife to request that he be brought to the clinic for treatment of his hypercalcemia.

Summary

Economic outcomes are increasingly important for all types of healthcare, including palliative care. There are substantial opportunities for improvement by using disease management strategies and care pathways. Directed, ethically motivated interventions about futile care appear to produce significant cost savings. The use of advance directives or hospice care may be good medical care, but have not been shown to produce major economic benefit. Most recently, integrated palliative care teams have been shown to reduce hospital and end of life care costs for seriously ill patients.

The cost of care is rising due to the increasing age of the population, more cancer cases and chronic diseases, increased demand for treatment, and new and expensive technologies. Our limited resources must be rationed wisely so that we can provide both curative and palliative care. The ethical implications of using economic and management outcomes rather than traditional health outcomes include shifting emphasis from helping at all cost to helping at a cost society can afford, as well as how much society is willing to pay. The value of care to the dying versus those with curable illnesses, and tolerance of suboptimal care, are ethical and societal issues.

From the perspective of economics or health service research, the outcomes of palliative care do not differ from those of other cancer treatment or treatment of other chronic illnesses. For treatment to be justified, there must be some demonstrable improvement in disease-free or overall survival, toxicity, quality of life, or cost-effectiveness. Palliative care may improve survival, but it does not have a measurable cost-effectiveness ratio since it does not usually gain years of life.

Nurses clearly have the ability to impact the care and cost for this population and should be at the forefront of these issues. Economic issues are critical, and nursing is in a position to make an impact. The final caveat will however always be do the right thing.

References

1. Centers For Medicare And Medicaid Services, Office of the Actuary, National Health Statistics Group. National Health Care Expenditures Data. January 2012.

2. Robert Wood Johnson Foundation. High and Rising Health Care Costs: Demystifying U.S. Health Care Spending. October 2008. http://www.rwjf.org/content/dam/farm/reports/issue_briefs/2008/rwjf32704/subassets/rwjf32704_1 (accessed July 3, 2014).

3. Centers For Medicare And Medicaid Services. Projections of National Health Expenditures: Methodology and Model Specifications. Available at: http://www.cms.hhs.gov/nationalhealthexpenddata/downloads/projections-methodology.pdf (accessed June 10, 2013).

4. Kaiser Family Foundation and Health Research and Educational Trust. Employer Health Benefits 2012 Annual Survey. September 2012.

5. Kaiser Family Foundation. Medicare Chartbook, 2010. http://kff.org/medicare/report/medicare-chartbook-2010 (accessed October 22, 2013).

6. Martin AB, et al. Growth in US health spending remained slow in 2010; Health share of gross domestic product was unchanged from 2009. Health Affairs. 2012;31(1):208–219.

7. http://www.commonwealthfund.org/~/media/Files/Publications/Fund%20Report/2013/Apr/1681_Collins_insuring_future_biennial_survey_2012_FINAL.pdf

8. www.childrensdefense.org (accessed July 22, 2013).

9. Woolhandler S, Himmelstein D, Adams G, Almberg M. 2012 September 12. Despite Slight Drop in Uninsured, Last Year's Figure Points to 48,000 Preventable Deaths. Physicians for a National Health Program.

10. Riley GF, Lubitz JD. Long-term trends in medicare payments in the last year of life. Health Serv Res. 2010;45:565–576.

11. Teno JM, Gozalo PL, Bynum JPW, et al. Change in end-of-life care for Medicare beneficiaries: site of death, place of care, and health care transitions in 2000, 2005, and 2009. JAMA. 2013;309:470.

12. Kelley AS, McGarry K, Fahle S, Marshall SM. Out-of-pocket spending in the last five years of life. J Gen Intern Med. 2013;28:304–309.

13. SUPPORT Principal Investigators. A controlled trial to improve care for seriously ill hospitalized patients: the Study to Understand Prognoses and Preferences for Outcomes and Risks of Treatments (SUPPORT). JAMA. 1995;274:1591–1598.

14. Fisch MJ, Lee JW, Weiss M, et al. Prospective, observational study of pain and analgesic prescribing in medical oncology outpatients with breast, colorectal, lung, or prostate cancer. Ann Oncol. 2008;19(12):1985–1991.

15. Deandrea S, Montanari M, Moja L, Apolone G. Prevalence of undertreatment in cancer pain. A review of published literature. Ann Oncol. 2008;19(12):1985–1991.

16. Harrington SE, Smith TJ. The role of chemotherapy at the end of life: "When is enough, enough?" JAMA. 2008;299(22):2667–2678.

17. Frist W. 2012. How do you want to die? http://theweek.com//bullpen/column/233111/how-do-you-want-to-die.

18. Centers for Disease Control and Prevention (CDC). 2010. Infant Health. http://www.cdc.gov/nchs/fastats/infant_health.htm (retrieved July 5, 2013).

19. Parikh RB, Kirch R, Smith TJ, Temel J. Early Specialty Palliative Care: Translating Data in Oncology into Practice and Policy. N Engl J Med 2013;369:2347–2351.

20. Center for the Advancement of Palliative Care. CAPC 26. Berger JT, Rosner F. The ethics of practice guidelines. Arch Intern Med. 1996;156:2051–2056.

21. Callahan D. Controlling the costs of health care for the elderly—fair means and foul. N Engl J Med.1996;335:744–746.

22. Randall F. Palliative Care Ethics: A Good Companion. New York: Oxford University Press; 1996.

23. Daniels N. Just Health Care. New York: Cambridge University Press; 1985.

24. Sidgwick H. The Methods of Ethics. London: Macmillan; 1907.

25. Center for the Advancement of Palliative Care. CAPC State by State Report Card. http://reportcard capc org/pdf/state-by-state-report-card.pdf [serial online] 2011; Available from: capc.org (accessed October 10, 2013).

26. Trowman R, Chung H, Longson C, Littlejohns P, Clark P. The National Institute for Health and Clinical Excellence and its role in assessing the value of new cancer treatments in England and Wales. Clin Cancer Res. 2011;17(15):4930–4935. doi: 10.1158/1078-0432.CCR-10-2510. Epub 2011 Jul 26.

27. Matsuyama R, Reddy S, Smith TJ. Why do patients choose chemotherapy near the end of life?: A review of the perspective of those facing death from cancer. J Clin Oncol. 2006;24(21):3490–3496.

28. Slevin ML, Stubbs L, Plant HJ, et al. Attitudes to chemotherapy: comparing views of patients with cancer with those of doctors, nurses, and general public. BMJ. 1990;300:1458–1460.

29. Health Care Statistics. Available at: http://www.oecd.org/els/health-systems/oecdhealthdata2012-frequentlyrequesteddata.htm.

30. Central Intelligence Agency. The World Factbook. United States. Available at: https://www.cia.gov/library/publications/the-world-factbook/geos/us.html (accessed November May 3, 2013.

31. Smith TJ, Hillner BE, Desch CE. Efficacy and cost-effectiveness of cancer treatment: rational allocation of resources based on decision analysis. J Natl Cancer Inst. 1993;85:1460–1474.

32. Waugh N, Scott D. How should different life expectancies be valued? BMJ. 1998;1140–1316.

33. Laupacis A, Feeny D, Detsky AS, Tugwell PX. How attractive does a new technology have to be to warrant adoption and utilization?: Tentative guidelines for using clinical and economic evaluation. Can Med Assoc J. 1992;146:473–481.

34. Smith TJ. Which hat do I wear? JAMA. 1993;270:1657–1659.

35. Hillner BE, Smith TJ. Efficacy does not necessarily translate to cost effectiveness: a case study in the challenges associated with 21st-century cancer drug pricing. J Clin Oncol. 2009;27(13):2111–2113. doi: 10.1200/JCO.2008.21.0534.

36. Hughes M, Smith TJ. The future of palliative care. Annu Rev Public Health. 2014;35:459–475.

37. Pattenden J, Mason A, Lewin R. Collaborative palliative care for advanced heart failure: outcomes and costs from the 'Better Together' pilot study. Palliat Support Care. doi:10.1136/bmjspcare-2012-000251.

38. Higginson IJ, Costantini M, Silber E, Burman R, Edmonds P. Evaluation of a new model of short-term palliative care for people severely affected with multiple sclerosis: a randomised fast-track trial to test timing of referral and how long the effect is maintained. Postgraduate Medical Journal. 2011;87:769–775.

39. Brown M, Glick H, Harrell F, et al. Integrating economic analysis into cancer clinical trials: the National Cancer Institute–American Society of Clinical Oncology Economics Workbook. 1998:151–163.

40. Cassel J. Measurement issues for palliative care programs. In: Panke J, Coyne P (eds.), Conversations in Palliative Care. 3rd ed. Pittsburgh: Hospice and Palliative Nurses Association. 2011;329–334.

41. Temel JS, Jackson VA, Billings JA, et al. Phase II study: integrated palliative care in newly diagnosed advanced non-small-cell lung cancer patients. J Clin Oncol. 2007;25:2377–2382.

42. Connor SR, Pyenson B, Fitch K, Spence, C., Iwasaki K. Comparing hospice and non hospice patient survival among patients who die within a three year window. J Pain Symptom Manage. 2007;33(3):238–246.

43. Healthcare Payment Reform & Provider Reimbursement: A Summary of Strategies for Consideration by the Oregon Health Fund Board 43 43 http://www.oregon.gov/OHA/OHPR/hfb/delivery/payment_reform_provider_reimbursement_paper.pdf.

44. Swetz KM, Smith TJ. Palliative chemotherapy: when is it worth it and when is it not? Cancer J. 2010;16(5):467–472. doi: 10.1097/PPO.0b013e3181f28ab3. Review.

45. Neubauer MA, Hoverman JR, Kolodziej M, et al. Cost effectiveness of evidence-based treatment guidelines for the treatment of non-small-cell lung cancer in the community setting. J Oncol Pract. 2010;6:12–18.

46. Hoverman JR, Cartwright TH, Patt DA, et al. Pathways, outcomes, and costs in colon cancer: retrospective evaluations in two distinct databases. J Oncol Pract. 2011;7:52s–59s.

47. Brumley R, Enguidanos S, Jamison P, Seitz R, Morgenstern N, Saito S, et al. Increased satisfaction with care and lower costs: results of a randomized trial of in-home palliative care. J Am Geriatric Soc. 2007;55(7):993–1000.

48. Twaddle ML, Maxwell TL, Cassel JB, Liao S, Coyne PJ, Usher BM, et al. Palliative care benchmarks from academic medical centers. J Palliat Med. 2007;10(1):86–98.

49. Morrison RS, Penrod JD, Cassel JB, Caust-Ellenbogen M, Litke A, Spragens L, et al.; Palliative Care Leadership Centers' Outcomes Group. Cost savings associated with US hospital palliative care consultation programs. Arch Intern Med. 2008;168(16):1783–1790.

50. Smith T, Cassel JB. Cost and non-clinical outcomes of palliative care. J Pain Symptom Manage. 2009;38(1):32–44.

51. Morrison RS, Dietrich J, Ladwig S, et al. Palliative care consultation teams cut hospital costs for medicaid beneficiaries. Health Affairs. 2011;30:454–463.

52. Holloran SD, Starkey GW, Burke PA, Steele G Jr, Forse RA. An educational intervention in the surgical intensive care unit to improve ethical decisions. Surgery. 1995;118:294–298.

53. Dowdy MD, Robertson C, Bander JA. A study of proactive ethics consultation for critically and terminally ill patients with extended lengths of stay. Crit Care Med. 1998;26:252–259.

54. Smith TJ, Temin S, Alesi E, Abernethy A, Balboni T, Basch E, et al. American Society of Clinical Oncology provisional clinical opinion: the integration of palliative care into standard oncology care. J Clin Oncol. 2012;30(8):880–887.

55. Kelley AS, Deb P, Du Q, Aldridge Carlson MD, Morrison RS. The Care Span hospice enrollment saves money for medicare and improves care quality across a number of different lengths-of-stay. Health Affairs. 2013;32(3):552–561.

56. Aiken LS, Butner J, Lockhart CA, Volk-Craft BE, Hamilton G, Williams FG. Outcome evaluation of a randomized trial of the PhoenixCare intervention: program of case management and coordinated care for the seriously chronically ill. J Palliat Med. 20060;9(1):111–126.

57. Nicholas L, Langa KM, Iwashyna TJ, Weir DR. Regional variation in the association between advance directives and end-of-life medicare expenditures. JAMA. 2011;306(13):1447–1453. doi:10.1001/jama.2011.1410.

58. Coyne PJ. The case of Mrs. A. J Palliat Med. 2012;15(12):1397–1398.

59. Gaertner J, Drabik A, Marschall U, Schlesiger G, Voltz R, Stock S. Inpatient palliative care: a nationwide analysis. Health Policy. 2013;109(3):311–318.

60. Emanuel EJ, Cost savings at the end of life: WHAT do the data show? JAMA. 1996;275(24):1907–1914.

61. Lyckholm LJ, Coyne PJ, Kreutzer KO, Ramakrishnan V, Smith TJ. Barriers to effective palliative care for low income patients in late stages of cancer: report of a study and strategies for defining and conquering the barriers. Nurs Clin North Amer. 2010;45:399–409.

62. Coyne P, Dahlin C, Campbell M, Lentz J, Lynch M, Stahl D. Value of advanced practice nurse in palliative care: An HPNA position statement. J Hospice Palliative Nurs 2010 http://www.hpna.org/DisplayPage.aspx?Title1=Position%20Statements accessed 7/23/2013.

63. Coyne P, Panke J. Caring for the caregiver. In: Conversations in Palliative Care. 3rd ed. Pittsburgh: Hospice and Palliative Nurses Association; 2011:53–60.

CHAPTER 70

International palliative care initiatives

Stephen R. Connor

Over 1 million people die each week on our planet. In 2011 there were a total of 54,591,414 deaths from all causes according to the World Health Organization (WHO).[1] These causes are broken down into three major categories: (1) communicable, maternal, perinatal, and nutritional conditions (24.5%); (2) noncommunicable diseases (66.4%); and (3) injuries (9.1%). Palliative care is much more than end-of-life care; however, the mortality data help us to understand the scope of the need for global palliative care initiatives. The biggest palliative care need is for people living with noncommunicable diseases, followed by those with communicable diseases, such as HIV/AIDS and drug-resistant tuberculosis. Those dying suddenly of noncommunicable disease or injury or other infectious diseases or acute but potentially reversible illnesses are unlikely to be in a position to access palliative care.

There were close to 8 million deaths from cancer in 2011, and we believe at least 84% required palliative care.[2] Progress is being made in slowing the AIDS pandemic, but in 2011 there were still almost 1.6 million deaths, primarily in sub-Saharan Africa. There are also a large number of pediatric conditions that benefit from palliative care and a growing number of programs that are now providing neonatal palliative care. Palliative care is for all age groups and with the unprecedented rise in the proportion of elderly persons globally the need for palliative care is growing fast.

The WHO has recognized the immense and growing need to address noncommunicable disease morbidity and is calling for universal health coverage (UHC). The proposed definition of a health care continuum under UHC is promotion—prevention—treatment—rehabilitation—palliation. Thus palliative care is now considered to be a fundamental part of any national healthcare system and is increasingly being viewed as a human right.[3]

Still palliative care is only reliably available in Western Europe, North America, and Australia/New Zealand. The greatest needs for palliative care are in low- and middle-income countries where it is least available. A recent study[4] found that in 42% of countries no palliative care services are available. In 32% of countries there is no known palliative care activity at all, mainly in parts of Africa, Asia, and in the Middle East. In 10% of countries there was some interest in developing palliative care but no service delivery had started. Almost 40% of countries have some palliative care, but it is not yet widespread or integrated into the mainstream healthcare system. In only 19.3% of countries is palliative care somewhat integrated into the healthcare system, and in only 20 countries is it at a level of advanced integration.

A public health model is used to help foster the growth and development of palliative care.[5] The term "palliative care" is generally used internationally and includes hospice care. The public health model includes four components. The first is policy. Without policies that support palliative care nothing much can happen. These kinds of policies consist of inclusion of palliative care in relevant national healthcare laws and regulations, funding and service delivery models, development of national standards and clinical guidelines, and inclusion of palliative care as a recognized specialty or subspecialty.

The second component of the public health strategy is education and includes media and public advocacy, curricula and courses for health professionals, expert training, and family caregiver training and support. The third component of the public health strategy is medication availability, and this needs to be implemented parallel to education. Without access to essential palliative medicines clinical training is ineffective, as professionals need to see the efficacy of palliative treatment at the bedside. Medicine availability must include the oral opioids, incorporating both immediate and slow release morphine, as these are the most widely used medications for pain relief. Many other essential medicines are needed and are listed in a recent model list of essential palliative medicines by the WHO.[6]

There is a very serious problem globally with access to controlled substances that are required in the provision of palliative care. The International Narcotics Control Board has estimated that 80% of the world's population has very limited or no access to strong opioids. Australia, Canada, New Zealand, the United States, and several European countries account for more than 90% of the global consumption of opioid analgesics.[7] The Commission on Narcotic Drugs has called for a return to balance between policies that restrict access to narcotics to prevent illicit use and policies that ensure adequate availability of opioids for medical and scientific use.[8]

The fourth component of the public health strategy is implementation. While there are individual philanthropic programs that have emerged without government support in many countries, the widespread availability of palliative care does not happen without the preceding three components in place. Implementation often begins with pilot palliative care programs that demonstrate how palliative care can be implemented in a country and serve as centers for bedside training. Implementation should also be driven by the needs and involvement of the community.

The role of nursing is of major importance in the implementation of palliative care globally. Nursing is the most needed and utilized member of the interdisciplinary palliative care team. Unfortunately in many parts of the world professional nursing is underdeveloped or in early stages of development. For example, in many of the former Soviet republics physicians perform functions that are typically conducted by nurses in Western countries, while nurses are relegated to assistant roles that require less skill. This is not effectively using the training or focus of either profession, to the disadvantage of patients and professionals alike. Nursing education must teach greater independence and professionalism to fully use the skills of these clinicians. There is also a movement toward task shifting in developing countries so that community health workers can be trained to perform many nursing functions and nurses can be freed to perform more advanced, and greatly needed, care.

The following chapters offer useful studies in how hospice and palliative care can be initiated in many different settings including those with higher and lower resource levels. Palliative care in Canada, Australia and New Zealand, the United Kingdom, western and eastern Europe, Latin America, Africa, Japan, and the Philippines are all included in this section. There is also a chapter on palliative care in situations of conflict to highlight some of the special caring requirements and burdens for populations including refugees and those in conflict zones. There is also a new chapter on palliative care as a human right. While there is no substitute for personal connections and individual initiative, nurses interested in supporting the advancement of palliative care globally can do so through involvement in a variety of international initiatives including:

The Worldwide Palliative Care Alliance—www.thewpca.org

The International Association for Hospice and Palliative Care www.hospicecare.com
The Foundation for Hospices in sub-Saharan Africa www.fhssa.org
The International Children's Palliative Care Network www. icpcn.org

References

1. World Health Organization. Cause specific mortality: Regional estimates for 2000-2011. http://www.who.int/healthinfo/global_burden_disease/estimates_regional/en/index.html. Accessed 25 August 2013.
2. Connor S, Sepulveda C, (eds.). Global Atlas of Palliative Care at the End-of-Life. London, Geneva: Worldwide Palliative Care Alliance and World Health Organization; 2014.
3. Brennan F. Palliative care as an international human right. J Pain Symptom Manage 2007;33:494–499
4. Lynch T, Connor S, Clark D. Mapping levels of palliative care development: a global update. J Pain Symptom Manage. 2013;45(6):1094–1106.
5. Stjernsward J, Foley KM, Ferris FD. The public health strategy for palliative care. J Pain Symptom Manage. 2007;33:486–493.
6. World Health Organization. Model Lists of Essential Medicines. http://www.who.int/medicines/publications/essentialmedicines/en/. Accessed 26 August 2013.
7. International Narcotics Control Board. Report of the International Narcotics Control Board on the Availability of Internationally Controlled Drugs: Ensuring Adequate Access for Medical and Scientific Purposes. http://www.incb.org/documents/Publications/AnnualReports/AR2010/Supplement-AR10_availability_English.pdf. Accessed 26 August 2013
8. Commission on Narcotic Drugs. Promoting Adequate Availability of Internationally Controlled Narcotic Drugs and Psychotropic Substances for Medical and Scientific Purposes While Preventing Their Diversion and Abuse. Resolution. http://daccess-dds-ny.un.org/doc/UNDOC/LTD/V11/815/54/PDF/V1181554.pdf?OpenElement. Accessed August 26, 2013.

CHAPTER 71

Palliative care in Canada

Doris Howell and Ann Syme

Key points

◆ Development and service delivery of hospice and palliative care in Canada has further evolved in the past decade due to initiatives at federal, provincial, and local levels.

◆ Some of the current innovations in hospice palliative service delivery include integrated models of care, palliative home care including virtual and telehealth delivery, and a shift from exclusive specialist models of care to the application of palliative principles to address population needs across the healthcare system.

◆ Hospice palliative care nursing in Canada has evolved to a recognized nursing specialty, and new roles, for example, nurse practitioner, enable nursing to provide leadership in integrated models of interdisciplinary service delivery. There is also an emphasis on developing hospice palliative skills of the entire nursing work force.

Canadians are served by a publicly funded healthcare system and, when asked, state that quality end-of-life care is important to them. In the last decade there has been a national effort toward making quality end-of-life care an entrenched core value of Canada's healthcare system.[1] National healthcare policy for palliative care has been championed by the Canadian Hospice Palliative Care Association (CHPCA)[2] and a committed Senator, Sharon Carstairs, whose latest report calls for five elements necessary for Canadians to have access to quality palliative care services: (1) a culture of care, (2) sufficient capacity, (3) support for caregivers, (4) integrated services, and (5) leadership.[3]

The guiding definition for hospice palliative care in Canada was established by the CHPCA and acknowledges the need for hospice palliative care to be accessible across the trajectory of life-threatening illness wherever that patient/family is receiving care to reduce suffering and optimize quality of living and extending into bereavement. The definition for hospice palliative care in Canada includes a number of concepts that have guided development of services and emerging integrated and simultaneous models of care that are discussed later in this chapter. The full definition is as follows:

Hospice palliative care is aimed at relief of suffering and improving the quality of life of persons who are living with or dying from advanced illness or are bereaved.[4]

Hospice palliative care strives to help patients and families address physical, psychological, social, spiritual and practical issues, and their associated expectations, needs, hopes, and fears; prepare for and manage self-determined life closure and the dying process; and cope with loss and grief during the illness and bereavement.

Hospice palliative care aims to treat all active issues, prevent new issues from occurring, and promote opportunities for meaningful and valuable experiences, personal and spiritual growth, and self-actualization.

Hospice palliative care is appropriate for any patient and/or family living with, or at risk of developing, a life-threatening illness due to any diagnosis, with any prognosis, regardless of age, and at any time they have unmet expectations and/or needs and are prepared to accept care.

Hospice palliative care may complement and enhance disease-modifying therapy or it may become the total focus of care.

This chapter describes palliative and end-of-life care from national and provincial perspectives and the trends and innovations in hospice and palliative care service delivery in Canada and specifically the developments in nursing. To provide a context within Canada, factors that have influenced the development of hospice palliative care in Canada inclusive of geographic and population diversity; the three levels of government accountable for healthcare delivery—federal, provincial, and regional; and the advocacy role of the Canadian Hospice Palliative Care Association are also described.

Context of care in Canada

Canada is the biggest country in the Americas, and second in the world in regard to land mass, with 3,854,082 square miles.[5] The nation is divided into 10 provinces and three northern territories, has two official languages (English and French), and is geographically diverse with a mix of urban, rural, and remote areas. The population in Canada reached 35 million in 2012, and Canada continues to be one of the fastest growing nations in the group of nations with the largest economies in the world.[6] The majority (86%) of the population lives in the provinces of Ontario, Quebec, British Columbia, and Alberta, and mainly in urban cities. This continued growth in Canada is due to immigration; approximately 260,000 persons have been arriving annually since 2006.[7] Therefore, Canada comprises a rich variety of cultural groups. The four main cultural groupings include the Aboriginal peoples, British and French "founders" of Canada, and more recently, immigrants from Asia, Africa, and other non-European nations.[8] It is estimated that about 28% of the population is foreign born, with 55% expected to be born in Asia.[9] The fastest growing religion is Islam; its growth rate exceeds other religions in Canada with a recorded prevalence rate of 1 million Muslims in Canada.[9]

As in other countries such as Australia, there is also a large Aboriginal population in Canada, about 1.4 million persons.[10] The Aboriginal population is defined by the Constitution Act of 1982 and includes North American Indian, Inuit, and Métis.[10-11] Aboriginal persons represent just over 3% of Canada's total population.[8] The North American Indian makes up 62% of the Aboriginal population, the Métis 30%, and the Inuit 5%.[12] The Aboriginal population has the highest population growth rate, with half of the Aboriginal population under 25 years contrasted with half of the non-Aboriginal population under 38 years of age. The Aboriginal population faces significant health disparities as they face a disproportion burden of ill health and racism in access to healthcare and lack of sensitivity of providers in provision of relevant palliative care.

The unique cultural, end-of-life care needs of the Aboriginal population and the continued interest in Aboriginal hospice palliative care have been identified through several federal government, national organizations, and Aboriginal forums and papers.[13] In the report *Cross-Cultural Considerations in Promoting Advance Care Planning in Canada*, guidelines for caregiving in the aboriginal community were identified to include: (1) respect of individuals; (2) practice conscious communication; (3) use of interpreters; (4) involvement of family, including extended family; (5) recognition of alternatives to truth-telling; (6) practice of noninterference; and (7) allowing the practice of traditional medicine.[14] In addition to the areas of growth that have occurred in the past decade with regard to Aboriginal hospice palliative care, significant gaps need to be addressed.[1] These gaps include the acquisition of knowledge and evidence to inform program and policy development and service delivery; jurisdiction and policy clarity around service provision on and off reserve; limitations of Aboriginal issues in healthcare education curriculum; cultural competence; practical aspects of health service delivery on and off reserve settings and with vulnerable populations; fragmentation and effective funding and reporting models; Aboriginal grief and bereavement models and services; and basic housing, food, and clothing needs that impact daily Aboriginal living and dying. Recognition of the experience of living and dying in the Aboriginal population is fundamental to care that is sensitive to the needs of this population.[15]

This "Canadian Mosaic" of cultural, ethnic, and linguistic diversity has resulted in multiple perspectives in the development of hospice palliative care services and in the complexity of end-of-life issues that must be addressed by interprofessional teams and providers across care sectors. Respect for diversity and the identification of hospice palliative care needs and preferences for care in these diverse populations is a fundamental principle of palliative care in Canada, but it does create challenges in the development of relevant and appropriate services.

Influence of healthcare policy and national initiatives

Universality is the central premise of Canada's publicly funded healthcare system; mandated through federal legislation in The Medical Care Insurance Act of 1966.[16] In this Act all insured residents in Canada regardless of ability to pay "must be entitled to the insured health services provided by the provincial or territorial healthcare insurance plan on uniform terms and conditions."

The Canada Health Act of 1984 (CHA) followed to ensure reasonable access to health services without financial or other barriers through five key principles: public administration, comprehensiveness, universality, portability, and accessibility.[17] The CHA legislates criteria for insured and extended healthcare services that the provinces and territories must fulfill to receive federal cash transfer payments under the Canada Health Transfer (CHT) system.[18] Palliative care is not included as part of the CHA, and since healthcare services are provincially regulated, palliative care is not consistently identified as a core service in provincial healthcare budgets.[19] This has resulted in variations in the structure and funding of hospice palliative care services across Canada, particularly in home and community-based services.[20-21]

Variations in access to care have also occurred as a result of regionalization of healthcare in most provinces. Regionalization has been taking place since the 1990s as it allows for autonomous decision-making by healthcare regions in a province regarding service allocations. This sociopolitical context for healthcare delivery in Canada has been shown to result in disparities in equality of access to care and health outcomes. Equality in access to hospice palliative care services is problematic in Canada, with reports of over 70% of those dying in Canada not in receipt of care.[22]

As shown in Box 71.1, a number of healthcare legislative and other national initiatives have influenced the development of hospice palliative care services in Canada. The establishment of the Canadian Palliative Care Association (CPCA) in 1991 and its evolution to the Canadian Hospice Palliative Care Association (CHPCA),[23] to integrate hospice and palliative care service development, remains key to the development of hospice palliative care in Canada. The mandate of CHPCA is described in more detail in the next section.

Additionally, recommendations of the Kirby report and the Romanow commission[24] have been influential in the evolution of homecare as an essential service and the provision of benefits for time off work to support informal caregivers. The initial development of palliative care in Canada was mainly institution based. However, as a result of decreasing federal financing for healthcare, Canadian provinces have been focused on restructuring the delivery of their healthcare services to reduce reliance on national government–funded healthcare.[25] This has led to a shift to deinstitutionalize care to the home and community care sector,[26] which is desired by Canadians.[27]

The shift in care to home and community-based services was facilitated through funding investments by the federal, provincial, and territorial First Ministers in 2004[28] and the release of the Pan-Canadian Gold Standards for Palliative Home Care: Towards Equitable Access to High Quality Palliative and End-of-Life Care at Home by the CHPCA and the Canadian Home Care Association (CHCA) in December 2006.[29] This document identified gold-level standards for palliative home care to ensure its consistent development across Canada and equality in access to essential components including case management, nursing and personal support worker care, and palliative specific pharmaceuticals. The call for further development of a pan-Canadian home care strategy across all levels of government and particularly to increase access to palliative care in a broad range of settings, including residential hospices, and for the expansion of drugs and supplies to home care recipients was further recommended in the 2012 government report *A Time for Transformative Change: A Review of the 2004 Health Accord*.[30]

Box 71.1 Canadian healthcare legislation and initiatives

1991—Canadian Palliative Care Association deemed a national charitable organization

1994—White Paper

1995—Release of the Senate Committee report *Of Life and Death*

2000—Release of the Subcommittee of the Standing Senate Committee on Social Affairs, Science and Technology report *Quality End of Life Care: The Right of Every Canadian* (commonly referred to as Carstairs' report)

2001—Secretariat on Palliative and End-of-Life Care established; Senator Carstairs appointed as federal Minister with Special Responsibility for Palliative Care

—Canadian Palliative Care Association changes to Canadian Hospice Palliative Care Association (CHPCA)

2002—Release of the Model to Guide Hospice Palliative Care, CHPCA

2002—Release of the Kirby report *The Health of Canadians— The Federal Role*

—Release of the Romanow report *Commission on the Future of Health Care in Canada*

2004—Primary Care Health Transition Fund begins and funds Pallium Project (rural palliative care)

—Compassionate Care Benefit enacted

2006—Primary Health Care Transition Fund ends (Pallium enters evaluation phase)

—Compassionate Care Benefit expanded

2006—Accreditation Canada releases national standards and performance indicators

2007—Secretariat on Palliative and End-of-Life Care disbanded

2010—Quality End-of-Life Care as a Basic Right for all

2012—Senate Committee Report: *A Time for Transformative Change: A Review of the 2004 Health Accord*

2012—The Way Forward: Moving Toward Community-Integrated Palliative Care in Canada

---

Progress in the development of home and community-based care appears to have occurred as a result of these national initiatives. In May 2012, in the Fact Sheet for Hospice Palliative Care in Canada,[31] the CHPCA reported that all provinces now have some form of palliative drug coverage for home care patients. However, fewer (6 of 13 provinces) have policies on providing access to nursing and personal care services 24 hours a day, 7 days a week, and access to case managed care is unclear.

Deinstitutionalization and shifting of care to the home and community has not happened without criticism, as it has resulted in a significant emotional and financial burden being left on the shoulders of family caregivers.[32,33] For instance, federal funding for costs of end-of-life care are only 70% supported, with the remaining 2% being not-for-profit supported and 27% family-borne.[34] Caregiving by families is estimated to be worth $25–$26 billion and $80 million dollars annually in out-of-pocket costs.[35,36] A response to this issue, although considered far from adequate, was an amendment to the Canada Labour Code in 2004 to offer a Compassionate Care Benefit through the Employment Insurance program to provide 6 weeks (extended to 8 weeks, in 2006) paid leave to eligible Canadians to care for a dying loved one.[37] Multiple

stakeholder groups are engaged to ensure that family caregivers are not left with the burden of caregiving and adequate supports are available to assist them in this process as part of the quality agenda for hospice palliative word care in Canada.

In 2010, the Senate report *Quality End-of-Life Care as a Basic Right for all Canadians* was tabled and identified the goals for a change in the death-denying culture of care, increased capacity building, more focus on caregiver support, and the integration of services and leadership across Canada.[38] The report proposed 17 recommendations to serve as a roadmap (2010–2020) for the federal government, provincial and territorial governments, and the entire community to meet these goals, making it the responsibility of every Canadian to work together at all three levels of government (federal, provincial, regional). The CHPCA was charged with reporting on the progress in the nation regarding the recommendations in this report and continues to do so through its Fact Sheets disseminated across Canada and on its website.

In 2012, the federal government in Canada, announced an investment of over 3 million dollars to move forward a plan for the integration of hospice palliative care services across all sectors of healthcare service and community-based care. As a result, key organizations are working in partnership to develop strategic directions under the umbrella The Way Forward: Moving Toward Community-Integrated Palliative Care in Canada initiative. This initiative will focus on the following activities and outcomes: (1) describe the current environment and issues through scoping reviews and discussion documents as a basis for consultations; (2) consult with a wide range of partners and stakeholders; (3) develop and implement a framework for community-integrated palliative care models, which will include strategic directions, priorities for action, and a road map for implementation; (4) distribute the results to stakeholders who are in positions to implement the framework; and (5) evaluate the activities, outputs, and outcomes of the initiative.[39] The CHPCA provides leadership and works in partnership with multiple stakeholder groups in Canada to ensure progress and advocacy for change.

Canadian Hospice Palliative Care Association

The CHPCA has been the national voice for hospice palliative care in Canada, it is a charitable not-for-profit organization whose mission is to provide leadership and play a national advocacy role in hospice palliative care.[40] The CHPCA achieves this mission by supporting research, promoting education and training, improving public awareness of hospice palliative care, and advocating for increased programs and services, and works in close partnership with other national organizations. Priorities for the CHPCA over the past 5 years follow:

1. Promoting integration of hospice palliative and end-of-life care principles and practices into all health settings

2. Promoting education of healthcare providers in all health settings

3. Promoting evidence-informed policy

4. Building strong partnerships to improve hospice, palliative, and end-of-life care

5. Raising awareness about hospice palliative end-of-life care

6. Building the capacity of the Canadian Hospice Palliative Care Association

One of the key priorities of CHPCA has been to develop and reach consensus on national standards for palliative care to ensure consistency in the development of hospice palliative care services. Subsequently, the Model to Guide Hospice Palliative Care: Principles, Norms and Practices provided a conceptual framework to facilitate consistency in the development and delivery of palliative care services across Canada.[4] This document provides definitions, values, guiding principles, and foundational concepts that form the basis for hospice palliative care; a framework of population needs, principles, and norms of practice to guide patient/family care; and the application of the model to other activities such as education. Through a collaborative effort of the CHPCA and the Canadian Network of Palliative Care for Children and with support from Health Canada, a companion document, Pediatric Hospice Palliative Care: Guiding Principles and Norms of Practice was released in 2006 to promote consistent and quality palliative care for children.[41] The Model to Guide Hospice Palliative Care was fundamental to the development of standards for accreditation of hospice palliative care services in Canada and is part of national surveillance under cancer control.[42]

Accreditation for hospice palliative care services in Canada

Accreditation Canada has been conducting health services reviews for 50 years. Their goal is to "ensure that safe, efficient and reliable care is being delivered within health systems."[43] Accreditation Canada released their 2008 Canadian Health Accreditation Report stating that 977 service organizations were surveyed in 2007. To influence organization and health-system changes it was crucial to develop nationally accredited standards for palliative and end-of-life care. Accreditation Canada began to develop hospice palliative and end-of-life care standards in 2003. It identified its guiding principles as sustainability, timeliness, relevance, efficiency, rigor, specificity, client/family focus, flexibility, and adaptability. This project was funded through Health Canada's Secretariat on Palliative and End-of-Life Care and included the provision of a national set of standards, an accreditation program for hospice organizations, and a core set of performance measures or indicators.[44,45] These standards were released in May 2006. The standards focus on the following:

♦ Investing in hospice palliative and end-of-life services;

♦ Engaging prepared and proactive staff;

♦ Providing safe and appropriate services;

♦ Enhancing quality of life;

♦ Maintaining accessible and efficient clinical information systems; and

♦ Measuring quality and achieving positive outcomes.[46]

Although not inclusive, five initial core indicators that were developed include (1) availability of hospice palliative care 24/7; (2) continuity of care; (3) identification of the degree and management of distress (measured using Edmonton Symptom Assessment System[47]); (4) family/caregiver satisfaction with end-of-life care; and (5) documentation of client and family service goals.[45]

Present status of hospice palliative care

Access to quality care

In an international Quality of Death index released in 2010, the Economist's Intelligence Unit ranked Canada as ninth in comparison to other countries in regard to the quality of palliative and end-of-life care.[48] As noted by the CHPA, "the harsh reality is that 70% or more of Canadians currently do not have access to palliative care."[31] As described earlier, this is partly due to the overarching jurisdictional issues, but it is also attributable in part to other factors such as geographic remoteness, ongoing institutional restructuring, eligibility requirements (i.e., completion of active treatment still exists as eligibility for palliative care units), federal jurisdiction over particular groups, and the multiple points of entry into the healthcare system. While significant progress has been made in Canada toward ensuring equality of access to quality hospice palliative care services, continuing challenges include adequate and consistent funding of services across jurisdictions and geographies, capacity to deliver services across multiple cultures and faiths, the appropriate preparation of a knowledgeable healthcare workforce, and the growing unprecedented demand for services as the population ages and lives longer with chronic disease conditions and life prolongation occurs for those living with advanced and metastatic disease due to cancer.[20]

The movement in Canada has been toward specialization in palliative care, and while this may have drawn attention to the skills and principles that are required for quality palliative care, this movement has also contributed to a sequestering of care in programs and palliative care units where specialists practice. This has resulted in the labeling of Hospice Palliative Care in Canada as "urban centric" and has limited access to hospice palliative care services for those living outside of urban areas.[25]

In spite of universality of healthcare, disparities in access to healthcare do occur in the Canadian healthcare system on the basis of factors such as sex, age, socioeconomic status, ethnicity, and geography. The quality of hospice palliative care for ethnoculturally diverse populations in Canada was identified in this research[25] as an understudied area, and it is unclear whether the quality of hospice and palliative care in these populations is consistent with their values and preferences. The foundations of the modern palliative care/hospice movement are based on Christian tradition and teachings and a growing recognition of the futility and indignity of continuing expensive and intrusive treatments for people who are clearly dying. Guiding palliative care principles are based on the Western ethics of "truth-telling" and patient autonomy. These principles are often in direct conflict with the beliefs and values of many of the persons that we care for, resulting in culturally insensitive decision-making and health policies. For instance, South Asian populations may view terminal illness as "God's wish," and so they do not wish to discuss or plan for their death. Other authors suggest that there are more similarities than differences between ethnocultural groups' understanding of what palliative care should address and entail.[49] However, interdisciplinary providers of palliative care may be less experienced in negotiating the complex and difficult terrain of issues at end-of-life in caring for those with differing values and belief systems.[50] Additionally, the meaning and value focused on place of care and death in the home may not be of equal precedence to those with a diverse cultural background or who face socioeconomic or other health disparities.

In December 2000, the Quality End-of-Life Coalition (QELCC) was formed representing a broad group of 31 stakeholder organizations across Canada under the auspices of the CHPCA.[51] Quality coalitions now exist in most provinces and have been instrumental in advocating for better care at the provincial and regional levels to ultimately improve hospice palliative care for all.[52]

Place of death

In 2012, an annual death rate of 252,242 was reported for Canadians, a rate expected to increase to 432,000 by 2041.[53] Most Canadians die in old age, and of these a significant majority die due to chronic illnesses including cancer and cardio/cerebro-vascular and lower respiratory diseases, which are the leading causes of death in that order. The majority of Canadians express a desire to die at home or in their home communities.[27] Whether this goal can be realized is influenced by the diseases from which Canadians die, whether they live in a city or rural or remote area, the province in which they reside, cultural diversity, the nature of their private health insurance plans, provincial coverage of health services, access to informal caregivers, and their personal wealth.[4] However, research on location of death in Canada does suggest a trend toward an increasing number of out-of-hospital deaths, which is considered an indicator of the need for palliative home and community-based care and quality of care.

Wilson and colleagues in their research on location of deaths for 1,806,318 Canadians across the provinces except Quebec noted a decline in hospital deaths during 1994–2004 from 77.7% to 60.6 %.[46] Similarly, Statistics Canada reported that 68.6% of Canadians died in a hospital in 2008.[54] More recent reports suggest a reduction in the number of hospital deaths, at least for cancer patients. In 2013, the Canadian Institute for Health Information (CIHI) reported that about half (45%) of Canadian cancer deaths—excluding Quebec—occurred in acute care hospitals.[55] Wide variation by province was noted, with higher rates of hospital deaths for cancer patients in Manitoba (69%) and New Brunswick (66%) and the lowest rates noted for Ontario (40%) and British Columbia (39%). High rates of hospitalization and emergency room visits in the last weeks of life were also noted in this CIHI report and, including deaths in hospital, these are accepted indicators of poor quality of palliative care at the population level.[56]

As noted by the CHPCA, variations in place of death are likely explained by provincial differences in access to palliative care beds, the availability of community-based services such as home care or community-based hospice services, and low access to interdisciplinary palliative care expertise.[57] It is less clear where other patients with life-limiting chronic illness die, and there is an identified need to expand access to a range of palliative care services for those dying of conditions other than cancer. Even though cancer patients represent only 28% of Canadian deaths,[58] they make up 80%–90% of home-care clients receiving end-of-life care with the Community Care Access Centres in Ontario.[59] Individuals with diseases of the circulatory system (35% of deaths) and of the respiratory system (about 10% of deaths) are under-represented.[58] In Ontario, research has shown that home care in the last 6 months of life reduces emergency department visits,

hospitalizations, healthcare costs, and increases home as a place of death for a range of diagnoses.[60] However, differential access to palliative home care or other services in rural or remote areas is noted and higher rates of hospital death for those living in rural areas are well documented.[61] Several other factors may influence in-hospital death rates: cultural and spiritual beliefs; availability of integrated, interdisciplinary care; ability of family members to provide care; financial considerations (access to drugs, pain pumps, and oxygen); and education and reimbursement systems for providers, but these are not measured in administrative data used for estimating location of death in Canada.[62]

Nurses play an instrumental role in the provision of palliative care in rural and remote areas of Canada. Factors contributing to the complexity of nursing service delivery in these areas are low service volumes, lack of health services, human resources, and ability to reach remote areas due to seasonal variations in the Canadian climate.[63] The literature repeatedly identifies the needs for rural and remote nurses to be able to cross-train and be flexible in their knowledge and skills.[64] Consequently, a focus on primary healthcare reform and particularly the role of the primary care physicians and nurse practitioners in palliative care delivery has been an important direction as part of deinstitutionalization from acute care hospitals.

Models of care

Palliative care services have developed and are delivered according to differing models of care across Canada. In some jurisdictions, service has grown out of academic and healthcare organizations partnering and developing capacities. For instance, palliative care was initially focused in acute care hospitals with the establishment of palliative care units at the Royal Victoria Hospital in Montreal and the St. Boniface Hospital in Winnipeg in 1974.[65] These were modeled after the British system of palliative care, and specifically St. Christopher's Hospice, and emphasized an interdisciplinary, comprehensive approach to care with attention to symptom control and psychosocial-spiritual distress. In other areas of Canada, service has grown out of a community awareness of the lack of end-of-life care and capacity within mainstream services. And in most there is a combination of "top-down" and "bottom-up" approaches leading to blended models of community based and tertiary services. For instance, Hospice Victoria in British Columbia has its earliest beginnings as a grass-roots movement initiating services in the community in 1978.[66] This program has now expanded to receive 50% of its funding from provincial government and serves over 400 palliative patients at any given time in an integrated system of care that includes a 17-bed acute palliative care inpatient unit, 10 long-term palliative care beds, a 24 hour/7 days/week palliative rapid response program, and an inter-disciplinary consultation service with an annual operating budget of over 7 million dollars.[66]

Integrated models of care

Healthcare reform in Canada has had a strong emphasis on integrated service networks to address the separation of hospitals, primary care, home, and community-based care sectors. Currently, there is not an agreed on definition for integrated care but there are core concepts that are considered integral to this type of "organized system" of care, as follows: patient-centered (care is organized around patient needs as opposed to providers'), continuous (care follows the patient over time, creating seamless transitions throughout the care journey), and collaborative (brings together independent providers in health and social systems to provide personalized care to the patient).[67]

The expectation for seamless access to hospice palliative care services across care settings through integrated models of care has also been articulated by the Ontario College of Family Physicians and Cancer Care Ontario.[68] This model describes four levels of care with the understanding that patients move between these levels based on their needs across the end-of-life trajectory: Level 1, primary care, is required by the largest population of patients, and the expectation is that this is made available within the primary care sector by health providers including primary health care physicians and nurse practitioners trained in the provision of a palliative care approach; Level 2, secondary care, also assumes a level of expertise in hospice palliative care and includes access to specialists in symptom and emotional distress management; Level 3, complex care, is for patients that do not respond to established protocols that require specialist/tertiary hospice palliative care expertise; Level 4, tertiary interventions, may require specialized expertise such an acute palliative care bed in hospital (CCO Models). Integrated models of care are emerging in Canada and include many of the elements articulated by the Agency for Health Care Research and Quality (AHRQ).[69] Examples of integrated models of care in Canada include those in Manitoba, British Colombia, Alberta, and Nova Scotia and in some regions in Ontario. In general, the following elements are available or in development with mechanisms for governance or networking among the care elements[69]:

1. Inpatient palliative care (hospital-wide palliative care consults; acute tertiary level inpatient beds for those with complex symptoms)

2. Outpatient palliative care (includes palliative care consultation clinics)

3. Linkage to palliative home care (team communicates regularly with the inpatient unit)

4. Provider education and research (partnership with academic health center, internal conferences, and leadership provision to other organizations)

5. Family support (available through home care or volunteer hospice services)

6. Alternative care options for death at home (long-term care palliative beds or residential hospices with free-standing beds in a designated facility)

There are emerging pockets of excellence for integrated palliative home care pilot programs also emerging to address needs in rural areas. For instance, Marshall and colleagues described a model of shared care that integrated services between the home care program (case management, nursing, and allied health services), family physician group practices in three group practices, and an interdisciplinary palliative care team (palliative care advanced practice nurse, palliative medicine physician, bereavement counselor, psychosocial-spiritual advisor).[59] Key features of the program included systematic and timely identification of patients with palliative care needs using best-practice criteria (Would you be surprised if this patient were to die in the next 12 months? Does the patient have symptom or psychosocial care needs?), regular scheduled meetings among all team members for care planning, coordinated care facilitated by outcome-based assessment, common needs-assessment approach and communication exchange, access to specialists 24 hours/day/7 days/week, and counseling and bereavement support for patient and family. This model of palliative care has been shown to reduce symptom and psychosocial distress[70] and is still less costly than care in hospitals.[71] Integrated care systems may help to ensure that patients do not fall in the cracks in the transition between care settings and may facilitate continuity of care.[72]

Another program of excellence in integrated care provision is in Alberta. In Alberta, the Edmonton Zone Palliative Care Program (EZPCP) has been in operation since July 1995. Previously, access to palliative care services was inconsistent. Two palliative care units existed, one at the Edmonton General Hospital and one at the Misericordia Hospital. In 1992, 21% (290 patients), of all cancer patients dying in the region had access to these services. Palliative home care was also providing care in the community. In the 1999/2000 reporting year, access to palliative care consultation for cancer patients was 79.4%. The EZPCP has maintained this level of increased access through the community-based model of care every year since the program began. Although access to palliative care is reported for cancer patients, the program also supports patients with other diagnoses. In 1999/2000, 10% of patients seen (126/1273) were patients with other diagnoses.

Palliative care is often misconstrued with end-of-life care, and this has been a significant barrier to earlier access to palliative care in oncology programs from the perspective of both clinicians and patients, with referral often occurring in the final weeks of life. Thus, the integration of palliative care early in the course of life-threatening illness, specifically oncology programs, has been a goal of care in North America, based on level 1 evidence of benefit,[73] and in many provinces in Canada. In Ontario, an integrated care approach has been labeled a "simultaneous care approach."[68] A simultaneous approach to care embraces the concept of palliative care being applicable early in the course of the disease, in conjunction with other therapies that are intended to prolong life, such as chemotherapy or radiation therapy. The simultaneous approach supports the definition of "palliative care" being distinguished from that of "end-of-life care," which specifically refers to services provided to dying patients and their families. This model of care approach focuses on helping patients move through the trajectory of a progressive, life-threatening disease by enabling their changing goals of care to be met at all stages based on an interdisciplinary approach to care that attends to symptom management, psychosocial issues, and advance care planning.

In Ontario, a phase II Randomized Control Trial (RCT) demonstrated that earlier integration of palliative care with oncology care results in improvements in common symptoms such as pain, fatigue, nausea, anxiety, dyspnea, depression, drowsiness, constipation, and insomnia.[74] In oncology programs in Ontario, Manitoba, and Alberta this simultaneous approach to care has been facilitated through early identification of symptom and psychological distress using routine collection of patient-reported outcome measures for nine common symptoms using the Edmonton Symptom Assessment System (ESAS) or the revised version that provided better explanation to patients for completing some scales

(ESAS-r)[75] at every visit in all 14 regional cancer programs and by visiting nurses in home care programs using similar scales.[76, 77]

Given that most of these specialist models of care have largely been successful in large urban areas, for which there is increasing recognition, particularly with the unprecedented growth of the aging population[78] and the expected demand for palliative care services, a number of jurisdictions are exploring mechanisms to introduce a "palliative approach" in their care systems.[63] A palliative approach is one way of introducing palliative care principles to a wide range of patients in the health system earlier in the illness trajectory. A palliative approach recognizes that, although not all people with life-limiting illness require specialized palliative services, they do require care that is aimed at improving quality of life by preventing and relieving suffering through early identification, assessment, and treatment of physical, psychosocial, and spiritual concerns.[79] A palliative approach also introduces conversations about living well and being supported that lead to advance care planning for patients and their families. A palliative approach is introduced when the healthcare provider asks the following question: Is this person sick enough that death within the next year would not be surprising (not prognosis dependent)?[80] These questions are pivotal in the cancer clinic setting, as they identify patients earlier in the trajectory with palliative care needs.

The adoption of a palliative care approach is also considered to be fundamental to ensuring access to palliative care in long-term care facilities in Canada. The CHPCA in partnership with the Quality Palliative Care in Long Term Care Alliance (QPC-LTC) aims to develop the capacity for high-quality care in long-term care facilities to reach the following goals: expand advance care planning uptake in long-term care, enhance resources to allow long-term care facilities to create hospice palliative care programs, strengthen interprofessional collaboration with long-term care facilities and the community, and integrate hospice palliative care philosophy into resident-centered care.[81]

Virtual hospice and telehealth technology

Another highly successful model for reaching patients and family members in need of palliative support wherever they live has been virtual hospice approaches or the use of telehealth technology. This is essential given Canada's vast geography and the difficulty of winter travel to some rural and remote areas that would otherwise be unreachable. There is a great need for patient information and utilization data to flow between various healthcare providers, care settings, and across provincial settings and beyond. It has been vital to look for solutions that will strengthen the coordination of care through innovation and creativity and facilitate seamless patient movement regardless of the location of care delivery. The vision statement of the Canadian Society for Telehealth aims toward achieving "optimal health for all."[82]

Several recent Web-based innovations in Canada will help to address some of the challenges experienced in the provision of rural and remote areas in palliative care. In 2001, Health Canada announced funding to support the development of the Canadian Virtual Hospice (CVH).[83] The Canadian Virtual Hospice goals are to facilitate, via a Web-based forum, equitable distribution of mutual support, the exchange of information, communication, and collaboration between and among healthcare professionals, researchers, the terminally ill, and their families.

Another example is the rural palliative telehealth project funded by Alberta Health and Wellness in 2007. The project in Alberta determined that telehealth technology offers an e-health solution to the challenges faced with a widely dispersed rural population. This project demonstrated that there was improved access to secondary-level palliative care consultation, improved home support, reduced emergency visits and hospitalizations, reduced need for travel, and improved symptom management for rural and home-bound patients. The body of evidence continues to grow, demonstrating that telehealth visits are as effective as face-to-face consultations.[84]

Another example of telehealth solutions to improve access to care was led by nurses in British Columbia. Leaders in the Fraser Health regions of British Columbia identified the need to improve access for palliative and end-of-life care around the clock (i.e., 24/7), specifically to ensure the generalist nursing workforce who deals with a broad range of health problems could also address questions related specifically to hospice palliative care. The exploration of how information and communications technology could be used to achieve this kind of support for home-based palliative patients and their families begun. This was a collaboration between the Fraser Health Hospice Palliative Care Program and BC Nurse Line. A pilot project was conducted in which hospice palliative care content was incorporated into the provincial call system for after-hours calls. At any one time, 750 home-based hospice palliative care clients had access to after-hours telephone lines. "Healthwise Knowledge base triage protocols" that include specialized content specific to palliative care were added to enhance the existing tools. The results of the project demonstrated that 80% of calls met the needs of the patients and/or families. With this support, 91% of the patients were able to stay home throughout the night.[85] Only six home visits have been made in the 2 years since implementation of this after-hours service. The nurses involved in the project were able to leverage their experience and develop training tools, a resource manual for using the HPC protocols, and templates to enable other health authorities to develop these types of programs.

Palliative care nursing

Nurses have always cared for dying patients as part of their practice throughout history. The scopes of practice for healthcare providers are front and center in the evolution of healthcare practices. Licensed practical nurses (LPNs) have assumed several preexisting functions of the registered nurse (RN) and often work in collaborative practice models with an RN. Registered nurses, clinical nurse specialists, and nurse practitioners (NPs) have assumed functions that were within the scope of primary care physicians less than 2 decades ago or are delegated through medical directives.

Official recognition of the nurse's role in hospice palliative care in Canada began in 1993, in Winnipeg, where nurses met to form an interest group. This evolved into an official network and recognized group of the CHPCA and continues to provide a national voice to advance hospice palliative nursing care in policy development, education, and research. In 2002, the first Standards for Hospice Palliative Care Nursing were developed. These standards, based on the supportive care model, identified six dimensions that reflected the therapeutic role of hospice palliative nursing: valuing, connecting, empowering, doing for, finding meaning, and preserving integrity. Following the endorsement of these standards and competencies by hospice palliative care nurses in Canada, the Canadian Nurses Association (CNA), in conjunction with the CHPCA Nurses Interest Group, initiated the process of specialty certification for hospice palliative care nursing. Certification by the CNA "requires adherence to rigorous practice standards, a commitment to continuous learning."[86] The first sitting of the certification exam occurred in April 2004 with updates to the exam and related competencies in 2010. Since its inception as a Canadian Nurses Certification specialty in 2003, the number of nurses certified in hospice palliative care in 2008 alone was 20.4%. This was an increase from 916 to 1247 nurses certified to the 2012 figure of 1408 nurses with hospice palliative care certification.

Many Canadian universities offer education for the development of advanced nursing practice as either nurse practitioners or clinical nurse specialists with an opportunity to focus on palliative care. Postdiploma certificates have also been offered at several community colleges and range from single courses to full university credits. More recently, the results of a survey of nurse educators in a Canadian university faculty of nursing was undertaken to identify what nurse educators knew or did not know about end-of-life care.[87] The results of the survey indicated that although hospice palliative care education is being addressed in most programs that participated in the survey, there is a need to further develop palliative and end-of-life curricula. Challenges to do so include adding additional content to full curricula, the tension to balance generalist and specialist competencies in undergraduate education, faculty and organizational approval, and practicum placement sites.[88] The results of this survey were used to by the CHPCA's Nurses' Interest group partnering with the Canadian Association of Schools of Nursing (CASN) to create resources for baccalaureate educators to help their students to understand and apply palliative care principles in their care for patients and families facing a life-threatening disease. In 2011, CASN released the document Palliative and End-of-Life Care: Entry to Practice Competencies and Indicators for Registered Nurses to facilitate greater integration of this area of nursing in undergraduate curricula in Canada.[89] More recently, CASN also released a guide for faculty in the use of story for educating nurses about hospice palliative care nursing, *Palliative and End-of-Life Care Teaching and Learning Resources, 2012*.[90] This was followed by the Master's Diploma in Advanced Practice Oncology/Palliative Care Nursing at the University of Windsor for first entry of students in 2013.[91]

The most recent development to support the role of nurses in hospice and palliative care came in the form of legislation. In 2012, the federal Controlled Drugs and Substances Act was revised to permit nurse practitioners to prescribe opiates to their patients[92] This new legislation is now being adopted across Canada in the provincial regulations that oversee the practices of nurse practitioners, of which there were 1990 licensed in Canada in 2009.[93] This is an extremely important step in jurisprudence to allow nurse practitioners to participate in symptom control, a mainstay of palliative practice.

In planning for the future, the Canadian Nurses Association report *Toward 2020 Visions for Nursing* calls for nurses to provide leadership in this change by "setting an agenda to create a healthcare system that truly serves and reflects the priorities of Canadians. But no one will appoint them to the task."[94] This provides incredible opportunities and challenges for nursing staff as well as for those who specialize in hospice palliative care. This

report also identifies several scenarios for a preferred future that can be applied to hospice palliative care nursing, such as:

- Providing leadership in the education of nursing, interdisciplinary teams and the public as well as leading and/or participating in research regarding the impact of individual and family coping and decision-making;
- Increasing the knowledge, skill, and research to be able to respond to changing disease patterns;
- Identifying and supporting effective coping mechanisms as well as identifying at-risk individuals and families in order to contribute to the wellness trend with an expectation of increased education and engagement in personal health;
- Promoting advanced practice hospice palliative care nurses such as clinical nurse specialists and nurse practitioners who are well placed to provide increased integration of a holistic health movement into mainstream medicine;
- Identifying global environmental issues such as pollution and/ or radiation exposure that contribute to major health changes and life limiting conditions or disease which could benefit from palliative and end-of-life care.

Additionally, the future will consist of various health system trends that continue to see a shift to community-based services, use of technology, increased focus on long-term and end-of-life care, expectations and support for increased family involvements, and funding-ratio changes. It is clear, however, that if new delivery models are not developed, the current shortage of healthcare professionals will impact healthcare adversely. There is an urgent need to work differently. This provides an incredible opportunity for hospice palliative care nurses to engage in community development and enhancing the communities' capacities to provide compassionate and effective hospice palliative care services in the most appropriate settings of care.

Ethical issues: decision-making at the end of life and the euthanasia debate

Decision-making at the end of life

Decision-making at the end-of-life is a complex issue with many facets that need to be considered in supporting patients/families to make decisions that are consistent with their values and preferences.[95] In a recent editorial, Goodman suggested the solution to improving care was not to blindly drive systems toward greater use of hospice palliative care services but to improve decision quality so that patients can make an informed choice regarding active curative care, supportive care, or simultaneous care.[96] Shared-decision making is considered the mechanism by which patients define their own values, preferences, and the quality of palliative and end-of-life care desired.[97] Shared decision-making may be particularly important in Canada where the population is ethnoculturally diverse and differing views may be held about preferences for quality end-of-life care.

Advance care planning

Advance care planning is one aspect of shared-decision making at the end-of-life that is receiving significant attention in hospice palliative care in Canada. Advance care planning is generally described as a process of planning for a time when an individual does not have the mental capacity to make decisions about his/her own healthcare or treatment.[98] That planning may include the choice of someone to act, as substitute decision maker (SDM) or proxy, for that person should he or she become mentally incapable of giving or refusing consent to healthcare. Advance care planning may include a directive about a person's values and beliefs, likes and dislikes, how he or she generally wants to be cared for, where he or she wants to live, as well as communication of specific wishes about health treatments, medications, and end-of-life care. Identification and clarification of advance care planning concepts and terms understood by professionals and consumers is provided in the Health Canada *The Glossary Project* report.[99] A review of the status of advance care planning in Canada identified variation in the levels of expertise about advance care planning in some areas of the country, some areas where little knowledge exists, and differing legislation across Canada.[99]

Advance care planning was initially identified as a priority at a National Action Planning Workshop for End-of-Life Care held in 2002.[100] In 2012, the CHPCA with funding from Health Canada released a National Framework for Advanced Care Planning in Canada.[101] This document focuses on outlining all advance care planning activity, program development, and standards of practice across healthcare organizations. It outlines principles and a framework that includes a four-part model of essential elements for advance care planning and specific strategies within these elements:

1. Engagement of the legal system, healthcare system, healthcare professionals/providers, and the general public;

2. Education of the general public and education and training of professional providers;

3. System infrastructure including policy and program development and tools to support conversations and documentations;

4. Continuous quality improvement.

These four basic building blocks are linked to provincial/national policy, regulatory bodies such as accreditation and the environment in which it functions.[101] The CHPCA is taking a leadership role to advance this work and has established an Advanced Care Planning Task Group. This group's report identified the essential role of nurses in initiating communication with patients/families about advance care planning and in ensuring their wishes and preferences are acknowledged and advocated for within the healthcare system.[101]

Euthanasia and medical aid to dying

The issue of assisted death has been an undercurrent in discussions regarding access to quality palliative care in Canada, as has the continued realization that in spite of best practices in hospice palliative care there are some patients who experience unrelenting physical and existential suffering. However, assisted suicide and euthanasia remain prohibited activities under the Criminal Code of Canada.[102] The last major, Special Senate Committee report on assisted death and euthanasia in Canada was published in 1995.[103] It recommended that euthanasia should continue to be treated as murder under the Criminal Code of Canada. Again, in April 2010, in spite of public support for the decriminalization of assisted suicide and voluntary euthanasia, a private members bill to decriminalize assisted death and euthanasia was tabled in Parliament but defeated in the House of Commons.[104]

More recently, the issue of assisted death and euthanasia resurfaced in the spring of 2010 when a nonpartisan Committee of the Quebec National Assembly studied the issues and launched a public consultation process. This consultation process culminated in the report Living with Dignity written by the Select Committee on Dying with Dignity.[105] This report identified 24 recommendations necessary to improve palliative care in the province of Quebec, including training and education of healthcare professionals in palliative care, a practice guide on the use of terminal sedation, improvements to home palliative care, and creation of a palliative care unit under the Department of Health and Social Services. What's more, following consultation with experts from other countries with similar legislation and expert testimony that included patients/family members with a terminal illness, the Special Committee considered a further option ("medical aid in dying") to be necessary in end-of-life care in exceptional circumstances.

On June 12, 2013, this report culminated in the tabling of Right to Die Legislation in the National Assembly of Quebec. The headlines in national newspapers reported, "Quebec may be the first province in Canada to consider allowing patients to request a form of medically-supervised euthanasia."[105,106] This tabling of legislation has raised significant controversy in Canada and specifically from the palliative care community, since Canadians hold beliefs on both sides of this debate. In response the CHPCA, reiterated that the goals of hospice palliative care is to improve the quality of life for patients and families and intends to neither hasten nor postpone death and that more needs to be done to improve access to quality palliative care.[107] A survey of the Canadian Society of Palliative Care Physicians (CSPCP) showed that the majority (88%) of physicians are opposed to the legalization of euthanasia.[108] This development in Canada is a striking example of the provincial jurisdiction over healthcare services and the view that this is within the rights of the province to decide on this as part of provincial legislation.

Education in hospice palliative care

The need to develop hospice palliative care education for both the public and healthcare professionals has been described in most of the Senate reports and in reports of the CHPCA Quality Coalition. However, the development of hospice palliative care education for healthcare professionals has been a complex undertaking in Canada. To accomplish this there has been a need to develop collaboration and linkages with licensing or accrediting bodies, schools/faculties, and practicing professionals. In spite of these challenges, some progress in nursing curricula for hospice palliative care services has been achieved as described earlier in the section on nursing development. In addition, there are now 17 medical schools across the country that provide education in palliative care to new physicians and education programs for nurses, social workers, pharmacists, and pastoral care providers.[109] Some medical schools offer a 1-year fellowship with added competence in palliative medicine, accredited by the Royal College of Physicians and Surgeons of Canada and the College of Family Physicians of Canada.[110] The Royal College has also proposed a 2-year subspecialty in palliative medicine, with adult and pediatric training streams.[111]

Progress in hospice palliative care education in Canada has been supported in large part by the Canadian Pallium Project that was established in 2001 with a focus on the development and implementation of education of rural physicians, nurses, and pharmacists with a particular focus across western provinces in Canada.[112] This scope was broadened in 2003 to northern and eastern Canada, including Newfoundland and Nova Scotia. This renewed emphasis focused on courses for primary healthcare professionals, education programs for chaplains, and clinical decision support tools. This phase of the work also included a Pallium workshop for nurses and personal support workers (PSWs) working with First Nation peoples. In 2011, with additional funding, Pallium further developed its course, the LEAP—Learning Essential Approaches to Palliative Care courseware that is being implemented in regional networks across Canada and targeting palliative care training to healthcare professionals across care sectors and for those working with patients facing end-of-life due to chronic diseases other than cancer (i.e. dementia, COPD, CHF, renal, neurological [e.g., ALS]). A nationally based academic steering community is being established to further guide the development of training programs and educational curricula in hospice palliative care.

The Canadian Partnership Against Cancer, as part of the national cancer control strategy in Canada, has also provided funding to advance training in hospice palliative care for oncology healthcare professionals to support sequential models of care provision. The Palliative Care Working Group finalized its evaluation of the Education in Palliative and End-of-Life Care for Oncology (EPEC™-O) curriculum, which provides training for oncology professionals. The EPEC™-O curriculum was rolled out across the country through ongoing regional workshops held in 2011 and 2012.[113] In addition, a French version of the curriculum was completed. A planning toolkit for jurisdictions to host regional workshops was also completed, and the first of seven planned workshops was held in 2012.

Research in hospice palliative care

In 2012, a report from the Canadian Cancer Research Alliance (CCRA), *Investment in Research on Survivorship and Palliative and End-of-Life Care 2005–2008*, documented the country's investments in cancer research focused on palliative and end-of-life care.[114] The report indicates that between 2005 and 2008 survivorship and palliative and end-of -life research received 4.6% of the overall investment in cancer research across the country, approximately $18.5 million a year. In palliative and end-of-life research, much of the work involved healthcare delivery for cancer patients or studies of the physiological effects of cancer. The complexity of research in palliative care populations has been extensively documented, with emphasis on particular recruitment strategies and methodologies.[115]This has not dampened recognition of the urgent need for research in hospice palliative care. This need was acknowledged through national investments in palliative care research by the Canadian Institute of Health Research (CIHR) in 2003 with the development of a strategic initiative to encourage and stimulate either new investigators or investigators currently working and who have an interest in palliative and end-of-life care. The identified outcomes were to promote innovative pilot or feasibility studies, develop evidence necessary to determine viability of new research avenues, and build research

capacity.[116] As well, the CIHR determined in 2003 that palliative and end-of-life care is one of their most important strategic directions for research. There were three components to the initiative:

- One-year pilot projects to target and assess innovative approaches;
- Five-year New Emerging Team grants to build capacity and to promote new research teams or increase existing teams; and
- One-year career transition awards to attract new researchers into this area of specialty.

Since this initial investment, networks for research have continued to collaborate or new ones have been formed throughout Canada to conduct research to better understand the scope and care needs of palliative and end-of-life populations and their families. Examples of these networks include the Victoria Palliative Research Network (Victoria, British Columbia), the Division of Palliative Medicine (Edmonton, Alberta), and Network for End of Life Studies in Nova Scotia. Examples of research initiatives include the following:

- Network for End of Life Studies in Nova Scotia has identified its beginning steps for developing a surveillance strategy for its palliative population identified in *The End of Life Care in Nova Scotia Surveillance Report* (2008).[117]
- Research on family care-giving in Palliative and End-of-Life Care—initiated through CIHR funding in 2004, this group is focused on studying family caregiving.
- A research collaboration between four western provinces is reported in *Health Care Use at the End of Life in Western Canada*. Identified in this report is the use of hospital and pharmacy services specifically analyzing the location of death, hospital use in the last year of life, and use of community-dispersed drugs and supplies.
- Prognostication studies conducted through collaborative research projects with University of Victoria and University of Alberta.

Since the majority of Canadians die from nonmalignant causes, the Institute of Circulatory and Respiratory Health (ICRH) is also a key stakeholder in conducting research in this vital area as well.

Summary

There has been tremendous change in palliative and end-of-life care in Canada in the past decade. Numerous influences, national and provincial developments, and best-practice models have emerged to continually enhance care provision for Canadians. The establishment of the Health Canada Secretariat on Palliative and End-of-Life Care provided a mechanism for the palliative care community to collectively initiate key strategies to further enhance hospice palliative care nationally. The enhanced support for community-based services and family caregivers are significant in continuing to broaden the scope of palliative care services.

Further development of palliative and end-of-life care standards, measurable outcomes, and indicators to create common methods to be able to compare and measure various programs and services, along with quality coalitions across the country will be essential drivers of quality hospice palliative care in the next decade. With courage to look beyond traditional approaches of care delivery and to collectively develop the hospice palliative nursing voice within collaborative and interprofessional models, hospice palliative care nurses and the nursing work force are well positioned to provide leadership in the provision of exceptional integrated care, education, and research to further enhance and ensure quality palliative and end-of-life care to all Canadians.

Acknowledgments

We acknowledge Dennie Hycha and Lynn Whitten chapter, the authors of the 2000 edition of this chapter, which provided the foundation for this chapter. Sandy McKinnon was an original author of the 2000 chapter on Canada. Sandy died in 2000; her ongoing influence on the 2000 chapter is also acknowledged.

References

1. Health Council of Canada. Seniors in Need, Caregivers in Distress: What Are the Home Care Priorities for Seniors in Canada? April 2012. Available at: http://www.healthcouncilcanada.ca/rpt_det.php?id=348 (accessed May 29, 2013).
2. Canadian Hospice Palliative Care Association. It Depends on Where You Die! Settings of Care in Canada. June 2012. Available at: http://www.chpca.net/news-and-events/news-item-15.aspx (accessed May 29, 2013).
3. Standing Senate Committee on Social Affairs, Science and Technology. Raising the Bar: A Roadmap for the Future of Palliative Care in Canada. June 2010. The Senate of Canada. Available at: http://www.virtualhospice.ca/Assets/Raising%20the%20Bar%20June%202010_Senator%20Sharon%20Carstairs_20100608160433.pdf (accessed May 29, 2013).
4. Ferris FD, Balfour HM, Bowen K, Farley J, Hardwick M, Lamontagne C, et al. A Model to Guide Hospice Palliative Care: Based on National Principles and Norms of Practice. Canadian Hospice and Palliative Care Association, Ottawa, ON, 2002.
5. Statistics Canada. 2005. Land and Freshwater Area, by Province and Territory (2005). Available at: http://www.statcan.gc.ca/tables-tableaux/sum-som/l01/cst01/phys01-eng.htm (accessed June 12, 2013).
6. Statistics Canada. Portrait of the Canadian Population in 2012: National Portrait. Available at: http://www12.statcan.ca/english/census06/analysis/popdwell/NatlPortrait1.cfm (accessed May 20, 2013).
7. Annual Report on Immigration. Citizenship and Immigration Canada (CIC). Parliament of Canada, Ottawa, ON. November 2012. Accessed at: http:///wwwcicnews.com/2012/11/Canada-announces-immigration-levels-ear-111990.html (accessed on May 20, 2013).
8. Statistics Canada. National Household Survey (NHS). May 8, 2013. http://www23.statcan.gc.ca/imdb/p2SV.pl?Function-get Survey&SDDS=5178&Item_Id=75585&lang=en (accessed May 29, 2013).
9. Statistics Canada. 2007. Overview 2011—Aboriginal Peoples. Available at:http://www41.statcan.ca/2007/10000/ceb10000_000_e.(access May 20, 2013).
10. Aboriginal Self-Government. Aboriginal Affairs and Northern Development in Canada. June 9, 2012. Available at: http://www.aadnc.gc.ca/eng/1100100016293/1100100016294 (accessed June 12, 2013).
11. Statistics Canada. Aboriginal Peoples in Canada in 2011 National Household Survey: Aboriginal Peoples in Canada: First Nations People, Métis and Inuit 2011 Census. Available at: http://www12.statcan.ca/english/census06/analysis/aboriginal/surpass.cfm (accessed June 2013).
12. National Inventory of Hospice Palliative Care Resources and Tools for Aboriginal Peoples, Prepared for: First Nations and Inuit Health, First Nations and Inuit Home and Community Care Program, Health Canada, Canadian Hospice Palliative Care Association,

May 4, 2007. Available at: http://www.chpca.net/media/7712/Inventory_Aboriginal_Resources_2007.pdf (accessed May 20, 2013)
13. Con A. Cross-Cultural Consideration in Promoting Advance Care Planning, Prepared for the Palliative and End-of-Life Care Unit, Chronic and Continuing Care Division, Secretariat on Palliative and End-of-Life Care, Primary and Continuing Health Care Division of the Health Care Policy Directorate, Health Canada, p. 6, 2008. Available at: http://www.bccancer.bc.ca/NR/rdonlyres/39C930BB-1AAA-4700-98BB-9004835F3BD/28582/COLOUR030408_Con.pdf (accessed October, 2013).
14. Canadian Hospice Palliative Care Association. A Discussion Document on Aboriginal Hospice Palliative Care in Canada, Health Canada. Prepared for Canadian Hospice Palliative Care Association by Hanson and Associates; 2007. Available at: http://034fa33.netsol-host.com/ Resources/MovingForwardbyBuildingonStrengths%20A%20Discussion%20Document%20on%20Aboriginal%20Hospice%20PalliativeCareCanada.pdf and http://nshpca.ca/wp-content/uploads/2014/03/Moving-Forward.pdf (accessed May 20, 2013)
15. Castelden H, Crooks VA, Hanlon N, Schuurman N. Providers Perceptions of Aboriginal Palliative Care in British Columbia's Rural Interior. Health Soc Care Comm 2010;18(5):483–491.
16. Medical Insurance Act. R.R.O. 1990 Regulation 552. Government of Canada.
17. Canada Health Act, 1984, C.6, s.l., pp. 1–12.
18. Canada Health Transfer Act, Department of Finance Canada. What Is the Canada Health Transfer (CHT)? 2011. Available at: www.fin.gc.ca (accessed June 12, 2013).
19. Quality End-of-Life Care Coalition of Canada. Blueprint for Action 2010 to 2020. Ottawa, ON; 2010.Available at: http://www.qelccc.ca/media/3743/blueprint_for_action_2010_to_2020_april_2010.pdf (accessed May 20, 2013)
20. "Canadian Cancer Society's Steering Committee: Canadian Cancer Statistics 2010. Toronto: Canadian Cancer Society, 2010." Canadian Cancer Statistics 2010—Special Topic: End-of-Life Care. Released May 2010.
21. Rachlis M. Prescription for Excellence. Toronto, Canada: Harper Collins; 2004.
22. Canadian Institute for Health Information. Health Care Use at the End-of-Life in Western Canada. Ottawa, ON: CIHI; 2007.
23. Canadian Hospice Palliative Care Association (CHPCA). Strategic Plan and Progress Report. 2006–2009. Available at: http://www.chpca.net_us/CHPCA_Strategic_Plan_2006_2009.pdf (accessed May 13, 2013).
24. Reforming Health Protection and Promotion in Canada: Time to Act. The Standing Senate Committee on Social Affairs, Science and Technology. Chair: The Honourable Michael J.L. Kirby, November 2003, Parliament of Canada, Available at: http://www.parl.gc.ca/Content/SEN/Committee/372/soci/rep/repfinnov03-e.htm (accessed May 10, 2013).
25. Williams AM, Crooks VA, Whitfield K, Kelley ML, Richards J-L, DeMiglio L, et al. Tracking the evolution of hospice palliative care in Canada: A comparative case study analysis of seven provinces. BMC Health Serv. Res. 2010;10:147–158.
26. Canadian Home Care Association. 2008. Integration of Care: Exploring the Potential Alignment of Home Care with Other Health Care Sectors. Ottawa, ON: Author. Available at: http://www.cdnhomecare.ca/media.php?mid=1853&xwm=true (accessed on June 10, 2013).
27. Bacon J. Hospice Palliative Home Care in Canada: A Progress Report. Ottawa: Quality End-of-Life Care Coalition of Canada; 2008.
28. First Ministers Meeting on the Future of Health Care 2004: A Ten Year Plan to Strengthen Health Care in Canada. Ottawa, ON: Health Canada, Parliament of Canada; 2004.
29. Canadian Hospice Palliative Care Association. The Pan-Canadian Gold Standard for Palliative Home Care: Towards Equitable Access to High Quality Hospice Palliative and End-of-Life Care at Home. Ottawa, ON: Canadian Hospice Palliative Care Association, 2006

30. A Time for Transformative Change: A Review of the 2004 Health Accord. The Standing Senate Committee on Social Affairs, Science and Technology Senate, Ottawa, Ontario, Canada, March 2012. Available at: www.senate-senat.ca/social.asp (accessed June 1, 2013).

31. Canadian Hospice Palliative Care Association. Fact Sheet: Hospice Palliative Care in Canada. 2012. Available at: http://www.chpca.net/media/7622/fact_sheet_hpc_in_canada_may_2012_final.pdf (Accessed June 1, 2013)

32. Family Caregiving in Palliative and End-of-Life Care. Available at: http://www.coag.uvic.ca/eolcare/ (accessed June 12, 2013).

33. Canadian Hospice Palliative Care Association. Valuing Caregiving and Caregivers: Family Caregivers in the Integrated Approach to Palliative Care, The Way Forward Initiative: An Integrated Palliative Approach to Care, 2013.

34. Dumont S, Jacobs P, Fassbender K, Anderson D, Turcotte V, Harel F. Costs associated with resource utilization during the palliative phase of care: a Canadian perspective. Palliat Med. 2009 Dec;23(8) 708–717.

35. Parliamentary Committee on Palliative and Compassionate Care, Not to be Forgotten: Care of Vulnerable Canadians, November 2011. Available at: http://pcpcc-cpspsc.com/wp-content/uploads/2011/11/ReportEN.pdf (accessed May 20, 2013)

36. Hollander MJ, Guiping L, Chappell NL. Who cares and how much?: The imputed economic contribution to the Canadian healthcare system of middle-aged and older unpaid caregivers providing care to the elderly. Healthc Q. 2009;12(2):42–49.

37. Employment Insurance Compassionate Care Benefit, Government of Canada, Service Canada, January 2013. Available at: www.servicecanada.gc.ca/eng/sc/ei/benefits/compassionate.shtml (accessed October, 2013).

38. Subcommittee to Update "of Life and Death" of the Standing Senate Committee on Social Affairs Science and Technology. Quality End-of-Life Care: The Right of Every Canadian. Ottawa: Government of Canada; 2001.

39. The Way Forward: Moving Toward Community-Integrated Palliative Care in Canada. Toronto, ON: Quality Coalition of Canada, Canadian Partnership Against Canada; June 12, 2012.

40. Caring for Canadians at End-of-Life: A Strategic Plan for Hospice Palliative Care and End-of-Life Care in Canada to 2015, CHPCA, Ottawa, ON. Her Majesty the Queen in Right of Canada. May 4, 2007.

41. Pediatric Hospice Palliative Care: Guiding Principles and Norms of Practice. Canadian Hospice Palliative Care Association and the Canadian Network of Palliative Care for Children, Ottawa, ON. March 2006. Available at: http://www.chpca.net/media/7841/Pediatric_Norms_of_Practice_March_31_2006_English.pdf (accessed May 20, 2013)

42. Accreditation Canada. (2013). Safety in Canadian health care organizations: A focus on transitions in care and Required Organizational Practices. Ottawa, ON: Accreditation Canada. Available at: http://www.accreditation-canada.ca (accessed October 2013).

43. Accreditation Canada. Hospice Palliative and End-Of-Life Care. Available at: http://www.accreditation-canada.ca/default.aspx?page=58 (accessed October, 2103).

44. Accreditation Canada. Strategy. Available at: http://www.accreditation-canada.ca/default.aspx?page=47&cat=34 (accessed October, 2013).

45. Accreditation Canada. Qmentum Program 2009: Hospice, Palliative, and End-of-Life Services. Available at: http://www.accreditation-canada.ca (accessed October, 2013).

46. Wilson D, Cohen J, Deliens L, Houttekier D. The preferred place of last days: results of a representative population-based survey. J Palliat Med. 2013;16(5):502–508.

47. Bruera E, Kuehn N, Miller MJ, Selmser P, Macmillan K. The Edmonton Symptom Assessment System (ESAS): a simple method for the assessment of palliative care patients. J Palliat Care. 1991;7:6–9.

48. Economist Intelligence Unit (The Economist). The Quality of Death: Ranking End-of-Life Care Across the World. London, UK: Commisioned by the Lien Foundation. 2010.

49. Bosma H, Apland L, Kazanjian A. Cultural conceptualizations of hospice palliative care: more similarities than differences. Palliat Med. 2010;24(5):510–522.

50. Bowman KW, Singer PA. Chinese seniors' perspectives on end-of-life decisions. Soc Sci Med. 2001;53(44): 55–64.

51. CHPCA. Quality End-of-Life Care Coalition of Canada, History and Background of the Coalition. Available at: http://www.chpca.net/qelccc/information_and_resources/3_History_and_Mandate-nov2007.pdf (accessed October, 2013).

52. Implementing an Integrated Hospice Palliative Care System in Ontario: Recommendations from the Quality Hospice Palliative Care Coalition of Ontario, Quality End-of-Life Coalition, Brief to the Government. Nov. 29, 2010. Available at: http://www.qhpcco.ca/Hospice_Palliative_Care_Policy_Brief_to_Government.pdf (accessed: October, 2013).

53. Statistics Canada, Death Estimates by Province and Territory, CANSIM, Table 051-0004 and Catalogue no. 91-215-X. Ottawa, ON: Government of Canada. Available at: Canada.gc.ca (accessed June 1, 2013).

54. The Dartmouth Atlas of Health Care. Percent of Cancer Patients Dying in Hospital 2003–2007. Updated 2012. http://www.dartmouthatlas.org/data/table.aspx?ind=176&tf=20&ch=&loc=&loct=2&fmt=206 (accessed May 13, 2013).

55. Canadian Institute for Health Information. End-of-Life Hospital Care for Cancer Patients. 2013. Available at: https://secure.cihi.ca/free_products/Cancer_Report_EN_web_April2013.pdf (accessed May, 2013).

56. Seow H, Barbera L, Howell D, Dy SM. Using more end-of-life homecare services is associated with using fewer acute care services: a population-based cohort study. Med Care. 2009;48(12):

57. Policy Brief on Hospice Palliative Care. Quality End-of-Life Care?: It Depends on Where You Live…and Where You Die. Canadian Hospice Palliative Care Association, June 2010. Available at: http://www.chpca.net/media/7682/HPC_Policy_Brief_-_Systems_Approach_-_June_2010.pdf (accessed on May 20, 2013)

58. Tu J, Nardi L, Fang J, Liu J, Khalid L, Johansen H. National trends in rates of death and hospital admissions related to acute myocardial infarction, heart failure and stroke, 1994–2004. CMAJ: Can Med Assoc J. 2009;180(13):1–11.

59. Marshall D, Howell D, Brazil K, Howard M, Taniguchi A, Rush B. Enhancing family physician capacity to deliver quality palliative home care: The Niagara West end of life shared-care model. Can Fam Physician. 2008;54:1703–1703e7.

60. Seow H, Barbera L, Howell D, Dy S. How end-of-life homecare services are used from admission to death: a population-based cohort study. J Palliat Care. 2010;26(4):270–278.

61. Barbera L, Sussman J, Viola R, Husain A, Howell D, Librach L, et al. Factors associated with the end of life health service use in patients dying of cancer. Healthc Policy. 2010;5(3):125–143.

62. Howell D, Abernathy T, Cockerill R, Brazil K, Wagner F, Librach L. Predictors of home care expenditures and death at home for cancer patients in an integrated comprehensive palliative home care pilot program. Healthc Policy. 2011;6(3):e73–e92.

63. Pesut B, McLeod B, Hole R, Dalhuisen M. Rural nursing and quality end-of-life care palliative care…palliative approach…or somewhere in-between? Adv Nurs Sci. 2012;35(4):288–304.

64. Kelley ML, Sletmoen W, Williams AM, Nadin S, Puiras T. Integrating policy, research, and community development: a case study of developing rural palliative care. In: Kulig JC, Williams AM (eds.), Health in Rural Canada. Vancouver, BC: UBC Press; 2012:219–238.

65. Coyte P, Howell D. Appropriate Settings for Palliative Care. Report Prepared Under Grant 02709 from the Ministry of Health and Long-Term Care in Ontario. Toronto, ON: Home and Community Care Research and Evaluation Centre, University of Toronto; 2001.

66. Victoria Hospice. Palliative Care Research. Available at: http://www.victoriahospice.org/health-care-professionals/palliative-care-research/palliative-care-research-projects (accessed June 28, 2013).

67. Kodner, D. All together now: a conceptual exploration of integrated care. Healthc Q. 2009;13:7–11.

68. Von Roenn JH. The integration of palliative care and oncology: the evidence. J Natl Compr Canc Netw. 2013;11 Suppl 1:S11–S16.

69. Ceronsky L. Comprehensive, integrated palliative care reduces costs and improves satisfaction among patients and their families within a large health system. Agency for Healthcare Research and Quality. 2008. Available at: http://www.innovations.ahrq.gov/content. aspx?id=263 (accessed June 12, 2013).

70. Howell D, Marshall D, Brazil K, Taniguchi A, Howard M, Foster, G, et al. A shared care model pilot for palliative home care in a rural area: impact on symptoms, distress, and place of death. J Pain Symptom Manage. 2011;42(1):60–75.

71. Klinger C, Howell D, Zakus D, Marshall D, Zakus D, Brazil K, et al. Resource utilization and costs analyses of home-based palliative care service provision: The Niagara West end-of-life shared-care project. Palliat Med. 2013;27(2):115–122.

72. Cancer Journey Action Group. Cancer and Palliative Care: Integration and Continuity of Care. Toronto, ON: Canadian Partnership Against Cancer; 2009, March.

73. Smith TJ, Temin S, Alesi ER, Abernethy AP, Baloboni TA, et al. American Society of Clinical Oncology provisional clinical opinion: the integration of palliative care into standard oncology care. J Clin Oncol. www.jco.org. Feb 6, 2012. (accessed June 12, 2013).

74. Follwell M, Burman D, Le LW, Wakimoto K, Seccareccia D, Bryson J, et al. Phase II study of an outpatient palliative care intervention in patients with metastatic cancer. Clin Oncol. 2009;27(2):206–213.

75. Watanabe SM, Nekolaichuk C, Beaumont C, Johnson L, Myers J, Strasser F. A multi-centre comparison of two numerical versions of the Edmonton Symptom Assessment System in palliative care patients J Pain Symptom Manage 2011;41:456–468.

76. Dudgeon D, King S, Howell D, Green E, Gilbert J, Hughes E, et al. Cancer Care Ontario's experience with implementation of routine physical and psychological symptom distress screening. Psycho-Oncol. 2011;21(4):357–364.

77. Gilbert JE, Howell D, King S, Sawka C, Hughes E, Angus H, et al. Quality improvement in cancer symptom assessment and control: the Provincial Palliative Care Integration Project (PPCIP). J Pain Symptom Manage. 2012;43(4):663–678.

78. Canadian Hospice Palliative Care Association. 2013. Canadians Are Aging. We've Done the Math. Have You? Available at: http://www. chpca.net/news-and-events/news-item-33.aspx (accessed May, 2013).

79. Canadian Hospice Palliative Care Association. Caring for Canadians at End of Life: A Strategic Plan for Hospice, Palliative and End-of-Life Care in Canada to 2015. Available at: http://chpca.net/media/7562/chpca_strategic_plan_2010_2015.pdf (accessed May 2013).

80. Gold Standards Framework. Prognostication Framework. Available at: http://www.goldstandardsframework.org.uk/index.html (accessed May 2013).

81. Quality Palliative Care in Long Term Care: A Community-University Research Alliance (QPC-LTC Alliance). Thunder Bay, ON: Lakehead University Available at http://www.palliativealliance.ca (accessed May 29, 2013).

82. Praxia Information Intelligence and Gartner Inc. Telehealth Benefits and Adoption: Connecting People and Providers Across Canada. Commissioned by: Canada Health Infoway, May 30, 2011. Available at: https://www.infoway-inforoute.ca/index.php/resources/reports?start=5 (accessed: May 20, 2013)

83. Health Canada. Canadian Virtual Hospice: Knowledge Development and Support in Palliative Care. November 2001. Available at: http://www.hc-sc.gc.ca/english/media/releases/2001/2001_121ebk1.htm (accessed November 2008).

84. Sevean PS, Dampier S, Spadoni M, Strickland S, Pilatze S. Patients and families experiences with video telehealth in rural/remote communities in Northern Canada. J Clin Nurs. 2008;10:1365–2702.

85. Roberts D, Tayler C, MacCormack D, Barwich D. Canadian Nurse: Telenursing in Hospice Palliative Care. Can Nurse. 2007;103(5):24–7.

86. Canadian Nurses Association, Department of Regulatory Policy. Available at http://www.nurseone.ca/Default.aspx?portlct=StaticHtmlViewerPortlet&plang+1&ptdi+623 (accessed July 8, 2013).

87. Fothergill-Bourbonnais F, Brajtman S, Fiset V. A survey of educators; end-of-life care learning needs in a Canadian baccalaureate nursing program: we cannot teach what we do not know. J Palliat Care. 2009;25:3:233–240.

88. Final Report to Health Canada-Competencies for Palliative and End-of-Life Care, Ottawa, ON. Canadian Association of Schools of Nursing; 2008.

89. Palliative and End-of-Life Care: Entry-to-Practice Competencies and Indicators for Registered Nurses. Ottawa, ON. Canadian Association of Schools of Nursing; 2011.

90. Palliative and End-of-Life Care: Entry-to-Practice Competencies and Indicators for Registered Nurses: A Toolkit for Educators. Ottawa, ON. Canadian Association of Schools of Nursing; 2012.

91. Graduate Diploma in Advanced Practice Oncology/Palliative Nursing, University of Windsor, Windsor, Ontario. March 2013, Joint Press Release. Available at: http://www.desouzanurse.ca/files/resources/UWindsorDiploma.pdf (accessed May 29, 2013)

92. A Notice to Nurse Practitioners About Controlled Drugs and Substances. 2012. CNO (College of Nurses of Ontario), supported by the Ontario College of Pharmacists Available at http://www.cno.org/learn-about-standards-guidelines/educational-tools/nurse-practitioners/a-notice-to-nurse-practitioners-about-controlled-drugs-and-substances (accessed May 23, 2013)

93. Nurse Practitioners in Canada. 2012. Available at: http://health-carecoopscanada.files.wordpress.com/2012/07/2012-03-nurse-practitioners-in-canada-2.pdf (accessed May 29, 2013).

94. Canadian Nurses Association. Toward 2020 Visions for Nursing, Principal Investigators M. Villeneuve and J. MacDonald. 2006. Available at: www.cna-aiic.ca/CNA/documents/pdf/publications/Toward-2020-e.pdf (accessed December 2008).

95. The Royal Society of Canada Expert Panel: End of Life Decision-Making, RSC-Royal Society of Canada, The Academies of Arts, Humanities and Sciences of Canada. November. 2011.

96. Goodman D. End-of-life cancer care in Ontario and the United States: quality by accident or quality by design? Editorial. J Natl Cancer Inst. 2011;103(11):840–841.

97. Belanger E, Rodriguez C, Groleau D. Shared decision-making in palliative care: a systematic mixed studies review using narrative synthesis. Palliat Med. 2011;25(3):242–261.

98. Implementation Guide to Advance Care Planning in Canada: A Case Study of Two Health Authorities. March 2008. Available at: http://www.hc-sc.gc.ca/hcs-sss/alt_formats/pdf/pubs/palliat/2008-acp-guide-pps/acp-guide-pps-eng.pdf (accessed May 20, 2013).

99. Health Canada. Advance Care Planning the Glossary Project—Final Report, 2006. Available at: http://www.hc-sc.gc.ca/hcs-sss/pubs/palliat/2006-proj-glos/index-eng.php#Toc144091361 (accessed October, 2013).

100. Ipsos-Reid Survey. Hospice Palliative Care Study: Final Report. The GlaxoSmith Kline Foundation and the Canadian Hospice Palliative Care Association, Ottawa, January 2004, p. 31.

101. National Framework for Advanced Care Planning in Canada, Canadian Partnership Against Cancer and the Canadian Hospice Palliative Care Association, January 2012. Available at: http://www.advancecareplanning.ca/media/40158/acp%20framework%202012%20eng.pdf (access date: May 20, 2013)

102. Criminal Code of Canada, 1892, c.29

103. The Special Senate Committee on Euthanasia and Assisted Suicide, Parliament of Canada, Ottawa, Ontario. June 1995.

104. Ottawa, Ontario, April 21, 2010 (LifeSiteNews.com)—The Canadian Parliament overwhelmingly defeated today the private members bill

seeking to legalize euthanasia and assisted suicide. The House of Commons rejected Bill C-384, Parliament of Canada.

105. Dying with Dignity Report. Quebec, Quebec: National Assembly of Quebec. March 2012.

106. Schafer A. The great Canadian Euthanasia Debate. The Globe and Mail. August 23, 2012. http://www.theglobeandmail.com/life.health-and-fitness/the-great-canadian-euthanasia-debate/article4200477/ (accessed July 13, 2013).

107. Canadians Urged to Talk About Hospice Palliative Care First. Canadian Hospice Palliative Care Association and Canadian Society for Palliative Care Physicians, Canadian Hospice Palliative Care Association, Response to Bill 52. June 13, 2013.

108. Canadian Society of Palliative Care Physicians Oppose Euthanasia and Assisted Suicide. November, 2010, Alberta Health Services, Alberta, Canada.

109. Educating Future Physicians in Palliative and End-of-Life Care (EFPPEC), The Association of Faculties of Medicine in Canada, Ottawa, ON. Available at:www.efppec.ca. (accessed June 14, 2013).

110. College of Family Physicians of Canada (CFPC) and the Royal College of Physicians and Surgeons of Canada (RCPSC). Ottawa, ON. Available at: www.royalcollege.ca/credentials. (accessed on June 1, 2013)

111. Monette M. Palliative care subspecialty in the offing. CMAJ: Can Med Assoc J. 2012;184(12): 4255.

112. Pallium Canada. Working together to improve the quality of living and dying and Canada. http://www.pallium.ca/.

113. Education in Palliative and End-of-Life Care for Oncology (EPEC™-O) Curriculum. Toronto, ON:2011–12 Canadian Partnership Against Cancer Corporation.

114. Canadian Cancer Research Alliance. Investment in Research on Survivorship and Palliative and End-of-Life Care, 2005–2008: A Special Report from the Canadian Cancer Research Alliance's Survey of Government Voluntary Sector Investment in Cancer Research. Toronto: CCRA; 2011.

115. Bosma H, Johnston M, Cadell S, Wainwright W, Abernathy N, Feron A, et al. Canadian Social Work Competencies for Hospice Palliative Care: A Framework to Guide Education and Practice at the Generalist and Specialist Levels. Canadian Hospice Palliative Care Association. 2008. Available at: http://www.chpca.net/interest_groups/social_workers-counselors/socialwork_counsellors_competencies.html (accessed June 1, 2013).

116. Canadian Institute of Health Research. Available at: www.cihr-irsc.gc.ca/e/12874 (accessed December 2008).

117. End of Life Care in Nova Scotia Surveillance Report. Network for End of Life Studies (NELS) Interdisciplinary Capacity Enhancement (ICE), Dalhousie University, Halifax, Nova Scotia. Available at: http://nels.schoolofhealthservicesadministration.dal.ca/ (accessed October, 2013).

CHAPTER 72

Palliative care in Australia and New Zealand

Margaret O'Connor

Key points

- There are commonalities and differences between models of palliative care in Australia and New Zealand, based on aspects like geography, historical models, culture, and community involvement.

- Palliative care nurses in both countries are increasingly taking on advanced practice leadership roles in research, education, and policy.

Palliative care nursing in Australia and New Zealand shares many features with practice elsewhere in the world. The similarities between palliative care nursing from this part of the world and other countries are often highlighted through contributions to journals and in the adoption of texts written or coedited by Australians and accepted by international publishers.[1,2] The purpose of this chapter is both to profile palliative care in Australia and New Zealand and to provide insights into key innovations, focusing on developments in areas of education and training; research; policy and international links; and advanced practice roles education, policy, and international links.

Some essential differences between Australia and New Zealand

Australia and New Zealand (NZ) are often considered together—consistently labeled as "down under" and far away in world consciousness. Despite being close geographically and sharing a predominantly British heritage, these countries have significantly different cultures that are important to understand before exploring palliative care developments in the two countries.

New Zealand is a small country consisting of two large islands and one smaller, sparsely populated island, where industry is predominantly agricultural. The total population is 4.5 million, according to the 2006 census.[3] There was no Census conducted in 2011 due to the catastrophic earthquakes in Christchurch, and 2013 census data was not yet available at the time of this writing. The population is very young with the total average age being 33.1 years. About 1 in 7 New Zealanders are Māori, and today more than twice as many Māori are aged over 80 years than a decade ago. According to Statistics NZ's population estimates, on June 30, 2012, 682,200 people in the country identified as Māori and about 5,000 Māori were 80 years or older, almost double that of 10 years earlier. The population is unevenly spread between the two main islands, with almost 75% living in the North Island. European/Pakeha (white) make up almost 80% of the population; with 13.6% Maori and 6.4% Pacific Islanders.[3] People aged 65 years and over now make up 14% of New Zealand's total population.

Specialist health services are likely to be confined to large cities in each of the two main islands, but most general health services are available locally. However, New Zealand's population density, 16 people per cubic square kilometer (compared to 234.5 per km^3 in Britain), has some effect on access to health services, with those in less densely populated areas having less access to specialized services, including palliative care.[4]

In contrast, Australia is the smallest continent, but one of the largest countries in the world, comprising a large island and one very small island state of Tasmania. The population is about 23,000 million (www.abs.gov.au) with approximately 90% of the population living in about 3% of the coastal land area, making city living very dense. According to the 2011 census (www.abs.gov.au), indigenous Australians make up about 2.6% of the population, although the number of about ½ million individuals is projected to rapidly increase over the next 10 years. Australia has undergone significantly more migration than New Zealand, with 25% of the population born overseas at the 2011 census. The main countries where overseas-born Australians come from are the United Kingdom, New Zealand, China, Italy, Vietnam, and the Phillipines (www.abs.gov.au). Newer immigrant groups come from Nepal, the Sudan, India, Bangladesh, and Pakistan. This makes for a very diverse population with one dominant cultural group and many minorities.

Because of the size of its land mass, Australia's rural and remote populations may be very isolated, with the nearest neighbor a day's drive away; this has implications for models of health service. Despite the Aboriginal population constituting only a small percentage of the total population, they make up 30% of the population of central Australia, and in some communities are the main clients of health services.

It is clear, then, that Australia and New Zealand have similarities and differences. Both countries feature a predominance of people from Anglo-Celtic origins and were populated by these settlers at a similar time, although under different circumstances—Australia was established as a penal colony and New Zealand with free settlers. Both were colonialist settlements featuring disenfranchisement of the existing population—in Australia the native Aboriginal people, and in New Zealand the Maori. Since that time, New Zealand has remained largely bicultural despite limited migration from other parts of the world, while Australia is considered a complex and diverse multicultural society. Despite many languages being spoken in Australia, English is the only official language. In contrast, both English and Maori are recognized national languages in New Zealand, and significant effort has been made to maintain Maori cultural identity and influence at a national level. A resurgence in Maori nationalism over recent years has been more effective in influencing national policy than has similar indigenous nationalism in Australia.

Australian and New Zealand models of health and palliative care

Both countries have a long history of universal health insurance systems that provide basic healthcare to all people, supplemented by a system of private healthcare, which is more extensive in Australia. There is a consistent valuing of universal access to adequate healthcare within the two populations despite increasing trends toward user payment and an increasing proportion of individual contribution for some services.

Both countries feature a trend toward privatization of public facilities that affects healthcare services, perhaps most noticeable in residential aged care.[5] Privatization of residential aged care facilities has resulted in fewer not-for-profit providers and an increased need to profit from care of the elderly, with considerable potential impact on access to palliative care services,[6] when combined with the shift toward user payments. Despite this, healthcare remains at a high standard, with access to a range of generalist and specialist services at a level consistent with that of other countries with universal healthcare systems. Spending on health in both Australia and New Zealand is 8% to 9% of gross domestic product. In both countries, most generalist services are available to rural communities, but specialist services, such as radiotherapy, usually require travel to a large city. In remote areas of Australia, access to healthcare may be limited to a regular monthly clinic by the Royal Flying Doctor Service and limited access to outreach telephone or online services. In some remote settings, nursing care maybe provided through remote nursing stations where nurses are expected to serve as advanced generalists attending to a range of healthcare concerns within the community.

Structure and delivery of palliative care

In comparison with many parts of the world, hospice and palliative care developments in Australia and New Zealand are well advanced, with services required to meet established standards of service delivery.[7,8] In a 2010 study of 40 countries around the world, The Economist Intelligence Unit utilized a "Quality of Death" measure to assess end-of-life care; Australia listed as second and New Zealand third.[9] Models of palliative care delivery in both countries feature inpatient, home care, and hospital support teams, with New Zealand evidencing more use of daycare services than Australia. Urban cities tend to support all service elements, with home-care provision showing the most variation. In larger rural cities, small specialist services provide support and consultancy services to generalist nurses and local doctors. Palliative care developments in both countries are notable for their lack of homogeneity, with models of care dependent on historical factors,

financial support, population density, and the local community environment.

The first hospice service in New Zealand opened in 1979,[4] with services now operating in the main cities across the country (www.hospice.org.nz). Palliative care in New Zealand features the development of small community inpatient hospices that link strongly with local community nursing services in the provision of home care, and are highly dependent on local fundraising. The system is well organized through a national association that facilitates communication between members, including a biannual national conference. The Palliative Care Council of New Zealand was established in 2008 to provide independent and expert advice to the minister of health and to report on New Zealand's performance in providing palliative and end-of-life care.

The Boost Hospice Care funding was introduced in 2009 and gave hospices an additional $60 million over the 4 years to June 2013 to help them expand care and services and meet financial challenges. This increased the proportion of average hospice funding provided by the government from 50% to 70%. Boost Hospice Care funding was rolled over for a further 2 years and the $15 million per year would now continue until 2015.

In a document published in 2010 reflecting on the progress made on the palliative care strategy for New Zealand, a number of pressing concerns were raised, including a lack of data on the need for palliative care for New Zealand's population, current service provision and service utilization. Without evidence and data it was impossible to monitor and evaluate progress or to formulate strategic advice to the minister of health on initiatives to reduce inequalities in access to palliative care, or to improve the quality of the care provided. In response to this situation two national health needs assessments were undertaken: the Phase 1 Report, released in June 2011, provided the first estimates in New Zealand of the need for palliative care on a national and regional basis. The key drivers of palliative care need in New Zealand were examined and mortality and hospital discharge data were used to develop estimates of palliative care need on a population basis. These estimates indicated a 24% increase in the number of people who might benefit from palliative care over the next 15 years.

The Phase 2 report, released in 2013, deals with palliative care capacity and capability in New Zealand and presents a comprehensive description of specialist palliative care services provided by hospices, hospital-based teams, and primary palliative care providers (http://www.cancercontrolnz.govt.nz/sites/default/files/National-Health-Needs-Assessment-for-Palliative-Care%20Summary%20Jun13_0.pdf).

The first Australian hospices predate the opening of St. Christopher's in London (1969) by 79 years—the establishment by the Irish Sisters of Charity of hospices in Sydney (1890) and Melbourne (1938). These traditional large bed-based facilities followed the Irish model and philosophy of caring for dying people in a facility linked to, but separate from, an acute hospital.[10] Over time, the skills and expertise in caring for dying people were seen to be concentrated in the hospice, resulting in a separation of this knowledge from other healthcare settings.[1] Following the global spread of modern hospice, Australia's response during the 1980s and 1990s occurred largely through the development of community-based palliative care services with a particular emphasis on care in the home.[10] However, significant change has taken place in service delivery, with increased emphasis in both state and federal government health policy to improve access to palliative care by utilizing a primary healthcare framework to ensure equitable service distribution across the community and healthcare systems. To this end, Palliative Care Australia promotes a needs-based model of care, necessitating the significant involvement of primary care providers, which ensures people receive the right level of care, commensurate with their stage of illness, symptom burden, and other needs.[11,12] New inpatient developments are increasingly linked to acute services to assist in the availability of appropriate beds for people in acute settings. There is increasing recognition of the need for the expertise of palliative care being available across hospital systems and of the applicability of palliative care principles for people dying of any illness. Hospital-based palliative care consultancy teams, often nurse-led, have become increasingly utilized in acute hospitals.[13,14]

Palliative care services in both countries uphold the principle of supporting a person's decision to be cared for and to die where they choose. Australian government policy directions clearly support the care of people in their own homes[15]; this emphasis requires specific attention to respite care and 24-hour access to supportive advice.

Cultural issues

A key feature of New Zealand healthcare is its responsiveness to Maori nationalism, which calls for greater control over their own health and services compatible to cultural beliefs. Cultural safety is a feature of Maori demands for appropriate health service development, and is a concept that moves beyond cultural sensitivity, featuring both acknowledgment and respect for difference, toward implementation of strategies to promote and nurture the cultural identity of the person who is ill.[16] With growing ethnic diversity in the New Zealand population, it is increasingly important for health providers and practitioners to provide services that are responsive to the diverse cultural, linguistic, and religious groups that they serve. Cultural competence is now also required under the Health Practitioners Competence Assurance Act 2003,[17] with each professional regulatory body setting standards of cultural competence for their members.

In New Zealand, nurses have long taken the lead on cultural issues in health with the production in 1992 of guidelines,[16] which were then updated in 2011.[17] These guidelines define cultural safety as "an outcome of nursing and midwifery education that enables safe service to be defined by those who receive the service."[17(p. 5)] Ultimately, this means that people of one culture feel able to utilize a health service provided by another culture without feeling at risk. The New Zealand Palliative Care Strategy, released in February 2001,[18] specifically detailed expectations for Maori and Pacific people, including development of linkages with Maori organizations, local service plans, and the employment of care coordinators in conjunction with local Maori providers. Building on that, the New Zealand Cancer Control Strategy: Action Plan 2005–2010 provides more detail on actions arising from the objectives of the Strategy.[19]

In contrast, the Australian indigenous people remain a marginalized group with a health status significantly below that of other Australians, despite strong government programs to address their health issues. A long history of neglect and suffering as a result of earlier ethnocentric government policy has left a legacy of difficulties for indigenous peoples. And chronic illnesses like diabetes and kidney failure are endemic.

In 2004, Australia's peak health research body, the National Health and Medical Research Council (NHMRC) released ethical guidelines for conducting research with Aboriginal and Torres Strait Islanders, a move highly significant in raising the importance of respecting different values and ethics.[20] While the National Palliative Care Strategy of 2000 identified[21] a need for services "to cater sensitively and flexibly for the needs of Aboriginal and Torres Strait Islanders,"[21(p. 6)] the 2010 Strategy makes no mention of this group.[22] However the work of individual researchers continues, to support mainstream healthcare workers in providing culturally appropriate palliative care for Aboriginal and Torres Strait Islander peoples.[23]

Working with indigenous people, culturally responsive models of palliative care delivery are developing, to ensure that traditional practices that surround care of dying people and death are understood, respected, and incorporated into care. For example, an inpatient facility constructed in Darwin incorporated the ability to move a bed outside the room, so that a patient could be cared for and die in the open air. The facility is also able to undertake the traditional smoking ceremony, conducted in the facility after a person has died, to drive their spirit away.[23]

Important research[24] has challenged a dominant palliative care nursing belief in open discussion about death and dying and describing the rituals and traditions of other cultures. Open discussion is unacceptable in cultures where there is belief that even saying the word "dying" may precipitate the event.[24]

Of particular relevance in both Australia and New Zealand, are the expectations of people from Asian cultures living in both countries. In a multicultural country like Australia, the barriers of culture and language have been the basis for examining communication patterns and styles between health providers and patients, and a lack of effective communication may mean less than satisfactory exchanges between health providers, patients, and their families.[24] In particular, ways of breaking bad news, decision-making processes, and other forms of communication differ between cultures as to what is acceptable.[25] During the past decade, projects have developed culturally appropriate information on palliative care services for the particular cultural community, aimed at improving service provision and access[24]; but because information is most often introduced through service providers, it is limited to those who access such services. Systematic attention to cultural safety should move beyond access to interpreters, multilingual information, and liaison with ethnic community organizations and religious groups.

Rural and remote communities

Nurses working in rural areas suggest there is significant work needed to provide for the palliative care needs of rural communities.[26] Rural and remote communities in both Australia and New Zealand are not homogeneous; they offer various challenges to health delivery based on demographics, local culture, physical environment, and distance from health services. Rural nurses, providing palliative care as one aspect of a broader health role in the community, suffer significant professional isolation. In some settings, particularly in remote areas, the nurse may be the sole health practitioner in a community, receiving telephone support from a doctor located some distance away. The challenge is to develop sustainable models of palliative care provision in many of these communities.

One successful primary healthcare program has been the Program of Experience in the Palliative Approach (PEPA; http://www.pepaeducation.com). Supported by the Australian government under the National Palliative Care Program, the program aims to improve access and quality of services across Australia, through the up-skilling of mainly primary healthcare providers. The program has three components to develop the knowledge and skills of participants: funded clinical workforce placements, integration of learning into the workplace, and networks of support. Travel, accommodation, and funding to cover the replacement of the clinician for the time of the placement are also provided to ease the participation of clinicians, especially those in rural areas.

Models of after-hours service provision

Consistent with the standards of Palliative Care Australia is the requirement to plan coordinated care among service providers, so that patients and their caregivers are well supported, particularly in the home environment.[8] In many places this will include provision of 24-hour access to support. The nature of this support differs across services and between rural and metropolitan areas and maintaining the after-hours service can place significant strain on small services in terms of small numbers of nurses sharing after-hours responsibilities. Two main models of metropolitan after-hours provision have developed that address this strain. The first consists of a triage model where a related inpatient service receives calls from patients or family members at home regarding their needs. In an evaluation of this model,[27] the triage nurse was able to manage 30% (192 calls) of calls alone. The remaining 70% (437 calls) were transferred to the specialist community palliative care nurse on call. Of these, a further 43% (186 calls) were managed by the specialist nurse with telephone support. The remaining 57% (251 calls) required a home visit. Importantly, the identity of the triage nurse was significantly related to whether the call could be managed alone, suggesting improvements in training and support for the triage nurse could increase the number of calls managed in this way and further reduce burden on the specialist community palliative care nurse.

The second model consists of sharing after-hours responsibilities between specialist palliative care services and generalist community nursing services, either within one geographic area or across a city-rural area. In Australian metropolitan areas generalist community nursing services offer after-hours care and are already available to visit patients at home requiring palliative care. All nurses are provided with basic palliative care knowledge and skills and have access to updated information about the specific palliative patients seeking after-hours support on a daily basis. In some settings this service is supplemented by telephone support after hours by a specialist palliative care nurse, increasing the capacity of the general community nurse to meet the patients' needs. In rural areas, there are successful models where support is provided by a city-based specialist service by telephone.[28]

Night respite can be another means of improving after-hours support. An Australian study undertaken by Kristjanson and colleagues,[29] described the benefits of night respite for patients receiving a home palliative care service and their families. The investigators developed and tested a brief assessment tool to determine those patients and families most in need of night respite. Care aides were then specifically trained to provide night respite support, and 53 patients received this support over an 11-month period. Results indicated that the assessment tool was reliable and feasible for use in practice. Findings from this study revealed that the types of patients most in need of night respite support were confused, agitated, or incontinent. As well, families with high levels of caregiver fatigue were particularly in need of this type of respite. Patients and family caregivers reported high levels of satisfaction with the night-respite service, and 70% of patients who died during the study were able to die at home. Cost estimates indicated that the home-care and night-respite service was delivered for approximately one-third the cost for an equivalent period of inpatient palliative care.

Palliative care in aged care settings

During the last two decades, research has indicated that the proportion of people dying in Australian residential aged care facilities has steadily increased. The increased number of residents dying in residential aged care facilities has focused attention on the need for a palliative approach that may enhance the care already provided to both residents and the families. A palliative approach[30] aims to improve the quality of life for individuals facing the end stage of their life, by reducing their suffering, treating pain, and assessing other physical, cultural, psychological, social, and spiritual needs. The palliative approach should be able to be provided by all health professionals in all settings of care, with referral to specialist palliative care services where patient needs require this.[6]

In response to the developing recognition of the needs of people dying in residential aged care, in 2002 the Australian Government Department of Health and Ageing commissioned the development of evidence-based *Guidelines for a Palliative Approach in Residential Aged Care* (www.caresearch.org). Revised in 2006, the Guidelines have been widely distributed to aged care settings throughout the country; in 2011 similar guidelines were developed for use in the community. Companion training packages have also been developed.

The Guidelines provide all levels of staff working in these facilities with evidence-based criteria against which their services can be monitored. They also assist in the identification of local strengths and weaknesses in the provision of a palliative approach in residential aged care facilities, providing a mechanism by which changes in service delivery maybe evaluated over time. A related project has also commenced to engage medical practitioners in their work in residential aged care environments (www.palliativecare.org.au).

In early 2008, the Australian Government introduced a new Aged Care Funding Instrument (ACFI) to allocate an additional subsidy for residents with additional care needs like those requiring palliative care. The ACFI is based on an assessment of a resident's care needs and is intended to better match funding to the increasing complex care needs of residents as they approach their end of life. Residents in aged care facilities with palliative care needs are eligible for the maximum funding assessment rating under ACFI's Complex Health Care Supplement, where ratings on medications and complex healthcare questions are used to determine a resident's suitability for the supplement.

In New Zealand in 2009 the Ministry of Health and Hospice New Zealand considered the results of a national stock-take into palliative care service provision and subsequent funding was provided to develop a national education resource comprising nine learning packages. One package was assisted in development through collaboration with the residential aged care and health for older people sectors, ensuring the learning packages are "fit for purpose." The packages are taught collaboratively by members of the multidisciplinary teams from both hospice and aged care, allowing the best of specialist palliative care knowledge and gerontology care to be taught. In 2013 a generic version of the Fundamentals of Palliative Care will be developed in order to provide education across all care settings. In 2014 a blended e-learning version is planned for development.

Research

Increasingly, palliative care research in Australia is led from a multidisciplinary team of investigators with nurses commonly taking lead roles. The National Health and Medical Research Council, Australia's peak research body, has previously acknowledged the importance of palliative care and allocated specific funding in a way that targets improvements in research outputs and building research capacity, although this has not continued.

Several states in Australia have active multidisciplinary academic palliative care centers. There is an increasing trend toward formalized research collaborations to maximize research outcomes, and palliative care research in Australia is no exception. The Centre for Palliative Care Education and Research (St Vincent's and The University of Melbourne) has worked to discern optimal ways of promoting research collaboration in order to avoid duplication, and promote capacity building. As part of this project, 95% of respondents to a statewide survey ($n = 76$), many of whom were nurses, reported a desire for a structured research collaboration. The top two responses in other key areas related to palliative care research are noted in Box 72.1.

The Palliative Care Clinical Studies Collaborative (PaCCSC) is a research collaboration of a number of universities that aims to improve quality of care for patients through access, awareness, and quality use of palliative care medicines in the community through clinical studies (www.caresearch.com.au).

The Psycho-Oncology Co-operative Research Group (PoCoG) is, again, a national collaboration that aims to improve the outcomes of patients experiencing a diagnosis of cancer, their families, and their caregivers through evaluation and implementation of psychosocial and supportive care interventions for patients, caregivers, health professionals, and the healthcare system. Although its focus is not specifically palliative care research, some activities are related, and therefore, worth highlighting in this review (www.pocog.org.au).

The International Palliative Care Family Carer Research Collaboration (IPCFRC) under the auspices of the European Association of Palliative Care but operating out of Australia, was established by two nurses.[31] This group aims to develop a strategic approach to palliative care research planning related to family caregivers of people requiring palliative care by establishing international partnerships and promoting information exchange (www.ipcfrc.unimelb.edu.au).

One nationally funded initiative to assist with the transfer of knowledge to practice is CareSearch (www.caresearch.com.au).

Box 72.1 Research priorities, enablers, and barriers in Victoria, Australia

Research priorities

1. Symptom management
2. Rural settings

Enablers to undertaking palliative care research

1. Funded research positions
2. Ability to combine clinical work with research

Barriers to undertaking palliative care research

1. Funding
2. Lack of research experience/expertise

Enablers to dissemination of research findings

1. Funding to attend palliative care conferences
2. Palliative care peer-reviewed journals

Barriers to dissemination of research findings

1. Time
2. Lack of knowledge regarding the process surrounding publishing research findings

Enablers to translation of research results to clinical care

1. Close partnerships between researchers and service care providers
2. Organizational culture

Barriers to translation of research results to clinical care

1. Lack of time to keep up to date with literature
2. Lack of organizational support

This is an electronic evidence-based online resource of palliative care literature not typically available in existing anthologies, which was developed for palliative care practitioners, educators, and researchers.[32] Indexed and reviewed literature includes unpublished abstracts, government- and organization-sponsored documents, theses from Australian universities, and international published palliative care literature missing from standard electronic databases.

Given the global environment in which nursing and healthcare is informed, several Australian and New Zealand nurses are actively participating in international palliative care initiatives. Typical organizations in which nurses are involved on boards include the International Association of Hospice and Palliative Care, the Asia Pacific Palliative Care Network, the IPCFRC, and the Worldwide Palliative Care Alliance. In addition, palliative care nurses in Australian and New Zealand are regularly invited to present their work at international palliative care congresses.

Policy

As indicated in various sections of this chapter, over the last 10 years or so, Australia has enjoyed a period of healthy development of service-related palliative care policy, many of which were developed by the Australian government in partnership with peak bodies and service providers, but which now require revision (www.health.gov.au/palliativecare).

Palliative care nurses in New Zealand have been actively involved in Ministry of Health policy work in both cancer and palliative care. Of particular note is the National Cancer Control and Action Strategy Plan (http://www.moh.govt.nz/moh.nsf/indexmh/cancercontrol-strategyandactionplan), providing direction in this area of health for the country for the next 5 years. In response to this plan, District Health Boards, which include membership of nurses, have provided their regional implementation responses.

As part of developing the New Zealand nursing workforce, the National Professional Development Framework for Palliative Care Nursing in Aotearoa, New Zealand, (www.moh.govt.nz), aims to develop palliative care nursing in order to improve end-of-life care for patients. A set of competency indicators together with resource materials to help nurses acquire these competencies have been developed.

Of note in the last few years has been the development of national palliative care special interest groups for nurses in both countries. This has provided a vehicle for the voice of nursing to be heard in this discipline and an opportunity to promote nursing work in policy development, education, and research, through nursing-specific conferences. Governments have utilized these groups to seek advice on particular issues.

In New Zealand, a lack of a common understanding of what makes up specialist palliative care services has impacted the strategic development of palliative care services, contributing to variable access to services for people with a palliative care need. In 2012, hospices described the minimum range of professionals in the multidisciplinary specialist palliative care team, and the qualification requirements of each of these professional groups. The team description was adopted by the Ministry of Health and translated across into the specialist palliative care services indicative staffing profiles in a Resource and Capability Framework for Adult Palliative Care Services in New Zealand. Commissioned in 2011, this Framework is a resource for district health boards, designed to provide guidance to funders and policymakers, informs strategic planning and purchasing of accessible and equitable palliative care services for New Zealanders. The Framework describes the levels of palliative care required in New Zealand including the resources and capabilities needed to support service delivery and was released in 2013.[33]

In New Zealand the palliative care needs of children and young people and their families/whānau have been recognized since 1998; however, a corresponding development of services has not occurred. There is only one specialist pediatric palliative care service, which is based at Starship Children's Health in Auckland. The service is not recognized or funded as a national resource, and access to specialist palliative care is inequitable. At the local level, the delivery of pediatric palliative care services is highly variable. Teams of public health service providers are sometimes supported by hospice services, and primary care providers are rarely involved in a systematic way.

The Ministry of Health commissioned a project to provide implementation-focused guidance to improve the integration of palliative care service delivery to children and young people in New Zealand. It examines pediatric palliative care services, both in New Zealand and internationally, and uses the results as the basis for a proposed framework for developing a coherent, integrated, and coordinated system of pediatric palliative care service delivery. The report *Guidance for Integrated Paediatric Palliative Care Services in New Zealand* was released in September 2012, proposing a framework that includes the Starship Paediatric Palliative Care Team. This team would be situated as the national specialist service, with national consultative and service development responsibilities; nurse coordinators and lead pediatricians in each health region would lead service development.[34]

Education, training, and advanced practice

Although almost all nurses are exposed to end-of-life and palliative care issues, undergraduate nursing education in palliative care remains inconsistent within both countries. There remains significant work to routinely include palliative care in the core undergraduate curriculum and the National Palliative Care Strategies,[20,22] of both Australia and New Zealand include the fostering of education of palliative care professionals. In Australia, the government funded a suite of resources for use in all undergraduate health science curricula. Named PCC4U (Palliative Care Curriculum for Undergraduates), the resources have been widely distributed, with nursing courses especially responsive. In April 2013, of the 220 health sciences courses identified, there were 85 courses actively implementing the project resources in their curriculum and 70 reviewing or planning to implement the resources (http://www.pcc4u.org/).

It is apparent that most palliative care education occurs at postgraduate level and, as such, is optional and self-directed.[35] Of note are the online and distance courses that have developed, probably partly in response to the isolation of many rural work environments in both countries. There are a variety of continuing education (short course) and postgraduate (university auspiced) courses available in Australia (http://www.caresearch.com.au/caresearch/Education). There has also been a recent focus on establishing specialist multidisciplinary education initiatives, which have demonstrated effectiveness.[36] Such initiatives have been used as the basis for developing a university-accredited specialist training program that seeks to become the minimum requirement for health professionals to work in specialist palliative care settings (http://www.mccp.unimelb.edu.au/courses/award-courses/specialist-certificate/palliative-care).

In New Zealand, palliative care nursing has seen an increased focus on multidisciplinary teamwork, shared care in the community, and nurse specialists in hospital consultancy and plans to recognize nurse practitioners with limited prescribing rights. Nursing competencies had been incorporated into the main tertiary courses for hospice nurses by 2002.[36]

Regarding scope of practice, numerous senior roles have developed in both countries. Clinical nurse consultants, clinical nurse specialists, and nurse practitioners undertake consultative roles in a variety of settings like acute hospitals, specialist palliative care units, aged care, and the community. Perceived constraints on practice include workload, a lack of available time for the number of patients, resistance from medical colleagues, limited prescribing rights, and fear of litigation. Despite these difficulties, advanced practice roles continue to develop. The minimal education requirement for endorsement is a completed Masters of

Nurse Practitioner (MNP) and includes a therapeutic medication module(s) and a clinical internship.

In New Zealand in 2009 the Ministry of Health and Hospice New Zealand considered the results of a national evaluation of palliative care service provision. Nationally, there were two areas of need:

- Nationally consistent education programs that support generalist palliative care providers; and

- Revised palliative care standards and an ongoing implementation program to ensure consistency in the quality of service regardless of locality.

The Minister of Health then allocated a portion of the funding that was available to address difficulties in accessing palliative care services to Hospice NZ for the two projects. This funding commenced on January 1, 2010.

As noted above, some funding was utilized to develop learning packages in collaboration with the residential aged care and health for older people sectors. Additionally, in 2012 the Hospice NZ Standards for Palliative Care were developed to ensure consistency in the quality of service delivered regardless of locality. The Standards are supported by a quality palliative care review program. Peer mentors support continuous improvement and assist services to ensure they have carried out a robust self-assessment (the peer review).

Current issues and looking to the future

There are a number of current issues impinging on future development in both countries. In relation to workforce, the aging and retirement of nurses with expertise in palliative care may leave inexperienced staff to carry more and more caseloads. This has implications for planning models of healthcare, including palliative care, into the future.

Funding, together with increased workloads, is an ongoing concern. In Australia, the model is imminently changing from block funding to activity-based funding; the implications of this change are yet to be demonstrated. With more care being planned to be delivered in people's homes, funding models will need to maintain community-focused priorities, to enable people not only to die in their place of choice but also, to save unnecessary hospital admissions. In relation to nursing roles, the community-based and consultative aspects are likely to continue to develop into the future, in line with developing health policy.

Conclusion

Palliative care nursing in Australia and New Zealand continues to develop and grow. Nurses now perform significant leadership roles in both countries, evident in clinical practice, education, and research. Academic positions in palliative nursing provide sector leadership and are increasingly successful in attracting competitive research funding. These academic positions have continued to be established with close relationships with clinical facilities, maintaining a research agenda that is clinically relevant.

Looking to the future, workforce issues will continue to impact on the shape of palliative care. Issues like the aging of the health workforce and the need to continually up-skill generalist staff by making education readily available are significant. Continuing to work closely with both government policies and the peak bodies will influence the further development of palliative care and particularly the work in primary healthcare environments that makes palliative care equitably available across regions, settings, and populations. Improvements in community awareness and understandings of palliative care are regarded as essential in future planning.

This chapter demonstrates that nurses are at the forefront of developing service systems able to meet the needs of people requiring palliative care in our communities and are committed to sustainable models of palliative care delivery. Mainstreaming and primary healthcare models, together with the important integration of policy, research, and practice, will allow palliative care nurses in Australasia to continue their leadership roles in advancing palliative care practice and ensuring its place in healthcare.

Acknowledgments

I acknowledge the former work of colleagues (and friends) Sanchia Aranda, Linda Kristjanson, and Peter Hudson, who permitted my building on their foundational content in developing this chapter. Anne Morgan, Practice Advisor, Hospice New Zealand, provided an update of the relevant aspects of this chapter.

References

1. O'Connor M, Aranda S, eds. Palliative Care Nursing: A Guide to Practice. 3rd ed. Oxford: Radcliffe Medical Press; 2012.
2. Hudson PL, Payne S, eds. Family Care and Palliative Care: A Guide for Health and Social Care Professionals. Oxford: Oxford University Press; 2008.
3. New Zealand Population Census. 2006. Available at: www. stats.gov. nz/statsweb.nsf (accessed December 2, 2008).
4. Payne S. To supplant, supplement or support?: Organizational issues for hospices. Soc Sci Med. 1998;46:1495–1504.
5. Duckett S, Willcox S. The Australian Health Care System. 4th ed. Melbourne: Oxford University Press; 2011.
6. O'Connor M. Decrepit death as a discourse of death in older age: implications for policy. Intl J of Older People Nurs. 2009;4:263–271.
7. Hospice New Zealand Standards for Palliative Care. Quality Review Programme and Guide. Wellington: Hospice New Zealand; 2012.
8. Standards for Palliative Care Provision. 4th ed. Canberra: Palliative Care Australia; 2005.
9. The Economist Intelligence Unit. The quality of death: ranking end-of-life care across the world. London: Economist Intelligence Unit; 2010.
10. Allen S, Chapman Y, O'Connor M, Francis K. The evolution of palliative care and the relevance to residential aged care: understanding the past to inform the future Collegian. 2008;15(4):165–171.
11. Palliative Care Australia. A Guide to Palliative Care Service Development—A Population-Based Approach. Canberra: Palliative Care Australia; 2005.
12. Palliative Care Service Provision in Australia: A Planning Guide. 2nd ed. Canberra: Palliative Care Australia; 2003.
13. O'Connor M, Chapman Y. The palliative care clinical nurse consultant: an essential link. Collegian. 2008;15:151–157.
14. O'Connor M, Peter L, Walsh K. Palliative care nurse consultants in Melbourne, Australia: a "snap shot" of their clinical role. Int J Palliat Nurs. 2008;14/7:350–356.
15. Australian Government, Department of Health and Ageing. Community Attitudes to Palliative Care Issue. Canberra: Australian Government; 2003.
16. Ramsden I. Kawa Whakaruruhau: Guidelines for Nursing and Midwifery Education. Wellington: Nursing Council of New Zealand; 1992.
17. Guidelines for Cultural Safety, the Treaty of Waitangi, and Maori Health in Nursing and Midwifery Education and Practice. Wellington: Nursing Council of New Zealand; 2011.

18. The New Zealand Palliative Care Strategy. Wellington: New Zealand Ministry of Health; 2001.

19. Cancer Control Taskforce, 2005. Available at: http://cancercontrolnz.govt.nz/sites/default/files/Positioning%20Palliative%20care%20in%20NZ.pdf.

20. National Health and Medical Research Council. Values and Ethics: Guidelines for Ethical Conduct in Aboriginal and Torres Strait Islander Health Research. Canberra: National Health and Medical Research Council; 2003.

21. Australian Government, Department of Health and Ageing National Palliative Care Strategy: A Framework for Palliative Care Service Development. Canberra: Australian Government; 2000.

22. Australian Government, Department of Health and Ageing. Supporting Australians to Live Well at the End of Life. National Palliative Care Strategy. Canberra: Australian Government; 2010.

23. McGrath P, Phillips E. Insights on end of life ceremonial practices of Australian Aboriginal peoples. Collegian. 2008;15:125–133.

24. Hsu C, O'Connor M, Lee S. Understandings of death and dying for people of Chinese origins. Death Stud. 2009;33:153–174.

25. O'Connor M, O'Brien A, Griffiths D, Poon E, Chin J, Payne S, Nordin R. What is the meaning of palliative care in the Asia-Pacific Region? Asia-Pacific J Clin Oncol. 2010;6(3):1–6.

26. Phillips J, Davidson P, Jackson D, Kristjanson L, Bennett M, Daly M. Enhancing palliative care delivery in a regional community in Australia. Austral Health Rev. 2006;30(3):370–379.

27. Palliative Care Research Team, Monash University. What happens after dark?: Improving "After Hours" Palliative Care Planning in Urban and Rural Victoria, for Patients, Their Carers and Health Professionals. Report to the Commonwealth Department of Health and Ageing. Monash University, 2009.

28. Ciechomski L, Tan H, O'Connor M, Miles G, Klein B, Schattner P. After hours palliative care provision in rural and urban Victoria, Australia. Asia-Pacific J Health Manage. 2009;4(1):57–63.

29. Kristjanson L, Cousins K, White K, et al. Evaluation of a night respite community palliative care service. Int J Palliat Nurs. 2004;10(2):84–90.

30. O'Connor M, Davis M, Abernathy A. Language, discourse and meaning in palliative medicine. Prog Palliat Care. 2010;18(2):1–6.

31. Hudson P, Zordan R, Trauer T. Research priorities associated with family caregivers in palliative care: international perspectives. J Palliat Med. 2011, 14(4) 397–401

32. Tieman J. Multiple sources: mapping the literature of palliative care. Palliat Med. 2009;23:425–431.

33. Resource and Capability Framework for Adult Palliative Care Services in New Zealand. Available at: http://www.health.govt.nz/publication/resource-and-capability-framework-integrated-adult-palliative-care-services-new-zealand.

34. Guidance for Integrated Paediatric Palliative Care Services in New Zealand. Availab at: http://www.health.govt.nz/publication/guidance-integrated-paediatric-palliative-care-services-new-zealand.

35. Spruyt O, Macleod R, Hudson P. Australia and New Zealand. In: Wee B, Hughes N (eds.), Palliative Care Education: Building a Culture of Learning. Oxford: Oxford University Press; 2007:59–67.

36. Quinn K, Hudson AM, Thomas K. "Palliative care the essentials": evaluation of a multidisciplinary education program. J Palliat Med. 2008;11(8):1122–1129.

CHAPTER 73

Palliative care in the UK

Nancy Preston and Katherine Froggatt

The historical context

In the United Kingdom (UK), the establishment of specific institutions for the care of dying people began in the 1890s. The Hostel of God in Clapham (now Trinity Hospice), was established in 1891. This was closely followed by St. Luke's Hospice in Battersea (1892) and St. Joseph's Hospice in Hackney (1895). Subsequently, there was little significant development in numbers of hospices until the 1960s, when the rapid expansion of the hospice movement occurred in response to the changing social climate and the increasing incidence of deaths from cancer.[1]

The first modern hospices were established both in the United Kingdom and the United States in the 1960s, a period when there was widespread criticism of institutional care. The hospice provided an alternative to the dominant medical model of cure. Dying had become an isolating experience because of the increasing use of technology within medicine, while the cultural value of individualism meant that dying was no longer a communal event.[2] The dying person was often left to experience death on their own amid indefinite, and often unrealistic, technological intervention.[3] The hospice movement aimed to respond in areas where the healthcare system was seen to be failing, particularly with respect to people dying of cancer—a major cause of death in men and women.[4]

The experiences arising from these deaths from cancer, generally occurring in acute hospitals, with patients dying alone in side rooms alienated from their family, often with inappropriate technological intervention, was an impetus for the hospice movement, which offered an alternative to this way of dying. It provided care in which relationships were central and people did not die alone; people found others alongside them at the end of their lives.

The needs of these dying people were met by the emerging hospice movement, Abel[5] suggests, in the following ways: control by doctors was minimized, equal weight was placed on the skills of diverse professionals through the presence of a multidisciplinary team, the gap between the experts and nonexperts was bridged through the use of volunteers, the course of nature as ending in death was increasingly accepted, and the bureaucratization and institutionalization of modern medical care was challenged, particularly the regimentation of the delivery of care. It was suggested that hospice care avoided these disadvantages, and the traditional boundaries of medical concern were crossed, by seeing the family, rather than the individual, as the unit of care. The philosophy of the hospice movement was, and is, concerned with normalizing life, so that death is reduced to an ordinary and natural event[2] and, ideally, control is moved into the patient's own hands, another aspect of the increasing emphasis placed on the individual in contemporary (postmodern) society.

The modern hospice movement

The name that is synonymous with the modern hospice movement is that of Dame Cicely Saunders. She trained as a nurse, social worker, and doctor, and her interest in terminal care was consolidated when she went to St. Joseph's Hospice in 1958. Here she confronted issues to do with pain control, truth and honesty among the dying, and the role of the family, concerns that are still important to the movement today. Her personal experience of watching individuals dying in pain and patients not knowing they were dying, the norm within hospital care at that time, motivated Dame Cicely Saunders to find alternatives. In 1967, she was instrumental in opening the first purpose-built hospice at St. Christopher's Hospice in South London. It had an emphasis on research and teaching as well as patient care. Two years later in 1969, the home care work started. In 1971, the bereavement services commenced, and day care services began in 1974.[6]

The development of bereavement services arose out of lay and professional concern at the lack of support for people who had been bereaved. Cruse, a charity started in 1959, took the lead, offering support to bereaved widows and widowers.[7] In the 1970s, Colin Murray Parkes, a psychiatrist at the Tavistock Centre for Human Relations, studied the bereavement experience of widows, and his work was the stimulus for the bereavement service at St Christopher's Hospice. St Christopher's Hospice, and many other hospices, later diversified their services into home care, day care, and bereavement services, away from purely inpatient units.[8,9]

While hospices continue to provide inpatient services to patients, there is an increase in hospice specialist palliative care services, with the majority being provided by hospices in the community.[9] There has been a growing debate in the UK about the ideal place of death, with patients identifying the home as the preferred setting.[10] This has been supported by government policy in the National End of Life Care Programme, and it seems this goal is being realized for some patient groups. In a recent report on place of death for cancer patients, while the hospital remains the most common place of death (48% of deaths), 24.5% of deaths occurred at home, and 16.4% of deaths in hospices, which is an increase over home and hospice deaths since 2005.[11]

Political developments

Much of the political development within UK palliative care has its origins in developments within cancer care. The Calman Hine report, in 1985, changed the way cancer services were operated in the UK.[12] There was a recognition that cancer specialists and specialist treatments were often limited to certain geographical regions of the UK, resulting in patients receiving less-than-optimum local care or needing to travel long distances for treatments such as radiotherapy. Cancer centers were initiated to provide more local treatment, and guidelines developed for the optimum treatment of different cancers, which sometimes included specific sections on palliative care.[13]

Palliative care first became recognized as a medical specialty in the UK in 1987, when a 4-year training program was introduced. The English National Board for Nursing then introduced their first course, Care of the Dying.[6]

In 2000, Cancer Networks were established through the National Cancer Plan.[14] This gave hospices and palliative care units an opportunity to engage more formally with mainstream cancer services and have their work commissioned. In the 2008 Department of Health Report,[15] there was a desire to create a "set of new voluntary agreements between the government, private and third sector organisations on actions to improve health outcomes."[15(p. 3)] There was also recognition in the National Institute for Clinical Excellence (NICE) that the kind of palliative services they recommended were dependent on funding. These developments potentially provided more financial resilience for hospices, which were vulnerable to changes in the level of giving from the general population to support their work. The government aimed that the state would provide 50% of the funding for hospices; however 13 years later hospices were still funded predominantly from the voluntary sector.[9]

The culmination of numerous frameworks by the Department of Health was the first UK National End of Life Care Strategy in 2008, for England,[17] which was a milestone for the UK. End-of-life care could refer to the last year of a patient's life and was an umbrella term. Building on previous statements, the strategy envisioned end-of-life care as not solely focused on cancer patients. It also addressed the issue that the majority of end-of-life care is delivered by nonspecialist teams including general healthcare staff as well as untrained staff. These staff were seen as needing support and education but gauged at their level of practice and degree of specialization. Surveys had highlighted that the majority of patients want to die at home or in their usual place of care such as a nursing home.[10] One of the key goals of this strategy was to help patients to die in their preferred place of death, and an analysis of death figures shows that increasingly patients are dying at home or in their usual place of care, although the hospital death remains the most common.[11]

The English strategy describes the challenges of end-of-life care in the context of death, dying and society; outlines an end of life care pathway; and considers care in different settings, support for carers and families, workforce issues, measurement and research, and how to make change happen. The end-of-life care pathway as outlined in the strategy provides the structure for the provision of resources, tools, educational material, case studies, and publications to support the provision of end-of-life care in England.[17] Three specific approaches have been promoted: an integrated care pathway (Liverpool Care Pathway); Gold Standards Framework; and advance care planning (such as the Preferred Priorities for Care document). The linear pathway that underpins the English End of Life Care Strategy has been challenged,[18] and a model of service provision based on service journeys has been proposed but this has yet to be acted on.

As the delivery of healthcare has been devolved down to the four countries—England, Scotland, Wales, and Northern Ireland there are therefore differences in budgets, priorities, and regulatory processes that shape how palliative care is delivered. Each of the other three nations in the United Kingdom has also developed its own palliative care strategy that reflects these differences,[19–21] and they commonly promote the use of the three tools and approaches mentioned earlier.

The Liverpool Care Pathway

The Liverpool Care Pathway (LCP) was designed by Professor John Ellershaw and his team at the Marie Curie Institute, Liverpool, to deliver hospice type care to patients in nonspecialist palliative care units such as general medical wards and the community.[22] It is an integrated care pathway. Pathways were initially developed in the United States as a means of delivering care within the constraints of the insurance system. Indeed there are similar systems in the United States that have had not been so widely adopted and have had less evaluation.[23] In the UK, integrated care pathways were championed and developed in key areas such as stroke and then promoted in palliative care.

One of the aims of the LCP was to prevent unnecessary invasive treatment during the last hours of a patient's life, similar to the care experienced in a hospice. The LCP has a particular emphasis on symptom control in the last 48 hours of life, to promote comfort and encourage planning for anticipated symptoms. Part of this planning includes anticipatory prescribing of analgesia and sedatives that are commonly used at the end of life. However, one of the key challenges is identifying that patients are in a nonreversible state and where death is likely. Indeed prognostication is known to be an inexact science and so identifying patients through a multidisciplinary team was seen as one method of helping identify patients.[24]

In the UK there has been widespread adoption of the LCP, and it has been introduced to a number of other countries worldwide. However, since 2012, in the UK there has been an ongoing media debate about the use of the LCP.[25] Part of the issue seems to have come from how the pathway has been implemented by staff with patients being wrongly diagnosed as being in the last 48 hours of life and a lack of communication with relatives about what is happening. This has led to the LCP being seen as a death pathway and a means to facilitate death and has provoked anxiety about why these patients were placed on the pathway. In response to this public outcry a rapid review of the evidence was commissioned; this resulted in a recommendation to withdraw the pathway as there was insufficient evidence to recommend its safe implementation.[26] There are indications that the pathway improves symptom control, documentation of care, continuity of care, lower levels of bereavement, staff confidence, and communications with staff and relatives.[27–32] However, the research underpinning its use is often of a less robust research design. A cluster randomized controlled trial in Italy[33] showed that only breathlessness was improved in patients receiving care under the pathway, although insufficient patients had been recruited to the study to make definitive recommendations.[34] Existential issues are less well addressed on the LCP and indeed are not differentiated out of from the experience of symptoms and pain. The LCP is a tool health professionals can employ to assist in how they deliver care, and ultimately, how the pathway is implemented is down to the individuals in a unit.

The Gold Standards Framework

The Gold Standards Framework (GSF) is a framework for a planned system of care that provides staff with a structure to deliver palliative care, in consultation with the patient and family. The aim is to promote better coordination and organization of care through collaboration between health professionals, optimize out-of-hours care, and prevent inappropriate hospital admissions.

The framework was developed by a GP with a special interest in palliative care (Dr. Keri Thomas), and was initially developed for use in primary care. It has subsequently been adapted for the care home, acute hospital, community hospital, and domiciliary care settings, and more recently for dementia care. Seven key areas are addressed within the framework: communication, coordination of care, control of symptoms, continuity of care in the out-of-hours period, continued learning of staff, carer support for family members and friends, care in the dying phase. Addressing these areas leads to three underlying processes:

1. Identification of a patient in need of palliative care

   In primary care, discussions take place between the GP and nursing staff, who decide, with the help of specially produced prognostic indicators,[35] which patients might be expected to live for less than a year. These patients are entered onto a supportive care register, which is used to plan, record, and monitor patient care at regular healthcare team meetings in the GP practice. In care homes, the nursing team meet, ideally with the GP(s), to have a similar discussion about their residents.

2. Assessment of an individual's need

   This is undertaken to consider physical and psychological symptoms and social or spiritual needs. Any preferences and choices that are important to the patient and family are also considered.

3. Planning ahead

   Planning ahead is required, particularly for the "out-of-hours" situation. This means ensuring that handover forms have been sent to ambulance services and that medications that might be needed are available in the home or care home.

Within a GP practice or care home a GSF coordinator is appointed and is responsible for implementing and maintaining the framework. The whole program is overseen by the central National Gold Standards Framework team, which provides training for the GSF coordinators.

To date 95% of GP practices (8500) have achieved Foundation level use of the GSF.[36] This reflects the embedding of the program in the palliative care quality measures used to assess English GP practices, so ensuring a high use of the intervention. A further level of investment, the "Going for Gold" training program is also being implemented, with seven GP practices achieving accreditation in 2012. In the care home sector, 2300 care homes, mainly those offering nursing care, have undertaken the training. A smaller number have achieved accreditation (*n* = 395).[37] The other developments in acute hospitals, community hospitals, and domiciliary care are much more recent, and the level of involvement limited to date.

There is some evidence of positive outcomes from the use of GSF. In primary care, introduction of the GSF has led to greater use of processes to support palliative care delivery and some evidence of improvements in the quality of palliative care.[38] In care homes, a number of small-scale evaluations have been published.[39–41] These show perceived benefits for residents of paying greater attention to giving residents choice and better symptom control. For staff, benefits identified were increased staff confidence, improved team communication, and greater engagement with external support and expertise, with the added benefit of a better reputation for the home.[40]

The role of nurses in the delivery of this framework is key. They often take on the role of facilitators and coordinators for the program in GP practices and for the care home program.

Advance Care Planning

Advance care planning (ACP) has been implemented internationally and in the UK. In the UK, the Preferred Priorities of Care[42] document has been proposed as an appropriate tool in the End of Life Care Strategy.[17] Advance care planning is understood to be a process of discussion and review between an individual and others (health and social care staff and/or family) in order to enable individuals to express, and, if they wish, record information about their views, their values, and even specific treatment choices. This can then be used to inform decisions about their future care. While the English End of Life Care Strategy proposes the use of the Preferred Priorities of Care, it is recognized that other advanced planning tools can be used.[43]

In the US, ACP is rooted in public empowerment and self-determination,[44] whereas in the UK it builds on initiation by healthcare providers.[45] Such a model for ACP depends on communication by healthcare staff, namely physicians and nurses.[46] However, it is widely recognized that healthcare staff often find it challenging to initiate discussions about death and dying with patients who are approaching the end of their lives and their families[47–49] and that to do so requires skillful and thoughtful communication.[50–54]

In 2003, an ACP tool called Preferred Place of Care (PPC) was developed in the northwest of England in order to help healthcare staff to initiate potentially difficult conversations and allow patients' wishes and preferences regarding end-of-life care to be communicated and documented. The PPC contains three key questions that provide a framework for end-of-life discussions. It was revised in 2007 and renamed Preferred Priorities for Care,[42] to reflect its broader focus on wishes and preferences at the end of life, rather than just place of care.

The PPC is a patient-held document that can be transferred between care settings with the patient as necessary. Although it is patient held, it is important that the wishes and preferences for care that are documented in the PPC are communicated to others, especially family members and healthcare staff, in order that the preferences may be fulfilled.[55] In practice, the PPC tool is usually facilitated by a member of healthcare staff (most frequently a community-based nurse),[56,57] and its use and implementation is often dependent on this member of staff.

Despite its widespread promotion through the National Health Service (NHS), little published evidence exists about PPC and its use.[42,57,58] Research is ongoing about both public and nurses' views on the use of PPC, and preliminary research findings indicate that people would welcome the opportunity to talk about planning their care and assumptions about people's nonwillingness to engage with the topic of death and dying need to be challenged.[55]

Current palliative care provision

Palliative care can be provided at different levels: a palliative care approach and specialist palliative care.[59] A palliative care approach is provided by staff without a specialist role in palliative care in settings and services where few palliative care patients are cared for. In contrast, a specialist palliative care service comprises a multidisciplinary team of nurses, doctors, and allied health professionals offering care for physical, emotional, social, and spiritual needs of people with life-limiting illness or chronic illness.[59] Nurses have a role to play in both settings either as providers of palliative care or as specialists in palliative care working in a specialist setting or service with engagement in more generalist settings, usually based externally to the setting.

Settings of care

Palliative care can be provided where ever people live or are requiring care.

Hospices in the UK are usually located in specialist buildings offering either inpatient care and/or day care services. The number of inpatient hospices and palliative care units is 220 (Table 73.1), with approximately 5.5 beds per 100,000 population.[60]

In England, 5% of all deaths occur in hospices,[61] but a larger number of people are supported as they die, through hospice at home and home care teams. There is increasing engagement and support for people with conditions other than cancer, although these tend to be defined diagnostic groups, such as neurological conditions, heart failure, chronic pulmonary disease, and some attention to people with dementia.

Acute hospitals are generalist palliative care settings, yet are the place of death for over half the population. In 2010, 54% of the English population died in hospitals.[61] Many hospitals host specialist palliative care teams who support patients with palliative care needs within the hospital's wards. Currently, 308 specialist teams exist in hospitals.[62] Although the teams are often multidisciplinary, nurses have been key to the membership of the team, providing specialist advice and support for generalist nurses in the setting. In a small number of hospitals (*n* = 31; 248 beds),[62] specialist palliative care units exist, providing palliative care for people with specialist palliative care needs.

Table 73.1 Hospice and palliative care provision

	Adult services	Children services
Hospice and palliative care units	220	42
Inpatient beds	3175	334
Homecare units	288	NA
Hospice at home	127	NA
Day centers	272	NA

Source: Reference 60.

Palliative care is also provided in *day care* settings—clinics and centers, either stand-alone or located alongside other palliative care services, such as hospices. In the UK there are 272 day hospices/day care services.[62] They offer social support alongside medical, nursing, and rehabilitative care. Different models for day care exist with different emphases placed on these different types of care. There has been much discussion about the benefits and impact of day hospice care. A recent review indicated patients describe attendance as a valuable experience, with respect to the opportunity to engage with other people and the provision of support. However, the evidence about the impact on well-being for these individuals is not yet present.[63]

Care homes in the UK refers to long-term care facilities that are a collective institutional setting where care is provided for people who live there, 24 hours a day, 7 days a week, for an undefined period of time. The care provided includes on-site provision of personal assistance with activities of daily living; nursing and medical care may be provided on-site or by nursing and medical professionals working from an organization external to the setting.

With different figures available for each of the four nations (England, Scotland, Wales and Northern Ireland) we report on the data from England, and anticipate the same trends across the four countries. In England, there are 18,255 care homes providing 459,448 registered places.[64] Of the care homes, 75% were residential care homes (with no on-site nursing), but these institutions provided care to only 56% of the care home population.[64] Of the population, in England, 18% die in care homes.[61] Care provision in this sector is complex, with differences in type (residential or nursing), size, and ownership. The average size of residential care homes is 18 beds, and for nursing homes just under 47 beds. Nursing homes are more likely to site in the private sector (88%), with some voluntary sector ownership (10%). A higher proportion of voluntary- (22%) and council- (7%) sector-run residential care homes exist, although 69% of these care homes still sit in the private sector.[64]

A number of initiatives have been undertaken to develop palliative care in this sector, from national, regional, and local programs. The Gold Standards Framework program has already been described for care homes, but other programs have been developed by the English end-of-life care program specifically for care homes (Table 73.2).

As with the GSF program, these initiatives draw on nurses as specialist facilitators to ensure successful implementation of the programs, working to support care home staff.

People also receive palliative care in their own *domestic homes*. By "home" we refer to people's domestic homes, but this also includes sheltered housing and assisted living settings where people hold a tenancy for their accommodation. There has been great emphasis placed on supporting people to remain and die in their own homes over a number of years in the United Kingdom.[17] There are increases in recent years of the proportion of people being enabled to die in their own homes (now 21%), although there are regional variations.[10] Specialist community palliative care support teams exist (337 services),[62] to provide support for people with palliative care needs in their own homes. Again, often multidisciplinary in their structure, they work to advise and support general care providers (district nurses, general practitioners) and family carers to support the person in their own home.

Table 73.2 Care home palliative care development

Program	
The route to success in end of life care—achieving quality in care homes	Provides information about the interventions required to meet the six steps identified in the End of Life Care Strategy in order to deliver high quality end of life care in care homes.
Six Steps to Success Training Programme for Care Homes	Developed in the northwest of England, this initiative uses a facilitator to provide seven workshops and training to help care home staff implement a framework for end-of-life care. It also addresses the six steps in the nationally identified pathway to quality end-of-life care.

Nursing roles

Palliative nursing is core to the different types of palliative care provision provided in all the UK care contexts described above. Palliative nursing roles can be identified in the UK that reflect the increasing level of palliative care specialization.

As there is an expectation that nurses in all settings provide a palliative care approach, all registered general nurses (RGNs) are expected to be able to provide this level of care and identify when there is a need to refer to a specialist for assistance in complex situations. One aspect of care that all nurses need to be able to provide concerns Last Offices. This final aspect of care for a patient also has implications for the bereavement experience of family members.[65]

Clinical nurse specialists were the earliest palliative care role present in the UK. Their presence in palliative care reflected wider specialist development in oncology nursing.[12] The aspects of work clinical nurse specialists cover in palliative care includes: clinical work, consultation with others, teaching, leadership, and research. Core to this specialist palliative nursing practice is working with three groups of people[66]: patients and families, health and social care professionals and managers, policymakers, and planners.

The UK evidence regarding the impact of these specialist roles is limited and now dated, but it does show some positive outcomes for patients with respect to quality of life and emotional and cognitive functioning.[67,68]

Nurse consultants

A more significant development within palliative nursing has been the development of the nurse consultant role. Their establishment arose from recognition of the need to keep experienced skilled nursing staff in clinical practice rather than career development through a move to either managerial or educational roles. The original guidance on the role identified four core functions[69]:

◆ Expert practice function

◆ Professional leadership and consultancy function

◆ Education training and development function

◆ Practice and service development, research, and evaluation.

The relative importance of these different areas of responsibility was never prescribed, although clinical practice working with patients, families, and communities was identified as being key. Appointments can be made within the NHS and the voluntary sector, of particular relevance for palliative care. Levels of education, training, experience, or function required for nurse consultants have not been agreed. Nurse consultants exist in palliative care in different contexts—hospital, hospice, care home, and community settings with posts in both pediatric and adult palliative care.

A further development in the UK regarding advanced nurse practitioners has had some influence on palliative nursing. Advanced level practice is defined as that which "encompasses aspects of education, research and management but is firmly grounded in direct care provision or clinical work with patients, families and populations."[70(p. 7)] The elements of work within the role concern clinical or direct care practice, leadership and collaborative practice, improving quality and developing practice, developing self, and others. They are able to diagnose, order investigations, prescribe, and admit or discharge patients.[71] The advanced nurse practitioner elements may be integrated into clinical nurse specialist or nurse consultant level posts, subject to appropriate training and demonstration of competencies.

Linked to the advanced practice roles is the issue of nurse prescribing. The extent of medications that can be nurse-prescribed has increased over time, and palliative care was an area identified where nurses could prescribe, within their competency. The extent to which palliative care clinical nurse specialists prescribe is limited.[72] Only 11% of 1575 respondents were trained as independent nurse prescribers, and only half ($n = 88$) of these were actually prescribing. Factors identified that explained this low level of prescribing activity included deficits in training with respect to its length and focus. A lack of medical mentorship was also noted. Further development with respect to training and implementation was required at this time.

The future of palliative care in the UK

Four key areas are considered in terms of the future of palliative care provision in the UK: context for change, increasing diversification, service integration, and increased demand for evidence.

The current context for change in palliative care service provision in the UK from 2010 onward has been dominated by financial constraints. Financial issues are affecting both the public sector and voluntary sector, and these roles are under review. With cuts in public spending and reduced charitable giving, challenges to continue to provide current levels of services in the same ways can be questioned. More fundamentally, Demos also highlighted seven key problems in delivery of personalized end-of-life care[18]:

◆ Delayed identification of the dying phase

◆ Gaps in discussing, recording, and acting on end-of-life preferences

◆ Difficulties in triggering appropriate care after diagnosis

◆ Perverse incentives in the assessment of eligibility for support

◆ Problematic or delayed discharge into the community

The move to community-based services not only reflects an ideological shift to allow people to die at home but also has a cost basis. Hospices providing inpatient beds are still seen as synonymous with palliative care provision by the general public in the UK. There is a challenge to maintain the same profile through more community-based services. However, it is likely that the provision of hospice at home services will increase.

Meanwhile, there are encouraging signs that palliative care will continue to move beyond just meeting the needs of people with cancer, to include other people with a noncancer diagnosis. This raises similar questions about the demands and ability of services to meet them. Linked to this is how services are integrated to accommodate for this, which needs to be explored; a project is underway that aims to assess best practice in delivering integrated palliative care services across Europe including the UK.[73] Diversification also continues into other settings where care is delivered, with new initiatives in prisons.[74] Finally, one of the main areas of change will occur as palliative care begins to embrace research in general to provide excellent evidence-based care through research, practice development, and evaluation. Nurses are key to these changes as providers of general and specialist palliative care, and their up-skilling to work creatively and flexibly in new systems of care will continue.

References

1. Clark D. History and culture in the rise of palliative care. In: Payne S, Seymour J, Ingleton C (eds.), Palliative Care Nursing. 2nd ed. Buckingham, England: Open University Press; 2011.

2. Moller DW. On Death Without Dignity: The Human Impact of Technological Dying. Amityville, NY: Baywood; 1990.

3. Rinaldi A, Kearl MC. The hospice farewell: ideological perspectives of its professional practitioners. Omega. 1990;21(4):283–300.

4. James N, Field D. The routinization of hospice: charisma and bureaucratization. Soc Sci Med. 1992:34(12):1363–1375.

5. Abel EK. The hospice movement: institutionalizing innovation. Int J Health Serv. 1986;16(1):71–85.

6. Hansford P. Palliative care in the UK. In: Ferrell BR, Coyle N (eds.), Oxford Textbook of Palliative Nursing. 3rd ed. New York: Oxford University Press; 2010:1265–1274.

7. History of Cruse. Available at: http://www.kvg.pwp.blueyonder.co.uk/History%20of%20Cruse.htm. Accessed June 28, 2013.

8. The Hospice History Programme. available at: http://www.hospice-history.org.uk/byoralsurname?id=0086&search=p&page=0 Accessed June 28, 2013.

9. National Council for Palliative Care. National Survey of Patient Activity Data for Specialist Palliative Care Services. MDS Full Report for the Year 2011–2012. Public Health England, 2013.

10. Gomes B, Calanzani N, Higginson IJ. Local Preferences and Place of Death in Regions Within England, 2010. London: Cicely Saunders Institute; 2011.

11. Gao W, Ho YK, Verne J, Glickman M, Higginson IJ, on behalf of the GUIDE Care project. Changing Patterns in Place of Cancer Death in England: A Population-Based Study. PLOS Medicine. 2013;10(3):e1001410.

12. Department of Health. A Policy Framework for Commissioning Cancer Services. A Report by the Expert Advisory Group on Cancer to the Chief Medical Officer of England and Wales. London: Department of Health; 1985.

13. Department of Health. Guidance on Commissioning Cancer Services Improving Outcomes in Gynaecological Cancer The Manual. Crown Copyright; 1999.

14. Department of Health. The NHS Cancer Plan: A Plan for Investment, a Plan for Reform. London: Department of Health; 2000.

15. Department of Health. NHS Next Stage Review—What It Means for the Third Sector. London: Department of Health; 2008.

16. National Institute for Clinical Excellence (NICE). Improving Supportive and Palliative Care for Adults with Cancer. London: National Institute for Clinical Excellence; 2004.

17. Department of Health. End of Life Care Strategy: Promoting High Quality for all at the End of Life. London: Department of Health; 2008.

18. Paget A, Wood C. "People's final journey must be one of their choosing...": Ways and Means. London: Demos; 2013.

19. Scottish Government. Living and Dying Well: A National Action Plan for Palliative and End-of-Life in Scotland. Edinburgh: Scottish Government; 2008.

20. Wales Palliative Care Planning Group. Report to the Minister for Health and Social Services. Cardiff: Wales Palliative Care Planning Group; 2008.

21. Department of Health, Social Services and Public Safety. Living Matters: Dying Matters: A Palliative and End of Life Care Strategy for Adults in Northern Ireland. Belfast: Author; 2010.

22. Ellershaw J, Wilkinson S. Care of the Dying: A Pathway to Excellence. Oxford, England: Oxford University Press; 2003.

23. Bookbinder M, Blank AE, Arney E, et al. Improving end-of-life care: development and pilot-test of a clinical pathway. J Pain Symptom Manage. 2005;29(6):529–543.

24. Stevinson C, Preston N, Todd C; Cancer Experiences Collaborative (CECo). Defining priorities in prognostication research: results of a consensus workshop. Palliat Med. 2010;24(5):462–468.

25. http://www.dailymail.co.uk/news/article-2225009/The-medical-professions-lethal-arrogance-Liverpool-Care-Pathway.html Accessed October 25, 2013.

26. Costantini M, Romoli V, Di Leo S, et al. Liverpool Care Pathway for patients with cancer in hospital: a cluster randomised trial. 2014;383(9913):226–237.

27. Ellershaw J, Smith C, Overill S, Walker SE, Aldridge J. Care of the dying: setting standards for symptom control in the last 48 hours of life. J Pain Symptom Manage. 2001;21:12–17.

28. Verbeek L, Van Zuylen L, Gambles M, et al. Audit of the Liverpool care of the dying patient in a Dutch cancer centre. J Palliat Care. 2006;22:305–308.

29. Verbeek L, Van Zuylen L, Swart SJ, et al. The effect of the Liverpool Care Pathway for the dying: a multi centre study. Palliat Med. 2008;22:145–151.

30. Gambles M, Stirzaker S, Jack BA, Ellershaw JE. The Liverpool Care Pathway in hospices: an exploratory study of doctor nurse perceptions. Int J Palliat Nurs. 2006;12:414–421.

31. Jack BA, Gambles M, Murphy D, Ellershaw JE. Nurses' perceptions of the Liverpool Care Pathway for the dying patient in the acute hospital setting. Int J Palliat Nurs. 2003;9:375–381.

32. Van der Heide A, Veerbeek L, Swart S, Van Der Rijt C, Van Der Maas PJ, Van Zuylen L. End-of-life decision making for cancer patients in different clinical settings and the impact of the LCP. J Pain Symptom Manage. 2010;39:33–43.

33. Parry R, Seymour J, Whittaker B, Byrd L, Cox K Rapid Evidence review: pathways focused on the dying phase in end of life care. 2013. Accessed online October 25, 2013.

34. Currow DC, Abernethy A. Lessons from the Liverpool Care Pathway—evidence is key. Lancet. 2014;383(9913):192–3.

35. Gold Standards Framework. Prognostic Indicator Guidance. www.goldstandardsframework.org.uk/cd-content/uploads/files/General%20Files/Prognostic%20Indicator%20Guidance%20October%202011.pdf. Accessed June 29, 2013.

36. www.goldstandardsframework.org.uk/accredited-gp-practices. Accessed June 29, 2013.

37. www.goldstandardsframework.org.uk/accredited-care-homes. Accessed June 29, 2013.

38. Dale J, Petrova M, Munday D, Koistinen-Harris J, Lall R, Thomas K. A national facilitation project to improve primary palliative care: impact of the Gold Standards Framework on process and self-ratings of quality. Qual Saf Health Care. 2009;18:174–180.

39. Badger F, Plumridge G, Hewison A, Shaw KL, Thomas K, Clifford C. An evaluation of the impact of the Gold Standards Framework on collaboration in end-of-life care in nursing homes: a qualitative and quantitative evaluation. Int J Nurs Stud. 2012;49(5):586–595.

40. Hall S, Goddard C, Stewart F, Higginson IJ. Implementing a quality improvement programme in palliative care in care homes: a qualitative study. BMC Geriatr. 2011;11:31. doi: 10.1186/1471-2318-11-31.

41. Hockley J, Watson J, Oxenham D, Murray SA. The integrated implementation of two end-of-life care tools in nursing care homes in the UK: an in-depth evaluation. Palliat Med. 2010;24(8):828–838.

42. Preferred Priorities for Care. Available from: http://www.endoflifecareforadults.nhs.uk/tools/core-tools/preferredprioritiesforcare. Accessed June 28, 2013.

43. Brinkman-Stoppelenberg A, Rietjens JA, van der Heide A Effects of advance care planning on end of life care: an overview. 2012. Manuscript submitted for publication.

44. Sabatino CP. The evolution of health care advance care planning law and policy. Milbank Q. 2010;88(2):211–239.

45. Stein GL, Fineberg IC. Advance care planning in the U.S. and U.K.: a comparative analysis of policy, implementation, and the social work role. Br J Soc Work. 2013. doi: 10.1093/bjsw/bct013vb

46. Samanta A, Samanta J. Advance care planning: the role of the nurse. Br J Nurs. 2010;19(6):1060–1061.

47. National End of Life Care Programme. Capacity, Care Planning and Advance Care Planning in Life Limiting Illness: A Guide for Health and Social Care Staff. National End of Life Care Programme, 2011. Available from: http://www.endoflifecareforadults.nhs.uk/publications/pubacpguide. Accessed September 7, 2012.

48. Reynolds J, Croft S. Applying the Preferred Priorities for Care document in practice. Nurs Stand. 2011;25(36):35–42.

49. Almack K, Cox K, Moghaddam N, Pollock K, Seymour J. After you: conversations between patients and healthcare professionals in planning for end of life care. BMC Palliat Care. 2012;11:15. http://www.biomedcentral.com/1472-684X/11/15.

50. Cox K, Moghaddam N, Almack K, Pollock K, Seymour J. Is it recorded in the notes?: Documentation of end-of-life care and preferred place to die discussions in the final weeks of life. BMC Palliat Care. 2011;10:18. doi: 10.1186/1472-684x-10-18. http://www.biomedcentral.com/1472-684X/10/18.

51. Clayton JM, Butow PN, Tattersall MHN. When and how to initiate discussion about prognosis and end-of-life issues with terminally ill patients. J Pain Symptom Manage. 2005;30(2):132–144.

52. Field D, Copp G. Communication and awareness about dying in the 1990s. J Palliat Med. 1999;13:459–468.

53. Wiener JS, Cole SA. Three principles to improve clinician communication for advance care planning: overcoming emotional, cognitive and skill barriers. J Palliat Med. 2004;7(6):817–829.

54. Froggatt K, Vaughan S, Bernard C, Wild D. Advance care planning in care homes for older people: an English perspective. Palliat Med. 2009;23:332–338.

55. Fineberg IC, O'Connor L. Evaluation of Preferred Place of Care (PPC): Towards Quality Improvement. Report, Lancaster University, July 2011. Available from: http://www.lancs.ac.uk/shm/research/ioelc/programmes/service-models-archive.php#ppceval. Accessed July 25, 2012.

56. Seymour J, Almack K, Kennedy S. Implementing advance care planning: a qualitative study of community nurses' views and experiences. BMC Palliat Care. 2010;9(4). http://www.biomedcentral.com/1472-684X/9/4.

57. Wood J, Storey L, Clark D. Preferred place of care: an analysis of the 'first 100' patient assessments. Palliat Med. 2007;21:449–450.

58. Preston H, Fineberg IC, Callagher P, Mitchell DJ. The preferred priorities for care document in motor neurone disease: views of bereaved relatives and carers. Palliat Med. 2012:26(2):132–138.

59. Radbruch L, Payne S; EAPC Board of Directors. White paper on standards and norms for hospice and palliative care in Europe: part 1. Eur J Palliat Care. 2009;16(6):278–289.

60. Help the Hospices: Facts and Figures available at: http://www.helpthehospices.org.uk/about-hospice-care/facts-figures/ Accessed June 28, 2013.

61. Office for National Statistics. Mortality Statistics—Deaths Registered in 2010. [unpublished provisional data to these published by the ONS in the autumn 2011]. Office for National Statistics; 2011.

62. Centeno C, Lynch T, Donea O, Rocafort J, Clark D. EAPC Atlas of Palliative Care in Europe 2013—Full Edition. Milano: EAPC (European Association for Palliative Care); 2013.

63. Stevens E, Martin CR, White CA. The outcomes of palliative care day services: a systematic review. Palliat Med. 2011;25(2):153–169.

64. Care Quality Commission. The Adult Social Care Market And The Quality of Services. London: Care Quality Commission; 2010.

65. Henry C, Wilson J. Personal care at the end of life and after death. Nurs Times. 2012;108: online issue.

66. Payne S, Ingleton C, Sargeant A, Seymour J. The role of the nurse in palliative care settings in a global context. Cancer Nurs Pract. 2009:8(5): 21–26.

67. Clark D, Seymour J, Douglas HR, et al. Clinical nurse specialists in palliative care. Part 2: Explaining diversity in the organization and costs of Macmillan nursing services. Palliat Med. 2002;16(5):375–385.

68. Corner J, Clark D, Normand C. Evaluating the work of clinical nurse specialists in palliative care. Palliat Med. 2002;16(4):275–277.

69. Department of Health. Health Service Circular 29th September 1999. HSC 1999/217: Nurse Midwife and Health Visitor Consultants: Establishing Posts and Making Appointments. London: Department of Health; 1999.

70. Department of Health. Advanced Level Nursing: A Position Statement. London: Department of Health; 2010.

71. Royal College of Nursing Advanced Nurse Practitioners. An RCN Guide to Advanced Nursing Practice, Advanced Nurse Practitioners and Programme Accreditation. London: RCN; 2012.

72. Ryan-Woolley B, McHugh G, Luker K. Prescribing by specialist nurses in cancer and palliative care: results of a national survey. Palliat Med. 2007;21(4):273–277.

73. See www.insup-c.eu/. Downloaded June 29, 2013.

74. Turner JM, Payne S, Barbarachild Z. Care or custody?: An evaluation of palliative care in prisons in North West England. Palliat Med. 2011;25(4)370–377.

CHAPTER 74

Palliative care in Europe

Marianne Jensen Hjermstad and Stein Kaasa

Key points

- The diversity in economy, culture, and health policy in today's Europe represent a challenge for the development of palliative care (PC), and does not permit the implementation of one particular PC model everywhere.

- The need for palliative care will rise because of the increasing cancer incidence and an elderly population, and accentuates the need for professional education and sufficient core competencies for delivery of high quality care at basic, intermediate, and specialist levels.

- Many cancer patients with incurable disease live much longer than before thanks to novel therapeutic agents, and often experience acute or chronic side effects which call for an early introduction of PC to provide adequate and systematic symptom management and follow-up care.

Palliative care begins from the understanding that every patient has his or her own story, relationship, and culture and is worthy of respect as an individual. This implies that palliative care should be patient oriented, guided by the needs of the patient and taking into account his or her values and preferences, and that ethical issues are considered with cultural variation in needs and values.

Both the former and most recent definition of palliative care from the World Health Organization (WHO) stated that palliative care is "an approach that improves the quality of life of patients and their families facing the problems associated with life-threatening illness, through the prevention and relief of suffering by means of early identification and impeccable assessment and treatment of pain and other problems, physical, psycho-social, and spiritual."[1,2] Recommendations on the organization of palliative care to meet these aspects were also emphasized in a document on palliative care from the Council of Europe in 2003.

Palliative care should be offered at all levels in the healthcare system and should be regarded as an integral part of all medical services; it is multidimensional and interdisciplinary. The WHO definition also emphasizes that "palliative care is applicable early in the course of illness, in conjunction with other therapies that are intended to prolong life."[2]

There has been a remarkable development of palliative care in Europe during the last decade in particular, which is a result of the systematic and continuous work from the European Association of Palliative Care (EAPC) in close collaboration with important stakeholders from a variety of healthcare disciplines.[3] The vision is to achieve professional excellence in palliative care that meets the needs of patients and caregivers. The work toward consensus-based treatment guidelines and standardized outcome measurements represent two of several steps in this direction.[4–8]

Typical components of palliative care in parts of Europe today include proactive, multidimensional and quantitative symptom-assessment, communication interventions emphasizing both preparation for the dying process and maintaining hope, alongside tumor-directed and symptomatic treatment.[9] Quite often specialist palliative care is delivered by specialized palliative care interdisciplinary teams in designated units and is therefore not available to all who may need this level of professional care.[10–13] This has led to international discussions on how to achieve a professional integration of oncology and specialist palliative care, with an ongoing EAPC project focusing on care delivery models in general oncology centers as a start.[14]

Based on the above, it is obvious that palliative care has its own special characteristics that are not entirely covered by the competence, organization, and structure as of today's mainstream healthcare system. Thus, there has been a considerable development in recognizing palliative care as a medical and nursing specialty, and palliative medicine and nursing have increasingly being acknowledged in many countries as a medical specialty beyond the basic level.[15,16] In many European countries palliative medicine is now a mandatory subject in the medical schools, as in Germany since 2013. In the Nordic countries, a 2-year specialist training program for physicians working in palliative medicine was started in 2003, and attracted huge interest.[17] The course is offered every other year, lasts 21 months, and is composed of six 1-week slots of teaching with working assignments in the intervals. All participants conduct a small research project, and many write a paper for publication, preferably for international journals. More than 150 participants had completed the course in the spring of 2013.

Cancer causes 20% of deaths in the European Region. With more than 2.4 million new cases and 1.3 million deaths each year, cancer is the most important cause of death and morbidity in Europe after cardiovascular diseases, accounting for 26% of all deaths in 2008.[18]

The cancer incidence rate is steadily increasing every year in most European countries.[19] The cancer mortality rates have shown a gradual decrease in many western European countries, and in Norway a demonstrated improved survival is seen in all the major cancers: breast, prostate, lung, and colorectal.[19] Nevertheless, the steadily aging population and improved treatment mean that more patients are living longer with metastatic disease. The most recent EUROCARE 4 analyses[20] showed slight increases in survival and decreases in geographic differences over time compared with the figures from the previous EUROCARE study for all cancer studied. This was interpreted as a result of improvements in healthcare services in countries with poor survival and taken as an indication of better cancer care.

Because palliative care goes far beyond opioid availability and pain treatment and encompasses all the key elements of the holistic nursing approach—the care needs, the suffering, and the dignity and the quality of life of patients and relatives toward the last stages of life—it seems inappropriate to draw artificial lines between disease-modifying therapy and palliative care. This becomes even more evident when we know that many cancer patients are not cured from their disease but will live much longer even when diagnosed with incurable malignancies thanks to novel therapeutic agents. This has led to remarkable changes in oncology practice,[11] and once again emphasizes the need to introduce palliative care early in the stage of disease to provide the necessary support and important elements of this care to all patients. Thus, the development and improvement of palliative care is an important, growing, and large public health issue across nations and cultures regardless of diagnoses.

The purpose of this chapter is to present some of the European experiences with respect to the development, organization, and delivery of palliative care, educational issues, and research.

The situation in Europe

Because of the increasing life expectancy and declining birth rates, the age distribution in many European nations is skewed toward a larger proportion of older people. It is well known that the overall cancer incidence rises with advanced age, and statistics show that three out of four new cancers arise in people above the age of 60 in some European countries.[19] Because this proportion is likely to increase due to an increasing cancer incidence, an aging population, and maybe also lifestyle changes, more people with cancer are expected in the near future. Predictions for causes of death in Europe over a 20-year period from 1990 to 2020 show a changing pattern (Table 74.1), with more people living with and dying from chronic diseases.[1,21]

Palliative care is often associated with cancer, but the principles and definitions of palliative care are universal for several diseases.[2] Although different diseases present with various symptoms along the illness trajectory, epidemiological studies show that many symptoms and problems in the last year of life are similar.[22] Most often this represents a challenge to the healthcare systems in the

Table 74.1 Predicted causes of death in Europe for 2020 compared with the 1990 figures

Disorder	Predicted ranking 2020	Previous ranking 1990
Ischemic heart disease	1	1
Cerebrovascular disease (including stroke)	2	2
Chronic obstructive pulmonary disease	3	6
Lower respiratory infections	4	3
Lung, trachea, and bronchial cancer	5	10

Sources: Davies and Higginson (2004), reference 1; Murray and Lopez (1997), reference 21.

delivery of effective and adequate end-of-life care to an increasing number of people. However, in many, if not most, specialized palliative care units (PCUs) more than 90% of the patients suffer from advanced cancer, [6] and early provision of professional palliative care improves quality of life and may also increase survival.[23] Reports show that such evidence from quality palliative care is not yet available for dementia.[24] This diagnosis now represents a huge health challenge with more than 35.6 million people living with this disease, a number that is expected to double by 2013.[25] To extend and promote palliative care beyond the field of oncology, EAPC has launched several initiatives focusing on palliative care to other groups, for example the elderly, patients with neurological diseases, and children,[26] and for people on the African continent.[27]

Europe has gone through great political changes in the last 20 years and particularly so during the last decade, economically and culturally. From 2004, 12 new countries have become members of the European Union (EU), counting 28 membership states by July 2013. The new states are primarily former eastern European states, with Bulgaria and Romania as new members in 2007 and Croatia as the most recent in July 2013, with another five candidates on the list. Despite an economic growth in Europe in general, there is still great diversity related to industrial, economic, cultural, and health policy aspects, as well as significant differences in population size, from 5 million in Norway to more than 83 million people in Germany and 105 million people in Russia. These diversities represent a challenge for the development of palliative care across Europe, which is shown in the recently launched EAPC Atlas of Palliative Care in Europe 2013[28] suggesting a relationship between the establishment of palliative care programs and the Human Development Index (HDI) or other indicators related to national expenditure on health. Specific initiatives have been launched that focus on the development of palliative care in eastern Europe, with respect to education and clinical training, establishing of services, and improved access to opioids.[3,28] Also, the Open Society Institute (OSI), now known as the Open Society Foundations (OSF)[29] has played a major role in the development of palliative care in eastern European countries. The OSF is a grant-making operation founded in 1993 aimed to shape public policy to promote democratic governance, human rights, and economic, legal, and social reform. Locally, OSF implements a range of initiatives to support the rule of law, education, public health, and independent media to raise the awareness of basic human rights, such as healthcare. This has resulted in an improved availability of palliative care in eastern Europe in general over the last 5 years despite the relatively poor living standards in that part of the continent, although huge differences still remain.

The continuously increasing medical and scientific collaboration across borders has led to the development of various models for palliative care. Some European centers are influenced by the Canadian model in Edmonton, Alberta,[30] the Beth Israel Medical Center program in New York City, New York,[31] or by the WHO project on palliative care implementation that influenced the development of palliative medicine throughout Spain.[32] However, directly adopting a model from another nation with a different healthcare system is not always feasible. An example of this is the integration of the departments of pain service and palliative medicine into one, as has been successfully done at Beth Israel in New York. The pain programs in Europe are most often closely linked to anesthesiology, and, as such, not only are caring for palliative care patients but also taking care of patients with postoperative pain, chronic nonmalignant pain, chronic back pain, acute pain conditions, and so forth. Although pain treatment is an essential part of palliative care, the linkage between departments in Europe is more often based on cooperation and consultation services and, to some extent, translational research. Several services in Europe have begun either from pain/anesthesiology and/or oncology teams. It seems that the most successful programs have been able to combine the skills and knowledge across specialties and disciplines. This, together with today's clear recommendation from the WHO, EAPC, and other organizations of an early introduction of palliative care in the disease trajectory, is a strong argument in the discussion of a stronger integration of oncology and specialized palliative care. This may also indicate that it is time is to merge small departments of palliative care with departments of pain management.

The EAPC Atlas[28] "gives a comprehensive overview of the development of palliative care in Europe. The work is one of the outcomes of the EAPC Task Force on the Development of Palliative Care in Europe, initiated in 2003. The aims were "to provide an updated, reliable and comprehensive analysis on the development of palliative care within each European country, in order to generate and disseminate an 'evidence base' of clear and accessible research-based information concerning the current provision of the discipline across the WHO European region."[28]

The work was based on (1) an expert survey in which 89 "key persons" from 49 countries of the WHO European region were identified to complete the quantitative Facts Questionnaire asking about factual data on palliative care provision in each country. The qualitative Eurobarometer Survey was also completed, which places the quantitative Facts data within a sociocultural context, a wider milieu of healthcare policy, and in relation to social, ethical, and cultural factors; (2) a peer-review process of the data; (3) an update of the literature review from the former Atlas from 2007; and (4) additional information from the EAPC Head Office on national activities, attendance to conferences, website hits, plus assistance from the cartography department.[28] Data from 46 of the 53 countries in the WHO European region is included in the Atlas.

This gives information about the national palliative care activities with respect to implementation of palliative programs, finances and funding, and delivery of care through PCUs/hospices/home care, as well as education, specialist training, and research. There has been a gradual growth in this medical field during the last 3 decades, with significant innovations in the last 10 years. The first national PCUs were opened in Great Britain in 1967, in Cyprus in 1974, and in Norway in 1993. Germany, France, Poland, and Finland followed before 1999. After this, Romania, the Netherlands, Belgium, Hungary, Portugal, Austria, Switzerland, Slovakia, Denmark, and Luxembourg all established their units before the change of the millennium. However, as can be seen in Figure 74.1, there are huge differences across countries with respect to the number of PC beds and PCU services per million inhabitants across countries. Ireland, Iceland, and Belgium have the highest concentration of PCUs, with almost 18–20 units per million inhabitants, with the United Kingdom, Sweden, Netherlands, Poland, and Austria in the second category with 12-16 units per million. We can find the United Kingdom, Sweden,

the Netherlands, Poland, and Austria in a second group of countries with 12–16 units per million. A total of 23 services were identified in Czech Republic, where the density of services is still low.[28] An EAPC position paper on standards and norms for hospice and palliative care in Europe claims that the original estimate of 50 palliative care beds per million inhabitants should be upgraded to 80–100 beds per million inhabitants.[33,34] It should be remembered however, that the differences displayed in the numbers presented here in part represent a real difference but are also in part due to a report bias in that there are differences in definitions of what constitutes a palliative care bed and a PCU across Europe.

To place palliative care on the health policy agenda, strategic interventions based on evidence-based knowledge and consensus among international experts in the field are mandatory to gain the necessary influence. This can be achieved through the establishment of professional organizations, such as the EAPC (www.eapc-net.eu),[3] development of pan-European research networks such as the INTERDEM (Early detection and INTervention in DEMentia)[35] and the European Palliative Care Research Centre (PRC)[36] in Trondheim, Norway, and formal collaborations between related associations and networks within clinical work and research.

The EAPC was established in 1988 with 42 members, on the initiative of Professor Ventafridda and the Floriani Foundation in Italy. The aim of the EAPC is to promote palliative care in Europe at the scientific, clinical, and social levels. In 1998, the EAPC was awarded the status of nongovernmental organization (NGO) of the Council of Europe and was transformed to "Onlus" (nonprofit organization with social utility). By 2013, the EAPC had individual members from 47 nations across the world, and collective members from 54 national associations in 32 European countries (Figure 74.2), representing not only professionals but also volunteers contributing to palliative care.[3]

The activities of the EAPC have grown exponentially since its foundation 25 years ago, in order to develop and promote palliative care in Europe through information, education, and research using multiprofessional collaboration, while engaging with stakeholders at all levels. The work is mainly focused on six areas: policy, organization, education, ethics, clinical and care, and research, supplemented by a special section on specific target groups (children, people with intellectual disabilities, neurological diseases, family carers, etc.).[3]

The activities generally involve either task forces—time-limited international working groups often involving leading experts in the field and focusing on specific objectives—or white papers, which are specific remits that are agreed to by the board. A variety of task forces have been established (Figure 74.3), primarily within the areas of policy, education, and clinical and care and for the specific target groups.[3] Results from this work have been disseminated as several important position papers or statements, clinical guidelines, recommendations on educational curricula or consensus, and are regarded as important for informing policy, practice and education in Europe and beyond.

The EAPC first participated in two Expressions of Interest presented to the European community for the sixth and seventh Framework Research Programs within the EU. As a result of this work, research programs related to palliative care and advanced cancer have been brought to the forefront of the agenda for advanced research and have led to the initiation of several subsequent palliative care projects that have also received funding

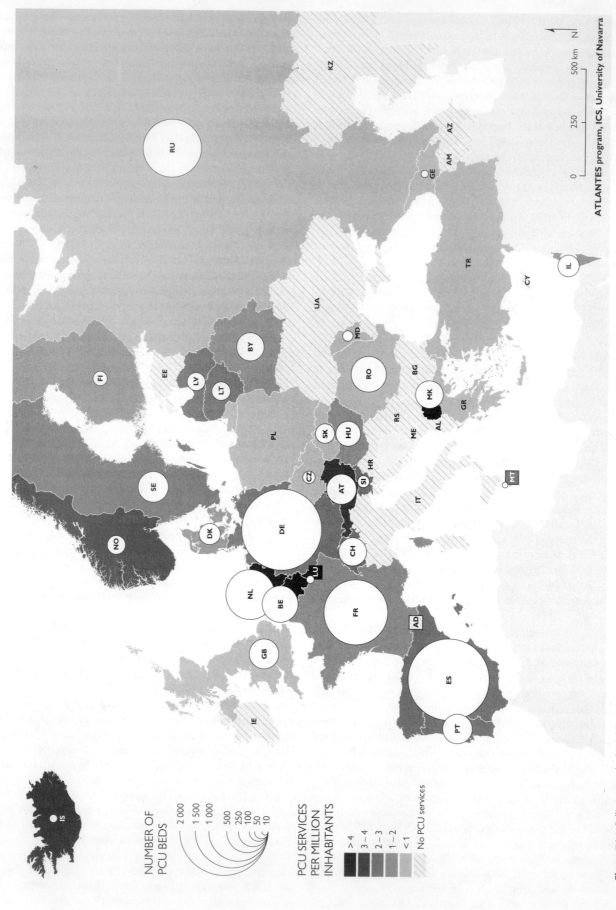

Figure 74.1 Palliative care beds and units. Source: Adapted with permission, EAPC Atlas of Palliative Care in Europe 2013, reference 28.

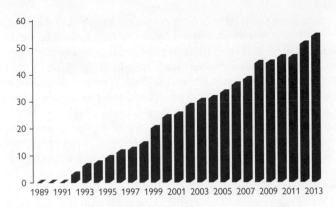

Figure 74.2 Development of collective member associations in the EAPC, 1989 to 2013.

from the Framework Research Programs of the EU.[37] This has improved the scientific level in palliative care research, has substantially increased the European collaboration in the field, and has also led to more multidisciplinary research.

The European Palliative Care Research Collaborative (EPCRC; 2006–2010)[38] was the first major palliative care project within the Framework Programs of the EU.[39] The project engaged 60 coworkers at 11 centers in 6 European countries and collaborators from Canada and Australia. The EPCRC had close links to the EAPC and the EAPC Research Network (EAPC RN). Workshops run by the EPCRC were arranged at all EAPC congresses, 2007–2010.[38]

The EPCRC addressed three main areas in three main symptoms: genetics, assessment and classification, and guidelines in pain, depression, and cachexia. The major objectives were to develop novel genetic methods for the prediction of opioid responses and individual variation in cachexia, in addition to developing consensus and evidence-based methodology for assessment and classification of pain, cachexia, and depression. Examples of important results from the work of the EPCRC include the update and publication of European evidence-based guidelines for opioid analgesics for cancer pain in close collaboration with the EAPC RN.[3] Also, a new, European Clinical Guideline[5] on the Management of Depression in Palliative Care was developed under the EPCRC umbrella.[38] The guideline development is based on a comprehensive process involving expert and public consultations and literature reviews, also including a Cochrane review[40] for the depression guidelines on the use of antidepressants for depression in physically ill people.

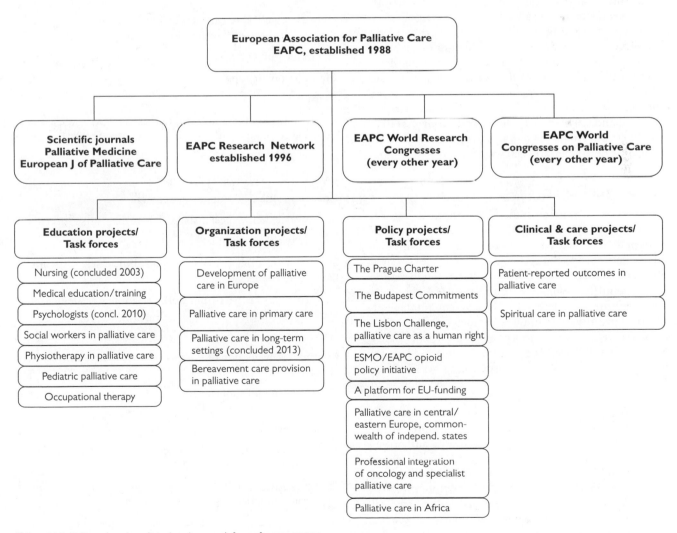

Figure 74.3 Policy, education, clinical, and care task forces for core groups.

The EPCRC cachexia work team has produced new European, clinical guidelines on the management of cancer cachexia in advanced cancer patients, with a focus on refractory cachexia.[38] This has been a comprehensive process involving expert and public consultations and literature reviews. For all of these guidelines, patient-friendly summaries (leaflets) in five European languages can be downloaded from the EPCRC website.[38]

The European Commission's Executive Agency for the Public Health Program (PHEA) received funding for the development of mechanisms for reporting and analysis of health issues and producing public health reports, focusing on best practices and models in palliative care—that is, the provision of specialist versus basic palliative care as dependent and integrated approaches.[3] Subsequent to the funding of the EPCRC project, two other initiatives, the PRISMA[41] (reflecting the positive diversities of European priorities for research and measurement in end-of-life care) and a European collaboration to optimize research for the care of cancer patients in the last days of life (OPCARE9)[42] were also recently funded by the European Union.[37] More recently the ATOME project (Access to Opioid Medication in Europe),[43] the IMPACT[44] and the EUROIMPACT[45] projects received funding from the seventh Framework Program for Research of the European Union,[39] focusing on opioid availability, improving dementia and cancer palliative care, and developing a multidisciplinary and intersectorial educational research framework in Europe aimed at monitoring and improving palliative care respectively. Another newly financed project, the Integrated Palliative Care—InSup-c[46] focuses on the best way to deliver care to people who have advanced cancer, heart failure, or lung disease toward the end of life.

An ultimate goal is to ensure that palliative care research is represented at national and international palliative care congresses. For Europe as a whole, the promotion and financing of palliative care research within the EU framework represents a major step forward.

Criteria for excellence

At present, there is no uniform European consensus regarding the minimum set of indicators that constitutes a center of excellence in palliative care. Although this is a universal problem that also exists outside Europe, a major challenge is related to the agreement on a definition of these criteria. Furthermore, the conceptual definitions of home care and hospice differ across countries and cultures. The latter has negative connotations in southern European cultures,[16] and it is obvious that the definition of hospice care meets with much less consensus than the definition of palliative care. There seem to be fundamental differences in the understanding of hospice care, which probably reflect the different ways that hospices are used in western Europe.[33]

The national models for delivery of palliative care are not identical, and they are not equally prioritized in each country, either economically or politically. In Norway, the health authorities launched a national palliative care program with clinical guidelines in 2008, which was recently updated (2012).[47] Also, the Norwegian Directorate of Health has started a development project of formalizing palliative medicine as an accredited medical specialty. The intention is to stimulate recruitment and secure a more universal national palliative care service.

Because of the relatively large economic, political, and cultural diversities across Europe, it might not be feasible to aim for the implementation of one particular model of excellence everywhere. In 2003, the European Society for Medical Oncology (ESMO) initiated an accreditation program, the ESMO Designated Centres of Integrated Oncology and Palliative Care, in which cancer centers can receive special recognition for achieving a high standard of integration of medical oncology and palliative care.[48] This means that the centers must provide comprehensive services in supportive and palliative care as part of their routine care, but other criteria also apply, such as expert medical and nursing care in the evaluation and relief of pain and other physical symptoms, continuity of care, expert care in relief of psychological and existential distress, emergency care of inadequately relieved symptoms, clinical education, and participation in basic or clinical research.[48] Although many centers do not fulfill all of these criteria due to various reasons, there are nevertheless certain key criteria that can be used in all models of palliative care to ensure the sufficient comprehensive provision and quality of care. These criteria include the following:

Delivery and Content of Care

- Inpatient professional palliative care services in PCUs or hospices
- Outpatient palliative care services or home care, organized by the PCU or through the established healthcare services
- Size of the unit and patient case mix
- Multidisciplinary approach
- Consultation services
- A systematic approach to symptom assessment and classification, and common indicators for the quality of care

Education and Advanced Training

- Basic levels, medical/nursing schools
- Continuing medical/nursing education
- Palliative medicine specialists, palliative care nurse specialists
- University chairs of palliative medicine
- Systematic training of clinicians and clinical scientists in palliative care research
- Opportunities for part-time work assignments, 50/50 clinical work and research

Research

- Continuous evaluation of the quality of palliative care services (structure, process, delivery)
- Consensus of indicators for the classification and assessment of subjective patient-reported outcomes
- Evidence-based knowledge to provide guidelines for treatment
- National and international multicenter studies, and the development of formal research collaboratives
- Translational research to close the gap between basic sciences and clinical practice
- National and international networking, such as the EAPC RN and other formal structures

Integration of Palliative Medicine and Care in Public Healthcare

◆ Policy, advocacy, lobbying

◆ Earmarked funding to palliative care research on a national level, possibly similar to the British or Canadian models, preferably with incentives for national and international collaboration

At the University Hospital in Trondheim, Norway, a fully integrated model has been developed during the last decade (Figure 74.4). The program started with the development of a 12-bed inpatient unit (acute palliative care) and an outpatient program, including a consultation service at the various wards and departments at the University Hospital. The staff composition is interdisciplinary with highly trained nurses and doctors. A close collaboration with the municipality of Trondheim has been organized as an integrated part of the palliative care program. This has resulted in establishment of designated PCUs or beds in several nursing homes, combined with specialist palliative care service in patients' homes in collaboration with the general practitioners (GPs) and home-care nursing services in the community. The outpatient clinics, both for cancer patients and for chronic nonmalignant pain, and the palliative medicine unit have succeeded in joining forces regarding their clinical, educational, and research-related activities.

The European Association of Palliative Care activities: an example of international networking

European Association of Palliative Care initiatives

The EAPC serves as a catalyst for international collaboration and networking with respect to distribution and delivery of care, clinical collaborative work, and research. As previously mentioned, there is a steadily growing number of activities, task forces (Figure 74.3), and individual and collective members (Figure 74.2).

An important priority of the EAPC during the last decade has been the development of high-quality palliative care in Eastern Europe. The EAPC coordination center at Stockholm's Sjukhem Foundation in Stockholm, Sweden, was established in 2002,[49] supported by the Open Society Institute.[29] The major aims of the EAPC East project, which was established as a task force in 2001, were to support and improve the development of palliative care and to coordinate the activities and initiatives in eastern Europe. In most of these countries, the care is unevenly distributed and poorly developed, and drugs such as opioids are not readily accessible everywhere.[50,51] For example, a recent report covering 21 eastern European and 20 western European countries shows that many patients do not receive adequate relief of pain because of excessive regulatory restrictions on the availability and accessibility of opioids,[52] previously demonstrated by huge variation of access to medication depending on geographical area in Albania[53] and a lack of certain formulas in Romania.[54] Some national laws and regulations prohibit the prescription of opioids for use outside of the hospitals[55] and only allow treatment for a limited period.[50–52,56] Through international networks and collaboration with people and organizations interested in and working with palliative care in eastern Europe, palliative care is put on the health policy agenda, a prerequisite for funding and change of practice. The first peak in this work was in the fall of 2004. Media campaigns, seminars, and discussions occurred in order to disseminate the recommendations from the Council of Europe documents, that "legislation should make opioids and other drugs accessible in a range of formulations and dosages for medical use," as well as the recommendations from EAPC and national organizations.

Unlike the United States, the EU is not a federation, but an assembly of countries ("member states") that remain independent sovereign nations. However, some of their decision-making power is delegated to shared institutions they have created, so that decisions on specific matters of joint interest can be made democratically at European level, for example, the European Council.[57] This makes consensus-based policy statements and collaborative efforts from

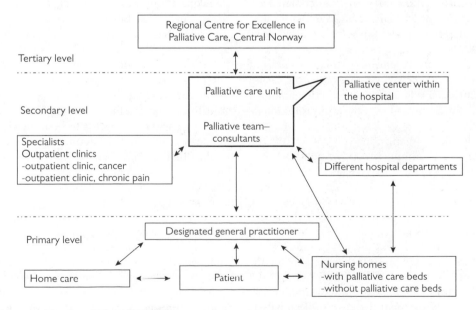

Figure 74.4 The Trondheim organizational model for palliative care.

professional organizations important assets in order to influence the policymaking. One example is the Budapest Commitments,[58] an initiative launched in 2007 in which the EAPC joined forces with the International Association for Hospice and Palliative Care (IAHPC)[59] and the Worldwide Palliative Care Alliance (WPCA)[60] to initiate a framework for palliative care development. The goal was to use a framework to help individuals and national palliative care organizations to identify and establish development goals in five major areas—drug availability, policy, education, quality, and research—by choosing commitments from a list of proposals or drafting their own among these five areas.[61]

More recently, another initiative was launched in collaboration with the IAHPC[59] and the Human Rights Watch (HRW)[62]: the Lisbon challenge,[63] emphasizing the access to adequate palliative care as a human right. The four main objectives challenge the national governments to check how well they perform in relation to (1) ensuring access to essential medicines, including opioid medications, to all who need them; (2) developing health policies that address the needs of patients with life-limiting or terminal illnesses; (3) ensuring that healthcare workers receive adequate training on palliative care and pain management at undergraduate levels; and (4) ensuring, through the development of structures and processes, the implementation of palliative care. Partner support is provided from leading international organizations, such as the Council of Europe, the World Health Association, the World Medical Association, and the International Council of Nurses, an important strategy for promoting palliative care throughout countries and regions in Europe.

The Prague Charter (palliative care as a human right)[64] represents a step related to the Lisbon challenge. This declaration urges governments to relieve suffering and recognize palliative care as a human right, with the intention of improving access to palliative care worldwide. The petition can be signed directly on the Internet,[65] thereby supporting the initiative.

Today, information is disseminated through a variety of channels. The official EAPC website, www.eapcnet.eu,[3] is an important communication tool for members and nonmembers, providing continuously updated information on activities, conferences, publications, and reports. Also, social media like Twitter and Facebook are gaining increasing importance in spreading news and promoting engagement palliative care worldwide. The two journals of the EAPC, the *European Journal of Palliative Care* and the peer-reviewed *Palliative Medicine*, with a steadily increasing impact factor (2.6 in 2012), have gained wide attention among a variety of researchers, clinicians, and other health professionals working in palliative care.

The EAPC RN is a daughter organization of the EAPC.[66] The EAPC RN was founded in 1996, aiming to conduct pan-European prospective studies, based on the fact that collaborative research is a key issue for palliative care. A cross-sectional survey of palliative care in Europe was organized by the EAPC RN, covering 143 centers in 21 countries.[67] An important result from this study, besides the clinical data, was the great potential for establishing palliative care research networks across different countries and cultures. The first two large research projects that were initiated—the European Pharmacogenetic study (EPOS)[68] and PAT-C,[69] the precursor of the EPCRC project[38]—were also important in order to consolidate the fruitful environment within European palliative care research.

The EAPC RN has organized several expert working groups on topical issues in palliative care for which common European positions or recommendations are needed, for example, symptom assessment and management,[69-78] prognostication,[79] consensus-based guidelines,[4-5] and so forth.

The EAPC RN extends an open invitation to all healthcare professionals to take part in developing a platform for this palliative care research within the EAPC RN. The network offers an established structure for collaborative research as well as an infrastructure for taking care of data handling, organization of studies, and so forth.[66]

Recently, the Junior International Forum (JIF)[80,81] was established adjacent to the EAPC RN, with the intention of fostering international collaboration and providing a meeting place for PhD and postdoctoral students and other young scientists in the field of palliative care. The first meeting was held during the fifth EAPC Research Forum in Norway, 2008.

Two major activities by the EAPC are the EAPC Forum on Research in Palliative Care and the EAPC congresses. These are each held every other year and hosted by different European countries. The 7th Research Forum was organized in Trondheim, Norway, in 2012. There were 1172 participants from 49 countries compared with 342 participants representing 35 nations in the first Forum in Berlin in 2000. The last EAPC congress in Prague, Czech Republic, in 2013 attracted 2295 participants from 87 countries, and the 1092 submitted abstracts represented 72 different countries, showing a steady increase of participating nations.

European Association of Palliative Care projects, taskforces, and white papers

As previously mentioned, and depicted in Figure 74.3, the EAPC has initiated several task forces, which have a limited time scope and are constituted with specific missions. Some of these also function as expert groups or advising bodies to the EAPC board of directors. The EAPC task force on palliative care and euthanasia is one example and represents the official EAPC position on these issues.[82] The European perspective includes quite different laws on euthanasia and patient assisted suicide, and most states uphold a ban. The major aim of this task force was to revise the EAPC's statement and judgment of palliative care and euthanasia. The work was started in 2001 and ended in 2005, created much debate, and resulted in a position paper published in 2009[77] and guidelines in several European languages.

More people are expected to be in need of palliative care; for example, in high-income countries, 69%–82% of those who die need palliative care.[83] This means that in the years to come, provision of adequate palliative care will increasingly be provided also outside the hospital settings and to a larger extent in primary care. This represents a major challenge in relation to education and training. Although some aspects of education and training are discipline specific, there are clearly elements of palliative care training and core competencies for practice that are relevant to all professional groups involved in palliative care. The recent EAPC white paper on core competencies presents expert opinion on global core competencies for professional practice, irrespective of discipline, and is intended as a resource for practitioners and educators alike.[84,85]

One of the reasons for the increased demand for palliative care is the changing practice represented by an extension of palliative care to more noncancer conditions.[83] Dementia is one of these conditions, and the EAPC white paper on palliative care in dementia[6] provides a model of dementia progression, suggests prioritizing of care goals, and defines optimal palliative care grouped in domains with a total of 57 recommendations for practice, policy, and research.

Patient-reported outcome measurement plays an increasingly important role in palliative care, being used to assess patients, evaluate the effectiveness of interventions, or audit existing services.[1] Several instruments exist for a variety of outcome measures in palliative care. In order to improve outcome measurement in palliative care, a taskforce on patient-reported outcome measurements in palliative care was initiated in 2011.[86]

Delivery of palliative care models

As pointed out earlier in this chapter, the organization and delivery of palliative care services in Europe is diverse and unevenly distributed. A German survey from the beginning of the decade, for example, showed not only that the quality and availability of palliative care beds had developed rapidly but also that only a minority of the units surveyed had a ratio of nursing staff to inpatient beds of 1.4:1 or more, as recommended by the German Association for Palliative Medicine.[87] A Spanish survey conducted about the same time from region of Catalonia, showed that this region had about 46% of the nation's palliative care programs but only 15% of the entire Spanish population.[88] Since then, a positive development has taken place, as shown in Figure 74.1 and depicted in the EAPC Atlas of Palliative Care,[28] although there are still differences across and within countries.

Palliative care is delivered through various channels, and the degree to which it is integrated, coexisting, or separated from the formal healthcare system varies considerably. In many countries, health professionals, as well as volunteers and private, charitable, and religious organizations, in primary care and through general hospitals, carry out much palliative care. In Spain, for example, private organizations are providing home-based palliative care to a substantial number of people, and care is likewise provided through volunteers in countries such as Hungary, Italy, and France. However, there is little tradition for volunteer work as a separate workforce in the Nordic countries. With the increasing knowledge and recognition of the complexity in the symptomatology of incurable diseases, a common model of providing care in Europe has been to concentrate expertise in multiprofessional teams. These teams work in hospitals, inpatient units, hospices, or in the community in direct patient care or acting as consultants. To fully integrate palliative care into the general healthcare system, political guidelines from the healthcare authorities are necessary. In 2001, the Italian National Health Service passed a law saying that palliative care programs should be provided free to patients and families. This built on a previous law on hospice development that was followed by a budget allocation to the regional administrations. Several other European countries, for example, the United Kingdom, France, Norway, and Spain, also have health policy directives on palliative care implementations and delivery of services.

An all-inclusive and comprehensive overview of all European centers is difficult to present. Because the statistical and reporting guidelines vary so much within each country, it is difficult to obtain sufficient documentation for valid comparisons across countries. Also, the basis for making statistical predictions for care needs varies,[83] as does the availability of updated uniform and nationwide registries on diagnoses, services, and care delivery. In addition, the field is rapidly developing, which may be taken as a quality criterion in itself! The EAPC Atlas of Palliative Care,[28] however, presents a very good overview of the palliative care services on a country-by-country basis, with several maps quantifying, for example, types of PCUs across the European continent (Figure 74.5) and the distribution and existence of home care teams (Figure 74.6).

Nevertheless, the individual centers within or across nations may adhere to the previously mentioned criteria of excellence in varying degrees. Table 74.2 presents the activities of 18 centers in Europe according to the previously mentioned criteria, based on an e-mail survey conducted by one of the authors of this chapter.

Delivery and content of care

Comprehensive care

Most studies on delivery of care uncover the importance that patients and families place on receiving a well-organized package of care.[86] Quite often these professional teams take care of the most advanced patients with complex symptomatology and rapidly changing needs. Despite this, there is evidence that such specialized teams are effective in relieving distressing symptoms and can improve the quality of life of the patients and families toward the end of life.[89,90] Research studies concerning patient preferences in relation to end-of-life care show that the majority of respondents (43%–84%) would prefer to die at home.[91–93] However, preferences may change as the disease progresses.[92] Scandinavian trials on different ways of coordinating palliative care services across the different settings of hospital, home, and community have found that a higher proportion of people can be helped to remain and to die at home as they wish to, and to spend less time in nursing homes.[94]

Palliative care models encompass the provision of comprehensive care, and most centers presented in Table 74.2 also have outpatient/daycare facilities and home care services. However, there is no universal way of delivering palliative care, because the national health services are organized and reimbursed for this work in different ways. In many PCUs, the hospital palliative care teams provide direct patient care after discharge (see Table 74.2). In certain parts of Spain, private organizations have a car service to take palliative experts from the hospital to the patients' homes. In Norway, there was no tradition for physicians to leave the hospital to take care of the patients at home. The financial system was prohibitive of such activities, with no reimbursement for extramural activities. Through intense and evidence-based lobbying, however, local politicians were convinced that the hospitals, not the individual physicians, should be reimbursed for this work. Thus, the Trondheim model was implemented in one region, enabling more people to stay in their homes.[94] In the Netherlands, on the other hand, the home care services are generally well functioning, and the hospital palliative care teams basically serve as a facilitator and consultant to ease the transition between the PCU and the home. A Dutch evaluation showed that the team served the needs of the professional caregivers in a variety of settings and

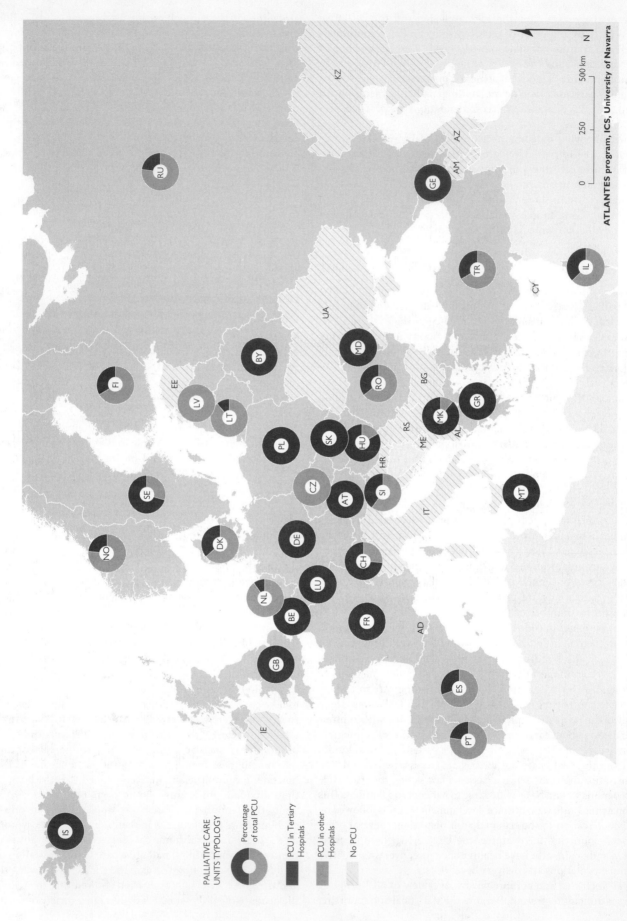

**PALLIATIVE CARE
UNITS TYPOLOGY**

Percentage
of total PCU

PCU in Tertiary
Hospitals

PCU in other
Hospitals

No PCU

ATLANTES program, ICS, University of Navarra

N

500 km

250

0

Figure 74.5 Types of palliative care units. Source: Adapted with permission, EAPC Atlas of Palliative Care in Europe 2013, reference 28.

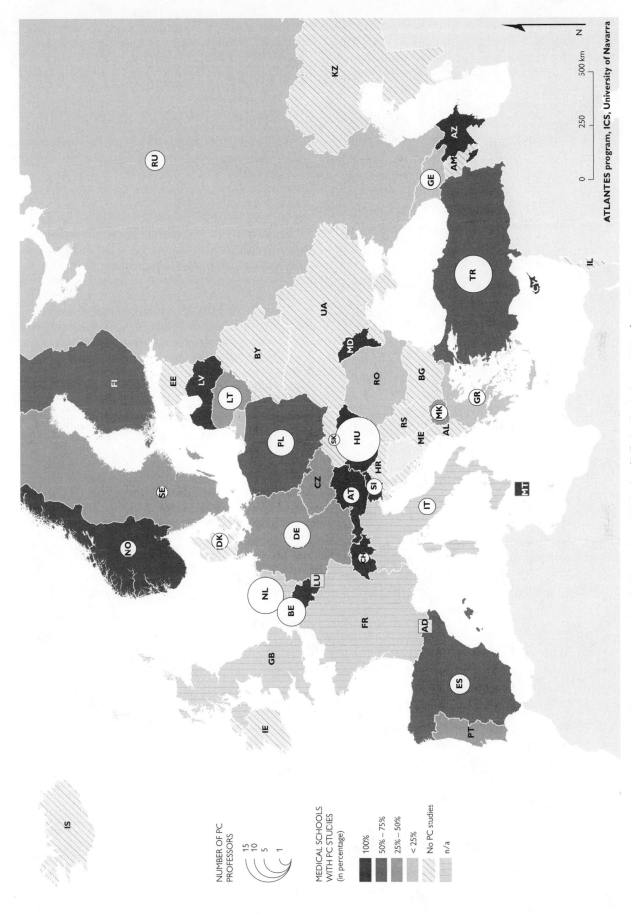

NUMBER OF PC PROFESSORS

- 15
- 10
- 5
- 1

MEDICAL SCHOOLS WITH PC STUDIES
(in percentage)

- 100%
- 50% – 75%
- 25% – 50%
- < 25%
- No PC studies
- n/a

ATLANTES program, ICS, University of Navarra

Figure 74.6 Professors and curricula in palliative care. Source: Adapted with permission, EAPC Atlas of Palliative Care in Europe 2013, reference 28.

Table 74.2 Description of some European palliative care (PC) centers in relation to certain quality criteria

Country	Name	Palliative care unit (PCU), size, team composition[a]	Outpatient unit	Home care[b]	Patients	Education/training consultation services	Research	Specific activities
Denmark, Copenhagen	Department of Palliative Medicine Bispebjerg Hospital	Acute PCU, 12 beds. Multidisciplinary team: doctors, nurses, social worker, physical and occupational therapists, psychologists, chaplains	Yes	Yes	All cancer patients	Collaborating with the medical and nursing schools and the university. Postgraduate/specialist training for nurses and doctors. Consultants in other units and home care	Clinical intervention research and psychosocial research. Multidisciplinary, PhD students	Continuous quality monitoring. In charge of establishing a national palliative care quality and research database
Germany, Bonn	Hospital of Bonn and Centre of Palliative Medicine, Malteser Hospital Bonn/ Rhein-Sieg	Acute PCU, 8 beds (in Malteser hospital). Multidisci-plinary team: doctors, nurses, psychologist, physical therapist, social worker, chaplain from hospital	Yes, integrated in Centre of Integrated Oncology (CIO)	Specialist home care team with doctors and nurses (in Malteser hospital)	95% cancer patients	Collaborating with the medical and nursing schools and universities. Undergraduate education with lectures and seminars, (20 hours are mandatory), post-graduate 40 hours course, advanced PC course. Involved in development of PC curriculum in Germany. Consultation services for other units and home care, other professionals. Undergraduate education with lectures and seminars, (28 hours are mandatory), post-graduate 40 hours course, advanced PC course. Leadership and train-the-trainer courses	Clinical drug trials, epidemiological studies, qualitative research, case reports, research on outcome and quality assurance and on guideline development. Research on pain assessment. Multidisciplinary	Active in political activities to advance PC, through, for example, media to inform patients, relatives, and medical staff
Germany, Munich,	Department of Palliative Medicine, Munich University Hospital	Acute PCU, 10 beds, multiprofessional team: doctors (oncologists, neurologists, anesthesiologists), nurses, social worker, chaplain, psychologist, physiotherapist, breathing therapist	No, but planned	Yes (specialist palliative home care team)	80% cancer, 20% noncancer (predominantly MND, Parkinson's, multisystem atrophy	Undergraduate training with lectures and mainly small group seminars (15 students) Postgraduate education center with palliative care courses on different levels for doctors, nurses, pharmacists, social workers, etc.	Research on breathlessness, outcome measurement and complexity, neurological disease, spirituality, pharmacy consultation	National guideline development; palliative care pharmacy consult service; involvement in national and international policy development

Hungary, Budapest	Budapest Hospice House	Acute PCU (Sept. 2004), 10 beds. Multidisciplinary team: doctors, nurses, physical therapist, social worker, psychologist, psychiatrist, bereavement counselor	Yes, pain clinic and psychooncology and bereavement services	Yes	Primarily cancer patients	Continuous PC training of staff, and several courses for other professionals and the public. Accredited 1-week training for nurses. Organizing international courses with other former Eastern European states	New psychooncology research program (2008), focusing on anxiety/depression and distress, first Hungarian protocol on these issues	
Italy, Milan	Cure Palliative, Terapia del dolore e Riabilitazione. Fondazione IRCCS Istituto Nazionale dei Tumori	Hospice (10 beds), PC day-hospital (4 beds). Multidisciplinary team: doctors, nurses, social worker, physical therapists, volunteers	Yes	Yes	All cancer patients	Collaborating with postgraduate education for doctors (master's courses, specialty schools). Pain and PC consulting service for other units	Assessment and treatment strategies for difficult cancer pain: neuropathic, chronic iatrogenic, breakthrough, bone pain, management of end-of-life care. Multidisciplinary, PhD students	EAPC coordinating office located here
Netherlands, Amsterdam	VUmc	Acute PCU (Sept. 2004), 4 beds in close collaboration with hospice, 10 beds for terminally ill. Multidisciplinary	Yes. Multidisciplinary Anesthesiology/pain clinic and palliative oncology clinic	PC team serves as consultants in close collaboration with home care	90% cancer patients	Consultation services and regional courses for professionals	Government-funded research program in PC, public health and extramural medicine, symptom management. PhD students	Partner in Network Palliative Care Amsterdam. Organized a regional Helpdesk with PC help team for professionals
Netherlands, Groningen	UMC Groningen	Acute PCU, 2 beds in Dept. of Internal Medicine. Multidisciplinary team: physicians (medical oncologist, pulmonary oncologist, anesthesiologist, psychiatrist, gastroenterologist, internal medicine), nurse specialists, social worker, home care technology expert, dietitians, chaplain	Yes, integrated in pain clinic and in the department of oncology.	Yes	Majority cancer patients	Collaborating with the medical and nursing schools and the university. Postgraduate/specialist training for nurses and physicians. Consultants in other units and home care.	Symptom management, transition of care. Multidisciplinary, PhD students.	Partner in Network Palliative Care Groningen Central. Participant in a regional Helpdesk with PC help team for professionals.

(Continued)

Country	Name	Palliative care unit (PCU), size, team composition[a]	Outpatient unit	Home care[b]	Patients	Education/training consultation services	Research	Specific activities
Netherlands, Maastricht	MUMC+	Acute PCU, two beds in the Oncology unit. Multidisciplinary team: doctors, nurses, social worker, chaplain	Yes,	PC team serves as consultants in close collaboration with home care	85% Cancer patients, 15% noncancer patients	Continuous PC education/training for oncologists, nurses and general practitioners. Participation in postgraduate courses for physicians, oncology nurses, others.	Clinical and translational research in neuropathic pain and dyspnea	Partner in Network Palliative Care Limburg. "The Palliative Care Formulary"
Netherlands, Nijmegen	UMC St Radboud	PCU in Dept. of Oncology, 5 beds. Multidisciplinary team: doctors, nurses, supported by specialist nurses, psychologist	Yes. Multidisciplinary through the PC team	PC team serves as consultants in close collaboration with home care	Majority cancer patients	Continuous PC education/courses for staff. Consultation services for other units and home care, other professionals	Symptom management, improvement of PC, ethics. Multidisciplinary, PhD students	
Netherlands, Rotterdam	Erasmus MC	Acute PCU, 13 beds. Multidisciplinary team: doctors (medical oncologist, neurooncologist, anesthesiologist, psychiatrist), nurse-specialists, social worker, home care technology expert, dieticians, chaplain	No	Program for home care technology in close collaboration with home care institutes	All cancer patients	Continuous PC education/training for oncologists, nurses and general practitioners. Participation in postgraduate courses for physicians, oncology nurses, others. Specific focus on development and implementation of intervention programs	Clinical and epidemiological research: symptom prevalence, development of clinical interventions, end-of-life care and end-of-life decision-making, organizational aspects of PC. Multidisciplinary, PhD students	Partner in Network Palliative Care Rotterdam. A multidisciplinary regional PC team is coordinated for phone consultations
Netherlands, Leiden	Leiden University Medical Centre	Multidisciplinary team: doctors (internal medicine/radiation oncology/anesthesiology and GP/geriatric specialist), nurses and nurse specialists, social worker, chaplains. Close collaboration with hospice	Yes	No	90% cancer, 10% noncancer	Continuous PC education/courses for staff, oncologists, nurses, and general practitioners. Consultation services for other units and home care, other professionals. Specialist training for residents and nurses	Clinical research: symptom prevalence, development of clinical interventions. Initiation of randomized radiotherapy trials on pain management. Multidisciplinary, PhD students	Active partner in meetings of several national palliative care developments

Norway, Oslo	Avdeling lindrende behandling	Acute PCU, 12 beds, outpatient clinic, ambulant team within the hospital and the local catchment area. Multidisciplinary team: doctors, nurses, social worker, physical therapists, chaplain, dieticians, psychologist	Yes	No	99% cancer patients	Continuous PC education and training for medical students, physicians and nurses in collaboration with the University. Consultants in other units	Link to the University through the Regional Center for Excellence in Palliative Medicine, which holds a chair in palliative medicine. PhD/master's students
Norway, Trondheim	Seksjon lindrende behandling (SLB)	Acute PCU, 16 beds + up to 16 in a designated nursing home. Multidisciplinary team: doctors, nurses, social workers, physical therapists, dieticians, chaplains	Yes	Yes, as a project from 2013	95% cancer patients	Continuous PC education and training for medical students, physicians, and nurses in collaboration with the University. Regular internal education, courses and training on basic/specialist levels. Consultants in other units, home care and the nursing homes	Close link to the University, chair in palliative medicine. Specific research seminars, high degree of translational research, substantial number of scientific publications on PC every year. Multidisciplinary, several postdoc/phD and master's students
Scotland, Edinburgh	Edinburgh Cancer Centre. Edinburgh Cancer Research Centre	No PCU, but access to oncology beds. Multidisciplinary team of consultants, nurses, social worker, with access to physiotherapy, occupational therapy, and chaplaincy	Yes. General, research and complex pain clinics	No. Provided by local hospices	90% cancer and 10% nonmalignant patients	Formal program of education for palliative medicine. Postgraduate MSc in Palliative Care	University Chair of Palliative Medicine. Coordinator of National Research Program, including multicenter RCTs. Several MD and PhD students. Local links with oncology and hospices. National links through NCRI. EU links through EAPC.
Spain, Barcelona	Institut Català d'Oncologia	Acute PCU, 16 beds. Multidisciplinary team: doctors, nurses, social workers, psychologist, psychiatrist, physical therapist, nutritionist	Yes. Difficult cancer pain clinic Collaborative Multiple Myeloma Clinic Collaborative Radiation Oncology Clinic	Yes	All cancer patients	University hospital support team to serve other units. Individually based continuous education and training for staff. Master in PC located on site, doctors/nurses. Pre- and postgraduate training for physicians and nurses in collaboration with the university	Active research department, center-based and multicenter studies. Multidisciplinary research. Two university chairs. Master in PC, and several PhD students. CATPAL (Catalan multicenter cooperative group), 1998, design of studies and trials Grupo de Cuidados Paliativos en el seno de la Red Temática de Investigación Cooperativa en Cáncer (RTICC) OMS Collaborative Centre

(Continued)

Country	Name	Palliative care unit (PCU), size, team composition[a]	Outpatient unit	Home care[b]	Patients	Education/training consultation services	Research	Specific activities
Sweden, Stockholm	Palliativt Sentrum, Stockholms Sjukhem (SSH)	Acute PCU, 36 beds (20 + 16). Multidisciplinary team: specialist doctors in oncology, geriatrics, pain, neurology, internal medicine, hematology nurses, social workers, physical therapists, occupational therapists, chaplains	No	Yes	90% cancer patients	Continuous PC education and training for medical students, physicians, and nurses in collaboration with the Karolinska Intitutet, University Hospital. Several medical training positions. Educational unit. Continuous education and courses for team members at the unit and other healthcare professionals. Consultation services for other units and acute hospitals	Collaborating with the University, chair in palliative medicine and nursing. Specific research seminars. Substantial no. of scientific publications on PC every year. Multidisciplinary research, several PhD students. Translational research and development projects. International collaboration. A Web-based multicenter research network including the research tool PANIS. Starting clinical drug trials. Research based on the national quality registry in palliative care	The Swedish Palliative Network (SPN), a Web-based information service developed and based here Executive office for the Swedish National Swedish National Council for Palliative Care, NRPV
UK Lancaster,	St Johns Hospice and Lancaster University	Hospital and community teams, full multidisciplinary membership	Yes	Yes	Majority cancer patients (85%), but increasing number of other diagnoses	Regular undergraduate teaching and postgraduate training for specialist doctors, regional teaching program for clinical nurse specialists and general practitioners	Clinical studies on pain, end-of-life care decisions. Lead unit for regional network of research active hospices	
UK, Leeds	Academic Unit of Palliative Care, University of Leeds	Hospital and community teams, full multidisciplinary membership	Yes	Yes	Majority cancer patients (85%), but increasing number of other diagnoses	Regular undergraduate teaching and postgraduate training for specialist doctors, regional teaching program for clinical nurse specialists and general practitioners	Clinical studies on pain, end-of-life care decisions. Lead unit for regional network of research active hospices	

that most consultations concerned physical and pharmacological problems.[95]

Some of the PCUs shown in Table 74.2 are closely collaborating with nursing homes, for example, in the Netherlands and Norway, as recommended by Norwegian governmental committees.[96] Extending intensive services to sites of more traditional care represents a challenge on the political, personal, organizational, economical, and educational arenas. Hospitals and nursing homes often have different budgets,[4] and cost containment might be difficult when expensive drugs, fluids, and transfusions become part of daily care. This also increases the workload for the PCU care teams with respect to direct out-of-hospital patient care, extended consultation services, and specifically designed educational programs at basic and advanced levels.

Multidisciplinary approach and consultation services

The increasing complexity of the tasks involved in palliative care makes it clear that multidisciplinary teams are necessary for the identification and interventions needed to meet the rapidly changing needs of patients and families. Professionals in specialist palliative care settings may form relatively permanent teams, as is the case in most of the European centers presented in Table 74.2. Physicians, nurses, physical therapists, and social workers are included in most teams, supplemented by psychologists, psychiatrists, dietitians, bereavement counselors, chaplains, and others. Depending on the context of care, the individual team professionals also may serve as expert consultants for palliative patients in other hospital units, the home-care service, and nursing homes. The situation may also be the opposite, with palliative care teams seeking specialist services in disciplines such as neurology, anesthesiology, and pharmacology. Continuity of care across the PCU/hospice/home-care interface is more easily achieved through a multidisciplinary team composition if the responsibilities and strategies for the care plan are agreed on. Again, the earlier the patients are seen with this holistic multiprofessional approach, the more adequately their needs might be met. Another major advantage of the multidisciplinary teamwork is the aspect of bereavement care of staff in cases with bereavement overload, an area traditionally better managed by professions other than physicians. The increasing number of professions involved in palliative care is directly reflected in the membership of palliative care organizations. The German Association for Palliative Medicine was founded by 17 physicians in 1994. There were 50% physicians and 40% nurses among the 1100 members in 2003. At the EAPC 2013 Congress in Prague, Czech Republic, around 50% of the 1092 submitted abstracts were from physicians and about 10% from nurses. Altogether, the abstract submitters represented more than 25 professions in contrast to almost 100% of the abstracts coming from physicians at the first Research Forum in 2000.[3]

As previously mentioned in this chapter, we think that palliative care should become more integrated in the main healthcare system in the future, and that basic and intermediate levels of palliative care should be delivered by all healthcare providers in different sectors. An important implication however, is the need to increase the general and specific competence, among all professions, with specific emphasis on doctors and nurses. There may also be a need to reorganize the work and responsibilities of today's specialized multidisciplinary teams, in order to disseminate the advanced knowledge.

Education and advanced training

Rapid progress in the growth of professionals interested in palliative care began from 1995/96 and onward. This is evidenced by the steadily increasing number of members in the EAPC, from around 8300 in 1996 to more than 50,000 in 2008, the increasing number of collective member associations (Figure 74.2), and the fact that there are now 38 national palliative care associations in Europe.[28]

As previously mentioned, the increased need for palliative care and the many channels of delivery represent a major challenge in relation to professional education and the core competencies that are necessary to deliver high quality care. The EAPC white paper on palliative care education[84,85] suggests a three-tier framework to prepare practitioners academically, consisting of education on the principles and practices of palliative care related to the healthcare professionals' initial training: (1) the palliative care approach, toward an integration of palliative care methods in general care settings; (2) general palliative care that is intended for professionals frequently involved with palliative care patients; and (3) specialist palliative care. The paper is a strong argument for education, institutional collaboration, shared learning, and curricula design in line with Frenk et al.[97]

However, the link between academics and palliative care has only progressed slowly by establishing palliative medicine as a formal part of the medical programs at a university level.[15] A review from 2006 showed that academic positions in this field were found in 10 European countries (Belgium, United Kingdom, Germany, Finland, Greece, Norway, Poland, Sweden, Netherlands, Italy).[16] This review also showed that teaching in palliative medicine was on the curricula for medical students in the following 10 countries: Germany, Norway, Sweden, Finland, France, Greece, United Kingdom, Poland, Spain, and Hungary.[16] Some new programs incorporating palliative care have been developed at various undergraduate or graduate curricula in Croatia, Romania, Turkey, Lithuania, and Switzerland. University affiliations also vary throughout Europe, as shown in Figure 74.6, showing the distributions of professors in palliative care.

The review reported that formal training as palliative medicine specialists was less common and only existed in United Kingdom, Romania, Poland, Germany, Norway, Sweden, Denmark, Iceland, and Finland,[16] with specialized palliative textbooks in indigenous languages in 12 countries. Fortunately, the situation has improved somewhat since this review, and according to the EAPC Atlas, 13 countries have specialist programs in palliative medicine, while eight have a certification in process.[28]

The situation is basically the same for the nursing curricula, with few countries having palliative care as formal parts of the graduate or postgraduate levels or as an accredited specialization. The United Kingdom has been in the forefront regarding palliative care nursing; all basic nurse education (advanced diploma level) includes teaching about core palliative care knowledge and skills. At a post-basic qualification level, there are approximately 10 university-based courses offering master's-level courses in palliative care and psychosocial palliative care. These courses are usually taught in a multidisciplinary context. According to Larkin,[98] the United Kingdom remains a beacon of palliative care learning, offering not only theoretical but clinical learning. These opportunities are less readily available in many European countries and are essential to the translation of theory to practice.

The recent extension of the EU has led to a more flexible employment market, with less restriction on crossing borders for work. A priority of the EU to facilitate this flexibility is the process toward more universal educational programs. Revising the different medical school curricula and the postgraduate specialist education programs to make them more standardized is an example of this.

Palliative care research

Palliative care had its origin in the hospice movement emerging in the United Kingdom in the late 1960s. For quite some time, it was erroneously believed that research had no priority in this context. The development of palliative care in most countries in the 1960s and 1970s took place outside of the mainstream healthcare system and outside academic institutions. It was primarily directed toward developing different clinical programs in hospitals, hospices, and consultant team activities.[37] However, many of the European stakeholders in palliative care at the time, Vittorio Ventafridda (Italy), Cicely Saunders, Geoffrey Hanks, and Robert Twycross (UK), as well as Kathey Fowley in the United States were conducting high-quality palliative care research. This research makes it clear that palliative care ideology is based not "only on compassion but equally on skills preferably founded on scientific evidence."[99,100]

The need for research

Research is indispensable for the further development and improvement of palliative medicine and nursing and is necessary to increase the evidence base for practice.[15,101,102] We have witnessed an increased interest and development in interdisciplinary palliative care research during the last decade. For example, within the United Kingdom there is recognition of the importance of palliative care nursing research and involvement of nurses in multidisciplinary research teams. In addition, there is evidence of the growth in scholarship and publication of research from a bibliometric analysis[103] although there remain concerns about the number of small-scale studies in many palliative care research studies, for example, on symptom assessment.[104,105] Although nursing in general makes a very small contribution to UK National Health Service (NHS) research in comparison to the number of nurses involved in delivering care, palliative care represents one area of research that nurses have readily engaged with.[105] The steadily increasing number of international collaborative efforts in clinical and translational research in palliative care and advanced cancer are promising, yet there are many challenges ahead.[106,107]

Research is poorly embedded in the clinical work with patients in advanced stages of disease. This may partly result from the traditional focus on compassion and the perceptions of the healthcare providers that patients should not be bothered with interventions or self-report questionnaires for assessment of symptoms, the so-called "gate-keeping." Despite reports that the lack of standardized symptom assessment prohibits optimal symptom management,[107–110] that cancer patients do not receive adequate

symptom management or palliative care during the course of their illness,[74,70,108–113] and that collection of patient-reported outcomes positively influences the doctor-patient communication and is endorsed by patients,[114–117] systematic, standardized assessment of symptoms as a step toward better pain and symptom management has continued to have low priority in routine clinical activity.[15,98] Furthermore, a significant proportion of the palliative care research, maybe in relation to nursing in particular, has focused on examining the prevalence of frequent symptoms in cancer patients with advanced disease. It is well known that patients with advanced cancer experience multiple symptoms at the time[67,109] with studies reporting a median of 7.1 symptoms (range 0–12) for outpatients, 7.9 (range 1–13) for inpatients, or even higher.[111,118–121] However, prevalence data differs greatly across studies, which is due to a number of factors. Three of the most important are listed here:

1. There is no common understanding of how to describe and characterize a palliative care population, including which variables to use on a detailed level.[122–124]

2. It is generally agreed that the information needs to be elicited directly from the patient whenever possible,[70,104,107,125] but this is not systematically adhered to. The use of subjective assessments, however, accentuates the importance of using a standardized assessment system to validly describe, quantify, monitor, and compare symptoms at a given point or over time,[107,126] a work that has gained wide attention within the palliative care research community over the past few years resulting in papers with specific recommendations.[5,8,78,107,126,127]

3. Use of different research methods has contributed to the diverging results across studies. Most prevalence studies based on self-report of symptoms are cross-sectional studies in palliative care or advanced cancer patients with relatively small samples similar to other clinical studies in palliative care.[128,129]

Although there are many obstacles to the prioritization of research in palliative care—methodological, clinical, attitudinal, and ethical—these problems can be overcome. Based on experience, most patients are willing to participate in various types of palliative care research, including randomized trials on, for example, the impact of palliative care services,[130,131] evaluation of pain programs,[132] palliative radiotherapy,[133] and randomized intervention studies on physical training.[134,135] However, a recent study by Stone et al.[136] demonstrated that in a carefully planned, noninterventional study with rather simple assessments less than one-tenth of the patients admitted to the relevant units were included, due to many different reasons. The main implications from this are that the study results may reflect the situation for a minor group of the patients only, that it raises concerns about the generalizability of findings and concern that little is known about the patients who did not participate, once again a reminder of the need to characterize the study sample in a standardized manner.

Funding still remains a major obstacle for research. Despite the fact that about 50% of cancer patients eventually die from their disease, less than 0.05% of funding goes to research in palliative care. In the best-case scenario, only 0.18% of the oncology research budget is invested in palliative care, relative to 0.9% in the United States.[137] Nevertheless, Canadian and British national programs have funded the establishment of long-lasting,

Table 74.3 Examples of basic and clinical research topics for multidisciplinary research

Areas	Content—some examples
Biomedical—Basic	Pain, cachexia, anorexia, fatigue
Biomedical—Basic and clinical	Mechanisms of drug actions: Interindividual variability—adverse effects Pharmacokinetics—the elderly
Biomedical—Clinical	Controlled clinical trials Symptom control/medical interventions
Psychological—Clinical	Classification and assessment of pain Prognostication of pain relief Classification and assessment of cachexia Classification and assessment of anxiety/depression Cognitive function (in palliative care)
Sociological	Family Bereavement Areas for delivery of care
Healthcare provision	Standards for palliative care Consensus on a minimum set of indicators present in a center of excellence in palliative care Quality assurance
Philosophical	Euthanasia/patient assisted suicide

multidisciplinary groups covering a broad spectrum of palliative care research[138] (Table 74.3). Because a sound body of scientific research increases the chances of receiving funding for research projects, it is important that national and international research collaboratives be able to rely on predictable and sustainable funding over time.

Despite the difficulties involved in palliative care research, there is general consensus that the benefits of conducting research outweigh the many clinical and ethical challenges. The future looks bright, however, as evidenced in a recent EAPC European survey, displaying great enthusiasm for research in the palliative care community across Europe.[28]

Evidence-based medicine and palliative care

A definition of evidence-based medicine (EBM) states that it is the conscientious, explicit, judicial use of the best available evidence in order to offer the patient the most optimal individual care.[139] Thus, retrieving and applying the best available evidence is important to every clinician in the diagnostic workup and treatment of patients.[140] There are no contradictions between the philosophy of palliative care and EBM, although this debate has been going on for decades.

Many of the decisions made in palliative care are based on inferior quality studies, clinical experience, or extrapolation from studies performed in other populations, as seen, for example, in pain management. The need for EBM in palliative care is evident. Treatment of patients with a complex pathophysiology depends on research that focuses on the specific patient population and their problems.

There are at present two major areas in palliative care research that deserve particular attention. The first is to work toward achieving consensus on how to assess and classify the most prevalent symptoms experienced by patients in advanced stages of cancer.[37,107] Recent reviews have shown that more than 80 different assessment tools were used to measure pain,[126] and that the development of new tools is a continuously ongoing process without a defined rationale for doing so.[104,127] Furthermore, agreed on definitions are of the utmost importance for making comparisons across studies, providing a valid basis for drawing conclusions about selection of medication or other treatment options. As already pointed out, it is a major problem in clinical palliative care trials that study populations vary considerably in several characteristics associated with the symptom being studied; this is also the case in randomized controlled trials.[124,141] Stringent definitions of patient characteristics and observations are required to identify to which class or subclass the patient belongs. Agreement on a minimum set of characteristics for a palliative care population is necessary to increase the evidence base of research.[142] Currently an International Delphi Process has been conducted to achieve consensus on a set of basic medical and sociodemographic variables for use in clinical trials in palliative care—The EAPC Basic Dataset with a multicenter study being underway to pilot the dataset.[143] Other areas that need more in-depth studies are related to cancer and noncancer pain and symptoms, barriers to accessing care, and differences in the social, psychological, cultural, and spiritual aspects of palliative care from the point of patients, relatives, and caregivers (Table 74.3). One example is related to the fact that most patients in palliative care are elderly. This is in contrast to most studies in mainstream oncology, internal medicine, and even in pain treatment, where the upper age limit often is 70 to 75 years. The validity of extrapolating data from these age groups into older populations is questionable, and the need for appropriate research programs in the elderly is warranted,[144] as acknowledged by the IMPACT project[44] among others.

Research collaboration

In palliative care research, national or international multicenter collaborative studies are usually prerequisites for obtaining sufficiently large samples, which in turn makes it necessary to consolidate collaboratives in clinical research.[106,107] The way of doing this within the EAPC RN has been successful, and has led to several ongoing projects in the area of clinical palliative care, and as already mentioned, funding from the European Community; these are important steps in the right direction to foster international collaboration.

To succeed in achieving consensus with respect to assessment and classification of symptoms and on how to define a palliative care population, a systematic, stepwise approach in a multiprofessional and international collaborative composed of clinicians, researchers, and basic scientists is necessary. An example of this is the stepwise systematic work of the EPCRC[38] toward a better method for symptom assessment, as shown in Box 74.1.[107] In relation to pain, the overall goal of the ECPCR was to develop a computer-based symptom assessment tool that is both for and by the patient and the clinician, with a software content that is based on international consensus and is applicable for clinical work and research with a high degree of user friendliness.

Box 74.1 The EPCRC stepwise approach

Step 1. Definition of content and selection of items based on systematic literature review

♦ Determine the content of the measure based on the literature, the content of widely used forms, the clinical expert experience, and advice from an expert panel.

♦ Generate an item pool for pain assessment, primarily based on existing pain assessment tools and reflecting the recommended dimensions.

Step 2. Data collection number 1

Step 3. Analyses of data and functional specification of a computerized pain assessment tool

Step 4. International expert evaluation II

Step 5. Patient involvement, qualitative interview, and focus groups to document qualitative evidence of content and face validity

Step 6. Development of a computerized analyses model (software based on collected data)

Step 7. International data collection number 2

Step 8. Data analysis

Step 9. Programming of first version of the computer-based pain assessment tool

Source: Adapted from Kaasa et al. (2008), reference 107.

Computers used interactively have the potential to process, report, and communicate results reliably, efficiently, and cost-effectively between people. The use of electronic devices for symptom assessment offers several benefits compared with the traditional paper and pencil method. These include advantages with respect to data collection and storage, instant calculation and immediate presentation of scores, data quality, and tracking of symptoms over time. Rapid transfer of results may also facilitate follow-up of patients outside hospitals. Moreover, computerized assessment may be targeted to the individual if programmed to automatically select or skip questions based on the patient's previous answers, thereby reducing the respondent burden. Such processes may also allow tailor information to be provided to patients and their caregivers. Computerized versions of frequently used assessment tools for patient-reported outcomes such as the SF-36[145] have been developed for use with different digital devices and platforms, among others by the QualityMetric group,[146] and the PROMIS system[147] and for the EORTC QLQ-C30.[148,149] To develop the appropriate and user-friendly software, the EPCRC placed great emphasis on design, input, and review by patients and clinicians during the development process meetings, steps 1 and 5 (Box 74.1), and during the data collection process, steps 2 and 7.

As part of the EPCRC project, a clinical study testing a computerized symptom assessment tool; the EPCRC-CSA (European Palliative Care Research Collaborative—Computerized Symptom Assessment study) was conducted in 17 centers in eight countries between 2007 and 2009.[38] All patient- and clinician-reported data were directly entered on touch-screen laptop computers, providing 1017 records from patients with incurable metastatic or locally advanced cancer for analyses.[150] The entire assessment was completed by 95% of the patients, but lower performance status reduced compliance and increased need for assistance. More than 50% preferred computerized assessment to the paper and pencil version, regardless of prior experience with computers. The promising results from this study have led to new projects related to computerized symptom assessment—one that is primarily focusing on a computerized pain body map[151] and another that combines preconsultation systematic symptom assessment on iPads with a support system for clinical decision-making.

The European way to promote research

To further develop and improve the assessment and classification of cancer pain in general, the initiatives taken within the European and international palliative care community should be continued. Many of the European centers presented in Table 74.2 were engaged in research activities on various levels. To successfully integrate multidisciplinary research in a palliative care program, certain criteria have to be accomplished:

♦ Professional leadership

♦ Agreement on and promotion of a clear strategy and research agenda

♦ Parallel development of clinic and research

♦ An infrastructure that ensures interaction with scientists not working in the palliative field

♦ Translational research

♦ Multicenter national and international cooperation

♦ Research programs at all levels: undergraduate, PhD students, postdoctoral, and researchers

♦ Continuous application for funding at all levels

♦ Dissemination of results

♦ Leading journals

♦ Conferences

♦ Involvement of the public

The former pain and palliation research group in Trondheim, Norway,[101] is an example of a multiprofessional group that was active in international collaborative research from the start. The main research areas—pharmacogenetics, genetic variability related to pain control, pain management, subjective symptom assessment, development and use of computer technology for symptom reporting, physical function, ethical issues, communication, and symptom palliation—were subsequently carried forward into the European Palliative Care Research Centre (PRC)[36] based at the Faculty of Medicine and Trondheim University Hospital in Norway. The PRC was established in 2009 with recommendations and support from the EAPC,[3] the Norwegian Cancer Society, and other international bodies such as the Open Society Foundations in the United States and the Floriani Foundation in Italy. The PRC coordinates groups and individual researchers across Europe along with researchers in North America and Australia, and consists of 13 core collaborating centers. The PRC coordinates and participates in a variety of studies, both national and international. An important aim of the work within the PRC is to organize large international multicenter studies, and from

2012 and onward the recruitment of patients has started or is in the pipeline for several studies.[36] Some of these studies are prospective trials following the disease trajectory, symptom development, and treatment effects and side effects for a long period of time. On example is the European Palliative Care Cancer Symptom study (EPCCS) that is being conducted in 30 centers in 12 countries. Other studies employ a randomized controlled study design and have a close collaboration with basic scientists focusing on different biomarkes related to the primary study outcomes. These studies primarily focus on specific symptoms such as metastatic bone pain, the Palliative Radiotherapy of Bone Metastases Study; cachexia, the MENAC study (Multimodal Exercise/Nutrition/Anti-inflammatory treatment for Cachexia); and different approaches to pain relief: patient-controlled nasal fentanyl versus oral morphine and the TVT-study examining a two-step versus three-step approach to cancer pain relief.[152]

The PRC aims to improve the knowledge about palliative care among all health professionals. To increase the scientific competence, a biomedical-focused international PhD program in palliative care has been established by the PRC. The program is formally established at Norwegian University of Science and Technology, but all core collaborating institutions contribute to the program[153] Several PhD students from many of the EU-funded research programs such as the IMPACT[44] and EUROIMPACT[45] are currently pursuing their degrees, with parts of their study being an exchange between Norway and other international institutions, such as the Cancer Institute in Milan, the Dutch university hospitals, and King's College in the UK.

The challenges

Although palliative care in Europe has undergone a remarkable development from its start in the 1960s and into the second decade of a new millennium, there are still challenges ahead. As we have demonstrated in this chapter, there are still major differences within Europe, on the social, political, financial, and developmental levels, all of which impact on the distribution, delivery, and access to palliative care. One problem relevant to the collection of survey data on palliative care is that there is no clear definition of the minimum number or set of indicators characterizing a palliative care program, a hospice, or a PCU in a nursing home. To be able to describe and compare programs across countries, it is urgent to agree on minimum criteria for developing a palliative care program at various levels of the healthcare system.

Nevertheless, the challenges appear to be universal. The first is related to the total integration of palliative care into the general healthcare system both in the inpatient and outpatient sector and the policy implications of such integration. This would include education and specialist training at basic and advanced levels through universities and medical associations and a multidisciplinary approach. In addition, special national and EU research programs in palliative care have started on the road of evidence-based palliative medicine. Striving for these goals is evidence-based practice with compassion—the cornerstone in the professional encounter with patients.

Acknowledgments

The following persons have contributed specific information for this chapter:

RG Helgås, Trondheim, Norway
S Lindström, Stockholm, Sweden
J Porta-Sales, Barcelona, Spain
M Groenvold, Copenhagen, Denmark
K vd Rijt, Amsterdam, Netherlands
A Pigni, Milan, Italy
L Radbruch, Bonn, Germany
C Bausewein, Munich, Germany
MI Bennett, Leeds, UK
A Giordano, Milan, Italy
S Payne, Lancaster UK
B Laird, Edinburgh, UK
K Pardon, Belgium

References

1. Davies E, Higginson IJ, eds. Palliative Care. The Solid Facts. WHO Regional Office for Europe, Copenhagen 2004. Available at: http://www.euro.who.int/document/e82931.pdf (accessed June 25, 2013).
2. World Health Organization. Homepage. Available at: http://www.who.int/cancer/palliative/definition/en/ (accessed June 25, 2013).
3. European Association for Palliative Care. Homepage. Available at: http://www. eapcnet.eu (accessed June 25, 2013).
4. Caraceni A, Hanks G, Kaasa S, et al. Use of opioid analgesics in the treatment of cancer pain: evidence-based recommendations from the EAPC. Lancet Oncol. 2012;13:e58–e68.
5. Rayner L, Price A, Hotopf M, Higginson IJ. The development of evidence-based European guidelines on the management of depression in palliative cancer care. Eur J Cancer. 2011;47(5):702–712.
6. van der Steen JT, Radbruch L, Hertogh CMPM, et al. White paper defining optimal palliative care in older people with dementia: a Delphi study and recommendations from the European Association for Palliative Care. Palliat Med. 2014;28(3):197–209.
7. Cherny NI, Radbruch L. European Association for Palliative Care (EAPC) recommended framework for the use of sedation in palliative care. Palliat Med. 2009;23(7):581–593.
8. Janberidze E, Hjermstad MJ, Haugen DF, Sigurdardottir KR, Løhre ET, Lie HC, Loge JH, Kaasa S, Knudsen AK; EURO IMPACT How Are the Patient Populations Characterized in Studies Investigating Depression in Advanced Cancer? Results From a Systematic Literature Review. J Pain Symptom Manage. 2014 Mar 28. pii: S0885-3924(14)00134-1. doi: 10.1016/j.jpainsymman.2013.11.013. [Epub ahead of print].
9. Jacobsen J, Jackson V, Dahlin C, et al. Components of early outpatient palliative care consultation in patients with metastatic non-small cell lung cancer. J Palliat Med. 2011;14(4):459–464.
10. Centeno C, Clark D, Lynch T, et al. Facts and indicators on palliative care development in 52 countries of the WHO European region: results of an EAPC Task Force. Palliat Med. 2007;21(6):463–471.
11. Greer JA, Jackson VA, Meier DE, Temel JS. Early integration of palliative care services with standard oncology care for patients with advanced cancer. CA Cancer J Clin. 2013;63(5):349–363.
12. Gaertner J, Weingärtner V, Wolf J, Voltz R. Early palliative care for patients with advanced cancer: how to make it work? Curr Opin Oncol. 2013;25(4):342–352.
13. Kaasa S. Integration of general oncology and palliative care. Lancet Oncol. 2013;14(7):571–572.
14. European Association for Palliative Care. Professional Integration. Homepage. Available at http://www.eapcnet.eu/Themes/Policy/Professionalintegration.aspx (accessed June 25, 2013).
15. Kaasa S, Hjermstad MJ, Loge JH. Methodological and structural challenges in palliative care research: how have we fared in the last decades? Palliat Med. 2006;20:727–734.
16. Rocafort J, Centeno C. EAPC Review of Palliative Care in Europe. European Association for Palliative Care. Milan, Italy: EAPC Head Office; 2008.
17. Nordic Specialist Course in Palliative Medicine. Homepage. Available at: www.nscpm.org (accessed June 30, 2013).
18. OECD Health at a Glance. Homepage. Available at: http://www.oecd-ilibrary.org/social-issues-migration-health/health-at-a-glance-

europe-2010/cancer-incidence_9789264090316-18-en (accessed June 30, 2013)

19. The Norwegian Cancer Registry. Homepage. Available at: http://www.kreftregisteret.no/no (accessed July 2, 2013)

20. Berrino F, De Angelis R, Sant M, et al. Survival for eight major cancers and all cancers combined for European adults diagnosed in 1995–99: Results of the EUROCARE-4 study. Lancet Oncol. 2007;8(9):773–783.

21. Murray CJL, Lopez AD. Alternative projections of mortality and disability by cause 1990–2020: Global burden of disease study. Lancet. 1997;349:1498–1504.

22. Edmonds P, Karlsen S, Khan S, Addington-Hall J. A comparison of the palliative care needs of patients dying from chronic respiratory diseases and lung cancer. Palliat Med. 2001;15(4):287–295.

23. Temel JS, Greer JA, Muzikansky A, et al. Early palliative care for patients with metastatic non-small cell lung cancer. N Engl J Med. 2010;363(8):733–742.

24. van der Steen JT. Dying with dementia: what we know after more than a decade of research. J Alzheimers Dis. 2010;22(1):37–55.

25. World Health Organization. Dementia: A Public Health Priority. Switzerland, Geneva: WHO; 2012.

26. European Association for Palliative Care. Specific Groups. Homepage. Available at http://www.eapcnet.eu/Themes/Specificgroups.aspx (accessed July 3, 2013).

27. European Association for Palliative Care. Policy. Homepage. Available at http://www.eapcnet.eu/Themes/Policy/PalliativeCareinAfrica.aspx (accessed July 3, 2013).

28. EAPC Atlas of Palliative Care in Europe 2013—Cartographic Edition. EAPC European Association for Palliative Care, 2013. Available at: http://www.unav.es/centro/cultura-y-sociedad/ (accessed June 22, 2013).

29. Open Society Foundations. Homepage. Available at http://www.opensocietyfoundations.org (accessed August 7, 2013).

30. Bruera E, Sweeney C. Palliative care models: international perspective. J Palliative Med. 2002;5:319–327.

31. Portenoy R, Heller KS. Developing an integrated department of pain and palliative medicine. J Palliat Med. 2002;5(2):623–633.

32. Gòmez-Batiste X, Porta J, Tuca A, et al. Spain: the WHO demonstration project of palliative care implementation in Catalonia: results at 10 years (1991–2001). J Pain Symptom Manage. 2002;24(2):239–244.

33. Radbruch L, Payne S; on behalf of EAPC Board of Directors. White Paper on Standards and Norms for Hospice and Palliative Care in Europe. Recommendations from the European Association for Palliative Care—part 1. Eur J of Palliative Care. 2009;16(6):278–289.

34. Radbruch L, Payne S; on behalf of EAPC Board of Directors. White Paper on Standards and Norms for Hospice and Palliative Care in Europe. Recommendations from the European Association for Palliative Care—part 2. Eur J of Palliative Care. 2010;17(1):22–33.

35. Early detection and INTervention in DEMentia (INTERDEM). Homepage. Available at: http://www.interdem.org/ (accessed July 5, 2013).

36. European Palliative Care Research Centre (PRC). Homepage. Available at: http://www.ntnu.edu/prc/ (accessed July 23, 2013)

37. Kaasa S, Radbruch L. Palliative care research: priorities and the way forward. Eur J Cancer. 2008;44(8):1175–1179.

38. European Palliative Care Research Collaborative (EPCRC). Homepage. Available at: http://www.epcrc.org (accessed July 5, 2013).

39. European Commission's Directorate-General for Research, Seventh Framework Programme (FP7). Homepage. Available at: http://cordis.europa.eu/fp7/projects_en.html (accessed July 9, 2013).

40. Rayner L, Price A, Evans A, Valsraj K. Antidepressants for depression in physically ill people. Editorial Group: Cochrane Depression, Anxiety and Neurosis Group. Cochrane Database Syst Rev. 2010 Mar 17;(3):CD007503. doi: 10.1002/14651858.CD007503.pub2. Review.

41. PRISMA. Reflecting the Positive Diversities of European Priorities for Research and Measurement in End of Life Care. Homepage. Available at: http://www.prismafp7.eu (accessed July 10, 2013).

42. OPCARE-9. Homepage. Available at: http://www.liv.ac.uk/opcare9/index.htm (accessed July 10, 2013).

43. ATOME (Access to Opioid Medication in Europe). Homepage. Available at: http://www.atome-project.eu (accessed July 10, 2013).

44. IMPACT (Implementation of Quality Indicators in Palliative Care Study). Homepage. Available at: http://www.impactpalliativecare.eu/ (accessed July 10, 2013).

45. EUROIMPACT (The European Intersectorial and Multi-disciplinary Palliative Care Research Training). Homepage. Available at: http://www.euro-impact.eu/ (accessed July 10, 2013).

46. InSup-c (Integrated Palliative Care). Homepage. Available at: http://www.insup-c.eu// (accessed July 10, 2013).

47. Norwegian Directorate of Health. [Nasjonalt handlingsprogram for Palliasjon, Norwegian version] National Palliative Care Program with Clinical Guidelines. Available at: http://www.helsedirektoratet.no/publikasjoner/nasjonalt-handlingsprogram-med-retningslinjer-for-palliasjon-i-kreftomsorgen-/Publikasjoner/nasjonalt-handlingsprogram-for-palliasjon-i-kreftomsorgen.pdf.

48. ESMO (European Society for Medical Oncology). Available at: http://www.esmo.org/Patients/Designated-Centres-of-Integrated-Oncology-and-Palliative-Care (accessed August 9, 2013).

49. Fürst CJ. The European Association for Palliative Care initiative in Eastern Europe. J Pain Symptom Manage. 2002;24(2):134–135.

50. Clark D, Wright M. Transitions in End of Life Care. London: Open University Press; 2003.

51. Lynch T, Clark D, Centeno C, et al. Barriers to the development of palliative care in the countries of Central and Eastern Europe and the Commonwealth of Independent States. J Pain Symptom Manage. 2009;37(3):305–315.

52. Cherny NI, Baselga J, de Conno F, Radbruch L. Formulary availability and regulatory barriers to accessibility of opioids for cancer pain in Europe: a report from the ESMO/EAPC Opioid Policy Initiative. Ann Oncol. 2010 Mar;21(3):615–626. doi: 10.1093/annonc/mdp581.

53. Newton M. The development of terminal care in Albania. Eur J Palliat Care. 2001;8(6):246–249.

54. Mosoui D, Andrews CC, Perrols G. Palliative care in Romania. Palliat Med. 2000;14(1):65–67.

55. Costello J, Gorchakova A. Palliative care for children in the Republic of Belarus. Int J Palliat Nurs. 2004;10(4):197–200.

56. Salmon I. A British nurse's view of palliative care in Russia. J Palliat Nurs. 2001;7(1):37–43.

57. The European Council. Homepage. Available http://www.european-council.europa.eu/home-page.aspx (accessed July 15, 2013).

58. Radbruch L, Foley K, De Lima L, Praill D, Fürst CJ. The Budapest Commitments: setting the goals a joint initiative by the European Association for Palliative Care, the International Association for Hospice and Palliative Care and Help the Hospices. Palliat Med. 2007;21(4):269–271.

59. International Association for Hospice and Palliative Care (IAHPC). Homepage. Available at: http://hospicecare.com/home/ (accessed July 15, 2013).

60. Worldwide Palliative Care Alliance (WPCA). Homepage. Available at: http://www.thewpca.org/ (accessed July 15, 2013).

61. Fürst CJ, de Lima L, Praill D, Radbruch L. An update on the Budapest Commitments. Eur J Pall Care. 2009;16(1):22–25.

62. Human Rights Watch (HRW). Homepage. Available at: http://www.hrw.org/ (accessed July 11, 2013).

63. The Lisbon Challenge. European Association for Palliative Care. Homepage. Available at: http://www.eapcnet.eu/Themes/Policy/Lisbonchallenge.aspx (accessed July 15, 2013).

64. The Prague Charter. European Association for Palliative Care. Homepage. Available at: http://www.eapcnet.eu/Themes/Policy/PragueCharter.aspx (accessed July 15, 2013).

65. The Prague Charter Petition. Homepage. Available at: http://www.avaaz.org/en/petition/ The_Prague_Charter_Relieving_Suffering (accessed July 15, 2013).

66. EAPC Research Network (EAPC RN). Homepage. Available at: http://www.eapcnet.eu/Themes/Research/AbouttheEAPC ResearchNetwork.aspx (accessed July 15, 2013).

67. Laugsand EA, Kaasa S, de Conno F, Hanks G, Klepstad P; Research Steering Committee of the EAPC. Intensity and treatment of symptoms in 3,030 palliative care patients: a cross-sectional survey of the EAPC Research Network. J Opioid Manage. 2009;5(1):11–21.

68. Klepstad P, Fladvad T, Skorpen F, et al. European Palliative Care Research Collaborative (EPCRC); European Association for Palliative Care Research Network. Influence from genetic variability on opioid use for cancer pain: a European genetic association study of 2294 cancer pain patients. Pain. 2011;152(5):1139–1145.

69. Fyllingen EH, Oldervoll LM, Loge JH, et al. Computer-based assessment of symptoms and mobility in palliative care: feasibility and challenges. J Pain Symptom Manage. 2009;38(6):827–836.

70. Caraceni A, Cherny N, Fainsinger R, et al. Pain measurement tools and methods in clinical research in palliative care: recommendations of an expert working group of the European Association of Palliative Care. J Pain Symptom Manage. 2002;23:239–255.

71. Mercadante S, Radbruch L, Caraceni A, Cherny N, et al. The Steering Committee of the European Association for Palliative Care (EAPC) Research Network. Episodic (breakthrough) pain: consensus conference of an expert working group of the European Association for Palliative Care. Cancer. 2002;94(3):832–839.

72. Klepstad P, Kaasa S, Cherny N, Hanks G, De Conno F; the Research Steering Committee of the EAPC. Pain and pain treatments in European palliative care units: a cross sectional survey from the European Association for Palliative Care Research Network. Palliat Med. 2005;19(6):477–484.

73. Stiefel F, Die Trill M, Berney A, Olarte JMN, Razavi D. Depression in palliative care: a pragmatic report from the Expert Working Group of the European Association for Palliative Care. Support Care Cancer. 2001;9(7):477–488.

74. Radbruch L, Strasser F, Eisner F, et al. Fatigue in palliative care patients—an EAPC approach. Palliat Med. 2008;22(1):13–32.

75. Ripamonti C, Twycross R, Baines M, et al. Clinical-practice recommendations for the management of bowel obstruction in patients with end-stage cancer. Support Care Cancer. 2001;9(4):223–233.

76. Cherny N, Ripamonti C, Pereira J, Davis C, Fallon M, McQuay H, et al., for the Expert Working Group of the EAPC Network. Strategies to manage the adverse effects of oral morphine: an evidence-based report. J Clin Oncol. 2001;19(9):2542–2554.

77. Cherny NI, Radbruch L; Board of the European Association for Palliative Care. European Association for Palliative Care (EAPC) recommended framework for the use of sedation in palliative care. Palliat Med. 2009;23(7):581–593.

78. Knudsen AK, Brunelli C, Klepstad P, Aass N, et al. Which domains should be included in a cancer pain classification system?: Analyses of longitudinal data. Pain. 2012;153(3):696–703.

79. Maltoni M, Caraceni A, Brunelli C, et al. Prognostic factors in advanced cancer patients: evidence-based clinical recommendations—a study by the steering committee of the European association for palliative care. J Clin Oncol. 2005;23(25):6240–6248.

80. EAPC Junior Forum. Homepage. Available at: http://www.eapcnet.eu/Themes/Research/JuniorForum.aspx (accessed July 15, 2013).

81. Gretton SK, Droney J, Branford R, Stene GB, Knudsen AK, Kaasa S. EAPC Research Network: The Junior Forum. Eur J Palliat Care. 2009;16:232–235.

82. EAPC PC and Euthanasia Taskforce. Homepage. Available at: http://www.eapcnet.eu/Themes/Ethics/PCeuthanasiataskforce.aspx (accessed July 15, 2013).

83. Murtagh FE, Bausewein C, Verne J, Groeneveld EI, Kaloki YE, Higginson IJ. How many people need palliative care?: A study developing and comparing methods for population-based estimates. Palliat Med 2013 Palliat Med. 2014;28(1):49–58.

84. Gamondi C, Larkin P, Payne S. Core competencies in palliative care: an EAPC White Paper on palliative care education—part 1. Eur J Pall Care. 2013;20(3):86–92.

85. Gamondi C, Larkin P, Payne S. Core competencies in palliative care: an EAPC White Paper on palliative care education—part 2. Eur J Pall Care. 2013;20(3):140–145.

86. EAPC Taskforce on Palliative Care Outcomes. Homepage. Available at: http://www.eapcnet.eu/Themes/Clinicalcare/Outcomemeasurement.aspx (accessed July 20, 2013).

87. Radbruch L, Nauck F, Fuchs M, Neuwohner K, Schulenberg D, Lindena G. What is palliative care in Germany?: Results from a representative survey. J Pain Symptom Manage. 2002;23(6):471–483.

88. Centeno C, Hernansanz S, Flores LA, Rubiales AS, Lopez-Lara F. Spain: palliative care programs in Spain, 2000: a national survey. J Pain Symptom Manage. 2002;24(2):245–251.

89. Higginson IJ, Finlay I, Goodwin DM, et al. Do hospital-based palliative teams improve care for patient and families at the end of life? J Pain Symptom Manage. 2002;23(2):96–106.

90. Higginson IJ, Finlay IG, Goodwin DM, et al. Is there evidence that palliative care teams alter end-of-life experiences of patients and their caregivers? J Pain Symptom Manage. 2003;25(2):150–168.

91. Beccaro M, Costantini M, Giorgi Rossi P, et al. Actual and preferred place of death of cancer patients: results from the Italian survey of the dying of cancer (ISDOC). J Epidemiol Community Health. 2006;60(5):412–416.

92. Agar M, Currow DC, Shelby-James TM, Plummer J, Sanderson C, Abernethy AP. Preference for place of care and place of death in palliative care: are these different questions? Palliat Med. 2008;22(7):787–795.

93. Gomes B, Higginson IJ, Calanzani N, et al. PRISMA Preferences for place of death if faced with advanced cancer: a population survey in England, Flanders, Germany, Italy, the Netherlands, Portugal and Spain. Ann Oncol. 2012;23(8):2006–2015.

94. Jordhøy MS, Fayers P, Saltnes T, Ahlner-Elmqvist M, Jannert M, Kaasa S. A palliative care intervention and death at home: a cluster randomised trial. Lancet. 2000;356(9233):888–893.

95. Schrijvemaekers V, Courtens A, van den Beuken M, Oyen P. The first 2 years of a palliative care consultation team in the Netherlands. Int J Palliat Nurs. 2003;9(6):252–257.

96. Kaasa S, Breivik H, Jordhoy M. Norway: development of palliative care. J Pain Symptom Manage. 2002;24(2):211–214.

97. Frenk J, Chen L, Bhutta ZA, et al. Health professionals for a new century: transforming education to strengthen health systems in an interdependent world. Lancet. 2010;376(9756):1923–1958.

98. Larkin P. Education and scholarship in palliative care. In: Payne S, Seymour J, Ingleton C, eds. Palliative Care Nursing: Principles and Evidence for Practice. 2nd ed. Maidenhead: McGraw-Hill Press; 2008:591–607.

99. Saunders C. Watch with me. Nurs Times. 1965;61:1615–1617.

100. Saunders C. A personal therapeutic journey. BMJ. 1996;313:1599–1601.

101. Kaasa S, Dale O. Pain and Palliative Research Group. Building up research in palliative care: an historical perspective and a case for the future. Clin Geriatr Med. 2005;21(1):81–92.

102. Kaasa S. Palliative care research: time to intensify international collaboration. Palliat Med. 2008;22(4):301–302.

103. Payne S, Turner M. Research methodologies in palliative care: a bibliometric analysis. Palliat Med. 2008;22(4):336–342.

104. Hjermstad MJ, Gibbins J, Haugen DF, Caraceni A, Loge JH, Kaasa S. On behalf of the EPCRC, European Palliative Care Research Collaborative. Pain assessment tools in palliative care: an urgent need for consensus. Palliat Med. 2008;22(8):895–903.

105. Rafferty AM, Traynor M. Assessing research quality. J Adv Nurs. 2006;56(1):2–4.

106. Fainsinger RL. Global warming in the palliative care research environment: adapting to change. Palliat Med. 2008;22(4):328–335.

107. Kaasa S, Loge JH, Fayers P, et al. Symptom assessment in palliative care: a need for international collaboration. J Clin Oncol. 2008;26(23):3867–3873.

108. Von Roenn JH, Cleeland CS, Gonin RR, et al. Physician attitudes and practice in cancer pain management: a survey from the Eastern Cooperative Oncology Group. Ann Intern Med. 1993;119(2):121–126.

109. Meuser T, Pietruck C, Radbruch L, Stute P, Lehmann KA, Grond S. Symptoms during cancer pain treatment following WHO-guidelines: a longitudinal follow-up study of symptom prevalence, severity and etiology. Pain. 2001;93(3):247–257.

110. Patrick DL, Ferketich SL, Frame PS, Harris JJ, Hendricks CB, Levin B, et al. National Institutes of Health State-of-the-Science Conference Statement: symptom management in cancer: pain, depression, and fatigue, July 15–17, 2002. J Natl Cancer Inst. 2003;95(15):1110–1117.

111. Chang VT, Hwang SS, Feuerman M, Kasimis BS. Symptom and quality of life survey of medical oncology patients at a veterans affairs medical center: a role for symptom assessment. Cancer. 2000;88(5):1175–1183.

112. Deandrea S, Montanari M, Moja L, Apolone G. Prevalence of undertreatment in cancer pain: a review of published literature. Ann Oncol. 2008;19(12):1985–1991.

113. Cleeland CS, Gonin R, Hatfield AK, et al. Pain and its treatment in outpatients with metastatic cancer. N Engl J Med. 1994;330:592–596.

114. Velikova G, Booth L, Smith AB, et al. Measuring quality of life in routine oncology practice improves communication and patient well-being: a randomized controlled trial. J Clin Oncol. 2004;22(4):714–724.

115. Velikova G, Keding A, Harley C, Cocks K, Booth L, Smith AB, Wright P, Selby PJ, Brown JM. Patients report improvements in continuity of care when quality of life assessments are used routinely in oncology practice: secondary outcomes of a randomised controlled trial. Eur J Cancer. 2010;46(13):2381–2388.

116. Detmar SB, Muller MJ, Schornagel JH, Wever LD, Aaronson NK. Health-related quality-of-life assessments and patient-physician communication: a randomized controlled trial. JAMA. 2002;288(23):3027–3034.

117. Brundage M, Leis A, Bezjak A, et al. Cancer patients' preferences for communicating clinical trial quality of life information: A qualitative study. Qual Life Res. 2003;12(4):395–404.

118. Caraceni A, Portenoy RK. An international survey of cancer pain characteristics and syndromes. IASP Task Force on Cancer Pain. International Association for the Study of Pain. Pain. 1999;82(3):263–274.

119. Hickok JT, Morrow GR, Roscoe JA, et al. Occurrence, severity, and longitudinal course of twelve common symptoms in 1129 consecutive patients during radiotherapy for cancer. J Pain Symptom Manage. 2005;30(5):433–442.

120. Portenoy RK, Thaler HT, Kornblith AB, et al. Symptom prevalence, characteristics and distress in a cancer population. Qual Life Res. 1994;3(3):183–189.

121. Walsh D, Donnelly S, Rybicki L. The symptoms of advanced cancer: relationship to age, gender, and performance status in 1,000 patients. Support Care Cancer. 2000;8(3):175–179.

122. Boisvert M, Cohen SR. Opioid use in advanced malignant disease: why do different centers use vastly different doses?: A plea for standardized reporting. J Pain Symptom Manage. 1995;10(8):632–638.

123. Borgsteede SD, Deliens L, Francke AL, et al. Defining the patient population: one of the problems for palliative care research. Palliat Med. 2006;20(2):63–68.

124. Van Mechelen W, Aertgeerts B, De Ceulaer K, et al. Defining the palliative care patient: a systematic review. Palliat Med. 2013;27(3):197–208.

125. Jensen MP. The validity and reliability of pain measures in adults with cancer. J Pain. 2003;4(1):2–21.

126. Holen JC, Hjermstad MJ, Loge JH, et al. Pain assessment tools: is the content appropriate for use in palliative care? J Pain Symptom Manage. 2006;32(6):567–580.

127. Hjermstad MJ, Fainsinger R, Kaasa S. Assessment and classification of cancer pain. Curr Opin Support Palliat Care. 2009;3(1):24–30.

128. Quigley C. Hydromorphone for acute and chronic pain. Cochrane Database Syst Rev. 2002(1):CD003447. PMID:11869661.

129. Wiffen PJ, McQuay HJ. Oral morphine for cancer pain. Cochrane Database Syst Rev. 2007(4):CD003868. PMID:17943804.

130. Jordhøy MS, Kaasa S, Fayers P, Overness T, Underland G, Ahlner-Elmqvist M. Challenges in palliative care research; recruitment, attrition and compliance: experience from a randomised controlled trial. Palliat Med. 1999;13(4):299–310.

131. Jordhøy MS, Fayers P, Loge JH, Ahlner-Elmqvist M, Kaasa S. Quality of life in palliative cancer care: results from a cluster randomised trial. J Clin Oncol. 2001;19(18):3884–3894.

132. Hanks G, Robbins M, Sharp D, et al. The IMPACT study: a randomised controlled trial to evaluate a hospital palliative care team. Br J Cancer. 2002;87(7):733–739.

133. Sundstrøm S, Bremnes R, Aasebø U, et al. Hypofractionated palliative radiotherapy (17 Gy per two fractions) in advanced non-small-cell lung carcinoma is comparable to standard fractionation for symptom control and survival: a national phase III trial. J Clin Oncol. 2004;22(5):801–810.

134. Oldervoll LM, Loge JH, Paltiel H, et al. The effect of a physical exercise program in palliative care: a phase II study. J Pain Symptom Manage. 2006;31(5):421–430.

135. Oldervoll LM, Loge JH, Lydersen S, et al. Physical exercise for cancer patients with advanced disease: a randomized controlled trial. Oncologist. 2011;16(11):1649–1657.

136. Stone PC, Gwilliam B, Keeley V, et al. Factors affecting recruitment to an observational multi-centre palliative care study. BMJ Support Pall Care. 2013;3(3):318–323.

137. Higginson IJ. End-of-life care: lessons from other nations. J Palliat Med. 2005;8(Suppl 11):S161–S173.

138. Payne S, Addington-Hall J, Sharpe M. Supportive and palliative care research collaboratives in the United Kingdom: an unnatural experiment. Prog Palliat Care. 2007;21:663–665.

139. Sackett D, Richardson WS, Rosenberg W, Haynes B. Evidence Based Medicine. London: Churchill Livingstone; 1996.

140. McQuay HJ, Moore A, Wiffen P. Research in palliative medicine: the principles of evidence-based medicine. In: Doyle D, Hanks G, Cherny N, Calman K, eds. Oxford Textbook of Palliative Medicine. 3rd ed. Oxford, England: Oxford University Press; 2003:119–128.

141. Sigurdardottir KR, Oldervoll L, Hjermstad MJ, et al. How are palliative care cancer populations characterized in randomized controlled trials?: A literature review. J Pain Symptom Manage. 2013;47(5):906–914.

142. Currow DC, Wheeler JL, Glare PA, et al. A framework for generalizability in palliative care. J Pain Symptom Manage. 2008;37:373–386.

143. Sigurdardottir K, Haugen DF, Bausewein C, Rosland JH, Kaasa S. The EAPC Basic Dataset. Results from an International Delphi Process. Palliat Med. 2014;28(6):463–473.

144. Davies E, Higginson IJ. eds. 2004. Better Palliative Care for Older People. Copenhagen: WHO Regional Office for Europe. Available at http://www.euro.who.int/document/ E82933.pdf (accessed December 20, 2008).

145. Ware JE. SF 36 Health Survey Manual and Interpretation Guide. 1st ed. Boston: New England Medical Center; 1993.

146. Quality Metric Incorporated. Generic Health Surveys. Available from: http://www qualitymetric com/WhatWeDo/GenericHealth Surveys/tabid/184/Default aspx (accessed July 21, 2011).

147. PROMIS. Patient-Reported Outcomes Measurement Information System. Available from: http://www nihpromis org (accessed July 23 2013).

148. Erharter A, Giesinger J, Kemmler G, Schauer-Maurer G, Stockhammer G, et al. Implementation of computer-based quality-of-life monitoring in brain tumor outpatients in routine clinical practice. J Pain Symptom Manage. 2010;39(2):219–229.

149. Holzner B, Giesinger JM, Pinggera J, Zugal S, et al. The Computer-based Health Evaluation Software (CHES): a software for electronic patient-reported outcome monitoring. BMC Med Inform Decis Mak. 2012;9(12):126.

150. Hjermstad MJ, Lie HC, Caraceni C, et al. Computer based symptom assessment is feasible in patients with advanced cancer—results from an international multi-centre study, the EPCRC-CSA. J Pain Sympt Manage. 2012;44(5):639–654.

151. Jaatun EAA, Hjermstad MJ, Gundersen OE, Oldervoll L, Kaasa S, Haugen DF. Development and testing of a computerized pain body map in patients with advanced cancer. J Pain Symptom Manage. 2013. Epub ahead of print. PMID:23856098, doi:pii: S0885-3924(13)00306-0. 10.1016/j.jpainsymman.2013.02.025.

152. European Palliative Care Research Centre (PRC). Projects. Homepage. Available at http://www.ntnu.edu/web/prc1/projects (accessed July 23, 2013).

153. Palliative Care Research Centre (PRC). International PhD. Homepage. Available at http://www.ntnu.edu/prc/phdprogramme (accessed July 23, 2013).

CHAPTER 75

Palliative care in Latin America

Tania Pastrana, Denisse Ruth Parra Giordano, Miguel Antonio Sánchez Cárdenas, Xiomara Carmona Montoya, and Beatriz Montes de Oca

Key points

- Latin America is undergoing similar demographic changes affecting other parts of the world, namely an aging population and increasing prevalence of chronic disease. These changes will create greater need for palliative care services.

- Palliative care is in the nascent phases of development in many countries within Latin America, making access to care limited for many patients.

- Barriers include restricted opioid availability, limited education regarding palliative care for healthcare professionals, and inadequate funding for these services.

- Despite these obstacles, nurses in many countries in Latin America are leading efforts to improve access to palliative care.

Overview

Latin America corresponds to 15% of the land area on the earth's surface (19,197.0 km^2)[1] with a population of approximately 581 million in 2012.[2] There are huge differences between the countries regarding size, political history, and geography as well as a vast social, ethnic, and demographic diversity. This chapter focuses on 18 Spanish-speaking countries and one Portuguese-speaking country (Brazil) (countries included are Argentina, Bolivia, Brazil, Chile, Colombia, Costa Rica, Cuba, Dominican Republic, Ecuador, El Salvador, Guatemala, Honduras, Mexico, Nicaragua, Panama, Paraguay, Peru, Uruguay, and Venezuela).

As with other regions in the world, Latin America is undergoing a demographic and epidemiological transition. The population is aging and the prevalence of chronic diseases represents this trend, including the need for palliative care. The beginning of palliative care in Latin America was relatively isolated and carried out by pioneers motivated by experts in Europe and North America.[3] Its origin can be traced back to the 1980s, when teams from Colombia and Argentina started to work in inpatient and outpatient services, respectively. At the end of the decade there were already six countries with some form of palliative care service.[4] Currently all countries in Latin America have some form of palliative care with more in development.

Palliative care policy in Latin America

There are national palliative care laws in only three countries (Chile, Colombia, and Mexico) and national plans/programs in seven countries (two countries are still in the implementation stage).[4] Following the global trend, the initial palliative care models of care were linked to cancer programs or pain clinics (usually run by anesthesiologists).[4] This fact has on the one hand favored the growth of palliative care, but on the other hand it has limited the development of palliative care as an independent discipline and hindered the provision of palliative care for patients with conditions other than cancer.[5] The access to palliative care service and medications is dependent on geographic location (most are located in large urban centers) and income category, reflected in the insurance system and affordability of medicines.[4]

Adequate opioid availability

The consumption of opioids in Latin America is 4.8 morphine equivalent (ME) mg per capita, far below the world average (58.11 ME mg), with Argentina, Brazil, and Chile having the highest consumption with over 10 mg per capita.[6] The limited collaboration in some countries among those who prescribe and those who regulate opioids is an important contributing factor in these low doses.[4] Other factors are the limited availability and, particularly, cost issues[7]; however, recently there have been important improvements in access to these medication.[8]

Models of care provision

According to the Palliative Care Atlas, Latin America has a total of 922 palliative care services (1.63 services per million people), ranging from 0.024 services per million in Honduras to 14.65 per million in Costa Rica. Almost half (46%) of the existing services in the region are located in Argentina and Chile, which account for 10% of the population[4] (see Figure 75.1).

Forty-three percent of the services in the region are located exclusively at secondary- and tertiary-level hospitals (WHO classification of levels of service is applied [primary, secondary, and tertiary] in this review), where the support team is the most frequent model of palliative care. This type is common in Argentina, with 80 teams. Almost 80% of the countries have two or less support teams. Eighty-four percent of the countries have two or less palliative care services working

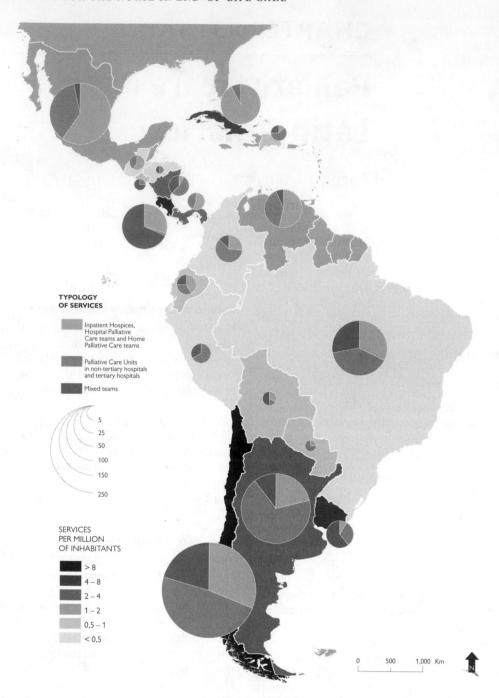

TYPOLOGY OF SERVICES

Inpatient Hospices, Hospital Palliative Care teams and Home Palliative Care teams

Palliative Care Units in non-tertiary hospitals and tertiary hospitals

Mixed teams

5
25
50
100
150
250

SERVICES PER MILLION OF INHABITANTS

> 8
4 – 8
2 – 4
1 – 2
0,5 – 1
< 0,5

0   500   1,000 Km

N

Figure 75.1 Palliative care services in Latin America.[9]

exclusively in secondary-level hospitals. Chile and Argentina have the majority of services in tertiary-level hospitals, while 42% have two or less palliative care services working at this level.[4]

Approximately one-third of the services in Latin America are provided only at the primary level, home care teams being the most frequent type. Six countries have no hospices, eight do not have home care teams, and 13 do not have palliative care service at community centers (multilevel teams are excluded).[4]

The provision of palliative care is often carried out by teams working at the tertiary level who also work in primary care centers; these "multilevel services" account for 20% of all services of the region in this category. This mixed form is most frequent in

Costa Rica, Uruguay, and Chile; three-fourths of the countries have at least two multilevel services.[4]

Most of the services are tailored to the adult population, while a few programs exist for pediatric patients.[10] The qualification of the teams is heterogeneous. While some teams have experienced qualified palliative care specialists, others have completed short seminars and/or online training courses.[4]

Education in palliative care

Education regarding palliative care has been concentrated predominantly on medical personnel. It is estimated that fewer than 15% of physicians working in palliative care received any palliative care–specific education and training during their undergraduate years.[11]

The number of palliative care teachers is very limited. The regional average is 14 teachers per country and totals range from 0 (Bolivia and Honduras) to 45 (Mexico). The number of nonmedical teachers is much lower (1.5 regional average).[4]

In only 10 countries are there postgraduate courses, mostly for physicians.[4] In these countries palliative care is also accredited as a specialty/subspecialty (four countries) or certificate (six countries). Exceptions are Chile, where palliative care is recognized, without any active courses, and Paraguay, which has a postgraduate course but no accreditation. Argentina is the only country with accreditation for palliative care nursing, since 2010.[4]

Research groups are located in 42% of the countries; however, their contribution to palliative care research in the region has been scarce. As of 2011, a total of 106 original papers from Latin America and the Caribbean had been published. Authors from only 10 countries of 45 had published papers in peer-reviewed journals, and of these, more than half were from Brazil.[12]

Eleven countries in the region have at least one palliative care association. In 2001 the Latin American Association for Palliative Care (ALCP, for its name in Spanish) was founded to support the development of palliative care in the region.[13]

Chile

This section discusses the professional development of nursing in Chile. It focuses on four areas: clinical, management, education, and research highlighting nursing's relationship with palliative care.

Chile is a long and narrow country that stretches between the Los Andes Mountain Range and the Pacific Ocean to the southeast of South America. It has several special geographic features as it has territory in Polynesia with the Easter Islands, in the Antarctic, and in the South American continent. In 2010, Chile had a population of 17.1 million inhabitants, with an index poverty of 11.5% and with 36% of the population categorized as indigent. Ninety-eight percent of the population is literate and projected life span is 78.8 years; both are indicators of strong socioeconomic and health levels within the region.[14] These demographic changes have led to a progressive decrease in the birth rate, with an increase in both birth rate and survival, all generating a population pyramid with an increase in the number of aged and a proportional decrease in the number of young people to care for these older Chileans.[15] The problems and challenges related to the gradual aging of the population include a considerable increase in the prevalence of chronic illnesses and an increased number of ill elderly people who are living longer and demand the use of palliative care, not only those with cancer but also those with other life-threatening illnesses.[16]

Nursing in Chile

The first course in nursing in Chile was given in 1902, in the Children's Hospital Roberto del Río. The first School of Nursing at the University of Chile, the first in Latin America, was founded in 1906.[17] The School of Sanitary Nursing began in 1927. In 1938 the Association of University Nurses of Chile was started. The College of Nurses of Chile with public rights was founded, and in 1963 the Chilean Society of Education in Nursing was convened.[18–20]

Legally, the profession of nursing was incorporated through the reform of article 113 of the Sanitary Code in 1997. "The professional services of nurses include care management in regard of promotion, maintenance and restoration of health and illnesses or injuries."[21] The next sections describe palliative care nursing in Chile through characterization of nursing's role in its four areas of development.

Palliative care in Chile

Halfway through the 1990s palliative care arrived in Latin America, including Chile. In 1994 the National Program of Relief of Pain Due to Terminal Cancer and Palliative Care was created, within the auspices of the Explicit Guarantees in Health; since the year 2005 the program has aimed to improve the quality of life of those with cancer, mainly through the improvement of the management of pain, in different centers of public assistance.[22]

Palliative care nursing in Chile

Within the team, nursing has an important role, as the nurse is the clinician who spends the most time at the bedside. Nurses provide support to people by addressing basic needs to obtain the highest degree of well-being and quality of life. Palliative care nursing includes providing care to patients and their families in the face of advancing illness. Therefore, nurses, together with the team, work to help patients and families adjust to the reality of advanced illness; to relieve symptoms; to communicate well with the patient, family, and other team members; and to collaborate with the other professionals who might be involved.[23]

According to the Chilean Health Ministry, the main aims for nurses working with patient-family unit are

- To educate about the patient/family present situation, treatments, daily care.
- To maintain and improve of the patient's quality of life.
- To preserve the autonomy of the patient.
- To prevent adverse effects that may occur from the analgesics or other treatments implemented for the control of pain and other symptoms.
- To identify early risk factors for symptoms or other complications of cancer and other life-threatening illnesses.
- To facilitate the auto-administration of simple techniques of relaxation to favor the rest during sleep and the activity during the vigil.
- To favor the healthy family dynamics.

(Adapted from *Management of the Administrative Role of Nursing in Palliative Care*.)

The administrative area refers not only to the positions of leadership held by the professional nurse in the palliative care team but also, at the secondary level, to a nurse coordinating the service of relief of pain and palliative care, or at the primary level, to a person in charge of the plan of care for patients in the home. This task is characterized as performing the following objectives:

- Providing and coordinating resources.
- Implementing systems of registration and interprofessional communications.
- Coordinating the interventions of the interdisciplinary team.
- Supervising the interventions and therapeutic treatments, as well as the quality of the care.

Palliative care nursing in Chile: direct care

The direct service provided by nursing depends on the level of care where service is provided as well as the position held by the nurse. Chile has numerous levels of palliative care:

Primary care of health: 3 residential hospices and 83 teams of exclusive home services.

Secondary level: 32 palliative care services that operate in centers of the secondary level.

Tertiary level: 28 palliative care units that operate exclusively in hospitals of the tertiary level.

Multilevel: 57 services with multilevel teams (56 in the public area)

Team of hospital support: 74 exclusive teams of hospital support.

Palliative care nursing in Chile: education

Nurses in Chile educate patients and families as well as colleagues. The National Program of Relief of Pain Due to Cancer and Palliative Care has established the importance of teaching about subcutaneous or parenteral hydration and drug delivery and administration of home oxygen, as well as other assessment, treatment, safety, and hygiene topics.[24,25]

Palliative care is included at several levels of professional nursing education:

Pregraduate: In at least 12 of the 21 faculties of medicine, palliative care is included in the curriculum as courses or as an isolated class.

Postgraduate: The official university accreditation in palliative care existed from 2006 to 2009 given by a private university in agreement with the Ministry of Health. Since 2000, the Ministry of Health has a plan for training the primary, emergency, and secondary service teams. There is also binational training in Spain and Chile. Some universities offer rotations for residents of internal medicine in the palliative care program and intensive courses of palliative medicine to physicians and other professionals.

Teachers: There are 30 teachers for the palliative care curricula in faculties of medicine and more than 40 teachers for nonmedical faculties.

Palliative care nursing in Chile: research

Nursing, the official journal of the College of Nurses of Chile, was first published in 1965 and continues today. Since 1990 the Pontifical Catholic University of Chile has edited the scientific magazine *Horizon of Nursing*, and in 1995 the University of Concepción began publishing the journal *Science and Nursing*.[26,27] In 1968 the Scientific Societies of Nursing was formed; nurses play an active role in the numerous national and international societies. These include the Chilean Association of Palliative Medicine (SOCHIMEDPAL), which is in the process of formation and in assessing its dependence on the Society of Cancerology or on the Chilean Association for the Study of Pain.

National program of relief of pain and palliative care in Chile

Regarding the development of this program, the Technical Report of 2009 reported developments in three areas:

- The program achieved a reduction in the prevalence of pain (associated with an improvement in quality of life) in terminally ill patients; in 2000, 80% were admitted with pain rated as moderate to severe, compared with 34.5% in 2009. Also, among the dying, the prevalence of moderate to severe pain decreased from 39.8% in 2000 to 16% in 2009.

- From 1999 to 2009, the percentage of patients who died at home with palliative care increased from 55% to 96%.

- The therapeutic consumption of morphine has gradually increased.

Colombia

In Colombia, nursing is recognized as a profession that cares for the person, the family, and the community. The profession addresses sociocultural characteristics, needs, and rights, as well as the physical and social environment that influences health and welfare. State organizations that provide guidance include the National Association of Nurses of Colombia, the Colombian Association of Faculties of Nursing, the National Ethical Tribunal of Nursing, and the National Technical Council of Nursing, a permanent organization that provides advice and consultancy to the national government and to nursing organizations with regard to the policies and practice of the nursing profession within Colombia.

Nurses have historically been involved in many settings of care, including hospitals, public health care, and primary care. Nursing has contributed to the management and assurance of the individual and society's health through direct care as well as formulation of public policies within health ministries and through nongovernmental work.[28] Nursing has traditionally been involved in the care of persons with terminal illness, and therefore, has been intimately involved in the development of palliative care in Colombia.

Palliative care in Colombia

Palliative care started in Colombia in the 1980s with the creation of the first Unit of Pain, in the University of Antioquia. Services for the care of the terminally ill subsequently developed to control symptoms common in the advanced stages of the illness. Demographic changes in Colombia include greater longevity, with an increase in chronic conditions requiring end-of-life care. In Colombia, the development of palliative care has been strongly linked to the field of oncology, where significant results have been obtained with the implementation of the National Policy for the Control of Cancer. Oncological illnesses are the third leading cause of death, with a high prevalence of breast, cervical, esophageal, and stomach tumors, which are often diagnosed at later stages.[29]

The development of palliative care nursing in Colombia

Colombia initiated several regulations to enhance palliative care, which, combined with the existing legal regulations for the practice of nursing, make up the legal framework for the practice of palliative care.

Law 1384 of 2010 (the Sandra Ceballos Law) explicitly guarantees palliative care as part of the integral management of patients with cancer and their families in Colombia. This law states that palliative care is directed at the improvement of quality of life of the patient and survivors of cancer and their caregivers, ensuring the provision of palliative care and relief of pain at the different settings of care, and ensures access to and availability of opioids in the country.[30]

On May 6, 2013, this law was modified by Resolution 1419 of the Ministry of Social Protection; this established conditions for the organization and integral management of the networks of cancer care services, guaranteeing quality care for all persons with cancer in all the stages of the disease. Likewise, there is currently a revision of the bill in the House of Representatives of Congress of the Republic that seeks to regulate the rights of persons with chronic, degenerative, and irreversible illnesses to receive palliative care, and to allow individuals to decline extraordinary therapeutic procedures that do not fulfill the principles of therapeutic proportionality and improvement of quality of life.

Within the existing regulations regarding palliative care, the importance of the practice of nursing is recognized. For example, Article eight of the Sandra Ceballos Law recognizes the need to train nurses in palliative care and describes the type of care provided by nurses. The law supports the implementation of training measures for nurses to improve the delivery of palliative care for those with life-threatening illnesses.

On December 28, 2011, Agreement 029 of the Regulating Committee of Health updated the Colombian Health Compulsory Plan to support diagnosis of and treatment for illnesses seen in palliative care for the health of members of the General System of Social Security.[31] The same administrative act authorizes the inclusion of alternative and supplementary therapies by institutions that provide health services, which are part of the network of Entities that Promote Health, and emphasizes the need to see patients with terminal illness who are experiencing pain or impaired function and provide interventions and psychological care to support the patient and family.

Nurses have been recognized as crucial members of healthcare teams. This importance is supported by Law 911 of 2004, which dictates regulations regarding practice of the nursing profession in Colombia, establishing principles for the development of practice, teaching, and research regarding the different stages of the life cycle and the precise moment of death.[32]

Palliative care nursing education in Colombia

There are many programs to train nurses regarding curative treatment of illness and physical recovery, but only a few programs are directed to the treatment and care of persons with terminal illnesses. At the present time, the Colombian Association of Faculties of Nursing (ACOFAEN) has 36 members, located throughout the country, who are developing a curriculum to address the needs of patients with a terminal stage of illness.[33]

A plan of development for 2009–2018 established by the ACOFAEN, along with outlines set forth by the National Ethical Tribunal of Nursing, states that the training of professional nurses must begin during pregraduate courses to facilitate the integral understanding of palliative care and its application. This training should include care of the person with cancer and of those with dementia and Alzheimer's disease, as well as end-stage heart and renal disease.

At the present time, because few programs are available, nurses often attend sessions developed for physicians—internal medicine, neurology, pain medicine, or oncology—relying on academic programs of specialization that train professionals to offer medical care to patients with oncological illness. In Colombia, the first postgraduate programs to include palliative care nursing in their curricula have focused on the care of the person with cancer. Currently there are three programs of disciplinary specialization (two in the city of Medellín and one in Bogotá) in this field. Likewise, there are university institutions that offer programs at a specialization level in palliative care that are interdisciplinary (patients, social workers, and psychologists) and programs of continuing education for graduates with an average of 120 hours of instruction. At the present time, a master's degree in palliative care nursing is being developed to provide a curriculum that guarantees suitable professionals with excellent academic quality.

In Colombia the provision of health services is organized by levels: the first level is primary care, with a focus on promotion of health and prevention of illness; the second level includes hospitalization and outside consultation of medium complexity; and the third level is directed at specialized services of high complexity. At the present time, palliative care is found at all levels of care, including programs devoted to home care and hospices.

At the present time, palliative care services are available in 13 institutions of care; however, nursing participation is found in only three of them. Regarding the location of these services, 38% are in Bogotá D.C., 30% are in Medellín, 23% are in the city of Cali, and 7% in the city of Pasto, with little access to palliative care in intermediate cities.

The first level of care has 63 programs of home care for the patient who, due to his or her functional condition, cannot be cared for in an ambulatory program. Nursing personnel play key roles in the coordination and provision of this kind of care.

Care of palliative care patients may be provided by assistants under the supervision of nursing professionals. This care may include activities of daily living and instrumental tasks, particularly when the patient has reduced function or the family caregiver is unable to assume this care.

Nursing research in palliative care

The National System of Science and Technology of Colombia is organized through the state agency Colciencias, which is in charge of management of the data derived from research conducted within the country. Currently there are 22 research groups associated with nursing care, and 3 of these are research groups investigating care of the chronically ill patient, oncological nursing, and care at the end of life.

It is important to acknowledge the work carried out in research on family caretakers, including characterization of this phenomenon as well as an intervention called Taking Care of the Caretaker. This program has been recognized nationally and regionally for its contribution to decreasing family/caregiver burden.

For palliative care nursing to develop as a field in Colombia, several developments are needed.

◆ Programs of palliative care must be included at the level of primary care in health, incorporating nurses with specialized training into this field. This will guarantee control of symptoms, training of family caretakers, and monitoring of opioids and medications of special control. Palliative care programs must be developed at the master's and doctorate levels.

- Publication of experiences from the provision of services and of research in palliative care nursing needs to be promoted, and practices that foster professional development need to be described.

- To consolidate the nursing chapter of the Colombian Association of Palliative Care, participation of the profession in the formulation of public policies needs to be improved.

Mexico

Mexico is the 11th most populated country in the world, with more than 112 million people. The states with the greatest number of inhabitants are the State of Mexico (15,175,862), the Federal District (8,851,080), and Veracruz de Ignacio de la Llave (7,643,194). The least populated states are Baja California Sur (637,026), Colima (650,555), and Campeche (822,441). During the last 60 years, Mexico's population has grown five times, from 25.8 million people in 1950 to the current population of more than 112 million, representing a yearly growth rate of 1%.[34]

Mexico has made great strides in education in the last 20 years. In 2004 general literacy was 92% and youth literacy ages (15–24) was 96%. Primary and secondary education is free and compulsory throughout the country according to Mexican law. Bilingual programs have been established, and some indigenous communities also have intercultural education. Mexico was one of the first countries taking the lead during the 1970s in establishing a system of distance education in the secondary schools of rural communities. In 2005 this system counted more than 30,000 connected schools with 1 million students receiving this education program through videoconferences and teleconferences transmitted via satellite. These schools are known in Mexico as "telesecundarias." This system is also used in some countries of Central America and Colombia, as well as in the southern parts of United States, as a teaching method for bilingual education.

Palliative care in Mexico

The first state to initiate the beginning of palliative care was Jalisco, Mexico. In February, 2013; changes to the federal law covering pain and palliative care were realized by the secretary of health, Dr. Alfonso Paterson Fara, with hospice coordination by Hospice Cristina.[35] The history of this achievement is important to describe.

At the end of his term in 2006, Senator Felipe Vicencio Alvarez of Jalisco introduced a bill for general health on palliative care; in April 2007 Senator Lazaro Mazon Alonso introduced a controversial initiative that proposed to modify the codes of criminal law and decriminalize assisted suicide, as well as a general law of voluntary termination of curative treatment allowing ample opportunity for euthanasia. A week later, Deputy Jorge Quintero Belo took up the issues raised by Senator Philip Vicencio, again proposing reforms to the palliative care initiative, which opened the door to advancing palliative care.

This took 6 months, and in October of the same year (2007) Senators Teresa Ortuno Gurza and Judith Delgado Diaz introduced another initiative to the Health Act to guarantee the rights of the terminally ill, which became a pivotal issue of controversy in opposition to previous proposals. In November 2007, a month after the previous initiatives, Senator Federico Doring Cesar carried a bill to the tribunal attempting to decriminalize active euthanasia, but this was not passed into the General Health Law.

By January 2008 the president of the Senate Health Commission, Ernesto Saro Boarman, extended an invitation to attend a general meeting in Mexico City to discuss palliative care. Dr. Susana Lua Nava of Bioethics, Dr. Bistre Goen, and his assistant Beatriz Montes de Oca participated.[36] After the meeting, the Senator was fully impressed regarding pain and palliative care, promising that during his office he would try to include them in the health system. Later that month, Deputy Ector Jaime Ramirez Barba presented an integration of the major elements of each aforementioned initiative, with the participation of Senator Ernesto Saro Boarman, Guillermo Tamborrel Suarez, and Deputy Samuel Aguilar Solis. And on September 3, 2008, Senator Teresa Ortuno Gurza introduced the 16th of October as National Observance day of Palliative Care, which was approved by the Chamber. After considerable lobbying by various fronts, the Reforms to the General Health Laws relating to Palliative Medicine were published in the official Federal Journal of General Health Law Reform on January 5, 2009.

In 2009, the Ministry of Health introduced the "OFFSET" program to four or five states, coordinated by Health Control, led by Dr. Guadalupe Perez Cabello. In each of these states round tables with experts from the pain and palliative care field were gathered to achieve the following goals:

1. List the different palliative care programs that exist in Mexico.

2. Create working groups of experts in palliative care.

3. Create a charter for the working group.

4. Develop outlines and clinical guidelines for management throughout the republic.

5. Support and advise existing palliative care groups and encourage the creation of new programs in the various health units.

On January 15, 2010, the second congregation of Experts on Palliative Care was held, and a constitutional act was finally signed. A directory was published of all of the centers offering palliative care. Unfortunately, after this date no mention was made of the work developed by the working groups, and no one knew what had transpired. It is disheartening to have seen this law abandoned years after having been approved. The universities, notwithstanding the fact that it is a requirement under the law to introduce palliative care as part of undergraduate medical training, as well as within schools of nursing and social work, have not been included in these schools.

Palliative care nursing in Mexico

Nurses obtain training through two different educational tracts: a professional degree that requires 3 years of study and a dissertation followed by a professional examination (accounting for less than 10% of all nurses), or a program that includes 2 years of study and 6 months of service resulting in the designation of general nurse (less than 20% of nurses). Nursing assistants have 1 year of study with 500 hours of service and they account for 70% of all nurses.

There are numerous challenges facing nurses in Mexico. Salaries are very low, requiring many nurses to work overtime to be able to provide for their families. Nurses are often not recognized as professionals, either by medical colleagues or by the public. Challenges also exist for palliative care nursing. Few universities offer courses on palliative care within basic nursing programs, and continuing education courses are limited.

Palliative nursing is a young profession in Mexico. Dedicated nurses with knowledge, skill, and vision for the future will help advance the field in Mexico to benefit citizens of this dynamic country.

Conclusion

Despite important efforts being made in different Latin American countries to improve access to palliative care, palliative care is far from accessible and affordable to the population that could benefit from this care. The development is focused mostly in the medical sector. Palliative nursing care is further underdeveloped, being isolated to a few countries such as Argentina and Cuba, where there is a strong interest in training and/or accreditation.

The challenge for palliative care in Latin America is to develop a model of care appropriate to the sociocultural context and integrated to public health including suitable policies, education, and implementation of palliative care programs to all levels of society.

References

1. World Bank. World Development Indicators: Rural Environment and Land Use. 2013. http://wdi.worldbank.org/table/3.1 Accessed September 10, 2013.
2. World Bank. Latin America and Caribbean. 2011. http://data.worldbank.org/region/latin-america-and-caribbean. Accessed September 10, 2013.
3. Bruera E. Palliative care in Latin America. J Pain Symptom Manage.1993;8(6):365–368.
4. Pastrana T, De Lima L, Wenk R, et al. Atlas de Cuidados Paliativos de Latinoamérica. 1st ed. Houston: IAHPC Press; 2012.
5. Pastrana T, Eisenchlas J, Centeno C, De Lima L. Status of palliative care in Latin America: looking through the Latin America Atlas of Palliative Care. Curr Opin Support Palliat Care. 2013;7(4):411–416
6. Pain and Policy Studies Group. Opioid Consumption Data. 2010. http://www.painpolicy.wisc.edu/opioid-consumption-data. Accessed September 16, 2013.
7. Wenk R, Bertolino M, De Lima L. Analgésicos opioides en Latinoamérica: la barrera de accesibilidad supera la de disponibilidad. Medicina Paliativa. 2004;11(3):148–151.
8. Leon MX, De Lima L, Florez S, et al. Improving availability of and access to opioids in Colombia: description and preliminary results of an action plan for the country. J Pain Symptom Manage. 2009;38(5):758–766.
9. Pastrana T, De Lima L, Pons J, Centeno C. Edición Cartográfica del Atlas de Cuidados Paliativos en Latinoamérica. Houston: IAHPC; 2013.
10. Varela AMS, Dussel V, Barfield R, Bidegain M, De Lima L, Dellon E. Perceived resources and barriers to pediatric palliative care among healthcare practitioners attending the V Latin American palliative care association (ALCP) meeting (755). J Pain Symptom Manage. 2011;41(1):306.
11. Wenk R, Bertolino M. Palliative care development in South America: a focus on Argentina. J Pain Symptom Manage. 2007;33(5):645–650.
12. Pastrana T, De Lima L, Eisenchlas J, Wenk R. Palliative care research in Latin America and the Caribbean: from the beginning to the Declaration of Venice and beyond. J Palliat Med. 2012;15(3):352–358.
13. Eisenchlas J, Monti C. Development of the Latin America association for palliative care. Prog Palliat Care. 2012;20(4):227–229.
14. The Official Travel Guide to Chile. Where We Are. 2013. http://www.chile.travel/es/acercade-chile/donde-estamos.html. Accessed June 20, 2013.
15. Panamerican Organization of Health. Health in Chile 2010. Outlook of the Situation of Health and the System of Health in Chile. Santiago, Chile: 2011. http://www.pano.org/chi/images/PDFs/salud%20chile%202010.pdf.
16. Pastrana T, De Lima L, Wenk R, Eisenchlas J, Monti C, Rocafort J, et al. Atlas de Palliative Care in Latin America Chile. Houston: IAHPC Press; 2012. http://cuidadospaliativos.org/uploads/2012/10/atlas/07_Chile.pdf.
17. Muñoz, Mendoza CL, Isla Lund X, Alarcón Sanhueza S. Historical evolution and professional development of nursing in Chile. Cult. Los Cuid. Año III N 5 1 Semester. 1991:45–51. http://193.145.233.67/dspace/handle/10045/5184. Accessed April 21, 2013.
18. College of Nurses of Chile. History. http://www.colegiodeenfermeras.cl/historia.html. Accessed June 2, 2013.
19. Martín FH, del Gallego Lastra R, González SA, Ruiz JMG. Nursing in history: analysis from the professional perspective. Cult Los Cuid Rev Nursing Humanities. 1997;(2):21–35. http://rua.ua.es/dspace/bitstream/10045/5239/1/CC_02_05.pdf.
20. University of Chile School of Nursing. History. http://enfermeria.med.uchile.cl/School.html. Accessed June 2, 2013.
21. Ministry of Public Health (CL). Sanitary Code of the Republic of Chile of December 16, 1997: Article 113, regulates the professional practice of the Nurse. Santiago (CL): MINSAL; 1997.
22. Del Río PMI, Palma A. Palliative care: history and development. Bulletin Esc Med Pontif. Catholic University Chile. 2007;32(1):16–22. http://escuela.med.puc.cl/publ/boletin/20071/CuidadosPaliativos.pdf.
23. Junin M. Rol of Nursing in Palliative Care. First Virtual Symposium of Pain, Palliative Medicine and Advances in Pharmacology of Pain. Argentina; 2001.
24. Ministry of Health. Rule National Program of Relief of Pain due to Cancer and Palliative Care. 5th ed. Santiago, MINSAL; 2009.
25. Ministry of Health. Clinic Guide AUGE: Relief of Pain due to Advanced Cancer and Palliative Care. Santiago, MINSAL; 2011.
26. Pontificial Catholic University of Chile: School of Nursing. Horizon of Nursing. 2010. http://revistahorizonte.uc.cl/. Accessed June 2, 2013.
27. Editorial University of Conception. Science and Nursing. http://www2.udec.cl/~webpubl/enfermeria/index.html. Accessed June 2, 2013.
28. Gómez C. The professionalization of nursing in Colombia. In: The Art and the Science of the Care. Bogotá: National University of Colombia; 2002.
29. Latin American Association of Palliative Care. Latin American Atlas of Palliative Care. Buenos Aires; 2012. http://cuidadospaliativos.org/uploads/2012/10/atlas/Atlas%20de%20Cuidados%20Paliativos%20en%20Latinoamerica.pdf.
30. Colombia. Congress of the Republic. Law 1384 of 2010, by which the actions for the integral care of cancer in Colombia are regulated. Bogotá; 2010. http://www.secretariasenado.gov.co/senado/basedoc/ley/2010/ley_1384_2010.html.
31. Colombia. Congress of the Republic. Agreement 029, by which the modifications to the Obligatory Plan of Health are established. Bogotá; 2011. http://www.secretariasenado.gov.co/senado/basedoc/ley/2011/ley_1438_2011.html.
32. Colombia. Ministry of Education. Law 911 of 2004, by which the odontological code of the profession of Nursing Colombia and other regulations are regulated. Bogotá; 2004. http://www.mineducacion.gov.co/1621/articles-105034_archivo_pdf.pdf.
33. Colombian Association of Faculties of Nursing. Plan of development Acofaen 2009-2018. Bogotá; 2009. http://acofaen.org.co/.
34. Wikipedia. Demographics of Mexico. 2013. http://wikipedia.org/wiki/Demographics_of_Mexico. Accessed December 2, 2013.
35. Hospice Cristina. A Hand for Help and a Listening Heart. 2009. http://hospicecristinaac.com.mx/. Accessed December 2, 2013.
36. Bistre S. New Legislation on Palliative Care and Pain in Mexico. Pain Palliat Care Pharmacother. 2009;23(4):419–425. doi: 10.3109/15360280903332153.

CHAPTER 76

Palliative care in Africa

Faith N. Mwangi-Powell, Julia Downing, Richard A. Powell, Fatia Kiyange, and Henry Ddungu

Key points

- Originating in Africa 35 years ago, provision of palliative care on the continent has generally been inconsistent, often provided from isolated centers with limited geographic coverage. Recent efforts have centered on governments working closely with these centers to integrate palliative care into mainstream healthcare systems. Despite these advances, there remain countries with no palliative care service provision.

- The primary mode of palliative care service delivery is home-based care. Predominantly dependent on volunteers, this has implications for staff recruitment and retention and the maintenance of an acceptable standard of patient care.

- Pain in Africa is disturbingly undertreated among adults and children, with opioid analgesic consumption remaining extremely low in relation to medical need. There is an emerging trend to alter existing legal provisions to enable other specially trained cadres (e.g., nurses) to prescribe opioids for patients in moderate-to-severe pain.

- Nurses have a pivotal role in palliative care provision on the continent given they are present at all levels of the healthcare system, from the facility to the community.

- Traditionally, children have been neglected by palliative care service development in Africa. Recently there has been an emphasis on developing pediatric services in several countries.

The second-largest continent, stretching across five time zones, Africa covers an area of 30.2 million square kilometers (11.7 million square miles), including its adjacent islands, approximately 20% of the global land area. Its estimated 1,072 million inhabitants, amounting to 15.2% of the world's total population,[1] are distributed across five regions and 54 independent nations, including the newly established South Sudan: Eastern Africa (17 nations); Central Africa (9); Northern Africa (7); Southern Africa (5); Western Africa (16) (Figure 76.1).

In general terms, the vast expanse of the Sahara desert acts as a natural geographic separator between the predominantly Arabic coastal north and the African south. However, there is a rich heterogeneity of ethnic groups (including non-African groups) populating the continent. This diversity is partly indicated by the estimated 1,000 to 2,000 indigenous languages, based around four major linguistic families: the Afro-Asiatic languages; Nilo-Saharan languages; the Niger-Congo languages; and the click consonants-based Khoisan languages. Postcolonial governmental attempts to forge national unity from such linguistic variation have meant that, in many countries, English, French, Portuguese, and Spanish are used for official public discourse.

Political and socioeconomic situation

Following increasing commercial and missionary interest in the "Dark Continent" among mid-19th-century explorers, the territorial "scramble for Africa" occurred in the late 19th century among European powers. With the exception of Liberia and Ethiopia, between 1880 and 1912 colonial nation-states were established across the continent. For many nations, this caused artificial delineation of national boundaries, exerting a socially destabilizing effect. In those countries with numerically significant colonizing populations, however, the effects of the "scramble" were more significant: systems were established that ensured disproportionate political influence to Europeans over indigenous Africans.

Confronted by rising nationalism in the 1950s and 1960s, European powers granted independence to most territories. In the postcolonial 1970s and 1980s, however, many African states were characterized by episodes of sociopolitical instability, corruption, violence, and authoritarian rule. In the late 1980s and early 1990s, some states attempted to initiate democratic reforms. However, this ongoing democratic transition has proven problematic, and the negative political and social narrative persists in stereotyping the continent. Political instability and civil strife have continued to taint some countries; for example, nearly 1 million people were killed in the Rwandan genocide of 1994, while successive wars in the Democratic Republic of the Congo have killed millions.

Economically, despite extensive natural resources (e.g., oil, gold, diamonds), Africa remains an overwhelmingly underdeveloped continent, with the vast majority of its predominantly rural population engaged in cash crop production. Indeed, 37 of the bottom 46 ranked countries (from 142nd to 186th) reported in the 2013 *United Nations' Human Development Report* were African.[2]

Health systems in Africa

Following independence, many African countries sought to address the social inequities of colonization. As such, improving people's well-being by overcoming the discriminatory restrictions underpinning colonial social policy and advancing social development were prioritized.[3] Up to the end of the 1970s many African health systems, as well as education sectors, expanded as a result of centralized funding, with an increase in trained health professionals. Despite this expansion, inequitable access to health services persisted, as did unmet health needs given capacity

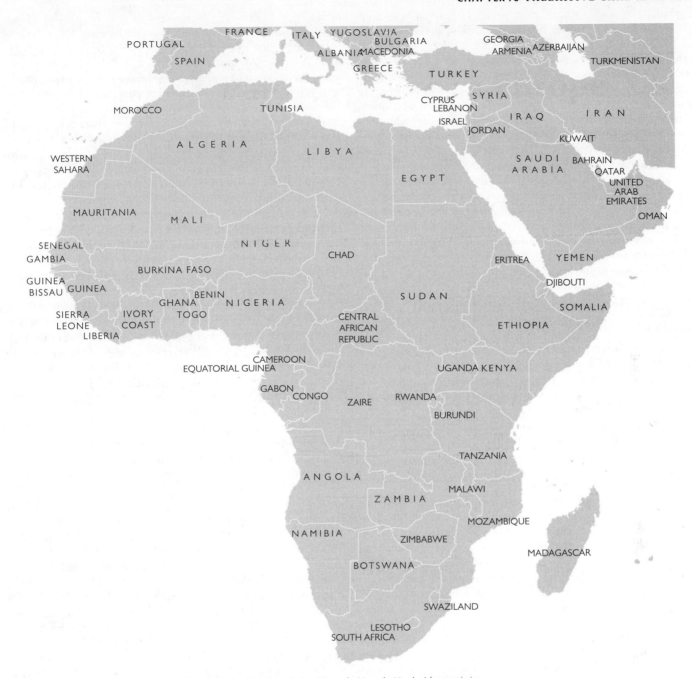

Figure 76.1 Countries of Africa. Source: African Palliative Care Association, Kampala, Uganda. Used with permission.

limitations. Additionally, during this period there was recognition of the qualitative difference in service provision in urban and rural health settings, with the former receiving greater resources. Consequently, primary healthcare systems were introduced in many nations to address this healthcare imbalance, an agenda embodied in the Declaration of Alma-Ata in 1978.[4]

By the 1980s, economic crises across Africa resulted in inequities in health systems reentering public discourse. In response, governmental austerity measures, and externally driven structural adjustment programs, entailed commitments to cost recovery and user charges, as well as the introduction of marketization as the principle determining policy and practice. The diminution of the public sector, compounded by reductions in real income occasioned by repeated currency devaluations, meant that health cadres relocated from the public health sector to more financially rewarding employment, while reduced public funding resulted in deterioration of the physical infrastructure and equipment of public health facilities.

Today, and generally, there are three different types of health systems: the *public system*, which is based around specialist, regional, district and home-based care (HBC) providers, with services provided free to inpatients and outpatients; an *insurance-based system*, which is either based around individual, private contributions or around an employer-related health scheme; and the *private-sector system*, which is for a relatively small percentage of the population with sufficient financial resources.

In most African countries, however, health inequalities and differential service access continue to pose a considerable challenge, with impoverished households excluded from accessing affordable quality healthcare services resorting to self-medicating (sometimes with counterfeit medicines), home-based health-seeking behaviors as a consequence.[3] Health systems across the continent remain weak, with more than 20% of total health expenditure in nearly half of the 46 countries in the WHO African Region provided by external sources.[5] This weakness in part arises from poverty; the overwhelming communicable and noncommunicable disease (NCD) burden; inadequate institutional capacity (e.g., for cancer treatment); inefficient use of potential national expertise; weak coordination of health development partners; frequent and often inconsistent changes in government policies; inadequate legislation; weak accountability and lack of transparency; poor implementation of international agreements and regulations; and a crisis in human health resources.

The historical perspective and current status of palliative care

The disease burden in sub-Saharan Africa is significant. The region remains most severely affected by HIV and AIDS, with nearly 1 in every 20 adults (4.9%) living with HIV, accounting for 69% (23.5 million) of the people living with the disease globally.[6] Some positive trends have been reported latterly, with the number of people dying from AIDS-related causes in the region dropping from 1.3 million in 2009 to 1.2 million in 2011.[7]Additionally, in 2010 there were 259,500 new cases of tuberculosis (TB) and 2.1 million TB-related deaths,[8] with the continent accounting for 80% of all TB cases among people living with HIV.[8]

Cancer is an emerging public health problem regionally.[9] In 2008, there were 542,000 cancer-related deaths and 715,000 new cancer cases, projected to nearly double (970,000 deaths and 1.28 million new cases) by 2030;[10] 36% of cancers are infection related, twice the global average.[11] Furthermore, with expectations of projected increases in NCDs caused by demographic and epidemiological transitions, evidence exists of a rising burden of chronic diseases (such as hypertension and diabetes) in countries like Cameroon[12] and South Africa.[13]

The development of palliative care in Africa originated 35 years ago, when Island Hospice was founded in Harare, Zimbabwe, in May 1979.[14] Many of its pioneer services were advanced by highly motivated individuals with minimal financial resources. Today, although provision of palliative care on the continent is inconsistent, often provided from isolated centers rather than integrated into the mainstream healthcare system, there are signs of positive developments.[15,16] For example, a survey of hospice and palliative care services on the continent in 2006 found not only that 44.7% (21 of 47) of African countries had no identified hospice or palliative care activity but also that only 8.5% (n = 4) could be classified as having services approaching some measure of integration with mainstream service providers,[14] while this number was even lower for children's services, with 81% of surveyed countries having no identified palliative care activity.[17] In contrast, a follow-up review of developments undertaken by the World Palliative Care Alliance in 2011 revealed that sub-Saharan Africa has shown the most notable changes in service development, with nine countries moving from group 1/2 (no known activity/capacity building) to group 3a (isolated provision).[18] This development was primarily attributed to the work of the African Palliative Care Association (APCA), a pan-African organization established in 2004 to promote the scale-up of palliative care across the continent. Recent efforts have centered on governments working closely with established care centers to integrate palliative care into governmental health services. However, despite advances, there are still some countries without any palliative care service provision.

Historically, and despite reported need among care providers, the evidence base underpinning much of palliative care service provision has been inadequate.[19] Indeed, although donor demands (primarily led by the President's Emergency Plan for AIDS Relief [PEPFAR]) for the proven impact of funded projects impelled monitoring and evaluation onto the African palliative care agenda, palliative care research remains relatively formative,[20] despite some positive advances (e.g., the number of publications on palliative care in Africa has increased from 9 prior to 1990, to 82 between 2006 and 2010).[16]

Responding to this need, the APCA established the African Palliative Care Research Network (APCRN), whose mandate is to support the development of evidence for palliative care through research and research skills transfer to inform the discipline's further development.[21] With regional hubs in Eastern, Western, Northern and Southern Africa, linked to academic centers in Europe and North America, the work of APCRN will be vital in addressing the current evidence gap.

The obstacles to undertaking research in Africa include limited palliative care research skills and the resources to undertake it, as well as researchers operating in isolation from a community of like-minded peers in often unsupportive work environments.[22] The APCRN aims to overcome these challenges and build a methodologically strong evidence base for palliative care on the continent. Part of its early work has been the development of a region-wide, prioritized research agenda.[23] This infrastructure has been augmented by linking the network to the European Association of Palliative Care's Task Force on Palliative Care in Africa.

Part of the APCRN includes established academic centers like Makerere University, in Uganda, and the University of Cape Town, in South Africa, with both organizations running formal courses and workshops on research methods, as well as engaging in research itself. Research conducted to date by these and other bodies across the continent is diverse, ranging from the physical, including the multidimensional nature of the disease burden and its correlates,[24–27] to the spiritual domains of patients' experiences,[28,29] to their information and communication preferences[30] and needs in the dying process,[31,32] from the role of traditional healers in identifying the care needs and cultural practices of patients[33] to the roles of volunteers in service provision[34,35] and including methodological research to develop age- and culture-appropriate, validated patient-level outcome tools.[36,37]

Research into children's palliative care across the region has, however, been minimal, with an appraisal of the evidence showing just five papers published in peer-reviewed journals.[38] Research is urgently needed to provide evidence for children's palliative care.[39] The International Children's Palliative Care Network (ICPCN) is therefore currently working in collaboration with other stakeholders (such as APCA, UNICEF and the Foundation for Hospices in sub-Saharan Africa) to develop this evidence base.

Studies underway include a Delphi study to identify research priorities, a three-country study to quantify the need for children's palliative care, and an evaluation of what makes children's palliative care services successful.

The public health approach to palliative care in Africa

Based on earlier guidance to national governments, the World Health Organization (WHO) recently revealed an enhanced model of palliative care provision. For the public health approach—which is population and risk-factor oriented rather than symptom- or disease-oriented—to work, it must be founded on appropriate government policies, adequate drug availability, the education of health professionals, and implementation of palliative care at all levels (see Figure 76.2) and must be integrated into national healthcare systems.[40] Additionally, while it is not included within the enhanced model of palliative care provision, there has been a call for research to be recognized as the fifth pillar of the model in order to stimulate further improvements in care.[41]

Government policy

The adoption and promotion by government of appropriate health policies is the cornerstone of an effective healthcare system. These include a national health policy, an essential medicines policy, and education policies.

National health policy

The failure of the Declaration of Alma-Ata (1978), which formally adopted primary healthcare as the means for bringing comprehensive, universal, equitable, and affordable healthcare services closer to people, and the Bamako Initiative (1987), among others, to improve access and quality of healthcare in Africa, was ultimately replaced by the United Nations' Millennium Development Declaration and its eight Millennium Development Goals

(MDGs) to be realized by 2015: (1) eradicate extreme poverty and hunger; (2) achieve universal primary education; (3) promote gender equality and empower women; (4) reduce child mortality; (5) improve maternal health; (6) combat HIV/AIDS, malaria, and other diseases; (7) ensure environmental sustainability; and (8) develop a global partnership for development.[42] This declaration has been underpinned by a plethora of funding initiatives—not least being the Global Fund against AIDS, TB, and Malaria, the US President's Malaria Initiative, and PEPFAR—resulting in new rounds of national health policies and strategic plans in the health sector or revision of existing ones.

The MDG framework has helped galvanize development efforts and guide global and national development priorities since 2000. While three of the eight goals have been achieved prior to the 2015 deadline, progress has been uneven within and across countries and, to date, Africa has been one of the regions struggling to meet the health-related MDGs. As the world approaches 2015, work has been initiated on advancing the global development agenda beyond that date, providing further opportunities for advocating for palliative care under the universal health coverage agenda.[43] The year 2011 also provided policy opportunities for addressing the burden of NCDs, with a UN High Level Summit on their prevention and control producing a political declaration with palliative care included as a core response, together with an agreed indicator in the monitoring and evaluation framework of the resulting Global NCD Action Plan.[44,45]

However, a review of the extent of integration of palliative care into health systems showed that out of 54 African countries, only 7 have palliative care incorporated into either their health or cancer strategic plans (Democratic Republic of the Congo, Kenya, Mauritius, Namibia, South Africa, Tanzania, and Uganda), while only three (Mozambique, Rwanda, and Swaziland) have developed stand-alone national palliative care policies.[46] Some countries, such as Malawi, are implementing national palliative care guidelines while others (Botswana, Ethiopia, Nigeria, Zambia,

Policy
• Palliative care part of national health plan,
policies, related regulations
• Funding/service delivery models support palliative care delivery
• Essential medicines
(Policy makers, regulators, WHO, NGOs)

Drug Availability
• Opioids, essential
medicines
• Importation quota
• Cost
• Prescribing
• Distribution
• Dispensing
• Administration

(Pharmacists, drug
regulators, law
enforcement agents)

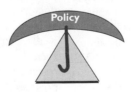

Policy

Implementation
• Opinion leaders
• Trained manpower
• Strategic & business
plans – resources,
infrastructure
• Standards, guidelines
measures
(Community & clinical leaders,
administrators)

Education
• Media & public
advocacy
• Curricula, courses—
—professionals,
trainees
• Expert training
• Family caregiver
training & support

(Media & public,
healthcare providers &
trainees, palliative care
experts, family caregivers)

Figure 76.2 Enhanced WHO public health model. Source: Reprinted from Sternsward et al. (2007), reference 40, with permission from Elsevier.

and Zimbabwe) are drafting policies, strategies, and guidelines. As such, nongovernmental, faith, or community-based organizations with no inherent financial sustainability remain key players in the provision of palliative care services on the continent.[47]

Essential medicines policy

Currently, 99% of deaths with untreated pain from cancer and HIV are in low- and middle-income countries[48] and 80% of the world's population live in countries with low or no access to medicines for severe to moderate pain.[49] Access to medication is crucial to high-quality and effective pain and symptom management. African governments are urged by the WHO to institute a policy on essential medicines for adults and children that embraces palliative care medicines (including opioids, such as oral morphine) for effective pain management and is supported by a policy on their importation to ensure that all in need can access medications that are affordable and effective.[50]

In many African countries, however, access to even the simplest pain-relieving medication is limited, while strong analgesics (e.g., opioids), are overly restricted.[51] A policy on essential medicines should ensure that systemic challenges in the opioid supply chain are addressed to ensure a balanced distribution framework.

Education policies

In 2004, the WHO recommended that governments develop policies that include palliative care in training curricula for health workers at all levels, equipping them with the discipline's knowledge and core competencies.[52] Currently, only seven countries have palliative care integrated in the curriculum of health professionals (Botswana, Kenya, Malawi, Namibia, South Africa, Tanzania, and Uganda) and have recognized palliative care as an examinable subject.[53]

Drug availability

Access to palliative care medicines is crucial to ensure effective pain and symptom management, especially opioids (such as morphine) for moderate-to-severe pain. However, despite its prevalence among cancer and HIV/AIDS patients, pain in Africa is disturbingly undertreated among adults and children.[54] For example, according to the WHO data,[55] approximately 552,100 people died of cancer in sub-Saharan Africa in 2009, with studies showing that 80% of people dying with cancer need pain treatment.[56] Opioids are also critical in treating pain in AIDS patients. However, of the 1.84 million people who died from HIV/AIDS in the region in 2009, approximately 50% had no access to appropriate pain medication.[57] Based on these numbers, in 2009 effective pain treatment in sub-Saharan Africa was needed by about 441,680 people who died of cancer and about 920,000 people who died of HIV/AIDS.[57]

The US-based Wisconsin Pain Policy Studies Group report very low morphine consumption for Africa, with only South Africa in 2010 reporting morphine consumption above the global mean (Figure 76.3).[58] Governments in sub-Saharan Africa reported an overall annual consumption of 720 kg of opioids annually across the whole region for the years 2007–2009.[59] Based on the estimation that, on average, patients who need pain treatment at the end of life consume 67.5 mg of morphine daily for 3 months,[57] 720 kg is enough to provide treatment for about 116,600 people (i.e., about 8.6% of the total number of painful deaths from cancer or HIV/AIDS).[59]

Barriers to opioid analgesic supply on the continent include, among others: insufficient training of healthcare professionals in the use of opioids; misperceptions of healthcare professionals, policy makers, and patients and their families regarding the safety of opioids; exaggerated fears about the development of dependence syndrome; unduly harsh sanctions for unintentional mishandling of opioids by heath workers; practical issues, such as not enough prescribers; and overly restrictive laws and regulations on the trade, distribution, and use of opioids.[60] Indeed, a recent global study investigating the availability and accessibility of opioids for the management of cancer pain reported most African countries were found to be using a wide number of regulatory restriction types to limit the accessibility of opioids, ranging from two in Botswana and Namibia, to seven in Egypt and Mauritius.[61]

The United Nations' Economic and Social Council has called on Member States to remove such barriers to the medical use of opioid analgesics, and the International Narcotics Control Board has requested governments to promote the rational use of opioids for pain management. In April 2013 the African Union Commission on Controlled Substances and Access to Pain Management Drugs resolved to address impediments to adequate access to opioid analgesics for pain management and take steps to improve the availability of narcotic drugs and psychotropic substances for the relief of pain.[62] Given that such appeals require supplementary advocacy with national policy makers, APCA has undertaken policy-influencing work across Eastern, Southern, and Western Africa to promote the availability and accessibility of pain-relieving medicines, especially opioids. Additionally, substantial international developments have laid the groundwork for coordinated global action between governments, intergovernmental organizations, and civil society, including two resolutions of the UN Commission on Narcotic Drugs, the Political Declaration's recognition of palliative care, and major UN reports.[63,64] Progress has been made in many countries, including Uganda, Kenya, and Nigeria, through the joint efforts of ministries of health, healthcare workers, national palliative-care associations, regional networks, international nongovernmental organizations and supporters, the Global Access to Pain Initiative (GAPRI), and the WHO Collaborating Centre–designated Pain and Policy Studies Group.[59]

Despite the challenges, progress is being made on the continent to make pain medicines accessible to patients. The relative lack of doctors on the continent means that there is a growing acceptance of "task-shifting," enabling other appropriately trained specialist health cadre (e.g., nurses) to prescribe opioids. For example, in Uganda in 2002, a statutory instrument on drug prescription was revised to allow specially trained nurses and clinical officers to prescribe oral morphine and other palliative care medicines without supervision from a doctor.[65] However, task shifting does not negate the imperative to educate doctors in the need for effective pain management, and address the "opiophobia" that perceives such medicines as addictive and that renders health workers vulnerable to legal prosecution. Moreover, there is a need for African governments to use cheaper, but still effective, generic opioids (including reconstituted morphine sulfate powder) that governments can afford without fear of running out. Countries such as Swaziland and Nigeria have reviewed their local systems and mechanisms to make morphine available and accessible to their

AFRO Consumption of Morphine, 2010

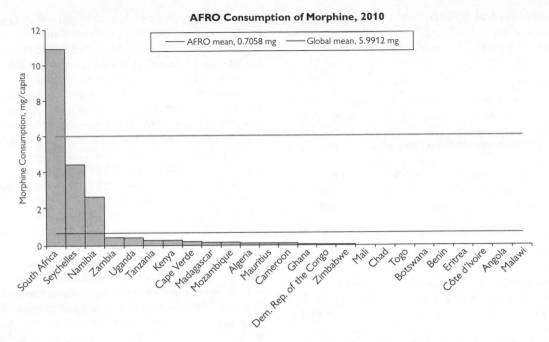

Figure 76.3 Consumption of morphine, Africa, 2010, mg/capita. Source: Copyright Pain and Policy Studies Group, Pain and Policy Studies Group University, University of Wisconsin, home of the/WHO Collaborating Centre for Pain Policy and Palliative Care (2013). Reprinted with permission from Pain and Policy Studies Group, University of Wisconsin, USA, AFRO region 2006 consumption, www.painpolicy.wisc.edu/internat/AFRO/index.htm. Reprinted with permission: University of Wisconsin Pain and Policy Studies Group.

patients in need. Indeed, the government of Swaziland had its first supply of morphine powder at the end of 2012.

Education

Palliative care education should target diverse audiences (e.g., policy makers, healthcare workers, and the general public) to increase their awareness, skills, and knowledge of, and change their attitudes toward, care for those with life-threatening illness. One critically important group, however, is national leaders (both clinical and academic) responsible for education, and it is vital that palliative care professionals work collaboratively with them to change existing, and develop new, palliative care educational curricula.

There are numerous educational initiatives in Africa that seek to address the holistic needs of patients and their families, with an emphasis on pain and symptom management and psychosocial, cultural, and spiritual needs. These programs range from short certificate courses to diploma, undergraduate, and master's-level degrees. In South Africa, for example, there is a multidisciplinary master's course conducted at the University of Cape Town,[66] while a master's program is being planned in Uganda and a new program is under development in Tanzania.

Several countries (including Botswana, Kenya, Malawi, Swaziland, Tanzania, Uganda, and Zambia) have developed and are implementing national palliative care training programs, while other countries (such as Mozambique and Namibia) are adapting similar programs. Recently the APCA developed educational materials and resources to support national palliative care programs that include: a palliative care core curriculum and a framework of core competencies for palliative care providers in Africa. Additional materials (such as a monitoring and evaluation framework for palliative care education and a palliative care training methodology guide) have been finalized by the APCA, along with e-learning modules, and will be made available for use in Africa.

Recently, palliative care has received some academic recognition within the region with the appointment of three honorary professors, two in Uganda at Makerere University and one in South Africa at the University of Cape Town, an important step forward in the advancement of palliative care in the academic setting.

Implementation

Without effective implementation, the other components of the enhanced WHO public health model are redundant. As mentioned, the profile of palliative care in the region has been increasing over the past decade, with 16 African countries establishing national palliative care associations and seven countries including palliative care in national plans and policies.[47] Regardless of these developments, palliative care is still not fully integrated into national health systems but is instead delivered through diverse service models, with the primary mode of palliative care service delivery being HBC, which is predominantly dependent on volunteers. Consequently, most African governments need to ensure there are sufficient funding and appropriate service delivery models in place to support the expansion of palliative care in their respective countries.

In addition to addressing the issues of staff recruitment and retention, it is imperative that African palliative care providers ensure HBC services provide acceptable standards of patient care. Of particular importance in this respect is the development and adherence to national quality care standards, based on criteria developed by the APCA.[67] Moreover, to ensure widespread implementation, it is important that palliative care be integrated into all levels of the healthcare system, including the specialist, regional, and district (as well as HBC) facilities. To date, many countries (including Botswana, Democratic Republic of the Congo, The Gambia, Kenya, Malawi, Mozambique, Namibia, Nigeria, Rwanda, South

Africa, Swaziland, Tanzania, Uganda, Zambia, and Zimbabwe) are actively integrating palliative care into their health systems by supporting palliative care development in public hospitals.[53]

Case study—Kenya

One of the recent success stories of palliative care integration into health systems on the continent is from Kenya. Founded in 2006, the Kenya Hospice and Palliative Care Association, with its member hospices, has been spearheading palliative care development in the country through advocacy, education and health systems strengthening. Through this work, palliative care has been included in several national strategy documents, including the national cancer control strategy and the HIV/AIDS strategy. More importantly, palliative care has been included in the curriculum of higher institutions of learning for doctors and nurses. At the implementation level, and with support from the Ministry of Health, palliative care has been integrated into services across 11 provincial government hospitals. Plans are underway to scale-up this integration into district hospitals. These developments have resulted in the establishment of public hospital palliative care units that are linked with local hospices thereby increasing access to palliative care for patients who need it in Kenya.

The multidisciplinary team and palliative care

In Africa, where there are limited numbers of health professionals, the multidisciplinary team should include whomever is considered most appropriate (e.g., nurses, doctors, social workers, counselors, and allied health professionals) working alongside others such as traditional, religious and community leaders, teachers, and community health workers.

Despite the theoretical ideal, the reality in rural Africa is that the team may comprise only one or two members (e.g., a nurse and community volunteer working alongside family members). The precise nature of the team will vary according to the care model provided, be that a specialist palliative care unit, a hospital, a roadside clinic, or HBC service. A number of public hospitals have established functional palliative care teams and units, including Mulago National Referral Hospital in Uganda, Kenyatta National Referral Hospital in Kenya, Mulanje District Hospital in Malawi, the Kibagabaga District Hospital in Rwanda, and the Livingstone General Hospital in Zambia, as well as several hospitals in South Africa. For the majority of African countries, however, without dedicated palliative care teams, it is important that services network effectively with other services to ensure that patients are able to receive care in a home and facility setting.

The nurse's role in palliative care in Africa

Nurses have a pivotal role in palliative care provision on the continent given they are present at all levels of the healthcare system, from the facility to the community. The merits of the holistic focus and broad skills base of the nursing profession are supplemented by the fact that for the vast majority of African patients—especially in rural areas—nurses are the only healthcare professionals available. For example, in Tanzania, there is one doctor per 100,000 people and 24 nurses; in Mozambique, there are three

doctors per 100,000 people and 34 nurses; and in Côte d'Ivoire, there are 14 doctors per 100,000 and 48 nurses.[68]

Nurses' roles within palliative care in Africa are varied, including vital ones in the development of teamwork assessment, communication, counseling, treatment and prescribing as appropriate, training and supervision, advocacy, and health promotion.[69] Liaising with other professional and nonprofessional caregivers is crucial and an often unrecognized part of their roles.

As outlined above, to ensure accessibility to palliative care services (particularly in the rural areas) some countries are changing existing legislation so that palliative care–trained nurses are enabled to prescribe medications such as oral morphine. Following Uganda's work in this area, other countries (e.g., Malawi, Namibia, South Africa, Swaziland, and Zimbabwe) are attempting to emulate that country's innovation.

Education and mentorship, for the patient, family, community health workers, and other nurses, is another vital part of the nurses' role in palliative care in Africa. Training family members to care for their loved ones and providing them with support and mentorship to accomplish this, is an important part of enabling HBC delivery. Additionally, the significant workforce role played by community-based volunteers means that nurses also have a pivotal role to play in equipping the former with the necessary skills and supporting them through supervision.

The important role of research in African palliative care development is now recognized. Nurses are increasingly trained to develop and implement research programs, with several dedicated research nurses appointed across the region providing much needed leadership in this area. This is an important advance not only in the development of palliative care in the region but also in the valuation of the nurses' role. However, despite this positive development, the inadequate incorporation of palliative care into preservice (undergraduate) training for nurses, the lack of clear career pathways for nurses interested in specializing in palliative care, and the lack of recognition of palliative care qualifications by local ministries of health and education, continue to be a challenge.

Sociocultural, religious, and spiritual issues influencing palliative care

Africa has a rich diversity of cultures providing people with a framework to understand their experiences and influence the way palliative care is delivered to patients and their families. Common social, cultural, religious, and spiritual needs of the patient and their family include: overwhelming social needs; communication around issues of death, grief, and bereavement; and perceptions and beliefs and practices surrounding illness and death, among others.

Deprivation for many in Africa means that social needs are central to palliative care provision, with patients concerned for the welfare of their children (including their school fees, care arrangements when death comes, and their inability to afford their basic needs).

Patients and their families experience the common phases of grief, including denial, anger, depression, bargaining, and acceptance. They additionally experience understandable fear and anxieties and sometimes self-blame for contributing to the disease's cause, especially HIV/AIDS. Many African patients who are in denial do not prioritize their medical treatment, but instead resort to traditional healing in the belief that their ancestors could be angry with them. Moreover, the taboo that surrounds death in most African countries means that communication regarding this important topic is problematic, a fact that is compounded by the overwhelming number of patients presenting at health facilities that render meaningful discussion of sociocultural, religious, and spiritual issues nearly impossible.

Although variation exists for the preferred location of death (i.e., home or facility-based), for many patients, a home death is the desired choice, provided appropriate care is accessible.[70] However, recent research among the public in Windhoek, Namibia, showed that palliative care needs to be available across the continuum of care, because while many identify home as the preferred place of care, others prefer to receive care in hospital.[71] Although there is a need to sensitize communities and healthcare workers to respect such dying patients' priorities, there is also recognition that the facility-based alternative to a domiciliary death is unaffordable for the majority of patients. Consequently, training programs for family caregivers and community volunteers are widely implemented to ensure the provision of basic HBC, supplemented with support and supervision from professional teams.

Africa is characterized by multiple religious denominations, with most following Christianity (45%) or Islam (40.6%), the adherents of which can also simultaneously practice traditional African religions.[72] These religious and spiritual beliefs and practices can prove very important to the terminally ill as they influence their attitude and insight toward illness and death.[73]

Many Africans believe there are four main categories of diseases: African disease, foreign disease, chronic disease, and plague.[74] Consequently, some diseases are primarily addressed using indigenous African medicines and traditional healers (which are extensively used on the continent), whereas others are treated using modern scientific medicine and medical professionals. However, given that many pharmaceutical products currently remain largely unaffordable and inaccessible to the majority of Africans, many patients interact with their local traditional healers, whose dispensed herbal medicines can interact negatively with medically prescribed treatments. As a result, some African countries have established collaborative medical programs (e.g., for HIV/AIDS) between traditional and modern health practitioners to nurture an environment of joint learning and care provision.[75] Moreover, given the lack of healthcare providers trained in assessing patients' psychosocial, religious, and spiritual needs, some palliative care organizations recruit social and spiritual care professionals to support clinical teams with complex cases, and train their team members.

Special populations

For some patients, palliative care service provision can be problematic because of multiple factors (e.g., stigma, especially for HIV/AIDS, and various financial, social, or legal barriers). This is especially the case in Africa for internally displaced persons (IDPs), prisoners, and the armed forces, among others.[76]

Internally displaced persons

Defined as "someone who has been forced to flee his or her home, but who has not reached a neighboring country and therefore, unlike a refugee, is not protected by international law and is not eligible to receive many types of aid,"[77] there is in excess of an estimated 10.4 million IDPs across sub-Saharan Africa (a third of the world's internally displaced population) who have fallen through the safety net provided to many ordinary citizens and also not receiving palliative care.[78]

Prisoners

Millions of people are imprisoned across Africa, in conditions that are commonly extremely basic, often characterized by deficient sanitation, poor nutrition, limited access to medical services, and heightened risk of infection (e.g., in 2006 the HIV prevalence in South African prisons was 45%, much higher than the general population).[79] For released prisoners, poor discharge planning and follow-up, compounded by the stigmas of illness and being an ex-convict, mean that accessing care can remain problematic. In South Africa, pioneering work undertaken by the Hospice Palliative Care Association of South Africa (HPCA) has introduced palliative care to the Department of Correctional Services in line with the provisions of the Constitution to ensure sound policies and best practices in palliative care in the correctional services environment. Similar work is being undertaken in Kenya, Uganda, and Zimbabwe. A key concern for these populations, particularly in South Africa, is the development of multidrug-resistant TB.

Armed forces

The armed forces (i.e., army, navy, air force, presidential guard, police, etc.) are another unique subpopulation for African palliative care services. Often members are forced to live apart from their families for considerable durations of time (often exposing them to risky health behaviors; e.g., unprotected sex with commercial sex workers), while the suspicion that a diagnosis of ill health will impact adversely on their career prospects and living situation means that they can often present in the advanced stages of life-threatening illnesses. It is important that armed forces recognize and integrate palliative care within their military health system. This approach has been followed in Uganda, where members of the Ugandan People's Defence Force have established their own branch of the country's national palliative care association, and work to identify and treat soldiers and their families.

Key to the provision of palliative care among such subpopulations is the establishment of trust, adapting services to ensure that those who feel marginalized, stigmatized and are distrustful of society can receive the benefits of its healthcare system.

Children's palliative care

Approximately 42% of the population of Africa is under 15 years old, with countries such as Uganda having 48% of the population in 2011 below that age.[68] In 2010, an estimated 3.1 million children under 15 in sub-Saharan Africa were living with HIV/AIDS, with 230,000 dying in that year alone.[80] Additionally, despite the deficiencies of existing systems to enumerate its incidence and prevalence, in 2008, 22,647 (5%) of the 420,978 cancer related deaths in sub-Saharan Africa were in children under 15 years of age.[81] Assessment of the need for children's palliative care is complex, however a systematic review of children's palliative care provision around the world showed that there is a great need for the development of pediatric palliative care in sub-Saharan Africa.[82]

The palliative care needs of children differ from those of adults. For example, children's differential development stages will affect their understanding of their illness; they are not legally competent to consent to medical treatment; they may have deficient skills to verbalize their needs, or express their pain and discomfort; and they may protect their parents or loved ones at their own expense.

Traditionally, children have been relatively neglected by palliative care service development on the continent, despite the fact they may have already experienced parental and sibling deaths and now face their own mortality. This neglect is exacerbated by the limitations of existing community and health service physical and human resources, including: restricted access to pediatric medical formulations; lack of understanding of the disease process in children; limited access to affordable and accessible chemotherapy and antiretroviral therapy services, which are often centered around urban areas; societal myths concerning whether children can neurologically feel pain; and familial financial destitution that forces parents to make exacting decisions on who among their needy should receive their finite resources (i.e., the dying child or their caregiver). However, the growing awareness of the positive impact that it can exert on children has resulted in an increasing demand that pediatric palliative care should no longer be the "orphan" of its adult equivalent. This demand manifested itself in the ICPCN's charter of rights for children with life-limited and life-threatening illnesses, which promises to be an important advocacy tool for the development of children's palliative care on the continent.[83]

There is also a recognition that, given it is often the same nurse (particularly in rural areas, in the absence of specialist children's hospitals and palliative care services) who has responsibility for delivering care to adults and children, the distinct differences that characterize children mean it is imperative that pediatric palliative care is integrated into all palliative care trainings where a small number of health professionals can receive specialist children's palliative care training to enable them to provide support and mentorship to others. This should be supplemented by effective networking and collaboration between organizations involved in children's palliative care (e.g., general home-based programs, children's daycare programs, inpatient programs, and hospital-based programs).

Much work has been done over the past few years in strengthening children's palliative care across the region, with developments in service provision, education, drug availability, and research. The Beacon Centre program, established in 2009, set out to improve access to children's palliative care in South Africa, Tanzania, and Uganda. The focus was on education and service delivery, and "beacon centres" have been formed to provide ongoing clinical training and supervision. It is hoped that the lessons learned from this project can be used in developing services elsewhere in the region.[84]

There has been an expansion in training on children's palliative care, with training in part being provided through the ICPCN in several countries, including Malawi, Sudan, Tanzania, Uganda, and Zambia. Plans are also underway for a diploma in children's palliative care to be run by Mildmay Uganda, which will be available for participants from around the region. Work on access to medications has continued in an integrated manner for both adults and children, with children accessing opioids in services where previously it was unavailable (e.g., at the University Teaching Hospital in Lusaka, Zambia). The APCA is also leading the way, along with its partners, in the development of a pediatric palliative outcome scale—the APCA African Children's Palliative Outcome Scale—promising to be an important tool for clinical practice, audit, and research, it was due to be finalized in 2015.[85]

Ethical and legal issues

In most African countries, legal and ethical frameworks for palliative care are in their infancy or indeed nonexistent. Latterly the international community has embraced the notion that denial of palliative care and pain and symptom control is an infringement of an individual's human rights.[86] Indeed, recently at the United Nations Human Rights Council, the UN Special Rapporteur on Torture noted that denial of essential pain relief medications, including lack of access to oral morphine, due to policies that prioritize strict drug control regulations over patient care, or inadequate domestic provision of medications, constitute torture and ill-treatment.[87]

For the vast majority of countries in the region, however, this remains an ideal; restricted healthcare budgets and multiple competing demands mean that populations cannot access even basic public health requirements, such as clean water, sanitization, or rudimentary healthcare. Consequently, for many palliative care professionals in the region, advocating for palliative care as a right of every adult and child is tempered by the need to advocate for other more basic human rights that will also improve the quality of life of those with life-limiting illnesses.

Generic palliative care ethical issues include truth-telling, informed consent, patient autonomy, and doing no harm to patients. However, specific ethical challenges exist in Africa resulting from its varied cultures, and the high prevalence of HIV/AIDS, which compounds usual ethical considerations around stigma, disclosure, and blame. Additionally, many African health professionals believe that human life must be preserved at all costs, resulting in terminally ill patients being transported back to their local hospital for medical procedures they neither need nor can afford. The APCA, in collaboration with the Ministry of Health in Uganda, the Palliative Care Association of Uganda and the Uganda Network of Law Ethics and HIV/AIDS (UGANET), is addressing these by exploring legal and human rights issues for palliative care patients. To this end they have developed materials that include user guides and educational materials for patients, families, and healthcare providers. Similar work has been undertaken in Kenya and South Africa, with manuals and guidelines by both countries' national palliative care associations.

Beyond legal issues, there is also widespread disparity in gender power relations that can affect women not only in sexual issues but also in terms of adequate access to information regarding their illness, their economic dependency, loss of inheritance property following their spouse's death, and lack of control over end-of-life treatment preferences. In palliative care, respect for patient autonomy entails the individual making their own decisions, something that is premised on adequate information regarding potential treatment and care options. However, this premise is undermined in those parts of Africa where sociocultural norms dictate that the needs of the family and community supersede those of the individual. For example, in some cultures any decisions regarding treatment will be made by the senior familial male member, sometimes at the patient's expense. This situation can be compounded by the paternalistic nature of heathcare systems, where women and girls may be discouraged from asking questions and healthcare workers may be reluctant to discuss illness, death, and dying.[88]

Although advance directives and living wills are gradually being introduced and discussed in the region (mainly in southern Africa),[89] they remain in many areas embryonic concepts and philosophical discussion points, as does that of euthanasia.

Challenges to palliative care in Africa

◆ *Delayed health-seeking behavior:* Palliative care has traditionally been viewed as an "end-stage" intervention, signaled by the conclusion of the need for curative treatment, despite clinical evidence that patients need pain, symptom management, and psychosocial care throughout the disease trajectory.[90] With the advent of highly active antiretroviral therapy (HAART), this perception was further misplaced. However, the fact remains that large numbers of people infected by HIV/AIDS and cancer delay seeking medical assistance (e.g., because of the stigma associated with HIV/AIDS and the cost of treatment).

◆ *Lack of trained palliative care professionals:* Not only is there a worldwide health workforce crisis, as noted at the second Global Forum on Human Resources for Health in 2011—characterized by widespread global shortages, maldistribution of personnel within and between countries, migration of local health workers, and poor working conditions[91]—but also there is a significant deficit in skilled palliative care professionals (with limited opportunities for health workers to acquire palliative care training). The preponderant reliance on HBC volunteers also raises questions regarding the quality and sustainability of services significantly dependent on their contribution.[92]

◆ *Unfavorable drug environments:* As stated earlier, despite the overwhelming medical need, access to even the simplest pain-relieving medication—not to mention the strong painkillers (i.e., opioids)[93]—and antibiotics to treat opportunistic infections in many African countries is provided within very restrictive policy and operational environments (e.g., limited legitimate prescribers).

◆ *Logistical challenges to service provision:* The geographical and topographical challenges facing effective palliative care provision cannot be understated. Given the relatively low level of urbanization in many African countries (e.g., 2.2 people per km² in Namibia), services sometimes have to be provided to low-density populations across vast rural areas. Additionally, the preference of many health professionals to work in urban locations means that rural healthcare provision is primarily left to community- and home-based volunteers, offering care that is often no more than supportive in nature.

◆ *Limitations of existing service models in an era of HAART:* Although HAART is pivotal to effective HIV/AIDS management, the extent to which current African HBC models are able to integrate it into their existing services is a challenge. Many current models are, to varying degrees, largely nonmedicalized. However, efforts to address this challenge have shown that HAART can be provided as part of a palliative care service by community-based indigenous healthcare workers as long as training and resource needs are adequately addressed.[94]

◆ *Other challenges include* lack of rigorous research evidence indicating the benefits of palliative care; poor public awareness and understanding of the discipline; uncommitted national governments; lack of government funding as part of national health programs; entrenched attitudes within the medical profession; cultural taboos surrounding death and the disclosure of diagnosis; and the absence of a consensus that regards palliative care as a basic human right.

Summary

The discipline of palliative care started relatively late in Africa and advanced over the preceding three decades by highly committed individuals with access to limited resources to meet an overwhelming need. The agenda for the coming years is significant, encompassing the need to overcome government indifference and effect high-level policy change, training for its primarily volunteer cadre as well as orthodox pre- and inservice health workers (to include recruitment, training, and retention issues), improving societal and medical understanding and use of opioids for effective pain management, building effective linkages between relevant stakeholders (e.g., academics, oncologists, pediatricians, those working with the aged, etc.), and developing and utilizing a methodologically rigorous research base to inform service development, policy development and, ultimately, maximize the quality of patients' lives.

References

1. Population Reference Bureau. 2012 World Population Data Sheet. New York: Population Reference Bureau; 2012.
2. United Nations Development Programme. Human Development Report 2013. The Rise of the South: Human Progress in a Diverse World. New York: United Nations Development Programme; 2013.
3. Council for the Development of Social Science Research in Africa. 2005. Access and Equity in African Health Systems. http://www.codesria.org/spip.php?article290 (accessed July 5, 2013).
4. World Health Organization. Alma-Ata 1978: Primary Health Care, HFA Sr. No. 1. Geneva: World Health Organization; 1978.
5. Kirigia JM, Diarra-Nama AJ. Can countries of the WHO African region wean themselves off donor funding for health? Bull World Health Org. 2008;86:889–892.
6. Joint United Nations Programme on HIV/AIDS (UNAIDS). UNAIDS Report on the Global AIDS Epidemic. Geneva: UNAIDS; 2012.
7. United Nations. The Millennium Development Goals Report 2012. New York: United Nations; 2012.
8. World Health Organization (WHO). Global Tuberculosis Report. Geneva: WHO; 2012.
9. Jemal A, Bray F, Forman D, et al. Cancer burden in Africa and opportunities for prevention. Cancer. 2012;118:4372–4384.
10. Ferlay J, Shin H-R, Bray F, et al. Estimates of worldwide burden of cancer in 2008: GLOBOCAN 2008. Int J Cancer. 2010;127:2893–2917.
11. Parkin DM. The global health burden of infection-associated cancers in the year 2002. Int J Cancer. 2006;118:3030–3044.
12. Echouffo-Tcheugui JB, Kengne AP. Chronic non-communicable diseases in Cameroon—burden, determinants and current policies. Global Health. 2011;7:44.

13. Mayosi BM, Flisher AJ, Lalloo UG, et al. The burden of non-communicable diseases in South Africa. Lancet. 2009;374:934–947.

14. Wright M, Clark D. Hospice and palliative care in Africa: a review of developments and challenges. Oxford, England: Oxford University Press, 2006.

15. Powell RA, Mwangi-Powell FN, Kiyange F, et al. Palliative care development in Africa: How we can provide enough quality care? BMJ Support Palliat Care. 2011;1:113–114.

16. Grant L, Downing J, Namukwaya E, Leng M, Murray SA. Palliative care in Africa since 2005: good progress, but much further to go. BMJ Support Palliat Care. 2011;1:118–122.

17. Knapp C, Woodworth L, Wright M, et al. Pediatric palliative care provision around the world: a systematic review. Pediatr Blood Cancer. 2011;57:361–368.

18. Lynch T, Connor S, Clark D. Mapping levels of palliative care development: a global update. J Pain Symptom Manage. 2013;45:1094–1106.

19. Harding R, Powell RA, Downing J, et al. Generating an African palliative care evidence base: the context, need, challenges and strategies. J Pain Symptom Manage. 2008;36:304–309.

20. Powell RA, Downing J, Radbruch L, et al. Advancing palliative care research in Africa: from Venice to Nairobi. Palliat Med. 2008;22:885–887.

21. APCA. Strategic Plan, 2011–2010. Kampala, Uganda: APCA; 2011.

22. Powell RA, Harding R, Namisango E, et al. Palliative care research in Africa: an overview. Eur J Palliat Care. 2013;20:162–167.

23. Powell RA, Harding R, Namisango E. et al. Palliative care research in Africa: consensus building for a prioritized agenda. J Pain Symptom Manage. 2014;47(2):315–324.

24. Wakeham K, Harding R, Bamukama-Namakoola D, et al. Symptom burden in HIV-infected adults at time of HIV diagnosis in rural Uganda. J Palliat Med. 2010;13:375–380.

25. Harding R, Selman L, Agupio G, et al. The prevalence and burden of symptoms amongst cancer patients attending palliative care in two African countries. Eur J Cancer. 2011;47:51–56.

26. Harding R, Selman L, Agupio G et al. Prevalence, burden, and correlates of physical and psychological symptoms among HIV palliative care patients in sub-Saharan Africa: an international multicenter study. J Pain Symptom Manage. 2012;44:1–9.

27. Simms VM, Gikaara N, Munene G, et al. Multidimensional patient-reported problems within two weeks of HIV diagnosis in East Africa: a multicentre observational study. PLoS ONE 2013;8:e57203.

28. Selman L, Siegert RJ, Higginson IJ, et al. The "Spirit 8" successfully captured spiritual wellbeing in African palliative care: factor and Rasch analysis. J Pain Sympt Manage. 2011;47:51–56.

29. Kale SS. Perspectives on spiritual care at Hospice Africa Uganda. Int J Palliat Nurs. 2011;17:177–182.

30. Selman L, Higginson IJ, Agupio G, et al. Meeting information needs of patients with incurable disease and their families in South Africa and Uganda: multicentre qualitative study. BMJ. 2009;338: b1326.

31. Murray SA, Grant E, Grant A, et al. Dying from cancer in developed and developing countries: lessons from two qualitative interview studies of patients and their carers. BMJ. 2003;326:368.

32. Kikule E. A good death in Uganda: survey of needs for palliative care for terminally ill people in urban areas. BMJ. 2003;327:192–194.

33. Graham N, Gwyther L, Tiso T, Harding R. Traditional healers' views of the required processes for a "good death" among Xhosa patients pre- and post-death. J Pain Symptom Manage. 2013;46:386–394.

34. Emanuel RH, Emanuel GA, Reitschuler EB, et al. Challenges faced by informal caregivers of hospice patients in Uganda. J Palliat Med. 2008;11:746–753.

35. Jack BA, Kirton JA, Birakurataki J, et al. The personal value of being a palliative care Community Volunteer Worker in Uganda: a qualitative study. Palliat Med. 2012;26:753–759.

36. Harding R, Selman L, Agupio G, et al. Validation of a core outcome measure for palliative care in Africa: the APCA African Palliative Outcome Scale. Health Qual Life Outcomes. 2010;8:10.

37. Downing J, Ojing M, Powell RA, et al. A palliative care outcome measure for children in sub-Saharan Africa: early development findings. Eur J Palliat Care. 2012;19:292–295.

38. Downing J, Simon ST, Mwangi-Powell FN, et al. Outcomes 'Out of Africa': The selection and implementation of outcome measures for palliative care in Africa. BMC Palliat Care. 2012;11:1.

39. Harding R, Albertyn R, Sherr L, et al. Pediatric palliative care in sub-Saharan Africa: a systematic review of the evidence for care models, interventions, and outcomes. J Pain Symptom Manage. 2014;47:642–651.

40. Stjernsward J, Foley K, Ferris F. The public health strategy for palliative care. J Pain Symptom Manage. 2007;33:486–493.

41. Harding R, Selman L, Powell RA, et al. Cancer control in Africa 6: research into palliative care in sub-Saharan Africa. Lancet Oncol. 2013;14:e183–188.

42. WHO. Cancer PAIN Relief and Palliative Care. Technical Report Series 804. Geneva: World Health Organization; 1990.

43. United National Social Economic Development Council. Millennium Development Goals and post-2015 Development Agenda, 2013. http://www.un.org/en/ecosoc/about/mdg.shtml (accessed December 16, 2013).

44. Hogerzeil HV, Liberman J, Wirtz VJ, et al.; Lancet NCD Action Group. Promotion of access to essential medicines for non-communicable diseases: practical implications of the UN political declaration. Lancet. 2013;381:680–689.

45. Payne S, Leget C, Peruselli C, et al. Quality indicators for palliative care: debates and dilemmas. Palliat Med. 2012;26:679–680.

46. APCA. Palliative Care in Southern Africa: Review of Current Policies and Opportunities for Scaling Up Care. Kampala: APCA; 2012.

47. Mwangi-Powell FN, Powell RA, Harding R. Models of delivering palliative and end-of-life care in Sub-Saharan Africa: a narrative review of the evidence. Curr Opin Support Palliat Care. 2013;7:223–228.

48. GAPRI. 2012. Access on Essential Pain Medicines Brief—2010 Data. www.gapri.org/sites/default/files/private/Fact%20sheet_0.pdf (accessed March 2013).

49. WHO. Ensuring Balance in National Policies on Controlled Substances: Guidance for Availability and Accessibility of Controlled Medications. Geneva: WHO; 2011.

50. WHO. World Health Organization supports global effort to relieve chronic pain. http://www.who.int/mediacentre/news/releases/2004/pr70/en/index.html (accessed July 7 2013).

51. Powell RA, Kaye R, Ddungu H, Mwangi-Powell FN. Brief Global Reports—advancing drug availability: experiences from Africa. J Pain Symptom Manage. 2010;40:9–12.

52. A Community Health Approach to Palliative Care for Cancer and HIV/AIDS Patients in Sub-Saharan Africa. Geneva: World Health Organization; 2004.

53. Mwangi-Powell FN. APCA's role in the development of palliative care in Africa. Prog Palliat Care. 2012;20:230–233.

54. Harding R, Easterbrook P, Dinat N, Higginson IJ. Pain and symptom control in HIV disease: under-researched and poorly managed. Clin Infect Dis. 2005;40:491–492.

55. WHO. Global Health Observatory Data Repository. http://apps.who.int/ghodata/ (accessed July 5, 2013).

56. Foley KM, Wagner JL, Joranson DE, Gelband H. Pain control for people with cancer and AIDS. In: Jamison DT, Breman JG, Measham AR, et al., (eds.), Disease Control Priorities in Developing Countries. 2nd ed. New York: Oxford University Press; 2006:981–994.

57. INCB. Narcotic Drugs: Estimated World Requirements for 2011—Statistics for 2009 (E/INCB/2010/2). Vienna: United Nations International Narcotics Control Board; 2011.

58. Consumption of Morphine, Africa, 2010 mg/capita. Pain and Policy Studies Group, University of Wisconsin/WHO Collaborating Centre. 2012.

59. O'Brien M, Mwangi-Powell FN, Soyannwo O, et al. Improving access to analgesics for patients with cancer in Sub-Saharan Africa. Lancet. 2013;14;e176–e182.

60. Harding R, Powell RA, Kiyange F, et al. Provision of pain- and symptom-relieving drugs for HIV/AIDS in sub-Saharan Africa. J Pain Symptom Manage. 2010;40:405–415.

61. Cleary J, Powell RA, Munene G, et al. Formulary availability and regulatory barriers to accessibility of opioids for cancer pain in Africa: a report from the Global Opioid Policy Initiative (GOPI). Ann Oncol. 2013;24(Supplement 11):xi14–xi23.

62. Report of the Proceedings of the experts Meeting on The Impact of Non-communicable Diseases (NCDs) and Neglected Tropical Diseases (NTDs) on development in Africa: Sixth session of Ministers of Health 22–24 April 2013, Addis Ababa, Ethiopia.

63. Commission on Narcotic Drugs. Resolution 53/4: Promoting Adequate Availability of Internationally Controlled Licit Drugs for Medical and Scientific Purposes While Preventing Their Diversion and Abuse. March 2010. http://www.unodc.org/documents/commissions/CND-Res-2000-until-present/CND53_4e.pdf (accessed June 2013).

64. Commission on Narcotic Drugs. Resolution 54/6: Promoting Adequate Availability of Internationally Controlled Narcotic Drugs and Psychotropic Substances for Medical and Scientific Purposes While Preventing Their Diversion and Abuse. Resolution 54/6. March 2011. http://www.unodc.org/documents/commissions/CND-Res-2011to2019/CND54_6e1.pdf (accessed June 2013).

65. Jaqwe J, Merriman A. Uganda: delivering analgesia in rural Africa: opioid availability and nurse prescribing. J Pain Symptom Manage. 2007;33:547–551.

66. Ens CD, Chochinov HM, Gwyther E, et al. Postgraduate palliative care education: evaluation of a South African program. S Afr Med J. 2011;101:42–44.

67. APCA. Standards for Providing Quality Palliative Care Across Africa. Kampala: APCA; 2011.

68. WHO. World Health Statistics. Geneva: WHO; 2013.

69. Downing J, Finch L, Garanganga E, et al. Role of the nurse in resource-limited settings. In: Gwyther L, Merriman A, MpangaSebuyira L, et al., (eds.), A Clinical Guide to Supportive and Palliative Care for HIV/AIDS in Sub-Saharan Africa. Kampala, Uganda: African Palliative Care Association; 2006:345–56.

70. World Health Organization. A Community Health Approach to Palliative Care for HIV/AIDS and Cancer Patients in sub-Saharan Africa. Geneva: World Health Organization; 2004.

71. Powell RA, Namisango E, Gikaara N, et al. Public priorities and preferences for end-of-life care in Namibia. J Pain Symptom Manage. 2014;47:620–630.

72. McLaughlin A. In Africa, Islam and Christianity are growing—and blending. The Christian Science Monitor, January 26, 2006. www.csmonitor.com/2006/0126/p01s04-woaf.html (accessed July 7, 2013).

73. Powell RA, Selman L, Galimaka-Kabalega D. Perspectives on end-of-life care in global context: Africa. In: Lazenby M, McCorkle R, Sulmasy D (eds.), Safe Passage: A Global Spiritual Sourcebook for Religion at the End of Life. Oxford: Oxford University Press; 2014:20–35.

74. Waliggo JM, Gwyther L, Mguli E, et al. Spiritual and cultural care. In: Gwyther L, Merriman A, MpangaSebuyira L, et al. (eds.), A Clinical Guide to Supportive and Palliative Care for HIV/AIDS in Sub-Saharan Africa. Kampala, Uganda: African Palliative Care Association; 2006:233–248.

75. Hills SY, Finch L, Garanganga E. Traditional medicine. In: Gwyther L, Merriman A, MpangaSebuyira L, et al. (eds.), A Clinical Guide to Supportive and Palliative Care for HIV/AIDS in Sub-Saharan Africa. Kampala, Uganda: African Palliative Care Association; 2006:219–232.

76. Downing J. Special populations. In: Gwyther L, Merriman A, MpangaSebuyira L, et al. (eds.), A Clinical Guide to Supportive and Palliative Care for HIV/AIDS in Sub-Saharan Africa. Kampala, Uganda: African Palliative Care Association; 2006:323–334.

77. United Nations High Commission on Refugees. Refugees by Numbers. Geneva: United Nations High Commission on Refugees; 2004.

78. Internal Displacement Monitoring Centre (iDMC) Global Overview 2012: People Internally Displaced by Conflict and Violence. Geneva: IDMC; 2013.

79. UNAIDS. HIV and prisons in sub-Saharan Africa: Opportunities for Action. Geneva: UNAIDS; 2007.

80. GLOBOCAN 2008. Sub-Saharan Africa—Both Sexes Estimated Mortality by Age. http://globocan.iarc.fr/age-specific_table_n_html.asp?selection=185960&title=Sub-Saharan+Africa&sex=0&type=1&stat=1&window=1&sort=0&submit=%A0Execute%A0 (accessed July 2, 2013).

81. UNAIDS. World AIDS Day Report. New York: UNAIDS; 2011.

82. Knapp C, Woodworth L, Wright M, et al. Pediatric palliative care provision around the world: a systematic review. Pediatr Blood Cancer. 2011;57: 361–368.

83. ICPCN 2008. The ICPCN Charter of Rights for Life Limited and Life Threatened Children. October 2008. http://www.icpcn.org.uk/page.asp?section=000100010014&sectionTitle=Charter (accessed July 2, 2013).

84. Downing JD, Marston J, Selwyn C, et al. Developing children's palliative care in Africa through beacon centres: lessons learnt. BMC Palliat Care. 2013;12:8.

85. Downing J, Atieno M, Powell RA, et al., and the APCA AIDSTAR Project Advisory Group. Development of a palliative care outcome measure for children in sub-Saharan Africa: findings from early phase instrument development. Eur J Palliat Care. 2012;19:292–295.

86. Brennan F. Palliative care as an international human right. J Pain Symptom Manage. 2007;33:494–499.

87. Mendez J. Report of the Special Rapporteur on Torture and Other Cruel, Inhuman or Degrading Treatment or Punishment. Human Rights Council Twenty-second Session Agenda item 3 A/HRC/22/53, Feb 1, 2013.

88. Sebuyira LM, Gwyther L. Ethical and human rights issues. In: Gwyther L, Merriman A, MpangaSebuyira L, et al. (eds.), A Clinical Guide to Supportive and Palliative Care for HIV/AIDS in Sub-Saharan Africa. Kampala, Uganda: African Palliative Care Association; 2006:309–322.

89. Stanford J, Sandberg DM, Gwyther L, et al. Conversations worth having: the perceived relevance of advance care planning among teachers, hospice staff, and pastors in Knysna, South Africa. J Palliat Med. 2013;16:762–767.

90. Breitbart W, McDonald MV, Rosenfeld B, et al. Pain experience in ambulatory AIDS patients—I: Pain characteristics and medical correlates. Pain. 1996;68:315–321.

91. WHO. 2011. Report on the Prince Mahidol Award Conference 2011. 2nd Global Forum on Human Resource for Health. www.who.int/workforcealliance/knowledge/resources/SecondHRHForum_report_en.pdf (accessed July 2, 2013).

92. Powell RA, Mwangi-Powell FN. Improving palliative care in Africa: selection, training, and retention of community-based volunteers is a priority. Br Med J. 2008;337:1123–1124.

93. Harding R, Higginson IJ. Palliative Care in Sub-Saharan Africa: An Appraisal. London: The Diana, Princess of Wales Memorial Fund; 2004.

94. Campbell C, Nair Y, Maimane S, Sibiya Z. Home-based carers: a vital resource for effective ARV roll-out in rural communities? AIDS Bull. 2005;14:22–27.

CHAPTER 77

Palliative care in Japan

Sayaka Takenouchi and Keiko Tamura

Key points

◆ It was 33 years ago when the first hospice inpatient facility was opened in Japan. There has been increasing attention given to hospice and palliative care by both the government and the public since then.

◆ Facilities offering hospice/palliative care are increasing year by year. However, there was still an inadequate number of facilities available for patients with life-threatening illnesses. In response to the unmet needs of those patients, the Cancer Control Act was implemented in April of 2007.

◆ There are notable differences in the field of medicine and cultural background in Japan. Culturally sensitive educational programs need to be established so that medical professionals can learn not only sophisticated palliative care contents but also how to assist their patients in advance care planning with their own unique cultural background.

Transition of palliative care in Japan

Establishment of hospice

The modern hospice movement began with the establishment of St. Christopher's Hospice in the suburbs of London, United Kingdom, in 1967. Thereafter, the hospice movement spread from the United Kingdom to the United States and around the world. The hospice concept was introduced in Japan in the 1970s, and the discussion of the need for hospice programs was started. In 1981, the first in-hospital independent hospice inpatient facility was founded within Seirei Mikatahara General Hospital of Shizuoka prefecture. This was followed in 1984 by the creation of an in-hospital hospice floor at Yodogawa Christian Hospital in Osaka City. Since their establishment, not only medical professionals but also the public has shown great interest in topics relating to death and dying. This has led to a growing implementation of hospice care services within medical facilities in Japan.[1] Table 77.1 outlines the history of palliative care in Japan from 1973 to 2013.

Governmental approach

In an effort to improve the quality of end-of-life care and palliative care in Japan, the Ministry of Health and Welfare released a report, the *Investigative Committee for the Role of Terminal Care*, in June 1989. This report was followed in April 1990 by the introduction of the Palliative Care Unit Admission Fee.[1] This new system allocated a fixed amount of money to cover medical services provided in palliative care facilities as long as the stipulated criteria were met. This resulted in an increased number of facilities providing hospice or palliative care in Japan. However, the Palliative Care Unit Admission Fee applied only to end-of-life care provided to patients with illnesses such as cancer and AIDS. In addition, it only applied to medical care provided within the facilities that fulfilled the stipulated criteria.[2] As a result, many patients who were desperate for quality palliative care did not have the opportunity to benefit from this political measure.

To solve this problem, the Remuneration for Medical Services was revised in 2002 to include an Additional Medical Fee for Palliative Care. This was a significant step in the development of hospice and palliative care in Japan. In addition to the in-hospital medical services within the hospice/palliative care facilities, the fee revision provided additional medical service fees for palliative care provided in general floors by a full-time team of staff that engaged in alleviation of symptoms. This provided an incentive to expand hospice and palliative care consultation services to the general units as well as home-based services including outpatient care and home visits. Box 77.1 shows the criteria for facilities that can provide inpatient hospice/palliative care within the current Japanese healthcare coverage.

Facilities offering hospice/palliative care are increasing annually, as can be seen in Figure 77.1, with 274 hospice/palliative care units (5475 beds) country wide as of February 2013.[4]

However, in 2002, only 4% of the patients who died from cancer spent the last days of their lives receiving hospice or palliative care. It was obvious that there was still an inadequate number of facilities available for those patients. The government added requirements for palliative care facilities to be authorized in 2002. One of those requirements was the need to be approved by the Japan Council for Quality Health Care (JCQHC).

Some organizations failed to qualify by the JCQHC standard and could not register their new palliative care facilities. This led to a decline in facilities in 2003 (Figure 77.1). A further decline of facilities in 2007 is considered to be due to the Remuneration for Medical Services, which was revised in 2006. Each facility has struggled to ensure a nurse-to-patient ratio of a minimum of one RN for every seven patients in general medical or postsurgical care units. This nurse-to-patient ratio was required in order to obtain the increase in revenues as outlined in the revision. This resulted in a delay of plans to open new palliative care facilities.

Cancer Control Act

In response to the unmet needs of cancer patients, the Cancer Control Act was approved in June 2006 and implemented in April 2007. The aim was to create a nationwide structure for providing specialized medical treatment for cancer patients. The Act was a response to a particular social problem—many cancer patients seeking desirable cancer treatment had to "roam" around many medical facilities; those patients were called "cancer refugees."

Table 77.1 The history of hospice/palliative care in Japan

1973	Activities by the Organized Care of Dying Patients (OCDP) started at Yodogawa Christian Hospital.
1977	Activities at St. Christopher's Hospice in the UK were introduced in the newspaper.
	The first meeting of the Japanese Association for Clinical Research on Death and Dying was held.
1981	The first Japanese hospice was opened at Seirei Mikatahara General Hospital.
1984	A hospice was opened at Yodogawa Christian Hospital.
1989	Ministry of Health, Labor, and Welfare announced a report by the Investigative Committee for the Role of Terminal Care.
1990	Ministry of Health, Labor, and Welfare introduced the Palliative Care Unit Admission Fee as the remuneration for medical services under health insurance.
1991	Japan Hospice Palliative Care Foundation (presently, a nonprofit organization, Hospice Palliative Care Japan) was founded.
1996	The first meeting of the Japanese Society of Palliative Medicine was held.
	The Japanese Nursing Association launched accreditation of Oncology Certified Nurse Specialist.
1999	The Japanese Nursing Association launched accreditation of Certified Nurse for palliative care, cancer pain management nursing, etc.
2002	Additional Charge for Palliative Care was started as remuneration for medical services under health insurance. (2,500 yen/day).
2006	The Cancer Control Act was enacted.
2007	The Cancer Control Act was enforced.
2008	Additional Charge for Palliative Care increased to 3,000 yen/day.
2009	The number of palliative care units reached over 200 facilities.
2010	Additional Charge for Palliative Care increased to 4,000 yen/day.
2014	The number of palliative care units reached 308 facilities, 6182 beds (as of June, 15th).

Source: Adapted from reference 2.

Box 77.1 Facility criteria for palliative care unit admission fee

1. Patients mainly with malignant tumors or AIDS shall be admitted to the palliative care unit, and palliative care should be provided in the unit as a team.

2. Within this unit, care must be always provided by a minimum of no less than one RN for every 7 patients. However, if the number of RNs is higher than the specified number above, the number of RNs on night shift shall be two or more.

3. Sufficient equipment and structure must be prepared to provide the adequate treatment.

4. Physicians who completed training in palliative care should be assigned, provided, however, that this shall only apply when providing care for patients with malignant tumors who are eligible for calculating palliative care unit admission fee.

5. Sufficient building and facilities must be prepared to provide adequate treatment.

6. Structure to determine the hospitalization/discharge of patients must be in place.

7. The ratio of hospital rooms must be appropriate for providing special treatment environment as optional medical treatment, as stipulated in subparagraph 4 of paragraph 2 of Article 63 of the Health Insurance Law and subparagraph 4 of paragraph 2 of Article 64 of the Act for the Assurance of Medical Care for the Elderly.

8. The facility must be a designated cancer care hospital or a medical facility evaluated by Japan Council for Quality Health Care, or an equivalent thereof.

9. Training must be provided to physicians and nurses of related medical institutions.

Source: 2012 Ministry of Health, Labor, and Welfare Notification No. 77: Facility Criteria, etc., for Basic Medical Service Fee Excerpt from "Facility Criteria for Palliative Care Unit Admission Fee."[3]

Increasing demands from the patients and citizens to improve this situation resulted in this Cancer Control Act.

The Cancer Control Act focused on three areas: (1) prevention and early detection of cancer; (2) equalization of cancer medical services; and (3) research. The second area—equalization of cancer medical services—stipulated that palliative care be promoted in order to maintain and improve the quality of life of cancer patients under medical treatment.

In addition, in June 2007, based on the Cancer Control Act, the Japanese government formulated the Basic Plan to Promote Cancer Control Programs. Feedback from the Cancer Control Promotion Council, which included cancer patients and their families as its members, was taken into account. The Basic Plan to Promote Cancer Control Programs placed "initiation of palliative care at an early stage of treatment" as a priority.[5,6] The Act stipulated that alleviation of physical symptoms and support for psychological issues be provided, not only in the terminal phase of the disease but also from the early stages of treatment. The goal was for cancer patients and their families to maintain their quality of life as much as possible. Thus, the foundation was laid to seamlessly provide palliative care to patients and their families in various situations of life-threatening illness.

Modes of hospice care/palliative care

In Japan, hospice care and palliative care are provided in many forms: in-hospital independent type, in-hospital floor type, in hospital segmented type, home care, and free-standing type.[1]

The in-hospital floor type uses one of the units of a general hospital as a hospice or a palliative care unit, while the in-hospital segmented type has no independent building or unit but has a palliative care team to provide consultations of palliative care at the request from the staff or patients of the floor. The home care type

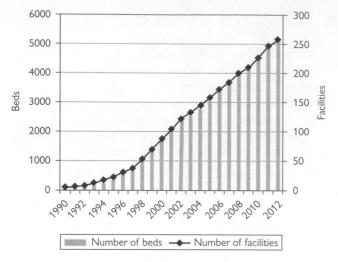

Figure 77.1 Number of registered/approved facilities for palliative care unit admission fee and number of beds, 1990 to 2012. Source: Hospice Palliative Care Japan (2013), reference 4.

has no inpatient care facility (or has only a short-term inpatient care facility) and practices mainly home-based hospice/palliative care. Finally, the free-standing type is independent of any general hospitals in terms of relationship and location. There are only a few free-standing facilities offering hospice/palliative care in Japan. An example is the Life Planning Center Foundation Peace House Hospice in Kanagawa prefecture.[7]

Training of medical professionals with specialized knowledge regarding palliative care

Opioid consumption in Japan for medical use remains less than one-tenth of that of the developed Western countries (Table 77.2). This reflects a lack of appreciation of the critical importance of opioid availability and use in the relief of suffering and the control of pain and dyspnea, especially at the end of life.[8]

When the Basic Plan to Promote Cancer Control Programs was approved by the cabinet on June 15, 2007, a goal was set that "within 10 years, all doctors engaging in cancer treatment would acquire basic knowledge about palliative care through training." The prime minister announced that he would work to realize the goal "within 5 years" so as to be ahead of schedule for the "within 10 years" plan. The Japanese government strongly encouraged doctors working with cancer patients to complete their palliative care training as quickly as possible to meet the goal of "completing within 5 years."[6]

In this way, in addition to preparing a structure to provide comprehensive palliative care to patients and their families, specialized education and training in this field are being promoted. The goal is to increase the number of doctors with specialized knowledge and skills in palliative care at the same time as establishing a number of medical institutions that offer cancer treatment through palliative care teams.[6]

Nurse specialists in palliative care

Following the revision of the Medical Service Fee in 2002, the number of nurse specialists working in clinical settings increased (Figure 77.2). With support and encouragement from their departments, many of these nurses received training on "how to organize a palliative care team."[9]

There are two types of credentialing systems in hospice/palliative care nursing. Certification fields especially relevant to this area are; Certified Nurse Specialists (CNSs) in Cancer Nursing, Palliative Care Certified Nurses (CNs), and Cancer Pain Management CNs. The roles of CNSs are excellent nursing practice, consultation with care providers including nurses, coordination among the concerned parties, ethical coordination to protect the rights of individuals, education of nursing personnel, and research activities at clinical settings. They are certified as CNSs by completing a master's program at a graduate school after obtaining a national license for nurses, and then passing the credentialing examination given by the Japanese Nursing Association (JNA) after accumulating a certain amount of experience. CNSs are required to renew the certification every 5 years. A credentialing system for Oncology CNS was introduced in Japan in 1996, and there were 514 CNSs specializing in oncology nursing as of October 2014.[10]

On the other hand, a credentialing system for CNs was introduced by JNA for palliative care certified nurses and cancer pain management certified nurses in 1999. The roles of CNs are nursing practice at high level, instruction of nurses, and consultation with nurses. They are certified as CNs by accumulating a certain amount of experience after obtaining a national license for nurses, and then passing the credentialing examination given by JNA after completing the required education program for certification. It is required to renew the certification every 5 years. Currently there are 21 certification fields for CNs in Japan, and 1,295 palliative care CNs and 638 cancer pain management CNs had been certified as of January 2013.[10]

Apart from the educational structure, to train specialists in particular fields there is a wide variance in palliative care education within basic nursing training programs and for new staff or generalists working on hospice/palliative care units. There was recognition that for nurses this was an important issue to be addressed[11] and palliative care training within basic nursing education/continuing nursing education was reevaluated. The need to train instructors that provide the palliative care education was identified.[12] To this end, in 2007, the educational program End-of-Life Nursing Education Consortium (ELNEC) developed by the American Association of Colleges of Nursing (AACN) and the City of Hope National Medical Center in the United States, was translated into Japanese and adapted to fit the present situation in Japan. This resulted in the ELNEC-Japan Faculty Development Program. The expectation was that with this training, nurse educators would improve the quality of palliative nursing care and end-of-life care for practicing nurses as well as nursing students in Japan. To date, over 997 nurses representing all 47 prefectures have certified as ELNEC-Japan trainers by attending national programs. They returned to their institutions or regions to train other nurses and members of interdisciplinary teams. The evaluation of the ELNEC-Japan Faculty Development Program demonstrated positive changes in self-rated confidence in teaching, preparing to teach, and leading initiatives in end-of-life care. Participants evaluated the program highly and also reported increases in the length and frequency of their educational sessions related to palliative care after completing the program. They also reported using new strategies in their teaching, including practical work, case studies, and role plays.[13]

Table 77.2 International comparisons of usage of medical narcotics morphine, fentanyl, and oxycodone in total (morphine equivalent g/day per million population)

	2000–2002	2001–2003	2002–2004	2003-2005	2004–2006	2005–2007	2006–2008	2007–2009
Austria	472.3	548.5	632.1	735.5	882.1	1,102.5	1,315.0	1,504.5
Canada	498.8	635.5	817.4	916.5	1,090.3	1,273.4	1,387.7	1,644.4
Australia	271.6	307.4	343.7	375.9	427.3	516.4	639.8	780.6
USA	743.8	910.3	1,072.6	1,249.5	1,403.4	1,567.2	1,694.3	1,792.6
France	274.6	306.0	330.3	378.5	460.1	558.1	603.9	640.7
UK	153.3	152.7	186.4	254.5	298.5	272.8	291.1	330.9
Germany	354.3	428.5	584.9	732.4	1,088.7	1,343.7	1,531.3	1,422.7
Japan	25.9	38.8	49.2	61.0	69.1	77.5	83.8	97.9
Italy	46.6	72.2	94.6	123.3	140.3	157.8	192.5	267.5
Korea	21.2	21.2	18.4	23.0	36.7	56.8	85.4	125.7

Note: (1) No data for oxycodone in 2003 or earlier.

(2) Data before 2000 cannot be compared because of changes in method.

(3) Fentanyl 0.6mg = Oxycodone 75mg = morphine 100mg (INCB, defined daily doses for statistical purposes).

Source: Consumption of Narcotic for Medical Use, reference 8.

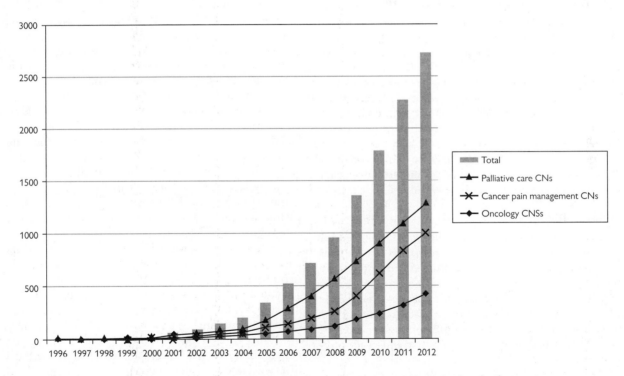

Figure 77.2 Growing numbers of nurse specialists in palliative care, 1996 to 2012. Source: Japanese Nursing Association (2013), reference 10.

Dissemination and awareness of palliative care to the general public

With governmental and professional activities in place to strengthen the overall quality of palliative care, the next step was to disseminate this information to patients and their families so that quality care could be accessed if needed. However, the concept of palliative care has not been widely known or fully accepted by the Japanese general public as part of comprehensive medical and nursing care.

Since 2007, a project for dissemination and awareness of palliative care has been in effect. The goal is to increase public awareness and understanding of hospice and palliative care and what these have to offer. According to a survey conducted by the government in January 2013, 34.3% of adults knew the term "palliative care" very well, and 29% knew the word "palliative care" only, but the rest, 35.7% of the population, had never heard of the word. This result shows that these educational activities and publicity campaigns might have not been effective. The beliefs that palliative care is medical care for patients that have "given up and simply await their death" or that opioids, even when medically indicated, are "dangerous" are still fairly common.[14] These results show that the concept of palliative care remains unfamiliar to most Japanese. To increase public awareness and send accurate information about palliative care, the Ministry of Health, Labor, and Welfare, in April 2007, developed plans for the Dissemination and Awareness Project. The project called "The Orange Balloon Project" was entrusted to the Japanese Society for Palliative Medicine.[15] This project has been continued and various educational events have been conducted for the public by several societies related to palliative care in Japan. Increasing numbers of patients and their family members from patient advocacy groups have also been actively involved in this project and cooperating with medical and nursing societies.[16] The project continues to send the message that agonizing symptoms of life-threatening illnesses can be palliated and medical professionals are striving to help those patients.

Challenges for palliative care in Japan

Challenges related to sociocultural background

There is a social trend to avoid conversations about death and facing death or dealing with death-related situations within the sociocultural background of Japan.[1] This barrier creates delays in introducing palliative care to the patients and their families early on in the disease process based on need not prognosis. Another challenge for Japanese nurses to practice quality palliative/end-of-life care is that the Ministry's criteria for admission and staffing and space regulation for hospice and palliative care units. Regrettably those criteria limit payment for hospice and palliative care to patients with progressive cancer or AIDS. This result in Japanese dying from other illnesses unfortunately are not given opportunities to benefit from palliative and hospice care.

Educational challenges

Although the previously described activities to educate medical and nursing professionals who engage in palliative care are well under way, many patients and their families continue to report experiencing feelings of hurt or abandonment when the focus of their care shifts from cancer treatment to palliative care. There is an urgent need to include communication skills as an essential skill to be taught to all medical and nursing professionals, especially for those participating in palliative care and end-of-life care.

Enhancement of home care

The Basic Plan to Promote Cancer Control Programs includes as one of the objectives "accommodating the wishes of cancer patients, by increasing the number of patients that can choose to receive treatment in the comfort of their home or region with which they are familiar."[6] This objective requires preparation for a structure and environment to provide palliative care, not only in hospitals but also in the homes of cancer patients. Coordination and cooperation between sites of care, depending on the changing needs of the patient, will be necessary to achieve this objective. In addition, it is important that each region take into consideration characteristics of their particular demographics so that a systematic approach to initiating home medical treatment and to constructing a regional alliance that can support the patients and their families will be in place.

Expansion of the role of hospice/palliative care units

Today in Japan, hospice/palliative care facilities are not only expected to control symptoms that are difficult to manage within general floors or at home, but also to support home-care teams visiting patients at end-of-life. In the future, it is envisioned that hospices and palliative care facilities will be able to offer specialized care to alleviate the patients' sufferings at various stages of disease and treatment. In addition, these medical facilities would function as a base for the regional alliance and work toward providing training to medical and nursing professionals in palliative care. In this way, the quality of palliative care would be enhanced throughout the entire region.

Summary

Since 1990, the Japan Ministry of Health, Labor, and Welfare has actively advocated to facilitate palliative care by designating palliative care as eligible for national health insurance. Because of the significant suffering experienced by cancer patients and using that as an impetus—the Ministry of Health, Labor, and Welfare has launched multiple nationwide projects to facilitate the dissemination of palliative care. In 2007, one of these actions of great significance was to change the criteria of palliative care admissions to include all cancer patients with a considerable level of suffering irrespective of stage of the disease. The Ministry also mandated that all 353 regional cancer centers throughout Japan establish palliative care teams, and approved palliative care teams as eligible for national health coverage.[17] These are all big steps, which are applicable to other chronic and debilitating life-threatening illnesses. With the implementation of these measures, palliative care provided to patients and their families in Japan is expected to steadily improve.

There are notable differences in the field of medicine and cultural background in Japan. The palliative care approach to patients and families also differs from the approach to care provided by other departments. For example, in palliative care, medical professionals are expected to be sensitive toward the family and patients' cultural background since it plays a significant role in planning their care.

Culturally sensitive educational programs need to be established so that medical professionals could learn not only sophisticated palliative care contents, but also how to assist their patients in advance care planning with their own unique cultural background. Even if palliative care at home becomes well developed, there will always be patients who will choose to spend the last days of their lives in the general hospitals. It is therefore essential to offer chances for any medical professionals who provide care to patients and families facing life-threatening illness to be educated so that they can offer high quality palliative care for those in need.

References

1. The Japanese Association for Clinical Research on Death and Dying. Clinical Approaches on Death and Dying, IV: Future Terminal Care. Tokyo, Japan: Chuo Seihan; 1995:12.
2. Yasuo Shima. Future hospice/palliative care: establishing expertise and community dissemination. In: Japan Hospice Palliative

Care Foundation. Hospice/Palliative White Paper 2007. Specialty in Palliative Care-Palliative Care Team and Palliative Care Unit. Tokyo, Japan: Seikaisha; 2007:10–16.

3. Ministry of Health, Labor, and Welfare. Notification, etc., Regarding 2012 Revision of Medical Service Fee. Facility Criteria, etc., Applied for Basic Treatment Fee. Ministry of Health, Labor, and Welfare Notification No. 77, 2012. Available at: http://www.mhlw.go.jp/bunya/iryouhoken/iryouhoken15/dl/5-1.pdf (accessed June 13, 2013).

4. Hospice Palliative Care Japan. Available at: http://www.hpcj.org/what (accessed June 14, 2013).

5. Ministry of Health, Labor, and Welfare. Health Service Bureau General Affairs Division Cancer Control Promotion Office. 2007. The first Conference of Dissemination and Awareness Regarding Cancer. Data: Cancer-Related Statistics. Available at: http://www.mhlw.go.jp/shingi/2008/10/s1024-9.html (accessed July 08, 2014).

6. Masashi Kato. Yasuhisa Takeda. The structure of Japanese medical services and palliative care movements in Japan's cancer control and the future directions for palliative care—based on the plans of the "Basic plan to promote cancer control programs." In: Japan Hospice Palliative Care Foundation. Hospice/Palliative White Paper, 2008. Structure of Medical Services and Regional Networks for Palliative Care. Tokyo, Japan: Seikaisha; 2008:6–13.

7. Tetsuo Kashiwagi. Hospice/Palliative Care Definitive Edition. Tokyo, Japan: Seikaisya; 2006:140–148.

8. Center for Cancer Control and Information Services of National Cancer Center. Cancer Statistics 2008 Data Section. Consumption of Narcotic for Medical Use. 2012; 93. Available at: http://ganjoho.jp/data/professional/statistics/backnumber/2012/cancer_statistics_2012.pdf (accessed June 13, 2013).

9. Toshiko Matsumoto. The present situation and foresight into postgraduate training of nurses for palliative care certified nurses. In: Japan Hospice Palliative Care Foundation. Hospice/Palliative White Paper, 2006. Education and Human Resource Development for Palliative Care. Tokyo, Japan: Seikaisha; 2006:17–19.

10. Japanese Nursing Association. Credentialing System. Available at: http://www.nurse.or.jp/jna/english/nursing/education.html (accessed October 7, 2014).

11. Futami N. Present situation and issues of nursing education in palliative treatment for cancer. Palliat Med. 2006;8:27–33.

12. Sakamoto S, Asai A, Kosugi S. Evaluation of ethical teaching method in terminal care using the education program of End-of-Life Nursing Education Consortium (ELNEC) by Japanese nurse-practitioners engaging in end-of-life phase treatments. Kumamoto University Press. Adv Ethics Res. 2007;2:54–65.

13. Takenouchi S, Miyashita M, Tamura K, Kizawa Y, Kosugi S. Evaluation of the end-of-life nursing education consortium— Japan faculty development program: validity and reliability of the "End of life nursing education questionnaire." J Hosp Palliat Nurs. 2011;13(6):368–375.

14. Minister's Secretariat, Public Relations Office. Survey on Cancer Control. Summary of Results. Cancer Information 2012. Available at: http://www8.cao.go.jp/survey/h24/h24-gantaisaku/2-4.html (accessed June 14, 2013).

15. Japanese Society for Palliative Medicine. Orange Balloon Project. Entrusted Survey on Palliative Care in Cancer Treatment in 2007. Available at: http://www.kanwacare.net/(accessed June 14, 2013).

16. Eguchi K. Development of palliative medicine for cancer patients in Japan: from isolated voluntary effort to integrated multidisciplinary network. Jpn J Clin Oncol. 2010;40(9):870–875.

17. Morita T, Miyashita M, Tsuneto S, et al. Palliative care in Japan: shifting from the stage of disease to the intensity of suffering. J Pain Symptom Manage. 2008;6:e6–e7.

CHAPTER 78

Palliative care in South Korea

Hyun Sook Kim and Boon Han Kim

Key points

♦ Cancer became the first leading cause of death in Korea in 1983.

♦ The most important issues in Koreans' perception about the end-of-life care were 'giving no burden of care to others' and 'staying with family and significant others'. In reality, however, many Koreans still receive futile treatment even after their conditions are diagnosed as terminal; the number of Koreans who died in their home decreased substantially, while in hospitals increased.

♦ The concept of hospice was introduced to Korea about 50 years ago, but not consolidated yet firmly within Korean society. Compared with the advancement in education and research, systematization of hospice palliative care in Korea is progressing slowly.

♦ Advanced Practice Nurses (APN) in hospice palliative care are educated with Master's degree since 2003. The role of APN in Korea is similar to that in the United States except that Korean APN are not allowed to issue prescription.

♦ Currently, hospice care in Korea is targeting only terminal cancer patients and their family members, while the demand for expanding the service for non-cancer terminal patients is rapidly increasing in the healthcare community.

Located at the crossroads of Northeast Asia, Korea lies between Japan, the Russian Far East, and China. After World War II, a republic government was set up in the southern half of the Korean Peninsula while a communist-style government occupied the northern half of the Korean Peninsula. The Korean Demilitarized Zone serves as the buffer between North Korea and South Korea. South Korea rose out of absolute poverty but became one of the most economically successful countries among developing countries since the Korean War (1950–1953).

As of the end of 2012, South Korea's total population was estimated at 50 million with a density of about 500 people per square kilometer (Korea National Statistical Office, 2012; http://www.index.go.kr). Although the population grew by about 3% annually during the 1960s, the rate decreased to below 1% over the decades that followed due to aggressive government-driven family planning. The rate was 0.21% in 2005 and is expected to be 0.02% by the year 2020. In the 1960s, the population distribution of Korea was pyramidal with a high birth rate and relatively short life expectancy. Today the age-group distribution is more bell shaped

due to the low birth rate and extended life expectancy. People who are 15 and younger will make up a decreasing portion of the total, while those 65 and older will account for 15.7% of the total by the year 2020 (http://www.korea.net). As of 2012, life expectancy at birth was 77.9 years for males and 84.6 years for females, which is 20 years longer than the life expectancy in 1960 (Korea National Statistical Office, 2012; http://www.kostat.go.kr).

Attitudes toward death

In 2011, there were 257,396 deaths (705 per day on average). The primary causes of mortality and morbidity have shifted from acute, infectious disease to chronic disease over the last half century. By 2011, the top five causes of death in Korea were cancer, cerebral vascular accident (CVA), cardiovascular diseases, suicide, and diabetes mellitus (Korea National Statistical Office, 2012). Every year, approximately 190,000 people are diagnosed with cancer in Korea and 72,000 die from the disease (Korea National Statistical Office, 2012; http://www.kostat.go.kr). Cancer became the first leading cause of death in Korea in 1983. Cancer mortality has been steadily increasing over the last two decades, and cancer deaths accounted for 28% of all deaths in 2011. Leukemia is the leading among cancer causes of death for those under 20, stomach cancer for people in their 30s, liver cancer for ages 40–50, and lung cancer for those over 60. Cancer in the circulatory system is a main cause of death for Koreans 40 and under, while CVA is a common cause of death in people 50 and over. About 20% of these deaths are acute and sudden, while the rest occur following chronic illness.

A national study conducted in 2004 showed that over half of Koreans (54.8%) chose their home as the preferred place of death.[1] And a recent study also showed that most Korean adults chose their home (46%) or long-term care facilities (37.7%) over hospitals (10.8%) as the preferred place for the end-of-life period if they have a life-threatening illness.[2] Despite their preferences, the number of Koreans who died in their home decreased substantially from 72.9% in 1992 to 18.8% in 2012, while those who died in hospitals increased from 16.6% in 1992 to 70.1% in 2012 (Korea National Statistical Office, 2013; http://www.kostat.go.kr).

Most Koreans would prefer to withdraw from medically futile life-sustaining treatment.[1,3] A recent survey revealed the most important issues in Koreans' perception about end-of-life care were (1) giving no burden of care to others (36.7%) and (2) being with family and significant others (30.0%).[4] In reality, however, many Koreans still receive futile treatment even after their conditions are diagnosed as terminal. Furthermore, Korean law does not allow doctors to remove life-sustaining treatment, regardless of the patient's condition or desires or those of family members. The limited hospice palliative care that is offered often demands a high degree of family responsibility; the caregivers of terminal patients are usually immediate family members or private caregivers hired by the family. For these reasons, Korean family members of terminally ill patients experience heavy physical, emotional, and social stresses—much more so than families in the West.[5-6] The family caregivers of patients with terminal cancer will take care of the patient in "enduring with a headstall: suffering or responsibility."[6] In 2009, the Supreme Court granted the right to die to a 77-year-old patient, identified by her surname Kim, who had been in a coma for 456 days. The decision was that all medical treatment to prolong her life would be stopped and the respirator was taken off line on June 24, 2009. Kim first visited the hospital for a bronchial endoscopy in February 2008 for suspected lung cancer. During the biopsy, Kim suffered unexpected profuse bleeding and lapsed into a coma. Kim's family sued for permission to let her die in peace on the grounds that living on a respirator would not be her wishes. The core question was how to confirm that this was Kim's opinion while she was in coma. The Supreme Court said Kim's case satisfied four conditions to die with dignity: that the patient must be examined by a third medical party to prove that he or she has no chance of recovery, that the patient should have expressed a strong desire to halt life-sustaining treatment, that the only means of death is to remove life-sustaining treatment, and that only medical doctors have the right to stop treatment.[1]

This was the first recognized case in Korea of a person's right to die with dignity, and the case led to heated debate. A discussion is ongoing within the medical society to reach consensus and to establish guidelines on the withdrawal of life-sustaining treatment. The importance of hospice palliative care has been brought to the public's attention. However despite such ruling, the Advance Directives (ADs) Act has still not been passed. A recent study showed that patients with chronic diseases preferred to have their healthcare decisions made by their spouse (41.6%) or their son/daughter (27.2%) on their behalf when they could no longer make those decisions.[3] These patients also reported that they had no living wills (96.4%) and had not heard of ADs (91.45). Therefore, serious conflicts are common among patients, family members, and health professionals over the end-of-life treatment decisions. A report from The Economist Intelligence Unit in 2010 ranked South Korea 32 out of 40 countries in the End of Life Care Index.[7]

History of hospice palliative care

Hospice care in Korea began in 1965 at the Calvary Hospice in Gangneung City by the Sisters of the Little Company of Mary. The societal chaos and turmoil in a post–Korean War environment made it almost impossible to build new facilities for terminal patient care. Even during these trying times, the Calvary Hospice and the Australian Sisters of the Little Company of Mary persisted in providing care for terminally ill patients by following the mission provided by founder Mary Potter: "Tomorrow will be too late. Let us pray for those dying today."

The concept of hospice care was introduced to Korea in the 1970s, as the entire nation strived to work toward a better future.

Hospice care expanded in the 1980s through the revolutionary care provided for the terminally ill by the Catholic University of Korea at Seoul St. Mary's Hospital. The first physician to introduce hospice care in South Korea was Kyung-Shik Lee, a hematology/oncology specialist who was an assistant professor in internal medicine at the Catholic University School of Medicine in 1981. Most of the academic focus in the early 1980s was on prolonging the life span of patients, and thus hospice care was not a widely discussed topic. However, Dr. Lee's experiences showed him that some patients would become terminally ill and pass away regardless of technological advances. Dr. Lee believed that the process of dying was as important as the process of living and surviving in many of his cancer patients.[1,8] Student hospice care began in September 1981 under the supervision of Catholic University medical and nursing students, and the concept of hospice care was further advanced and implemented through an oncology conference in June 1982 at St. Mary's Hospital. A department dedicated to hospice care centered on the nursing staff was established at St. Mary's Hospital, and began operation in March 1987. The first hospice units (10 beds total) were established at St. Mary's Hospital in October 1988. A program for home hospice care was also initiated in the oncology department of Severance Hospital in 1988, while another project on home hospice care began that same year in the nursing department of Ewha Women's University under the supervision of a resident nurse. Saint Columban Hospice opened its doors in 1989 by providing house calls that eventually evolved into home hospice care. Thereafter, hospice programs largely provided by religious social services or volunteer activities blossomed around the nation: the three hospice programs available in 1965–1980 grew to 17 in 1980–1990; 73 in 1990–2000; 125 in 2000–2004; and 130 in 2007.[9]

The increase of hospice facilities led to the establishment of the Korean Hospice Association in 1991 and the Korean Catholic Hospice Association in 1992. These two associations have greatly influenced the expansion of hospice care in Korea, despite the religious undertones that were inextricably linked to their missions.

In 1995, So Woo Lee, a professor of the Seoul National University College of Nursing conducted a study, The National Hospice Care Service Development in Korea[5] (outsourced by the Ministry for Health and Welfare), reporting on the status of terminal patients and their family caregivers. Professor Lee then developed the Internet-based hospice information service system.[10] That same year (1995), The Catholic University of Korea's nursing school was selected as WHO's Collaborating Center for Hospice and Palliative Care, and the school began medical training for structured hospice and palliative care, focusing on nursing (http://hospice.catholic.ac.kr).

The researchers who participated in "The National Hospice Care Service Development in Korea" realized the need for establishing an academic society. Some of the researchers and the medical cadres of the Catholic University of Korea who were operating the hospice inpatient unit at the time joined forces to form an eight-member steering committee (Chair Kyung-Shik Lee and three nurses were included). After 3 months of preparation, the Korean Society for Hospice and Palliative Care (KSHPC) was established in 1998 (www.hospicecare.co.kr). The purpose for the establishment of the KSHPC was to advance academics pertaining to hospice palliative care in Korea; to increase the quality of life for terminal cancer patients, factoring in the public health policies and medical regulations that would help them to lead a comfortable life; to interact with the international hospice palliative care academic societies and associations; and to exchange information. Professor Lee, a nurse and one of the steering committee members, served as the second president of this academic society. In 1998, hospice and palliative care were unfamiliar to many doctors. In fact, there were many who held negative views about hospice. Thus, it is not surprising that nursing is the leading occupation among members of the KSHPC.[1]

The KSHPC hosted a hearing session on the hospice systemization in 1999 along with the Korean Catholic Hospice Association and Korea Hospice Association at the National Assembly Member Center. In 2002, it published *Guidance for Cancer Patient Pain Management* jointly with the Korean Cancer Study Group. In 2003, it organized a symposium on the Korean Hospice and Palliative Care Systemization jointly with the National Cancer Center, and submitted a draft hospice law to the Ministry for Health, Welfare, and Family Affairs. The Korean society is trying hard to systemize hospice palliative care. On March 2005, it supervised the Asia Pacific Hospice Conference (APHC) that is held every 2 years. Likewise, it is involved heavily in the interchange with foreign nations. Moreover, KSHPC published the *Korean Journal of Hospice and Palliative Care*, first edition, volume 1, in December 1998—the year when the academic society was established. It published the journal at least once a year until 2001, twice a year from 2002 to 2006, and quarterly since 2007, contributing to the academic development of the hospice and palliative care scholars, including the nurses.

However, nurses were very passionate about the organizations that define their inherent roles and that can help them increase their knowledge. Thus, the Korean Hospice Palliative Nurses Association (KHPNA) was established on August 29, 2003. Professor Lee of the Seoul National University, who was the chair of the steering committee for the launch of the society, served as the first president of KHPNA. The author, Professor Boon Han Kim of the Hanyang University, served as the president following Professor Lee. Due to the effort made by the KHPNA, nurses in the area of hospice palliative care are now recognized as specialized nurses. In March 2004, graduate-level training for nurses (advanced practice nurses, or APNs) specializing in hospice palliative care began. As of 2012, more than 400 nurses were active as members of the KSHPC and KHPNA.

The establishment of academic organizations has served as a turning point in increasing interaction between Korean experts on hospice and palliative care with overseas institutions. The APHC agreed to develop a hospice palliative care model that is appropriate for our culture along with the people of the Asia Pacific region. The medium used is the academic conference that is hosted every 2 to 3 years in the Asia Pacific region. The sixth APHC was held in 2005 in Seoul, Korea, with the theme of Changing Society and Human Life with Hospice and Palliative Care. The sixth APHC promoted the advancement of the hospice palliative care system in Korea, and stimulated related academic researches. Moreover, it publicized the need to increase attention to terminal cancer patients' quality of life. This international trend will advance hospice palliative care. In 2001, the Asia Pacific Hospice Palliative Care Network (APHN) was established as an academic forum for hospice palliative care professionals of the Asia Pacific region; Hong Kong, Japan, Taiwan, Singapore, Indonesia, India,

Thailand, Malaysia, Vietnam, Myanmar, Nepal, Pakistan, Sri Lanka, Australia, New Zealand, and Korea subscribed as member nations. After the establishment of the APHN, the network was in charge of the APHC. Dr. Young Sun Hong represented Korea from the establishment of the academic society, and he eventually served as the president for years (2007-2009). In 2009, Hyun Sook Kim, a nurse and an author, was recommended as a council member to represent Korea in the APHN council, which is made up primarily of medical doctors.

Systemization is continuing slowly compared with the academic advancement of hospice palliative care. The National Cancer Center sponsored several studies that provided evidence to support Korean standardization of hospice palliative care services.[9–11] Systemization at the government level involves creating and submitting guidelines on the standards and regulations pertaining to hospice palliative care.

In March 2005, representatives of hospice-related organizations in the nation gathered to declare a day of global palliative care and presented a declaration on this occasion. The Korea declaration, which calls for the expansion of the government's support on the policy level, was based on the Barcelona Declaration on the Hospice and Palliative Care, which was published in the Worldwide Global Summit for National Association of Hospice Palliative Care on December 9, 1995. It is used as a symbol to encourage medical service targeting the terminal cancer patients from different parts of the world.[8]

In 2003, the central government began supporting institutions that offer hospice service to terminal cancer patients to provide necessary support under the Cancer Control Act, thanks to the incessant efforts of the academic society and the National Cancer Center. In 2006, there were 23 institutions offering hospice palliative care for 2060 terminal cancer patients, and by 2010 support was increased to provide for 6564 terminal cancer patients in 40 institutions. In June 2011, through amendments to the Cancer Control Act, the government established more concrete hospice palliative care systems to improve quality of life for terminally ill cancer patients and their families. Since 2009, the Ministry for Health and Welfare Affairs (www.mw.go.kr) has been processing a pilot project for developing a medical health insurance policy for hospice palliative care. Home hospice palliative care also has been processed as a demonstrative project (National Cancer Information Center, www.cancer.go.kr). The Cancer Control Act also set a requirement for physicians, nurses, and social workers working in hospice palliative care settings to complete over 60 hours of mandatory education in hospice palliative care beginning in 2012 (Health Insurance Review & Assessment Service, http://www.hira.or.kr; Ministry of Health & Welfare, http://www.mw.go.kr).

Hospice palliative care nursing education

Master's program: advanced practice nurse in hospice palliative care

The Ministry of Education and Human Resources Development is the government body responsible for the formation and implementation of educational policies. The government provides guidance on basic policy matters as well as financial assistance. The Ministry of Health and Welfare affairs regulate the number of students admitted to heath-related fields (medicine, nursing, physical therapy, etc.) in Korea. The Korean Accreditation Board of Nursing, founded in 2004, is the body responsible for the nursing education accreditation, APN education institution appointment and evaluation, national certification examination for APNs, and the national licensing examination for nurses (www.Kabon.or.kr).

The "specialized nurse" was changed to "APN" by a revised medical law on January 2000. The areas of APN have expanded from 4 areas to 10 areas in 2003 and to 13 areas in 2006. The APN program became a masters program, and an APN in hospice palliative care program started in March 2004.

As of 2008, 11 graduate nursing schools had been appointed as the APN in hospice palliative care. Seventy-five students per each year are admitted to become APNs in hospice palliative care. As of 2012, 286 out of 12,518 APNs were specialized in hospice palliative care in Korea (Korean Nurses Association, http://koreanurse.or.kr/).

To qualify as an APN in hospice palliative care, students must complete at least 13 credits in the basic core curriculum, 10 credits in classes in their major that address theories, and 10 credits in practicum classes. In all, they must complete at least 33 credits to be eligible to take the nationally administered board examination for APN, including at least 220 hours of basic core classes, at least 160 hours of classes essential for their major, and at least 300 hours of practical training in their major. Thus, this is handled by the

individual schools. A detailed curriculum is shown in Table 78.1. The APN certification examination is operated by the Ministry for Health and Welfare Affairs, and the Korean Nurses Association (KNA) acts as a proxy. National certification is granted to those who pass both the first test (written) and the second test (practical).

The roles of the APN in hospice palliative care are divided into 9 duties and 46 tasks, and the classes on the theories and on the practical training and test on the practical training are formed according to the analysis of these roles. The role of the APN in Korea is very similar to that of the APN in the United States, except that by 2013 the Korean APN did not yet have prescription privileges.

Certified program for generalist hospice palliative care nurses

The Catholic University of Korea College of Nursing was authorized as Collaborating Centre for Hospice Palliative Care by the WHO on September 28, 1995. The following year, the Research Institute for Hospice Palliative Care was established within The Catholic University of Korea College of Nursing. The institute directs the hospice, where research and training are conducted to plan for and implement structured work. This research institute offered over 300 hours of education programs for generalist

Table 78.1 Curriculum for APN in hospice palliative care

Classification	Subject	Credit	Hour	Remarks
Core curriculum for APN in all areas	Nursing theory	2	32	
	Advanced nursing role	2	32	
	Pharmacology	2	32	
	Advanced physical examination & practice	3	64	
	Thesis research	2	32	
	Pathophysiology	2	32	
	Subtotal	**13**	**224**	
Theory education for APN in hospice palliative care only	Introduction to hospice palliative nursing	2	32	
	Pain & symptom management	2	32	
	Psychosocial spiritual nursing care	2	32	
	Bereavement, family care, and counseling	2	32	
	Hospice management	2	32	
	Subtotal	**10**	**160**	
Practical training	Hospice palliative nursing practicum I-1	1	32	Home hospice
	Hospice palliative nursing practicum II-1	1	32	Bereaved family
	Hospice palliative nursing practicum III	2	64	Community health center
	Hospice palliative nursing practicum IV	2	64	Hospice unit
	Hospice palliative nursing practicum I-2	2	64	Hospice unit
	Hospice palliative nursing practicum II-2	2	64	Hospice unit
	Subtotal	**10**	**320**	
Total		**33**	**704**	

Source: Graduate School of Information in Clinical Nursing, *Hanyang University Bulletin* (2012). Hanyang University Press.

hospice palliative care nurses beginning in 1996. There were 588 graduates of this education program as of 2008 (http://hospice. catholic.ac.kr). Besides these institutions, short-term and ad hoc training programs (which range in length from 1 to 6 months) take place at nursing schools or hospice institutions.

Moreover, the need to supply specialists was raised in the academic community prior to the systemization of the hospice palliative care. At the Korean National Cancer Center, a minimum of 60 hours training was suggested[12] in order for the nurses to work in the hospice and palliative care institutions. Based on this criterion, a pilot program for the hospice of terminal cancer patients was conducted during 2004 and 2005. This basic training program was developed for physicians, nurses, social workers, clergy, and volunteers working in hospice and palliative care, and the training was conducted around the nation for 2 years. Moreover, the demands of the nurses who participated in this training were factored in to suggest a 78-hour long training curriculum for nurses.[12]

While conducting these diverse educational programs, it was necessary to train the trainers who were to be responsible for the development of basic standard hospice palliative education program that use standardized training materials and who would be responsible for training in individual regions. To this end, the National Cancer Center with the backing of the government selected nurses, doctors, and social workers to attend the Education on Palliative and End-of-Life Care (EPEC) training (http://www. epec.net) in 2006–2007. They then developed a 60-hour-long basic standard education program for all interdisciplinary team in hospice palliative care based on the EPEC project.[9,12]

The National Cancer Center had a further plan for development of an advanced level curriculum for each interdisciplinary team, and the first work was for the nurses (Table 78.2).

In March 2009, a task force team (TFT) for developing a curriculum for certified generalist hospice palliative care nurses was established and developed the curriculum collaborating with the KHPNA. That organization developed guidelines for certified generalist hospice palliative care nurses. The guidelines identified 8 duties, 36 tasks, and 137 task elements. The education and training subcommittee of the National Cancer Center, the Cancer Control

Table 78.2 Professional development aims in hospice palliative care from the government's second-term 10-year plan for cancer control

	Year 2006	Year 2010	Year 2015
Train-the-trainer	20 (2007)	120	200
Physician	Develop course	130	260
◆ Palliative medicine diploma certification			
Nurse	Develop course	900	1,800
◆ APN in hospice palliative care (100/year)			
Social worker	Develop course	65	130
Clergy	Develop course	65	130
Volunteer	Develop course	10,000	20,000

Source: The Ministry for Health, Welfare and Family Affairs (2005). National Cancer Control.

Institute, developed the curriculum. The TFT developed over 130 hours (98 hours in theory and 32 hours in practice) of educational programming based on the KHPNA guidelines (Table 78.3)[13]: palliative nursing care (6 hours), understanding life and death (4 hours), pain and symptom management (23 hours), psychosocial care (7 hours), spiritual care (6 hours), complementary intervention (8 hours), communication (8 hours), final hours and bereavement (9 hours), hospice management (11 hours), end-of-life care for special populations (10 hours), and practicum (32 hours). The materials of the End-of-Life Nursing Education Consortium (ELNEC) international training program (http://www.aacn.nche.edu/elnec/) were translated into Korean and incorporated into this curriculum with permission from the ELNEC project. The content of this curriculum was developed in 2009, the pilot course was operated in 2010, and now a Web-based certified hospice palliative nurse education program is operating (http://hospice.el.or.kr/).

End-of-Life Nursing Education Consortium train-the-trainer program

An ELNEC core train-the-trainer program was held August 20–21, 2009, in Seoul by the City of Hope National Medical Center (COH), the American Association of Colleges of Nursing (AACN) and ELNEC Project-Korea collaborating with KHPNA. The ELNEC Project is a national end-of-life education program administered by COH and AACN designed to enhance palliative care in nursing. The ELNEC Project-Korea team consists of four nurses who were trained as ELNEC trainers in the United States and two nurses who are key board members of KHPNA. The faculties of the courses were ELNEC principal investigator Dr. Betty Ferrell, ELNEC consultant Dr. Judith Paice, and four Korean nurses who were trained in the United States. One hundred seventy-eight nurses and other interdisciplinary team members attended the course, and 145 nurses, who represented all provinces of South Korea, were certified as ELNEC trainers with satisfactory outcomes.[14]

In July 2010, a 2-day ELNEC-Geriatric train-the-trainer program was held in Seoul. A total of 203 participants, including physicians, nurses, and social workers, were certified as ELNEC-Geriatric trainers, and this course contributed to increasing the nurses' knowledge for palliative care in long-term care.[15] Then in July 2012, a 2-day ELNEC-Pediatric Palliative Care (PPC) train-the-trainer program was held, and 191 participants were certified as ELNEC-PPC trainers in Seoul, Korea. The successful implementation of these programs aided in increasing the nurses' knowledge and led to educating and training other nurses and health professionals to improve quality of end-of-life care that is not confined to terminal cancer but rather addresses all life-threatening illness.

Hospice palliative care setting

In Korea, the institutions that provide hospice palliative care can be divided into three major groups: inpatient hospice palliative care unit of hospitals or free-standing hospice institutions, home hospice palliative care, and home-based cancer patient hospice through regional public health centers.

As of 2007, there were 113 hospice palliative care institutions in Korea, including 21 home hospice institutions, 19 palliative care units, 19 mixed types, 12 free-standing hospice institutions, and 42 other type institutions. In June 2011, through amendments

Table 78.3 Job analysis for role identification of generalist hospice palliative care nurses: frequency, criticality, and difficulty of each task

Duty		Task		Frequency*		Criticality*		Difficulty*	
				Mean	SD	Mean	SD	Mean	SD
A	Data collection	A1	Pain assessment	3.64	0.69	3.92	0.27	2.77	0.64
		A2	Assess physical symptoms related to terminal disease	3.26	0.78	3.67	0.51	2.69	0.62
		A3	Collect data through diagnostic tests & labs	3.30	0.73	3.43	0.61	2.53	0.79
		A4	Identify psychosocial needs of patients and family	3.17	0.86	3.72	0.52	2.81	0.70
		A5	Identify spiritual needs of patients and family	3.21	0.85	3.74	0.49	3.11	0.87
		A6	Assess needs related to impending death	3.24	0.86	3.81	0.42	2.80	0.72
		A7	Assess the bereaved family	2.81	0.89	3.60	0.55	2.93	0.69
		Total		3.23	0.77	3.53	0.47	2.76	0.69
B	Clinical decision-making: diagnosis, planning, evaluation	B1	Formulate nursing diagnoses	2.94	0.86	3.66	0.53	2.73	0.74
		B2	Develop care plans	2.96	0.88	3.68	0.55	2.76	0.72
		B3	Evaluate the effectiveness of nursing intervention	2.99	0.86	3.68	0.52	2.76	0.76
		B4	Modify nursing care based on evaluation	2.77	0.86	3.55	0.59	2.85	0.72
		Total		2.92	0.87	3.65	0.55	2.77	0.74
C	Therapeutic intervention & nursing care	C1	Implement pain intervention	2.90	0.92	3.60	0.57	2.58	0.76
		C2	Implement symptom management care	3.04	0.85	3.69	0.52	2.57	0.76
		C3	Provide psychosocial support	3.02	0.80	3.66	0.50	2.79	0.74
		C4	Provide spiritual support	2.82	0.89	3.67	0.49	2.82	0.78
		C5	Implement end-of-life care	2.96	0.89	3.68	0.52	2.76	0.76
		C6	Implement care for the bereaved family	2.54	0.95	3.53	0.59	2.91	0.74
		Total		2.88	0.89	3.63	0.54	2.73	0.76
D	Coping in the emergency situation	D1	Assess emergency status	2.78	0.90	3.75	0.53	2.81	0.83
		D2	Clinical decision-making: diagnosis, planning, & evaluation	2.81	0.88	3.68	0.52	2.86	0.75
		D3	Emergency care	2.79	0.94	3.67	0.54	2.73	0.75
		D4	Utilize resources and transfer	2.93	0.93	3.61	0.61	2.41	0.82
		Total		2.81	0.91	3.70	0.54	2.75	0.80
E	Education & counseling	E1	Educate patients, family, & caregivers	2.88	0.88	3.66	0.51	2.74	0.69
		E2	Therapeutic communication	3.16	0.86	3.78	0.49	2.81	0.75
		E3	Counseling	2.84	0.91	3.71	0.50	2.77	0.74
		Total		2.93	0.89	3.70	0.50	2.76	0.75
F	Environment and resource management	F1	Manage documents and information	3.13	0.97	3.66	0.55	2.31	0.79
		F2	Human resource management	2.89	1.07	3.68	0.54	2.82	0.81
		F3	Manage facility/resource	2.74	1.02	3.47	0.66	2.38	0.79
		F4	Manage public finance	2.36	1.06	3.48	0.67	3.33	0.72
		F5	Manage safety & environment	2.50	1.13	3.63	0.66	2.79	0.74
		F6	Infection control	2.73	1.04	3.62	0.56	2.74	0.72
		F7	Public relations	2.71	0.96	3.63	0.56	2.81	0.72
		Total		2.74	1.02	3.59	0.60	2.65	0.75

(continued)

Table 78.3 Continued

Duty		Task		Frequency*		Criticality*		Difficulty*	
				Mean	SD	Mean	SD	Mean	SD
G	Consultation, regulation, & collaboration	G1	Consultation	2.54	0.91	3.62	0.54	2.95	0.77
		G2	Establish and maintain collaborative relations	2.86	0.93	3.64	0.55	2.48	0.85
		Total		2.75	0.92	3.63	0.54	2.63	0.82
H	Quality control & participation in professional development	H1	Participate in policy development	2.56	0.92	3.68	0.56	2.77	0.74
		H2	Implement legal and ethical affairs	2.87	0.93	3.77	0.44	2.74	0.71
		H3	Educate personnel related to hospice palliative care	2.82	0.96	3.62	0.65	2.64	0.78
		Total		2.75	0.93	3.72	0.51	2.74	0.73

*Frequency, criticality, and difficulty of duty or task were measured with a 4-point scale.

Source: Kim et al. (2010), reference 13

of the Cancer Control Act, a standard requirement was set for authorization of inpatient palliative care units for terminal cancer patients and their family, and as of October 2013, 55 palliative care units had been authorized nationally (National Cancer Information Center, http://www.cancer.go.kr). However, home hospice palliative care has not yet been authorized and is at a demonstration project stage that relies heavily on support from charity organizations, government or local government funding, and volunteers. As of 2011, 29 home hospice palliative care facilities had been reported in South Korea: 11 (37.9%) hospital-based facilities, 4 (13.8%) hospital-independent-center-based care facilities, and 10 (34.5%) home-based care only.[16] Thus, the impact of the amendment to the Cancer Control Act is that the inpatient palliative care unit for terminal cancer patients and their family has increased while the other charity facilities have been steadily declining.

Hospice team members can include physicians, nurses, social workers, clergies, volunteers, pharmacists, nutritionists, physical therapists, art therapists, music therapists, and speech therapists. From these interdisciplinary members, physicians, nurses, social workers, and volunteers are required to establish a palliative care unit and the other members are included according to the setting. In Korea, the nurses act as coordinators for the hospice setting but the role of the physicians is considered to be more important. Issues such as lack of trained physicians and social worker participation, lack of financial support, and lack of interdisciplinary team members' awareness of home hospice palliative care[16] are making the system slow to change; but change is definitely occurring.

Systemization of hospice palliative care

Policy development of hospice palliative care

Compared with the advancement in education and research, systemization is progressing slowly in Korea. Systemization of the Korean government's hospice palliative care has been conducted only for patients suffering from cancer, considered the number

one cause of death, and their family members. In response to the growing cancer burden at the government level, the Cancer Control Division was established within the Bureau of Health Promotion, Ministry of Health and Welfare, in 2000. Also, the National Cancer Center was founded in March 2000 as a government-funded institution devoted to research, patient care, education, and training in cancer. The Cancer Control Act, another important legal framework for controlling cancer in Korea, was legislated in 2003 and revised in 2010. This law authorizes the health and welfare minister to formulate and implement cancer control programs including supportive palliative care and to promote international collaboration as well. In early 2006, the comprehensive second-term cancer control plan for the next 10 years (2006–2015) was forged to strengthen the cancer control efforts at the government level. The government's second-term 10-year plan to conquer cancer plans to secure 2,500 beds by 2015—thereby providing hospice palliative care to 40,000 terminal cancer patients (about 50% of the target population). The Ministry of Health and Welfare, through the revision of the Cancer Control Act in 2010 that took effect in 2011, has been implementing the following:

1. Formulate and disseminate guidelines on pain control or symptom care for terminal cancer patients to improve quality of life.

2. Foster palliative medical facilities and train professional healthcare workers for palliative care.

3. Execute the home visiting program for terminal cancer patients.

4. Develop a palliative care education program for patients and families.

5. Implement other tasks that are needed to improve palliative care.

A survey collected from 1,000 participants from Korean general population aged from 19 to 69 years showed that 91% of the population agreed that a 5-year national strategy for end-of life care should be implemented by the central government (45.5%), the National Assembly (20.2%), or civic groups (10%).[4]

Future of hospice palliative care

Since the concept of hospice was introduced to Korea 50 years ago, it has not yet consolidated its position firmly within Korean society. The institutionalization of hospice palliative care for terminal cancer patients and their families began in 2011. There are many issues to be resolved.

A system of financial support should be systemized as a first measure. Current fee-for-service based Korean national health insurance (KNHI) system is not suitable for the terminal patients who need comprehensive care daily, and the Korean government plans to introduce per-diem rate that covers all aspects of hospice palliative services as an alternative option. The KNHI per-diem rate proposition prepared by the government based on the two pilot studies (period: 2009–2010, 2011–2013) with selected hospital based palliative care units for terminal cancer patients has not been accepted due to a large difference in the estimation of per-diem rate between the government and service providers. It is strongly suggested that a mutually agreeable per-diem rate system of KNHI be introduced soon for improving the quality of life for the terminal patients and their families. This medical charge system should be applied not only to patients who are in palliative care while hospitalized but also to home hospice patients. Second, it is necessary to vitalize home hospice, and to turn the current focus from palliative care based on hospitalization to a home-hospice-centered policy. Moreover, a service delivery system needs to be developed so that hospice palliative care while hospitalized and home hospice can be offered as a continuum. In Korea, people prefer to benefit from hospice palliative care while at home, which in turn increases satisfaction level. People prefer to spend their final hours at home due to strong feelings of affinity with family members. Third, standardization of training and operation of advanced training programs are required not only for nurses but for people from all types of professions who participate in the interdisciplinary team. Fourth, hospice palliative care, which is currently targeting only terminal cancer patients and their family members, needs to be offered to noncancer terminal patients as well. Moreover, it is necessary to provide service to special groups such as pediatric or geriatric palliative care. Fifth, hospice palliative care should be provided under special circumstances, such as for patients dying in the emergency room due to acute illness or accident or in the intensive care unit, as well as their family members.

Because death is an unavoidable part of life, it is necessary to provide hospice palliative care to anyone in need, from any place.

References

1. Kim HH, Kim BH. Palliative care in South Korea. In: Ferrell BR, Coyle N (eds.), Oxford Textbook of Palliative Nursing. 3rd ed. New York: Oxford University Press; 2010:1339–1346.
2. Park J. Home health care serves for terminally ill patients and dying at home. Dissertation. Seoul: Yonsei University; 2011. Korean.
3. Yu SJ, Chae YR, Choi YS, et al. Patients' perceptions of advanced directives and preferences for medical care near the end of life in South Korea. J Hosp Palliat Nurs. 2013;15(4):233–243.
4. Lee SH, Shin DE, Sim JA, et al. Public perception and acceptance of the national strategy for well-dying. Korean J Hosp Palliat Care. 2013;16(2):90–97.
5. Lee SW, Lee EO, Ahn HS, et al. The national hospice care service development in Korea. Korean Nurse. 1997;36(3):49–69.
6. Choi ES, Kim KS. Experiences of family caregivers of patients with terminal cancer. J Korean Acad Nurs. 2012;42(2):280–290.
6. Economist Intelligence Unit. The quality of death ranking end-of-life care across the world. London: Economist Intelligence Unit; 2010.
7. Korean Society for Hospice and Palliative Care. History of Korean Society of Hospice and Palliative Care for 10 Years. Seoul: Korean Society for Hospice and Palliative Care; 2008.
8. National Cancer Center. Basic Level Standard Curriculum for the Hospice Palliative Interdisciplinary Team. Ilsan: National Cancer Center; 2009.
9. Lee SW, Lee EO, Park HA, et al. Development of Internet based hospice information service system. J Korean Soc Med Inform. 1999;5(1):109–118.
10. Kang J, Koh SJ, Yoo YS, et al. Development of the standard hospice and palliative care education program in Korea: results from the demonstration project. J Palliat Med. 2010;13(6):703–710.
11. Choi ES, Yoo YS, Kim HS, et al. Curriculum development for hospice and palliative care nurses. Korean J Hosp Palliat Care. 2006;9(2):77–85.
12. Kim BH, Choi SO, Chung BY, et al. Job analysis for role identification of general hospice palliative nurse. Korean J Hosp Palliat Care. 2010;13(1):13–23.
13. Kim HS, Kim BH, Yu SJ, et al. The effect of an end-of-life nursing education consortium course on nurses' knowledge of hospice and palliative care in Korea. J Hosp Palliat Nurs. 2011;13(4):222–229.
14. Kim BH, Kim HS, Yu SJ, et al. Evaluation of End-of-Life Nursing Consortium-Geriatric Train-the-Trainer Program in Korea. Korean J Adult Nurs. 2012;24(4):390–397.
15. Park C-S, Yoon S, Jung Y. The status of home-based hospice care in Korea. Korean J Hosp Palliat Care. 2013;16(2):98–107.

CHAPTER 79

Palliative care in Eastern Europe

Nicoleta Mitrea and Daniela Mosoiu

This chapter is divided into several sections, including a general introduction, where demographic data, cultural aspects, and common characteristics of countries in Eastern Europe are presented, as well as a review of individual countries in the region with examples of success stories presented by leaders from those countries.

In the process of implementing palliative care in Eastern Europe a commonly used framework has been the World Health Organization's Model for Public Heath.[1] According to this model there is a need for specific *policies* supporting palliative care integration into national strategic plans, including:

♦ **educational** programs for healthcare providers as well as authorities, media, family caregivers, and the general public,

♦ **implementation programs** to bring care to those in need

♦ **available drugs** with special attention given to opioids as essential medications to relieve pain

Description of the Eastern European region

There are different perspectives regarding the countries that belong to Eastern Europe, depending on numerous factors: geographic, political, economic, and cultural.

Geographically, Eastern Europe is the eastern part of the European continent, between the Ural and Caucasian Mountains at the eastern border, with an arbitrary line chosen to define the western border (Figure 79.1).

Politically, for almost 30 years, the Berlin Wall represented the barrier between East and West in Europe. After its fall in 1989, countries under the communist regime fought to obtain independence from the influence of the United Soviet Socialist Republic (USSR) and to become democratic republics.

Economically, most of these countries have an agricultural background, with industry and factories collapsing after the fall of communism, as the USSR was the primary market for their products. The impact of communism is now seen in these countries through the industrial architectural style of the blocks of flats in urban cities, the economic decline resulting in significant poverty and unemployment, and centralized politico-administrative systems that go hand-in-hand with rigid bureaucracy.

Culture is what makes us strangers when we are not at home.[2] Some authors describe Eastern Europe from a cultural perspective as the region in Europe with influences of Byzantine, Orthodox, and some Turk-Islamic cultures.[3,4]

Eastern Europe is a region where ethnic, national, social and political, religious, and cultural diversities have led to tensions, hostilities, and clashes, and also to wars, massacres, deportation, and "ethnic cleansing"; diversity in all its richness has been the target of deliberate destruction here.[5] Fifty years of communism put a strong mark on the lives of generations that lived under the principals of dictatorship, in centralized systems characterized by a lack of freedom of speech, spiritual belonging, and cultural inheritance, and complete prohibition of ownership.[6]

The Eastern European nations share several cultural and economical behaviors:

♦ A long-term orientation, which means they are more likely to save and value thrift

♦ A hunger for new products and learning new skills

♦ A preference for communication involving nonverbal cues

♦ A tendency to pay attention to social branding and personal recommendation

♦ A keenness toward self-service.[7]

According to the United Nations Statistic Division, the following 10 countries were classified as being located in Eastern Europe: Belarus, Bulgaria, Czech Republic, Hungary, Republic of Moldova, Poland, Romania, Russia, Slovakia, and Ukraine.[8,9]

For this chapter we use the above classification and have added three other countries: Albania, Greece, and Serbia. The long-term collaborative relationship between the authors and palliative care leaders in these countries in southeastern Europe, and their obvious commitment to the relief of suffering in patients and families, are reasons for presenting their situation and accomplishments.

The 13 countries included in our discussion here have a population of approximately 318 million inhabitants, with 4.3 million deaths per year (Figure 79.2). Noncommunicable diseases as a cause of death represent between 82% of deaths in Russia and 94% in Bulgaria. In this region cancer mortality is higher in countries like Greece, Czech Republic, Poland, and Hungary.

From a socioeconomic point of view, these countries are not a homogeneous group. Health expenditure ranges from $386 per capita in Moldova to $2918 per capita in Greece. However, palliative care in these countries has frequently developed outside the public system (through donations and private funding) and as a result, there is no linear correlation between health expenditure and advancement of palliative care in these countries (Table 79.1).

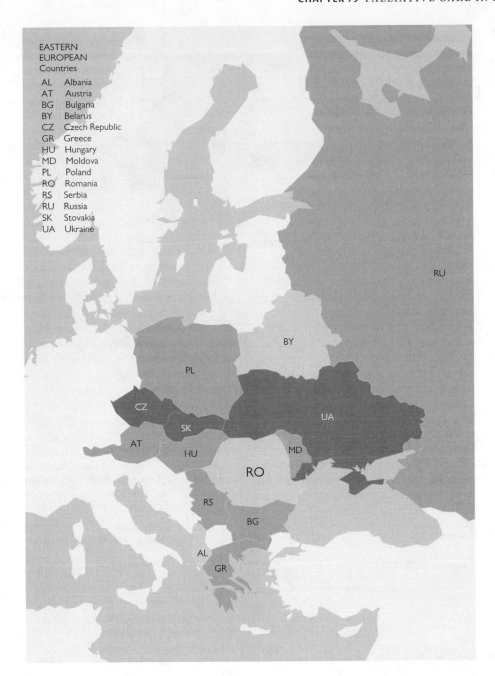

EASTERN
EUROPEAN
Countries

AL   Albania
AT   Austria
BG   Bulgaria
BY   Belarus
CZ   Czech Republic
GR   Greece
HU   Hungary
MD   Moldova
PL   Poland
RO   Romania
RS   Serbia
RU   Russia
SK   Slovakia
UA   Ukraine

Figure 79.1 Map of Eastern Europe.

Impact of Communist heritage on the development of palliative care in Eastern Europe

The common communist background has had a direct influence on the development of palliative care services in these countries. The centralized systems, including healthcare decision-making, are still in place today, more than 20 years after the fall of the Berlin Wall. As a result, some countries in the region, like Moldova[10] and Russia,[11] have taken a top-down approach in the development of their services by putting into place regulations for the development of services based more on international expertise than on the needs and realities of the country.

Social and medical services are split and exist under distinct umbrellas: the Ministry of Social Welfare and the Ministry of Health provide different funding for social and medical aspects of care, making it difficult to provide holistic care. Some programs, like day care and bereavement services, fall between these two funding streams.

The old Semasko communist healthcare model was heavily reliant on inpatient care, with little attention given to community care.[12] Even today these countries have a high percentage of beds/1000 inhabitants[13] and are struggling to reform their healthcare to make it more efficient. This model of delivering healthcare becomes a barrier in developing home-based palliative care services, a very valuable setting of care for societies where home is the

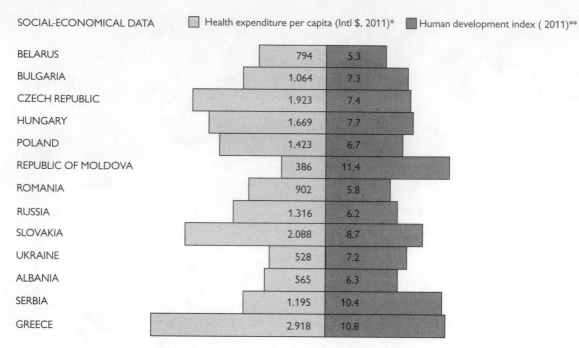

	Health expenditure per capita (Intl $, 2011)*	Human development index (2011)**
BELARUS	794	5.3
BULGARIA	1.064	7.3
CZECH REPUBLIC	1.923	7.4
HUNGARY	1.669	7.7
POLAND	1.423	6.7
REPUBLIC OF MOLDOVA	386	11.4
ROMANIA	902	5.8
RUSSIA	1.316	6.2
SLOVAKIA	2.088	8.7
UKRAINE	528	7.2
ALBANIA	565	6.3
SERBIA	1.195	10.4
GREECE	2.918	10.8

*http://www.who.int/countries/en/-accessed August 13th, 2013 | **http://www.who.int/countries/en-accessed August 13th, 2013

Figure 79.2 Socioeconomic data.

Table 79.1 Demographic and epidemiological data

	Country	Population 2012[a]	Number of deaths 2008[b]	NCD* proportional mortality 2008[c]		Cancer proportional mortality 2008[d]	
				Number	(%)	Number	(%)
1	ALBANIA	3,227,373	27,978	24,900	89	5,036	18
2	BELARUS	9,527,498	131,379	114,300	87	17,097	13
3	BULGARIA	7,397,873	110,425	103,800	94	15,460	14
4	CZECH REPUBLIC	10,565,678	103,000	92,700	90	27,810	27
5	GREECE	11,418,878	97,363	88,600	91	27,262	28
6	HUNGARY	9,949,589	127,419	118,500	93	31,855	25
7	POLAND	38,317,090	382,921	340,800	89	99,559	26
8	REPUBLIC OF MOLDOVA	3,519,266	45,172	39,300	87	6,324	14
9	ROMANIA	21,387,517	248,901	226,500	91	47,291	19
10	RUSSIA	142,703,181	2,095,488	1,718,300	82	272,413	13
11	SERBIA	9,846,582	123,895	117,700	95	24,779	20
12	SLOVAKIA	5,480,332	53,000	47,700	90	12,190	23
13	UKRAINE	44,940,268	754,535	648,900	86	82,999	11

*NCD—noncommunicable diseases
[a] Centeno C, Pons JJ, Lynch T, Donea O, Rocafort J, Clark D. EAPC Atlas of Palliative Care in Europe 2013—Cartographic Edition. Milan: EAPC Press; 2013.
[b] http://www.who.int/nmh/countries/en/, accessed August 13, 2013. The figure for deaths has been calculated by the authors from the WHO mortality database and is not attributed to the WHO.
[c] http://www.who.int/nmh/countries/en/, accessed August 13, 2013. The figure for NCD (noncommunicable diseases) mortality has been calculated by the authors from the WHO database and is not attributed to the WHO.
[d] http://www.who.int/nmh/countries/en/, accessed August 13, 2013. The figure for cancer mortality has been calculated by the authors from the WHO database and is not attributed to the WHO.

preferred place for death[14] and where traditional values require that the family be involved in the care of their dying relative.[15]

Another trait inherited from communism is the hierarchical structure of medical and healthcare professions. It is common for health systems in all the countries included in this chapter to have nurses subordinate to physicians. This is partially related to the different educational levels for these professionals, but even in countries where nurses are educated at a university level, the recognition of each role remains an issue. For palliative care, where teamwork is a core principle, overcoming this attitude is a huge challenge.

Overview of palliative care development in Eastern Europe

The World Wide Palliative Care Alliance characterizes global development of palliative care into six categories as follows[16]:

- Level 1: **No Known Activity**
- Level 2: **Capacity Building** (countries where there is no palliative care service established but there is evidence of wide-ranging initiatives designed to create the capacity for hospice-palliative care services to develop)
- Level 3a: **Isolated Provision** (the development of palliative care is patchy, often home-based in nature, and not well supported, with limited availability of morphine)
- Level 3b: **Generalized Provision** (the development of palliative care in a number of locations with the growth of local support in those areas, multiple sources of funding, availability of morphine, provision of some training and education initiatives)
- Level 4a: **Preliminary Integration** (the development of a critical mass of palliative care in a number of locations, a variety of palliative care providers and types of services, availability of morphine and some other strong pain-relieving drugs, limited impact of palliative care on policy, provision of a substantial number of training and education initiatives by a range of organizations)
- Level 4b: **Advanced Integration** (the development of a critical mass of palliative care in a wide range of locations, comprehensive provision of all types of palliative care by multiple service providers, broad awareness of palliative care, unrestricted availability of morphine and all other strong pain-relieving drugs, substantial impact of palliative care on policy, in particular on public health policy, the development of recognized education centers, academic links forged with universities, the existence of a national palliative care association)

The countries in the Eastern European region are included in following categories:

- Level 3a: Bulgaria, Greece, Moldova, Russia, and Ukraine,
- Level 3b: Albania, Belarus, Czech Republic,
- Level 4a: Hungary Serbia, Slovakia
- Level 4b: Poland, Romania

Palliative care services in the region

The numbers of specialized palliative services in the countries in this region are represented in Table 79.2. The information in the table combines data from the European Association of Palliative Care Atlas[17] and responses from questionnaires provided by key persons in the respective countries. In all countries, services are directed toward both cancer and noncancer patients.

Bulgaria: Vratsa—a designated European Society for Medical Oncology (ESMO) center for integration of oncology and palliative care

Vratsa, although not one of the largest cities in the country, has made significant contributions to the development of palliative medicine in Bulgaria. The Vratsa Comprehensive Cancer Center was founded in 1952 and is an important part of the specialized oncology network in Bulgaria. In 1996 the first hospital team and outpatient clinic for the treatment of cancer pain was established, and, based on the work of these teams, the first hospital palliative care department was founded in the country in 1998. The palliative care team comprises doctors, nurses, a psychologist, social worker, lawyer, priest, and volunteers. These individuals provide specialized care for patients with uncontrolled symptoms, especially pain, and management of patients in crisis. The department consists of an inpatient unit with 13 beds, a day center, an outpatient consulting unit, and a center for psychological and social support for patients and families. A school for cancer patients and their families was organized in the palliative care department in 2010, and in 2011 a hotline was established to provide support for crisis management of cancer patients and their families.

From January 7, 2007, to March 6, 2013, there were 2952 hospitalizations with 28,728 hospital days; the average length of a hospital stay was 9.75 days. During this period 372 patients died in the department, and the hospital mortality was 12.6% for the period.

Through a joint international project between Bulgaria and Holland, a postgraduate education program for nurses in palliative care was developed and the department became a place for clinical training for medical students and also a training ground for postgraduate education for nurses studying for a master's degree. Beginning in 2013 the Palliative Care Department in Vratsa became the main organizer of courses for postgraduate training in palliative care for the country. Clinical trials of drugs, especially for the treatment of pain and other symptoms common in advanced cancer, are conducted in this center. As a result of these efforts the Comprehensive Cancer Center in Vratsa was accredited as a designated center for integration of oncology and palliative care by ESMO in 2011. (Personal communication from Nikolay Yordanov.)

Romania: Hospice Casa Sperantei—a beacon center in the region

Started in 1992 as a palliative care home-based service in Brasov at the initiative of Graham Perolls, Hospice Casa Sperantei (HCS) has quickly moved toward developing and delivering education programs by building in 1997 the Princess Diana Study Centre for Palliative Care. This was possible due to a European grant that has fostered transfer of expertise from British partners at the University of Greenwich and the Ellenor Foundation to HCS and by preparing not just educational materials and curricula but also clinical training to future palliative care trainers. The educational program has been subsequently supported by the Open Society Foundation. Presently, HCS is playing a major role in education in

Table 79.2 Palliative care services in the region

Country	Services																				
	Inpatient units				Palliative home care teams				Ambulatory				Day centers				Palliative care hospital teams			
	No.	Location	Members of the id team	Eligible diagnoses	No.	Location	Members of the id team	Eligible diagnoses	No.	Location	Members of the id team	Eligible diagnoses	No.	Location	Members of the id team	Eligible diagnoses	No.	Location	Members of the id team	Eligible diagnoses
BELARUS	15 for adults, 5 for children	Minsk and 6 other regions	Physician, nurse, psychologist	Cancer & noncancer	5	Minsk	Physician, nurse, psychologist	Cancer patients	—	—	—	—	—	—	—	—	—	—	—	—
BULGARIA	48	—	—	Cancer & noncancer	11		—	—	—	—	—	—	—	—	—	—	3	—	—	—
CZECH REPUBLIC	17 (430 beds)	—	Physician, nurse, social worker, psychologist	Cancer & noncancer	10		Physician, nurse, social worker, psychologist, volunteers	Cancer & noncancer	—		Physician, nurse, social worker, psychologist	Cancer & noncancer	9		Phisician, nurse, social worker, psychologist	Cancer & noncancer	2		Phisician, nurse, social worker, psychologist	Cancer & noncancer
HUNGARY	11	—	A total of 1541 persons in Hungary	Cancer & noncancer	72		A total of 1541 persons in Hungary	Cancer & noncancer	3		A total of 1541 persons in Hungary	Cancer & noncancer	—			Cancer & noncancer	4	—	A total of 1541 persons in Hungary	Cancer & noncancer
POLAND	145		Multiprofessional and voluntary	Cancer & noncancer	408		Multiprofessional and voluntary	Cancer & noncancer	8		Physician, nurse, social worker, psychologist	Cancer & noncancer	7		Phisician, nurse, social worker, psychologist	Cancer & noncancer	8		Phisician, nurse, social worker.	Cancer & noncancer
REPUBLIC OF MOLDOVA	2	Chisinau Zubresti		Cancer & noncancer	5	Chisinau Zubresti Taraclia Ocnita Cimislia		Cancer & noncancer	5	Chisinau Zubresti Taraclia Ocnita Cimislia		Cancer & noncancer	1	Zubresti		Cancer & noncancer	1	Chisinau		Cancer
ROMANIA	36	Free-standing or hospital departments, charitable/public/private	Physician and nurse	Cancer & noncancer	19	Free-standing or hospital departments, charitable/public/private	Physician, nurse and social worker	Cancer & noncancer	3	Free-standing or hospital departments, charitable/public/private	Physician and nurse	Cancer & noncancer	4	Free-standing or Hospital departments, charitable/public/private	Nurse, assistant nurse, volunteers	Cancer & noncancer	2	Free-standing or Hospital departments, charitable/public/private	Physician, nurse and social worker	Cancer & noncancer

Country	No.	Location	Patient type	Team	No.	Location	Patient type	Team	No.	Location	Patient type	Team	No.	Location	Patient type	Team
RUSSIA	62 (1763 beds)	–	Cancer & noncancer	Physician and nurse	–	–	–	–	–	–	–	–	–	–	–	–
SLOVAKIA	11 (277 beds)	–	Cancer & noncancer	Physician and nurse	–	–	–	–	–	–	–	–	–	–	–	–
UKRAINE	58	Most of the regions	Cancer & noncancer	3–5 members	8	Zhytomir, Ivano-Frankivs, Mykolaiv, Ternopil, Kharkiv, Cherkassy, and 2 other regions (no specific confirmation)	Cancer & non-cancer	3–5 members (depending on the region)	–	in all regions of the country	–	1 nurse and often either a general practitioner or family doctor who is responsible for first visit	7	Volyn, Zhytomir, Zaporozhie, Ivano-Frankivsk, Lviv, Kharkiv, Kherson	Any, except pediatric care	3–5 members
ALBANIA	–	–	–	–	1	KORCA	Cancer	–	1	KORCA	–	6	1	KORCA	Cancer	–
GREECE	–	–	–	–	2	ATTICA AREA	a) Adult patients with cancer b) Children and teenagers with cancer & non-cancer chronic patients	Nurse, physician, social worker, physiotherapist, occupational therapist, psychologist, priest and Volunteers	2	ATTICA AREA	Adult patients with cancer & non-cancer chronic diseases	6 Nurse, physician, psychologist	1	ATTICA AREA	4 Adult patients with cancer	Nurse, physician, social worker, physiotherapist, occupational therapist, psychologist, priest, and volunteers
SERBIA	3	Sombor Zrenjanin Leskovac	All patients in need of PC	doctor, nurses, social worker (where available)	57	Belgrade (BELhospice) 56 HC services in different cities of Serbia	All patients in need of PC	BELhospice: doctors, nurses, social worker. Psychologist and chaplain are available if needed. Other services mostly consist of doctor and nurses, occasionally a social worker is available	1	BELGRADE (Institute for Oncology and Radiology of Serbia)	Cancer	Doctors, nurses, social worker, psychologist				

palliative care not just in Romania but also in the whole Eastern European region.

In 1998, HCS was the initiator of the Romanian National Association having the vision of uniting the voices of the few existing palliative care services at that time and building a network and support group for those interested in palliative care.

In 1999, HCS organized the first consensus palliative care meeting, inviting all relevant stakeholders in education (medical university representatives, nursing school leaders, representatives of the education department in the Ministry of Health), media, regulators, authorities, representatives of professional bodies (college of doctors, nursing association). The meeting addressed steps necessary to the development of palliative care in Romania according to the WHO model for public health approach. As a result of the meeting, palliative care was recognized as a medical subspecialty in 1999.

In 2001 through a USAID grant, with support from National Hospice and Palliative Care Association in the United States, the first Romanian standards for palliative care were developed.

In 2002 HCS opened the first comprehensive palliative care service, comprising inpatient services, outpatient clinics, and day centers for adults and children in Brasov. These services were added to the existing home-based services and the education programs.

In research conducted evaluating palliative care services in Eastern Europe,[18] Romania was found to be fulfilling the criteria for being a beacon country for palliative care development, and HCS was named as one of the five centers of excellence in palliative care in Eastern Europe. This role has continued over the years through the active involvement of HCS in the support of developing services throughout Romania, but also assisting programs in surrounding countries (e.g., Moldova), as well as advocating for legal changes to allow access to pain medications and inclusion of financial provisions for palliative care within the funding system.

At present HCS offers services to around 2000 patients annually in both Brasov and Bucharest and in the rural area of Brasov County, has trained over 12,000 professionals, and is in the process of opening a new hospice in Bucharest while working with the government to advance a national palliative care program.

Slovenia: milestones in the development of palliative care

The development of palliative care in Slovenia goes back as far as 1995, when the first hospice was created. In 2004 the first palliative hospital teams and first inpatient units were opened. With the help of WHO experts, a draft of the National Program of Palliative Care was produced in 2007 and was later tested in 2009 with support from the Ministry of Health in a pilot project in three Slovenian regions. In 2010 the successful results of this pilot project led the government to adopt the program for the entire country. This was followed by the formation of the Slovenian Palliative Medicine Society in 2011.

Together with education of health professionals, public awareness about the importance of and advances in palliative care has risen. There are many nongovernmental organizations (NGOs) that support the development of palliative care in Slovenia. Internationally two units have been granted the Certification for Excellence in Medical Oncology and Palliative Care. (Personal communication from Maja Ebert Moltara, Mateja Lopuh.).

National policies

For the countries in the region, except Greece, Ukraine, and Slovakia, a national palliative care strategy is approved or in the process of approval. New legislation and policies have been developed to include palliative care in the public healthcare system. Provisions were made for education of both doctors and nurses, approval of service regulations and standards, and funding of services. Belarus is the only country in the region that has developed special provisions for pediatric palliative care.

Serbia: toward a national strategy

The Ministry of Health recognized the need for the development of palliative care services as one of the priorities in the healthcare sector and asked for European Union (EU) support, which materialized through the project Development of Palliative Care Services in Serbia, begun in March 2001. The project is implemented by an international consortium led by Oxford Policy Management (UK), along with BELhospice (Serbia), Hospices of Hope (UK), and Casa Sperantei (Romania).

As a result of the work conducted by members of this project, many changes have happened to advance palliative care in Serbia:

- Continuous medical education (CME) training in palliative care (Level I—two days and Level II—four days) has been developed and accredited by the Serbian Health Council. To date 1023 staff employed in health institutions and gerontology centers have received Level I and Level II training provided through the scope of this EU-funded project. The Level III clinical training is planned for newly opened palliative care units (PCUs) and started for some units in April 2013.

- A curriculum has been developed and accepted for undergraduate medical training. A student handbook for the undergraduate medical curriculum for the course has been developed, accepted by four medical schools in Serbia (Belgrade, Nis, Novi Sad, and Kragujevac) as a handbook for undergraduate students, and launched on March 26, 2013.

- Similarly, an academic curriculum for undergraduate nursing training has been developed and approved. Training materials were translated and sent to higher nursing schools for comments and endorsement. Four of the higher nursing schools have confirmed that they officially agree with the proposed teaching materials and will introduce the course. The palliative care course will be provided to nursing students starting in the next academic year.

- The first specialty course for social workers involved in the delivery of palliative care services was accredited by the Republican Institute for Social Protection and delivered to a number of social workers working in health institutions. This is currently the only European government-accredited course in palliative care for generalist social workers. Work has also begun with the faculty of political science to integrate palliative care into the undergraduate curriculum for social workers.

- The process of developing a comprehensive design for the model of care and service delivery appropriate to Serbia began in August 2012. The work is focused on a detailed specification of the model of palliative care delivery including resource and organizational requirements. The final documents will address issues such as assessment of human and other resource input requirements, assessment of workload, operational procedures, quality standards, referral protocols, performance indicators, etc.

◆ Government funds for refurbishment of PCUs were disbursed in December 2011 to seven of 13 sites planned for the first phase of funding as per the palliative care strategy. Three of these institutions (Sombor, Zrenjanin, and Leskovac) are open and caring for patients. An additional five institutions were scheduled to receive the funds by the end of July 2013.

◆ The essential medicines list for palliative care based on recommendations from the WHO and the International Association for Hospice and Palliative Care (IAHPC) has been developed by the Republican Expert Committee for palliative care and is being put forward for adoption by the Health Insurance Fund.

◆ A review of legislation governing palliative care service provision was completed and recommendations for change drafted. In February, the Ministry of Health established a palliative care working group to work on the legislative changes required for the improvement of palliative care services in Serbia.

◆ An assessment of the need for children's palliative care was undertaken, and the first training program on children's palliative care took place in April 2013. The International Children's Palliative Care Network developed an online e-learning module on pain in children, linked to the new WHO pain guidelines; this has been translated into Serbian and is now available online.

(Personal communication from Natasa Milicevic, Julia Downing.)

Russia: palliative care for children

On December 24, 2012, an order of the Government of the Russian Federation (№2511-p) was approved, called Program: Development of Health, including Subprogram 6—Palliative Care, Including Children.

Since 2012, there has been a working group for the development of the Order of Provision of Palliative Care for Children; the group includes representatives of the Ministry of Health and various community organizations. The draft of the Order has been uploaded onto the website of the Ministry of Health for public comment.

As a result, in the regions of the Russian Federation there are approximately 30 services that currently provide palliative care for children in hospital and at home (palliative care units, children's hospices, and palliative care centers for children).

In 2013, for the first time, the Committee of Public Relations of the Moscow government allocated a grant for the provision of palliative care for children and young adults. The recipient was the Foundation for the Development of Palliative Care for Children, created in 2011. Currently, under the patronage of the Foundation there are more than 50 children with terminal illnesses in dire need of palliative care. The Foundation provides professional palliative care for children, aimed at improving their quality of life, and addressing the negative effects of the disease while supporting the entire family. The mobile team of palliative care services for children and young adults includes certified physicians, nurses, a psychologist, and social workers. The Foundation also implements a number of research projects and social development programs for children in Russia. (Personal communication from Kumirova Ella, Savva Natalia.)

Access to medication

The types and formulations of pain medication are variable in the countries in the region. Oral morphine, especially in immediate-release formulations, is not available in Belarus, Moldova, and Russia. Cost is a significant barrier, along with prescribing regulations that limit access to these medications for patients in need (Poland is a notable exception). See Tables 79.3 and 79.4. The total morphine equivalent dose per capita is as low as 1.6 mg per capita in Russia and goes up to 91 mg per capita for Greece.

Greece: reviewing Access to Opioid Medication—the ATOME Project

Greece participated in the Access to Opioid Medication in Europe (ATOME) project, aiming to improve opioid legislation in 12 European countries with low morphine consumption rates. At the National ATOME Conference that was conducted in Athens, palliative care forces in Greece joined their efforts to promote the rights of patients with chronic illnesses. Representatives from scientific societies, palliative care services, and patient organizations agreed on amendments to the law on controlled substances and presented them to the Ministry of Justice and the Greek Parliament. Some of the suggestions were endorsed and, for the first time, there has been a distinction in the law between opioid use for medical reasons and drug abuse. Additionally a physician specialized in palliative care was included in the National Drugs Committee, a government body responsible for developing regulations regarding opioid availability and other restrictions. Finally, an amendment was passed permitting doctors to prescribe, on an emergency basis, opioids at a dose higher than the one defined by the law. (Personal communication from Patiraki Elisabeth, Katsaragakis Stylianos, Tserkezoglou Aliki.)

A win for palliative care in Ukraine

In order to prescribe morphine to a terminally ill cancer patient, a physician in the Ukraine needed a panel of three additional doctors to confirm this need. In May 2013, terminally ill patients and their families in Ukraine received a long-awaited piece of good news. After decades of restrictive drug policies severely limiting access to opioids for pain relief, the Cabinet of Ministers finally lifted burdensome prescription procedures. Decree #333 is a lesson in how doctors, patients, families, and advocacy organizations can work together to improve end-of-life care. The idea of drug control has driven drug policies in Ukraine since Soviet times. Authorities focused on illicit drug use, paying little or no attention to access to opioids like morphine for pain and symptom control. With each new piece of legislation, the doctors and patients faced more and more restrictions and requirements making pain control and management next to impossible in the country.

Doctors were only allowed to prescribe patients 50 milligrams of morphine per day—an arbitrary amount with no basis in medical evidence. In fact, in countries where access to pain relief is a reality, a typical patient with late-stage cancer might get 2,000 mg or more of morphine per day, or whatever is needed to manage his or her pain symptoms. To address these unnecessary restrictions, in mid-2010 the Open Society Foundation launched a joint

Table 79.3 National policies

Country	Palliative care (PC) part of the national health program		Funding available to support PC delivery	
	Y/N	Details	Y/N	Details
BELARUS	YES	PC is part of the Public Health Law: PC for adults with cancer is included in the National Program of Oncology for 2011–2015; PC for children is included in the National Plan for the Advancement of Children's Rights for 2012–2016.	YES	—
BULGARIA	YES	PC is part of national anticancer policy and strategic planning and a national program for HIV/AIDS.	YES	Funding from national health insurance fund only for cancer patients
CZECH REPUBLIC	YES	National Strategy for Palliative Care	YES	—
HUNGARY	YES	—	YES	—
POLAND	YES	Since 1981, voluntary hospices; in 1998 the Program for Palliative Care was introduced by the Ministry of Health; in 1999 palliative medicine was introduced as a medical specialty; since 2004 palliative nursing has been a nursing specialty.	YES	In 2008, based on the Ministry of Health Order, public expenditure on palliative care increased by approximately 30% (in 2011, by approximately 4%–8%). Since 2004 each citizen is allowed to donate 1% of their annual tax for nonprofit organizations (including hospice-palliative-care-related ones).
REPUBLIC OF MOLDOVA	YES	*Order nr. 234 on June 9, 2008, about development of palliative care service in the Republic of Moldova *Order nr. 154 on June 1, 2009, about organization of palliative care services	YES	*Order nr. 875 on December 27, 2010, about cost approval of an assisted case in medical palliative care provided in hospital/hospice for 2011 *National Insurance Company from Moldova for inpatient units and home-based palliative care services *Order nr. 884 on December 30, 2010, about approval of the National Standard in Palliative Care *Other projects and grants
ROMANIA	YES	New legislation was adopted concerning prescribing of opioid medication, patients' rights to include access to palliative care, recognition of palliative care as a medical subspecialty, compulsory palliative care module for nursing schools, funding for palliative care as part of the National Frame Contract. Palliative care is in the process of being introduced in the National Health Care Program.	YES	Inpatient units and home-based palliative care services are funded through the insurance fund. Services offering day care can apply for funds for the social services they provide. 2% of taxes can be directed toward charitable work by citizens. Funding is also through charitable donations and international grants.
RUSSIA	YES	The federal law of the Russian Federation, number 323, on November 21, 2011: "On the basis of health protection in the Russian Federation"	YES	The budget and extrabudgetary funds
SLOVAKIA	NO	—	YES	There is no payment required for palliative care consultation or hospitalization.
UKRAINE	NO	—	YES	Minimal funding is available at the regional level. No funding at the national level
ALBANIA	YES	The organization is part of National Working Group for Palliative Care	YES	The donators are LCM (Little Company of Mary), DAI (Dorcas Aid International), SOROS Foundation, VAF (Vodafone Albania Fondation).
GREECE	NO	—	NO	—
SERBIA	YES	Palliative care strategy was adopted by government in 2009	YES	For patients treated by governmental services. HIF does not fund BELhospice (charity organization) and its work.

Table 79.4

Country	Drug availability		Do patients pay? (Y/N)	Limitation to prescribing? (Y/N)	Total morphine equivalence mg/capita (1)
	Opioid name	**Form of presentation**			
BELARUS	1. Tramadol 2. Morphine 3. Fentanyl 4. Hydromorphone	1. Short-acting tablets, vials 2. Vials 3. Patches, sublingual tablets 4. Sustained-release tablets	NO	YES	15.8736
BULGARIA	1. Morphine Ampules 2. Morphine Tablets 3. Oxycodone Tablets 4. Oxycontin 5. Targin (Oxicodone /Naloxone MR) MR 6. Victanyl (Fentanyl TDS) Patch 7. Tramadol Caps; AMP 8. Dihidrocodeine Tablets 9. Methadone (for substitution) 10. Buprenorphine 11. Lydol (Pethidine) 12. Fentanyl Injection (for acute therapy) 13. Sufentanyl Injection (for acute therapy) 14. Tilidine Injection (synthetic opioid, in a fixed combination with naloxone) 15. Paracetamol + Codeine 16. Paracetamol + Tramadol	1. Vials—10 mg, 20 mg; 2. 10 mg, 30 mg, 60 mg, 120 mg 3. 10 mg; 20 mg; 4. 10 mg; 20 mg; 40 mg; 80 mg 5. 10/5; 20/10; 40/20 mg 6. 20 mcg; 50 mcg; 75 mcg; 100 mcg 7. 50 mg 8. 60 mg, 90 mg 9. Solution 10. Tablets 11. Vials 12. Vials 13. Vials 14. 1 mL/50 mg 15. Tablets 16. Tablets	NO—opioids are free of charge for the treatment of pain in cancer and HIV/AIDS patients. YES, for terminally ill patients with diagnoses other than HIV/AIDS and cancer, opioids are not free of charge; therefore patients are forced to pay full price of the drugs.	YES. There are no limits on the type and amount of prescribed opioids; however, there remain some limitations. Opioids are still prescribed on a special form and may be obtained only from a pharmacy that has a license to dispense opioids.	57.3825
CZECH REPUBLIC	Most opioids are available		YES	YES	78.2486
HUNGARY	1. Morphine 2. Hydromorphone 3. Oxycodone 4. Fentanyl 5. Buprenorphine 6. Methadone 7. Codeine 8. Tramadol 9. Dihydrocodeine 10. Dextropropoxyphene	1. Vials, Tablets 2. Tablets 3. Tablets 4. Patch 5. Patch 6. Tablets 7. Tablets 8. Tablets, vials, solution, suppositories 9. Tablets 10. Tablets	NO Cancer patients pay only box fee (about 1 €)	YES *Lack of short-acting opioids *Legal regulations has changed—easier prescribing	67.87'19
POLAND	1. Morphine 2. Oxycodone 3. Buprenorphine 4. Fentanyl	1. Vials, tablets, controlled-release tablets 2. Vials, tablets, controlled-release tablets 3. Patches, tablets, vials 4. Patches, transmucosal formulations	Oxycodone; Fentanyl—those medications received full reimbursement status. Other drugs: copayment by patients at very low level	NO	33.0828

(continued)

Table 79.4 Continued

Country	Drug availability		Do patients pay? (Y/N)	Limitation to prescribing? (Y/N)	Total morphine equivalence mg/capita (1)
	Opioid name	**Form of presentation**			
REPUBLIC OF MOLDOVA	1. Tramadol 2. Morphine 3. Omnopon (also Pantopon, a mixture of hydrochlorides of opium alkaloids, containing about 50% morphine)	1. Immediate-release tablets (50 mg); slow-release tablets (100 mg); solution (100 mg) for parenteral administration 2. Long-acting tablets (10 mg) and immediate-release solution (1%–1 mL containing 8.6 mg of pure substance) for parenteral administration 3. Immediate-release solution (2%–1 mL containing 13.4 mg of pure substance) for parenteral administration	YES	YES	7.9308
ROMANIA	1. Morphine 2. Hydromorphone 3. Oxycodone 4. Dihydrocodeine 5. Codeine 6. Pethidine 7. Fentanyl 8. Pentazocine 9. Tramadol 10. MethadonE	1. Vials: 20 mg/1 mL; immediate-release tablets: 10 mg, 20 mg; slow-release tablets: 10 mg, 30 mg, 60 mg, 100 mg, 200 mg 2. Vials: 0.02%/1 mL 3. Slow-release tablets: 10 mg, 20 mg, 40 mg, 40 mg 4. Long-acting tablets: 60 mg, 90 mg, 120 mg 5. Tablets: 15 mg 6. Vials: 10 mg/2 mL 7. Patches: 20, 50, 75, 100 µg/h; sublingual tablets: 100, 200, 300, 400, 600, 800 µg/h; amp: 0.05 mg/mL 8. Vials: 30 mg/mL; tablets: 50 mg 9. Vials: 50 mg/mL, 100 mg/2 mL; immediate-release tablets: 50 mg; slow-release tablets: 100 mg, 150 mg, 200 mg; suppositories: 100 mg 10. Tablets: 2.5 mg	NO for cancer patients where cost is 100% or 90% covered by the state. YES for noncancer patients, where just tramadol and oxycodone can be prescribed 50% compensated	Major improvement with the changes in legislation that have taken place since 2007	—
RUSSIA	1. Morphine 2. Tramadol 3. Trimeperidine (analog of prodine, related to pethidine) 4. Fentanyl 5. Codeine in combined preparations	1. Vials and sustained-release tablets 2. Vials 3. Vials 4. Patch, vials 5. Tablets	NO	YES	1.6015
SLOVAKIA	Essential medications are generally available throughout Slovakia		YES	YES	67.2112
UKRAINE	1. Morphine 2. Buprenorphine 3. Omnopon (papaverine, morphine, codeine) 4. Methadone 5. Fentanyl 6. Thiopental 7. Propofol 8. Tramadol	1. Vials and tablets 2. Vials and tablets 3. Vials 4. Tablets and syrup 5. Vials and patch 6. Vials 7. Vials 8. Vials and capsules	—	YES	9.0964

(continued)

Table 79.4 Continued

Country	Drug availability				
	Opioid name	Form of presentation	Do patients pay? (Y/N)	Limitation to prescribing? (Y/N)	Total morphine equivalence mg/capita (1)
ALBANIA	1. Morphine	1. Morphine sulfate tablets 10 mg; morphine hydrochloride 10 mg/mL	NO Free of charge only for cancer patients	YES	7.3623
GREECE	1. Morphine 2. Codeine (+ paracetamol) 3. Tramadol 4. Fentanyl 5. Pethidine Hydrochloride 6. Nalbuphine Hydrochloride	1. Powder, vials 2. Tablets, suppositories 3. Tablets, oral solution, suppositories, vials 4. Patch, sublingual tablets, inhaler 5. Vials 6. Vials	NO	YES Morphine tablets (slow and immediate release) are not available. All opioids need special prescriptions and permission from the local prefecture. Morphine and fentanyl have limitations, by law, in the maximum daily dose.	91.5176
SERBIA	1. Morphine 2. Fentanyl 3. Tramadol	1. Morphine hydrochloride vials 10 and 20 mg/mL; morphine solution 20 mL (20 mg/mL); morphine unit dose vials 10 mg/5 mL and 30 mg/5 mL 2. 25 mcg/h, 50 mcg/h, 75 mcg/h and 100 mcg/h 3. Vials: 50 mg/mL, 100 mg/2mL; capsules: 50 mg; SR tablets: 100, 150, 200 mg	NO	YES SR oral morphine is not available. The total amount of controlled substances to be prescribed is limited, designated controlled substances can only be prescribed for a period of 14 days.	37.1569

campaign aimed at reviewing the Ukrainian legislative and regulatory barriers that limit the supply of opioids in health facilities and pharmacies. The review found that in order to prescribe morphine to a terminally ill cancer patient, a physician would need a panel of three additional doctors to confirm this recommendation. Any change in dosage or route needed to be verified by the same panel. Burdensome regulations also surrounded the process for destroying empty morphine vials. Once again, a commission of officials including police officers had to verify that every single vial was accounted for and destroyed.

In effect, these requirements prevented many terminally ill patients from receiving any pain relief. Patients were told that it was too early to start morphine or that by starting morphine they were risking addiction. Doctors resorted to relying on weak analgesics to treat chronic pain. As a result, many terminally ill patients in Ukraine lived with uncontrolled severe pain.

Despite these hurdles, NGO's working in palliative care and human rights were determined to find a solution that could bring about change quickly and prevent patients from experiencing inhumane and degrading treatment. The Ministry of Interior and

State Service for Drug Control were attentive to these concerns and soon joined a working group to review and develop changes to the existing legislation. The working group quickly decided that rather than change old documents it would be more strategic to push for a new policy that would override the old policies and establish new, more progressive norms.

This work was backed up by two reports: a 2010 publication from the International Narcotics Control Board called *Availability of Internationally Controlled Drugs: Ensuring Adequate Access for Medical and Scientific Purpose*, which highlighted the disproportionately small use of opioids for medical purposes in Ukraine, and the World Health Organization's *Ensuring Balance in National Policies on Controlled Substances*, which called on governments to ensure balance between control and access measures. These publications informed the draft legislation, but it still took more than 2 years of intensive advocacy at different levels to push the ministries and other state bodies to agree to these fundamental regulation changes.

During this time advocacy efforts continued, including the Human Rights Watch report *Uncontrolled Pain*, which sparked national and international media interest. The short film *50 Milligrams Is Not Enough* was launched as part of a larger awareness campaign featuring a 27-year-old cancer patient in terrible pain whose mother went to extreme effort in order to get pain relief for her bed-ridden son. This work culminated in the All-Ukrainian League for Palliative Care continually lobbying government officials to change the existing law. Finally, on May 13, 2013, the Cabinet of Ministers passed Decree #333, lifting burdensome procedures for prescribing and accessing opioids. Now:

- individual physicians can prescribe opioids to patients without panel review;
- empty vials can be destroyed without commission oversight;
- per the discretion of chief doctors, facilities can stock up to 1 month's supply of drugs;
- physicians must ensure that a patient receives an adequate supply of opioid medications through a prescription that can be filled in local or hospital pharmacies;
- patients and/or family members can pick up their medication directly from healthcare facilities and store these at home.

This huge change came on the heels of another recent win where the government signed MOH Order #77, allowing use of oral morphine in Ukraine. Of course, this new legislation is not perfect, especially for Ukrainians living in rural areas. In a country that is home to almost 2.4 million people, there are only four pharmacies certified to carry controlled medications such as morphine. Healthcare providers also need education on how to prescribe morphine and other controlled medications, in addition to education for pharmacists about filling such prescriptions. Finally, there is still much work to be done in order to dispel myths about opioid use among patients and families. But at least for now, the realization of true palliative care has made great strides in Ukraine. (Personal communication from Victoria Tymoshevska and Kseniya Shapoval.)

Education in palliative care

Poland and Hungary have palliative care recognized as a subspecialty both for doctors and nurses, whereas Romania and Czech Republic have it officially accredited just for doctors, and Bulgaria and Greece only for nurses. There are more training programs available for continuous medical education for doctors and nurses; countries in the region, excepting Moldova and Russia, are able to provide local continuing education courses. All countries run awareness campaigns for the sensitization of the general public (Table 79.5).

Poland—social education about end-of-life care and call for volunteering

Social support of hospice and palliative care through volunteering are important parts of the modern hospice movement in Poland, but with professionalization of palliative care there was less attention given to voluntary and nonmedical aspects of holistic care.

In 2004 the National Chaplain of Hospices, along with the Hospice Foundation, started a national awareness campaigns regarding end-of-life care, called Hospice Is Life, Too. With participation of the main TV stations and most of the national and regional media, during one month there were around 1000 media events regarding hospice-palliative care and end-of-life issues. Collaborating with over 100 hospice-palliative care centers, all the hospices noticed the following: breaking the taboo of discussing end-of-life issues; promotion of voluntary services for those in need; and increasing fundraising at the national and local levels. As a result of this first campaign, a website was created, serving as the first source of information regarding hospice and palliative care in Poland (www.hospicja.pl).

The second campaign was developed through the participation of 118 hospice-palliative care units, focusing on conversations with patients and families regarding wishes at the end of life. This campaign included public debates and concerts, and was launched during the first International Day of Hospice and Palliative Care Around the World in 2005. Subsequent nationwide campaigns have addressed loss, grief, and bereavement in the mass media and in local meetings. Every campaign has concluded with practical textbooks and monographs regarding the discussed issues, and these have been donated to all hospice-palliative care centers and have been made available for students and the general public.

From 2007 to 2010 educational campaigns have been devoted to hospice volunteering. Hospice Foundation received a grant to train volunteer coordinators from hospices throughout Poland, and more than 100 centers have started this program. Most of them were from rural areas, which wanted to improve the level of their service by involving more trained volunteers.

"I Like to Help"—the training of hospice coordinators—has helped to return vital elements of hospice-palliative care to the existing system in Poland. Information, promotion, and regular recruitment to the voluntary service have been proposed along with training of volunteer coordinators. One of the results of this program has been a number of publications for the coordinators and hospice volunteers. They have been recognized as a great help for volunteers but also for family members and other people who help elderly and handicapped people in their homes. This program has connected schools and universities with local volunteer coordinators and has reached out to these young students. Coordinators have created educational programs with teachers, training about end-of-life issues and recruiting candidates for hospice volunteers. Important volunteer groups, called Volunteers 50+, have emerged while hospice-palliative care centers have reached out to local communities, parishes, and organizations for pensioners with information about possibilities for voluntary service. Centers have noticed an increase in the number of volunteers from this age group, adding their knowledge and experience to existing teams.

The "I Like to Help" program has been a success in teaching local communities and the entire society in Poland about end-of-life issues and also about the need for unifying formal and informal care. In 2012 two books were published analyzing the various activities' impact on patients and their families, the hospice-palliative care teams, and the local communities. The influence of these efforts on the general public has also been researched. Findings of these scientific publications demonstrate the positive effects of the "I Like to Help" program, regarding hospice-palliative care in Poland, especially nonmedical care, teamwork, and volunteer engagement.

The book *The Role of Volunteering in Care at the End of Life* reveals possibilities for further development of care for people

Table 79.5

Country	Education										
	PC a specialty/subspecialty			CME Courses			PC module included in basic training			PC in media & public advocacy programs (Y/N)
	For physicians	For nurses	For other professionals (please name)	For physicians	for nurses	For other professionals (please name)	For physicians	For nurses	For other professionals (name it)	
BELARUS	NO	NO	NO	YES	YES	NO	NO	NO	NO	YES
BULGARIA	NO	YES	YES 40 h for psychologists	YES 40 h postgraduate training	NO	NO	NO	YES 40 h	NO	YES
CZECH REPUBLIC	YES	NO	NO	YES GPs and oncologists	YES, ELNEC courses	NO	YES, oncologists only	NO	NO	YES
HUNGARY	YES Licence exam	YES Specialty 1 year, 1200 h	NO	YES	YES Postgraduate courses 40 h	YES Psychologist	YES Elective subject in basic training	YES (20–40 h)	YES Psychotherapist (20 h)	YES
POLAND	YES	YES	YES—Psychologists	YES	YES	YES	YES	YES	YES—Social workers	YES
REPUBLIC OF MOLDOVA	NO	NO	NO	NO	NO	NO	YES 40 h	YES	NO	YES
ROMANIA	YES	NO	NO	YES	YES	YES	YES	YES	NO	YES
RUSSIA	NO	NO	NO	NO	NO	NO	NO	NO	NO	YES
SLOVAKIA	NO	NO	NO	YES	YES	NO	NO	NO	NO	YES
UKRAINE	NO	NO	NO	YES Varies from 16 to 80 h of training, both clinical and theoretical, in some cases up to 168 h	YES Varies from 16 to 80 h of training, both clinical and theoretical	YES Social workers, psychologists—varies from 8 to 40 h of training, both clinical and theoretical	YES	YES	YES Social workers, psychologists	
ALBANIA	NO	NO	NO	YES 40 h	YES 40 h	NO	YES 10 h	YES 10 h	NO	YES
GREECE	NO	YES	YES	YES	YES	YES	YES Elective 26 h	YES 26 h	NO	NO
SERBIA	NO	NO	NO	YES	YES	YES Social workers	YES 30 h	YES 45 h	NO Accreditation in progress for social workers	YES

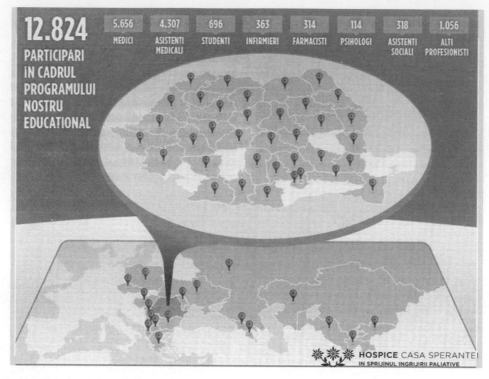

Figure 79.3 Participants in the palliative care education program.

at the end of life in Poland, using good practices of hospice-palliative care in Poland, that can be extended toward all people dying in institutions and in home care. Expertise in palliative care and a tradition of social support, volunteering, and holistic care could be an answer to the future challenges of an aging society and limited resources for health and social care in Poland and Eastern Europe. (Personal communication from Piotr Krakowiak.)

Romania: education is a drive for change

Palliative care education started in Romania with the opening in 1997 of the Princess Diana Study Centre as part of Hospice Casa Sperantei. Since its founding, this education center has played a pivotal role in preparing the workforce in palliative care in Romania and in the region. Over 12,800 participants from Romania and 18 other countries in the region have attended introductory courses, advanced training programs, and subspecialty courses at the Centre (Figure 79.3). The education center works with over 100 accredited trainers from all over Romania and is a partner with the University of Transylvania in running the multidisciplinary palliative care master course since 2010.

Since 2012 an online program has been launched for general practitioners with the aim of spreading palliative care approaches within the community. Courses are available in Romanian and in Russian (http://www.studiipaliative.ro/educatie/cursuri-on-line-ro) and an information center offers access to written and video material to lay caregivers (www.infopaliatie.ro).

Conclusion

Eastern Europe is a diverse group of countries, most having been under the rule of the Soviet Republic until the early 1990s. Each country has faced unique challenges in the provision of quality hospice and palliative care, ranging from limited opioid availability to economic hardship. Programs are developing through the dedication and extraordinary efforts of committed professionals. Patients and their families are benefiting from these efforts and many more will continue to receive excellent end-of-life care as education, policy, and clinical advances progress.

References

1. Stjernsward J, Foley K, Ferris F. The public health strategy for palliative care. J Pain Symptom Manage. 2007;33(5).:486–493.
2. ELNEC. 2010. International Training Program, Module 5: Cultural and Spiritual Consideration in End-of-Life Care.
3. Applebaum A. Iron Curtain: The Crushing of Eastern Europe, 1944–1956. 2012.
4. Berend, Ivan T. Decades of Crisis: Central and Eastern Europe before World War II. 2001.
5. Ellmeier A, Rásky B. Differing Diversities: Eastern European Perspectives, Transversal Study on the Theme of Cultural Policy and Cultural Diversity, phase 2. Culture and Cultural Heritage Department, Council of Europe Publishing; 2006.
6. http://www.studylecturenotes.com/management-sciences/economics/470-what-are-the-important-characteristics-of-communism. Accessed July 31, 2013.
7. Intersperience. Cultures Diverge Across Eastern European Boundaries. http://www.intersperience.com/knowledge_more.asp?know_id=43. Accessed august 13, 2013.
8. United Nations Statistics Division—Standard Country and Area Codes Classifications (M49).
9. Population Division, DESA, United Nations. World Population Ageing 1950–2050.
10. Mosoiu D. European insight: developing palliative care in Moldova: a top-down approach. Eur J Palliat Care. 2011;18(1):46–49.
11. Vvedenskaya E. Changing the Legislation: An Example from Russia: Free Communication. Prague: EAPC World Congress; 2013.

12. European Observatory on Health Care Systems and Policies. 2005. Health Care Systems in Transition. Berlin. http://www.euro.who. int/__data/assets/pdf_file/0008/75149/E86823sum.pdf. Accessed August 30, 2013.

13. OECD. Health at a Glance: Europe 2010: 87. http://www.oecd-ilibrary. org/docserver/download/8110161e.pdf?expires=1380195437&id=id&a ccname=guest&checksum=2A06B933E23911CEE0D5BE46E3E281EF. Accessed August 30, 2013.

14. IMAS.

15. Horeica R, Mosoiu D, Anania P. Assessment of Quality in Palliative Home Care with FEHC. Poster EAPC World Congress. Prague, 2013.

16. Lynch T, Connor S, Clark D. 2013. Mapping levels of palliative care development: a global update. J Pain Symptom Manage. 45(6): 1094–1106.

17. Centeno C, Lynch T, Donea O, Rocafort J, Clark D. EAPC Atlas of Palliative Care in Europe 2013—Full Edition. European Association for Palliative Care. http://hdl.handle.net/10171/29291. Accessed August 30, 2013.

18. Clark D, Wright M. Transition in End of Life Care. Buckingham: Open University Press; 2003:180–194.

CHAPTER 80

Palliative care in the Philippines

Ayda G. Nambayan and Henry U. Lu

Key points

◆ The Philippines consists of an archipelago of 7101 islands

◆ Health care varies widely and poverty is a serious problem

◆ Rural health care is provided by folk healers or medicine men

◆ Hospice care was introduced to the Philippines in the 1980's—currently 34 palliative care organizations provide end-of-life care to Filipinos, most of them in urban areas

◆ Culture, traditions beliefs and religion play an important part in attitudes towards death and suffering—discussions about death is usually avoided

◆ Family is central in health care decisions and caring for family members

Country background

The Philippines (Pilipinas, Republic of the Philippines, Republika ng Pilipinas) is a sovereign state located in Southeast Asia, west of the Pacific Ocean. It is an archipelago, containing 7107 islands, with a total land area, inclusive of the inland bodies of water, of approximately 300,000 square kilometers (120,000 sq mi), making the country the 73rd largest independent nation in the world. It also boasts the fifth longest coastline in the world with 36,289 kilometers or 22,549 miles.[1] Although there are 7,107 islands, the country is mainly divided into three main geographical regions: Luzon, Visayas, and Mindanao. The capital city is Manila, which also has the most dense population.

The Philippines' geographical relationship with other Southeast Asian countries is defined by bodies of water; the Luzon Strait to the north separates the Philippines from Taiwan, and Vietnam is located to the west, across the South China Sea. A few hundred kilometers southwest of the Philippines lies the island of Malaysia, across the Sulu Sea. The Celebes Sea separates the southern region of the Philippines from Indonesia, while the Philippine Sea binds the eastern area with Palau as the closest island neighbor.

The tropical location of the archipelago, being on the Pacific Ring of Fire, makes the Philippines prone to earthquakes and typhoons. It has been recorded that every day the country experiences approximately 20 seismic activities, which are generally very weak. The islands also experience five to six strong typhoons every year that often cause serious destruction and death.[2]

The Philippines has a total population of 92.34 million people, making it the seventh-most populated country in Asia and 12th in the world. In addition, it is estimated that 11 million Filipinos

are living outside the country, the majority are Overseas Filipino Workers (OFWs). Metro Manila is the most populous city with approximately 11 million people.[3] The Philippines is a secular nation with a constitution that separates church and state; however, 90% of the population is Christian and predominantly Roman Catholic. Muslims make up about 5% to 10% of the population, mostly living in the Mindanao, Palawan, and the Sulu areas, commonly known as the Moro region.[4] There are also several aboriginal and tribal groups who practice the Philippine traditional religions blended with Christianity and Islam.

The geographical location of the Philippines creates some differences in the way that death and dying are perceived and dealt with in the country. Although there are some central beliefs, practices and traditions related to death and dying vary between the three main island regions where most of the population resides. These differences are further complicated by urban or rural locality and by inclusion of the tribal groups, which are still an important part of Philippine society. For example, it is traditional that a 4- to 7-day wake follows a death. The wake serves not only to honor the dead but also as a way to start the family's bereavement process. However, the location, and how the wake is conducted, varies. In the urban areas, the wake is usually held in a funeral home, whereas in rural areas the wake is generally located in the family home. For the T'boli tribe, the number of days of the wake depends on the position of the dead within the tribal society; the higher the position, the longer the wake.[5]

Healthcare

Healthcare in the Philippines varies widely, from the very sophisticated, world-class care in the major metropolis to almost non-existent care in remote rural municipalities. Poverty is a serious problem in the Philippines, with 51% of the population living on less than $2.00 per day.[6] Thus, for most Filipinos, healthcare is generally episodic with low priority given to preventive care. Poverty is more pronounced in rural areas, and with more limited resources available healthcare in these areas of the country is highly deficient. In most cases, rural healthcare is provided by the *arbularyo* (folk healer or medicine man), who often uses *tawas* (alum) and candle drippings as diagnostic tools and herbs, coconut oil, prayers, chants, and "supernatural cures" for healing practices.

Medical care in the Philippines is paid for through a combination of public and private funds, which include health insurance plans and out-of-pocket payments. Private health insurance, although available, is generally unaffordable to many Filipinos; in addition to high premiums, the full cost of medical expenses is not often covered by insurance and many people are still unable to pay the difference. In 1995, the Philippine Health Insurance Corporation (Phil Health) was established to administer the National Health Insurance Program. The premiums depend on income levels and may be co-shared with employers. For indigent Filipinos, the entire premium is shared by the national and local governments. However, in its country profile on the Philippines, the World Health Organization (WHO) stated, "under the current health care financing arrangements, low income families are being pushed into poverty due to payments for health care."[7] For the poor, there is an additional schema through charitable disbursement of funds raised through the Philippine Charity Sweepstakes (PCSO), intended to sustain free medical and health services to the poorest of the poor Filipinos.

In 2006, healthcare expenditure was only 3.8% of the gross domestic product (GDP); 67.1% came from private entities (self-pay and other healthcare payors), while 32.9% was from the government. Currently, there is a steady decline in the governmental share for healthcare and, with the current population growth, it is projected that there will be less to spend per person. In 2010, the allocation for the healthcare budget was approximately Php 310.00 ($8.00) per person.[6] This reality translates into more episodic than preventive models of care. Late diagnosis in advanced stages of disease is common, creating high mortality rates. Because cancer is often diagnosed in its late stage, even with available treatment options, the Philippine mortality rate from cancer is currently at 50%.[8]

There are 1921 hospitals in the Philippines (total bed capacity of 93,183; 1 bed per 900 people), 719 are government supported and 1,202 are privately owned. There are an estimated 90,370 physicians, 480,910 nurses, and 43,220 dentists.[8] The uneven geographical distribution of these healthcare providers between rural and urban areas further creates inequities in the provision of healthcare. In addition, Filipino healthcare professionals, especially nurses, are one of the most common labor commodity exported by the Philippines.[9] Being one of the major donor countries has its impact on the healthcare of this island nation.

The island nation is administratively divided into autonomous regions, provinces, municipalities, and barangays. The barangays are the smallest administrative division and very similar to a village, district, or ward. It can be an inner city or a suburban neighborhood. To date, there are 42,028 barangays in the Philippines.[10] A category of healthcare provider called the barangay health volunteer (also called barangay health worker) renders primary care services in the communities they live and serve. They undergo 5 weeks training, and their functions include providing information, education, and services for primary healthcare, family planning, and nutrition. These health workers can be trained to be hospice volunteers to meet the needs of the patients and families especially in remote areas of the country.

Big industrial companies often have their own clinic, employing physicians and nurses to provide the first line of care. When employees need hospitalization, these companies often have mutual agreements with major hospitals for inpatient care. In most cases the company covers all or part of the medical costs as part of employee benefits.

Although there is a pharmacy regulatory law related to prescriptive dispensing of medications, many medications like antibiotics can still be bought over the counter without a physician's prescription. The community pharmacy is either a single branch store independently owned and operated by a registered pharmacist, generally located in rural areas, or a chain pharmacy, owned by a corporation. Chain pharmacy accounts for about 60% of pharmaceutical outlets in the country. It has an overall advantage of better storage practices and a larger stock of drugs that are often from reliable sources. In both types of community pharmacies, the current practice is mainly dispensing with minimal (if any) patient medication counseling.[11] In the Philippines, expenditures in medicines are mostly out-of-pocket because they are not covered by health insurance benefits.

Filipino life expectancy is also increasing from 53.4 in the 1960s to 71.4 in 2010. Coronary heart disease leads the causes of death, accounting for approximately 25%.[8] However, since there is no requirement for the cause to be medically determined prior to a death registration (especially in remote areas where registries may not even exist), the data cannot be accurately substantiated. Table 80.1 shows the 2009 morbidity and mortality rates in the country.

Culture

The historical development and the geographical location of the country shaped many of the cultural practices and beliefs in the Philippines. The Filipino culture is a blending of both Eastern and Western cultures. The country's beliefs and practices show attributes found in other Asian countries with Malay and Chinese heritage, yet, it also displays a considerable degree of Spanish and American influences. The Filipinos are known for their festivals (known as barrio fiestas), generally to commemorate/honor the feast days of the town's patron saint.

The festive nature of the Filipinos is often regarded as the most likely basis for the merriment during the weeklong wakes for the deceased. The embalmed body is placed in a coffin for viewing surrounded by funeral lights, flowers, and other objects favored by the deceased. The wake is often held at the house of the deceased or at a funeral home. The family, relatives, friends, and acquaintances of the deceased participate in the vigil, often lasting around the clock. Food and drinks are customarily served to the guests and viewers. Besides offering condolences, the guests often contribute money (called *abuloy* or *ambag*) to help defray the cost of the funeral and the burial. Usual activities during the

Table 80.1 Ten leading causes of death in the Philippines (2009)

Cause of death	Total deaths
1. Diseases of the heart	100,908
2. Diseases of the vascular system	65,489
3. Malignant neoplasms	47,732
4. Pneumonia	42,642
5. Accidents	35,990
6. Tuberculosis, all forms	25,470
7. Chronic lower respiratory diseases	22,755
8. Diabetes mellitus	22,345
9. Nephritis, nephrotic syndrome, and nephrosis	13,799
10. Certain conditions originating in the perinatal period	11,514

Source: Department of Health, Philippines. www.doh.gov.ph.

wake include singing, guitar, and card and game playing such as Mahjong, Bingo, and *Sakla* (local card game).

Death in the Philippines is often a crisis, born out of little or no preparation for death. Like their neighboring countries of China and Malaysia, Filipinos avoid talking about death and dying. It is a common belief that "if one talks about it, it may actually happen to them", or if someone else like a family member, talks about death and dying, they may actually be wishing it on the patient. Although death is generally considered to be part of living, most Filipinos are not prepared when death occurs. In addition, the characteristic that is very much part of the Filipino psyche is the "Bahala Na" (come what may) attitude, as God will always provide. In the face of difficult circumstances such as a life-threatening illness, the "Bahala Na" attitude somehow sustains the Filipino.

Filipinos also have the habit of "saving face" when challenged with adversity. Filipinos want to project an image that "everything is alright," often making it difficult to hold meaningful conversations especially when one is nearing death. Most Filipinos seldom complain about their symptoms, often suffering in quiet desperation. A contributing factor is the deep-seated faith that a higher power (God or Allah) will provide and that suffering is a way of being close to a Higher Power and of attaining eternal salvation. In addition, the practice of saving face could very well be one of the underlying factors influencing patients' and families' decisions to conceal the seriousness of their situation to one another. This practice creates a dichotomy between the needs and wishes of both the patient and the family, which often places healthcare providers at a difficult position when caring for a dying patient.

Although there is a paucity of sociological research on these cultural beliefs and practices as they relate to the Filipino experiences of death and dying, the authors believe that the Filipino culture has a great impact on the care of the dying in the Philippines. Further, this is a challenge that needs to be prioritized to advance palliative and end-of-life care in the Philippines.

Historical development of palliative and hospice in the Philippines

Competing national and societal priorities characterized the early development of palliative and hospice care in the Philippines. Hospice care first began with a variety of programs that provide care to patients with debilitating, advanced, or life-limiting conditions. These supportive programs are often tied with home care services, since most Filipinos prefer to care for ailing family members or delegate the care to someone they know. In 1988, Dr. Josefina Magno, a Filipino oncologist and one of the pioneers for the hospice movement in the United States, returned to the Philippines and began to organize and champion the hospice movement in the country. Box 80.1 shows the stepwise development of hospice and palliative care in the country.

In 1989, the Philippine Cancer Society (PCS) released a study indicating that 73% of Filipino cancer patients had cancer-related pain, 60% of which was persistent.[12] As an outcome, a governmental policy was established, through the Department of Health (DOH)–sponsored Philippine Cancer Control Program (PCCP), that identified cancer pain relief as a priority activity. Alongside this priority, DOH also implemented measures to improve accessibility and availability of oral morphine. In 1991, then-PCS-president Dr. Mita Pardo de Tavera introduced the concept of

---

Box 80.1 Development of hospice and palliative care in the Philippines

- 1988—Dr. Josefina Magno came back to Manila to pioneer establishment of hospice care and education

- 1989—Pain control became an essential component of cancer care

- 1991—First home hospice established by the Philippine Cancer Society

- 1994—First hospice seminar at the Cancer Institute of the Philippines—Philippine General Hospital; followed by a series of training programs initiated by PCS

- Founding of Madre de Amor and Ayala Alabang Hospice Care Foundation, providing free and compassionate care to patients with life-threatening illness

- 1995—First hospice convention sponsored by the PCS and DOH

- 2000—University of the Philippines-Philippine General Hospital established hospice and palliative care training in the Department of Family Medicine

- 2004—National Hospice Palliative Care Council of the Philippines (NHPCCP), later known as Hospice Philippines, was launched

- 2008—Invitational summit for stakeholders from the Philippines, Indonesia, and Thailand to identify problems of opioid use, to assure availability and accessibility of the drug for pain control in palliative care, and to identify achievable targets for implementation strategy and action plan

- 2010—CHED mandate for inclusion of palliative/hospice care in all healthcare curricula

- 2010, 2012—Makati Medical Center Pain and Palliative Care Conference, cosponsored by the Pain Society of the Philippines, International Union Against Cancer, Open Society Institute, and ELNEC of the City of Hope/American Association of Colleges of Nursing

- 2013—Development of the Center for Palliative Care Education and Research, Makati Medical Center, in collaboration with ELNEC, City of Hope, and American Association of Colleges of Nursing

---

the Hospice Home Care Program. The program implemented the modified WHO analgesic ladder (cutting the ladder down to two steps, using opioid-like tramadol in the second step. Although these measures demonstrated the efficacy of the WHO Method of Cancer Pain Relief among Filipino patients, data also showed that pain relief alone did not significantly improve overall quality of life, further demonstrating the need for comprehensive palliative care services.[13]

In the mid-1990s, Dr. Josefina Magno returned to the Philippines, bringing a wealth of experience related to hospice care. She worked tirelessly to convince the medical community that hospice care is an alternative to futile treatment and to the common belief of death as a medical failure. Dr. Magno was challenged by the minister of health to demonstrate hospice care in Manila and if successful, the Department of Health will encourage provision of hospice care to every region, municipality, and barangay of the country. Within 4 months, Dr. Magno obtained commitments from two medical schools to introduce hospice in their curricula and convinced the biggest private hospital in Manila to establish a hospice program. The degree of enthusiasm fueled by government support resulted in the establishment of numerous hospice services, both in the private and governmental sector.

In January 1994, the first hospice seminar was held at the Cancer Institute of the University of the Philippines-Philippine General Hospital (UP-PGH) auditorium. It was a 2-day course on hospice care for healthcare providers. This training was followed in 1995 by the first National Convention on Hospice, again sponsored by the Philippine Cancer Society and the Department of Health. It was also during this time that a comprehensive manual, covering all aspects of supportive care, was nationally released in both English and Tagalog (Filipino language). The training and increased awareness of the need for hospice care, along with government support, resulted in the creation of both hospital- and community-based hospice programs.

Hospice and palliative care training is ongoing in the Philippines with both professional and lay volunteer training being offered on a regular basis. In 2000, the UP-PGH Department of Family and Community Medicine created the first postresidency and fellowship program in hospice and palliative care. Originally, the training in hospice care was limited to medical students and family medicine residents. Over time, the program expanded to include nurses, yet, the program is still primarily geared toward the training of physicians who are specializing in palliative care medicine. Lay volunteer training is regularly conducted by two hospice foundations, namely Madre de Amor and PALCARE. Madre de Amor Hospice, the longest running hospice program in the country, conducts volunteer training on a regular basis. PALCARE on the other hand, partners with other institutions to provide training to both lay and professional providers.

In 2002, a change in government administration resulted in a reordering of priorities, causing weakened governmental support, and many of these institutions have closed or are barely surviving. At this time, the interest in palliative and hospice care also waned. In spite of declining governmental support, palliative care activists formed the National Hospice and Palliative Care Council of the Philippines (now known as Hospice Philippines) in 2004, to be the organization that unites and coordinates various hospice and palliative care institutions in the country. Aiming to promote networking activities between its members, it became the link in delivering hospice care resulting in effective cross referral of patients, and ensuring the best quality of life for the terminally ill.[14] In 2006, then President Gloria Macapagal-Arroyo declared the first week of October of each year as National Hospice and Palliative Care Week. Currently, this week is being jointly celebrated with various activities such as themed fun walks and religious activities.

In 2010, the Commission on Higher Education (CHED) mandated that palliative and end-of-life care content be included in all healthcare curricula. Various implementation strategies were suggested by the Board of Nursing, including the development of an elective course with clinical practicum and integrating the concepts in each nursing course. The clinical practicum includes a visit to the home for the aged and exposure to hospice programs.

Politically, there are pending legislative bills in the Philippine congress that advocate for provision of hospice and palliative care. Known as the Palliative and End-of-Life Care Act 2009, 2010, 2011, and 2012 (SB 3366, Hon. A. Pimentel; HB 2542, Hon. J.V. Ejercito; HBO 4627, Hon. G.M. Arroyo and D.M. Arroyo; SB 3342, Hon. F. Marcos, Jr.), the bill provides mandates for the establishment of a palliative care trust fund to financially support palliative and end-of-life care services in all private and governmental hospitals, healthcare provider education and training, research, and compassionate care leave benefits for caregivers and families of patients with a life-threatening illness.

Although the Philippines is categorized by the International Observatory on End of Life Care Typology as a country in Group 3 (one with localized palliative care provision), palliative and end-of-life care is still far from ideal. Where terminally ill patient spend their last days depends on such factors as one's economic means, the family's support network, and the facilities available. Many nurses perceived dying patients still experienced suffering and were in a state of helplessness and powerlessness at their death.[15]

Opportunities and challenges

Education

In the Philippines, there are a variety of venues for palliative and end-of-life care education. Training opportunities such as international conferences, local conferences sponsored by professional organizations, integration into the healthcare curricula, institutional initiatives such as in-service training, and governmental and nongovernmental organization-sponsored seminars abound. On the other hand, there is a pervasive lack of public awareness when it comes to palliative and end-of-life care. Contributing factors may include the culture of ignoring death and the firm religious belief in a higher power or the strong family support that makes Filipinos disregard this important aspect of living.

Although healthcare curricula is standardized by the Commission on Higher Education (CHED) and regulated by professional boards, still, there are school to school variations in the amount of content and in the curricular implementation. Factors such as faculty expertise, school interests, and resources often influence content selection and implementation. The 2010 CHED mandate for curricular inclusion of palliative care concepts was implemented differently and independently by each school of nursing. As an example, in order to abide with the mandate, most schools followed suggested curricular implementation of a palliative care elective course. Although this is a good measure of curricular integration, the nature of an elective course limits it to students who have interest in palliative care. Clinical resources may also be limited, as most of the 139 hospice programs are centrally located in major cities and are privately owned, reducing the opportunities for direct clinical practice.

Since 1989, the hospice approach has been an integral part of the Family/General Medicine training at the UP-PGH residency program. Clinical experiences in supportive, family, and hospice care occurs during the second year of a 3-year residency program. In 2000, UP-PGH offered a 1-year fellowship program in hospice and palliative care, the first program in the Philippines. Using a holistic approach to care and a variety of care settings (home, clinics, institution), the training is designed to educate physicians in the assessment and management of physical symptoms as well as psychospiritual and social aspects. Although a well-intended program, this training only graduated a handful of palliative care specialists since its inception, a minimal number compared with other specialties.

Other educational opportunities are easily available. Continuing education on palliative and end-of-life care abound, as it is one of the more commonly offered and well-attended topics for such professional activities. The Philippine Nurses Association placed palliative and hospice care nursing as one of its priorities and has been very supportive in cosponsoring such programs. In many instances, the End-of-Life Nursing Education Consortium (ELNEC) program has been presented in Manila and in the other major islands of the country mostly by foreign speakers invited by interested organizations. However, in spite of many educational opportunities, it is interesting to note that Wright indicated low credibility and interest in palliative care as one of the major challenges in the Philippines.[16]

Since 2010, Makati Medical Center (MMC) has been collaborating with several professional organizations (Philippine Nurses' Association, Pain Society of the Philippines, International Union Against Cancer, and Open Society Institute) to hold a 2-day international conference on palliative and end-of-life care. Although the conference was well attended with approximately 450 participants and with very positive program evaluations, when the organizers looked at long-term outcomes of behavior change and increased palliative care referral, it appeared to have had minimal impact, especially within MMC. In response, the MMC administration agreed to establish a Center for Palliative Care Education and Research (CPCER) after yet another workshop in 2012. The Center is a component of the MMC Supportive Care Service and will serve as the educational and research segment of the service. The CPCER is designed primarily to be the focal point of palliative and end-of-life care education and research for multidisciplinary healthcare providers within and outside Makati Medical Center. Collaborating with the City of Hope/American Association of Colleges of Nursing ELNEC project in the United States, the educational arm uses the ELNEC modules as the base curriculum and adapted it into the Philippine culture and multidisciplinary clinical practice. The research arm aims to reach out as a resource to schools of nursing as well as the hospital medical residency program for undergraduate and graduate research. The 5-year strategic plan for the Center includes collaboration with the Department of Health to train the barangay healthcare workers, both in urban and rural areas of the country. Box 80.2 lists the purposes of the Center, while Figure 80.1 shows the schematic diagram of the Center's purposes and activities. Program evaluations are tightly embedded in each of the Center's activities for purposes of improvement and outcome measures.

Although it may seem that educational opportunities are easily available to improve palliative and end-of-life care delivery, there is a need to look at the outcomes of such activities. Despite certain successes and important progress in many areas of palliative care in the country, large disparities still exist. To date, there is minimal evidence of the integration of palliative care in clinical activities, such as palliative care referrals, funding to support activities,

Box 80.2 Purposes of the Center for Palliative Care Education and Research

- Serve as the educational component of the MMC Supportive Care Service
- Provide quality palliative care education within and outside of MMC
- Collect and disseminate updated information in palliative and end-of-life care
- Act as resource for palliative care investigations both in-house and interinstitutionally
- Advance palliative care through political, societal, and academic advocacy

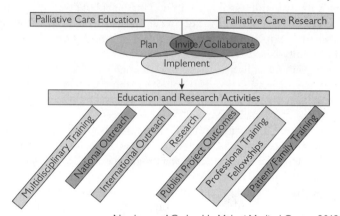

Nambayan, AG., Lu, H., Makati Medical Center, 2012

Figure 80.1 Schematic diagram of the functions and activities of the center for palliative care education and research at Makati Medical Center, Makati City, Philippines.

and others. Seemingly, there is also a lack of deep awareness related to end-of-life care needs of patients and families. Could this reticence be brought about by sociocultural, economic, geographical, or other factors inherent in this country? In a country where there is a paucity of research, this is not only a challenge but an opportunity as well.

Clinical practice

In most instances, both the medical and lay communities use the terms "hospice" and "palliative care" synonymously to mean that the patient is nearing death, generally within 6 months or less. The indistinguishable use of the terms often creates confusion and reluctance to accept or ask for the service. There is also a perception that palliative care is mainly focused on pain control/alleviation, most probably from the historical links to the Pain Society of the Philippines, while hospice care is often associated with dying and support for the bereaved.[16]

In a country where medical reimbursement is generally an out-of-pocket expense, patients and families may opt to not be referred to another specialist like a palliative care physician. Patients and families continue to be cared for by their primary physician/specialist who may not have adequate training in managing the symptoms experienced by terminally ill patients. It is not uncommon to find terminally ill patients being intubated or prescribed futile treatments because of the physician's lack of training in symptom management. In addition, the cultural value of "Never giving up" and the healthcare provider's attitude of "need to cure/death is defeat" often results in futile and burdensome care. Along the same lines, there are reports of reluctance or unwillingness among physicians to refer patients for palliative care, believing that they can manage patient's symptoms just as they have managed the patient's disease.[16]

Pain is a common symptom experienced by dying patients; in the Philippines, it was estimated that 75% of cancer patients who are terminally ill experienced intense pain.[12,13] This study caused social alarm, resulting in collaborative efforts to facilitate access to opioids. Although provisions were made for opioid availability for pain relief, studies have shown that even if there is an adequate awareness of the WHO analgesic ladder among physicians, there is widespread reluctance to prescribe strong opioids such as morphine.[17] The low prescription rate and nonuse of morphine caused overstocking and withdrawal of funds from the Department of Health, further compromising patient care.

Another issue related to opioid prescription includes regulatory difficulties in obtaining prescriptive privileges. Philippine physicians are required to have an S2 license to be able to prescribe regulated drugs such as opioids and also to use yellow prescription pads. Because of rampant illegal usage of regulated drugs, it is an arduous task to secure an S2 license and to get the yellow prescription pads. Physicians have to deal with three governmental agencies: the Dangerous Drugs Board (DDB), being the policymaking entity; the Philippine Drug Enforcement Agency (PDEA), as the implementing unit; and the Department of Health (DOH), being the dispensing body. Physicians report that besides a personal appearance, it generally takes 1 day to apply for the S2 license, and the yellow pad is only available for purchase in a few DOH-selected hospitals in the major cities. Further, the physician is required to hand over the used prescription pads when procuring new ones and is limited to a maximum of five pads per procurement. In addition, there is a threat of death penalty/life imprisonment, with substantial financial consequences and license revocation, for unlawful prescription of dangerous drugs.[18,19] As a result, only 4% of all Filipino practicing physicians have an S2 license and are eligible to prescribe narcotics, which further corroborates the reluctance to prescribe strong opioids to manage and control the dying patients' pain.[17]

Opioid availability is also influenced by the uneven distribution of drugstores that dispense regulated drugs. Regulated drugs are not customarily stocked by all drugstores; smaller, privately owned pharmacies generally do not stock regulated drugs for safety reasons and because these drugs do not move as fast as the others like antibiotics. The same is true for even big franchised pharmacies; only selected drugstores located in big cities generally carry regulated drugs.[20] Further, data from DDB showed that 43% of the national opioid importation was bought by six major hospitals in the country, leaving only half to supply the rest of the country.[21]

The other factor is cost. Although morphine is relatively cheap, it still becomes a major expense when prescribed on a regular basis. For families whose average daily income is Php 300.00, even the cheapest morphine becomes a financial burden. Table 80.2 shows the comparative retail prices of opioids in the more populated, urban city (Metro Manila) and the less populated city (Davao) of the islands. Recently, the DOH allocated free morphine through government hospitals for the indigent patients who need them; however, there are reports that for various reasons, the patients still are not getting them.[22]

In 2008, an invitational summit was sponsored by the Open Society Institute and the Pain and Policy Studies Group of the University of Wisconsin. Chaired by Dr. Henry Lu, the meeting was attended by stakeholders (clinicians, pharmaceutical companies, PDEA and DDB personnel from the Philippines, Thailand, and Indonesia). The goal was to identify common problems relating to use of opioids and also to assure availability and accessibility of opioid analgesics to control pain in palliative care and to identify achievable targets for each country with an implementation strategy and action plan. As a result, the then–secretary of health pledged 10 million pesos ($238,000.00) worth of morphine per year to be given free to all indigent cancer patients. Unfortunately, the program lasted only a year due to administrative changes within the Department of Health and amid irregularities in distribution, storage, monitoring, and dispensing of the opioids. There were reported cases that in some government hospital pharmacies, the free morphine was being sold or was kept unused.[18]

Healthcare providers' experiences with those who are terminally ill also influences the types of interventions they deemed as important to promote a dignified death for Filipino patients. In a study to validate the appropriateness of the International Classification for Nursing Practice (ICNP), *Palliative Care for Dignified Dying* catalog for palliative nursing in the Philippines, Doorenbos et al. reported that nurses who "work often" with dying patients identified interventions that are appropriate for dealing with patients' states of helplessness and powerlessness.

Table 80.2 2013 comparative retail prices of opioids in Metro Manila and Davao City, Philippines

Drug brand and preparation	Price (Philippine Peso) Metro Manila, Luzon Island (US dollars)	Price (Philippine Peso) Davao city, Mindanao Island (US dollars)
Morphine immediate-release 10 mg tablet	21.00 (0.48)	25.00 (0.57)
MST Continus (controlled-release) 10 mg tablet	23.15 (0.53)	24.70 (0.57)
Oxycontin 10-mg tablet	105.00 (2.41)	105.45 (2.41)
Oxycodone immediate-release 5 mg tablet	129.00 (2.96)	107.97 (2.47)
Buprenorphine 5 mcg/h patch	834.00 (19.12)	780.00 (17.88)
Fentanyl 25 mcg/h patch	1,308.50 (29.00)	1,173.04 (26.89)
Tramadol controlled-release 100 mg tablet	91.00 (2.09)	82.35 (1.91)

Nurses who "work less often" with dying patients identified physiological interventions such as provisions for fluids and electrolytes as important interventions to support the dignity of dying patients.[15] The discrepancy between the nurses who "work often" and those who "work less" suggests the importance of education and experience in helping patients maintain dignity while dying.

Culture

The Filipino's perspective on death and dying centers around cultural values and beliefs related to religion, family, and interpersonal harmony. In Philippine society, family plays a fundamental role in the lives of its members and is rated as the most important source of happiness and the social unit that binds Filipinos together.[23] In the context of a terminal illness, values that may affect interactions between healthcare providers, patients, and families include a strong respect for elders, a strong reliance on family as decision-makers in case of illness, and a strong expectation of care by the family. In addition, Filipinos are deeply religious people and even though they believe in personal responsibility, they tend to ascribe illness to reasons of God or a higher power, often believing in "God's will."

When a disclosure of "bad news" is given to Filipino patients and families, it is not uncommon that in the confusion of the moment, attempts to maintain harmony include protecting each other from the bleak reality of the inevitable loss. Patients would ask the healthcare provider to not inform their family about the prognosis or the other way around (family not wanting to inform patient). This practice often puts the healthcare provider in a difficult position when caring for the patient and their families.

Filipinos also believe that suffering has redemptive qualities, making them closer to their God or higher power. Most often, patients would be reluctant to report pain or other symptoms, and would suffer in quiet desperation. Other reasons why patients and families may not report distressing symptoms such as pain include fear of addiction or opioid tolerance and misconceptions about other opioid side effects. Altogether, these create a problem for the healthcare provider whose goal is to alleviate suffering. Nurses often do not rely on subjective reports of pain and distress, rather, they rely on their assumptions; thus, the need for further training on symptom management.

Geography

The Philippines is an archipelago of 7,107 islands, separated by vast body of waters. The geographical make-up of the Philippine islands poses a problem for national initiatives such as palliative care. In addition, there is a large disparity of resources between big urban cities like Metro Manila and rural areas like the small towns of the province of Batangas, approximately 100 km from Manila. The geographical challenge created a problematic provision of palliative care in remote areas and patchy throughout the country. The implementation of a national initiative such as palliative and end-of-life care will need to be taken into the community level, with emphasis on training and support of not only the barangay healthcare workers but also the public health nurses employed by the Department of Health. Currently, these healthcare providers are focused on maternal and child health, infections, and nutrition.

Socioeconomic conditions

Just as the geographical layout of the Philippines is as sharply divided between urban and rural, so is the socioeconomic stratum of the Filipino people. Because of national calamities such as typhoons and flooding, the WHO predicted an uncertain track for the Philippines to reach the Millenium Development Goal (MDG) target of 22.7% below the national poverty threshold by 2015.[24] Although economic growth in the Philippines averaged 4.5% in 2010, in the last decade, poverty has worsened, further widening the gap between the poor and the rich. The availability of palliative care in both the government and private hospitals does not guarantee equitable care delivery. Resources, level of personnel training, and accessibility to medications for symptom management vary between these two types of hospitals. The reality is that patients who have money are attracted to private care with better resources while the poor tend to go to government facilities with minimal resources and a payment schema that is usually scaled according to the patient and family's ability to pay. The wide variation in healthcare distribution presents unique challenges to equitable healthcare delivery in general and to palliative and end-of-life care in particular.

The other alternative is the community and/or foundation-based hospice organizations that usually provide free care for patients who are admitted to their programs. However, even in these alternative facilities, the care is not 100% free, for these hospice organizations have administrative staff, physicians, nurses, social workers, and caregivers who are on the payroll.[25] In addition, needed supplies and medications are generally bought by the families. Patients and families still have to buy necessary supplies and medications or do without.

Summary

Culture, traditions, beliefs, and religion play an important part in every Filipino's life and death. In addition, the family is central and carries a significant importance especially in healthcare decisions. Families are generally very involved in caring for their loved ones who are dying and equally expect healthcare providers to do the same. These are the hospice/palliative care activists who, against all odds, continuously try to improve their patients' quality of life and provide them with elements of dignity.

The movement toward palliative and hospice services in the Philippines began in the 1980s and gathered momentum with collaborations in many sectors of the Philippine society. However in 2000, the enthusiasm for palliative care waned when funding was cut due to the reordering of governmental priorities. To date, only 34 palliative care organizations provide end-of-life care to Filipinos, most of them situated in populous urban areas. In spite of training and the rich history of palliative care development in the Philippines, much has yet to be done before it can be said that palliative and end-of-life care is alive and well in the 7,107 islands of the Philippine archipelago.

References

1. Philippines Information Agency. http://www.pia.gov.ph/news/index. php. Accessed April 2, 2013.
2. The Philippines. http://www.philippines.hvu.nl/climate2.htm. Accessed April 3, 2013.
3. National Statistics Office of the Philippines. www.census.gov.ph/. Accessed April 3, 2013.

4. US Department of State. The Philippine International Religious Report. 2008. http://www.state.gov/j/drl/rls/irf/2008/108421.htm. Accessed March 30, 2013.

5. Burial on Tribal Land. http://www.euntes.com/burial.html. Accessed March 20, 2013.

6. World Bank. http://search.worldbank.org/data?qterm=poverty%20philippines&language=EN. Accessed March 30, 2013.

7. World Health Organization. 2007. Country Cooperation Strategy: WHO/Philippines.

8. Department of Health, Republic of the Philippines. www.doh.gov. Accessed April 3, 2013.

9. Nurses in the Philippines. http://en.wikipedia.org/wiki/Nursing_in_the_Philippines. Accessed March 2013.

10. Philippine National Statistical Coordination Board (NCSB). www.nscb.gov.ph.

11. Ocampo LM. Address given at the Annual Convention of the Philippine Pharmaceutical Association. Manila, Philippines, 2012.

12. Ngelangel CA, Wang HM. Cancer and the Philippine Cancer Control Program. Jpn J Clin Oncol. 2002;32(suppl 1):S52–S61.

13. Laudico AD. The Philippines: status of cancer pain and palliative care. J Pain Symptom Manage. 1996;12(2):133–134.

14. Kalalo A. Hospice Care in the Philippines. St. James COPA Foundation.http://stjames-copa.com/news-page4-vol4-issue4.html. Accessed May 30, 2013.

15. Doorenboos AZ, Abaquin C, Ferrin ME, et al. Supporting dignified dying in the Philippines. Int J Palliat Nurs. 2011;17(3):125–130.

16. Wright M, Hamzah E, Phungrassamy T, Bausa-Claudio A. Hospice and Palliative Care in Southeast Asia. 1st ed. New York; Oxford University Press; 2010.

17. Javier, FO, Magpantay, LA, Espinosa, EL. Harder, SM. and Unite, MA. Opioid use in chronic pain management in the Philippines. Eur J Pain. 2001;5(Suppl A):83–85.

18. Lu HU. Personal observations.

19. Dangerous Drug Boards. www.ddb.gov.ph/. Accessed April 3, 2013.

20. Republic Act 9165. http://www.senate.gov.ph/lisdata/81856680!.pdf. Accessed June 26, 2013.

21. Beltran, J. Pain Management Issues in Low Resource Countries. Presented at the 25th Annual Conference of the Pain Society of the Philippines, Tagaytay City, Philippines, April, 2013.

22. Vilches C. Pain Management Issues in Low Resource Countries. Presented at the 25th Annual Conference of the Pain Society of the Philippines, Tagaytay City, Philippines, April, 2013.

23. Virola R. What Makes Women Happy? National Statistical Coordination Board: Philippines' Policy Making and Coordinating Body on Statistical Matters. 2010. www.nscb.gov.ph/headlines/StatsSpeak/2010/110810_rav_joe_happiness.asp. Accessed May 29, 2013.

24. Index Mundi. http://www.indexmundi.com/philippines/economy_overview.html. Accessed May 30, 2013.

25. Kalalo A. Hospices Offer Compassionate Care. Inquirer/Opinion/Talk of the Town. Posted September 16, 2007. http://opinion.inquirer.net/inquireropinion/talkofthetown/view/20070916-88809/Hospices_offer_compassionate_care. Accessed May 30, 2013.

CHAPTER 81

Palliative care in situations of conflict

Nathan I. Cherny

Key points

♦ Incurable, life-threatening illness is endemic and it often occurs in places of conflict. In these circumstances, care delivery is often compromised or complicated.

♦ People on different sides of a political conflict share a common traumatized existence.

♦ Geneva Convention clearly recognizes the special status of the wounded or sick, be they civilians or combatants, and emphasizes the separation of medical care from the military conflict.

♦ One need not love a foe, but their suffering can be acknowledged and should be relieved when possible.

♦ Through this process, new opportunities for understanding and for mitigating enmity can be developed.

Situations of political conflict are characterized by enmity and potential for, or actual, violence. Conflict of this ilk may be manifested as outright war, a cycle of terror and reprisals, or a grumbling enmity between religious, national, ethnic, or cultural groups.

Incurable, life-threatening illness is endemic and it often occurs in places of conflict. In these circumstances, care delivery is often compromised or complicated. Situations of conflict occur in many places in the world and, at any time, a substantial proportion of the world population is involved in conflict of one sort or other. Conflicts, such as war or terror, traumatize the involved populations.[1-3] The nature of conflict has changed particularly with regard to the likelihood of civilian casualty, which from around 5% at the beginning of the century has risen to as high as 90% in some ongoing conflicts.[4] In this situation, bereavement, fear, anxiety, and depression become commonplace. Persistent conflicts may generate feelings of hopelessness and helplessness.

These observations are derived from my experience in working with Palestinian and Israeli patients in a Jewish hospital in Jerusalem since 1994.

Our context

Jerusalem is a city that has existed in a situation of conflict over the past 100 years. Historically this has been the ancient capital of the Jewish people and currently it is the capital of the modern state of Israel. Jerusalem, however, is also claimed by the Palestinian Arab population as their capital. Indeed, Palestinians and Jews have been in conflict over the destiny of this small strip of land between the Mediterranean and the Jordan River since the inception of the plan to reestablish a Jewish state in the area.

Attempts to achieve some form of rapprochement between the Jewish and Palestinian peoples have been intensified since the Oslo accords in 1993. The breakdown of negotiations in 2000 was accompanied by a violent Palestinian uprising characterized by a wave of terror against Israeli citizens with subsequent restrictions on Palestinian movements and reprisals against terror organizations and their supporters. Thousands of peoples have been killed on both sides.[5]

In the midst of this, the Cancer Pain and Palliative Medicine Service, in the Department of Oncology at Shaare Zedek Medical Center, has provided palliative care for both Israeli and Palestinian patients. Shaare Zedek Medical Center is a Jewish general hospital that serves the entire population of Jerusalem. Reflecting the demographics of the city, 20% of the population is made up of Palestinian Arabs, most of whom are Muslims.

The Cancer Pain and Palliative Medicine service is an integral part of the oncology service and it is based in the oncology day hospital. The service consists of 2 physicians, a palliative care nurse coordinator and education and research coordinator, four social workers (Hebrew, Arabic, and Russian), a chaplain and liaison psychiatrist, and a psychologist. The service provides ambulatory and inpatient care. Community care is provided in cooperation with a number of home hospice services. Although most of the clinicians are Jewish, both of the Arabic-speaking social workers, many of the junior medical officers, and the thoracic surgeon (who works very closely with the service) are Palestinian.

Uniting and dividing experiences

Peoples on different sides of a political conflict of this ilk share a common traumatized existence.[2,3,6,7] Both sides suffer from risk of violent death or injury; both sides are vexed by injustices wrought by the other. Two peoples with different readings of history and different cultures may yet have a common home, a common homeland, often common cities, neighborhoods, and healthcare services.[8]

Conflict breeds bias, and this is often manifested among both patients and healthcare providers.

Illness is a unifying experience. The experiences of physical and psychological distress and fear of deterioration or death are universal. Similarly, the desire to care for the ill and to alleviate suffering is, fundamentally, universal. Indeed, even in the situation of very awful conflict, heathcare can provide opportunities to bridge between communities and peoples.

Nurses have a very special role to play in this situation. Given the greater opportunity for intimate contact and often, greater time for dialogue and compassionate care, their role is critical. This is true both in regard to care delivery and also for the critical role of developing bonds of trust. Communication is critical to the success of this endeavor, and this will often require the use of a translator to ensure that the patient is understood and that they understand the care provider.

Barriers to care in situations of conflict

Infrastructural

Conflicts commonly disrupt the flow of persons (patients and healthcare providers), the availability of care and the delivery of healthcare. Often patients are unable to get to the needed health-care facilities and healthcare providers may be hampered in their ability to get to their patients. Physical resources may be limited by diversion of resources for other purposes, lack of free movement of goods, or use of limited healthcare resources by the combatants or victims. In times of war or conflicts, medications, sterile dressings, hospital beds, and healthcare providers may be in short supply. Often, the cost of medications may be inflated due to the collapse of health insurance arrangements or shortage.

Bias and access

Both patients and healthcare providers may be affected by bias against persons on the other side of the conflict barrier. This bias may be generated by resentment, fear, cultural misunderstanding, or demonization. Bias may hinder patients from seeking healthcare that may involve contact with healthcare providers or other patients from the other side of the conflict. Similarly bias may influence healthcare providers in their attitudes or in delivery of care to persons on the other side of the divide. This can be as mild as personal distaste or as severe as overt hostile neglect or sabotage of treatment.

Distrust and enmity

Neither patients nor healthcare providers are protected from the political and social environment. Both parties may carry and project distrust and/or enmity that may be manifest in the carer-patient interaction. Distrust or enmity can interfere with all aspects of care delivery. Distrust and/or enmity may also affect other relationships: patients sharing the same waiting room or adjacent hospital beds, healthcare providers from different sides of the conflict, or patient's family members' relationships with the healthcare providers.

Safety

Death or injury to healthcare providers is, sadly, common in war and conflict. Beneficently minded healthcare providers often feel naively protected by the nature of the humanitarian work that they undertake. The enmity of conflict is often such that it is stronger than any compunction about the killing of carers.[9] Similarly, patients seeking medical assistance may be endangered en route to care; they may be confused for combatants, suspected of malice, or may simply be traversing a conflict zone.[10,11]

Narrative: "I almost killed a patient today"

Monday night; 11 PM. I almost killed a patient with methadone today. She was (and thankfully still is) a 68-year-old lady who came to see me from Natanya. She has a huge inoperable cancer deep in her abdomen and, even with high doses of morphine, her pain hadn't been adequately relieved.

Under close supervision I gave her two doses of methadone. Over the next 2 hours her pain subsided. She was able to get up and walk about. She seemed to have good relief without excessive drowsiness, confusion, or sleepiness.

Methadone is not widely available and, in Jerusalem, there is only one pharmacy that carries it. At 3.15 this afternoon, I wrote out a prescription and sent this lady and her husband to buy the methadone before they headed back to Natanya. To avoid parking problems, they went to the pharmacy by cab.

The pharmacy is in the middle of town . . . on Jaffa road near Zion Square. Half an hour later I was called to the emergency room. A terrorist had shot some 30 people in the center of town . . . exactly outside the pharmacy. I was quietly panicked. They didn't arrive in our emergency room. I checked with the emergency coordination center. They weren't on any of the emergency room lists. That meant that they were both alive and well or, possibly, dead but unidentified.

It was a very long hour until they returned to hospital to ask where else that could possibly get the methadone. The shooting had broken out as they approached the area and their cab driver was diverted.

Few things scare physicians, and particularly physicians relieving pain with opioids, than almost killing a patient with a medication intended to help. I am an expert in the side effects of methadone, but this would have been a new side effect for me. These are strange and evil times.

Abuse

In some instances healthcare resources are seconded or abused to facilitate violence.[12] The harboring of combatants or weapons in hospitals or clinics and the ferrying of arms or combatants in ambulances or disguised as doctors, medics, or nurses undermines the assumption of benevolence.[13] In order to be respected, it is essential that the credibility of the beneficence of healthcare providers be maintained. Without the assumption of benevolence, ambulances, healthcare providers, or even patients may be submitted to justifiable suspicion, which may cause delays in genuine care delivery due to security concerns and suspicion of potentially hostile intentions.[14]

Why provide care in conflict?

Medicine is a fusion of humanity, science, and compassion. Humanity and compassion dictate that the suffering of illness must be addressed, and, when possible, relieved. This holds true for all who suffer, be they friends or foes. One need not love a foe, but their suffering can be acknowledged and should be relieved when possible. Through this process, new opportunities for understanding and for mitigating enmity can be developed. The Geneva Convention clearly recognizes the special status of the wounded or sick, be they civilians or combatants, and emphasizes the separation of medical care from the military conflict.[15]

Depersonalization and dehumanization of the enemy are common processes in conflict.[16] Often members of the "enemy" are demonized such that they are perceived as fundamentally hostile, evil, and unworthy, or even worthy of harm (such as abuse, torture, and punishment without due process).[16] These processes of depersonalization, dehumanization, and demonization are reinforced by lack of intimate contact between peoples. Social contacts are limited by perceived or real issues of fear, risk of harm, distrust, and enmity. All of these processes make the possibility of cooperation or conflict resolution more difficult.

Medicine has the potential to be a positive agent of change. Provision of care across lines of enmity creates the potential to reverse some of these processes.[17] Given that suffering at the end of life is universal, there is a very special opportunity for palliative care clinicians working in regions of conflict. Where end-of-life care is so often ignored or neglected, palliative care emphasizes humanity and respect for human dignity in a very special way. This focus on humanity stands in stark contrast to the disregard for the value of human life that is so much part of war and terror. Through the delivery of care, there is a potential to break barriers of suspicion and hatred and to reverse the processes of depersonalization, dehumanization, and demonization.[18]

Case study 1

Mr. A was a 40-year-old husband of a young Palestinian woman with metastatic colon cancer. Together they had four children and they lived in East Jerusalem. In September 2000 he had been at the site of a violent clash between Palestinian protesters and the Israeli armed services. The young man who stood beside him was shot and killed, and he carried the body away from the battle scene.

When he initially came with his wife to an Israeli hospital he was full of anger at Israelis and Jews and he had little reservation about hiding his hostility. The treating oncologist was an orthodox Jewish Israeli, Dr. S. They communicated with the help of a Palestinian social worker.

Over 2 years, Dr. S. cared for this young family. Mrs. A underwent several lines of chemotherapy; some were successful, others less so. When she developed a bowel obstruction, Dr. S. arranged for a diverting colostomy and supported the family through the ordeal. The treating nurses would hold her hands and stroke her hair and extended the same care and support that they would to any other patient.

Slowly, enmity faded and Mr. A, his wife, and family became a part of the routine in the oncology day hospital. As her illness progressed she became increasingly dependent on help from the palliative care nurse. Because they lived in an area that had become increasingly unsafe for Israelis, and in the absence of a Palestinian home care program, we had to make do with telephone support and hospital-based ambulatory care.

Mrs. A ultimately developed severe pain with lumbosacral plexopathy. She was admitted for pain stabilization. She did not achieve adequate relief with Patient Controlled Analgesia (PCA) morphine, and she was switched to methadone, which provided reasonable relief. It became clear however that she would not be able to return home, and she died in the oncology/palliative care ward, surrounded by her family and friends and her mainly Israeli doctors and nurses.

A week after her death her husband returned with his four children with gifts and thanks for the staff. To Dr. S he said, "You are now my brother."

Facilitating care delivery across lines of enmity

Advertise availability and neutrality

Unless it is known that care is available irrespective of conflict and irrespective of "sex, race, nationality, religion, political opinion or other similar criteria,"[15] many potential patients may not seek help. Advertisement can be in the form of letters to doctors, commercial advertisements, or the print or electronic media.[19]

Demilitarize hospitals and clinics

It is absolutely unacceptable for hospitals to be militarized by any party in the conflict; they must be respected neutral territory. When this principle is not adhered to, those in need of help may be too afraid to seek care. The abuse of hospitals either as bases for attack or as asylum for health combatants undermines impartiality and potentially invites incursion or conflict. As stated in the Geneva Convention I: Art. 2, "No persons residing, in whatever capacity, in a hospital zone shall perform any work, either within or without the zone, directly connected with military operations or the production of war material."[15] This is further highlighted in the Convention for the Amelioration of the Condition of the Wounded in Armies in the Field which states, "Ambulances and military hospitals shall be recognized as neutral, and as such, protected and respected by the belligerents as long as they accommodate wounded and sick."[20]

Finances and payment

Healthcare provision costs money and, unless supported by charity, costs must be covered to ensure ongoing ability to provide care. Emergency care should be available to all presenting need, irrespective of ability to pay. For patients without insurance or financial resources, providing ongoing care can present logistic challenges. Several options are possible: provision of care at cost, arranging for care to be provided by healthcare services across the divide of conflict, or providing subsidized or charitable care. Arranging care, at lesser expense to the patient, across the lines of conflict requires the development and maintenance of lines of communications with healthcare practitioners on the other side of the conflict. In our experience, even in the setting of political animosity and differences, this sort of humanitarian cooperation has been possible and positive.

Physical access

Patients, their carers, and their family members may need specific permits to enable them to reach healthcare facilities across lines of enmity. Members of the healthcare team are often able to liaise directly with civic or military authorities to facilitate the granting of permits. In doing so, there is an element of responsibility insofar as the clinicians need to be adequately convinced that these permits will not be abused to ferry either arms or combatants. Because the authorities at check posts may, sometimes, be hostile to the patients or their families, it is helpful to provide them with written testimony to the fact that they are seeking healthcare, with a specific contact name and telephone number for verification purposes. This is often a challenging situation, as medical practitioners may be doubtful about exposing themselves to the risks of misuse of this kind of request.

Cost containment

To protect the interests of the patient and the healthcare provider, the clinician has a duty to try to contain costs of care provision as far as possible. This concern reflects itself in clinical decision-making in regard to both diagnostic investigations and therapeutics. One needs to be aware of the cost of medications and the most effective formulations to provide ongoing care. Commonly available formulations of controlled-release opioids may be prohibitively expensive, and cheaper options such as immediate release morphine or methadone may be preferred.

Clinician liaison and cooperation

Professionals caring for individuals on both sides can initiate dialogue between the factions. Often patients can get adequate care without enduring all of the logistic barriers involved in crossing lines of enmity. It is often useful to liaise with physicians and nurses across the lines of enmity, to evaluate the availability of care and the limits of care resources. In suggesting to a patient that they not cross lines of enmity and that they seek care locally, one must first be sure that there is a real possibility of receiving adequate care. In so doing, it is appropriate to invite open lines of communication to address any medical issues that may arise. This approach requires effort in creating and maintaining an efficient medical network, based on reciprocal respect of a common ethical framework and commitment to quality of care. Telemedicine and phone consultations are often useful to maintain clinical follow-up despite movement restrictions.

Address the needs of children

War and conflict inflicts a very severe price on the psychological and physical well-being of children.[3,17,21–25] Building on the axiom that children need to be protected from the effects of war, clinicians can work together in promoting child health. This can take the form of collaborative research, shared patient management, and joint conferences focusing on child welfare.[17]

Create a bank of returned medications

Returned and unused medications are usually discarded or destroyed. When there are potential patients who do not have the resources to pay for medication, this is wasteful and inappropriate. Returned medications should be stored appropriately and may be used in the care of patients who do not have resources to pay for them. In our setting we have successfully done this with cytotoxics, analgesics, antiemetics, and other potentially expensive medications.

Creative improvisation

Often, normal care structures, such as home hospice services or day clinic availability will be unavailable or inaccessible. In such cases the available care resources need to be evaluated to explore the possibility of some form of improvisation, which may be suboptimal, but at least fills a modicum of care needs. This may involve a compromise on the care plan; for example when a PCA could not be maintained at home because home care staff could not safely visit, we switched the patient to methadone suppositories, which were both cheap and effective. Often family members, or sometimes friends and neighbors will need to be trained to provide for care needs or even to do simple procedures such as tube feeding, suction, and wound care.

Case study 2

Mrs. FW was a 60-year-old Palestinian woman from a small village just outside Jerusalem who presented to an Israeli hospital with metastatic breast cancer with liver and bone metastases. She received palliative antitumor therapies in two Israeli hospitals. She was regularly reviewed in the day hospital by the palliative care service, who managed her pain with transdermal fentanyl and oral morphine.

Her condition deteriorated just as the conflict in Jerusalem worsened. Because of excessive personal risk, home hospice services were unable to attend her. The danger was understood by the patient and her family, who not only accepted this with sorry resolve but also actively discouraged staff from placing themselves at risk.

Contact was made with a local doctor and nurse; with the support and instruction of the palliative care service they undertook a program of home care. When she was unable to take oral medication, a PCA pump was provided and serviced by the local medical team with daily telephone support from the palliative care service. This arrangement was successfully maintained until the patient's death at home.

International organizations

Several international organizations have created special infrastructures to assist in the provision of care in situations of conflict. It is very helpful to know and to develop relationships with those services and agencies active locally.

The World Health Organization (WHO)

Sponsored by the United Nations, this international organization has widely accepted and acknowledged credibility that usually crosses all lines of conflict. Indeed, the WHO is mandated by its Constitution (article 2) to "furnish appropriate technical assistance and, in emergencies, the necessary aid upon the request or acceptance of Governments." In such situations, national authorities have the prime responsibility to respond to the needs of the affected population, but in protracted conflict situations the situation can often deteriorate to a degree that undermines the capacity of the local authorities to meet the urgent public health needs. Through its presence in all countries, its regional structure, its technical units and programs at headquarters, its use of the existing health partnerships (such as the well-established polio network), and its system of collaborating centers, the WHO is well structured to deliver its technical advisory support to national and local authorities, sister agencies, the donor community, international nongovernmental organizations (NGOs), and local self-help groups.

Médecins Sans Frontières

Médecins Sans Frontières (also known as Doctors Without Borders, DWB, or MSF)[26] is a private, nonprofit organization that is at the forefront of emergency healthcare as well as care for populations suffering from endemic diseases and neglect. Healthcare professionals working for Médecins Sans Frontières deliver emergency aid to victims of armed conflict, epidemics, and natural and man-made disasters, and to others who lack healthcare due to social or geographical isolation. They provide primary healthcare, perform surgery, rehabilitate hospitals and clinics, run nutrition and sanitation programs, train local medical personnel, and provide mental healthcare.

Physicians for Human Rights

Physicians for Human Rights[27] is less involved with providing actual care but can contribute to health are provision in the world by protecting human rights.[28] When the ability to provide care has been hampered by bias, malice, or draconian rule, they have been helpful as an international advocate. They provide teams of experts to investigate and expose violations of human rights.

International Medical Corps

Similar to Doctors Without Borders, the International Medical Corps[29] is a global nonprofit organization dedicated to providing care in places of distress and conflict through healthcare training and relief and development programs. By offering training and healthcare to local populations and medical assistance to people at highest risk, and with the flexibility to respond rapidly to emergency situations, the International Medical Corps rehabilitates devastated healthcare systems and helps bring them back to self-reliance.

Narrative: me and Muhammad

Dr. Muhammad Natshe is dying. A father of five, a devout Muslim, he is a sweet man of peace who has lived almost all of his life through the tumult of Middle East Conflict. Tonight, as I write these words, he lies in a three-bed room in Internal Medicine A at Shaare Zedek Medical Center (an Orthodox Jewish Hospital In West Jerusalem). He is weak and tired. Three of his sons were at his bedside when I bid him farewell tonight. As I left, I saw his eldest son prostrate and barefoot on his prayer mat, face to Mecca, deep in prayer.

Formerly a handsome man with a strong resemblance to the late King Hussein of Jordan, Dr. Natshe is now withered and prematurely aged. The whites of his eyes are yellow, tinged with an early jaundice from his now failing liver. His abdomen is distended with fluid; his legs are bloated by edema. His eyes are bright and his broad loving smile breaks through the misery, sadness, and fear of his current circumstances. Like many Palestinian men, he has smoked most of his adult life. Now the lung cancer, which presented 9 months ago, has erupted through the brief response to chemotherapy and threatens the function of his vital organs.

Today, I am Muhammad's doctor; his oncologist and palliative medicine physician. That was not always the case. I first encountered him as a colleague. He was a highly respected general practitioner in East Jerusalem. There, close to the spectacular hubbub of the Damascus Gate of the Old City of Jerusalem, he tended to a large practice. Patients he referred were among the first Palestinians that I treated when I arrived in Jerusalem some 7 years ago. He was a caring and involved family doctor. I was impressed and touched by his devotion: be it visiting his patents when they were admitted to our hospital, or caring, alongside the home hospice service, for his patients who were approaching their deaths.

Dr. Natshe was a general practitioner by default. He had initially wanted to be a surgeon and had, indeed, started a surgical residency at Hadassah Hospital in early 1973. Shortly after it began, his residency was interrupted by the surprise attack of the Yom Kippur War. The Jewish world was shocked and outraged at the surprise attack. Most Palestinians supported the Egyptian/Syrian alliance. Dr. Natshe took leave from Hadassah during the war and, in the aftermath, he felt too embarrassed to return to his residency in surgery. After 3 years of general practice, he applied and was accepted back to Hadassah as a radiology resident. The medical world of Israel, the West Bank, and Jordan is small, and word of Dr. Natshe's appointment quickly reached Amman. The Jordanian Medical Association dispatched a strongly worded letter of reprimand, intimating that it would be treasonous to work in an Israeli hospital. Thus, Muhammad returned to his general practice, where he worked until the toll of the lung cancer and the adverse effects of its treatment made it impossible to continue.

Faith and pragmatism: Dr. Natshe's eyes twinkle with enthusiasm as he explains his love of Islam and the word of The Prophet. He is a deeply religious man and, in the encroaching shadow of death, his faith in God's ultimate beneficence underscores his inner strength and courageous coping. His sons are dapper, deferential, and attentive to their frail father. Even in his ill-fitting hospital pajamas, I can see his tired chest rise with pride at the sight of them. He tells me that he insisted that each of them learn a trade before entering tertiary education. He has successfully assured them of short- and long-term economic opportunity. His eldest son, a part-time hairdresser, studies computer engineering at an Israeli Technical School; the second, a part-time truck driver, studies industrial chemistry at the Hebrew University. The boys speak to me in Hebrew and English. He tells them that they will need to look after their mother, as he will soon be gone.

Tomorrow, I plan to discharge Dr. Natshe back to his home in East Jerusalem. After 3 days in hospital, his pain and vomiting are now controlled. He is very weak. In a week, I anticipate I will need to again drain his abdomen of the reaccumulating fluids that painfully distend his abdomen and compress his viscera. By then, he will probably be too weak to return to the hospital, so I will attend to him at home.

Dr. Muhammad Natshe, Palestinian physician, man of Islam, man of God, father and husband, is my colleague, my patient, and my friend. I will care for him and his family with all of the skill and devotion that I can muster. I have promised him my commitment and my service as long as it is needed. Sadly, that won't be long.

That I am a Jew, that I am Israeli, that our peoples are in conflict in an awful time of violence and hatred, are irrelevant to the humanity that binds us. I will miss him when he's gone.

Behind the headlines, behind the shocking and awful images of violence, death, cruelty, and humiliation small acts of caring, cooperation, and love play themselves out daily. This is another reality of the Intifada. Gladly, this is part of my reality, my source of hope and strength.

Regional initiatives to promote palliative care in the Middle East

The Middle East Cancer Consortium

The Middle East Cancer Consortium (MECC) is part of project between the United States and the ministries of health of Cyprus, Egypt, Israel, Turkey, and Palestine. The organization has been instrumental in promoting regional cancer registries and joint projects in medical genetics and, in particular, palliative care.[30]

Palliative care has been the major focus of its educational and regional initiatives.[31,32] Under the auspices of MECC there have been multiple meetings and training programs bringing together clinicians who often come across the lines of conflict. This has been a unique opportunity to create dialogue and interaction between clinicians from Israel with their colleagues from many parts of the Middle East with whom they would not have regular contact such as those from Palestine, Lebanon, Iraq, Afghanistan, and other countries in the region.

In 2009 the first meeting of the MECC Palliative Care Steering Committee (MPCSC) was held.[33] The goals of this group are "to develop and implement a shared strategy to build palliative care capacity in MECC and other Middle Eastern countries." At their inaugural meeting the participants reviewed the situation in each of the participating countries as well as strategies for integrating palliative care into existing healthcare. The overall plan of this initiative is to develop "One Voice to guide the implementation of palliative care services to respond to the multiple needs of patients and families living with cancer and other life-threatening illnesses across the Middle East."

Most recently, MECC has been one of the collaborating organizations in the international collaborative study to evaluate the availability and accessibility of opioids for the management of cancer pain in Africa, Asia, the Middle East, India, Latin America, and the Caribbean.

Cross-conflict training and educational opportunities at Shaare Zedek Medical Center

With the support of the Middle East Cancer Consortium, the Shaare Zedek Medical Center in Jerusalem has provided educational resources and opportunities to help in the development of palliative medicine in Palestine. This creates the opportunity for Israeli and Palestinian clinicians to work side-by-side in the care of both Jewish and Palestinian patients. This sort of opportunity not only helps in the development of skills but also promotes the understanding of the common humanity shared between peoples living across the divide of unresolved political conflict.

Conclusions

War and conflict are among the major challenges to humanity. The provision of palliative care in times and places of conflict is fraught with personal and infrastructural difficulty. In meeting these challenges, healthcare providers have the potential to be positive agents of change. The challenges are great, but the potential rewards even greater.

References

1. Shalev AY, Freedman S. PTSD following terrorist attacks: a prospective evaluation. Am J Psychiatry. 2005;162(6):1188–1191.
2. Lavi T, Solomon Z. Palestinian youth of the Intifada: PTSD and future orientation. J Am Acad Child Adolesc Psychiatry. 2005;44(11):1176–1183.
3. Solomon Z, Lavi T. Israeli youth in the Second Intifada: PTSD and future orientation. J Am Acad Child Adolesc Psychiatry. 2005;44(11):1167–1175.
4. Downes AB. Targeting Civilians in War. Ithaca, NY: Cornell University Press; 2008.
5. Statistics, Fatalities 29.9.2000–30.11.2008. 2008. http://www.btselem.org/English/Statistics/Casualties.asp. Accessed December 2008.
6. Shuter J. Emotional problems in Palestinian children living in a war zone. Lancet. 2002;360(9339):1098.
7. Khamis V. Post-traumatic stress and psychiatric disorders in Palestinian adolescents following intifada-related injuries.Soc Sci Med. (1982). 2008;67(8):1199–1207.
8. Minear L, Weiss TG, eds. Humanitarian Action in Times of War—A Handbook for Practitioners. Boulder and London: The Humanitarianism and War Project; 1993.
9. Siegel-Itzkovich J. David Applebaum. BMJ. 2003;327(7416):684.
10. Giacaman R, Husseini A, Gordon NH, Awartani F. Imprints on the consciousness: the impact on Palestinian civilians of the Israeli Army invasion of West Bank towns. Eur J Public Health. 2004;14(3):286–290.
11. Miranda JJ. Ambulances and curfews: delivering health care in Palestine. Lancet. 2004;363:176.
12. Pearl MA. Ambulances and curfews: delivering health care in Palestine. Lancet. 2004;363(9412):895; author reply 895–896.
13. Cohn JR, Romirowsky A, Marcus JM. Abuse of health-care workers' neutral status. Lancet. 2004;363(9419):1473.
14. Viskin S. Shooting at ambulances in Israel: a cardiologist's viewpoint. Lancet. 2003;361(9367):1470–1471.
15. Geeva Conventions. Geneva Convention (I) for the Amelioration of the Condition of the Wounded and Sick in Armed Forces in the Field. Geneva, Switzerland: Geneva Conventions; 1949.
16. Vetter S. Understanding human behavior in times of war. Military Med. 2007;172(12 Suppl):7–10.
17. Wexler ID, Branski D, Kerem E. War and children. JAMA. 2006;296(5):579–581.
18. Ashkenazi T, Berman M, Ben Ami S, Fadila A, Aravot D. A bridge between hearts: mutual organ donation by Arabs and Jews in Israel. Transplantation. 2004;77(1):151–155; discussion 156–157.
19. Rees M. Amid the killing, E.R. is an oasis. Time. 2003;161(25):36–38.
20. Geneva Conventions. Convention for the Amelioration of the Condition of the Wounded in Armies in the Field, Article 1. 1864.
21. Qouta S, Punamaki RL, Montgomery E, El Sarraj E. Predictors of psychological distress and positive resources among Palestinian adolescents: trauma, child, and mothering characteristics. Child Abuse Neglect. 2007;31(7):699–717.
22. Elbedour S, Onwuegbuzie AJ, Ghannam J, Whitcome JA, Abu Hein F. Post-traumatic stress disorder, depression, and anxiety among Gaza Strip adolescents in the wake of the second Uprising (Intifada). Child Abuse Neglect. 2007;31(7):719–729.
23. Berger R, Pat-Horenczyk R, Gelkopf M. School-based intervention for prevention and treatment of elementary-students' terror-related distress in Israel: a quasi-randomized controlled trial. J Trauma Stress. 2007;20(4):541–551.
24. Abdeen Z, Greenough PG, Chandran A, Qasrawi R. Assessment of the nutritional status of preschool-age children during the second Intifada in Palestine. Food Nutr Bull. 2007;28(3):274–282.
25. Espie E, Gaboulaud V, Baubet T, et al. Trauma-related psychological disorders among Palestinian children and adults in Gaza and West Bank, 2005–2008. Int J Ment Health Syst. 2009;3(1):21.
26. Doctors Without Borders. http://www.msf.org/. Accessed July 2013.
27. Physician for Human Rights. http://physiciansforhumanrights.org/. Accessed July 2013.
28. Shauer A, Ziv H. Conflict and public health: report from Physicians for Human Rights-Israel. Lancet. 2003;361(9364):1221.
29. International Medical Corps. https://internationalmedicalcorps.org/. Accessed July 2013.
30. Silbermann M, Khleif A, Tuncer M, et al. Can we overcome the effect of conflicts in rendering palliative care? An introduction to the Middle Eastern Cancer Consortium (MECC). Curr Oncol Rep. 2011;13(4):302–307.
31. Bingley A, Clark D. A comparative review of palliative care development in six countries represented by the Middle East Cancer Consortium (MECC). J Pain Symptom Manage. 2009;37(3):287–296.
32. Zeinah GF, Al-Kindi SG, Hassan AA. Middle East experience in palliative care. Am J Hosp Palliat Care. 2013;30(1):94–99.
33. Moore SY, Pirrello RD, Christianson SK, Ferris FD. Strategic planning by the palliative care steering committee of the Middle East Cancer Consortium. J Pediatr Hematol Oncol. 2011;33(Suppl 1):S39–S46.

CHAPTER 82

Palliative care as a human right

Frank Brennan, Liz Gwyther, Diederik Lohman, Fatia Kiyange, Tamar Ezer, and Faith N. Mwangi-Powell

Key points

- There are significant gaps in the provision of palliative care around the world.

- Many national and international palliative care associations consider palliative care a basic human right.

- Various international human rights conventions recognize the right to health. Governments that have ratified these conventions are obliged to guarantee the rights contained in them.

- Palliative care is an integral part of healthcare.

- According to the United Nations:

  1. The right to healthcare is "the right of everyone to the enjoyment of the highest attainable standard of physical and mental health."

  2. That right contains four "interrelated and essential elements"[1]: availability, accessibility, acceptability, and quality.

  3. The obligations related to the right to health are expressed as general principles that can be applied to various health services, including palliative care. There are certain "core obligations" of all signatory nations, irrespective of their resources. Those obligations, as they relate to palliative care, include:

     (a) to adopt and implement a national policy on palliative care;

     (b) to ensure access to health facilities, goods, and services on a nondiscriminatory basis;

     (c) to provide essential medications, including opioid analgesics. An obligation of "comparable priority" is to ensure relevant training in palliative care for healthcare workers.

- Senior UN human rights officials and organizations have expressly and repeatedly recognized access to palliative care and pain management as a human right.

- Nurses, individually and collectively, can use human rights arguments to advocate for governments to develop national policies on palliative care, reform unnecessarily restrictive drug control laws, and promote the development of palliative care services. That advocacy can be strengthened by alliances with national and international pain and palliative care associations and human rights organizations.

Introduction

Human beings are mortal. How we die is a matter of universal concern. The quality of death in the context of life-limiting illnesses—the level of suffering endured, the capacity of carers, whether professional or family, and the resources available to them—varies greatly around the world. For some, there are excellent services that are accessible, skilled, and adequately resourced to provide care and support for the patient and their family throughout their illness. For most, there are significant deficits in such services. Indeed, for many, such professional services simply do not exist. Approximately 58 million people die every year, or more than 1 million every week. At least 35 million of these people will die of chronic life-limiting illnesses and, if one includes family and carers who need help and assistance, it means that at least 100 million people worldwide would benefit from hospice and palliative care each year. Unfortunately, it has been estimated that only about 10% of those that need it receive it.[2] In 2011 only 136 of world's 234 countries (58%) had established one or more hospice–palliative care services, and 159 countries (68%) were actively engaged in either delivering a hospice–palliative care service or developing the framework within which such a service could be delivered. Therefore, 75 nations—a significant number of countries—still have no hospice or palliative care provision.

The discipline of palliative care arose in response to these questions and the needs of patients with life-limiting illnesses. While palliative care services continue to grow and develop, significant deficiencies remain. Far too many nations have no public policy on the provision of palliative care, unnecessarily restrictive drug control laws, limited service provision, and little if any education of nursing and medical undergraduates on the care of patients with life-limiting illnesses.

Nurses working in palliative care or exposed to its ethos understand its value in both tangible and intangible ways. To relieve someone of severe pain or nausea, to calm a delirious patient, to console a grieving family, to make the dying process dignified and loving rather than tumultuous and agonizing is of immediate and long-lasting benefit. Those acts will enter the narrative of the family and be thought about forever. Indeed such acts represent the essence of nursing.

With such knowledge, and conscious of both and the enormous disparities in the provision of palliative care globally and the significant benefits that flow from its provision, the palliative care community began articulating a profound but challenging idea—that palliative care should be seen as a human right. There have been many such statements, from both the perspective of pain management and palliative care. For a summary of these declarations see Box 82.1. This chapter explores how this proposition can be justified, what this proposition means in reality, and how using these concepts can be tools of advocacy and change.

Box 82.1 International statements articulating pain management and/or palliative care as human rights and their sponsoring organizations

Pain management

Global Day Against Pain (2004)—IASP, EFIC, WHO

The Panama Proclamation—Proclamation of Pain Treatment and the Application of Palliative Care as Human Rights (2008)—Latin American Federation of IASP Chapters, Foundation for the Treatment of Pain as a Human Right.

Joint Declaration of and Statement of Commitment to Pain Management and Palliative Care as Human Rights (2008)—IAHPC, WPCA

The Declaration of Montreal (2011)—IASP

Council of the World Medical Association (WMA) (2011)

The Morphine Manifesto (2012)—Pallium India, IAHPC, PPSG, and 60 other organizations.

Palliative care

The Cape Town Declaration (2002)—African Palliative Care educators

International Working Group (European School of Oncology) (2004)

The Korea Declaration (2005)—second Global Summit of National Hospice and Palliative Care Associations

The Panama Proclamation—Proclamation of Pain Treatment and the Application of Palliative Care as Human Rights (2008)—Latin American Federation of IASP Chapters, Foundation for the Treatment of Pain as a Human Right.

World Hospice Day (2008)—IAHPC

The Lisbon Challenge (2011)—EAPC, IAHPC, HRW

The Prague Charter (2013)—EAPC, IAHPC, WPCA, HRW

EAPC—European Association of Palliative Care; EFIC—European Chapters of the IASP; HRW—Human Rights Watch; IAHPC—International Association of Hospice and Palliative Care; IASP—International Association for the Study of Pain; PPSG—Pain and Public Policy Studies Group, University of Wisconsin/WHO Collaborating Center for Pain Policy and Palliative Care; WPCA—Worldwide Palliative Care Alliance; WHO—World Health Organization.

The basic argument

While it may be obvious to state that there is a moral obligation to relieve suffering at the end of life, can one argue that the provision of palliative care is a basic human right? Governments may or may not be swayed by moral arguments. They will be more likely to be persuaded where there is a legal and, more especially, an international legal foundation for their response.

All governments in the world have signed at least one international convention on human rights that includes the right to health.[3] The provision of care to patients with life-limiting illnesses up to and including their death is part of healthcare. Indeed, the WHO has stated that "the fundamental responsibility of the health profession to ease the suffering of patients cannot be fulfilled unless palliative care has priority status within public health and disease control programmes; it is not an optional extra."[4] What does this responsibility involve for those governments who have signed and ratified these conventions? The UN Committee overseeing the implementation of the International Covenant on Economic, Social and Cultural Rights (ICESCR), the convention that contains the first binding articulation of the right to health, stated that the right to health contained four "interrelated and essential elements": availability, accessibility, acceptability, and quality.[1] In the original Covenant, each State party was asked to progressively realize the contained rights "to the maximum of its available resources."[5] In their General Comment on the right to health the Committee set out in detail what were "core obligations" expected of governments irrespective of their resources. They included obligations to ensure access to health facilities, goods, and services on a nondiscriminatory basis, the provision of essential drugs, as defined by the World Health Organization (WHO), and the adoption and implementation of a national public health strategy.[6] Interpreting this Comment in the context of palliative care, this would oblige nations to ensure access to services without discrimination; the provision of basic medications for symptom control and terminal care, including analgesics; and the adoption and implementation of national pain and palliative care policies.

In addition to the "core obligations" the Committee also enumerated obligations "of comparable priority."[7] These included "To provide education and access to information concerning the main health problems in the community" and "To provide appropriate training for health personnel, including education on health and human rights." In the context of palliative care, a "main health problem" in all countries, this would obligate governments to ensure the education of health professionals in the principles and practice of palliative care and, further, provide access to information regarding palliative care for the general community.

From principles to practice

How does theory meet practice? What issues confront governments in the provision of palliative care and to what extent can an argument based on human rights be made? This section of the chapter contains a series of case studies and commentaries linking the theoretical arguments made above with the daily practice of palliative care.

Nation A

Nation A, a country of 1.5 million people, gained independence 15 years ago. Approximately 50% of the population are under 15 years of age. It has one of lowest per capita incomes in the world. It has one major hospital in its capital city and four provincial hospitals. There are no designated palliative care health professionals in the country. There is no national policy on palliative or end-of-life care. If patients deteriorate they are often taken home to die. There is a small stock of morphine in the main hospital, but it is rarely used. Despite being encouraged to do so, the nation does not report its estimated annual opioid requirements to the International Narcotics Control Board (INCB), a body that oversees the licit and illicit use of opioids around the world. The nation is a signatory of the International Covenant of Economic, Social and Cultural Rights (ICESCR), which contains a recognition of the right to health.

This is a nation that is clearly struggling with all aspects of governance. The provision of healthcare is one aspect of that struggle. Nevertheless, as a signatory to a UN convention that articulates a right to health, the national government has a set of responsibilities that it must meet. In terms of palliative care there are two basic initial steps. The first is to formulate a national policy on palliative care so as to ensure its integration into the healthcare system. The second is to ensure the availability and accessibility of morphine and other essential palliative care medications, engage with the INCB, and commence a process of estimating the quantity of opioid medications that the country may require. The INCB, recognizing the struggle of many nations to make these calculations has published clear guidelines on this process.[8] In order to be effective, those steps need to be taken concurrently with the development of an efficient system of opioid availability and the education of nurses and doctors in all aspects of palliative care, including the safe and appropriate use of opioids.

Nation B

Nation B has a population of 55 million. The nation's drug control laws were drawn up in the colonial era and have not been amended. The laws place considerable restrictions on opioid availability, which means that the only available analgesics are nonopioids. In a provincial hospital a 53-year-old woman with metastatic cervical cancer cries out in pain most of the day and night. The medications available to her—paracetamol and ibuprofen—cannot control her pain.

Accessibility to opioid medications is a human right. It has been recognized in two principal ways by the United Nations. The denial or restriction of access to opioids for medical purposes may violate the right to healthcare as well as the prohibition of cruel, inhuman, or degrading treatment.

Access to essential medications is one of the "core obligations" of signatory governments. By restricting the availability and accessibility of an essential medication in pain management, the current national drug control laws are a breach of the right to health. Examples of nations that have entered a process of opioid law reform are Romania and the Ukraine. Romania changed its very restrictive drug control laws in 2005, following a collaboration between the Ministry of Health and the Pain and Policy Studies Group (PPSG) at the University of Wisconsin.[9] Following a 2011 report by Human Rights Watch on palliative care in the Ukraine, the National Drug Control Service there convened a working group that drafted new drug control regulations. Those regulations were adopted in 2013.[10]

The second pathway of recognition emerged from the right not to be treated in a cruel, inhuman, or degrading manner.[11] In a 2009 report to the Human Rights Council the UN Special Rapporteur on Torture and Cruel, Inhuman or Degrading Treatment stated, "all measures should be taken to ensure full access [to pain treatment and opioid analgesics] and to overcome current regulatory, educational and attitudinal obstacles to ensure full access to palliative care."[12] The two pathways were synthesized in a joint statement made by the UN Special Rapporteurs on the Right to Health and on Torture to the Chairperson of the UN Commission on Narcotic Drugs in 2008: "The failure to ensure access to controlled medicines for the relief of pain and suffering threatens fundamental rights to health and to protection against cruel inhuman and degrading treatment. International human rights law requires that governments must provide essential medicines—which include, among others, opioid analgesics—as part of their minimum core obligations under the right to health.... Lack of access to essential medicines, including for pain relief, is a global human rights issue and must be addressed forcefully."[13]

The INCB has also expressly linked the accessibility of controlled medications to human rights. In its report *Availability of Internationally Controlled Drugs: Ensuring Adequate Access for Medical and Scientific Purposes* (2011)[14] it stated that the "[l]ack of availability of narcotic drugs...may deprive patients of their fundamental rights and the opportunity to have relief from physical pain and suffering."[14] The Report emphasized the importance of balance in the approach of all nations between the availability and appropriate use of controlled medications and the prevention of diversion and abuse of opioids.

For a nurse working in such a nation a practical measure would be to contact their national or regional palliative care association to create or add to local efforts to improve access to opioids.

Nation C

Nation C has a population of 70 million. Opioids are available in three major cancer hospitals. In those hospitals a limited number of doctors are authorized to prescribe opioids for cancer pain. Morphine is not available in other centers. A 48-year-old father of four daughters is diagnosed with lung cancer and tuberculosis. He lives in a remote area. His condition deteriorates. He experiences a sudden onset of severe pain in his midback. An X-ray reveals a vertebral fracture. The doctors feel the fracture is most likely to be metastatic in origin. Radiotherapy is unavailable locally. He can barely walk and cannot travel the significant distance over mountains to the cancer hospital. To obtain morphine for his pain, he would have to travel for hours to the country's capital, which he cannot afford.

Here the nation might argue: "We have morphine available. Therefore, we are in compliance with our responsibilities under the international right to health." This statement is incorrect. Availability does not equal accessibility. In this case morphine may be available but it is not accessible for the patient because only doctors at the main cancer centres are allowed to prescribe it. This restriction therapeutically disenfranchises those patients—and their clinicians—who do not meet these criteria. One argument that emerges from human rights law is discrimination. The right to nondiscrimination and equality is entrenched in the ICESCR,[6] and the Committee overseeing the Covenant considered that nondiscrimination is a critical dimension of the accessibility of healthcare.[15] Discrimination may be direct or indirect. An example of direct discrimination would be a national law denying opioid access to prisoners or refugees. The above scenario is an example of indirect or de facto discrimination: a nation deliberately restricts the availability of opioids to a limited number of hospitals so that geographical distance and poverty means that only a small proportion of the population will realistically have access to these medications.

In addition to failing to fulfill obligations derived from the right to healthcare, the UN Special Rapporteur on Torture argued that "the de facto denial of access to pain relief, if it causes pain and suffering, constitutes cruel, inhuman or degrading treatment or punishment."[12]

A notable example of a country expanding the accessibility of opioids is Uganda. Recognizing that a significant shortage of doctors, especially in the rural areas, compounded a lack of access to opioids, a law was passed authorizing the prescribing of opioids by nurses with the requisite training.

At a practical level, as with the previous example, all the above arguments could be used as part of local advocacy to improve accessibility of opioids. Nurses could join or support hospice or home-based care organizations that could lobby for changes including better access to opioids and permitting hospice workers to carry opioids to people in their homes.

Nation D

Nation D is a nation of 45 million people. While most palliative care services are provided by nongovernment organizations, the government provides some services. The department of health places express restrictions on eligibility for these services. The services are only available for two groups of patients—those with cancer and those with HIV/AIDS. A 56-year-old man with end-stage tuberculosis lives at home. He is deteriorating. Other adults in the family have died. His family is struggling enormously. They live some distance from a nongovernment clinic. He asks his family to take him to a government hospital to die.

Nation E

Nation E is a nation of 28 million. There is a national cancer control program. The program addresses the needs only of patients undergoing curative care. In this country the most recent data reveals that 70% of cancer patients are diagnosed when their disease is metastatic.

These are examples of discriminatory government policy that violates the right to health. The Committee overseeing the right to health in the ICESCR stated that "States are under an obligation to respect the right to health by . . . refraining from denying or limiting equal access for all persons . . . to preventive, curative and palliative health services."[16]

Regarding the patient with tuberculosis there is another practical response. If health professionals, including nurses, are trained in palliative care they may be able to deliver the care required as part of comprehensive healthcare without needing to refer the patient to a palliative care service. In addition, they could also participate in lobbying for an extension of services. Certainly the restrictions placed on the provision of palliative care by these nations is contrary to the WHO definition of palliative care, in which care is not confined to those with certain diagnoses but is extended to all those with life-limiting illnesses.

Nation F

Nation F has a universal health insurance scheme. Palliative care services are not covered under this scheme. Oral morphine is not included in the medicines list of the insurance package. Compounding this, pharmacies participating in the insurance scheme do not stock opioids. An 82-year-old woman lives alone with limited resources. She has metastatic breast cancer with rib metastases. She requires opioids to relieve her pain. She can afford a small supply of opioids, but they quickly run out. She is told that oral morphine is not included in her package, and she cannot afford other preparations of opioids.

A critical issue here is the lack of integration of palliative care into public health insurance policies. The effect of these policies is that those citizens who rely entirely on universal health insurance and who cannot afford private insurance will need to pay for palliative care services. As the patient deteriorates, these services would inevitably increase the financial burden on the family. According to the Committee overseeing the ICESCR, one of the essential elements of healthcare is accessibility. That includes economic accessibility: "Payment for health care-services . . . has to be based on the principle of equity, ensuring that these services, whether privately or publicly provided, are affordable to all, including socially disadvantaged groups."[15] The Committee also stated: "States have a special obligation to provide those who do not have sufficient means with the necessary health insurance and health care facilities."[17] Palliative care should be integrated into the insurance scheme.

Nation G

In Nation G, palliative care is a relatively new concept for health professionals. After much lobbying, the government provides funding for services but expressly states that this funding extends only to adults. There is no government funding for pediatric palliative care. The provision of pediatric palliative care is not included in the national palliative care policy. The nation is a signatory to the UN Convention on the Rights of the Child.

The Convention on the Rights of the Child contains a clear statement on the rights of children and adolescents to the provision of healthcare.[18] The Committee overseeing the Convention identified the responsibility of signatory nations to support the palliative care of children.[19] They expressed concern that, in a particular country, "the majority of palliative care is provided by non-government organizations without sufficient financial support" and "recommends that the State party establish a funding mechanism for the provision of palliative care for children and support the palliative care services provided by non-government organizations."[19]

The promotion of palliative care through human rights—a nurse's perspective

Nurses have a pivotal role in the provision of palliative care. Nurses are aware that simple interventions can make a significant difference to their patients. Equally, their flexibility, capacity, and expertise are frequently tested by the challenges of ill patients and their families. It is that experience and skill that allow nurses to speak with credibility, both individually and collectively, to policy makers. Advocacy, born of practical knowledge, can be greatly strengthened by and, indeed, founded on, an argument based on international human rights and the obligations that flow from those rights.

The source, form, and content of that advocacy may vary. It may arise from nursing associations directly advocating to governments. Equally, that advocacy may arise from alliances formed with national, regional, and international pain and palliative care associations. Those international bodies include the International Association of Hospice and Palliative Care (IAHPC), the International Association for the Study of Pain (IASP) and the Worldwide Palliative Care Alliance (WPCA). In addition, fruitful sources of support reside in bodies such as the Pain and Public Policy Group, in Wisconsin, with their record in assisting governments in opioid law reform, and major human rights organizations such as Human Rights Watch.

The content of that advocacy, simple and direct, should be constantly tied to the core obligations of signatory nations under the international human rights conventions. Those obligations include ensuring a universal access to services; the provision of basic medications for symptom control and terminal care, including analgesics; and the adoption and implementation of national pain and palliative care policies.

Conclusion

The concept that access to the provision of palliative care is a fundamental right has foundations in international human rights law. Governments who sign conventions that contain a right to health have obligations that are directly relevant to palliative care. An argument based on human rights is a potentially strong one that can be made to governments by all health professionals, including nurses, promoting the formation of national palliative care policies, the assurance of access to essential medications, and the provision of services.

References

1. Committee on Economic, Social and Cultural Rights. 2000. General Comment 14, The Right to the Highest Attainable Standard of Health. 2000. Article 12. UN Doc. E/C.12/2000/4.
2. Lynch T, Clark D, Connor SR. Mapping levels of Palliative Care Development: A Global Update 2011. Worldwide Palliative Care Alliance, 2011. Accessible at: www.thewpca.org/resources/.
3. United Nations Declaration of Human Rights (UNDHR), 1948; International Covenant on Economic, Social and Cultural Rights (ICESCR), 1966; Convention on the Elimination of Discrimination Against Women (CEDAW), 1979; Convention on the Rights of the Child (CRC), 1989; and International Convention on the Elimination of Racial Discrimination (ICERD), 1965.
4. World Health Organization. National Cancer Control Programmes—Policies and Managerial Guidelines. 2nd ed. Geneva: WHO; 2002:86.
5. International Covenant on Economic, Social and Cultural Rights (ICESCR), 1966. Article 2.
6. Committee on Economic, Social and Cultural Rights. 2000. General Comment 14, The Right to the Highest Attainable Standard of Health. 2000. Article 43. UN Doc. E/C.12/2000/4.
7. Committee on Economic, Social and Cultural Rights. 2000. General Comment 14, The Right to the Highest Attainable Standard of Health. 2000. Article 44. UN Doc. E/C.12/2000/4.
8. INCB, WHO, UN. Guide on Estimating Requirements for Substances Under International Control. 2012. Accessible at: http://www.who.int/hiv/oub/idu/est_requirements/en/index.html.
9. Mosulu D, Mungiu OC, Gigore B, Landon A. Romania: changing the regulatory environment. J Pain Sympt Manage. 2007;33:610–614.
10. Human Rights Watch: Defending Human Rights Worldwide. Accessible at: http://www.hrw.org/news/2013/02/13/ukraine-breakthrough-cancer-pain.
11. International Covenant on Civil and Political Rights (ICCPR), 1966. Article 7.
12. Nowak M. Report by Manfred Nowak, Special Rapporteur on Torture and Other Cruel, Inhuman or Degrading Treatment or Punishment. Promotion and Protection of All Human Rights, Civil, Political, and Economic, Social and Cultural Rights, Including the Right to Development. Human Rights Council, Seventh Session, Agenda Item 3. A/HRC/10/44. January 14. 2009.
13. Nowak M, Hunt P. Special Rapporteurs on the Question of Torture and the Right of Everyone to the Highest Attainable Standard of Physical and Mental Health. Letter to Mr D. Best, Vice-Chairperson of the Commission on Narcotic Drugs, December 10 2008. Accessible at: http://www.ihra.net/Assets/1384/1/Special RapporteursLettertoCND012009.pdf.
14. International Narcotics Control Board (INCB). Availability of Internationally Controlled Drugs: Ensuring Adequate Access for Medical and Scientific Purposes. 2011. E/INCB/2010/1/Supp.1. Accessible at: http://www.incb.org.
15. Committee on Economic, Social and Cultural Rights. 2000. General Comment 14, The Right to the Highest Attainable Standard of Health. 2000. Article 12(b). UN Doc. E/C.12/2000/4.
16. Committee on Economic, Social and Cultural Rights. 2000. General Comment 14, The Right to the Highest Attainable Standard of Health. 2000. Article 34. UN Doc. E/C.12/2000/4.
17. Committee on Economic, Social and Cultural Rights, General Comment 14, The right to the highest attainable standard of health. 2000. Article 19. UN Doc. E/C.12/2000/4 (2000).
18. Convention on the Rights of the Child (CRC), 1989. Article 24.
19. Committee on the Rights of the Child (CRC), 2011.Fifty-Sixth Session. 17 January–4 February 2011. Consideration of Reports Submitted by States Parties Under Article 44 of the Convention. Concluding Observations: Belarus. CRC/C/BLR/CO/3-4.

CHAPTER 83

A good death

Gay Walker

As we reflect on the chapters of this textbook, we are grateful for the significant and measureable advances that have been made in hospice and palliative care nursing to make possible "a good death." Thanks to the outstanding contributions of many palliative and hospice "pioneers" and caregivers, tens of thousands of adults and their family members are experiencing something more than mere end-of-life comfort. As Dr. Cicely Saunders stated, "although a terminal illness may be perceived or experienced primarily as negative or devastating, for many persons it becomes an opportunity for personal growth and healing." Clearly, we can readily envision these end-of-life principles applied to adults, particularly the elderly, but as we consider these principles applied to children, there is a hesitation in our hearts. A "good death" for a child whose life is just beginning? Whose parents have the hopes and dreams that every parent has for that child's future and boundless potential? It seems counterintuitive that a "good death" could even seem possible, which is precisely why the field of pediatric hospice and palliative care nursing requires a specialized approach. An approach that takes into consideration that children are not just little adults. They have unique physical, emotional, and psychosocial needs. Compound that with the unique and often extreme needs of parents, siblings, friends, and community, and it becomes clear that moving from a "negative or devastating" experience to an "opportunity for personal growth and healing" is truly challenging.

Having helped hundreds of terminally ill children and their families navigate through their complex journey at end of life and beyond, it is my conviction that with specialized pediatric palliative care, children can indeed experience a "good death" and family and friends can indeed experience peace and opportunity.

Maddie's story

No ordinary day

This was no ordinary day. Maddie was no ordinary 5-year-old. In her typical fashion she charged into that day with all the joy and anticipation of a much awaited "snow day." Someone had figured out how to bring snow from the mountains to a group of children living in a balmy Southern California beach city in the middle of January. She seemed a little tired, but it had been a long week at school and Christmas break had been filled with activities. Nevertheless, as a precaution her mom, Kajsa, had had a blood test done the previous week, as Maddie was never tired! The results came back normal—nothing to be concerned about. Still, her speech on that eventful morning was a little slurred. Oh well, she would be in full gear soon. The snow and her beloved twin cousins were waiting! Later that day, amid flying snow balls and sledding, Maddie started slowing down; it appeared that her foot was dragging. Not only was she having trouble walking but also now she could not get her words out. This was very troubling because Maddie was typically very verbal and articulate. A frantic call to her doctor resulted in a direct visit to the emergency room at the local Children's Hospital. Maddie's mom and dad, Collie, had been divorced for the last year and a half and had shared their homes and hearts with their beloved daughter. Collie raced to the ER to meet them. Tests were done, and Kajsa and Collie were told that Maddie needed to be immediately transferred to the intensive care unit. It was Saturday, January 15, 2011—no ordinary day.

Difficult decisions

The next morning, they were brought into a small private room to review the findings of the scans by the neurologist. They both recalled thinking it must be bad news if the chaplain and two social workers were also present. They were told clearly that Maddie had the most feared and lethal of all pediatric brain tumors, a diffuse intrinsic pontine glioma (DIPG) and that it was incurable, inoperable. With this knowledge and understanding, fear and grief immediately gripped them both. The world stood still as they sought some glimmer of hope. Then Collie asked the excruciating questions:

"Is our daughter going to die?"
"I am so sorry but she will."
"How long does she have?"
"4 to 6 months at best."

It all seemed unreal, unthinkable, as they considered the treatment options. A 5-week course of radiation was a possibility but surely no guarantee of quality of life and it could at best merely postpone the inevitable. Overwhelmed, Kajsa dropped to her knees and crouched in the corner of that small room. When she stood up, she and Collie strangely knew what their next decision was. They would bring Maddie home safe and protected, away from fear and strange hospital machines and treatments. Had they been told there was even a 1% chance for cure they would have "climbed any mountain" to find it. When cure was not an option, comfort and quality of life became the goal. Hope would need to be redefined. Their job as parents was to protect Maddie, if not from the ravages of the cancer, at least from the fear it could bring. It was at this time that they were told about the option of hospice. Fortunately, there was a pediatric hospice and palliative care agency in their community. Immediately, Monday January 17, a referral was made. They brought Maddie home that very day, not wanting to waste any precious time. So, as they began this painful journey, they agreed that their home was to become a "no cry house." Maddie disliked crying for any reason, life was "way too beautiful." She had from the youngest age loved the ocean and all the creatures in it and could rival the best oceanographer with her knowledge. So she settled into her ocean-themed room.

Her parents chose not to tell her the full extent of her disease except to say that she had "an owie in her head" and that maybe she would need some medicine. "When she starts asking more questions we will answer to the best of our ability and her understanding," they decided. They felt that if she had been older they would have been obligated to be more truthful, but that the best course at her age was to protect her from unnecessary fears. Nevertheless, her parents perceived that somehow, she understood the truth. At her age her understanding of death was unique to the mind of a 5-year-old living in a "magical world." They soon discovered that what Maddie really wanted was clear, simple answers to her questions about her illness. Once that was accomplished, Maddie then moved on with the fun of the day. Kajsa tells this story of a conversation that took place shortly after Maddie's diagnosis. I had just given her a bath and as she had her arms wrapped around me while I dried off her warm, sweet-smelling skin, Maddie said,

"Mommy, I want to be with you forever and ever, because I love you."

"Well thank goodness for that, because I will be your mommy forever and ever."

"Even when I die?"

"Even when you die. We will be angels together and play hide and seek in the sky and have dinner parties in the fluffy clouds."

"OK, but let's definitely not have ketchup so we don't get our white wings messy."

Specialized care

That week I met Maddie and her parents at their home where they would all be living. Amid Scooby Doo cartoons, doing the hula, and getting a lesson from her on how dolphins swim, we began planning her care.

As the care manager, we talked about the pediatric interdisciplinary team available to them 24 hours a day, 7 days a week. Whether their needs were medical, emotional, spiritual, or social, they had a team of dedicated pediatric specialists available to them. "We may not always need to call but it is such a relief to know someone is there for us," they stated. As I listened, I began to enter into their world and understand their unique situation. Our loving relationship began. Witnessing their tremendous sorrow and yet their clarity regarding the plan of care they desired was a privilege. They had a set of beliefs and values that guided all the difficult decisions they had to make. Looking ahead to the inevitable, life would be unbearable without their precious Maddie, but until that time they had a lot to do! The Make-a-Wish trip to Hawaii, swimming in her beloved ocean, frolicking with the sea turtles, home schooling with her favorite teachers, playing with friends, dancing, art projects, grandparent visits, Scooby Doo cartoons, and many more of her favorite activities—life to be lived, memories to be made! "She became our inspiration," said her parents. "If Maddie could go through all of this so could we."

As it turned out, one of the key members of the team for this family was the social worker. Specially trained in pediatric hospice and palliative care, she was able to provide timely, practical and lasting input for both Kajsa and Collie that ultimately had a positive impact on Maddie's end-of-life care.

By request, the social worker met with each parent separately every week enabling them to "pour their hearts out and gain important perspective." They were always willing to resolve conflicts or tensions in their relationship so they could better care for their daughter. Stress seemed to be coming at them from all sides, and they needed an outlet that was objective and yet compassionate to their situation. Having a resource with this combined experience and skill set who would come to them in their home and have the time to listen as they worked through "this dark world" was a special gift. In addition to Maddie's parents, there was the need to help her grandparents, cousins, and church and school friends make sense of her illness. The entire community had an active place in her life, and consequently, needed support during this devastating time.

Although a chaplain was available to them through the hospice team, the family preferred the support of the priest from Maddie's school, whom she really loved. We often wonder about what children Maddie's age think concerning spiritual concepts. Although difficult to quantify, undoubtedly, children have a profoundly unique connection to the spiritual world. Maddie's dad, Collie, communicated this amazing experience. Shortly after his daughter was diagnosed, Maddie began having very active dreams. Actually, they may be better characterized as conversations. While asleep, she would be mumbling, not in a distressed way, but more like she was having a vibrant conversation. This went on every night for quite some time. In the morning she would say, "Daddy I am so tired I can't get any good sleep because they all want to talk with me." He asked her if she wanted to tell him what they were saying and she looked at him thoughtfully and said, "I don't think I should tell you yet." As the end came closer the conversations increased until on one memorable night she awoke from a sound sleep and cried out "Daddy, daddy can you see it? It's so beautiful, it's so beautiful…I feel like I am floating just like they told me I would—this is fun!…" Collie composed himself and looking up to the ceiling said softly, "I don't know who you are but I think you are here to help my daughter not be afraid through this process. Thank you, please take care of her." As soon as Collie whispered these words, Maddie instantly fell into a sound sleep. No more conversations. Perhaps the innocence of children opens up other worlds.

As Maddie's health declined, the hospice team was able to prepare her parents for what to expect in her last days. It was crucial at this stage that her parents understood and were involved in the clinical component of pain and symptom management. With the support of a highly trained pediatric palliative care medical director and certified hospice and palliative nurse at the bedside, this goal was accomplished. During this time of physical decline and as the clinical care was modified and intensified, Collie, her father, felt great purpose and comfort in being meaningfully involved—"doing something and not just standing by helplessly." Faithfully, every 6 hours, he gently and carefully gave her the medicines she needed to be pain free. Her seizures began to intensify, and pediatric dosing of medicines was adjusted for their control. The level of care was changed from routine to continuous care, and a nurse was assigned 24 hours a day until these progressive symptoms were managed. Throughout this time of transition, Maddie's parents felt as if they could "ask every nightmare question" they needed in order to prepare them for each stage of Maddie's dying while maintaining her dignity. Throughout the entire ordeal, Maddie's mother was never gone from her side. This reminded me of what Maddie taught me about dolphins, "the baby dolphin sleeps with both eyes closed and the mommy sleeps with one eye open to always protect her baby."

Maddie died in her bed at home on March 13, 2011, at 9 PM. She lived 57 days from the time of her diagnosis.

Shortly before she died, Collie told his sweet Maddie that "it was time to go to heaven and become an angel," and that "mommy and daddy would be all right," and that "being her parent was the most special thing he ever done."

In Maddie's final moments, Kajsa whispered to her precious daughter that "it was time to go, it is going to be so beautiful, we will be OK." Then Kajsa sang her the night-night songs she had loved her whole life, kissed her cheek, and said "Sov gott," which means "sleep well" in Swedish.

Among the many supports that the hospice team provided, one of the most important for this family was contacting the mortuary and assisting in the arrangements after Maddie's death. Collie was so overcome with grief that he said "it would have broken me if I had to make that call."

From the very beginning Maddie's parents realized that there would be no miracle cure for their daughter. But what they came to realize during Maddie's final days was that "the biggest miracle of all was to see how comfortably she died."

The importance of legacy

Maddie's ashes were spread over the beautiful Pacific Ocean that she so loved. And although there were so many things she would never do, become a teenager, fall in love, get married, have a career, and children of her own, her wonderful impact lives on. Kasja was inspired shortly after Maddie's diagnosis to create a lasting legacy worthy of her amazing daughter, and together they created a foundation that would fund the construction and ongoing operation of a world-class learning center for children at the Ocean Institute in her memory. Maddie was even one of the very first donors: Shortly before she died, Maddie won a photo contest, winning $500 for a picture of her and her mother sharing a sweet kiss under a rainbow in Hawaii. She gave the entire sum to the Ocean Institute, saying with some of her last words that it was "for the kids." Maddie's spirit energized an entire community to raise over a million dollars in 3 short months and on June 11, 2011, what would have been her 6th birthday, the Maddie James Seaside Learning Center (MJSLC) was officially dedicated. Now generations of children will learn to care for the ocean and all its creatures that Maddie loved so well. Her classmates continue to support this legacy and in so doing keep her memory alive. Children of all ages want to give back!

The legacy of a child reminds us not just of their presence with us, but that they made a difference, they changed our world no matter how many days or years they were here. It is the promise that they will always be remembered.

Bereavement

We have no word to describe a parent who has lost a child, not "widow" or "widower," just bereaved parent. The grief that began the moment she was diagnosed has taken many forms for Maddie's parents in the years since her death. Being a "bereaved parent is like living in a world that has stopped when everyone else's world keeps going, and you've been left behind." Collie personally describes it this way: "A black hole is in my heart that will exist until I die. Nothing will ever fill that space; the best I can do is grow some beautiful flowers around the edge. I can anticipate

the first birthday without her or the holidays without her laughter and prepare for them, but unexpectedly having a small, blonde girl with glasses run by in the grocery store stops my heart and my world once again. And it probably always will."

His journey of grief, however, has taught him that there is some meaning and purpose. "Maddie taught me to genuinely love…to forget the small stuff that doesn't matter. To look at the world like a big beautiful ocean. Out of a great tragedy has come awesome blessing."

Maddie's mom tells us, "I've come to accept that sorrow will be my companion for the rest of my life. I have learned to embrace it and not feel wrong about having it as a friend. There have been moments of happiness this year…happiness is laced with a little bit of sorrow, and that's OK. It won't be the life that I wanted, but it can still be a good life. A life surrounded by Maddie's spirit. In a time of horrific tragedy and loss, a lot of beauty has come of it. I choose a life of remembering that beauty."

Her grandparents remind us that we expect our children to bury us. "We never imagine that we will have to watch our own children suffer their loss and help them bury our grandchildren."

Perhaps the following poem that Kajsa wrote expresses it best:

TWO YEARS
It's two years to the day since I kissed you goodnight
Watched your last breath as your wings took first flight
Waking up since then in a too quiet house
No lunch to pack, no after school snack, no visits to Mickey Mouse
I go from angry, to sad, to wanting someone to fault
Amazed the pain in my heart hasn't caused a complete halt
Yes, there's the story of strength, support, and unprecedented giving
But I would give it all back to spend just one more day with you living
To hear your laugh, to see you dance, to feel those hugging arms around me
To be called the most beautiful name in the world just one more time,
"mommy"
As I did last year, and will do every year on this day
I went out on the ocean and I brought you a lei
Orchids of purple and white, two strands joined together
Like the ones worn kissing under our rainbow, an image I will cherish
forever
So, until I am faced with getting through this day next year
Know that every moment in between will be filled with your memory
near.

Grief will be a lifelong companion for Maddie's parents. The hospice bereavement team walked with them for the first 13 months making sure they were connected to support and resources. Our friendship endures, and when I spoke to them to hear the story "one more time" for the writing of this chapter, time once again stood still and it was as if Maddie was with us. The window of suffering had begun to open to a window of peace and opportunity.

Principles learned

When children die, they deserve the best of care at the end of life just as we have lavished care on them at the beginning and throughout their lives. Maddie's story instructs us on these key pediatric palliative principles:

1. Children experience a unique variety of complex life-threatening illnesses not seen in adults. Often similar illness proceeds very differently in children. Their causes and the way children die are very different as a result.

2. Children, by their nature, experience their illness within the context of growth and development.

3. Referral to pediatric palliative care should be at time of diagnosis of a life-limiting or life-threatening disease. Regardless whether the anticipated outcome is cure or death.

4. Clear, honest communication by the doctor with the parents faced with difficult decisions directly impacts the quality of life of the child. Weighing the benefits of medical technology or the burden it can bring requires practiced communication and listening skills.

5. The multidisciplinary team for a child includes not only the traditional core team of doctor, nurse, chaplain, social worker, and volunteer but also other pediatric specialties such as child life, child psychology, art therapy, music therapy, therapeutic touch, pediatric pharmacological interventions, and other integrative services.

6. Support and implementation of palliative and end-of-life specialty within the heathcare settings of hospital and community are crucial.

7. Being involved in building a child's legacy is our promise that we will never forget them.

8. The members of the healthcare team helping a child to "die well" need intentional support and care—as they give themselves to this sacred work.

9. Bereavement and grief support are not optional. They are a fundamental component of excellent palliative care for children. Serving not only the child but the family, siblings, school, church, and entire communities.

10. The family is always the unit of care.

Resource for end-of-life care education

http://endoflife.northwestern.edu/religion_spirituality/pain.cfm. Accessed October 10, 2013.

Appendix
Palliative care resource list
Rose Virani and Licet Garcia

Bibliographies/texts

Panke JT, Coyne PJ, eds. Conversations in Palliative Care. 3rd ed. Pittsburgh, PA: Hospice and Palliative Nurses Association; 2011.

Puchalski CM, Ferrell B. Making Health Care Whole: Integrating Spirituality into Patient Care. West Conshohocken, PA: Templeton Press; 2010.

Wolfe J, Hinds PS, Sourkes BM, eds. Textbook of Interdisciplinary Pediatric Palliative Care. Philadelphia, PA: Elsevier Saunders; 2011.

Oxford University Press

http://www.oup-usa.org

Armstrong-Dailey A, Zarbock S, eds. Hospice Care for Children. 3rd ed. New York, NY: Oxford University Press; 2009.

Beattie J, Goodlin S, eds. Supportive Care in Heart Failure. New York, NY: Oxford University Press; 2008.

Benjamin M, Curtis J. Ethics in Nursing: Cases, Principles, and Reasoning. New York, NY: Oxford University Press; 2010.

Berlinger N, Jennings B, Wolf SM, eds. The Hastings Center Guidelines for Decisions on Life-Sustaining Treatment and Care Near the End of Life. 2nd ed. New York, NY: Oxford University Press; 2013.

DeSandre PL, Quest TE, Portenoy RK, eds. Palliative Aspects of Emergency Care. New York, NY: Oxford University Press; 2013.

Ferrell BR, Coyle N. The Nature of Suffering and the Goals of Nursing. New York, NY: Oxford University Press; 2008.

Hanks G, Cherney NI, Christakis NA, Fallon M, Kaasa S, Portenoy RK, eds. Oxford Textbook of Palliative Medicine. 4th ed. New York, NY: Oxford University Press; 2011.

Lynn J, Schuster JL, Wilkinson A, Simon LN, eds. Improving Care for the End of Life: A Sourcebook for Health Care Managers and Clinicians. New York, NY: Oxford University Press; 2008.

Miller FG, Truog RD. Death, Dying, and Organ Transplantation: Reconstructing Medical Ethics at the End of Life. New York, NY: Oxford University Press; 2012.

Rocker G, Puntillo KA, Azoulay E, Nelson JE, eds. End of Life Care in the ICU: From Advanced Disease to Bereavement. New York, NY: Oxford University Press; 2010.

Strada AE, Portenoy RK, eds. Grief and Bereavement in the Adult Palliative Care Setting. New York, NY: Oxford University Press; 2013.

Wittenberg-Lyles E, Goldsmith J, Ferrell B, Ragan S. Communication in Palliative Nursing. New York, NY: Oxford University Press; 2013.

Yennurajalingam S, Bruera E, eds. Oxford American Handbook of Hospice and Palliative Medicine. New York, NY: Oxford University Press; 2011)=.

References/resource centers/databases

American Academy of Hospice and Palliative Medicine AAHPM-UNIPAC Self Study Program
http://www.aahpm.org/resources/default/unipac-4th-edition.html

- ◆ *UNIPAC One:* The Hospice/Palliative Medicine Approach to Care
- ◆ *UNIPAC Two:* Alleviating Psychological and Spiritual Pain in the Terminally Ill
- ◆ *UNIPAC Three:* Assessing and Treating of Pain
- ◆ *UNIPAC Four:* Managing Non-Pain Symptoms
- ◆ *UNIPAC Five:* Communication and the Physician's Role on the Interdisciplinary Team
- ◆ *UNIPAC Six:* Ethical and Legal Decision-Making When Caring for the Terminally Ill
- ◆ *UNIPAC Seven:* The Hospice/Palliative Medicine Approach to Caring for Patients with HIV/AIDS
- ◆ *UNIPAC Eight:* The Hospice/Palliative Medicine Approach to Caring for Pediatric Patients
- ◆ *UNIPAC Nine:* Caring for Patients with Chronic Illness, Dementia, COPD, and CHF

City of Hope Pain/Palliative Care Resource Center
http://prc.coh.org

Clinical Communication Collaborative: Centering Communication in Palliative Care
http://www.clinicalcc.com

End-of-Life Nursing Education Consortium (ELNEC)
http://www.aacn.nche.edu/ELNEC/ELNEC

Shaare Zedek Cancer Pain and Palliative Care Reference Database
http://www.chernydatabase.org

US Department of Veterans Affairs

http://www.va.gov/GERIATRICS/Guide/LongTermCare/Hospice_and_Palliative_Care.asp

Guidelines

Agency for Healthcare Research and Quality (AHRQ) Pain Guidelines (formerly Agency for Health Care Policy and Research [AHCPR])
http://www.ahrq.gov/clinic/cpgsix.htm

"Fast Facts"/Palliative Care-EPERC-End of Life Palliative Education Resource Center http://www.eperc.mcw.edu/EPERC/Factsandconcepts

National Comprehensive Cancer Network (NCCN)—Palliative Care Clinical Practice guidelines
http://www.nccn.org/professionals/physician_gls/PDF/palliative.pdf

National Consensus Project for Quality Palliative Care, 3rd edition
http://www.nationalconsensusproject.org

National Framework and Preferred Practices for Palliative and Hospice Care Quality
http://www.qualityforum.org/Publications/2006/12/A_National_Framework_and_Preferred_Practices_for_Palliative_and_Hospice_Care_Quality.aspx

World Health Organization (WHO)
http://www.who.int/medicines/areas/quality_safety/Scoping_WHOGuide_malignant_pain_adults.pdf

Journals/newsletters

American Journal of Hospice and Palliative Medicine
http://ajh.sagepub.com

Cancer Care News Newsletter
http://www.cancercare.org

Hayward Medical Communications
http://www.haywardpublishing.co.uk/ejpc_.aspx

International Association for Hospice and Palliative Care
http://www.hospicecare.com

International Journal of Palliative Nursing
http://www.markallengroup.com/healthcare

Journal of Hospice and Palliative Nursing
http://www.jhpn.com

Journal of Pain and Palliative Care Pharmacotherapy
http://informahealthcare.com/ppc

Journal of Pain and Symptom Management
http://www.elsevier.com

Journal of Palliative Care
http://www.criugm.qc.ca/journalofpalliativecare/

Journal of Palliative Medicine
http://www.liebertpub.com

Journal of Psychosocial Oncology
http://www.tandfonline.com/toc/wjpo20/current#.UaY9bNJON2A

Journal of Supportive Oncology
http://www.supportiveoncology.net

National Comprehensive Cancer Network (NCCN)
http://www.nccn.org

National Hospice and Palliative Care Organization (NHPCO) Newsline
http://www.nhpco.org

Oncology Nursing Form (ONF)
http://www.ons.org

Pain: Clinical Updates International Association for the Study of Pain
http://www.iasp-pain.org

Palliative and Supportive Care
http://journals.cambridge.org/action/displayJournal?jid=pax

Palliative Medicine
http://pmj.sagepub.com/

Psycho-Oncology
http://www.wiley.com

Progress in Palliative Care

http://www.leeds.ac.uk/lmi

Southern California Cancer Pain Initiative (SCCPI) Newsletter
http://sccpi.coh.org

Supportive Care in Cancer
http://rd.springer.com/journal/520

Organizations and websites (patient, professional, and state pain initiatives)

AARP (American Association of Retired Persons)
http://assets.aarp.org/external_sites/caregiving/end/internal_resources.html

Aging with Dignity
http://www.agingwithdignity.org

American Academy of Hospice and Palliative Medicine (AAHPM)
http://www.aahpm.org

American Academy of Pain Medicine (AAPM)
http://www.painmed.org

American Academy of Pediatrics (AAP)
http://www.aap.org

American Association for Therapeutic Humor
http://www.aath.org

American Board of Hospice and Palliative Medicine
http://www.abhpm.org

American Cancer Society (ACS)
http://www.cancer.org

American Geriatrics Society (AGS)
http://www.americangeriatrics.org

American Holistic Nurses Association
http://www.ahna.org

American Hospice Foundation
http://www.americanhospice.org

American Medical Association (AMA)
http://www.ama-assn.org

American Nurses Association (ANA)
http://nursingworld.org

American Pain Society (APS)
http://www.ampainsoc.org

American Society for Bioethics and Humanities
http://www.asbh.org

American Society for Pain Management Nursing (ASPMN)
http://www.aspmn.org

American Society of Clinical Oncology (ASCO)
http://www.asco.org

American Society of Law, Medicine and Ethics
http://www.aslme.org

Association for Death Education and Counseling (ADEC)
http://www.adec.org

Association of Oncology Social Work (AOSW)
http://www.aosw.org

Association of Pediatric Hemotology/Oncology Nurses (APHON)
http://www.aphon.org

Before I Die: Medical Care and Personal Choices
http://www.thirteen.org/bid

Beth Israel Medical Center, Department of Pain Medicine and Palliative Care
http://stoppain.org

Candlelighters: Childhood and Cancer Family Alliance
http://www.candle.org

Caregiver Regional Resources
http://www.caregiver.com/regionalresources/
Catholic Health Association of the United States
http://www.chausa.org
Center for Applied Ethics and Professional Practice (CAEPP)
http://caepp.edc.org
Center for Palliative Care (Harvard Medical School)
http://www.hms.harvard.edu/cdi/pallcare
Center for Palliative Care Studies (formally known as Center to Improve Care of the Dying)
http://medicaring.org
Center for Practical Bioethics
http://www.practicalbioethics.org/
Center to Advance Palliative Care
http://www.capc.org
Children's Hospice International (CHI)
http://www.chionline.org
Children's Project on Palliative/Hospice Services (CHIPPS)
http://www.nhpco.org
City of Hope Pain/Palliative Care Resource Center (COHPPRC)
http://prc.coh.org
Compassion in Dying Federation
http://www.compassionandchoices.org
The Compassionate Friends, Inc. (TCF)
http://www.compassionatefriends.org
Department of Health and Human Services, Healthfinder
http://www.healthfinder.gov
Edmonton Regional Palliative Care Program
http://www.palliative.org
End-of-Life Care for Children
http://www.childendoflifecare.org
End-of-Life Nursing Education Consortium (ELNEC)
http://www.aacn.nche.edu/ELNEC
End-of-Life Palliative Education Resource Center (EPERC)
http://www.eperc.mcw.edu
European Association for Palliative Care (EAPC)
http://www.eapcnet.org
Family Caregiver Alliance
http://www.caregiver.org
Grief.Net
http://www.griefnet.org
GriefShare
http://www.griefshare.org
GROWW: Grief Recovery Online for All Bereaved
http://www.groww.org
Gundersen Lutheran
http://www.respectingchoices.org
Hospice Association of America
http://www.nahc.org/haa/
Hospice Foundation of America
http://www.hospicefoundation.org
Hospice Net
http://hospicenet.org
Hospice and Palliative Nurses Association (HPNA)
http://www.hpna.org
Hospice Resources.Net
http://www.hospiceresources.net
International Association for the Study of Pain (IASP)
http://www.iasp-pain.org/

The International Work Group on Death, Dying and Bereavement
http://www.iwgddb.org
The Joint Commision/Palliative Care Certification
http://www.jointcommision.org/certification/palliative_care_program_benefits.aspx
Kidney Supportive Care
http://www.kidneysupportivecare.org/Home.aspx
Long Term Care Planning Network
http://www.ltcplanningnetwork.com
Medical College of Wisconsin Palliative Care Center
http://www.mcw.edu/pallmed
Mom, Always-Helpful Mothers Facing a Terminal Diagnosis
http://www.MomAlways.com
National Association for Home Care (NAHC)
http://www.nahc.org
National Cancer Institute (NCI)
http://www.cancer.gov
   ◆ Factsheet: Palliative Care in Cancer
National Consensus Project (NCP)
http://www.nationalconsensusproject.org
National Hospice and Palliative Care Organization (NHPCO)
http://www.nhpco.org
National Institute of Aging
http://www.nia.nih.gov
National Institute of Health
http://www.nih.gov
   ◆ Fact Sheet: End-of-Life
National Institute of Nursing Research (NINR)
http://www.ninr.nih.gov
   ◆ Because of Nursing Research: End-of-Life Care in the ICU
   ◆ Palliative Care: The Relief You Need When You're Experiencing the Symptoms of Serious Illness (Also available in Spanish)
   ◆ NINR Focus: End-of-Life Issues
National Quality Forum Framework for Palliative Care
http://www.qualityforum.org/Publications/2006/12/A_National_Framework_and_Preferred_Practices_for_Palliative_and_Hospice_Care_Quality.aspx
National Prison Hospice Association
http://www.npha.org
Oncology Nursing Society (ONS)
http://www.ons.org
   ◆ Oncology Nursing Society and Association of Oncology Social Work Joint Position on Palliative and End-of-Life Care
Open Society Foundations
http://www.opensocietyfoundations.org
Oregon Health Sciences University, Center for Ethics in Health Care
http://www.ohsu.edu/ethics
Pain and Policy Studies Group University of Wisconsin
www.painpolicy.wisc.edu
Patient Education Institute
http://www.patient-education.com
Pediatric Pain
http://pediatricpain.ca
Physicians Orders for Life Sustaining Treatment
http://www.polst.org
Promoting Excellence in End-of-Life Care
http://www.promotingexcellence.org
Resource Center of the Alliance of State Pain Initiatives
http://trc.wisc.edu

The Robert Wood Johnson Foundation (RWJF)
http://www.rwjf.org
Southern California Cancer Pain Initiative (SCCPI)
http://sccpi.coh.org/
Supportive Care Coalition
http://www.supportivecarecoalition.org
State Pain Policy Advocacy Network: SPPAN
http://sppan.aapainmanage.org
University of Wisconsin Pain and Policy Studies Group
http://www.painpolicy.wisc.edu
US Department of Veteran Affairs/Guide to Long Term Care
http://www.va.gov/geriatrics/guide/longtermcare/Hospice_
and_Palliative_Care.asp
Wisconsin Cancer Pain Initiative
http://aspi.wisc.edu/wpi

Position statements

American Nurses Association (ANA)
http://nursingworld.org/MainMenuCategories/
EthicsStandards/Ethics-Position-Statements

◆ Euthanasia, Assisted Suicide, and Aid in Dying

◆ Nursing Care and Do Not Resuscitate (DNR) and Allow Natural Death Decisions

◆ Foregoing Nutrition and Hydration

◆ Registered Nurses' Roles and Responsibilities in Providing Expert Care And Counseling at the End of Life

◆ The Nurses's Role in Ethics and Human Rights: Protecting and Promoting Individual Worth, Dignity, and Human Rights in Practice Settings

American Nursing Leaders
http://www.dyingwell.com/downloads/apnpos.pdf

◆ Advanced Practice Nurses Role in Palliative Care

American Society of Pain Management Nurses (ASPMN)
http://www.aspmn.org

◆ Assisted Suicide

◆ Pain Management at the End of Life

◆ Authorized and Unauthorized ("PCA by Proxy") Dosing of Analgesic Infusion Pumps

◆ Pain Assessment in the Patient Unable to Self-Report

◆ Pain Management in Patients with Substance Abuse Disorders

◆ Use of Placebos in Pain Management

◆ Joint Statement: The Use of As Needed Range Orders for Opioid Analgesics in the Management of Acute Pain

◆ Promoting Pain Relief and Preventing Abuse of Pain Medications: A Critical Balancing Act

Hospice and Palliative Nurses Association (HPNA)
http://www.hpna.org

◆ Complementary Therapies in Palliative Care Nursing Practice

◆ Evidence-Based Practice

◆ Legalization of Assisted Suicide

◆ Pain Management

◆ Palliative Sedation

◆ Role of Palliative Care Nursing in Organ and Tissue Donation

◆ Shortage of Registered Nurses

◆ Spiritual Care

◆ The Ethics of Opiate Use Within Palliative Care

◆ Value of Advanced Practice Nurse in Palliative Care

◆ Value of Licensed Practical/Vocational Nurse in Palliative Care

◆ Value of the Nursing Assistant in End-of-Life Care

◆ Value of Nursing Certification

◆ Value of the Professional Nurse in End-of-Life Care

◆ Withholdings and/or Withdrawing Life Sustaining Therapies

Oncology Nursing Society (ONS)
http://www.ons.orgp

◆ Cancer Pain Management

◆ End-of-Life Care

◆ The Impact of the National Nursing Shortage on Quality Cancer Care

◆ The Nurse's Responsibility to the Patient Requesting Assisted Suicide

◆ ONS and Association of Oncology Social Work Joint Position on End-of-Life Care

◆ Use of Complementary and Alternative Therapies in Cancer Care

Reports

Center for Palliative Care Studies
http://medicaring.org/ whitepaper

◆ Living Well at the End of Life: Adapting Health Care to Serious Chronic Illness in Old Age

Institute of Medicine/National Academies Press
http://www.nap.edu or http://www.iom.edu/Reports.aspx

◆ Approaching Death: Improving Care at the End of Life (1997)

◆ Improving Palliative Care for Cancer (2001)

◆ Working Together: We Can Help People Get Good Care When They Are Dying (2002)

◆ Improving Palliative Care: We Can Take Better Care of People with Cancer (2003)

◆ When Children Die: Improving Palliative and End-of-Life Care for Children and Families (2003)

◆ Describing Death in America: What We Need to Know (2003)

◆ Complementary and Alternative Medicine in the United States (2005)

◆ Organ Donation: Opportunities for Action (2006)

◆ Ensuring Quality Cancer Care Through the Oncology Workforce: Sustaining Care in the 21st Century: Workshop Summary (2009)

◆ Relieving Pain in America: A Blueprint for Transforming Prevention, Care, Education, and Research (2011)

- The Future of Nursing: Leading Change, Advancing Health (2011)
- Delivering Affordable Cancer Care in the 21st Century: Workshop Summary (2013)

Means to a Better End
http://www.rwjf.org/files/publications/other/meansbetterend.pdf
National Hospice and Palliative Care Organization (Children's International Project on Palliative/Hospice Services-ChIPPS)
http://www.nhpco.org/files/public/ChIPPSCallforChange.pdf

- A Call for Change: Recommendations to Improve the Care of Children Living with Life-Threatening Illness
- NHPCO's Standards for Pediatric Care

Precepts of Palliative Care
http://www.sgna.org/resources/statements/statementiob.html
Precepts of Palliative Care for Children, Adolescents, and Their Families
http://www.apon.org/files/public/last_acts_precepts.pdf
Promoting Excellence in End-of-Life Care
http://www.promotingexcellence.org/apn

- Advanced Practice Nursing: Pioneering Practices in Palliative Care

Robert Wood Johnson Foundation Funded Reports
http://www.rwjf.org/pr/product.jsp?id=20792

Research instruments

Brown University Center Toolkit of Instruments to Measure End-of-Life Care (TIME)
http://www.chcr.brown.edu/pcoc/toolkit.htm
Center to Improve Care of the Dying/Toolkit of Instruments to Measure End of Life
http://www.gwu.edu/~cicd/toolkit/toolkit.htm
City of Hope Pain/Palliative Care Resource Center
http://prc.coh.org
(refer to Research Instruments section)
Edmonton Assessment Tools
http://www.palliative.org/PC/ClinicalInfo/AssessmentTools/AssessmentToolsIDX.html
National Palliative Care and Research Center
http://www.npcrc.org/resources/resources_show.htm?doc_id=376168
Patient-Reported Outcome and Quality-of-Life Instruments Database
http://www.proqolid.org
Promoting Excellence in End-of-Life Care
http://www.promotingexcellence.org/i4a/pages/index.cfm?pageid=3276
State of the Art Review of Tools for Assessment of Pain in Non-verbal Older Adults
http://prc.coh.org
(refer to Pain in the Elderly section)
Supportive Care Coalition System Assessment Tool
http://www.supportivecarecoalition.org/images/reports/supportive%20care%20coalition%20system%20assessment%20.pdf

Media/videos

A Beautiful Death
http://www.abeautifuldeath.net/living-with-death/excellent-videos-about-palliative-care-hospice
Center to Advance Palliative Care/Audio Conferences
http://www.capc.org/?gclid=CL3n1KCt3LcCFTFgQgodzwIATQ
City of Hope Pain/Palliative Care Resource Center
http://prc.coh.org
(refer to End-of-Life/Palliative Care section for extensive video listings)
David's Cancer Video Blog
http://dbocancerjourney.blogspot.com/2013/02/video-17-cancer-and-palliative-care.html
Fanlight Productions
http://www.fanlight.com
The End of Life: Exploring Death in America
http://www.npr.org/programs/death
Get Palliative Care
http://www.getpalliativecare.org/videos-podcasts-livechats
Hospice Basics Video Service
http://www.nhpco.org/about-hospice-and-palliative-care/hospice-basics-video-series
Initiative for Pediatric Palliative Care (IPPC)
http://www.ippcweb.org/video.asp
On Our Own Terms
http://www.pbs.org/wnet/onourownterms
Palliative Care Assessment Video
http://www.ohsu.edu/xd/education/continuing-education/center-for-ethics/comfort-care-education/continuing-education/video.cfm
Palliative Care Video
http://www.palliativecarevideo.com
PBS Home Video
http://www.pbs.org
University of Michigan (Evan Mayday)
http://www.med.umich.edu/nursing/EndOfLife/mayday.htm

Blogs

American Academy of Hospice and Palliative Medicine
http://www.aahpm.org/apps/blog
GeriPal/Geriatrics and Palliative Care
www.geripal.org
Hospice and Palliative Care Community Blog Directory
http://www.nhpco.org/contact-us/hospice-and-palliative-care-community-blog-directory
Journal of Palliative Medicine
http://palliativejournal.stanford.edu/
Pallimed
http://www.pallimed.org
Practical Bioethics
http://practicalbioethics.blogspot.com

Index